D1552410

DIAGNOSTIC IMAGING
CARDIOVASCULAR

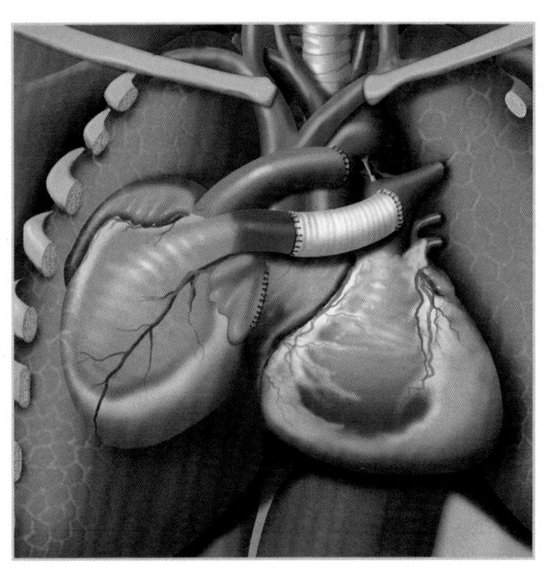

DIAGNOSTIC IMAGING
CARDIOVASCULAR

Suhny Abbara, MD

Assistant Professor of Radiology, Harvard Medical School
Director, Cardiovascular Imaging Section, Massachusetts General Hospital
Director of Education, MGH Cardiac MRCT Program
Boston, MA

T. Gregory Walker, MD

Associate Radiologist
Massachusetts General Hospital
Instructor of Radiology
Harvard Medical School
Boston, MA

Steven G. Imbesi, MD

Professor of Radiology and Neurosurgery
Department of Radiology
University of California, San Diego Medical Center
San Diego, CA

Perry P. Ng, MBBS (Hons), FRANZCR

Assistant Professor, Department of Radiology
Interventional Neuroradiologist
University of Utah Health Sciences Center
Salt Lake City, UT

Anne Roberts, MD

Professor of Radiology
Chief of Interventional Radiology
University of California, San Diego Medical Center
and Veteran Administration Hospital, San Diego
San Diego, CA

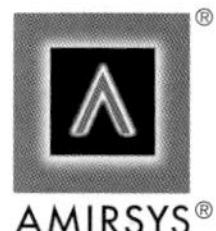

AMIRSYS®

Names you know, content you trust®

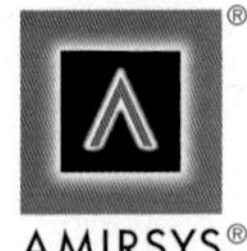

AMIRSYS®

Names you know, content you trust®

First Edition

Composition by Amirsys Inc, Salt Lake City, Utah

Printed in Canada by Friesens, Altona, Manitoba, Canada

ISBN-13: 978-1-4160-3340-0
ISBN-10: 1-4160-3340-8
ISBN-13: 978-0-8089-2383-1 (International English Edition)
ISBN-10: 0-8089-2383-8 (International English Edition)

Notice and Disclaimer

Library of Congress Cataloging-in-Publication Data

Diagnostic imaging. Cardiovascular / [edited by] Suhny Abbara, T. Gregory Walker, Steven G. Imbesi. -- 1st ed.
p. ; cm.
Includes bibliographical references and index.
ISBN-13: 978-1-4160-3340-0 (alk. paper)
ISBN-10: 1-4160-3340-8 (alk. paper)
ISBN-13: 978-0-8089-2383-1 (international ed. : alk. paper)
ISBN-10: 0-8089-2383-8 (international ed. : alk. paper)
1. Cardiovascular system--Imaging--Handbooks, manuals, etc. I. Abbara, Suhny. II. Walker, T. Gregory (Thomas Gregory), 1953- III. Imbesi, Steven G. IV. Title: Cardiovascular.
[DNLM: 1. Cardiovascular Diseases--diagnosis--Handbooks. 2. Cardiovascular System--pathology--Handbooks. 3. Diagnostic Imaging--Handbooks. WG 39 D536 2008]

RC683.5.I42D53 2008
616.1'0754--dc22

2008026707

To my beloved wife Amanda and our son Tyler. Their love and never wavering support makes it all possible.

Also, to my parents, Marlene and Yasser, and my sisters, Mona and Susu, with great appreciation for their love, friendship and their encouragement.

Finally, to all of our residents and fellows, as their enthusiastic thirst for knowledge drives us to teach and to perpetually learn.

SA

To Jimmy, Jack, Sonya, Cinde, and Gordon with love. And to Papa McGuire, Baba, and Winston; they would have loved this.

TGW

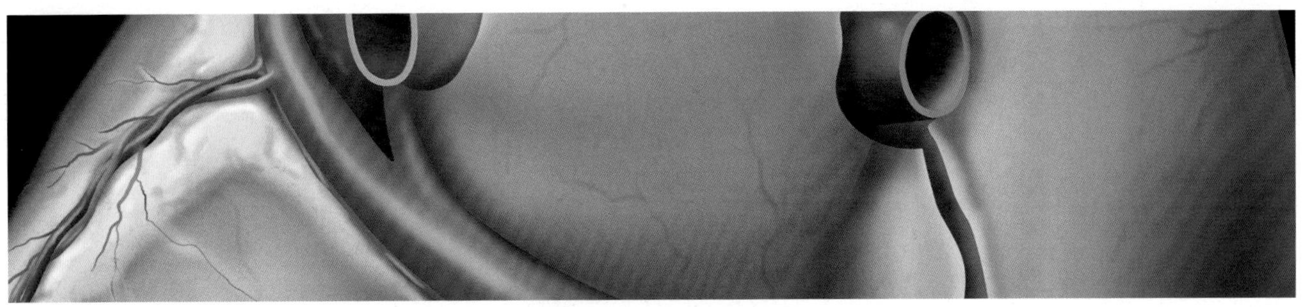

AUTHORS

Jonathan D. Dodd, MB MSc, MRCPI, FFR(RCSI)
Consultant Radiologist and Clinical Lecturer
Diagnostic Cardiac CT/MRI Program and Thoracic Imaging
Department of Radiology
St. Vincent's University Hospital and
University College Dublin
Dublin, Ireland

Ricardo C. Cury, MD
Medical Director of Cardiac MRI and CT
Baptist (Miami) Cardiac & Vascular Institute
Miami, FL
Consultant Radiologist, Massachusetts General Hospital
Assistant Professor of Radiology, Harvard Medical School
Boston, MA

Sjirk J. Westra, MD
Pediatric Radiologist
Pediatric Radiology Fellowship Director
Massachusetts General Hospital
Associate Professor, Radiology
Harvard Medical School
Boston, MA

Mayil S. Krishnam, MD, MRCP(UK), DMRD(UK), FRCR(UK)
Assistant Clinical Professor of Radiology
Diagnostic Cardiovascular & Thoracic Imaging
Department of Radiological Sciences
University of California, UCLA Medical Center
Los Angeles, CA

Allene Salcedo Burdette, MD
Assistant Professor of Interventional Radiology
Department of Radiology
University of Utah Hospitals and Clinics
Salt Lake City, UT

Douglas Green, MD
Assistant Professor of Radiology
Department of Radiology
University of Washington
Seattle, WA

Sanjeeva P. Kalva, MBBS, MD
Assistant Radiologist
Division of Cardiovascular Imaging & Intervention
Department of Radiology
Massachusetts General Hospital
Assistant Professor of Radiology
Harvard Medical School
Boston, MA

Alexander S. Urioste, MD
Clinical Instructor
Department of Radiology
University of California, San Diego Medical Center
San Diego, CA

Anand V. Soni, MD
Clinical and Research Fellow
Cardiac MR PET CT Program
Massachusetts General Hospital
Boston, MA

William G. Bradley, Jr, MD, PhD, FACR
Professor and Chair
Department of Radiology
University of California, San Diego Medical Center
San Diego, CA

Contributing Authors

Pablo Abbona, MD
Shalin J. Amin, MD
Veronica Arteaga, MD
Chad Barker, MD
Michael Anthony Bolen, MD
Christine Chao, MD
Aqeel A. Chowdhry, MD
Michael Grant, MD
Simon S.M. Ho, MBBS, FRCR
Darlene M. Holden, MD
Gabriella Iussich, MD
Praveen Jonnala, MD
Gudrun M. Feuchtner, MD
Derek Lohan, MD
Ricardo Loureiro, MD
Laxmi Mantrawadi, MD
Tan-Lucien H. Mohammed, MD, FCCP
Dirceu S.B. Neto, MD
Boris Nikolic, MD
Jeffrey Olpin, MD
Andrew Picel, MD
Ammar Sarwar, MD
Amar B. Shah, MD
Daniel Sommers, MD
Anderanik Tomasian, MD
Carol Wu, MD

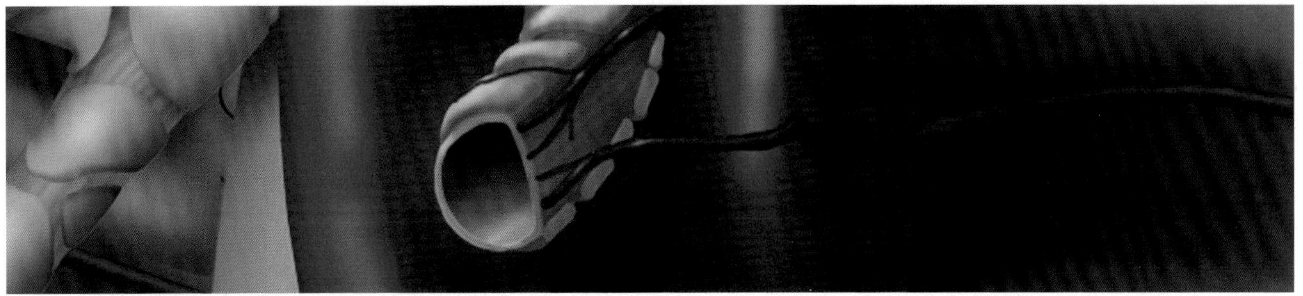

DIAGNOSTIC IMAGING: CARDIOVASCULAR

We at Amirsys and Elsevier are proud to present Diagnostic Imaging: Cardiovascular, the final volume in our acclaimed Diagnostic Imaging (DI) series. We began this precedent-setting, image- and graphic-rich series with David Stoller's Diagnostic Imaging: Orthopaedics. The next volumes, DI: Brain, DI: Head and Neck, DI: Abdomen, DI: Spine, DI: Pediatrics, DI: Obstetrics, DI: Chest, DI: Breast, DI: Ultrasound, DI: Pediatric Neuroradiology, DI: Nuclear Medicine, DI: Emergency, and DI: Gynecology are now joined by Suhny Abbara and Greg Walker's fabulous new textbook, DI: Cardiovascular.

Cardiovascular imaging, once the exclusive domain of radiology, was largely taken over by cardiologists in the days of invasive coronary angiography. With the advent of the newest multi-detector-row CT angiography, 3D workstation rendering of large datasets, and cardiac MR, cardiovascular imaging has once again become of interest to radiologists. Noninvasive cardiac and vascular imaging in many institutions is now a shared activity, much to the benefit of our patients. And it isn't just the heart, it's all blood vessels that come into the purview of this exciting, innovating technology. Minimally invasive procedures are hot, HOT, HOT!!! DI: Cardiovascular shows you not just what to look for (it includes both common and less common presentations of many diseases that can be quickly and accurately diagnosed using the popular new modalities), it also elegantly covers procedure-related issues.

Again, the unique bulleted format of the DI series allows our authors to present approximately twice the information and four times the images per diagnosis compared to the old-fashioned traditional prose textbook. All the DI books follow the same format, which means that our many readers find the same information in the same place—every time! And in every body part! The innovative visual differential diagnosis "thumbnail" provides you with an at-a-glance look at entities that can mimic the diagnosis in question and has been highly popular (and much copied). "Key Facts" boxes provide a succinct summary for quick, easy review.

In summary, Diagnostic Imaging: Cardiovascular is a product designed with you, the reader, in mind. Today's typical practice settings demand efficiency in both image interpretation and learning ever-evolving procedures. We think you'll find this new volume a highly efficient and wonderfully rich resource that will significantly enhance your practice—and find a welcome place on your bookshelf. Enjoy!

Anne G. Osborn, MD
Executive Vice President & Editor-in-Chief, Amirsys, Inc.

H. Ric Harnsberger, MD
CEO & Chairman, Amirsys, Inc.

Paula J. Woodward, MD
Senior Vice President & Medical Director, Amirsys, Inc.

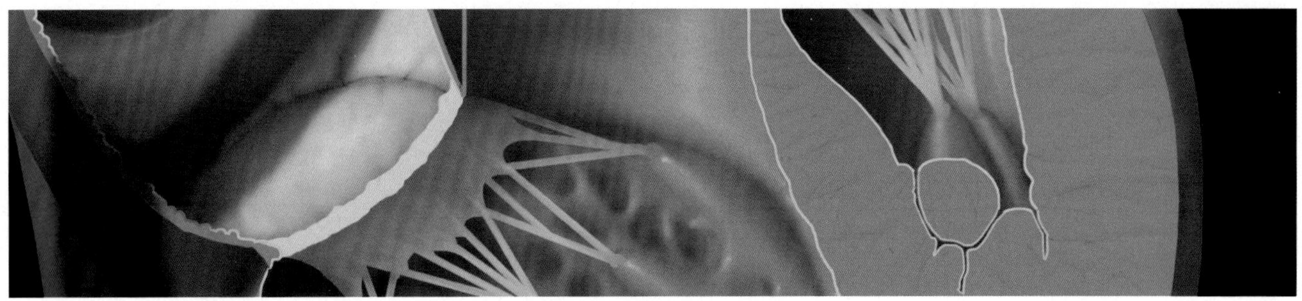

FOREWORD

Diagnostic Imaging: Cardiovascular addresses an important emerging aspect of current clinical practice, cardiovascular imaging with emphasis on CT and MR. As befits the goals of these volumes, the authors have provided an encyclopedic kaleidoscope of all the important imaging diagnoses, distilled to the essential findings in each of the appropriate imaging modalities. As in other volumes, emphasis is placed on imaging findings, pathology and clinical aspects of the disease to allow the diagnostician to have an intelligent and directed consultation with different referring clinical services. In addition to the key role of CT and MR in most diagnostic categories, additional imaging pertinent to particular diagnoses (including radiography, echocardiography, digital subtraction angiography and isotope imaging), are frequently referenced.

This volume is divided into two major sections, the first dealing with cardiac imaging diagnoses and the second with non-cardiac vascular diagnoses, both arterial and venous. Illustrations have been carefully selected to highlight the critical imaging findings, the importance of which is understood by references to the pathology and the clinical aspects of the disease. A concise differential diagnosis is provided together with "imaging pearls". All sections contain a summary statement of "key facts", a list of the most critical information which the reader can reference both prior to and subsequently following the reading of each individual clinical entity, and its diagnosis.

This volume by its design is a teaching summary of fundamental facts and inferences that are gleaned from careful observation of different imaging modalities. The authors do not seek to educate the reader in the physics and nuances of imaging technology or in the techniques employed. That is for other textbooks with different aims and methods. Rather, in this book, the diagnostician, already armed with an understanding of imaging technology, is guided into both the definitive diagnostic points and the subtleties of imaging interpretation as they apply to modern imaging technology.

The authors are to be congratulated on a concise, informative and up to date analysis of imaging and its role in the diagnosis of increasingly prevalent cardiovascular diseases. By using this volume, the diagnostician can approach each patient study with the appropriate background information to enable useful and productive interchange of information with referring services, particularly cardiology, cardiothoracic surgery, and vascular surgery. A copy of this volume should be in every department that provides cardiovascular imaging services to its referring clinician population.

W. Dennis Foley, MD
Professor of Radiology
Director of Digital Imaging
Medical College of Wisconsin
Milwaukee, WI

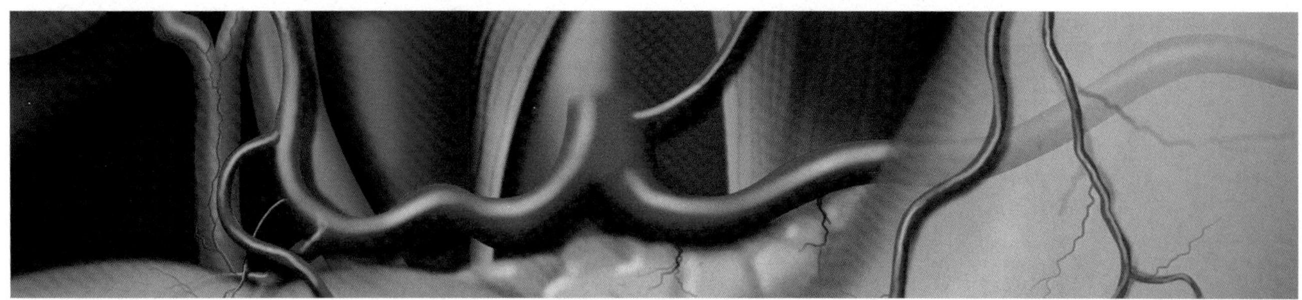

PREFACE

The significant maturation of cardiovascular medicine over the past 30 years has lead to substantial reductions in cardiovascular morbidity and mortality. While the fight against cardiovascular disease has lead to improvements in prevention and treatment strategies, advances in cardiovascular imaging have played important roles in more targeted and effective implementation of these strategies. The past decade in particular has been characterized by an unprecedented pace of technical developments in cardiovascular imaging. Since Kim et al showed remarkably good correlation between the presence of infarcted myocardium in pathologic specimens and the presence of delayed hyper-enhancement of myocardium on MRI in 1999, there has been an explosion of original research papers investigating the use of MRI for defining the extent of myocardial scar and myocardial fibrosis from other causes. As a consequence, manufacturers have made cardiac MRI technology more robust and thereby have enabled many imaging sites to include cardiac MRI into their clinical repertoire.

In the late 1980s and the 1990s electron beam CT scanners allowed us a first noninvasive glimpse of the coronary arteries. Electron beam CT was then succeeded by a new type of mechanical CT, the multi detector row CT scanners (MDCT). MDCT allowed more detailed imaging of the walls and lumens of the coronary vasculature. Over the last ten years we have witnessed a technological explosion leading to a rapid evolution of MDCT scanners: 2, 4, 8, 12, 16, 20, 32, 40, 64, 256, and most recently 320 detector rows. Recently dual source CT scanning was introduced which utilizes two X-ray tubes mounted on one gantry. In the same time period, the temporal resolution has improved from 250 ms to 83 ms and cardiac scan times shortened from approximately 40 second breathholds down to 1 single heart beat. In the first half of the past 10 years coronary MDCT was nearly exclusively performed in research settings at a select number of academic centers, however, over the past 5 years a large number of centers are using this imaging technology clinically. Paralleling this growth, cardiac CT imaging has been embraced by a number of medical organizations and imaging societies. A new cardiac imaging society that is dedicated solely to cardiovascular CT, the Society of Cardiovascular CT, was founded recently, and a new peer reviewed Journal, The Journal of Cardiovascular Computed Tomography, emerged in the summer of 2007. Clinical training guidelines and a first multi-society statement on appropriateness of clinical indications have been published.

Given continued improvements in MR and CT imaging technology, it is up to cardiovascular imagers to continue to progress and understand how new types of available imaging data can be acquired and applied to better characterize cardiovascular disease. We have to learn how and when to use these advanced imaging techniques. We have developed new ways of displaying cardiovascular anatomy, and we now have to learn to recognize and interpret never before encountered findings i.e. the 'new look' of familiar pathology (and normal variants).

This book aims to aid the cardiovascular imager in these efforts. Diagnostic Imaging: Cardiovascular is divided into two parts: a cardiac part that covers acquired and congenital coronary, cardiac and pericardial pathology, and a vascular part that covers thoracic, abdominal, extremity and neurovascular entities.

The book follows the format of the Diagnostic Imaging series. Text is presented in a bulleted format to allow for large amounts of information to be presented in a structured, comprehensive and easy to read manner. This format has proven useful, especially when it comes to quickly finding exact information needed at the reading workstation. Unlike other cardiovascular imaging textbooks this text does not focus on just one imaging modality. Rather, this book highlights the appropriate roles for all currently available imaging modalities and the resulting imaging findings pertinent to individual cardiovascular diagnoses. Although the major focus of this text is on state of the art MRI/MRA, MDCTA and gated CT imaging of cardiovascular pathology, this image collection also includes relevant radiographs, angiograms, ultrasounds, echocardiograms and nuclear medicine images.

The authors contributing to this text are committed to presenting you with the best examples of imaging of individual cardiovascular disease entities including typical appearances and variants, images of mimickers, and comprehensive differential diagnoses. I am grateful to the devotion of this fine group of experts. In addition to the authors and the editorial team at Amirsys, there are many people that have contributed to this work in one way or another. We are grateful to Christopher Sigakis, MS, Drs. Rodrigo Pale, Joe Hsu, Matthew Gilman, Dirceu Barbosa, and especially to Dr. Godtfred (Fred) Holmvang.

We truly hope that you will enjoy this book and will find it useful in your practice.

Suhny Abbara, MD
Assistant Professor of Radiology, Harvard Medical School
Director Cardiovascular Imaging Section, Massachusetts General Hospital
Director of Education, MGH Cardiac MRCT Program
Boston, MA

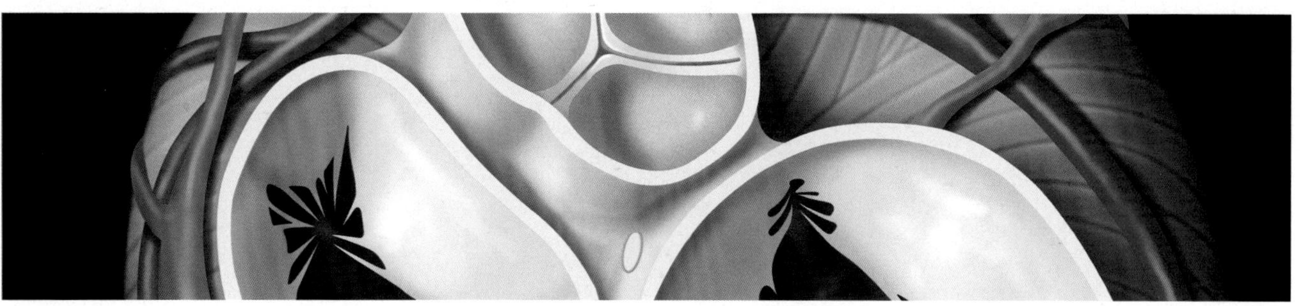

ACKNOWLEDGMENTS

Illustrations

Richard Coombs, MS
Lane R. Bennion, MS
Wes Price, MS

Image/Text Editing

Douglas Grant Jackson
Amanda Hurtado
Kaerli Main

Medical Text Editing

Henry J. Baskin, Jr., MD

Case Management

Roth LaFleur
Jeffrey J. Marmorstone

Production Lead

Melissa A. Hoopes

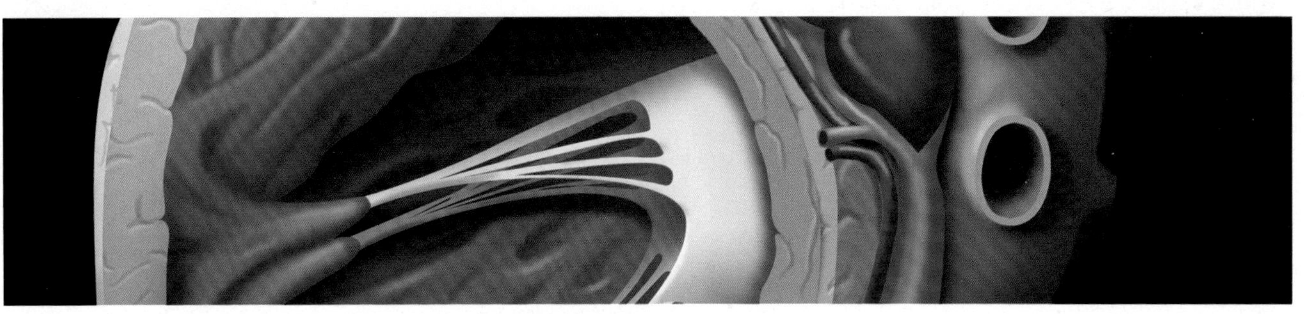

SECTIONS

PART I
Cardiac

PART II
Vascular

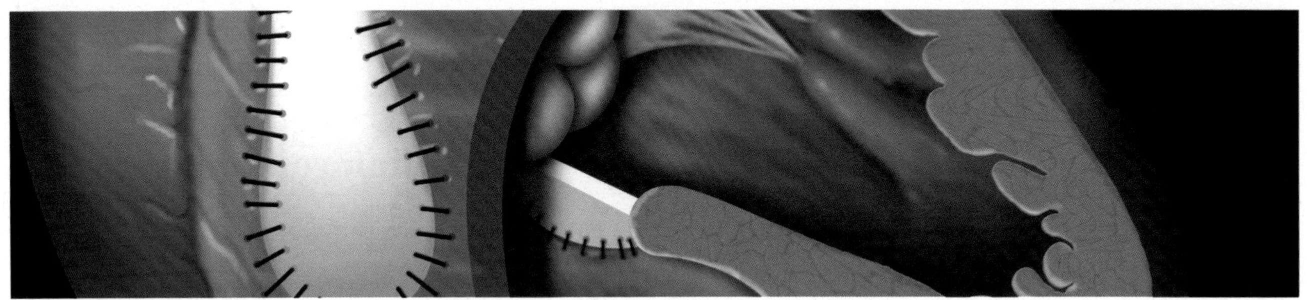

TABLE OF CONTENTS

PART I
Cardiac

SECTION 1
Congenital

SECTION 2
Valvular

Introduction and Overview

Valvular

SECTION 3 Pericardial

Introduction and Overview

Pericardial

SECTION 4 Neoplastic

SECTION 5 Cardiomyopathy

SECTION 6 Coronary Artery

Introduction and Overview

Coronary Artery

SECTION 7 Heart Failure

SECTION 8 Hypertension

SECTION 9 Electrophysiology

PART II Vascular

SECTION 1 Brain

Introduction and Overview

Brain

SECTION 2
Head & Neck

Introduction and Overview

Head & Neck

SECTION 3 Spine

SECTION 4 Thorax

Introduction and Overview

Thorax

SECTION 5 Abdominal

Introduction and Overview

Aorta

Visceral Arteries

Portal Hypertension

Venous

SECTION 6
Renal

Introduction and Overview

Renal

SECTION 7
Extremities

Upper Extremities

Pelvis

Lower Extremities

DIAGNOSTIC IMAGING
CARDIOVASCULAR

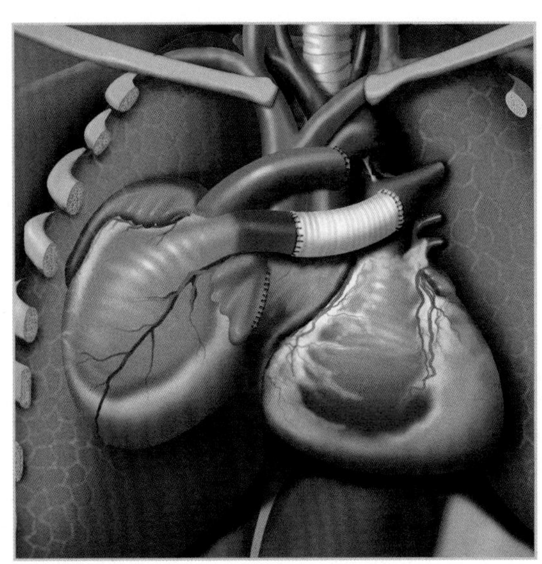

PART I

Cardiac

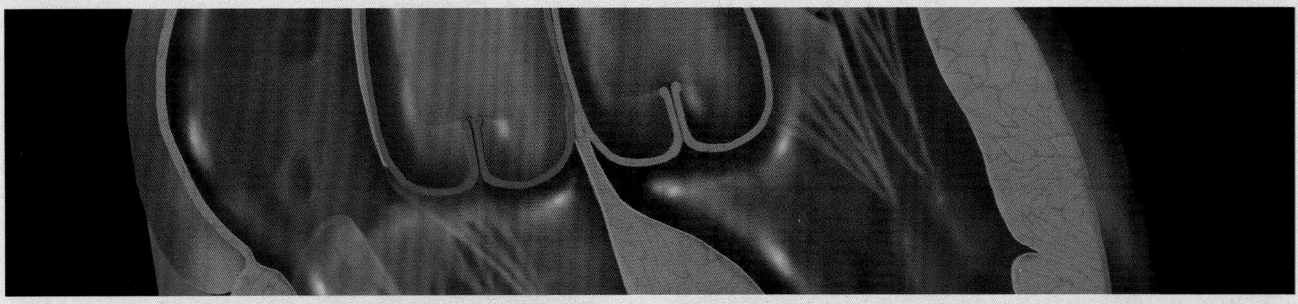

SECTION 1: Congenital

COARCTATION OF AORTA

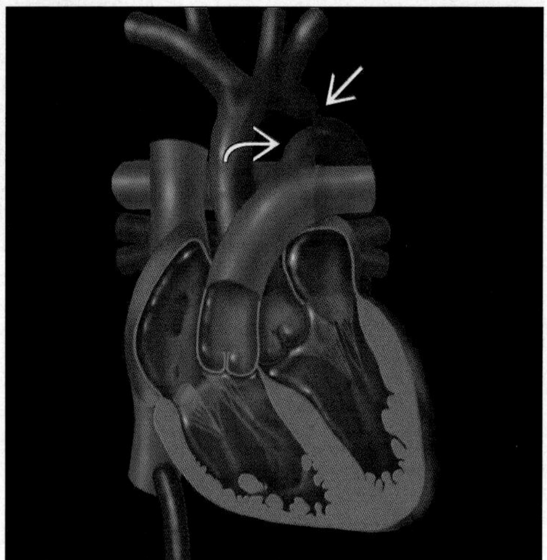

Coronal graphic shows preductal coarct ➔ with PDA ➔ and right to left shunt resulting in decreased oxygenation in the descending aorta only.

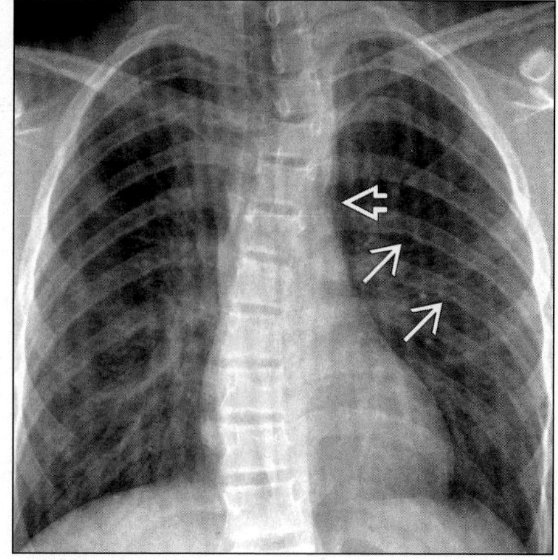

Anterior posterior radiograph shows abnormal aortic knob contour ➔ ("3" sign). Bilateral rib notching is present ➔, indicating enlarged intercostal arteries.

TERMINOLOGY

Abbreviations and Synonyms

- Coarc, coarct (CoA)

Definitions

- Narrowing of the aortic lumen with obstruction to blood flow
- May be discrete or associated with arch and isthmus hypoplasia

IMAGING FINDINGS

General Features

- Best diagnostic clue
  - Classic plain film appearance: Rib notching, "figure 3" sign
  - Focal aortic narrowing, presence of collaterals
- Location
  - Major types
    - Preductal (infantile), juxtaductal & postductal (adult)
    - Simple (isolated) and complex (associated with other malformations such as atrial septal defect [ASD], ventricular septal defect [VSD] and mitral stenosis)
    - Significant (> 20 mmHg gradient ± proximal hypertension)

Radiographic Findings

- Radiography
  - Chest radiography findings
    - Rib notching (above age 5 years)
    - Scalloped posterior sternal contour due to enlarged internal mammary collaterals
    - Post-stenotic dilatation of proximal descending aorta, "figure 3" sign
    - Left ventricular (LV) hypertrophy: Rounded elevated apex
    - Esophagram: Impression by dilated descending aorta, "reversed 3" sign
  - Pulmonary venous hypertension in preductal newborns
    - Cardiomegaly in complicated coarct due to L-R shunt from VSD, ASD or patent ductus arteriosus (PDA)

DDx: Coarctation

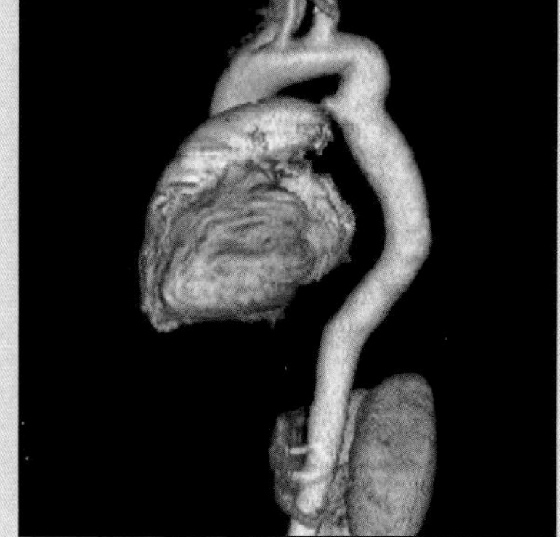

Pseudocoarctation

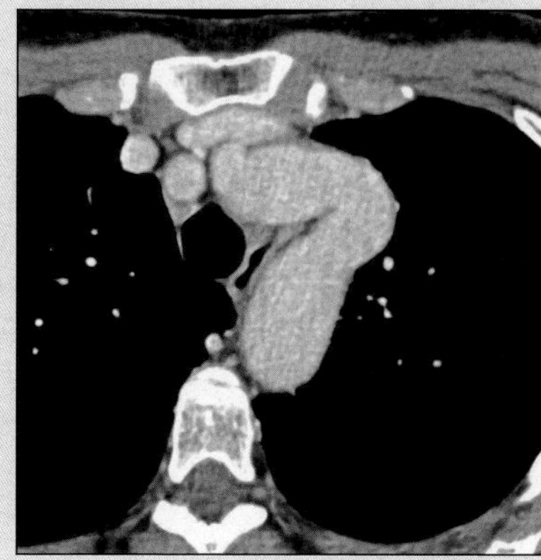

Pseudocoarctation

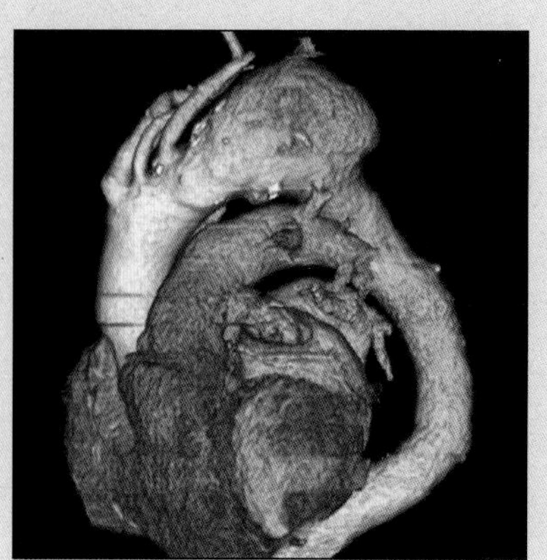

Arch Aneurysm

COARCTATION OF AORTA

Key Facts

Terminology

- Narrowing of the aortic lumen with obstruction to blood flow
- May be discrete or associated with arch and isthmus hypoplasia

Imaging Findings

- Preductal (infantile), juxtaductal & postductal (adult)
- Simple (isolated) and complex (associated with other malformations such as atrial septal defect [ASD], ventricular septal defect [VSD] and mitral stenosis)
- Rib notching (above age 5 years)
- Post-stenotic dilatation of proximal descending aorta, "figure 3" sign
- Esophagram: Impression by dilated descending aorta, "reversed 3" sign
- Gated CT may reveal bicuspid aortic valve ± ascending aortic aneurysm
- Phase-contrast MR: For estimate of flow velocities, gradient and collateral flow

Pathology

- Frequently associated with bicuspid aortic valve (50-85%)
- Associated with Turner syndrome (13-36% have coarctation)

Clinical Issues

- Frequently asymptomatic, incidentally found
- Older child, adult: Hypertension, diminished femoral pulses, differential blood pressure between upper and lower extremities (arm-leg gradient)

CT Findings

- CTA
    - CT angiography with volume rendered 3D reconstruction depicts coarctation and collaterals
        - Oblique view along long-axis of stenotic segment best for localization of minimal luminal diameter and perpendicular views for cross-sectional diameter measurements
        - Candy cane arch views best for measuring distance of coarct from left subclavian artery
    - May demonstrate ectatic/aneurysmatic left subclavian artery
    - Excellent tool to detect collaterals (internal mammaries, intercostal)
    - Dilated brachiocephalic vessels and aorta proximal to lesion
    - Gated CT may reveal bicuspid aortic valve ± ascending aortic aneurysm
    - CTA best tool to noninvasively depict treatment complications
        - Restenosis after balloon angioplasty/stenting
        - Aneurysm after angioplasty or subclavian artery patch or other patch repair
        - Mycotic aneurysm distal to coarct
- Cranial CTA may reveal berry aneurysms

MR Findings

- MRA: MR angiography with volume rendered 3D reconstruction depicts morphology of coarctation and collaterals
- Cardiac-gated T1WI (black blood)
    - Sagittal-oblique plane through aortic arch shows location of coarctation
    - Perpendicular views for cross-sectional diameter measurements
- Gradient-echo (GRE) cine (white blood)
    - In sagittal-oblique (candy cane) plane for anatomy
    - Length of systolic (dark) flow jet - hemodynamic significance
    - Aortic regurgitation (bicuspid aortic valve)
- Phase-contrast MR: For estimate of flow velocities, gradient and collateral flow
    - Phase contrast images at coarctation site determine peak velocities and gradient
    - Axial aortic phase-contrast images immediately distal to coarct and at diaphragmatic crura allows for quantification of collateral flow
    - Increased flow at diaphragm is due to collateral inflow distal to coarct

Echocardiographic Findings

- Echocardiogram
    - Imaging of aortic arch and branches in suprasternal long axis view
    - Relationship of coarctation with PDA
    - May depict bicuspid aortic valve
- Pulsed Doppler: Doppler used to estimate gradient across coarctation

Angiographic Findings

- Cardiac catheterization with angiography findings
    - Can determine location and type of coarct
    - Direct measurement of gradient
    - Balloon angioplasty and stenting
    - Coronary angiography is performed pre-operatively due to premature atherosclerosis

Imaging Recommendations

- Echocardiography for primary diagnosis in infancy
- Older child: MR for pre-operative work-up and post-operative surveillance for re-coarctation, aneurysms
- Catheterization reserved for gradient measurement and intervention

DIFFERENTIAL DIAGNOSIS

Hypoplastic Left Heart Syndrome

- Congestive heart failure in newborn
- Hypoplastic LV
- Ductus-dependent systemic perfusion
- Retrograde flow in hypoplastic ascending aorta

Interrupted Aortic Arch

- Flow to descending aorta via PDA

COARCTATION OF AORTA

Pseudocoarctation

- Elongation with kinking of aorta without obstruction to blood flow

Takayasu Arteritis

- Acquired inflammatory condition
- Acute phase: Aortic wall enhancement
- Chronic phase: Narrowing/occlusion of aorta and branch vessels

PATHOLOGY

General Features

- General path comments
  - Frequently associated with bicuspid aortic valve (50-85%)
  - Other associations: VSD (33%), PDA (66%), transposition, subaortic and mitral stenosis ("parachute" deformity, Shone syndrome), Taussig-Bing anomaly, endocardial fibroelastosis
  - Embryology
    - Postnatal contraction of fibrous ductal tissue in aortic wall
    - Abnormal fetal hemodynamics (e.g., hypoplastic left heart associated with preductal coarctation)
  - Pathophysiology
    - Increase in systemic vascular resistance (left ventricular afterload)
    - Hypertension due to renal hypoperfusion
    - Congestive heart failure (newborn, associated complex heart disease)
    - LV hypertrophy
    - Development of collaterals to bypass the stenosis (internal mammary, intercostal, superior epigastric arteries)
- Genetics
  - Usually sporadic
  - Associated with Turner syndrome (13-36% have coarctation)
- Epidemiology
  - Incidence: 2-6 per 10,000 live births
  - More common in males (2:1), Caucasians

Gross Pathologic & Surgical Features

- Focal shelf or waist lesion
- Diffuse narrowing of a segment of aortic arch (isthmus)
- Post-stenotic dilatation of descending aorta

CLINICAL ISSUES

Presentation

- Most common signs/symptoms
  - Often asymptomatic
  - Headaches from hyperperfusion
  - Claudication from hypoperfusion
  - Symptomatic critical coarct (1st week of life)
    - Congestive heart failure (CHF): Second most cause of CHF in infancy after hypoplastic left heart
    - Lower extremity cyanosis
    - Pulmonary edema
- Category: Acyanotic, normal heart size and normal pulmonary vascularity
- Hemodynamics: LV pressure overload
- Frequently asymptomatic, incidentally found
- Infancy: Congestive heart failure (due to associated anomalies)
- Older child, adult: Hypertension, diminished femoral pulses, differential blood pressure between upper and lower extremities (arm-leg gradient)
- Bacterial endocarditis

Natural History & Prognosis

- Re-coarctation (< 3%, higher when operated in infancy)
- Post-operative aneurysms (24% after patch angioplasty)
- Long term survival decreased (late hypertension, coronary artery disease)

Treatment

- Resection and end-to-end anastomosis or interposition graft
- Prosthetic patch, subclavian flap aortoplasty
- Balloon angioplasty

DIAGNOSTIC CHECKLIST

Image Interpretation Pearls

- Aortic cross-sections through narrowest segment helpful to differentiate pseudo coarctation from coarctations

SELECTED REFERENCES

1. Shih MC et al: Surgical and endovascular repair of aortic coarctation: normal findings and appearance of complications on CT angiography and MR angiography. AJR Am J Roentgenol. 187(3):W302-12, 2006
2. Mahadevan V et al: Endovascular management of aortic coarctation. Int J Cardiol. 97 Suppl 1:75-8, 2004
3. Massey R et al: Surgery for complex coarctation of the aorta. Int J Cardiol. 97 Suppl 1:67-73, 2004
4. Duke C et al: Aortic coarctation and recoarctation: to stent or not to stent? J Interv Cardiol. 14(3):283-98, 2001
5. Bogaert J et al: Follow-up of patients with previous treatment for coarctation of the thoracic aorta: comparison between contrast-enhanced MR angiography and fast spin-echo MR imaging. Eur Radiol. 10(12):1847-54, 2000
6. Jenkins NP et al: Coarctation of the aorta: natural history and outcome after surgical treatment. QJM. 92(7):365-71, 1999
7. Riquelme C et al: MR imaging of coarctation of the aorta and its postoperative complications in adults: assessment with spin-echo and cine-MR imaging. Magn Reson Imaging. 17(1):37-46, 1999
8. Muhler EG et al: Evaluation of aortic coarctation after surgical repair: role of magnetic resonance imaging and Doppler ultrasound. Br Heart J. 70(3):285-90, 1993

IMAGE GALLERY

Typical

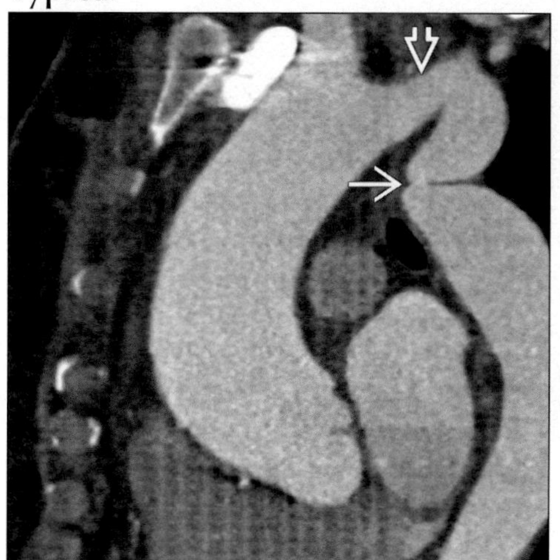

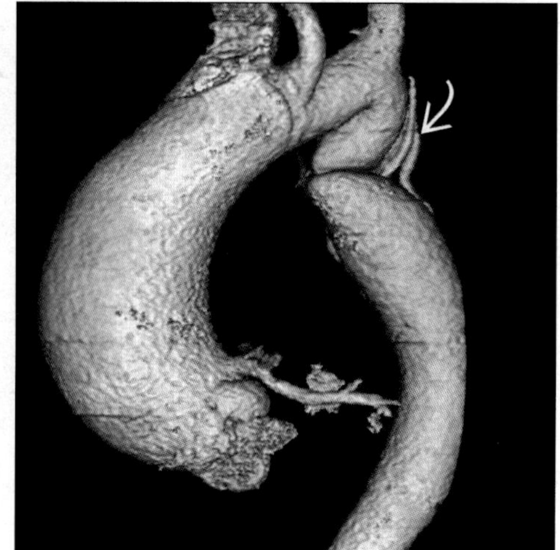

(Left) *Oblique CTA shows coarctation with high grade stenosis distal to left subclavian artery origin. Note, hypoplastic distal arch.* ***(Right)*** *Oblique CTA volume rendering in same patient as previous image shows coarctation with hypoplastic arch and collaterals.*

Variant

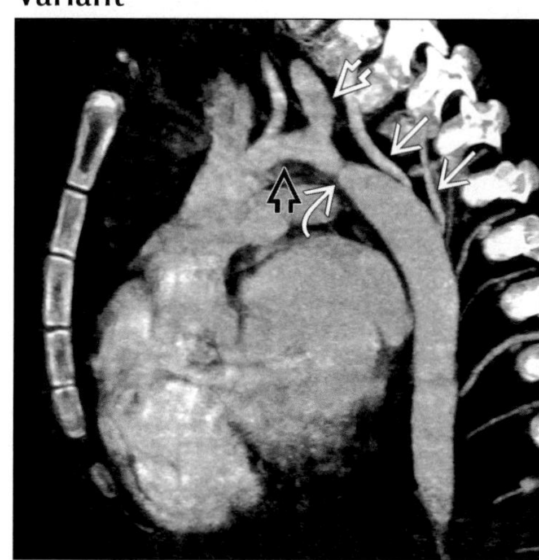

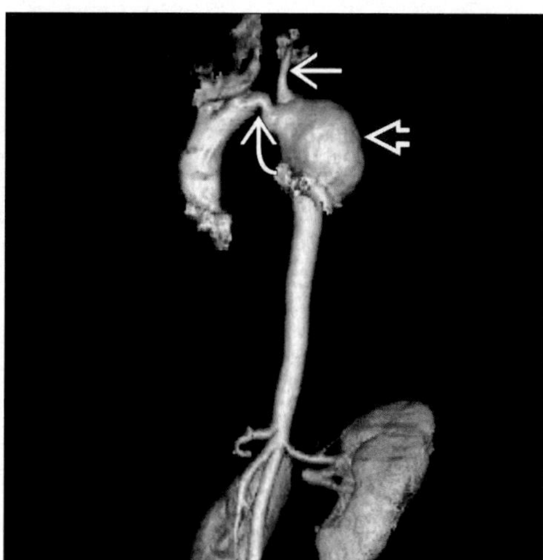

(Left) *Oblique CTA shows hypoplastic arch and coarctation with large collaterals and ectatic left subclavian artery.* ***(Right)*** *Oblique CECT volume rendering shows coarctation proximal to the left subclavian artery with a mycotic aneurysm distal to the coarctation.*

Variant

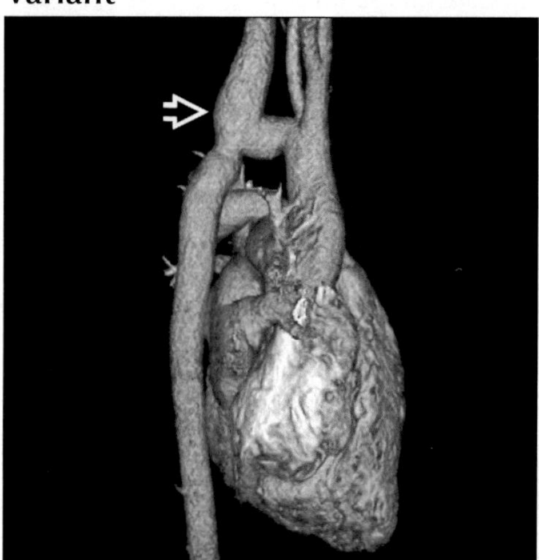

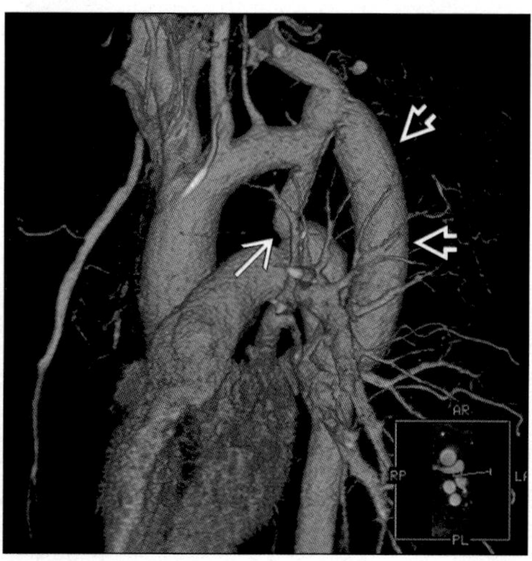

(Left) *Oblique CTA volume rendering shows aneurysm of proximal left subclavian artery and mild coarctation immediately distal to its origin.* ***(Right)*** *Oblique MRA surface rendering shows coarctation with bypass graft repair from left subclavian artery to descending aorta distal to coarctation.*

DOUBLE AORTIC ARCH

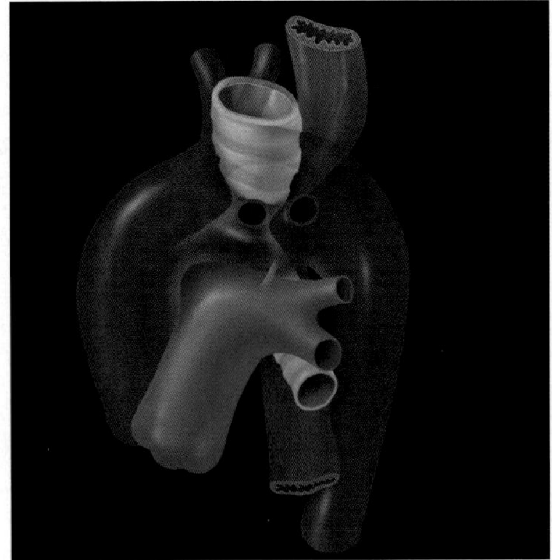

Graphic shows double aortic arch anomaly, with complete vascular ring encircling and compressing trachea and esophagus.

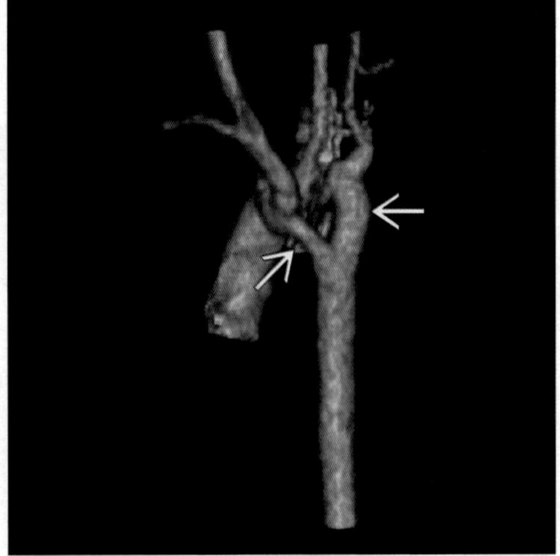

3D coronal CTA, posterior view, shows the complete vascular ring ➡. The dominant right-sided arch is higher in position than the smaller left-sided one.

TERMINOLOGY

Definitions

- Congenital aortic arch anomaly related to persistence of both the left and right fourth aortic arches

IMAGING FINDINGS

General Features

- Best diagnostic clue: Severe compression of trachea with evidence of right and left aortic arches
- On cross-sectional imaging, both left and right arches are identified arising from ascending aorta
- Each arch gives rise to a ventral carotid and a dorsal subclavian artery (symmetric "four artery sign")
- Right arch often larger and more superior than left
- Right arch runs behind esophagus to join left arch
- Part of left arch may be atretic but patent portions remain connected by compressing fibrous band

Radiographic Findings

- Radiography
  - Prominent soft tissue on either side of the trachea
  - Bilateral tracheal indentations, mid-tracheal stenosis
  - Trachea is deviated from dominant arch, or may be in abnormal midline position (normally trachea is slightly deviated to right by left arch)
  - Right arch indentation commonly somewhat higher and more prominent than left
  - On lateral view, anterior and posterior compression of trachea at level of arch
  - Symmetric aeration, no unilateral air trapping

Fluoroscopic Findings

- Anteroposterior view: Bilateral indentations on contrast-filled esophagus, often at different levels
- Lateral view: Prominent oblique or nearly horizontal posterior indentation

CT Findings

- CTA
  - Four artery sign: Symmetric take-off of four aortic branches on axial image at thoracic inlet: 2 ventral carotids and 2 dorsal subclavians
  - Two arches encircling trachea and esophagus, leading to severe mid-tracheal compression
  - Smaller of two arches may be partially atretic
  - Severe tracheal compression at level of double arch

DDx: Arch Anomalies

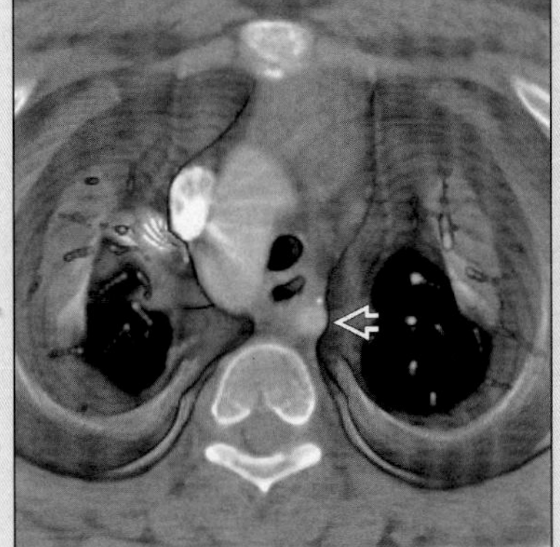

Right Arch, Aberrant LSA

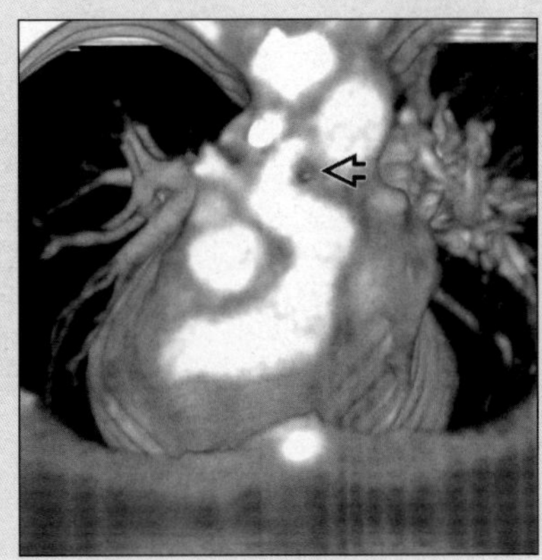

Left PA Sling

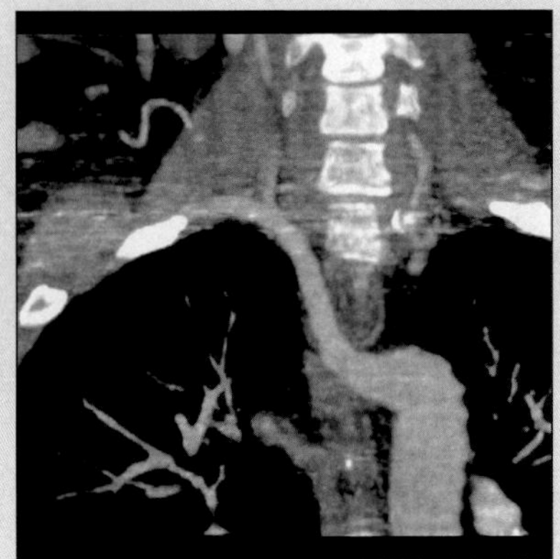

Left Arch, Aberrant RSA

DOUBLE AORTIC ARCH

Key Facts

Terminology

- Congenital aortic arch anomaly related to persistence of both the left and right fourth aortic arches

Imaging Findings

- On cross-sectional imaging, both left and right arches are identified arising from ascending aorta
- Each arch gives rise to a ventral carotid and a dorsal subclavian artery (symmetric "four artery sign")
- Right arch often larger and more superior than left
- Trachea is deviated from dominant arch, or may be in abnormal midline position (normally trachea is slightly deviated to right by left arch)

Pathology

- Epidemiology: Most common symptomatic vascular ring (55%)
- True complete vascular ring with trachea and esophagus encircled
- Dominant right arch, left descending aorta: 75%
- Dominant left arch, right descending aorta: 20%

Clinical Issues

- Most common signs/symptoms: Inspiratory stridor, worsening with feeding
- Determination of which arch is smaller on cross-sectional imaging will determine on which side thoracotomy is performed

Diagnostic Checklist

- Look for signs of atretic segments of the double arch anomaly (will not be opacified on CTA or MRA, and show no flow voids on spin echo MR)

  - Coronal 3D images helpful to show arch anatomy
  - Dynamic airway evaluation with multidetector CT

MR Findings

- Axial and coronal images most helpful
- Findings comparable with CTA

Echocardiographic Findings

- Echocardiogram
  - Suprasternal notch view most helpful, showing two separate aortic arches, each giving rise to separate carotid and subclavian arteries (no brachiocephalic trunk)
  - Often insufficient for pre-operative diagnosis (does not show airway compression)

Angiographic Findings

- Conventional: Rarely required with use of CT, MR

Imaging Recommendations

- Best imaging tool
  - Radiography remains primary diagnostic test
    - If radiography demonstrates lack of tracheal compression, vascular ring excluded
  - Barium swallow rarely obviates need for cross-sectional imaging
    - However many asymptomatic arch anomalies are first diagnosed by barium swallow
  - Cross-sectional imaging (CT or MR) performed to confirm diagnosis and define anatomic variations
- Protocol advice
  - Axial and coronal images/reformations
  - Multidetector-row CTA faster to perform that MR, with generally no need for sedation and endotracheal intubation
  - CT shows airway compromise better than MR

DIFFERENTIAL DIAGNOSIS

Right Arch with Aberrant Left Subclavian Artery (LSA) and Other Arch Abnormalities

- Differentiate with cross-sectional imaging

Left Pulmonary Artery (PA) Sling

- Compression on anterior aspect of esophagus and posterior aspect of trachea on radiography
- Often associated with tracheomalacia

Innominate Artery Compression Syndrome

- Anterior tracheal, no esophageal compression

Nonvascular Masses

- Small middle mediastinal masses or larger anterior or posterior masses that compress trachea

PATHOLOGY

General Features

- General path comments
  - Related to embryological persistence of the right and left fourth aortic arches
  - Pathophysiology: Severe airway and esophageal compression by vascular ring
  - Underlying tracheomalacia is frequently associated
  - Hemodynamics: No hemodynamic sequelae, unless associated with congenital heart disease
- Genetics: No specific genetic defect identified
- Epidemiology: Most common symptomatic vascular ring (55%)
- Associated abnormalities
  - Typically an isolated lesion
    - 20% associated with congenital heart disease (tetralogy of Fallot, ventricular septal defect, coarctation, patent ductus arteriosus, transposition of great arteries, truncus arteriosus)

Gross Pathologic & Surgical Features

- True complete vascular ring with trachea and esophagus encircled
  - Dominant right arch, left descending aorta: 75%
  - Dominant left arch, right descending aorta: 20%
  - Arches equal in size: 5%
- Smaller of two arches may be partially atretic

DOUBLE AORTIC ARCH

CLINICAL ISSUES

Presentation

- Most common signs/symptoms: Inspiratory stridor, worsening with feeding
- Other signs/symptoms: Apneic attacks, noisy breathing, "seal bark" cough

Demographics

- Age: Typically presents early in life, soon after birth

Treatment

- Thoracotomy with division of smaller of two arches, atretic segments and ligamentum arteriosum
  - Rare complication: Aortoesophageal fistula
- Determination of which arch is smaller on cross-sectional imaging will determine on which side thoracotomy is performed
- < 30% of post-operative patients: Persistent airway symptoms, due to tracheobronchomalacia and/or persistent extrinsic airway compression
  - Caused by midline/circumflex descending aorta or previously ligated arch
- 11% of patients require a second operation to relieve airway symptoms: Aortopexy or other vascular suspension procedures, cartilaginous tracheal ring resection followed by airway reconstruction

DIAGNOSTIC CHECKLIST

Consider

- Look for signs of atretic segments of the double arch anomaly (will not be opacified on CTA or MRA, and show no flow voids on spin echo MR)

Image Interpretation Pearls

- "Four artery sign" on axial slice at thoracic inlet

SELECTED REFERENCES

1. Cerillo AG et al: Sixteen-row multislice computed tomography in infants with double aortic arch. Int J Cardiol. 99(2):191-4, 2005
2. Chan MS et al: Angiography and dynamic airway evaluation with MDCT in the diagnosis of double aortic arch associated with tracheomalacia. AJR Am J Roentgenol. 185(5):1248-51, 2005
3. Greil GF et al: Diagnosis of vascular rings and slings using an interleaved 3D double-slab FISP MR angiography technique. Pediatr Radiol. 2005
4. Schlesinger AE et al: Incomplete double aortic arch with atresia of the distal left arch: distinctive imaging appearance. AJR Am J Roentgenol. 184(5):1634-9, 2005
5. Backer CL et al: Pediatric cardiac surgery. 3rd ed. Philadelphia, Mosby. 234-50, 2003
6. Subramanyan R et al: Vascular rings: an important cause of persistent respiratory symptoms in infants and children. Indian Pediatr. 40(10):951-7, 2003
7. Yilmaz M et al: Vascular anomalies causing tracheoesophageal compression: a 20-year experience in diagnosis and management. Heart Surg Forum. 6(3):149-52, 2003
8. Fleck RJ et al: Imaging findings in pediatric patients with persistent airway symptoms after surgery for double aortic arch. AJR Am J Roentgenol. 178(5):1275-9, 2002
9. Park SC et al: Pediatric cardiology. Vol 2. 2nd ed. London, Churchill Livingstone. 1559-75, 2002
10. Skinner LJ et al: Complete vascular ring detected by barium esophagography. Ear Nose Throat J. 81(8):554-5, 2002
11. Brockes C et al: Double aortic arch: diagnosis missed for 29 years. Vasa. 29(1):77-9, 2000
12. Gustafson LM et al: Spiral CT versus MRI in neonatal airway evaluation. Int J Pediatr Otorhinolaryngol. 52(2):197-201, 2000
13. McMahon CJ et al: Double aortic arch in D-transposition of the great arteries: confirmation of dominant arch by magnetic resonance imaging. Tex Heart Inst J. 27(4):398-400, 2000
14. Krinsky GA et al: Thoracic aorta: comparison of single-dose breath-hold and double-dose non-breath-hold gadolinium-enhanced three-dimensional MR angiography. AJR Am J Roentgenol. 173(1):145-50, 1999
15. Beghetti M et al: Double aortic arch. J Pediatr. 133(6):799, 1998
16. Donnelly LF et al: The spectrum of extrinsic lower airway compression in children: MR imaging. AJR Am J Roentgenol. 168(1):59-62, 1997
17. Fattori R et al: Intramural posttraumatic hematoma of the ascending aorta in a patient with a double aortic arch. Eur Radiol. 7(1):51-3, 1997
18. Hopkins KL et al: Pediatric great vessel anomalies: initial clinical experience with spiral CT angiography. Radiology. 200(3):811-5, 1996
19. Murdison KA: Ultrasonic Imaging of Vascular Rings and Other Anomalies Causing Tracheobronchial Compression. Echocardiography. 13(3):337-356, 1996
20. Othersen HB Jr et al: Aortoesophageal fistula and double aortic arch: two important points in management. J Pediatr Surg. 31(4):594-5, 1996
21. Ito K et al: A case of the incomplete double aortic arch diagnosed in adulthood by MR imaging. Radiat Med. 13(5):263-7, 1995
22. Katz M et al: Spiral CT and 3D image reconstruction of vascular rings and associated tracheobronchial anomalies. J Comput Assist Tomogr. 19(4):564-8, 1995
23. Simoneaux SF et al: MR imaging of the pediatric airway. Radiographics. 15(2):287-98; discussion 298-9, 1995
24. Tuma S et al: Double aortic arch in d-transposition of the great arteries complicated by tracheobronchomalacia. Cardiovasc Intervent Radiol. 18(2):115-7, 1995
25. van Son JA et al: Demonstration of vascular ring anatomy with ultrafast computed tomography. Thorac Cardiovasc Surg. 43(2):120-1, 1995
26. van Son JA et al: Imaging strategies for vascular rings. Ann Thorac Surg. 57(3):604-10, 1994
27. Kramer LA et al: Rare case of double aortic arch with hypoplastic right dorsal segment and associated tetralogy of Fallot: MR findings. Magn Reson Imaging. 11(8):1217-21, 1993
28. Chun K et al: Diagnosis and management of congenital vascular rings: a 22-year experience. Ann Thorac Surg. 53(4):597-602; discussion 602-3, 1992
29. Formanek AG et al: Anomaly of the descending aorta: a case of persistent double dorsal aorta. AJR Am J Roentgenol. 156(5):1033-5, 1991
30. Jaffe RB: Radiographic manifestations of congenital anomalies of the aortic arch. Radiol Clin North Am. 29(2):319-34, 1991
31. Lowe GM et al: Vascular rings: 10-year review of imaging. Radiographics. 11(4):637-46, 1991

DOUBLE AORTIC ARCH

IMAGE GALLERY

Typical

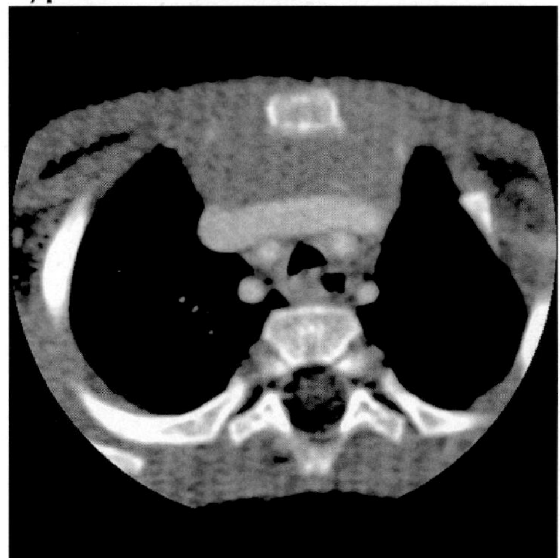

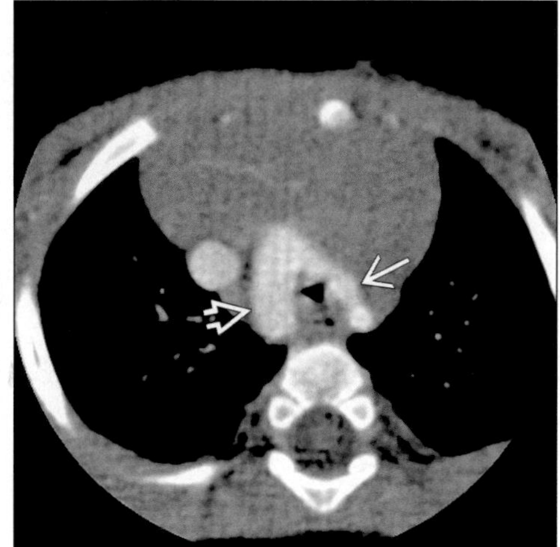

*(**Left**) Axial CTA shows "4 artery sign" in upper mediastinum, due to symmetrical take-off of brachiocephalic arches from ipsilateral aortic arch. (**Right**) Axial CTA shows dominant right arch ➡, smaller left arch ➡ and tracheal compression.*

Typical

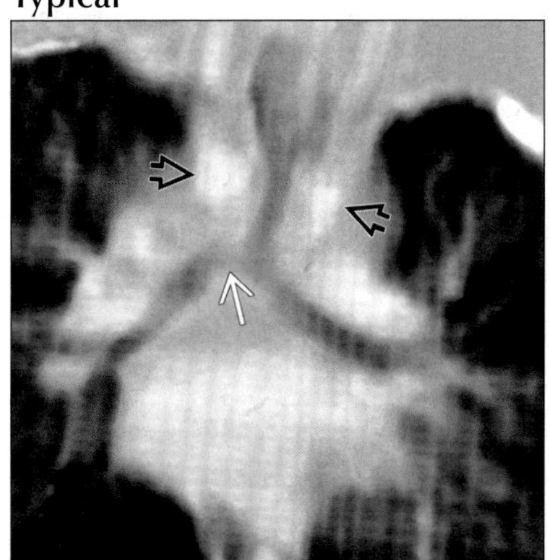

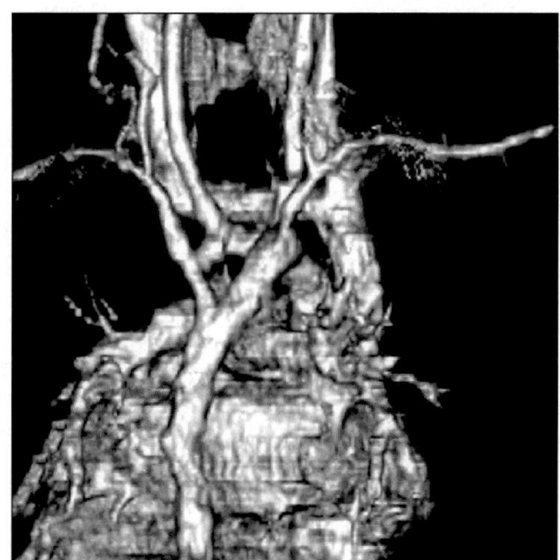

*(**Left**) Coronal CTA shows mild tracheal compression by both arches ⇨, and additional area of stenosis in left mainstem bronchus ➡ not related to vascular ring and likely representing bronchomalacia. (**Right**) Right posterior-oblique view, 3D shaded surface rendition CTA shows both arches meeting posteriorly to form the descending aorta.*

Variant

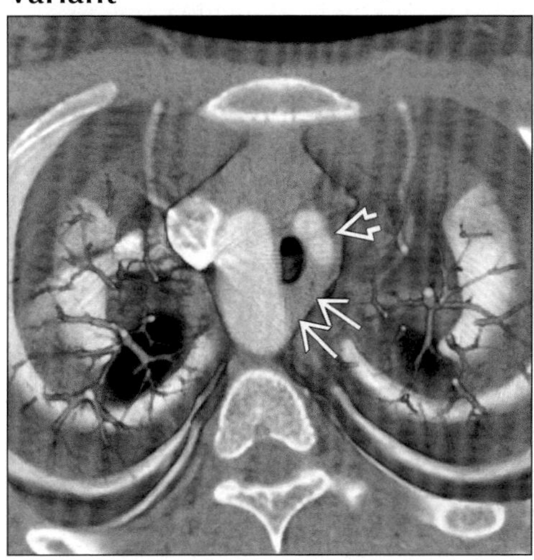

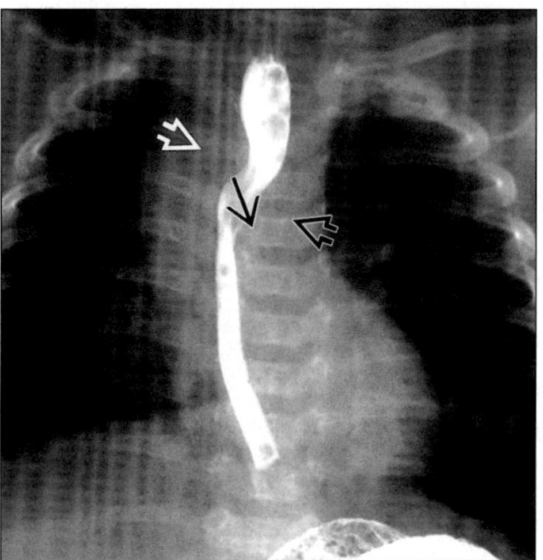

*(**Left**) Axial CTA shows dominant patent right arch and smaller left arch ➡ with atretic distal segment of left arch. Area of atresia is indicated by ➡. (**Right**) Frontal view of esophagram shows typical indentations from higher dominant right arch ➡, lower left arch ⇨ and oblique retro-esophageal impression →, which is best seen on a lateral view (not shown).*

RIGHT AORTIC ARCH

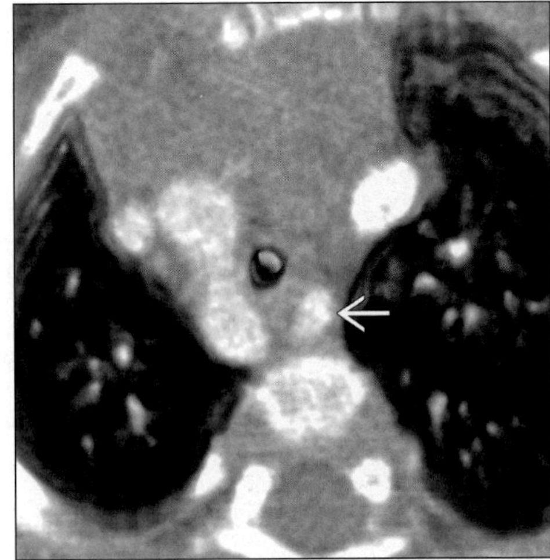

Axial CTA in asymptomatic young infant with stridor shows right aortic arch and aberrant LSA ➡. Note mild tracheal narrowing and also bilateral superior venae cavae.

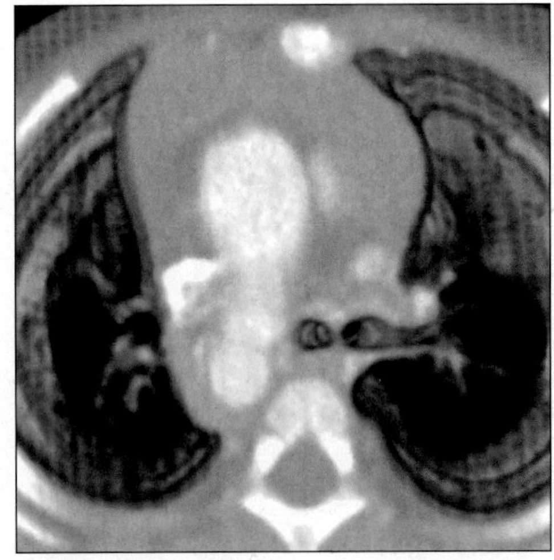

Axial CTA shows right aortic arch with mirror image branching in patient with tetralogy of Fallot.

TERMINOLOGY

Definitions

- Aortic arch located to right of trachea

IMAGING FINDINGS

General Features

- Best diagnostic clue
  - Left-sided tracheal deviation by right arch
  - Arch courses over right main stem bronchus
- Morphology
  - Right arch with mirror image branching: Associated with cyanotic congenital heart disease (CHD)
  - Right arch with aberrant left subclavian artery (LSA): Isolated anomaly, not often associated with CHD
    - In 60% there is dilatation of the origin of the aberrant LSA (aortic diverticulum of Kommerell)
    - May be associated with airway compression: Left ligamentum arteriosum completes vascular ring

Radiographic Findings

- Radiography
  - Aortic arch indentation on right of trachea, which is deviated to the left
  - More soft tissue over right pedicle than over left
  - Right-sided descending aorta line
  - If aneurysmal dilatation of aortic diverticulum or LSA: Prominence of left mediastinum

Fluoroscopic Findings

- Barium swallow: Indentations only seen when aberrant LSA is present
  - Frontal view: Oblique filling defect coursing from right-inferior to left-superior
  - Lateral view: Posterior indentation
  - Large posterior indentation: Aortic diverticulum

CT Findings

- Axial images: Patency and branches of arch segments
- Coronal recons: Tracheal compression (if present)

MR Findings

- Axial and coronal images show branching pattern of arch and effect on tracheobronchial tree
- Coronal thin-section images through the junction of the transverse and descending aorta demonstrate origin and proximal aspect of aberrant LSA

DDx: Right Aortic Arch

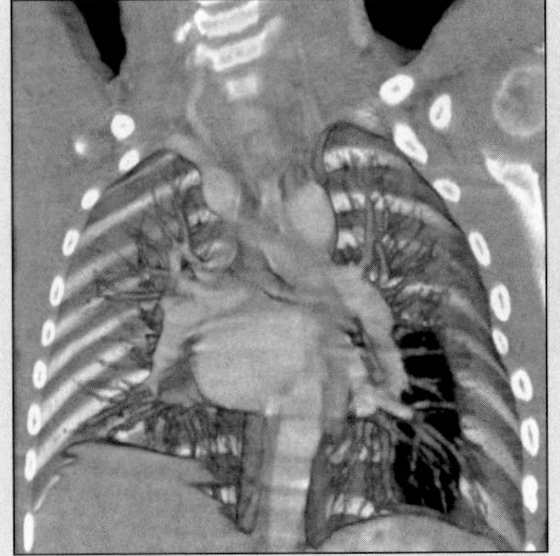

Double Aortic Arch

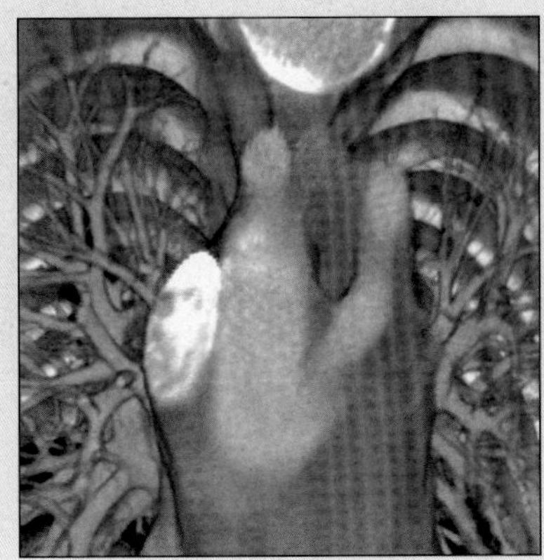

Double Arch, Atretic Left Arch

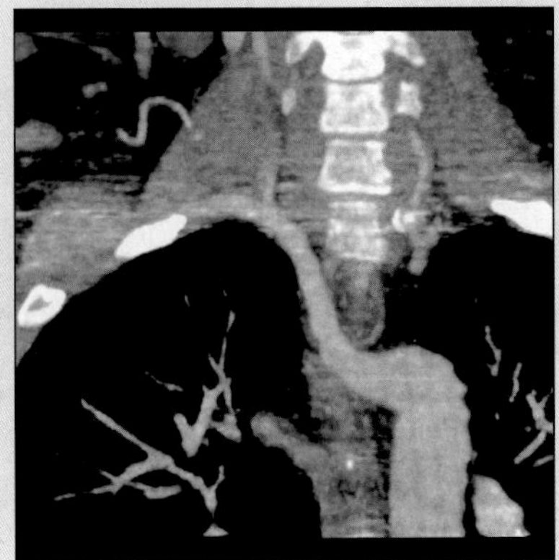

Left Arch, Aberrant RSA

RIGHT AORTIC ARCH

Key Facts

Imaging Findings

- Left-sided tracheal deviation by right arch
- Arch courses over right main stem bronchus
- Right arch with mirror image branching: Associated with cyanotic congenital heart disease (CHD)
- Right arch with aberrant left subclavian artery (LSA): Isolated anomaly, not often associated with CHD
- Barium swallow: Indentations only seen when aberrant LSA is present

Pathology

- All arch anomalies result from interruption of the hypothetical double arch model of Edwards
- Most common congenital anomaly of aortic arch in asymptomatic population

Clinical Issues

- Right arch with aberrant LSA: Incidental finding, often asymptomatic (only symptoms in 5%)
- Right arch with aberrant LSA and constricting left ligamentum arteriosum: Division of ligamentum via left thoracotomy

Diagnostic Checklist

- Right arch, no airway compression on radiograph, aberrant LSA on esophagram: No further work-up needed (non-constricting ring)
- Right arch with airway compression and aberrant LSA on esophagram: Perform cross-sectional imaging
- Right arch, mirror image branching pattern: Evaluate for cyanotic CHD

Echocardiographic Findings

- Echocardiogram
  - Defines arch pattern (mirror image vs. aberrant LSA)
  - Origin of aberrant LSA is well seen, especially in the presence of an aortic diverticulum of Kommerell

Imaging Recommendations

- Best imaging tool
  - Multidetector-row CTA with 3D reconstruction
    - Advantages: Fast, generally no need for sedation/anesthesia, no need for intubation, and therefore better evaluation of airway compression
    - Disadvantage: Radiation dose
  - Multiplanar MR
    - Advantage: No radiation dose
    - Disadvantages: Takes longer to perform than CT, more artifacts (metal, motion)
- Protocol advice
  - Axial thin slices through tracheobronchial tree and proximal descending aorta, to show arch branching pattern and presence of aberrant LSA
  - Coronal imaging depicts airway compression

DIFFERENTIAL DIAGNOSIS

Double Aortic Arch

- Left arch often not well seen, atretic segment and not left ligamentum arteriosum maintains fibrous continuity of vascular ring
- Characterized by tracheal narrowing, is nearly always symptomatic (stridor)

Left Aortic Arch with Aberrant Right Subclavian Artery

- Mirror image of right aortic arch with aberrant LSA
- Oblique posterior esophageal indentation from left-inferior to right-superior
- Isolated abnormality, incidentally found and usually without airway compression
- Rarely symptomatic from esophageal compression (dysphagia lusoria)

PATHOLOGY

General Features

- General path comments
  - All arch anomalies result from interruption of the hypothetical double arch model of Edwards
    - Normal development: Interruption distal to right subclavian artery (RSA)
    - Right arch, mirror image branching: Interruption distal to left subclavian artery
    - Right arch, aberrant LSA: Interruption between left common carotid and LSA
    - Left arch, aberrant RSA: Interruption between right common carotid and RSA
  - Aberrant LSA rarely lies anterior to the trachea (5%)
  - When associated with coarctation, aberrant subclavian artery can serve as a major collateral when it arises distally to coarctation
  - Embryology-anatomy
    - Embryological persistence of the right 4th arch
    - Retroesophageal (Kommerell) diverticulum: Remnant of embryonic left fourth aortic arch and connects to left ductus ligament
    - LSA can arise directly from the descending aorta or can arise from an aortic diverticulum
    - Left ductus persists as ligamentum arteriosum, which completes vascular ring
    - Right ductus is obliterated
  - Arch anomalies rarely cause dysphagia, and more frequently cause stridor from airway compression by complete vascular ring, part of which may be fibrotic (atretic segments, ligamentum arteriosum)
    - Left ligamentum arteriosum connects to subclavian artery ⇒ loose vascular ring
    - Left ligamentum arteriosum connects to aortic diverticulum of Kommerell ⇒ tight vascular ring
  - Pathophysiology
    - Airway compression only when complete tight vascular ring is present
    - Symptomatic esophageal compression in the absence of airway compression is rare
    - No hemodynamic disturbance (unless with CHD)

RIGHT AORTIC ARCH

- Genetics
  - Right or left arch with aberrant subclavian artery: No specific genetic defect identified
  - Right arch with mirror image branching: As with associated congenital heart lesion
- Epidemiology
  - Most common congenital anomaly of aortic arch in asymptomatic population
    - Left arch with aberrant RSA: 0.5%
    - Right arch with aberrant LSA: 0.1%
    - 14% of patients with right arch have aberrant LSA
- Associated abnormalities
  - CHD in 10-15% of cases with right arch
    - Tetralogy of Fallot, pulmonary atresia with ventricular septal defect: 25% has right arch
    - Truncus arteriosus: 30-40% has right arch
    - Transposition of great arteries
  - Cyanotic heart lesion with right arch: Tetralogy is most likely (truncus and pulmonary atresia are rare)

CLINICAL ISSUES

Presentation

- Most common signs/symptoms
  - Right arch with aberrant LSA: Incidental finding, often asymptomatic (only symptoms in 5%)
    - May cause symptoms in infancy, provoked by airway infection (mucosal edema), improves with age and growth of child
    - When associated with tightly constricting left ligamentum arteriosum: Congenital stridor
    - Symptoms may develop when aberrant artery is tortuous or aneurysmal
    - Posterior esophageal indentation by aberrant subclavian artery rarely causes dysphagia (lusoria)
  - Right arch with mirror image branching: Determined by associated cyanotic cardiac anomaly
- Other signs/symptoms: Chronic cough, "asthma"

Natural History & Prognosis

- Determined by natural history of co-existing CHD
- Symptoms from tracheomalacia, residual stenosis and vascular compression are common after repair, which most children eventually outgrow, but some require additional surgery

Treatment

- Right arch with aberrant LSA and constricting left ligamentum arteriosum: Division of ligamentum via left thoracotomy
  - Aortopexy may be needed additionally
  - When associated with complete cartilaginous tracheal ring: Resection and tracheal reconstruction
- Otherwise dependent on associated heart lesion

DIAGNOSTIC CHECKLIST

Consider

- Right arch, no airway compression on radiograph, aberrant LSA on esophagram: No further work-up needed (non-constricting ring)
- Right arch with airway compression and aberrant LSA on esophagram: Perform cross-sectional imaging
- Right arch, mirror image branching pattern: Evaluate for cyanotic CHD

Image Interpretation Pearls

- Determine branching pattern of the right arch
- Look for subclavian vessel running behind esophagus on cross-sectional studies

SELECTED REFERENCES

1. Holmes KW et al: Magnetic resonance imaging of a distorted left subclavian artery course: an important clue to an unusual type of double aortic arch. Pediatr Cardiol. 27(3):316-20, 2006
2. Malik TH et al: The role of magnetic resonance imaging in the assessment of suspected extrinsic tracheobronchial compression due to vascular anomalies. Arch Dis Child. 91(1):52-5, 2006
3. Salanitri J: MR angiography of aberrant left subclavian artery arising from right-sided thoracic aortic arch. Br J Radiol. 78(934):961-6, 2005
4. Cina CS et al: Kommerell's diverticulum and right-sided aortic arch: a cohort study and review of the literature. J Vasc Surg. 39(1):131-9, 2004
5. Backer CL et al: Pediatric cardiac surgery. 3rd ed. Philadelphia, Mosby. 234-50, 2003
6. Rosa P et al: Aberrant right subclavian artery syndrome: a case of chronic cough. J Vasc Surg. 37(6):1318-21, 2003
7. Subramanyan R et al: Vascular rings: an important cause of persistent respiratory symptoms in infants and children. Indian Pediatr. 40(10):951-7, 2003
8. Donnelly LF et al: Aberrant subclavian arteries: cross-sectional imaging findings in infants and children referred for evaluation of extrinsic airway compression. AJR Am J Roentgenol. 178(5):1269-74, 2002
9. Zachary CH et al: Vascular ring due to right aortic arch with mirror-image branching and left ligamentum arteriosus: complete preoperative diagnosis by magnetic resonance imaging. Pediatr Cardiol. 22(1):71-3, 2001
10. Midiri M et al: Right aortic arch with aberrant left innominate artery: MR imaging findings. Eur Radiol. 9(2):311-5, 1999
11. McLeary MS et al: Magnetic resonance imaging of a left circumflex aortic arch and aberrant right subclavian artery: the other vascular ring. Pediatr Radiol. 28(4):263-5, 1998
12. Newman B: MR of right aortic arch. Pediatr Radiol. 26(5):367-9, 1996
13. Katz M et al: Spiral CT and 3D image reconstruction of vascular rings and associated tracheobronchial anomalies. J Comput Assist Tomogr. 19(4):564-8, 1995
14. Schlesinger AE et al: MR of right aortic arch with mirror-image branching and a left ligamentum arteriosum: an unusual cause of a vascular ring. Pediatr Radiol. 25(6):455-7, 1995
15. Kleinman PK et al: Left-sided esophageal indentation in right aortic arch with aberrant left subclavian artery. Radiology. 191(2):565-7, 1994
16. Turkenburg JL et al: Case report: aneurysm of an aberrant right subclavian artery diagnosed with MR imaging. Clin Radiol. 49(11):837-9, 1994
17. van Son JA et al: Imaging strategies for vascular rings. Ann Thorac Surg. 57(3):604-10, 1994
18. McNally PR et al: Dysphagia lusoria caused by persistent right aortic arch with aberrant left subclavian artery and diverticulum of Kommerell. Dig Dis Sci. 37(1):144-9, 1992

RIGHT AORTIC ARCH

IMAGE GALLERY

Typical

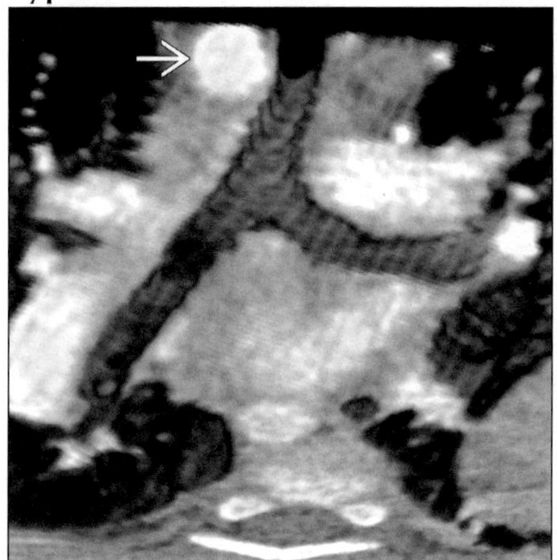

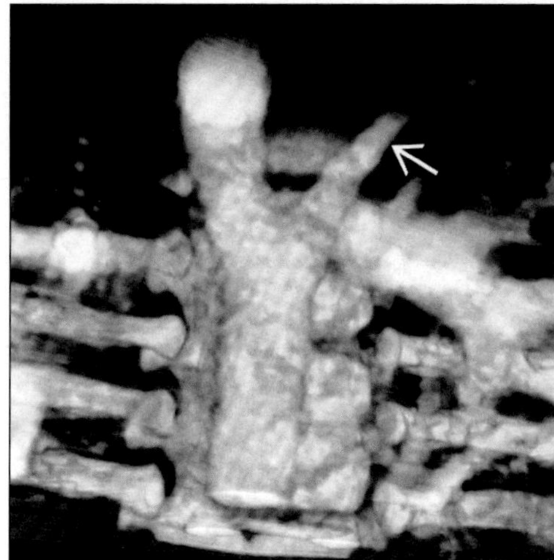

(Left) *Coronal volume rendition of CTA shows right aortic arch ➔, with no tracheal compression.* ***(Right)*** *Changing the opacity setting of this rendition reveals the presence of an aberrant LSA ➔.*

Variant

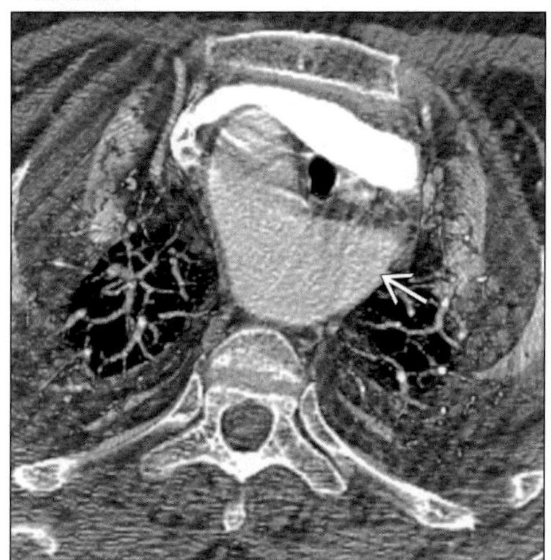

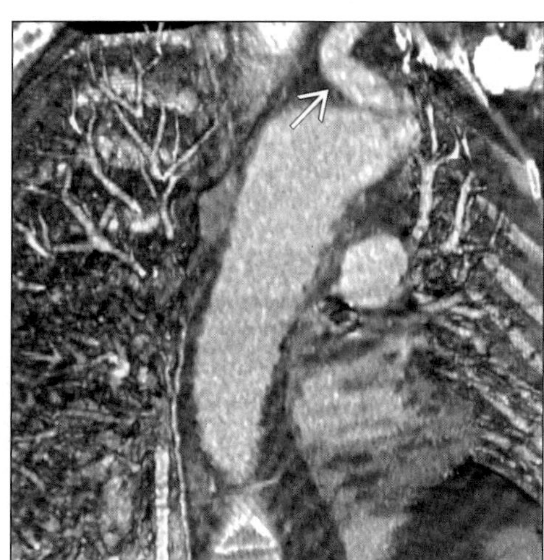

(Left) *Axial CTA in asymptomatic 49 year old woman shows right aortic arch and aneurysmally dilated diverticulum of Kommerell ➔.* ***(Right)*** *Coronal rendition in same patient as previous image shows take-off of LSA ➔ from this aortic diverticulum of Kommerell.*

Typical

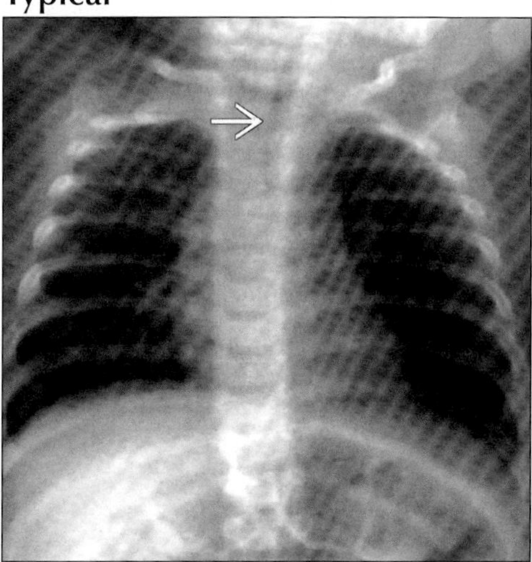

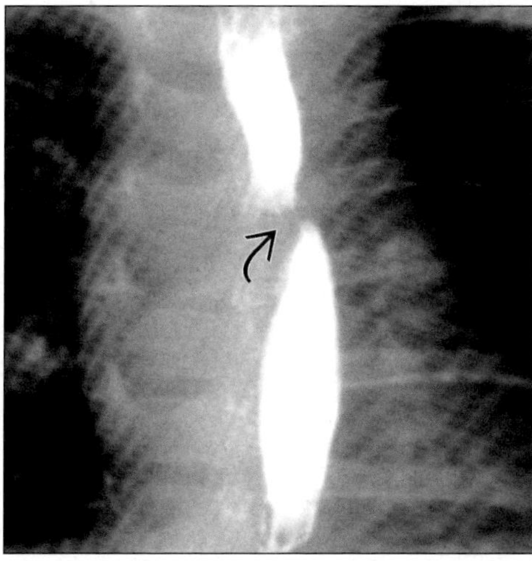

(Left) *Radiograph shows shows leftward position of the trachea ➔ in this patient who is rotated to the left.* ***(Right)*** *Esophagram depicts an oblique indentation ➔ on the esophageal lumen, caused by the aberrant left subclavian artery.*

PULMONARY SLING

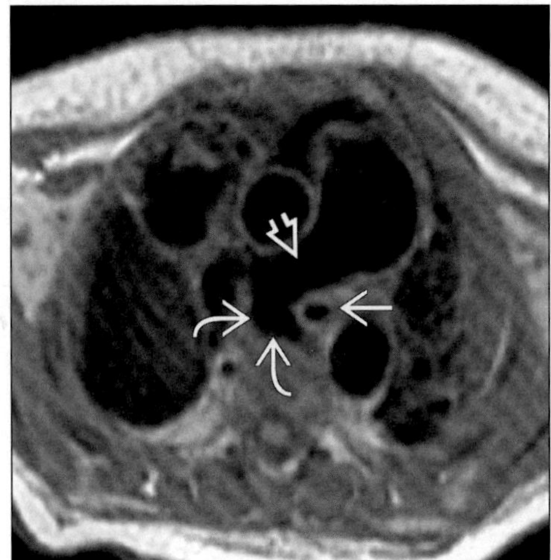

Axial T1WI MR shows type 1A left pulmonary artery sling ➡, originating from the proximal right pulmonary artery ➡ and encircling and compressing the distal trachea ➡.

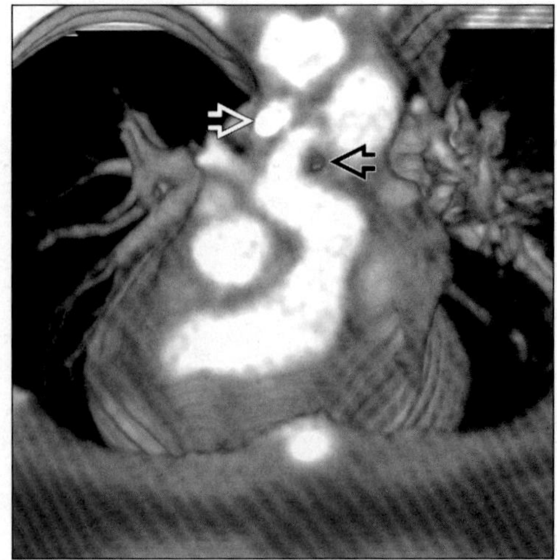

Superior view, cut plane volume rendition CTA shows an anomalous origin of the left pulmonary artery, which courses between the esophagus (identified by nasogastric tube, ➡) & the stenosed distal trachea ➡.

TERMINOLOGY

Abbreviations and Synonyms

- Anomalous origin of the left pulmonary artery (PA)
- Aberrant left pulmonary artery

Definitions

- Left branch PA originates from proximal right PA forming a "sling" around distal trachea as it passes leftward between trachea and esophagus

IMAGING FINDINGS

General Features

- Best diagnostic clue
  - Asymmetric lung inflation, narrowing of distal trachea which is displaced towards the left, anterior impression on mid-esophagus
  - Only vascular ring to course between the trachea and esophagus
- Morphology
  - Type I: Carina in normal location at T4-5 ⇒ predominant hyperinflation of right lung
    - With normal ("eparterial") right upper lobe bronchus
    - With tracheal bronchus (bronchus suis = "pig bronchus") to right upper lobe
  - Type II: Low carina (T6), with "ring-sling" complex: Diffuse stenosis of intermediate left bronchus (ILB), complete cartilage rings, multi-level absence of membranous portion of trachea ⇒ bilateral hyperinflation
    - Initial bifurcation at T4 into right upper lobe bronchus and ILB, which bifurcates at T6 into bridging right lower lobe bronchus and left mainstem bronchus
    - Lower ILB bifurcation is compressed by sling
    - Absent or abortive right upper lobe bronchus
    - Diffusely stenosed ILB (as in IIA) bifurcates at T6 into bridging right and left mainstem bronchus (low "inverted T" airway bifurcation)

Radiographic Findings

- Radiography
  - Only vascular ring associated with asymmetric lung inflation and aeration

DDx: Tracheal Compression by Vascular Ring

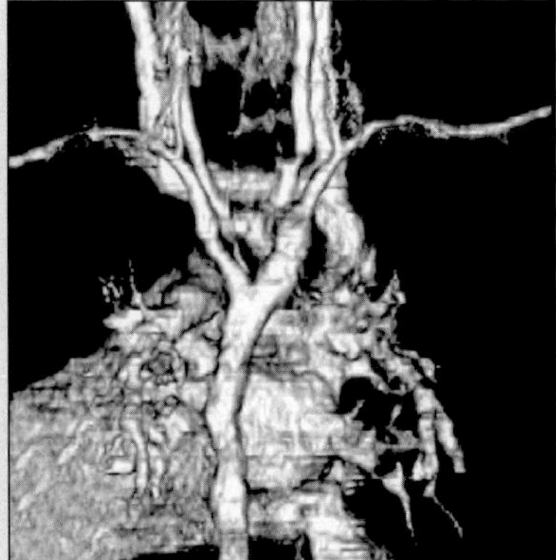

Double Aortic Arch

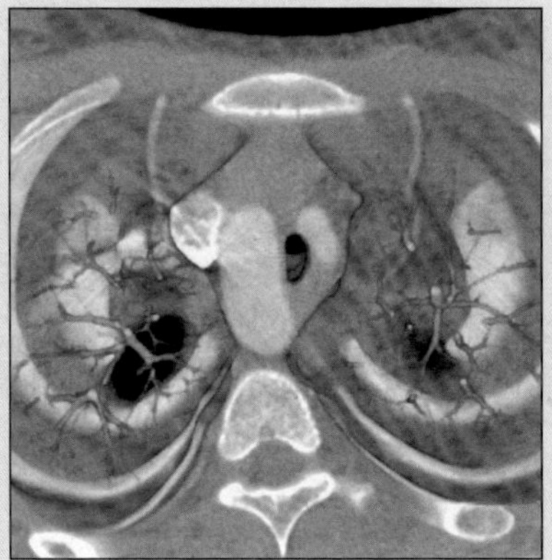

Double Arch, Atretic Left Arch

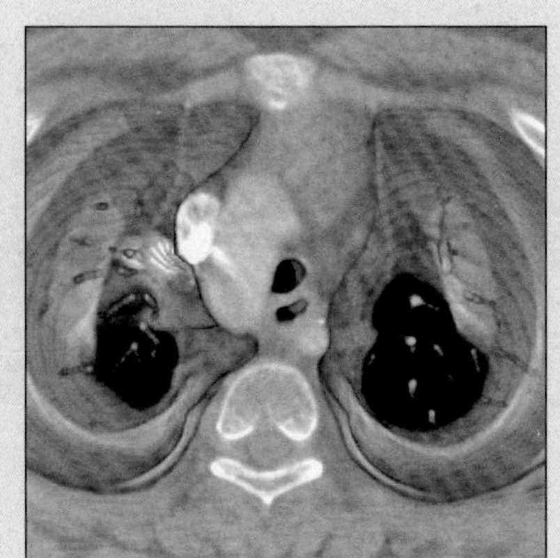

Right Arch, Aberrant LSA

PULMONARY SLING

Key Facts

Terminology

- Left branch PA originates from proximal right PA forming a "sling" around distal trachea as it passes leftward between trachea and esophagus

Imaging Findings

- Only vascular ring to course between the trachea and esophagus
- Type I: Carina in normal location at T4-5 ⇒ predominant hyperinflation of right lung
- Type II: Low carina (T6), with "ring-sling" complex: Diffuse stenosis of intermediate left bronchus (ILB), complete cartilage rings, multi-level absence of membranous portion of trachea ⇒ bilateral hyperinflation
- Only vascular ring associated with asymmetric lung inflation and aeration
- Lateral view: Round soft tissue density between distal trachea and esophagus
- Barium swallow: Pulmonary sling is the only vascular ring that leads to an anterior indentation on the esophagus
- Left PA arises from the right, rather than the main PA
- Degree of tracheal compression typically severe
- When complete tracheal rings are present, the trachea will have a very round (rather than oval) appearance with an abnormally small diameter
- Best imaging tool: CTA faster and logistically easier than MR in critically ill infants on a ventilator

Clinical Issues

- Most common signs/symptoms: Severe stridor, hypoxia, ventilator dependency

  - Lateral view: Round soft tissue density between distal trachea and esophagus

  - Posterior compression of the trachea, typically distally at the level of the distal trachea or carina
  - Distal trachea or right main bronchus may be bowed anteriorly
  - Low position of the left hilum

Fluoroscopic Findings

- Barium swallow: Pulmonary sling is the only vascular ring that leads to an anterior indentation on the esophagus
- Trachea is compressed at same level from posteriorly

Echocardiographic Findings

- Echocardiogram
  - Absence of normal PA bifurcation
  - Anomalous origin of left PA from proximal right pulmonary artery
  - Associated other cardiac anomalies

Other Modality Findings

- CT and MR features
  - Cross sectional imaging obtained to confirm diagnosis and delineate anatomy prior to surgery
  - Pulmonary sling and tracheal compression typically best demonstrated on axial CT or MR images
  - Left PA arises from the right, rather than the main PA
  - Left PA forms a "sling" around the trachea as it passes leftward between trachea and esophagus
  - Degree of tracheal compression typically severe
  - Distal trachea and carina often displaced to the left
  - Often findings of coexisting congenital heart disease evident
  - When complete tracheal rings are present, the trachea will have a very round (rather than oval) appearance with an abnormally small diameter

Imaging Recommendations

- Best imaging tool: CTA faster and logistically easier than MR in critically ill infants on a ventilator
- Protocol advice
  - Thin axial slices and multiplanar reconstructions are most helpful to depict sling anatomy
  - Coronal images or 3D reconstructions display effect of sling on tracheobronchial tree

DIFFERENTIAL DIAGNOSIS

Middle Mediastinal Mass

- Lymphadenopathy
- Bronchogenic cyst
- Esophageal duplication cyst

Primary Bronchial Malformation

- Congenital lobar emphysema/bronchial atresia
- Tracheobronchomalacia
- Complete cartilaginous ring

Midline Descending Aorta Carina Compression Syndrome

- Aorta immediately anterior to spine, leading to "mediastinal crowding": Posterior compression on carina or left main stem bronchus
- May be isolated, or associated with right lung hypoplasia, arch anomalies

PATHOLOGY

General Features

- General path comments
  - Frequently associated with hypoplasia/dysplasia of distal trachea and main stem bronchi
  - Hemodynamics: Determined by associated cardiac anomaly
  - Pulmonary hypertension from severe hypoxia
- Genetics: No specific genetic defect identified
- Etiology
  - Embryology
    - Agenesis or obliteration of the left sixth aortic arch, which normally forms the left branch PA
    - Arterial supply of left lung via persistent primitive artery originating from right PA

PULMONARY SLING

- ○ Pathophysiology: Severe stridor secondary to
  - ▪ Compression of distal trachea, carina, main stem bronchi: Uneven inflation of the lungs (obstructive emphysema > atelectasis)
  - ▪ Associated tracheobronchomalacia
  - ▪ Associated intrinsic airway narrowing (complete cartilaginous rings): Types IIA and IIB
- Associated abnormalities: Other congenital malformations (50%), lung hypoplasia, horseshoe lung

Gross Pathologic & Surgical Features

- Left PA arises from the right, rather than the main PA
- Left PA forms a "sling" around the trachea as it passes leftward between the trachea and esophagus
- It enters hilum of left lung posteriorly to left main stem bronchus
- Severe compression of distal trachea and right main stem bronchus
- Main stem bronchi have abnormal horizontal course ("inverted T"), with abnormal branching patterns to upper and lower lobes (types IIA and IIB)
- Often associated with with complete tracheal cartilaginous rings (50%)

CLINICAL ISSUES

Presentation

- Most common signs/symptoms: Severe stridor, hypoxia, ventilator dependency
- Other signs/symptoms: Noisy breathing, "seal bark" cough, apneic spells, recurrent pulmonary infections early in life

Demographics

- Age: Typically presents in neonatal period

Natural History & Prognosis

- Type II: Less favorable than other vascular rings, due to associated anomalies (60-80%)
  - ○ Intrinsic tracheobronchial anomalies (complete rings, absent membranous portion of trachea), tracheomalacia
  - ○ Congenital heart disease: Aortic arch anomalies, ventricular septal defect (10%), atrial septal defect (20%), patent ductus arteriosus (25%), single ventricle, tetralogy of Fallot, partial anomalous pulmonary venous return, persistent left superior vena cava (20%)
  - ○ Pulmonary and systemic anomalies: Hypoplastic right lung, horseshoe lung, tracheo-esophageal fistula, imperforate anus, absence of gallbladder, Meckel diverticulum, biliary atresia, Hirschsprung disease

Treatment

- Surgical division of left PA from its anomalous origin, with implantation to its normal location of origin, from main PA
- Tracheobronchial reconstruction if there are complete cartilaginous rings or other associated tracheobronchial malformation (types IIA and IIB)

DIAGNOSTIC CHECKLIST

Image Interpretation Pearls

- Anterior indentation on esophagus = left pulmonary artery sling

SELECTED REFERENCES

1. Choo KS et al: Atelectasis of the left lung induced by subcarinal pulmonary artery sling. Pediatr Radiol. 35(5):543-5, 2005
2. Backer CL: Vascular rings and pulmonary artery sling. In: Mavroudis C et al, ed. Pediatric cardiac surgery. 3rd ed. Philadelphia, Mosby. 234-50, 2003
3. Eichhorn J et al: Images in cardiovascular medicine. Time-resolved three-dimensional magnetic resonance angiography for assessing a pulmonary artery sling in a pediatric patient. Circulation. 106(14):e61-2, 2002
4. Hwang HK et al: Horseshoe lung with pseudo-ring-sling complex. Pediatr Pulmonol. 34(5):402-4, 2002
5. Park SC et al: Vascular ring and pulmonary artery sling. In: Anderson RH et al, ed. Pediatric Cardiology. vol. 2. 2nd ed. London, Churchill Livingstone.1559-75, 2002
6. Bove T et al: Tracheobronchial compression of vascular origin. Review of experience in infants and children. J Cardiovasc Surg (Torino). 42(5):663-6, 2001
7. Hodina M et al: Non-invasive imaging of the ring-sling complex in children. Pediatr Cardiol. 22(4):333-7, 2001
8. Lee KH et al: Use of imaging for assessing anatomical relationships of tracheobronchial anomalies associated with left pulmonary artery sling. Pediatr Radiol. 31(4):269-78, 2001
9. Woods RK et al: Vascular anomalies and tracheoesophageal compression: a single institution's 25-year experience. Ann Thorac Surg. 72(2):434-8; discussion 438-9, 2001
10. Berdon WE: Rings, slings, and other things: vascular compression of the infant trachea updated from the midcentury to the millennium--the legacy of Robert E. Gross, MD, and Edward B. D. Neuhauser, MD. Radiology. 216(3):624-32, 2000
11. Di Cesare E et al: Pulmonary artery sling diagnosed by magnetic resonance imaging. Magn Reson Imaging. 15(9):1107-9, 1997
12. Donnelly LF et al: The spectrum of extrinsic lower airway compression in children: MR imaging. AJR Am J Roentgenol. 168(1):59-62, 1997
13. Siripornpitak S et al: Pulmonary artery sling: anatomical and functional evaluation by MRI. J Comput Assist Tomogr. 21(5):766-8, 1997
14. Newman B et al: Left pulmonary artery sling: diagnosis and delineation of associated tracheobronchial anomalies with MR. Pediatr Radiol. 26(9):661-8, 1996
15. Pu WT et al: Diagnosis and management of agenesis of the right lung and left pulmonary artery sling. Am J Cardiol. 78(6):723-7, 1996
16. Katz M et al: Spiral CT and 3D image reconstruction of vascular rings and associated tracheobronchial anomalies. J Comput Assist Tomogr. 19(4):564-8, 1995
17. Phillips RR et al: Pulmonary artery sling and hypoplastic right lung: diagnostic appearances using MRI. Pediatr Radiol. 23(2):117-9, 1993
18. Vogl TJ et al: MRI in pre- and postoperative assessment of tracheal stenosis due to pulmonary artery sling. J Comput Assist Tomogr. 17(6):878-86, 1993
19. Berdon WE et al: Vascular anomalies and the infant lung: rings, slings, and other things. Semin Roentgenol. 7(1):39-64, 1972

PULMONARY SLING

IMAGE GALLERY

Typical

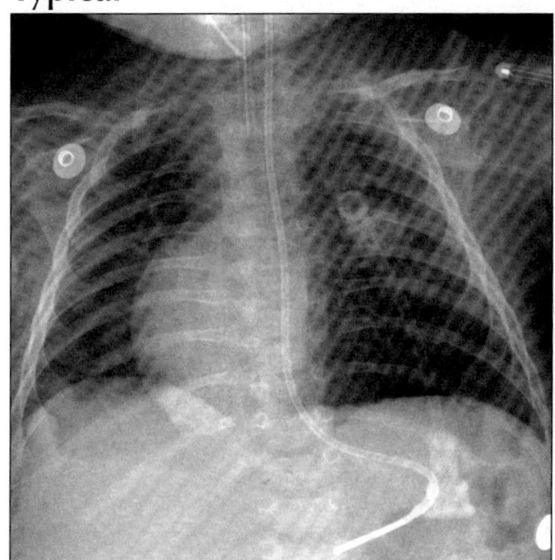

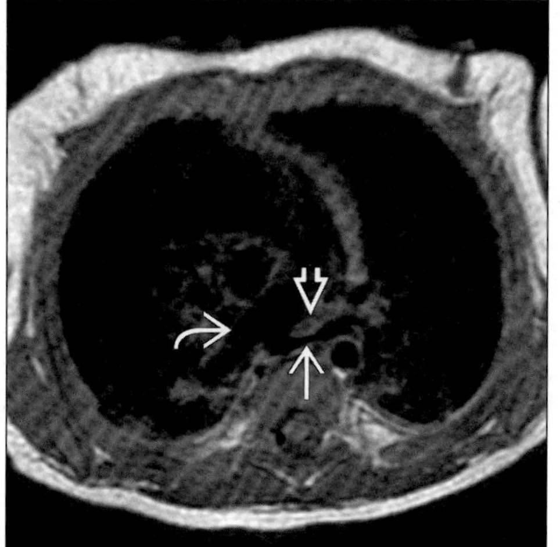

(Left) *Radiograph shows asymmetric lung volumes (R < L) with shift of the heart and mediastinum into the right hemithorax.* ***(Right)*** *Axial T1WI MR shows the pulmonary sling, anomalous origin of the left pulmonary artery from the right pulmonary artery. Note pinpoint stenosis of distal trachea.*

Variant

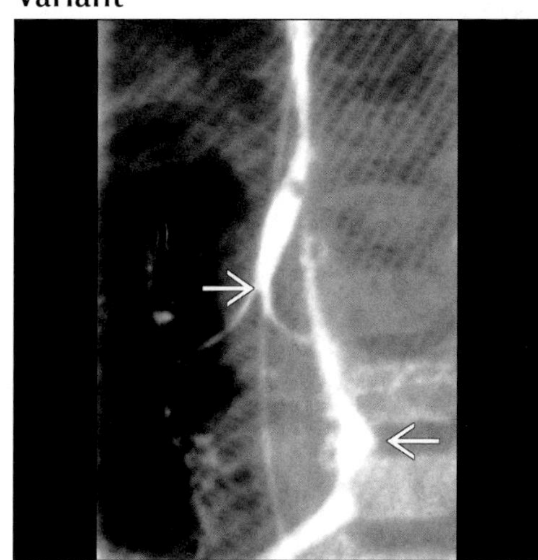

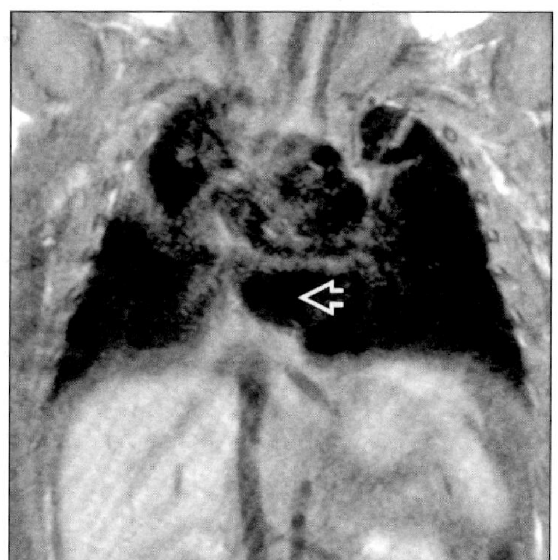

(Left) *Bronchogram demonstrates anomalous branching patterns of the tracheobronchial tree, with two separate tracheas and carinae, with lack of filling of bronchi in atelectatic left lower lobe.* ***(Right)*** *Coronal T1WI MR in the same patient as previous image, shows horseshoe lung segment in the retrocardiac area.*

Variant

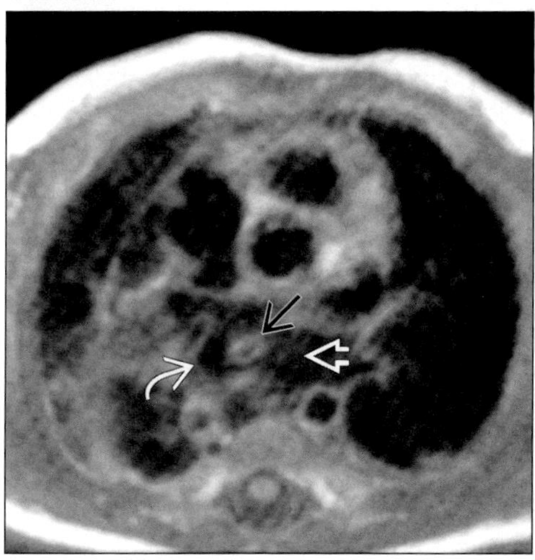

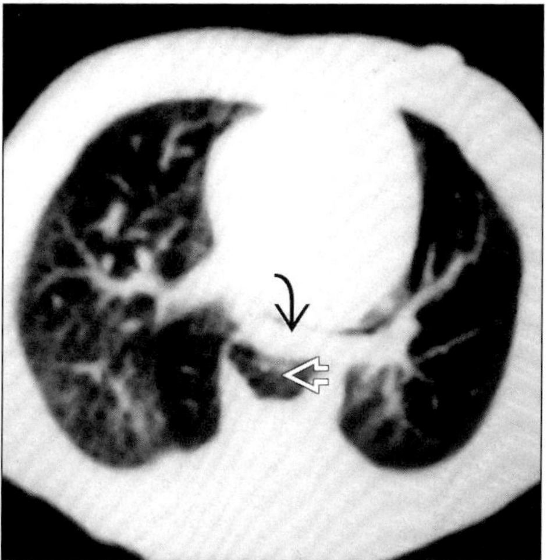

(Left) *Axial T1WI MR in the same patient as previous image shows a horseshoe lung segment in the retrocardiac area and the left pulmonary artery circling around the lower-most of the tracheal carinae.* ***(Right)*** *Axial NECT in the same patient as previous image, shows distal aspect of LPA sling, traveling to the left lung, and horseshoe lung segment in the posterior mediastinum.*

D-TRANSPOSITION

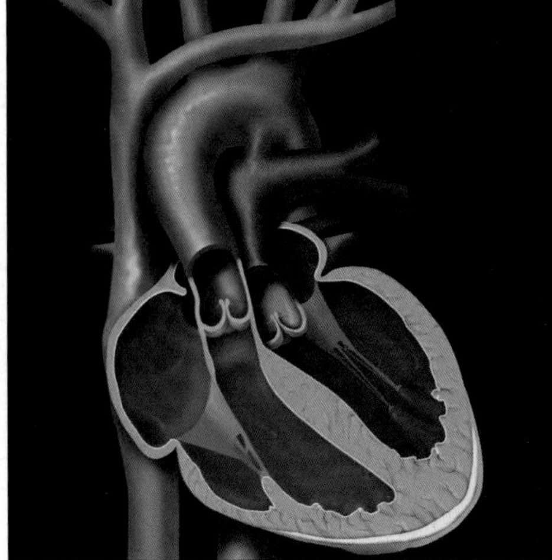

Graphic shows anteriorly-placed aorta, connected via infundibulum to right ventricle, and posteriorly-placed pulmonary artery, directly connected to left ventricle.

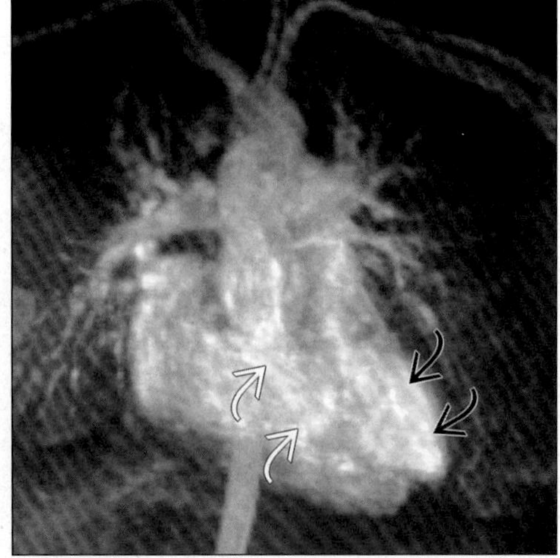

Coronal MIP MRA demonstrates the malposition of the ventricles relative to the great vessels. The right ventricle ➡ is related to the ascending aorta and the left ventricle ➡ gives origin to the pulmonary artery.

TERMINOLOGY

Abbreviations and Synonyms

- Ventriculoarterial discordance with atrioventricular concordance

Definitions

- Aorta arises from right ventricle (RV) and pulmonary artery from left ventricle (LV)
- Category: Cyanotic, cardiomegaly, increased pulmonary vascularity
- Hemodynamics
  - RV → systemic circulation: Pressure overload
  - LV → pulmonary circulation: Volume overload
  - Incompatible with life without flow admixture

IMAGING FINDINGS

General Features

- Best diagnostic clue: Great vessels lie parallel and almost in the same sagittal plane, aortic valve in anterior position and to right (D-loop) of pulmonary valve

Radiographic Findings

- Radiography
  - May be normal in neonates
  - Cardiomegaly
  - Narrow mediastinum ("egg-on-side" heart)
  - Increased pulmonary vascularity

CT Findings

- CTA
  - Post-op CTA: Anteriorly-positioned pulmonary artery (PA) and posterior aorta in same sagittal plane
    - Traction on both branch PAs may lead to stenosis
    - Anterior tracheal or left mainstem bronchus compression by ascending aorta
    - Cardiac-gated multi-detector cine CT: Ventricular function (when contra-indication for MR)
  - CTA is preferred modality after placement of metallic stents for branch pulmonary artery stenosis

MR Findings

- T1WI
  - Cardiac-gated axial images for segmental cardiac analysis: Atrioventricular concordance and ventriculoarterial discordance

DDx: Cyanosis with Increased Pulmonary Vascularity

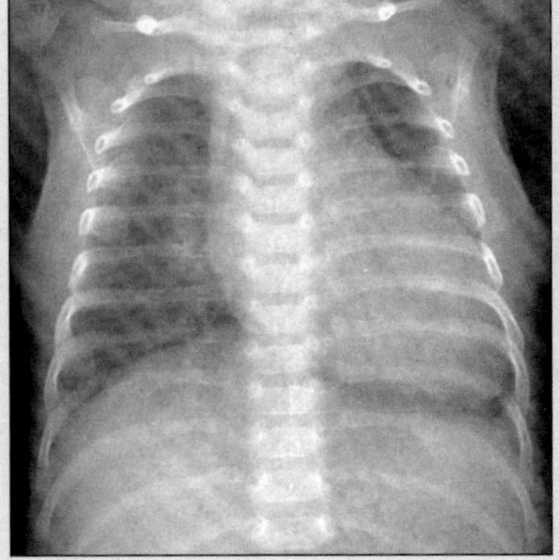

Truncus Arteriosus

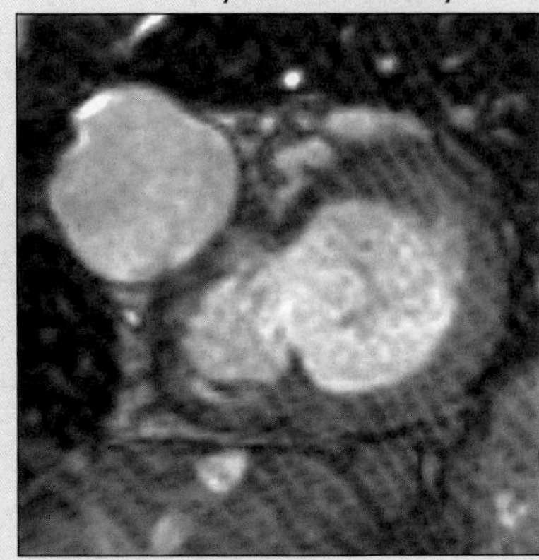

Tricuspid Atresia

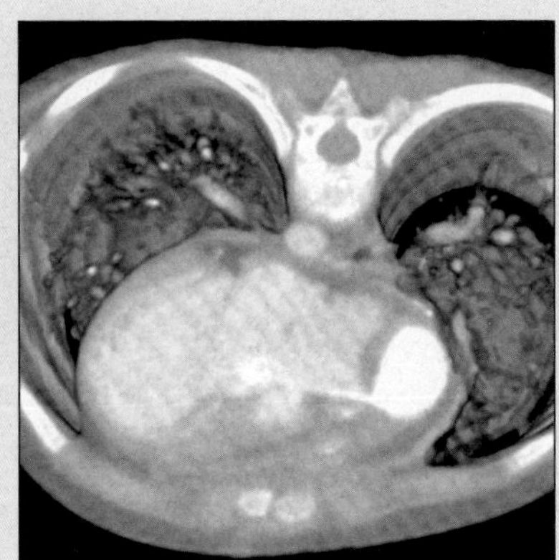

Single Ventricle

D-TRANSPOSITION

Key Facts

Terminology
- Ventriculoarterial discordance with atrioventricular concordance
- Aorta arises from right ventricle (RV) and pulmonary artery from left ventricle (LV)
- Category: Cyanotic, cardiomegaly, increased pulmonary vascularity

Imaging Findings
- Best diagnostic clue: Great vessels lie parallel and almost in the same sagittal plane, aortic valve in anterior position and to right (D-loop) of pulmonary valve
- Narrow mediastinum ("egg-on-side" heart)
- CTA is preferred modality after placement of metallic stents for branch pulmonary artery stenosis
- Multiplanar steady-state free precession cine is the gold standard for cardiac function evaluation, ventricular volume measurements
- Conventional: Cardiac catheterization only for Rashkind procedure (emergency balloon atrial septostomy)

Pathology
- Coronary anomalies are frequent
- Survival dependent on admixture: PFO, VSD, PDA

Clinical Issues
- Complication of arterial switch: Traction on branch PAs by anteriorly transposed main PA, leading to branch origin stenosis
- Mustard/Senning procedures: RV failure, atrial thrombosis, arrhythmias

---

    - Patent foramen ovale (PFO), ventricular septal defect (VSD), (sub-) pulmonary stenosis
    - Post-operative assessment of PA stenosis
    - If metal artifact from stents: Double inversion sequence
- T2* GRE
  - Multiplanar steady-state free precession cine is the gold standard for cardiac function evaluation, ventricular volume measurements
    - RV dysfunction following atrial switch procedures, not able to sustain systemic circulation
    - Baffle obstruction after Mustard/Senning
- T1 C+: Delayed-enhancement myocardial MR to detect ischemia complicating coronary transposition
- MRA
  - Gadolinium-enhanced MRA for post-op PA stenosis
  - MR coronary angiography with navigator-echo respiratory gating: Patency transposed coronaries
  - Velocity-encoded phase contrast MRA with flow velocity measurements, allowing calculations of gradients across stenoses (PAs, atrial baffles)

Echocardiographic Findings
- Segmental cardiac analysis: Identification of atria, ventricles, great arteries and their connections
- Identification of PFO, VSD, patent ductus arteriosus (PDA)
- Proximal coronary artery anatomy

Angiographic Findings
- Conventional: Cardiac catheterization only for Rashkind procedure (emergency balloon atrial septostomy)

Imaging Recommendations
- Echocardiography allows for complete pre-operative diagnosis in majority
- CT or MR for post-operative complications of pulmonary arteries, atrial baffle

DIFFERENTIAL DIAGNOSIS

Complex Transposition
- Associated (sub-) pulmonary stenosis, VSD

Associated Preductal Coarctation with PDA
- Small RV and aorta; large LV and pulmonary artery

Truncus Arteriosus, Aortopulmonary Window, Tricuspid Atresia, Single Ventricle with Unobstructed Pulmonary Flow
- All have cardiomegaly with increased vascularity

PATHOLOGY

General Features
- General path comments
  - Atria and ventricles are morphologic normal
  - Coronary anomalies are frequent
    - Right coronary artery dominance
    - Circumflex branch originates from right coronary
    - Single coronary ostium
  - Embryology
    - Single embryological error: Faulty separation of aorta and pulmonary artery from primitive bulbus cordis (cono-truncus)
    - Heart is otherwise structurally normal
  - Pathophysiology
    - Separation of pulmonary and systemic circulations
    - Survival dependent on admixture: PFO, VSD, PDA
- Genetics
  - No genetic factors identified
  - Not associated with extracardiac malformations or chromosomal abnormalities
- Epidemiology
  - Incidence: 1 in 3,000 live births
  - 5% of congenital heart disease
  - Males > females

D-TRANSPOSITION

Gross Pathologic & Surgical Features

- Infundibulum of RV connected to aortic valve, anterior and slightly to right of midline (D-loop)
- LV connected without infundibulum to pulmonary valve, posterior and slightly to left of aortic valve

CLINICAL ISSUES

Presentation

- Severe cyanosis not improving with oxygen, little respiratory distress

Natural History & Prognosis

- Early death without communicating shunt
- Large VSD: Congestive heart failure in neonatal period
- Patients with large VSD and (sub-) pulmonic stenosis: Mild symptoms, may survive without treatment
- Transposition with early switch: Good prognosis
- Complication of arterial switch: Traction on branch PAs by anteriorly transposed main PA, leading to branch origin stenosis
- Long-term prognosis determined by potential coronary abnormalities
- Complex transposition: Dependent on associated anomalies
- Mustard/Senning procedures: RV failure, atrial thrombosis, arrhythmias

Treatment

- Prostaglandin E1 to keep ductus arteriosus open
- Emergency balloon atrial septostomy (Rashkind)
- Surgical early: Arterial switch with transposition of coronaries (Jatene)
  - Late arterial switch not possible (pressure drops in LV connected to pulmonary circulation, which is then no longer able to sustain systemic pressures)
- Surgical late: Re-routing of venous flow in atria with pericardial baffle (Mustard) or reorientation of the atrial septum (Senning)

SELECTED REFERENCES

1. Laffon E et al: Quantitative MRI comparison of pulmonary hemodynamics in mustard/senning-repaired patients suffering from transposition of the great arteries and healthy volunteers at rest. Eur Radiol. 16(7):1442-8, 2006
2. Mohrs OK et al: Time-resolved contrast-enhanced MR angiography of the thorax in adults with congenital heart disease. AJR Am J Roentgenol. 187(4):1107-14, 2006
3. Warnes CA: Transposition of the great arteries. Circulation. 114(24):2699-709, 2006
4. Raman SV et al: Usefulness of multidetector row computed tomography to quantify right ventricular size and function in adults with either tetralogy of Fallot or transposition of the great arteries. Am J Cardiol. 95(5):683-6, 2005
5. Taylor AM et al: MR coronary angiography and late-enhancement myocardial MR in children who underwent arterial switch surgery for transposition of great arteries. Radiology. 234(2):542-7, 2005
6. Tops LF et al: Intraatrial repair of transposition of the great arteries: use of MR imaging after exercise to evaluate regional systemic right ventricular function. Radiology. 237(3):861-7, 2005
7. Lissin LW et al: Comparison of transthoracic echocardiography versus cardiovascular magnetic resonance imaging for the assessment of ventricular function in adults after atrial switch procedures for complete transposition of the great arteries. Am J Cardiol. 93(5):654-7, 2004
8. Roest AA et al: Cardiovascular response to physical exercise in adult patients after atrial correction for transposition of the great arteries assessed with magnetic resonance imaging. Heart. 90(6):678-84, 2004
9. Fogel MA et al: Mid-term follow-up of patients with transposition of the great arteries after atrial inversion operation using two- and three-dimensional magnetic resonance imaging. Pediatr Radiol. 32(6):440-6, 2002
10. McMahon CJ et al: Preoperative identification of coronary arterial anatomy in complete transposition, and outcome after the arterial switch operation. Cardiol Young. 12(3):240-7, 2002
11. Tulevski II et al: Usefulness of magnetic resonance imaging dobutamine stress in asymptomatic and minimally symptomatic patients with decreased cardiac reserve from congenital heart disease (complete and corrected transposition of the great arteries and subpulmonic obstruction). Am J Cardiol. 89(9):1077-81, 2002
12. Gutberlet M et al: Arterial switch procedure for D-transposition of the great arteries: quantitative midterm evaluation of hemodynamic changes with cine MR imaging and phase-shift velocity mapping-initial experience. Radiology. 214(2):467-75, 2000
13. Lidegran M et al: Magnetic resonance imaging and echocardiography in assessment of ventricular function in atrially corrected transposition of the great arteries. Scand Cardiovasc J. 34(4):384-9, 2000
14. Sidi D: Complete transposition of the great arteries. In: Moller JH, Hoffman JIE ed. Pediatric cardiovascular medicine, 1st ed. Philadelphia, Churchill Livingstone. 351-62, 2000
15. Tulevski II et al: Dobutamine-induced increase of right ventricular contractility without increased stroke volume in adolescent patients with transposition of the great arteries: evaluation with magnetic resonance imaging. Int J Card Imaging. 16(6):471-8, 2000
16. Chen SJ et al: Three-dimensional reconstruction of abnormal ventriculoarterial relationship by electron beam CT. J Comput Assist Tomogr. 22(4):560-8, 1998
17. Lorenz CH et al: Right ventricular performance and mass by use of cine MRI late after atrial repair of transposition of the great arteries. Circulation. 92(9 Suppl):II233-9, 1995
18. Blakenberg F et al: MRI vs echocardiography in the evaluation of the Jatene procedure. J Comput Assist Tomogr. 18(5):749-54, 1994
19. Hardy CE et al: Usefulness of magnetic resonance imaging for evaluating great-vessel anatomy after arterial switch operation for D-transposition of the great arteries. Am Heart J. 128(2):326-32, 1994
20. Beek FJ et al: MRI of the pulmonary artery after arterial switch operation for transposition of the great arteries. Pediatr Radiol. 23(5):335-40, 1993
21. Theissen P et al: Magnetic resonance imaging of cardiac function and morphology in patients with transposition of the great arteries following Mustard procedure. Thorac Cardiovasc Surg. 39 Suppl 3:221-4, 1991
22. Chung KJ et al: Cine magnetic resonance imaging after surgical repair in patients with transposition of the great arteries. Circulation. 77(1):104-9, 1988
23. Campbell RM et al: Detection of caval obstruction by magnetic resonance imaging after intraatrial repair of transposition of the great arteries. Am J Cardiol. 60(8):688-91, 1987
24. Matherne GP et al: Cine computed tomography for diagnosis of superior vena cava obstruction following the Mustard operation. Pediatr Radiol. 17(3):246-7, 1987

D-TRANSPOSITION

IMAGE GALLERY

Typical

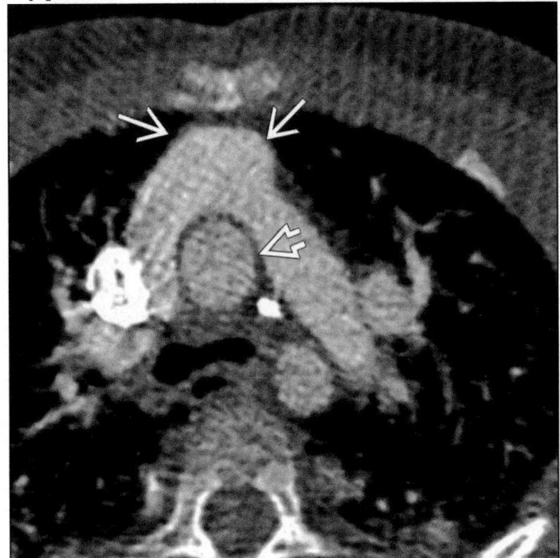

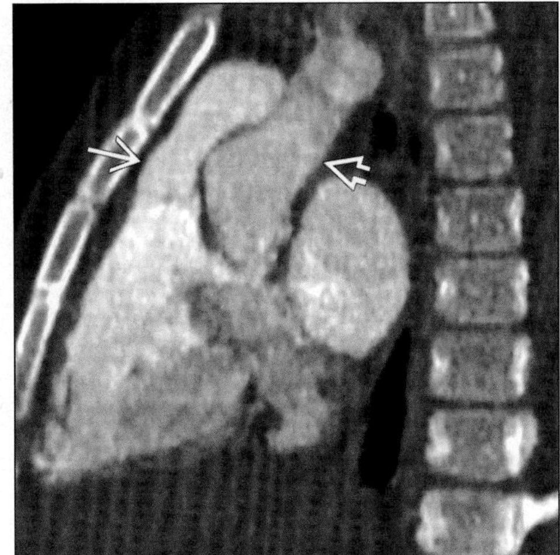

(Left) *Axial cardiac CT in patient who underwent the arterial switch operation shows the typical post-operative anatomy, with the main pulmonary artery anteriorly to the ascending aorta.* ***(Right)*** *Sagittal cardiac CT in same patient, shows the typical antero-posterior relationship of the pulmonary artery and the ascending aorta, which are running in the same sagittal plane, with lack of normal spiraling around each other.*

Typical

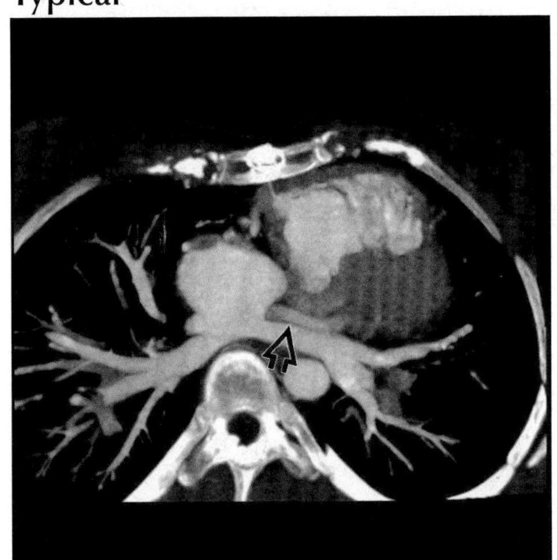

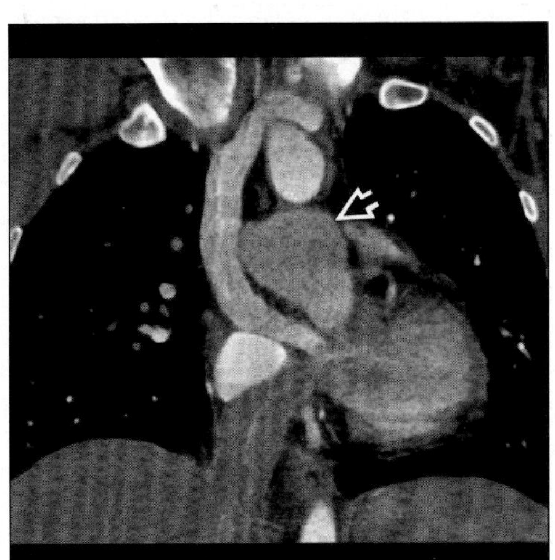

(Left) *Axial cardiac CT shows atrial baffle in patient with Mustard repair. The flow from the pulmonary veins is directed to the right atrium → right ventricle → aorta (not shown).* ***(Right)*** *Coronal cardiac CT shows systemic venous return baffled to posteriorly-placed left ventricle → pulmonary artery.*

Typical

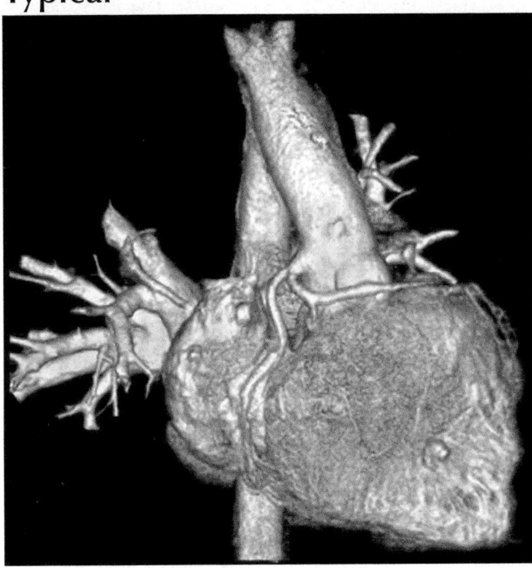

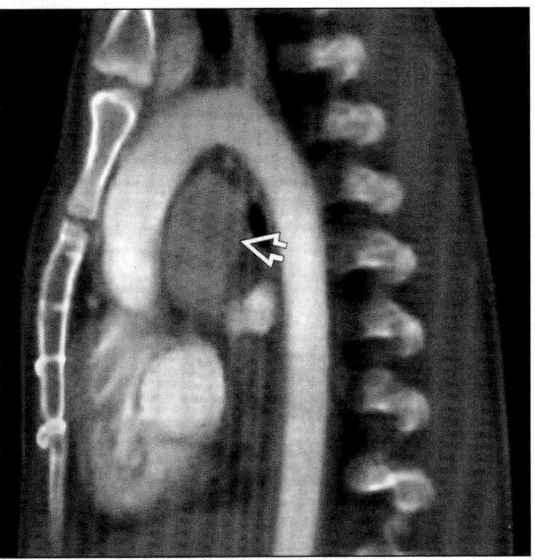

(Left) *Coronal cardiac CT shows anteriorly-placed D-loop aorta, which is connected with right ventricle.* ***(Right)*** *Sagittal CTA shows anteriorly-placed aorta, which is connected with right ventricle, and posteriorly placed pulmonary artery, which is connected to left ventricle (not shown).*

L-TRANSPOSITION

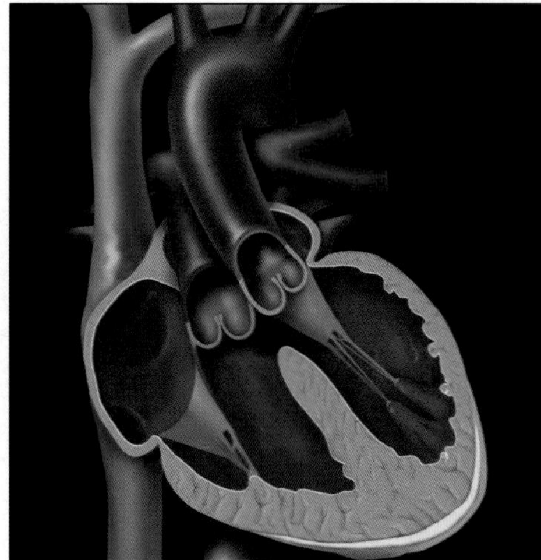

Graphic shows left-sided ascending aorta, connected to left-sided morphological right ventricle (trabeculated). Right-sided pulmonary artery is connected to right-sided left ventricle. Note high VSD.

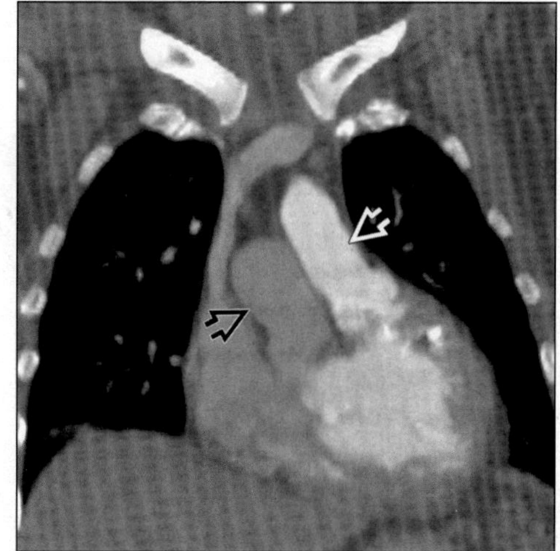

Coronal CTA shows L-loop ascending aorta ➡ arising from trabeculated right ventricle, and the abnormal side-by-side relationship with the pulmonary artery ➡, with no spiraling around each other.

TERMINOLOGY

Abbreviations and Synonyms

- "Congenitally corrected transposition" (misnomer)
- Discordant transposition

Definitions

- Inversion of ventricles and great arteries: Atrioventricular and ventriculoarterial discordance
- Category: Dependent on associated anomalies
  - Ventricular septal defect (VSD, 60-70%): Acyanotic, increased pulmonary vascularity
  - Left ventricular outflow tract (subpulmonary) obstruction (30-50%): Cyanotic
  - Dysplasia (Ebstein anomaly) with regurgitation of left-sided atrioventricular (AV) valve: Pulmonary venous congestion/hypertension
  - Conduction abnormalities, heart block
  - Only 1% have no associated anomalies: True congenitally corrected transposition
- Hemodynamics
  - Right atrium → mitral valve → right-sided morphologic left ventricle (LV) → pulmonary circulation
  - Left atrium → tricuspid valve → left-sided morphologic right ventricle (RV) → systemic circulation
  - Hemodynamics dependent on associated anomalies
- Segmental analysis of atrial, ventricular and great vessel morphology, relationship and connections for complete description of this complex disorder

IMAGING FINDINGS

General Features

- Best diagnostic clue: Great vessels lie parallel and almost in the same coronal plane, aortic valve anterior and slightly to the left (L-loop) of pulmonary valve
- Morphology
  - {S, L, L} heart: Atrial situs solitus, L-loop, L-transposed great arteries
    - Right-sided morphologic LV characterized by associated mitral valve, smooth wall and absent outflow chamber to pulmonary valve
    - Left-sided morphologic RV characterized by tricuspid valve, trabeculated wall, moderator band and infundibulum below aortic valve

DDx: L-Transposition: Associated Anomalies

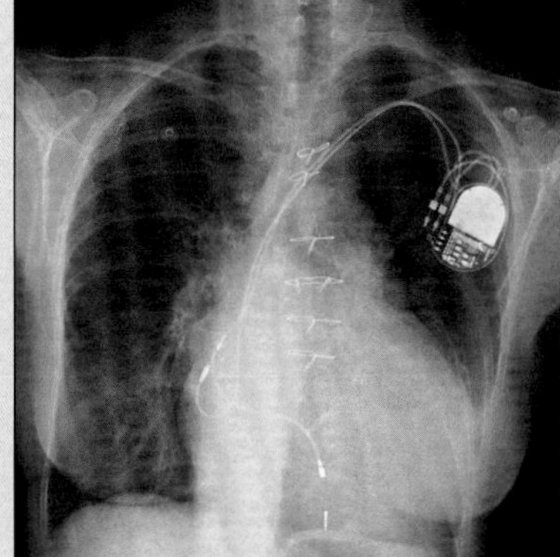

Cardiomegaly

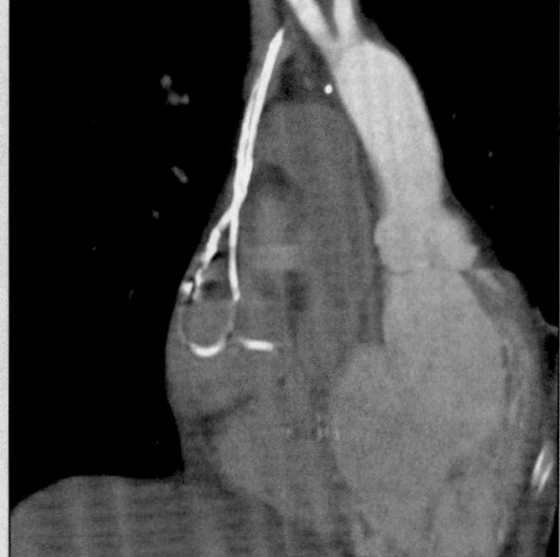

Pacemaker

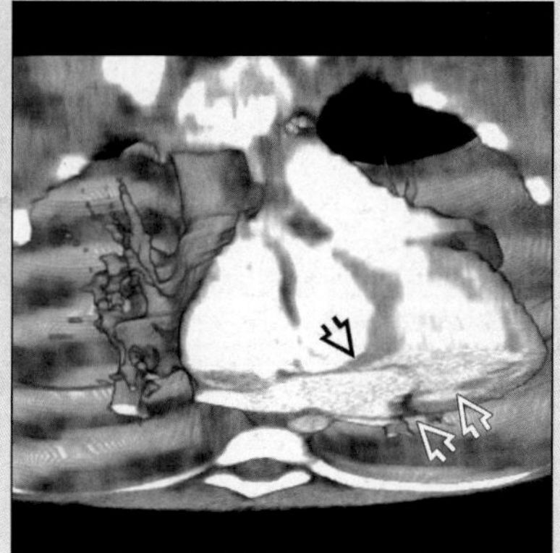

Ebstein L Tricuspid

L-TRANSPOSITION

Key Facts

Terminology

- Inversion of ventricles and great arteries: Atrioventricular and ventriculoarterial discordance
- Category: Dependent on associated anomalies
- Ventricular septal defect (VSD, 60-70%): Acyanotic, increased pulmonary vascularity
- Left ventricular outflow tract (subpulmonary) obstruction (30-50%): Cyanotic
- Dysplasia (Ebstein anomaly) with regurgitation of left-sided atrioventricular (AV) valve: Pulmonary venous congestion/hypertension
- Only 1% have no associated anomalies: True congenitally corrected transposition
- Segmental analysis of atrial, ventricular and great vessel morphology, relationship and connections for complete description of this complex disorder

Imaging Findings

- Best diagnostic clue: Great vessels lie parallel and almost in the same coronal plane, aortic valve anterior and slightly to the left (L-loop) of pulmonary valve
- T1WI: Multiplanar cardiac-gated T1WI and 3D gadolinium MRA for segmental cardiac analysis and anatomic evaluation
- Segmental cardiac analysis: Identification of atria, ventricles, great arteries and their connections
- Echocardiography allows for complete pre-operative diagnosis in majority of cases

Clinical Issues

- Double switch operation to prevent late systemic ventricular (RV) failure

---

- {I, D, D} heart: Atrial situs inversus, D-loop, D-transposed great arteries
  - Mirror image of {S, L, L} heart
  - Almost always associated with cardiac malposition: Mesocardia, dextroversion, true dextrocardia (25%)

Radiographic Findings

- Radiography
  - Classic: Straight upper left heart border
  - Other findings from associated anomalies

CT Findings

- 3D CT angiography can depict abnormal atrioventricular and ventriculoarterial relationships

MR Findings

- T1WI: Multiplanar cardiac-gated T1WI and 3D gadolinium MRA for segmental cardiac analysis and anatomic evaluation
- T2* GRE: Dobutamine stress short-axis steady-state free precession cine MR for functional evaluation of RV: Can it sustain the systemic circulation?

Echocardiographic Findings

- Echocardiogram
  - Segmental cardiac analysis: Identification of atria, ventricles, great arteries and their connections
  - Continuity between right-sided mitral and pulmonary valve annulus
  - Discontinuity between left-sided tricuspid and aortic valve annulus
  - Abnormally straight, vertical course of interventricular septum

Imaging Recommendations

- Protocol advice
  - Echocardiography allows for complete pre-operative diagnosis in majority of cases
  - CT or MR as complementary noninvasive cross-sectional tests for more complex abnormalities

DIFFERENTIAL DIAGNOSIS

Congestive Heart Failure, Increased Pulmonary Blood Flow

- Isolated VSD
- Double inlet ventricle
- Tricuspid atresia with increased pulmonary blood flow
- Double outlet right ventricle with subaortic VSD

Cyanosis, Decreased Pulmonary Blood Flow

- Tetralogy of Fallot

Atrioventricular Discordance with Ventriculoarterial Concordance

- Isolated ventricular inversion, with each ventricle connected to its appropriate great artery, and physiology resembling D-transposition

PATHOLOGY

General Features

- General path comments
  - Ventricular arrangement is not simply the mirror image of normal
  - Ventricles and great arteries form an L-loop
  - Interventricular septum is more vertical in orientation than normal
  - Coronary distribution is mirror image of normal (right-sided coronary bifurcates into circumflex and anterior descending arteries)
  - Embryology: Primitive cardiac tube loops to the left (L-loop), leading to ventricular inversion and left-sided position of ascending aorta
  - Pathophysiology
    - Determined by associated anomalies: VSD, subpulmonary stenosis, AV valve dysfunction
    - Late sequel: Left-sided RV is not able to sustain systemic circulation
- Genetics
  - No genetic factors or chromosomal abnormalities

L-TRANSPOSITION

  - Not commonly associated with extracardiac malformations
- Epidemiology: Incidence: 1 in 13,000 live births, 1% of congenital heart disease, males > females
- Associated abnormalities
  - VSD: 80%
  - LV outflow tract (subpulmonary) obstruction: 30%
  - Left-sided tricuspid valve dysplasia, Ebstein anomaly, regurgitation: 30%
  - Can be associated with atrial situs inversus: Dextrocardia {I, D, D}
  - Rare: Ventricular hypoplasia, AV canal, straddling AV valves, aortic atresia, coarctation or interruption

Gross Pathologic & Surgical Features

- Right-sided morphologic LV connected without infundibulum to pulmonary valve, which is slightly posterior and to right of aortic valve
- Infundibulum of left-sided morphologic RV connected to aortic valve, which is slightly anterior and to left of pulmonary valve (L-loop)
- Pulmonary artery and ascending aorta lie nearly parallel in same coronal plane
- Interruption of conduction system of heart due to malalignment between atrial and ventricular septa: Disconnection between atrioventricular node and bundle of His → third degree heart block

CLINICAL ISSUES

Presentation

- Most common signs/symptoms
  - Heart failure (VSD, systemic AV valve dysfunction)
  - Cyanosis (subpulmonary stenosis)
  - Rarely completely asymptomatic, presenting as incidental finding on chest radiograph (straight upper left heart border)
- Other signs/symptoms
  - Conduction disturbances: Bradycardia (heart block) and tachydysrhythmia
  - Decreased exercise tolerance due to dysfunction of systemic ventricle (RV)

Natural History & Prognosis

- Determined by presence of AV valve dysfunction
- Guarded prognosis due to progressive systemic AV valve and RV dysfunction after corrective surgery: 50% mortality after 15 years
- Patients with true congenitally corrected transposition may have a normal life expectancy

Treatment

- Surgical treatment focused on associated abnormalities
  - Congestive heart failure from VSD shunt: PA banding or VSD closure
  - Cyanosis from subpulmonary stenosis: Systemic to PA shunt (Blalock) or LV to PA conduit (Rastelli)
  - Pulmonary venous hypertension from tricuspid valve dysfunction: Tricuspid valvuloplasty
- Double switch operation to prevent late systemic ventricular (RV) failure
  - Venous switch (Senning) re-routes the atrial blood into the appropriate ventricles
  - Ventricular (Rastelli) or arterial switch: Morphologic LV becomes systemic ventricle
- Pacemaker insertion

SELECTED REFERENCES

1. Chang DS et al: Congenitally corrected transposition of the great arteries: imaging with 16-MDCT. AJR Am J Roentgenol. 188(5):W428-30, 2007
2. Dorfman AL et al: Magnetic resonance imaging evaluation of congenital heart disease: conotruncal anomalies. J Cardiovasc Magn Reson. 8(4):645-59, 2006
3. Kantarci M et al: Congenitally corrected transposition of the great arteries: MDCT angiography findings and interpretation of complex coronary anatomy. Int J Cardiovasc Imaging. 2006
4. Mohrs OK et al: Time-resolved contrast-enhanced MR angiography of the thorax in adults with congenital heart disease. AJR Am J Roentgenol. 187(4):1107-14, 2006
5. Warnes CA: Transposition of the great arteries. Circulation. 114(24):2699-709, 2006
6. Sorensen TS et al: Operator-independent isotropic three-dimensional magnetic resonance imaging for morphology in congenital heart disease: a validation study. Circulation. 110(2):163-9, 2004
7. Tulevski II et al: Regional and global right ventricular dysfunction in asymptomatic or minimally symptomatic patients with congenitally corrected transposition. Cardiol Young. 14(2):168-73, 2004
8. Karl TR et al: Congenitally corrected transposition of the great arteries. In: Mavroudis C, Backer CL, ed. Pediatric cardiac surgery. 3rd ed. Philadelphia, Mosby. 476-95, 2003
9. Dodge-Khatami A et al: Comparable systemic ventricular function in healthy adults and patients with unoperated congenitally corrected transposition using MRI dobutamine stress testing. Ann Thorac Surg. 73(6):1759-64, 2002
10. Tulevski II et al: Usefulness of magnetic resonance imaging dobutamine stress in asymptomatic and minimally symptomatic patients with decreased cardiac reserve from congenital heart disease (complete and corrected transposition of the great arteries and subpulmonic obstruction). Am J Cardiol. 89(9):1077-81, 2002
11. Schmidt M et al: Tc-99m MIBI SPECT correlated with magnetic resonance imaging for cardiac evaluation of a patient with congenitally corrected transposition of the great arteries (L-TGA). Clin Nucl Med. 26(8):714-5, 2001
12. Freedom RM. Congenitally corrected transposition of the great arteries. In: Moller JH, Hoffman JIE ed. Pediatric cardiovascular medicine, 1st ed. Philadelphia, Churchill Livingstone. 391-408, 2000
13. Schmidt M et al: Congenitally corrected transposition of the great arteries (L-TGA) with situs inversus totalis in adulthood: findings with magnetic resonance imaging. Magn Reson Imaging. 18(4):417-22, 2000
14. Reddy GP et al: Case 15: Congenitally corrected transposition of the great arteries. Radiology 213:102-6, 1999
15. Chen SJ et al: Three-dimensional reconstruction of abnormal ventriculoarterial relationship by electron beam CT. J Comput Assist Tomogr. 22(4):560-8, 1998
16. Formanek AG: MR imaging of congenitally corrected transposition of the great vessels in adults. AJR Am J Roentgenol. 154(4):898-9, 1990
17. Park JH et al: MR imaging of congenitally corrected transposition of the great vessels in adults. AJR Am J Roentgenol. 153(3):491-4, 1989

L-TRANSPOSITION

IMAGE GALLERY

Typical

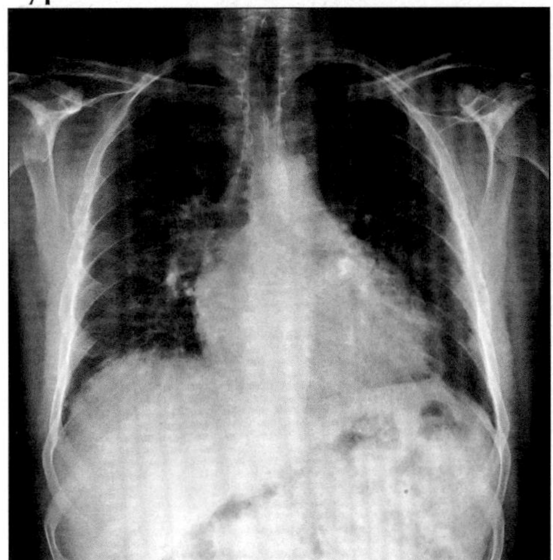

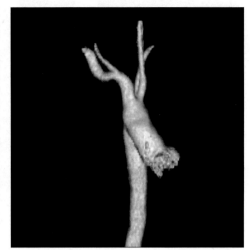

(Left) *Posteroanterior radiograph shows abnormal straightening of the left upper heart border.* ***(Right)*** *Coronal cardiac CT in the same patient as previous image, shows L-loop configuration ascending aorta, leading to the abnormality on plain film.*

Typical

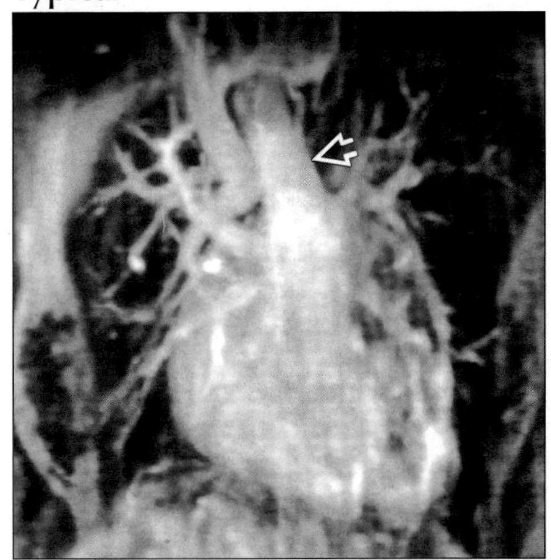

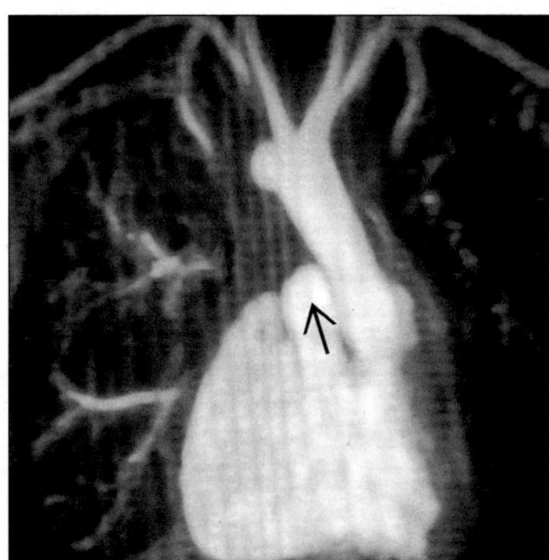

(Left) *Coronal MRA MIP reconstruction, shows L-loop of ascending aorta ➡ in a patient with complex cyanotic congenital heart disease (double-outlet right ventricle, cor tri-atriatum).* ***(Right)*** *Coronal MRA in the same patient as previous image, shows pulmonary artery ➡ to lie to the right of the ascending aorta.*

Typical

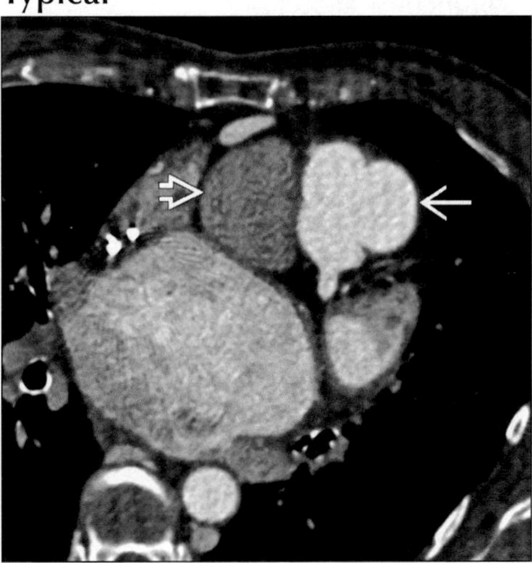

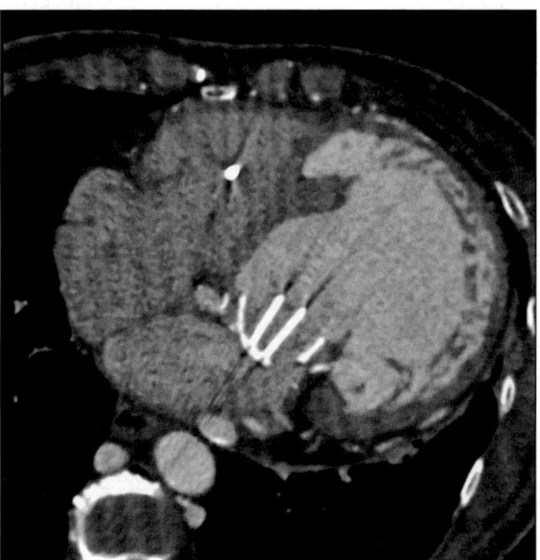

(Left) *Axial cardiac CT shows pulmonary artery ➡ to lie to the right of the L-looping ascending aorta ➡. Note dilated left atrium.* ***(Right)*** *Axial cardiac CT shows right-sided left ventricle, dilated left-sided right ventricle (with trabeculations), and replacement of left-sided tricuspid valve.*

TRUNCUS ARTERIOSUS

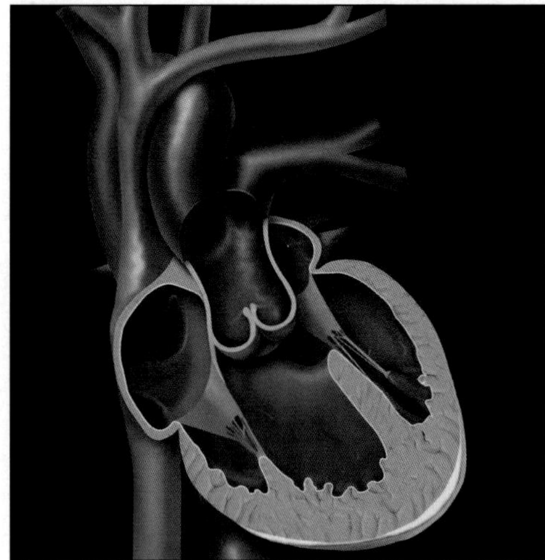

Graphic shows type 1 truncus with common truncal valve, overriding high VSD, giving rise to aorta (note right aortic arch) and main pulmonary artery. Cyanosis is due to flow admixture within ventricles and truncus.

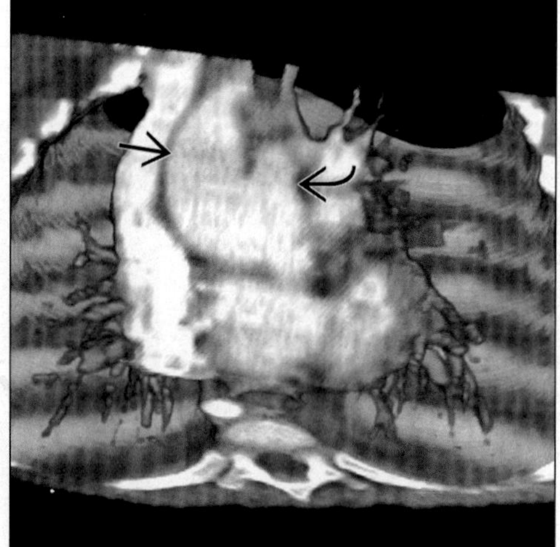

Coronal CTA shows common trunk, giving rise to right-sided aortic arch ➔ and pulmonary artery ➔.

TERMINOLOGY

Abbreviations and Synonyms

- Common arterial trunk

Definitions

- Common arterial vessel arising from the heart, giving rise to aorta, pulmonary arteries (PAs) and coronaries

IMAGING FINDINGS

General Features

- Best diagnostic clue
  - Common arterial trunk arising from both ventricles
  - Classic plain film appearance: Cardiomegaly, increased pulmonary vascularity, narrow mediastinum, right aortic arch
  - Category: Cyanotic, cardiomegaly, increased pulmonary vascularity
  - Hemodynamics
    - Both ventricles connected with pulmonary and systemic circulation
    - Flow admixture across ventricular septal defect (VSD) and within truncus → cyanosis
    - Postnatal drop in pulmonary vascular resistance → relative increase in pulmonary blood flow → volume overload of pulmonary circulation
  - Truncus arteriosus is the heart lesion most commonly associated with right aortic arch (30-40%)
  - Frequently associated with absent thymus and parathyroid glands: DiGeorge syndrome

Radiographic Findings

- Radiography
  - Cardiomegaly
  - Active pulmonary vascular congestion (shunt vascularity)
  - Right aortic arch common
  - Narrow mediastinum due to thymic agenesis
  - Dilated pulmonary arteries may compress neighboring bronchi → atelectasis

CT Findings

- CTA
  - Relationship of branch PAs with truncus
  - Coronary anatomy

DDx: Cyanosis, Increased Pulmonary Vascularity

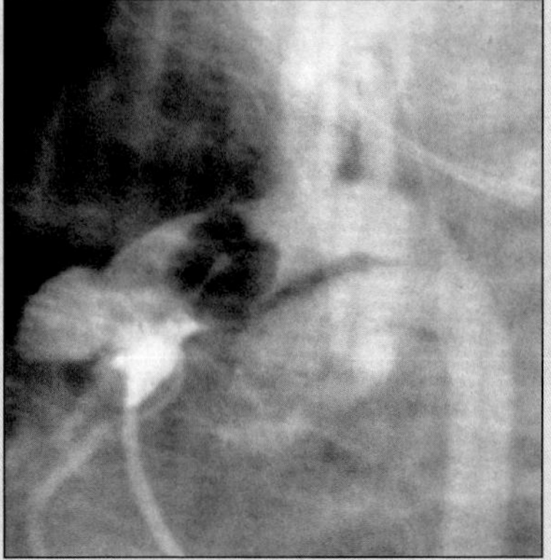

Transposition

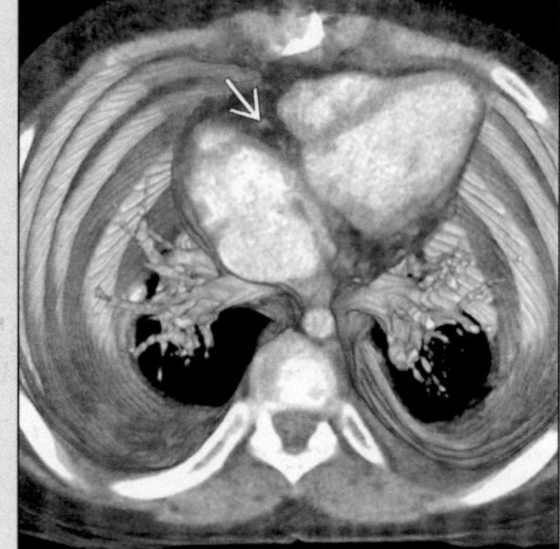

Tricuspid Atresia

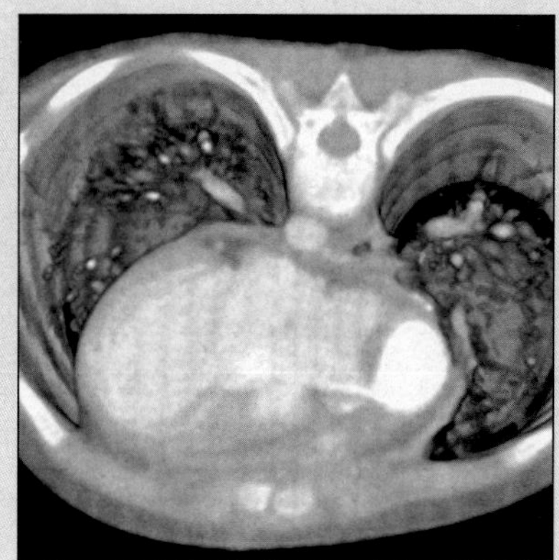

"T(s)ingle" Ventricle

TRUNCUS ARTERIOSUS

Key Facts

Terminology
- Common arterial vessel arising from the heart, giving rise to aorta, pulmonary arteries (PAs) and coronaries

Imaging Findings
- Classic plain film appearance: Cardiomegaly, increased pulmonary vascularity, narrow mediastinum, right aortic arch
- Category: Cyanotic, cardiomegaly, increased pulmonary vascularity
- Both ventricles connected with pulmonary and systemic circulation
- Truncus arteriosus is the heart lesion most commonly associated with right aortic arch (30-40%)
- Frequently associated with absent thymus and parathyroid glands: DiGeorge syndrome
- MR/CTA for post-operative assessment of conduit stenosis, stent placement

Pathology
- Pathophysiology: Congestive heart failure versus cyanosis (degree of cyanosis is determined by balance of pulmonary and systemic resistance)

Clinical Issues
- Progressive congestive heart failure with drop in pulmonary vascular resistance in young infant
- Increasing cyanosis due to shunt reversal with development of pulmonary hypertension
- Surgical repair, with placement of conduit between right ventricle and PA, and closure of VSD
- Conduit revisions are frequently necessary throughout patient's life time

  - Post-operative: Patency and size of conduit, calcification and stenosis
  - CTA is best technique to evaluate stent placement

MR Findings
- T1WI
  - Cardiac-gated axial images for pre-operative definition of PA anatomy
  - Post-operative: Conduit stenosis, anastomotic pseudoaneurysm
- T2* GRE: Steady-state free precession cine MR: Truncal valve regurgitation, ventricular function
- MRA: Gadolinium-enhanced MRA for global anatomy, patency of PA conduit

Echocardiographic Findings
- Echocardiogram
  - Common arterial trunk originating from both ventricles
  - High (outlet) VSD immediately below truncal valve
  - Common truncal valve with 2 (5%), 3 (60%) or 4 (25%) cusps
- Color Doppler
  - Bidirectional flow across VSD
  - Truncal valve regurgitation

Angiographic Findings
- Conventional
  - Cardiac catheterization with angiography
    - To define the exact type of truncal anatomy
    - Truncal valve insufficiency
    - Hemodynamic study is gold standard for calculation of pulmonary vascular resistance

Imaging Recommendations
- Protocol advice
  - Primary diagnosis made with echocardiography
  - MR/CTA for pre-operative delineation of PA anatomy
  - MR/CTA for post-operative assessment of conduit stenosis, stent placement

DIFFERENTIAL DIAGNOSIS

Transposition of the Great Arteries
- Presents earlier in life with more severe cyanosis, ductus-dependent

Aortopulmonary Window
- Congenital fenestration between ascending aorta and PA, with separate aortic and pulmonary valves

Common Atrioventricular (AV) Canal
- When unbalanced (right or left dominant): Cyanosis frequently occurs due to admixture

PATHOLOGY

General Features
- General path comments
  - Common outflow tract of both ventricles, over non-restrictive VSD
  - No separate outflow portion (infundibulum) of right ventricle
  - Right-sided aortic arch with mirror-image branching (30-40%)
  - Embryology
    - Lack of separation of primitive bulbus cordis into aorta and main PA
    - Associated persistence of primitive aortic arches
  - Pathophysiology: Congestive heart failure versus cyanosis (degree of cyanosis is determined by balance of pulmonary and systemic resistance)
    - Marked increase in pulmonary blood flow in early neonatal period, due to drop in pulmonary vascular resistance → slight improvement in cyanosis but worsening congestive heart failure
    - Development of pulmonary vascular obstructive disease leads to improvement in congestive heart failure but worsening in cyanosis
- Genetics
  - Strong association with deletion on the long arm of chromosome 22 (22q11 syndrome)

TRUNCUS ARTERIOSUS

- CATCH-22: Conofacial anomaly, absent thymus, hypocalcemia, heart defect
- Velocardiofacial (Shprintzen) syndrome
- Theory: Abnormal migration of neural crest tissue that interferes with development of cardiac tube
- Epidemiology: 2% of all congenital cardiac anomalies
- Associated abnormalities
  - Agenesis of thymus and parathyroid glands
  - Persistence of primitive aortic arches

Gross Pathologic & Surgical Features

- Many variations exist, involving interruption of the aortic arch (11-14%), absence of a branch PA (hemitruncus) and patent ductus arteriosus
- Position of common trunk with respect to VSD
  - Predominantly positioned over right ventricle (42%)
  - Predominantly positioned over left ventricle (16%)
  - Equally shared (42%)

Staging, Grading or Classification Criteria

- Classification of Collett and Edwards
  - Type 1: Separation of common trunk into ascending aorta and main PA
  - Type 2: Common take-off of branch PAs from trunk, with no main PA
  - Type 3: Both branch PAs originate separately from posterolateral aspect of ascending aorta
  - Type 4: "Pseudotruncus", pulmonary arterial supply from major aortopulmonary collateral arteries (MAPCAs), arising from descending aorta; controversial entity, misnomer for pulmonary atresia with VSD and MAPCAs
- Classification of Van Praagh
  - Type A1: Same as Collett and Edwards type 1
  - Type A2: Collet and Edwards types 2 and 3
  - Type A3: Unilateral pulmonary artery with collateral supply to contralateral lung
  - Type A4: Truncus with interrupted aortic arch

CLINICAL ISSUES

Presentation

- Most common signs/symptoms
  - Progressive congestive heart failure with drop in pulmonary vascular resistance in young infant
  - Increasing cyanosis due to shunt reversal with development of pulmonary hypertension
- Other signs/symptoms
  - T-cell immunodeficiency (thymic agenesis - DiGeorge syndrome)
  - Neonatal tetany (absent parathyroid glands)

Natural History & Prognosis

- Untreated: 65% 6 month and 75% 1 year mortality
- Intractable congestive heart failure
  - Marked increase in pulmonary flow after drop in pulmonary vascular resistance
  - Aggravated by presence of truncal valve regurgitation (in 50% of cases)
- Eventual shunt reversal with progressive cyanosis and sudden death
  - Pulmonary vascular obstructive disease with Eisenmenger physiology can develop as early as 6 months of age
- Post-operative course determined by function of PA conduit and morbidity of conduit replacement

Treatment

- Palliative: Banding of main PA
  - Initial palliation with PA banding often unsatisfactory, with early development of pulmonary arterial hypertension
  - Early complete repair (at 2-6 weeks of life) is favored by most surgeons
- Surgical repair, with placement of conduit between right ventricle and PA, and closure of VSD
  - Conduit revisions are frequently necessary throughout patient's life time
    - Patient outgrows fixed conduit size
    - Calcification
    - Stenosis, neointimal hyperplasia
    - Anastomotic pseudoaneurysm
    - Conduit valve dysfunction (regurgitation)
  - Truncal valve dysfunction (regurgitation) is common → need for valvuloplasty, prosthesis

SELECTED REFERENCES

1. Dorfman AL et al: Magnetic resonance imaging evaluation of congenital heart disease: conotruncal anomalies. J Cardiovasc Magn Reson. 8(4):645-59, 2006
2. Muhler MR et al: Truncus arteriosus communis in a midtrimester fetus: comparison of prenatal ultrasound and MRI with postmortem MRI and autopsy. Eur Radiol. 14(11):2120-4, 2004
3. Razavi R et al: Diagnosis of hemi-truncus arteriosis by three-dimensional magnetic resonance angiography. Circulation. 109(3):E15-6, 2004
4. Mavroudis C et al: Truncus arteriosus. In: Mavroudis C , Backer CL ed. Pediatric cardiac surgery. 3rd ed. Philadelphia, Mosby. 339-52, 2003
5. Lim C et al: Truncus arteriosus with coarctation of persistent fifth aortic arch. Ann Thorac Surg. 74(5):1702-4, 2002
6. Murashita T et al: Giant pseudoaneurysm of the right ventricular outflow tract after repair of truncus arteriosus: evaluation by MR imaging and surgical approach. Eur J Cardiothorac Surg. 22(5):849-51, 2002
7. Taylor JFN: Persistent truncus arteriosus. In: Moller JH, Hoffman JIE ed. Pediatric cardiovascular medicine. 1st ed. Philadelphia, Churchill Livingstone. 499-510, 2000
8. Rajasinghe HA et al: Long-term follow-up of truncus arteriosus repaired in infancy: a twenty-year experience. J Thorac Cardiovasc Surg. 113:869-78, 1997
9. Donnelly LF et al: MR imaging of conotruncal abnormalities. AJR Am J Roentgenol. 166(4):925-8, 1996
10. Levine JC et al: Anastomotic pseudoaneurysm of the ventricle after homograft placement in children. Ann Thorac Surg. 59(1):60-6, 1995
11. Engle MA et al: Endocarditis with aneurysm involving an aortic homograft used to correct a truncus arteriosus: medical-surgical salvage. Br Heart J. 67(5):409-11, 1992
12. Chrispin A et al: Echo planar imaging of normal and abnormal connections of the heart and great arteries. Pediatr Radiol. 16(4):289-92, 1986
13. Chrispin A et al: Transectional echo planar imaging of the heart in cyanotic congenital heart disease. Pediatr Radiol. 16(4):293-7, 1986

TRUNCUS ARTERIOSUS

IMAGE GALLERY

Typical

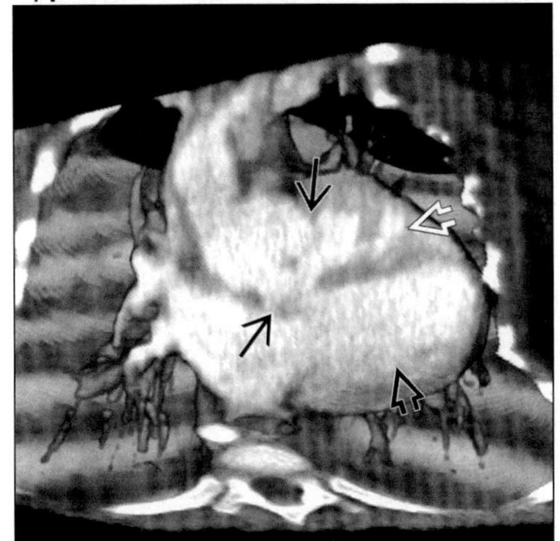

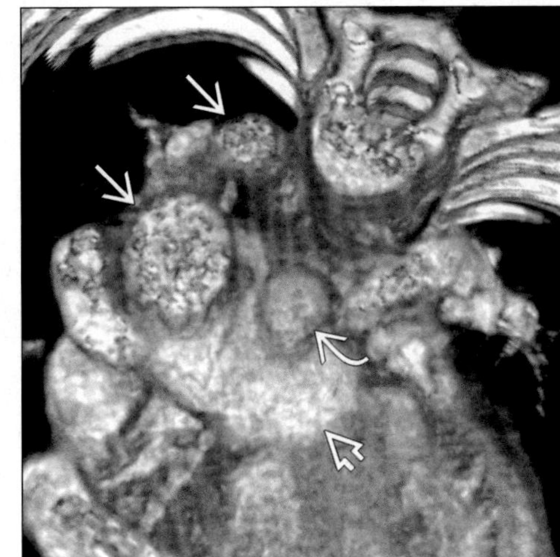

(Left) *Coronal CTA shows truncal valve → overriding both right ⇨ and left ➡ ventricles. Note right aortic arch.* ***(Right)*** *Oblique CTA shows truncus ➡, giving rise to right aortic arch ➡ and pulmonary trunk ↪.*

Typical

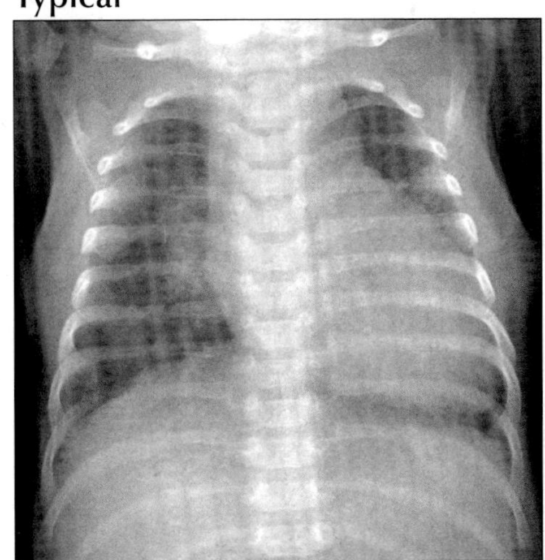

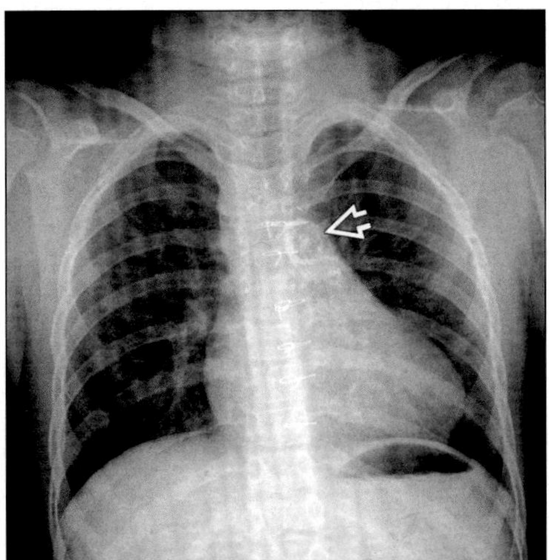

(Left) *Anteroposterior radiograph shows cardiomegaly, pulmonary venous congestion and hyperinflation. This patient has a left aortic arch.* ***(Right)*** *Anteroposterior radiograph shows calcified pulmonary artery conduit ➡ after truncus repair. Note right aortic arch.*

Variant

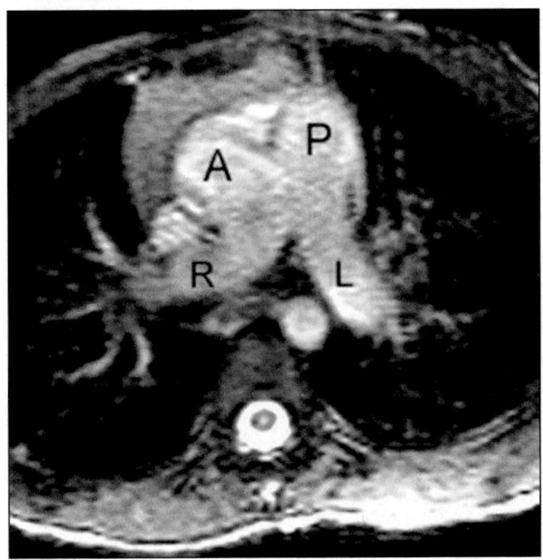

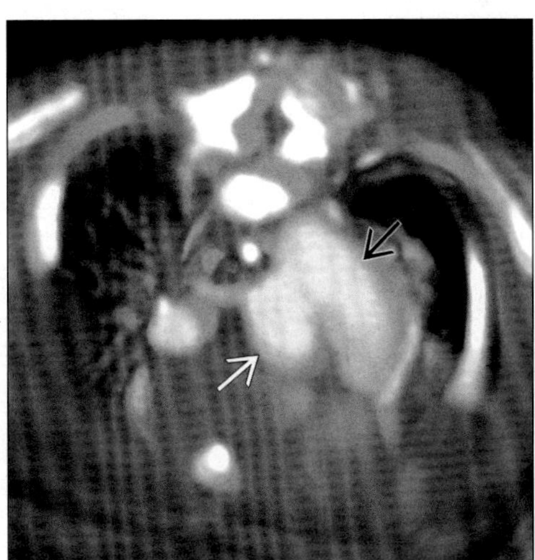

(Left) *Axial MR cine shows large connection between aorta (A) and pulmonary artery (P), consistent with aortopulmonary window. R = right branch pulmonary artery; L = left branch pulmonary artery.* ***(Right)*** *Oblique CTA shows connection between aorta → and pulmonary artery ➡ in this 3 day old infant with aortopulmonary window.*

PULMONARY ATRESIA

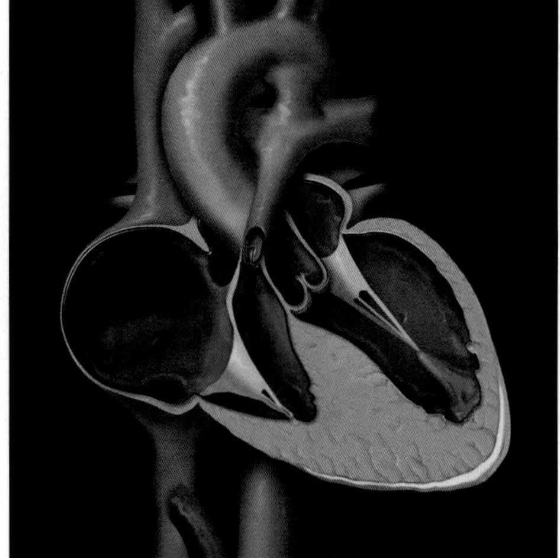

Graphic shows pulmonary atresia with intact ventricular septum. Note patent foramen ovale, dilatation of right atrium and right ventricular hypertrophy. Pulmonary arteries are perfused via patent ductus arteriosus.

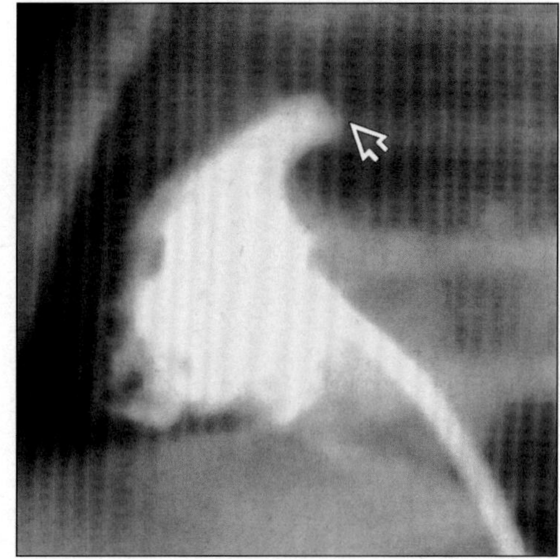

Lateral angiography, right ventricular injection, shows occlusion at the pulmonary valve ➡.

TERMINOLOGY

Abbreviations and Synonyms

- Pulmonary atresia (PAt) with VSD and multiple aortopulmonary collateral arteries (MAPCAs)
  - Also sometimes referred to as "truncus arteriosus type 4" or "pseudotruncus" (misnomers)
- PAt, intact VS: Pulmonary atresia with intact ventricular septum

Definitions

- Two distinct entities, differentiated by presence or absence of a ventricular septal defect (VSD)
  - PAt, VSD, MAPCAs: Hypoplastic/absent pulmonary arteries (PAs), MAPCAs supply one or both lungs
  - PAt, intact VS: Normal-sized PAs supplied by ductus arteriosus, patent foramen ovale (PFO)
- Both are characterized by underdevelopment of right ventricular outflow tract (RVOT) and pulmonary valve
  - PAt, VSD, MAPCAs: At extreme end of the spectrum of RVOT-obstructive (Fallot-type) heart lesions, with complex and highly variable PA anatomy
- Category: Cyanotic, cardiomegaly, decreased and/or irregular pulmonary vasculature
- Hemodynamics: Extreme outflow obstruction of right ventricle (RV), (almost) entire cardiac output goes into dilated overriding ascending aorta

IMAGING FINDINGS

General Features

- Best diagnostic clue: Atresia of RVOT and/or pulmonary valve

Radiographic Findings

- Radiography
  - Extreme "boot-shaped" appearance of heart
  - Right-sided aortic arch common
  - Diminutive hilar shadows
  - Irregular branching patterns of MAPCAs
  - PAt, intact VS: Severe cardiomegaly from massive right atrial dilatation

CT Findings

- CTA
  - Better than echocardiography for PA anatomy
  - CTA best used to provide anatomic road-map for subsequent catheterization

DDx: Cyanosis, Decreased Pulmonary Vascularity

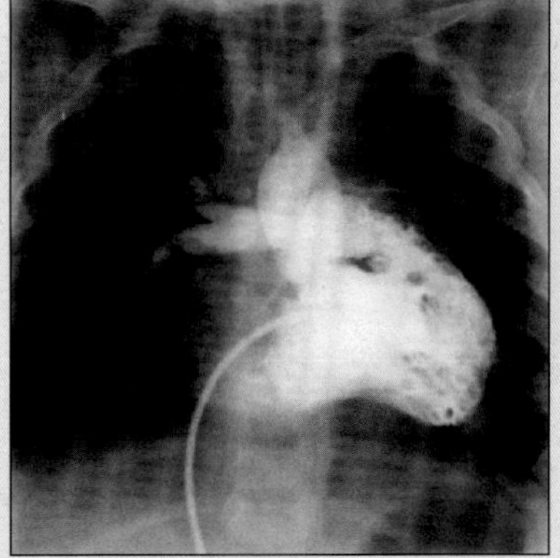

Tetralogy of Fallot

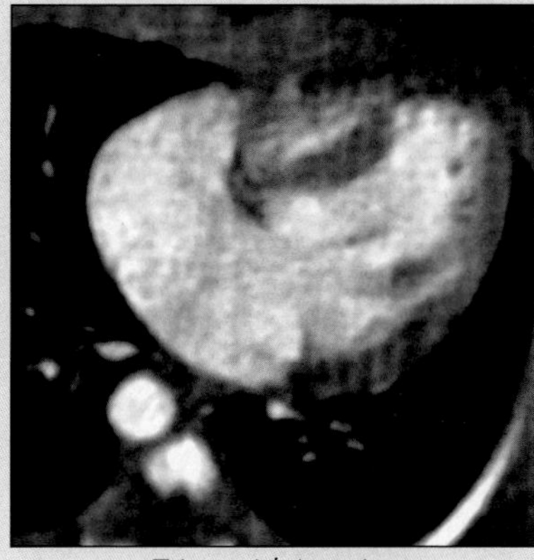

Tricuspid Atresia

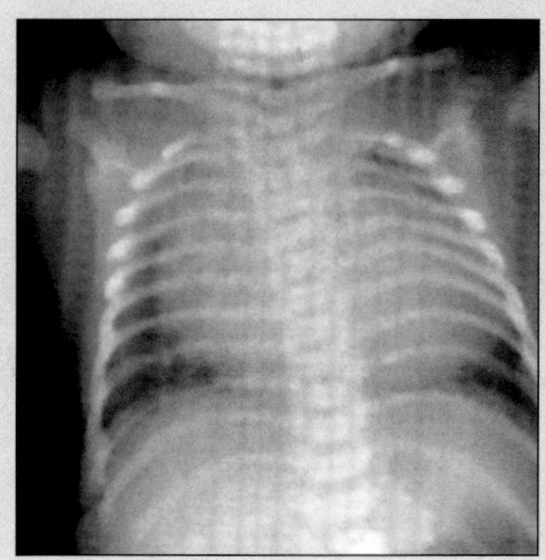

Ebstein Anomaly

PULMONARY ATRESIA

Key Facts

Terminology

- Two distinct entities, differentiated by presence or absence of a ventricular septal defect (VSD)
- Both are characterized by underdevelopment of right ventricular outflow tract (RVOT) and pulmonary valve
- Category: Cyanotic, cardiomegaly, decreased and/or irregular pulmonary vasculature
- Hemodynamics: Extreme outflow obstruction of right ventricle (RV), (almost) entire cardiac output goes into dilated overriding ascending aorta

Imaging Findings

- Best diagnostic clue: Atresia of RVOT and/or pulmonary valve
- CTA best used to provide anatomic road-map for subsequent catheterization

Pathology

- Pathophysiology of PAt, VSD, MAPCAs: Balance between flow though PAs and MAPCAs determines pulmonary perfusion
- Pathophysiology of PAt, intact VS: Obligatory right → left shunt through PFO
- Hilar arteries = true PAs
- Presence and confluence of central portions of true PAs important for surgical repair

Clinical Issues

- Progressive cyanosis after birth with closure of ductus arteriosus
- Prognosis is guarded, depends on feasibility of surgery
- PAt, VSD, MAPCAs: Staged complete repair
- PAt, intact VS: Type of repair dependent on RV size and RV-dependency on coronary circulation

    - Saves overall radiation, contrast, procedure time
  - CTA is excellent modality for unstable post-operative patients

MR Findings

- T1WI: PAt, VSD, MAPCAs: Cardiac-gated axial images for pre-operative definition of PA anatomy
- T2* GRE: Short- and long-axis steady-state free precession (SSFP) cine MR for functional assessment, tricuspid regurgitation
- MRA: Coronal gadolinium-enhanced MRA for detailed analysis of PA anatomy and MAPCAs

Echocardiographic Findings

- Echocardiogram
  - PAt, VSD, MAPCAs
    - Characterizes intracardiac anatomy, position and size of VSD, aortic root override
    - Development of branch PAs, their confluence
  - PAt, intact VS
    - Morphology of interatrial septum: Is there any restriction to flow across PFO?
    - Size of RV and tricuspid annulus (expressed as a "z-score"), degree of tricuspid regurgitation: Important for planning of surgical repair

Angiographic Findings

- Conventional
  - PAt, VSD, MAPCAs
    - Selective injection with pressure recordings of all MAPCAs, imaging of true PAs
    - Pulmonary venous wedge injections for retrograde filling of diminutive PAs
  - PAt, intact VS
    - Suprasystemic pressure recordings in RV
    - Detailed imaging of coronary anatomy through RV and aortic root injections: RV to coronary communications, stenoses, interruptions

Imaging Recommendations

- Protocol advice
  - PAt, VSD, MAPCAs
    - Initial diagnosis with echocardiography
    - CT or MR for assessment of PA anatomy, post-operatively for shunt/conduit patency
    - Cardiac catheterization for hemodynamic assessment, selective injection studies and catheter-based interventions

DIFFERENTIAL DIAGNOSIS

Tetralogy of Fallot

- At least partial patency of RVOT

Complex Cyanotic Heart Lesions with Component of (Sub)pulmonary Stenosis

- Double outlet right ventricle
- Transposition of great arteries with VSD
- Single ventricle
- Tricuspid atresia

Ebstein Anomaly

- May mimic PAt, intact VS with large tricuspid annulus and massive tricuspid regurgitation

PATHOLOGY

General Features

- General path comments
  - Embryology (PAt, VSD, MAPCAs)
    - RVOT obstruction → hypoplasia of PAs
    - Persistence or hypertrophy of primitive arterial connections to lungs
    - Hypertrophy of bronchial arteries
  - Pathophysiology of PAt, VSD, MAPCAs: Balance between flow though PAs and MAPCAs determines pulmonary perfusion
    - PA flow at sub-systemic pressures, restricted by narrow caliber and eventual closure of ductus arteriosus
    - MAPCA flow leads to increased lung perfusion at systemic pressures (unless restricted by stenosis)
    - Degree of cyanosis determined by intracardiac admixture and amount of pulmonary flow

   - Large amount of pulmonary blood flow through unrestricted MAPCAs → congestive heart failure
 - Pathophysiology of PAt, intact VS: Obligatory right → left shunt through PFO
   - Pulmonary arteries supplied by PDA
   - Small heavily trabeculated right ventricle with suprasystemic pressures
   - Depending on size of tricuspid valve annulus: Severe tricuspid regurgitation, leading to massive right atrial dilatation (comparable to Ebstein)
   - Transmyocardial sinusoids connecting right ventricular cavity with coronary artery system cause coronary flow reversal during diastole, leading to myocardial ischemia and infarction
- Epidemiology: Rare congenital cyanotic heart lesions, often classified together with tetralogy of Fallot

Gross Pathologic & Surgical Features

- Hilar arteries = true PAs
- Presence and confluence of central portions of true PAs important for surgical repair
- MAPCAs originating from
  - Ascending aorta
  - Brachiocephalic or intercostal arteries
  - Ductus arteriosus
  - Descending aorta (most common)

Microscopic Features

- Pulmonary vascular disease develops in vascular bed of high-flow MAPCAs → increase in cyanosis

CLINICAL ISSUES

Presentation

- Most common signs/symptoms
  - Progressive cyanosis after birth with closure of ductus arteriosus
  - Congestive heart failure with large unobstructed high-flow MAPCAs
- Other signs/symptoms: Failure to thrive, polycythemia, finger clubbing

Natural History & Prognosis

- Progressive cyanosis due to development of pulmonary vascular disease → irreversible pulmonary hypertension
- Life expectancy when untreated less than 10 years
- Survival into adulthood now possible: "Adult congenital heart disease"
  - Need for lifelong follow-up with multiple imaging tests
- Prognosis is guarded, depends on feasibility of surgery

Treatment

- Prostaglandin E1 to keep ductus arteriosus open
- Palliative: Systemic-to-PA shunt (Blalock-Taussig, central), initial banding of high-flow MAPCAs
- PAt, VSD, MAPCAs: Staged complete repair
  - Unifocalization of MAPCAs and true PAs (if existent, to allow for PA growth)
  - Early one-stage repair in infancy, with incorporation of all MAPCAs in PA conduit, may be feasible
  - Complete repair with incorporation of MAPCAs and PAs in conduit, connected to reconstructed RVOT, closure of VSD (may not be possible due to high pressure in pulmonary system from residual stenosis/hypoplasia and pulmonary vascular disease)
  - Catheter-based interventions (balloon angioplasty with stenting of stenoses, coil embolization of small superfluous and/or bleeding MAPCAs)
- PAt, intact VS: Type of repair dependent on RV size and RV-dependency on coronary circulation
  - Restriction in flow across PFO: Balloon atrial septostomy
  - Catheter-based or surgical pulmonary valvotomy
  - Sudden decompression of RV through valvotomy, RVOT repair or transannular patch may lead to myocardial ischemia/infarction
  - When RV is too hypoplastic for bi-ventricular repair: Cavopulmonary (Glenn) shunt, staged completion of univentricular repair (Fontan)

SELECTED REFERENCES

1. Greil GF et al: Imaging of aortopulmonary collateral arteries with high-resolution multidetector CT. Pediatr Radiol. 36(6):502-9, 2006
2. Boechat MI et al: Cardiac MR imaging and MR angiography for assessment of complex tetralogy of Fallot and pulmonary atresia. Radiographics. 25(6):1535-46, 2005
3. Roche KJ et al: Assessment of vasculature using combined MRI and MR angiography. AJR Am J Roentgenol. 182(4):861-6, 2004
4. Baque J et al: Evaluation of pulmonary atresia with magnetic resonance imaging. Heart. 87(2):159, 2002
5. Okada M et al: Modified Blalock-Taussig shunt patency for pulmonary atresia: assessment with electron beam CT. J Comput Assist Tomogr. 26(3):368-72, 2002
6. Holmqvist C et al: Pre-operative evaluation with MR in tetralogy of fallot and pulmonary atresia with ventricular septal defect. Acta Radiol. 42(1):63-9, 2001
7. Doyle TP et al: Tetralogy of Fallot and pulmonary atresia with ventricular septal defect. In: Moller JH, Hoffman JIE ed. Pediatric cardiovascular medicine, 1st ed. Philadelphia, Churchill Livingstone. 391-408, 2000
8. Freedom RM: Pulmonary atresia and intact ventricular septum. In: Moller JH, Hoffman JIE ed. Pediatric cardiovascular medicine. 1st ed. Philadelphia, Churchill Livingstone. 442-60, 2000
9. Powell AJ et al: Accuracy of MRI evaluation of pulmonary blood supply in patients with complex pulmonary stenosis or atresia. Int J Card Imaging. 16(3):169-74, 2000
10. Ichida F et al: Evaluation of pulmonary blood supply by multiplanar cine magnetic resonance imaging in patients with pulmonary atresia and severe pulmonary stenosis. Int J Card Imaging. 15(6):473-81, 1999
11. Westra SJ et al: Cardiac electron-beam CT in children undergoing surgical repair for pulmonary atresia. Radiology. 213(2):502-12, 1999
12. Choe YH et al: MR imaging of non-visualized pulmonary arteries at angiography in patients with congenital heart disease. J Korean Med Sci. 13(6):597-602, 1998
13. Frank H et al: Magnetic resonance imaging of absent pulmonary valve syndrome. Pediatr Cardiol. 17(1):35-9, 1996
14. Taneja K et al: Comparison of computed tomography and cineangiography in the demonstration of central pulmonary arteries in cyanotic congenital heart disease. Cardiovasc Intervent Radiol. 19(2):97-100, 1996

PULMONARY ATRESIA

IMAGE GALLERY

Typical

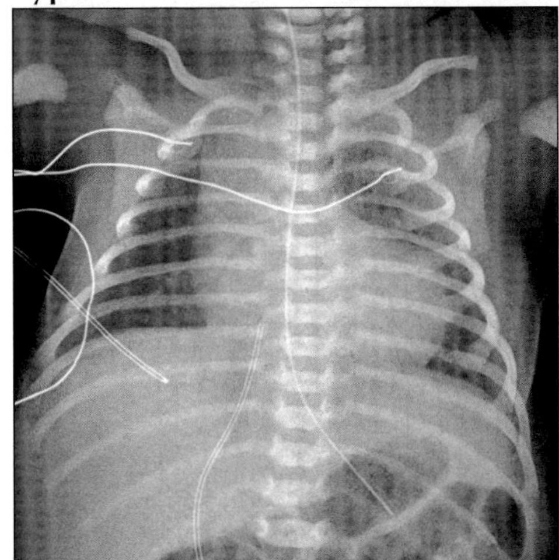

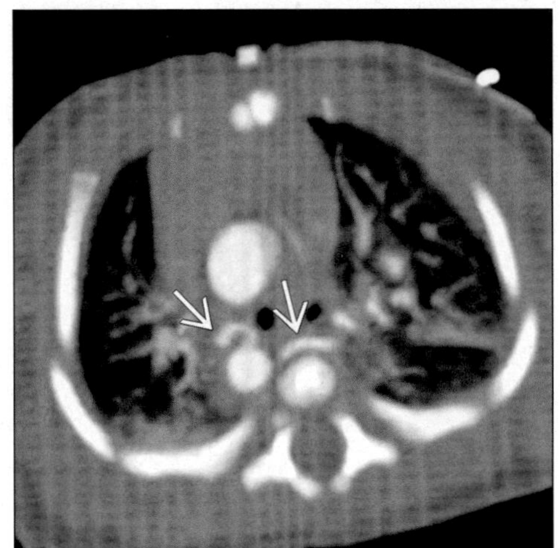

(Left) *Anteroposterior radiograph in a cyanotic newborn with pulmonary atresia-VSD-MAPCAs shows cardiomegaly, concave pulmonary artery segment and mild pulmonary edema.* ***(Right)*** *Axial cardiac CT shows right aortic arch and aortopulmonary collateral arteries ➡.*

Typical

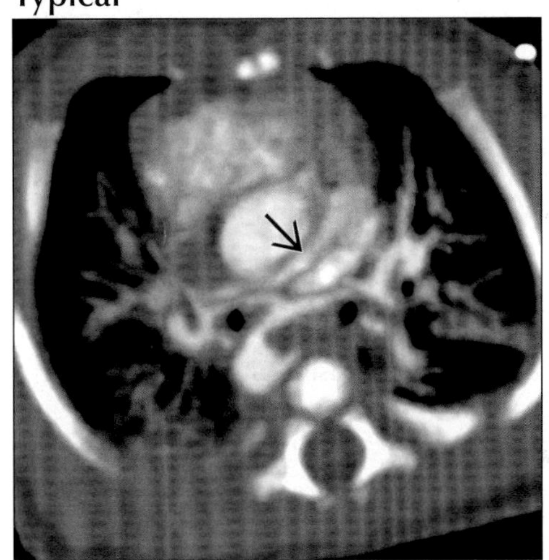

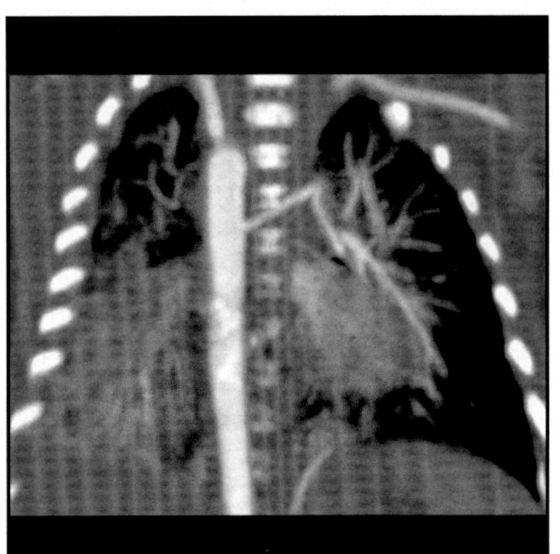

(Left) *Axial cardiac CT shows aortopulmonary collaterals in posterior mediastinum, and hypoplastic right branch pulmonary artery ➡, originating from atretic pulmonary valve.* ***(Right)*** *Coronal cardiac CT shows right aortic arch, prominent aortopulmonary collateral supplying the left lung.*

Typical

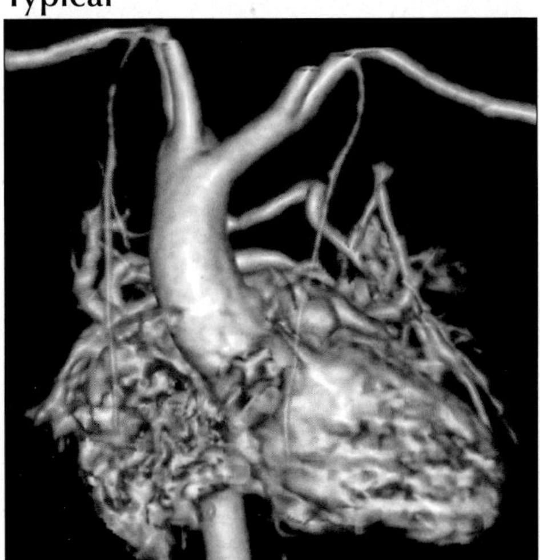

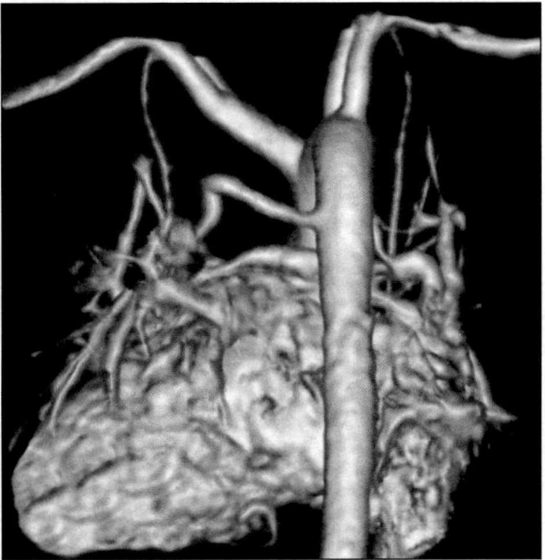

(Left) *Coronal cardiac CT (anterior view of shaded surface rendition) shows right aortic arch, MAPCAs supplying the left lung.* ***(Right)*** *Coronal cardiac CT (posterior view of shaded surface rendition) shows distribution of the MAPCAs, with larger vessels supplying the left lung than the right.*

TOTAL ANOMALOUS PULMONARY VENOUS RETURN

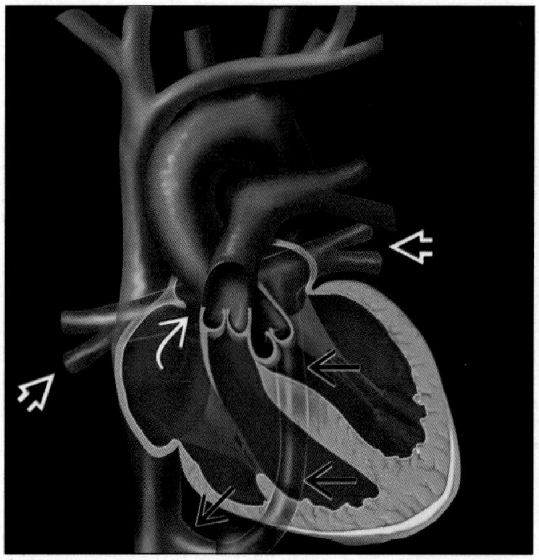

Graphic shows pulmonary veins forming retrocardiac common vein that descends below diaphragm to drain into IVC. (Left to to right shunt) note: ASD causing right to left shunt.

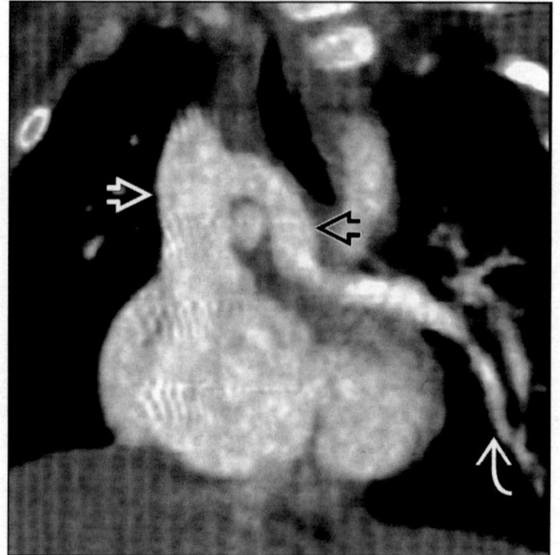

Oblique gated CTA shows left inferior pulmonary vein draining into common vein which arches over right pulmonary artery to connect to enlarged SVC. Note enlarged right atrium.

TERMINOLOGY

Abbreviations and Synonyms

- Total anomalous pulmonary venous return (TAPVR), total anomalous pulmonary venous connection

Definitions

- Embryologic failure of common pulmonary vein to connect to left atrium
  - Abnormal connection of pulmonary veins to right atrium, coronary sinus, systemic veins or their tributaries resulting in left to right shunt
  - Atrial septal defect of varying size present (right to left shunt) resulting in admixture lesion

IMAGING FINDINGS

General Features

- Best diagnostic clue: No pulmonary veins connecting to left atrium

Radiographic Findings

- Radiography
  - Type I: "Snowman" heart appearance on plain film
  - Type II: Indistinguishable from atrial septal defect (ASD) on plain film
  - Type III: Small heart, reticular pattern in the lungs: Edema on plain film
  - Cardiomegaly (types I and II), small heart (type III)
  - Shunt vascularity (types I and II), pulmonary edema (type III)
  - Wide mediastinum (type I, "snowman heart"), narrow mediastinum (types II and III, thymic atrophy)
  - Left vertical vein may be visible in type I

CT Findings

- 3D CT angiography: For pre- and post-operative pulmonary vein caliber measurements
  - Excellent for pre-operative determination of anatomy and drainage site
  - May demonstrate atrial septal defect (ASD)
  - Enlarged right atrium (RA) and right ventricle (RV)
- Thickened interlobular septa, peribronchial cuffing and ground-glass opacities suggest post-operative anastomotic pulmonary venous stenosis

DDx: TAPVR

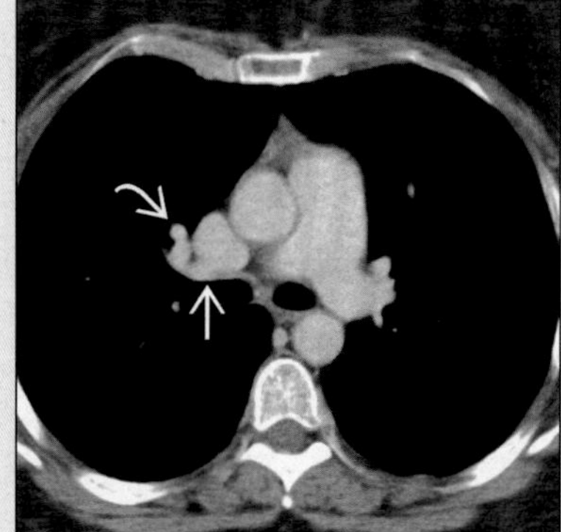

Right Sided PAPVR

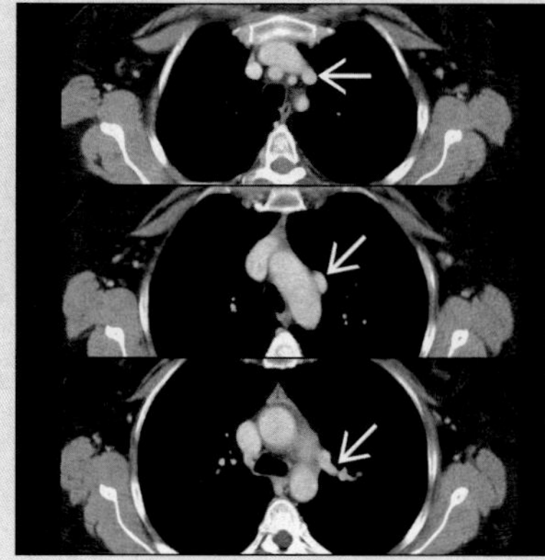

Left Sided PAPVR

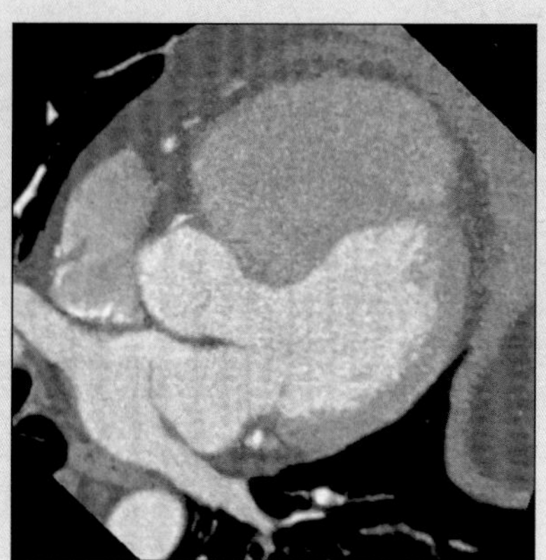

Cor Triatriatum

TOTAL ANOMALOUS PULMONARY VENOUS RETURN

Key Facts

Terminology
- Total anomalous pulmonary venous return (TAPVR), total anomalous pulmonary venous connection
- Embryologic failure of common pulmonary vein to connect to left atrium

Imaging Findings
- Type I: "Snowman" heart appearance on plain film
- Type II: Indistinguishable from atrial septal defect (ASD) on plain film
- Type III: Small heart, reticular pattern in the lungs: Edema on plain film
- Cardiomegaly (types I and II), small heart (type III)
- Shunt vascularity (types I and II), pulmonary edema (type III)
- Wide mediastinum (type I, "snowman heart"), narrow mediastinum (types II and III, thymic atrophy)

Pathology
- Supracardiac TAPVR (type I): "Vertical" common pulmonary vein carries blood from both lungs and joins left innominate vein
- Cardiac TAPVR (type II): Common pulmonary vein joins coronary sinus or right atrium directly
- Infracardiac TAPVR (type III): Common pulmonary vein traverses diaphragm to join portal vein, ductus venosus or inferior vena cava
- All pulmonary venous return to R heart (extracardiac L → R shunt)
- Intracardiac R → L shunt through ASD or PFO
- All types are admixture lesions
- Category: Cyanotic; heart size and pulmonary vascularity depend on type

MR Findings
- Cardiac-gated T1WI: Anomalous connection best seen in axial plane
- Gadolinium enhanced MRA: Allows for multiplanar reformations and volume-rendered 3D imaging
  - Best pulse sequence to define anatomy
- Cine-MR: For functional cardiac assessment, flow jets, regurgitation
  - May demonstrate ASD, enlarged RA and RV
- Phase-contrast MRA: For detection of pulmonary vein anastomotic stenosis (flow velocities > 100 cm/sec are diagnostic)

Echocardiographic Findings
- Echocardiogram
  - Lack of connection of pulmonary veins to left atrium
  - Right-sided chamber enlargement in types I and II
  - Patent foramen ovale (PFO)
  - Associated cardiac and abdominal situs abnormalities
  - Limited for assessment of post-operative venous obstruction

Ultrasonographic Findings
- Abdominal ultrasound in type III may demonstrate large infradiaphragmatic vascular channel from thorax with flow towards abdomen
  - Variable intrahepatic or extrahepatic connection
    - Eventually drains into IVC
  - May demonstrate area of narrowing with flow acceleration

Angiographic Findings
- Conventional
  - Seldom required for primary diagnosis
  - After repair: For diagnosis and treatment of anastomotic pulmonary venous stenosis

Imaging Recommendations
- Primary diagnosis with echocardiography
- CT, MR for post-operative pulmonary vein anastomotic stenosis

DIFFERENTIAL DIAGNOSIS

Cor Triatriatum
- Pulmonary venous connection occurred but remains stenotic

Hypoplastic Left Heart Syndrome
- Pulmonary blood return to left atrium, atretic or hypoplastic mitral valve causes shunting via ASD into RA
- Small left ventricle and ascending aorta, persistent ductus arteriosus with retrograde aortic flow towards arch vessels

Persistent Fetal Circulation Syndrome, Primary Pulmonary Hypertension
- Associated with severe hyaline membrane disease, meconium aspiration

PATHOLOGY

General Features
- General path comments
  - Three types
    - Supracardiac TAPVR (type I): "Vertical" common pulmonary vein carries blood from both lungs and joins left innominate vein
    - Cardiac TAPVR (type II): Common pulmonary vein joins coronary sinus or right atrium directly
    - Infracardiac TAPVR (type III): Common pulmonary vein traverses diaphragm to join portal vein, ductus venosus or inferior vena cava
  - Hemodynamics
    - All pulmonary venous return to R heart (extracardiac L → R shunt)
    - Intracardiac R → L shunt through ASD or PFO
    - All types are admixture lesions
  - Low systemic blood flow may lead to associated hypoplasia of left-sided cardiac chambers
  - Embryology

TOTAL ANOMALOUS PULMONARY VENOUS RETURN

- Lack of normal incorporation of primitive common pulmonary vein into posterior wall of left atrium
- Persistence and enlargement of embryological pathways for pulmonary venous return via umbilicovitelline and cardinal veins
  - Pathophysiology
    - All types have PFO to allow for obligatory R → L flow, leading to varying degrees of cyanosis (less severe in types I, II: Pulmonary hypercirculation)
    - Non-obstructive TAPVR (types I and II): ASD physiology, pulmonary plethora, congestive heart failure
    - Obstructive TAPVR (type III): Common pulmonary vein is obstructed by diaphragmatic hiatus → pulmonary venous congestion and edema
- Genetics
  - No specific genetic defect found
  - Occasionally associated with other complex cyanotic heart disease, asplenia syndrome, atrioventricular canal
- Epidemiology
  - 1-3% of congenital heart disease, more frequent in neonatal period
    - 2% of deaths due to congenital heart disease in first year of life

Gross Pathologic & Surgical Features

- Corrective surgery connects common pulmonary vein via window with left atrium and all other abnormal pulmonary venous connections are ligated

Staging, Grading or Classification Criteria

- Category: Cyanotic; heart size and pulmonary vascularity depend on type

CLINICAL ISSUES

Presentation

- Clinical Profile: Symptom severity depends on interatrial connection size and pulmonary resistance
- Types I, II: Initially asymptomatic, followed by congestive heart failure
- Type III: Severe cyanosis at birth
- Patent ductus arteriosus: Persistent fetal circulation

Natural History & Prognosis

- Highly variable
- No patients survive without surgical treatment
- Type I, II: Initially asymptomatic, with gradual development of congestive heart failure (ASD physiology)
- Type III, obstructive forms: Death within a month
- After surgical repair: Determined by associated cardiac anomalies and development of pulmonary vein anastomotic stenosis

Treatment

- Prostaglandin E1 to improve systemic perfusion in pulmonary hypertension
- Early surgical anastomosis of pulmonary venous confluence to left atrium

DIAGNOSTIC CHECKLIST

Consider

- Volume rendered 3D imaging to define anatomy
- Look for anastomotic pulmonary vein stenoses on post-operative CTA or MRA
- Look for connection with left atrium to exclude cor triatriatum (if no connection to RA) or unroofed coronary sinus (if coronary sinus collects pulmonary veins and drains into RA)

SELECTED REFERENCES

1. Gallego C et al: Congenital hepatic shunts. Radiographics. 24(3):755-72, 2004
2. Chen SJ et al: Validation of pulmonary venous obstruction by electron beam tomography in children with congenital heart disease. Ann Thor Surg. 71:1690-2, 2001
3. Videlefsky N et al: Magnetic resonance phase-shift velocity mapping in pediatric patients with pulmonary venous obstruction. Am J Cardiol. 87:589-93, 2001
4. Kim TH et al: Helical CT angiography and three-dimensional reconstruction of total anomalous pulmonary venous connections in neonates and infants. AJR Am J Roentgenol. 175(5):1381-6, 2000
5. Livolsi A et al: MR diagnosis of subdiaphragmatic anomalous pulmonary venous drainage in a newborn. J Comput Assist Tomogr. 15(6):1051-3, 1991
6. Duff DF et al: Infradiaphragmatic total anomalous pulmonary venous return. Review of clinical and pathological findings and results of operation in 28 cases. Br Heart J. 39(6):619-26, 1977

TOTAL ANOMALOUS PULMONARY VENOUS RETURN

IMAGE GALLERY

Typical

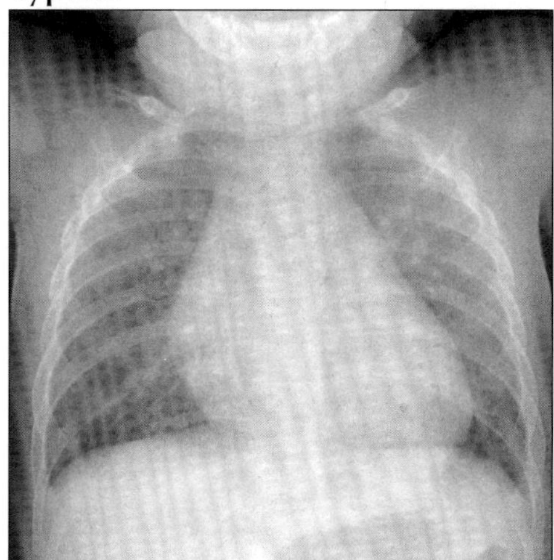

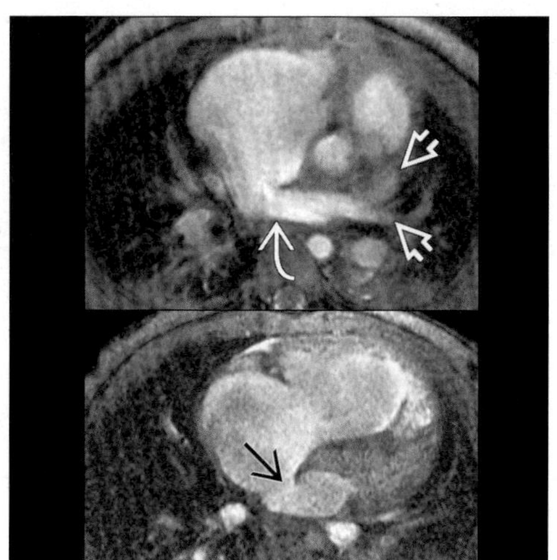

(Left) *AP radiograph shows enlarged right heart without pulmonary obstruction in patient with cardiac TAPVR.* ***(Right)*** *Axial MR cine show pulmonary veins ➡ draining into posterior common vein ➡ which drains into right atrium (cardiac TAPVR). Note: Enlarged right atrium and ventricle, large ASD ➡.*

Typical

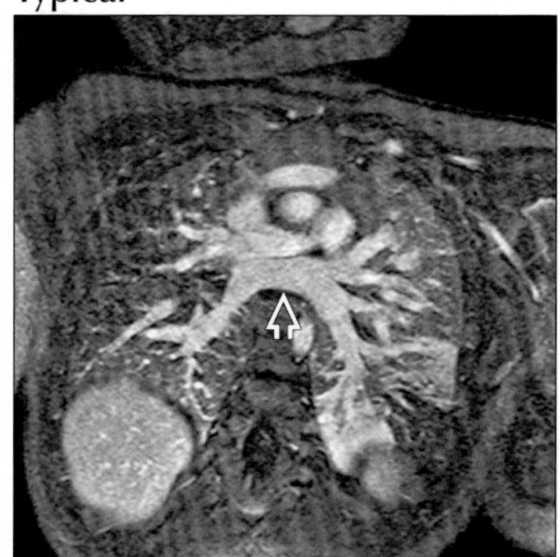

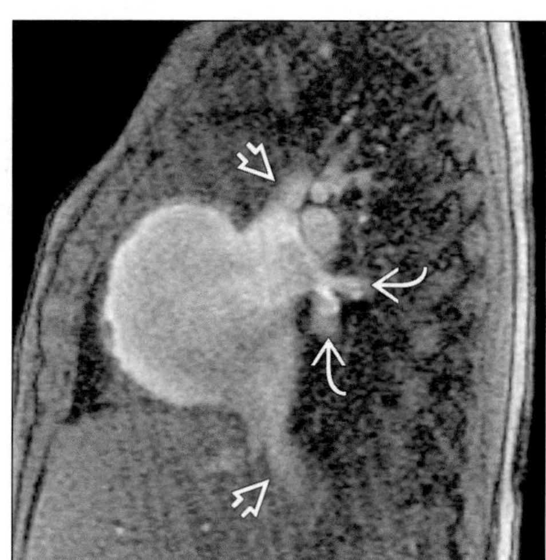

(Left) *Coronal MRA shows all four pulmonary veins collecting in common vein ➡ posterior to left atrium.* ***(Right)*** *Oblique MR cine shows enlarged right atrium and ventricle. Note superior and inferior venae cava ➡. Superior and inferior right pulmonary veins ➡ drain into RA via common vein.*

Variant

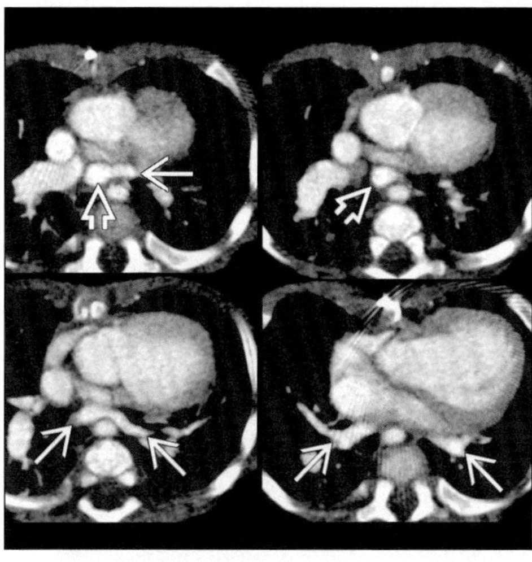

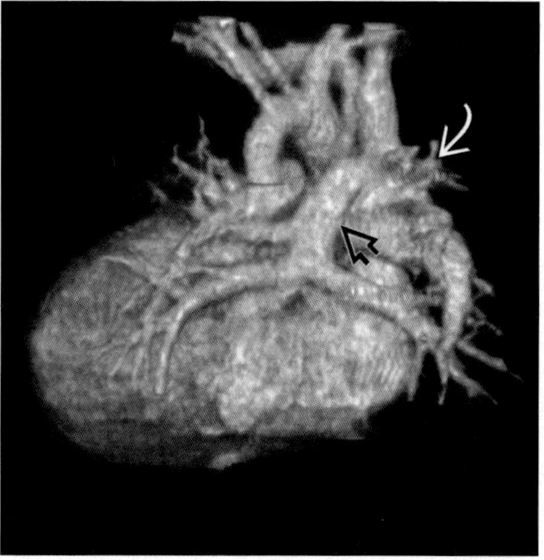

(Left) *Axial CECT shows pulmonary veins (PV) ➡ forming common retrocardiac vein ➡. Note: Single ventricle.* ***(Right)*** *Posterior volume rendered 3D CTA in same patient as previous image shows common vein draining into SVC ➡. Note: Right upper PV ➡ drains directly into SVC therefore this is considered "mixed" anomalous pulmonary return.*

SCIMITAR SYNDROME

Posteroanterior radiograph shows cardiac shift to the right and narrowed intercostal spaces due to pulmonary hypoplasia, and characteristic shadow from scimitar vein in right lung base →.

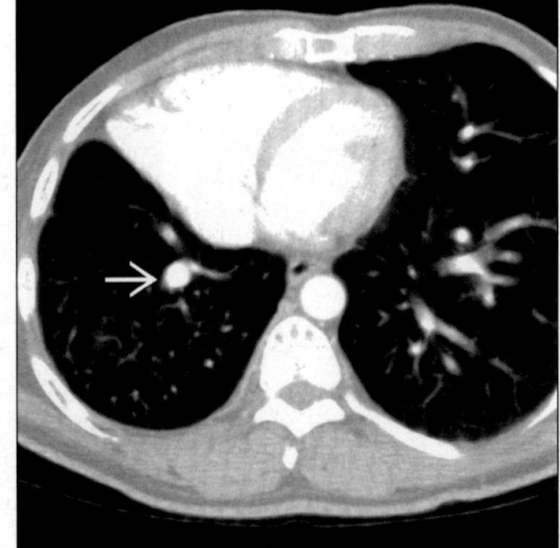

Axial CECT shows tubular round structure from scimitar vein in right lung base →, which could be traced down to inferior vena cava. Note right lung hypoplasia and shift of mediastinum towards right.

TERMINOLOGY

Abbreviations and Synonyms

- Hypogenetic lung/pulmonary venolobar syndrome

Definitions

- Right lung hypoplasia, anomalous right pulmonary venous connection to inferior vena cava (IVC)
- Often associated: Anomalous systemic arterial supply
- Category: Acyanotic, right-sided cardiac chamber enlargement, increased pulmonary vascularity (partial anomalous pulmonary venous return)
- Hemodynamics: Venous flow from right lung returns to right atrium ⇒ volume overload of right heart [atrial septal defect (ASD) equivalent]

IMAGING FINDINGS

General Features

- Best diagnostic clue: Scimitar sign = curved anomalous venous trunk, resembling a Turkish sword, in right medial costophrenic sulcus near right heart border, that increases in caliber in a caudad direction

Radiographic Findings

- Radiography
  - Right lung hypoplasia
  - Dextroversion of heart (no dextrocardia: Apex is still directed towards the left)
  - Prominent right atrium, active pulmonary vascular congestion: Shunt vascularity
  - Scimitar vein in right medial costophrenic sulcus

Fluoroscopic Findings

- Normal excursions of both hemidiaphragms, no air trapping

CT Findings

- Axial images show scimitar vein joining IVC
- CT angiography with 3D reconstruction most helpful to demonstrate anomalous systemic arterial supply, right pulmonary and mainstem bronchus hypoplasia

MR Findings

- Cardiac-gated T1WI: Anomalous pulmonary venous connection best seen in axial and coronal planes
- Phase-contrast MRA for shunt flow calculation

DDx: Anomalous Pulmonary Venous Return

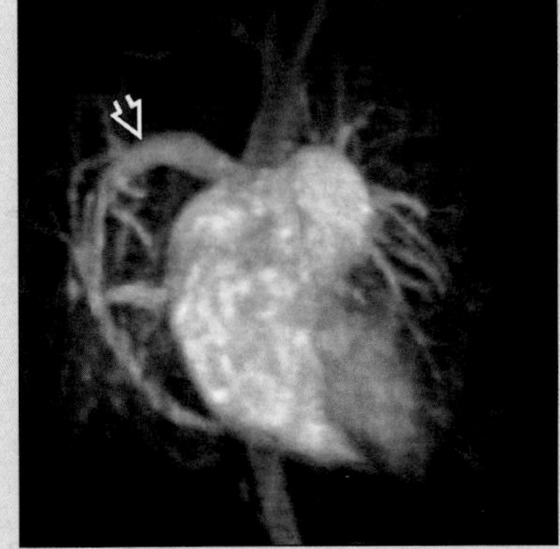

R Lung → Brachiocephalic Vein

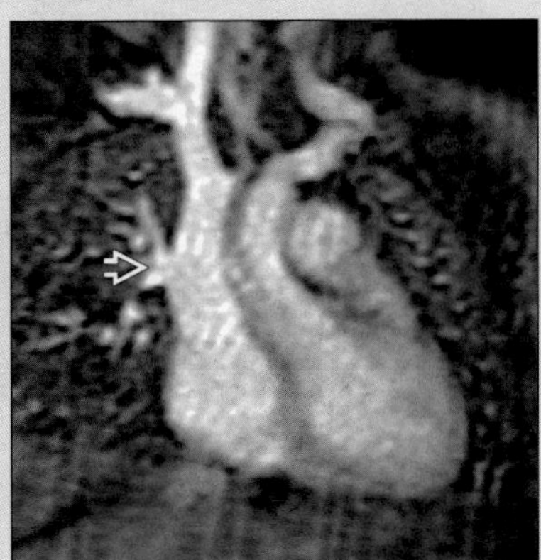

R Upper Lobe → SVC

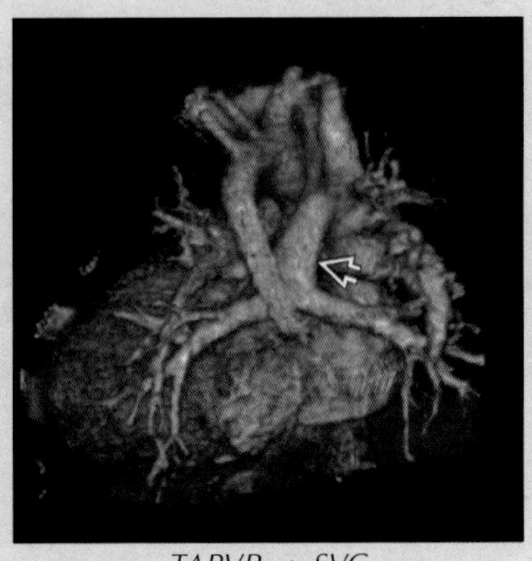

TAPVR → SVC

SCIMITAR SYNDROME

Key Facts

Terminology

- Right lung hypoplasia, anomalous right pulmonary venous connection to inferior vena cava (IVC)
- Category: Acyanotic, right-sided cardiac chamber enlargement, increased pulmonary vascularity (partial anomalous pulmonary venous return)
- Hemodynamics: Venous flow from right lung returns to right atrium ⇒ volume overload of right heart [atrial septal defect (ASD) physiology]

Imaging Findings

- Best diagnostic clue: Scimitar sign = curved anomalous venous trunk, resembling a Turkish sword, in right medial costophrenic sulcus near right heart border, that increases in caliber in a caudad direction
- CT angiography with 3D reconstruction most helpful to demonstrate anomalous systemic arterial supply, right pulmonary and mainstem bronchus hypoplasia
- CTA or MRA are better than echocardiography for complete assessment, and can replace diagnostic angiocardiography
- Angiography reserved for coil embolization

Clinical Issues

- Depending on age at presentation and size of left to right shunt
  - Newborn: Congestive heart failure, right heart volume overload, pulmonary hypertension
  - Young child: Recurrent infections in right lung base
  - Older child and adult: Often asymptomatic (incidental finding on chest radiograph)

- Gadolinium-enhanced MRA, coronal acquisition with 3D reconstruction for anomalous right pulmonary venous and arterial development

Echocardiographic Findings

- Echocardiogram
  - No right pulmonary veins entering left atrium
  - Scimitar vein connecting to IVC

Angiographic Findings

- Conventional
  - Scimitar vein opacifies during venous phase of pulmonary artery injection
  - Injection of abdominal aorta: Anomalous systemic arterial supply to right lung base (originating from celiac axis, right phrenic artery, descending aorta)
    - Road map for embolization of systemic artery

Imaging Recommendations

- CTA or MRA are better than echocardiography for complete assessment, and can replace diagnostic angiocardiography
- Angiography reserved for coil embolization

DIFFERENTIAL DIAGNOSIS

Other Forms of Partial Anomalous Pulmonary Venous Connection

- Right pulmonary vein(s) to azygous vein, superior vena cava, right atrium (with sinus venosus atrial septal defect)

True Dextrocardia with Abdominal Situs Solitus

- Other complex cardiac anomalies

Isolated Right Pulmonary Hypoplasia

- Normal right pulmonary venous connection to left atrium

Pulmonary Sequestration

- Mass in right lung base not connected to bronchial tree, systemic arterial supply and venous drainage to pulmonary (intralobar) or systemic (extralobar) veins

PATHOLOGY

General Features

- General path comments
  - Associated in 25% with other anomalies
    - Sinus venosus atrial septal defect most common
    - Ventricular septal defect, tetralogy of Fallot, patent ductus arteriosus
    - Diaphragmatic abnormalities: Accessory hemidiaphragm, hernia
    - Horseshoe lung (lung segment crossing over midline in posterior mediastinum)
  - Embryology
    - Primary abnormality in development of right lung, with secondary anomalous pulmonary venous connection
  - Pathophysiology
    - Obligatory left to right shunt to right atrium: ASD physiology
- Genetics: No specific genetic defect identified
- Associated abnormalities
  - Major
    - Absence of right pulmonary artery
    - Accessory diaphragm (duplication of diaphragm)
    - Absence or interruption of inferior vena cava
  - Minor: Tracheal trifurcation, diaphragmatic eventration or (partial) absence, phrenic cyst, horseshoe lung, esophageal or gastric lung, anomalous superior vena cava, absent left pericardium
  - Cardiac and spinal abnormalities

Gross Pathologic & Surgical Features

- Right lung (including pulmonary artery and bronchus) hypoplasia or agenesis
  - Most commonly affecting right upper/middle lobes

SCIMITAR SYNDROME

- Anomalous right pulmonary venous drainage to IVC (most frequent) or right atrium, superior vena cava, azygous vein, portal vein, hepatic vein
- Systemic arterialization of right lung base (without sequestration)

Microscopic Features

- Normal parenchyma in right lung base (as opposed to sequestration)
- Systemic artery branches anastomose with right pulmonary artery vascular bed in right lung base
- Long-standing shunt: Pulmonary vascular disease, leading to irreversible pulmonary hypertension (Eisenmenger physiology)

CLINICAL ISSUES

Presentation

- Most common signs/symptoms
  - Depending on age at presentation and size of left to right shunt
    - Newborn: Congestive heart failure, right heart volume overload, pulmonary hypertension
    - Young child: Recurrent infections in right lung base
    - Older child and adult: Often asymptomatic (incidental finding on chest radiograph)

Natural History & Prognosis

- Large shunt: Development of irreversible pulmonary hypertension
- Moderate to poor prognosis with neonatal presentation
- May be asymptomatic for many years with small shunt

Treatment

- Embolization of systemic arterial supply
- Baffling of common right pulmonary vein onto left atrium
- Surgical repair indicated when L-R shunt > 2:1

DIAGNOSTIC CHECKLIST

Consider

- Pre-operative identification of systemic arterial supply followed by embolization is important to avoid bleeding complications

Image Interpretation Pearls

- Recognize anomalous vessel in medial costophrenic sulcus
  - Runs perpendicular to expected course of right inferior pulmonary vein
  - Increases in caliber in caudad direction (as opposed to normal pulmonary vein)

SELECTED REFERENCES

1. Tsitouridis I et al: Scimitar syndrome versus meandering pulmonary vein: evaluation with three-dimensional computed tomography. Acta Radiol. 47(9):927-32, 2006
2. Yoo SJ et al: The relationship between scimitar syndrome, so-called scimitar variant, meandering right pulmonary vein, horseshoe lung and pulmonary arterial sling. Cardiol Young. 16(3):300-4, 2006
3. Khan MA et al: Usefulness of magnetic resonance angiography for diagnosis of scimitar syndrome in early infancy. Am J Cardiol. 96(9):1313-6, 2005
4. Berrocal T et al: Congenital anomalies of the tracheobronchial tree, lung, and mediastinum: embryology, radiology, and pathology. Radiographics. 24(1):e17, 2004
5. Sinha R et al: Scimitar syndrome: imaging by magnetic resonance angiography and Doppler echocardiography. Indian J Chest Dis Allied Sci. 46(4):283-6, 2004
6. Konen E et al: Congenital pulmonary venolobar syndrome: spectrum of helical CT findings with emphasis on computerized reformatting. Radiographics. 23(5):1175-84, 2003
7. Kramer U et al: Scimitar syndrome: morphological diagnosis and assessment of hemodynamic significance by magnetic resonance imaging. Eur Radiol. 13 Suppl 4:L147-50, 2003
8. Marco de Lucas E et al: Scimitar syndrome: complete anatomical and functional diagnosis with gadolinium-enhanced and velocity-encoded cine MRI. Pediatr Radiol. 33(10):716-8, 2003
9. Vanderheyden M et al: Partial anomalous pulmonary venous connection or scimitar syndrome. Heart. 89(7):761, 2003
10. Reddy R et al: Scimitar syndrome: a rare cause of haemoptysis. Eur J Cardiothorac Surg. 22(5):821, 2002
11. Vaes MF et al: Scimitar syndrome. JBR-BTR. 85(3):160-1, 2002
12. Zylak CJ et al: Developmental lung anomalies in the adult: radiologic-pathologic correlation. Radiographics. 22 Spec No:S25-43, 2002
13. Do KH et al: Systemic arterial supply to the lungs in adults: spiral CT findings. Radiographics. 21(2):387-402, 2001
14. Gilkeson RC et al: Gadolinium-enhanced magnetic resonance angiography in scimitar syndrome: diagnosis and postoperative evaluation. Tex Heart Inst J. 27(3):309-11, 2000
15. Huddleston CB et al: Scimitar syndrome presenting in infancy. Ann Thor Surg. 67:154-60, 1999
16. Henk CB et al: Scimitar syndrome: MR assessment of hemodynamic significance. J Comput Assist Tomogr. 21(4):628-30, 1997
17. Baran R et al: Scimitar syndrome: confirmation of diagnosis by a noninvasive technique (MRI). Eur Radiol. 6(1):92-4, 1996
18. Vrachliotis TG et al: Hypogenetic lung syndrome: functional and anatomic evaluation with magnetic resonance imaging and magnetic resonance angiography. J Magn Reson Imaging. 6(5):798-800, 1996
19. Boothroyd AE et al: Shoe, scimitar or sequestration: a shifting spectrum. Pediatr Radiol. 25(8):652-3, 1995
20. Woodring JH et al: Congenital pulmonary venolobar syndrome revisited. Radiographics. 14(2):349-69, 1994
21. Figa FH et al: Horseshoe lung--a case report with unusual bronchial and pleural anomalies and a proposed new classification. Pediatr Radiol. 23(1):44-7, 1993

SCIMITAR SYNDROME

IMAGE GALLERY

Typical

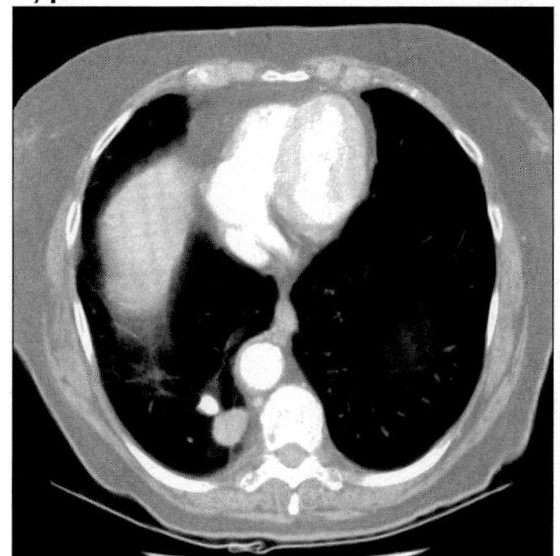

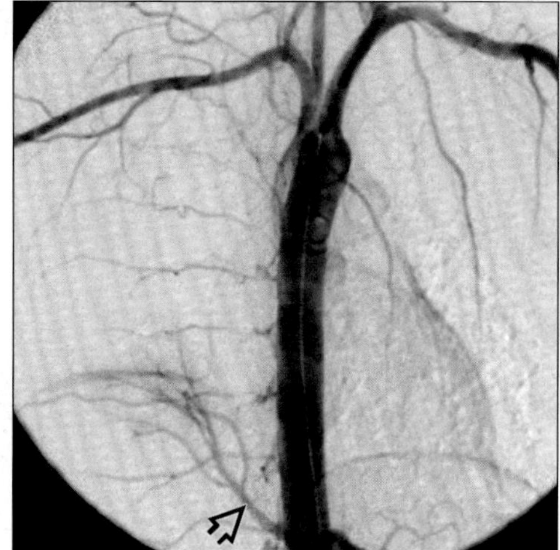

(Left) Axial CECT in asymptomatic adult shows tortuous pulmonary veins in medial right lung base, that could be traced down to inferior vena cava. *(Right)* Anteroposterior arteriogram shows systemic artery ⇨ supplying the right lung base in a patient with venolobar syndrome. This artery is invariably present and usually requires pre-operative embolization.

Typical

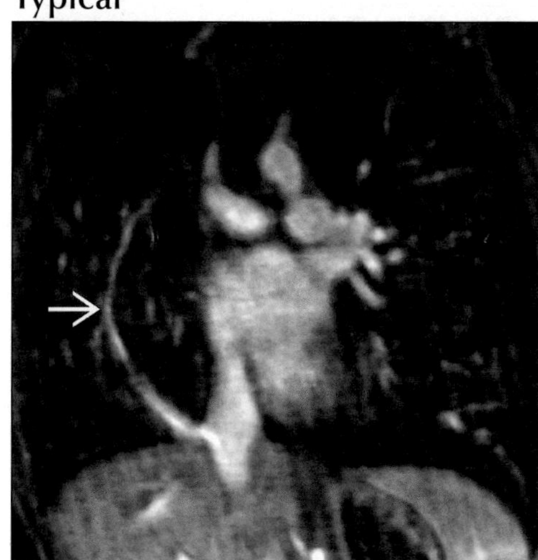

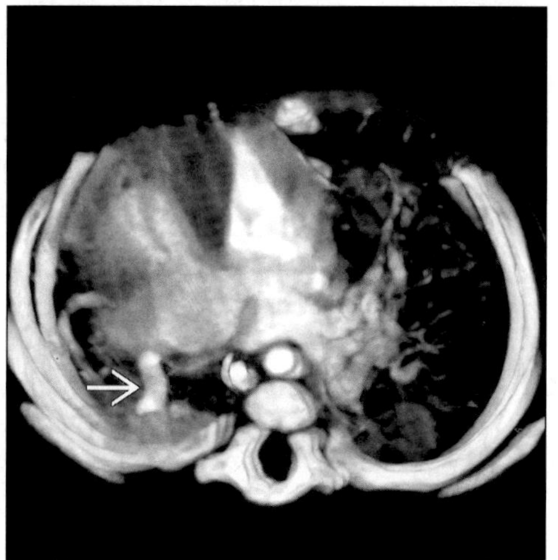

(Left) Coronal MR cine shows right medial lung base scimitar vein ➡ joining the inferior vena cava. *(Right)* Axial CECT thick slab rendition in young infant with heart failure, shows cardiac shift and scimitar vein ➡, which could be traced directly to right atrium.

Typical

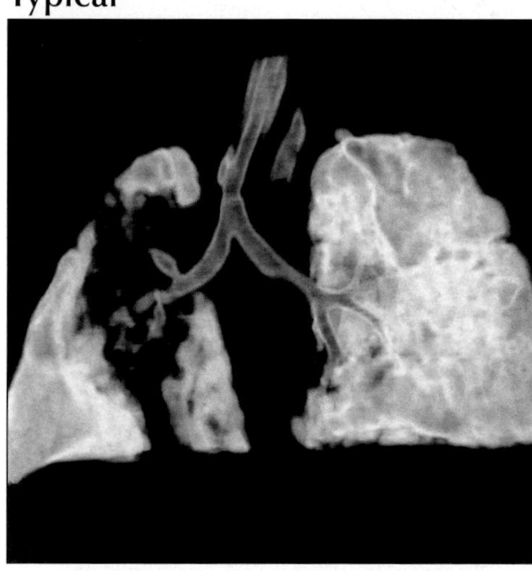

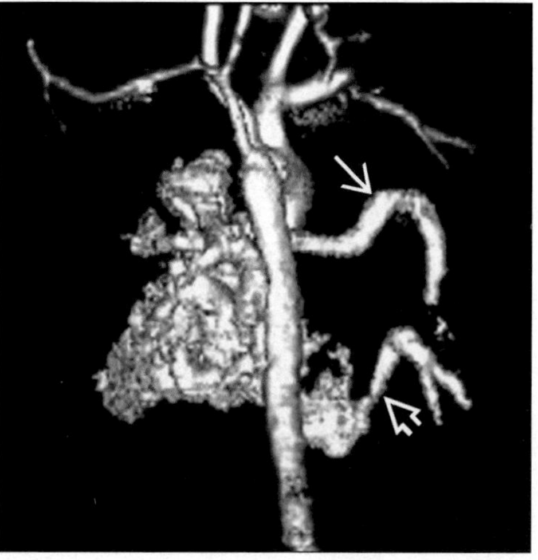

(Left) Coronal volume rendition of chest CT in same infant as previous image, shows relative right lung hypoplasia. *(Right)* Posterior view of surface rendition shows dilated right pulmonary artery ➡ and scimitar vein ⇨ connecting to right atrium in infant with pulmonary hypertension and heart failure.

HYPOPLASTIC LEFT HEART SYNDROME

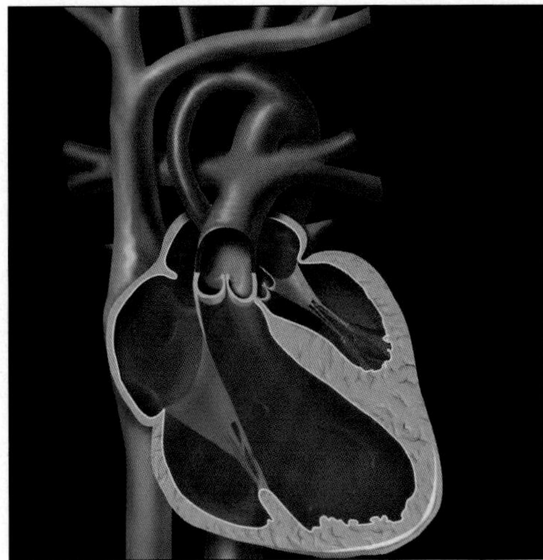

Graphic shows hypoplasia of LA, LV, aortic valve and ascending aorta. Systemic flow depends on patency of ductus arteriosus.

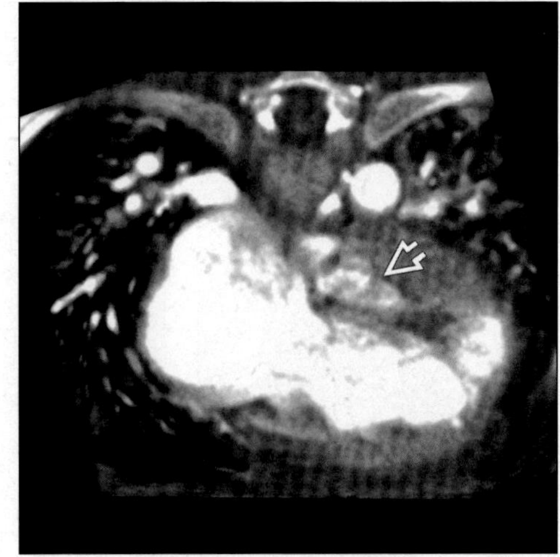

Oblique CTA shows hypoplastic left ventricle ➡ and dilated right-sided cardiac chambers.

TERMINOLOGY

Abbreviations and Synonyms

- Hypoplastic left heart syndrome (HLHS)
- Aortic atresia

Definitions

- Hypoplasia/atresia of the ascending aorta, aortic valve, left ventricle (LV) and mitral valve
  - Secondary findings: Patent ductus arteriosus (PDA), juxtaductal coarctation
- Most severe congenital heart lesion presenting in neonatal period with congestive heart failure, cardiogenic shock and cyanosis
- Category: Cyanotic, cardiomegaly, increased pulmonary vascularity
- Hemodynamics
  - Severe obstruction to flow to systemic circulation = ductus-dependent
  - Retrograde flow in hypoplastic aortic arch and ascending aorta for cranial and coronary perfusion
  - Volume overload in pulmonary circulation
  - Left-to-right shunting through patent foramen ovale
  - Flow admixture in right atrium → severe cyanosis

IMAGING FINDINGS

General Features

- Best diagnostic clue: Hypoplasia of ascending aorta, LV

Radiographic Findings

- Radiography
  - Cardiomegaly
  - Pulmonary venous congestion with interstitial fluid
  - Hyperinflation
  - Narrow mediastinum due to thymic atrophy

CT Findings

- CTA
  - Patency of aortopulmonary (Blalock-Taussig) and cavopulmonary (Glenn) shunts
  - Seroma associated with Blalock-Taussig shunt
  - Airway compression by dilated neo-aortic arch following Norwood repair

MR Findings

- T2* GRE
  - Short-axis steady-state free precession (SSFP) cine MR for functional assessment of univentricular heart, to determine suitability for Fontan operation

DDx: Left Heart Obstructive Lesions

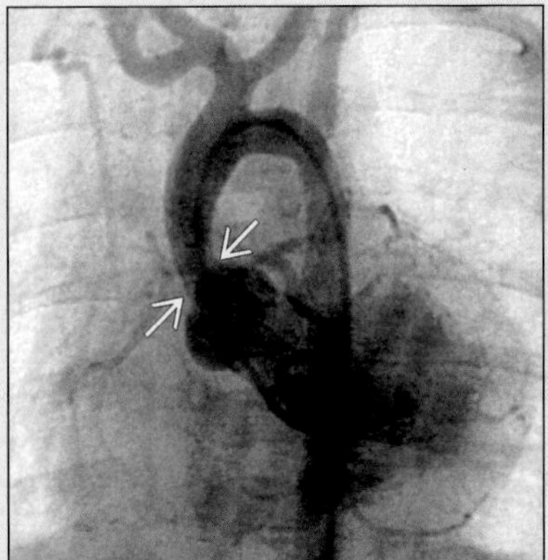

Aortic Stenosis

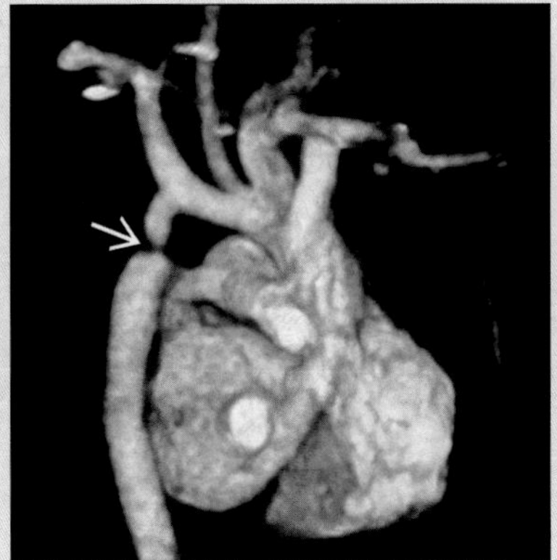

Infantile Coarctation

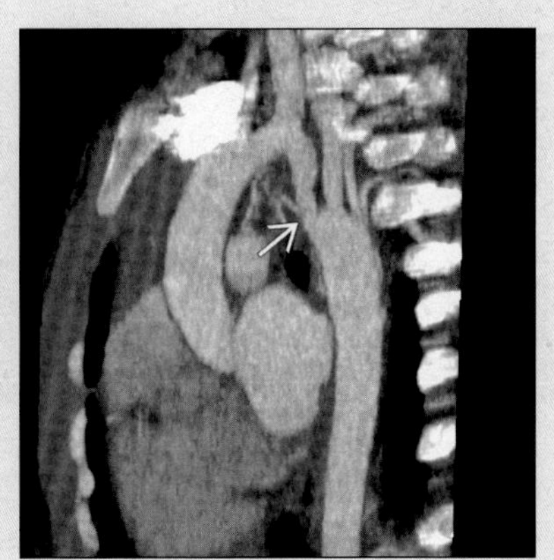

Postductal Coarctation

HYPOPLASTIC LEFT HEART SYNDROME

Key Facts

Terminology

- Hypoplasia/atresia of the ascending aorta, aortic valve, left ventricle (LV) and mitral valve
- Most severe congenital heart lesion presenting in neonatal period with congestive heart failure, cardiogenic shock and cyanosis
- Category: Cyanotic, cardiomegaly, increased pulmonary vascularity
- Severe obstruction to flow to systemic circulation = ductus-dependent
- Retrograde flow in hypoplastic aortic arch and ascending aorta for cranial and coronary perfusion
- Flow admixture in right atrium → severe cyanosis

Imaging Findings

- Primary diagnosis made with echocardiography in majority of cases
- Post-operative: Functional MR and interventional catheterizations for residua/sequelae of Fontan operation

Clinical Issues

- Medical: Prostaglandin E1 to keep PDA open
- Norwood: Atrial septectomy, construction of neo-aorta from pulmonary artery, Blalock-Taussig shunt for pulmonary perfusion (3 weeks)
- Conversion to hemi-Fontan (Glenn shunt between superior vena cava and right PA, 4-6 months)
- Fontan: Fenestrated venous conduit through right atrium of inferior caval flow to right PA (1.5-2 years)
- In some centers: Cardiac transplantation

  - SSFP cine MR for ventricular volume measurements in marginally hypoplastic left heart, to determine feasibility of bi-ventricular repair
- MRA
  - Velocity-encoded phase contrast (PC-) MRA for measurements of flow through aortic isthmus, PDA and foramen ovale
    - Can predict response to intra-operative test closure of ASD and PDA to determine feasibility of bi-ventricular repair

Echocardiographic Findings

- Echocardiogram
  - HLHS increasingly diagnosed prenatally
    - Retrograde flow in diminutive ascending aorta
    - LV growth arrest only becomes manifest between 18-22 weeks of gestation
  - Postnatal diagnosis with echo sufficient for treatment planning
    - Diminutive ascending aorta < 5 mm
    - Small, thick-walled LV
    - Mitral valve size is expressed as a Z-score: Important parameter to decide whether a bi-ventricular repair is possible in marginally hypoplastic LVs
    - Dilatation of right-sided chambers and pulmonary artery (PA)
    - Size and location of ductus arteriosus
    - Patency of foramen ovale or presence of atrial septal defect
    - Abnormal ventricular wall motion (ischemic damage, fibroelastosis)
- Color Doppler
  - Hemodynamics of aortic root
  - Left-to-right shunt through foramen ovale
  - Tricuspid regurgitation

Other Modality Findings

- CTA, MR: Occasionally performed after staged Norwood or Stanzel procedures
  - Residual stenosis of neo-aortic arch, coarctation
  - Functional assessment of marginally hypoplastic left heart with cine MR and velocity-encoded phase contrast MRA, prior to Fontan operation

Angiographic Findings

- Conventional
  - Cardiac catheterization with angiography; can be done via umbilical artery catheter
    - Retrograde flow in hypoplastic ascending aorta, filling of pulmonary arteries via ductus arteriosus

Imaging Recommendations

- Primary diagnosis made with echocardiography in majority of cases
- Post-operative: Functional MR and interventional catheterizations for residua/sequelae of Fontan operation

DIFFERENTIAL DIAGNOSIS

Critical Aortic Stenosis, Infantile Coarctation, Interrupted Aortic Arch

- Pressure overload of normally-developed left ventricle

Cranial (Vein of Galen) or Hepatic Arteriovenous Malformation

- Structurally normal heart, volume overload of all chambers

Cardiomyopathy, Endocardial Fibroelastosis

- Globally enlarged, structurally normal heart, myocardial dysfunction

Coronary Arteriovenous Fistula

- Left coronary originates from PA, LV infarction

Severe Arrhythmias: Paroxysmal Supraventricular Tachycardia

- Characteristic electrocardiogram

HYPOPLASTIC LEFT HEART SYNDROME

PATHOLOGY

General Features

- General path comments
  - Underdevelopment of left-sided cardiac structures
    - Hypoplasia or atresia of aortic and mitral valves
    - Hypoplasia of LV and ascending aorta
  - Compatible with normal fetal hemodynamics → no fetal compromise
  - Embryology
    - Abnormal partitioning of primitive conotruncus into left and right ventricular outflow tracts → hypoplasia/atresia of aortic valve
    - Diminished prenatal antegrade flow through aorta → underdevelopment of LV and ascending aorta
  - Pathophysiology
    - Severe obstruction to outflow of diminutive LV
    - Pulmonary venous flow shunts through foramen ovale into right atrium
    - Dilated right-sided cardiac chambers and PA
    - Systemic perfusion via PDA
- Genetics
  - No clear genetic defect demonstrated in majority
  - Not commonly associated with extracardiac malformations
- Epidemiology
  - 1-3 per 10,000 live births, M:F = 2:1
  - Fourth most common congenital heart lesion presenting under 1 year (7-9%)

Gross Pathologic & Surgical Features

- Severe hypoplasia of left-sided cardiac chambers and ascending aorta
- Large main pulmonary artery, ductus arteriosus
- Localized aortic coarctation (80%)
- Endocardial fibro-elastosis in small, thick-walled LV

CLINICAL ISSUES

Presentation

- Most common signs/symptoms
  - No circulatory symptoms immediately at birth but rapid deterioration
    - Congestive heart failure (volume overload pulmonary circulation)
    - Cardiogenic shock after closure of PDA
    - Cyanosis (flow admixture in right heart)
    - Hypoxia → pulmonary hypertension, persistent fetal circulation
- Other signs/symptoms
  - Poor systemic perfusion, metabolic acidosis
    - Acute tubular necrosis, renal failure
    - Necrotizing enterocolitis

Natural History & Prognosis

- Death within days/weeks when untreated
- Poor prognosis without treatment; has improved substantially in recent years
- Determined by complications, residua and sequelae of staged Norwood repair and Fontan operation (right ventricular dysfunction, venous hypertension)
- Significant tricuspid regurgitation after surgical palliation correlates with poor outcome

Treatment

- Medical: Prostaglandin E1 to keep PDA open
- Prenatal: US-guided balloon dilatation of aortic valve in mid/late fetal period is now possible
  - Change in fetal hemodynamics may enhance prenatal growth of left-sided cardiac structures
- Rashkind balloon atrial septostomy (in case of flow restriction across foramen ovale)
- Palliative repair
  - Norwood: Atrial septectomy, construction of neo-aorta from pulmonary artery, Blalock-Taussig shunt for pulmonary perfusion (3 weeks)
  - Damus-Kaye-Stanzel anastomosis: Variation of Norwood with side-to-side anastomosis between PA and hypoplastic ascending aorta
  - Conversion to hemi-Fontan (Glenn shunt between superior vena cava and right PA, 4-6 months)
  - Fontan: Fenestrated venous conduit through right atrium of inferior caval flow to right PA (1.5-2 years)
- Marginally hypoplastic LV: Bi-ventricular repair may be feasible
  - LV volume is commonly underestimated with echocardiography
  - Functional MR (SSPE-cine: Ventricular volumes and function; PC-MRA: Flow volumes) is more reliable
- In some centers: Cardiac transplantation

SELECTED REFERENCES

1. Sundareswaran KS et al: Impaired power output and cardiac index with hypoplastic left heart syndrome: a magnetic resonance imaging study. Ann Thorac Surg. 82(4):1267-75; discussion 1275-7, 2006
2. Muthurangu V et al: Cardiac magnetic resonance imaging after stage I Norwood operation for hypoplastic left heart syndrome. Circulation. 112(21):3256-63, 2005
3. Oye RG et al. Hypoplastic left heart syndrome. In: Mavroudis C, Backer CL ed. Pediatric cardiac surgery. 3rd ed. Philadelphia, Mosby. 560-74, 2003
4. Bardo DM et al: Hypoplastic left heart syndrome. Radiographics. 21(3):705-17, 2001
5. Cheatham JP: Intervention in the critically ill neonate and infant with hypoplastic left heart syndrome and intact atrial septum. J Interv Cardiol. 14(3):357-66, 2001
6. Herman TE et al: Special imaging casebook. Hypoplastic left heart, prostaglandin therapy gastric focal foveolar hyperplasia and brown-fat necrosis. J Perinatol. 21(4):263-5, 2001
7. Rosenthal A et al: Hypoplastic left heart syndrome. In: Moller JH, Hoffman JIE ed. Pediatric cardiovascular medicine, 1st ed. Philadelphia, Churchill Livingstone. 594-605, 2000
8. Fellows KE et al: MR imaging and heart function in patients pre- and post-Fontan surgery. Acta Paediatr Suppl. 410:57-9, 1995
9. Fogel MA et al: A study in ventricular-ventricular interaction. Single right ventricles compared with systemic right ventricles in a dual-chamber circulation. Circulation. 92(2):219-30, 1995
10. Kondo C et al: Nuclear magnetic resonance imaging of the palliative operation for hypoplastic left heart syndrome. J Am Coll Cardiol. 18(3):817-23, 1991
11. Norwood WI et al: Hypoplastic left heart syndrome. Ann Thorac Surg. 1991:688-95, 1991

IMAGE GALLERY

Typical

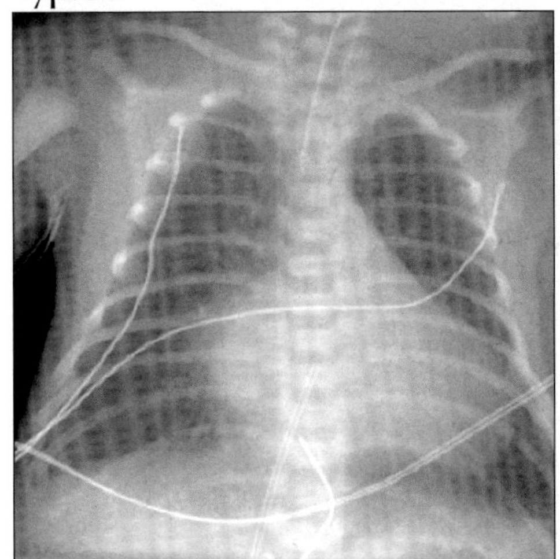

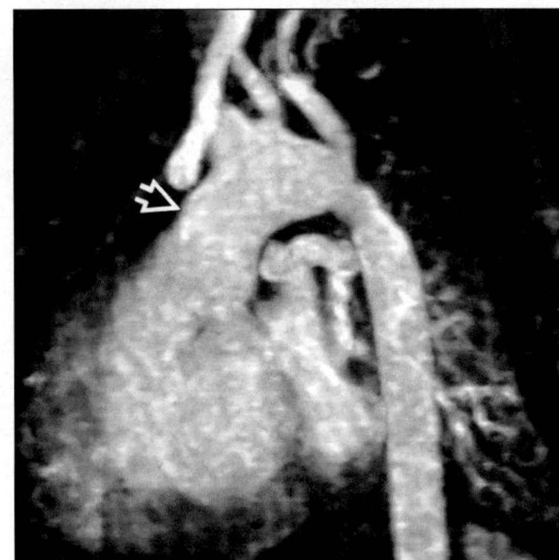

(Left) *Anteroposterior radiograph shows cardiomegaly, vascular congestion and hyperinflation. The upper mediastinum is narrow, indicative of thymic involution secondary to stress.* ***(Right)*** *Oblique MRA shows dilated main pulmonary artery ➡, which is the main cardiac outflow channel.*

Typical

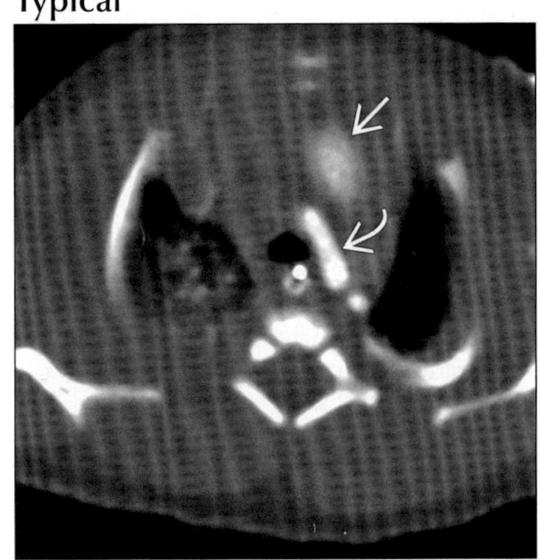

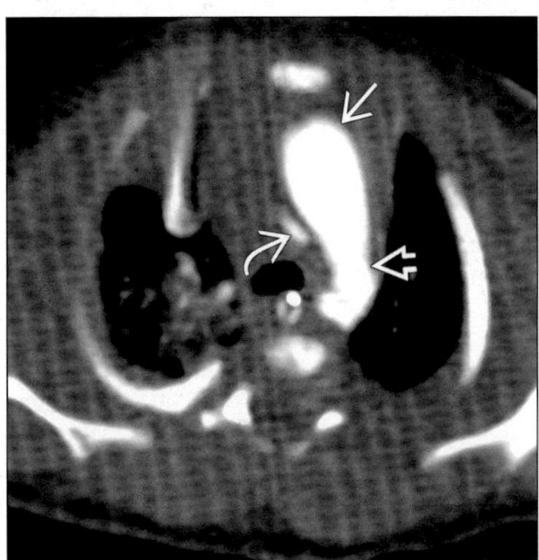

(Left) *Axial CTA demonstrates hypoplastic aortic arch ➡ and dilated main pulmonary artery ➡.* ***(Right)*** *Axial CTA shows hypoplastic ascending aorta ➡. The enlarged main pulmonary artery ➡ connects to the descending aorta via a large patent ductus arteriosus ➡.*

Typical

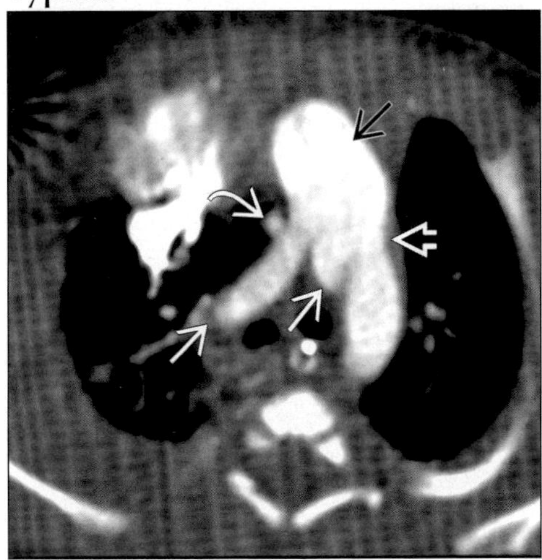

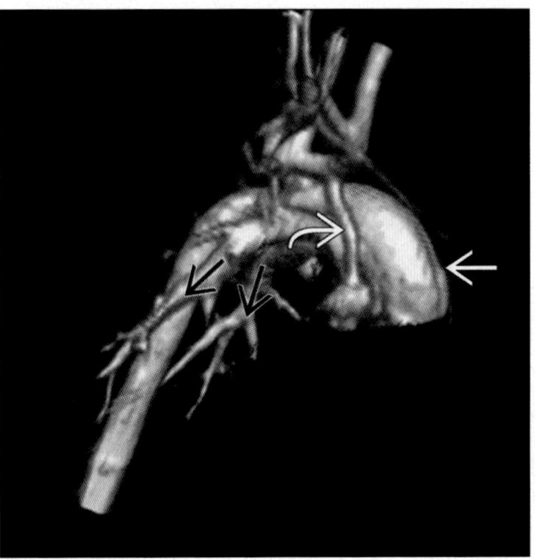

(Left) *Axial CTA shows hypoplastic ascending aorta ➡. The large main pulmonary artery → connects via the ductus arteriosus ➡ to the descending aorta. Notice take-off of both branch pulmonary arteries ➡ from the main pulmonary artery.* ***(Right)*** *3D CTA shows enlarged main pulmonary artery ➡, right and left branch pulmonary arteries → and hypoplastic ascending aorta ➡.*

HETEROTAXIA SYNDROMES

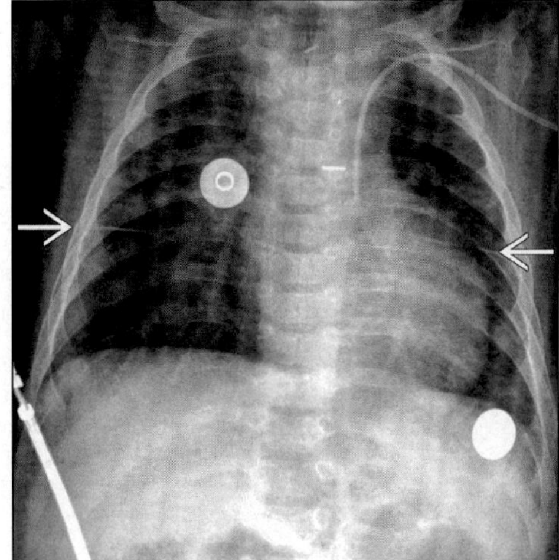

Anteroposterior radiograph in an infant with asplenia shows a right bronchial isomerism, bilateral minor fissures ➡, catheter in left SVC, and transverse liver. (Courtesy R. Kishnamurthy, MD).

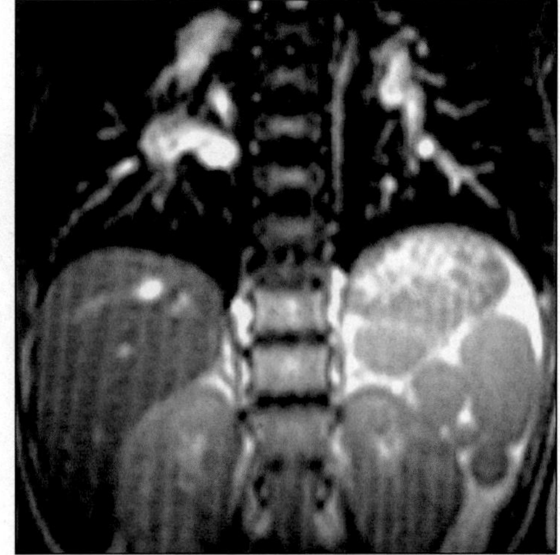

Coronal T2WI MR in an infant with a left isomerism (polysplenia syndrome) shows multiple spleens in the left upper abdomen. (Courtesy R. Kishnamurthy, MD).

TERMINOLOGY

Abbreviations and Synonyms

- Situs ambiguous, right/left isomerism, cardiosplenic syndromes, Ivemark syndrome

Definitions

- Disturbance of the normal left-right asymmetry in the position of thoracic and abdominal organs

IMAGING FINDINGS

General Features

- Best diagnostic clue: Abnormal symmetry in chest and abdomen

Radiographic Findings

- Radiography
  - Bilateral left- or right-sidedness in chest, findings of congenital heart disease (CHD), transverse liver, cardiac apex and stomach not on same side
  - Asplenia syndrome
    - Bilateral minor fissures
    - Symmetrical short mainstem bronchi with right-sided morphology (narrow carinal angle)
    - Pulmonary artery courses anterior to mainstem bronchus (eparterial bronchus)
    - Cardiomegaly, pulmonary edema
  - Polysplenia syndrome
    - No minor fissure on either side
    - Symmetrical long mainstem bronchi with left-sided morphology (wide carinal angle)
    - Pulmonary artery courses over and behind mainstem bronchus (hyparterial bronchus)
    - Absent IVC shadow on lateral film, prominent azygous shadow on AP
  - Both syndromes
    - Cardiac malposition (40%: Meso-/dextrocardia)
    - Transverse liver
    - Right-sided stomach with levocardia, left-sided stomach with dextrocardia, or midline stomach

CT Findings

- CTA
  - Rapid examination of chest and abdomen: Situs abnormalities, systemic and pulmonary venous connections, tracheobronchial anatomy

DDx: Situs Abnormalities

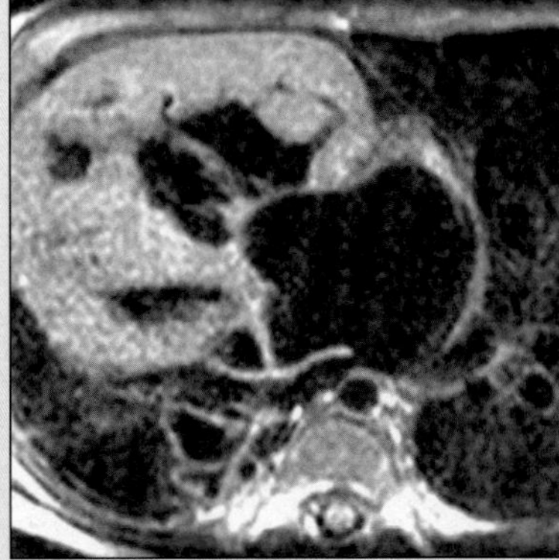

Dextrocardia, Common Atrium

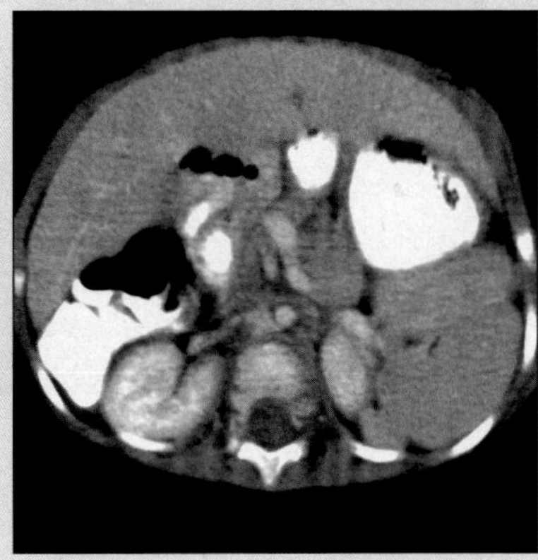

Transverse Liver, Polysplenia

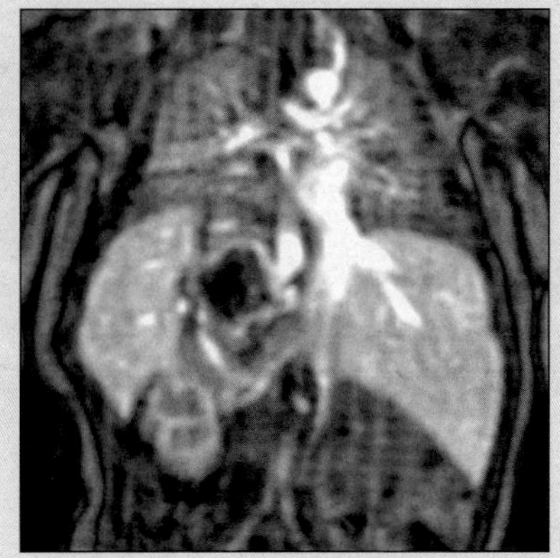

Transverse Liver, Asplenia

HETEROTAXIA SYNDROMES

Key Facts

Terminology
- Disturbance of the normal left-right asymmetry in the position of thoracic and abdominal organs

Imaging Findings
- Best diagnostic clue: Abnormal symmetry in chest and abdomen
- Classic plain film appearance: Transverse midline liver, discrepancy between position of cardiac apex and stomach, bilateral left- or right-sidedness in the chest, findings of congenital heart disease (CHD)
- Rapid examination of chest and abdomen: Situs abnormalities, systemic and pulmonary venous connections, tracheobronchial anatomy
- T1WI: Multiplanar imaging (coronal, axial) for segmental analysis of intracardiac connections and defects
- T2* GRE: Cine MR for ventricular volumes and function, to determine suitability for biventricular versus univentricular (Fontan) repair
- Gadolinium-enhanced 3D MRA: Comparable to CTA, better spatial resolution in coronal plane

Pathology
- Segmental approach to analysis of complex cardiac anomalies with cardiac malposition
- Any arrangement other than situs solitus or inversus is termed situs ambiguous (heterotaxia)

Clinical Issues
- Asplenia: Male neonate with severe cyanosis, susceptibility for infections
- Polysplenia: More variable, often presents later

  - Best for post-op patients (metallic clips, coils, stents)
  - Can replace and often provide more anatomic information than diagnostic angiocardiography

MR Findings
- T1WI: Multiplanar imaging for segmental analysis of intracardiac connections and defects
- T2* GRE: Cine MR for ventricular volumes and function, to determine suitability for biventricular versus univentricular (Fontan) repair
- MRA
  - Gadolinium-enhanced 3D MRA: Comparable to CTA
  - Ultrafast time-resolved Gd-MRA with repeated acquisitions allows for dynamic circulation study
  - Phase contrast MRA for flow quantification

Echocardiographic Findings
- Echocardiogram: Often definitive test for characterization of intracardiac anomalies, abnormal systemic and/or pulmonary venous connections

Other Modality Findings
- Upper GI study: Malrotation is frequently associated

Imaging Recommendations
- Protocol advice
  - Echocardiography, followed by MR
  - CTA for anatomic study in post-operative patients

DIFFERENTIAL DIAGNOSIS

Situs Inversus Totalis {I, L, L}
- Mirror image of normal
- Low association with CHD (3-5%); may be associated with immotile cilia syndrome (Kartagener): Sinusitis, bronchiectasis, infertility

True Dextrocardia, Abdominal Situs Solitus and Levocardia, Abdominal Situs Inversus
- Both have a high association with CHD (95-100%)

Dextroversion of the Heart
- Heart is positioned in right chest with apex and stomach still directed toward the left
- In right pulmonary hypoplasia (scimitar syndrome), left-sided mass lesions (diaphragmatic hernia, cystic adenomatoid malformation of lung)

PATHOLOGY

General Features
- General path comments
  - Heterotaxy syndrome represents a spectrum, with overlap between classic asplenia and polysplenia manifestations, and other anomalies
  - Embryology
    - Early embryological disturbance (5th week of gestation), leading to complex anomalies
  - Pathophysiology
    - Determined by complexity of associated CHD
    - Asplenia syndrome with anomalous pulmonary venous connections: Findings of pulmonary venous outflow obstruction may be masked when there is restriction to pulmonary arterial inflow at the same time (pulmonary atresia)
- Genetics: No specific genetic defect in majority
- Epidemiology
  - Prevalence 1 per 22,000 to 24,000; 1-3% of CHD
  - Asplenia is more common in boys; equal sex ratio for polysplenia

Staging, Grading or Classification Criteria
- Segmental approach to analysis of complex cardiac anomalies with cardiac malposition
  - Viscero-atrial situs designated by S (solitus = normal) or I (inversus = mirror image of normal)
  - Always associated on same side are
    - Major lobe of liver, IVC, anatomic right atrium, tri-lobed lung, eparterial bronchus
    - Spleen, stomach, descending aorta, anatomic left atrium, bi-lobed lung, hyparterial bronchus

HETEROTAXIA SYNDROMES

  - Any arrangement other than situs solitus or inversus is termed situs ambiguous (heterotaxia)
  - Ventricular loop: D (normal) or L (inverted)
  - Orientation of great arteries (presence of transposition) also designated by D or L
  - Segmental analysis summarized by 3-letter code: {S, D, D}, {I, L, L}, {S, D, L}
  - Connections: Concordant or discordant
  - Associated abnormalities: Transposition of great arteries (TGA), double outlet right ventricle (DORV), total anomalous pulmonary venous return (TAPVR)
- Two major subtypes
  - Asplenia syndrome = double right-sidedness
    - Absence of a spleen
    - IVC and aorta on same side
    - Bilateral SVC (36%), absent coronary sinus
    - Right isomerism of atrial appendages
    - Common atrium with band-like remnant of septum crossing atria in anteroposterior direction
    - Bilateral tri-lobed lungs
    - Bilateral eparterial bronchi
    - Associated with severe cyanotic CHD (atrioventricular septal defect, common AV valve, DORV, TGA, pulmonary stenosis/atresia)
    - Abnormalities of pulmonary venous connections: TAPVR (> 80%); often obstructed, below diaphragm (type III)
  - Polysplenia syndrome = double left-sidedness
    - Multiple spleens, anisosplenia, multilobed spleen
    - Abnormalities of systemic venous connections: Azygous continuation of IVC (> 70%), hepatic veins drain separately into common atrium
    - Bilateral SVC (41%), connect to coronary sinus
    - Left isomerism of atrial appendages
    - Common atrium or large ostium primum ASD
    - Bilateral bi-lobed lungs
    - Bilateral hyparterial bronchi
    - Associated with less severe CHD [common atrium, ventricular septal defect (VSD)]

CLINICAL ISSUES

Presentation

- Most common signs/symptoms
  - Asplenia: Male neonate with severe cyanosis, susceptibility for infections
  - Polysplenia: More variable, often presents later
- Other signs/symptoms: Malrotation, volvulus, preduodenal portal vein, absent gallbladder, extrahepatic biliary atresia, short pancreas

Natural History & Prognosis

- First year mortality: 85% asplenia, 65% polysplenia

Treatment

- Supportive, prostaglandins, antibiotic prophylaxis
- Asplenia/polysplenia with pulmonary overcirculation: Pulmonary artery banding
- Asplenia with obstructed pulmonary flow and TAPVR: Delicate balance between pulmonary arterial inflow and venous outflow
  - Placement of palliative systemic to pulmonary artery (Blalock-Taussig or central) shunt increases inflow
  - TAPVR repair needs to be done at the same time, to reduce outflow obstruction
- Early biventricular repair, if possible
- Univentricular repair, step 1: Glenn or hemi-Fontan
- Polysplenia: Incorporation of azygous vein to cavopulmonary anastomosis (Kawashima operation)
  - Post-operative: Development of pulmonary to systemic venous collaterals, arteriovenous malformations, pulmonary vein stenosis
- Completion of modified Fontan operation, if possible
  - One or more hepatic veins may have to be excluded from Fontan shunt → veno-venous collaterals
  - CTA or MRA prior to catheterization as road map for coil embolization of collaterals

DIAGNOSTIC CHECKLIST

Image Interpretation Pearls

- Rigorous application of segmental analysis on cross-sectional study will resolve any complex case

SELECTED REFERENCES

1. Maier M et al: Annular pancreas and agenesis of the dorsal pancreas in a patient with polysplenia syndrome. AJR Am J Roentgenol. 188(2):W150-3, 2007
2. Maldjian PD et al: Approach to dextrocardia in adults: review. AJR Am J Roentgenol. 188(6 Suppl):S39-49; quiz S35-8, 2007
3. Fulcher AS et al: Abdominal manifestations of situs anomalies in adults. Radiographics. 22(6):1439-56, 2002
4. Hong YK et al: Efficacy of MRI in complicated congenital heart disease with visceral heterotaxy syndrome. J Comput Assist Tomogr. 24(5):671-82, 2000
5. Marino B et al: Malposition of the heart. In: Moller JH, Hoffman JIE, ed. Pediatric cardiovascular medicine, 1st ed. Philadelphia, Churchill Livingstone. 621-41, 2000
6. Applegate KE et al: Situs revisited: imaging of the heterotaxy syndrome. Radiographics. 19(4):837-52; discussion 853-4, 1999
7. Gayer G et al: Polysplenia syndrome detected in adulthood: report of eight cases and review of the literature. Abdom Imaging. 24(2):178-84, 1999
8. Chen SJ et al: Usefulness of electron beam computed tomography in children with heterotaxy syndrome. Am J Cardiol. 81(2):188-94, 1998
9. Oleszczuk-Raschke K et al: Abdominal sonography in the evaluation of heterotaxy in children. Pediatr Radiol. 25 Suppl 1:S150-6, 1995
10. Winer-Muram HT: Adult presentation of heterotaxic syndromes and related complexes. J Thorac Imaging. 10(1):43-57, 1995
11. Bakir M et al: The value of radionuclide splenic scanning in the evaluation of asplenia in patients with heterotaxy. Pediatr Radiol. 24(1):25-8, 1994
12. Geva T et al: Role of spin echo and cine magnetic resonance imaging in presurgical planning of heterotaxy syndrome. Comparison with echocardiography and catheterization. Circulation. 90(1):348-56, 1994
13. Niwa K et al: Magnetic resonance imaging of heterotaxia in infants. J Am Coll Cardiol. 23(1):177-83, 1994
14. Wang JK et al: Usefulness of magnetic resonance imaging in the assessment of venoatrial connections, atrial morphology, bronchial situs, and other anomalies in right atrial isomerism. Am J Cardiol. 74(7):701-4, 1994
15. Winer-Muram HT et al: The spectrum of heterotaxic syndromes. Radiol Clin North Am. 27(6):1147-70, 1989

HETEROTAXIA SYNDROMES

IMAGE GALLERY

Typical

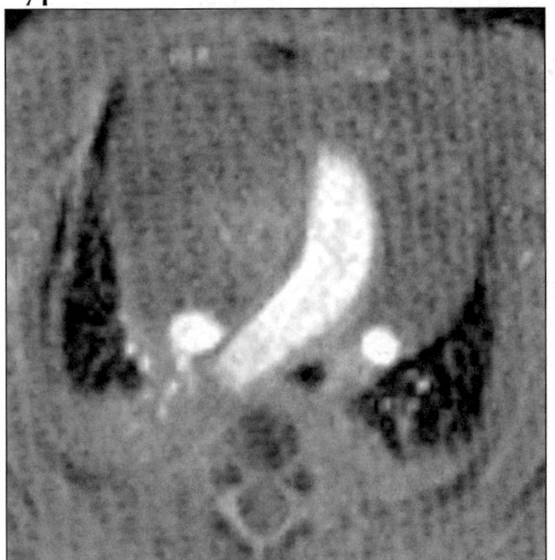

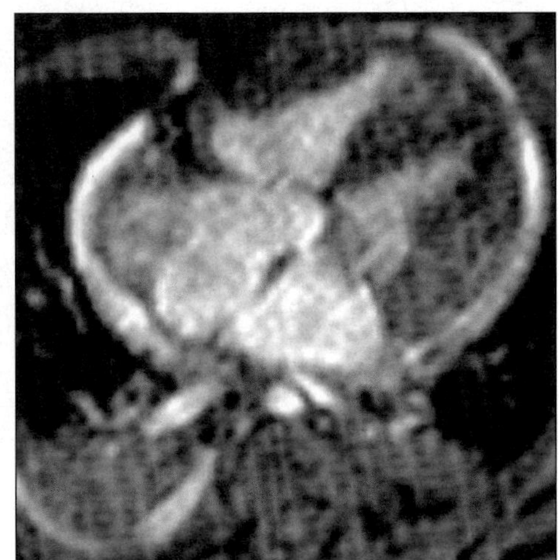

(Left) *Axial FGRE in a patient with right isomerism (asplenia) shows bilateral SVC. (Courtesy R. Krishnamurthy, MD).* ***(Right)*** *Axial FGRE in the same patient as previous image, shows balanced complete AV canal, with a rudimentary atrial septum. (Courtesy R. Krishnamurthy, MD).*

Typical

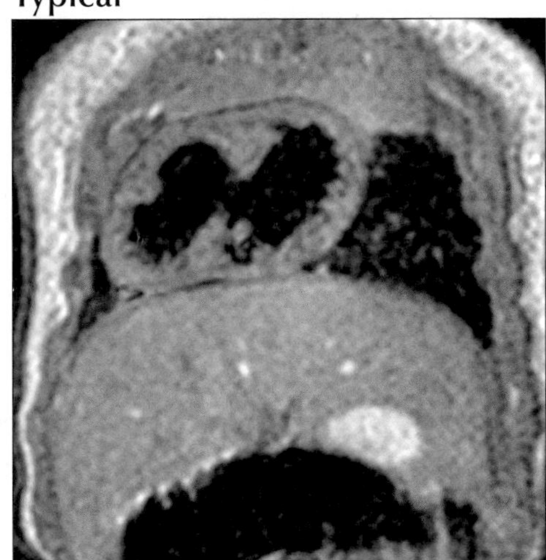

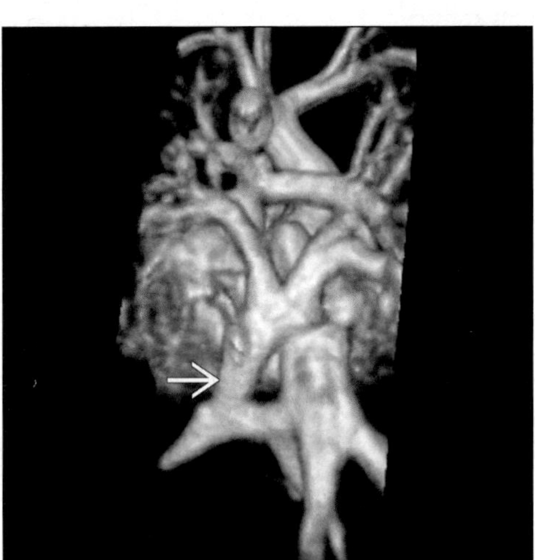

(Left) *Coronal FGRE in an infant with right isomerism (asplenia) shows dextrocardia, transverse liver, absence of spleen and midline stomach. (Courtesy R. Krishnamurthy, MD).* ***(Right)*** *Coronal FGRE MR angiogram, posterior view, shows infradiaphragmatic anomalous pulmonary venous return ➔ to left hepatic vein. (Courtesy R. Krishnamurthy, MD).*

Typical

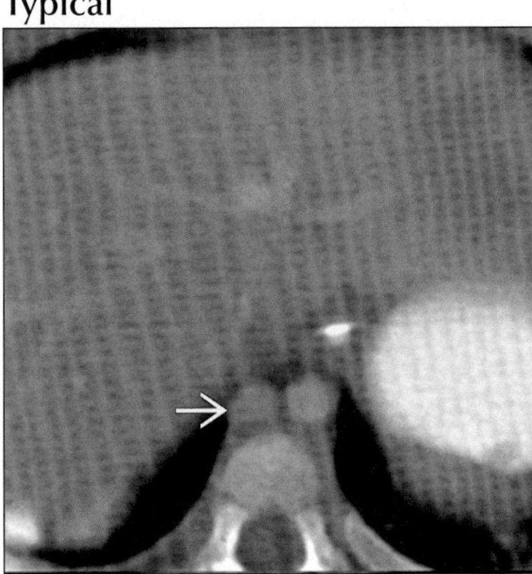

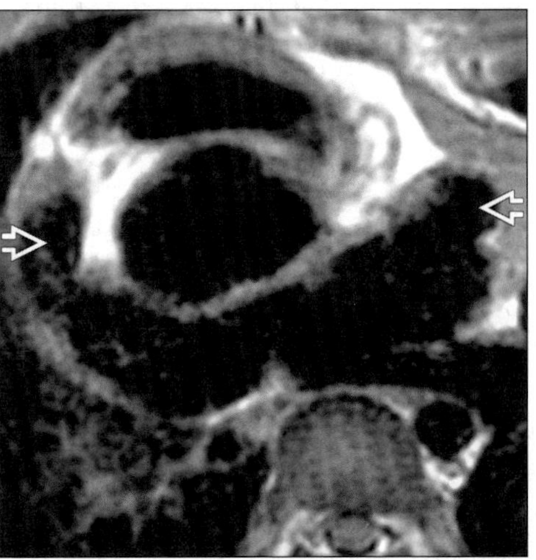

(Left) *Axial CECT shows azygous continuation ➔ of IVC in patient with left isomerism (polysplenia syndrome). (Courtesy R. Kishnamurthy, MD).* ***(Right)*** *Axial T1WI MR shows common atrium with left isomerism: Bilateral tubular finger-shaped atrial appendages ➲. (Courtesy R. Kishnamurthy, MD).*

SEPTAL DEFECTS

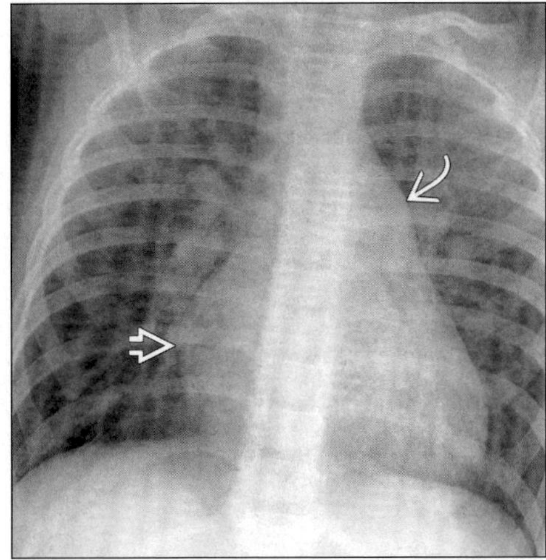

Anteroposterior radiograph in patient with ASD shows cardiomegaly, enlarged main pulmonary artery ➔ and increased pulmonary vascularity (overcirculation pattern). There is mild right atrial enlargement ➔.

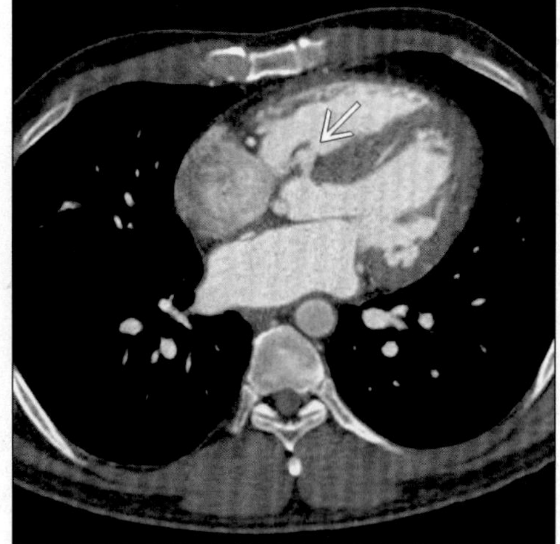

Axial cardiac CT shows small membranous septal VSD ➔, located just below aortic root.

TERMINOLOGY

Abbreviations and Synonyms

- Atrial septal defect (ASD)
- Ventricular septal defect (VSD)
- Atrioventricular septal defect (AVSD)

Definitions

- Cardiac anomalies characterized by defects in the septa dividing the right- from the left-sided chambers

IMAGING FINDINGS

General Features

- Best diagnostic clue
  - Category: Acyanotic, cardiomegaly, increased pulmonary vascularity
    - Shunt location → specific chamber enlargement
    - All intracardiac shunt lesions have small aorta
  - Hemodynamics: Volume overload leading to enlargement of receiving cardiac segment (and all segments distally to that)
    - ASD: Right atrium enlarged, **not** left atrium
    - VSD: Right ventricle and left atrium
    - AVSD: Right atrium and ventricle, **not** left atrium
- Location
  - ASD
    - Septum primum defect: Anterior/inferior septum
    - Septum secundum defect: Oval defect bordered by the fossa ovalis
    - Patent foramen ovale (PFO)
    - Sinus venosus defect: Superior, posterior to fossa ovalis, near superior vena cava
  - VSD
    - Inlet septal defect (associated with AVSD): 8-10%
    - Muscular or trabecular septal defect: 5-10%
    - Outlet or supracristal septal defect: 5%
    - Perimembranous septal defect: 75%
  - AVSD involves atrial and ventricular parts of septum
- Size: Variable, and may involve adjacent structures
- Morphology
  - PFO
    - Limbus is a thick muscular ridge which borders the foramen ovale
    - After birth, left atrial (LA) pressure rises and a thin flap on the LA side is forced against the limbus, achieving closure

DDx: Congenital Heart Disease with Left-to-Right Shunts

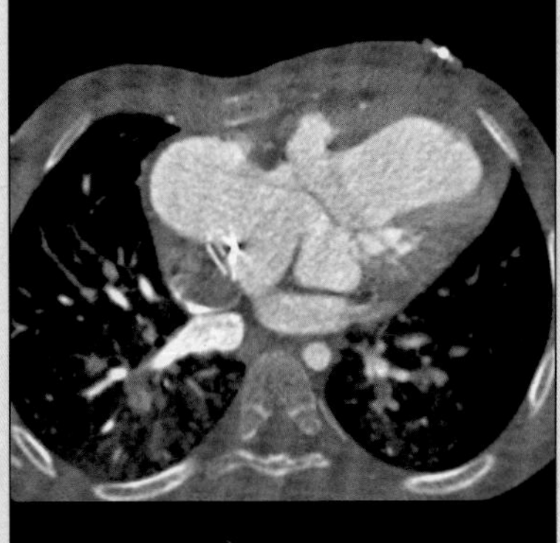

Unbalanced AVSD

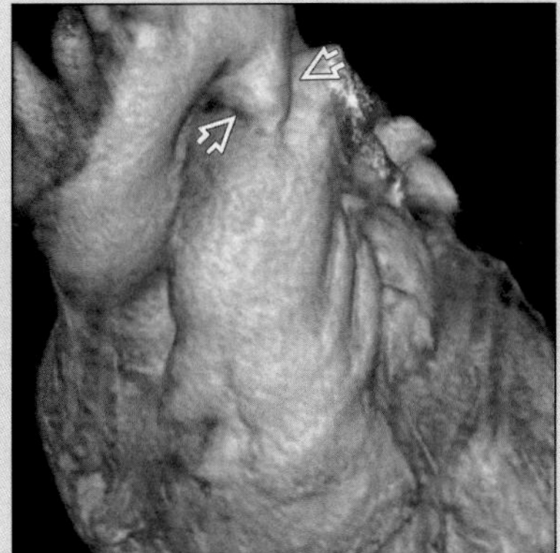

Patent Ductus

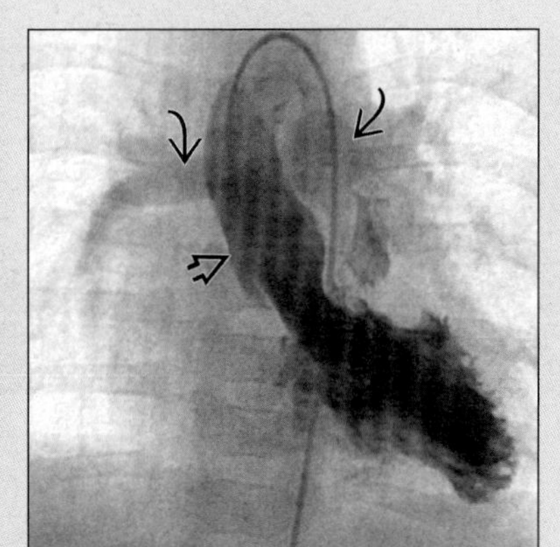

Double Outlet Ventricle

SEPTAL DEFECTS

Key Facts

Terminology
- Cardiac anomalies characterized by defects in the septa dividing the right- from the left-sided chambers

Imaging Findings
- Category: Acyanotic, cardiomegaly, increased pulmonary vascularity
- Hemodynamics: Volume overload leading to enlargement of receiving cardiac segment (and all segments distally to that)
- Classic plain film appearance: Cardiomegaly, convex pulmonary artery segment, active pulmonary vascular congestion = shunt vascularity
- Gradient echo or velocity encoded cine-MR: For functional cardiac assessment, flow jets, regurgitation
- Characterizes type, location and number of septal defect(s), hemodynamics

Pathology
- Volume overload to pulmonary circulation
- ASD: Low pressure shunt
- VSD, AVSD: Size of shunt determined by size of defect and pressure differential between ventricles
- Long term increase in pulmonary flow is associated with vessel injury
- Most common congenital cardiac lesions

Clinical Issues
- Moderate to large, high pressure shunts: Congestive heart failure (tachypnea, dyspnea, tachycardia, diaphoresis, failure to thrive, hepatomegaly)
- Untreated large shunt: Development of irreversible pulmonary hypertension (Eisenmenger)
- Untreated with pulmonary hypertension: Shunt reversal, paradoxical embolus, stroke and abscess

- Ostium primum ASD
  - Simplest form of AVSD, may exist in isolation, or with a cleft the in anterior leaflet of mitral valve
- Secundum ASD
  - Bordered by the edge of the fossa ovalis and the exposed circumference of the ostium secundum
- Sinus venosus ASD
  - Almost always associated with connection of the right upper pulmonary vein into SVC
- VSD
  - Variable morphology, dependent on location
  - Multiple defects occur, especially in trabecular septum ("maladie de Roger": Swiss cheese disease)
- Unroofed coronary sinus (CS)
  - Defect between roof of CS and inferior wall of LA

Radiographic Findings
- Radiography
  - Frequently normal in small shunts
  - Classic plain film appearance: Cardiomegaly, convex pulmonary artery segment, active pulmonary vascular congestion = shunt vascularity
  - When congestive heart failure: Venous (passive) congestion and interstitial fluid
  - Hyperinflation due to abnormal lung compliance and bronchial compression by dilated vessels
  - Sinus venosus ASD: Abnormal horizontal position of right upper pulmonary vein

CT Findings
- CTA: Performed to evaluate tracheo-bronchial compression by dilated pulmonary arteries

MR Findings
- ECG-gated T1WI: Defects best seen on long axis views
- Gradient echo or velocity encoded cine-MR: For functional cardiac assessment, flow jets, regurgitation
  - Can evaluate shunt severity by quantifying ratio of pulmonary to systemic flow
  - Used to evaluate for feasibility and sizing of endovascular occluder device placement
- Gadolinium MRA: Three-dimensional evaluation of vasculature
  - Time-resolved contrast-enhanced MR imaging (TRICKS): Real-time tracking of contrast bolus

Echocardiographic Findings
- Echocardiogram
  - Characterizes type, location and number of septal defect(s), hemodynamics
  - Transesophageal echo used in older patients and for placement of closure devices

Angiographic Findings
- Cardiac catheterization and angiography findings
  - Seldom required for primary diagnosis
  - For hemodynamic assessment of associated more complex heart lesions
    - Left anterior oblique view to show VSDs
    - Aortogram: Aortic regurgitation in outlet VSDs
  - For ASD closure with Amplatz device

Imaging Recommendations
- Primary diagnosis with echocardiography in children
- Catheterization is needed when pulmonary hypertension is suspected, and for interventions

DIFFERENTIAL DIAGNOSIS

Normal Chest
- Main pulmonary artery can be prominent normally between ages 8-12 years

Pulmonary Hypertension
- Primary, or secondary to congenital heart disease with shunting and/or chronic lung disease

Patent Ductus Arteriosus
- Large aorta

Double Outlet Right Ventricle (DORV)
- Pulmonary overcirculation due to lower pressures

Scimitar Syndrome
- Right pulmonary vein → right atrium: ASD physiology

SEPTAL DEFECTS

High-Output Conditions: Global Cardiomegaly, Wide Vascular Pedicle

- Extracardiac arteriovenous malformation/fistula
- Anemias

Myocardial Dysfunction: Global Cardiomegaly, Narrow Vascular Pedicle

- Cardiomyopathies
- Arrhythmias

PATHOLOGY

General Features

- General path comments
  - Embryology
    - Complex, dependent on location of defect and associated anomalies
    - Foramen ovale is the normal in-utero interatrial communication allowing flow from IVC to LA
  - Pathophysiology
    - Volume overload to pulmonary circulation
    - ASD: Low pressure shunt
    - VSD, AVSD: Size of shunt determined by size of defect and ventricular pressure differential
    - Increased flow increases work of right ventricle and increases venous return to left heart
    - Long term increase in pulmonary flow is associated with vessel injury
    - Pulmonary hypertension through complex interaction between endothelium and smooth muscle reaction (Eisenmenger physiology)
- Genetics
  - No specific genetic defect in majority
  - Holt Oram syndrome (ASD with upper extremity anomalies): Familial occurrence
  - Primum, AVSD associated with trisomy 21 in 65%
- Epidemiology
  - Most common congenital cardiac lesions
    - VSD: 20% of all congenital heart lesions
    - ASD: 10% of congenital heart lesions in children, yet 30% of congenital heart lesions in adults
  - Most common lesion associated with other lesions
  - True incidence of septal defects > reported (many close spontaneously)
- Associated abnormalities
  - VSD as intrinsic part of congenital heart lesion: Tetralogy of Fallot, truncus arteriosus, DORV
  - VSD and ASD are frequently associated with other lesions: Coarctation, tricuspid atresia
  - PFO is essential component of certain anomalies
    - R → L shunt: Ebstein anomaly, tricuspid atresia, hypoplastic right ventricle, TAPVR type III
    - L → R shunt: Hypoplastic left heart, mitral atresia

CLINICAL ISSUES

Presentation

- Most common signs/symptoms
  - Small, low pressure shunts: Asymptomatic murmurs
  - Moderate to large, high pressure shunts: Congestive heart failure (tachypnea, dyspnea, tachycardia, diaphoresis, failure to thrive, hepatomegaly)
  - Other symptoms depend on associated cardiac lesion
- Other signs/symptoms: Neurological symptoms from paradoxical emboli, atrial dysrhythmias

Demographics

- Age: AVSD < VSD < ASD
- Gender
  - Secundum ASD: M:F = 2:1
  - VSD: M:F = 1:1

Natural History & Prognosis

- Small muscular VSDs and PFOs close spontaneously
- Untreated large shunt: Development of irreversible pulmonary hypertension (Eisenmenger)
  - May be reversible initially: Need for early closure
- Reversal of shunt (R → L): Late onset cyanosis
- Associated cardiac anomalies determine final outcome
- Untreated with pulmonary hypertension: Shunt reversal, paradoxical embolus, stroke and abscess
- Lifetime risk of bacterial endocarditis

Treatment

- Temporizing procedure: Pulmonary artery banding
- ASD
  - Percutaneous catheter closure is treatment of choice
    - Not possible for ostium primum defects due to proximity of the atrioventricular valve
  - Large defects: Dacron patch or direct suture closure
  - Sinus venosus defect: More complex repair (right superior pulmonary vein directed to left atrium)
- VSD
  - Medical therapy (diuretics and afterload reduction)
  - Surgical closure: Technique depends on site of VSD
    - Perimembranous VSD: Through right atrium
    - Outlet (supracristal) VSD: Early closure to prevent sinus prolapse, damage to aortic valve leaflet
    - Muscular VSD: Repair via ventriculotomy, placement of closure device (experimental)

SELECTED REFERENCES

1. Beerbaum P et al: Atrial septal defects in pediatric patients: noninvasive sizing with cardiovascular MR imaging. Radiology. 228(2):361-9, 2003
2. Lapierre C et al: Evaluation of a large atrial septal occluder with cardiac MR imaging. Radiographics. 23 Spec No:S51-8, 2003
3. Wang ZJ et al: Cardiovascular shunts: MR imaging evaluation. Radiographics. 23 Spec No:S181-94, 2003
4. Varaprasathan GA et al: Quantification of flow dynamics in congenital heart disease: applications of velocity-encoded cine MR imaging. Radiographics. 22(4):895-905; discussion 905-6, 2002
5. Parsons JM et al: Morphological evaluation of atrioventricular septal defects by magnetic resonance imaging. Br Heart J. 64(2):138-45, 1990
6. Baker EJ et al: Magnetic resonance imaging at a high field strength of ventricular septal defects in infants. Br Heart J. 62(4):305-10, 1989

IMAGE GALLERY

Variant

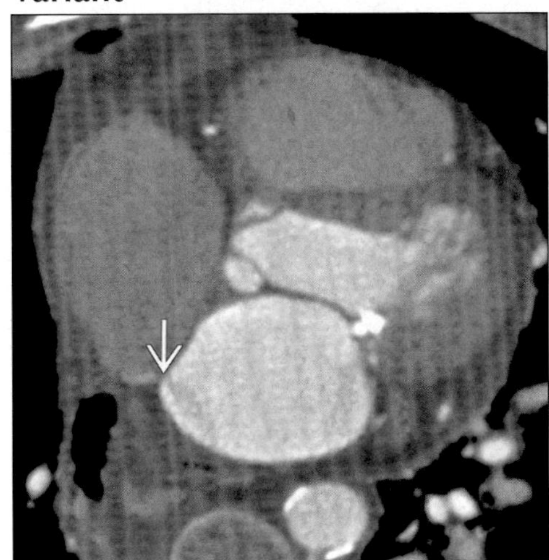

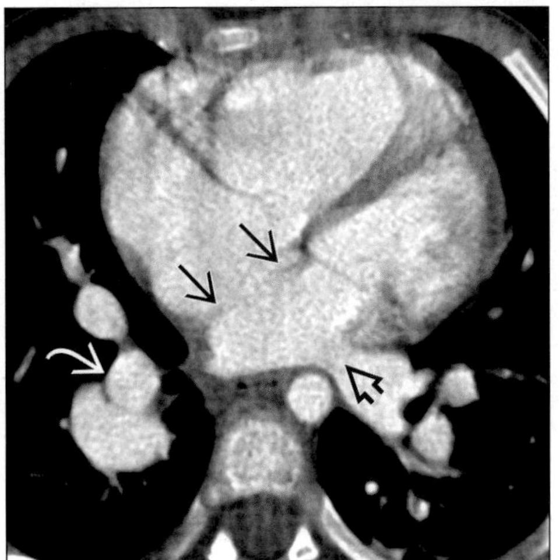

(Left) *Axial cardiac CT shows tiny ASD located in posterior wall of atrial septum ➡, allowing for bidirectional shunting. Note "positive" contrast flow jet in right atrium, and "negative" jet in left atrium.* ***(Right)*** *Axial CECT shows moderate-sized ASD ➡. The left lower lobe pulmonary vein drains normally into the left atrium ➡, whereas the congested right pulmonary veins ➡ were noted to drain anomalously into the azygos vein. Note right-sided chamber enlargement.*

Typical

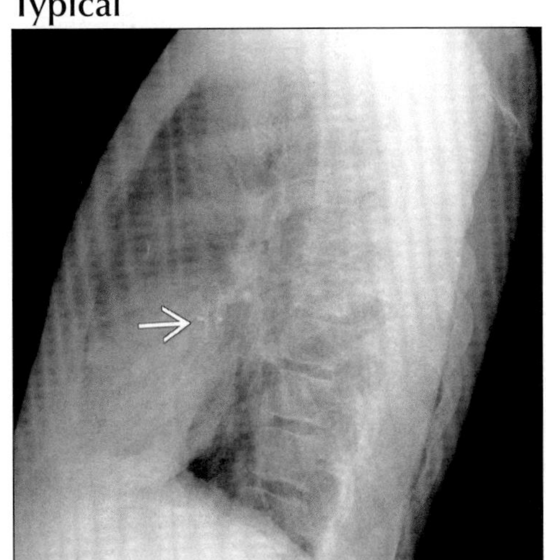

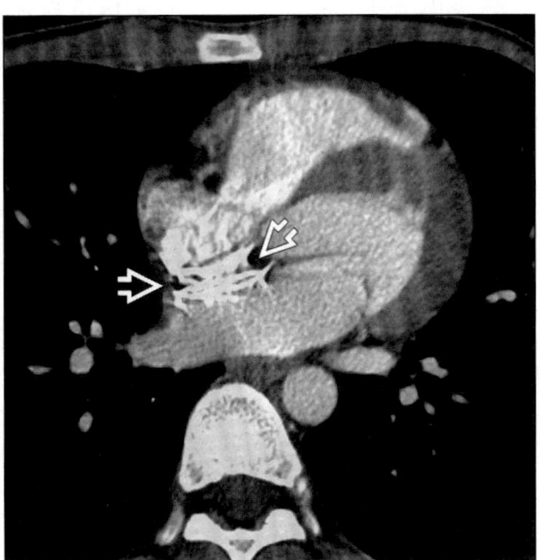

(Left) *Lateral radiograph shows typical appearance of an Amplatzer closure device ➡, that was placed to close an ASD. This device is usually better seen on a lateral than on a frontal view, where it projects over the spine.* ***(Right)*** *Axial CECT shows streak artifact from the closure device ➡ in the atrial septum.*

Typical

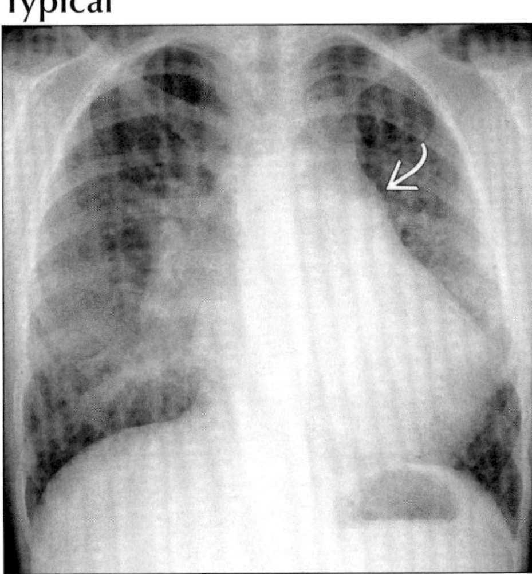

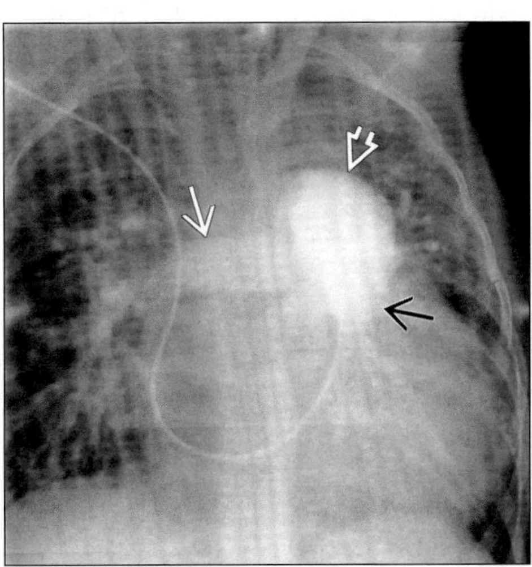

(Left) *Posteroanterior radiograph in cyanotic child with untreated VSD and irreversible pulmonary hypertension (Eisenmenger physiology) shows right ventricular prominence and a convex pulmonary artery segment ➡.* ***(Right)*** *Anteroposterior angiography in the same child as previous image, shows marked central dilatation of main ➡, right ➡ & left ➡ pulmonary arteries. Note "pruned" appearance of the peripheral pulmonary arteries.*

PATENT DUCTUS ARTERIOSUS

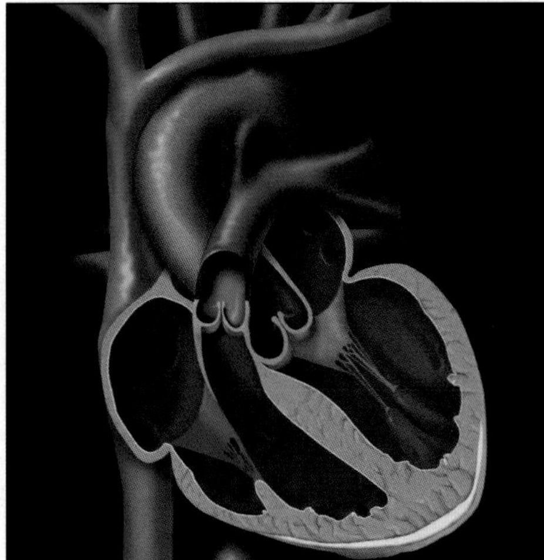

Graphic shows dilated left ventricle and enlargement of the ascending aorta compared to the pulmonary artery, indicative of volume overload of the left heart from aortic to pulmonary (left to right) shunt through PDA.

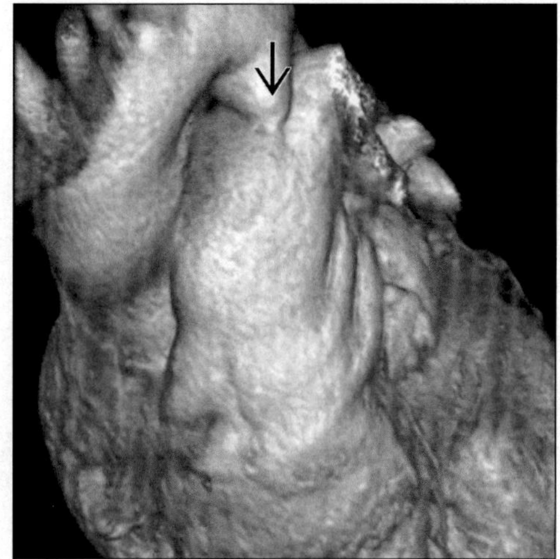

Oblique cardiac CT shows typical small PDA ⇒: Triangular in shape, larger on aortic side. Enlarged main pulmonary artery from volume overload.

TERMINOLOGY

Abbreviations and Synonyms

- Patent ductus arteriosus (PDA), persistent arterial duct, patent ductus Botalli

Definitions

- Persistent postnatal patency of the normal prenatal connection from the pulmonary artery to the proximal descending aorta
- Category: Acyanotic, increased pulmonary blood flow
- Hemodynamics: L → R shunt between aorta and pulmonary artery
- PDA is frequently an essential part of complex congenital heart disease
  - Hypoplastic left heart syndrome, preductal coarctation, interrupted aortic arch: Conduit for systemic perfusion (R → L flow)
  - D-Transposition: Necessary for admixture between systemic and pulmonary circuits (L → R flow)
  - Pulmonary atresia and other severe cyanotic heart disease with right-sided obstruction: Conduit for pulmonary perfusion (L → R flow)
- PDA is part of persistent fetal circulation syndrome: R → L flow
  - Severe lung disease (meconium aspiration, surfactant deficiency disease, neonatal pneumonia)
  - Primary pulmonary hypertension of neonate

IMAGING FINDINGS

General Features

- Best diagnostic clue: Ductus bump connecting to pulmonary artery

Radiographic Findings

- Radiography
  - Cardiomegaly (left atrium and left ventricle)
  - Increased pulmonary vascularity
  - Wide vascular pedicle (large aortic arch with "ductus bump")

CT Findings

- CTA
  - Excellent for sizing of ductus prior to cardiac catheterization for placement of occluder device
  - Volume renditions of aortic arch depict PDA

DDx: Ductus Arteriosus Associated with Other Heart Lesions

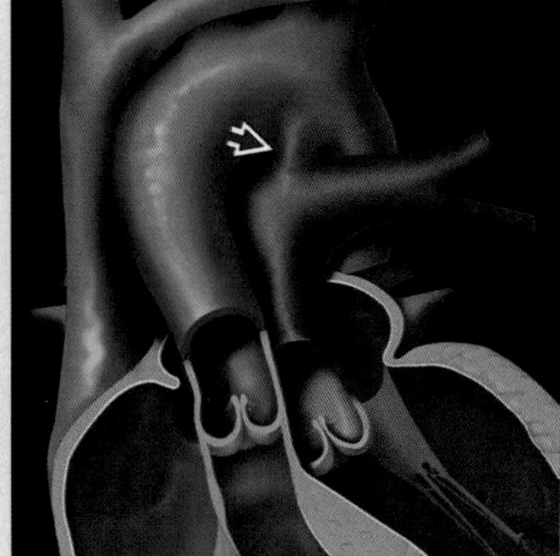

D-Transposition

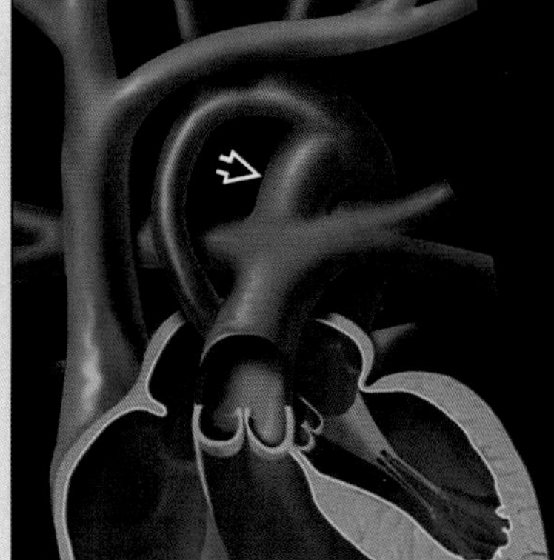

Hypoplastic Left Heart

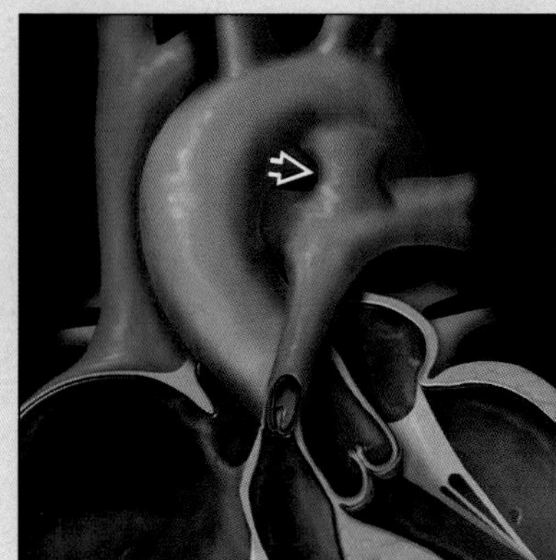

Pulmonary Atresia

PATENT DUCTUS ARTERIOSUS

Key Facts

Terminology

- Persistent postnatal patency of the normal prenatal connection from the pulmonary artery to the proximal descending aorta
- Category: Acyanotic, increased pulmonary blood flow
- Hemodynamics: L → R shunt between aorta and pulmonary artery
- PDA is frequently an essential part of complex congenital heart disease
- PDA is part of persistent fetal circulation syndrome: R → L flow

Pathology

- With pulmonary hypertension pressure overload of right ventricle, reversal of shunt (R → L), leading to cyanosis (Eisenmenger physiology)
- When closed: Forms ligamentum arteriosum, which may calcify (incidental calcification in aortopulmonary window on chest radiograph or CT)

Clinical Issues

- Irreversible pulmonary hypertension (Eisenmenger physiology) resulting in shunt reversal, development of cyanosis
- To close ductus in premature infants: Indomethacin
- To keep ductus open (cyanotic heart disease): Prostaglandin E1
- Term infants, older children: Surgical clipping or ligation
- Endovascular closure with duct occluder devices and/or coils

MR Findings

- Cardiac-gated T1 weighted (black blood) imaging
  - Sagittal oblique plane through aortic arch depicts ductus
- Gradient echo steady-state free precession cine MR for right ventricular function in cases with Eisenmenger pulmonary hypertension
- 3D gadolinium MRA with multiplanar reformations and volume rendered reconstructions

Echocardiographic Findings

- Echocardiogram: Suprasternal notch view: Direct visualization of ductus
- M-mode: Increased left-atrium-to-aorta ratio (> 1.2:1)
- Pulsed Doppler
  - Diastolic flow reversal in descending and abdominal aorta (ductus steal)
  - Flow acceleration across a constricting ductus: Transductal velocity ratio (TVR)
- Color Doppler: For flow direction through ductus

Angiographic Findings

- Conventional
  - Cardiac catheterization only needed for associated complex cyanotic heart disease, and to determine reversibility of pulmonary hypertension
  - Placement of PDA closure device

Imaging Recommendations

- Protocol advice: Treatment decisions based on echocardiographic findings only in majority of cases

DIFFERENTIAL DIAGNOSIS

Other Causes of L → R Shunting

- Septal defects, atrioventricular canal

Persistent Fetal Circulation Syndrome

- Pulmonary hypertension (primary or secondary to severe lung disease)
- Patent foramen ovale, PDA secondary to profound irreversible hypoxia

PATHOLOGY

General Features

- General path comments
  - In normal neonate ductus arteriosus closes functionally 18-24 hours after birth, anatomically at 1 month of age
  - PDA is postnatal persistence of normal prenatal structure
  - Embryology
    - Ductus originates from primitive sixth aortic arch
  - Pathophysiology (for simple PDA)
    - L → R shunt to pulmonary artery
    - Volume overload of left-sided cardiac cambers
    - With pulmonary hypertension pressure overload of right ventricle, reversal of shunt (R → L), leading to cyanosis (Eisenmenger physiology)
    - Diastolic flow reversal in aorta can lead to renal and intestinal hypoperfusion: Renal dysfunction, necrotizing enterocolitis
- Genetics: No specific genetic defect identified in most cases of isolated PDA
- Etiology
  - Prematurity: Persistent postnatal hypoxia → failure of contraction of ductus
  - Term infant: Associated with maternal rubella
- Epidemiology
  - 10-12% of congenital heart disease
  - 1 per 2,500-5,000 live births
  - Slightly more common in females
  - Associated with prematurity (21-35%)

Gross Pathologic & Surgical Features

- Patent arterial duct, most often wider on aortic side
  - Length: 2-8 mm; diameter 4-12 mm
  - Makes an acute angle with aorta in simple PDA; blunt angle with associated congenital heart disease
- Contractile tissue mainly on pulmonary side, spirally arranged muscle bundles in media
  - Prostaglandin E1 present in fetal life maintains relaxation
  - Increased oxygen pressure causes constriction

PATENT DUCTUS ARTERIOSUS

- Thickening of intima with mucoid degeneration
- When closed: Forms ligamentum arteriosum, which may calcify (incidental calcification in aortopulmonary window on chest radiograph or CT)
- Can be right-sided

CLINICAL ISSUES

Presentation

- Most common signs/symptoms
  - Characteristic machinery-like murmur
  - Bounding peripheral pulses
  - Congestive heart failure
  - Special situation: Premature infant recovering from surfactant deficiency disease
    - Decrease in hypoxia
    - Drop in pulmonary vascular resistance
    - Shunt flow through ductus arteriosus increases
    - Clinical and radiographic signs of congestive heart failure (cardiomegaly, pulmonary edema)
- Other signs/symptoms
  - Subacute bacterial endocarditis
    - Need for treatment of clinically "silent" PDA (incidentally detected with echo) is controversial
  - Ductal aneurysm
    - Can result from premature narrowing of ductus on pulmonary side

Natural History & Prognosis

- Irreversible pulmonary hypertension (Eisenmenger physiology) resulting in shunt reversal, development of cyanosis
- Isolated PDA: Excellent prognosis with early closure
- When associated with complex heart disease: Prognosis determined by underlying disorder
- Persistent fetal circulation, pulmonary hypertension: Treatment with extracorporeal membrane oxygenation (ECMO) is often necessary to disrupt vicious circle
  - Hypoxia → pulmonary vasoconstriction → decreased pulmonary flow → more severe hypoxia

Treatment

- To close ductus in premature infants: Indomethacin
  - Side effects: Renal failure, intestinal perforation, intracranial hemorrhage
- To keep ductus open (cyanotic heart disease): Prostaglandin E1
- Term infants, older children: Surgical clipping or ligation
  - Can be performed at bedside under video-assisted thoracoscopic and/or robotic guidance
  - Complications: Inadvertent ligation of aortic isthmus, pulmonary artery, recurrent laryngeal nerve injury
- Endovascular closure with duct occluder devices and/or coils
  - Small ductus (< 4 mm): Gianturco coils
  - Large ductus (> 4 mm): Ivalon plug, Rashkind and Amplatz duct occluders
  - Complications: Protrusion of occluder device into left pulmonary artery orifice (→ decreased left lung perfusion), peripheral embolization
  - Incomplete closure in 10-20%

SELECTED REFERENCES

1. Goitein O et al: Incidental finding on MDCT of patent ductus arteriosus: use of CT and MRI to assess clinical importance. AJR Am J Roentgenol. 184(6):1924-31, 2005
2. Cannon JW et al: Application of robotics in congenital cardiac surgery. Semin Thorac Cardiovasc Surg Pediatr Card Surg Annu. 6:72-83, 2003
3. Hillman ND et al: Patent ductus arteriosus. In: Mavroudis C, Backer CL, ed. Pediatric cardiac surgery. 3rd ed. Philadelphia, Mosby. 223-33, 2003
4. Morgan-Hughes GJ et al: Morphologic assessment of patent ductus arteriosus in adults using retrospectively ECG-gated multidetector CT. AJR Am J Roentgenol. 181(3):749-54, 2003
5. Wang ZJ et al: Cardiovascular shunts: MR imaging evaluation. Radiographics. 23 Spec No:S181-94, 2003
6. Anil SR et al: Coil occlusion of the small patent arterial duct without arterial access. Cardiol Young. 12(1):51-6, 2002
7. Jan SL et al: Isolated neonatal ductus arteriosus aneurysm. J Am Coll Cardiol. 39(2):342-7, 2002
8. Day JR et al: A spontaneous ductal aneurysm presenting with left recurrent laryngeal nerve palsy. Ann Thorac Surg. 72(2):608-9, 2001
9. Thanopoulos BD et al: Patent ductus arteriosus equipment and technique. Amplatzer duct occluder: intermediate-term follow-up and technical considerations. J Interv Cardiol. 14(2):247-54, 2001
10. Davies MW et al: A preliminary study of the application of the transductal velocity ratio for assessing persistent ductus arteriosus. Arch Dis Child Fetal Neonatal Ed. 82(3):F195-9, 2000
11. Gersony WN, Apfel HD: Patent ductus arteriosus and other aortopulmonary anomalies. In: Moller JH, Hoffman JIE, ed. Pediatric cardiovascular medicine, 1st ed. Philadelphia, Churchill Livingstone. 323-34, 2000
12. Alva C et al: Aneurysm of the pulmonary trunk with patent arterial duct. Cardiol Young. 9(1):70-2, 1999
13. Sandstede J et al: [Magnetic resonance imaging in persistent ductus arteriosus of Botalli] Rofo. 171(5):405-6, 1999
14. Schmidt M et al: Magnetic resonance imaging of ductus arteriosus Botalli apertus in adulthood. Int J Cardiol. 68(2):225-9, 1999
15. Acherman RJ et al: Aneurysm of the ductus arteriosus: a congenital lesion. Am J Perinatol. 15(12):653-9, 1998
16. Arora R et al: Transcatheter coil occlusion of persistent ductus arteriosus using detachable steel coils: short-term results. Indian Heart J. 49(1):60-4, 1997
17. Evangelista JK et al: Effect of multiple coil closure of patent ductus arteriosus on blood flow to the left lung as determined by lung perfusion scans. Am J Cardiol. 80(2):242-4, 1997
18. Dessy H et al: Echocardiographic and radionuclide pulmonary blood flow patterns after transcatheter closure of patent ductus arteriosus. Circulation. 94(2):126-9, 1996
19. Sharma S et al: Computed tomography and magnetic resonance findings in long-standing patent ductus. Case reports. Angiology. 47(4):393-8, 1996
20. Strouse PJ et al: Magnetic deflection forces from atrial septal defect and patent ductus arteriosus-occluding devices, stents, and coils used in pediatric-aged patients. Am J Cardiol. 78(4):490-1, 1996
21. Chien CT et al: Potential diagnosis of hemodynamic abnormalities in patent ductus arteriosus by cine magnetic resonance imaging. Am Heart J. 122:1065-73, 1991

PATENT DUCTUS ARTERIOSUS

IMAGE GALLERY

Typical

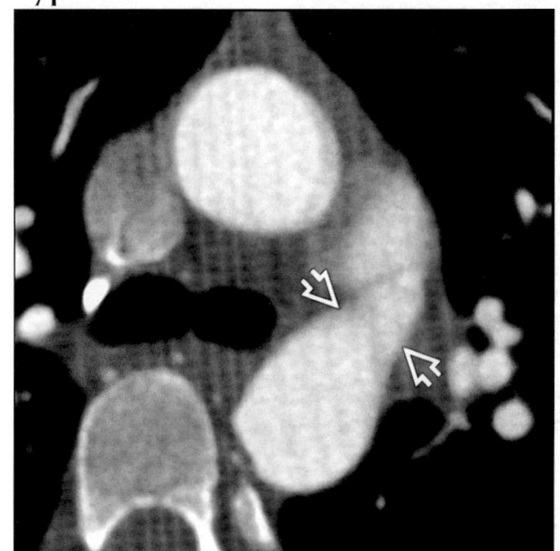

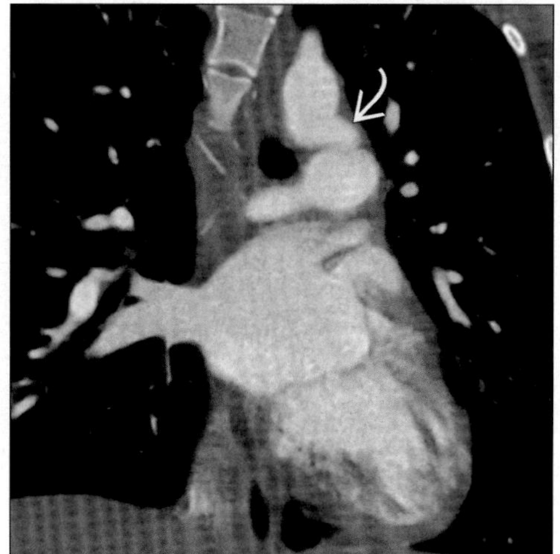

*(**Left**) Axial cardiac CT shows PDA ⯈, which has a broad connection to the proximal descending aorta. (**Right**) Coronal cardiac CT shows typical small PDA ⯈, connecting aorta to main pulmonary artery. Study was done for calibration of endovascular closure device.*

Typical

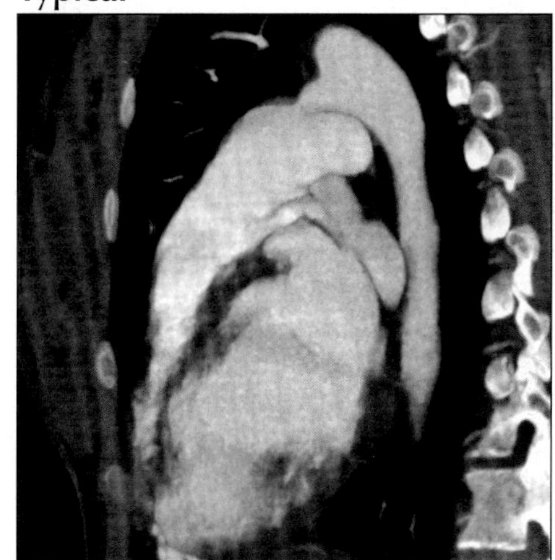

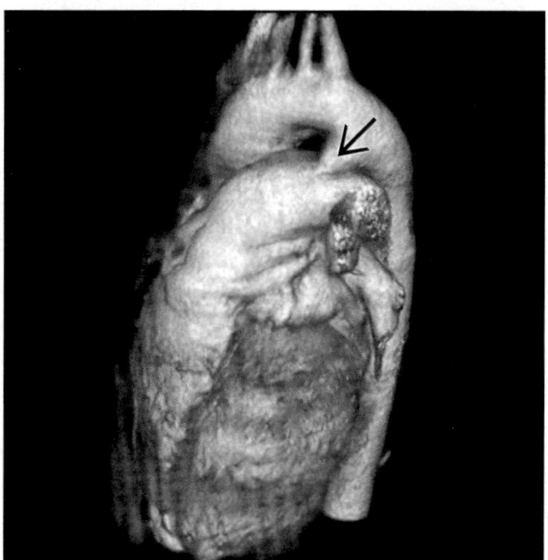

*(**Left**) Sagittal cardiac CT shows a broad connection of ductus with proximal descending thoracic aorta with a relative narrow connection with pulmonary artery. These images facilitated endovascular treatment. (**Right**) Oblique cardiac CT surface rendition provides global overview of ductus anatomy →.*

Typical

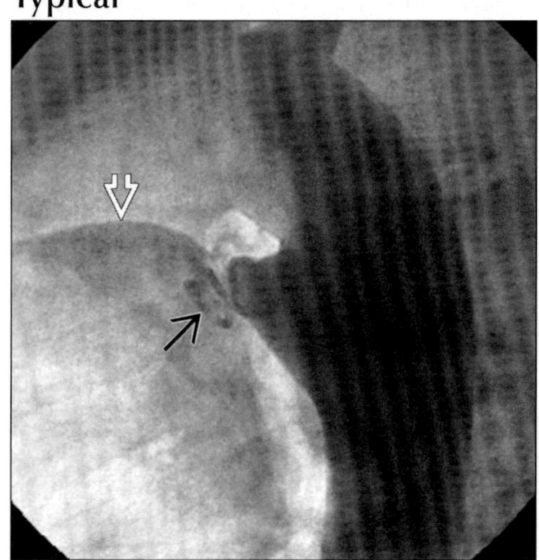

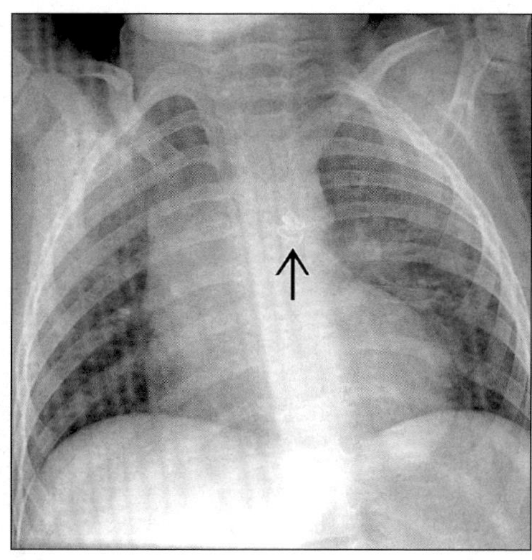

*(**Left**) Lateral catheter angiography shows endovascular coil → within the PDA with some contrast filling the main pulmonary artery ⯈. (**Right**) Anteroposterior radiograph shows normal pulmonary vascularity after closure of ductus with a coil →.*

EBSTEIN ANOMALY

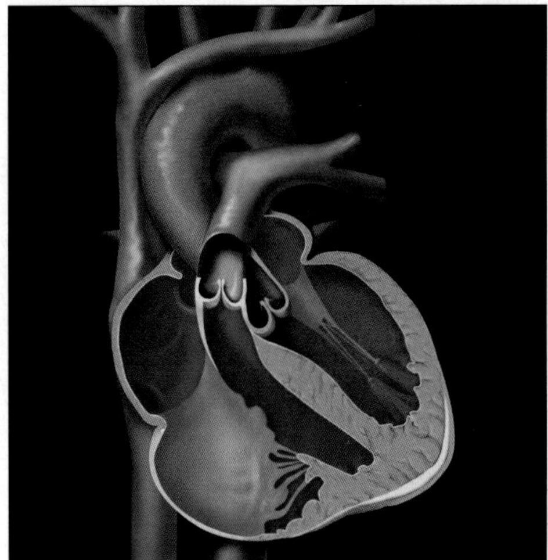
Graphic depicts downward displacement of the posterior tricuspid valve leaflet, which has become incorporated into the RV wall, leading to "atrialization" of the inflow portion of the RV.

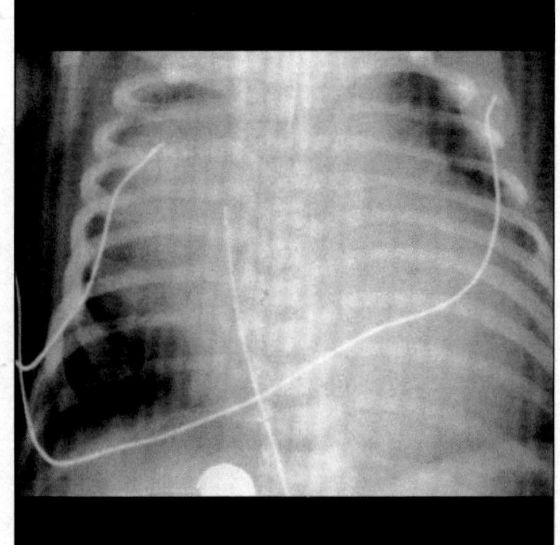
Anteroposterior radiograph shows global cardiomegaly in cyanotic infant. Echocardiography demonstrated right-sided chamber dilatation and left to right shunting through patent foramen ovale.

TERMINOLOGY

Definitions

- Downward displacement of the septal and posterior leaflets of the tricuspid valve
- Classic plain film appearance: Massive right-sided cardiomegaly ("box-shaped" heart)
- Category: Cyanotic, (severe) cardiomegaly, normal or decreased pulmonary vascularity
- Hemodynamics: Severe tricuspid valve regurgitation
  - Volume overload to right heart
  - Right-to-left shunting through patent foramen ovale (PFO) → cyanosis

IMAGING FINDINGS

General Features

- Best diagnostic clue: Downward displacement of septal tricuspid leaflet (≥ 8 mm/m² body surface area)
- Location: Tricuspid valve

Radiographic Findings

- Radiography
  - Severe right-sided cardiomegaly
    - Heart size can be near normal in newborn period but also can be massively enlarged at birth
    - Heart increases gradually in size over time, reaching massive proportions in untreated cases during adulthood
    - Cardiothoracic ratio used as follow up parameter
  - Small vascular pedicle
  - May mimic large pericardial effusion

CT Findings

- Electron beam cine CT has been used for functional analysis of ventricular contraction

MR Findings

- T1WI: Right chamber best seen on long axis imaging
- T2* GRE
  - Cardiac-gated steady-state free precession cine-MR
    - Ventricular volumes, ejection fraction of each ventricle, tricuspid regurgitation fraction
    - Left ventricular function affected by right ventricular (RV) dilatation, bowing of septum, mitral valve prolapse

DDx: Right-Sided Obstructive Cyanotic Heart Lesions

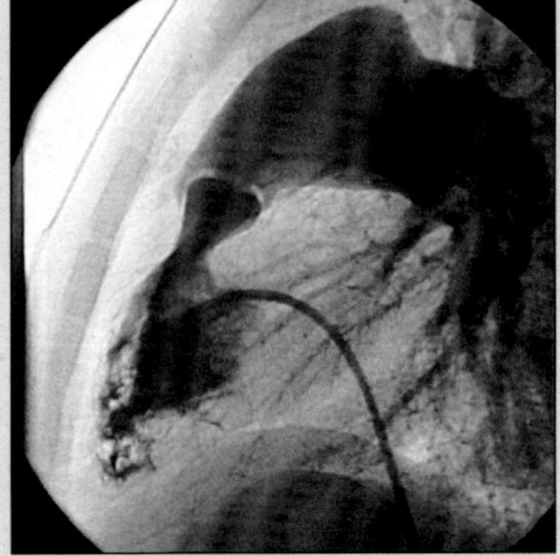
Critical Pulmonary Stenosis

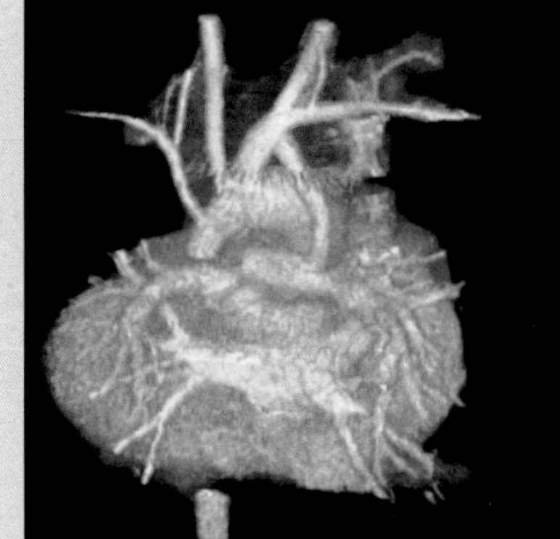
Tetralogy of Fallot

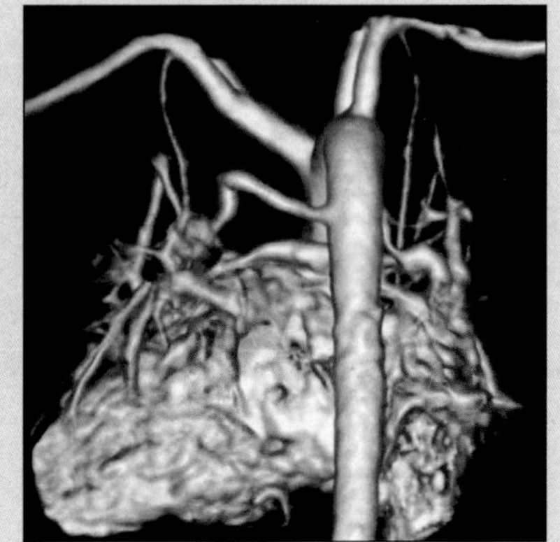
Pulmonary Atresia

EBSTEIN ANOMALY

Key Facts

Terminology

- Downward displacement of the septal and posterior leaflets of the tricuspid valve
- Classic plain film appearance: Massive right-sided cardiomegaly ("box-shaped" heart)
- Category: Cyanotic, (severe) cardiomegaly, normal or decreased pulmonary vascularity
- Hemodynamics: Determined by severe tricuspid valve regurgitation
- Volume overload to right heart
- Right-to-left shunting through patent foramen ovale (PFO) → cyanosis

Imaging Findings

- Best diagnostic clue: Downward displacement of septal tricuspid leaflet (≥ 8 mm/m^2 body surface area)
- Severe right-sided cardiomegaly
- Cardiac-gated steady-state free precession cine-MR
- Ventricular volumes, ejection fraction of each ventricle, tricuspid regurgitation fraction

Clinical Issues

- Wide spectrum of findings and ages at first presentation; some patients are asymptomatic
- Chronic right heart failure
- Presence of cyanosis depends on balance between right and left atrial pressure
- Prognosis is highly variable, dependent on hemodynamic significance of tricuspid regurgitation, presence of cyanosis
- Tricuspid valve replacement and/or reconstruction (valvuloplasty) is the definitive repair procedure

Nuclear Medicine Findings

- Radionuclide imaging
  - Decreased left ventricular ejection fraction in 50%

Echocardiographic Findings

- Echocardiogram
  - Right chamber enlargement, "atrialized" portion of right ventricle
  - Enlarged tricuspid annulus (expressed in z-score)
  - Apical displacement of septal tricuspid leaflet (> 15 mm in children < 14 year; > 20 mm in adults)
- Color Doppler
  - Tricuspid regurgitation
  - PFO with right-to-left shunting

Angiographic Findings

- Conventional
  - Characteristic notch at inferior RV border at insertion of displaced anterior tricuspid leaflet
  - Seldom required for primary diagnosis

Imaging Recommendations

- Protocol advice
  - Anatomic and functional assessment with echocardiography in infants
  - Cine MR in (young) adults

DIFFERENTIAL DIAGNOSIS

Large Atrial Septal Defect (ASD)

- Acyanotic
- Increased pulmonary vascularity
- Left-to-right flow through ASD

Pericardial Effusion

- Acyanotic
- Easy differentiation with echocardiography

Tricuspid Insufficiency

- Primary, due to dysplastic valve
- Often secondary to pulmonary atresia with intact ventricular septum

Uhl Anomaly and Arrhythmogenic Right Ventricular Dysplasia (ARVD)

- Similar but distinct entities with congenital absence (Uhl) or fatty infiltration (ARVD) of RV myocardium
- May be differentiated from Ebstein anomaly with spin-echo and cine MR

Right-Sided Obstructive Cyanotic Heart Lesions with Decreased Pulmonary Vascularity

- Tetralogy of Fallot
- Pulmonary atresia
  - With ventricular septal defect and aortopulmonary collaterals
  - With intact ventricular septum
    - Ebstein anomaly and pulmonary atresia with intact ventricular septum are the two lesions that cause the most severe cardiomegaly
- Tricuspid atresia
- Transposition of the great arteries (TGA) with pulmonary stenosis
- Double outlet RV with pulmonary stenosis

PATHOLOGY

General Features

- General path comments
  - Massive right-sided chamber enlargement
  - Three compartments: Right atrium, atrialized non-contracting inlet portion and functional outlet portion of RV
  - Ebstein anomaly frequently involves the left-sided tricuspid valve in congenitally corrected (L) transposition of the great arteries
  - Embryology
    - Insufficient separation of tricuspid valve leaflets and chordae tendineae from right ventricular endocardium
  - Pathophysiology
    - Massive tricuspid regurgitation

EBSTEIN ANOMALY

- Volume overload to right side of heart
- Right-to-left shunt through PFO → cyanosis
- Left ventricular diastolic dysfunction may result from massive right-sided cardiac enlargement
- Arrhythmias due to conduction abnormalities

- Genetics: Most often sporadic
- Epidemiology
  - < 1% of congenital cardiac anomalies, incidence 1/210,000 live births
  - M:F = 1:1
- Associated abnormalities: PFO, secundum ASD in 90%

Gross Pathologic & Surgical Features

- Thickened valve leaflets, adherent to underlying myocardium
- Downward displacement of septal and posterior tricuspid leaflets
- Normally placed, redundant "sail-like" anterior tricuspid leaflet
- May occur on left side of the heart with congenitally corrected (L) transposition

CLINICAL ISSUES

Presentation

- Most common signs/symptoms
  - Wide spectrum of findings and ages at first presentation; some patients are asymptomatic
  - Chronic right heart failure
    - Decreased exercise tolerance (classified as New York Heart Association class I-IV)
  - Presence of cyanosis depends on balance between right and left atrial pressure
    - Physiological drop in pulmonary vascular resistance in neonatal period → decrease in right-to-left shunting through PFO → gradual improvement in cyanosis in first weeks of life
    - Polycythemia
- Other signs/symptoms
  - Hydrops fetalis in neonatal cases
  - Severe cardiomegaly in fetal life → pulmonary hypoplasia
  - Thrombosis, paradoxical embolus
  - Arrhythmias
    - Atrial fibrillation, atrial flutter
    - Accessory atrioventricular conduction pathways (pre-excitation) → tachy-arrhythmias, which can be unexpected and fatal

Demographics

- Age: First presentation can range from newborn period through old age (average: 14 years)

Natural History & Prognosis

- Sudden death due to fatal atrial arrhythmias
- Uncomplicated pregnancies possible in women with hemodynamically well-balanced lesions
- Prognosis is dependent on hemodynamic significance of tricuspid regurgitation, presence of cyanosis

Treatment

- Supportive treatment in cyanotic neonate: Oxygen, nitric oxide ventilation to lower pulmonary resistance
- Systemic to pulmonary (Blalock-Taussig and central) shunts are ineffective
- Some patients benefit from total right-sided heart bypass procedures (Glenn → Fontan surgical treatment pathway)
- Tricuspid valve replacement and/or reconstruction (valvuloplasty) is the definitive repair procedure
  - Valvuloplasty and bioprosthesis placement are preferable to mechanical valve (allow growth; no need for life-long anticoagulation)
  - Valvuloplasty uses tissues from the existing valve (redundant anterior tricuspid leaflet)
  - Bioprosthesis: Homograft or xenograft (porcine valve)
- Indications for valve repair
  - NYHA class III and IV
  - NYHA class I and II with cardiothoracic ratio > 0.65
  - Significant cyanosis (arterial saturation < 80%) and/or polycythemia (Hb > 16 g/dL)
  - History of paradoxical embolus
  - Arrhythmia due to accessory atrioventricular pathway
- Arrhythmia treatments
  - Anti-arrhythmic drugs
  - Permanent pacemaker implantation
  - Radiofrequency ablation

SELECTED REFERENCES

1. Beerepoot JP et al: Case 71: Ebstein anomaly. Radiology. 231(3):747-51, 2004
2. Chauvaud S et al: Ebstein's anomaly: repair based on functional analysis. Eur J Cardiothorac Surg. 23(4):525-31, 2003
3. Dearani JA et al: Ebstein's anomaly of the tricuspid valve, In: Mavroudis C, Backer CL ed. Pediatric cardiac surgery. 3rd ed. Philadelphia, Mosby. 524-36, 2003
4. MacLellan-Tobert SG et al: Ebstein anomaly of the tricuspid valve. In: Moller JH, Hoffman JIE ed. Pediatric cardiovascular medicine, 1st ed. Philadelphia, Churchill Livingstone. 461-8, 2000
5. Ammash NM et al: Mimics of Ebstein's anomaly. Am Heart J. 134(3):508-13, 1997
6. Choi YH et al: MR imaging of Ebstein's anomaly of the tricuspid valve. AJR Am J Roentgenol. 163(3):539-43, 1994
7. Eustace S et al: Ebstein's anomaly presenting in adulthood: the role of cine magnetic resonance imaging in diagnosis. Clin Radiol. 49(10):690-2, 1994
8. Farb A et al: Anatomy and pathology of the right ventricle (including acquired tricuspid and pulmonic valve disease). Cardiol Clin. 10(1):1-21, 1992
9. Lau MK et al: Magnetic resonance imaging of Ebstein's anomaly: report of two cases. J Formos Med Assoc. 91(12):1205-8, 1992
10. Saxena A et al: Late noninvasive evaluation of cardiac performance in mildly symptomatic older patients with Ebstein's anomaly of tricuspid valve: role of radionuclide imaging. J Am Coll Cardiol. 17(1):182-6, 1991
11. Kastler B et al: Potential role of MR imaging in the diagnostic management of Ebstein anomaly in a newborn. J Comput Assist Tomogr. 14(5):825-7, 1990
12. Link KM et al: MR imaging of Ebstein anomaly: results in four cases. AJR Am J Roentgenol. 150(2):363-7, 1988

EBSTEIN ANOMALY

IMAGE GALLERY

Typical

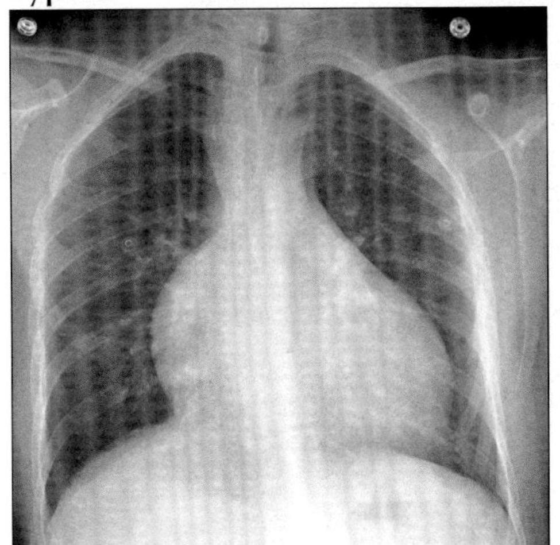

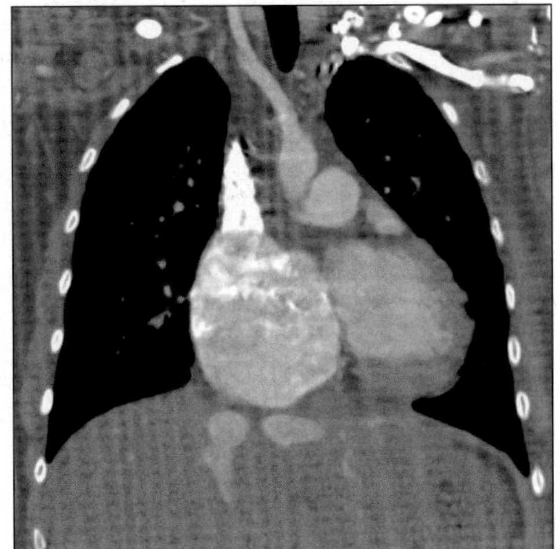

(Left) *Posteroanterior radiograph shows right-sided chamber enlargement.* ***(Right)*** *Coronal CECT confirms massive dilatation of the right atrium, as well as congestion of hepatic veins.*

Typical

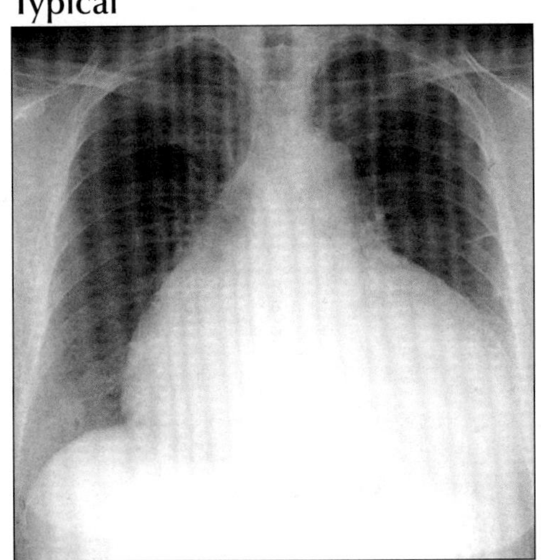

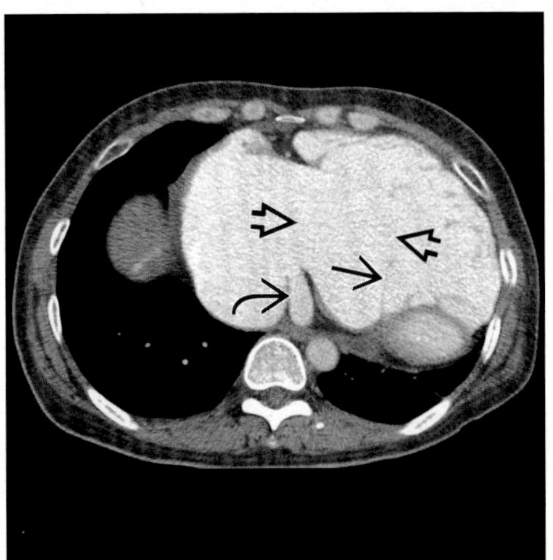

(Left) *Posteroanterior radiograph of a 48 year old woman with Ebstein anomaly shows massive right-sided cardiomegaly.* ***(Right)*** *Axial NECT shows apical displacement of septal tricuspid valve leaflet ➙, with atrialized portion of right ventricle (between ➪). Note dilatation of coronary sinus ↷.*

Typical

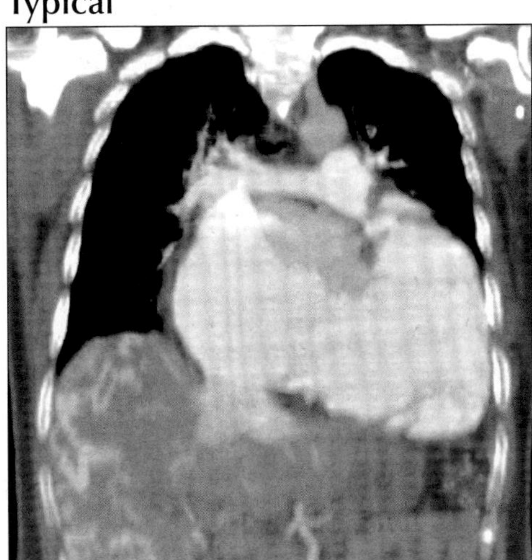

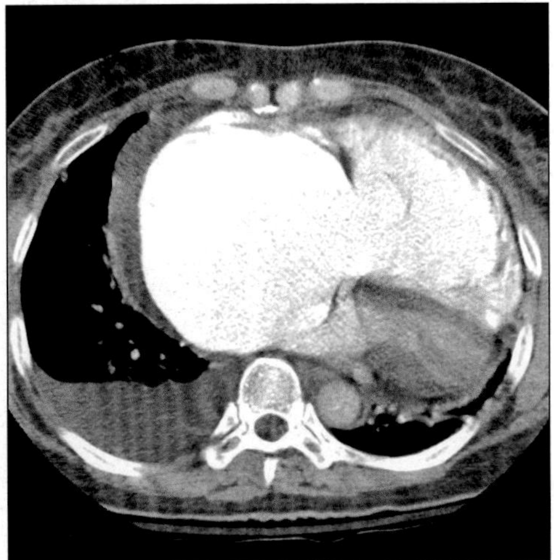

(Left) *Coronal CTA depicts massive dilatation of right-sided cardiac chambers. Note reflux of contrast into congested hepatic veins and parenchyma, due to tricuspid regurgitation.* ***(Right)*** *Axial CECT shows right-sided pleural effusion in Ebstein patient with right-sided heart failure.*

PARTIAL ANOMALOUS PULMONARY VENOUS RETURN

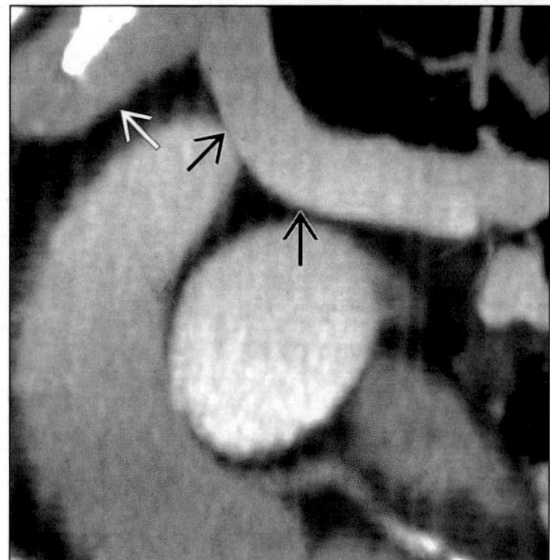

Oblique CECT shows the left upper lobe pulmonary vein draining to the left vertical vein ⇒, and then to the left subclavian vein ➡.

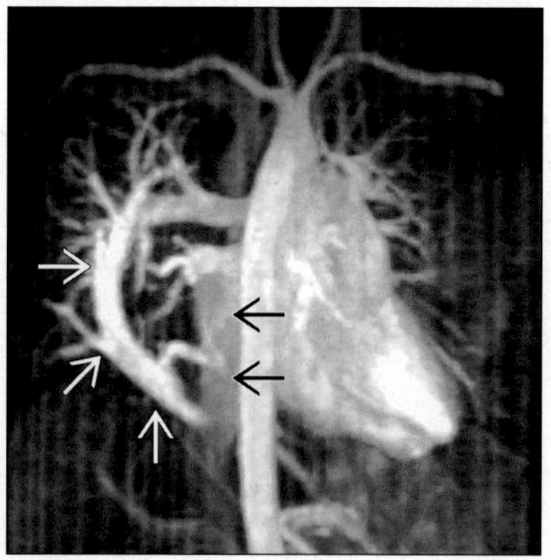

Coronal FGRE shows a scimitar vein draining ➡ into the inferior vena cava ⇒. (Courtesy J. Speckman, MD).

TERMINOLOGY

Abbreviations and Synonyms

- Partial anomalous pulmonary venous return (PAPVR)

Definitions

- Congenital anomaly where pulmonary veins (PV) drain into systemic veins rather than left atrium (LA)
  - Scimitar syndrome is right sided PAPVR draining into IVC, hypoplasia of right lung, dextroposition of heart

IMAGING FINDINGS

General Features

- Best diagnostic clue: Demonstration of abnormal PV drainage on cross-sectional imaging modality
- Location
  - On the right side, drainage to SVC, azygous vein, right atrium, coronary sinus, IVC
    - Scimitar vein courses from right middle lung downward to below diaphragm
  - On the left side, drainage into brachiocephalic vein

Radiographic Findings

- Radiography
  - Rare to identify abnormal vein
    - Scimitar vein is a curvilinear tubular opacity coursing downward from middle right lung
    - If obstructive venous drainage can cause pulmonary congestion
  - If significant left-to-right shunt, cardiomegaly, plethoric pulmonary vasculature

CT Findings

- CECT
  - Abnormal PV drainage
  - Right sided PAPVR associated with sinus venosus atrial septal defect (ASD)
    - In scimitar syndrome = vein with infradiaphragmatic drainage, hypoplastic right lung, cardiac dextroposition

MR Findings

- Double IR FSE can show ASD, phase contrast imaging can quantify L:R shunts

DDx: Other Structures

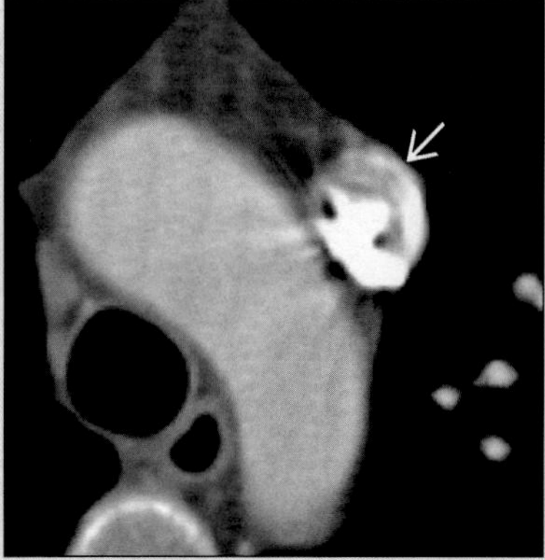

Left-Sided SVC

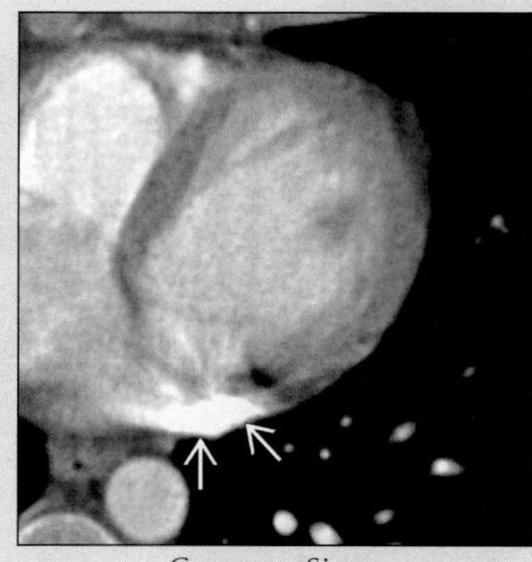

Coronary Sinus

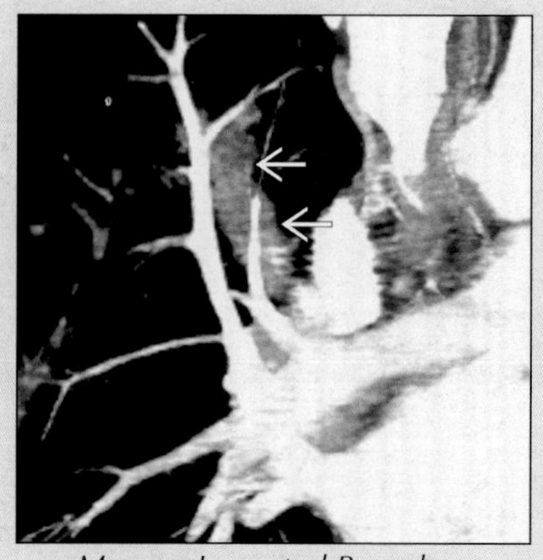

Mucous Impacted Bronchus

PARTIAL ANOMALOUS PULMONARY VENOUS RETURN

Key Facts

Terminology

- Congenital anomaly where pulmonary veins (PV) drain into systemic veins rather than left atrium (LA)

Top Differential Diagnoses

- Left Superior Vena Cava (SVC)
- Pulmonary Varix
- Left Superior Intercostal Vein

Clinical Issues

- Inadvertent clipping causes persistent lobar edema
- Contralateral pneumonectomy: PAPVR shunt may now account for majority of cardiac output
- Consider surgical or percutaneous closure of ASD

Diagnostic Checklist

- Discovery of PAPVR, look carefully for ASD: Cause of paradoxical emboli and stroke

DIFFERENTIAL DIAGNOSIS

Left Superior Vena Cava (SVC)

- 2 vessels ventral to the left upper lobe bronchus: Left superior vena cava and left superior PV
  - Drains into coronary sinus, right SVC may be absent

Pulmonary Varix

- Acquired or development dilatation of PV at its entrance to LA

Left Superior Intercostal Vein

- Aortic "nipple" on chest radiograph

PATHOLOGY

General Features

- Etiology: Persisting embryologic systemic venous connections
- Epidemiology: Incidence 0.5%
- Associated abnormalities
  - Right PAPVR into SVC: Sinus venosus ASD
  - Scimitar syndrome: ASD, systemic blood supply to the lung, extralobar sequestration, horseshoe lung, and pulmonary arteriovenous malformation

CLINICAL ISSUES

Presentation

- Most common signs/symptoms
  - Usually incidental radiographic finding
  - Scimitar syndrome
    - Infants can have severe CHF and pulmonary HTN
    - Older children have less severe symptoms

Natural History & Prognosis

- Shunt less than 2:1, normal life span

Treatment

- Options, risks, complications
  - Inadvertent clipping causes persistent lobar edema
  - Contralateral pneumonectomy: PAPVR shunt may now account for majority of cardiac output
    - May require reimplanting aberrant vein into LA appendage
  - Consider surgical or percutaneous closure of ASD

DIAGNOSTIC CHECKLIST

Image Interpretation Pearls

- Discovery of PAPVR, look carefully for ASD: Cause of paradoxical emboli and stroke

SELECTED REFERENCES

1. Demos TC et al: Venous anomalies of the thorax. AJR Am J Roentgenol. 182(5):1139-50, 2004
2. Remy-Jardin M et al: Spiral CT angiography of the pulmonary circulation. Radiology. 212(3):615-36, 1999

IMAGE GALLERY

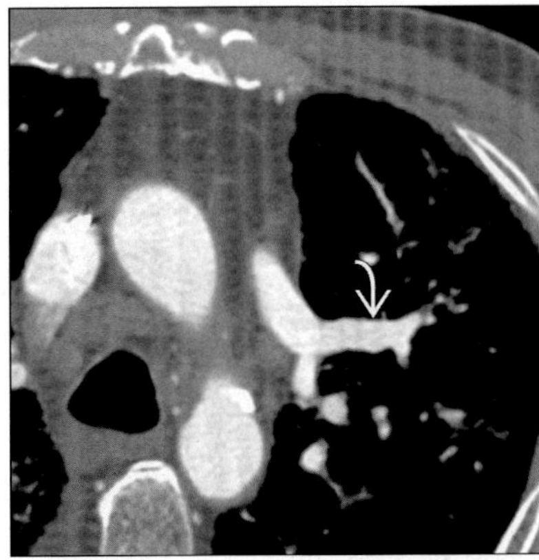

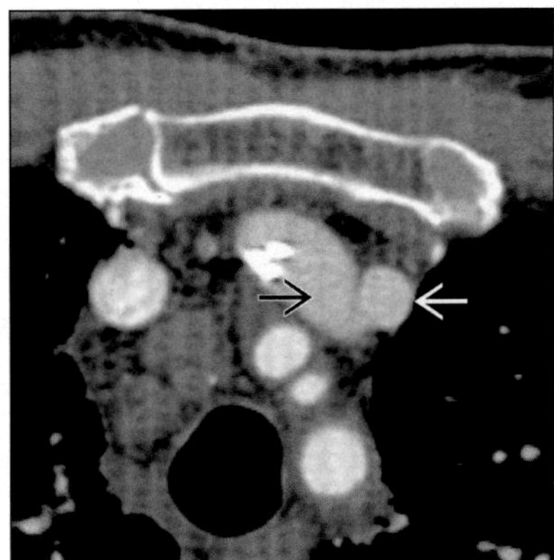

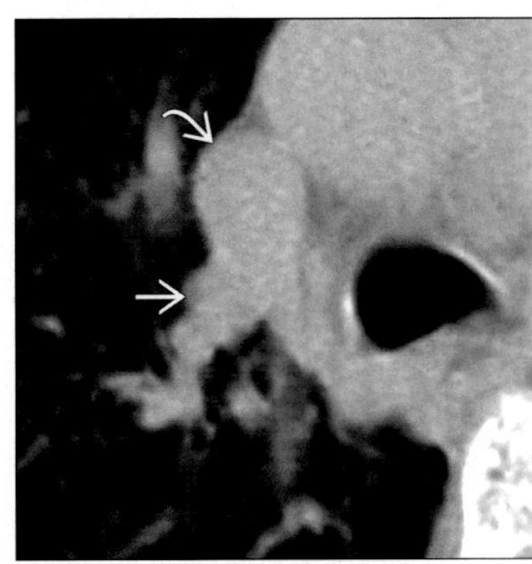

(Left) *Axial CECT shows anomalous left upper lobe pulmonary vein ➔ draining into the vertical vein.* ***(Center)*** *Axial CECT shows the left vertical vein ➔ draining into the left brachiocephalic vein ⇨.* ***(Right)*** *Axial NECT shows the right upper lobe pulmonary vein ➔ draining into the SVC ➔. (Courtesy J. Speckman, MD).*

COR TRIATRIATUM

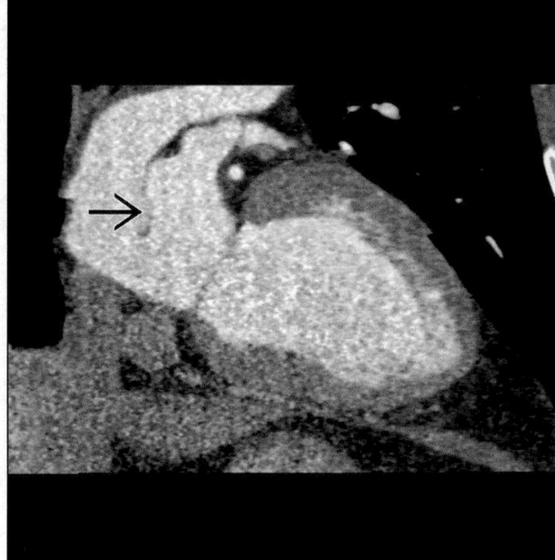

Oblique coronary CTA shows membrane ➔ dividing atrium into proximal, posterior receiving chamber and anterior, distal chamber. Membrane inserts between LAA and pulmonary vein ostium.

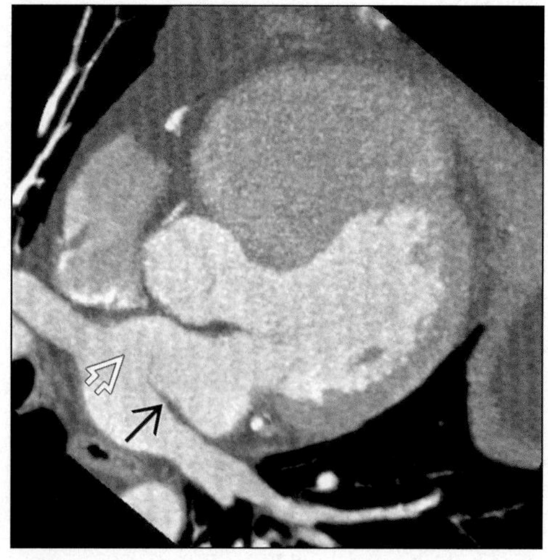

Oblique coronary CTA shows separating membrane ➔ and large defect ➡ allowing communication between posterior and anterior chambers.

TERMINOLOGY

Abbreviations and Synonyms

- Cor triatriatum sinister

Definitions

- Congenital anomaly with fibromuscular diaphragm or membrane dividing left atrium into posterior and anterior chambers
  - Posterior (proximal) chamber receives pulmonary veins, anterior (distal) chamber gives rise to left atrial appendage (LAA) and mitral valve
  - Communication between chambers through defect of varying size within membrane

IMAGING FINDINGS

General Features

- Best diagnostic clue: Membrane of varying size dividing left atrium into posterior and anterior chambers
- Location: Attaches between LAA and pulmonary vein ostia

CT Findings

- CECT
  - Membrane best seen on arterial phase gated CT
    - Paraseptal long axis reconstructions helpful in visualizing insertion site with respect to LAA ostium
  - Signs of pulmonary venous obstruction due to gradient across membrane (may mimic mitral stenosis)
    - Left atrium and right chambers may be dilated
    - Pulmonary venous hypertension (PVH) and interstitial edema
    - May develop main pulmonary artery enlargement secondary to chronic PVH

MR Findings

- Findings on black blood or cine images similar to CT
- Cine white blood or phase contrast images may demonstrate jet across membrane originating in mid left atrium

Echocardiographic Findings

- Echocardiogram

DDx: Cor Triatriatum Sinister

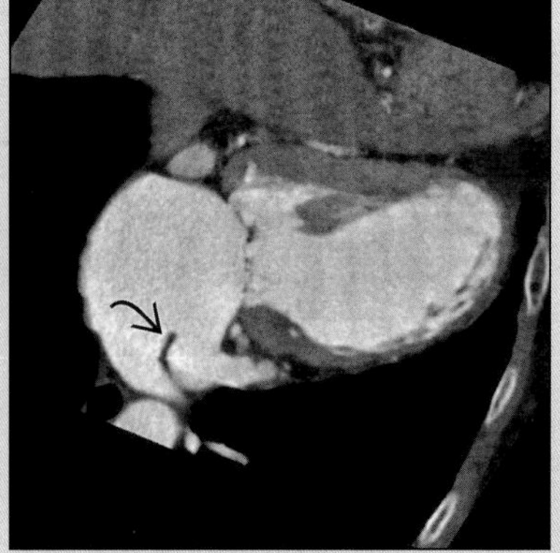

Coumadin Ridge

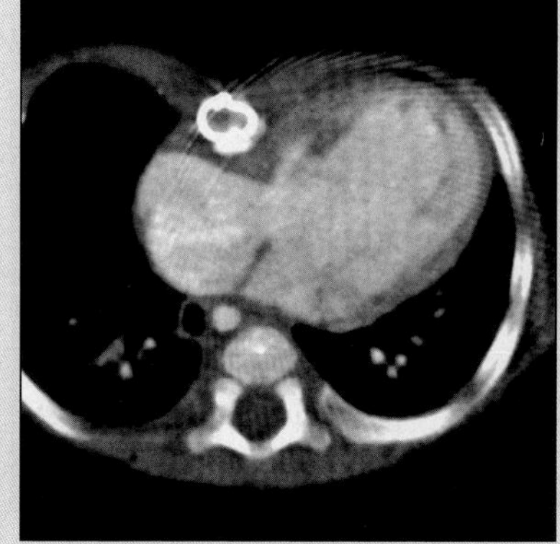

Single Atrium/Ventricle

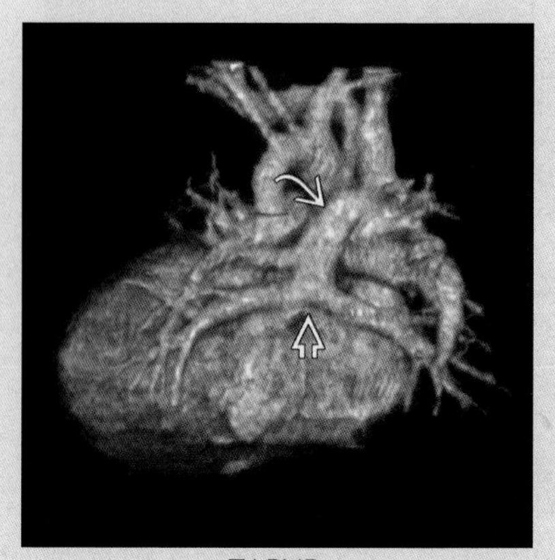

TAPVR

COR TRIATRIATUM

Key Facts

Terminology

- Congenital anomaly with fibromuscular diaphragm or membrane dividing left atrium into posterior and anterior chambers
- Posterior (proximal) chamber receives pulmonary veins, anterior (distal) chamber gives rise to left atrial appendage (LAA) and mitral valve
- Communication between chambers through defect of varying size within membrane

Imaging Findings

- Membrane best seen on arterial phase gated CT
- Paraseptal long axis reconstructions helpful in visualizing insertion site with respect to LAA ostium
- Signs of pulmonary venous obstruction due to gradient across membrane (may mimic mitral stenosis)
- Distinguished from supravalvular ring by being superior/posterior to left atrial appendage

- Trans esophageal ECHO preferred for membrane visualization
- High velocity Doppler flow in distal atrial chamber and at mitral orifice
- Diastolic fluttering of mitral valve leaflets
- Distinguished from supravalvular ring by being superior/posterior to left atrial appendage

Imaging Recommendations

- Protocol advice: Include left ventricular long axis planes to include membrane attachment site, mitral valve and LAA ostium

DIFFERENTIAL DIAGNOSIS

Submitral Ring or Web

- Web connects between left atrial appendage and mitral annulus

Total Anomalous Pulmonary Venous Return

- Common posterior collecting vein receives pulmonary veins and does not connect to left atrium
- Supracardiac, infracardiac or cardiac right sided drainage site may be identified

Cor Triatriatum Dextra

- Membrane dividing right atrium in anterior and posterior (receiving IVC and SVC) chambers

PATHOLOGY

General Features

- Etiology: Congenital malformation due to failure of incorporation of common pulmonary vein into left atrium

CLINICAL ISSUES

Presentation

- Symptoms may mimic mitral valve stenosis
- Signs of pulmonary venous hypertension
- Symptom severity depends on fenestration size
  - Larger defects have milder symptoms

Treatment

- Surgical resection

SELECTED REFERENCES

1. Modi KA et al: Diagnosis and surgical correction of cor triatriatum in an adult: combined use of transesophageal and contrast echocardiography, and a review of literature. Echocardiography. 23(6):506-9, 2006
2. Sarikouch S et al: Adult congenital heart disease: cor triatriatum dextrum. J Thorac Cardiovasc Surg. 132(1):164-5, 2006
3. Slight RD et al: Cor-triatriatum sinister presenting in the adult as mitral stenosis: an analysis of factors which may be relevant in late presentation. Heart Lung Circ. 14(1):8-12, 2005

IMAGE GALLERY

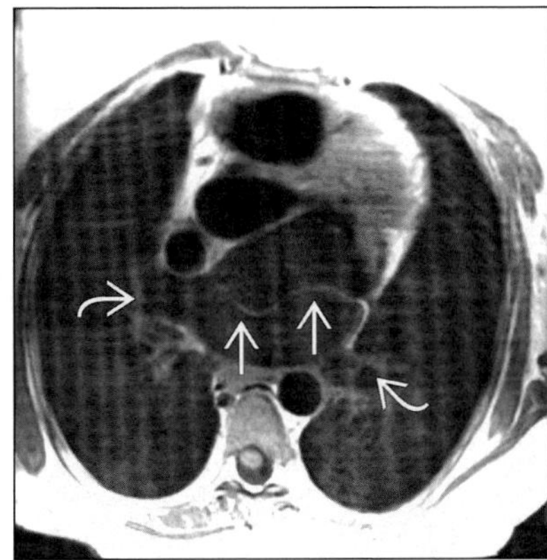

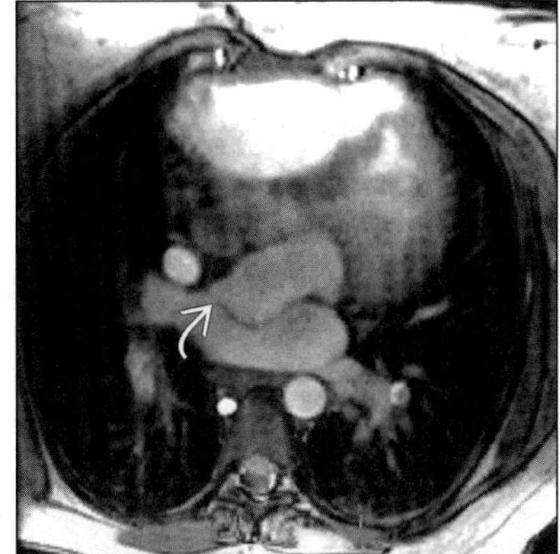

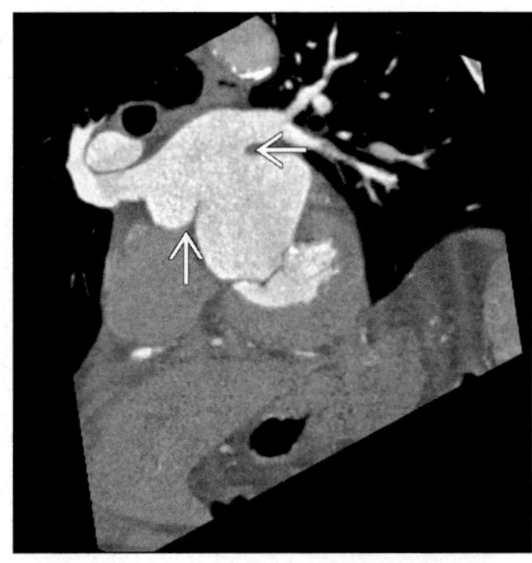

(Left) *Axial T1W SE MR shows membrane ➡ separating left atrium in posterior and anterior chambers. Posterior chamber receives pulmonary veins ➡.* ***(Center)*** *Axial MR cine shows same membrane and small defect ➡ connecting posterior and anterior chambers.* ***(Right)*** *Oblique coronary CTA in asymptomatic patient shows rudimentary membrane ➡ with very large connection of posterior and anterior chambers.*

ENDOCARDIAL CUSHION DEFECT

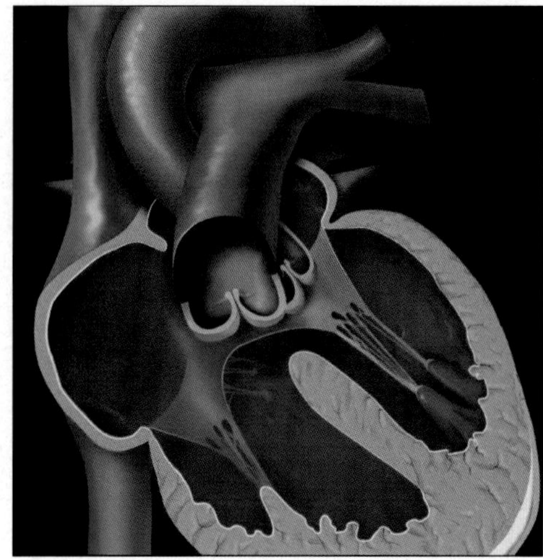

Graphic in complete AV canal shows typical location of defects in atrial and ventricular septum. Note the common AV valve, with straddling of the leaflets across the defects.

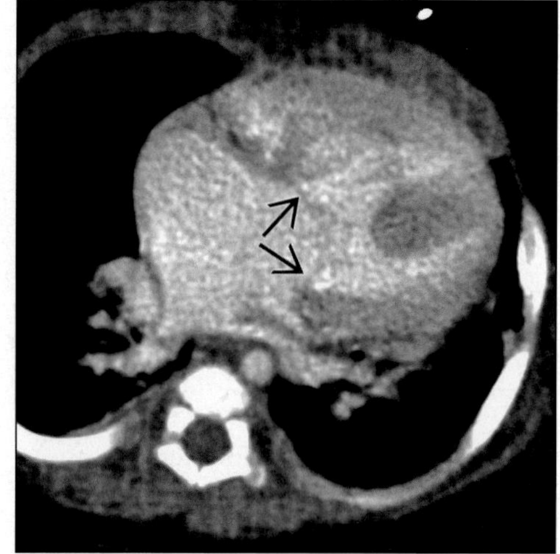

Axial CECT of complete atrioventricular canal shows absence of atrial septum and AV valve leaflets ➔ straddling over ventricular septum. Note enlargement of right-sided chambers.

TERMINOLOGY

Abbreviations and Synonyms

- Atrioventricular septal defect (AVSD)
  - Atrioventricular canal defect (AVC)
  - Endocardial cushion defect
  - Complete atrioventricular canal defect (CAVC)
- Ostium primum defect
  - Partial atrioventricular canal defect (PAVC)
  - Partial atrioventricular septal defect
  - Incomplete endocardial cushion defect

Definitions

- Broad spectrum of defects characterized by involvement in atrial septum, ventricular septum and atrioventricular-ventricular (AV) valves
  - Complete AVSD: Presence of both atrial and ventricular septal defects, common AV valve
  - Partial AVSD: Atrial septal involvement with separate mitral and tricuspid valve orifices
  - Unbalanced AVSD: One ventricular chamber is hypoplastic compared with the other
- 42-48% of Down syndrome or trisomy 21 have an AVC

IMAGING FINDINGS

General Features

- Best diagnostic clue
  - Chest radiograph
    - Large heart with large main pulmonary artery and increased pulmonary artery flow
    - Serial radiographs: Pulmonary hypertension
    - Mitral insufficiency: Pre and post-operative
    - When mitral insufficiency is severe, left atrium can be large and cause left lower lobe collapse
    - Children with large shunts: Increased incidence of upper respiratory infections, pneumonia
    - Pulmonary hypertension: Abnormal lung compliance and hyperinflated lungs (does not necessarily imply infection)
- Location
  - Complete atriventricular canal
    - Large defect in anterior inferior part of atrial septum
    - Large defect in ventricular septum
    - Common atrioventricular valve orifice
    - When AV valve opens towards one ventricle, unbalanced canal defect is present

DDx: Common Left-To-Right Shunts

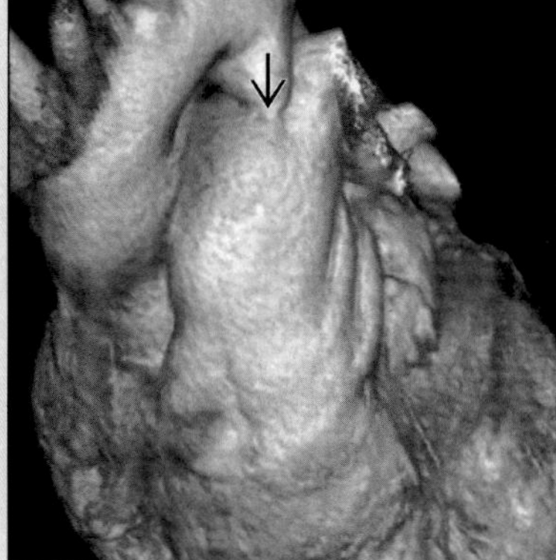

Patent Ductus Arteriosus

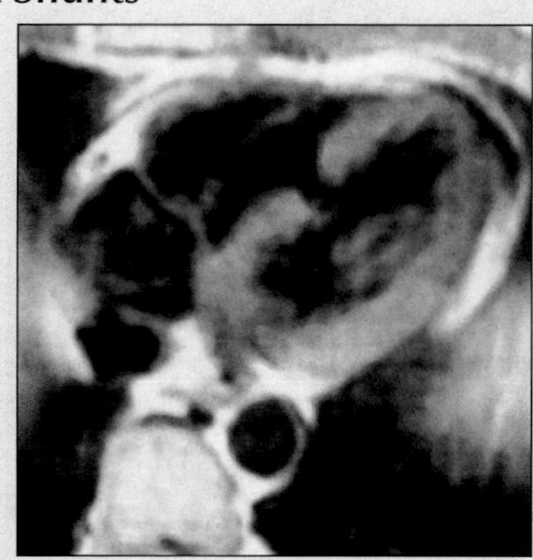

Ventricular Septal Defect

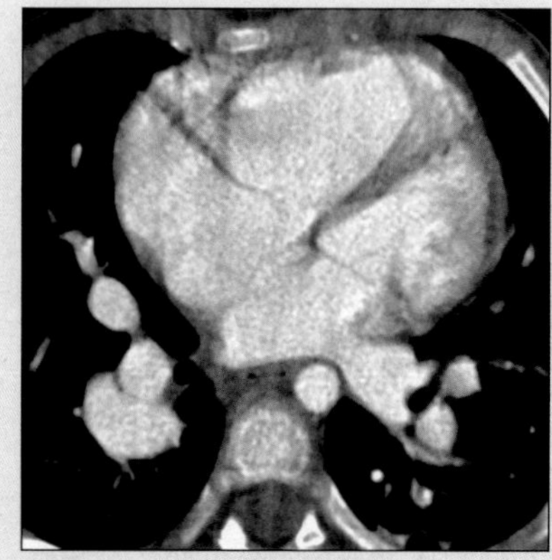

Atrial Septal Defect

ENDOCARDIAL CUSHION DEFECT

Key Facts

Terminology

- Atrioventricular septal defect (AVSD)
- Endocardial cushion defect
- Ostium primum defect
- Broad spectrum of defects characterized by involvement in atrial septum, ventricular septum and one or both of the atrioventricular-ventricular (AV) valves

Imaging Findings

- Large heart with large main pulmonary artery and increased pulmonary artery flow
- Echocardiography in infants and young children defines the lesion
- Demonstration of left-to-right shunt, severity of mitral regurgitation, tricuspid regurgitation

Top Differential Diagnoses

- Ventricular Septal Defect (VSD)
- Atrial Septal Defect (ASD)
- Patent Ductus Arteriosus (PDA)
- Sinus Venosus Atrial Septal Defect

Clinical Issues

- Large shunts present early with tachypnea, tachycardia, failure to thrive
- Small shunts: Well-tolerated through first decade and children may be asymptomatic
- Medical management until surgery depending on lesion and severity
- Elective repair in children 2-5 years, unless mitral regurgitation is present
- Single ventricle physiology: Staged single ventricle repair (Glenn, followed by Fontan)

        - Right ventricular or left ventricular dominance can occur
        - Results in single ventricle physiology
        - Unbalanced canal defect refers to hypoplasia of one ventricle
        - Hypoplasia of the inlet and outlet septum, resulting in hypoplasia of the chamber with malalignment of the ventricular septum
    - Ostium primum defect
        - Defect in anterior inferior aspect of atrial septum
        - May be isolated defect in atrial septum, but coexisting cleft in anterior leaflet of mitral valve is frequently present
        - 5 leaflet AV valve is present with separate valve orifices to right and left ventricle
        - Tricuspid and mitral valve leaflets adhere to the crest of the interventricular septum, mitral valve cleft
- Size: Broad spectrum of size of defects in AV septum and respective sizes of the ventricles
- Morphology
    - Complete atrioventricular canal
        - Defect in anterior inferior aspect of atrial septum
        - Defect in ventricular septum
        - Abnormal mitral valve attachments
    - Ostium primum defect: Defect in anterior inferior aspect of atrial septum

CT Findings

- CECT
    - Not done for diagnosis, but may identify the atrial and ventricular defects
    - Large heart with increased size of pulmonary arteries
    - Large right-sided structures such as right atrium right ventricle, pulmonary artery

Echocardiographic Findings

- Echocardiogram
    - Echocardiography in infants and young children defines the lesion
        - Primum defects have echo dropout in lower portion of the septum, cleft in mitral valve
        - Anterior and superior displacement of aorta, with elongation and narrowing of left ventricular outflow tract
- Color Doppler
    - Demonstration of left-to-right shunt, severity of mitral regurgitation, tricuspid regurgitation
        - Left ventricular outflow tract obstruction can be quantified

Angiographic Findings

- Conventional
    - Cardiac catheterization is not usually done for anatomy, but done to measure pulmonary vascular resistance
        - Left ventriculogram shows cleft in mitral valve, shunts, respective size of the ventricles and also left ventricular outflow tract obstruction

Imaging Recommendations

- Best imaging tool
    - Echocardiography in infants and young children defines the lesion
        - Primum defects have echo dropout in lower portion of the septum, mitral valve cleft
        - Complete AVSD demonstrate varying degree of absence of septum, size of defect and relative size of the ventricles

DIFFERENTIAL DIAGNOSIS

Ventricular Septal Defect (VSD)

- Most common congenital heart disease (CHD) with left-to-right shunt
- Most common CHD associated with other lesions
- Cardiac enlargement with increased pulmonary flow

Atrial Septal Defect (ASD)

- Defect is in the superior portion of the atrial septum
- Presents in older children
    - Usually asymptomatic from shunt
- Left-to-right shunt usually not large, but it can cause Eisenmenger physiology in adult if unrecognized

ENDOCARDIAL CUSHION DEFECT

Patent Ductus Arteriosus (PDA)

- Communication between the high pressure aorta with the lower pressure pulmonary artery
- Left-to-right shunt usually presents in infancy
- Closed by percutaneous occlusion devices

Sinus Venosus Atrial Septal Defect

- Defect high in the right atrial septum
- Usually associated with anomalous venous drainage of the right upper lobe vein
- Volume overloads the right atrium, the right ventricle and the pulmonary arteries

PATHOLOGY

General Features

- Genetics: Associated with trisomy 21 in 44-48%
- Etiology
  - Malformation occurring during the 5th week of gestation
  - Abnormal or inadequate fusion of the superior and inferior endocardial cushion
  - Abnormal fusion of the ventricular (trabecular) portion of the septum
- Epidemiology
  - 4-8 out of 1,000 live births have congenital heart defects
  - 5-8% have AVSD
- Associated abnormalities
  - Trisomy 21 children have constellation of clinical and radiographic findings
    - Chest radiograph may show 11 ribs, double manubrial ossification center in 80%
    - Many skeletal malformations, spectrum of retardation

CLINICAL ISSUES

Presentation

- Most common signs/symptoms
  - Complete atrial ventricular defect
    - Large shunts present early with tachypnea, tachycardia, and failure to thrive
    - Mitral insufficiency adds complexity and earlier symptoms
  - Partial atrial ventricular defect
    - Small shunts well-tolerated through first decade and children may be asymptomatic
    - Mitral insufficiency adds complexity and earlier symptoms
- Other signs/symptoms
  - Pathophysiology of lesions
    - Degree of left-to-right shunting is determined by size of defect and relative compliance of atria and ventricles
    - Right ventricular compliance reflects pulmonary vascular resistance
    - Infants have high pulmonary vascular resistance and therefore rarely have shunts
    - As pulmonary vascular resistance decreases, left-to-right shunting increases with age
    - Subsequent enlargement of right atrium, right ventricular enlargement and increase in pulmonary vascularity
    - Degree of regurgitation through mitral vale cleft depends on its size and also whether there are left-sided lesions such as coarctation
    - Cleft directs regurgitant blood through atrial defect

Demographics

- Age: Infants and children
- Gender: M = F

Natural History & Prognosis

- Complete atrioventricular canal presents in infancy with symptoms
- Children assessed for surgical repair
  - Post-operative course may be complicated by mitral insufficiency
  - Pulmonary hypertension occurs in unoperated children

Treatment

- Medical management until surgery depending on lesion and severity
- Surgical management: Partial AVSD
  - Closed by pericardial patch via right atrial approach
  - Percutaneous closure devices not usually done as the inferior attachment may injure AV valves
- Surgery for complete AVSD: 3% mortality
  - Elective repair in children 2-5 years, unless mitral regurgitation is present
  - Complications include mitral insufficiency which may require reoperation, valvuloplasty or replacement
  - Arrhythmias such as sinus node dysfunction or heart block
  - Single ventricle physiology: Staged single ventricle repair (Glenn, followed by Fontan)

SELECTED REFERENCES

1. Ferguson EC et al: Classic imaging signs of congenital cardiovascular abnormalities. Radiographics. 27(5):1323-34, 2007
2. Colletti PM: Evaluation of intracardiac shunts with cardiac magnetic resonance. Curr Cardiol Rep. 7(1):52-8, 2005
3. Ten Harkel AD et al: Development of left atrioventricular valve regurgitation after correction of atrioventricular septal defect. Ann Thorac Surg. 79(2):607-12, 2005
4. Formigari R et al: Better surgical prognosis for patients with complete atrioventricular septal defect and Down's syndrome. Ann Thorac Surg. 78(2):666-72; discussion 672, 2004
5. Beerbaum P et al: Atrial septal defects in pediatric patients: noninvasive sizing with cardiovascular MR imaging. Radiology. 228(2):361-9, 2003
6. Freeman SB et al: Population-based study of congenital heart defects in Down syndrome. Am J Med Genet. 80(3):213-7, 1998
7. Drinkwater DC Jr et al: Unbalanced atrioventricular septal defects. Semin Thorac Cardiovasc Surg. 9(1):21-5, 1997
8. van Son JA et al: Predicting feasibility of biventricular repair of right-dominant unbalanced atrioventricular canal. Ann Thorac Surg. 63(6):1657-63, 1997

ENDOCARDIAL CUSHION DEFECT

IMAGE GALLERY

Typical

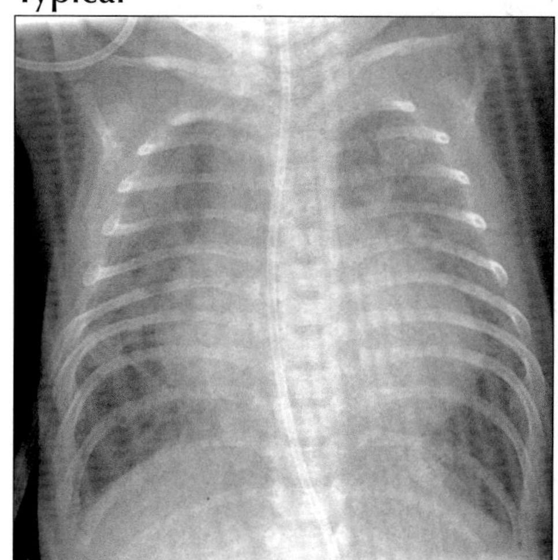

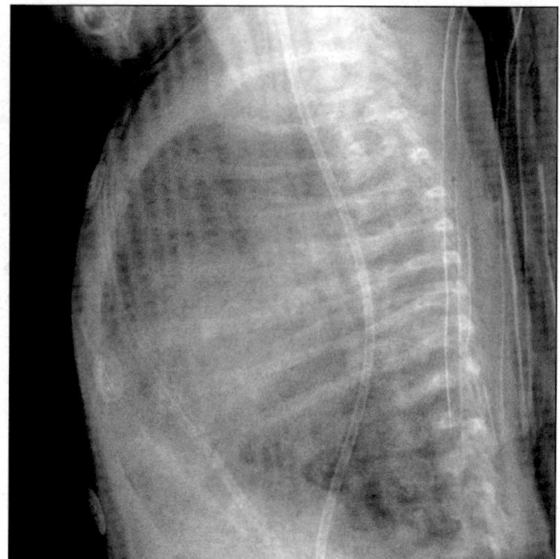

*(**Left**) Anteroposterior radiograph in infant with Down syndrome and endocardial cushion defects shows cardiomegaly and increased pulmonary artery flow. (**Right**) Lateral radiograph in the same patient as previous image, demonstrates marked hyperinflation of the lungs. The is a bifid manubrial ossification center.*

Typical

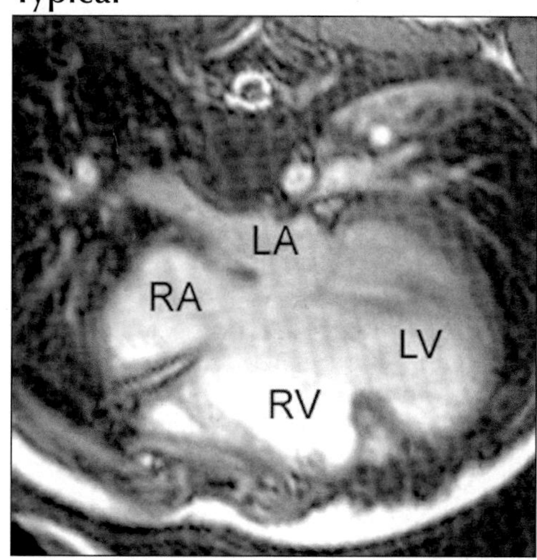

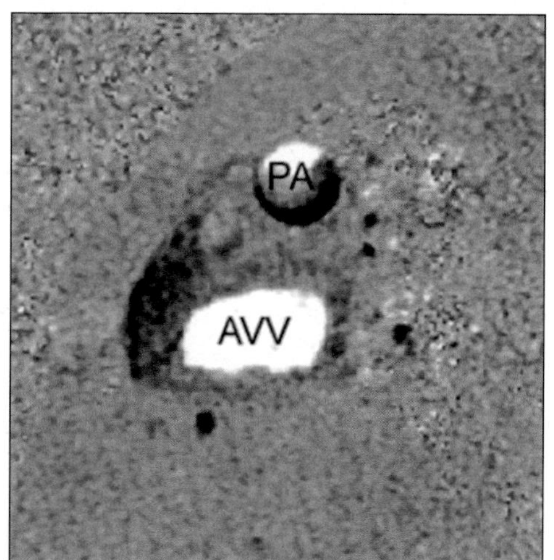

*(**Left**) Four chamber view (double oblique) MR cine shows a large common atrioventricular canal, with open communication between right atrium (RA), left atrium (LA), right ventricle (RV) and left ventricle (LV). (**Right**) Sagittal oblique phase-contrast MRA, magnitude image shows regurgitation across the common atrioventricular valve (AVV); pulmonary artery (PA).*

Typical

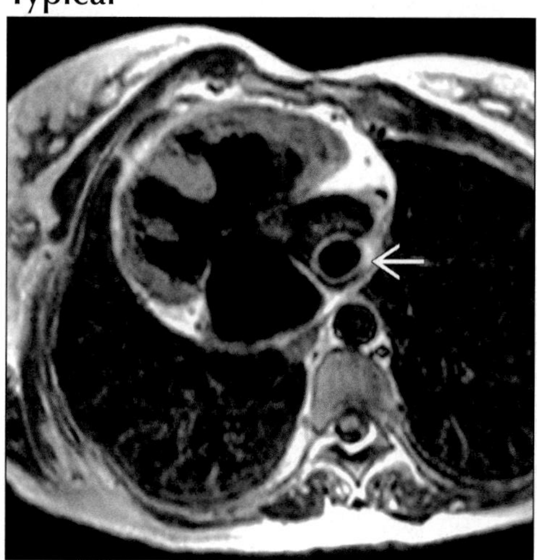

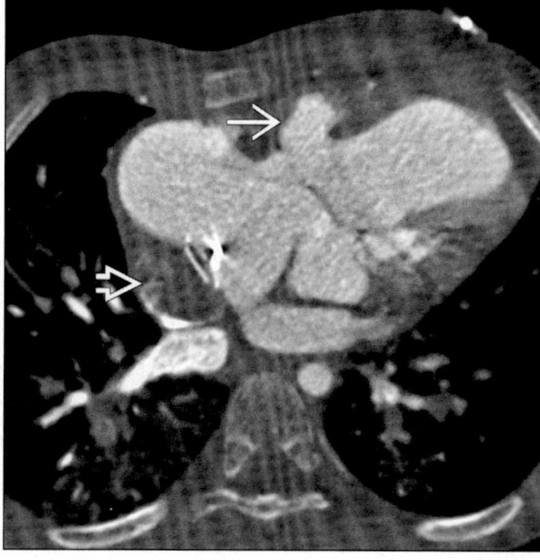

*(**Left**) Axial T1WI MR shows balanced AV canal, dextrocardia and intra-atrial Fontan conduit ➡ in patient with asplenia syndrome. (Courtesy R. Krishnamurthy, MD). (**Right**) Axial cardiac CT shows unbalanced AV canal, with common atrium and straddling AV valves and small right ventricle ➡. Note unopacified lateral tunnel Fontan conduit ➡.*

TETRALOGY OF FALLOT

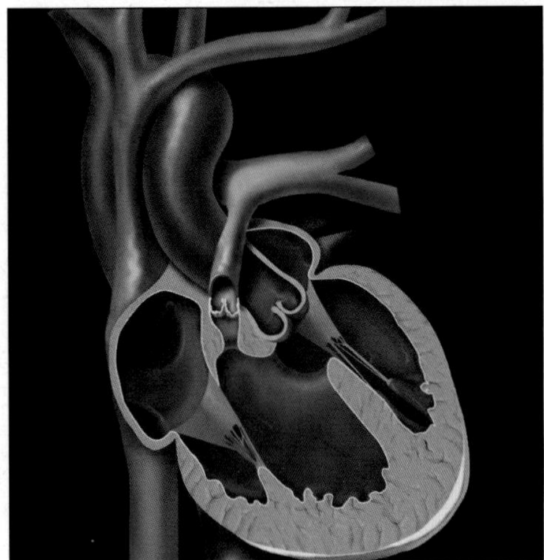

Graphic shows subvalvular and valvular pulmonary stenosis with hypoplastic pulmonary artery, VSD, muscular RV hypertrophy, and overriding aorta receiving mixed blood from RV and LV.

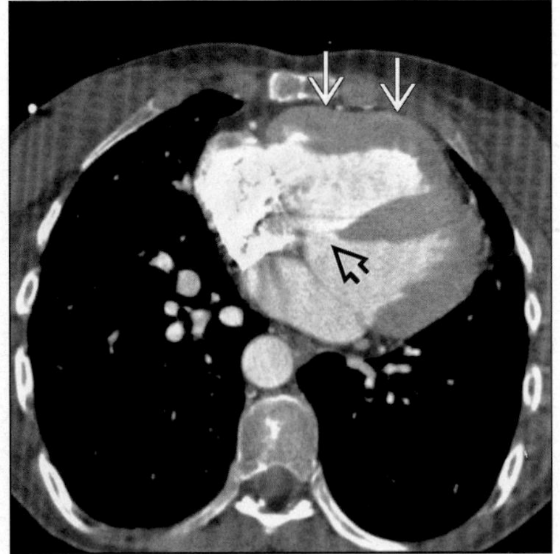

Axial coronary CTA shows marked right ventricular hypertrophy ➡ and membranous VSD ⇨. Other views demonstrate aorta overriding the VSD and there was a remote pulmonary stenosis repair.

TERMINOLOGY

Abbreviations and Synonyms

- Tetralogy of Fallot (TOF), Tet

Definitions

- Underdevelopment of pulmonary infundibulum due to unequal partitioning of conal truncus resulting in subvalvular or valvular right ventricular (RV) outflow tract (RVOT) stenosis, subaortic ventricular septal defect (VSD), overriding aorta and RV hypertrophy

IMAGING FINDINGS

General Features

- Best diagnostic clue: Infundibular stenosis of RVOT

Radiographic Findings

- Radiography
  - Classic plain film appearance: "Boot-shaped" heart
  - Normal heart size
  - Right-sided aortic arch in 25%
  - RV hypertrophy, concave pulmonary artery segment: "Boot-shaped" heart = "coeur en sabot"
  - Decreased pulmonary vascularity (pulmonary oligemia)

CT Findings

- CT angiography with volume rendition depicts PA anatomy
- May demonstrate aorto-pulmonary systemic collateral arteries
- RV hypertrophy usually evident on non-gated CTA
- Gated CTA excellent tool for depicting prior surgical repairs ± potential complications in adults
  - Blalock-Taussig (BT) shunt: Subclavian artery take down to pulmonary artery or tube graft (modified BT); usually ligated at time of definitive repair
  - Pott shunt: Left pulmonary artery to descending aorta; no longer performed
  - Waterston-Cooley shunt: Ascending aorta to right pulmonary artery
  - Definitive repair: Infundibular patch or tube graft repair + VSD closure

MR Findings

- Cardiac-gated T1WI (axial views)

DDx: Tetralogy of Fallot

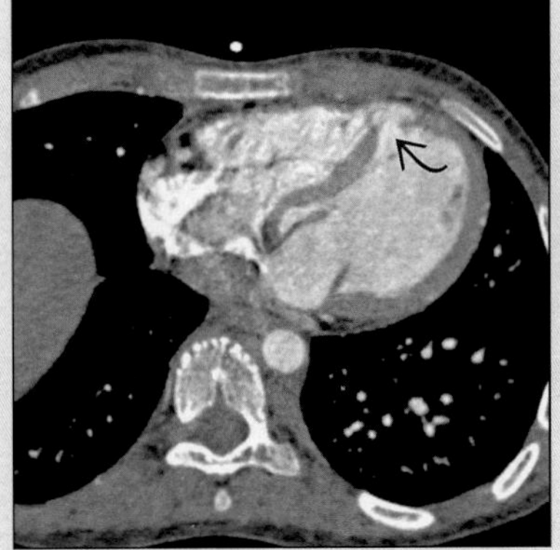

Isolated VSD

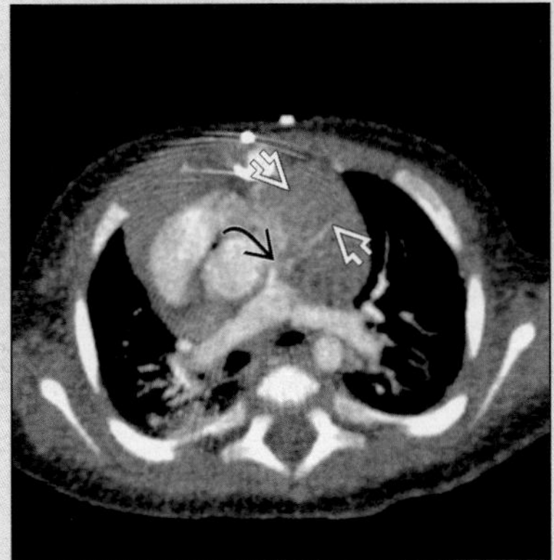

Pulmonary Atresia

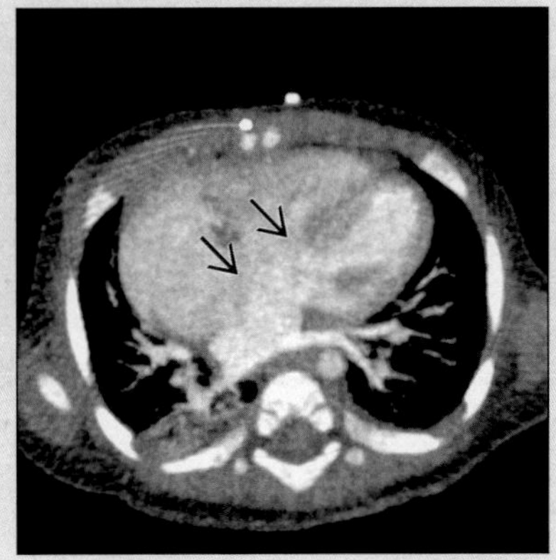

Endocardial Cushion Defect

TETRALOGY OF FALLOT

Key Facts

Terminology

- Underdevelopment of pulmonary infundibulum due to unequal partitioning of conal truncus resulting in subvalvular or valvular right ventricular (RV) outflow tract (RVOT) stenosis, subaortic ventricular septal defect (VSD), overriding aorta and RV hypertrophy

Imaging Findings

- Right-sided aortic arch in 25%
- RV hypertrophy, concave pulmonary artery segment: "Boot-shaped" heart = "coeur en sabot"
- Decreased pulmonary vascularity (pulmonary oligemia)
- Initial diagnosis with echocardiography
- CTA or MR for PA anatomy

Top Differential Diagnoses

- Trilogy of Fallot
- Pulmonary valvular stenosis, RV hypertrophy, and ASD with right to left shunt due to increased right-sided pressures
- Pentalogy of Fallot
- Tetralogy with additional atrial septal defect (ASD)

Pathology

- Right-sided aortic arch with mirror image branching (25%)
- Balance between RVOT obstruction and VSD
- Classic (blue) Tet = decreased pulmonary blood flow results in greater right to left shunting → cyanosis
- "Pink" Tet = normal or increased pulmonary flow → congestive heart failure

---

  - Pre-operative definition of PA anatomy, PA stenosis
  - Post-operative PA anatomy, patency of Blalock-Taussig shunts
- Gradient-echo (GRE) cine in short axis
  - RV function, ejection fraction
- Phase-contrast MRA: For estimate of RV function, regurgitation fraction
- 3D gadolinium MRA: For anatomy and depiction PA anatomy and MAPCAs

Echocardiographic Findings

- Echocardiogram
  - Location VSD, additional muscular VSDs
  - Degree of aortic override, position of arch
  - Degree of RVOT obstruction, function of pulmonary valve
  - Anatomy of branch pulmonary arteries (PAs)

Ultrasonographic Findings

- Grayscale Ultrasound
  - In utero: Dilated aorta overriding interventricular septum
  - No RV hypertrophy in second trimester
  - Perimembranous VSD and RVOT narrowing may be apparent

Angiographic Findings

- Cardiac catheterization and angiography findings
  - Coronary anatomy
  - PA branch stenosis: Balloon angioplasty with stent placement
  - Anatomy/distribution of MAPCAs

Imaging Recommendations

- Initial diagnosis with echocardiography
- CTA or MR for PA anatomy
- Cardiac catheterization for percutaneous interventions
- MR in older child with poor acoustic window for functional assessment of post-operative pulmonary regurgitation and RV dysfunction

DIFFERENTIAL DIAGNOSIS

Pulmonary Atresia with VSD

- Type A: Only native pulmonary arteries
- Type B: Pulmonary blood flow via both native pulmonary arteries and MAPCAs
- Type C: Only MAPCAs, no native pulmonary arteries

Tricuspid Atresia with VSD

- Muscular or membranous partition between right atrium and RV
- Obligatory shunting from right atrium → left atrium → LV → RV
- Decreased pulmonary flow → severe cyanosis at birth
- When associated with transposition increased pulmonary blood flow

Trilogy of Fallot

- Pulmonary valvular stenosis, RV hypertrophy, and ASD with right to left shunt due to increased right-sided pressures

Pentalogy of Fallot

- Tetralogy with additional atrial septal defect (ASD)

PATHOLOGY

General Features

- General path comments
  - Tetralogy of Fallot is most common heart lesion with right aortic arch
  - Frequently associated
    - PA branch stenosis or hypoplasia
    - Absence of pulmonary valve: Severe pulmonary regurgitation → aneurysmal dilatation of PAs → tracheobronchial compression
    - Patent foramen ovale
    - Right-sided aortic arch with mirror image branching (25%)
    - Coronary anomalies: Left anterior descending (LAD) arising from right coronary and crossing RVOT, with implications for surgical repair

TETRALOGY OF FALLOT

- Tracheo esophageal fistula
- Down syndrome
- Scoliosis, forked ribs
- Embryology
  - Abnormal bulbotruncal rotation and septation
  - Primary hypoplasia of infundibular septum
- Hemodynamics: RVOT obstruction leads to pressure overload
- Balance between RVOT obstruction and VSD
  - Classic (blue) Tet = decreased pulmonary blood flow results in greater right to left shunting → cyanosis
  - "Pink" Tet = normal or increased pulmonary flow → congestive heart failure
- Genetics
  - Associated with chromosomal abnormalities in 11% (chromosome 22)
  - Associated with other congenital anomalies in 16%; syndromal in 8%
- Epidemiology
  - Incidence: 3-5 per 10,000 live births
  - Fourth most common congenital heart anomaly
  - Most common cyanotic heart lesion

Staging, Grading or Classification Criteria

- Category: Cyanotic, normal heart size, decreased pulmonary vascularity

CLINICAL ISSUES

Presentation

- Varying degrees of cyanosis at birth
- Hypercyanotic spells with dyspnea on exertion relieved by typical "squatting position" when fatigued
  - Squatting pinches of femoral arteries resulting in increased systemic resistance which increases pulmonary flow
- Clubbing of fingers and toes
- Congestive heart failure (large VSD)
- After repair: Decreased exercise tolerance, RV dysfunction, arrhythmias
- Bacterial endocarditis, stroke due to paradoxical embolus to brain, hyperviscosity syndrome due to polycythemia

Natural History & Prognosis

- 10% of untreated patients live more than 20 years
- Short term: Excellent results after early complete repair
- Long term: Determined by right ventricular diastolic dysfunction

Treatment

- Palliative shunt
  - Classic Blalock-Taussig shunt: End-to-side subclavian artery to PA (opposite from aortic arch)
  - Modified Blalock-Taussig shunt: Interposition of Gore-Tex graft
  - Central shunt: Ductus-like connection between aorta and PA
- Complete repair: Enlargement of RVOT, closure of VSD
  - With transannular patch: Post-op pulmonary regurgitation

DIAGNOSTIC CHECKLIST

Consider

- MRA if MAPCAs are suspected in children
- CTA powerful tool in adults to detect treatment complication

SELECTED REFERENCES

1. Geva T et al: Magnetic resonance imaging-guided catheter interventions in congenital heart disease. Circulation. 113(8):1051-2, 2006
2. Geva T: Indications and timing of pulmonary valve replacement after tetralogy of Fallot repair. Semin Thorac Cardiovasc Surg Pediatr Card Surg Annu. :11-22, 2006
3. Prasad SK et al: Role of magnetic resonance angiography in the diagnosis of major aortopulmonary collateral arteries and partial anomalous pulmonary venous drainage. Circulation. 109(2):207-14, 2004
4. Haramati LB et al: MR imaging and CT of vascular anomalies and connections in patients with congenital heart disease: significance in surgical planning. Radiographics. 22(2):337-47; discussion 348-9, 2002
5. Holmqvist C et al: Pre-operative evaluation with MR in tetralogy of fallot and pulmonary atresia with ventricular septal defect. Acta Radiol. 42(1):63-9, 2001
6. Helbing WA et al: Clinical applications of cardiac magnetic resonance imaging after repair of tetralogy of Fallot. Pediatr Cardiol. 21(1):70-9, 2000
7. Reddy VM et al: Early and intermediate outcomes after repair of pulmonary atresia with ventricular septal defect and major aortopulmonary collateral arteries: experience with 85 patients. Circulation. 101:1826-32, 2000
8. Tchervenkov CI et al: Congenital Heart Surgery Nomenclature and Database Project: pulmonary atresia--ventricular septal defect. Ann Thorac Surg. 69(4 Suppl):S97-105, 2000
9. Greenberg SB et al: Magnetic resonance imaging compared with echocardiography in the evaluation of pulmonary artery abnormalities in children with tetralogy of Fallot following palliative and corrective surgery. Pediatr Radiol. 27(12):932-5, 1997
10. Greenberg SB et al: Tetralogy of Fallot: diagnostic imaging after palliative and corrective surgery. J Thorac Imaging. 10(1):26-35, 1995

TETRALOGY OF FALLOT

IMAGE GALLERY

Typical

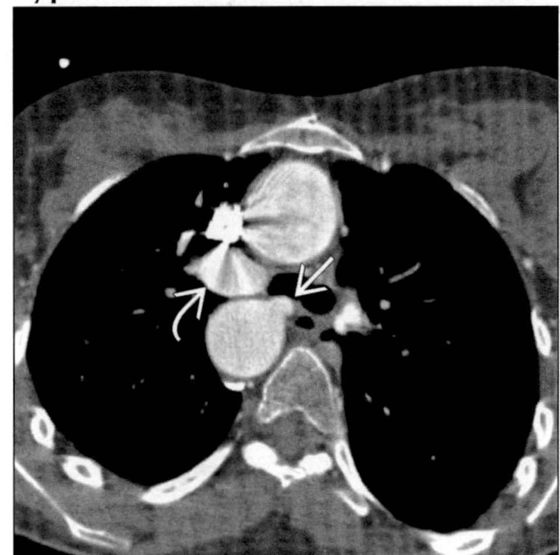

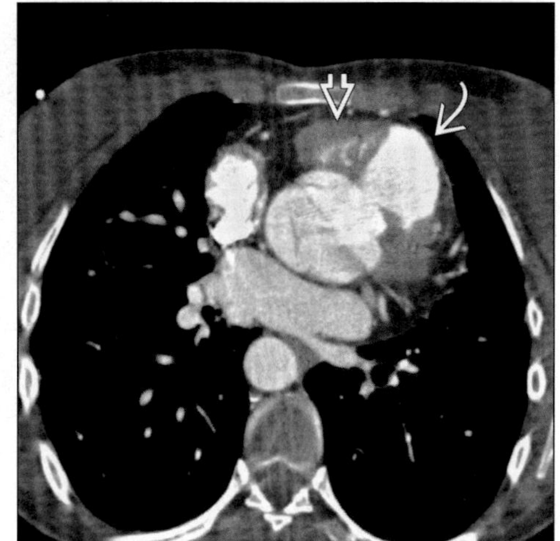

(Left) *Axial CTA shows right aortic arch with large anterior vessel origin ➡ and large vessel entering right lung ➡ above pulmonary hilum, both representing systemic aorto pulmonary collateral.* ***(Right)*** *Axial coronary CTA shows enlarged overriding aorta and right ventricular outflow tract with hypertrophic myocardium ➡ and very thin material representing RVOT patch repair ➡.*

Typical

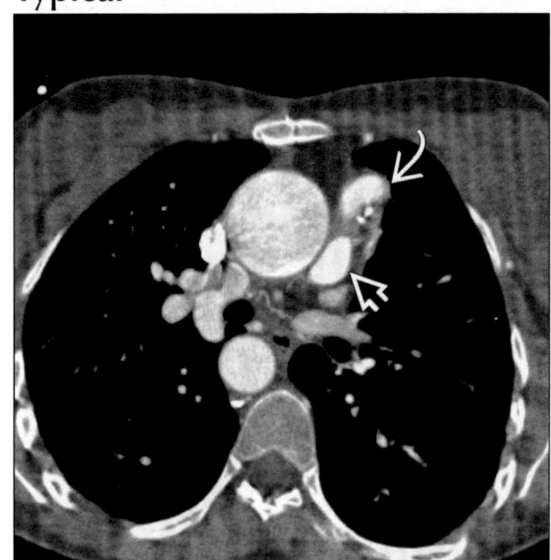

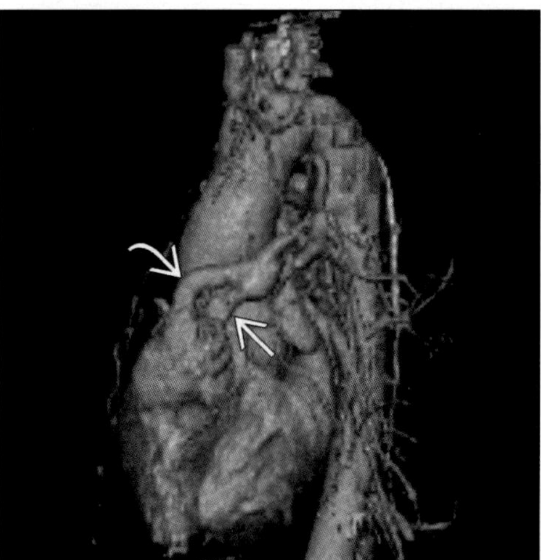

(Left) *Axial coronary CTA shows very small hypoplastic native main pulmonary artery ➡ and tubular structure ➡ more anterior representing bypass graft bridging pulmonary stenosis.* ***(Right)*** *Oblique coronary CTA volume rendering shows minute native pulmonary artery ➡ and bypass graft ➡ arising from RVOT with distal anastomosis at main pulmonary artery.*

Typical

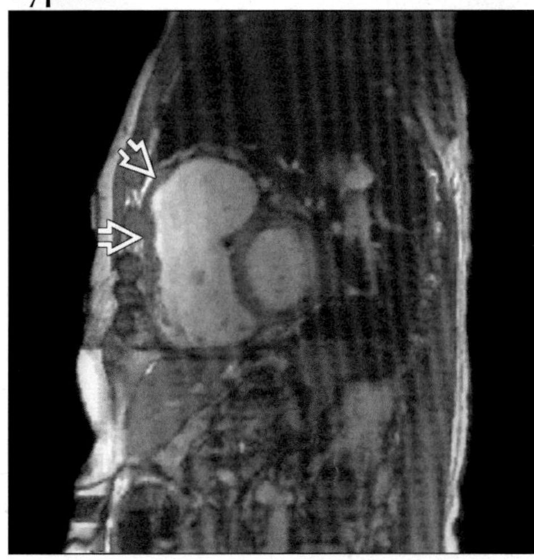

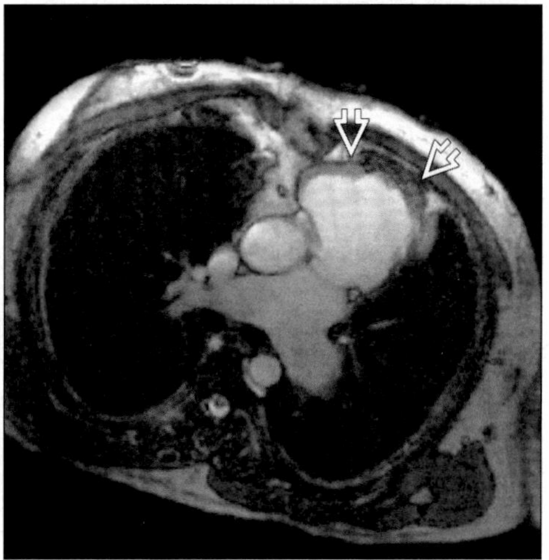

(Left) *Oblique MR cine in patient with repaired tetralogy and post repair pulmonary insufficiency shows markedly enlarged RV with filling of retrosternal clear space and markedly enlarged RVOT ➡.* ***(Right)*** *Oblique MR cine in same patient as previous image shows enlarged pulmonary arteries (compare to ascending aorta) and markedly enlarged RVOT ➡.*

TETRALOGY OF FALLOT PALLIATION: BT SHUNT

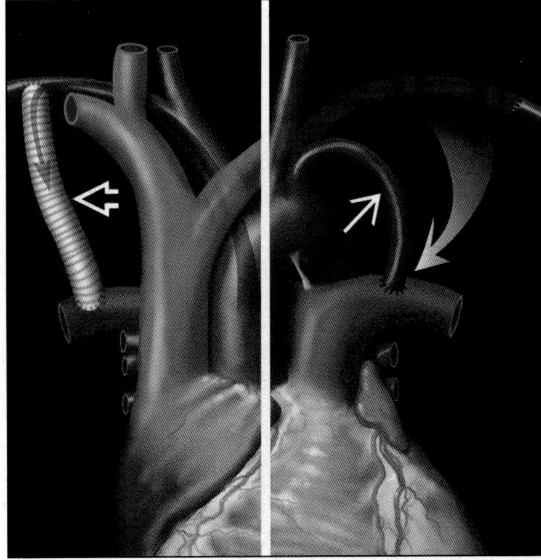

Graphic shows modified BT shunt ➡ connecting subclavian artery (SCA) and pulmonary artery. Left: Original BT shunt ➡ with distal ligated SCA. Mobilized proximal SCA is anastomosed to pulmonary artery.

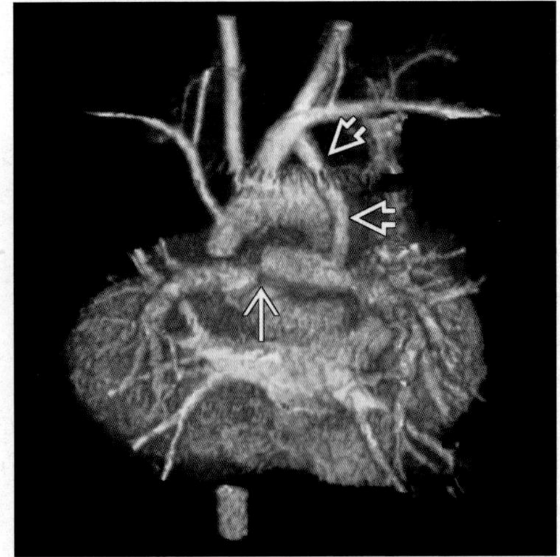

Posterior volume rendered CTA shows BT shunt ➡ connecting right brachiocephalic/subclavian artery and right pulmonary artery. Note left pulmonary artery stenosis ➡.

TERMINOLOGY

Abbreviations and Synonyms

- Blalock Taussig shunt, Blalock Taussig procedure, "blue-baby" operation

Definitions

- Palliative procedure to increase pulmonary blood-flow
- Original shunt sacrifices subclavian artery (distal ligation) proximal portion is routed downwards to end to side anastomosis with ipsilateral branch pulmonary artery
  - Named after Alfred Blalock (surgeon to first perform procedure, 1899-1964) and Helen Taussig (pediatric cardiologist, designed shunt, 1898-1986)
    - First performed November 1944 at Johns Hopkins University Hospital
- Modified BT shunt uses synthetic graft, usually polytetrafluoroethylene (Gore-Tex®)
  - Proximal anastomosis is end to side between graft (end) and subclavian artery or brachiocephalic trunk (side)
  - Distal anastomosis is end to side between distal graft (end) and ipsilateral pulmonary artery (side)

IMAGING FINDINGS

General Features

- Complications
  - Subclavian artery occlusion distal to graft anastomosis
  - Shunt occlusion in 11% of cases
    - More common in smaller grafts (4 mm)
  - Perigraft seroma in 2.5-9.5%
- Definitive repair usually follows in early childhood
  - VSD closure and Dacron patch relieving right ventricular outflow tract obstruction

Radiographic Findings

- Increased pulmonary blood-flow
- Rib notching ipsilateral to traditional shunt

CT Findings

- Tubular contrast-filled structure connecting subclavian and ipsilateral pulmonary artery
  - Occluded shunts difficult to visualize due to absence of contrast, multiplanar reconstructions helpful
- Excellent tool for detection of aortopulmonary collaterals prior to definitive repair

DDx: Blalock-Taussig Shunt

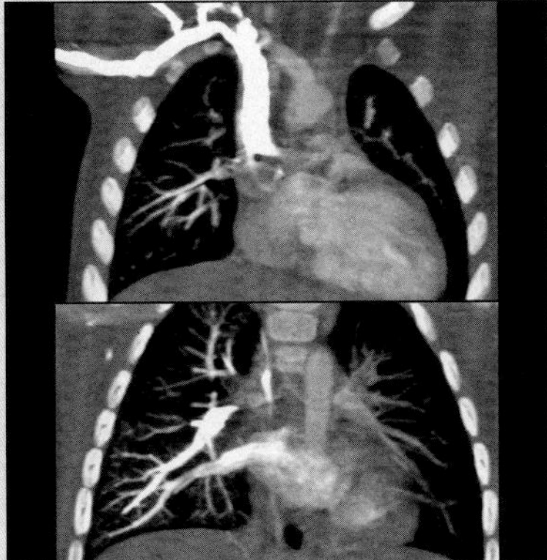

Glenn Shunt

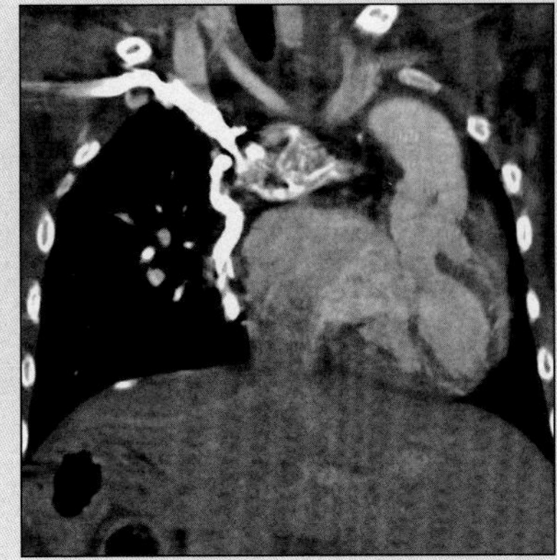

Glenn + Venous Collateral

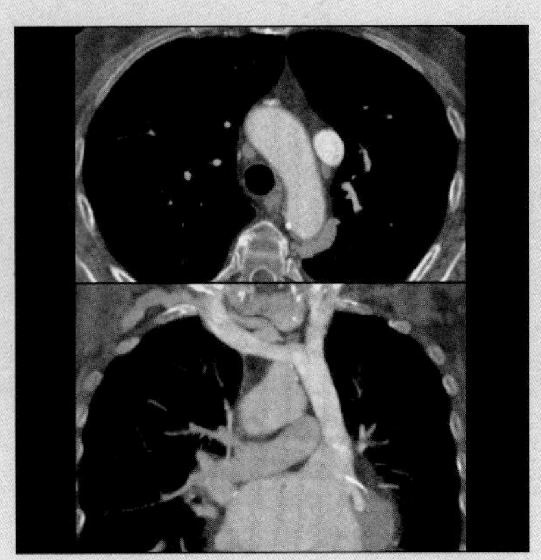

Left SVC

TETRALOGY OF FALLOT PALLIATION: BT SHUNT

Key Facts

Terminology

- Palliative procedure to increase pulmonary blood-flow
- Original shunt sacrifices subclavian artery (distal ligation) proximal portion is routed downwards to end to side anastomosis with ipsilateral branch pulmonary artery
- Modified BT shunt uses synthetic graft, usually polytetrafluoroethylene (Gore-Tex®)
- Proximal anastomosis is end to side between graft (end) and subclavian artery or brachiocephalic trunk (side)
- Distal anastomosis is end to side between distal graft (end) and ipsilateral pulmonary artery (side)

Imaging Findings

- Definitive repair usually follows in early childhood
- VSD closure and Dacron patch relieving right ventricular outflow tract obstruction

MR Findings

- Extra tubular flow void structure connecting subclavian and ipsilateral pulmonary artery
  - Bright signal on gradient echo or SSFP sequences
  - May contain high signal on spin echo or FSE or low signal on SSFP if occluded
- Perigraft seroma: T1 iso- and T2 hyperintense upper mediastinal collection with flow void (if patent shunt)
- May demonstrate chest wall collaterals if traditional BT or subclavian occlusion distal to graft anastomosis
- Phase contrast imaging allows quantification of flow dynamics

Echocardiographic Findings

- May demonstrate graft patency and pressure gradients across graft ± stenosis
- Turbulent flow entering right or left pulmonary artery

DIFFERENTIAL DIAGNOSIS

Other Forms of Tetralogy Palliation

- Waterston Cooley shunt
  - Ascending aorta to right pulmonary artery
- Potts shunt
  - Descending aorta to left pulmonary artery (no longer performed)

DIAGNOSTIC CHECKLIST

Consider

- Aorto-pulmonary collateral arteries may develop if otherwise insufficient pulmonary blood flow

SELECTED REFERENCES

1. van Rijn RR et al: Development of a perigraft seroma around modified Blalock-Taussig shunts: imaging evaluation. AJR Am J Roentgenol. 178(3):629-33, 2002
2. Coren ME et al: Complications of modified Blalock-Taussig shunts mimicking pulmonary disease. Arch Dis Child. 79(4):361-2, 1998
3. Hofbeck M et al: Color Doppler imaging of modified Blalock-Taussig shunts during infancy. Pediatr Cardiol. 15(6):163-6, 1994
4. Ichida F et al: [Magnetic resonance imaging: evaluation of the Blalock-Taussig shunts and anatomy of the pulmonary artery] J Cardiol. 22(4):669-78, 1992
5. Kastler B et al: Magnetic resonance imaging in congenital heart disease of newborns: preliminary results in 23 patients. Eur J Radiol. 10(2):109-17, 1990
6. Ullom RL et al: The Blalock-Taussig shunt in infants: standard versus modified. Ann Thorac Surg. 44(5):539-43, 1987
7. Sakuma I et al: [An application of X-ray computed tomography for complex cardiac anomalies] J Cardiogr. 13(3):699-713, 1983
8. Blalock A et al: The surgical treatment of malformation of the heart in which there is pulmonary stenosis or pulmonary atresia. JAMA. 128:189-202, 1945

IMAGE GALLERY

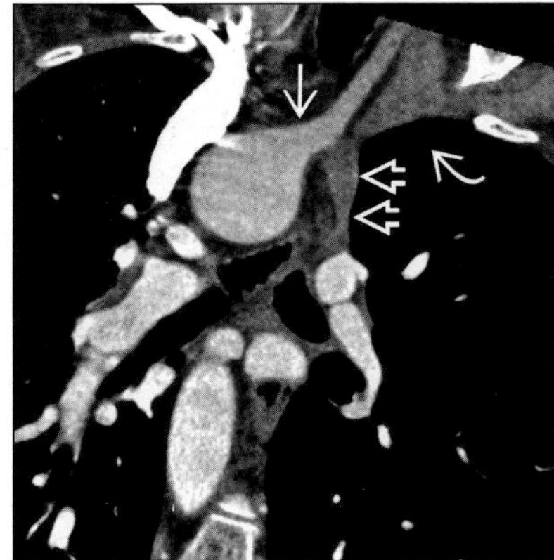

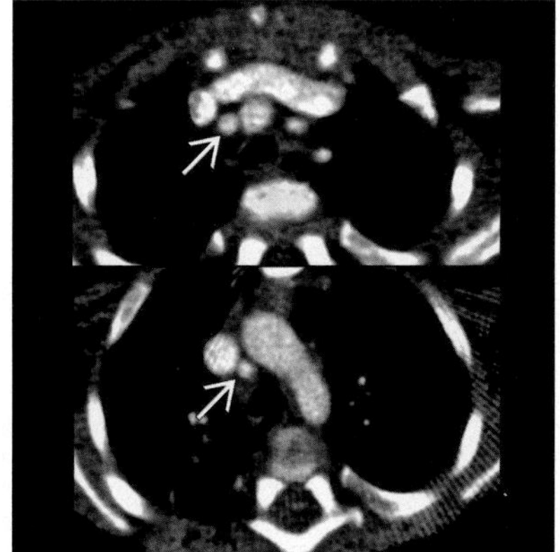

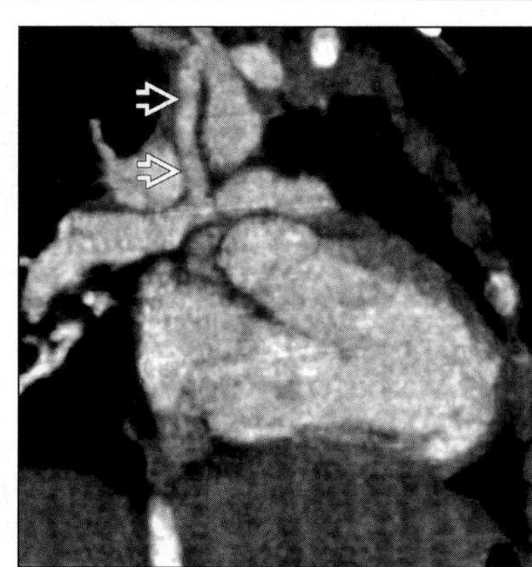

*(**Left**) Oblique CECT shows brachiocephalic trunk ➡ giving rise to left common carotid artery. Subclavian vein noted ➡ without accompanying artery. BT shunt ➡ occluded during definitive repair. (**Center**) Axial CECT shows "extra vessel" (BT shunt) ➡ adjacent to brachiocephalic trunk and aorta. (**Right**) Coronal CECT in same patient as previous image shows tubular synthetic graft ➡ connecting right subclavian artery and ipsilateral pulmonary artery.*

TETRALOGY OF FALLOT: DEFINITIVE REPAIR

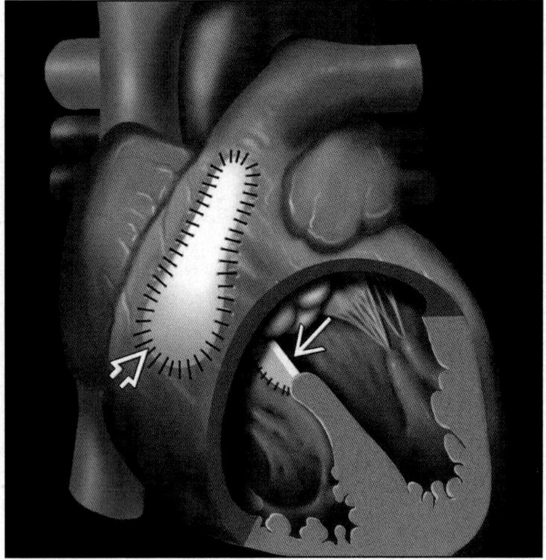

Graphic shows definitive Tetralogy of Fallot repair with ventricular septal defect patch ➡ and RVOT patch plasty ➡.

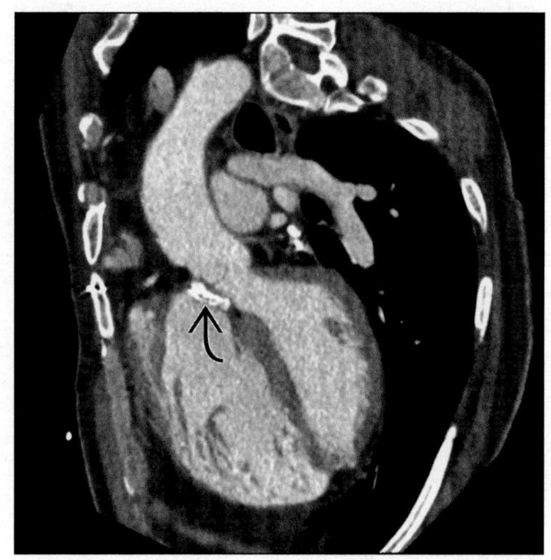

Oblique CECT shows densely calcified VSD patch repair ➚. Note overriding aorta and RV hypertrophy.

TERMINOLOGY

Abbreviations and Synonyms

- Tetralogy of Fallot (TOF) repair, complete repair

Definitions

- Closure of ventricular septal defect (VSD) and patch or graft repair of right ventricular outflow tract (RVOT) obstruction
  - Previous palliative shunts (Blalock-Taussig, Waterston-Cooley etc.,) usually taken down at time of definitive repair
  - VSD repair with prosthetic patch graft
  - RVOT obstruction (RVOTO) repair with RVOT or transannular patch ± division/resection of obstructing muscle bundles
    - Occasionally tube graft from RVOT patch or right atrium (RA) to pulmonary artery (PA) (Rastelli)
    - Semilunar pericardial allograft pulmonic valve repair or pulmonary valve sparing approaches may be chosen in some cases

IMAGING FINDINGS

General Features

- Best diagnostic clue
  - Calcified, nonenhancing patch between muscular ventricular septum and overriding aortic annulus (VSD repair)
    - Occasionally hyperdense pledgets may be noted
  - Thin and relatively deformed RVOT, potentially spanning into PA (± calcifications, hyperdense material)
    - Remainder of RA usually demonstrates thickened myocardium from RV hypertrophy
  - Occasionally hypoplastic PA with tube graft connecting RA to distal main PA

Radiographic Findings

- RV hypertrophy with filling of retrosternal clear-space
- May demonstrate calcifications along anterior RV wall on lateral radiograph
- May show systemic aorto-pulmonary collaterals

CT Findings

- CTA

DDx: Tetralogy of Fallot Repair

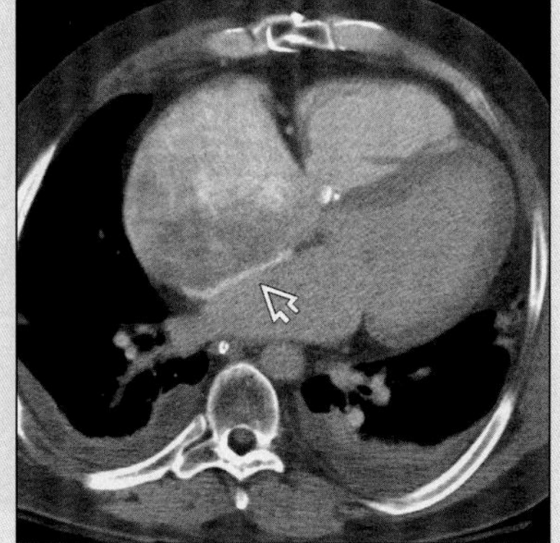

ASD Repair

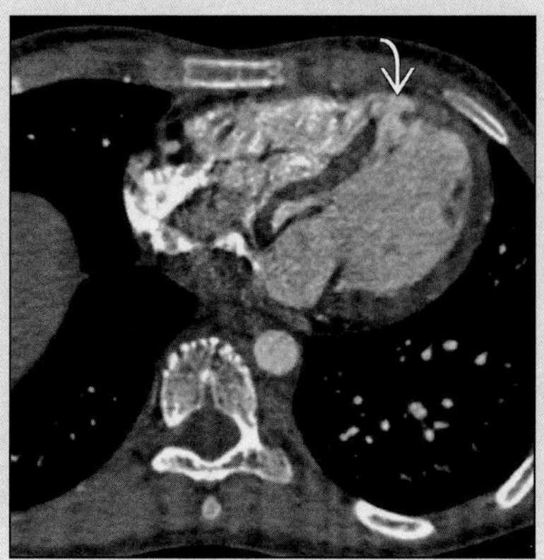

Isolated VSD

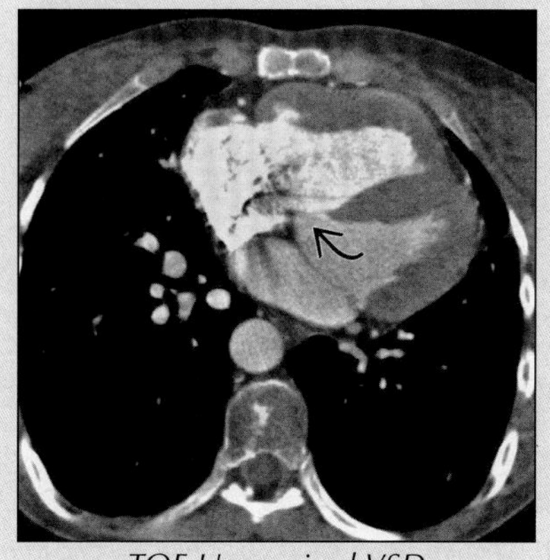

TOF Unrepaired VSD

TETRALOGY OF FALLOT: DEFINITIVE REPAIR

Key Facts

Terminology

- Closure of ventricular septal defect (VSD) and patch or graft repair of right ventricular outflow tract (RVOT) obstruction
- Previous palliative shunts (Blalock-Taussig, Waterston-Cooley etc.,) usually taken down at time of definitive repair
- VSD repair with prosthetic patch graft
- RVOT obstruction (RVOTO) repair with RVOT or transannular patch ± division/resection of obstructing muscle bundles

Imaging Findings

- Calcified, nonenhancing patch between muscular ventricular septum and overriding aortic annulus (VSD repair)
- RV hypertrophy with filling of retrosternal clear-space
- Calcified patch spanning malaligned ventricular septal defect from muscular septum to right aspect of aortic annulus
- CTA may show tube graft from RVOT patch or RA to distal main PA
- Gated CT preferred in adults because of motion free imaging of both intra and extracardiac structures
- MR is best tool for RV functional assessment
- **Phase contrast cine images**
- Can quantify pulmonic regurgitant fraction
- **Delayed enhancement**
- Fibrosis in adults correlates with markers of adverse clinical outcome, including ventricular dysfunction, exercise intolerance, and neurohormonal activation
- Isolated RV restriction late after repair in > 50% of patients
- Antegrade pulmonary flow during atrial systole

    - High density material at RVOT potentially transannular spanning into PA
        - May have pledgets at suture site
        - May calcify
        - Patch usually much thinner than native RV or RVOT tissue
    - RV dilatation + increased myocardial thickness
    - Aorta dextroposed overriding interventricular septum
    - Calcified patch spanning malaligned ventricular septal defect from muscular septum to right aspect of aortic annulus
        - Best seen on oblique left ventricular (LV) long axis view
        - May demonstrate hyperdense pledgets at suture sites
    - ± Native pulmonary artery stenoses
    - ± Aorto-pulmonary systemic collateral arteries
    - CTA may show tube graft from RVOT patch or RA to distal main PA
- Cardiac Gated CTA
    - Gated CT preferred in adults because of motion free imaging of both intra and extracardiac structures
    - Allows for calculation of RV function parameters

MR Findings

- MRA similar to CTA
- Perfusion MR shows patches as nonenhancing low intensity structures
- MR is best tool for RV functional assessment
    - Ejection fraction, end systolic and end diastolic volumes, muscle mass, and regional wall-motion abnormalities
- **Phase contrast cine images**
    - Can quantify pulmonic regurgitant fraction
- **Delayed enhancement**
    - Abnormal hyperenhancement indicates ventricular fibrosis
    - Fibrosis in adults correlates with markers of adverse clinical outcome, including ventricular dysfunction, exercise intolerance, and neurohormonal activation
    - Associated with arrhythmias

Echocardiographic Findings

- Routine imaging tool of choice for tetralogy repair follow-up
- Pulmonary regurgitation of varying degree
- Isolated RV restriction late after repair in > 50% of patients
    - A-wave contributes to pulmonary arterial forward flow and shortens duration of regurgitation resulting in relatively decreased cardiomegaly and improved exercise performance in patients with restriction
    - Antegrade pulmonary flow during atrial systole
    - Augmented during inspiration

Angiographic Findings

- Invasive but may allow interventions
    - Balloon angioplasty of branch pulmonary stenoses

Imaging Recommendations

- Best imaging tool
    - Depends on age and clinical question
    - ECHO best for intracardiac assessment of VSD
    - CTA best for detection of branch pulmonary stenosis and multiple aorto-pulmonary collateral arteries (MAPCA)

CLINICAL ISSUES

Natural History & Prognosis

- Long term complications include arrhythmias, RV function deterioration, pulmonary regurgitation and pulmonary artery stenoses
- Arrhythmias may be due to RVOT myotomies or muscle bundle resection or due to severe pulmonary regurgitation and RV dilatation
- Atrial flutter more common than atrial fibrillation
- Ventricular arrhythmias may be self limited but may require treatment
    - May lead to sudden cardiac death
    - Treatment may necessitate radiofrequency ablation
    - ± Implantable cardioverter defibrillator (ICD)

TETRALOGY OF FALLOT: DEFINITIVE REPAIR

- RV dilatation, functional and exercise deterioration usually due to pulmonary regurgitation
- Pregnancy may be feasible in some cases with modern TOF repairs

Treatment

- Pulmonary stenoses may be balloon dilated
  - MAPCAs occasionally coiled at same time
- Ventricular arrhythmia treatments include medical therapy, device/resynchronization therapy, and percutaneous intervention
- Severe pulmonary regurgitation may be repaired with elective pulmonary valve replacement
  - Benefit controversial
  - Should be performed before irreversible RV dysfunction ensues

DIAGNOSTIC CHECKLIST

Consider

- Volume-rendering of CTA or MRA for anatomic pulmonary arterial and RVOT anatomy assessment
- Gated CTA in adults
- Check for late complications
  - Branch pulmonary stenosis
  - Aorto-pulmonary systemic collaterals

SELECTED REFERENCES

1. Aboulhosn J et al: Management after childhood repair of tetralogy of fallot. Curr Treat Options Cardiovasc Med. 8(6):474-83, 2006
2. Babu-Narayan SV et al: Ventricular fibrosis suggested by cardiovascular magnetic resonance in adults with repaired tetralogy of fallot and its relationship to adverse markers of clinical outcome. Circulation. 113(3):405-13, 2006
3. Grothoff M et al: Pulmonary regurgitation is a powerful factor influencing QRS duration in patients after surgical repair of tetralogy of Fallot : A Magnetic Resonance Imaging (MRI) study. Clin Res Cardiol. 2006
4. Kleinveld G et al: Hemodynamic and electrocardiographic effects of early pulmonary valve replacement in pediatric patients after transannular complete repair of tetralogy of Fallot. Pediatr Cardiol. 27(3):329-35, 2006
5. Norton KI et al: Cardiac MR imaging assessment following tetralogy of fallot repair. Radiographics. 26(1):197-211, 2006
6. Buechel ER et al: Remodelling of the right ventricle after early pulmonary valve replacement in children with repaired tetralogy of Fallot: assessment by cardiovascular magnetic resonance. Eur Heart J. 26(24):2721-7, 2005
7. Hui W et al: Comparison of modified short axis view and apical four chamber view in evaluating right ventricular function after repair of tetralogy of Fallot. Int J Cardiol. 105(3):256-61, 2005
8. Oosterhof T et al: Corrected tetralogy of Fallot: delayed enhancement in right ventricular outflow tract. Radiology. 237(3):868-71, 2005
9. Therrien J et al: Optimal timing for pulmonary valve replacement in adults after tetralogy of Fallot repair. Am J Cardiol. 95(6):779-82, 2005
10. Geva T et al: Factors associated with impaired clinical status in long-term survivors of tetralogy of Fallot repair evaluated by magnetic resonance imaging. J Am Coll Cardiol. 43(6):1068-74, 2004
11. Li W et al: Doppler-echocardiographic assessment of pulmonary regurgitation in adults with repaired tetralogy of Fallot: comparison with cardiovascular magnetic resonance imaging. Am Heart J. 147(1):165-72, 2004
12. van Straten A et al: Right ventricular function after pulmonary valve replacement in patients with tetralogy of Fallot. Radiology. 233(3):824-9, 2004
13. Chien SJ et al: Idiopathic calcific constrictive pericarditis causing pulmonary stenosis associated with a ventricular septal defect mimicking tetralogy of Fallot. J Clin Ultrasound. 31(4):222-5, 2003
14. Duncan BW et al: Staged repair of tetralogy of Fallot with pulmonary atresia and major aortopulmonary collateral arteries. J Thorac Cardiovasc Surg. 126(3):694-702, 2003
15. Horstkotte D et al: [Congenital heart disease and acquired valvular lesions in pregnancy] Herz. 28(3):227-39, 2003
16. Kang IS et al: Differential regurgitation in branch pulmonary arteries after repair of tetralogy of Fallot: a phase-contrast cine magnetic resonance study. Circulation. 107(23):2938-43, 2003
17. Cho JM et al: Early and long-term results of the surgical treatment of tetralogy of Fallot with pulmonary atresia, with or without major aortopulmonary collateral arteries. J Thorac Cardiovasc Surg. 124(1):70-81, 2002
18. de Ruijter FT et al: Right ventricular dysfunction and pulmonary valve replacement after correction of tetralogy of Fallot. Ann Thorac Surg. 73(6):1794-800; discussion 1800, 2002
19. Promphan W et al: The right and left ventricular function after surgical correction with pericardial monocusp in tetralogy of fallot: mid-term result. J Med Assoc Thai. 85 Suppl 4:S1266-74, 2002
20. Vliegen HW et al: Magnetic resonance imaging to assess the hemodynamic effects of pulmonary valve replacement in adults late after repair of tetralogy of fallot. Circulation. 106(13):1703-7, 2002
21. Hirsch JC et al: Complete repair of tetralogy of Fallot in the neonate: results in the modern era. Ann Surg. 232(4):508-14, 2000
22. Waldman JD et al: Cyanotic congenital heart disease with decreased pulmonary blood flow in children. Pediatr Clin North Am. 46(2):385-404, 1999
23. McElhinney DB et al: Atrioventricular septal defect with common valvar orifice and tetralogy of Fallot revisited: making a case for primary repair in infancy. Cardiol Young. 8(4):455-61, 1998
24. Gatzoulis MA et al: Right ventricular diastolic function 15 to 35 years after repair of tetralogy of Fallot. Restrictive physiology predicts superior exercise performance. Circulation. 91(6):1775-81, 1995
25. Arciniegas E et al: Early and late results of total correction of tetralogy of Fallot. J Thorac Cardiovasc Surg. 80(5):770-8, 1980

TETRALOGY OF FALLOT: DEFINITIVE REPAIR

IMAGE GALLERY

Typical

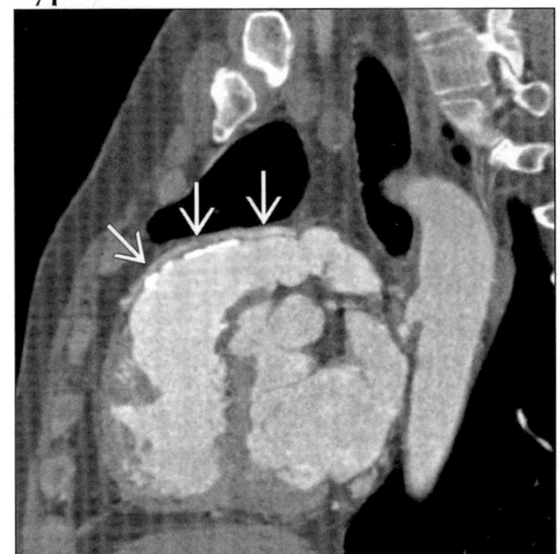

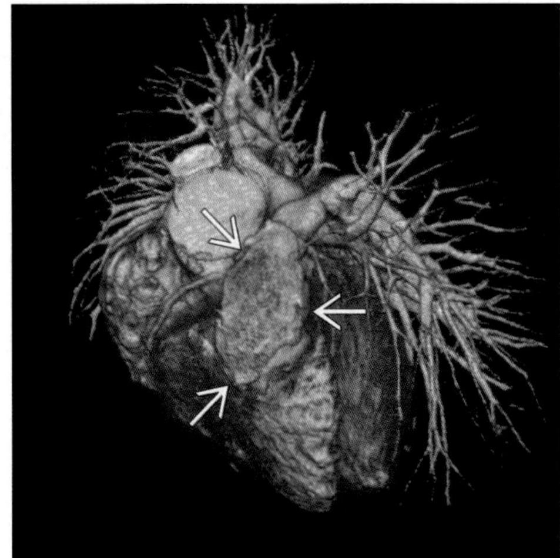

(Left) *Sagittal coronary CTA shows hyperdense synthetic material with calcifications spanning RVOT and proximal pulmonary artery, representing RVOT patch repair →. Note: Absent pulmonary valve leaflets.* ***(Right)*** *Oblique CTA volume rendering in same patient as previous image shows right ventricular outflow patch → extending into proximal pulmonary artery.*

Typical

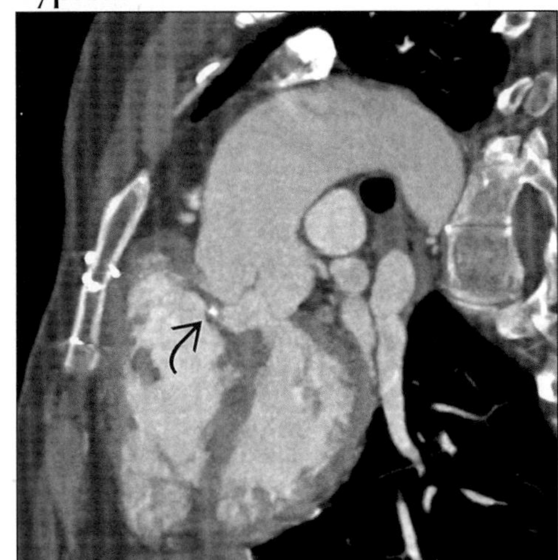

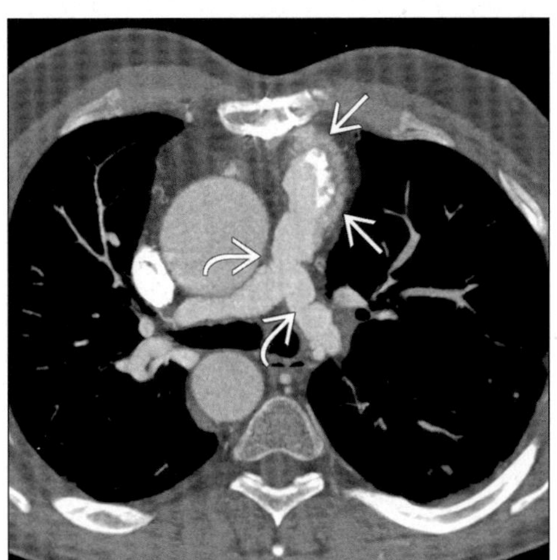

(Left) *Oblique cardiac CT shows dextroposed aorta overriding ventricular septum, RV hypertrophy and VSD patch repair with small calcification →.* ***(Right)*** *Axial CECT shows pulmonary artery with partially calcified RVOT patch →. Note: Pulmonary artery stenoses →.*

Variant

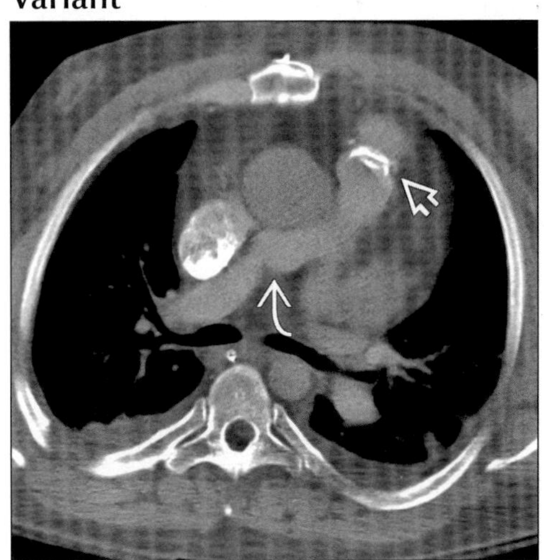

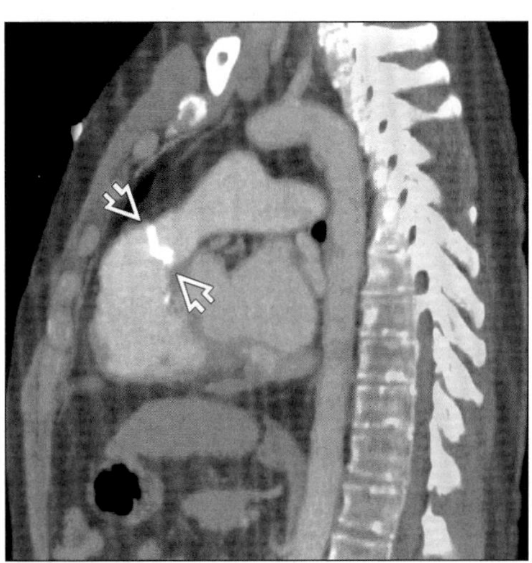

(Left) *Oblique CECT in adult patient with TOF shows pulmonary valve replacement →. Note: Right pulmonary artery distortion → due to previous Waterston shunt.* ***(Right)*** *Sagittal CECT in same patient as previous image shows prosthetic pulmonary valve →.*

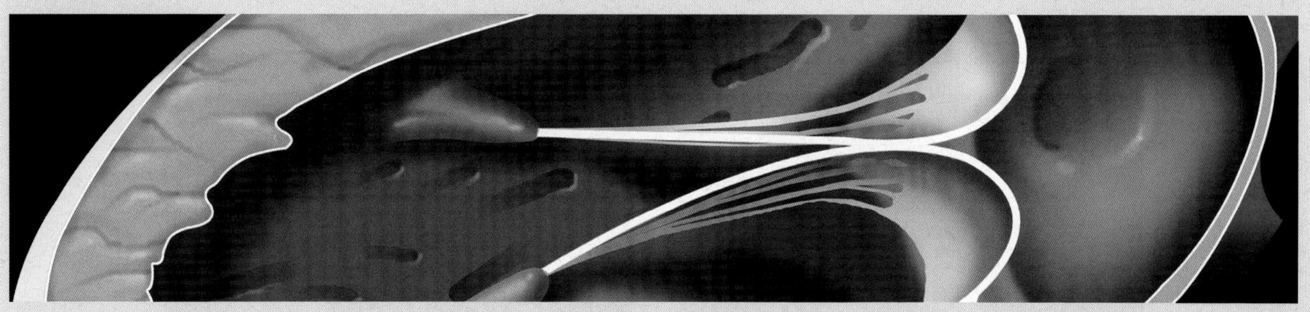

SECTION 2: Valvular

Introduction and Overview

Valvular

ANATOMY OF THE HEART

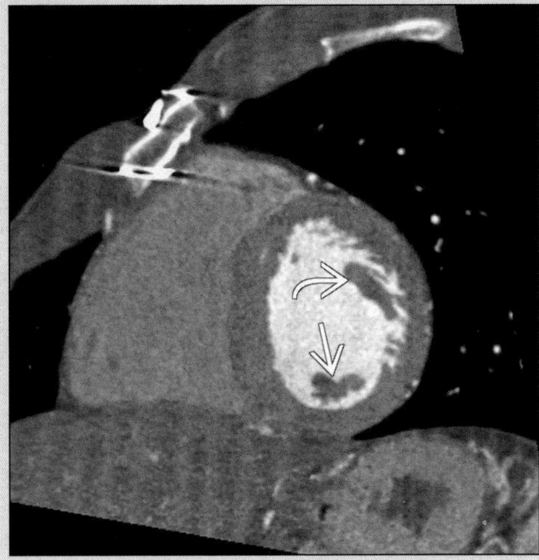

LV short axis cardiac CT shows LV as a round structure containing 2 papillary muscles (anterior-lateral ➡ and inferior medial ➡). Note: No trabecula or papillary muscles arise from LV septum.

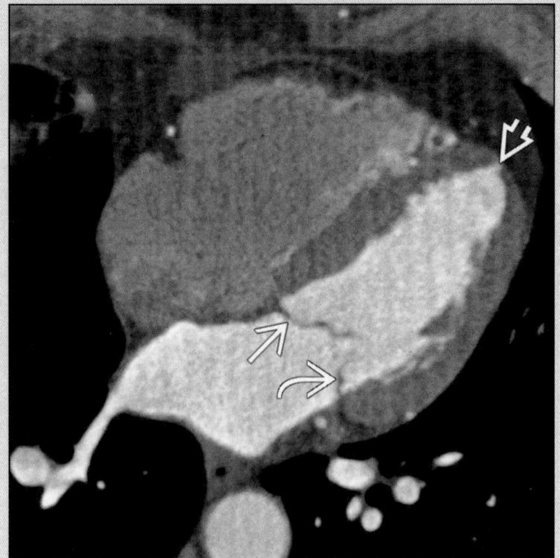

Four chamber view cardiac CT shows well opacified LA and LV with anterior ➡ and posterior ➡ MV leaflets. RA and RV are not opacified, rendering tricuspid valve invisible. Note: Normal LV thin-point ➡.

TERMINOLOGY

Abbreviations

- Left ventricle (LV)
- Left atrium (LA)
- Left atrial appendage (LAA)
- Right ventricle (RV)
- Right atrium (RA)
- Right atrial appendage (RAA)
- Aortic valve (AV)
- Mitral valve (MV)
- Right ventricular outflow tract (RVOT)
- Aorta (Ao)
- Pulmonary artery (PA)
- Pulmonary vein (PV)
  - Left inferior pulmonary vein (LIPV)
  - Left superior pulmonary vein (LSPV)
  - Right inferior pulmonary vein (RIPV)
  - Right superior pulmonary vein (RSPV)
- Superior vena cava (SVC)
- Inferior vena cava (IVC)
- Coronary sinus (CS)
  - Middle cardiac vein (MCV)
  - Great cardiac vein (GCV)
  - Marginal vein (MV) or lateral vein (LV)
  - Posterior vein of the left ventricle (PVLV), posterior left-ventricular vein (PLV)
  - Anterior interventricular vein (AIV)

IMAGING ANATOMY

General Anatomic Considerations

- Interpretation of anatomy is dependent on technology used as chamber lumen will be depicted based on various criteria
  - MR depiction of cavity lumen
    - White blood technique: Blood in motion is depicted as white, however flow artifact may cause signal dropout (black jets or lines across lumen)
    - Black blood techniques: Blood in rapid through-plane motion is depicted as black, however slower flowing, stagnant blood, or blood moving within the image plane may demonstrate high signal intensity
  - CT depiction of cavity lumen
    - Depends on level of contrast opacification
    - Often right-sided chambers without contrast and left-sided chambers contrast enhanced
    - If differential opacification of adjacent chambers is present, shunt across the chambers will be evident as high or low density jets
    - If slow filling of a chamber or part of a chamber is present, absence of enhancement may be due to thrombus or simply due to poor mixing of contrast enhanced blood with unenhanced blood (e.g., false-positive thrombus in LAA)

Critical Anatomic Structures

- **Right atrium**
  - Smooth-walled chamber that receives IVC, SVC, and coronary sinus and small anterior cardiac veins
    - Ridge between IVC and inferior RA is called Eustachian ridge
    - Eustachian ridge is remnant of eustachian valve
    - Eustachian valve function in utero: Directs arterialized blood (umbilical system/ductus venosus) from IVC through foramen ovale into LA
  - Thebesian valve at ostium of coronary sinus is visible in one third of cardiac CTAs
  - Contains a vertical ridge called "crista terminalis"
    - Connects SVC and IVC and contains fibers connecting sino atrial and atrioventricular nodes
    - Can be confused with mural thrombus or mass
  - Right atrial appendage is adjacent to SVC inflow
    - Broad-based, triangular shape
    - Contains pectinate muscles
  - Connects via tricuspid valve to RV
- **Right ventricle**
  - Anterior most chamber, triangular in shape
    - Anterior free wall of RV is immediately behind the sternum

ANATOMY OF THE HEART

Delayed Hyperenhancement (HE) Patterns

Subendocardial (= Ischemic)

- Confined to a coronary territory
- Acute or chronic myocardial infarcts demonstrate HE that is invariably based on the **subendocardium**
- Degree of transmurality is variable and ranges from a thin stripe of subendocardial HE to transmural HE
- Myocardium is thought to be "viable" (i.e., improvement of contractility after revascularization) if HE is less than 50% of wall thickness

Mid Myocardial HE (= Non-Ischemic)

- Linear within septum
  - Suggestive myocarditis or dilated cardiomyopathy
- Focal, at RV insertion sites
  - Hypertrophic cardiomyopathy (HCM)
- Patchy, non-coronary distribution
  - Non-specific, but **not** ischemic (sarcoid, HCM, Chagas disease, Myocarditis, etc.)

Subepicardial (= Non-Ischemic)

- Enhancement based on the outside border of LV myocardium, but not reaching endocardial surface
- Non-specific, but thought to be more typical for sarcoidosis and myocarditis [insufficient data available at this time]

Global Subendocardial HE

- Typically non-transmural enhancement of entire LV myocardium
  - Cardiac transplant
  - Amyloidosis

    - Does not contribute to the cardiac silhouette on frontal radiographs
  - Heavy trabeculations
  - Tricuspid valve is separated by a complete muscular ring (RVOT, infundibulum, conus) from the pulmonic valve
  - RV has trabecula and papillary muscles arising from the ventricular septum (LV does not!)
  - RV has three muscular bands that may contain conduction fibers (moderator band, parietal band, and septal band)
    - Moderator band is a prominent trabeculation that connects septum with apical portion of anterior RV free wall (inferior to parietal band)
    - Parietal band seen at junction of anterior RV free wall and RVOT
    - Septal band is difficult to see on MR or CT, runs between inlet and outlet portion of RV
- **Left atrium**
  - Receives typically 4 major pulmonary veins but PV anatomy is very variable
  - Common variants include
    - Common trunk of left superior and inferior PV
    - Separate origin of middle lobe PV
    - "Top pulmonary vein" = accessory vein that drains into LA superiorly and courses behind bronchus to superior segment of lower lobe (usually on left)
  - Junction of left superior PV and LAA forms a ridge (Q-tip sign) that on echocardiography can cause an reverberation artifact that projects echoes into the LAA and mimics thrombus
    - Because such false positive findings lead to unnecessary Coumadin therapy of affected patients, this normal structure is also referred to as the "Coumadin ridge"
    - This does not pose a diagnostic challenge for either CT or MR, but when correlating with a positive or questionable echocardiogram, presence of a prominent Coumadin ridge and absence of LAA thrombus may suggest false positive echo finding
  - Gives rise to LAA
    - Narrow ostium
    - Usually turns anterior and covers LM bifurcation and proximal LCX
    - Contains pectinate muscles that can be confused with thrombus
    - May contain filling defect or contrast gradient due to slow filling (poor LAA ejection fraction) which may mimic LAA thrombus on CT
    - Delayed focused scan helpful in demonstrating late filling of LAA (in absence of thrombus) or persistent filling defect (diagnostic of thrombus)
- **Left ventricle**
  - Bullet-shaped chamber, less trabeculated compared to RV
  - Contains two papillary muscles
    - Antero-lateral
    - Postero-medial
  - Chordae tendinae connect papillary muscles and edges of mitral valve (MV) leaflets
  - Mitral valve and semilunar valve (normally aortic, unless transposition of great vessels, then pulmonic) are always in fibrous continuity
  - LV wall consists of endocardium, myocardium, epicardial fat (contains coronary arteries) and epicardium (also known as visceral pericardium)
  - Ventricular septum normally does not give rise to trabeculations or papillary muscles
    - Basal most portion of interventricular septum is a short and thin segment called membranous septum (connects to aortic root)
  - Apical thin-point is at short segment at the apex where all fibers converge to a very thin fibrous plate (1-2 mm)
    - Width of the thin-point is only 1-3 mm, which differentiates it from chronic apical infarcts (usually > 1 cm width of thinned myocardium)
    - On cardiac CT the LV thin-point is visible in every individual
    - In MR, echocardiography and nuclear cardiology the LV thin-point is only occasionally observed due to poorer resolution and prospective prescription of slice orientation

ANATOMY OF THE HEART

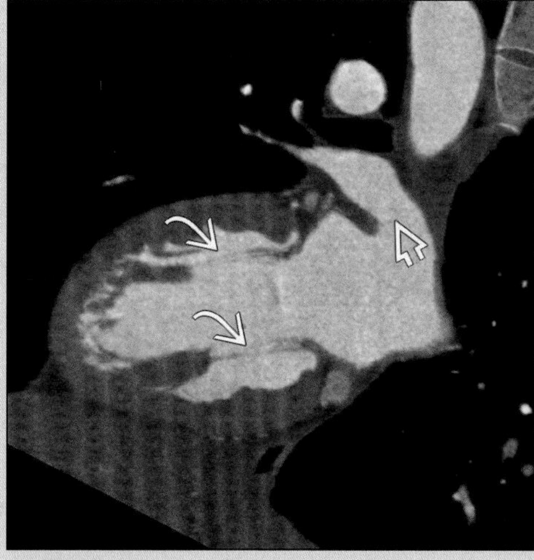

Paraseptal long-axis LV view of cardiac CTA shows bullet-shaped LV with papillary muscles and chordae tendinae ➔ connecting to MV. Note: Left superior PV ➔ always faces anteriorly.

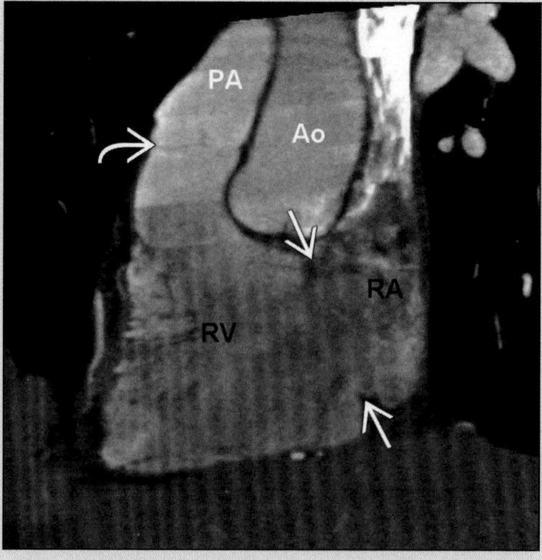

Paraseptal long-axis RV view of cardiac CTA shows triangular RV with RVOT separating the tricuspid annulus ➔ and pulmonic ➔ valve.

- Left ventricle is divided into 17 segments which are derived from 3 short axis LV levels (basal, mid and apical)
  - Basal (6 segments): Anterior, anterior septal, inferior septal, inferior, inferior-lateral, anterior-lateral
  - Mid (6 segments): Anterior, anterior septal, inferior septal, inferior, inferior-lateral, anterior-lateral
  - Apical (4 segments): Anterior, septal, inferior, lateral
  - Last segment is the "apex", best evaluated on 4 chamber or other LV long axis view
- Each segment is named by identifying the "level" (basal, mid, or apical) followed by the orientation
  - Examples: Mid antero-lateral segment, apical septal segment

Anatomic Relationships

- Thicker septum secundum and thinner septum primum for interatrial septum
  - Fossa ovalis contains only septum primum
  - Separation of septae can be seen in absence of patent foramen ovale (PFO)
  - PFO may be called if a contrast column can be followed from the higher density LA into the lower density RA (commonly through a channel between septum primum and secundum)

ANATOMY-BASED IMAGING ISSUES

Normal Measurements

- LV end diastolic volume (EDV) derived from MR
  - Men (mean [95% upper limit]): 114.9 mL [169.0 mL]
  - Women (mean [95% upper limit]): 84.4 mL [116.5 mL]
- LV end systolic volume (ESV)
  - Men (mean [95% upper limit]): 36.3 mL [65.0 mL]
  - Women (mean [95% upper limit]): 25.1 mL [40.9 mL]
- Ejection fraction (stroke volume [EDV-ESV] divided by EDV) = 55-75%
- Cardiac output (volume of blood ejected per minute) = 4-8 L/min at rest
- Stroke volume (volume of blood ejected with each cardiac cycle) = 60-100 mL/beat
- Cardiac Index (body size vs. cardiac output) = 2.5-4 L/min/m2
- LV myocardial thickness is measured only in end-diastole
  - Normal ≤ 12 mm
  - Basal septum may be slightly thicker
- LV mass
  - Men (mean [95% upper limit]): 155 g [201 g]
  - Women (mean [95% upper limit]): 103 g [134 g]

PATHOLOGY-BASED IMAGING ISSUES

Imaging Pitfalls

- Black blood techniques
  - Slowly moving blood, or blood moving within the image plane may have poor black blood effect which results in bright lumen
  - This may mimic intra cardiac or vascular thrombus or masses

RELATED REFERENCES

1. Mahrholdt H et al: Delayed enhancement cardiovascular magnetic resonance assessment of non-ischaemic cardiomyopathies. Eur Heart J. 26(15):1461-74, 2005
2. Shah et al. In: Edelman RR, et al., eds. Clinical Magnetic Resonance Imaging, 3rd ed. New York, Elsevier Press, 2005
3. Salton CJ et al: Gender differences and normal left ventricular anatomy in an adult population free of hypertension. A cardiovascular magnetic resonance study of the Framingham Heart Study Offspring cohort. J Am Coll Cardiol. 39(6):1055-60, 2002

IMAGE GALLERY

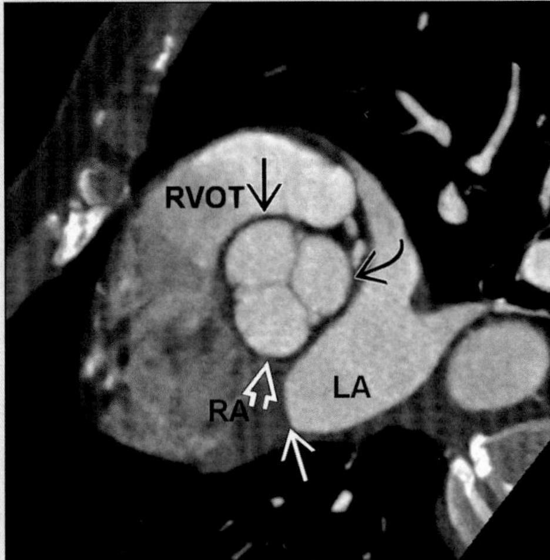

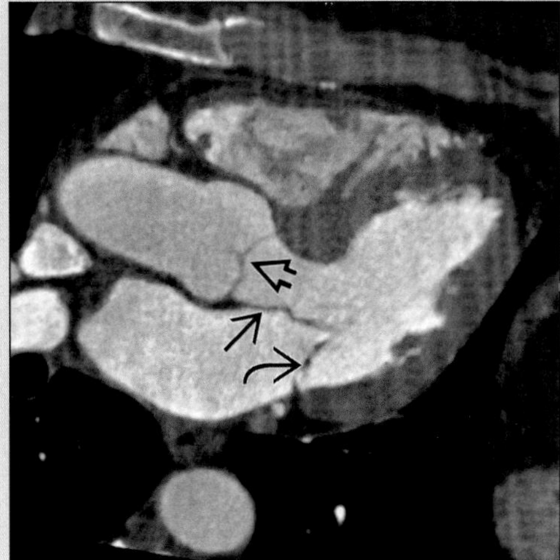

(Left) *Aortic valve short axis cardiac CT shows right coronary cusp → adjacent to RVOT, non-coronary cusp → adjacent to interatrial septum →, and left coronary cusp → adjacent to LAA.* ***(Right)*** *Three chamber view cardiac CT shows the atrioventricular valve (anterior → and posterior → mitral leaflets) and semilunar valve (aortic) → in fibrous continuity (as opposed to RV, where the RVOT separates the two).*

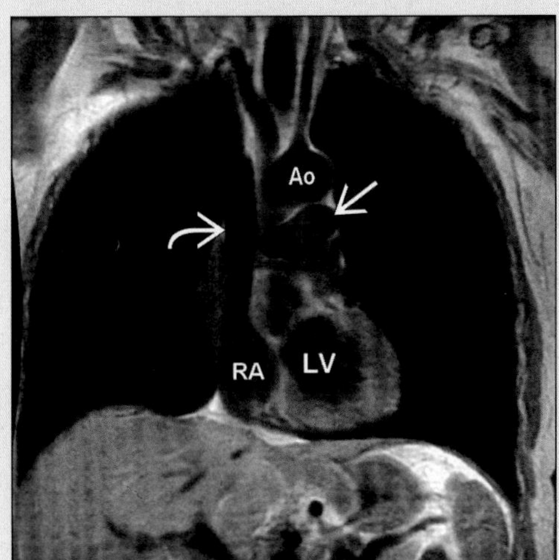

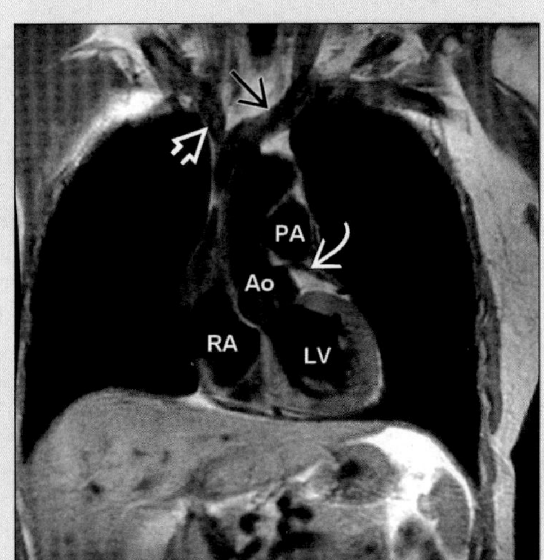

(Left) *Coronal T1WI FS MR shows RA receiving SVC →, aortic arch (Ao) giving rise to left common carotid artery, PA bifurcation → and LV.* ***(Right)*** *Coronal T2WI FSE MR (more anterior) shows aortic root originating from LV and giving rise to LM →. Note: Left → and right → innominate veins show blood as high signal intensity due to slow in-plane flow (mimics thrombus).*

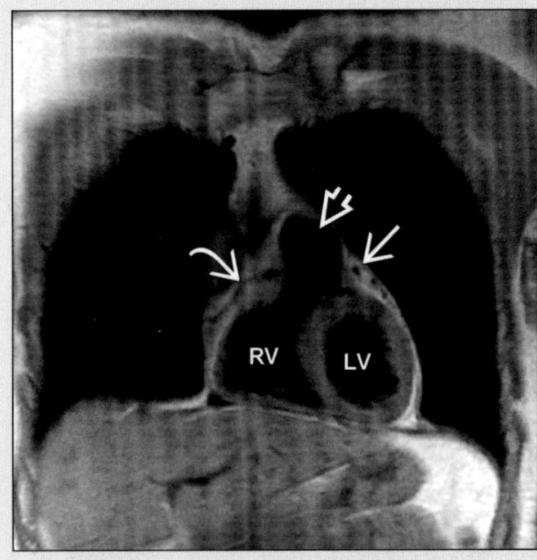

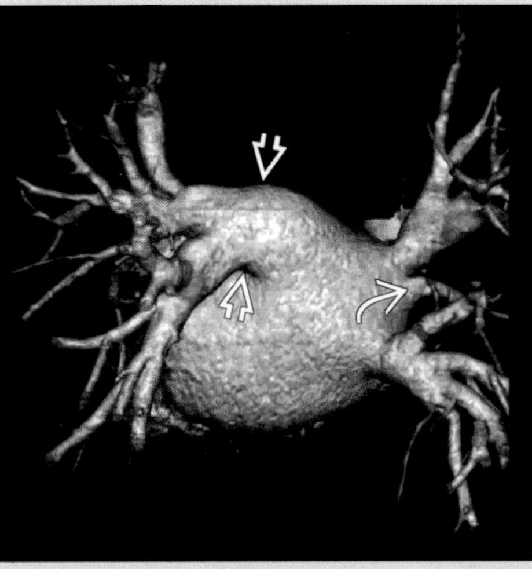

(Left) *Coronal T1WI FSE MR more anterior than previous shows RV and origin of PA → from RVOT. Note: Flow void from RCA →, and LAD →.* ***(Right)*** *Posterior VRT view cardiac CT shows normal variant anatomy of PVs with a common trunk → for left superior and inferior PV and a separate ostium of the right middle lobe PV →.*

AORTIC STENOSIS

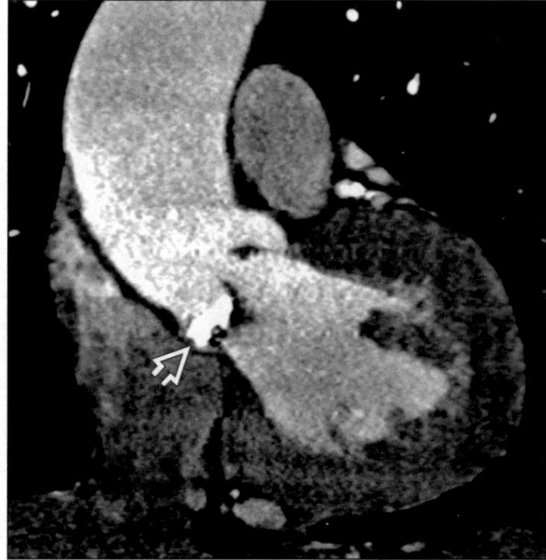

Coronal oblique cardiac CT shows a calcific ➡ aortic leaflet leading to restriction and stenosis of the aortic valve.

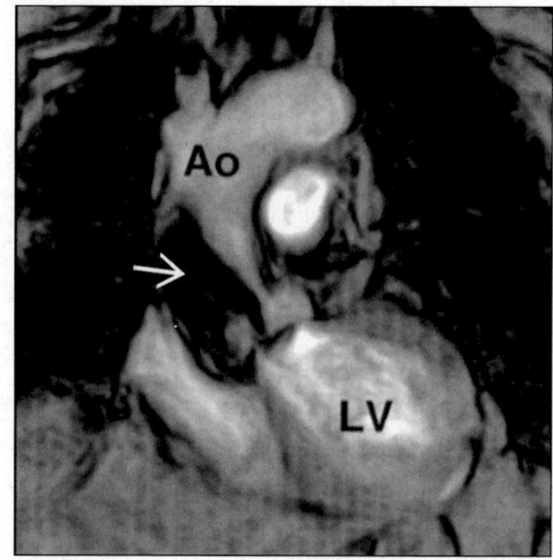

Coronal oblique MR cine shows a jet in the ascending aorta ➡ during LV systole, indicating aortic valve stenosis.

TERMINOLOGY

Abbreviations and Synonyms

- Aortic stenosis (AS)

Definitions

- Narrowing of the aortic outflow tract causing obstruction to flow from the left ventricle (LV) into the ascending aorta
  - Valvular (most common); subvalvular (rare); supravalvular (extremely rare)

IMAGING FINDINGS

General Features

- Best diagnostic clue: High velocity jet of blood ejected into left ventricular outflow during systole
- Morphology: Thickening, fusion and/or calcification of the aortic valve apparatus
- High peak systolic transvalvular pressure gradient
- Severe aortic stenosis (AS) may lead to concentric left ventricular hypertrophy (> 12 mm myocardium thickness)

Radiographic Findings

- Radiography
  - Chest X-ray
    - Enlarged cardiac silhouette with rounding of the left ventricular free wall and elevated apex
    - Calcification of the valve is frequent (best seen on lateral view)
    - Left ventricular enlargement may develop at late stage of chronic disease (LV failure)
    - Post-stenotic ascending aortic dilatation may be present

CT Findings

- NECT: Quantification of aortic valve calcification: > 1100 Agatston Score Units as cut-off for severe AS (93% sensitivity; 82% specificity)
- Cardiac Gated CTA
  - Fibrous leaflet thickening (hypodense) > 2 mm and calcification (hyperdense)
  - Concentric left ventricular hypertrophy (> 12 mm); later LV-dilatation and dysfunction
  - Planimetric measurement of the aortic valve orifice area (AVA) during mid-late systole
  - Post-stenotic dilatation of the ascending aorta

DDx: Types of Aortic Stenosis

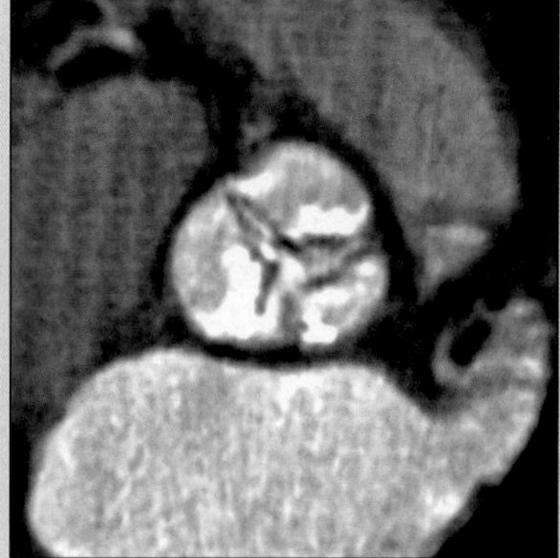

Degenerative AS (Tricuspid AV)

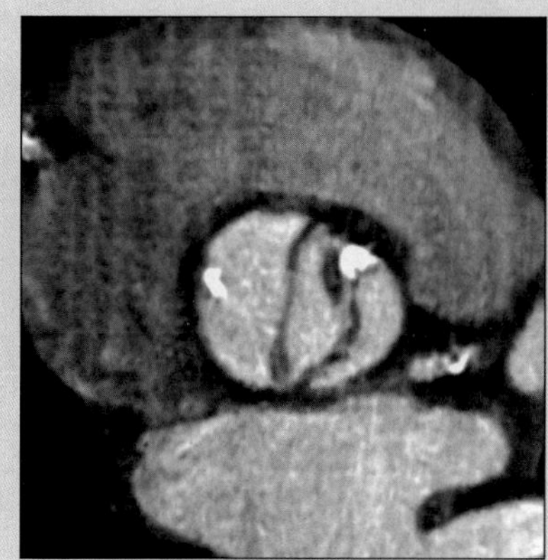

AS - Bicuspid Aortic Valve

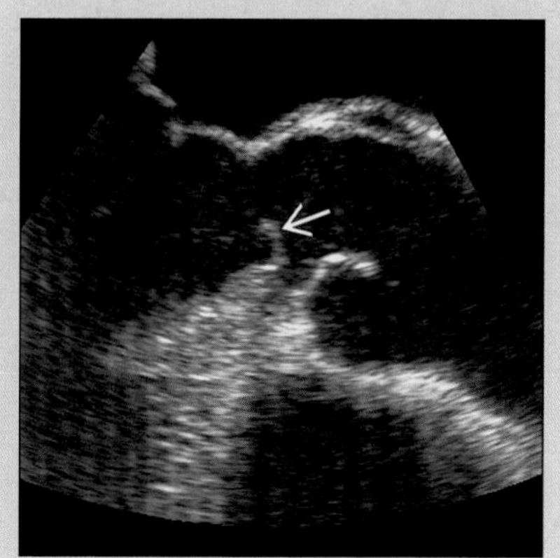

Subvalvular Membrane

AORTIC STENOSIS

Key Facts

Terminology

- Narrowing of the aortic outflow tract at valvular, or rarely at subvalvular levels

Imaging Findings

- Thickening, fusion and/or calcification of the aortic valve apparatus
- Severe aortic stenosis leads to concentric left ventricular hypertrophy
- LV-dysfunction (by Echo, CT or MR); MR is gold standard
- Best imaging tool: Echocardiography (high systolic transvalvular pressure gradient)
- Cardiac MR can calculate AVA (cine images) and peak systolic velocity and gradients (phase contrast)

Top Differential Diagnoses

- Degenerative/Calcific
- Rheumatic Disease
- Bicuspid Valve
- Subvalvular Aortic Stenosis

Clinical Issues

- Asymptomatic over long period ("mystery killer")
- LV-function is an important parameter to predict outcome and to define clinical management
- Surgical aortic valve replacement (AVR) is the standard treatment in patients with severe AS
- Surgical AVR significantly improves ventricular function and prognosis

  - Allows evaluation of coronary artery disease before valve surgery
  - Co-existent aortic regurgitation (usually mild-to-moderate) during diastole

MR Findings

- Systolic flow void (jet) into proximal aorta on bright blood cine imaging
- Left ventricular hypertrophy in severe AS, ± dilatation if LV failure occurs
- Calculation of the aortic valve area (AVA) has excellent correlation as compared to TEE
- Phase contrast MR allows for calculation of peak systolic velocity and gradients

Echocardiographic Findings

- Echocardiogram
  - Transthoracic echocardiography (TTE)
    - Calcified, thickened valve leaflets
    - Assessment of left ventricular function, left ventricular hypertrophy and enlargement
  - Transesophageal echocardiography (TEE)
    - Planimetry of the anatomic aortic valve orifice area (AVA) is highly accurate (but limited in the presence of severe calcification)
    - Better visualization of cusps and morphology (bicuspid vs. tricuspid)
  - Color and pulsed Doppler
    - Increased transvalvular pressure gradient (> 50 mmHg) and transvalvular velocity > 4 m/s indicates severe stenosis (if normal LV-function)
    - Calculation of the aortic valve orifice area (AVA) by continuity equation [velocity time integral (VTI)]
  - Transthoracic echocardiography is primary imaging modality for diagnosis and staging of disease severity

Angiographic Findings

- Conventional
  - Systolic jet into the aorta and severe calcification
  - Right and left catheterization allows valve aperture surface, cardiac function and pressure measurements in the pre-operative assessment
  - Valvular gradient measured during catheter pull-back and calculation of the aortic valve orifice area (by using Gorlin-formula)
  - Evaluation of coronary arteries before valve surgery

Imaging Recommendations

- Best imaging tool: Echocardiography, MR
- Protocol advice
  - ECG-gated cardiac CT
    - Image reconstruction during mid-systole (12-20% RR-interval); multiplanar reformations (MPR) for planimetry of the AVA

DIFFERENTIAL DIAGNOSIS

Degenerative Calcified Aortic Stenosis

- Marked fibrous/calcific thickening of all three leaflets
- Calcification more prominent at the base of leaflets
- Symptoms present in the 7th decade or beyond

Rheumatic Heart Disease

- Thickening predominately along the commissural edge
- Accompanies rheumatic mitral stenosis

Bicuspid Aortic Valve

- Two equal or unequal cusps
- Either "congenital" (fused raphe) or "secondary-degenerative" (cusp fusion)
  - Congenital
    - Prevalence 2%
    - Symptoms present in the 4th or 5th decade (due to early degeneration and leaflet thickening)
    - Association with coarctation and aneurysm of the aorta
  - Secondary-degenerative ("functional") in case of severe degenerative disease and fused leaflets

Subvalvular Aortic Stenosis

- Congenital subvalvular membrane

AORTIC STENOSIS

- Idiopathic hypertrophic subaortic stenosis (IHSS) caused by asymmetric thickening of the ventricular septum

Supravalvular Aortic Stenosis

- Extremely rare; associated with Williams-Beuren syndrome
- Hourglass narrowing above aortic bulbus

Rare Causes

- Infective endocarditis: Obstruction by vegetations
- Radiation valvulitis

PATHOLOGY

General Features

- General path comments: Thickening, fusion and calcification of aortic leaflets
- Etiology
  - Degenerative/calcific: Pathomechanism similar to atherosclerosis but with differences; calcification dominating
  - Bicuspid valve: Congenital with early degeneration
- Epidemiology: Prevalence of aortic valve calcification is 25% at age 65

Gross Pathologic & Surgical Features

- Stenotic cusps with nodular calcium depositions on the leaflets
- Calcification predominantly near the base of the valve

Microscopic Features

- Fibrous thickening and transvalvular calcification

Staging, Grading or Classification Criteria

- Mild, moderate and severe (grade I-III) by echocardiography
  - Mild: Aortic valve orifice area (AVA) > 1.5 cm²; mean pressure gradient < 25 mmHg
  - Moderate: AVA 1-1.5 cm²; transvalvular pressure gradient 25-40 mmHg
  - Severe: AVA < 1 cm²; transvalvular pressure gradient > 40 mmHg
    - Severe/critical (surgery indicated): AVA < 0.7 cm²

CLINICAL ISSUES

Presentation

- Most common signs/symptoms: Initially asymptomatic over long period ("mystery killer"), symptoms develop late
- Other signs/symptoms: Systolic heart murmur
- Chest pain (angina) simulating coronary artery disease (CAD) occurs in > 60% of patients with severe AS due to heart failure
- Exertional syncope secondary to fixed cardiac output
- Symptoms of left heart failure (dyspnea) late with progressive AS

Demographics

- Age: Prevalence increases with age: 2-5% if > 65 years

Natural History & Prognosis

- Bicuspid valve is the dominant cause below age 70 and calcific degenerative above 70
- Increased risk of sudden cardiac death, especially in symptomatic patients
- Left ventricular hypertrophy predicts the onset of symptoms

Treatment

- Surgical aortic valve replacement (AVR) is the standard treatment in patients with severe AS, associated with CABG if needed
- Mortality rate is ~ 4% for AVR; ~ 7% with accompanying CABG and ~ 10% with repair of another valve
- 10 year survival rate for AVR is ~ 85%

DIAGNOSTIC CHECKLIST

Consider

- Calcific aortic stenosis is predominant type (almost 100% of patients with aortic stenosis have calcification)
- Left ventricular function is an important parameter to predict outcome

Image Interpretation Pearls

- Valvular calcifications (seen on lateral X-ray, CT, Echocardiography)
- Echocardiography
  - Increased transvalvular pressure gradient and velocity
- ECG-gated cardiac CT and cardiac MR
  - Narrowing of aortic valve area (AVA) < 2 cm² during mid-systole
- Concentric LV-hypertrophy and dysfunction at late stage

SELECTED REFERENCES

1. Abbara S et al: Feasibility and optimization of aortic valve planimetry with MDCT. AJR Am J Roentgenol. 188(2):356-60, 2007
2. Pouleur AC et al: Aortic valve area assessment: multidetector CT compared with cine MR imaging and transthoracic and transesophageal echocardiography. Radiology. 244(3):745-54, 2007
3. ACC/AHA 2006 guidelines for the management of patients with valvular heart disease. Circulation. 114(5):e84-231, 2006
4. Alkadhi H et al: Aortic stenosis: comparative evaluation of 16-detector row CT and echocardiography. Radiology. 240(1):47-55, 2006
5. Feuchtner GM et al: Multislice computed tomography for detection of patients with aortic valve stenosis and quantification of severity. J Am Coll Cardiol. 47(7):1410-7, 2006
6. Rahimtoola SH: The year in valvular heart disease. J Am Coll Cardiol. 47(2):427-39, 2006
7. Braunwald E: Valvular Heart Disease. In: Braunwald E. Heart Disease: A Textbook of Cardiovascular Medicine 6th Ed. Philadelphia, W.B. Saunders Company, 2001

AORTIC STENOSIS

IMAGE GALLERY

Typical

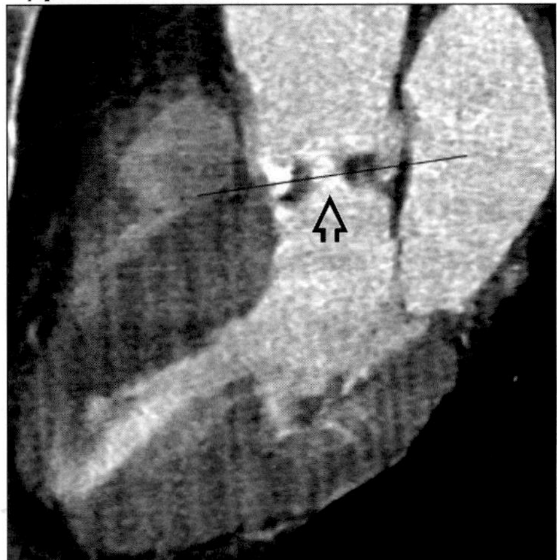

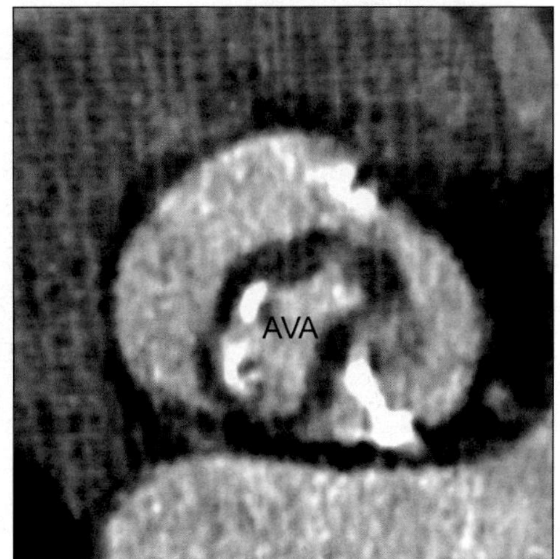

(Left) *Three chamber view cardiac CT shows thickened cusps with systolic orifice narrowing ⇨. Black line indicates level of short axis image.* ***(Right)*** *Short axis cardiac CT shows moderate-stenotic aortic valve area (AVA) of 1.2 cm². Round-shaped "fish-mouth" AVA is typical for bicuspid valve.*

Typical

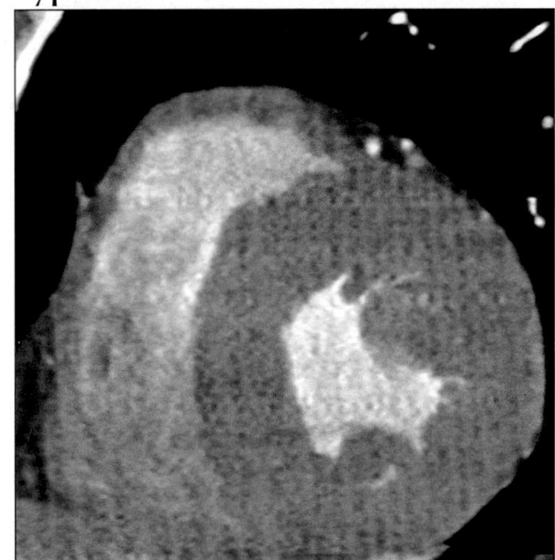

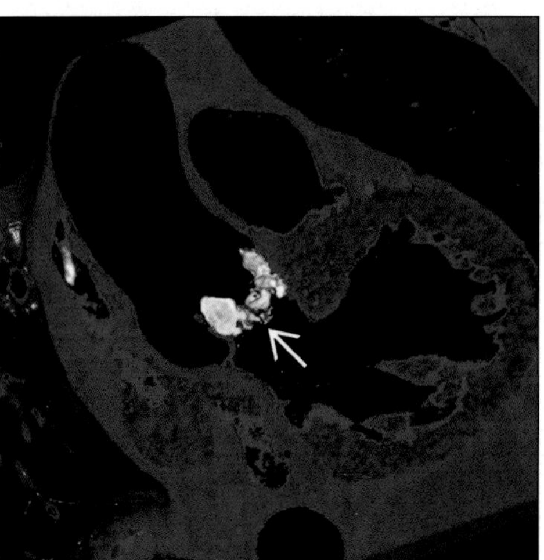

(Left) *LV short axis cardiac CT shows concentric thickening of the left ventricular myocardium.* ***(Right)*** *Coronal oblique cardiac CT shows heavy calcification ➡ in aortic stenosis (3D volume rendering technique).*

Typical

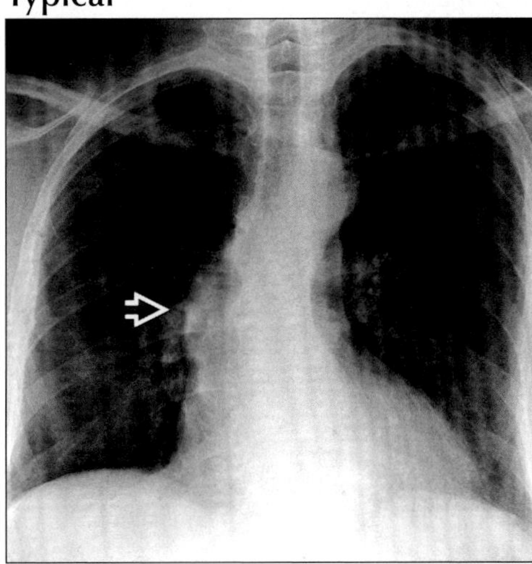

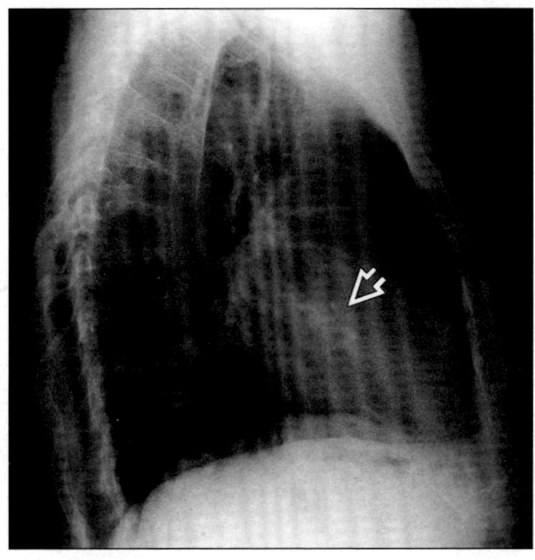

(Left) *Anteroposterior radiograph shows dilated ascending aorta ⇨.* ***(Right)*** *Lateral radiograph shows aortic valve calcification ⇨, which is highly suggestive of aortic valve stenosis if found on lateral radiograph. The association of aortic valve calcification detected by CT with functional aortic stenosis is less strong because CT may detect much smaller amounts of calcium.*

AORTIC REGURGITATION

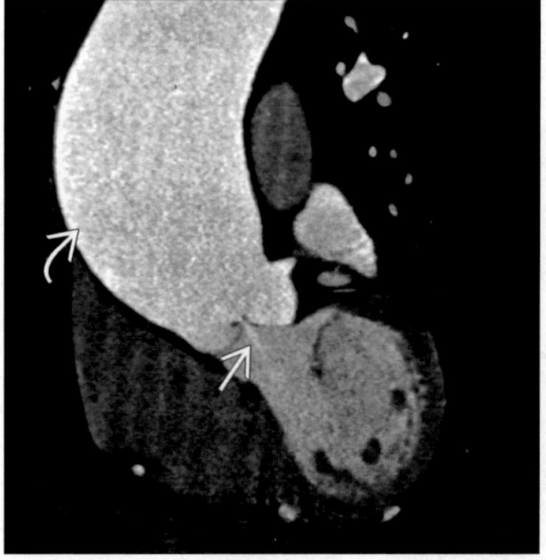

Coronal oblique cardiac CT shows ascending aortic aneurysm ➔, and incomplete coaptation of aortic valve cusps during diastole resulting in regurgitation. Note: Regurgitant jet ➔.

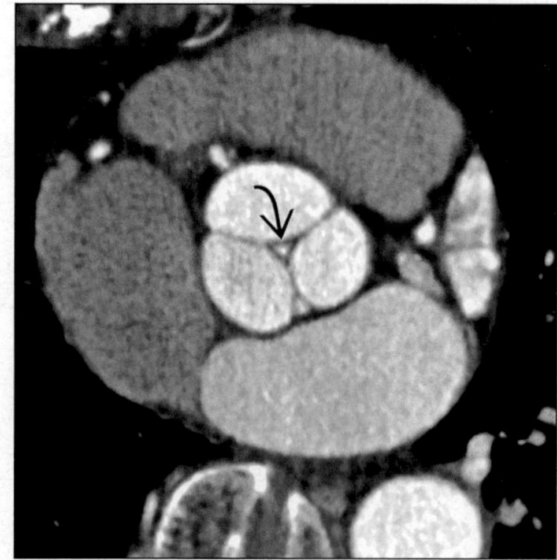

Short axis cardiac CT of the aortic valve demonstrates incomplete diastolic central coaptation of cusps ➔ resulting in a "triangular leakage area".

TERMINOLOGY

Abbreviations and Synonyms

- Aortic regurgitation (AR); aortic insufficiency (AI)

Definitions

- Incomplete closure of cusps during diastole leading to retrograde blood flow into left ventricle

IMAGING FINDINGS

General Features

- Best diagnostic clue: Retrograde blood flow into left ventricle by Doppler echocardiography
- Acute AR
  - No left ventricular dilatation
  - Pulmonary edema due to volume overload
- Chronic AR
  - Eccentric left ventricular hypertrophy and dilatation
  - Dilatation of the ascending aorta and the aortic root common
  - Valve calcification uncommon in pure aortic regurgitation

Radiographic Findings

- Chest Radiography
  - Acute AR
    - Normal left ventricle size
    - Pulmonary edema
  - Chronic AR
    - Minimal to massive left ventricle enlargement
    - Normal pulmonary vasculature until chronic severe left ventricular dysfunction and consecutive pulmonary venous hypertension
    - Dilatation of the ascending aorta

CT Findings

- CTA
  - Aortic root dilatation ± ascending aortic aneurysm frequent
  - Measurement of aortic annulus, maximal sinus of Valsalva diameter, sino-tubular (ST) junction diameters pre-operatively
  - Evaluation of sino-tubular junction effacement (indicates annuloaortic ectasia)
- Cardiac Gated CTA

DDx: Aortic Regurgitation

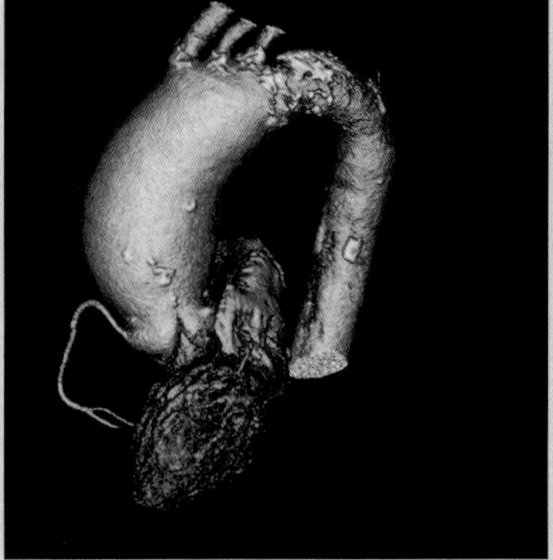

Ascending Aortic Aneurysm

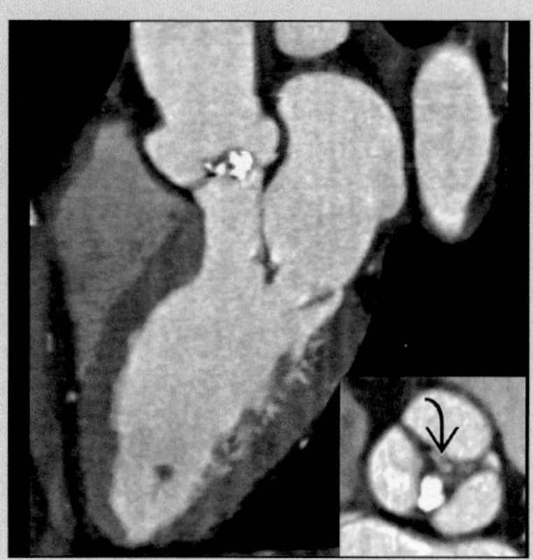

Calcific Aortic Stenosis

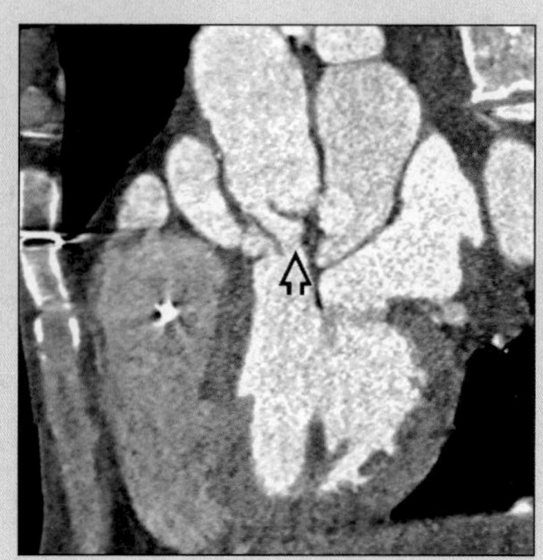

Infective Endocarditis

AORTIC REGURGITATION

Key Facts

Imaging Findings
- Best imaging tool: Doppler echocardiography
- Computed tomography
  - Aortic root dilatation/ascending aortic aneurysm
  - ECG-gated cardiac CT: Diastolic central regurgitant orifice is diagnostic for AR (moderate and severe)
- MR: Gold standard for accurate quantification of LV-function and regurgitant volume
- Radiograph: Dilated left ventricle ("boot-shaped") in severe chronic aortic regurgitation

Top Differential Diagnoses
- Aortic Root Disease/Dilatation
  - Most common cause of AR
- Rheumatic/Calcific Heart Disease
- Infective Endocarditis
- Trauma
- Bicuspid Valve

Pathology
- Acute AR, etiology: Infective endocarditis, ascending aortic dissection (type A Stanford)
- Chronic AR, etiology: Aortic root dilatation (degenerative; Marfan syndrome), rheumatic heart disease

Clinical Issues
- Acute AR
  - Signs of severe heart failure, normal LV- size
- Chronic AR
  - Asymptomatic at early stages, progressive signs of heart failure at late stage

  - Incomplete coaptation of cusps during diastole; "central valvular leakage" area visible on cross sectional transverse planes
  - Detects moderate and severe AR, but mild AR can be missed
  - Cusp morphology: Thickening, calcification or vegetations
  - Dilated left ventricle at late stage, gated CT allows calculation of LV-function/volumes

MR Findings
- Diastolic flow void (jet) area in left ventricle on flow-sensitive sequences (cine GRE) provides rough estimation of severity
- Ventricle dilatation in severe chronic AR
- Gold standard for functional assessment; ejection fraction, ventricular volumes and myocardial mass
- Calculation of the regurgitant volume with phase-contrast MR

Echocardiographic Findings
- Echocardiogram
  - 2D and transesophageal echocardiography (TEE)
  - Acute aortic regurgitation
    - Reduced opening motion and premature closure of valve
    - Delayed opening of mitral valve
    - Minimal dilatation of the LV cavity with normal function
  - Chronic aortic regurgitation
    - Marked dilatation of the LV cavity with decreased function
  - Estimation of LV-function
- M-mode: High frequency flutter of the anterior mitral valve leaflet is indirect sign
- Color Doppler
  - Most sensitive method for assessment of aortic regurgitation: Proximal jet-width ("vena contracta")
  - Central or eccentric retrograde jet
- Continuous wave (CW)-Doppler
  - Measurement of regurgitant jet velocity and calculation of pressure-half time (PHT)

Angiographic Findings
- Conventional
  - Left Ventriculogram
    - Regurgitant jet in LV following injection of contrast into aortic root

Imaging Recommendations
- Best imaging tool: Echocardiography followed by MR
- Protocol advice
  - ECG-gated cardiac CT
    - Coronary CT angiography examination protocol
    - Image reconstruction during diastole; oblique sagittal, coronal and perpendicular axial MPR for detection of incomplete coaptation of cusps

DIFFERENTIAL DIAGNOSIS

Aortic Root Disease
- Dilatation of aortic root (most common cause of pure aortic regurgitation) ± ascending aortic aneurysm
  - Etiologies: Degenerative/atherosclerotic, cystic medial necrosis, Marfan syndrome, aortitis
- Dissection

Rheumatic or Degenerative/Calcific Heart Disease
- Thickened and/or calcified leaflets prevent closure during diastole
- Associated with aortic stenosis and mitral valve disease

Infective Endocarditis
- Vegetations that prevent coaptation of the cusps
- Perforation of cusp

Trauma
- Rupture of the sinus of Valsalva
- Loss of commissural support producing prolapse
- Tear in ascending aorta or dissection

Bicuspid Valve
- Thickening of leaflets produces incomplete closure and/or prolapse

AORTIC REGURGITATION

PATHOLOGY

General Features

- General path comments
  - Valve leaflets
    - Thickening, shortening and retraction of one or more leaflets
    - Perforation of a valve leaflet or a vegetation that prevents coaptation of the leaflets
    - Traumatic destruction of a leaflet
  - Ascending aorta
    - Dilatation secondary to degeneration, dissection, hypertension and infection
- Etiology
  - Secondary to diseases of the aortic valve leaflets and/or the wall of the aortic root
  - Acute AR: Infective endocarditis, ascending aortic dissection, trauma
  - Chronic AR: Aortic root dilatation, rheumatic heart disease, bicuspid valve, very rare syphilis

Staging, Grading or Classification Criteria

- Mild, moderate and severe (grade I-III) by Doppler echocardiography
  - Severe: Proximal jet width > 6 mm (or > 65% of left ventricular outflow tract (LVOT); pressure-half-time (PHT) < 200 ms
  - Moderate: Proximal jet width 3-6 mm (or 25-65% of LVOT); PHT 200-500 ms
  - Mild: Proximal jet width < 3 mm (or < 25% of LVOT); PHT > 500 ms

CLINICAL ISSUES

Presentation

- Most common signs/symptoms: Chronic AR is asymptomatic over long period until signs of heart failure develops
- Other signs/symptoms: Decrescendo diastolic murmur
- Acute aortic regurgitation
  - Immediate signs of severe left heart failure due to volume overload
- Chronic aortic regurgitation
  - Progressive signs of left heart failure
  - Infectious endocarditis can exacerbate symptoms

Demographics

- Age
  - Variable age manifestation dependent on etiology
  - Prevalence: 4.9% (Framingham Heart Study, FHS)
  - Increasing prevalence with age: 8.5% females and 13% males at 54 years of age (FHS)
- Gender: 3:1 = M:F

Natural History & Prognosis

- Without surgery, patients with symptomatic AR live ~ 2-4 years
- LV-function is an important parameter to define clinical management and optimal time point of surgery
- If heart failure NYHA III-IV: High mortality with 25% annually

Treatment

- Acute aortic regurgitation
  - Intensive medical management to stabilize for aortic valve replacement surgery
  - Five year surgical survival: 85% survival in patients with EF > 45%, falling to 50% survival in patients with EF < 45%
- Chronic aortic regurgitation
  - Medical therapy: Antibiotic prophylaxis; vasodilators; calcium antagonists; arrhythmia control
  - 75% and 50% five and ten year survival
  - Surgical repair before severe left ventricular dysfunction occurs

DIAGNOSTIC CHECKLIST

Consider

- Acute and chronic AR can be distinguished by left atrial (LA) and left ventricle (LV) size (radiograph)
  - Acute: Normal LA-size (but often pulmonary edema and severe clinical symptoms)
  - Chronic: Enlarged LA and LV (symptoms late)
- Echocardiography is primary imaging modality
- ECG-gated cardiac CT
  - Detect moderate and severe AR (usually incidentally on coronary artery study)
  - Evaluate etiology (ascending aortic aneurysm, dissection, etc.)
- Cardiac MR to define best timing of surgery (regurgitant fraction and LV volume measurements)

Image Interpretation Pearls

- Radiograph: LA and LV-size enlarged
- Echocardiography: Retrograde Doppler flow during systole in left ventricle (prox. jet width and PHT-method)
- ECG-gated cardiac CT: Incomplete coaptation of cusps during diastole
- Cardiac MR: Regurgitant fraction and ventricular volumes

SELECTED REFERENCES

1. Alkadhi H et al: Aortic regurgitation: assessment with 64-section CT. Radiology. 245(1):111-21, 2007
2. Jassal DS et al: 64-slice multidetector computed tomography (MDCT) for detection of aortic regurgitation and quantification of severity. Invest Radiol. 42(7):507-12, 2007
3. Feuchtner GM et al: Diagnostic performance of MDCT for detecting aortic valve regurgitation. AJR Am J Roentgenol. 186(6):1676-81, 2006
4. Braunwald E: Valvular Heart Disease. In Braunwald E. Heart Disease: A Textbook of Cardiovascular Medicine 6th Ed. Philadelphia, W.B. Saunders Company, 2001
5. Singh JP et al: Prevalence and clinical determinants of mitral, tricuspid, and aortic regurgitation (the Framingham Heart Study). Am J Cardiol. 83(6):897-902, 1999

IMAGE GALLERY

Typical

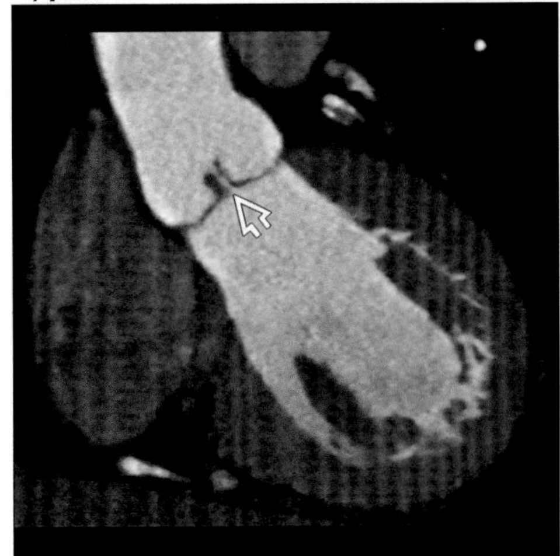

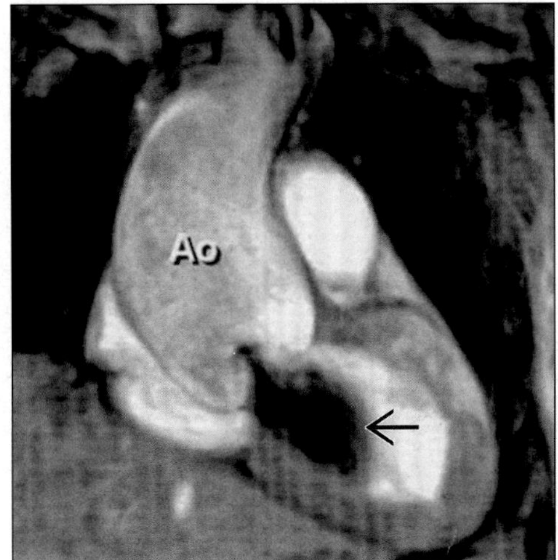

(Left) Coronal oblique cardiac CT shows incomplete closure of cusps during end-diastole resulting in an regurgitant orifice. *(Right)* Coronal oblique MR cine shows dark jet of regurgitant flow into the left ventricle during diastole. Note: Ascending aortic aneurysm.

Variant

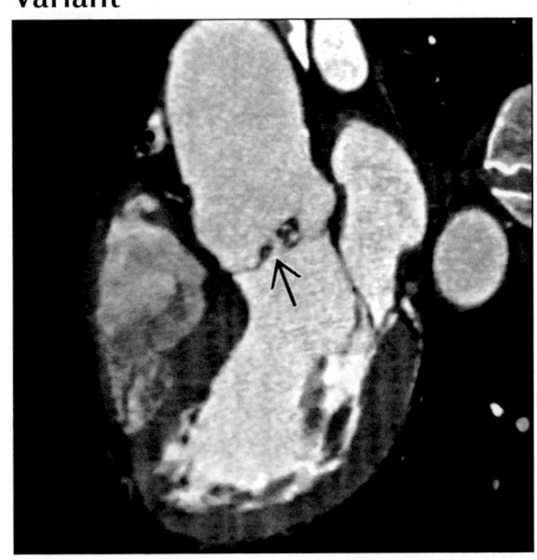

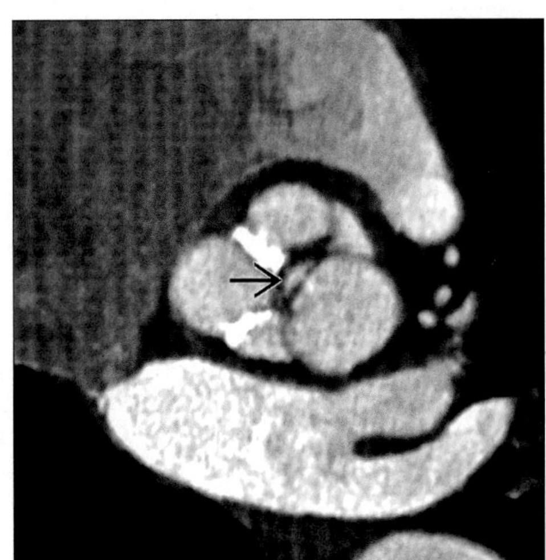

(Left) LVOT cardiac CT shows incomplete diastolic coaptation and very irregular thickened aortic valve cusps in a patient with rheumatic heart disease. *(Right)* Short axis cardiac CT revealed a "central leakage area", also known as the regurgitant orifice area in a patient with bicuspid aortic valve. Short axis CT images allow to planimeter (ROI) the regurgitant orifice area, which correlates with echocardiographic grading of AR severity.

Typical

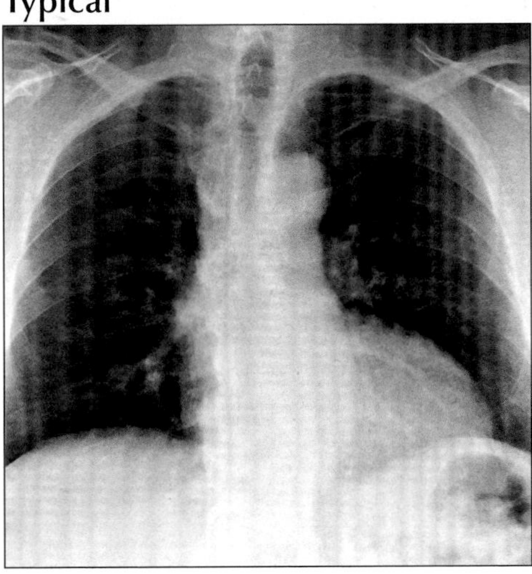

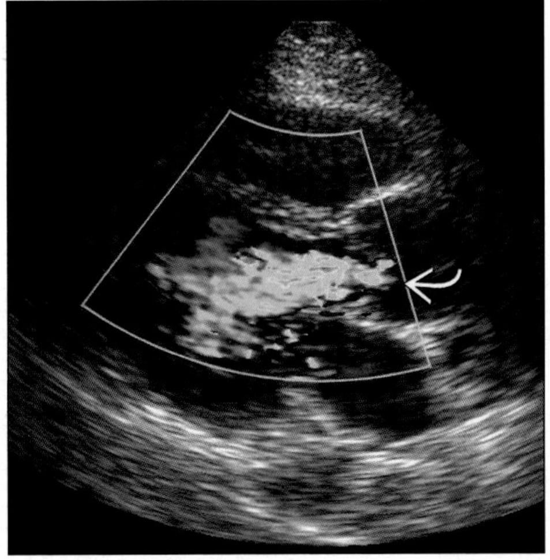

(Left) Posteroanterior radiograph of the chest shows dilated, rounded left ventricle ("boot-shaped") and enlarged cardiac silhouette due to isolated LV dilatation and normal pulmonary vasculature, consistent with chronic AR. *(Right)* Three chamber view color Doppler ultrasound (same patient as previous image) shows diastolic retrograde blood flow into left ventricle and large proximal jet of 8 mm representing severe aortic regurgitation.

BICUSPID AORTIC VALVE

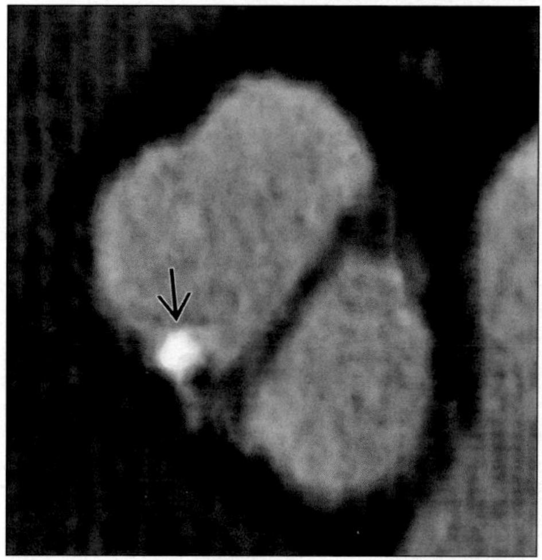

Short axis coronary CTA at the valve level in diastole shows a congenital bicuspid valve with two cusps. Note small piece of calcium ⇒. No malcoaptation to suggest aortic regurgitation.

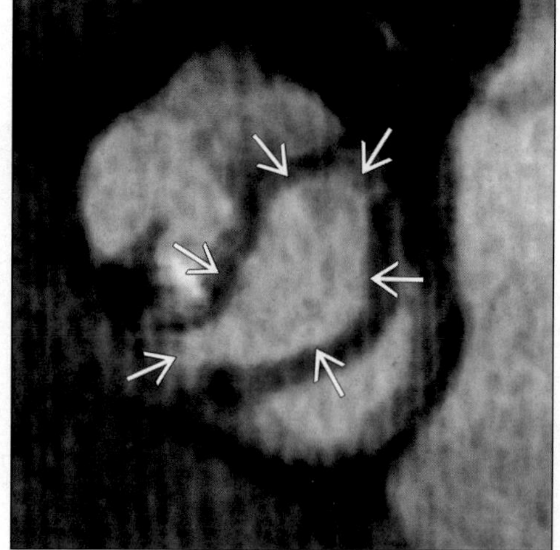

Short axis coronary CTA in systole in the same valve shows a non-stenotic congenital bicuspid valve. The opening area can be planimetered to quantify valve area ➡.

TERMINOLOGY

Abbreviations and Synonyms

- Bicuspid aortic valve (BAV)

Definitions

- Most common congenital cardiovascular malformation
  - Occurs in 1-2% of the population
  - There are 2 functional leaflets and most have 2 complete commissures
    - Less than half of cases have a fused raphe in the middle of one of the leaflets which may give the appearance of a trileaflet valve
- Acquired bicuspid valves result for inflammatory processes (i.e., rheumatic fever) or calcification of a normal trileaflet aortic valve

IMAGING FINDINGS

General Features

- Best diagnostic clue
  - Dilated aortic root with systolic doming and diastolic prolapse of a bicuspid aortic valve
  - Eccentric closure plane in systole
- Size
  - BAV are 2 cusps of generally unequal size
    - Occasionally a ridge or raphe lies across one cusp
- Morphology: Thickened leaflets with either an anteroposterior or horizontal orientation

Radiographic Findings

- Characteristic calcification along the valve commissures and annulus
- Frequently prominent calcified ridge along the raphe
- Cardiomegaly if the bicuspid aortic valve is accompanied by significant aortic regurgitation
- Prominence of the ascending aorta
  - May have post-stenotic ascending aortic aneurysm due stenotic jet

CT Findings

- NECT
  - Allows quantification of aortic valve calcium
    - Severity of valve calcium correlates with peak and mean aortic valve gradients in cases of stenosis
- Cardiac Gated CTA

DDx: Bicuspid Aortic Valve

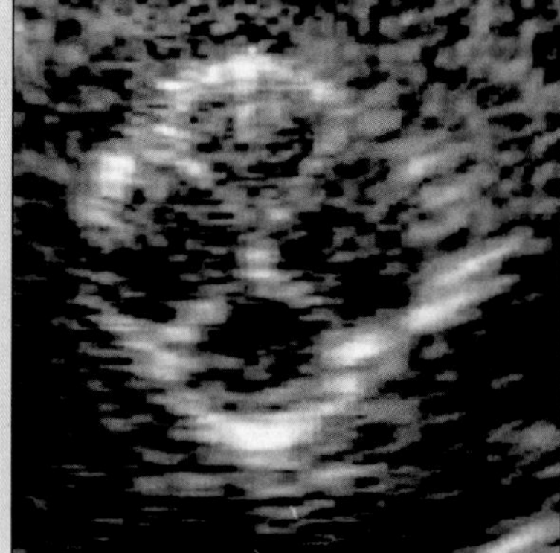

Quadricuspid Aortic Valve

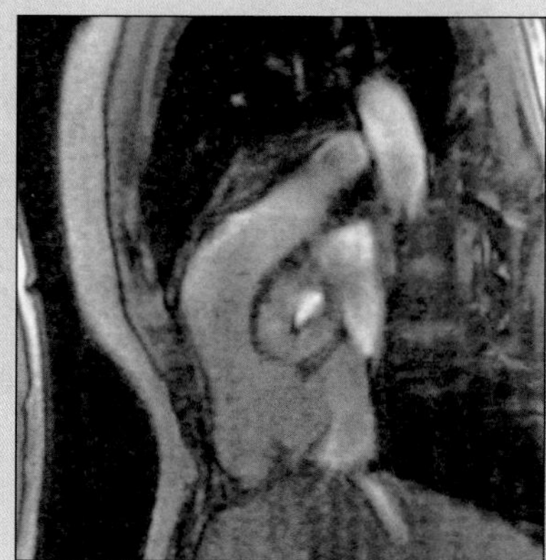

Unicuspid Aortic Valve

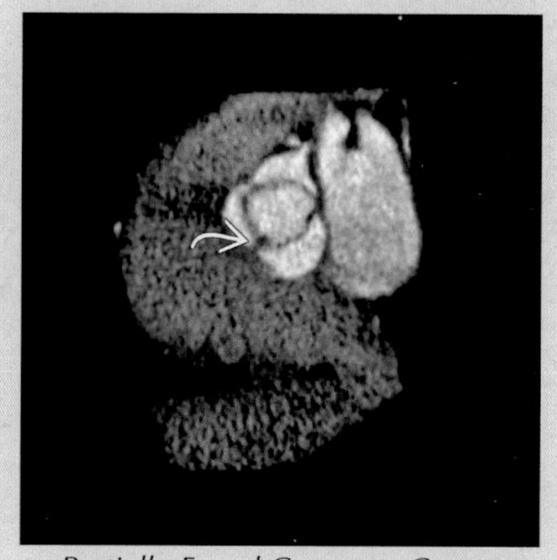

Partially Fused Coronary Cusps

BICUSPID AORTIC VALVE

Key Facts

Terminology

- Bicuspid aortic valve (BAV)
- Most common congenital cardiovascular malformation
- Acquired bicuspid valves result from inflammatory processes (i.e. rheumatic fever) or calcification of a normal trileaflet aortic valve

Imaging Findings

- Dilated aortic root with systolic doming and diastolic prolapse of a bicuspid aortic valve
- Eccentric closure plane in systole
- Best imaging tool: Echocardiography

Pathology

- Bicuspid aortic valves may be present in up to 1-2% of the population
- Highly associated with congenital left-sided obstructive lesions
- BAV is associated with aortic dilation, aneurysms, and dissection

Clinical Issues

- Generally asymptomatic
- Frequent incidental finding on echocardiography
- BAV are predisposed to infective endocarditis
- Aortic valve stenosis is the most frequent complication
- Serial assessment of the aortic valve to evaluate valvular function, chamber dimensions, and ventricular function
- Aortic valve replacement indicated for severe valve dysfunction, symptomatic patients, abnormal left ventricular dimensions and function

---

  - Accurately detects number of valve leaflets, valve motion, and valve calcium on cine CT
  - Quantify degree of aortic valve stenosis by valve area planimetry during systolic phase
  - Semiquantitatively grade aortic valve regurgitation by the size of the anatomic regurgitant orifice
  - Accurate assessment of associated aortic pathology

MR Findings

- MR Cine
  - Phase contrast cine MR (velocity-encoded) allows for flow quantification
  - Provides peak systolic flow and the valve gradient in cases of aortic stenosis
  - Provides regurgitant volume and regurgitant fraction in cases of aortic regurgitation
- SSFP White Blood Cine
  - Detect high velocity jet flow in cases of valve stenosis or retrograde flow across a regurgitant orifice by means of signal void
  - Quantification of left ventricular volume and function which are all essential for monitoring therapy or timing for surgical intervention
- Double IR FSE
  - Accurate morphological characterization of the valve cusps and their orientation (anterioposterior or right-left)
  - Complete assessment of the thoracic aorta

Echocardiographic Findings

- BAV shows a "doming" configuration in the long axis view when it opens during systole
- In the short axis view, the opening of the two leaflets creates a "fish-mouth" (oval) appearance
  - In some cases the valve may appear normal in diastole because a raphe in the larger leaflet may simulate a trileaflet valve
- Continuous wave Doppler measurements and estimate velocity and gradients in cases of aortic valve stenosis
- Color Doppler can be used to grade the severity of aortic regurgitation
- Transesophageal echocardiogram is useful to define valve commissures and vegetations

Angiographic Findings

- Two sinuses of Valsalva with two leaflets on anteroposterior 30 degree RAO projection
- Eccentric systolic jet of contrast with doming and thickening of the leaflets with left ventricular injections
- Dilated ascending aorta
- Aortic regurgitation on aortic root injections

Imaging Recommendations

- Best imaging tool: Echocardiography, MR

DIFFERENTIAL DIAGNOSIS

Other Valve Anomalies

- Unicuspid aortic valve, quadricuspid aortic valve

Aortic Stenosis

- Senile calcified aortic stenosis, subaortic stenosis, supravalvular stenosis

PATHOLOGY

General Features

- Genetics
  - Abnormal and inadequate production of microfibrillar proteins such as fibrillin-1
  - Abnormal endothelial nitric oxide synthase (eNOS) also implicated
  - Associated with familial clustering suggesting autosomal dominant inheritance with reduced penetrance
    - Incidence as high as 10-17% in first-degree relatives
    - Echocardiography is the recommended screening tool for offspring and first-degree relatives of patients identified as having a bicuspid aortic valve
- Etiology: Embryologic abnormality in the conotruncal channel

BICUSPID AORTIC VALVE

- Epidemiology
  - Bicuspid aortic valves may be present in up to 1-2% of the population
    - Since BAV may be silent through adulthood the incidence is likely underestimated
    - Incidence is not affected by geography or race
    - Male predominance is noted
- Associated abnormalities
  - Highly associated with congenital left-sided obstructive lesions
    - Coarctation of the aorta, supravalvular stenosis (Williams syndrome), interrupted aortic arch
  - BAV is associated with aortic dilation, aneurysms, and dissection
    - Aortic aneurysm is generally the result of post-stenotic dilation
    - Aortic root may also have inherent abnormal connective tissue with cystic medial necrosis similar to disorders such as Marfan syndrome
    - Even after valve replacement for BAV there is a risk of subsequent aortic dissection
  - Other associated congenital syndromes
    - Patent ductus arteriosus, familial aortic dissection, Turner syndrome (30% of patients have BAV)

Gross Pathologic & Surgical Features

- With aging, the valve is predisposed to sclerosis and calcification

Microscopic Features

- Early in the course is microscopic calcification and lipid deposition in the subendothelium and adjacent fibrosa
- With disease progression comes marked calcification and occasionally even cartilage deposition

CLINICAL ISSUES

Presentation

- Most common signs/symptoms
  - Generally asymptomatic
    - Frequent incidental finding on echocardiography
  - Symptoms result from the development of either valvular stenosis or regurgitation
- Other signs/symptoms
  - BAV are predisposed to infective endocarditis
    - Lifetime risk of developing infective endocarditis on a BAV is 10-30%
  - Symptoms may also develop secondary to associated aortopathies (i.e., aortic dilation and dissection)

Demographics

- Age: BAV may be identified in patients of any age
- Gender: M:F ratio 2:1 or greater

Natural History & Prognosis

- Aortic valve stenosis is the most frequent complication
  - BAV are present in the majority of patients presenting with aortic stenosis aged 15-65 y
  - Abnormalities where the right and noncoronary cusps are fused is more frequently associated with changes of stenosis or insufficiency in the pediatric population
  - Abnormalities where the right and left cusps are fused is less commonly associated with stenosis or insufficiency in children
    - This arrangement is much more commonly associated with coarctation of the aorta and a functionally normal valve
- Generally, the overall prognosis of BAV is good

Treatment

- Serial assessment of the aortic valve to evaluate valvular function, chamber dimensions, and ventricular function
- Infective endocarditis antibiotic prophylaxis prior to invasive procedures
- Modify coronary artery disease risk factors since their presence may accelerate BAV sclerosis and calcification
  - Treatment of hypercholesterolemia with a statin if present
- Balloon aortic valvuloplasty is the treatment of choice in pediatric cases
  - Later into childhood or adolescence there becomes a need for valve repair or replacement
  - Ross procedure (pulmonary autograft) considered in younger patients as an alternative to prosthetic valve replacement
- Aortic valve replacement indicated for severe valve dysfunction, symptomatic patients, abnormal left ventricular dimensions and function
- Aortic valve repair may be performed in cases of severe isolated aortic regurgitation
- Aortic root replacement is recommended in cases of BAV with aortic dilation at 4-5 cm

SELECTED REFERENCES

1. Lewin MB et al: The bicuspid aortic valve: adverse outcomes from infancy to old age. Circulation. 111(7):832-4, 2005
2. Cripe L et al: Bicuspid aortic valve is heritable. J Am Coll Cardiol. 44(1):138-43, 2004
3. Ward C: Clinical significance of the bicuspid aortic valve. Heart. 83(1):81-5, 2000
4. Arai AE et al: Visualization of aortic valve leaflets using black blood MRI. J Magn Reson Imaging. 10(5):771-7, 1999
5. Sabet HY et al: Congenitally bicuspid aortic valves: a surgical pathology study of 542 cases (1991 through 1996) and a literature review of 2,715 additional cases. Mayo Clin Proc. 74(1):14-26, 1999
6. Beppu S et al: Rapidity of progression of aortic stenosis in patients with congenital bicuspid aortic valves. Am J Cardiol. 71(4):322-7, 1993
7. Brandenburg RO Jr et al: Accuracy of 2-dimensional echocardiographic diagnosis of congenitally bicuspid aortic valve: echocardiographic-anatomic correlation in 115 patients. Am J Cardiol. 51(9):1469-73, 1983
8. Waller BF et al: Bicuspid aortic valve. Comparison of congenital and acquired types. Circulation. 48(5):1140-50, 1973

IMAGE GALLERY

Typical

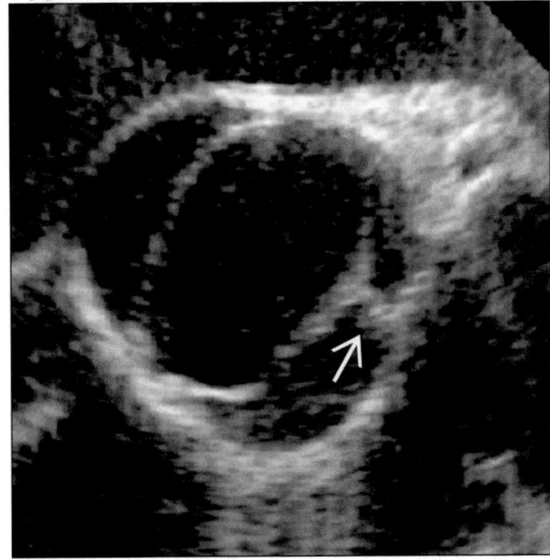

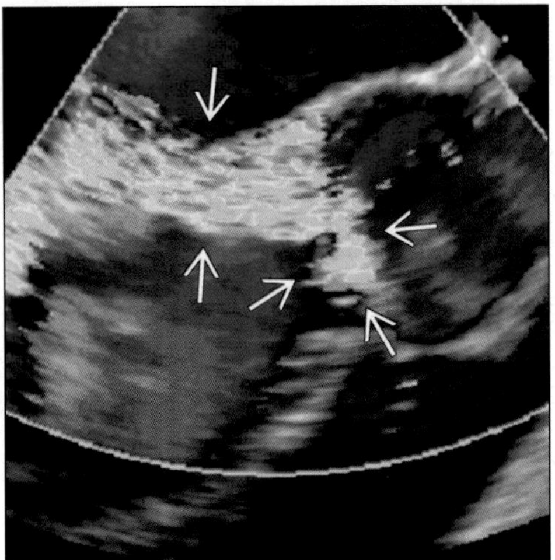

(Left) *Transesophageal short axis ECHO view of the aortic valve in systole shows a congenital bicuspid valve with typical "fish mouth" appearance. Note raphe ➔ in one of the cusps.* ***(Right)*** *Transesophageal long axis view of the aortic valve in the same patient with color Doppler shows a severe eccentric jet of aortic regurgitation ➔.*

Typical

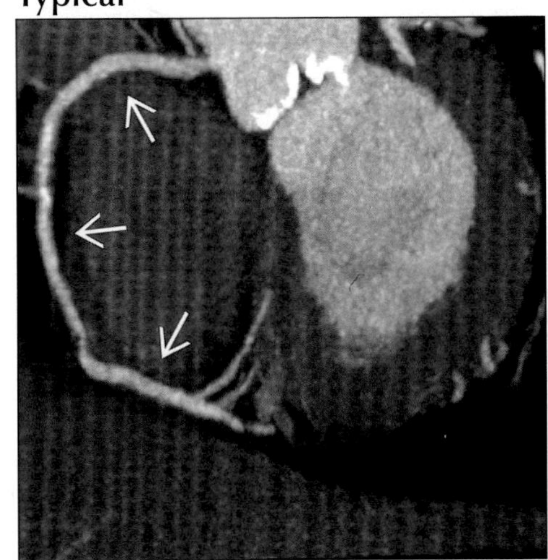

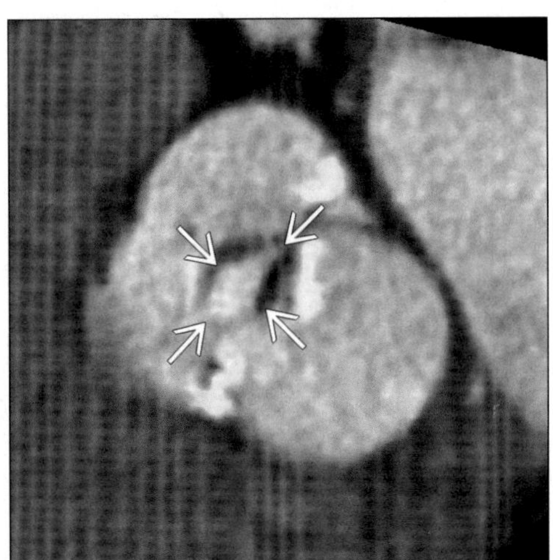

(Left) *Oblique coronary CTA shows heavily calcified aortic valve in a young patient prior to aortic valve surgery. The coronary CTA was performed for pre-operative assessment of CAD. Note the RCA ➔.* ***(Right)*** *Short axis coronary CTA at the valve level in systole in the same patient as previous image, shows reduced opening area ➔ indicating significant aortic stenosis.*

Typical

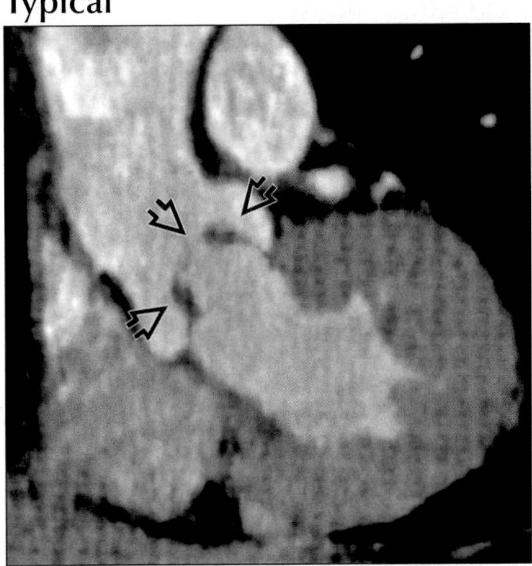

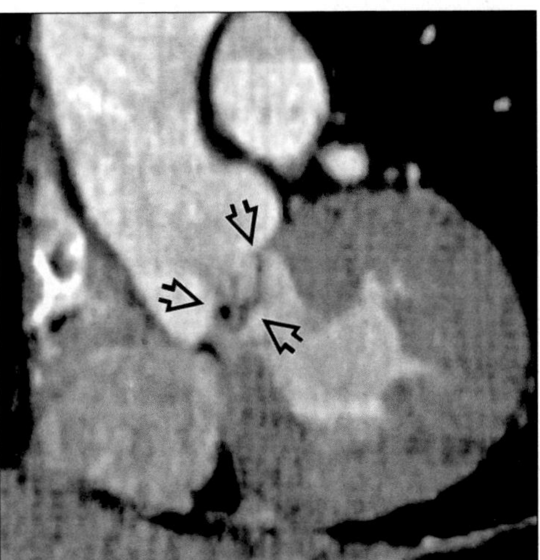

(Left) *Coronal oblique coronary CTA shows typical dooming of a bicuspid aortic valve cusps ⇨ in systole.* ***(Right)*** *Coronal oblique coronary CTA shows prolapse of the bicuspid valve cusps ⇨ in diastole in the same patient as previous image. Note thickening of the leaflets.*

MITRAL STENOSIS

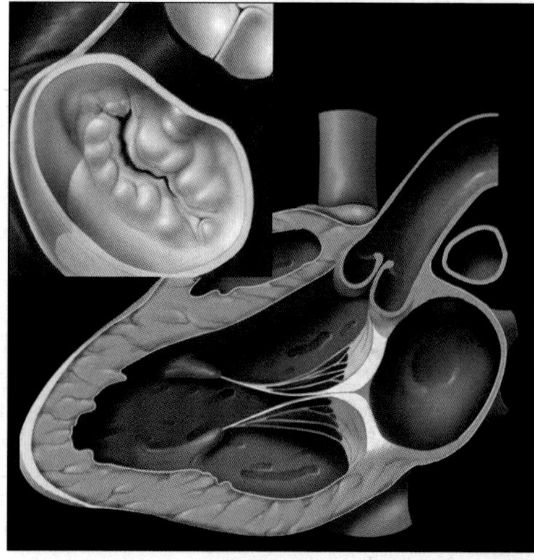

Three chamber view graphic shows severe thickening of mitral valve leaflets. Insert shows mitral valve in diastole from within left atrium. Note: Narrowed systolic mitral valve orifice caused by thick immobile leaflets.

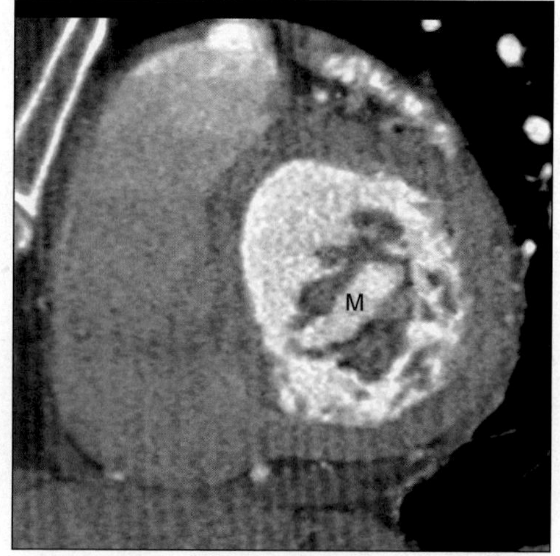

LV short axis cardiac CT shows stenotic mitral valve orifice (M) (1.2 cm²) and irregular nodular cusp thickening indicating rheumatic disease.

TERMINOLOGY

Abbreviations and Synonyms

- Mitral stenosis (MS)

Definitions

- Obstruction to left ventricular blood inflow at the level of the mitral valve (MV)

IMAGING FINDINGS

General Features

- Best diagnostic clue: Acceleration of flow at the mitral valve level during left ventricular diastole
- Morphology
  - Thickened and/or calcific leaflets; commisural fusion and/or chordal fusion
  - Left atrium dilatation

Radiographic Findings

- Chest Radiography
  - Left atrial enlargement
  - Pulmonary artery, right ventricle and right atrial enlargement
  - Pulmonary venous hypertension (redistribution, Interstitial edema with Kerley B lines, etc.)
  - If pulmonary arterial hypertension (chronic stage), descending right pulmonary artery diameter ≥ 16 mm

CT Findings

- Cardiac Gated CTA
  - "Doming" of anterior leaflet during diastolic opening and immobility of the posterior leaflet (4-D cine imaging)
  - Narrowing of mitral valve orifice
  - Thickening and/or calcification of valve leaflets, fusion of chordae tendinea
  - Left atrial enlargement and left atrial thrombi (hypodense, non-enhancing mass) frequent
  - Left atrial appendage (LAA) filling defects can cause false positive findings - delayed images are necessary to confirm thrombus
    - Normal arterial phase CTA excludes LAA thrombus
- NECT and CECT

DDx: Mitral Stenosis

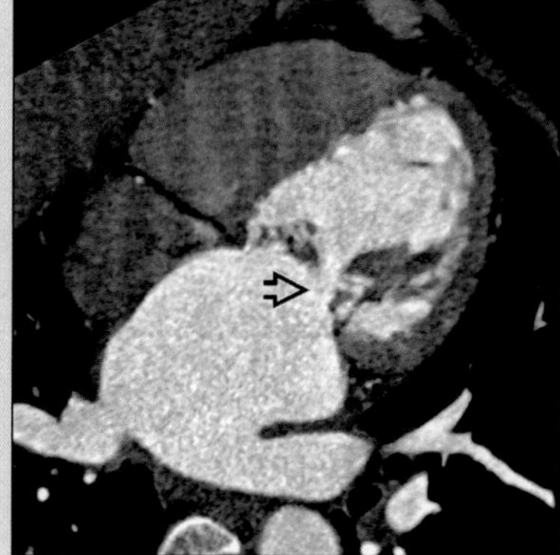

Rheumatic Heart Disease

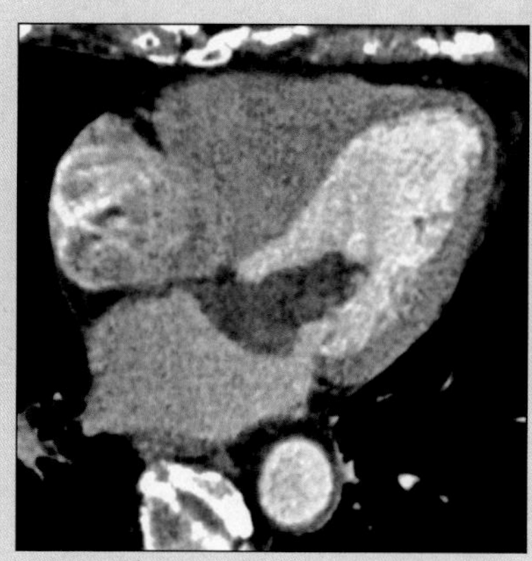

Obstruction by Myxoma

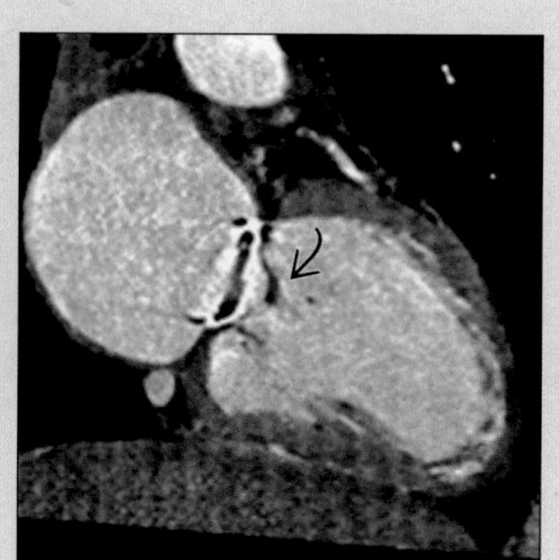

Prosthetic Valve Infection

MITRAL STENOSIS

Key Facts

Terminology
- Obstruction to left ventricular inflow at the level of the mitral valve

Imaging Findings
- Best imaging tool: Echocardiography
  - High systolic Doppler flow jet into left ventricle
  - "Doming" of anterior mitral valve leaflet
  - Left atrial enlargement
- CT and MR helpful to specify underlying disease in secondary mitral stenosis caused by obstruction of mitral valve
- CXR - Left atrial enlargement, pulmonary venous hypertension (redistribution, Kerley lines)

Top Differential Diagnoses
- Rheumatic Heart Disease (> 95%)
  - Irregular thickening and fusion of commissurae, and/or chordae tendinea
- Obstruction of Mitral Valve
  - Atrial myxoma
  - Vegetation in infective endocarditis
  - Ball-valve thrombus
- Other Causes: Rare
  - Congenital; malignant tumor (rhabdomyosarcoma, carcinoid); papillary fibroelastoma

Clinical Issues
- Dyspnea is the main clinical symptom (if orifice area < 1.5 cm^2)
- Frequent atrial fibrillation and associated left atrial thrombus
- Progressive disease leading to left atrial pressure increase and dilatation, and right heart failure

  - Mitral valve calcification: Prevalence 8% (age 60 years) causing mitral stenosis in 3.8%

MR Findings
- Diastolic flow void (jet) in left ventricle on CINE
- Left atrium enlargement
- Phase contrast can be used to calculate peak systolic velocity and gradients

Echocardiographic Findings
- Echocardiogram
  - 2D echocardiography
    - Increased acoustical impedance of stenotic valve
    - Fusion of leaflets with poor leaflet separation in diastole
    - Normal left ventricular function
    - Left atrial enlargement (> 45 mm)
    - "Doming" of anterior mitral valve leaflet
  - Transesophageal echocardiography
    - Detailed anatomy of the mitral valve
    - Better visualization of left atrial thrombus, in particular of left atrial appendage thrombus (flow measurement)
- Color Doppler
  - Increased transvalvular pressure gradient (CW-Doppler: Modified Bernoulli equation)
  - MV orifice area (by either continuity equation or PHT-method)
    - PHT method may be inaccurate in left ventricular compliance
  - High velocity flow jet in the left ventricle
  - Estimate pulmonary artery systolic pressure

Angiographic Findings
- Conventional
  - Determines the wedge pressure and indicates the degree of pulmonary hypertension, of MS and of regurgitation
  - Allows simultaneous right and left pressure measurements for direct curve comparison

Imaging Recommendations
- Best imaging tool
  - Echocardiography
    - Transthoracic as baseline examination
    - Transesophageal to clarify etiology, before surgery, and to rule out left atrial appendage thrombi
- Protocol advice
  - Cardiac ECG-gated CT
    - Systolic and diastolic image reconstruction with multiplanar reformations (MPR): Axial (4-chamber), sagittal (2-chamber) & short axis
    - 4D-cine imaging

DIFFERENTIAL DIAGNOSIS

Rheumatic Heart Disease
- Most frequent cause of mitral stenosis > 95%
- Irregular thickening and fusion of MV apparatus (chordal or commissural fusion), calcification

Obstruction of the Mitral Valve
- Atrial myxoma obstructing valve orifice (e.g., by diastolic prolapse)
- Infective endocarditis with vegetations obstructing valve orifice
- Ball-valve thrombus in the left atrium

Other Causes: Rare
- Congenital mitral stenosis
- Malignant carcinoid, rhabdomyosarcoma
- Severe annulus calcification
- Mucopolysaccharidoses including Hunter-Hurler, Whipple and Fabry disease
- Papillary fibroelastoma

PATHOLOGY

General Features
- General path comments
  - Rheumatic heart disease
    - Thickening, fusion and finally calcification of mitral leaflets, mitral annulus and proximal chordae tendineae

MITRAL STENOSIS

- Etiology: Rheumatic heart disease is the predominant cause (> 95%)
- Epidemiology: Prevalence 1.6% (females) and 0.4% (males)
- Associated abnormalities: Aortic regurgitation, tricuspid valve regurgitation

Gross Pathologic & Surgical Features

- Thickening and fusion of the mitral valve apparatus
  - Commissure thickening in 30%
  - Cusps thickening in 15%
  - Chordae in 10%
  - Combination of lesions in 45%
- Valve has funnel-shaped appearance
- Thickened, adherent leaflets inhibit opening and closing of the valve
- Orifice is frequently button-hole or "fish mouth-shaped"
- Calcium deposits in leaflets and occasional in annulus

Microscopic Features

- Fibrotic and calcific depositions in thickened leaflets

Staging, Grading or Classification Criteria

- Mild, moderate, severe (grade I-III) by echocardiography
  - Mild (grade I): Mitral valve orifice area > 1.5 cm^2; valvular pressure gradient < 5 mmHg
  - Moderate (grade II): Mitral valve orifice area 1.0-1.5 cm^2; valvular pressure gradient 5-10 mmHg
  - Severe (grade III): Mitral valve orifice area < 1.0 cm^2; valvular pressure gradient > 10 mmHg

CLINICAL ISSUES

Presentation

- Most common signs/symptoms: Dyspnea
- Clinical Profile
  - First symptoms during exercise even in mild mitral stenosis possible
  - Symptoms at rest develop if MV orifice area < 1.5 cm^2
- Exertional dyspnea frequently accompanied by cough and wheezing
- Stress-induced pulmonary edema (pregnancy)
- Progressive disease leading to left atrial pressure increase and dilatation, right heart failure
- Chest pain simulating coronary artery disease in 15% of patients
- High velocity jet of blood ejected into left ventricle during diastole (increased transmitral pressure gradient)
- Frequent atrial fibrillation & associated left atrial thrombus
  - Left atrial thrombi
    - Up to 30% in severe MS and atrial fibrillation
    - Anticoagulation is necessary to avoid risk of stroke

Demographics

- Age: 50-70 years (mean age of clinical presentation)
- Gender: Females:Males = 2:1

Natural History & Prognosis

- Symptoms appear 20-40 years after acute rheumatic fever in developed countries
- Progression more rapid in tropical and subtropical climates
- Severe disability (NYHA class II) 5-10 after initial symptoms
- 50-60% 10-year survival without surgery depending on clinical presentation; 0-15% 10-year survival if limiting severe clinical symptoms
- Mortality caused by progressive pulmonary and systemic congestion (60-70%) or pulmonary embolism (10%)

Treatment

- Medical therapy to reduce after-load and treat arrhythmias (most common atrial fibrillation)
- Percutaneous balloon mitral valvuloplasty with a mortality rate of 1-2% but relative high recurrence requiring surgery
- Surgical valvotomy with a mortality rate of 1-3% and five year survival rate > 90%
- Mitral valve replacement with a mortality rate of 3-8%

DIAGNOSTIC CHECKLIST

Consider

- Transthoracic echocardiography is primary imaging modality (increased transvalvular pressure gradient)
- Transesophageal echocardiography is standard to rule out left atrial appendage thrombi in AFIB
- ECG-gated cardiac CT and Cardiac MR useful
  - To clarify etiology of non-primary valvular MS (obstruction by myxoma, thrombus, etc.)

Image Interpretation Pearls

- "Doming" of anterior mitral valve leaflet
- Irregularly thickened leaflets with narrowing of the orifice area typically for rheumatic disease
- Enlargement of left atrium

SELECTED REFERENCES

1. Mahnken AH et al: MDCT detection of mitral valve calcification: prevalence and clinical relevance compared with echocardiography. AJR Am J Roentgenol. 188(5):1264-9, 2007
2. Bonow et al: ACC/AHA 2006 guidelines for the management of patients with valvular heart disease. Circulation. 114:124-138, 2006
3. Messika-Zeitoun D et al: Assessment of the mitral valve area in patients with mitral stenosis by multislice computed tomography. J Am Coll Cardiol. 48(2):411-3, 2006
4. Movahed MR et al: Increased prevalence of mitral stenosis in women. J Am Soc Echocardiogr. 19(7):911-3, 2006
5. Achenbach S et al: Electron beam computed tomography for the detection of left atrial thrombi in patients with atrial fibrillation. Heart. 90(12):1477-8, 2004
6. Braunwald E: Valvular Heart Disease. In: Braunwald E. Heart Disease: A Textbook of Cardiovascular Medicine 6th Ed. W.B. Saunders Company, Philadelphia, 2001
7. Otto CM: Mitral stenosis In: Otto CM. Valvular Heart Disease 1st Ed. W.B. Saunders Co. Philadelphia, 1999

MITRAL STENOSIS

IMAGE GALLERY

Typical

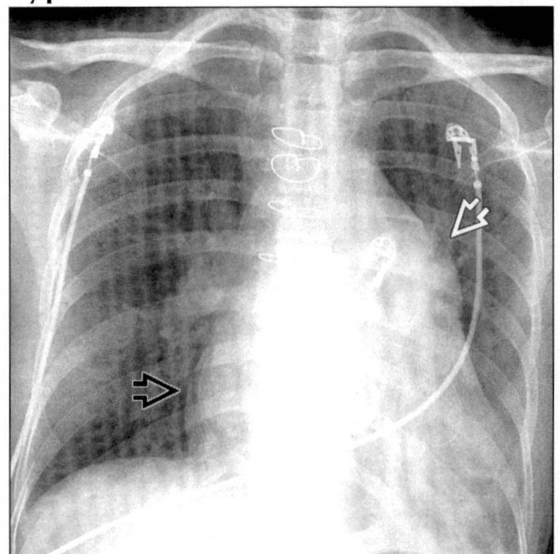

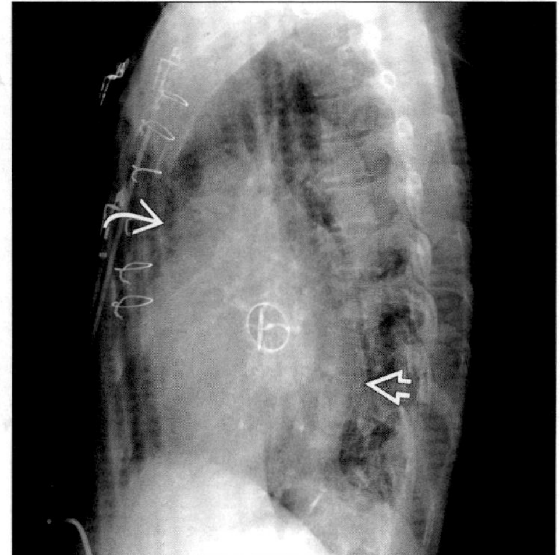

*(**Left**) Posteroanterior radiograph shows "bulging" of left atrium due to enlargement, right atrial enlargement, and PV redistribution. Note the dilatation of upper pulmonary venous vasculature. (**Right**) Lateral radiograph shows Medtronic Hall type tilting disc mitral valve replacement, enlargement of left atrium, and right ventricle (filled retrosternal space).*

Typical

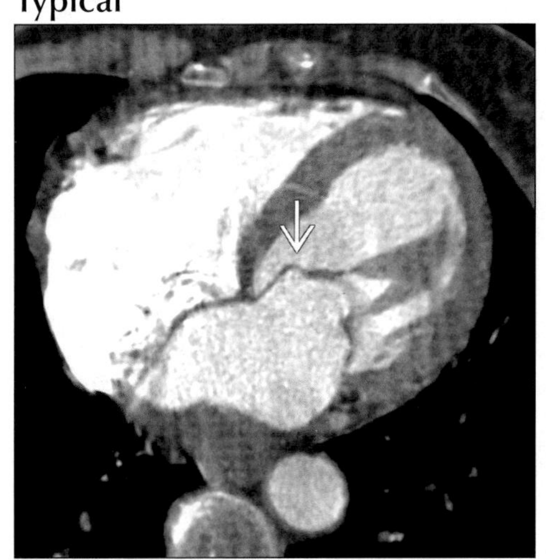

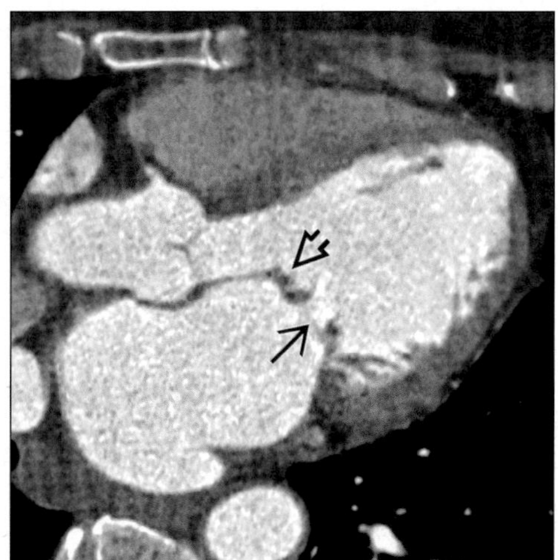

*(**Left**) Axial cardiac CT shows "doming" or hockey stick configuration of anterior mitral leaflet during diastole. (**Right**) Axial cardiac CT shows irregular thickening of the anterior mitral valve leaflet and diastolic narrowing of the orifice.*

Typical

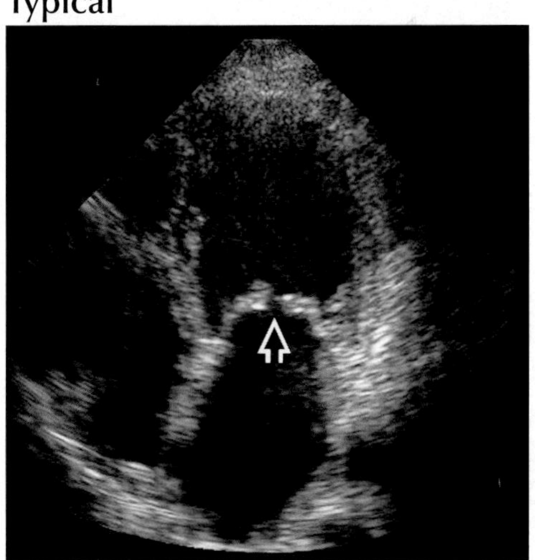

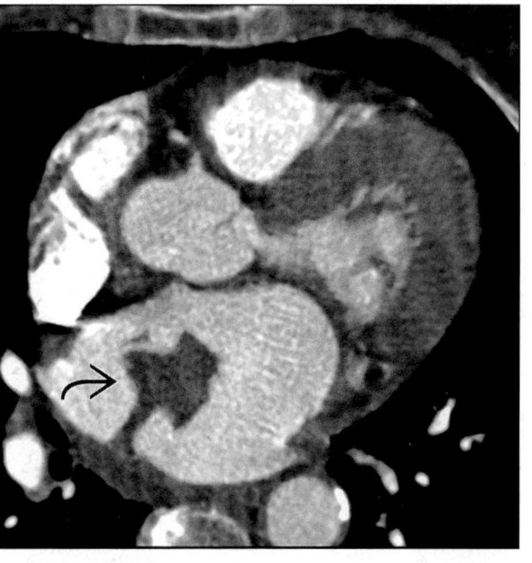

*(**Left**) Four chamber view B-mode echocardiography shows thickening of both mitral valve leaflets and narrowing of the orifice area. (**Right**) Axial cardiac CT shows a left atrial thrombus and left atrial enlargement in a patient with mitral valve stenosis.*

MITRAL VALVE PROLAPSE

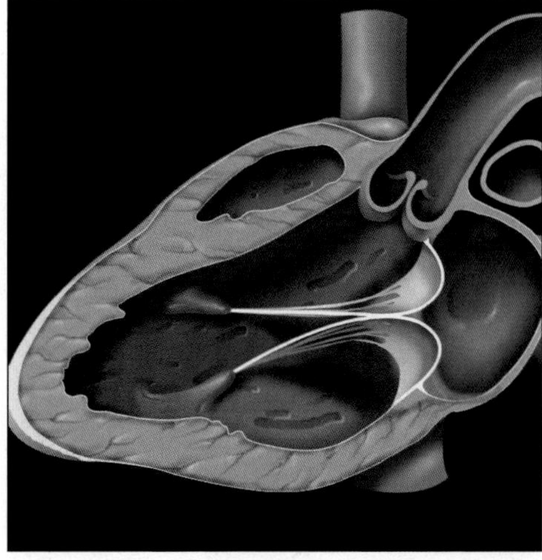

Three chamber view graphic shows bowing ("billowing") of mitral valve leaflets below annulus plane (flap backwards).

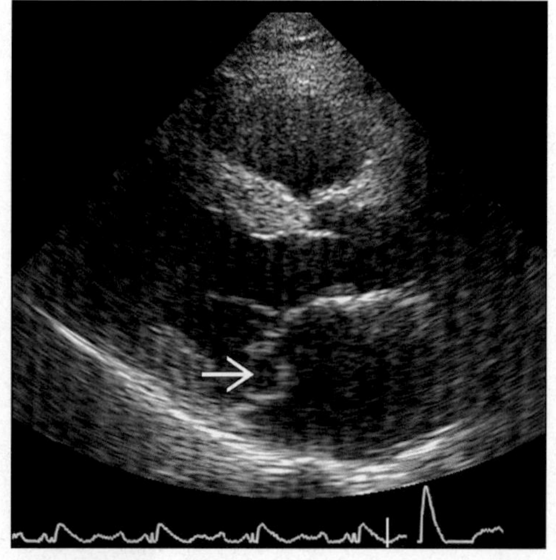

Three chamber view echocardiography shows systolic "bowing" ➡ of posterior mitral valve leaflet into left atrium.

TERMINOLOGY

Abbreviations and Synonyms

- Mitral valve prolapse (MVP)
- "Barlow syndrome"
- Click-murmur syndrome
- Floppy mitral valve syndrome

Definitions

- Systolic prolapse ("billowing" or "bowing") of 1 or both mitral leaflets > 2 mm below annulus into left atrium

IMAGING FINDINGS

General Features

- Best diagnostic clue: Midsystolic "bowing" (flap backwards) of thickened leaflets into the left atrium

Radiographic Findings

- Chest Radiography
  - Normal
  - If co-existent mitral regurgitation left atrial and left ventricle dilatation

CT Findings

- Cardiac Gated CTA
  - Thickened leaflets (3-5 mm) with systolic "bowing" > 2 mm into left atrium beyond the mitral annulus during systole
  - Incomplete closure of leaflets during ventricular systole if insufficiency

MR Findings

- MR Cine
  - Same criteria used in echocardiography - symmetrical bowing of valve leaflets > 2 mm behind the plane of the annulus
  - 3-chamber/LVOT tract view is the best view for the diagnosis of MVP
  - Co-existent mitral regurgitation as eccentric retrograde systolic flow jet
- Phase-contrast
  - Detect and quantify mitral regurgitation
  - Plane needs to be perpendicular to mitral valve regurgitant orifice

Nuclear Medicine Findings

- Stress Imaging Findings

DDx: Mitral Valve Prolapse

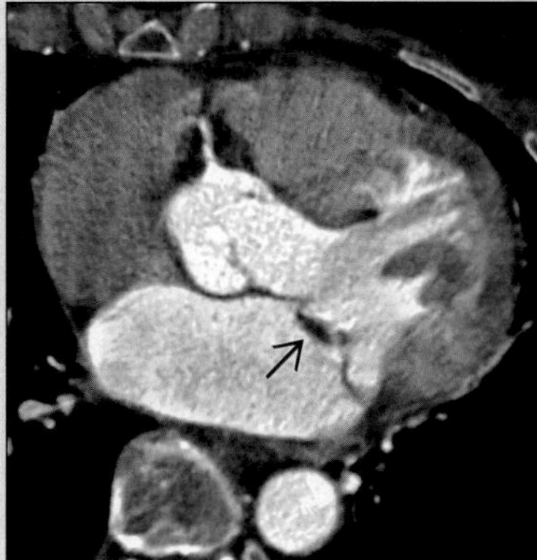

Idiopathic ("Billowing")

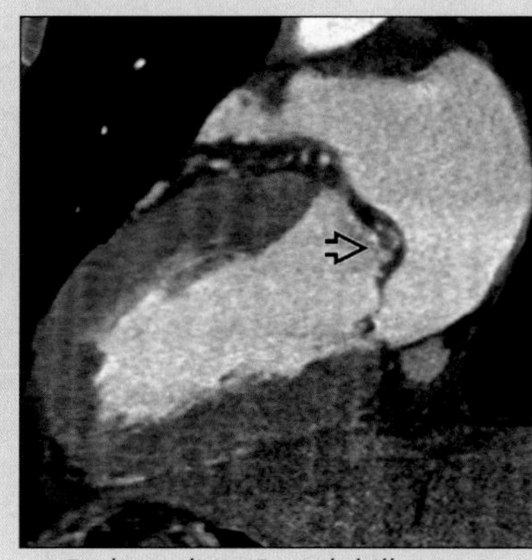

Endocarditis (Pseudobillowing)

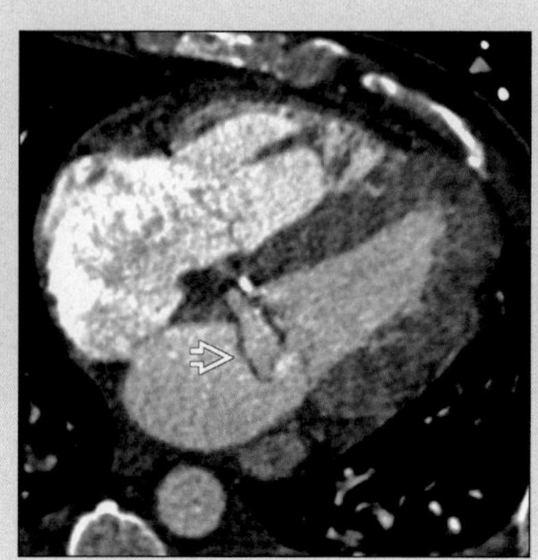

Endocarditis (Perforation)

MITRAL VALVE PROLAPSE

Key Facts

Imaging Findings

- Best imaging tool: Echocardiography
  - Systolic "bowing" of 1 or both leaflets > 2 mm into left atrium
  - Eccentric systolic high velocity regurgitant retrograde flow jet into the left atrium if mitral insufficiency
- ECG-gated cardiac CT may show MVP
- 3-chamber/LVOT tract view is the best view for the diagnosis of MVP

Top Differential Diagnoses

- Idiopathic; "Barlow Syndrome"
  - Strong hereditary component; most common form
- Hereditary Connective Tissue Disease (e.g., Marfan, Ehlers-Danlos Syndrome)
- Infective Endocarditis
  - Either true prolapse, free leaflet margin prolapse, or "pseudoprolapse" of vegetations
- Rheumatic Disease, Trauma
  - Diseased sub-valvular apparatus (ruptured chordae tendinea): Mostly free leaflet margin prolapse (flail leaflet)

Clinical Issues

- Spectrum from normal life to severe mitral regurgitation requiring surgery (moderate-severe MR in 10% of patients)
- Most prevalent cardiac valvular abnormality effecting 2-5% of the population

  - Normal in patients with MVP and chest pain

Echocardiographic Findings

- Echocardiogram
  - 2D echocardiography
    - Thickening (3-5 mm) of one or both valve leaflets
    - Symmetrical bowing of valve leaflets > 2 mm behind the plane of the annulus
    - Asymmetrical buckling of one or both leaflets into the left atrium
    - Prolapse of the aortic and tricuspid valves in 20% of patients
  - Transesophageal echocardiography
    - Detailed anatomy of the mitral valve and chordae
- Color Doppler: Eccentric systolic high velocity flow jet of mitral regurgitation (MR)

Angiographic Findings

- Conventional
  - Buckling of mitral valve
  - Scalloped valve edges reflecting redundant valve tissue
  - Retrograde systolic flow jet if mitral regurgitation

Imaging Recommendations

- Best imaging tool: Echocardiography
- Protocol advice
  - Echocardiography
    - Transthoracic and transesophageal approach if necessary
  - ECG-gated cardiac CT
    - Coronary CT angiography examination protocol
    - 4D-cine imaging; multiplanar reformations (MPR) (3-chamber, 2-chamber and 4-chamber view)
- Cardiac MR
  - Cine in the 3-chamber/LVOT view
  - Phase contrast to detect and quantify mitral regurgitation

DIFFERENTIAL DIAGNOSIS

Barlow Syndrome, MVP Syndrome

- Also referred to as MVP dysautonomia
- Most common form, not associated with other disease
- Myxomatous thickening and "billowing" of leaflets
- Concomitant mitral valve regurgitation may develop

Hereditary Connective Tissue Disease

- Marfan, Ehlers-Danlos syndrome
- Pseudoxanthoma elasticum
- Osteogenesis imperfecta
- Von Willebrand disease
- Periarteritis nodosa

Infectious Endocarditis (IE)

- Prolapse of perforated leaflets, free leaflet margins, or vegetations (mimicking leaflet prolapse)

Rheumatic Disease; Trauma

- Diseased sub-valvular apparatus (e.g., ruptured chordae) mostly leading to "flail" leaflet

PATHOLOGY

General Features

- General path comments
  - Thickened, redundant mitral valve (myxomatous connective tissue proliferation)
  - Systolic displacement of the valve > 2 mm above the annulus
  - Moderate or severe mitral regurgitation in 10% of patients
  - Fibrin deposits often form at the mitral valve left atrial angle
- Genetics: Several chromosomal loci have been identified for familial MVP
- Etiology
  - Primary (familial or non-familial) or secondary
  - Some people may inherit the condition, especially those associated with connective tissue disorders like Marfan syndrome

MITRAL VALVE PROLAPSE

- Epidemiology
  - Most prevalent cardiac valvular abnormalities effecting 2-5% of the population
  - Up to 40% of people have dysautonomia, an imbalance of the autonomic nervous system
- Associated abnormalities: Marfan syndrome, other connective tissue disease, Von Willebrand disease

Gross Pathologic & Surgical Features

- Myxomatous proliferation of valve leaflets

Microscopic Features

- Disordered arrangement of cells
- Fragmentation of collagen network
- Endothelial disruption is frequent

CLINICAL ISSUES

Presentation

- Most common signs/symptoms
  - Most patients are asymptomatic (60%) or experience syncope, palpitations or atypical chest pain
  - Atrial fibrillation due to progressive left atrial enlargement
  - Symptoms of heart failure develop in the presence of concomitant chronic mitral regurgitation and decreasing cardiac function
  - Irregular heartbeat or palpitations, especially while lying on the left side
  - May be associated with numerous symptoms of dysautonomia including
    - Panic attacks
    - Anxiety
    - Migraine
    - headaches
    - Depression
    - Fatigue
- Other signs/symptoms: Systolic "click" murmur
- Strong hereditary component for MVP
- 90% of Marfan syndrome and first degree relative effected
- Sudden cardiac death < 2% (most likely ventricular tachyarrhythmia), more frequent in familial form
- Fibrin emboli and increased risk of cerebrovascular accidents in patients < 45 years of age

Demographics

- Age: Manifestation usually between 20-40 years of age
- Gender: Females:males = 2:1

Natural History & Prognosis

- Spectrum from normal life to severe mitral regurgitation requiring surgery
- At risk for development of endocarditis, arrhythmias and spontaneous rupture of the chordae

Treatment

- Therapy directed toward specific symptoms
- Medical and surgical treatment for MVP patients with MR is the same as for patients with MR
- Most patients with mitral valve prolapse require no specific precautions
- To help prevent a heart valve infection, a person may need preventive antibiotics before certain dental or surgical procedures if a murmur of mitral insufficiency is present

DIAGNOSTIC CHECKLIST

Consider

- Echocardiography is primary imaging modality
- Cardiac ECG-gated CT may show MVP, most reliable in 3-chamber view
- Cardiac MR cine in the 3-chamber/LVOT tract view

Image Interpretation Pearls

- Systolic "bowing" of myxomatous thickened, redundant mitral valve leaflets
- Eccentric retrograde systolic jet in case of co-existent mitral regurgitation

SELECTED REFERENCES

1. Grau JB et al: The genetics of mitral valve prolapse. Clin Genet. 72(4):288-95, 2007
2. Hepner AD et al: The prevalence of mitral valve prolapse in patients undergoing echocardiography for clinical reason. Int J Cardiol. 2007
3. Pinheiro AC et al: Diagnostic value of color flow mapping and Doppler echocardiography in the quantification of mitral regurgitation in patients with mitral valve prolapse or rheumatic heart disease. J Am Soc Echocardiogr. 20(10):1141-8, 2007
4. Sharma R et al: The evaluation of real-time 3-dimensional transthoracic echocardiography for the preoperative functional assessment of patients with mitral valve prolapse: a comparison with 2-dimensional transesophageal echocardiography. J Am Soc Echocardiogr. 20(8):934-40, 2007
5. Mechleb BK et al: Mitral valve prolapse: relationship of echocardiography characteristics to natural history. Echocardiography. 23(5):434-7, 2006
6. Müller S et al: Comparison of three-dimensional imaging to transesophageal echocardiography for preoperative evaluation in mitral valve prolapse. Am J Cardiol. 98(2):243-8, 2006
7. Pepi M et al: Head-to-head comparison of two- and three-dimensional transthoracic and transesophageal echocardiography in the localization of mitral valve prolapse. J Am Coll Cardiol. 48(12):2524-30, 2006
8. Braundwald E. Valvular Heart Disease. In: Braundwald E. Heart Disease: A Textbook of Cardiovascular Medicine 6th Ed. W.B. Saunders Company, Philadelphia, 2001
9. Becker AE et al: Pathomorphology of mitral valve prolapse. In: Boudoulas H. Woolley CF (eds): Mitral Valve: Floppy Valve, Mitral Valve Prolapse and Mitral Regurgitation. 2nd Ed., Furuta, Armonk, NY, 2000
10. Boudoulas H et al: Natural History. In: Boudoulas H. Woolley CF (eds): Mitral Valve: Floppy Valve, Mitral Valve Prolapse and Mitral Regurgitation. 2nd Ed. Furuta, Armonk, NY, 2000

MITRAL VALVE PROLAPSE

IMAGE GALLERY

Typical

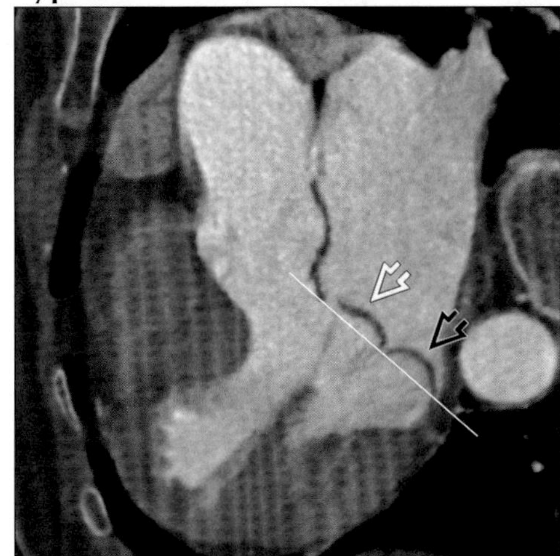

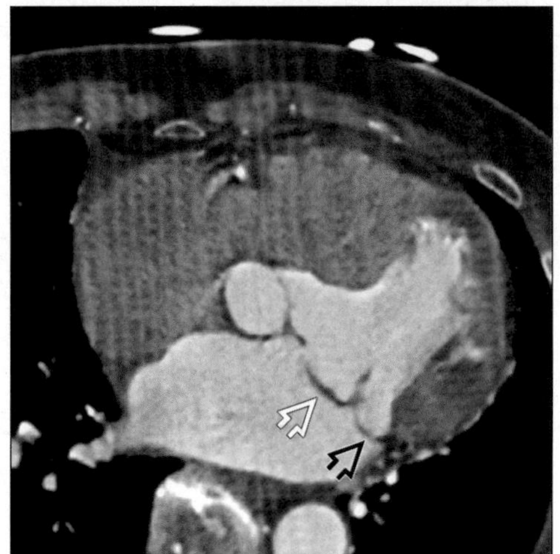

(Left) *Three chamber view cardiac CT shows "billowing" of the anterior and posterior leaflets below the annulus plane (line).* ***(Right)*** *Axial cardiac CT demonstrates mid-systolic "billowing" of the anterior and posterior leaflets.*

Typical

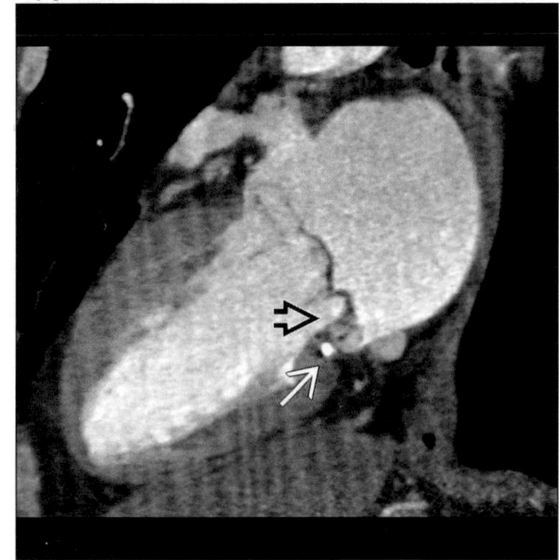

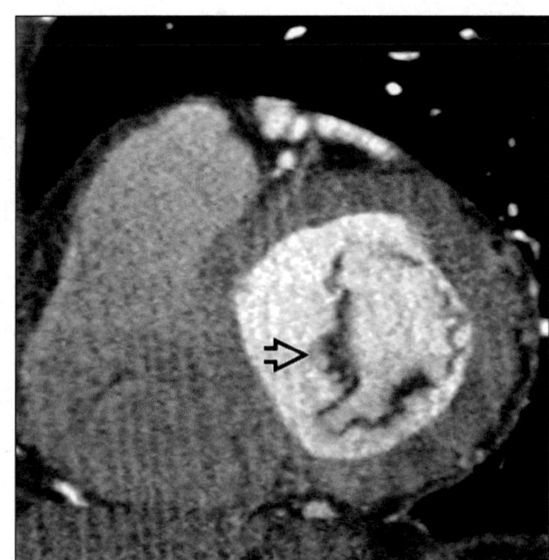

(Left) *2-Chamber view cardiac CT shows systolic "billowing" and mitral annular calcification.* ***(Right)*** *LV short axis cardiac CT shows myxomatous thickening of leaflets. Note open valve orifice during diastole.*

Typical

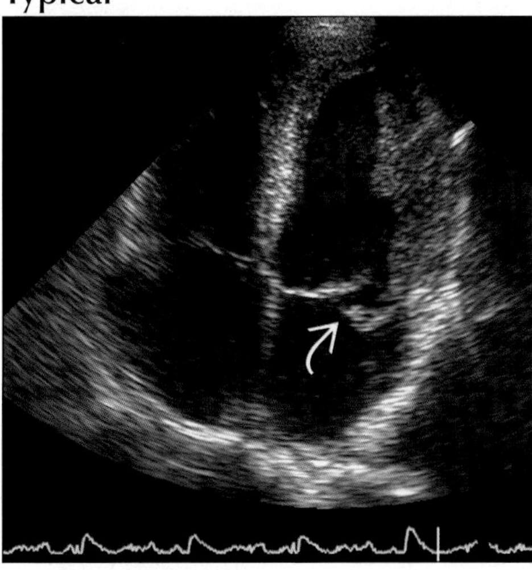

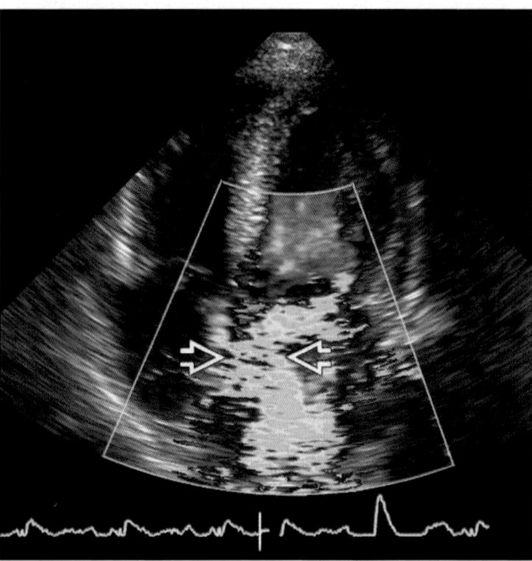

(Left) *Four chamber view echocardiography demonstrates posterior leaflet prolapse causing mitral regurgitation.* ***(Right)*** *Four chamber view color Doppler ultrasound confirmed eccentric retrograde Doppler flow jet into the left atrium indicating severe co-existent regurgitation.*

MITRAL REGURGITATION

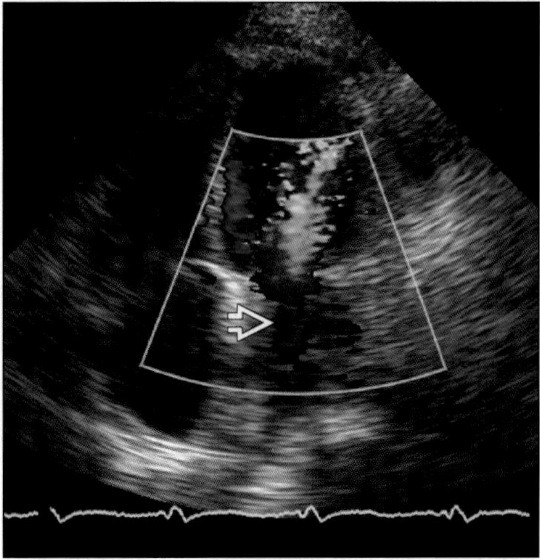

Four chamber view color Doppler ultrasound shows retrograde systolic Doppler flow jet into left atrium ➲.

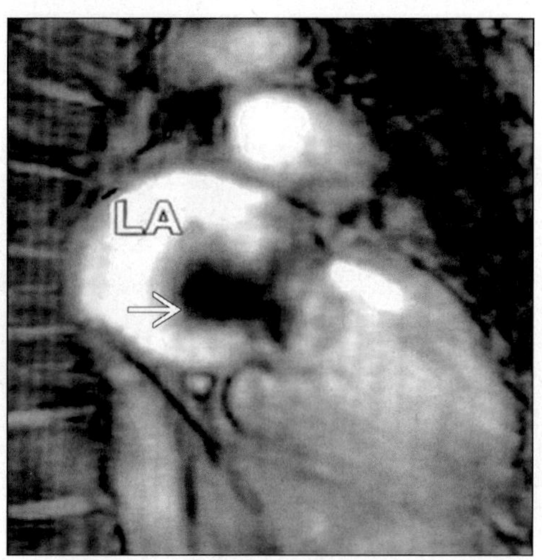

Long axis vertical MR cine shows signal void in the left atrium ➔ representing regurgitant jet during LV systole.

TERMINOLOGY

Abbreviations and Synonyms

- Mitral regurgitation (MR); mitral insufficiency (MI)

Definitions

- Incomplete closure of mitral valve during left ventricular systole leading to retrograde blood flow into left atrium

IMAGING FINDINGS

General Features

- Best diagnostic clue: Echocardiography: Retrograde Doppler flow jet during systole
- Acute MR
  - No left atrial enlargement
  - Sudden onset of pulmonary venous hypertension and edema
- Chronic MR
  - Left atrial (LA) and left ventricular (LV) enlargement
  - Calcification of mitral valve(MV) leaflets in the elderly

Radiographic Findings

- Radiography
  - Chronic MR
    - Cardiomegaly with LV and LA enlargement ("bulging" of left atrial appendage segment; splaying of carina, right double density)
    - Pulmonary vascular markings are typically normal, since pulmonary venous pressures are usually not significantly elevated
    - Right upper lobe pulmonary vascular congestion in 10% (late stage)
  - Acute MR
    - Interstitial edema with Kerley B lines (pulmonary venous hypertension) and pulmonary edema (volume overload)
    - Right upper lobe pulmonary edema due to direction of regurgitant jet

CT Findings

- Cardiac Gated CTA
  - Incomplete systolic coaptation of MV leaflets, planimetry (ROI) of regurgitant orifice area correlates with echocardiography grading of MR
  - LA and LV enlargement in chronic MR

DDx: Mitral Regurgitation

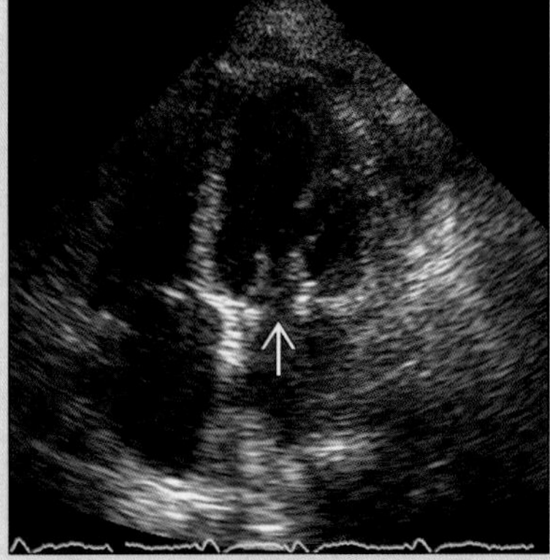

Rheumatic MV Disease

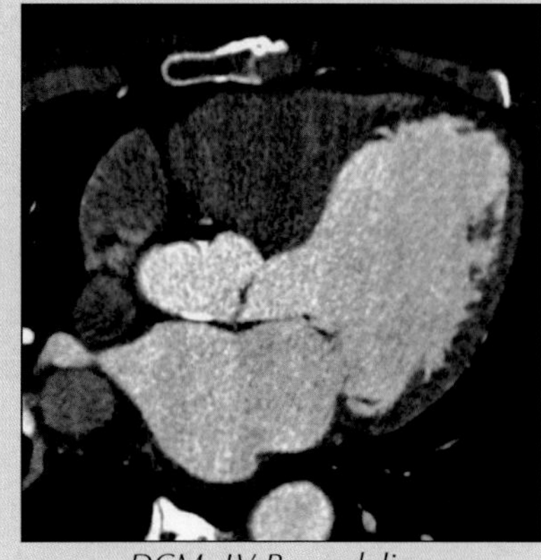

DCM: LV Remodeling

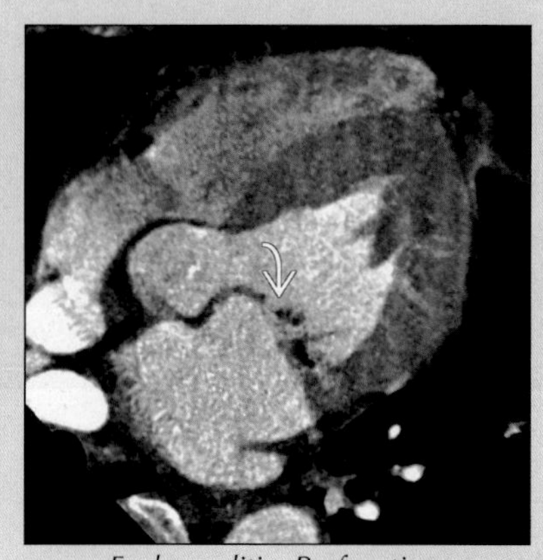

Endocarditis: Perforation

MITRAL REGURGITATION

Key Facts

Terminology
- Incomplete closure of mitral valve during left ventricular systole leading to retrograde blood flow into left atrium

Imaging Findings
- Best imaging tool: Echocardiography: Retrograde Doppler flow jet into left atrium during systole
- Acute MR: No left atrial enlargement, asymmetric pulmonary edema
- Chronic MR: Left atrial and left ventricular enlargement
- Rheumatic heart disease: Irregular cusp thickening and/or chordal fusion/rupture

Top Differential Diagnoses
- Rheumatic Heart Disease
- Infective Endocarditis
  - Perforation of leaflets or vegetations that prevent closure
- Dilated Cardiomyopathy
- Ischemic Heart Disease: Papillary muscle dysfunction

Pathology
- Acute MR, etiology: Ruptured papillary muscle or chordae tendinea (Inferior MI, trauma, rheumatic disease); cusp perforation (infective endocarditis)
- Chronic MR: Chronic infarct with LV remodeling, annular dilatation, rheumatic or myxomatous valve disease, mitral valve prolapse

Clinical Issues
- Clinical presentation depends on acuity of mitral regurgitation

  - Leaflet morphology
    - Rheumatic heart disease: Irregular cusp thickening and/or chordal fusion or rupture with or without calcification
    - Infective endocarditis: Perforation or prolapse of leaflets; vegetations

MR Findings
- Systolic flow void (jet) in left atrium
- Left atrium and ventricle dilation
- Gold standard for functional assessment; ejection fraction, LV volumes and mass
- Phase contrast MR can calculate the regurgitant fraction

Echocardiographic Findings
- Echocardiogram
  - 2D echocardiography
    - Chronic MR: Cardiomegaly with LV and LA enlargement
    - Estimation of left ventricular function: Increase in LV end diastolic and end systolic volumes; decrease in LV ejection fraction
  - Transesophageal echocardiography (TEE)
    - Detailed anatomy of the mitral valve pre-operatively (involved segments)
    - Preferred in acute MR, because TEE is more accurate to determine etiology and more accurate for quantification of regurgitant flow
    - Differentiation between prolapse or restrictive leaflet movement to define surgical technique
    - TEE can determine the area of the regurgitant flow at the level of the valve (regurgitant orifice area)
- Color Doppler: Systolic high velocity jet into LA: Quantification of severity (mild, moderate and severe: Grade 1-3) by measurement of jet width (vena contracta) and regurgitant volume

Angiographic Findings
- Left Ventricular Angiography Findings
  - Prompt appearance of contrast in LA following LV injection

Imaging Recommendations
- Best imaging tool: Echocardiography

DIFFERENTIAL DIAGNOSIS

Rheumatic Heart Disease
- Central regurgitant jet on Doppler echocardiography and left ventricular angiogram
- Irregular thickened leaflets that demonstrate reduced motion
- Usually chronic MR, but rupture of chordae can lead to acute MR

Infective Endocarditis
- Perforation of leaflets
- Vegetations may prevent complete leaflets coaptation

Cardiomyopathy
- Dilation of mitral annulus

Ischemic Heart Disease
- Papillary muscle dysfunction

Degenerative Heart Disease
- Calcific leaflets preventing complete closure

Mitral Valve Prolapse
- "Billowing" and eccentric regurgitant jet; caused by myxomatous thickening of leaflets, rather symmetric

Collagen Vascular Disease
- Scleroderma, lupus

PATHOLOGY

General Features
- General path comments
  - MR can occur with involvement of the mitral leaflets, mitral annulus, chordae tendineae or papillary muscle

MITRAL REGURGITATION

  - Deformation and retraction of one or both valve cusps
  - Retrograde systolic ejection of blood into left atrium
  - Associated LA and LV enlargement in chronic MR
  - Valve leaflets
    - Rheumatic heart disease with thickening, shortening and retraction of one or more leaflets and associated shortening of the chordae tendineae
    - Infectious endocarditis with perforation of a valve leaflet or a vegetation that prevents coaptation of the leaflets
    - Traumatic destruction of a leaflet
  - Mitral annulus
    - Dilation secondary to left ventricular enlargement
    - Degenerative calcification in diabetes, Marfan and Hurler syndromes: If severe, calcific spur can project into the left ventricle
  - Chordae tendineae
    - Rupture secondary to rheumatic fever, endocarditis and trauma
    - Posterior leaflet more frequently involved
  - Papillary muscle
    - Dysfunction associated with chronic ischemia and 20-30% of patients with myocardial infarction
    - Involvement or infiltration with abscess, neoplasm, sarcoid, granuloma
- Etiology
  - Acute MR: Ruptured papillary muscle or chordae tendinea (inferior MI, trauma, rheumatic disease); cusp perforation (infective endocarditis)
  - Chronic MR: Chronic infarct with LV remodeling, annular dilatation, rheumatic or myxomatous valve disease, mitral valve prolapse

Staging, Grading or Classification Criteria

- Mild, moderate, severe (grade I-III) by echocardiography
  - Mild: Vena contracta 1-3 mm, regurgitant volume < 30 mL
  - Moderate: Vena contracta 4-6 mm, regurgitant volume 30-59 mL
  - Severe: Vena contracta > 7 mm, regurgitant volume > 60 mL
- Regurgitant orifice area > 0.3 cm^2 = severe regurgitation

CLINICAL ISSUES

Presentation

- Most common signs/symptoms
  - Fatigue, exhaustion and right heart failure (late)
  - Chronic MR
    - Symptoms develop progressively
    - Depend on severity of lesion, rate of progression, pulmonary artery pressure and presence of associated coronary or myocardial disease
    - Left atrium is dilated
    - LV-eccentric hypertrophy and dilatation
  - Acute MR
    - Almost always severe symptoms
    - Left atrium is normal in size with an increase in pressure leading to pulmonary edema
    - Reduced forward output (shock) may develop due to LV volume overload
- Other signs/symptoms: In acute MR, a 3rd heart murmur or early diastolic flow rumble is characteristic, the typical holosystolic murmur may be absent
- Clinical Profile: Clinical presentation different in acute and chronic mitral regurgitation

Natural History & Prognosis

- Untreated: 40-60% mortality in 5 years

Treatment

- Medical therapy to reduce afterload, anticoagulation if atrial fibrillation
- Prophylaxis against endocarditis if anticipated bacteremia (dental extraction)
- Valve reconstruction or valve replacement surgery in patients with functional disability despite optimal medical management
- Indications for surgery for chronic mitral regurgitation include signs of left ventricular dysfunction
  - EF < 60% and a left ventricular end systolic dimension (LVESD) > 45 mm

DIAGNOSTIC CHECKLIST

Consider

- Jet of blood flowing from the left ventricle into the left atrium during ventricular systole
- Degree of severity of mitral regurgitation can be quantified by the regurgitant fraction

Image Interpretation Pearls

- Echo: Color Doppler showing regurgitant flow in the left atrium during systole
- Cardiac CT: Incomplete coaptation of leaflets during ventricular systole
- MR: Signal void in the left atrium during ventricular systole
- CXR: LV and LA (splaying of carina, right double density) enlargement

SELECTED REFERENCES

1. ACC/AHA 2006 guidelines for the management of patients with valvular heart disease. Circulation. 114:e84-231, 2006
2. Alkadhi H et al: Mitral regurgitation: quantification with 16-detector row CT--initial experience. Radiology. 238(2):454-63, 2006
3. Alkadhi H et al: Mitral regurgitation: quantification with 16-detector row CT--initial experience. Radiology. 238(2):454-63, 2006
4. Westenberg JJ et al: Accurate quantitation of regurgitant volume with MRI in patients selected for mitral valve repair. Eur J Cardiothorac Surg. 27(3):462-6; discussion 467, 2005
5. Braunwald E: Valvular Heart Disease. In: Braunwald E. Heart Disease: A Textbook of Cardiovascular Medicine 6th ed. Philadelphia, W.B. Saunders Company, 2001
6. Carabello B: Mitral Regurgitation. In: Rahimtolla SH (ed): Valvular Heart Disease and Endocarditis. Atlas of Heart Diseases. Vol. 11. Braunwald E (series editor). Current Medicine, Philadelphia, 1996

MITRAL REGURGITATION

IMAGE GALLERY

Typical

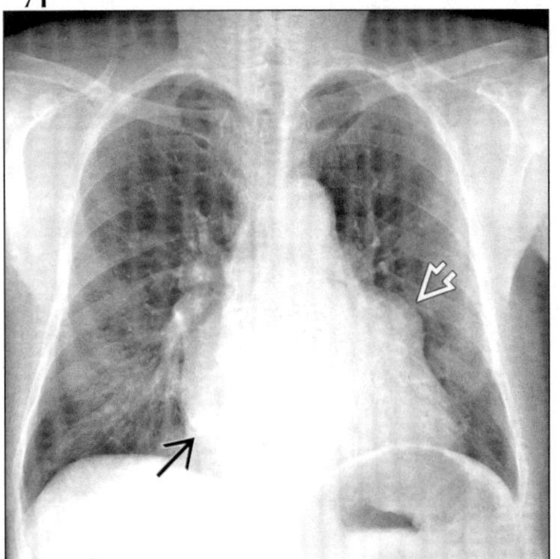

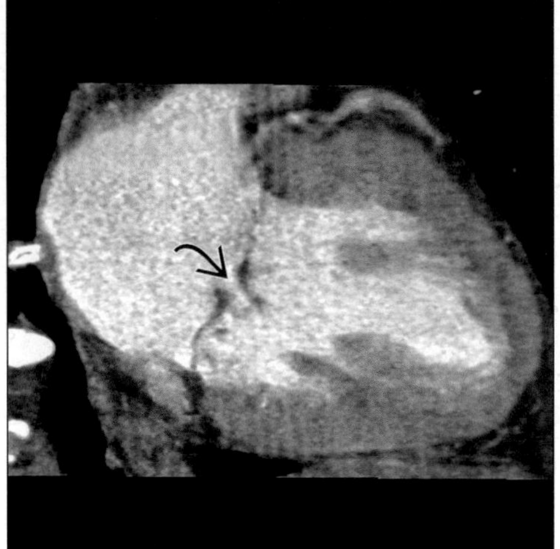

(Left) *Anteroposterior radiograph shows a typical configuration of the cardiac silhouette ➡ with "bulging" of the left atrial appendage segment and right double density ➡ due to left atrial enlargement, as well as splaying of the carina (combined mitral stenosis and regurgitation).* ***(Right)*** *Long axis vertical cardiac CT shows incomplete coaptation of leaflets ➡ during ventricular systole, resulting in an regurgitant orifice.*

Typical

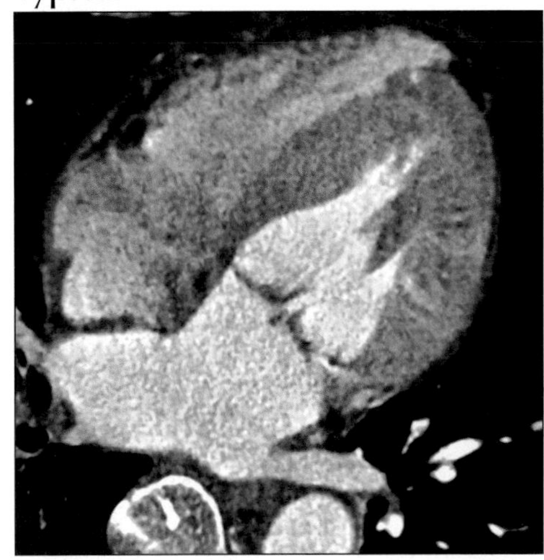

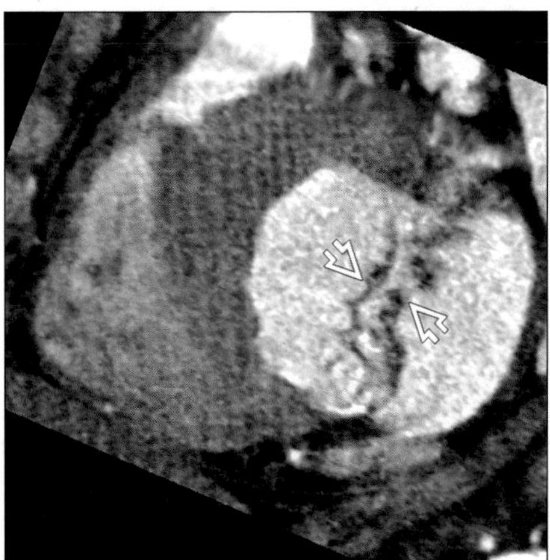

(Left) *Axial cardiac CT shows incomplete systolic closure of leaflets with small vegetation in orifice. Normal LA-size suggests acute AR in infective endocarditis.* ***(Right)*** *Short axis cardiac CT shows incomplete closure of valve and thickened leaflets ➡ in the same patient.*

Typical

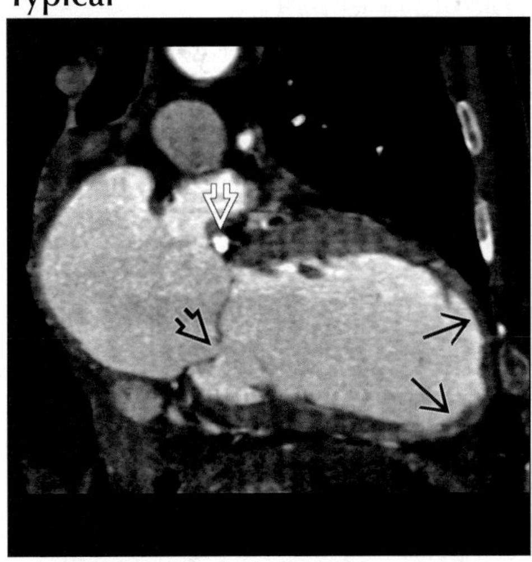

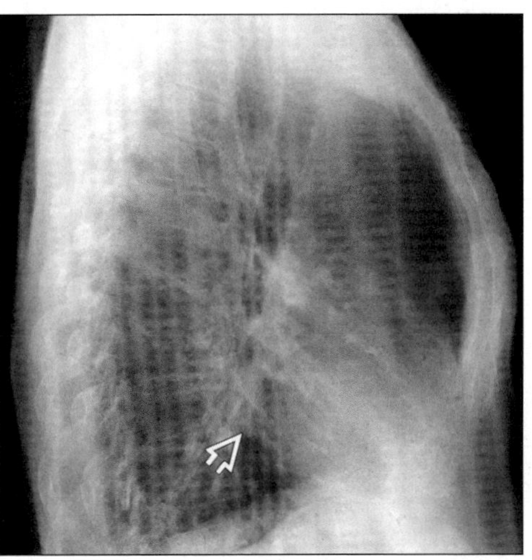

(Left) *Long axis vertical cardiac CT shows incomplete closure of mitral valve leaflets ➡ during diastole in ischemic dilated cardiomyopathy. Note severe left coronary artery calcification ➡, apical aneurysm ➡, and left atrial enlargement.* ***(Right)*** *Lateral radiograph shows left atrial enlargement ➡ in chronic severe mitral regurgitation.*

MITRAL ANNULAR CALCIFICATION

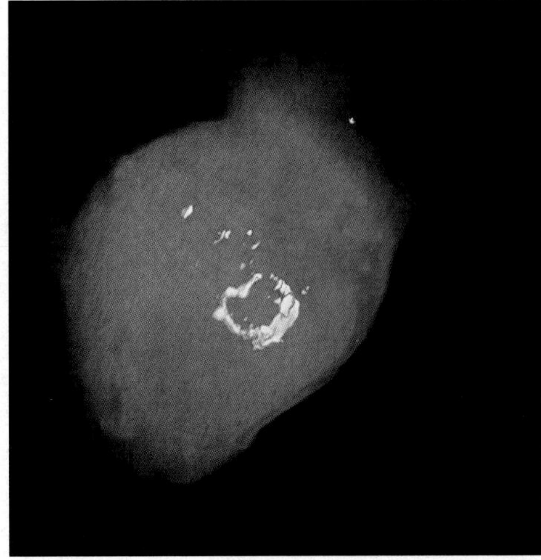

3D-VRT Cardiac CT shows almost circumferential mitral annular calcification.

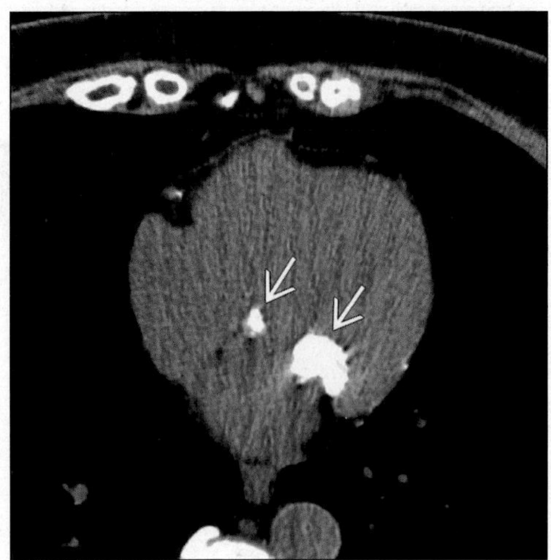

Axial NECT (calcium scoring) demonstrating prominent mitral annular calcification (MAC) ➡, particularly in the posterior leaflet.

TERMINOLOGY

Abbreviations and Synonyms

- Mitral annular calcification (MAC)
- Annular mitral valve calcification

Definitions

- Chronic degenerative calcification of the fibrous mitral valve annulus

IMAGING FINDINGS

General Features

- Best diagnostic clue: "J, C, U or O-shaped" mitral annular calcification
- Location: Posterior base (early stage) and full annulus (late stage)
- Morphology
  - Dense calcification
    - Rare variant: "Caseous calcification" (due to liquefaction necrosis)

Radiographic Findings

- Incomplete calcification of posterior annulus (forming a "J, C or U")
- Entire annulus calcified ("O-shape"); best seen on lateral projections

CT Findings

- NECT
  - Dense calcification within unenhanced cardiac tissue along expected location of posterior or entire annulus
  - Sparing of mitral valve leaflets

MR Findings

- Calcium usually dark on all pulse sequences
  - In expected location of mitral annulus
- Helpful for differential diagnosis of caseous calcification versus tumor

Echocardiographic Findings

- Echocardiogram
  - Hyperechogenic, dense calcification with acoustic shadowing
  - Uncommon, rare variant

DDx: Mitral Annular Calcification

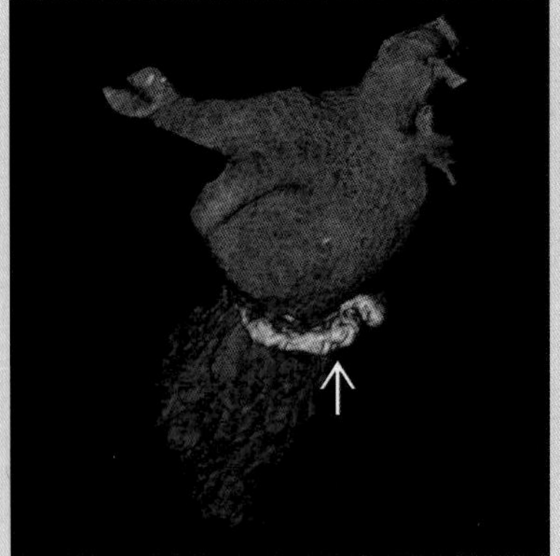

End-Stage Renal Disease

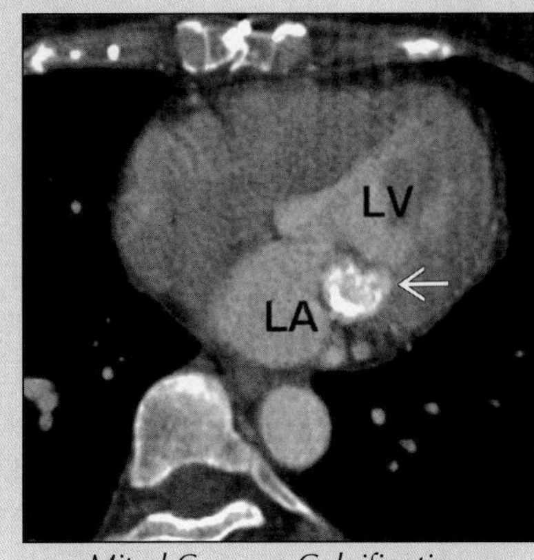

Mitral Caseous Calcification

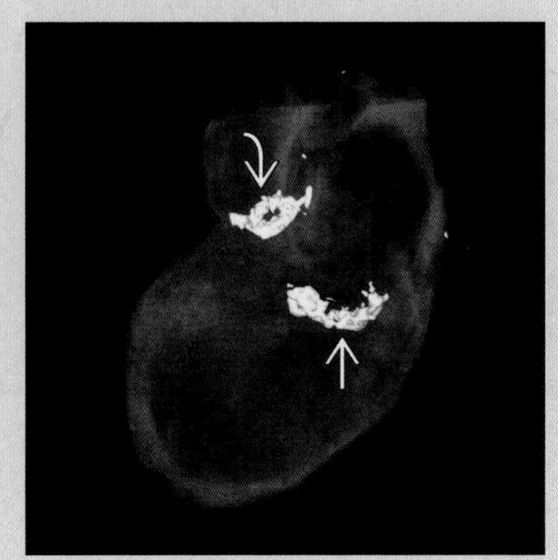

Multivalvular Calcification

MITRAL ANNULAR CALCIFICATION

Key Facts

Terminology
- Mitral annular calcification (MAC)
- Chronic degenerative calcification of the fibrous mitral valve annulus

Imaging Findings
- "C, J, U-shaped" posterior or "O-shaped" full mitral annulus calcification
- Imaging recommendations: X-ray (lateral projections), CT, echocardiography
- Rare variant: "Caseous MAC" ⇒ liquefaction necrosis
  - May mimic tumor or abscess

Top Differential Diagnoses
- End-stage renal disease (ESRD)
- Atherosclerosis
- Multivalvular Calcific Disease
- Caseous Calcification

Pathology
- Not associated with mitral valve stenosis or regurgitation

Clinical Issues
- Prevalence = 14% (FHS): 40% in patients with end-stage renal disease
- Slow progression, increasing prevalence with age
- MAC thickness correlates linearly with stroke risk (1 mm ⇒ 10%)
- Increased mortality in patients with chronic kidney disease
- Pre-disposing factor for infective endocarditis
- Marker for coronary artery disease in patients < 65 years

    - Caseous MAC = echodense mass with echolucent center (liquefaction necrosis)
    - May mimic tumor
- M-mode: Measurement of annulus thickness as predictor for stroke and cardiovascular disease
- Color Doppler: Concomitant regurgitation or stenosis (rare)

Imaging Recommendations
- Best imaging tool
  - Radiograph (lateral views)
  - Computed tomography
  - Echocardiography
- Protocol advice
  - CT
    - NECT is sufficient for diagnosis
    - Contrast-enhanced cardiac ECG-gated CT does not provide more diagnostic information
    - Cardiac CT may be useful for presurgical planning to assess myocardial involvement, to distinguish whether leaflets are calcified or not, and to distinguish caseous calcification from tumor
  - Transthoracic echocardiography
    - B-mode, M-mode and Doppler

DIFFERENTIAL DIAGNOSIS

End-Stage Renal Disease (ESRD)
- Extraosseous calcification develops due to secondary hyperparathyroidism
- Frequently combined with systemic vascular calcification (tunica media)

Atherosclerosis
- MAC is linked with aortic atheroma and coronary artery disease

Multivalvular Calcific Disease
- MAC is associated with aortic valve calcification, and aortic stenosis may develop

Caseous Calcification
- Solid, calcifying mass mimicking tumor

PATHOLOGY

General Features
- Genetics: May play a role; in patients with ESRD, genotype ENPP1 is associated with higher severity of systemic arterial calcification
- Etiology
  - End-stage renal disease
    - Secondary hyperparathyroidism and alterations in calcium metabolism leading to extraosseous calcium deposits
  - Atherosclerosis
    - Association with cardiovascular disease such as stroke, coronary artery disease and aortic atheroma
  - Multivalvular calcification: Association with MAC
  - Tuberculosis
  - May be a later stage of atherosclerotic disease
- Epidemiology
  - Prevalence = 14% in the Framingham Heart Study (FHS) population
  - Prevalence ~ 40% in end-stage renal disease (ESRD)
- Associated abnormalities: Not associated with mitral valve stenosis or regurgitation

Gross Pathologic & Surgical Features
- Calcification of the fibrous base of the mitral annulus
- Fibro-elastic deficiency
- If extensive calcification, myocardium may be involved (prevalence: 12% of surgical specimen)
- "Caseous calcification": Toothpaste-like, white material

Microscopic Features
- Calcium deposits
- Liquefaction necrosis (in case of caseous calcification)

CLINICAL ISSUES

Presentation
- Most common signs/symptoms
  - Usually asymptomatic

- Sometimes "mass-effect" if extensive calcium deposits, if AV-node is affected AV-block may develop
- Other signs/symptoms: In rare cases signs of co-existent mitral insufficiency or stenosis

Demographics

- Age
  - Increase with age
    - > 35% of the elderly population
- Gender: More common in females

Natural History & Prognosis

- Slow progression over time
- Increased risk of stroke
  - Dependent of MAC thickness measured by echocardiography
  - 1 mm increase ⇒ 10% increased risk
- In patients with chronic kidney disease: 3-fold increased mortality
- Pre-disposing factor for infective endocarditis
  - Bacterial endocarditis found in 19% of surgical specimen
- Marker for severe coronary artery disease in patients < 65 years of age
- Higher prevalence of coronary artery disease and aortic atheroma
- Association with incidental atrial fibrillation

Treatment

- Non-specific if asymptomatic (e.g., calcium metabolism regulation in ESRD)
- Surgery may be considered if symptoms due to mass effect
  - 5-year survival after surgery is 76%

DIAGNOSTIC CHECKLIST

Consider

- Mitral valve annulus calcification is a benign degenerative disease
- Most frequently an incidental finding on chest X-ray or CT
  - In particular in patients with end-stage renal disease or systemic atherosclerosis
- "Caseous calcification" is a rare variant which may mimic tumor, CT and MR imaging recommended

Image Interpretation Pearls

- Posterior annulus base calcification ("J, C, or U-shape") and full annulus ("O-shape") at late stage
- Best seen at lateral X-ray projections and CT

SELECTED REFERENCES

1. Eller P et al: Impact of ENPP1 genotype on arterial calcification in patients with end-stage renal failure. Nephrol Dial Transplant. 23(1):321-7, 2008
2. d'Alessandro C et al: Mitral annulus calcification: determinants of repair feasibility, early and late surgical outcome. Eur J Cardiothorac Surg. 32(4):596-603, 2007
3. Lubarsky L et al: Images in cardiovascular medicine. Caseous calcification of the mitral annulus by 64-detector-row computed tomographic coronary angiography: a rare intracardiac mass. Circulation. 116(5):e114-5, 2007
4. Poh KK et al: Prominent posterior mitral annular calcification causing embolic stroke and mimicking left atrial fibroma. Eur Heart J. 28(18):2216, 2007
5. Sharma R et al: Mitral annular calcification predicts mortality and coronary artery disease in end stage renal disease. Atherosclerosis. 191(2):348-54, 2007
6. Cury RC et al: Epidemiology and association of vascular and valvular calcium quantified by multidetector computed tomography in elderly asymptomatic subjects. Am J Cardiol. 94(3):348-51, 2004
7. Atar S et al: Mitral annular calcification: a marker of severe coronary artery disease in patients under 65 years old. Heart. 89(2):161-4, 2003
8. Fox CS et al: Mitral annular calcification predicts cardiovascular morbidity and mortality: the Framingham Heart Study. Circulation. 107(11):1492-6, 2003
9. Adler Y et al: Mitral annulus calcification--a window to diffuse atherosclerosis of the vascular system. Atherosclerosis. 155(1):1-8, 2001
10. Harpaz D et al: Caseous calcification of the mitral annulus: a neglected, unrecognized diagnosis. J Am Soc Echocardiogr. 14(8):825-31, 2001
11. Carpentier AF et al: Extensive calcification of the mitral valve anulus: pathology and surgical management. J Thorac Cardiovasc Surg. 111(4):718-29; discussion 729-30, 1996
12. Maher ER et al: Aortic and mitral valve calcification in patients with end-stage renal disease. Lancet. 2(8564):875-7, 1987

MITRAL ANNULAR CALCIFICATION

IMAGE GALLERY

Typical

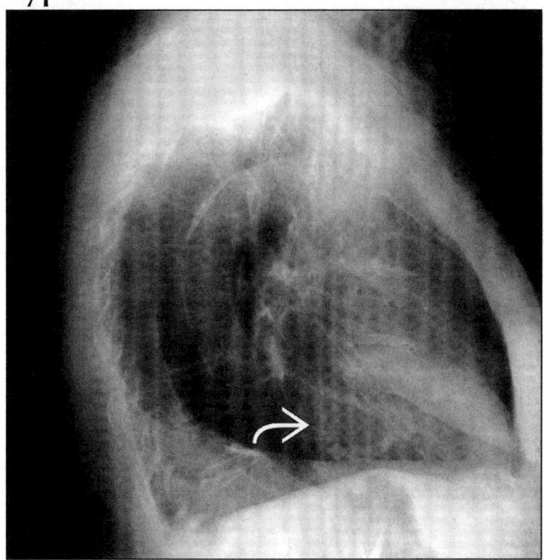

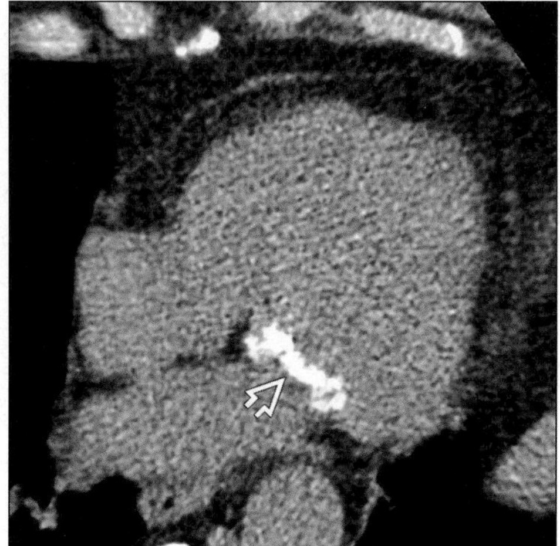

(Left) *Lateral radiograph demonstrates "O-shaped" mitral annular calcification.* ***(Right)*** *Axial NECT shows mitral annular calcification.*

Typical

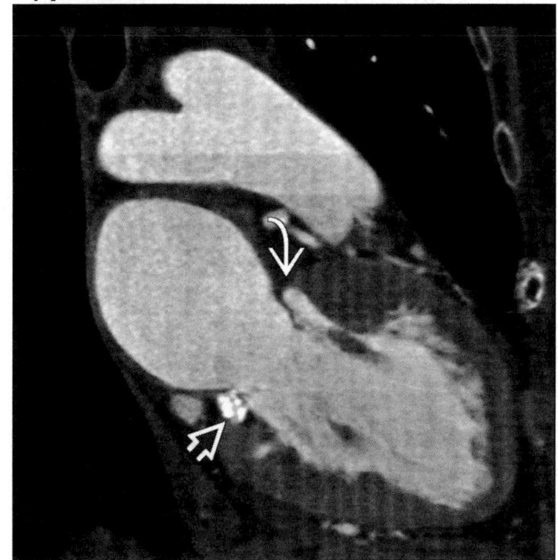

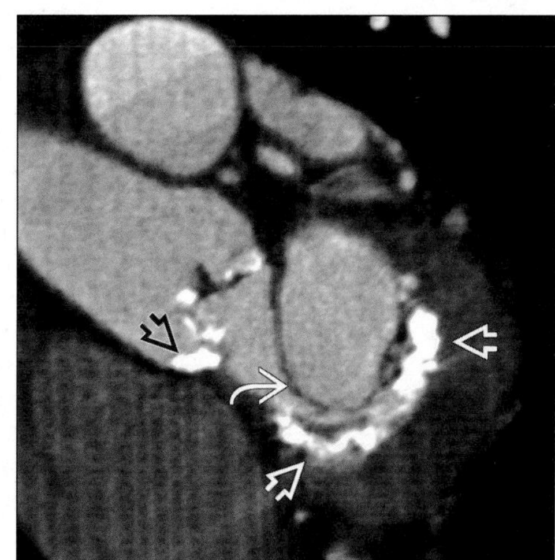

(Left) *Long axis vertical cardiac CT shows posterior annulus calcification. The anterior ring is spared.* ***(Right)*** *Coronal oblique CECT shows extensive posterior MAC with tender leaflets. Co-existent aortic valve calcium.*

Typical

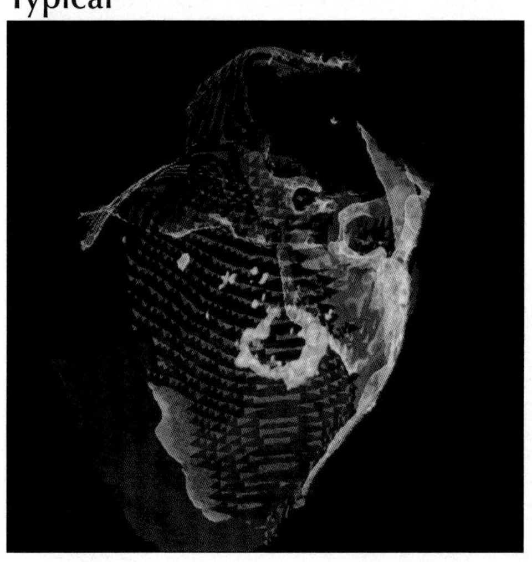

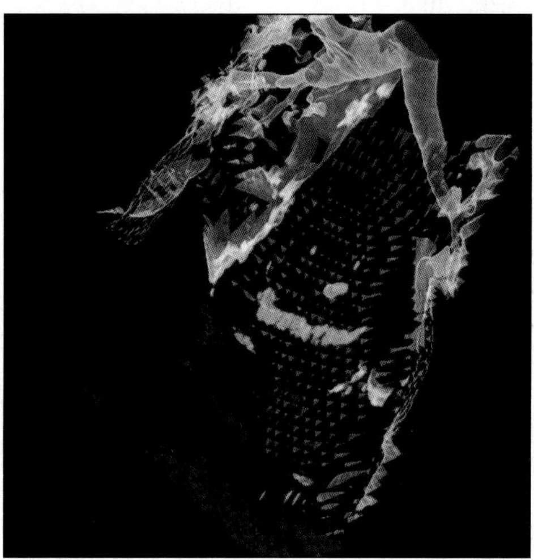

(Left) *Cardiac CT 3D-VRT anterior view shows "O-shaped" mitral annular calcification.* ***(Right)*** *Cardiac CT 3D-VRT shows "U-shaped" MAC.*

PULMONARY STENOSIS

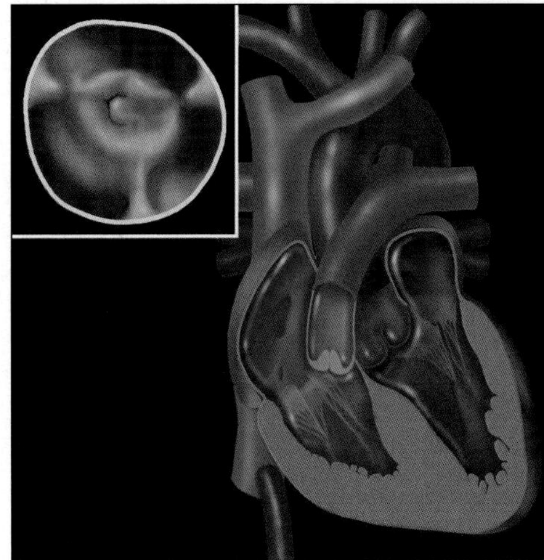

Graphic shows diffuse thickening of the pulmonary valve leaflets with a significantly diminished valvular orifice (inset).

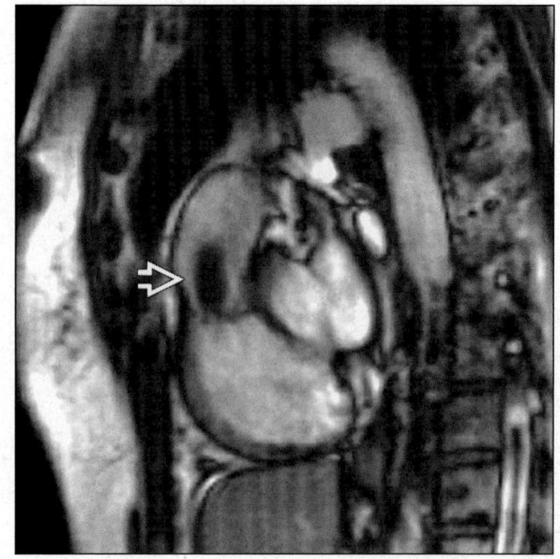

RVOT SSFP cardiac MR shows a focal area of signal dephasing ➪ emanating from the thickened pulmonary valve leaflets, consistent with high grade pulmonary valve stenosis.

TERMINOLOGY

Abbreviations and Synonyms

- Pulmonary stenosis (PS); pulmonic stenosis

Definitions

- Obstructive lesion (subvalvular, valvular, supravalvular or infundibular) of the right ventricular (RV) outflow tract with post-stenotic dilation of the pulmonary arteries

IMAGING FINDINGS

General Features

- Best diagnostic clue
  - Unilaterally enlarged left pulmonary artery (PA) on radiograph is highly suggestive of PS
    - PS jet frequently is directed towards the left PA and causes focal post-stenotic dilatation where the jet hits the arterial wall
    - Rarely a unilaterally enlarged right PA is present
- Morphology
  - Thickened and stenotic valve
  - Post-stenotic dilation of the pulmonary artery in > 80% of patients
  - Systolic flow jet into the pulmonary outflow tract
  - Right ventricular hypertrophy and dysfunction in severe pulmonary stenosis (PS)

Radiographic Findings

- Radiography
  - Chest radiography findings
    - Normal heart size with dilated pulmonary artery segment or left PA in ~ 80%
    - Pulmonary vascular markings may be decreased in pulmonary stenosis with an associated right-to-left shunt
    - Radiographic findings of congestive heart failure can be seen in severe stenosis with cardiomegaly, right atrial and right ventricular enlargement

CT Findings

- CTA: Currently plays little role in the assessment of pulmonary stenosis

DDx: Tetralogy of Fallot

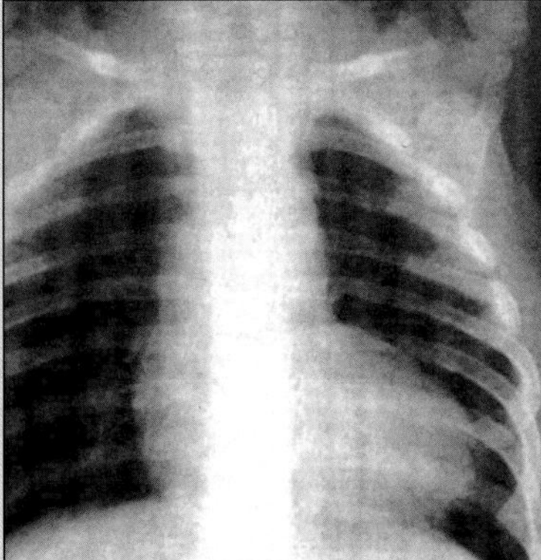

"Boot-Shaped" Cardiac Silhouette

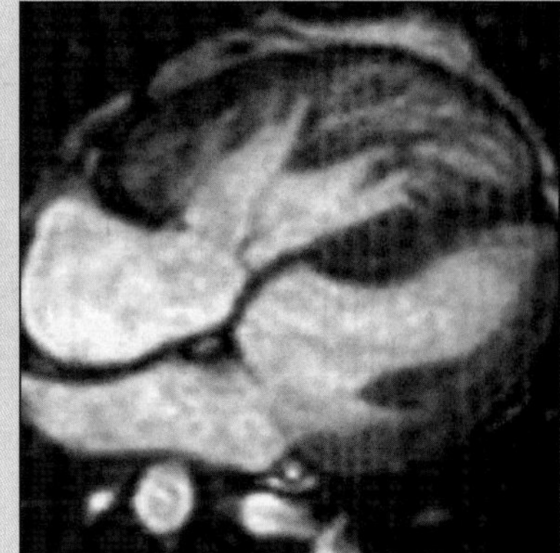

Right Ventricular Hypertrophy

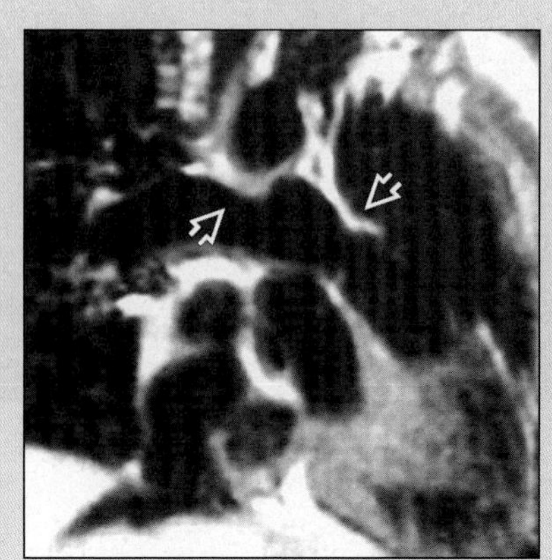

Stenoses of RV Outflow Tract

PULMONARY STENOSIS

Key Facts

Terminology

- Obstructive lesion (subvalvular, valvular, supravalvular or infundibular) of the right ventricular (RV) outflow tract with post-stenotic dilation of the pulmonary arteries

Imaging Findings

- Echocardiography remains the primary and most readily available modality in the assessment of valvular heart disease
- Thickened pulmonary valve with restricted systolic motion and reduced mobility of the valve leaflets
- Post-stenotic dilation of the pulmonary artery in > 80% of patients
- Phase contrast or velocity-encoding sequences provides instantaneous measurement of the spatial mean velocity in a region of interest
- MR with phase contrast imaging is rapidly becoming the most accurate and reproducible means for in vivo flow measurements

Pathology

- Pressure gradient across the lesion; severe > 80 mm Hg
- Epidemiology: Congenital form is most common > 90%
- Most common appearance is a conical, dome-shaped or windsock-like valve in which the leaflets protrude from their attachments into the pulmonary artery

Clinical Issues

- Treatment options include balloon valvuloplasty or surgical valvotomy in patients with right heart failure or gradients > 50 mm Hg

MR Findings

- T1WI: Normal valves are fast-moving, thin structures that are difficult to visualize with conventional T1 sequences
- T1WI FS: Newer fast spin echo "black blood" sequences provide improved spatial and temporal resolution of cardiac valves, particularly when valve leaflets are thickened and less mobile
- SSFP White Blood Cine
  - Moving valve leaflets are easily seen since flowing blood over the adjacent leaflets leads to signal loss from localized eddies and turbulence
  - Phase contrast or velocity-encoding sequences provides instantaneous measurement of the spatial mean velocity in a region of interest
    - Rapidly becoming the most accurate and reproducible means for in vivo flow measurements
    - Highly useful means of calculating pressure gradients across a stenotic valve

Echocardiographic Findings

- Echocardiogram
  - Remains the primary and most readily available modality in the assessment of valvular heart disease
    - Thickened pulmonary valve with restricted systolic motion and reduced mobility of the valve leaflets
    - Doming or windsock pulmonary valve
    - Post-stenotic dilation of pulmonary artery
    - Echocardiography provides an accurate means of measuring the pulmonary valve annulus in order to detect annular hypoplasia
  - Transesophageal echocardiography (TEE) is a valuable means of clarifying patients with suspected infective endocarditis or patients with poor acoustic windows
- Pulsed Doppler: Highly reproducible means of determining the velocity of flow across the stenotic valve, which can then be used to estimate the pressure gradient across the stenotic valve by applying the modified Bernoulli equation
- Color Doppler: Systolic high velocity flow jet in the pulmonary outflow tract

Angiographic Findings

- Conventional
  - Patients with ECG evidence of severe stenosis (> 50 mm Hg) usually undergo cardiac catheterization for confirmatory pressure assessment
    - Performed in concert with balloon pulmonary valvuloplasty
  - Catheterization is generally not indicated in mild or moderate pulmonary stenosis
  - Useful method of assessing the morphology of the right ventricle, pulmonary outflow tract and pulmonary arteries

DIFFERENTIAL DIAGNOSIS

Tetralogy of Fallot

- Cyanotic, congenital heart defect characterized by right ventricular outflow tract (RVOT) stenosis, right ventricular hypertrophy, ventricular septal defect and overriding aorta

Pulmonary Atresia

- Congenital atresia of the right ventricular outflow tract

Rheumatic Heart disease

- Usually associated with mitral and aortic valve disease

Carcinoid Syndrome

- High association of tricuspid valve disease

PATHOLOGY

General Features

- General path comments
  - Morphologic features of stenotic valve can vary

PULMONARY STENOSIS

- Valve most commonly described as a conical, dome-shaped or windsock-like structure in which leaflets protrude from their attachments into the pulmonary artery
- Orifice ranges from one to several millimeters
  - Hypoplasia of the pulmonary valve ring with associated dysplastic pulmonary valves can be occasionally seen
    - PV dysplasia results in nodular, thickened valve leaflets
- Genetics
  - PS is generally considered to be multifactorial in origin, although familial forms have been described
    - Recurrence rates amongst siblings are roughly 2-3%
    - Prevalence amongst offspring with a parent with PS is roughly 4%
  - May be associated with several genetic disorders
    - Primary valvular PS can be seen in association with Noonan syndrome
    - Supravalvular pulmonary stenosis can be seen in association with Rubella syndrome and Williams syndrome
- Etiology
  - Congenital heart disease (CHD) most common cause of PS
    - 80% isolated pulmonary valve stenosis
    - 20% associated with other forms of congenital heart disease
  - Rheumatic heart disease
    - Associated with mitral and aortic valvular disease
  - Carcinoid syndrome
    - Associated with tricuspid valvular disease
- Epidemiology
  - Pulmonary stenosis represents 8-12% of all congenital heart defects in children
    - Isolated PS with an intact ventricular septum is the second most common congenital cardiac defect
  - Prevalence among adults is 15% of all congenital heart defects
  - Patient's age at presentation varies with the severity of the obstruction
- Associated abnormalities
  - Atrial septal defect (ASD)
  - Ventricular septal defect (VSD)
  - Tetralogy of fallot

Gross Pathologic & Surgical Features

- "Dome-shaped" valve most common without calcification
- Thickened, fused leaflets, raphe extending from fused commissures
- Right ventricular hypertrophy can develop in cases of severe pulmonary valve stenosis

Microscopic Features

- Valve thickened with fibrous, myxomatous, and collagenous tissue

Staging, Grading or Classification Criteria

- Trivial pulmonary stenosis (gradient < 25 mm Hg)
- Mild pulmonary stenosis (gradient 25-50 mm Hg)
- Moderate pulmonary stenosis (gradient 50-80 mm Hg)
- Severe pulmonary stenosis (gradient > 80 mm Hg)

CLINICAL ISSUES

Presentation

- Most common signs/symptoms
  - Presentation depends on severity of symptoms
    - Patients with mild pulmonary stenosis are generally asymptomatic
    - Patients with moderate or severe may present with exertional dyspnea, as well as signs of systemic venous congestion which mimics congestive heart failure
- Other signs/symptoms: Cyanosis can occur in the setting of an associated right-to-left shunt due to a patent foramen ovale or atrial septal defect

Demographics

- Age: Patient's age at presentation is related to the severity of the obstruction
- Gender: M:F = 1:1

Natural History & Prognosis

- Severity of stenosis determines its relative morbidity and mortality
  - Mild-to-moderate valvar pulmonary stenosis is usually well-tolerated
  - Severe pulmonary stenosis can be associated with decreased cardiac output, right ventricular hypertrophy, early congestive heart failure and cyanosis

Treatment

- Observation, medical management and prophylaxis in patients with gradient < 50 mm Hg
- Balloon valvuloplasty or surgical valvotomy in patients with right heart failure or gradients > 50 mm Hg
- Recurrence of PS ~ 15% at 10 year; hemodynamically insignificant pulmonary regurgitation in > 80% of patients post treatment

SELECTED REFERENCES

1. Braundwald E: Valvular Heart Disease. In: Braundwald E. Heart Disease: A Textbook of Cardiovascular Medicine. 6th ed. Philadelphia, W.B. Saunders Company, 2001
2. Rao PS: Pulmonary Valve Disease. In: Alpert JS, Dalen JE and Rahimtoola SH (eds): Valvular Heart Disease. 3rd ed. Philadelphia, Lippincott William and Wilkin, 2000
3. Gielen H et al: Natural history of congenital pulmonary valvar stenosis: an echo and Doppler cardiographic study. Cardiol Young. 9(2):129-35, 1999
4. Otto CM: Right-sided Valve Disease. In: Otto CM: Valvular Heart Disease. 1st ed. Philadelphia, W.B. Saunders Company, 1999
5. Gikonyo BM et al: Anatomic features of congenital pulmonary valvar stenosis. Pediatr Cardiol. 8(2):109-16, 1987

PULMONARY STENOSIS

IMAGE GALLERY

Typical

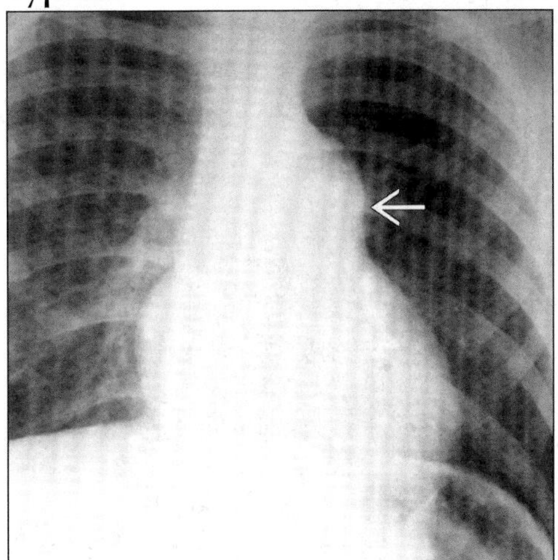

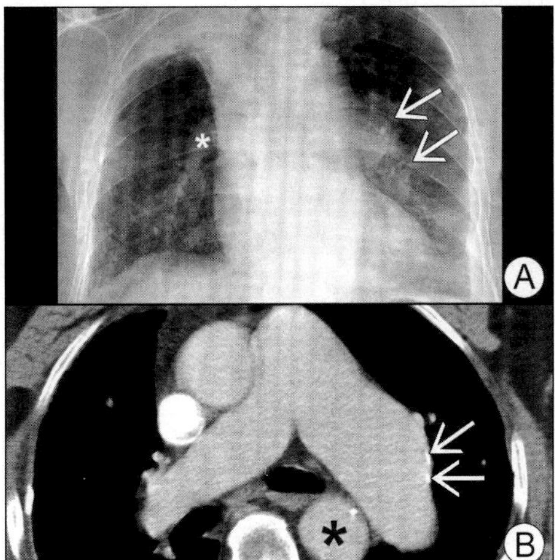

*(**Left**) Posteroanterior radiograph shows enlargement of the main pulmonary artery → consistent with post-stenotic dilatation of the main pulmonary artery. Pulmonary vascularity is somewhat reduced in this patient with a right-to-left shunt. (**Right**) Anteroposterior radiograph (A) shows enlarged left → and normal right (*) pulmonary artery (PA) due to PS. (B) Axial Chest CT shows enlarged left PA (compare to aorta [*]) with calcifications →.*

Typical

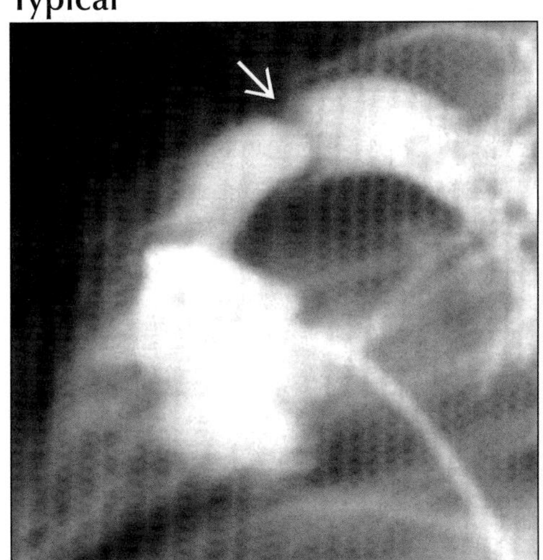

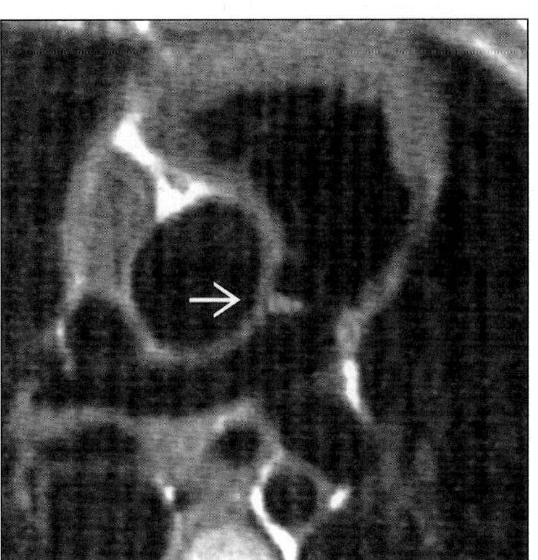

*(**Left**) Catheter angiography of the right ventricle shows an area of circumferential, high grade stenosis → of the pulmonary valve with mild post-stenotic dilatation of the main pulmonary artery. (**Right**) Oblique axial "black-blood" FSE through the main pulmonary artery shows diffuse thickening of a pulmonary valve leaflet →. Hypertrophic changes of the visualized right ventricle are likewise seen.*

Typical

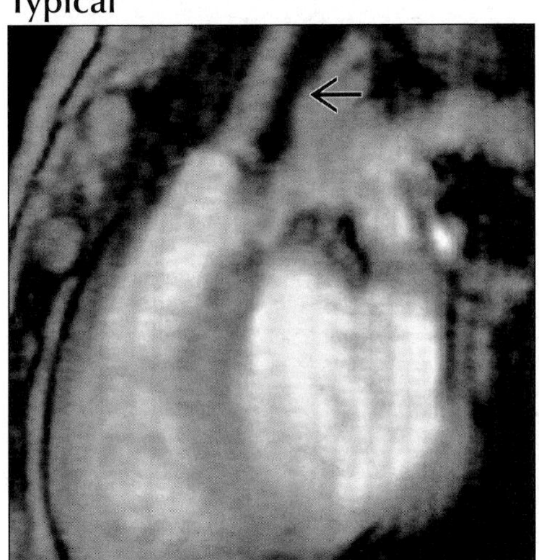

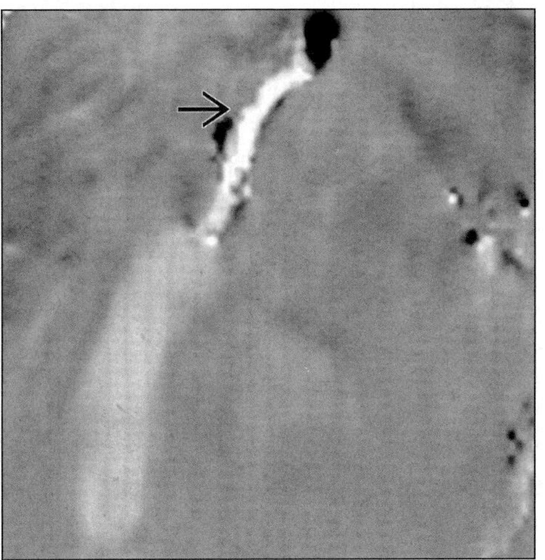

*(**Left**) RVOT magnitude image shows a narrow cone-shaped region of hypointense signal arising from the pulmonary valve →, consistent with severe pulmonary valve stenosis. (**Right**) Corresponding RVOT phase-contrast velocity map shows slit-like, turbulent flow through the pulmonary valve →, indicative of severe stenosis.*

PULMONARY REGURGITATION

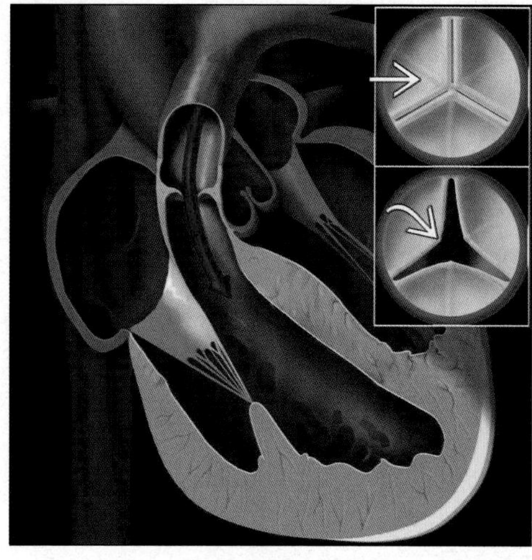

Graphic shows RV with the RVOT and main PA. The blue arrow indicates direction of PR jet. Inserts: Normal diastolic pulmonic valve ➔, and diastolic malcoaptation ➔ leading to PR.

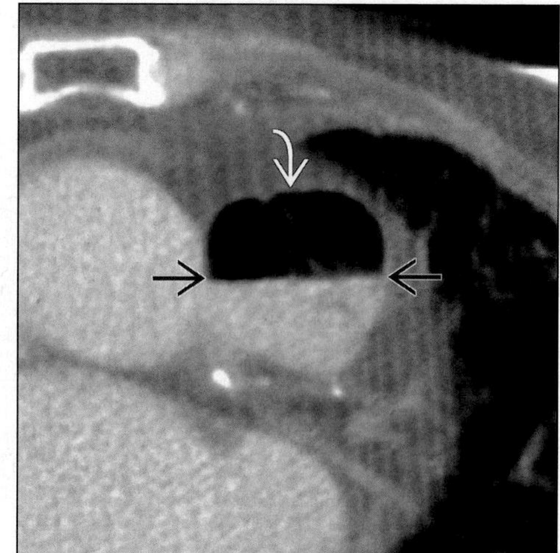

Axial CECT shows the pulmonic valve in short axis ➔. Note: Large amounts of inadvertently injected air causes an air-blood level ➔ and allows for unusually well-delineated valve cusps.

TERMINOLOGY

Abbreviations and Synonyms

- Pulmonary regurgitation (PR)
- Pulmonary insufficiency (PI)

IMAGING FINDINGS

General Features

- Morphology
  - Prominent pulmonary artery
  - Diastolic flow through pulmonary valve (PV) into right ventricle (RV)

Radiographic Findings

- Radiography
  - Dilated pulmonary artery
  - RV enlargement secondary to volume overload
  - Enlarged azygos vein, and vena cava

MR Findings

- Retrograde diastolic flow void (jet) into RV on SSFP or GRE cine exams
- Assessment of RV function
- Phase contrast study can calculate regurgitant volume

Echocardiographic Findings

- Echocardiogram: Dilated RV in severe PR
- Pulsed Doppler: Regurgitant flow detected
- Color Doppler
  - Diastolic flow jet into RV
  - Moderate-severe regurgitant jet on color Doppler reach 1-2 cm into the RV and last through ~ 75% of diastole

Angiographic Findings

- Conventional: Exclusion of other abnormalities of right heart failure

Imaging Recommendations

- Best imaging tool: Echocardiography

DIFFERENTIAL DIAGNOSIS

Surgical Complication

- Balloon valvuloplasty for congential pulmonary valve stenosis

DDx: Pulmonary Regurgitation

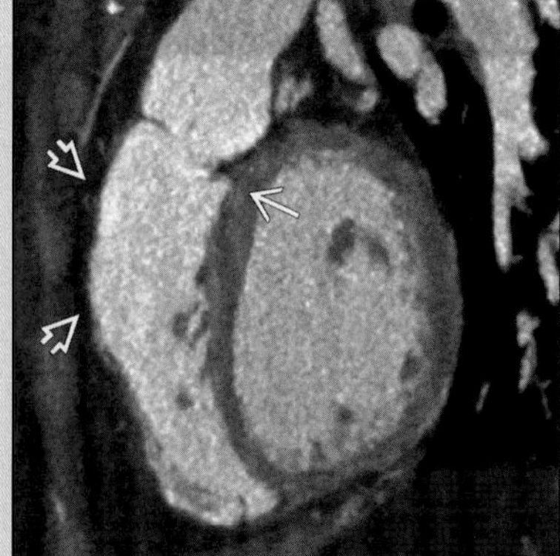

PV Sparing Tetralogy of Fallot Repair

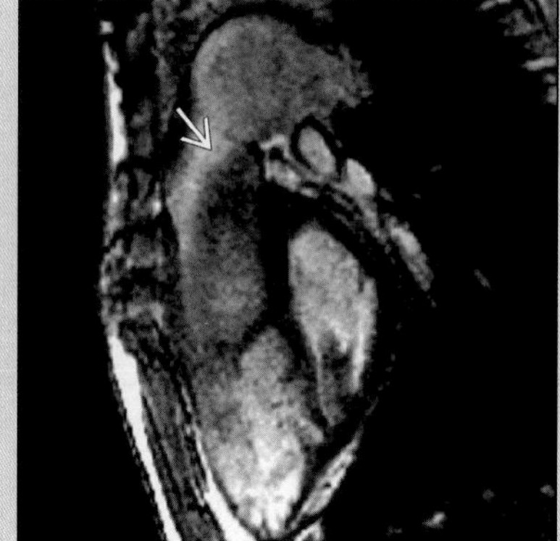

Congenital PS and PR

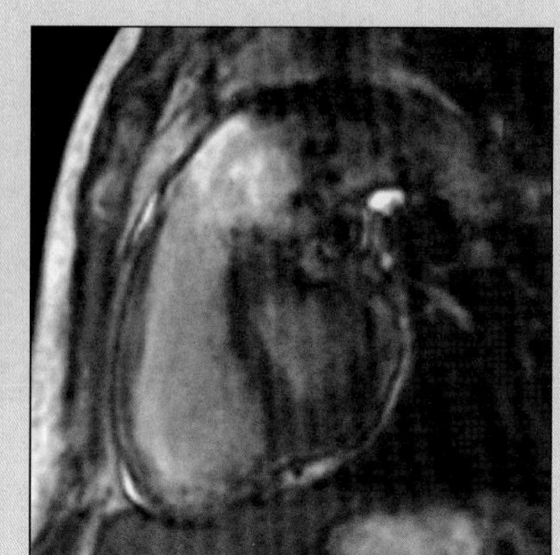

Severe Pulmonary Hypertension

PULMONARY REGURGITATION

Key Facts

Terminology
- Pulmonary regurgitation (PR)

Imaging Findings
- Prominent pulmonary artery
- Diastolic flow through pulmonary valve (PV) into right ventricle (RV)
- Moderate-severe regurgitant jet on color Doppler reach 1-2 cm into the RV and last through ~ 75% of diastole
- Best imaging tool: Echocardiography

Pathology
- Acquired causes are most common
- Pulmonary artery hypertension
- Endocarditis
- Primary congenital causes are rare
- Epidemiology: Usually benign condition

Congenital Heart Diseases
- Absence, malformed, or fenestrated leaflets

Normal Variant
- Mild PR is observed in the majority of normal subjects

Other Diseases
- Carcinoid syndrome, rheumatic heart disease, Marfan syndrome, infective endocarditis, iatrogenic (i.e., pulmonary artery catheter)

PATHOLOGY

General Features
- Etiology
  - Acquired causes are most common
    - Pulmonary artery hypertension
    - Endocarditis
  - Primary congenital causes are rare
- Epidemiology: Usually benign condition

CLINICAL ISSUES

Presentation
- Most common signs/symptoms: Right heart failure and dyspnea on exertion
- Usually asymptomatic
- Symptoms of right ventricle volume overload

Natural History & Prognosis
- Rare in adults
- Generally benign course

Treatment
- Primary pulmonary valve regurgitation is well-tolerated with a good prognosis
  - Valve replacement only if intractable heart failure
  - Valve treatment options consist of annulus repair or prosthetic valve replacement
- Secondary pulmonary valve regurgitation prognosis is related to underlying etiology (i.e., pulmonary arterial hypertension or chronic left sided inflow obstruction)
  - Treatment is directed towards the primary disorder

SELECTED REFERENCES

1. Braunwald E: Valvular Heart Disease. In: Braunwald E. Heart Disease: A Textbook of Cardiovascular Medicine. 6th ed. W.B. Saunders Company, Philadelphia, 2001
2. Rao PS: Pulmonary Valve Disease In: Alpert JS, Dalen JE and Rahimtoola SH (eds): Valvular Heart Disease. 3rd ed. Lippincott William and Wilkins, Philadelphia, 2000
3. Otto CM: Right-sided Valve Disease. In: Otto CM. Valvular Heart Disease. 1st ed. W.B. Saunders Co. Philadelphia, 1999

IMAGE GALLERY

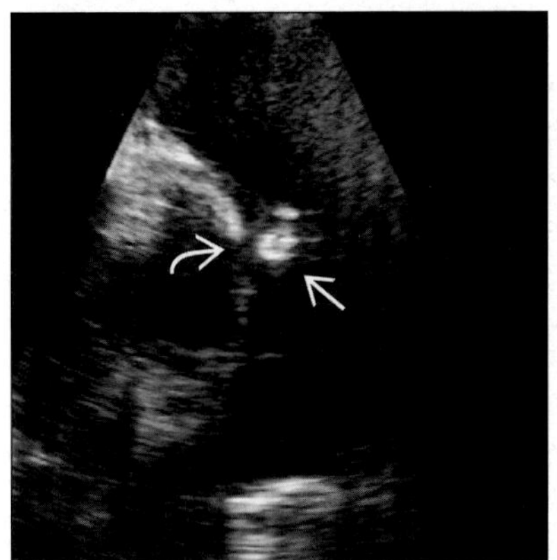

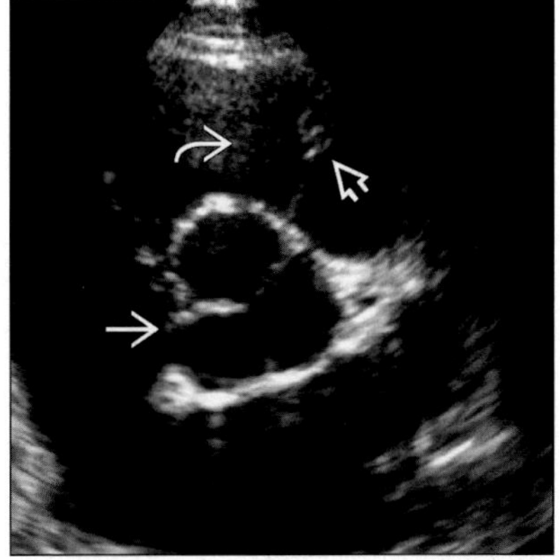

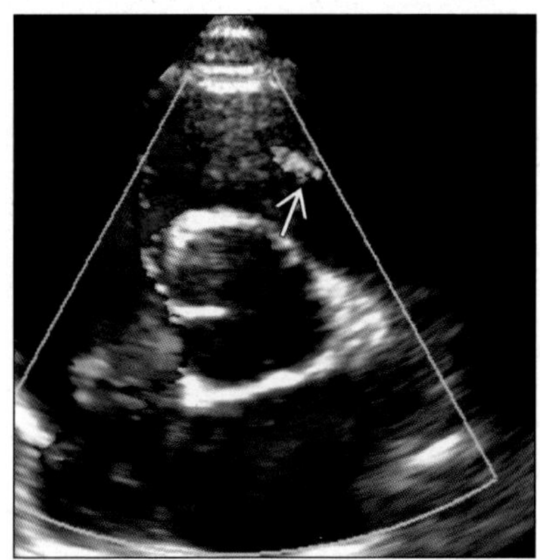

*(**Left**) Transthoracic echocardiogram shows the RVOT, pulmonic valve ➔ and bifurcation of the main PA. Note large circular echodensity on the leaflet ➔ consistent with endocarditis. (**Center**) Transthoracic parasternal short axis echocardiographic view shows the aortic valve ➔ with the RVOT and pulmonic valve ➔. Note rare presence of pulmonic valve papillary fibroelastoma ➔. (**Right**) Transthoracic echocardiogram short axis view with color Doppler in the same case of pulmonic valve papillary fibroelastoma shows mild-moderate jet of pulmonic regurgitation ➔.*

TRICUSPID STENOSIS

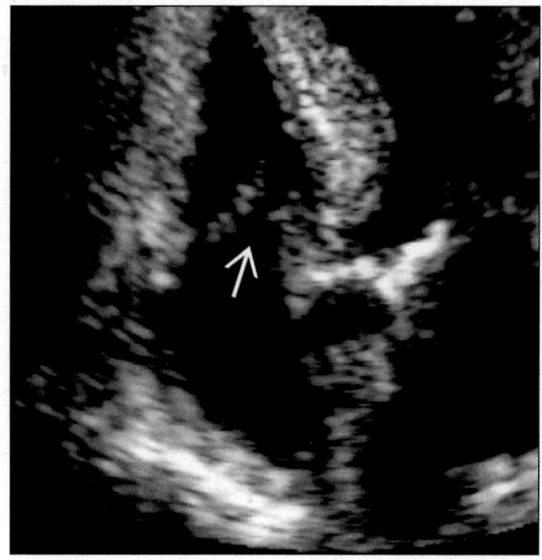

Apical five chamber view of transthoracic echocardiogram shows rheumatic tricuspid stenosis. Note restricted motion of the thickened tricuspid leaflets during diastole ➔.

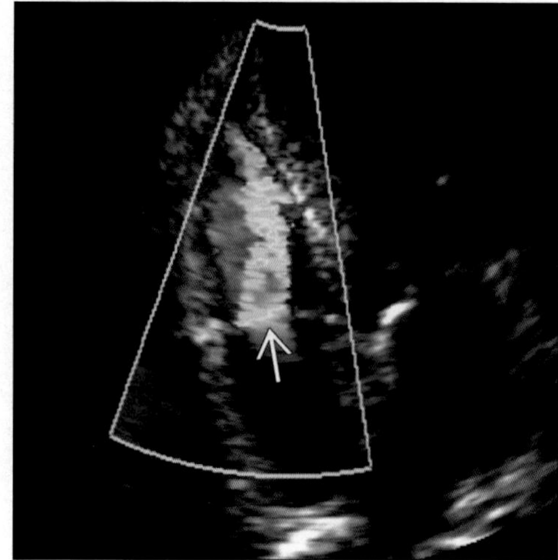

Apical five chamber view of transthoracic echocardiogram with color Doppler in same patient as previous image with rheumatic TS shows high inflow velocity with color aliasing ➔ at the valve orifice.

TERMINOLOGY

Abbreviations and Synonyms

- Tricuspid stenosis (TS)

Definitions

- Reduced valve area (< 2 cm^2 = severe TS)

IMAGING FINDINGS

General Features

- Best diagnostic clue: Mean Doppler gradient greater than 5 mm Hg across valve considered significant TS
- Morphology
  - Thickened and diastolic domed tricuspid leaflets
  - Right atrial enlargement
  - Dilated IVC

Radiographic Findings

- Radiography
  - Chest radiography findings
    - Marked right atrial (RA) enlargement
    - Dilatation of superior vena cava and azygos vein
    - Pulmonary arteries appear normal

CT Findings

- NECT: Calcified and thickened tricuspid valve leaflet with dilated RA (area greater than 20 cm^2)

MR Findings

- Diastolic flow void (jet) into right ventricle (RV)
- Right atrial enlargement

Echocardiographic Findings

- Echocardiogram
  - 2D echocardiography
    - Fused leaflets, diastolic doming, RA enlargement
    - Normal right ventricular function
  - Transesophageal echocardiography
    - Transgastric views best for valve anatomy
- Color Doppler
  - Diastolic high velocity turbulent flow across valve
  - High transvalvular pressure gradient on Doppler
  - Frequently associated tricuspid regurgitation

Angiographic Findings

- Conventional: Diastolic flow jet and decreased movement of valve leaflets

DDx: Tricuspid Stenosis

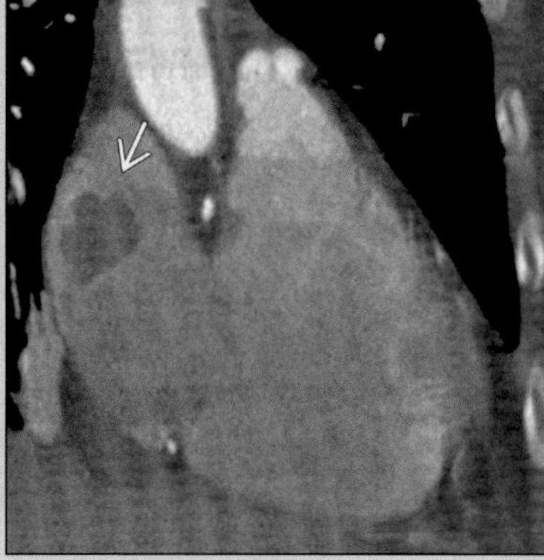

RA Mass with No Valve Obstruction

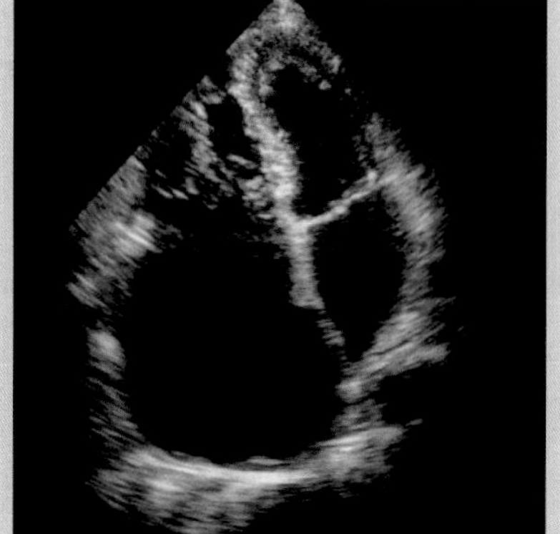

Epstein Anomaly

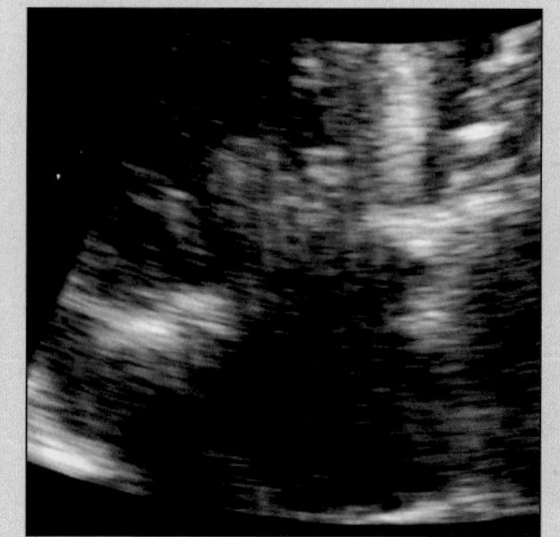

Tricuspid Valve Vegetation

TRICUSPID STENOSIS

Key Facts

Terminology
- Tricuspid stenosis (TS)

Imaging Findings
- Thickened and diastolic domed tricuspid leaflets
- Right atrial enlargement
- Best imaging tool: Echocardiography

Pathology
- Thickening and fusion of the tricuspid valve apparatus
- Rheumatic heart disease is the most common cause

Clinical Issues
- Most common signs/symptoms: Fatigue and edema related to low cardiac output

Imaging Recommendations
- Best imaging tool: Echocardiography

DIFFERENTIAL DIAGNOSIS

Rheumatic Heart Disease
- Most common cause of tricuspid stenosis
- 3% of rheumatic TS isolated, reminder associated with mitral stenosis
- 50% associated with functional tricuspid stenosis

Obstruction of the Tricuspid Valve
- Right atrial tumor/vegetation obstructing valve orifice
- Extracardiac neoplasm

Congenital Tricuspid Stenosis
- Tricuspid Atresia

Complication of Other Disease
- Carcinoid, medications (methysergide, ergotamine, fenfluramine ± phentermine), eosinophilic endomyocardial fibrosis, endomyocardial fibroelastosis

PATHOLOGY

General Features
- General path comments: Thickening and fusion of the tricuspid valve apparatus
- Etiology
  - Rheumatic heart disease is the most common cause
  - Carcinoid syndrome is second most common cause

CLINICAL ISSUES

Presentation
- Most common signs/symptoms: Fatigue and edema related to low cardiac output
- Other signs/symptoms: Fluttering sensation in the neck due to giant A waves in the jugular venous pulse
- Progressive fatigue and anorexia
- Hepatomegaly, ascites and peripheral edema

Natural History & Prognosis
- Symptoms develop over an extended period
- Most patients have co-existing mitral valvular disease

Treatment
- Salt restriction and diuretic therapy
- Balloon valvuloplasty
- Tricuspid valve replacement

SELECTED REFERENCES

1. Braunwald E: Valvular Heart Disease. In Braunwald E. Heart Disease: A Textbook of Cardiovascular Medicine. 6th ed. WB Saunders Company, Philadelphia, 2001
2. Ewy GA: Tricuspid Valve Disease. In Chatterjee K, et al [ed] Cardiology: Ann Illustrated Text Reference, vol 2. J.B. Lippincott, Philadelphia, 1991

IMAGE GALLERY

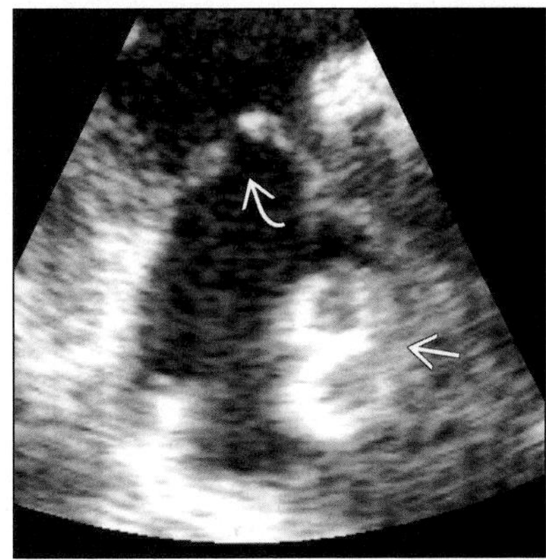

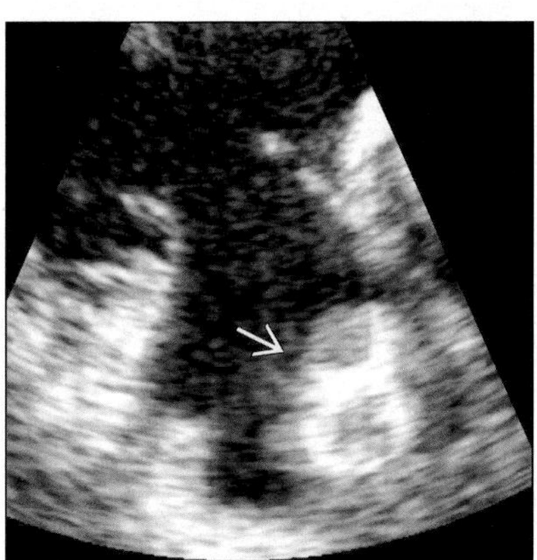

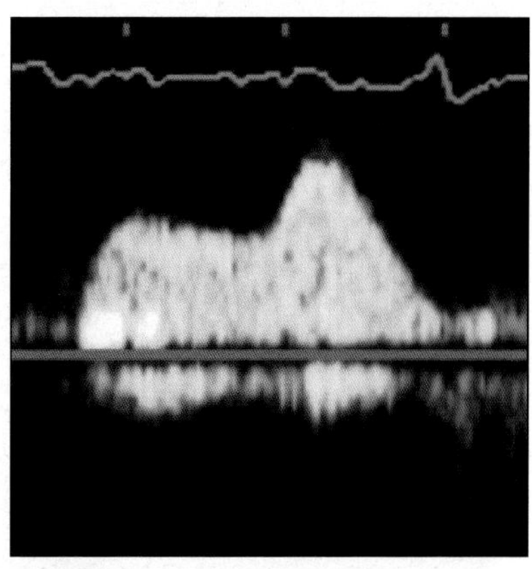

(Left) *Transthoracic echo RV inflow view in a patient with carcinoid shows thickened, retracted leaflets ➔ in systole. Note Amplatzer occluder device ➔ to repair an ASD.* ***(Center)*** *Transthoracic echo RV inflow view in same patient with carcinoid shows abnormal leaflets during diastole. Note ASD occluder device ➔ which was placed to prevent left-sided carcinoid valve disease.* ***(Right)*** *Continuous wave Doppler through tricuspid valve in case of stenosis shows elevated transvalvular velocity. From this the mean gradient can be determined.*

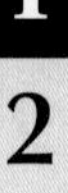

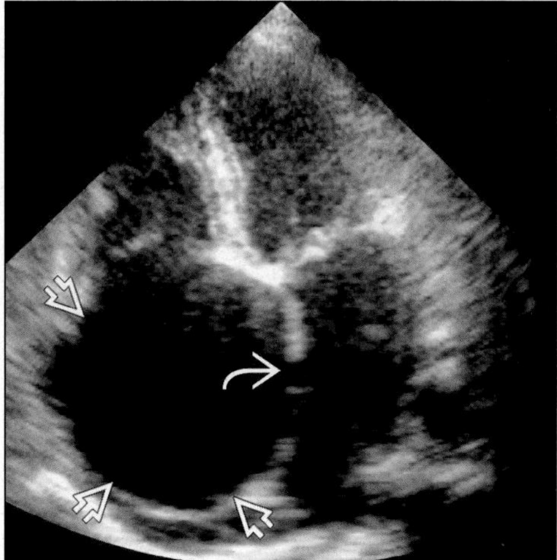

Transthoracic apical four chamber echo shows a dilated right atrium ➡. The interatrial septum bows to the left atrium consistent with elevated right atrial pressures ➡.

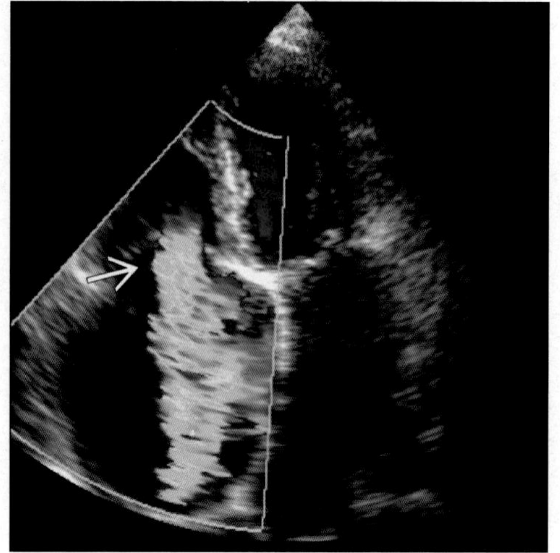

Four chamber view Color Doppler in the same four chamber view as previous image shows severe tricuspid regurgitation ➡.

TERMINOLOGY

Abbreviations and Synonyms

- Tricuspid regurgitation (TR)

IMAGING FINDINGS

Radiographic Findings

- Radiography
  - Chest radiography findings
    - Cardiomegaly with prominent right atrium and ventricle
    - Filling of retrosternal clear space
    - Distension of the azygous vein and superior vena cava (SVC) on frontal radiograph
    - Distended inferior vena cava (IVC) best seen on lateral radiograph

CT Findings

- NECT: Right atrial and ventricular dilation
- CECT: Dilated IVC and hepatic veins with systolic reflux of contrast
- Cardiac Gated CTA
  - Tricuspid valve usually not directly visualized on gated CT due to:
    - Presence of extensive mixing artifact from opacified SVC blood with non-opacified IVC blood
    - Saline flush may result in fluid density on both sides of leaflets rendering them invisible
  - Allows functional assessment of RV including determination of RV ejection fraction (RVEF) and volumes
  - Diastolic ventricular septal flattening due to volume overload
  - Dilated RA, RV, and systemic veins
  - Rarely delayed phase gated cardiac CT may show incomplete closure (regurgitant orifice) of tricuspid valve in ventricular systole

MR Findings

- Four chamber views and paraseptal long axis gradient echo or SSFP views most helpful
- Systolic flow void (jet) into right atrium
- Right atrium and ventricle dilation
- SVC, IVC, hepatic, and azygos vein dilatation ± systolic flow reversal

DDx: Tricuspid Regurgitation

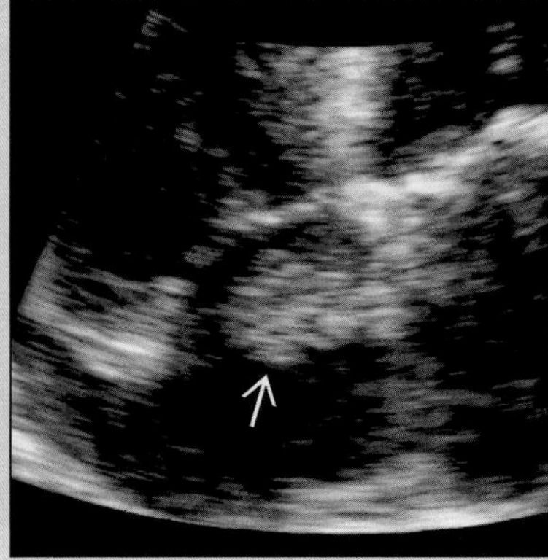

Large Vegetation

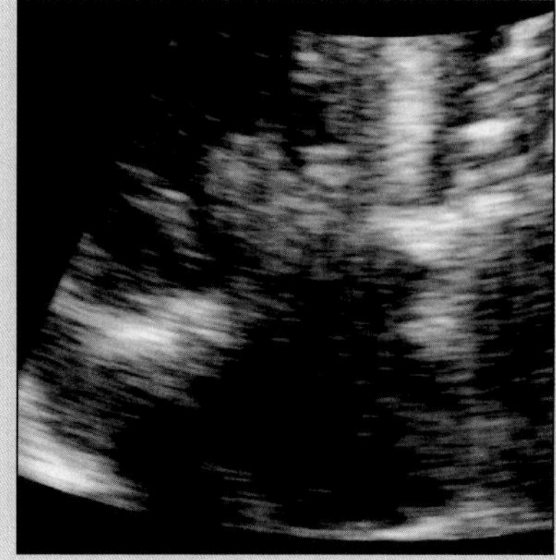

Large Prolapsing Vegetation

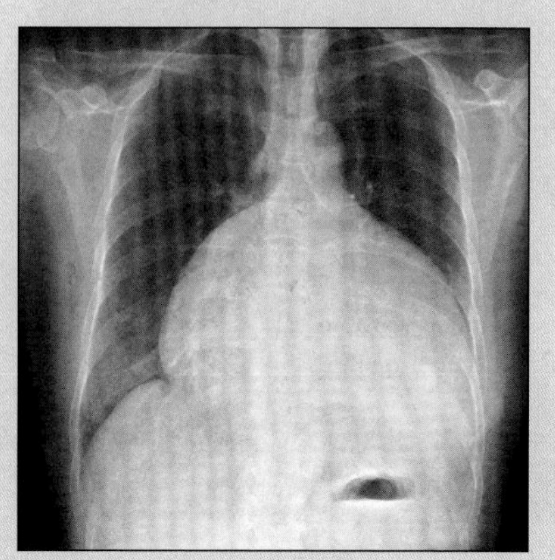

Epstein Anomaly

TRICUSPID REGURGITATION

Key Facts

Terminology
- Tricuspid regurgitation (TR)

Imaging Findings
- Tricuspid valve usually not directly visualized on gated CT due to:
- Presence of extensive mixing artifact from opacified SVC blood with non-opacified IVC blood
- Saline flush may result in fluid density on both sides of leaflets rendering them invisible
- Diastolic ventricular septal flattening due to volume overload
- Systolic high velocity flow jet in the right atrium
- Systolic flow reversal in the inferior vena cava or hepatic veins
- Best imaging tool: Echocardiography
- Protocol advice: Conventional MR gradient echo images demonstrate regurgitant jets better than newer SSFP pulse sequences

Pathology
- Deformation and retraction of valve cusps in primary diseases
- Myxomatous degeneration
- Any disease that causes abnormalities in the tricuspid valve apparatus (annulus, leaflets, chordae, and papillary muscles) can cause TR
- Trace to mild TR is common and detected by echocardiograph in more than 70% of patients

Clinical Issues
- Wide spectrum which depends on the severity and chronicity

- Diastolic ventricular septal flattening

Ultrasonographic Findings
- Grayscale Ultrasound
  - 2D echocardiography
    - Right ventricular volume overload pattern: RA enlargement, RV enlargement, diastolic ventricular septal flattening, dilated IVC and hepatic veins
    - These findings are not specific for severe TR and can be due to other entities
    - Thickened, myxomatous and retracted leaflets with increased echo reflectance
- Color Doppler
  - Systolic high velocity flow jet in the right atrium
  - Size of the regurgitant jet orifice at the valve and the the right atrium utilized in jet correlation to severity grades
  - Systolic flow reversal in the inferior vena cava or hepatic veins

Angiographic Findings
- Conventional
  - Right ventriculogram can visualize the regurgitant jet
    - Size of regurgitant contrast cloud in RA used for severity grading
  - Right heart pressure tracing reveal large V waves in the right atrial pressure curve

Imaging Recommendations
- Best imaging tool: Echocardiography
- Protocol advice: Conventional MR gradient echo images demonstrate regurgitant jets better than newer SSFP pulse sequences

DIFFERENTIAL DIAGNOSIS

Primary Tricuspid Regurgitation
- Endocardial cushion defects
- Rheumatic heart disease
  - Thickening of valve leaflets and/or cordae tendineae
- Ebstein anomaly
  - Excessive motion and delayed closure of the valve
  - Downward displaced septal leaflet
  - Atrialized portion of right ventricle
- Carcinoid syndrome
  - Stiffened and immobile leaflets
  - May involve left-sided valves in presence of ASD or PFO
- Infectious endocarditis
  - Vegetations on the valve leaflets
  - Predominantly in IV drug users
- Trauma, atrial tumors, pacemaker leads
  - Usually presence of secondary findings or history

Secondary Tricuspid Regurgitation
- Most common cause of TR
- Right heart failure of any etiology
- Right ventricular hypertension secondary to pulmonary stenosis
- Primary pulmonary hypertension and mitral valve disease
- RV systolic pressure gradients that exceed 55 mmHg produce functional TR

PATHOLOGY

General Features
- General path comments
  - Deformation and retraction of valve cusps in primary diseases
  - Myxomatous degeneration
- Etiology
  - Any disease that causes abnormalities in the tricuspid valve apparatus (annulus, leaflets, chordae, and papillary muscles) can cause TR
  - Posttransplantation
    - Moderate to severe TR in 15-20% of heart transplant recipients
    - May be avoided if modified inferior vena caval anastomosis is performed
  - Severe TR is occasionally idiopathic

- Proposed mechanism is annular dilatation due to aging, atrial fibrillation, or other causes
- Epidemiology
  - Trace to mild TR is common and detected by echocardiograph in more than 70% of patients
  - Considered physiologic when the jet does not extend greater than 1 cm into the atrium
- Associated abnormalities
  - Underlying cause of TR
    - Left ventricular failure
    - Chronic lung disease
    - Left ventricular inflow obstruction
  - Secondary findings of systemic venous hypertension
    - Hepatic congestion
- Valve leaflets
  - Rheumatic heart disease
    - Thickening
    - Shortening and retraction of one or more leaflets
    - Associate shortening of the chordae tendineae
  - Infectious endocarditis
    - Shortening and retraction of one or more leaflets
    - Associate shortening of the chordae tendineae
  - Traumatic destruction of a leaflet
  - Carcinoid syndrome
    - Fibrous plaques involving the leaflets
    - Primary carcinoid tumor
    - Hepatic carcinoid involvement
- Chordae tendineae
  - Thickening and retraction due to rheumatic fever

CLINICAL ISSUES

Presentation

- Most common signs/symptoms
  - Wide spectrum which depends on the severity and chronicity
    - In the absence of pulmonary hypertension trace to mild TR is common and well-tolerated and typically symptomatic
- Other signs/symptoms: Pulsations in the neck from prominent V waves in the jugular venous pulse
- Fatigue, exhaustion and right heart failure
- Hepatomegaly, ascites and peripheral edema

Treatment

- Medical therapy includes preload and afterload reduction in the setting of severe TR and right ventricular failure
- Surgical therapy more common in the setting of primary tricuspid regurgitation
- Secondary (functional) TR often treated surgically if another indication for cardiac surgery is also present, for example mitral or aortic valve surgery or coronary artery bypass graft
  - Annuloplasty most common procedure
    - 30-40% of patients have residual TR
    - < 5% require valve replacement in 5 years
  - Valve replacement surgery when annuloplasty is not feasible or failed
    - Survival post surgery ~ 70% in 5 years and ~ 40% in 10 years

DIAGNOSTIC CHECKLIST

Consider

- Gradient echo cine white blood sequences in four chamber views demonstrate regurgitant jet better than newer SSFP pulse sequences

Image Interpretation Pearls

- Regurgitation of contrast into enlarged hepatic veins suggestive of TR on non-gated CECT

SELECTED REFERENCES

1. Marelli D et al: Modified inferior vena caval anastomosis to reduce tricuspid valve regurgitation after heart transplantation. Tex Heart Inst J. 34(1):30-5, 2007
2. Mutlak D et al: Echocardiography-based spectrum of severe tricuspid regurgitation: the frequency of apparently idiopathic tricuspid regurgitation. J Am Soc Echocardiogr. 20(4):405-8, 2007
3. Ohye RG et al: Repair of the tricuspid valve in hypoplastic left heart syndrome. Cardiol Young. 16 Suppl 3:21-6, 2006
4. Yamasaki N et al: Severe tricuspid regurgitation in the aged: atrial remodeling associated with long-standing atrial fibrillation. J Cardiol. 48(6):315-23, 2006
5. Behm CZ et al: Clinical correlates and mortality of hemodynamically significant tricuspid regurgitation. J Heart Valve Dis. 13(5):784-9, 2004
6. Hannoush H et al: Regression of significant tricuspid regurgitation after mitral balloon valvotomy for severe mitral stenosis. Am Heart J. 148(5):865-70, 2004
7. Sadeghi HM et al: Does lowering pulmonary arterial pressure eliminate severe functional tricuspid regurgitation? Insights from pulmonary thromboendarterectomy. J Am Coll Cardiol. 44(1):126-32, 2004
8. Henein MY et al: Evidence for rheumatic valve disease in patients with severe tricuspid regurgitation long after mitral valve surgery: the role of 3D echo reconstruction. J Heart Valve Dis. 12(5):566-72, 2003
9. Braunwald E: Valvular Heart Disease. In: Braunwald E. Heart Disease: A Textbook of Cardiovascular Medicine. 6th ed. WB Saunders Company, Philadelphia, 2001
10. Ewy GA: Tricuspid Valve Disease. In: Alpert JS, Dalen JE and Rahimtoola SH (eds): Valvular Heart Disease. 3rd ed. Lippincott William and Wilkins, Philadelphia, 2000
11. Otto CM: Right-sided Valve Disease. In: Otto CM. Valvular Heart Disease. 1st ed. WB Saunders Company, Philadelphia, 1999

IMAGE GALLERY

Typical

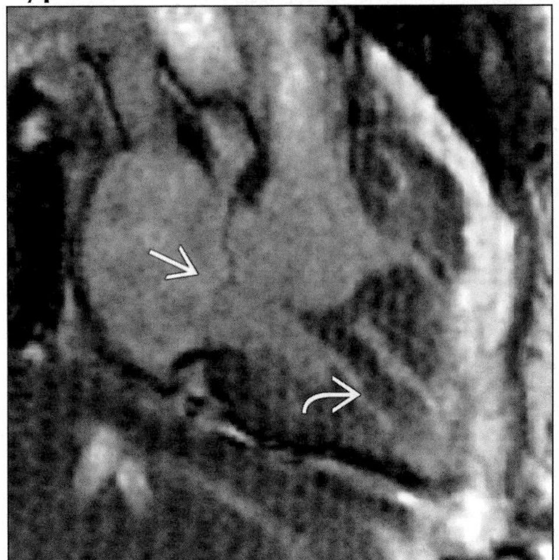

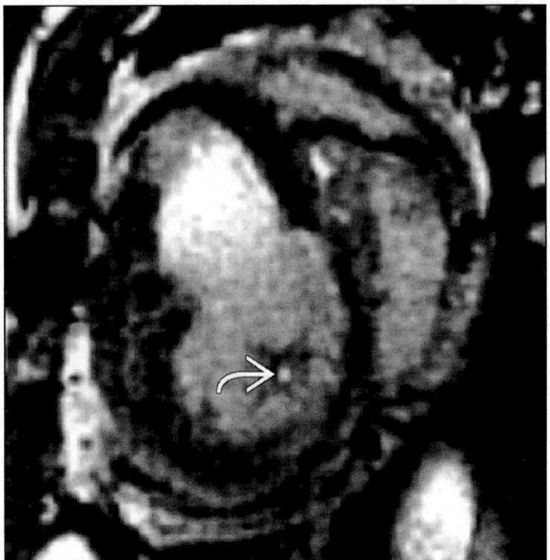

(Left) *RV paraseptal view SSFP MR sequence in a patient with D-TGA s/p atrial switch procedure shows a hypertrophied "systemic" ventricle ➔ and the tricuspid valve ➔.* ***(Right)*** *Short axis GRE view in the same patient with D-TGA s/p atrial switch shows malcoaptation of the tricuspid valve in systole with a regurgitant orifice ➔.*

Typical

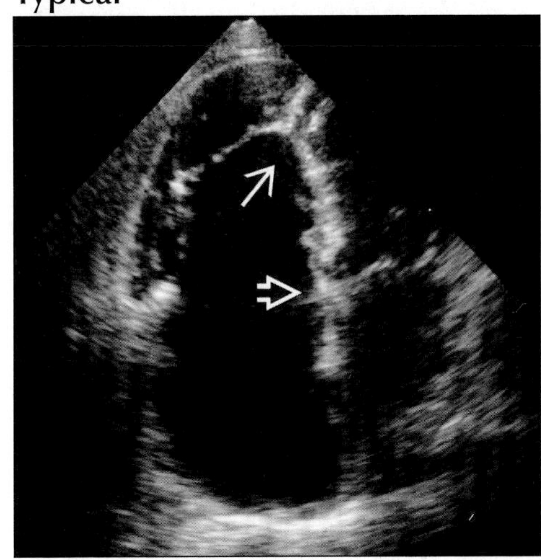

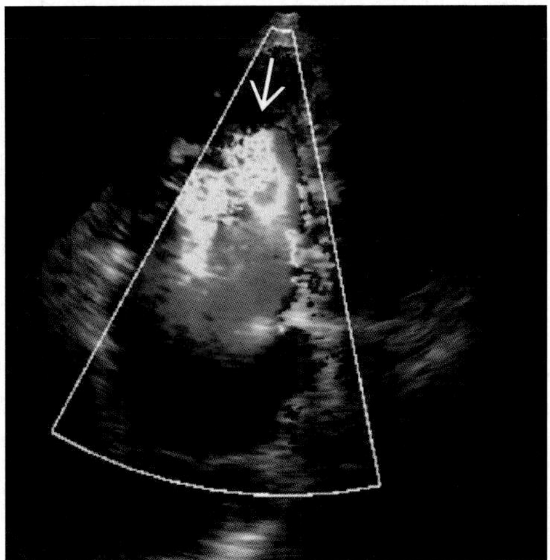

(Left) *Transthoracic echocardiographic apical four chamber view in a patient with Epstein anomaly shows severe apical displacement of the septal leaflet ➔ compared to the mitral valve leaflet origin ➔.* ***(Right)*** *Transthoracic apical four chamber view color Doppler in the same patient with Epstein deformity of the tricuspid valve shows severe tricuspid regurgitation ➔.*

Typical

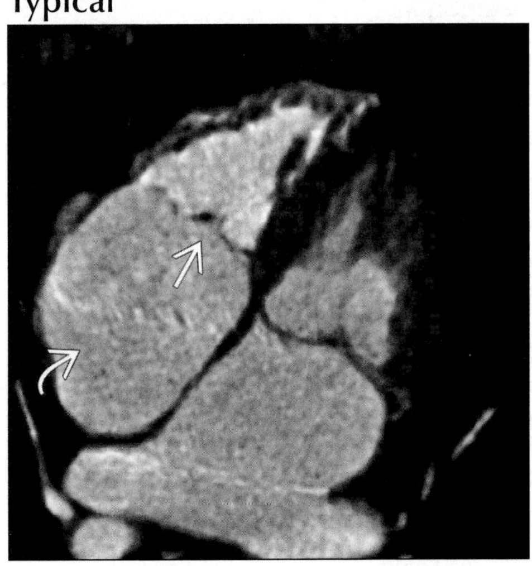

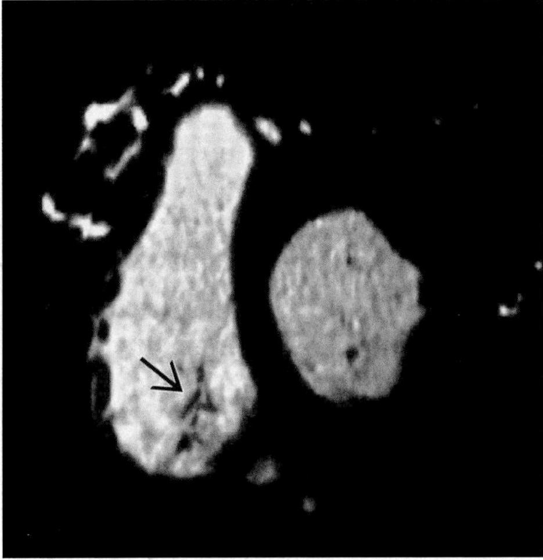

(Left) *Four chamber view coronary CTA delayed phase scan shows right atrial enlargement ➔ with malcoaptation of the septal and anterior tricuspid valve leaflets ➔.* ***(Right)*** *Oblique coronary CTA shows the tricuspid valve leaflets in short-axis during systole. Note the regurgitant orifice ➔.*

INFECTIVE ENDOCARDITIS (IE)

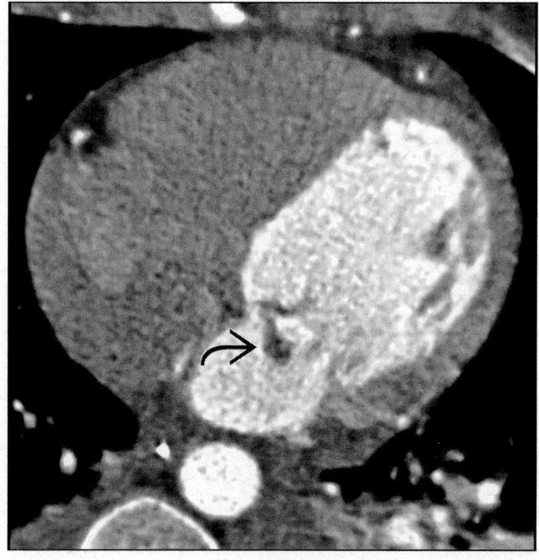

Axial cardiac CT shows ➚ vegetation at the anterior mitral leaflet.

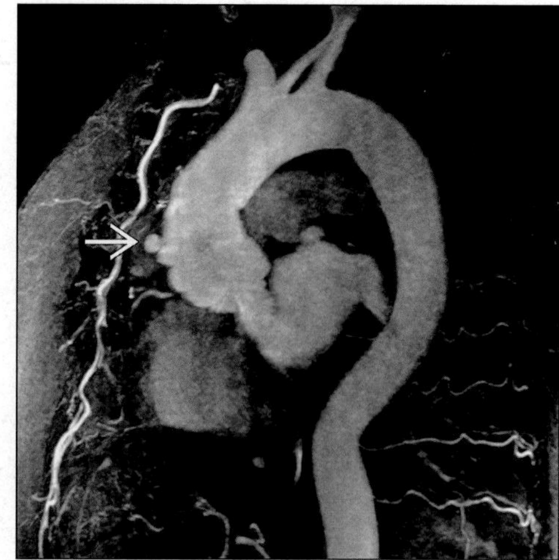

Gadolinium-enhanced MRA shows a dilated aortic root with multiple small pseudo-aneurysms ➡ in a patient who developed endocarditis and abscess formation after an aortic tube graft repair.

TERMINOLOGY

Definitions

- Inflammation of the endocardium most commonly affecting valves

IMAGING FINDINGS

General Features

- Best diagnostic clue
  - Valvular vegetations
  - Paravalvular abscess or pseudoaneurysm
- Location
  - Heart valves are the most common structure involved, less frequently cardiac chambers
  - Metallic devices (prosthetic valves, pacemakers, defibrillators)
- **Specific findings**
  - Vegetations: Irregularly shaped, oscillating masses adherent to the endocardium, may cause regurgitation
  - Paravalvular abscess: Irregularly shaped, inhomogeneous peri-valvular mass (e.g., peri-annular region, myocardium, pericardium) develops in up to 37%
  - Pseudoaneurysm: Space filled with contrast agent and communication with cardiac chambers or aortic root
  - Leaflet perforation: Discontinuity in a cusp
  - Fistula: Communication between cardiac chambers
  - Dehiscence: Rocking motion of prosthetic valve with excursion > 15% in any one plane
- **Non-specific findings**
  - Pericardial and/or pleural effusion
  - Septic bronchopneumonia

Radiographic Findings

- Chest Radiography
  - Septic pulmonary emboli especially in IV drug users
  - Pleural or pericardial effusion
  - Bronchopneumonia

CT Findings

- Cardiac Gated CTA
  - Vegetations and leaflet perforation may be seen
  - Perivalvular abscess and pseudoaneurysm involving

DDx: Infective Endocarditis

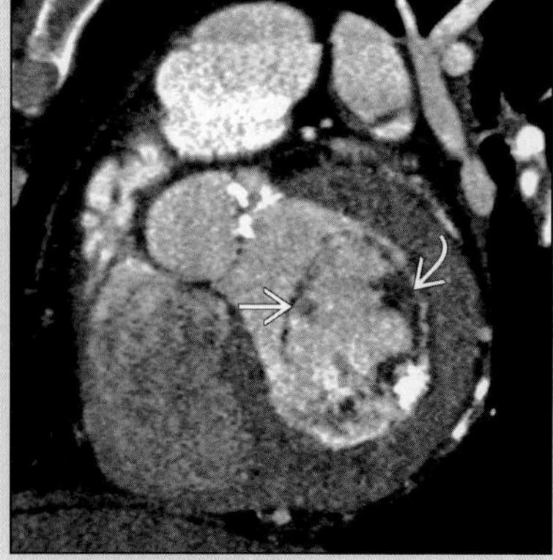

Mitral Valve Vegetations

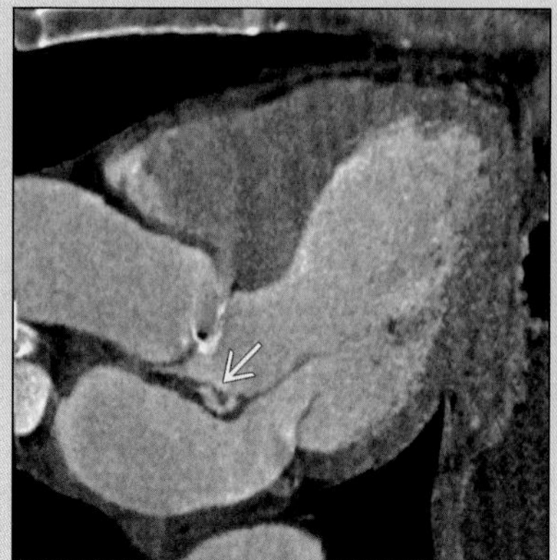

Mitral Valve Leaflet Perforation

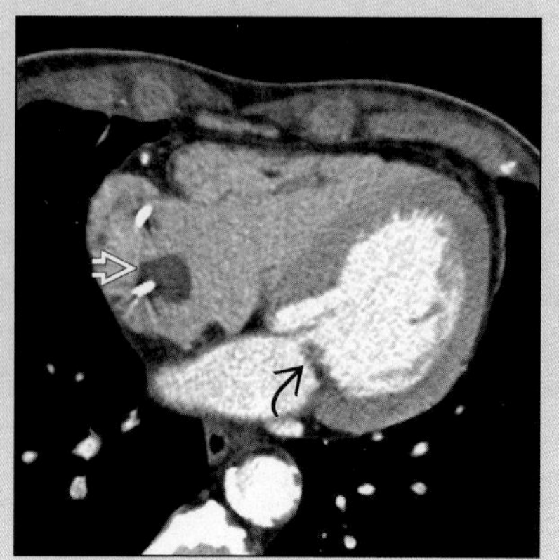

Guidewire Mass & Thickened MV

INFECTIVE ENDOCARDITIS (IE)

Key Facts

Terminology
- Bacterial infection of the endocardium

Imaging Findings
- Most commonly involving heart valves, less frequently cardiac chambers (e.g., left or right atrium)
- Specific lesions: Vegetations, cusp perforation, peri-valvular abscess/pseudoaneurysm, fistula
- New onset of valvular regurgitation is indirect sign
- Best imaging tool: Transesophageal echocardiography (TEE)
- ECG-gated cardiac CT useful before surgery for evaluation of
  - Peri-valvular abscess/pseudoaneurysm
  - Coronary artery disease and anatomical relationships
- Non-specific findings: Septic emboli (cerebral, systemic or pulmonary) frequent

Top Differential Diagnoses
- Degenerative or Rheumatic Valve Disease
- Prosthetic Valve Dysfunction

Clinical Issues
- Diagnosis is based on clinical and imaging findings according to modified Duke criteria (major and minor)
- Predisposing factors: Valvular disease, prostheses, pacemaker, ICD, IV-drug abuse, immunodeficiency
- Septic emboli and hematogenous seeding to remote sites frequent (mostly neurologic symptoms)
- Severe disease with high mortality up to 40%, mortality increases if peri-valvular abscess

    - Myocardium, pericardium
    - Annulus
    - Coronary sinus, coronary arteries
    - Aortic root pseudoaneurysm or abscess ("stranding" and/or effusion of peri-aortic fatty tissue)
  - Fistula
  - Regurgitation
  - Evaluation of coronary arteries before surgery (anatomical relationship to abscess and exclusion of significant coronary stenosis)
  - Assessment of left ventricular function before surgery

MR Findings
- In native valves can detect myocardial abscess, aortic root aneurysm and valve dysfunction; prosthetic valves produce artifacts
- Bright and black blood images are recommended
- Post-gadolinium images will show enhancement of the vegetation/abscess

Echocardiographic Findings
- Echocardiogram
  - 2D trans thoracic echocardiography (TTE)
    - Vegetation: Echodense irregular mass usually on the low pressure side of valve leaflet with oscillation during cardiac cycle and prolapse into chamber
  - Transesophageal echocardiography (TEE)
    - Detailed anatomy of vegetation; mobility
    - Paravalvular abscess
  - TEE is most sensitive imaging modality, TTE is less sensitive
- Color Doppler: Presence and severity of regurgitation (frequent) and stenosis (rare)

Angiographic Findings
- Left Ventricular Angiography
  - Can detect perivalvular abscess

Imaging Recommendations
- Best imaging tool
  - Transesophageal echocardiography (TEE)
  - ECG-gated cardiac CT before surgery (instead of invasive coronary angiography to avoid risk of embolization) for coronaries and peri-valvular involvement
- Protocol advice
  - ECG-gated cardiac CT
    - Coronary CT angiography scan protocol but homogeneous enhancement of right and left ventricle advantageous (biphasic contrast agent injection)
    - Image reconstruction: Multiplanar reformations of valves during diastole and systole; 4D-cine imaging

DIFFERENTIAL DIAGNOSIS

Degenerative or Rheumatic Valve Disease
- Thickened cusp (DD rather diffuse and symmetric) and calcification; not oscillating
- Cusp prolapse
- Ruptured chordae tendinea

Prosthetic Valve Dysfunction
- Pannus or thrombus
- Ruptured synthetic neo-chordae (DDx: High pressure side)

PATHOLOGY

General Features
- General path comments: Amorphous mass of thrombus and inflammatory products
- Etiology
  - Bacterial infection (common)
    - Staphylococcus aureus and streptococcus (80%), or enterococcus faecalis (10%)
    - HACEK-group (Hemophilus, Actinobacillus, Cardiobacterium, Eikenella, Kingella) may cause large vegetations > 1 cm
    - Mycobacterium tuberculosis (extremely rare)

INFECTIVE ENDOCARDITIS (IE)

- Fungal infection
  - Candida, aspergillus (especially in prosthetic valves or compromised immune system)
- Epidemiology
  - Predisposing factors
    - Degenerative or rheumatic valve disease
    - Prosthetic valves, pacemakers, defibrillators
    - IV drug abuses
    - Immunodeficiency

Gross Pathologic & Surgical Features

- Vegetation on valve leaflet or prosthetic valve
- Myocardial abscess

Microscopic Features

- Platelet and fibrin thrombus, inflammatory cells and bacteria

Staging, Grading or Classification Criteria

- Modified Duke criteria
  - Major criteria
    - Positive echocardiography (specific valvular lesions or new onset of regurgitation)
    - Positive blood culture with typical microorganism
  - Minor criteria
    - Fever (> 38 degrees Celsius)
    - Immunological phenomena (Osler nodes, positive rheumatoid factor, etc.)
    - Vascular phenomena (major arterial emboli, intercerebral hemorrhage, septic pulmonary embolism, etc.)
    - Predisposing cardiac condition (e.g., valvular disease, pacemaker, prosthesis, etc.) or IV drug abuses
- Diagnosis
  - Definite
    - Two major criteria or one major and 3 minor
    - Pathology or bacteriology of specific valvular lesions
  - Possible
    - One major and one minor or three minor
  - Rejected
    - Alternative firm diagnosis

CLINICAL ISSUES

Presentation

- Fever, anorexia, weight loss and changing heart murmur; signs of heart failure (dyspnea), petechiae
- Septic emboli with associated complaints, e.g., neurologic symptoms most common
- Diagnosis-based on clinical and imaging findings according to modified Duke criteria (major and minor)

Natural History & Prognosis

- 50-75% with prior conditions including mitral valve prolapse, rheumatic, congenital, degenerative valve disease, or prosthetic valves
- IE of prosthetic valve frequently extend to cause abscesses, fistulas and valve dehiscence resulting in paravalvular regurgitation
- Septic emboli and hematogenous seeding to remote sites frequent (mostly neurologic symptoms)
- Severe disease with high mortality up to 40%, mortality increases if peri-valvular involvement

Treatment

- Long term intravenous antibiotic therapy based on microbial profile
- Surgery is indicated if
  - Antimicrobial therapy failed
  - Risk of embolization (mobile vegetations and size > 1 cm)
  - Congestive heart failure (CHF) due to valvular dysfunction
  - Unstable prosthesis
  - Perivalvular invasion

DIAGNOSTIC CHECKLIST

Consider

- Severe disease with high mortality, best imaging tool is transesophageal echocardiography
- Cardiac CT useful before valve surgery to evaluate peri-valvular involvement and to exclude coronary artery disease

Image Interpretation Pearls

- Vegetations and cusp perforation
- Peri-valvular abscess, pseudoaneurysm

SELECTED REFERENCES

1. Feuchtner G. Multislice computed tomography in infective endocarditis. J Am Coll Card. in press, 2008
2. Panwar SR et al: Identification of tricuspid valve vegetation by computed tomography scan. Echocardiography. 24(3):272-3, 2007
3. ACC/AHA 2006 guidelines for the Management of Patients with Valvular Heart Disease. Circulation. 114:84-231, 2006
4. Christiaens L et al: Aortic valvular endocarditis visualised by 16-row detector multislice computed tomography. Heart. 92(10):1466, 2006
5. Meijboom WB et al: Pre-operative computed tomography coronary angiography to detect significant coronary artery disease in patients referred for cardiac valve surgery. J Am Coll Cardiol. 48(8):1658-65, 2006
6. Sachdev M et al: Imaging techniques for diagnosis of infective endocarditis. Cardiol Clin. 21(2):185-95, 2003
7. Karchmer AW: Infective Endocarditis. In: Braunwald E. Heart Disease: A Textbook of Cardiovascular Medicine 6th ed. W.B. Saunders Company, Philadelphia, 2001
8. Durack DT et al: New criteria for diagnosis of infective endocarditis: utilization of specific echocardiographic findings. Duke Endocarditis Service. Am J Med. 96(3):200-9, 1994
9. Bush LM et al: Clinical Syndrome and Diagnosis. In: Kaye D (ed): Infective Endocarditis. 2nd ed. Raven Press, New York, 1992
10. Sokil AB: Cardiac imaging in infective endocarditis. In: Kaye D (ed): Infective Endocarditis. 2nd ed. Raven Press, New York, 1992

INFECTIVE ENDOCARDITIS (IE)

IMAGE GALLERY

Typical

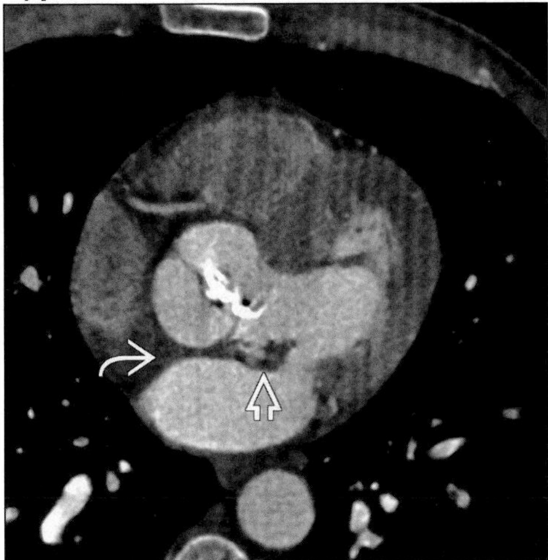

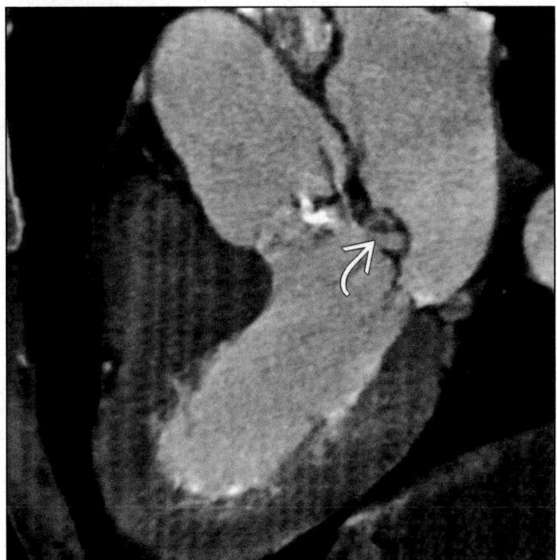

(Left) *Axial cardiac CT shows thickening of the anterior leaflet and aortic root abscess.* ***(Right)*** *Three chamber view cardiac CT shows perforated anterior mitral valve leaflet.*

Typical

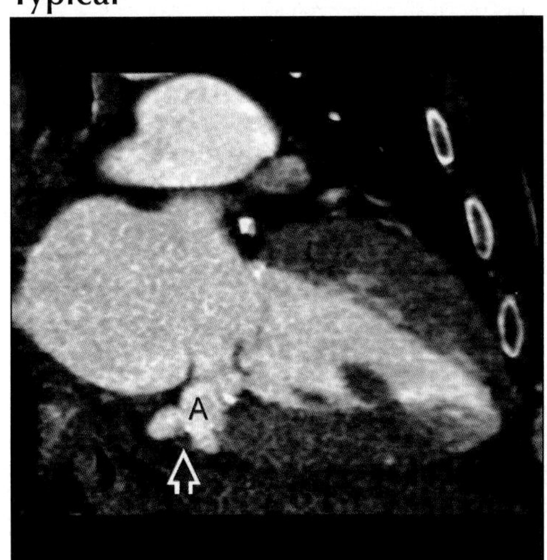

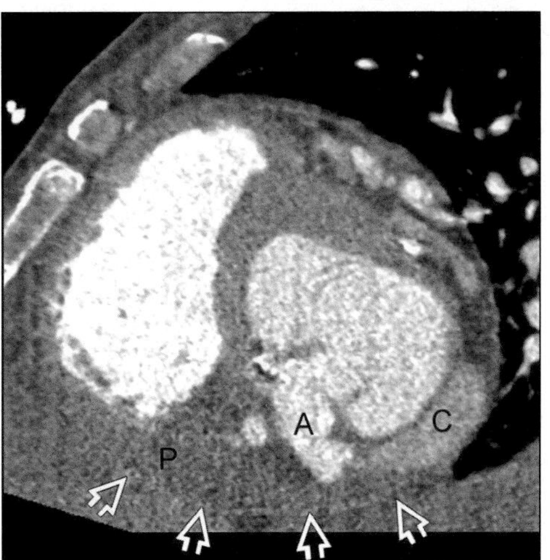

(Left) *Long axis vertical cardiac CT shows pseudoaneurysm (A) adjacent to the mitral valve due to infective endocarditis.* ***(Right)*** *LV short axis cardiac CT shows paravalvular abscess/pseudoaneurysm (A) with myocardial involvement, coronary sinus (C) obstruction and pericardial (P) abscess/effusion.*

Typical

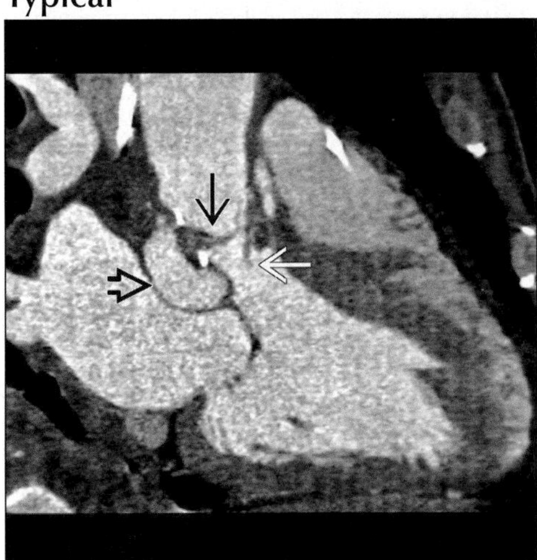

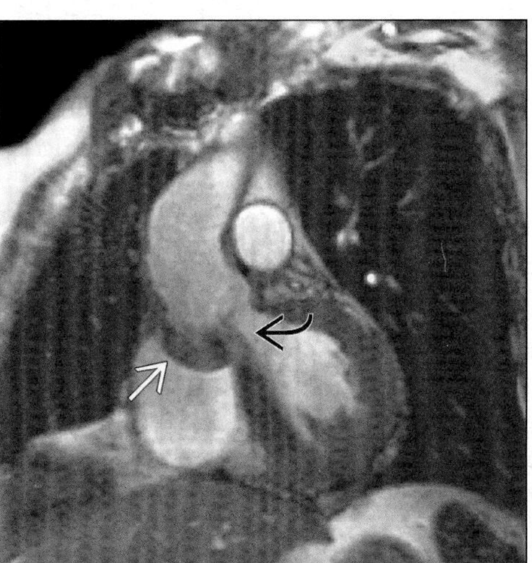

(Left) *Three chamber view cardiac CT shows aortic root pseudoaneurysm in setting of IE of bioprosthetic valve. Note: Thickened cusp and mobile vegetation causing diastolic regurgitation.* ***(Right)*** *Coronal oblique MR cine shows aortic root abscess due to infective endocarditis. Note also jet of aortic regurgitation.*

PROSTHETIC VALVE DYSFUNCTION

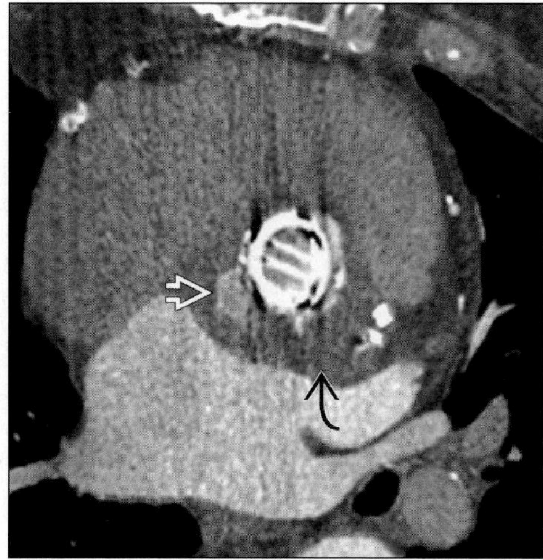

Axial cardiac CT shows paravalvular leakage and an aortic root abscess in an infected prosthetic valve.

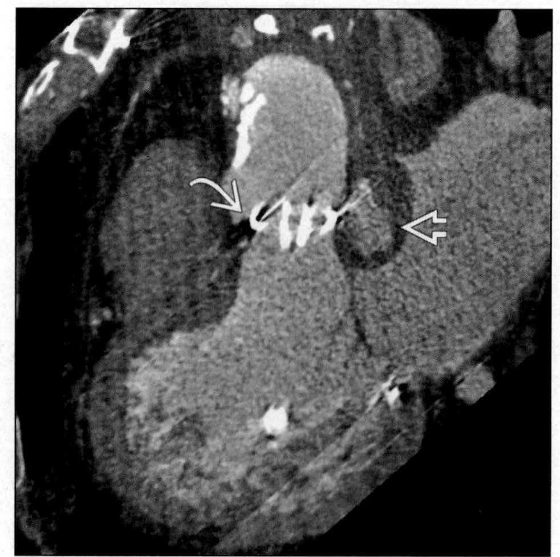

Three chamber view cardiac CT shows dehiscence, and paravalvular aneurysm of a mechanic prosthetic aortic valve.

TERMINOLOGY

Definitions

- Dysfunction depends on prosthesis type
  - **Mechanical prostheses**
    - Caged-ball valve (Starr-Edwards): Oldest
    - Tilting disc (Lillehei-Kaster; Björk-Shiley; Medtronic-Hall)
    - Bi-leaflet (St. Jude): Currently most commonly implanted, lowest thrombogenicity
  - **Bioprostheses ("tissue valves"):** Either stented or non-stented
    - Homograft
    - Xenograft-porcine: Hancock, Carpentier-Edwards, Medtronic-Intact
    - Autograft (Ross-procedure: Pulmonary valve into aortic position)

IMAGING FINDINGS

General Features

- **Dependent on type of prosthesis**
  - **All types**
    - Paravalvular leakage
    - Peri-valvular pseudoaneurysm
    - Dehiscence (rocking valve motion > 15° in any one plane)
    - Pannus/thrombus (rather mechanic)
    - Regurgitation (more common) or stenosis (less common)
    - Infective endocarditis (vegetations, abscess, cusp perforation) may or may not cause dysfunction
    - Frozen disc - causes severe regurgitation
  - **Mechanic valves, specific findings**
    - Broken or disrupted metallic leaflets
    - Impaired metallic leaflet motion due to pannus, thrombus or vegetation
    - Ball (Starr-Edwards) or disc dislodgement
  - **Bioprosthetic valve, specific findings**
    - Chronic degenerative tissue destruction, cusp perforation and calcification
  - **Percutaneous aortic valve prosthesis (stented), specific findings**
    - Proximal migration
    - Occlusion of coronary ostium if stent is placed too high, leading to fatal myocardial infarction
  - **Mitral valve annuloplasty, specific findings**

DDx: Prosthetic Valve Types

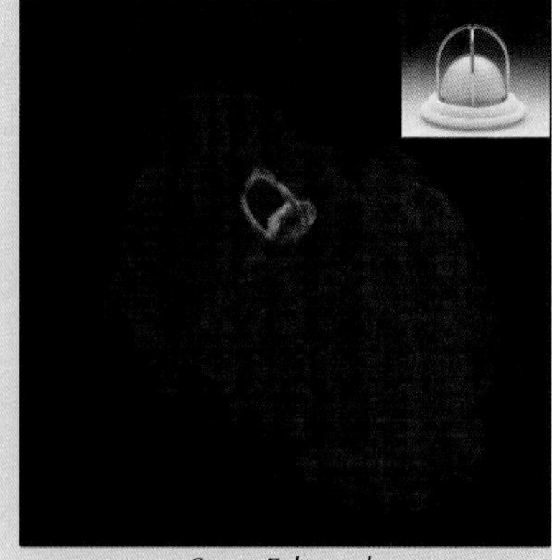

Starr-Edwards

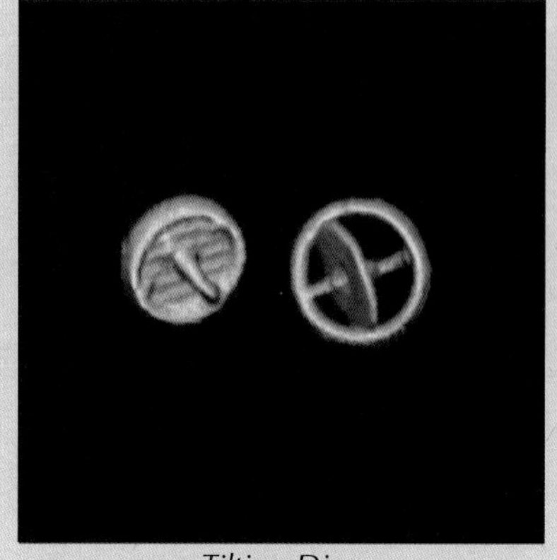

Tilting Disc

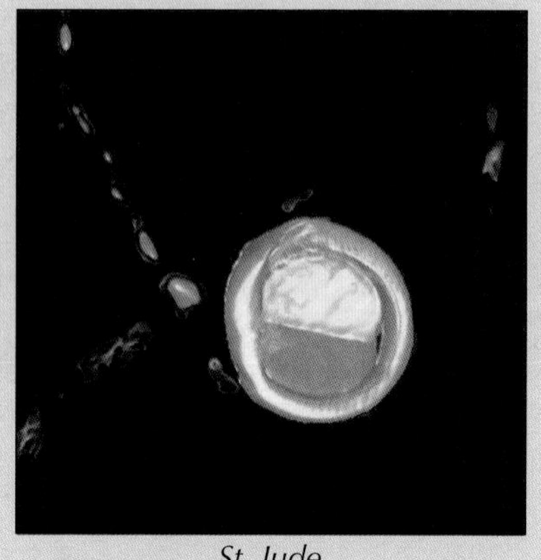

St. Jude

PROSTHETIC VALVE DYSFUNCTION

Key Facts

Imaging Findings
- Mechanical prosthesis dysfunction
  - Thrombus/pannus
  - Paravalvular leakage
  - Perivalvular pseudoaneurysm
- Bioprosthesis dysfunction
  - Chronic-degenerative tissue destruction (fibro-calcifying) and pseudoaneurysm
- All prostheses
  - Dehiscence
  - De-novo-regurgitation
  - Infective endocarditis (vegetations, leaflet perforation, peri-valvular abscess)

Clinical Issues
- Mechanical valve dysfunction is rare (thrombus, pannus, dehiscence, pseudoaneurysm)
- Bioprosthetic valve dysfunction is more common (30% after 10 years): Chronic-degenerative tissue destruction and calcification
- Increased risk of infective endocarditis

Diagnostic Checklist
- Transesophageal echocardiography is primary imaging modality
- Fluoroscopy for frozen disc
- ECG-gated cardiac CT useful for
  - Mechanic prostheses (4D-cine) if metallic artifacts limit echocardiography
  - Perivalvular abscess, pseudoaneurysm before surgery
  - Coronary arteries before surgery

- SAM: Systolic anterior movement of anterior mitral valve leaflet causing obstruction of LVOT
- Disruption of synthetic neo-chordae

Radiographic Findings
- Chest Radiography
  - Mechanical valve: Ball or disc dislodgement
  - Bioprosthetic valve: Calcification indicates chronic inflammatory process

Fluoroscopic Findings
- Fluoroscopy is gold standard for suspected frozen leaflet evaluation

CT Findings
- Cardiac Gated CTA
  - See general imaging features
  - Useful for pre-operative evaluation of perivalvular pseudoaneurysm
  - Useful for mechanic prosthesis if echocardiography is limited by massive metal artifacts
  - 4D-dynamic cine imaging for
    - Dehiscence
    - Mobility of disc or semi discs
    - Co-existent valvular regurgitation or stenosis
    - Mobility of vegetations, thrombus, pannus
    - Disruption of prosthetic valve leaflets
  - Coronary CT angiography
    - Exclusion of coronary artery disease (stenosis > 50%) before surgery

MR Findings
- Stenosis or regurgitation for specific valve
- Starr-Edwards: Not compatible for MR (steal ball)
- Metallic components may cause in artifacts resulting in signal void

Echocardiographic Findings
- Echocardiogram
  - Transesophageal better than transthoracic to clarify etiology, in particular for mitral valve prosthesis
    - See general imaging findings
- Color Doppler
  - De-novo regurgitation (more common) or stenosis (rare)
    - Mechanical prostheses: Mild regurgitation is normal, each type has a specific retrograde flow pattern (except Starr-Edwards: No regurgitation)
    - Bioprostheses: No regurgitation, but may develop if chronic-degenerative dysfunction
  - Paravalvular leakage
    - Eccentric Doppler jet, typically "half-moon" or "sickle-shaped"
  - Thrombus or pannus
    - Eccentric inflow pattern because leaflet motion is impaired
    - Thrombus: Lower echogenicity
    - Pannus: Higher echogenicity

Angiographic Findings
- Mechanic valve: Rocking of a dehiscing prosthesis, strut separation
- Paravalvular leakage, regurgitation and stenosis
- Exclusion of coronary artery disease before redo-surgery
- CAVE: Invasive catheter manipulation is associated with a high risk of embolization if mobile vegetations/thrombus

Imaging Recommendations
- Best imaging tool
  - Echocardiography (transesophageal preferred over transthoracic)
  - ECG-gated cardiac CT useful for
    - Metallic valve dysfunction if severe metal artifacts impair image quality on echocardiography
    - Peri-valvular abscess and pseudoaneurysm before surgery
    - Coronary artery disease before surgery
- Protocol advice
  - ECG-gated cardiac CT
    - Separate image evaluation during systole and diastole (for dehiscence and co-existent regurgitation or stenosis)

- 4D-dynamic cine imaging to evaluate prosthetic leaflet function or dysfunction and mobility of vegetations, thrombus
- 3D visualization of perivalvular pseudoaneurysm for pre-surgical planning

DIFFERENTIAL DIAGNOSIS

Infectious Endocarditis

- Vegetations may or may not cause dysfunction
- Peri-prosthetic valve abscess, pseudoaneurysm and tissue destruction involving myocardium, pericardium, coronary sinus

Thrombosis, Pannus

- Mechanical prosthesis
- Hypodense lesion or mass on CT
  - Thrombus ⇒ lower CT-density
  - Pannus ⇒ higher CT-density
- Can cause impaired movement of prosthetic valve leaflets
- ~ 20% of tricuspid valve replacement

PATHOLOGY

General Features

- Etiology
  - Mechanical valve failure is rare
  - Bioprosthetic valve failure is more common
- Epidemiology
  - Bioprostheses
    - Preferred in the elderly (males > 65 y, females > 70 y); Ross-procedure in children and adolescents
    - Limited long-term durability (in 30% dysfunction after 10 years; due to degeneration beginning in 4th-5th post-operative year)
    - Advantage: No long-term anticoagulation necessary
  - Metallic prosthesis
    - Excellent long-term durability (35 years for Starr-Edwards)

Microscopic Features

- Bioprostheses dysfunction
  - Fibrin deposition, calcification, fibrosis

CLINICAL ISSUES

Presentation

- Most common signs/symptoms
  - Dependent on whether acute or chronic dysfunction
    - Chronic: Gradual onset of congestive heart failure (CHF) symptoms
    - Acute: Acute heart failure symptoms; most common etiology infective endocarditis
- Clinical Profile
  - Severe clinical symptoms if prosthetic valve dysfunction is caused by acute infective endocarditis
    - Sepsis, thromboembolic events (stroke); systemic emboli (e.g., pulmonary)

Natural History & Prognosis

- Failure of mechanical valve apparatus is rare; consider thrombosis or pannus, and dehiscence
- Failure of bioprosthesis is more common with > 25% in 10 years (chronic-degenerative process)
- Increased risk of infective endocarditis

Treatment

- Medical therapy of infection, thrombosis and/or CHF
- Surgery indicated for severe dysfunction, non-responders or risk of complications (e.g., embolization)

DIAGNOSTIC CHECKLIST

Consider

- Transesophageal echocardiography is best imaging modality
- ECG-gated cardiac CT is useful for
  - Mechanic prostheses function by 4D-cine imaging: If metallic artifacts limit echocardiographic evaluation (commonly in aortic position)
  - Non-invasive exclusion of coronary artery disease before surgery
  - Visualization of peri-valvular abscess, pseudoaneurysm in particular before surgery

Image Interpretation Pearls

- Thrombus or pannus
- Paravalvular leakage
- Perivalvular pseudoaneurysm
- Dehiscence
- De-novo regurgitation

SELECTED REFERENCES

1. Bartel T, Müller S. Echocardiographie. 1st Ed. Elsevier Science Urban & Fischer. Munich, 2007
2. Leborgne L et al: Usefulness of ECG-gated multi-detector computed tomography for the diagnosis of mechanical prosthetic valve dysfunction. Eur Heart J. 27(21):2537, 2006
3. Mollet NR et al: High-resolution spiral computed tomography coronary angiography in patients referred for diagnostic conventional coronary angiography. Circulation. 112(15):2318-23, 2005
4. Teshima H et al: Detection of pannus by multidetector-row computed tomography. Ann Thorac Surg. 75(5):1631-3, 2003
5. Thai HM et al: Prosthetic Heart Valves. In: Alpert JS, Dalen JE and Rahimtoola SH (eds): Valvular Heart Disease. 3rd Ed. Philadelphia, Lippincott William and Wilkins, 2000
6. Otto CM: Prosthetic Valves. In: Otto CM. Valvular Heart Disease. 1st Ed. Philadelphia, W.B. Saunders Co. , 1999
7. Feuchtner G: Multislice computed tomography in infective endocarditis. JACC, 2008. In print.

PROSTHETIC VALVE DYSFUNCTION

IMAGE GALLERY

Typical

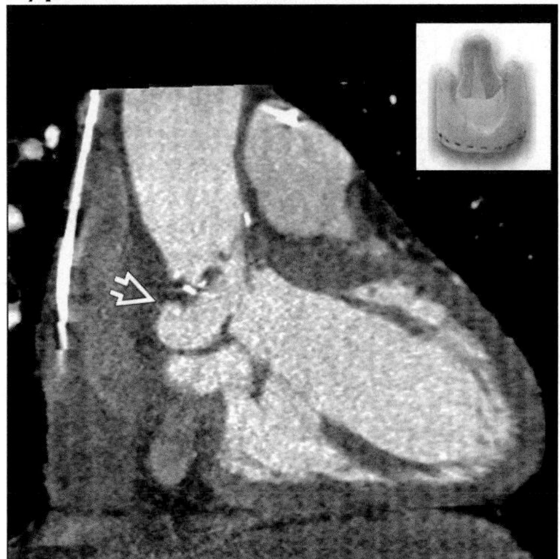

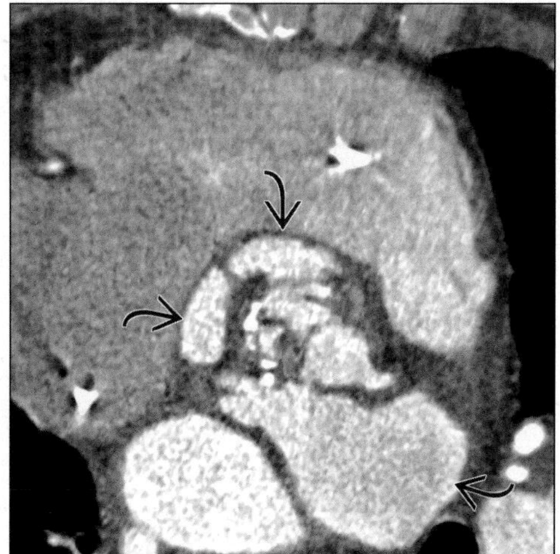

(Left) *Coronal oblique cardiac CT shows a dysfunctional bioprosthetic valve. Note: Perivalvular tissue destruction ➡, leaflet thickening and calcification.* ***(Right)*** *Axial cardiac CT shows three aortic root pseudoaneurysms ➡. Calcification of the aortic valve cusps and tissue proliferation indicating chronic inflammatory process.*

Typical

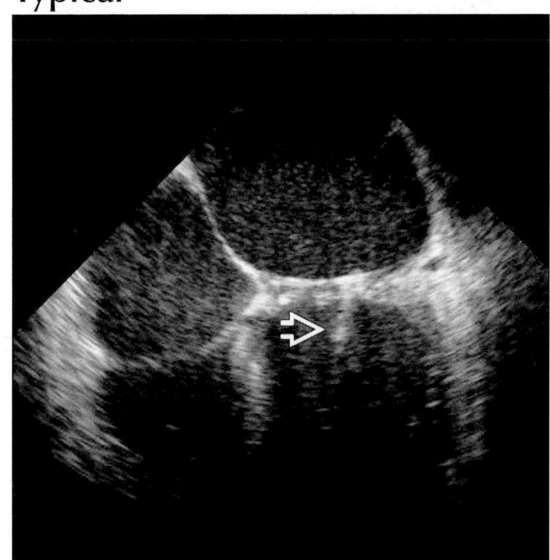

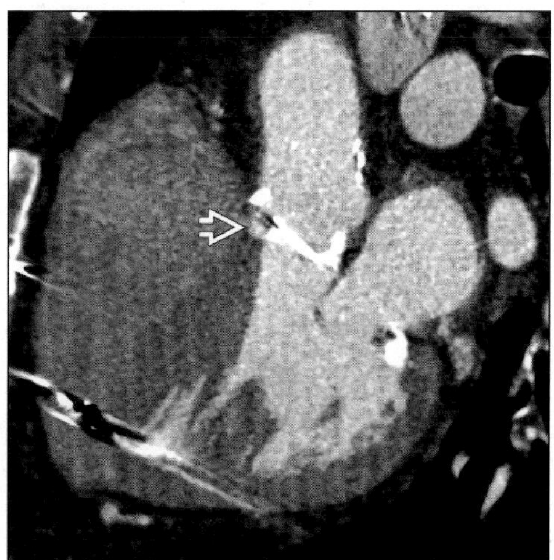

(Left) *Four chamber view B-mode echocardiogram shows prosthetic valve dysfunction due to vegetation ➡.* ***(Right)*** *Three chamber view cardiac CT shows paravalvular leakage ➡ of a mechanical, aortic, prosthetic valve.*

Typical

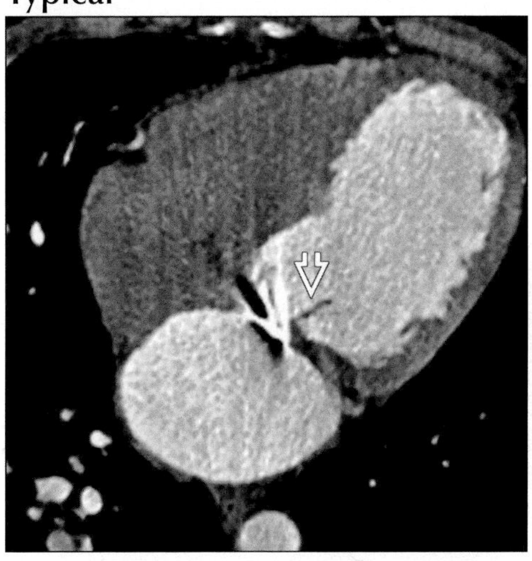

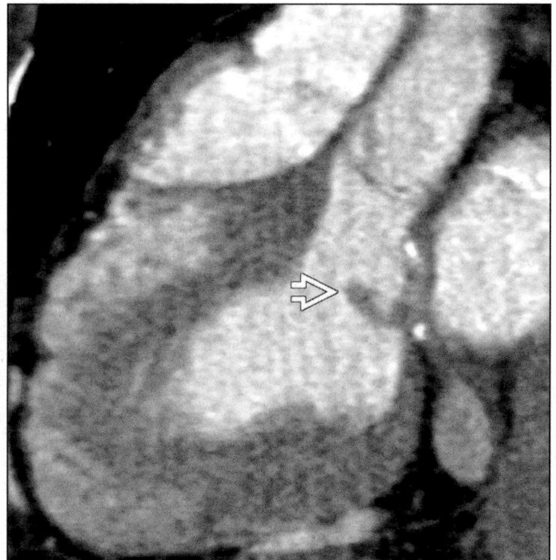

(Left) *Axial cardiac CT shows ruptured chordae tendinae ➡ from papillary muscle in a bioprosthetic mitral valve.* ***(Right)*** *Three chamber view cardiac CT shows ruptured chordae tendinae ➡ from papillary muscle in a patient with bioprosthetic mitral valve replacement.*

CARCINOID SYNDROME

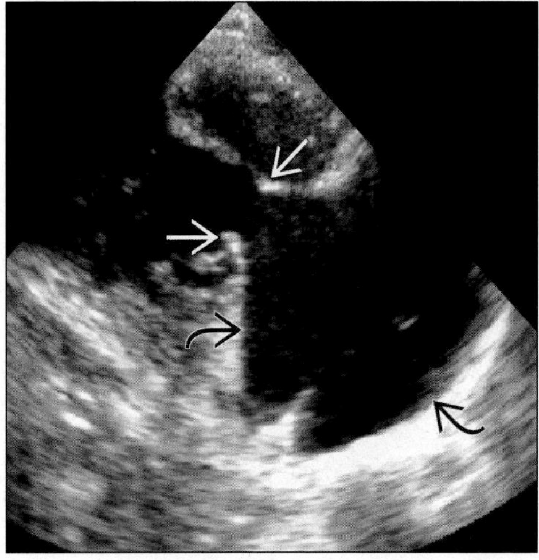

Echocardiogram (parasternal long axis right inflow tract) in a 50 year old male with carcinoid syndrome shows tricuspid leaflets ➔ which are thickened, retracted and hyperreflective. Note enlarged right atrium ↗.

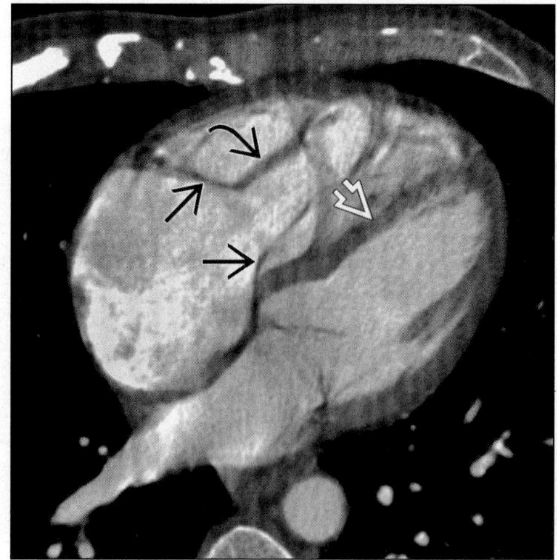

Axial CECT shows thickened tricuspid leaflets → and papillary muscles ↗ in cardiac carcinoid. Enlarged right atrium and ventricle from tricuspid regurgitation. Note flattening of interventricular septum ⇨.

TERMINOLOGY

Definitions

- Carcinoid tumor secretion of vasoactive substances (5-hydroxytryptamine, bradykinin and histamine) causing a clinical syndrome of flushing, diarrhea and bronchospasm
  - Most originate in the ileocecal region/appendix
    - Primary lung carcinoids secrete vasoactive substances directly into the pulmonary venous system, bypassing hepatic metabolism
  - Clinical symptoms occur when
    - Hepatic metastases overwhelm hepatic metabolism of tumour products, which are then secreted in high doses into the hepatic veins
    - Such substances cause cardiac valve leaflet fibrous endocardial plaques, classically on the tricuspid and pulmonary valves
    - Primary lung carcinoids secrete vasoactive substances directly into the pulmonary venous system, bypassing hepatic metabolism
  - Second most common cause of tricuspid stenosis (there is always concomitant regurgitation)

IMAGING FINDINGS

General Features

- Best diagnostic clue: Echocardiography shows thickened, retracted highly reflective tricuspid or pulmonary valve leaflets
- Location
  - Tricuspid and pulmonary valves are most commonly involved
  - Left-sided lesions can rarely occur in the presence of a patent foramen ovale, or primary pulmonary tumour
- Tricuspid regurgitation is the most common abnormality
- Thickened leaflets similar to rheumatic involvement
- Flow abnormalities related to degree of valve involvement

Radiographic Findings

- Radiography
  - Chest radiography findings
    - Enlarged cardiac silhouette
    - Right atrium enlargement

DDx: Other Causes of Tricuspid Valve Disease

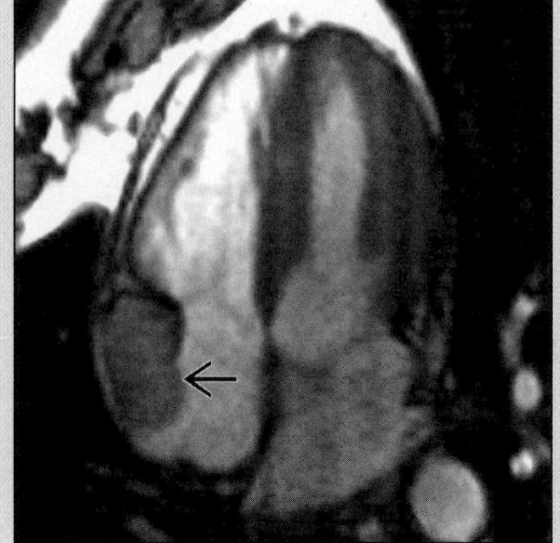

Malignancy (Angiosarcoma)

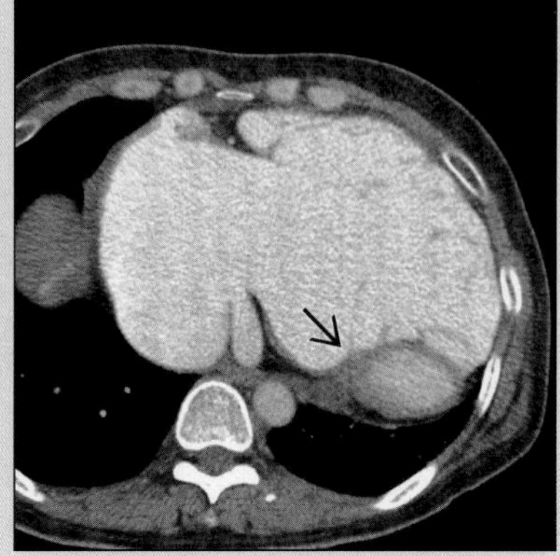

Ebstein Anomaly

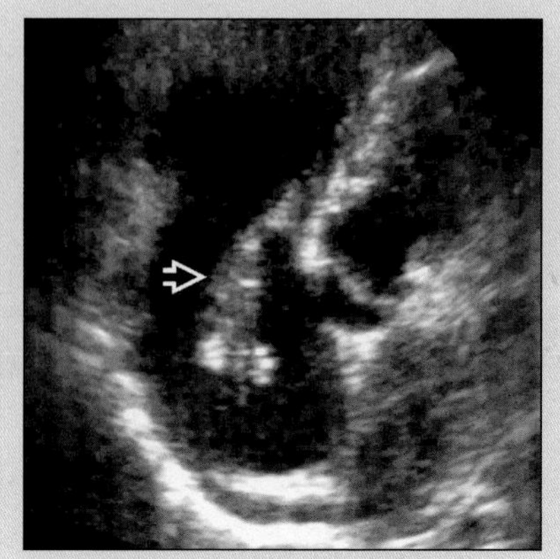

Tricuspid Endocarditis

CARCINOID SYNDROME

Key Facts

Terminology
- Carcinoid tumor secretion of vasoactive substances (5-hydroxytryptamine, bradykinin and histamine) causing a clinical syndrome of flushing, diarrhea and bronchospasm

Imaging Findings
- Best diagnostic clue: Echocardiography shows thickened, retracted highly reflective tricuspid or pulmonary valve leaflets
- Tricuspid and pulmonary valves are most commonly involved
- Tricuspid regurgitation is the most common abnormality
- Thickened leaflets similar to rheumatic involvement

Pathology
- Fibrous plaques are composed of smooth muscle cells mixed with mucopolysaccharide and collagen

Clinical Issues
- Most common signs/symptoms: Cutaneous flushing, diarrhea, bronchoconstriction and telangiectasia
- Progressive signs of right heart failure
- Cardiac involvement occurs in up to 50% of patients
- Medical therapy for right heart failure
- Balloon angioplasty in stenosis/surgical valve replacement in severe tricuspid regurgitation (on-table mortality high)
- Symptoms partially controlled with somatostatin analogues, serotonin antagonists, alpha-adrenergic blockers

    - Systemic venous hypertension (large azygos vein on AP film and superior vena cava on lateral film)
    - Pulmonary nodules in primary pulmonary disease
    - Decreased pulmonary vascularity in the presence of severe pulmonary stenosis

CT Findings
- CECT
  - Thickened, retracted tricuspid and pulmonary valves
    - Functional dataset may show fixed non-mobile leaflets
  - Enlarged right atrium, and ventricle
  - Pulmonary nodules in primary pulmonary disease
  - Decreased pulmonary vascularity in the presence of severe pulmonary stenosis

MR Findings
- Spin echo MR sequences show enlarged right atrium and thickening of tricuspid and pulmonary valve leaflets
- Bright blood steady state free precession cine sequences show functional tricuspid regurgitation and stenosis
- Phase-encoding sequences allow quantitative analysis of tricuspid regurgitation and stenosis

Nuclear Medicine Findings
- PET
  - Using
    - F-18-FDG
    - 18F-labeled somatostatin-receptor ligand ([18F]FP-Gluc-TOCA)
    - [68Ga]-DOTA-D-Phe(1)-Tyr(3)-Octreotide (DOTATOC)
- Octreoscan
  - Radiolabeled octreotide using either conventional scintigraphy or SPECT imaging

Echocardiographic Findings
- Echocardiogram
  - 2D, Doppler and transesophageal echocardiography (TEE)
    - Tricuspid valve: Regurgitation with or without stenosis
    - Pulmonary valve: Stenosis with regurgitation less common
    - Leaflets and papillary muscles may appear highly reflective
    - Tricuspid leaflets may be shortened, thickened, retracted and show incomplete coaptation
    - Pulmonary valve leaflets characteristically stay open in a fixed position
- Color Doppler
  - Shows a characteristic dagger-shaped Doppler signal with an early peak pressure and rapid decline
  - Biphasic flow pattern is seen in pulmonary insufficiency

Angiographic Findings
- Conventional
  - Enlarged right atrium and ventricle
  - Regurgitant jet of contrast into right atrium when contrast injected into right ventricle
  - Regurgitant jet of contrast into right ventricle when contrast injected into the pulmonary outflow tract

Imaging Recommendations
- Best imaging tool
  - Echocardiography
  - Cardiac MR

DIFFERENTIAL DIAGNOSIS

Rheumatic Heart Disease
- Presence of mitral and/or aortic valve disease required

Other Causes of Tricuspid or Pulmonary Valve Disease
- Right atrial tumor obstructing valve orifice
- Endocarditis
- Extracardiac neoplasm
- Fenfluramine and phentermine usage
- Ebstein anomaly

- Displacement of septal and posterior leaflets towards apex
- Large atrialized portion of right ventricle
- Sail-like anterior tricuspid leaflet

PATHOLOGY

General Features

- General path comments
  - Macroscopically the valves appear thickened and may be partly fused
    - Extensive diffuse infiltration from valves to myocardium may cause a restrictive cardiomyopathy

Gross Pathologic & Surgical Features

- Coaptation of nodular thickened valve leaflets
- Fibrous plaque coating the leaflets and papillary muscles

Microscopic Features

- Fibrous plaques are composed of smooth muscle cells mixed with mucopolysaccharide and collagen

CLINICAL ISSUES

Presentation

- Most common signs/symptoms: Cutaneous flushing, diarrhea, bronchoconstriction and telangiectasia
- Other signs/symptoms
  - Progressive signs of right heart failure
    - Elevated jugular venous pulse (JVP), prominent v wave
    - Edema
    - Ascites
  - Systolic murmur along left sternal border which shows inspiratory accentuation (regurgitation) and a diastolic rumble (stenosis)
- Rare cause of cardiac disease, yet cardiac complications are a significant cause of morbidity and mortality in this syndrome
- Although most common in the ileocecal valve region, can also be found in lung, biliary tract, pancreas, testis and ovary

Natural History & Prognosis

- Cardiac involvement occurs in up to 50% of patients
  - Progression is correlated to increased levels of serotonin
- Prognosis is poor: Mean survival is 1-2 years post diagnosis

Treatment

- Medical therapy for right heart failure
- Hepatic metastases
  - Systemic chemotherapy
  - Selective hepatic artery chemotherapy or embolization
  - Radiofrequency ablation
  - If small may be resectable
- Balloon angioplasty in stenosis/surgical valve replacement in severe tricuspid regurgitation (on-table mortality high)
- Symptoms partially controlled with somatostatin analogues, serotonin antagonists, alpha-adrenergic blockers

SELECTED REFERENCES

1. Park SB et al: Imaging findings of a primary bilateral testicular carcinoid tumor associated with carcinoid syndrome. J Ultrasound Med. 25(3):413-6, 2006
2. Strosberg JR et al: Selective hepatic artery embolization for treatment of patients with metastatic carcinoid and pancreatic endocrine tumors. Cancer Control. 13(1):72-8, 2006
3. Bastarrika G et al: Magnetic resonance imaging diagnosis of carcinoid heart disease. J Comput Assist Tomogr. 29(6):756-9, 2005
4. Halley A et al: Efficiency of 18F-FDG and 99mTc-depreotide SPECT in the diagnosis of malignancy of solitary pulmonary nodules. Eur J Nucl Med Mol Imaging. 32(9):1026-32, 2005
5. Seemann MD et al: Images in cardiovascular medicine. Cardiac metastasis: visualization with positron emission tomography, computed tomography, magnetic resonance imaging, positron emission tomography/computed tomography, and positron emission tomography/magnetic resonance imaging. Circulation. 112(21):e329-30, 2005
6. Collins N et al: Intrapericardial carcinoid metastasis. J Am Soc Echocardiogr. 17(6):675-6, 2004
7. Schaefer JF et al: Solitary pulmonary nodules: dynamic contrast-enhanced MR imaging--perfusion differences in malignant and benign lesions. Radiology. 232(2):544-53, 2004
8. Granberg D et al: Octreoscan in patients with bronchial carcinoid tumours. Clin Endocrinol (Oxf). 59(6):793-9, 2003
9. Gupta S et al: Hepatic artery embolization and chemoembolization for treatment of patients with metastatic carcinoid tumors: the M.D. Anderson experience. Cancer J. 9(4):261-7, 2003
10. Hoffmann U et al: Usefulness of magnetic resonance imaging of cardiac and paracardiac masses. Am J Cardiol. 92(7):890-5, 2003
11. Moller JE et al: Factors associated with progression of carcinoid heart disease. N Engl J Med. 348(11):1005-15, 2003
12. Mollet NR et al: MRI and CT revealing carcinoid heart disease. Eur Radiol. 13 Suppl 4:L14-8, 2003
13. Pickhardt PJ et al: Primary neoplasms of the appendix: radiologic spectrum of disease with pathologic correlation. Radiographics. 23(3):645-62, 2003
14. Farb A et al: Pathogenesis and pathology of valvular heart disease. In: Alpert JS, Dalen JE and Rahimtoola SH (eds): Valvular Heart Disease. 3rd Ed. Lippincott William and Wilkins, Philadelphia, 2000
15. Otto CM: Right-sided valve disease. In: Otto CM. Valvular Heart Disease.1st Ed. W.B. Saunders Company, Philadelphia, 1999
16. Mirowitz SA et al: MR and CT diagnosis of carcinoid heart disease. Chest. 103(2):630-1, 1993
17. Hanson MW et al: Carcinoid tumors: iodine-131 MIBG scintigraphy. Radiology. 172(3):699-703, 1989
18. Lund JT et al: Cardiac masses: assessment by MR imaging. AJR Am J Roentgenol. 152(3):469-73, 1989

CARCINOID SYNDROME

IMAGE GALLERY

Typical

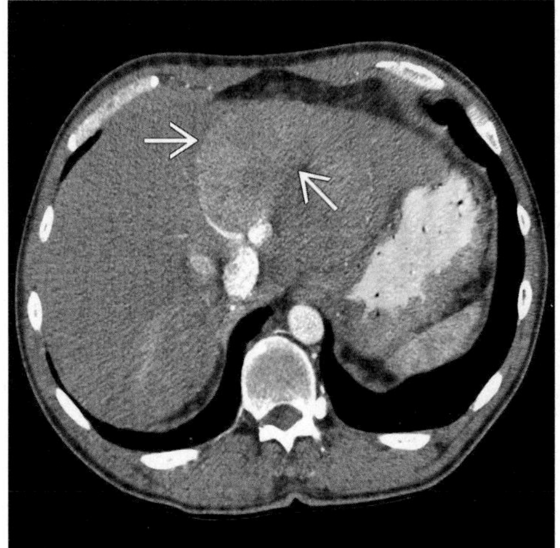

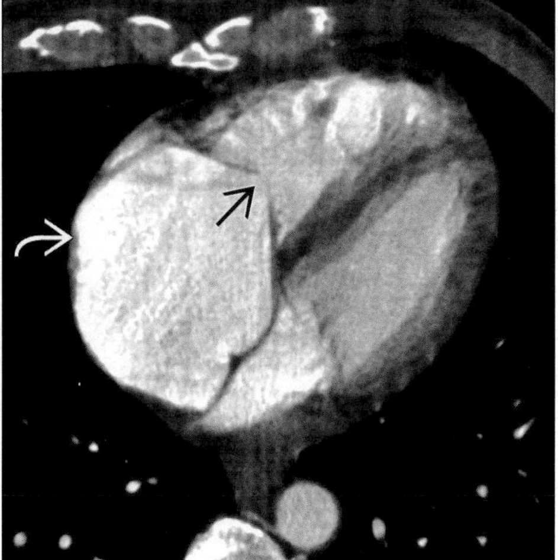

*(**Left**) Axial CECT shows enhancing mass in the right lobe of liver. Surgical biopsy confirmed carcinoid metastases. (**Right**) Corresponding CT shows markedly enlarged right atrium and severe tricuspid stenosis secondary to cardiac carcinoid.*

Typical

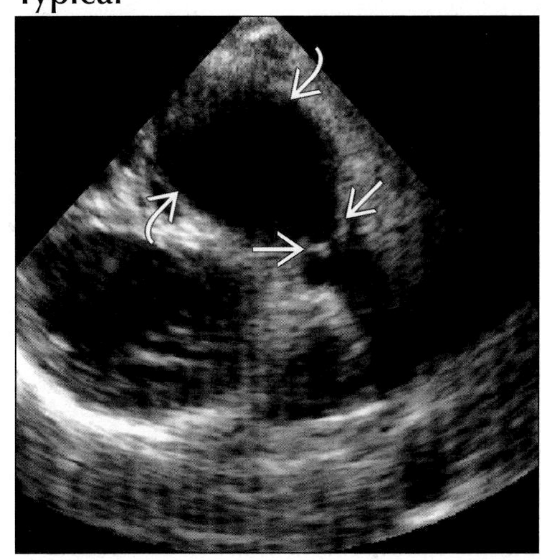

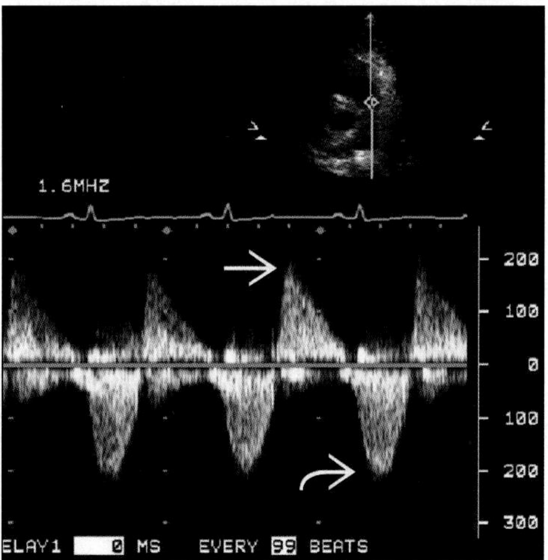

*(**Left**) Echocardiogram in a 61 year old male with carcinoid syndrome and severe pulmonary stenosis shows severely thickened and reflective pulmonary valves with secondary right ventricular enlargement. (**Right**) Corresponding pulsed Doppler shows biphasic flow pattern with high peak systolic pressure (pulmonary stenosis) and negative diastolic flow (pulmonary insufficiency).*

Typical

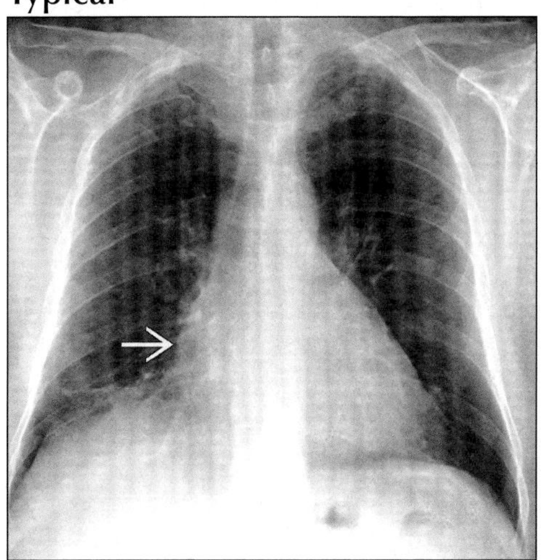

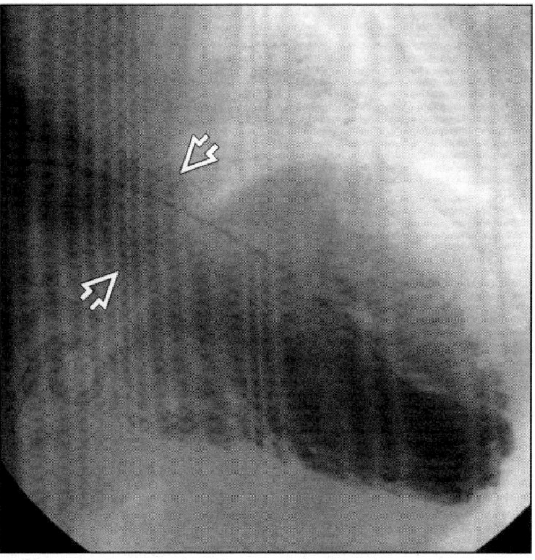

*(**Left**) PA radiograph in a 72 year old male with carcinoid syndrome shows an enlarged right atrium and decreased pulmonary vascularity secondary to pulmonary stenosis. (**Right**) Angiogram in 50 year old male with carcinoid syndrome shows a sharp jet of contrast passing retrogradely from the right ventricle into the right atrium secondary to tricuspid insufficiency.*

MULTIVALVULAR DISEASE

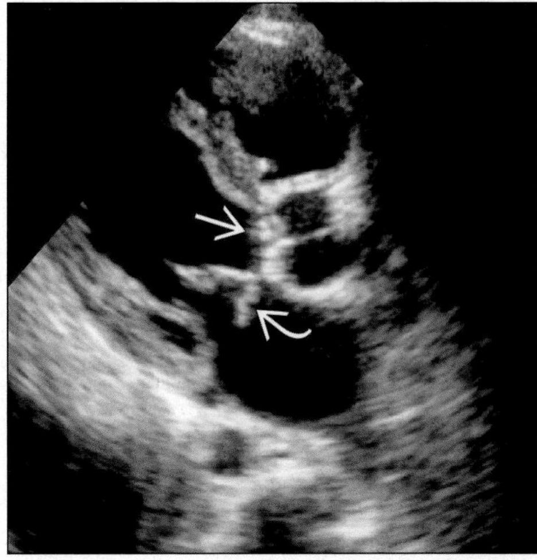

Parasternal long axis view transthoracic echo in diastole shows mitral and aortic valve endocarditis. Large mitral valve vegetation on the atrial side ➦. Vegetation coats the aortic valve ➡.

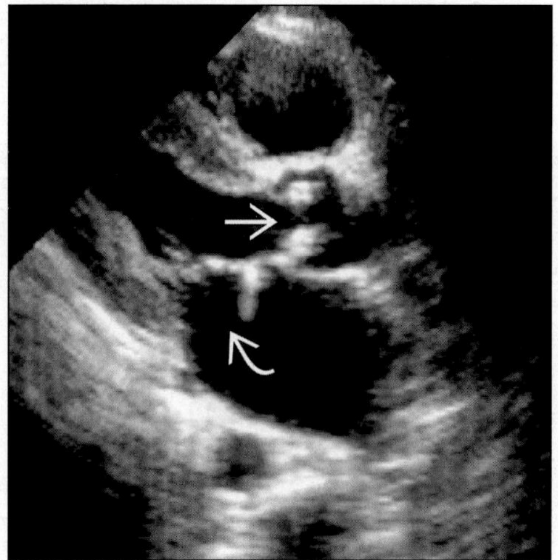

Transthoracic echo parasternal long axis view in systole in the same patient as previous image shows the mitral ➦ and aortic valve ➡ vegetations.

TERMINOLOGY

Abbreviations and Synonyms

- Tricuspid regurgitation (TR), pulmonic regurgitation (PR), aortic stenosis (AS), aortic regurgitation (AR), mitral stenosis (MS), mitral regurgitation (MR)

IMAGING FINDINGS

General Features

- See findings for specific valve disease

Imaging Recommendations

- Best imaging tool: Echocardiography

DIFFERENTIAL DIAGNOSIS

Rheumatic Heart Disease

- Most frequent cause of multivalvular disease

Infective Endocarditis

- Extension of the infection through mitral-aortic intervalvular fibrosa leads to MR and AR

Marfan Syndrome

- Bicuspid aortic valve with AS/AR and mitral valve prolapse with MR

Degenerative Calcification

- Frequently in MR and AS

Carcinoid

- Cause of combined tricuspid and pulmonic valve disease

PATHOLOGY

General Features

- General path comments
  - See findings for specific valve disease
  - Most common combination is MS with AS or AR
- Etiology
  - Rheumatic heart disease is the predominant cause
  - Primary single valve lesions can often cause secondary functional valve dysfunction in the distal downstream valve

DDx: Multivalvular Disease

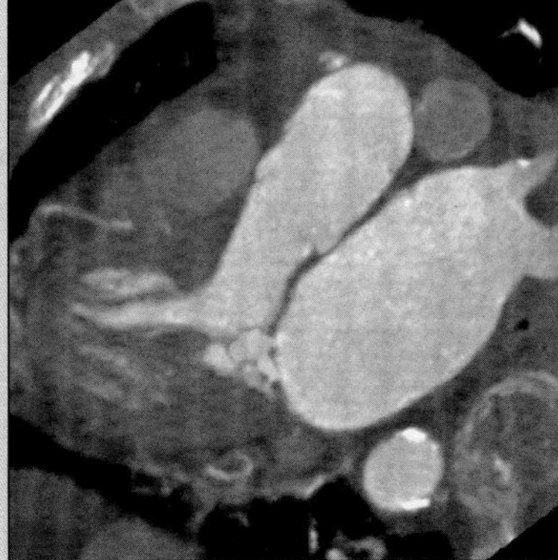

Mitral Annular Calcification

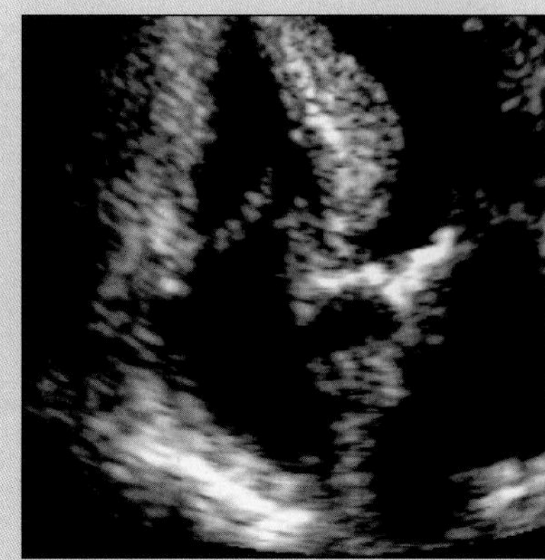

Rheumatic Heart Disease

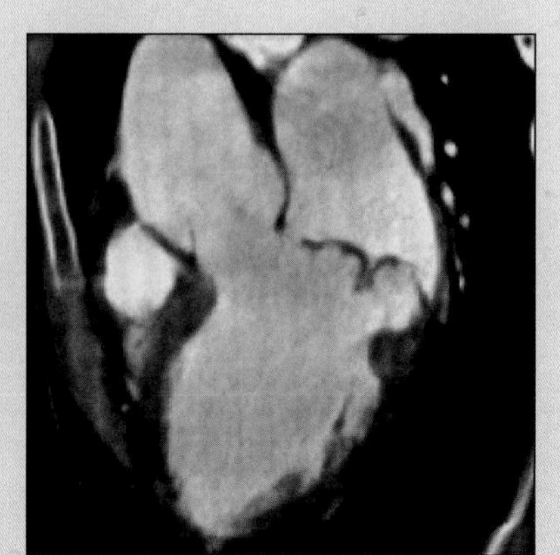

Marfan Syndrome with MVP

MULTIVALVULAR DISEASE

Key Facts

Imaging Findings
- See findings for specific valve disease
- Best imaging tool: Echocardiography

Top Differential Diagnoses
- Rheumatic Heart Disease
- Infective Endocarditis
- Marfan Syndrome
- Degenerative Calcification
- Carcinoid

Pathology
- Rheumatic heart disease is the predominant cause

Clinical Issues
- Symptoms dependent on combination of valve involvement
- Prominent signs in one valve can mask symptoms from other valve lesion

    - Aortic valve disease can lead to functional mitral regurgitation from elevated left ventricular end diastolic pressure
    - Mitral valve disease can lead to functional tricuspid regurgitation from pulmonary hypertension and right heart failure
  - Marfan syndrome and connective tissue disorders can cause multivalvular regurgitation

CLINICAL ISSUES

Presentation
- Most common signs/symptoms
  - Symptoms dependent on combination of valve involvement
  - Prominent signs in one valve can mask symptoms from other valve lesion
- Depends on the severity of each of the valve lesions
- In situation where valve damage is equal, proximal upstream valve determines symptoms and masks other distal lesion(s)

Natural History & Prognosis
- Combined aortic and mitral valve disease
  - MS with AS or AR is most frequent rheumatic valvular disease combination
    - Left ventricle is small, stiff, and hypertrophied in cases of AS and MS
    - Severe MS is usually accompanied by mild AR
    - Combination of MS and severe AR is uncommon
  - Myxomatous degeneration can cause AR and MR
  - AS and MR can produce severe pulmonary congestion
- Combined tricuspid and left-sided valve disease
  - Functional TR occurs in the majority of patients with significant MR due to elevated pulmonary arterial pressures and right ventricular dysfunction
  - TS occurs in approximately 30% of patients with MS
    - Women more likely to get TS with MS than men
- Significant triple valve disease is rare and usually is the result of rheumatic changes

Treatment
- Double valve replacement or replacement + valvuloplasty in severe cases
- Higher operative mortality: 10%
- Low 5 year survival rates; 80% with single valve replacement; 60% with double valve replacement
- Lower post-operative survival if pulmonary arterial hypertension, triple valve procedure, coronary artery disease, prior sternotomy, diabetes mellitus

SELECTED REFERENCES

1. Braunwald E: Valvular Heart Disease. In: Braunwald E. Heart Disease: A Textbook of Cardiovascular Medicine. 6th ed. WB Saunders Company, Philadelphia, 2001
2. Alpert JS, Dalen JE and Rahimtoola SH (eds): Valvular Heart Disease. 3rd ed. Lippincott William and Wilkins, Philadelphia, 2000

IMAGE GALLERY

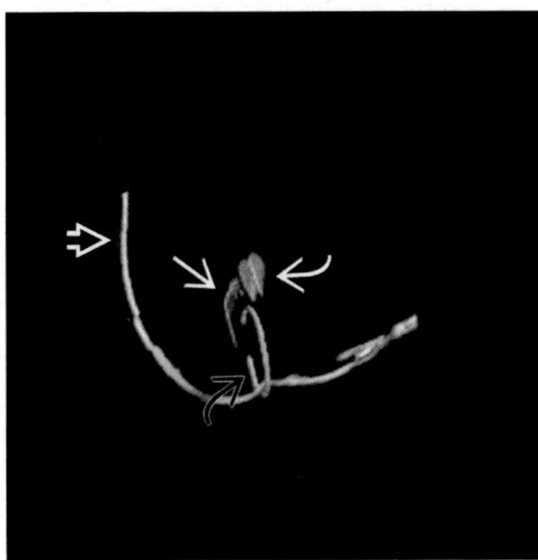

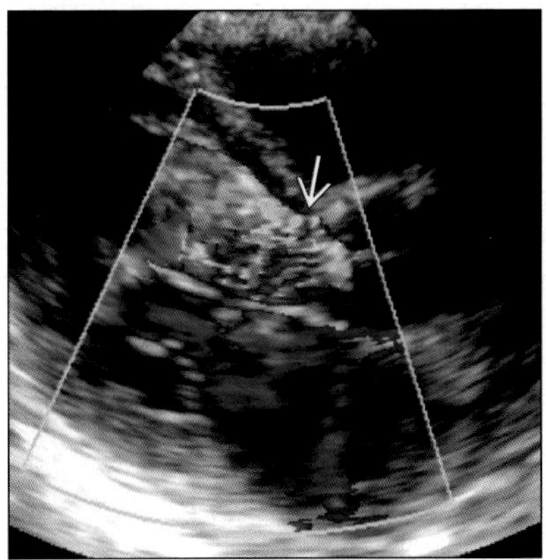

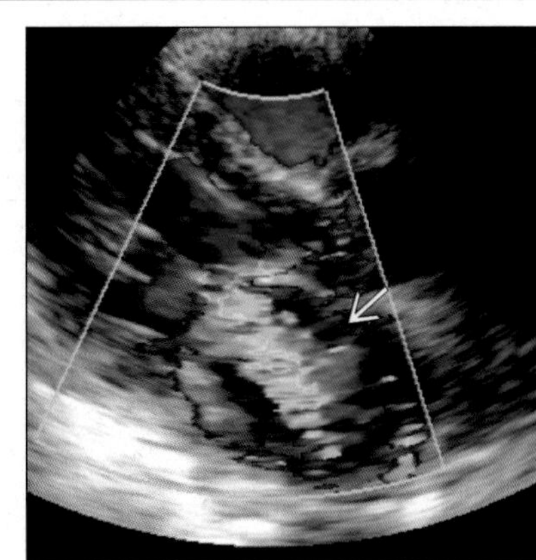

*(**Left**) Volume rendered cardiac CTA in systole shows bileaflet mechanical aortic valve ➡, bileaflet mechanical mitral valve ➡, and tricuspid valve ring ↗. Note pacemaker wire ➡. (**Center**) Transthoracic echo parasternal view with color Doppler in a patient with aortic and mitral valve endocarditis shows severe aortic regurgitation ➡. (**Right**) Transthoracic echo parasternal view during systole with color Doppler in the same patient with multivalvular endocarditis shows severe mitral regurgitation ➡.*

VALVULAR PROSTHESIS

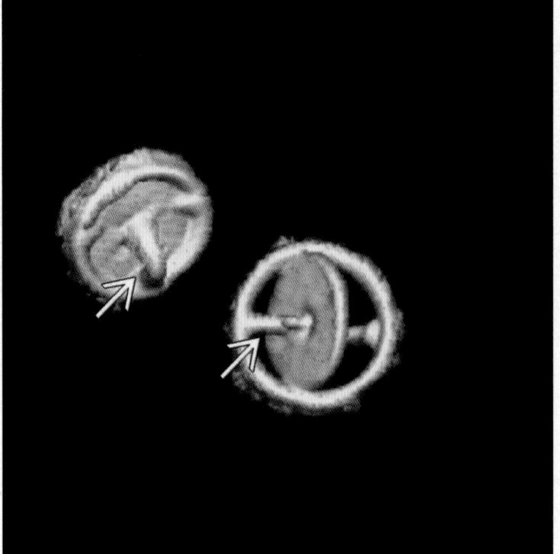

Oblique coronary CTA volume rendering shows normal closed aortic and open mitral Medtronic-Hall tilting disc valve replacements. Note: Single strut ➔ traverses central disc opening.

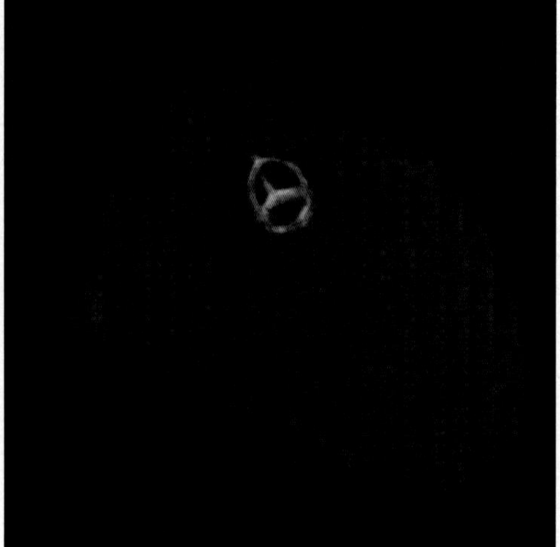

Oblique coronary CTA volume rendering shows typical appearance of Starr-Edwards aortic caged ball (3 prongs) valve replacement. Valves in mitral position typically have 4 prongs.

TERMINOLOGY

Definitions

- Replacement of diseased native cardiac valves with mechanical valve or tissue graft

IMAGING FINDINGS

General Features

- Location
  - Aortic valve or atrioventricular valves (mitral or tricuspid) rarely pulmonary in situ replacements
    - Tricuspid position: Bioprosthesis preferred because of higher risk of thrombus formation in mechanical valves (highest for tilting disc valves)
  - First ball valve was inserted in descending thoracic aorta to treat aortic insufficiency (AI) (Hufnagel valve)
  - Rarely apical left ventricular to descending thoracic aortic tube graft conduits are used to treat aortic stenosis (AS) if in situ aortic valve replacement is deemed too risky
- Morphology
  - Ball in cage valves
  - **Hufnagel valve**
    - First caged ball valve developed 1952
    - Implanted into descending aorta
    - ~ 200 valves implanted
  - **Harken-Soroff ball valve**
    - First in situ ball in cage valve - first implanted in March 1960
    - Less than 20 valves implanted (aortic only)
  - **Starr Edwards (1965) ball in cage valve**
    - Initial models used stellite alloy cage, later changed to bare metal cage
    - Silastic rubber ball
    - More than 80,000 implanted aortic and 100,000 mitral valves
    - Still in production
  - Other Ball in cage valves
    - Braunwald-Cutter: ~ 5,000 implanted, titanium cage covered with Dacron fabric (1968-1979)
    - Magovern-Cromie: ~ 7,300 aortic and ~ 200 mitral valves replaced (1962-1980)
    - Smeloff-Cutter: Double cage with "equator-seating" ball, 72,000 implanted (1966-1988)

DDx: Artificial Valve Replacements

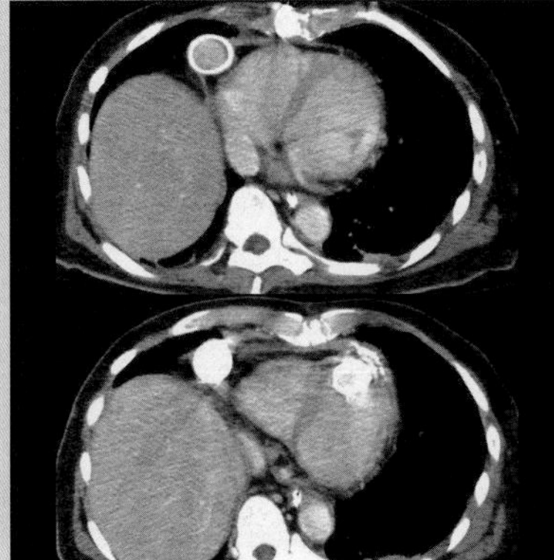

Ventricular Assist Device

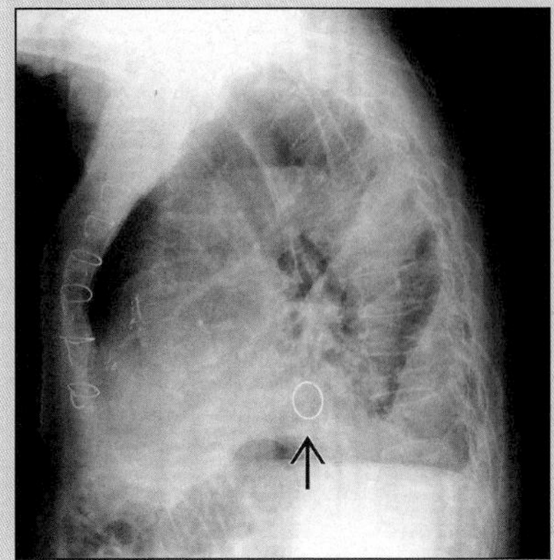

Apico-Aortic Conduit

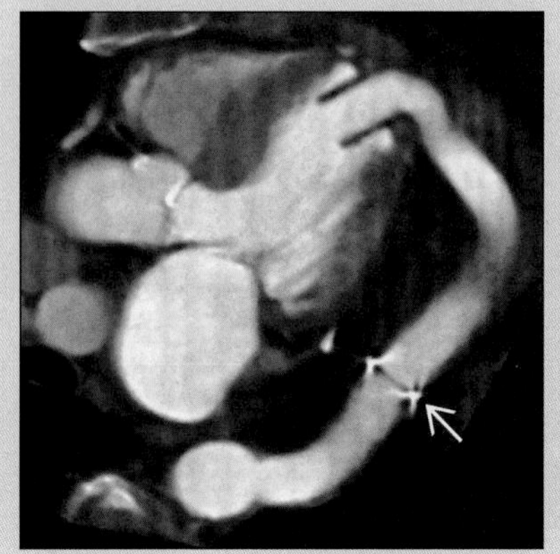

Apico-Aortic Conduit

VALVULAR PROSTHESIS

Key Facts

Imaging Findings

- Tricuspid position: Bioprosthesis preferred because of higher risk of thrombus formation in mechanical valves (highest for tilting disc valves)
- First ball valve was inserted in descending thoracic aorta to treat aortic insufficiency (AI) (Hufnagel valve)
- Smeloff-Cutter: Double cage with "equator-seating" ball, 72,000 implanted (1966-1988)
- **Bjork-Shiley flat disc (1969) and convexo-concave (1975) disc valves**
- Convexo-concave disc was developed to improve flow across valve but new design led to strut fractures in 2% of cases
- **Medtronic-Hall (previously Hall-Kaster valve) tilting disc valve (1977)**
- Strut traverses hole in disc
- **St. Jude Medical (1977)**
- First "all carbon" (pyrolyte) valve
- **Carbo-Medics (1986)**
- Housing can be rotated within sewing ring

Clinical Issues

- Thrombotic and bleeding complication rate with mechanical aortic prostheses (2-4%) is twice as high as with tissue prosthesis (1-2%)
- Fetal demise occurs in 25 to 30% of pregnant women with mechanical heart valves on warfarin or heparin
- Valve thrombosis occurs in 0.1% per year in aortic and 0.35% per year in mitral position
- Prosthetic valve endocarditis (PVE) occurs in 1.4-3.1% at 12 months and 3.2-5.7% at 5 years (cumulative)

- DeBakey-Surgitool: Pyrolyte ball ~ 1,200 aortic position only (1967-1984)
- Non-tilting disc valves
  - Kay-Shiley: Flat disc, widely used mitral valve replacement (MVR), ~ 12,000 mitral only (1965-1980)
  - Beall-Surgitool: Flat disc, initially Teflon, later pyrolyte disc ~ 4,800 mitral only (1967-1985)
  - Cooley-Cutter: Bi-conical silicone rubber disc later replaced with pyrolyte disc, 3,000 aortic and mitral implanted (1971-1978)
- Titling disc valves
- **Bjork-Shiley flat disc (1969) and convexo-concave (1975) disc valves**
  - Convexo-concave disc was developed to improve flow across valve but new design led to strut fractures in 2% of cases
  - Strut fractures have led to prophylactic valve replacements and a class action suit allowing patients for financial compensation for valve re-replacement
  - Consequently convexo-concave and even complication free flat disc valve production was terminated in 1986
  - ~ 300,000 Flat discs (aortic and mitral) and ~ 86,000 convexo-concave (aortic and mitral) disc valves implanted
- **Lillehei-Kaster tilting disc valve (1970-1987)**
  - Two side prongs hold valve in place
  - ~ 55,000 implanted
  - Omni-Science and Omni-Carbon valves are newer models and are still in production
- **Medtronic-Hall (previously Hall-Kaster valve) tilting disc valve (1977)**
  - Titanium housing with pyrolite disc
  - Strut traverses hole in disc
  - Wide spread use, > 300,000 aortic and mitral valves replaced
  - No mechanical failures reported, still in production
- Bileaflet valves
- **St. Jude Medical (1977)**
  - First "all carbon" (pyrolyte) valve
  - 1.3 million valves implanted predominantly in aortic and mitral positions
- **Carbo-Medics (1986)**
  - ~ 500,000 implanted in mitral and aortic positions
  - Housing can be rotated within sewing ring
  - Pyrolite housing and pyrolite discs
- Other bileaflet valves
  - Gott-Daggett: ~ 500 implanted in mitral and aortic position, flexible carbon coated leaflets (1963-1966)
  - Kalke-Lillehei: Only one implanted due to patient demise within 48 hours, first hingeless bileaflet valve (1968)
  - On-X: New carbon structure allows design modification that may allow for reduced anticoagulation levels (still investigational)
  - ATA open pivot valve: Bileaflet pyrolite valve with titanium lock ring
- Lifelong anticoagulation necessary for all mechanical heart valves
- In general longer durability of mechanical valves compared to tissue valves but more thrombogenic complications

- Tissue valves (bioprostheses)
  - Hancock porcine xenograft
    - Glutaraldehyde preserved porcine valve mounted on Dacron covered polypropylene strut
  - Carpentier-Edwards porcine xenograft
    - Pressure fixed and glutaraldehyde preserved and wire mounted porcine or pericardial valve
  - Ionescu-Shiley
    - Bovine xenograft
  - Cryopreserved homograft valve
  - Pulmonary autograft
- 3 months of anticoagulation required for tissue valves until sewing ring becomes endothelialized
  - No anticoagulation required thereafter

Imaging Recommendations

- Best imaging tool: Fluoroscopy or gated CT for assessment of leaflet function

VALVULAR PROSTHESIS

DIFFERENTIAL DIAGNOSIS

Aortic Calcifications

- Can mimic AVR on non-gated CT

Annuloplasty Ring

- Usually open ring on radiography or CT

CLINICAL ISSUES

Presentation

- Indications for mechanical valves
  - Age less than 40 years
    - Longer expected life → better durability of mechanical valves preferred but lifetime anticoagulation necessary
  - Aortic root and valve replacement needed (composite graft)
  - Anticoagulation required for other reasons anyway
  - Previous dysfunctional tissue valve
  - Dialysis
- Indications for bioprosthetic valves
  - Age ≥ 65 years
    - Shorter life expectancy → lower risk from thromboembolism and anticoagulation preferred
  - Previous thrombotic valve complication
  - Contraindication to anticoagulation
  - Possible pregnancy

Demographics

- Ethnicity: In contrast to coronary artery bypass surgery, race is not a significant predictor of operative mortality after isolated aortic or mitral valve replacement

Natural History & Prognosis

- Bleeding or thrombotic complications account for 50% of complications of tissue valves and for 75% of complications of mechanical valves
- Thrombotic and bleeding complication rate with mechanical aortic prostheses (2-4%) is twice as high as with tissue prosthesis (1-2%)
  - No difference in thrombotic and bleeding complications in mitral position (~ 4%)
- Mechanical prostheses usually cause subclinical mild chronic hemolysis
- Fetal demise occurs in 25 to 30% of pregnant women with mechanical heart valves on warfarin or heparin
- Valve thrombosis occurs in 0.1% per year in aortic and 0.35% per year in mitral position
- Prosthetic valve endocarditis (PVE) occurs in 1.4-3.1% at 12 months and 3.2-5.7% at 5 years (cumulative)
  - Commonly extends beyond valve annulus resulting in ring abscess and extravasation into abscess cavities
  - Fistulous tracts and septal tracts possible
  - Valve dehiscence may lead to significant paravalvular regurgitation
  - Myocardial abscess in ~ 30% in pathology series
- Prosthetic valve endocarditis (PVE) agents
  - Coagulase negative staphylococci → most common agent in first year (~ 30%) often agent in nosocomial PVE
  - Streptococci → more common after first year post implantation (~ 30%)
  - Staphylococcus Aureus → any time ~ 20% of PVE, 40-50% central nervous system complications
  - Enterococci → (~ 10% any time)
  - Poly microbial → ~ 5% of cases
  - Gram negative bacilli, Haemophilus, fungi, Candida, diphtheroids and other agents not uncommon
  - 5-8% are culture negative

DIAGNOSTIC CHECKLIST

Consider

- Check for paravalvular contrast collections and tissue stranding
  - May be only signs of paravalvular abscess

SELECTED REFERENCES

1. Gott VL et al: Mechanical heart valves: 50 years of evolution. Ann Thorac Surg. 76(6):S2230-9, 2003
2. Braunwald E: Valvular Heart Disease. In: Heart Disease: A Textbook of Cardiovascular Medicine. 6th ed. Philadelphia, WB Saunders Company, 2001
3. Karchmer AW: Infective Endocarditis. In: Heart Disease: A Textbook of Cardiovascular Medicine. 6th ed. Philadelphia, WB Saunders Company, 2001
4. DeWall RA et al: Evolution of mechanical heart valves. Ann Thorac Surg. 69(5):1612-21, 2000
5. Arom KV et al: Ten years' experience with the St. Jude Medical valve prosthesis. Ann Thorac Surg. 47(6):831-7, 1989
6. Nitter-Hauge S et al: Ten-year experience with the Medtronic Hall valvular prosthesis. A study of 1,104 patients. Circulation. 80(3 Pt 1):I43-8, 1989
7. Edmunds LH Jr: Thrombotic and bleeding complications of prosthetic heart valves. Ann Thorac Surg. 44(4):430-45, 1987
8. Björk V.O: Aortic valve replacement with the Björk-Shiley tilting disc valve prosthesis. Br Heart J. 33(suppl):42-6, 1971
9. Cruz AB Jr et al: A new caged meniscus prosthetic heart valve. Surgery. 58(6):995-8, 1965
10. HARKEN DE et al: Partial and complete prostheses in aortic insufficiency. J Thorac Cardiovasc Surg. 40:744-62, 1960
11. HUFNAGEL CA et al: Experiences with new types of aortic valvular prostheses. Ann Surg. 147(5):636-44; discussion 644-5, 1958
12. Taylor NE et al: Relationship between race and mortality and morbidity after valve replacement surgery.

VALVULAR PROSTHESIS

IMAGE GALLERY

Typical

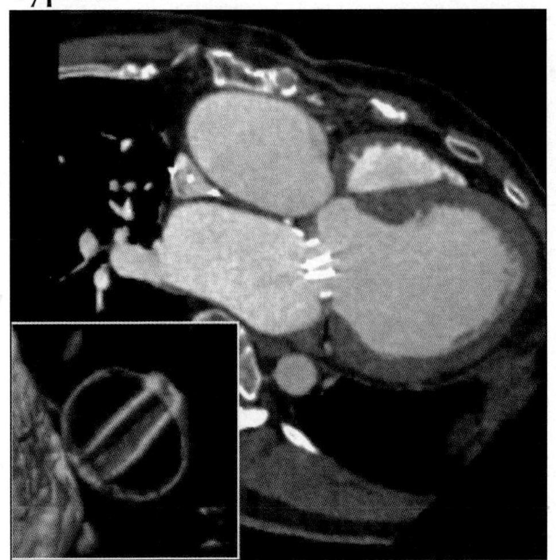

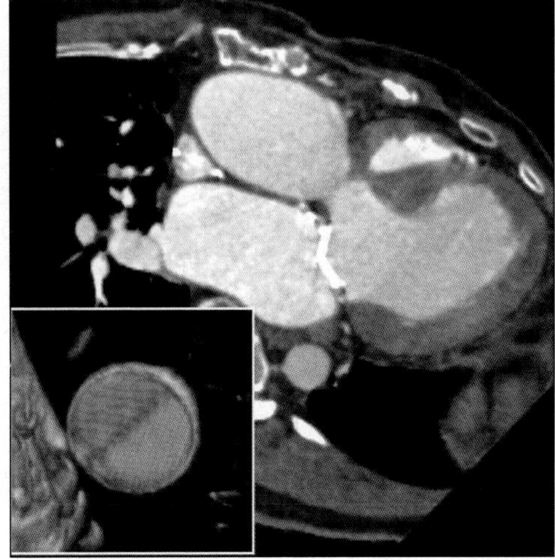

(Left) *Oblique coronary CTA shows mechanical bileaflet tilting disc valve replacement in mitral position during left ventricular filling. Insert shows volume rendering of open bileaflet valve.* ***(Right)*** *Oblique coronary CTA shows bileaflet mechanical valve prosthesis in mitral position during systole. Insert shows volume rendering of closed prosthesis.*

Typical

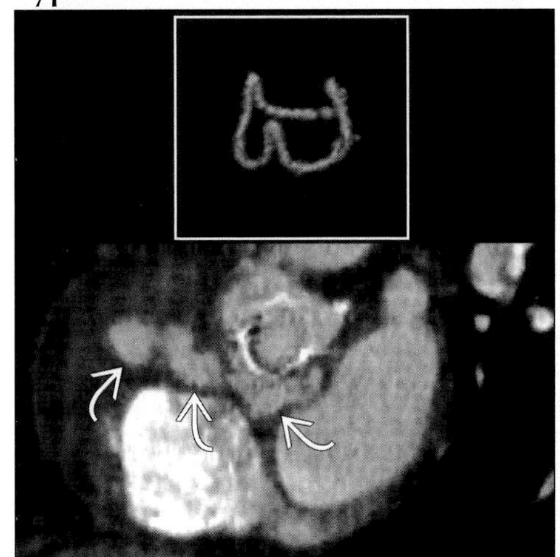

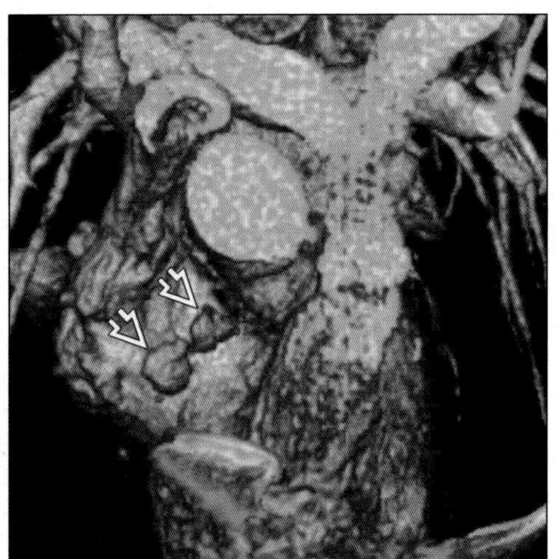

(Left) *Oblique CTA shows aortic Carpentier Edwards porcine tissue valve (insert shows volume rendering of valve frame). Three discrete extraluminal contrast cavities ➢ indicate PVE with paravalvular abscess.* ***(Right)*** *Oblique coronary CTA volume rendering shows two of the abscess cavities filled with contrast ➢.*

Typical

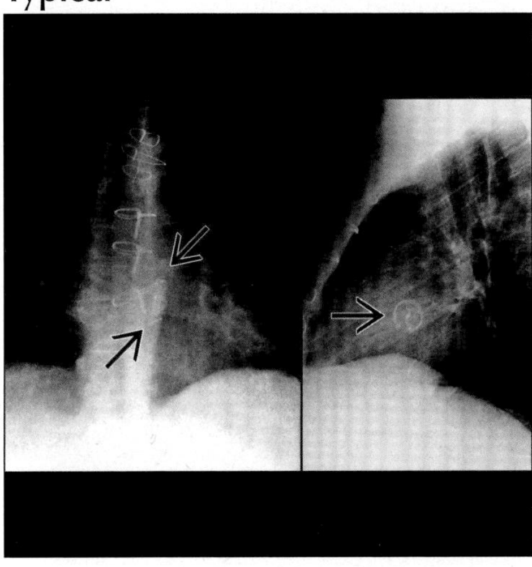

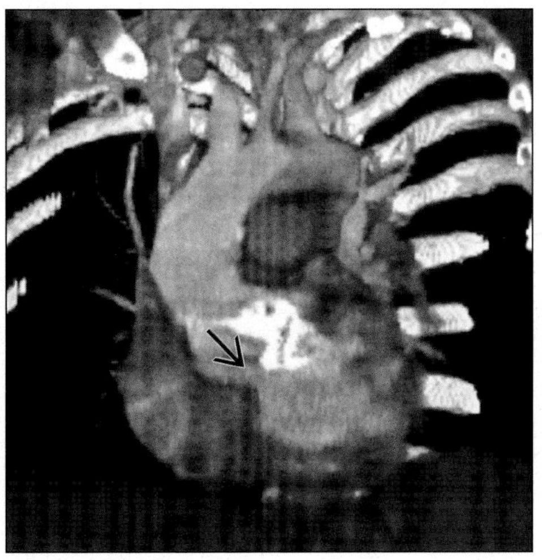

(Left) *PA and lateral radiograph shows tilting disc valve → in aortic position.* ***(Right)*** *Coronal CECT volume rendering in patient with endocarditis shows tilting disc valve not fully extending to aortic anulus indicating dehiscence. Note: Periprosthetic regurgitation → site.*

RHEUMATIC HEART DISEASE

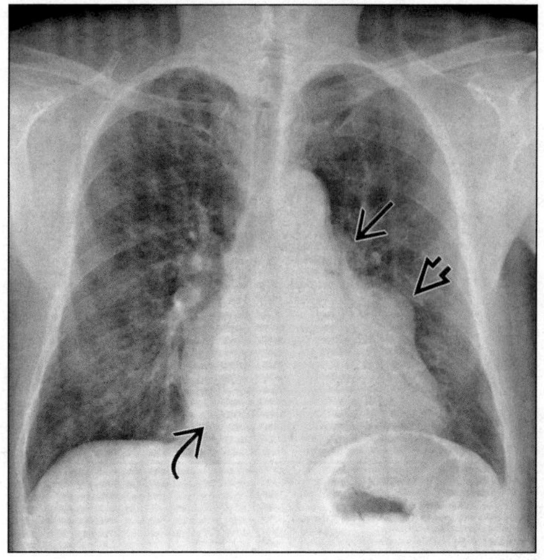

Posteroanterior radiograph shows pulmonary redistribution (PVH), convex LAA segment ⊳, convex PA segment → (2° PAH), and right double density ↗ (enlarged LA), consistent with rheumatic MS.

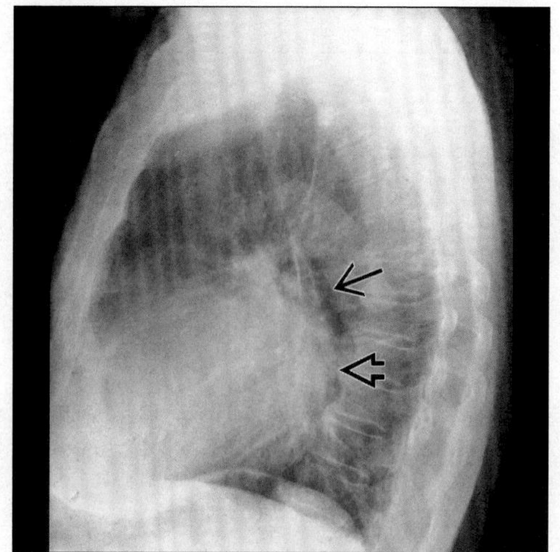

Lateral radiograph shows posteriorly displaced left main stem bronchus → due to an enlarged left atrium ⊳.

TERMINOLOGY

Definitions

- Rheumatic heart disease is a condition characterized by cardiac valve damage secondary to previous rheumatic fever
  - Rheumatic fever is a complication of group A beta-hemolytic streptococcal pharyngitis (strep throat) in children and adolescents
  - Rheumatic valve disease may first become apparent years or decades after initial infection
- May include valvular stenosis, regurgitation, left ventricular (LV) and left atrial (LA) enlargement, pericarditis and heart failure
- Most commonly affects mitral valve followed by aortic and tricuspid valve

IMAGING FINDINGS

Radiographic Findings

- Dilated left atrial appendage (LAA) and left atrium
  - Right-sided double density sign on frontal radiograph due to appearance of enlarged LA
  - Posterior displacement and slight elevation of the left mainstem bronchus
- Calcification of the left atrial wall
- Normal to slightly enlarged cardio-thoracic ratio
- Calcification of the mitral valve leaflets
- Interstitial pulmonary edema and/or pulmonary venous redistribution

CT Findings

- NECT
  - Enlarged left atrium
  - Calcification of the anterior and posterior leaflets of the mitral valve (NOT mitral annular calcification)
- Cardiac Gated CTA
  - Thickening of and incomplete opening of the mitral valve leaflets
    - Essential to perform multiphase imaging and reconstruction
    - Allows for mitral valve planimetry, though not commonly employed clinically
  - Allows assessment of additional valvular involvement
    - Aortic valve > tricuspid valve

DDx: Rheumatic Heart Disease

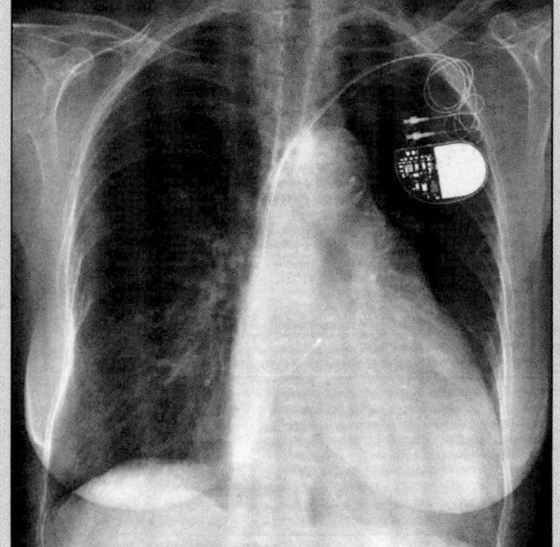

Dilated Cardiomyopathy

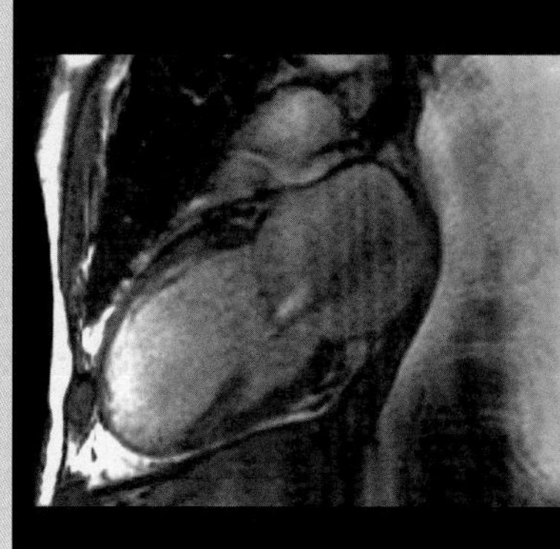

MR due to Myocardial Infarct

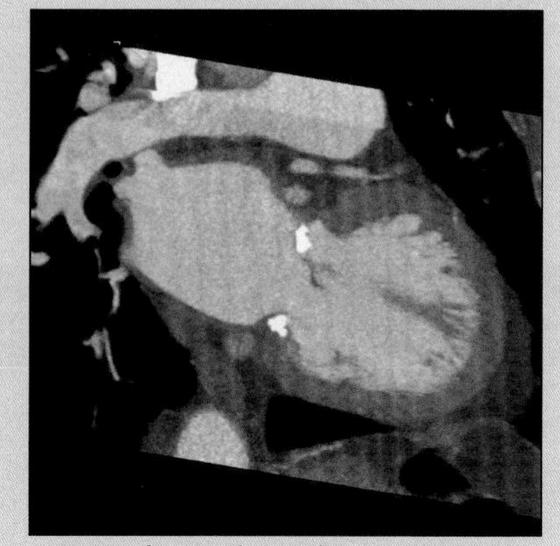

Mitral Annular Calcium (MAC)

RHEUMATIC HEART DISEASE

Key Facts

Terminology

- Rheumatic heart disease is a condition characterized by cardiac valve damage secondary to previous rheumatic fever
- Rheumatic fever is a complication of group A beta-hemolytic streptococcal pharyngitis (strep throat) in children and adolescents
- Rheumatic valve disease may first become apparent years or decades after initial infection
- Most commonly affects mitral valve followed by aortic and tricuspid valve

Imaging Findings

- Dilated left atrial appendage (LAA) and left atrium
- Right-sided double density sign on frontal radiograph due to appearance of enlarged LA
- Posterior displacement and slight elevation of the left mainstem bronchus
- Interstitial pulmonary edema and/or pulmonary venous redistribution
- Calcification of the anterior and posterior leaflets of the mitral valve (NOT mitral annular calcification)

Pathology

- Pathogenesis is believed to be due to an immune mediated reaction to the streptococcus bacterium
- Mitral valve may demonstrate a "fish mouth" or "button-hole" configuration

Clinical Issues

- Can prevent its development by giving antibiotics when strep throat is detected

---

- May demonstrate left atrial appendage (LAA) thrombus
    - Arterial phase CTA may be false positive if slow mixing of LA contrast with LAA
    - Delayed phase CT will demonstrate "filling in" of LAA if negative or persistent filling defect if positive for thrombus

MR Findings

- SSFP gradient echo images show mitral regurgitation and/or stenosis
    - Dephasing regurgitant jet indicates insufficiency
    - Antegrade jet indicates stenosis
- May demonstrate diastolic "doming" of the mitral valve, which indicates stenosis
- Evaluate entire mitral valve apparatus
    - May reveal thickening or retraction of chordae tendinae
- Use phase contrast technique to quantify the peak velocity of the stenotic jet and amount of mitral regurgitation
- May demonstrate enlarged LA ± left atrial appendage thrombus
    - Accuracy of MR for LAA thrombus detection is limited
    - Trans esophageal echocardiography (TEE) remains gold standard for LAA thrombus
- Assess ventricular function and quantify ejection fraction

Echocardiographic Findings

- Test of choice for initial evaluation and to assess for disease progression
- Doppler echocardiography used to calculate pressure half-time valve area and the trans valvular gradient
- Color Doppler can show both mitral stenosis and mitral regurgitation
- Severe stenosis is classified as having a transmural gradient > 10 mm Hg, pulmonary artery systolic pressure > 50 mm Hg and a mitral valve area < 1 cm^2
- Three-dimensional echocardiography is an emerging modality that allows for accurate planimetry of valve area
- Stress echocardiography is utilized if discordance between findings at rest and clinical findings with exercise
- Left atrial enlargement
- Valvular leaflet thickening, diastolic doming, and incomplete opening of the valve
- May demonstrate other valve involvement

DIFFERENTIAL DIAGNOSIS

Other Reasons for LA Inflow Obstruction

- Decreased LV compliance
    - Restrictive cardiomyopathy
    - Endomyocardial fibrosis
    - Dilated cardiomyopathy
- Chronic aortic stenosis
- Myxoma or other masses

Secondary Mitral Regurgitation

- Myocardial infarction

Carcinoid

- Presence of patent foramen ovale (PFO) may result in predominantly left-sided valve involvement

Medications

- Methysergide

Congenital

- Cor-triatriatum

Mucopolysaccharidoses

- Hunter-Hurler subtype

Autoimmune

- Systemic lupus erythematosus, rheumatic heart disease

RHEUMATIC HEART DISEASE

PATHOLOGY

General Features

- General path comments: End result of what is believed to be an autoimmune reaction to group A streptococcus leading to fibrinoid degeneration resulting in a verrucous appearance of the lesions on the valve
- Etiology: Pathogenesis believed to be an immune-mediated reaction to the streptococcus bacterium

Gross Pathologic & Surgical Features

- Mitral valve may demonstrate a "fish mouth" or "button-hole" configuration
- Pericardium and epicardium are thickened and may demonstrate fibrinous exudates
  - Pericardial adhesions may be present, however unlike in other settings, in this setting adhesions do not result in pericardial constriction

Microscopic Features

- Presence of Aschoff nodules that are characterized by monocyte-macrophage appearing cells and loss of normal adjacent myocardial muscle with fibrous tissue replacement

CLINICAL ISSUES

Presentation

- Other signs/symptoms
  - Systemic venous hypertension due to chronic severe MS and elevated pulmonary vascular resistance and right heart failure
    - Hepatomegaly
    - Edema, ascites
  - Disease may worsen in pregnant patients or may initially present during pregnancy because of increased cardiac output and heart rate
  - Typical murmur of mitral stenosis is a diastolic rumble at the apex
  - Atrial fibrillation
- Clinical Profile
  - Dyspnea, orthopnea, paroxysmal nocturnal dyspnea
  - Fatigue due to low cardiac output
  - Chest pain due to RV ischemia/failure in severe PAH
  - Syncope
  - Hemoptysis
  - Ortner syndrome (hoarseness due to left atrium compressing left recurrent laryngeal nerve)

Treatment

- Can prevent its development by giving antibiotics when strep throat is detected
- Control and treat elevated pulmonary venous pressure and heart failure
- Asymptomatic patients with
  - Severe mitral stenosis should undergo close clinical follow-up and a yearly echocardiogram
  - Moderate mitral stenosis should undergo an echocardiogram every 1-2 years
  - Mild mitral stenosis should undergo an echocardiogram every 3-5 years
- Symptomatic patients with moderate to severe mitral stenosis and/or pulmonary hypertension undergo intervention
  - Mitral valve replacement
  - Percutaneous mitral balloon valvuloplasty may be used in acute settings or prophylactic treatment for women of childbearing age
- Mitral valve annuloplasty has been proposed in patients with mitral regurgitation
  - Does not reduce mortality

DIAGNOSTIC CHECKLIST

Image Interpretation Pearls

- Convex left atrial appendage segment, right double density and pulmonary venous redistribution are classic findings of rheumatic MV disease
  - Convex pulmonary artery segment and large central pulmonary arteries may develop due to back pressure in chronic rheumatic MV disease

SELECTED REFERENCES

1. Carapetis JR: Rheumatic heart disease in developing countries. N Engl J Med. 357(5):439-41, 2007
2. American College of Cardiology/American Heart Association Task Force on Practice Guidelines; Society of Cardiovascular Anesthesiologists; Society for Cardiovascular Angiography and Interventions; Society of Thoracic Surgeons et al: ACC/AHA 2006 guidelines for the management of patients with valvular heart disease: a report of the American College of Cardiology/American Heart Association Task Force on Practice Guidelines (writing committee to revise the 1998 Guidelines for the Management of Patients With Valvular Heart Disease): developed in collaboration with the Society of Cardiovascular Anesthesiologists: endorsed by the Society for Cardiovascular Angiography and Interventions and the Society of Thoracic Surgeons. Circulation. 114(5):e84-231, 2006
3. Carapetis JR et al: Acute rheumatic fever. Lancet. 366(9480):155-68, 2005
4. Carapetis JR et al: The global burden of group A streptococcal diseases. Lancet Infect Dis. 5(11):685-94, 2005
5. Djavidani B et al: Planimetry of mitral valve stenosis by magnetic resonance imaging. J Am Coll Cardiol. 45(12):2048-53, 2005
6. Lin SJ et al: Quantification of stenotic mitral valve area with magnetic resonance imaging and comparison with Doppler ultrasound. J Am Coll Cardiol. 44(1):133-7, 2004
7. No authors listed: ACC/AHA guidelines for the management of patients with valvular heart disease. A report of the American College of Cardiology/American Heart Association. Task Force on Practice Guidelines (Committee on Management of Patients with Valvular Heart Disease). J Am Coll Cardiol. 32(5):1486-588, 1998
8. Wyttenbach R et al: Integrated MR imaging approach to valvular heart disease. Cardiol Clin. 16(2):277-94, 1998
9. Braunwald E: Valvular heart disease. In: Braunwald E, eds. Heart disease. 5th ed. Saunders, Philadelphia. 1007-76, 1997
10. Globits S et al: Assessment of valvular heart disease by magnetic resonance imaging. Am Heart J. 129(2):369-81, 1995

RHEUMATIC HEART DISEASE

IMAGE GALLERY

Typical

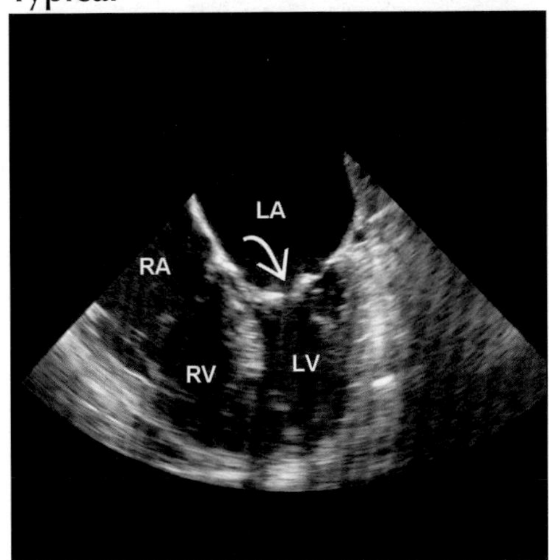

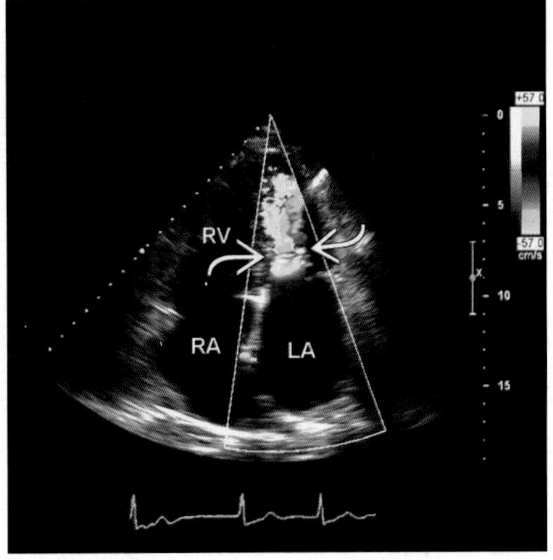

(Left) *TEE 4-chamber view shows markedly enlarged LA and thickened calcified mitral valve leaflets with diastolic doming ➔.* ***(Right)*** *TTE 4-chamber color coded Doppler image shows enlarged LA with diastolic flow convergence, aliasing and vena contracta ➔, indicating mitral valve stenosis. Note: Atrial fibrillation. (Courtesy R. Durst, MD).*

Typical

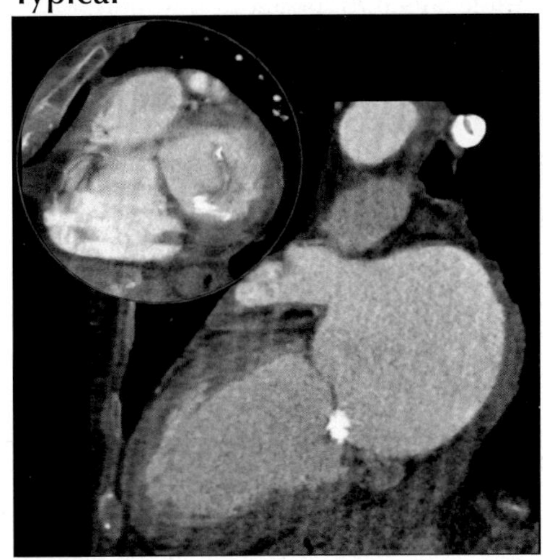

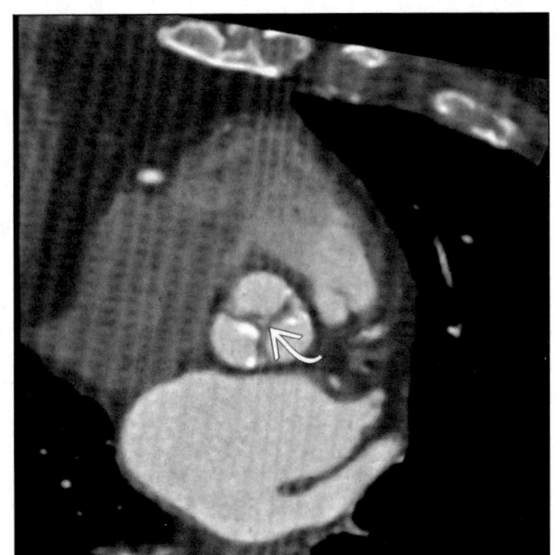

(Left) *LV long axis view and MV short axis views of coronary CT show rare case of mitral valve leaflet calcifications (not annulus) and enlarged left atrium.* ***(Right)*** *Aortic valve short axis cardiac CTA shows mild thickening and calcification of aortic cusps with incomplete coaptation. Note central aortic regurgitant orifice ➔.*

Typical

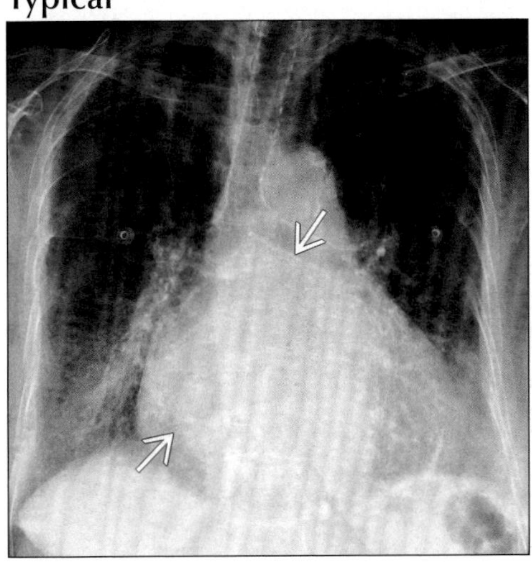

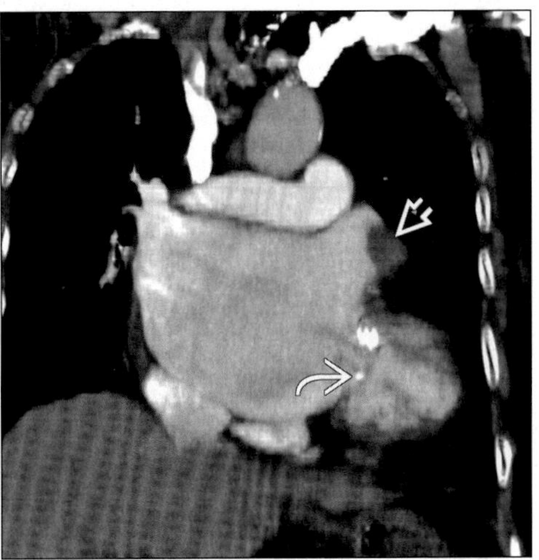

(Left) *Posteroanterior radiograph shows cardiomyopathy with right retrocardiac double density and splaying of carina, which indicate markedly enlarged left atrium ➔.* ***(Right)*** *Coronal CECT (same patient as previous image) shows markedly enlarged left atrium and normal sized ventricle. Note: Calcification of the posterior mitral leaflet ➔, and left atrial appendage thrombus ➔.*

LV APICAL AORTIC CONDUIT

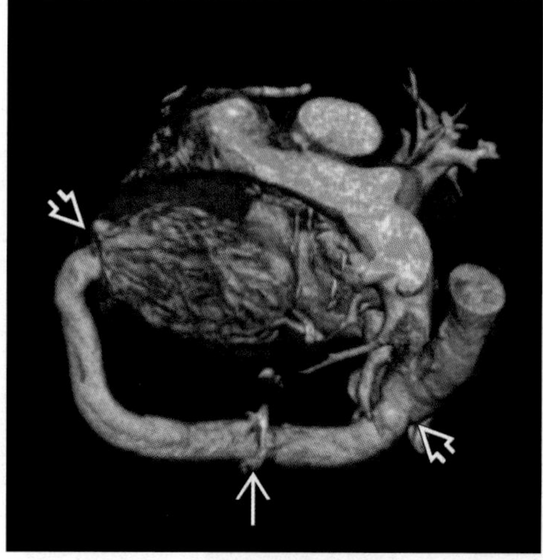

Oblique cardiac CT 3D volume rendering shows left ventriculogram with uncomplicated apicoaortic conduit. Note: Valve ➡, proximal and distal anastomoses ⇨.

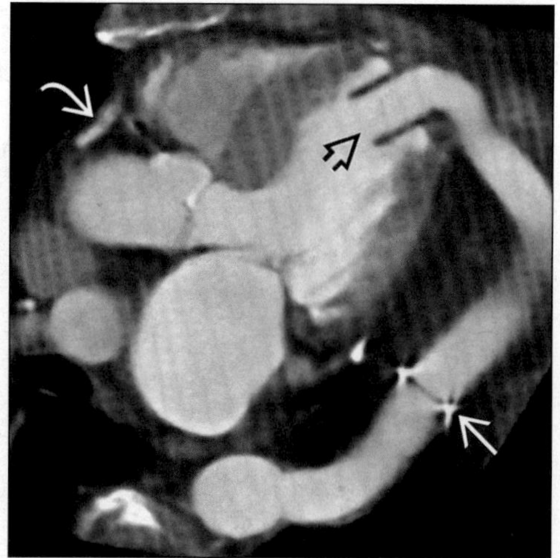

Three chamber view cardiac CT in same patient as previous image, shows unobstructed orifice of ventricular inflow component of conduit graft ⇨. Note: Conduit valve ➡ and aortocoronary bypass graft ➡.

TERMINOLOGY

Abbreviations and Synonyms

- Apical aortic conduit; apicoaortic conduit

Definitions

- Extra-anatomic valved graft connecting left ventricular (LV) apex to descending thoracic aorta
  - Typically used in patients with severe aortic stenosis and porcelain aorta or other condition precluding median sternotomy (retrosternal coronary grafts)
  - Complex congenital LV outflow tract anomalies ± hypoplastic ascending aorta and arch

IMAGING FINDINGS

General Features

- Best diagnostic clue: Graft connected proximally to apex of left ventricle and distally to descending thoracic aorta or rarely to great vessels
- Location
  - Complete metallic ring (conduit valve) usually in mid-portion of graft
    - May be visible lateral to the apex on frontal radiograph and in inferior middle mediastinum on lateral views

Imaging Recommendations

- Best imaging tool
  - Gated CT best to delineate graft course,implantation angle, proximal and distal anastomoses
  - MRA demonstrates graft course and may provide flow information
  - Echocardiography may not visualize entire conduit, but presence of Doppler gradients across the native LVOT indirectly suggest graft obstruction

DIFFERENTIAL DIAGNOSIS

Ventricular Assist Device

- Apical LV graft anastomosis but distal insertion into pump, not aorta
- Second tube graft from pump to usually ascending aorta

DDx: Apicoaortic Conduit

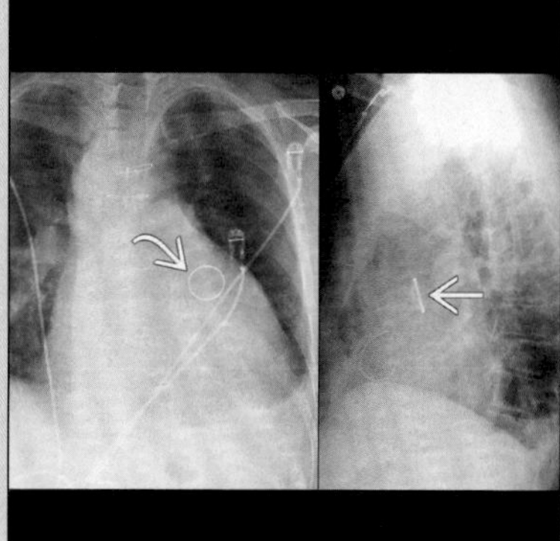

Pulmonary Valve Replacement

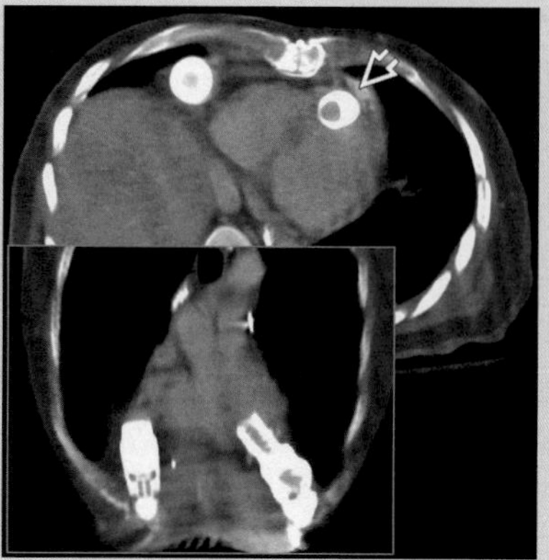

Ventricular Assist Device

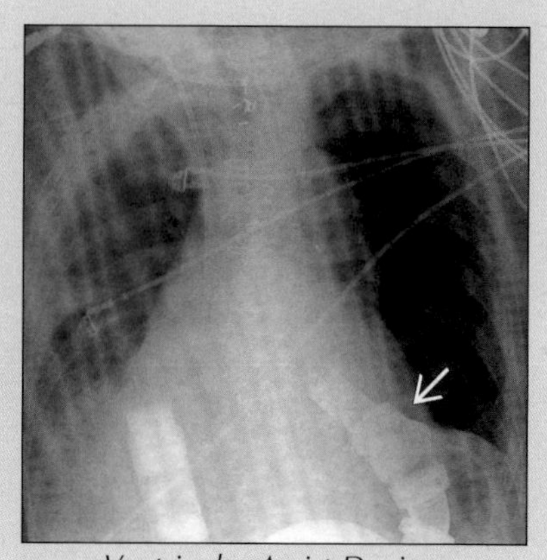

Ventricular Assist Device

LV APICAL AORTIC CONDUIT

Key Facts

Terminology

- Extra-anatomic valved graft connecting left ventricular (LV) apex to descending thoracic aorta
- Typically used in patients with severe aortic stenosis and porcelain aorta or other condition precluding median sternotomy (retrosternal coronary grafts)
- Complex congenital LV outflow tract anomalies ± hypoplastic ascending aorta and arch

Imaging Findings

- Gated CT best to delineate graft course,implantation angle, proximal and distal anastomoses
- MRA demonstrates graft course and may provide flow information
- Echocardiography may not visualize entire conduit, but presence of Doppler gradients across the native LVOT indirectly suggest graft obstruction

In Situ Valve Replacement

- May demonstrate complete metallic ring on radiograph, however location will correspond to that of replaced valve

PATHOLOGY

General Features

- Presence of conditions precluding median sternotomy or aortic disease (porcelain aorta) or congenital disease precluding in-situ valve replacement

CLINICAL ISSUES

Demographics

- Age
  - Utilized in two distinctly different population
    - 2 weeks to 19 years in congenital heart disease population
    - Elderly (~ 70) high risk patients with aortic valve disease and extensive aortic calcification ± prior surgery
- Gender: M = F (for congenital indications)

Natural History & Prognosis

- Longest known functioning conduit graft survival is 24 years and ongoing

DIAGNOSTIC CHECKLIST

Consider

- Extend range of gated CT from arch/great vessels to below diaphragm (distal anastomosis location varies)

Image Interpretation Pearls

- Evaluate angle of apical graft with respect to ventricular septum as this may be flow limiting

SELECTED REFERENCES

1. Faletra F et al: Multidetector computed tomography image of apical left ventricular descending aorta conduit. Heart. 93(4):449, 2007
2. Chiu KM et al: Images in cardiovascular medicine. Left ventricle apical conduit to bilateral subclavian artery in a patient with porcelain aorta and aortic stenosis. Circulation. 113(9):e388-9, 2006
3. Brown JW et al: Long-term results of apical aortic conduits in children with complex left ventricular outflow tract obstruction. Ann Thorac Surg. 80(6):2301-8, 2005
4. Freeman LJ et al: The longest functioning apical left ventricular to descending aortic valve conduit. Ann Thorac Surg. 79(4):1420, 2005
5. Fogel MA et al: Evaluation and follow-up of patients with left ventricular apical to aortic conduits with 2D and 3D magnetic resonance imaging and Doppler echocardiography: A new look at an old operation. Am Heart J. 141(4):630-6, 2001
6. Renzulli A et al: Long-term results of apico-aortic valved conduit for severe idiopathic hypertrophic subaortic stenosis. Tex Heart Inst J. 27(1):24-8, 2000

IMAGE GALLERY

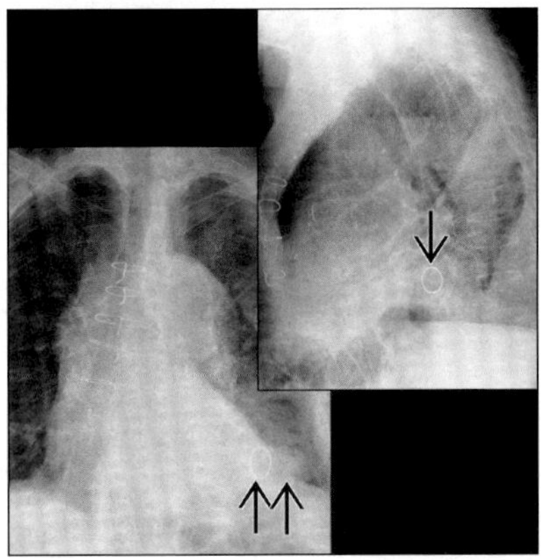

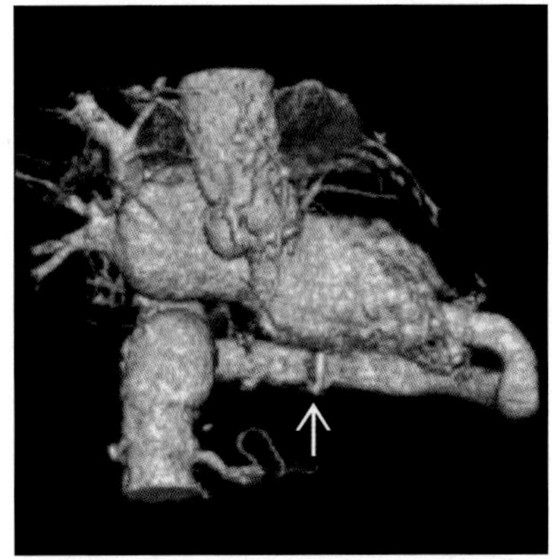

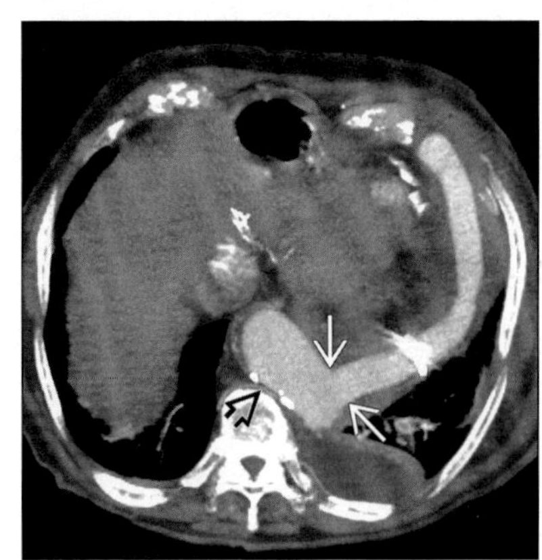

(Left) *Frontal and lateral radiographs show metallic complete ring and graft shadow ⇨ lateral to LV apex and in the middle mediastinum, corresponding to conduit valve.* ***(Center)*** *Oblique cardiac CT 3D volume rendering shows apicoaortic valved ➡ conduit and atherosclerotic calcification in aortic root and descending aorta.* ***(Right)*** *Oblique cardiac CT MIP image in same patient as previous image, shows unobstructed distal anastomosis ➡ to descending thoracic aorta ⇨.*

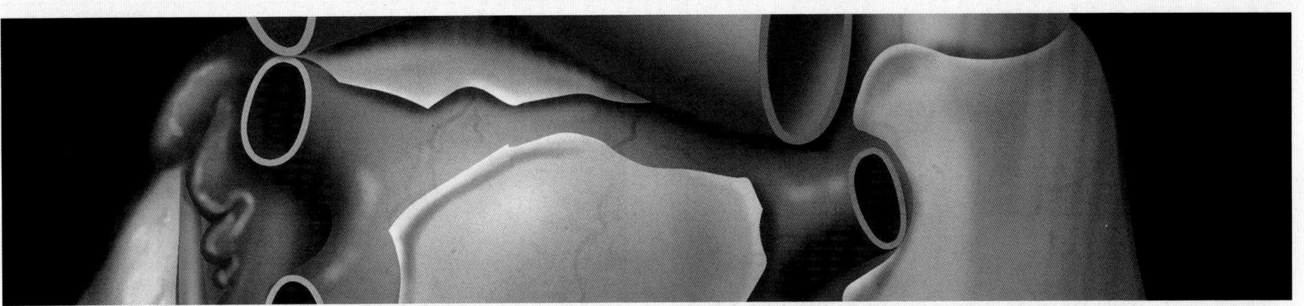

SECTION 3: Pericardial

Introduction and Overview

Pericardial

PERICARDIAL ANATOMY

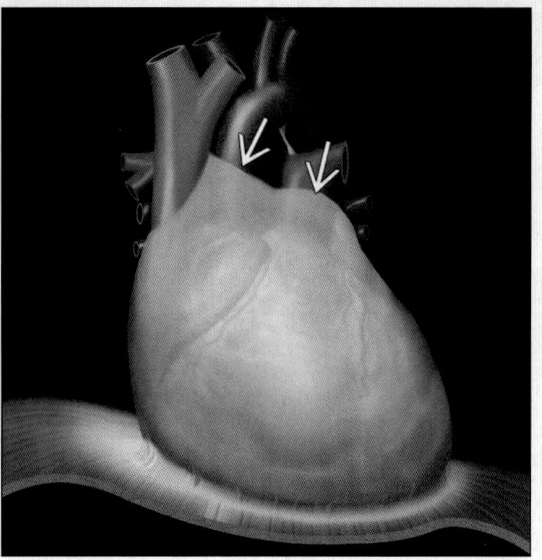

Anterior graphic shows the outer portion of the pericardial sac (parietal pericardium). Note: The proximal 2-3 cm of the aorta and pulmonary artery are intrapericardial. Pericardial reflection ➔.

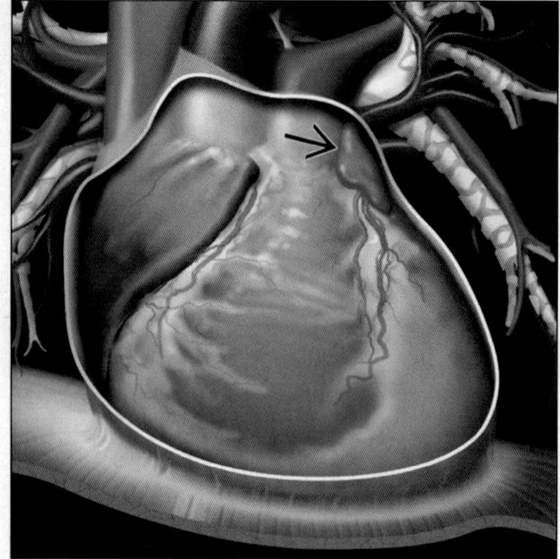

Anterior graphic with the parietal pericardium removed, shows glistening appearance of cardiac surface due to serous visceral pericardium covering the heart. Note: The left atrial appendage is intrapericardial ➔.

TERMINOLOGY

Abbreviations

- Pericardial effusion (PE)
- Constrictive pericarditis (CP)

Synonyms

- Visceral pericardium
  - Lamina visceralis pericardii
  - Epicardium
    - Epicardium only refers to those portions of the visceral pericardium that are in contact with the heart itself, not the great vessels
- Parietal pericardium
  - Pericardium
  - Pericardium fibrosum, fibrous pericardium
    - Technically this is only part of the parietal pericardium: Inner portion of the fibrous pericardium is covered with a layer of serous pericardium

Definitions

- Pericardium
  - Thin, double membranous sac that contains a small amount of serous fluid
  - Encloses heart and roots of arteries and veins leading to or arising from heart
  - Function of pericardium is to allow for friction free (minimized) movement of heart within mediastinum
- Pericardium consists of two layers
  - Visceral pericardium (= epicardium)
  - Parietal pericardium (commonly referred to as the "pericardium")
- Pericardial space: Space between the two layers of pericardium
  - Contains a small amount of fluid
- Pericarditis: Disorder due to inflammation of the pericardium
- Serous pericardium
  - Thin glistening membrane that lines the cardiac surface and inner surface of the pericardium
  - Innermost layer of the pericardium
  - Function is lubricating the pericardial sac to minimize friction
- Fibrous pericardium
  - Most superficial layer of parietal pericardium
  - Dense connective tissue that anchors the heart to the surrounding mediastinum
  - Embedded into mediastinal fat (immobile outer layer)
  - Lined with serous pericardium (to allow motion along its inner layer)

IMAGING ANATOMY

General Anatomic Considerations

- Pericardium covers all cardiac chambers, as well as approximately 3 cm of the aortic root and pulmonary trunk
- Pericardial reflections are the site where visceral and parietal pericardium are connected
  - Serous pericardium folds upon itself at the pericardial reflections
- Transverse sinus
  - Posteriorly above pulmonary vein ostia
  - Above oblique sinus (separated by horizontal pericardial reflection between superior pulmonary vein ostia)
  - Behind aortic root and pulmonary trunk, running from right (SVC) to left
- Oblique sinus
  - Posterior to left atrium, and anterior to esophagus and descending thoracic aorta
  - Extends superiorly behind the right pulmonary artery
  - Below transverse sinus
    - Transverse sinus and oblique sinus are separated by the horizontal pericardial reflection between the right and left superior pulmonary vein ostia
  - Extends medially to the bronchus intermedius (posterior pericardial recess)
- Pericardial sinus proper

PERICARDIAL ANATOMY

Differential Diagnosis of Pericardial Effusion

Serous (Transudate)
- Congestive heart failure
- Hypoalbuminemia
- Post radiation
- Myxedema

Fibrinous (Exudate)
- Uremia
- Collagen vascular disease
  - Systemic lupus erythematodes, scleroderma, rheumatoid arthritis, acute rheumatic fever
- Hypersensitivity
- Infection

Purulent
- Bacterial (staphylococcus, streptococcus, neisseria, pneumococcus)
- Viral
- Tuberculosis
- Fungal or parasitic

Hemopericardium
- Post myocardial infarct/rupture
- Coagulopathy
- Post surgical or catheter based procedure
- Cardiac malignancy
- Type A dissection
- Trauma

Lymphatic Effusion
- Congenital abnormalities
- Post-operative
- SVC obstruction
- Tumors

  - Consists of postcaval recess and left and right pulmonary venous recesses
- Superior pericardial recess
  - Synonym: Superior sinus of the pericardium
  - Immediately superior to right pulmonary artery on axial CT
  - Physiologic fluid within normal superior pericardial recess may mimic lymphadenopathy or cystic mass
  - "High-riding" superior pericardial recess refers to a recess that extended superiorly into the right paratracheal space
    - May mimic mediastinal lymphadenopathy or mass on CT or MR
    - Commonly appears rounded or oval-shaped
    - May be triangular, spindle-shaped, half-moon-shaped, or have an irregular border
- Pericardial sleeve
  - Recess of pericardium that covers pulmonary vein
    - Frequently misinterpreted as hilar adenopathy
    - Typically right inferior pulmonary vein

Critical Anatomic Structures
- The parietal pericardium is anchored within the mediastinal fat and is in direct connectivity to neighboring mediastinal structures
  - Anteriorly: Superior pericardio-sternal ligament
  - Inferiorly: Central tendon of diaphragm
  - Posteriorly: Esophagus, descending thoracic aorta
  - Laterally: Phrenic nerves (common site of traumatic pericardial rupture and cause for traumatic pneumopericardium)

Anatomic Relationships
- Phrenic nerves and accompanying pericardiophrenic arteries and veins
  - Run along right and left lateral pericardial surface in cranio-caudal direction
  - These structures are typically only faintly visible on newer MDCT scanners
  - Best visualized on volume rendered images
  - May be the source of nerve sheath tumors
  - Pericardiophrenic veins may enlarge due to collateral flow in case of SVC or IVC obstruction

ANATOMY-BASED IMAGING ISSUES

Key Concepts or Questions
- Pericardial neoplasms are typically metastases in the presence of systemic spread of extracardiac malignant tumors
  - Less commonly metastases of primary cardiac tumor
- Primary pericardial tumors are rare and include
  - Pericardial teratoma, may contain fat and dense calcifications or teeth
  - Hemangioma, enhancing multiloculated mass, bright on T1WI and T2WI
  - Solitary fibroma, may contain central calcifications
  - Pericardial mesothelioma
  - Primitive neuroectodermal tumor
- Pericardial cysts are common and typically found in the cardiophrenic angle
  - Bright on T2WI, dark or isointense on T1WI, no enhancement
- Other masses of the cardiophrenic angle are
  - Pericardial fat pad
  - Pericardial fat necrosis, typically increased density compared to normal fat
  - Thymoma or thymolipoma
  - Morgagni hernia, may contain fat, bowel, liver
  - Pleural cyst, bright on T2WI, dark on T1WI
  - Lymphadenopathy
  - Lymphangioma rare multicystic lesions may be intramural, epicardial, or pericardial

Imaging Approaches
- Echocardiography is first line test if pericardial effusion is suspected
  - High sensitivity for detecting pericardial fluid
  - Allows categorization of the size of effusions into small, moderate, and severe
  - Based on detection of sonolucent circumcardiac space of varying width
  - Important to differentiate diffuse from focal (loculated) effusions
  - Pericardial effusions may mimic pericardial effusion
- Best test for detection of pericardial calcification is CT

PERICARDIAL ANATOMY

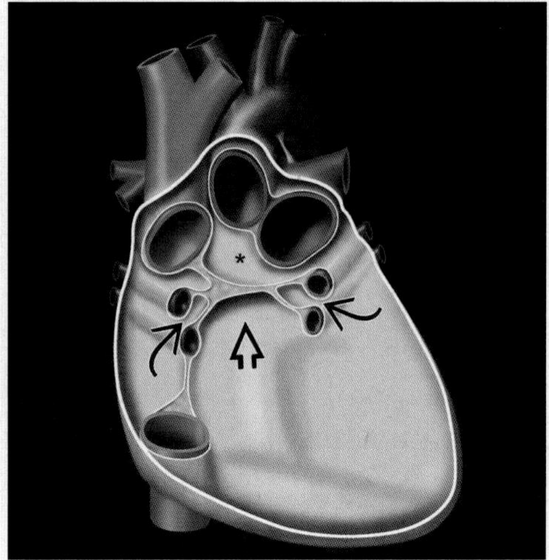

Anterior view graphic shows pericardial recesses covering proximal great vessel. The transverse (*) and oblique sinuses ⇨, and pulmonary venous recesses ↗ are separated by pericardial reflections.

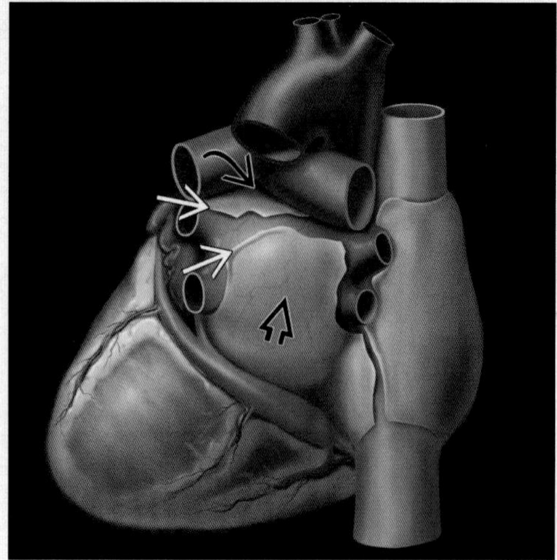

Posterior view graphic shows posterior surface of the heart. The parietal pericardium is removed at the pericardial reflections ➔. These separate the transverse sinus ↗ from the oblique sinus ⇨.

- Pericardial constriction typically worked up with echocardiography, occasionally followed by MR
  - May be difficult to differentiate from restriction
  - Pericardial thickening or calcification does not necessarily mean constrictive physiology is present
  - On the other hand, absence of pericardial thickening does not necessarily exclude pericardial constriction
- Pericardial masses are best characterized by MR
  - Often preceded by echocardiography

Imaging Protocols

- Pericardial adhesions are best proven with tagged cine MR
  - Tag lines are to be placed orthogonal to the portion of pericardium in question
  - If tag lines break into 2 along pericardium and pericardial portion, and epi-/myocardial portion of line separate freely during cardiac contraction, then absence of adhesion in that segment has been proven
  - If adhesions are present, the tag lines will appear to be distorted, but they do not separate along the pericardium

Imaging Pitfalls

- Normal thickness pericardium does not exclude pericardial constriction
- Pericardial sinuses and recesses such as pulmonic recess, postcaval recess and oblique sinus may mimic mediastinal lymphadenopathy or masses
- Superior aortic recess can mimic type A ascending aortic dissection
- Pulmonary vein recess or "pulmonary sleeves" may project into lung parenchyma and mimic pulmonary mass, or lymphadenopathy

Normal Measurements

- In absence of effusions pericardial thickness < 3 mm on CT or MR is considered normal

RELATED REFERENCES

1. Grizzard JD et al: Magnetic resonance imaging of pericardial disease and cardiac masses. Cardiol Clin. 25(1):111-40, vi, 2007
2. Pineda V et al: Lesions of the cardiophrenic space: findings at cross-sectional imaging. Radiographics. 27(1):19-32, 2007
3. Pepi M et al: Echocardiography in the diagnosis and management of pericardial disease. J Cardiovasc Med (Hagerstown). 7(7):533-44, 2006
4. Broderick LS et al: Anatomic pitfalls of the heart and pericardium. Radiographics. 25(2):441-53, 2005
5. Rienmüller R et al: CT and MR imaging of pericardial disease. Radiol Clin North Am. 42(3):587-601, vi, 2004
6. Truong MT et al: Pericardial "sleeve" recess of right inferior pulmonary vein mimicking adenopathy: computed tomography findings. J Comput Assist Tomogr. 28(3):361-5, 2004
7. Kodama F et al: Comparing thin-section and thick-section CT of pericardial sinuses and recesses. AJR Am J Roentgenol. 181(4):1101-8, 2003
8. Choi YW et al: The "High-Riding" superior pericardial recess: CT findings. AJR Am J Roentgenol. 175(4):1025-8, 2000
9. Groell R et al: Pericardial sinuses and recesses: findings at electrocardiographically triggered electron-beam CT. Radiology. 212(1):69-73, 1999
10. Kubota H et al: Fluid collection in the pericardial sinuses and recesses. Thin-section helical computed tomography observations and hypothesis. Invest Radiol. 31(10):603-10, 1996
11. Protopapas Z et al: Left pulmonic recess of the pericardium: findings at CT and MR imaging. Radiology. 196(1):85-8, 1995
12. Levy-Ravetch M et al: CT of the pericardial recesses. AJR Am J Roentgenol. 144(4):707-14, 1985

IMAGE GALLERY

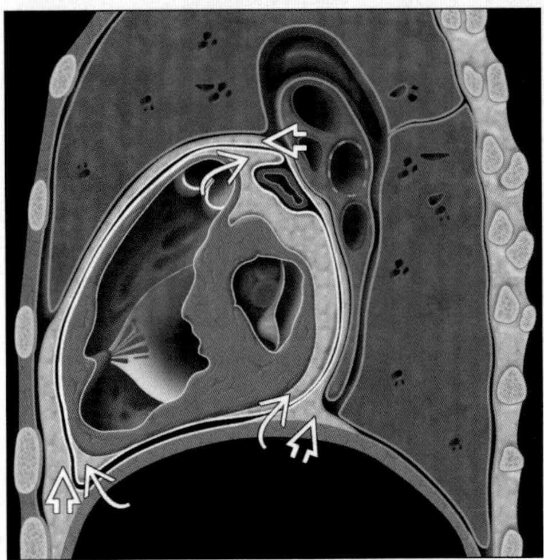

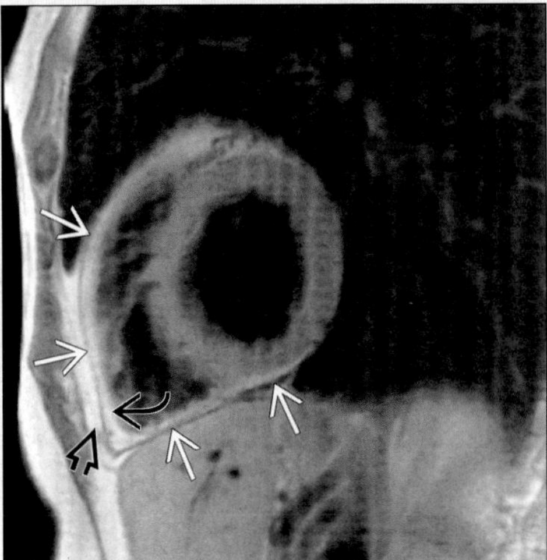

(Left) *Sagittal graphic shows pericardial fat separated from epicardial fat by the two layers of pericardium.* ***(Right)*** *Sagittal T1WI FSE MR shows pericardium along the anterior and inferior free walls of the right ventricle, clearly outlined by epicardial fat and pericardial fat. Visualization of the pericardium along the posterior and lateral LV walls is difficult because of little or no adjacent fat.*

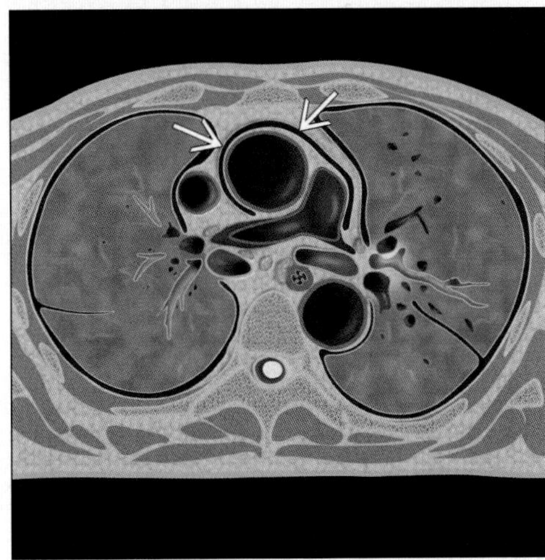

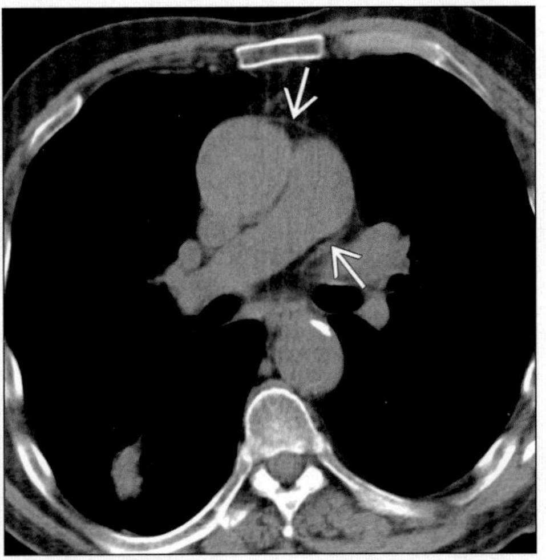

(Left) *Axial graphic shows pericardial recess covering the ascending aorta and proximal main pulmonary artery. Small amounts of fluid within the aortic recess may mimic a false lumen of aortic dissection.* ***(Right)*** *Axial NECT at a corresponding slice location shows normal thickness pericardial recess. Note: Identification of the pericardium may only be possible where fat is present between the pericardium and great vessels, as well as between pericardium & lung.*

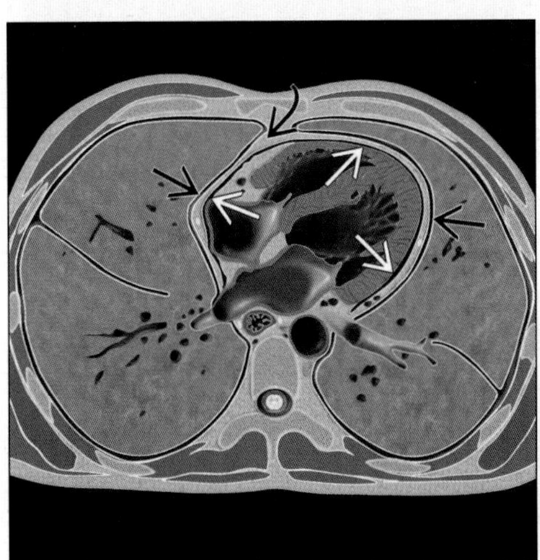

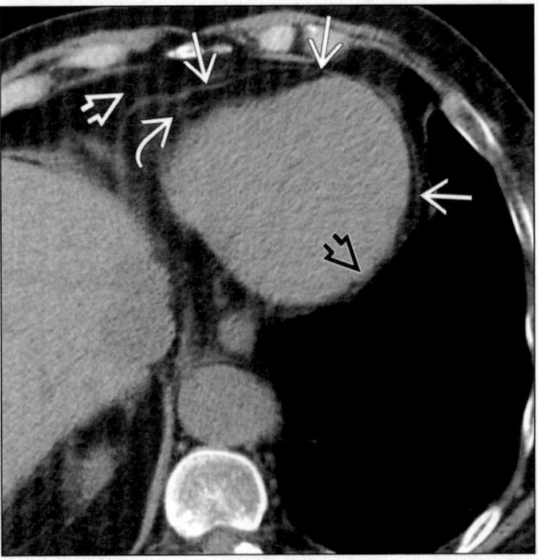

(Left) *Axial graphic shows a relationship between the pericardium and pleura, which are separated by a thin layer of pericardial fat.* ***(Right)*** *Axial NECT shows normal pericardium separating the anterior "pericardial fat" from the epicardial fat. The pericardium is rarely visible over the posterior and lateral LV.*

INFECTIOUS PERICARDITIS

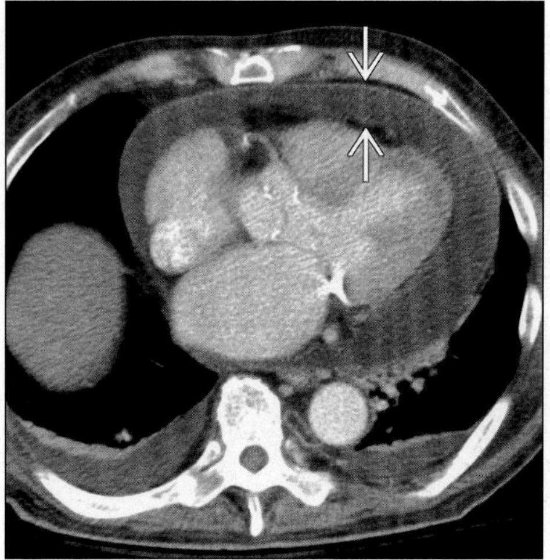

Axial CECT shows large pericardial collection measuring 17 HU. Note enhancing pericardium and epicardium ➡. Pericardiocentesis revealed purulent fluid.

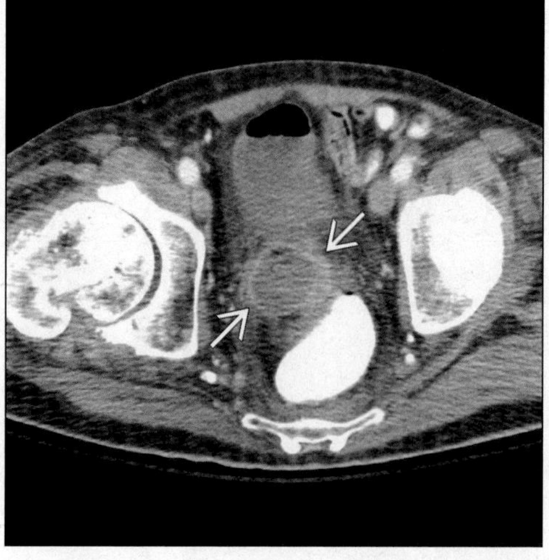

Axial CECT in same patient as previous image shows source of infection, a pelvic abscess ➡.

TERMINOLOGY

Abbreviations and Synonyms

- Pyopericardium, if bacterial

Definitions

- Pericarditis due to living agent

IMAGING FINDINGS

General Features

- Best diagnostic clue
  - Typical imaging characteristics of pericardial effusion
  - Thickened and enhancing pericardium and epicardium
  - Loculations with enhancing septation may be present
- Location: Diffuse involvement or focal loculated abscess
- Size
  - Varying size of pericardial fluid or purulent material
    - Up to 2 liters of fluid/pus

Radiographic Findings

- Radiography
  - Anterior posterior film
    - Flask-shaped cardiac silhouette
  - Lateral film
    - Fat pad sign: Separation of lower density retrosternal pericardial fat from cardiac epicardial fat by higher density effusion

CT Findings

- NECT
  - Thickened pericardial contour
  - Loculated effusion may mimic pericardial cyst
- CECT
  - Separation of epicardium and pericardium
  - Enhancing pericardium
  - Enhancing septation
  - Loculation
  - Rarely gas bubbles from gas producing organism or prior instrumentation
  - May demonstrate features of tamponade

MR Findings

- T1WI: Similar findings compared to CTA

DDx: Other Pericardial Disorders

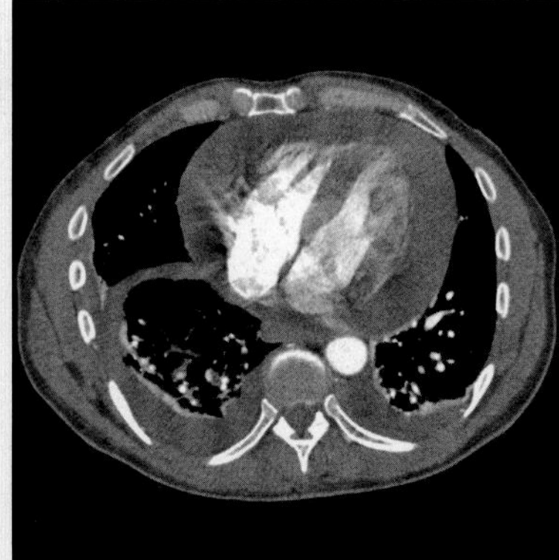

Tamponade

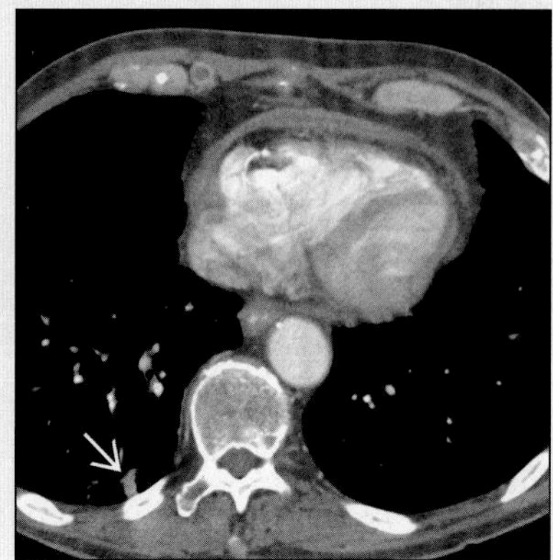

Malignant Effusion

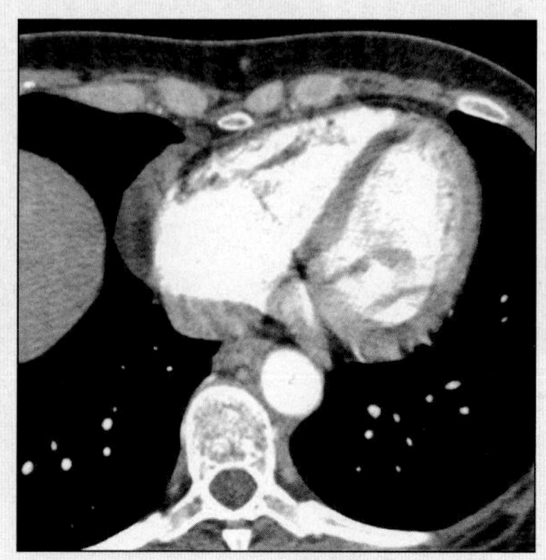

Pericardial Cyst

INFECTIOUS PERICARDITIS

Key Facts

Terminology
- Pericarditis due to living agent

Imaging Findings
- Typical imaging characteristics of pericardial effusion
- Thickened and enhancing pericardium and epicardium
- Loculations with enhancing septation may be present
- Flask-shaped cardiac silhouette
- Fat pad sign: Separation of lower density retrosternal pericardial fat from cardiac epicardial fat by higher density effusion
- Rarely gas bubbles from gas producing organism or prior instrumentation
- PET: FDG PET may demonstrate homogeneous uptake in pericardium if acute inflammation present

Top Differential Diagnoses
- Connective Tissue Disorders
- Metabolic Disorders
- Myocardial Infarction (MI)
- Aortic Dissection
- Neoplastic Pericarditis

Pathology
- Caused by bacteria, parasites, protozoa, viruses, or fungi
- Haemophilus influenza is a common cause in children

Diagnostic Checklist
- Examination of pericardial fluid imperative

- T2WI
  - May not demonstrate bright fluid as motion may dephase protons
  - For confirmation of pericardial fluid use phase contrast imaging
- T1 C+: Enhancing pericardium and septations
- Cine imaging may demonstrate signs of tamponade

Nuclear Medicine Findings
- PET: FDG PET may demonstrate homogeneous uptake in pericardium if acute inflammation present

Echocardiographic Findings
- Echocardiogram
  - Effusions of varied size
  - Tamponade in extreme cases
  - Rarely contrast echoes within pericardium from gas forming organisms
  - May demonstrate echogenic septations

Angiographic Findings
- Conventional
  - Invasive data usually acquired before percutaneous or open pericardiectomy
  - Features of tamponade

DIFFERENTIAL DIAGNOSIS

Connective Tissue Disorders
- Rheumatoid arthritis, systemic lupus, erythematosus, scleroderma

Metabolic Disorders
- Uremia

Myocardial Infarction (MI)
- 10-15% of acute MI
- Dressler syndrome

Drugs
- Procainamide, hydralazine, isoniazid, methysergide, phenytoin, anticoagulants

Aortic Dissection
- Rupture into the pericardium

Trauma
- After pericardiotomy (5-30% of cardiac operations)

Pericardial Cyst
- No enhancement of pericardium
- Usually grows outward from parietal pericardium with no mass effect on the heart

Neoplastic Pericarditis
- May demonstrate enhancing pericardial nodules and non-cardiac metastatic foci

Intrapericardial Teratoma
- May demonstrate lipid level and coarse calcification or teeth

PATHOLOGY

General Features
- General path comments
  - Caused by bacteria, parasites, protozoa, viruses, or fungi
  - Pyogenic pericarditis is uncommon
    - Bacterial infection is most often due to Streptococci, Staphylococci and gram-negative bacilli
    - Tuberculous pericarditis (< 5%) is insidious in onset and may exist without obvious pulmonary involvement
  - Acute pericarditis may be serous, fibrinous, sanguineous, hemorrhagic or purulent
  - Chronic pericarditis may be serous, chylous or hemorrhagic (effusive), fibrous, adhesive or calcific (may be constrictive)
- Etiology
  - May be hematogenous
  - Extension of myocardial abscess related to infectious endocarditis or mediastinal abscess

- Secondary to esophageal or lung cancer invasion and subsequent infection
- Bacterial
  - Staphylococcus, Streptococcus, Pneumococcus, Neisseria
  - Tuberculosis
  - Other mycobacteria
- Viral
  - Haemophilus influenzae
  - Coxsackie virus
  - Human immunodeficiency virus
  - Hepatitis B and A
- Fungal
- Parasitic
- Lymphogranuloma venereum
- Listeria

Gross Pathologic & Surgical Features

- Exudate: Fluid with large amount of protein and cellular debris
  - Specific gravity greater than 1020g/l
  - "Bread and butter" appearance on gross pathology

CLINICAL ISSUES

Presentation

- Most common signs/symptoms
  - Pericardial friction rub
    - Best heard with patient leaning forward
    - May disappear when effusion increases in size
  - Muffled heart sounds in larger effusions
  - Fibrosis and constriction may be a presenting sign of tuberculous pericarditis
  - Pain relieve when sitting up and leaning forward
  - Non productive cough
- Other signs/symptoms
  - Kussmaul sign: Paradoxical rise in jugular vein pressure with jugular vein distension
  - Pulsus paradoxicus: Prominent drop in systolic blood pressure and cardiac output
- Pleuritic chest pain, aggravated by thoracic motion, cough and respiration
- Abdominal pain may be presenting symptom
- Dyspnea, weakness, fever
- Tamponade
- ECG changes, triphasic or systolic and diastolic precordial friction rub

Demographics

- Age: All ages

Natural History & Prognosis

- Resolve with specific antimicrobial drugs
- May progress to chronic effusive pericarditis
- Viral myopericarditis, purulent pericarditis and cat-scratch disease may lead to pericardial constriction
- Purulent pericarditis almost always fatal if untreated
  - Mortality rate in treated patients: 40%

Treatment

- Antimicrobial drugs
- Aspirin, codeine or morphine, benzodiazepine for anxiety or insomnia
- Pericardiocentesis for relief of tamponade or purulent pericarditis

DIAGNOSTIC CHECKLIST

Consider

- Examination of pericardial fluid imperative
  - Cell count + differential, stains and culture for aerobic and anaerobic bacteria, acid-fasts and fungal
  - Viral cultures and viral nucleic acid detection assays
  - Cytology to exclude neoplasm
- Acute pericarditis may mimic acute myocardial infarction
  - Acute myocardial infarction must be excluded

Image Interpretation Pearls

- Enhancing pericardium separated by high density fluid of varying MR signal

SELECTED REFERENCES

1. Demmler GJ: Infectious pericarditis in children. Pediatr Infect Dis J. 25(2):165-6, 2006
2. Ha JW et al: Images in cardiovascular medicine. Assessment of pericardial inflammation in a patient with tuberculous effusive constrictive pericarditis with 18F-2-deoxyglucose positron emission tomography. Circulation. 113(1):e4-5, 2006
3. Abbara S et al. Pericardial and Myocardial Disease. In: Miller SW: Cardiac Imaging - The Requisites. Elsevier Mosby, Philadelphia, PA, 245-283, 2005
4. Pankuweit S et al: Bacterial pericarditis: diagnosis and management. Am J Cardiovasc Drugs. 5(2):103-12, 2005
5. Kirchhoff LV et al: Parasitic diseases of the heart. Front Biosci. 9:706-23, 2004
6. Ross AM et al: Acute pericarditis. Evaluation and treatment of infectious and other causes. Postgrad Med. 115(3):67-70, 73-5, 2004
7. Sagrista-Sauleda J et al: Effusive-constrictive pericarditis. N Engl J Med. 350(5):469-75, 2004
8. Troughton RW et al: Pericarditis. Lancet. 363(9410):717-27, 2004
9. Losik SB et al: Chemotherapy-induced pericarditis on F-18 FDG positron emission tomography scan. Clin Nucl Med. 28(11):913-5, 2003
10. Goyle KK et al: Diagnosing pericarditis. Am Fam Physician. 66(9):1695-702, 2002
11. Tsai WC et al: Morganella morganii causing solitary liver abscess complicated by pyopericardium and left pleural effusion in a nondiabetic patient. J Microbiol Immunol Infect. 35(3):191-4, 2002
12. Dhir V et al: Intrapericardial teratoma masquerading as pyopericardium. Indian J Chest Dis Allied Sci. 43(2):111-3, 2001
13. Spodick DH: The pericardium: A Comprehensive Textbook. Mercel Sekker, New York, 1997
14. Ku CS et al: Spontaneous contrast in the pericardial sac caused by gas-forming organisms. J Am Soc Echocardiogr. 4(1):67-8, 1991

INFECTIOUS PERICARDITIS

IMAGE GALLERY

Variant

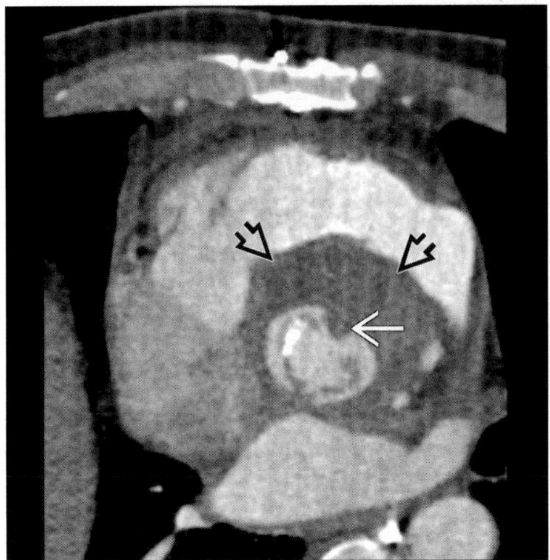

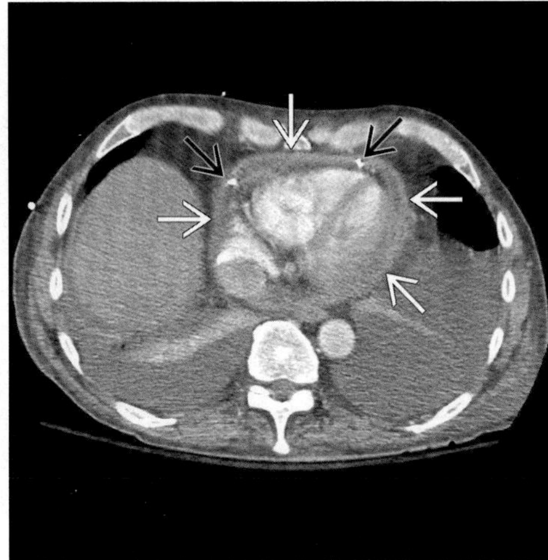

(Left) *Aortic valve short axis coronary CTA in septic patient shows bicuspid valve with vegetation ➡ ruptured into pericardium causing hematoma ⇨. Aortic valve replacement specimen grew Staphylococcus aureus.* ***(Right)*** *Axial CECT shows large pleural effusions, pericardial drain → with small effusion and enhancing pericardium ➡ in patient with pneumonia and viral pericarditis.*

Typical

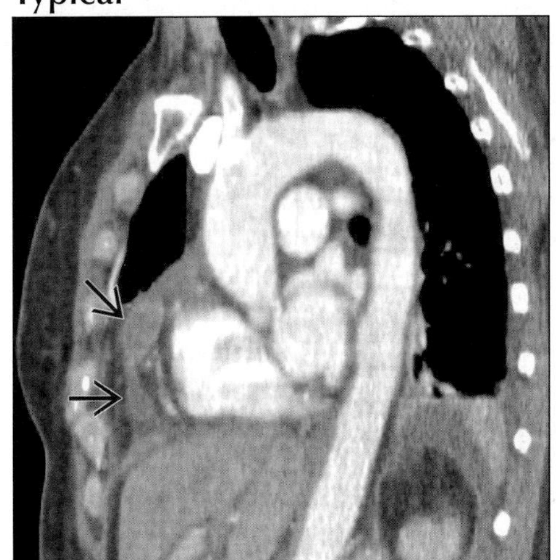

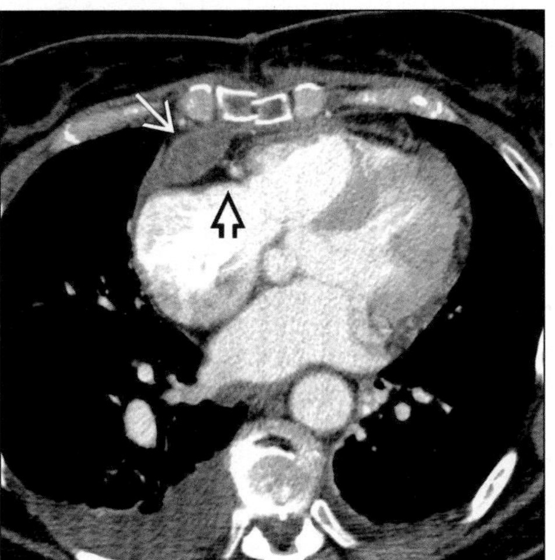

(Left) *Oblique CTA shows loculated pericardial effusions with pericardial enhancement → in a patient with post surgical pericardial infection.* ***(Right)*** *Axial CTA in same patient as previous image shows loculated effusion ➡ with enhancing epicardium and pericardium. Note mass effect on the right atrioventricular groove and RCA ⇨.*

Typical

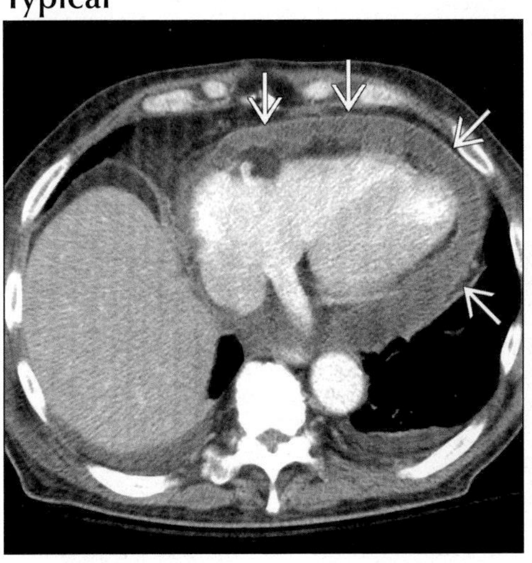

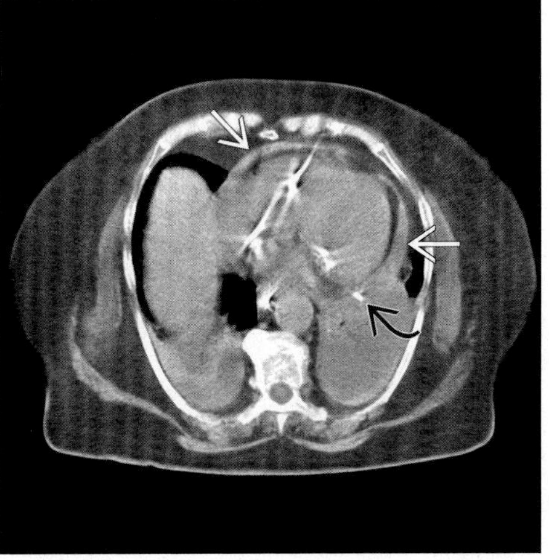

(Left) *Axial CECT in febrile patient shows large pericardial effusion with enhancing thickened pericardium ➡ and small pleural effusions. Pericardiocentesis revealed suppurative effusion.* ***(Right)*** *Axial NECT shows pericardial drain ↪ and thickened pericardial contour ➡ and pleural effusions in a patient with viral pericarditis.*

UREMIC PERICARDITIS

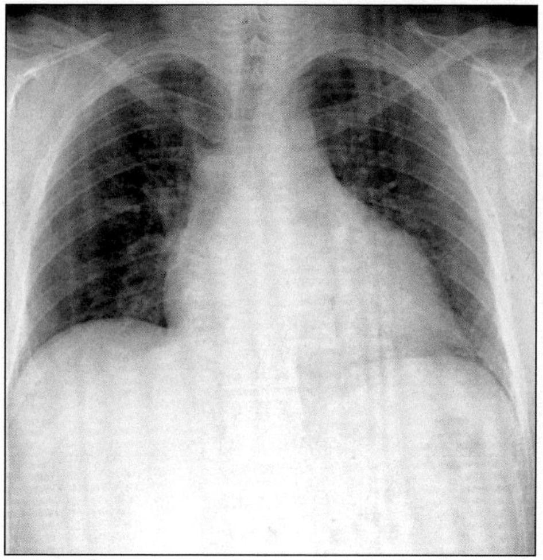

Coronal radiograph shows enlarged cardiac silhouette. (Courtesy Akram Shabaan, MBBCh).

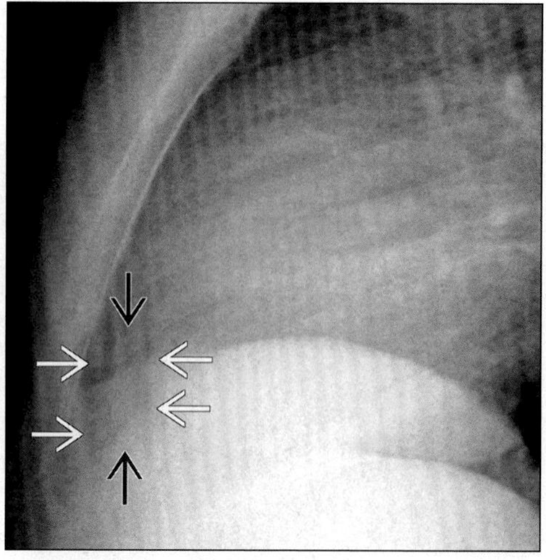

Sagittal radiograph shows effusion (bright ⇒) between pericardial fat (two dark layers ➡) epicardial fat, the "fat pad" or "Oreo Cookie™" sign. (Courtesy Akram Shabaan, MBBCh).

TERMINOLOGY

Definitions

- Nephrogenic pericarditis
  - Uremic patients who have not been dialyzed
  - Dialysis patients

IMAGING FINDINGS

General Features

- Best diagnostic clue: Thickened pericardium & effusion in renal patients

Radiographic Findings

- Radiography
  - Pericardial effusion
    - Flask or bottle shaped silhouette on AP
    - "Fat pad" or "Oreo Cookie™" sign on lateral

CT Findings

- Pericardial thickening (more than 1-2 mm) + effusion

Echocardiographic Findings

- Echocardiogram
  - Persistent echo-free space between parietal and visceral pericardium throughout cardiac cycle
    - May see fibrinous strands
  - Tamponade physiology in extreme cases

Other Modality Findings

- MR similar to CT + may show signs of tamponade

Imaging Recommendations

- Best imaging tool
  - Echocardiography
    - Detection of physiologic effects of effusion

DIFFERENTIAL DIAGNOSIS

Other Causes of Pericarditis

- Viral, bacterial, tuberculous pericarditis
  - Especially concerning in immunocompromised state

Aortic Dissection

- May cause hemorrhagic pericardial effusion and tamponade

DDx: Pericardial Effusions

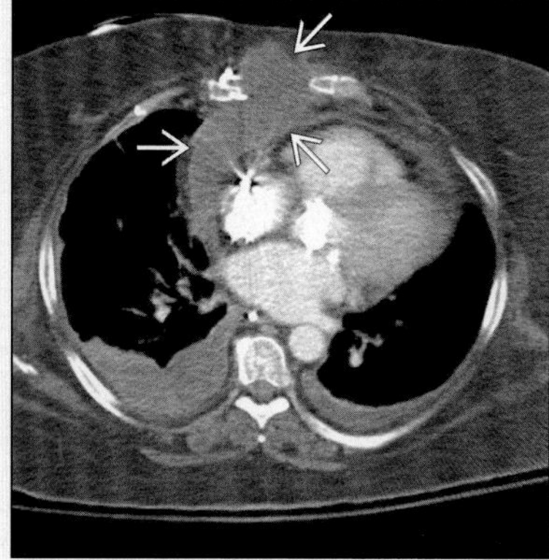

Wound Infection

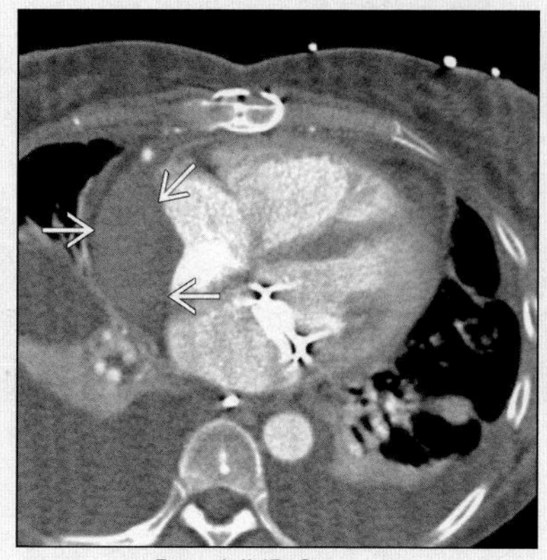

Post MVR Surgery

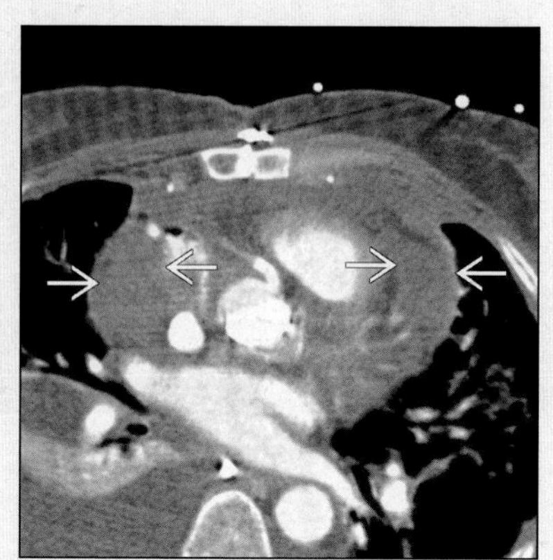

Post AVR Effusion

UREMIC PERICARDITIS

Key Facts

Terminology
- Nephrogenic pericarditis

Imaging Findings
- Best diagnostic clue: Thickened pericardium & effusion in renal patients

Pathology
- Acute fibrinous pericarditis, effusion, tamponade
- Epidemiology: 6-10% of patients with acute or chronic renal failure

Clinical Issues
- Quite variable, ranging from stable mild-moderate effusion without symptoms to frank tamponade
- Constriction is uncommon, though beginning to appear with long survival on dialysis
- Some effusions persist despite dialysis

Volume Overload
- Will produce transudative pericardial effusion

Myocardial Infarction
- Common in dialysis patients

Neoplastic Pericarditis
- Will not respond to dialysis

PATHOLOGY

General Features
- General path comments
  - Clinical manifestations
    - Acute fibrinous pericarditis, effusion, tamponade
- Etiology
  - Pathogenesis uncertain
    - May be related to retained metabolites; poor correlation with BUN
    - In some cases may result from viral infection
    - Related to hemorrhagic diathesis
- Epidemiology: 6-10% of patients with acute or chronic renal failure

Gross Pathologic & Surgical Features
- Thickened highly vascular pericardium, adhesions, serous or hemorrhagic pericardial effusion

CLINICAL ISSUES

Presentation
- Most common signs/symptoms: Pericarditis (sharp retrosternal pain aggravated by lying down and relieved by sitting up, friction rub), effusion (dyspnea if sizable), tamponade (tachycardia, hypotension, inspiratory jugular venous distention, paradoxical pulse)
- Other signs/symptoms: Fever, palpitations, confusion

Natural History & Prognosis
- Quite variable, ranging from stable mild-moderate effusion without symptoms to frank tamponade
- Constriction is uncommon, though beginning to appear with long survival on dialysis
- Some effusions persist despite dialysis

Treatment
- May respond to NSAIDS, corticosteroids, colchicine
- Intensified dialysis if hemodynamically insignificant
- Pericardiocentesis if persistent or progressive effusion
- Pericardial window for large, persistent, or recurrent effusion, purulent pericarditis, or tamponade

SELECTED REFERENCES

1. Sever MS et al: Pericarditis following renal transplantation. Transplantation. 51(6):1229-32, 1991
2. Spodick DH: Pericarditis in systemic diseases. Cardiol Clin. 8(4):709-16, 1990

IMAGE GALLERY

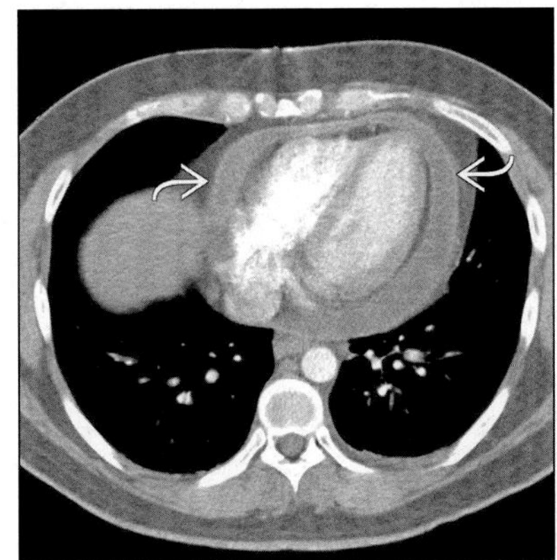

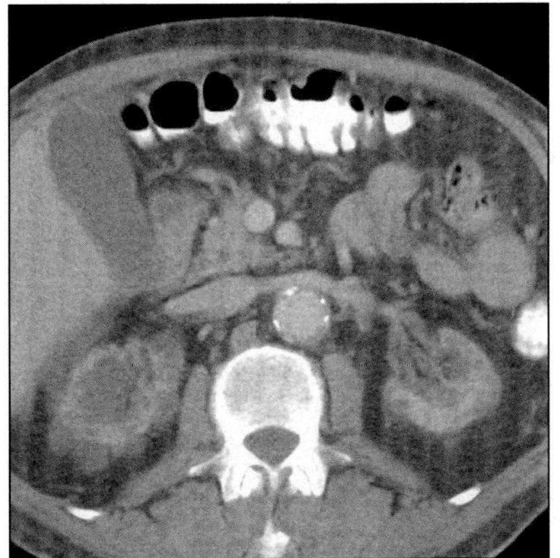

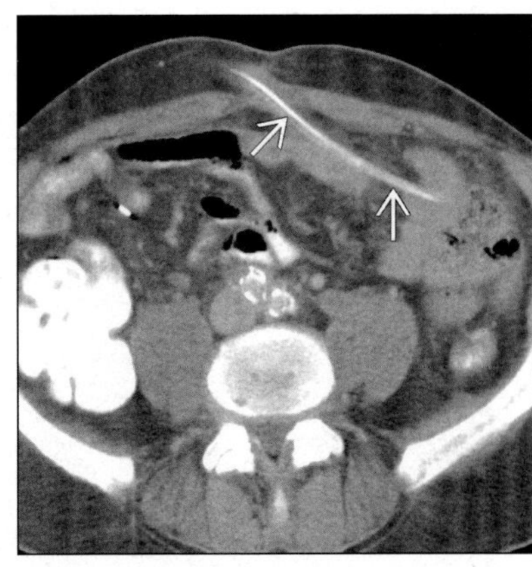

(Left) *Axial CECT shows pericardial effusion with thickened, enhancing pericardium ➡. (Courtesy A. Shabaan, MBBCh).* ***(Center)*** *Axial CECT shows weakly enhancing, small native kidneys with multiple cysts secondary to chronic renal failure.* ***(Right)*** *Axial CECT shows same patient as previous image, with peritoneal dialysis catheter ➡.*

NEOPLASTIC PERICARDITIS

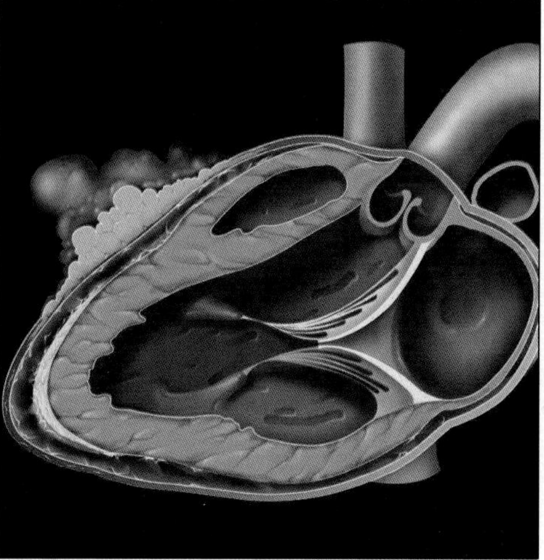

Graphic shows pericardial mass with pericardial effusion and adhesions.

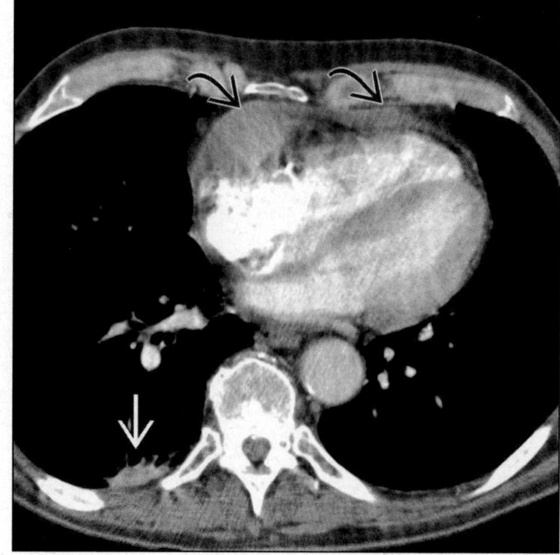

Axial CECT shows loculated effusion with mass effect on right atrium and ventricle and subtle pericardial enhancement ➩ in a patient with metastatic lung cancer ➡.

TERMINOLOGY

Definitions

- Pericardial involvement with primary or secondary neoplasm
  - Most frequently secondary neoplasm via direct invasion, lymphatic or hemorrhagic spread
- Pericardial effusion with diffuse or nodular pericardial thickening
  - Causes effusive-constrictive pericarditis
- Hemorrhagic effusion accompanying cardiac metastasis or primary cardiac tumor may be present without pericarditis

IMAGING FINDINGS

General Features

- Best diagnostic clue
  - Imaging studies will demonstrate effusion and/or enhancing mass lesions
  - May be by direct invasion of extracardiac mass or hematogenous spread directly to pericardium
  - Nodular enhancing pericardium
- Quite varied depending on tumor type
- Mass encasing heart
- Pericardial effusion evident by multiple imaging modalities

Radiographic Findings

- Radiography
  - Chest radiography findings
    - Flask-shaped cardiac silhouette in the presence of significant effusion
    - Soft tissue surrounding heart
  - Other evidence of primary or metastatic disease may be suggestive

CT Findings

- NECT
  - Thickening +/- irregularity of pericardial contour
  - High HU indicating hemorrhagic pericardial effusion
- CECT
  - Thickening of pericardial layers
  - Separation of thickened visceral and parietal pericardium by effusion
  - Invasion of epicardial or pericardial fat
  - Pericardial enhancement

DDx: Other Pericardial Disorders

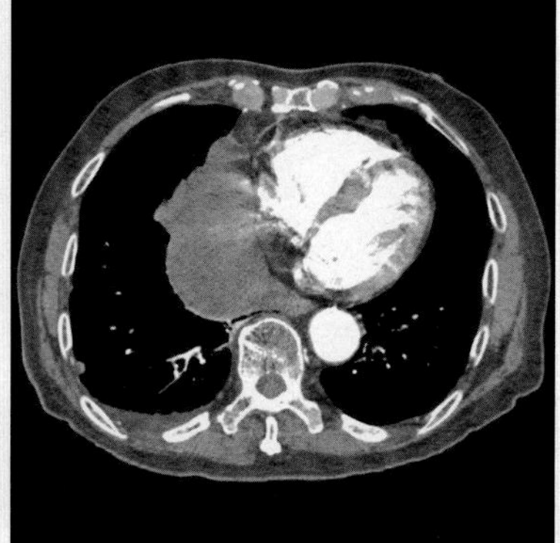

Pericardial Cyst

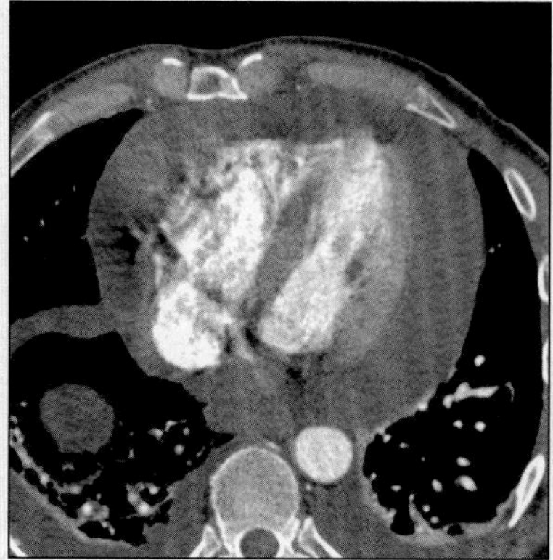

Benign Effusion

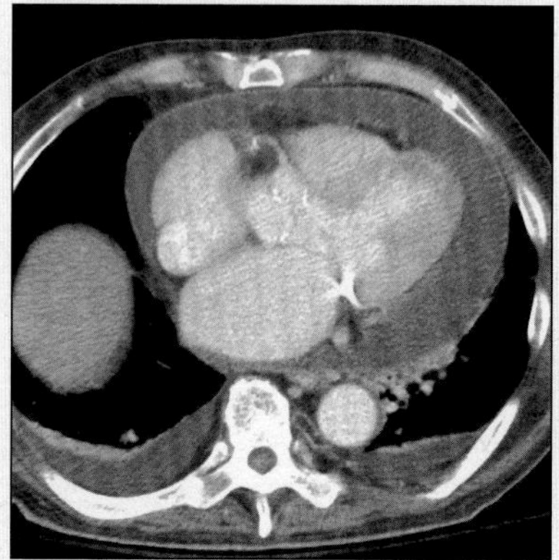

Pyopericardium

NEOPLASTIC PERICARDITIS

Key Facts

Terminology
- Most frequently secondary neoplasm via direct invasion, lymphatic or hemorrhagic spread
- Pericardial effusion with diffuse or nodular pericardial thickening
- Causes effusive-constrictive pericarditis

Imaging Findings
- Imaging studies will demonstrate effusion and/or enhancing mass lesions
- Cardiac MR or ECHO
- Ideal for functional analysis of constrictive physiology

Pathology
- Cells obtained through pericardiocentesis confirm diagnosis
- Pericardial biopsy frequently necessary

Clinical Issues
- Often asymptomatic
- Subacute effusive-constrictive pericarditis
- Acute pericardial tamponade may be presenting symptom
- Varied presentation from asymptomatic to tamponade
- Effusions reaccumulate
- Therapeutic pericardiocentesis, with complete drainage
- Pericardiotomy (percutaneous with balloon or surgical excision) to allow drainage into the pleural space
- Extensive pericardial excision

  - Evidence of primary malignancy within the myocardium or extracardiac anatomy
  - May demonstrate pericardial invasion of extracardiac tumor
  - Straightening of right ventricular and left ventricular heart borders
  - Dilated superior vena cava (SVC), azygos vein and inferior vena cava (IVC)
- CTA
  - Gated CTA may demonstrate septal bounce
  - Typical features of pericardial effusion, tamponade, or thickened pericardium
  - Enhancing mass may be visible
  - Image characteristics may suggest hemopericardium

MR Findings
- T1WI
  - Spin echo black blood images may demonstrate thickened nodular pericardium
  - Separation of visceral and parietal pericardium by fluid or blood
- T2* GRE
  - Functional images may demonstrate signs of pericardial constriction
    - Pericardial bounce
    - Flattening of right ventricle and shift of interatrial septum towards left ventricle
    - Dilated IVC and SVC
- T1 C+
  - Enhancement of irregular and thickened epicardium and pericardium
  - Enhancing mass may be visible
  - Delayed enhanced inversion recovery (IR) prepared imaging may demonstrate otherwise occult myocardial metastases

Nuclear Medicine Findings
- PET
  - May demonstrate high uptake within pericardium
    - May also identify remote noncardiac primary or other manifestations of metastases

Echocardiographic Findings
- Echocardiogram
  - Effusions of varied size
  - Tamponade physiology in extreme cases
  - Can demonstrate studding of pericardium with tumor
  - Fibrinous adhesions of pericardium

Angiographic Findings
- Conventional
  - Invasive data usually acquired before percutaneous or open pericardiectomy
  - Features of tamponade
  - Left ventriculogram may show flattening of left ventricular (LV) border

Imaging Recommendations
- Best imaging tool
  - Cardiac gated CTA
    - Best morphologic imaging, best spatial resolution in true 3D volume dataset
    - Will also allow limited functional assessment (septal bounce)
    - Best modality to demonstrate direct invasion from lung cancer or chest wall
  - Cardiac MR or ECHO
    - Ideal for functional analysis of constrictive physiology
    - ECHO may not visualize entire pericardium due to acoustic window restrictions

DIFFERENTIAL DIAGNOSIS

Constrictive Pericarditis
- Pericardial thickening and calcification

Pyopericardium
- Enhancing septations and loculations

Hemopericardium due to other Etiologies
- Traumatic
- Iatrogenic

- Ruptured type A dissection

Tuberculosis

- May lead to pericardial calcification and constriction

Post Surgical Pericarditis

- Benign effusion

Uremic Pericarditis

- Fibrinous aseptic pericardial inflammation
- Serosanguineous loculated effusion with fibrous adhesions

Extrapericardial Mediastinal or Pulmonary Mass Abutting Pericardium

- May eventually invade pericardium

Pericardial Cyst

- May mimic loculated effusion

PATHOLOGY

General Features

- General path comments
  - Cells obtained through pericardiocentesis confirm diagnosis
  - Pericardial biopsy frequently necessary
- Etiology
  - Primary tumors of the pericardium
    - Angiosarcoma and other less common sarcomas
    - Mesothelioma
    - Fibroma, lipoma
    - Pheochromocytoma, neurofibroma, neuroblastoma
    - Teratoma: Benign tumor in infants and children
    - Thymoma
  - Metastatic disease
    - Melanoma; 60% with pericardial involvement
    - Hodgkin and non-Hodgkin lymphoma
    - Leukemia, myeloma
    - Carcinoid
    - Direct invasion of mediastinal or pulmonary, chest-wall or breast tumors

CLINICAL ISSUES

Presentation

- Most common signs/symptoms
  - Often asymptomatic
  - Subacute effusive-constrictive pericarditis
  - Acute pericardial tamponade may be presenting symptom
- Varied presentation from asymptomatic to tamponade
- Pleuritic chest pain
- Dyspnea, edema, effusions
- Large pericardial effusions, tamponade
- Effusions reaccumulate
- Elastic constriction resulting from tumor encasement

Natural History & Prognosis

- Quite variable ranging from stable mild-moderate effusion without symptoms to frank tamponade
- Poor prognosis associated with widespread metastases (~ 4 months)
  - Lymphomas frequently respond to radiation or chemotherapy
- Primary malignant tumors have poor prognosis

Treatment

- Therapeutic pericardiocentesis, with complete drainage
- Pericardiotomy (percutaneous with balloon or surgical excision) to allow drainage into the pleural space
- Treatment of primary tumor
- Extensive pericardial excision
- Pericardial peritoneal shunt, or continuous percutaneous drainage
- Sclerosing treatment in rare cases

SELECTED REFERENCES

1. Little WC et al: Pericardial disease. Circulation. 113(12):1622-32, 2006
2. Abbara S et al. Pericardial and Myocardial Disease. In: Miller SW: Cardiac Imaging - The Requisites. Elsevier Mosby, Philadelphia, PA, 245-283, 2005
3. Bernhardt P et al: Cardiac magnetic resonance in outpatients in Germany-indications, complications and protocol suggestions from a high-volume center. Int J Cardiol. 2005
4. Imazio M et al: Relation of acute pericardial disease to malignancy. Am J Cardiol. 95(11):1393-4, 2005
5. Sagrista-Sauleda J et al: Effusive-constrictive pericarditis. N Engl J Med. 350(5):469-75, 2004
6. Troughton RW et al: Pericarditis. Lancet. 363(9410):717-27, 2004
7. Warren WH: Malignancies involving the pericardium. Semin Thorac Cardiovas Surg 12:119-29, 2000
8. Spodick DH: Neoplastic Pericardial Disease. In: Spodick DH: The Pericardium: A Comprehensive Textbook. Marcel Dekker, New York, 301-13, 1997
9. Cameron J et al. The etiologic spectrum of constrictive pericarditis. Am Heart J ; 113:354-360, 1987
10. Mann T et al: Effusive-constrictive hemodynamic pattern due to neoplastic involvement of the pericardium. Am J Cardiol. 41(4):781-6, 1978

NEOPLASTIC PERICARDITIS

IMAGE GALLERY

Typical

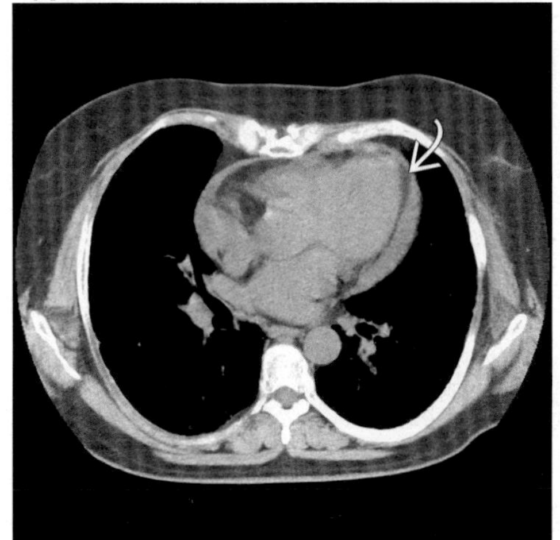

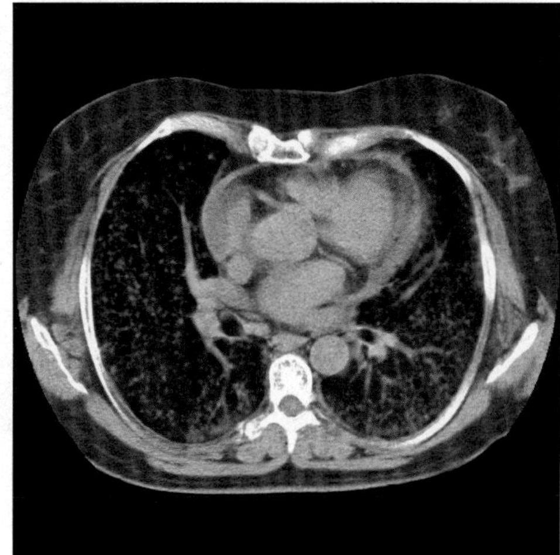

(Left) *Axial NECT shows thickened pericardial contour without definitive pericardial enhancement or hemopericardium ↪. Pathology positive for adenocarcinoma.* ***(Right)*** *Axial NECT lung windows of same patient as previous image shows pericardial effusion and miliary pulmonary metastasis. Pericardiocentesis revealed adenocarcinoma.*

Typical

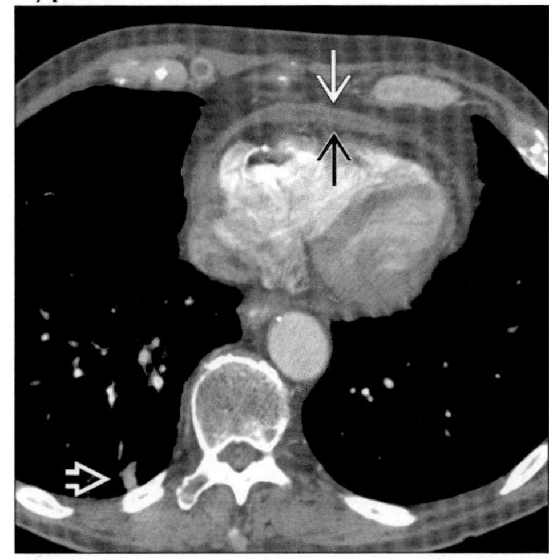

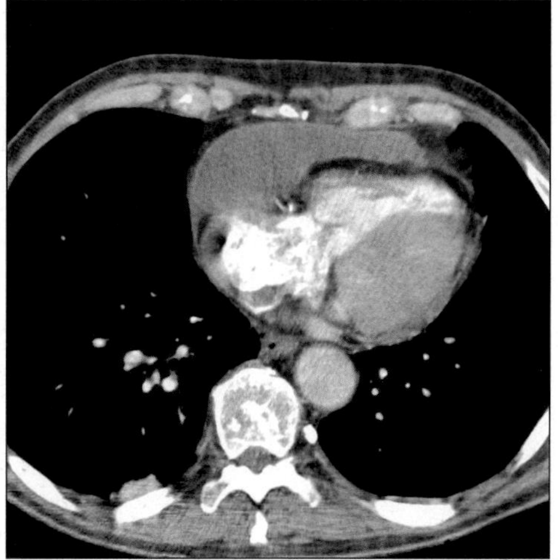

(Left) *Axial CECT shows thickened and enhancing epicardium → and pericardium → separated by a small effusion. A small pulmonary mass ⇨ and lymphangitic carcinomatosis are present.* ***(Right)*** *Axial CECT of same patient as previous image one month later shows progression of the effusion. Pericardiocentesis revealed malignant cells.*

Typical

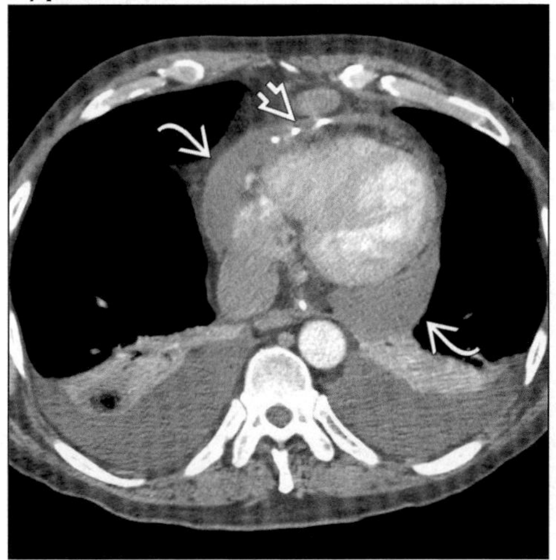

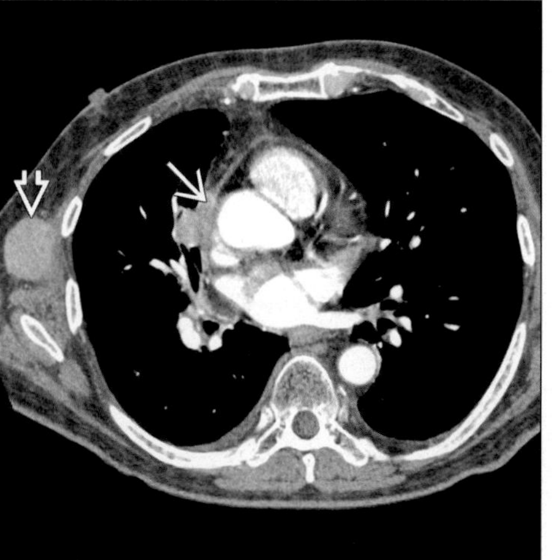

(Left) *Axial CECT shows loculated pericardial effusion with enhancing pericardium ↪. Pericardiocentesis revealed lymphoma. Note pericardial drain ⇨.* ***(Right)*** *Axial CECT shows a different patient with lymphoma and small pericardial effusion with enhancing pericardium and small solid implants →. Note other manifestations of lymphoma ⇨.*

CONSTRICTIVE PERICARDITIS

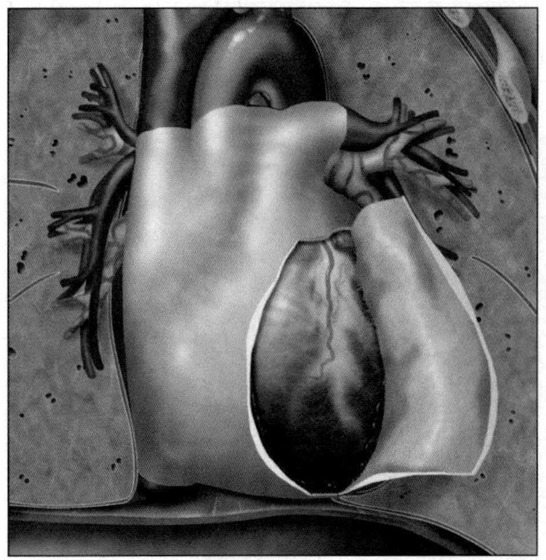

Coronal graphic shows opened parietal pericardium with pericardial thickening and inflammatory changes.

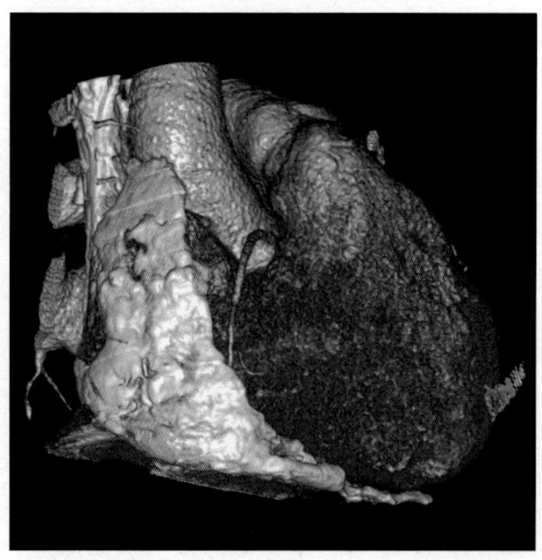

Oblique cardiac CT 3D volume rendering image shows extensive pericardial calcification in the lateral and inferior walls of the right atrium and part of the right ventricular inferior free wall.

TERMINOLOGY

Definitions

- Abnormal thickening of the pericardium resulting in impaired ventricular filling
  - Causes include postsurgical, postradiation, postinfectious, post-traumatic, postmyocardial infarction and idiopathic
  - Thickening does not necessarily indicate constrictive disease
  - Calcification suggests likelihood of constrictive physiology
  - At times isolated to the right side of the heart
- Associated findings: Tubular ventricular configuration and congestive heart failure

IMAGING FINDINGS

General Features

- Best diagnostic clue
  - Pericardial thickening in combination with heart failure
    - Pericardial calcifications highly suggestive
    - Thickness greater than 4-6 mm suggests but does not confirm pericardial constriction (normal 1-3 mm)
    - Associated signs of hepatic venous congestion, enlargement of atria, dilated superior/inferior vena cava and hepatic veins
    - Ascites, pleural effusions and pericardial effusion
- Location: Thickening may be diffuse or isolated over right atrium, right ventricle or right atrioventricular groove
- Morphology
  - Reduced volume and narrow tubular configuration of right ventricle
    - May see prominent leftward convexity or sigmoid-shaped septum
  - Echocardiography, cardiac MR or cardiac CT can demonstrate septal bounce on cine images

Radiographic Findings

- Radiography: Pericardial calcifications, bi-atrial enlargement and pleural effusions
- Calcification
  - Eggshell calcification predominantly inferior and right-sided

DDx: Constrictive Pericarditis

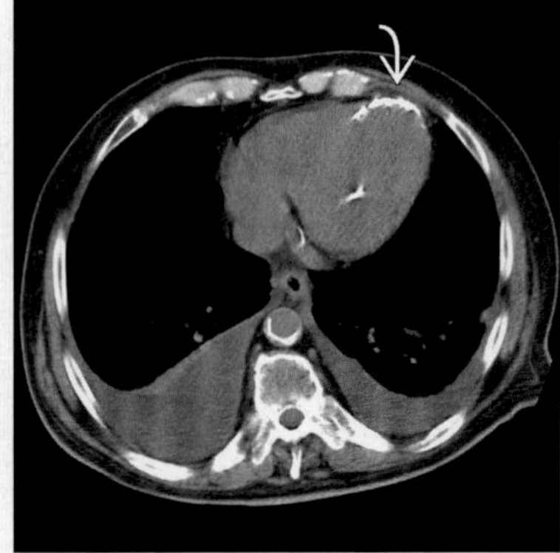

Myocardial Calcification

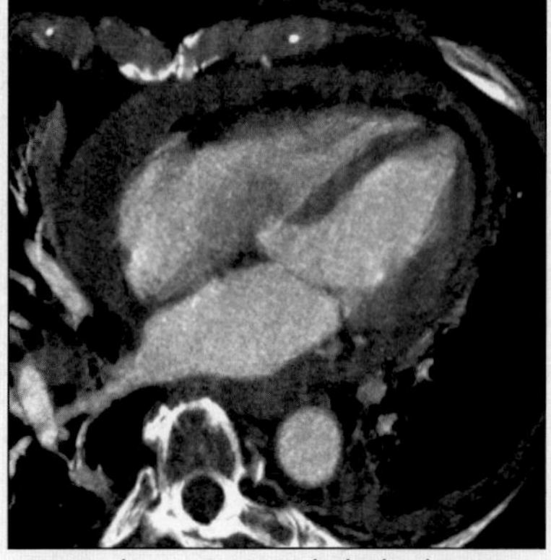

Neoplastic Pericardial Thickening

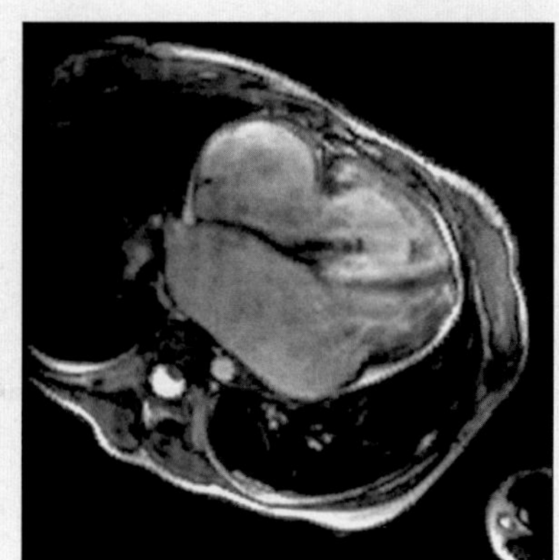

Restrictive Cardiomyopathy

CONSTRICTIVE PERICARDITIS

Key Facts

Terminology

- Causes include postsurgical, postradiation, postinfectious, post-traumatic, postmyocardial infarction and idiopathic
- Thickening does not necessarily indicate constrictive disease
- Calcification suggests likelihood of constrictive physiology
- Associated findings: Tubular ventricular configuration and congestive heart failure

Imaging Findings

- Thickness greater than 4-6 mm suggests but does not confirm pericardial constriction (normal 1-3 mm)
- Radiography: Pericardial calcifications, bi-atrial enlargement and pleural effusions
- CT: Best imaging modality to detect pericardial calcification
- Pericardial enhancement may indicate active inflammatory process
- MR more sensitive in distinguishing pericardial effusion from thickening
- MR: High sensitivity for distinguishing constrictive pericarditis from restrictive cardiomyopathy
- De-MR can detect pericardial hyper-enhancement

Top Differential Diagnoses

- Myocardial Calcification
- Pericarditis without Constriction
- Restrictive Cardiomyopathy
- Neoplasm
- Cardiac Tamponade

- With constrictive pericarditis
    - Widened superior mediastinum
    - Lack of pulmonary edema
    - Elevated diaphragms due to ascites

CT Findings

- NECT
    - Constrictive pericarditis findings
        - CT: Best imaging modality to detect pericardial calcification
        - Pericardial effusion/thickening (> 4-6 mm)
        - May be limited to the right side of the heart
    - Small effusion difficult to distinguish from thickening
        - Evaluate for attenuation characteristics of pericardial effusion
        - Exudative effusion as seen with infection, hemorrhage, neoplasm has increased attenuation
        - Transudative effusion has water attenuation (0-10 Hounsfield units)
- CECT
    - Pericardial enhancement may indicate active inflammatory process
        - Enhancement aids in distinguishing effusion from thickening
- Radiographic findings above not diagnostic of constrictive pericarditis without clinical scenario of physiologic constriction

MR Findings

- T1WI
    - Low signal intensity band > 4-6 mm encompassed by high signal intensity epicardial and pericardial fat
    - Pericardial effusion low signal intensity
    - Hemorrhagic effusion high signal intensity
- T2WI
    - Pericardium remains low signal intensity
    - Occasionally in subacute forms, thickened pericardium may have moderate to high signal intensity on spin echo images
    - Effusion very high signal intensity unless complicated by hemorrhage or proteinaceous material
- T1 C+: Pericardial enhancement may be seen with inflammatory process
- MR more sensitive in distinguishing pericardial effusion from thickening
    - Calcification seen only as signal void
    - Tagging lines can help detect pericardial adhesion
- MR: High sensitivity for distinguishing constrictive pericarditis from restrictive cardiomyopathy
- DE MR can detect pericardial hyper-enhancement
    - Related to acute/subacute inflammation or fibrous thickening
    - Also very useful to detect myocardial disease/restrictive cardiomyopathy

Echocardiographic Findings

- Primary diagnostic tool
    - Early diastolic filling becomes rapid with elevation and equalization of diastolic pressures in all cardiac chambers
    - Restriction of late diastolic filling
    - Septal bounce and inferior vena cava plethora with absent inspiratory collapse
- Suboptimal in demonstration of pericardial thickening
    - Transesophageal echo (TEE) allows better visualization of pericardium
        - TEE limited by small field of view and semi-invasive

Imaging Recommendations

- Best imaging tool
    - Echocardiography primary tool to investigate physiologic changes of pericardium, although limited in some cases
    - CT and MR useful to direct examine entire pericardium
    - MR more useful to distinguish constrictive pericarditis vs. restrictive cardiomyopathy
    - CT best tool to identify pericardial calcification
- Protocol advice: Perform MR and CT scans without and with contrast to assess for pericardial enhancement

CONSTRICTIVE PERICARDITIS

DIFFERENTIAL DIAGNOSIS

Myocardial Calcification

- Pericardial
  - Usually right-sided (less cardiac motion)
  - Diffuse and extensive
  - Spare left atrium and apex
  - Atrioventricular (AV) groove
- Myocardial
  - Usually left-sided
  - Focal
  - Apex typical location
  - Spares AV groove

Pericarditis without Constriction

- Distinction is made based on physiologic changes

Restrictive Cardiomyopathy

- Similar physiologic changes by echocardiography and cardiac catheterization
- Look for associated myocardial thickening and enhancement as seen with sarcoidosis, amyloidosis, hypertropic cardiomyopathy, lymphoma
- De-MRI is extremely helpful in detecting hyper-enhancement within the myocardium related to restrictive cardiomyopathy

Neoplasm

- Could cause restrictive physiology
- Metastases usually cause effusion, not masses
  - Focal or multifocal areas of enhancing pericardium consider metastatic disease, especially in face of known primary
- Primary tumors rare (sarcomas, large bulky tumors)

Cardiac Tamponade

- Large accumulation of fluid within the pericardium (hemorrhage, inflammatory process, effusion)

PATHOLOGY

General Features

- General path comments
  - Normal pericardial anatomy
    - Usually 2 mm thickness
    - Lies between variable amounts of epicardial and pericardial fat
    - Has fibrous and serous components
    - Fibrous elements attached to diaphragm, costal cartilage and sternum
    - Serous element thin mesothelial layer adjacent to the heart
    - Intervening potential space usually contains 15-50 mm fluid
- Etiology
  - Constrictive pericarditis caused by injury, iatrogenic, idiopathic processes
    - In developed countries, most common etiologies: Idiopathic (presumed viral) or post-CABG
    - In the developing world, infectious etiologies (TB has the highest total incidence)
  - Infectious: Viral (Coxsackie B, influenza); bacterial; tuberculosis; fungal or parasitic
  - Metabolic: Uremia
  - Inflammatory: Systemic lupus erythematosus; rheumatoid arthritis
  - Neoplastic: Metastasis

Gross Pathologic & Surgical Features

- > 50% with pericardial calcification will have constrictive pericarditis

CLINICAL ISSUES

Presentation

- Most common signs/symptoms
  - Symptoms are often vague and their onset is insidious
  - Physical examination: Jugular venous distention and Kussmaul sign
- Other signs/symptoms: Symptoms of heart failure

Treatment

- Surgical stripping of pericardium, difficult to remove entire pericardium
- Medical treatment is difficult and does not affect natural progression or prognosis of the disease
- May recur

DIAGNOSTIC CHECKLIST

Consider

- Assessing both morphologic (pericardial thickness) and physiologic parameters (septal bounce)

Image Interpretation Pearls

- Pericardial thickening, pericardial enhancement and presence of calcifications

SELECTED REFERENCES

1. Ha JW et al: Images in cardiology. Delayed hyperenhancement of the pericardium by magnetic resonance imaging as a marker of pericardial inflammation in a patient with tuberculous effusive constrictive pericarditis. Heart. 92(4):494, 2006
2. Gilkeson RC et al: MR evaluation of cardiac and pericardial malignancy. Magn Reson Imaging Clin N Am. 11(1):173-86, viii, 2003
3. Glockner JF: Imaging of pericardial disease. Magn Reson Imaging Clin N Am. 11(1):149-62, vii, 2003
4. Wang ZJ et al: CT and MR imaging of pericardial disease. Radiographics. 23 Spec No:S167-80, 2003
5. Breen JF: Imaging of the pericardium. J Thorac Imaging. 16(1):47-54, 2001
6. Rozenshtein A et al: Plain-film diagnosis of pericardial disease. Semin Roentgenol. 34(3):195-204, 1999
7. Watanabe A et al: A case of effusive-constructive pericarditis: an efficacy of GD-DTPA enhanced magnetic resonance imaging to detect a pericardial thickening. Magn Reson Imaging. 16(3):347-50, 1998
8. Masui T et al: Constrictive pericarditis and restrictive cardiomyopathy: evaluation with MR imaging. Radiology. 182(2):369-73, 1992

IMAGE GALLERY

Typical

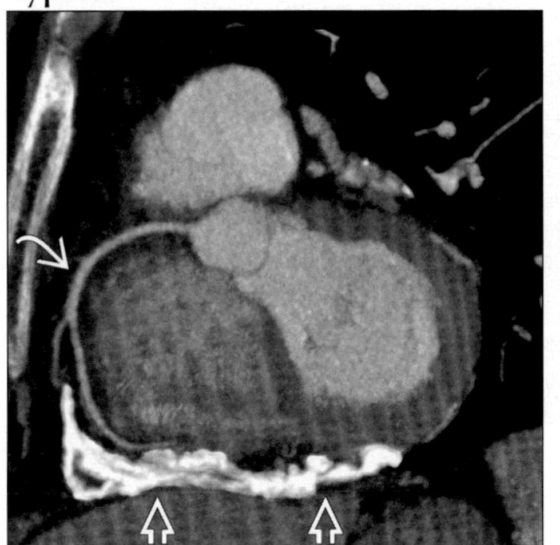

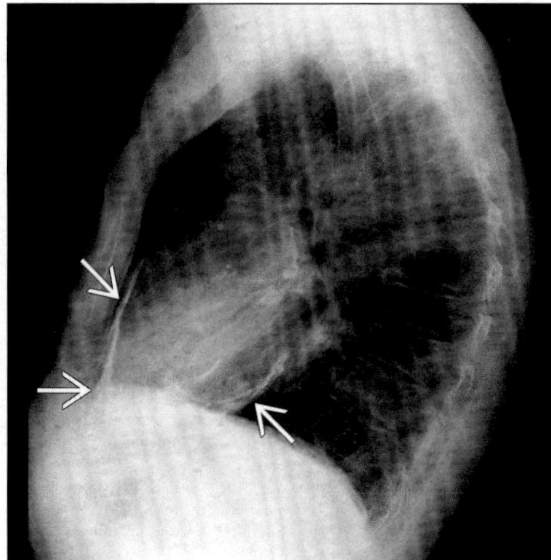

*(**Left**) Oblique coronary CTA image shows extensive calcification of the RV and LV inferior walls ➔. Note also patent right coronary artery with acute marginal branch take-off ➔. (**Right**) Lateral radiograph shows extensive pericardial calcification anteriorly and inferiorly ➔.*

Typical

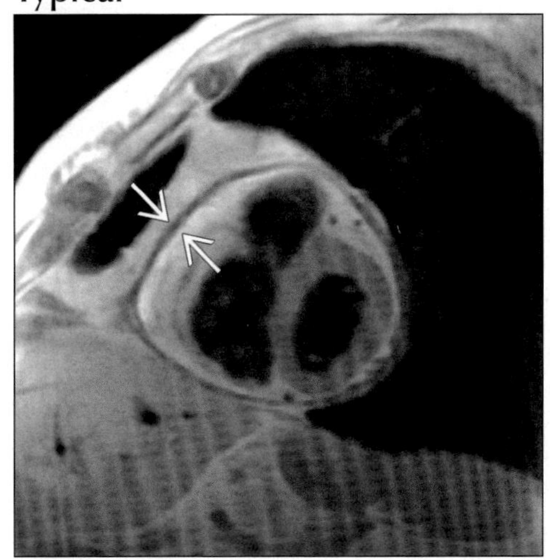

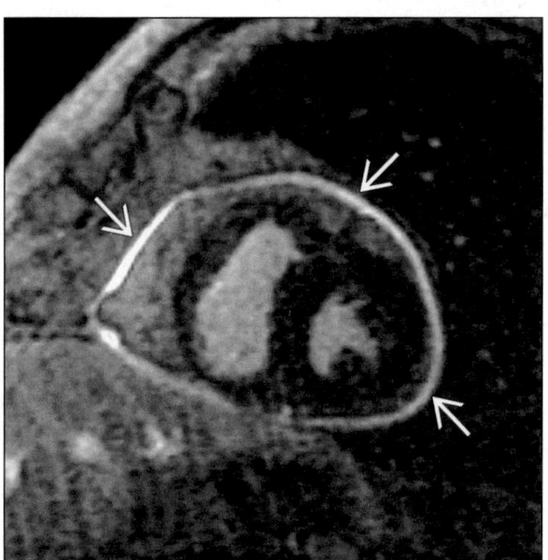

*(**Left**) Short axis view PDWI black blood image shows pericardial thickening up to 6 mm ➔. (**Right**) Short axis DE MR shows circumferential enhancement of the pericardium ➔ 10 minutes after gadolinium administration in a patient with subacute pericarditis.*

Typical

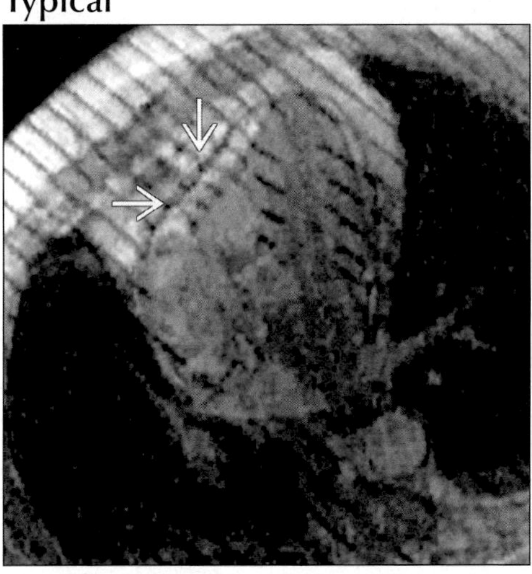

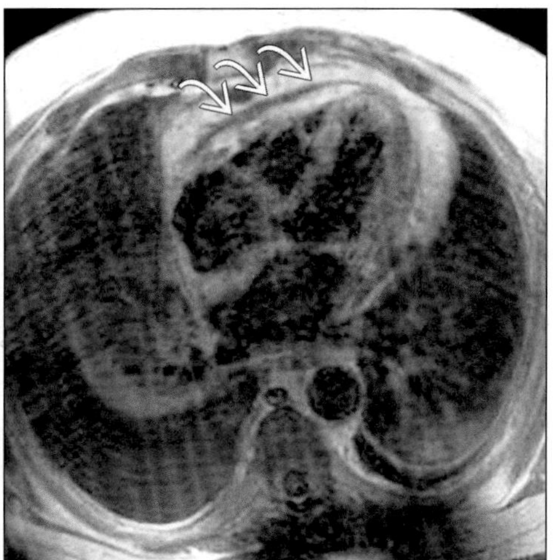

*(**Left**) Four chamber view tagging MR shows no break of the taglines along the pericardium of the RV anterior free wall ➔ suggesting pericardial adhesion. (**Right**) Four chamber view T1WI MR image post-gadolinium shows pericardial thickening and enhancement of pericardium in the RV free wall ➔. Note also bilateral pleural effusion, right > left.*

PERICARDIAL CYST

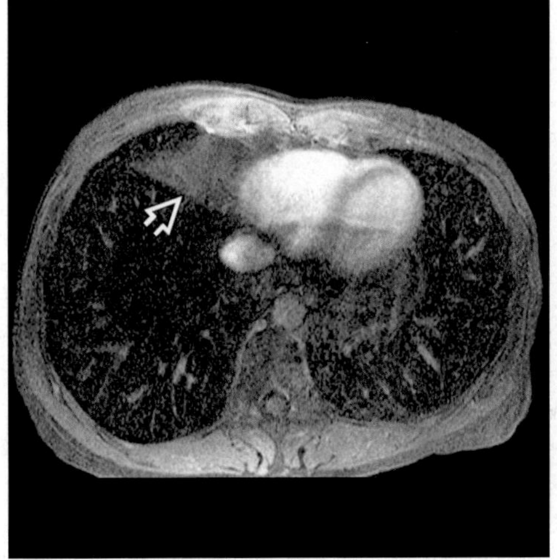

Axial T1WI MR shows low signal intensity mass ⇒ adjacent to the pericardium in the anterior right cardiophrenic angle, which extends into the major fissure.

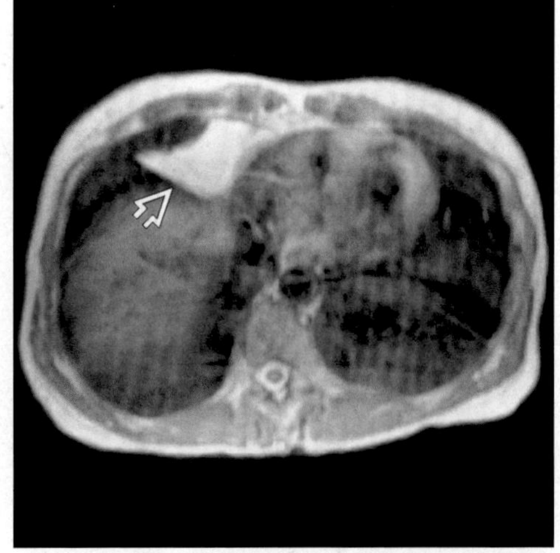

Axial T2WI MR of same patient as previous image shows homogeneous high signal intensity without septations ⇒, indicating the cystic nature of the mass.

TERMINOLOGY

Definitions

- Anomalous fluid containing mass of parietal pericardium
- Embryologic defect in coelomic cavity development or sequela of pericarditis

IMAGING FINDINGS

General Features

- Best diagnostic clue
  - Smoothly marginated
  - Adjacent to heart at right anterior costophrenic angle
  - Fluid density by CT
  - Water signal intensity by MR
  - Unilocular in 80-90%, multiloculated in 10-20%
- Location
  - Cardiophrenic (CP) angle
    - Right 70%
    - Left 10-40%
- Size: 2-30 cm in diameter
- Morphology
  - Well marginated rounded homogeneous mass
  - May change shape with cardiac cycle
  - May prolapse into pleural fissures

Radiographic Findings

- Radiography
  - Double density at right CP angle
  - Contour overlying the cardiac silhouette
  - Partly spherical with sharp smooth contours
  - May rarely occur in the mediastinum distant from the CP angle
    - In these cases, difficult to distinguish from bronchogenic or thymic cyst
  - May change shape with body positioning, respiration or cardiac cycle

CT Findings

- NECT
  - Smoothly marginated
  - Water attenuation (10 Hounsfield units), usually no septations
  - Non-calcified
  - Wall imperceptible
  - Usually at CP angle, especially on right

DDx: Other Cardiophrenic Pericardial Masses

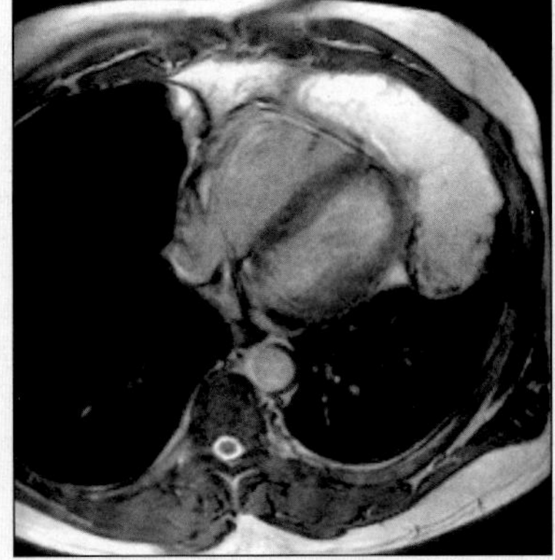

Lymphangioma

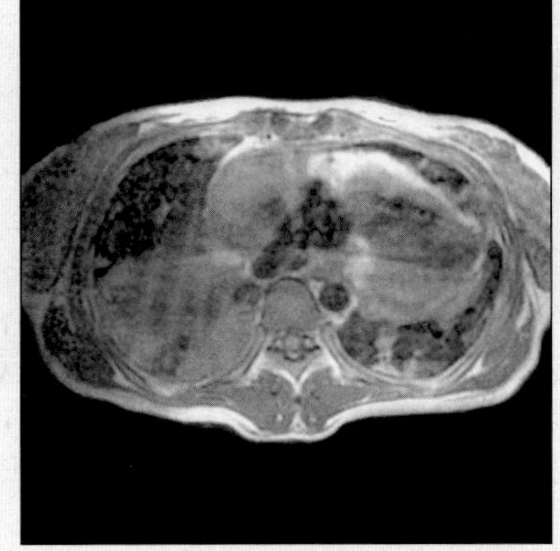

Angiosarcoma

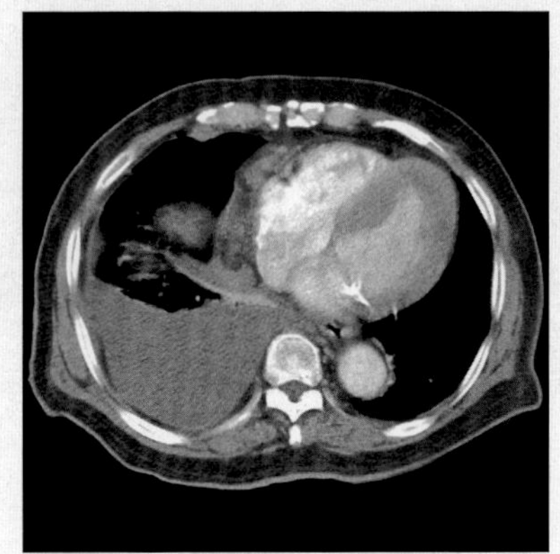

Lymphoma

PERICARDIAL CYST

Key Facts

Imaging Findings

- Smoothly marginated
- Adjacent to heart at right anterior costophrenic angle
- Fluid density by CT
- Water signal intensity by MR
- Unilocular in 80-90%, multiloculated in 10-20%
- Size: 2-30 cm in diameter
- May change shape with body positioning, respiration or cardiac cycle
- Homogeneous appearance
- No internal enhancement
- No enhancing wall
- Echocardiography primary tool to investigate pericardium
- Anechoic in appearance

Top Differential Diagnoses

- Loculated Pleural Effusion
- Bronchogenic Cyst
- Hematoma
- Esophageal Duplication Cyst
- Pericardial Metastases
- Hydatid Cyst

Pathology

- Invariably connected to pericardium
- Only a few show visible communication with pericardial sac

Clinical Issues

- Usually asymptomatic incidental finding

- CECT
  - Homogeneous appearance
  - No internal enhancement
  - No enhancing wall

MR Findings

- T1WI
  - Uniform low or intermediate signal intensity (SI)
  - Occasionally may contain highly proteinaceous fluid, which may have high SI on T1WI
- T2WI
  - Homogeneous
  - High signal intensity (follows that of water)
- T1 C+
  - No internal enhancement
  - No rim-enhancement
- MR imaging findings are diagnostic, generally requiring no further intervention
- Phase contrast imaging may detect slow internal flow if communicating with pericardial space

Echocardiographic Findings

- Anechoic space between epicardium and parietal pericardium

Imaging Recommendations

- Best imaging tool: Echocardiography or MR
- Protocol advice
  - Limited protocol needed
    - Axial and coronal T1WI and T1 C+
    - Axial and coronal T2WI
    - Coronal imaging helpful to demonstrate relationship to heart and pericardium
    - Short axis and 4 chamber planes not necessary
- Echocardiography primary tool to investigate pericardium
  - Anechoic in appearance
  - High sensitivity and ability to differentiate solid from cystic masses
  - Defines relationships with cardiac chambers
- CT and MR useful to
  - Examine entire pericardium
  - Distinguish myocardial from pericardial disease
  - Further characterize pericardial masses

DIFFERENTIAL DIAGNOSIS

Loculated Pleural Effusion

- Fluid density at CT
- Look for other loculations or free effusion
- Enhancing septations may be present
- History pertinent; more common post-operatively

Bronchogenic Cyst

- Same imaging characteristics as pericardial cyst
- Most commonly located in middle mediastinum around carina
- When infected or contain secretions, may appear as solid tumor or may have air-fluid level

Hematoma

- MR particularly useful
- Acutely demonstrates homogeneous high signal intensity on T1WI and T2WI
- Subacutely shows heterogeneous signal intensity, areas of high SI on T1WI and T2WI
- Chronically may show dark peripheral rim and low SI areas that may represent calcification, fibrosis, or hemosiderin deposition on T1WI
- High SI areas on T1WI or T2WI may correspond to hemorrhagic fluid
- No enhancement on T1 C+

Pericardial Fat Pad

- Echo-free space may be seen by echocardiography; may be difficult to distinguish from pericardial fluid
- Fat density by CT distinguishing feature

Morgagni Hernia

- Bowel or mesenteric fat in anterior hernia sac

Enlarged Pericardial Lymph Nodes

- Mantle radiation therapy: Cardiac blockers used to protect heart, area may be under treated
  - "Fat pad" sign: Enlarging recurrent nodes from lymphoma in under treated pericardial lymph nodes

- Appearance or enlargement of "fat pad" heralds the development of adenopathy
- Nodes may be irradiated since field was blocked initially
- May fill CP angle on frontal chest radiograph
- On lateral view may be retrosternal or at level of inferior vena cava or phrenic nerve

Thymic Cysts or Thymolipoma
- Cysts have fluid density at CT or MR
- Thymolipoma contains fat
- Thymus usually separable from pericardium

Esophageal Duplication Cyst
- Imaging characteristics identical to pericardial cyst
- Adjacent to esophagus, majority are cervical

Bronchogenic Carcinoma
- Separate from pericardium at CT
- Bronchogenic carcinoma can directly extend into pericardium
- Effusion and irregularly thickened pericardium or pericardial mass

Pericardial Metastases
- Lung and breast cancer most common
- Effusion and irregularly thickened pericardium or pericardial mass
- Enhancement common by CT or MR
- Most have low SI on T1WI and high SI on T2WI

Neurofibroma
- May cause CP angle mass
- Generally solid, but may have cystic components
- Enhancement internally with CT or MR

Hydatid Cyst
- Cystic mass with well-defined edges
- Internal trabeculations correspond to daughter membranes
- May be pericardial or intramyocardial
- May appear as solid mass if cyst replaced by necrotic matter
  - Contains membrane residues and granulomatous foreign-body inflammatory reaction

Pancreatic Pseudocyst
- History pertinent
- Look for peripancreatic inflammatory changes and fluid collections
- Usually extends through esophageal hiatus

PATHOLOGY

General Features
- General path comments: Benign cyst of mediastinum
- Etiology
  - Anomalous outpouching of parietal pericardium
  - Occurs by 4th week of gestation
  - Occurs as coalescing spaces form intraembryonic body cavity

Gross Pathologic & Surgical Features
- Invariably connected to pericardium
- Only a few show visible communication with pericardial sac

Microscopic Features
- Fibrous tissue lined by single layer of bland mesothelium
- Differentiate from bronchogenic cysts and esophageal duplication cyst by cell lining
  - Absence of bronchial or gastrointestinal epithelium respectively

CLINICAL ISSUES

Presentation
- Most common signs/symptoms: Usually asymptomatic incidental finding
- Other signs/symptoms
  - Occasionally may have chest pain
  - Pericardial tamponade may rarely occur

Treatment
- Generally incidental radiographic finding requiring no treatment
- Surgery if complicated by
  - Chest pain
  - Tamponade
  - Mistaken for malignancy
- No literature to support percutaneous drainage

DIAGNOSTIC CHECKLIST

Consider
- CT often diagnostic
- MR considered imaging gold standard

Image Interpretation Pearls
- T2 bright, T1 dark mass without septations in right costophrenic angle is diagnostic of pericardial cyst

SELECTED REFERENCES

1. Nijveldt R et al: Pericardial cyst. Lancet. 365(9475):1960, 2005
2. Guven A et al: A case of asymptomatic cardiopericardial hydatid cyst. Jpn Heart J. 45(3):541-5, 2004
3. Heirigs R et al: Images in cardiology: Pericardial cyst. Clin Cardiol. 27(9):507, 2004
4. Oyama N et al: Computed tomography and magnetic resonance imaging of the pericardium: anatomy and pathology. Magn Reson Med Sci. 3(3):145-52, 2004
5. Walker MJ et al: Migrating pleural mesothelial cyst. Ann Thorac Surg. 77(2):701-2, 2004
6. Glockner JF: Imaging of pericardial disease. Magn Reson Imaging Clin N Am. 11(1):149-62, vii, 2003
7. Gossios K et al: Mediastinal and pericardial hydatid cysts: an unusual cause of circulatory collapse. AJR Am J Roentgenol. 181(1):285-6, 2003
8. Kim JH et al: Cystic tumors in the anterior mediastinum. Radiologic-pathological correlation. J Comput Assist Tomogr. 27(5):714-23, 2003
9. Wang ZJ et al: CT and MR imaging of pericardial disease. Radiographics. 23 Spec No:S167-80, 2003
10. Breen JF: Imaging of the pericardium. J Thorac Imaging. 16:47-54, 2001

PERICARDIAL CYST

IMAGE GALLERY

Typical

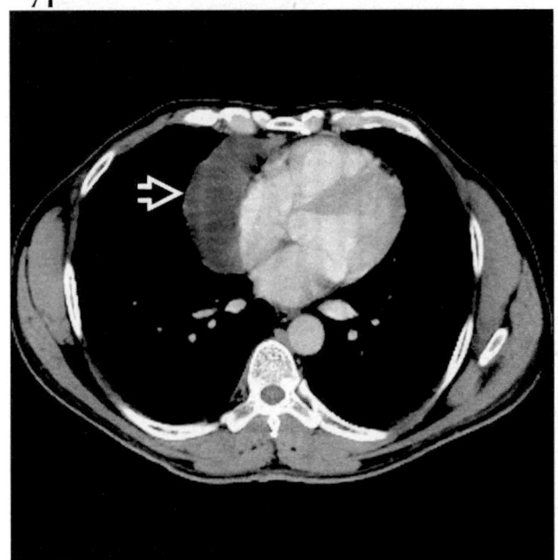

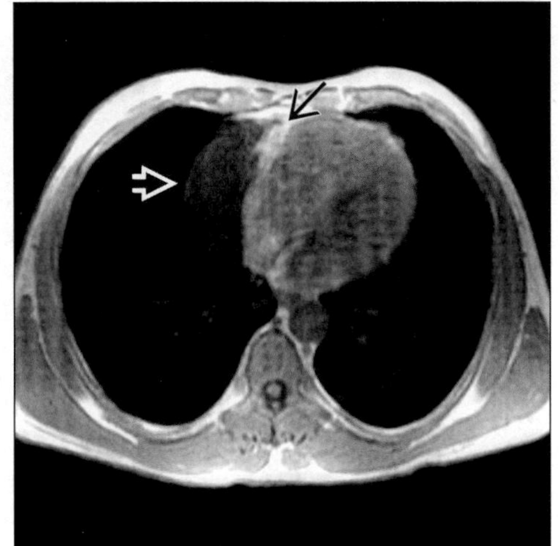

(Left) *Axial CECT shows fluid attenuation mass adjacent to the lateral wall of the right atrium ⇨, without evidence of enhancing walls or septations and without evidence of invasion.* ***(Right)*** *Axial T1WI MR shows low signal intensity of same mass in previous image ⇨. Note separation of the mass and heart by epicardial fat layer →.*

Typical

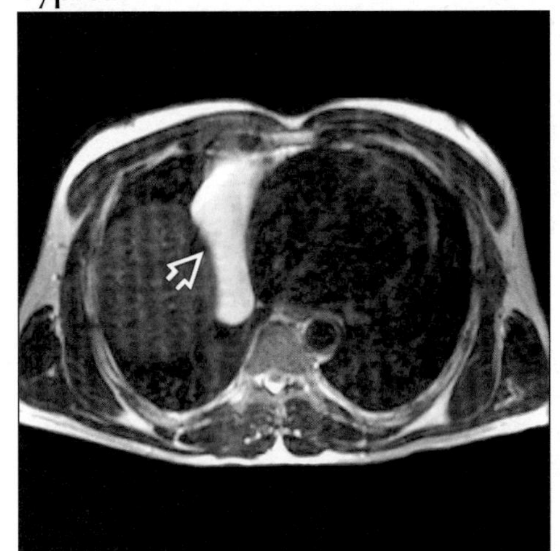

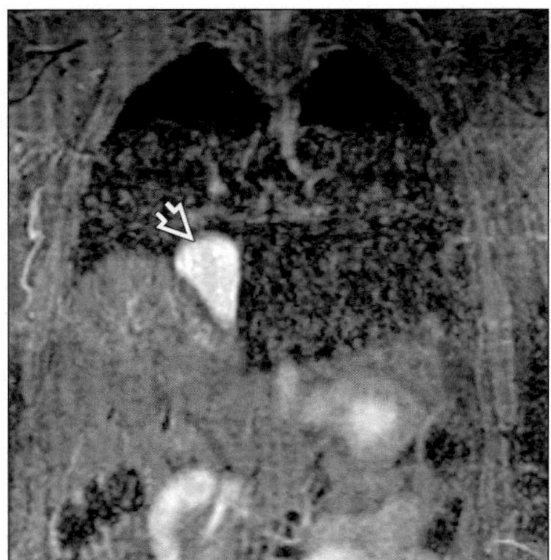

(Left) *Axial T2WI MR at a slightly lower level than then previous image shows homogeneous bright T2 signal of cardiophrenic mass without septations ⇨, indicating simple cystic nature.* ***(Right)*** *Coronal T2WI MR shows bright pericardial cyst ⇨ in the right cardiophrenic angle. Note signal loss of the heart and phase encoding artifact (horizontal image degradation) due to non-gated acquisition.*

Typical

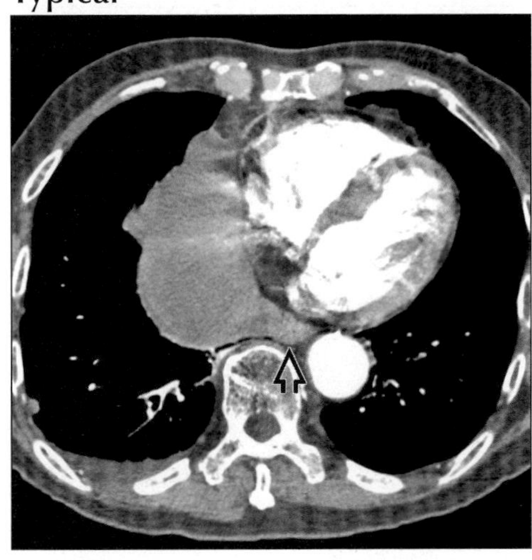

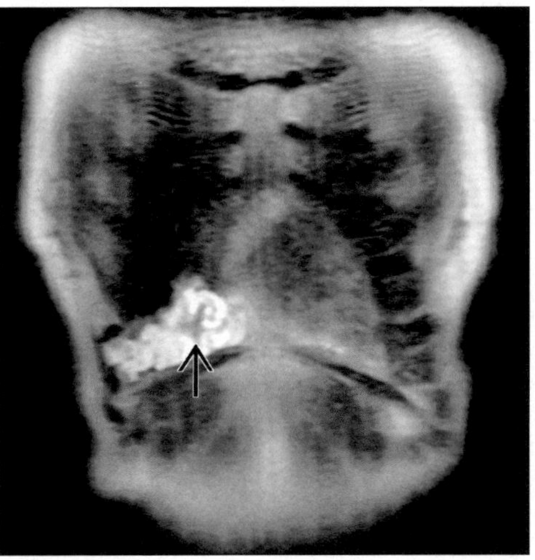

(Left) *Axial CECT shows unusually large right cardiophrenic angle pericardial cyst extending into the posterior mediastinum and abutting descending aorta ⇨.* ***(Right)*** *Coronal T2WI MR shows multilobulated pericardial cyst within right cardiophrenic and costophrenic angles. Note multiple septations are present →.*

ABSENT PERICARDIUM

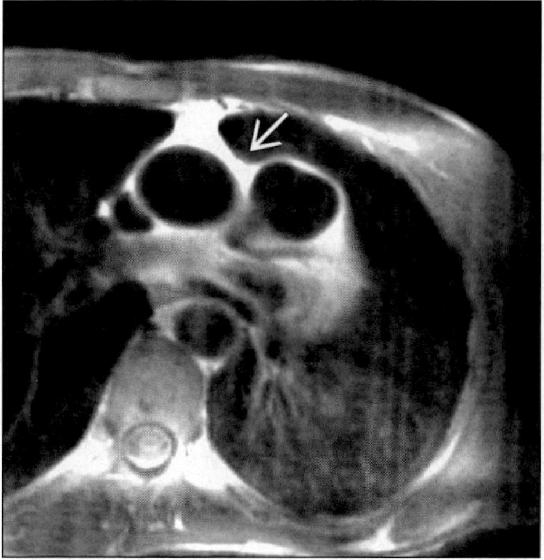

Axial T1WI MR shows that without the pericardium, the lung ➔ is able to herniate between the ascending aorta and pulmonary artery.

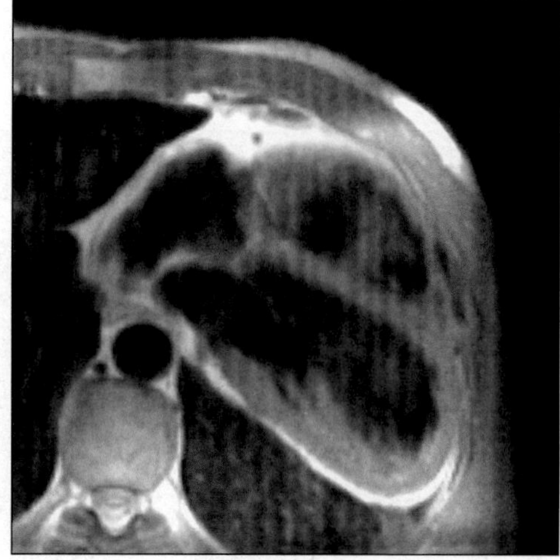

Axial T1WI MR shows the cardiac axis is rotated leftward. Note that both ventricles abut the lateral chest wall. Patient had completely absent left pericardium.

TERMINOLOGY

Definitions

- Absence of all or portions of pericardium

IMAGING FINDINGS

General Features

- Location: Absence of entire left side of pericardium, partial absence of left pericardium, complete absence, absent right pericardium

Radiographic Findings

- Radiography
  - **Partial absence of left pericardium**
    - Prominence of left atrial appendage
  - **Complete absence**
    - Levoposition of the heart
    - Flattening & elongation of left heart border
    - Lucent area between diaphragm and heart or aorta and pulmonary artery due to interposed lung

CT Findings

- NECT
  - Partial absence of left pericardium
    - Left atrial appendage herniation
  - Complete absence of pericardium
    - Lung between main PA and aorta
    - Rotation of the heart toward the left

MR Findings

- Double IR FSE: Same as CT

Echocardiographic Findings

- Echocardiogram: Cardioptosis, cardiac hypermobility, abnormal swinging motion, paradoxical or flat systolic septal motion

Imaging Recommendations

- Best imaging tool: CT or echocardiography

DIFFERENTIAL DIAGNOSIS

Complete Absence of Pericardium

- Rotation from RV chamber enlargement

DDx: Absent Pericardium

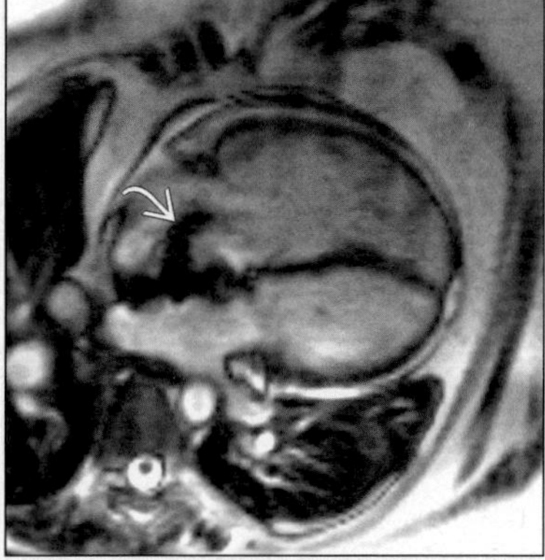

ASD, RV Enlarged

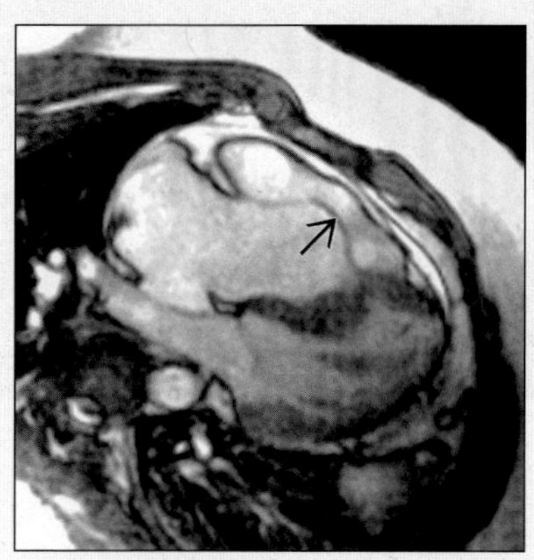

Ebstein Anomaly

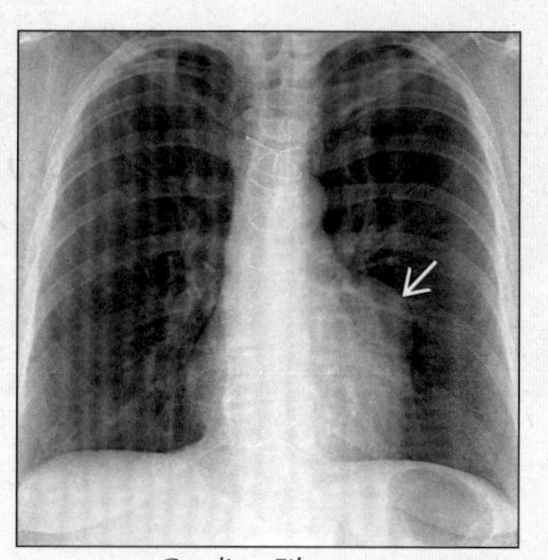

Cardiac Fibroma

ABSENT PERICARDIUM

Key Facts

Terminology
- Absence of all or portions of pericardium

Imaging Findings
- **Partial absence of left pericardium**
- Prominence of left atrial appendage
- **Complete absence**
- Levoposition of the heart
- Flattening & elongation of left heart border

Clinical Issues
- Usually asymptomatic incidental finding at surgery
- Non-exertional paroxysmal stabbing chest pain (partial absence)
- Complete absence of entire pericardium or absence of whole left or right side has excellent prognosis
- Partial absence more dangerous because of herniation
- Partial defects may require pericardiectomy or pericardioplasty and excision of herniated LAA

Focal Absence of Pericardium
- Pericardial fat pad or cyst, masses, Morgagni hernia, loculated pleural effusion, LV aneurysm

PATHOLOGY

General Features
- Etiology
  - Congenital absence due to premature atrophy of left common cardiac vein
  - Agenesis of pleuropericardium from poor blood supply
- Associated abnormalities
  - 30% have congenital cardiac abnormalities
    - Atrial septal defect, bicuspid aortic valve, patent ductus arteriosus, tetralogy of Fallot
  - Extracardiac defects
    - Bronchopulmonary sequestration, bronchogenic cysts
  - Other syndromes
    - VATER, Marfan, Pallister Killian (tetrasomy 12p)

CLINICAL ISSUES

Presentation
- Most common signs/symptoms
  - Usually asymptomatic incidental finding at surgery
  - Non-exertional paroxysmal stabbing chest pain (partial absence)
    - Herniation of left ventricle through defect → compression of coronary branches by rim of defect
  - Dyspnea, trepopnea (dyspnea when lying on one side but not the other), displaced apical impulse, murmurs, increased splitting of second heart sound due to associated RBBB
  - ECG may have RBBB, poor R-wave progression

Demographics
- Gender: M:F = 3:1

Natural History & Prognosis
- Complete absence of entire pericardium or absence of whole left or right side has excellent prognosis
  - Small increase in preload may lead to ventricular dilatation because of loss of ventricular constraint
- Partial absence more dangerous because of herniation
  - Herniation and strangulation of atria, appendages
  - Edge of defect compresses great vessels, coronaries

Treatment
- Partial defects may require pericardiectomy or pericardioplasty and excision of herniated LAA

SELECTED REFERENCES

1. Abbas AE et al: Congenital absence of the pericardium: case presentation and review of literature. Int J Cardiol. 98(1):21-5, 2005

IMAGE GALLERY

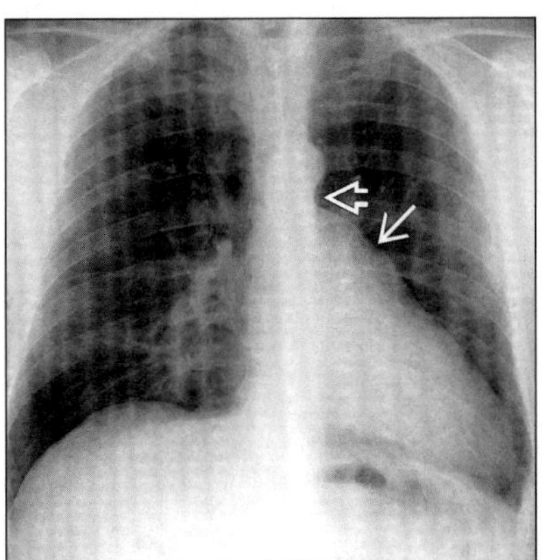

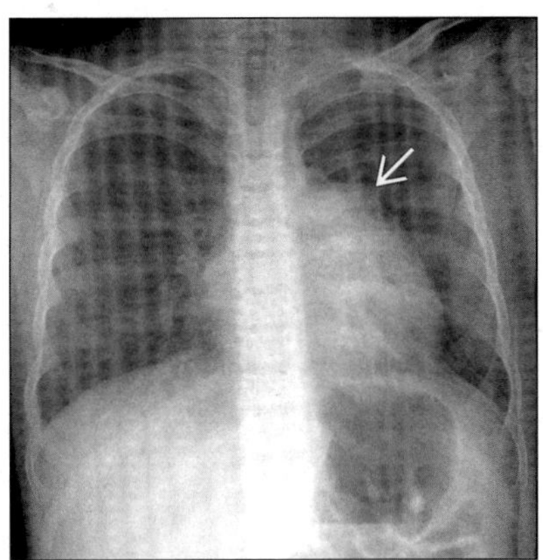

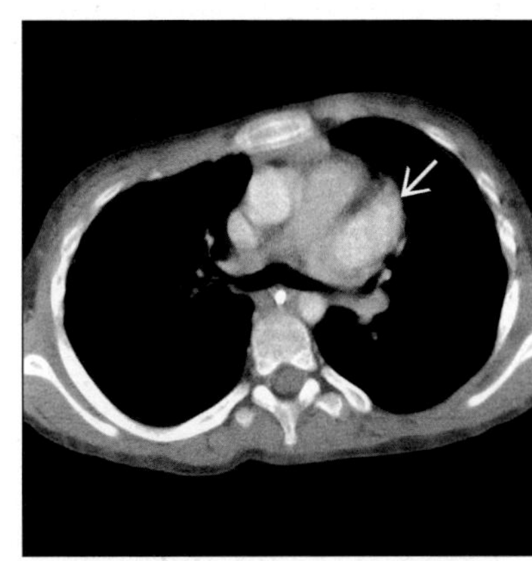

(Left) *Posteroanterior radiograph shows absence of the pericardium with herniated left atrial appendage ➡ and lung ➡ interposed between aortic arch and pulmonary artery.* ***(Center)*** *Posteroanterior radiograph shows partial absence of the pericardium with herniated left atrial appendage ➡. (Courtesy N. Dobos, MD).* ***(Right)*** *Axial CECT shows partial absence of the pericardium with herniated left atrial appendage ➡. (Courtesy N. Dobos, MD).*

PERICARDIAL EFFUSION

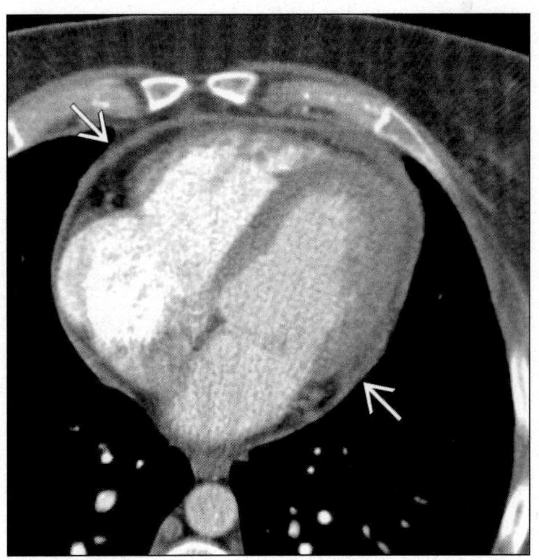

Axial CECT shows small circumferential pericardial effusion ➔.

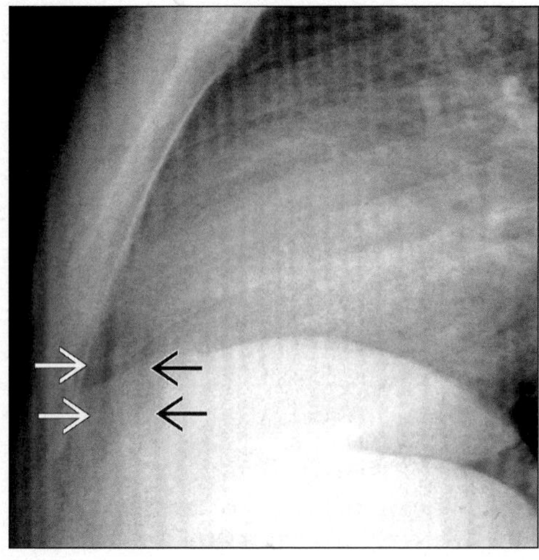

Lateral radiograph shows effusion between epicardial ➔ fat and pericardial fat ➔. The effusion lies in-between and appears more opaque. (Courtesy A. Shabaan, MD).

TERMINOLOGY

Definitions

- Transudate, exudate, or blood in pericardial sac

IMAGING FINDINGS

General Features

- Best diagnostic clue: Fluid in pericardial sac

Radiographic Findings

- "Fat pad" sign on lateral film is not sensitive
- Flask-shaped enlargement of cardiac silhouette is nonspecific, difficult to recognize

CT Findings

- CECT
  - CT may assess size and distribution of effusion
  - Can characterize blood, exudate, chyle, serous fluid
  - Can determine if associated pleural thickening

MR Findings

- Can also characterize nature of effusion
- Can depict associated pericardial thickening

Imaging Recommendations

- Best imaging tool
  - Echocardiography
    - Persisting echo-free space between parietal and visceral pericardium throughout the cardiac cycle
    - Frond-like, band-like, or shaggy intrapericardial echoes in complicated effusions

DIFFERENTIAL DIAGNOSIS

Fibrinous Pericarditis

- Thickening of pericardium more than 1-2 mm
- Enhancing pericardium

Pericardial Tamponade

- Effacement of epicardial fat
- Compression of ventricles, deformation of atria

PATHOLOGY

General Features

- Etiology

DDx: Complicated Effusions

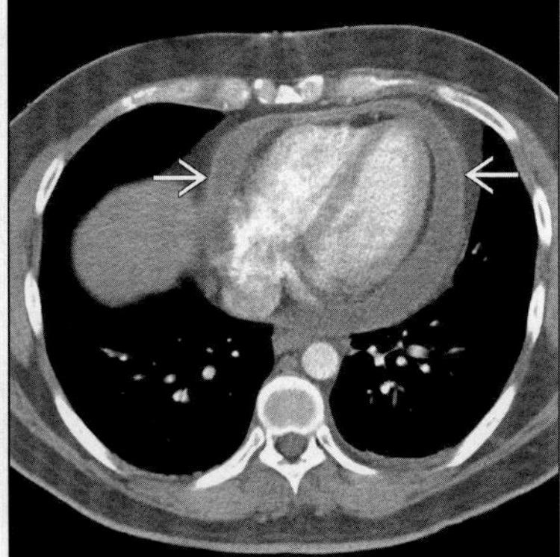

Exudative Effusion

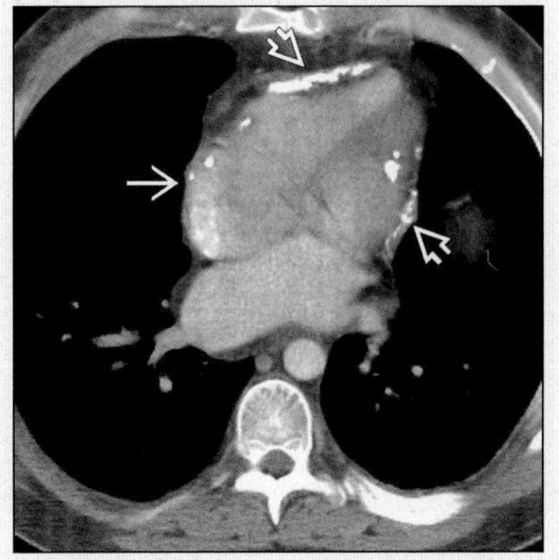

Constriction

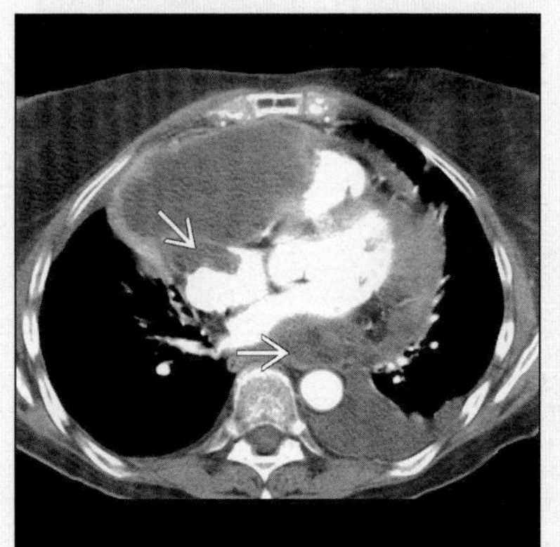

Metastatic Disease

PERICARDIAL EFFUSION

Key Facts

Terminology

- Transudate, exudate, or blood in pericardial sac

Imaging Findings

- CT may assess size and distribution of effusion
- Can characterize blood, exudate, chyle, serous fluid
- Can determine if associated pleural thickening

Pathology

- May develop post myocardial infarction
- Acute MI
- Dressler syndrome

Clinical Issues

- Symptoms dependent on rate of fluid accumulation
- Cardiovascular: Chest pain, pressure, discomfort, light-headedness, syncope, palpitations
- Conservative management if asymptomatic
- Pericardiocentesis
- Pericardial window

- ○ Congestive heart failure
- ○ Valvular heart disease
- ○ May develop post myocardial infarction
  - ▪ Acute MI
  - ▪ Dressler syndrome
- ○ Nephrogenic pericarditis
  - ▪ Uremia in patient who has not been dialyzed
  - ▪ Dialysis patient
- ○ Connective tissue disorders
  - ▪ RA, SLE, PSS
- ○ Drugs
  - ▪ Procainamide, hydralazine, isoniazid, methysergide, phenytoin, anticoagulants
- ○ Aortic dissection
  - ▪ Rupture into pericardium resulting in hemopericardium and tamponade
- ○ Trauma
- ○ Neoplasm
  - ▪ May be solid pericardial nodules
- ○ Myxedema
- ○ Radiation
- ○ Chylopericardium
- Epidemiology: 3.4% of necropsies

Gross Pathologic & Surgical Features

- Thickening of pericardium
- May be transudative, exudative, hemorrhagic
- Aspirate can be nonspecific

CLINICAL ISSUES

Presentation

- Most common signs/symptoms
  - ○ Symptoms dependent on rate of fluid accumulation
  - ○ Cardiovascular: Chest pain, pressure, discomfort, light-headedness, syncope, palpitations
  - ○ Respiratory: Cough, dyspnea, hoarseness

Demographics

- Gender: No gender predilection

Natural History & Prognosis

- Depends on etiology

Treatment

- Conservative management if asymptomatic
  - ○ NSAIDS, corticosteroids, colchicine
- Pericardiocentesis
  - ○ Can be deferred if suspected viral pericarditis or in uremic or dialysis patients
  - ○ Diagnostic procedure if suspected infection
  - ○ Therapeutic procedure if progressive or persistent effusion, tamponade
- Pericardial window

SELECTED REFERENCES

1. Rienmuller et al: CT and MR imaging of pericardial disease. Radiol Clin N Am. 42:587-601, 2004

IMAGE GALLERY

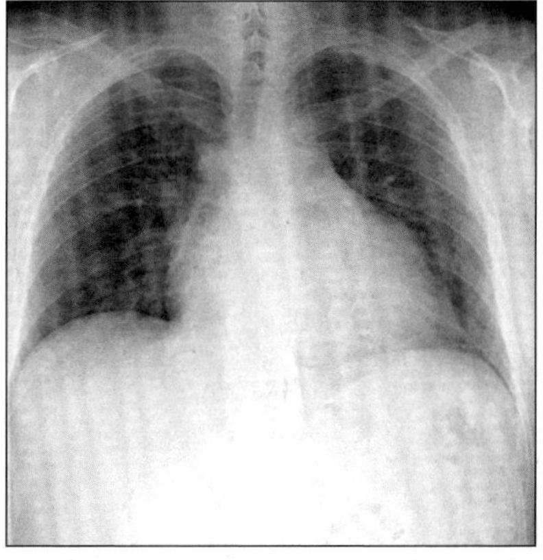
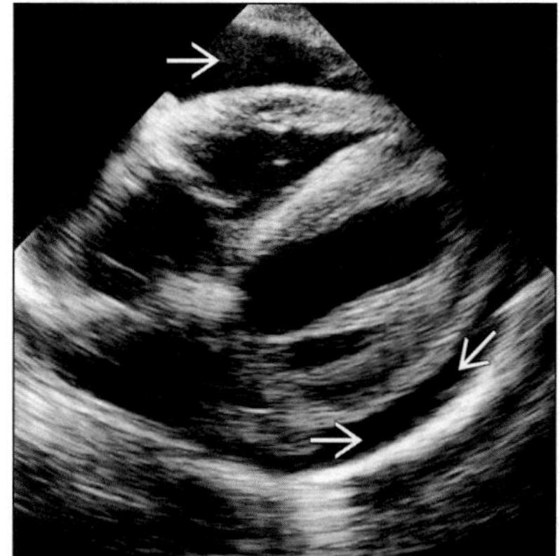
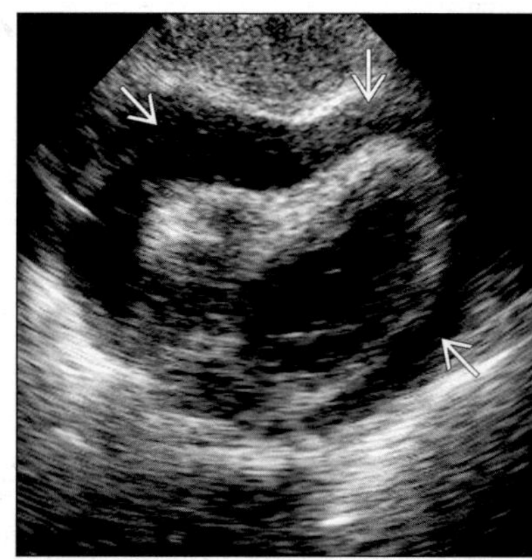

(Left) *Posteroanterior radiograph shows "water bottle" heart. (Courtesy A. Shabaan, MD).* ***(Center)*** *Four chamber view shows a large hypoechoic collection surrounding the heart representing a pericardial effusion ➔. (Courtesy B. Wilson, MD).* ***(Right)*** *Axial shows another large effusion in a patient with tamponade physiology ➔. (Courtesy B. Wilson, MD).*

PERICARDIAL TAMPONADE

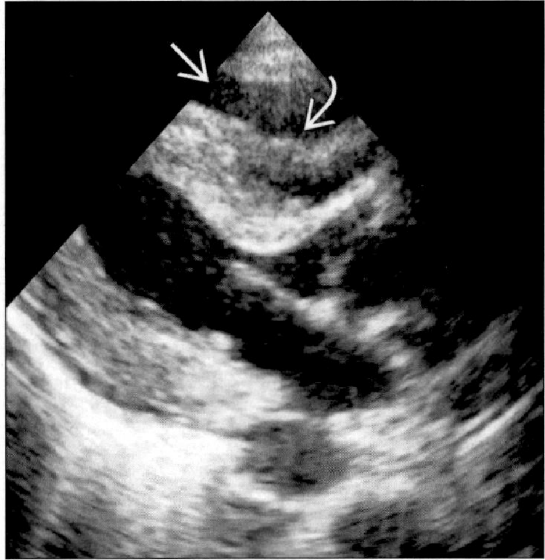

Parasternal long-axis echocardiogram in a 40 year old female with viral pericarditis shows pericardial effusion ➔ and diastolic inversion of the right ventricular free wall ➔.

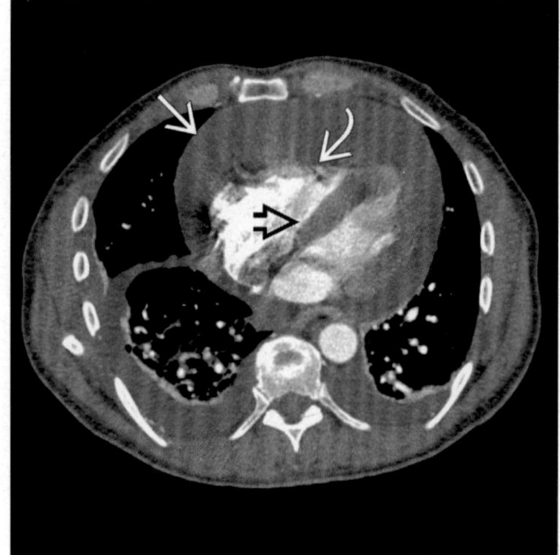

Axial CT in a 60 year old male with gastric cancer shows pericardial effusion ➔, compression of the right ventricular free wall ➔ and straightening of the interventricular septum ➔.

TERMINOLOGY

Definitions

- Fluid accumulation > 50 ml in the pericardial space resulting in impaired diastolic ventricular filling
  - Because this is a finite space, rapidly increasing fluid volumes can lead to cardiac compression
  - Small increases in intrapericardiac fluid may be well tolerated until a critical intrapericardial volume is reached
  - At this point, intrapericardiac pressure rises sharply, and cardiac output drops
- Presentation is related to chronicity of effusion: Slowly developing effusions are better tolerated than rapidly accumulating effusions
  - Treatment for acute tamponade involves pericardiocentesis

IMAGING FINDINGS

General Features

- Best diagnostic clue: Rapid increase in cardiac silhouette on serial chest radiographs
- Location: Pericardial space between the visceral (adjacent to the heart) and parietal (adjacent to the mediastinum) pericardium

Radiographic Findings

- Rapid increase in cardiac silhouette on serial chest radiographs
- "Water bottle configuration" with symmetrically enlarged silhouette
- Loss of retrosternal clear space
- "Fat pad sign": Separation of the retrosternal from the epicardial fat line
- "Differential density sign": Increased lucency around the heart margin secondary to effusion
- Normal lung parenchyma

Fluoroscopic Findings

- Pericardiocentesis is traditional gold standard for treatment
  - Often right catheterization is performed in addition
  - Allows monitoring of right heart pressures as pericardial fluid is removed

DDx: Possible Causes of Pericardial Effusion

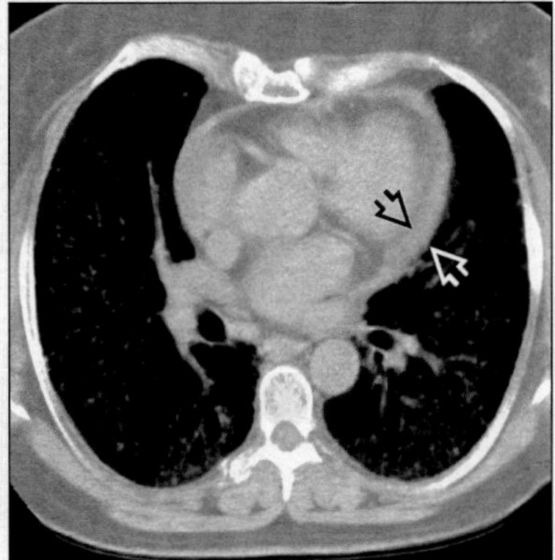

Malignant

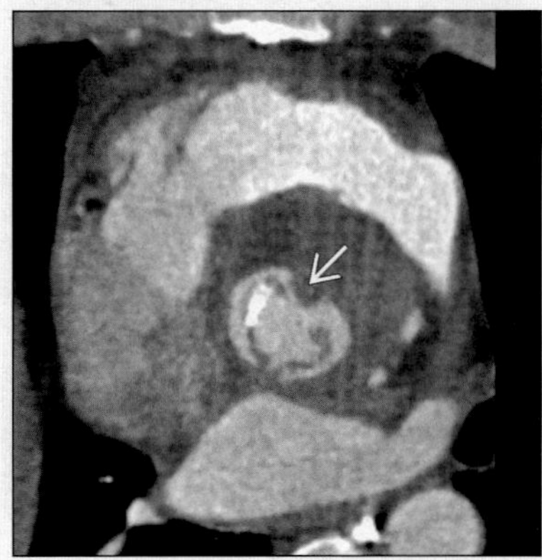

Infective Endocarditis

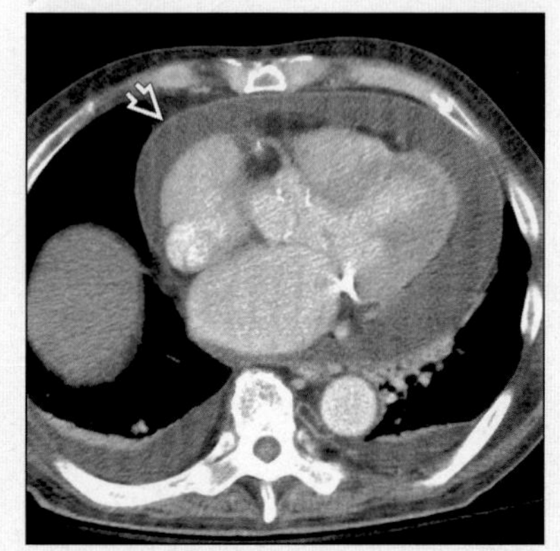

Pyopericardium

PERICARDIAL TAMPONADE

Key Facts

Terminology

- Fluid accumulation > 50 ml in the pericardial space resulting in impaired diastolic ventricular filling
- Presentation is related to chronicity of effusion: Slowly developing effusions are better tolerated than rapidly accumulating effusions

Imaging Findings

- Best diagnostic clue: Rapid increase in cardiac silhouette on serial chest radiographs
- Pericardiocentesis is traditional gold standard for treatment
- Allows monitoring of right heart pressures as pericardial fluid is removed
- Best imaging tool: Echocardiography showing > 50 ml that has accumulated over a short space time period

Top Differential Diagnoses

- Serous Pericardial Effusion
- Hemorrhagic Pericardial Effusion
- Fibrinous Pericardial Effusion
- Lymphatic Pericardial Effusion

Clinical Issues

- Spectrum of severity, ranging from asymptomatic to mild cardiac decompensation to complete cardiovascular collapse
- Pulsus paradoxus is a hallmark of cardiac tamponade: Defined as an inspiratory drop of > 10 mm Hg in systolic blood pressure
- Pericardiocentesis for acute tamponade

  - Initial elevated right atrial pressures with large X descent and diminished Y descent: As fluid is drained intrapericardial fluid decreases below interatrial pressure
  - If it does not, constrictive pericarditis should be considered

CT Findings

- Presence of > 50 ml pericardial fluid
- Dilated inferior vena cava and superior vena cava
- Deformed ventricular contour
- Angulation of interventricular septum
- Effusion density > 35 Hounsfield units is suggestive of hemorrhagic effusion
- Mediastinal lymphadenopathy is suggestive of tuberculous or neoplastic etiology
- Reflux of contrast into an enlarged azygous vein is a sensitive but nonspecific sign of tamponade
- Congestive hepatomegaly with periportal edema

MR Findings

- Presence of > 50 ml pericardial effusion
- Functional images may demonstrate
  - Collapse of right atrium and ventricle and enlarged systemic veins
- May demonstrate septations or enhancement, suggesting
  - Infection
  - Neoplasm
- May demonstrate pericardial masses, indicating neoplastic etiology
- Sensitive for blood clots

Echocardiographic Findings

- Presence of > 50 ml pericardial fluid accumulating over a short time period
- Right atrial and ventricular collapse
- Presence of loculations may suggest infection

Imaging Recommendations

- Best imaging tool: Echocardiography showing > 50 ml that has accumulated over a short space time period

DIFFERENTIAL DIAGNOSIS

Serous Pericardial Effusion

- Congestive heart failure
- Any cause of hypoalbuminemia

Hemorrhagic Pericardial Effusion

- Iatrogenic (most common cause)
- Trauma
- Acute myocardial infarction
- Neoplasm
  - Metastases (lung, breast, melanoma, leukemia, lymphoma)
  - Mesothelioma
  - Angiosarcoma
  - Teratoma

Fibrinous Pericardial Effusion

- Infection
  - Viral
  - Pyogenic
  - Tuberculosis (TB)
- Uremia
- Connective tissue disease
  - Rheumatoid arthritis
  - Systemic lupus erythematosus (SLE)
  - Acute rheumatic fever

Lymphatic Pericardial Effusion

- Neoplasm
- Congenital
- Iatrogenic

PATHOLOGY

General Features

- Etiology
  - Viral pericarditis
    - Most commonly echo or coxsackie virus
  - Hemorrhagic
    - Dissecting aortic aneurysm rupture into pericardial space

        - Traumatic or iatrogenic
    - Acute myocardial infarction
    - Renal failure
    - Neoplastic

CLINICAL ISSUES

Presentation

- Most common signs/symptoms
    - Spectrum of severity, ranging from asymptomatic to mild cardiac decompensation to complete cardiovascular collapse
    - In acute tamponade early features include
        - Tachycardia
        - Dyspnea
        - Edema
        - Elevated venous pressure
        - As volumes increase, intrapericardiac pressure rises and profound cardiovascular collapse and shock occur
    - In subacute or chronic tamponade signs of right heart failure predominate which include
        - Edema
        - Hepatomegaly
        - Ascites
        - Pleural effusions
- Other signs/symptoms
    - Pulsus paradoxus is a hallmark of cardiac tamponade: Defined as an inspiratory drop of > 10 mm Hg in systolic blood pressure
        - Falling blood pressure
        - Distant heart sounds
        - Pericardial friction rub
    - Distended jugular veins, and dyspnea may be only clinical clue
    - EKG shows
        - Reduced voltage
        - ST elevation
        - PR depression
        - Does not differentiate between tamponade and non-compressive effusions

Treatment

- Pericardiocentesis for acute tamponade
    - If effusion large, pericardial window
    - If effusion recurrent, pigtail drainage catheter

SELECTED REFERENCES

1. Cheng MF et al: Cardiac tamponade as manifestation of advanced thymic carcinoma. Heart Lung. 34(2):136-41, 2005
2. Hussain SM et al: Superior vena cava perforation and cardiac tamponade after filter placement in the superior vena cava--a case report. Vasc Endovascular Surg. 39(4):367-70, 2005
3. Klein SV et al: CT directed diagnostic and therapeutic pericardiocentesis: 8-year experience at a single institution. Emerg Radiol. 11(6):353-63, 2005
4. Weich HS et al: Large pericardial effusions due to systemic lupus erythematosus: a report of eight cases. Lupus. 14(6):450-7, 2005
5. Chang K et al: Infective endocarditis of the aortic valve complicated by massive pericardial effusion and rupture of a sinus of valsalva into the right atrium. J Am Soc Echocardiogr. 17(8):910-2, 2004
6. Cherian G et al: Tuberculous pericardial effusion: features, tamponade, and computed tomography. Angiology. 55(4):431-40, 2004
7. Collins D: Aetiology and management of acute cardiac tamponade. Crit Care Resusc. 6(1):54-8, 2004
8. Gulati GS et al: Pericardial abscess occurring after tuberculous pericarditis: image morphology on computed tomography and magnetic resonance imaging. Clin Radiol. 59(6):514-9, 2004
9. Habashy AG et al: The electrocardiogram in large pericardial effusion: the forgotten "P" wave and the influence of tamponade, size, etiology, and pericardial thickness on QRS voltage. Angiology. 55(3):303-7, 2004
10. Imazio M et al: Clinical management of acute pericardial disease: a review of results and outcomes. Ital Heart J. 5(11):803-17, 2004
11. Kabukcu M et al: Pericardial tamponade and large pericardial effusions: causal factors and efficacy of percutaneous catheter drainage in 50 patients. Tex Heart Inst J. 31(4):398-403, 2004
12. Oyama N et al: Computed tomography and magnetic resonance imaging of the pericardium: anatomy and pathology. Magn Reson Med Sci. 3(3):145-52, 2004
13. Tsolakis EJ et al: Cardiac tamponade rapidly evolving toward constrictive pericarditis and shock as a first manifestation of noncardiac cancer. J Card Surg. 19(2):134-5, 2004
14. Hsu LF et al: Transcardiac pericardiocentesis: an emergency life-saving technique for cardiac tamponade. J Cardiovasc Electrophysiol. 14(9):1001-3, 2003
15. Sievers B et al: Cardiovascular magnetic resonance of imminent cardiac tamponade due to postpericardiotomy syndrome. Int J Cardiol. 91(2-3):241-4, 2003
16. Spodick DH: Acute cardiac tamponade. N Engl J Med. 349(7):684-90, 2003
17. Kuvin JT et al: Postoperative cardiac tamponade in the modern surgical era. Ann Thorac Surg. 74(4):1148-53, 2002
18. Wintermark M et al: Blunt trauma of the heart: CT pattern of atrial appendage ruptures. Eur Radiol. 11(1):113-6, 2001
19. Aikat S et al: A review of pericardial diseases: clinical, ECG and hemodynamic features and management. Cleve Clin J Med. 67(12):903-14, 2000
20. Atar S et al: Bloody pericardial effusion in patients with cardiac tamponade: is the cause cancerous, tuberculous, or iatrogenic in the 1990s? Chest. 116(6):1564-9, 1999
21. Harries SR et al: Azygos reflux: a CT sign of cardiac tamponade. Clin Radiol. 53(9):702-4, 1998
22. Kirchner J et al: Primary congenital pulmonary lymphangiectasia--a case report. Wien Klin Wochenschr. 109(23):922-4, 1997
23. Duvernoy O et al: CT-guided pericardiocentesis. Acta Radiol. 37(5):775-8, 1996
24. Hernandez-Luyando L et al: Tension pericardial collections: sign of 'flattened heart' in CT. Eur J Radiol. 23(3):250-2, 1996
25. Goldstein L et al: CT diagnosis of acute pericardial tamponade after blunt chest trauma. AJR Am J Roentgenol. 152(4):739-41, 1989
26. Wolverson MK et al: Demonstration of unsuspected malignant disease of the pericardium by computed tomography. J Comput Tomogr. 4(4):330-3, 1980

PERICARDIAL TAMPONADE

IMAGE GALLERY

Typical

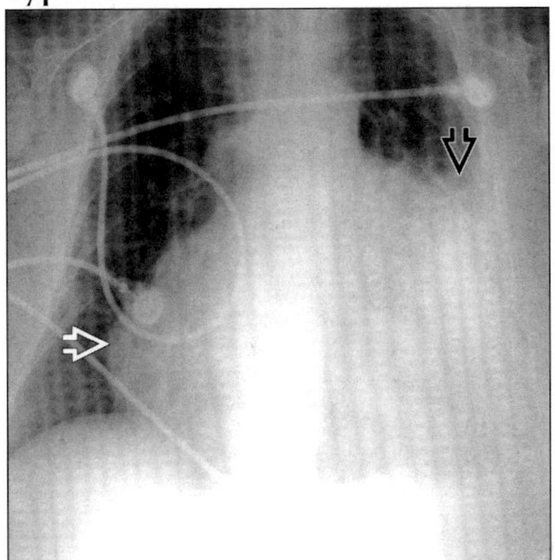

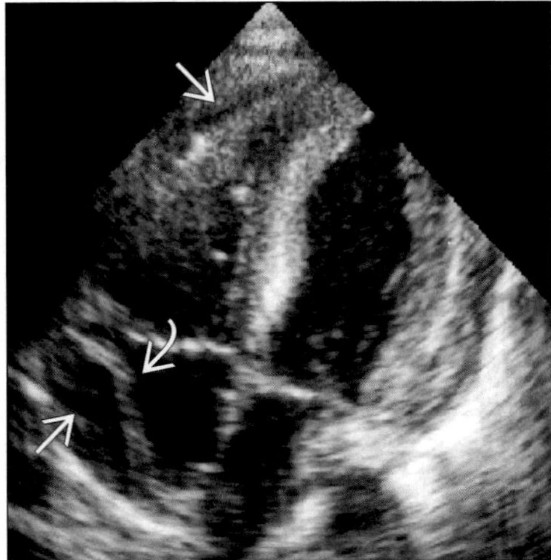

(Left) *Chest radiograph in 72 year old female with viral pericarditis shows enlarged, globular cardiac silhouette consistent with large pericardial effusion. Note also the left-sided pleural effusion.* ***(Right)*** *Echocardiogram shows pericardial effusion and right atrial inversion suggesting acute tamponade.*

Typical

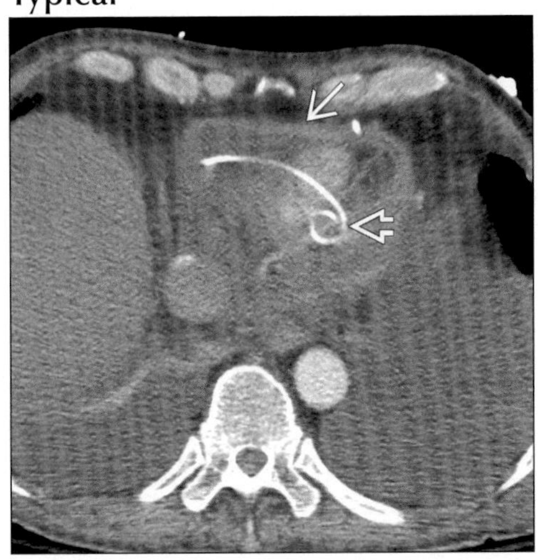

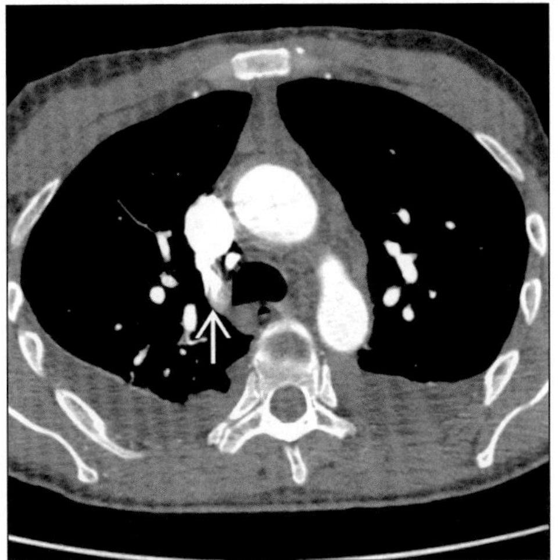

(Left) *Axial CECT in a 72 year old female with end stage renal failure shows an enhancing thickened pericardium and pericardial effusion. Pericardial pigtail drain was required for acute tamponade.* ***(Right)*** *Axial CECT in 60 year old male with pericardial effusion shows enlarged superior vena cava and reflux of contrast into azygous vein, a sensitive sign of tamponade in the setting of large pericardial effusion.*

Typical

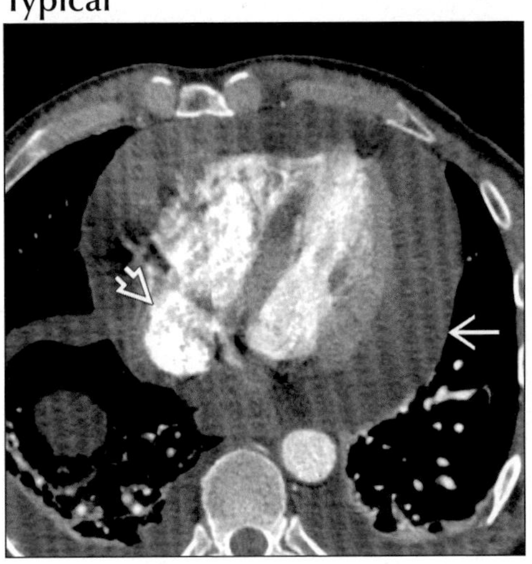

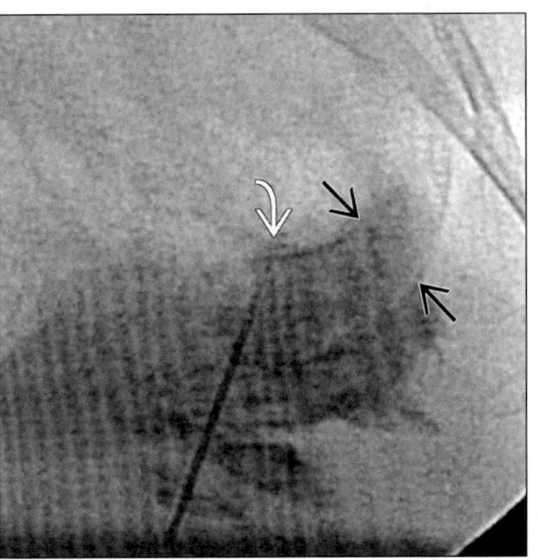

(Left) *Axial CECT shows enlargement of the inferior vena cava, a sensitive sign of tamponade in the setting of large pericardial effusion.* ***(Right)*** *Fluoroscopy shows an iatrogenic pericardiocentesis injury in a 47 year old female with end stage renal disease. Note contrast injection into the myocardium resulting in hemorrhagic tamponade.*

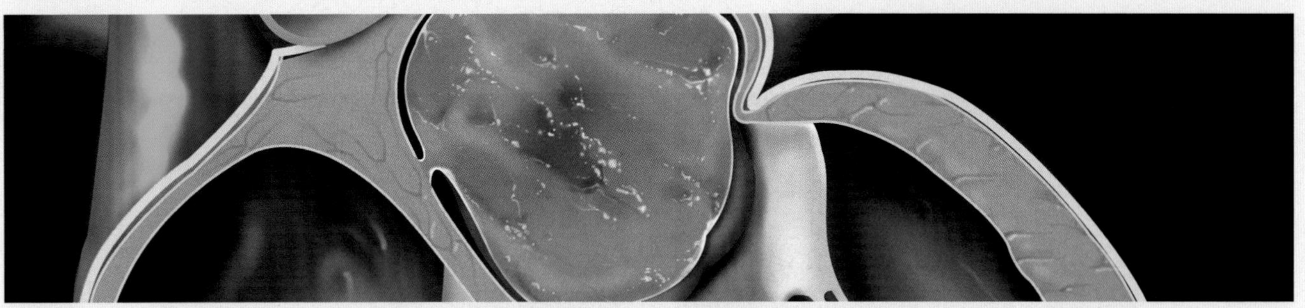

SECTION 4: Neoplastic

ATRIAL MYXOMA

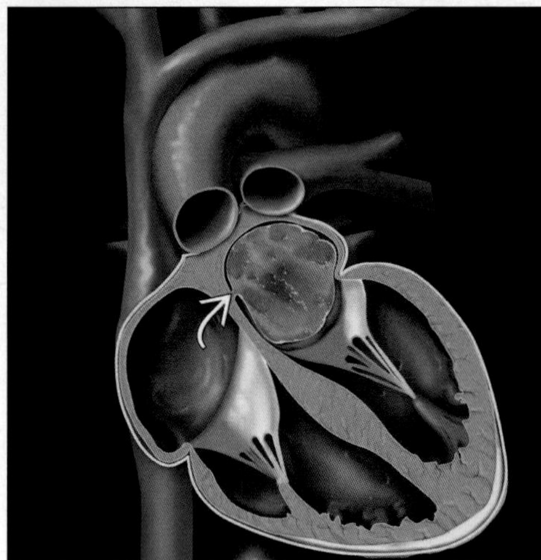

Four chamber view graphic shows typical left atrial myxoma with thin short stalk ➡ connecting to atrial septum. Note heterogeneous composition and mitral inflow obstruction.

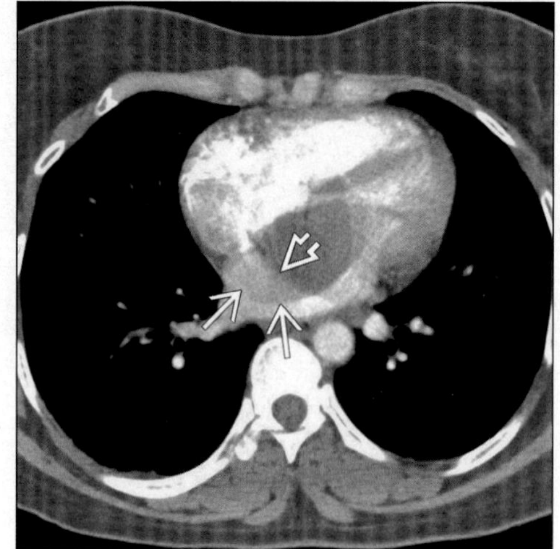

Axial non-gated CT shows atrial myxoma. Double contour represents tumor outline in diastole ➡ and systole ➡, and provides limited functional information (prolapse in and out off mitral anulus).

TERMINOLOGY

Abbreviations and Synonyms

- Myxoma

Definitions

- Most common primary tumor of the heart

IMAGING FINDINGS

General Features

- Best diagnostic clue
  - Generally requires cross-sectional imaging to visualize
  - Chest radiograph generally normal
    - Unless tumor obstructs valve (mitral or tricuspid), then findings consistent with valvular stenosis
- Location
  - Approximately 85% are located in the left atrium attached to atrial septum, usually at fossa ovalis
  - Most of the rest are in the right atrium
  - Occasionally biatrial
  - Rare sites
    - Inferior vena cava
    - Left ventricle
    - Right ventricle
    - Valve leaflets
- Size: 1-15 cm diameter
- Morphology
  - Usually single, may be multiple in familial forms
  - About 2/3 are smooth surfaced
  - About 1/3 are villous
    - Villous tumors are more likely to develop embolic complications

Radiographic Findings

- Radiography
  - Generally no abnormality of contour of heart on plain films
    - May be calcified, especially if origin right atrium
  - If tumor obstructs mitral valve, findings may mimic mitral stenosis
    - Enlarged left atrium
    - Pulmonary vascular congestion
    - May prolapse across mitral or tricuspid valve

CT Findings

- NECT

DDx: Atrial Myxoma

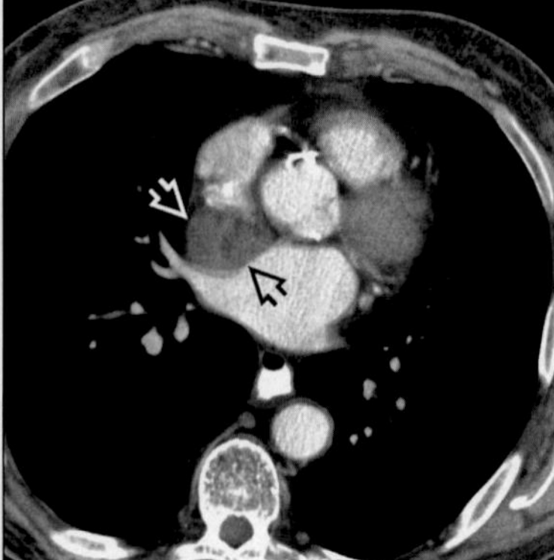

Metastasis

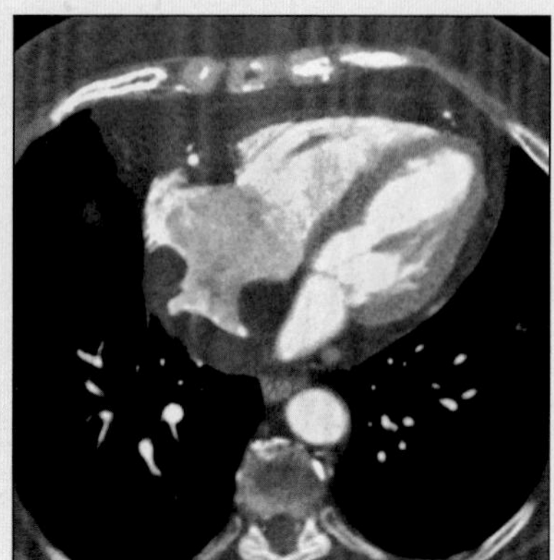

Lipomatous Hypertrophy

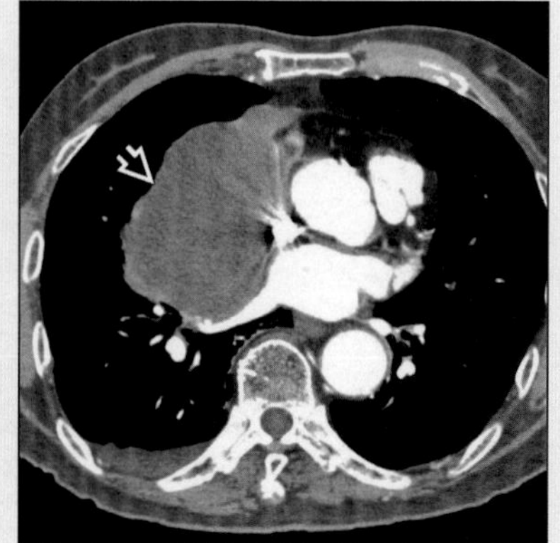

Squamous Cell Carcinoma

ATRIAL MYXOMA

Key Facts

Terminology
- Most common primary tumor of the heart

Imaging Findings
- Approximately 85% are located in the left atrium attached to atrial septum, usually at fossa ovalis
- Size: 1-15 cm diameter
- Villous tumors are more likely to develop embolic complications
- If tumor obstructs mitral valve, findings may mimic mitral stenosis
- Calcification is seen in about half of tumors in the right atrium
- Cardiac ultrasound can be useful to assess mobility of tumor
- Best imaging tool: Echocardiography

Top Differential Diagnoses
- Intracardiac Thrombosis
- Cardiac Metastasis
- Cardiac Lipoma
- Primary Cardiac Malignancies
- Cardiac Lymphoma

Clinical Issues
- Symptoms of valvular obstruction (40%)
- Constitutional (30%): Fatigue, weight loss, fever
- Peripheral embolization (50% to brain causing stroke or mycotic aneurysms)
- Gender: Approximately 60% female
- May become infected, producing fever, weight loss and septic emboli
- May recur after removal in 5%

- Tumor may not be visible without intravenous contrast
- May be hypodense compared to blood
- Calcification is seen in about half of tumors in the right atrium
- Calcification is rare in left atrial tumors

- CECT
  - Filling defect in cardiac chamber
    - Ovoid lesion with lobular (75%) or smooth (25%) contour
    - About 80% are low attenuation on CT
    - Generally no contrast-enhancement
    - Occasionally cystic
    - May have stalk
    - May change in position during cardiac cycle
    - May prolapse through mitral or tricuspid valve
  - Generally no associated adenopathy
  - Generally no pericardial effusion

MR Findings
- Similar to CT
- Majority are inhomogeneous on MR
  - Iso- or hypointense on T1WI
  - Usually hyperintense on T2WI
  - Positive enhancement with gadolinium (low to moderate)
- Calcification not as well identified as on CT
- May be well visualized without gadolinium using bright blood imaging

Nuclear Medicine Findings
- Positron emission tomography (PET) can show the tumor
- Most have low mitotic rate, not very metabolically active
  - If very active uptake is seen, consider other diagnoses: Angiosarcoma, lymphoma
- May be detected with gated cardiac blood pool scanning

Echocardiographic Findings
- Generally the initial imaging modality
- Hyperechogenic tumor
- Cardiac ultrasound can be useful to assess mobility of tumor
  - Can assess hemodynamic degree of obstruction, myxoma often prolapse through mitral valve
  - Stalk often well visualized

Imaging Recommendations
- Best imaging tool: Echocardiography

DIFFERENTIAL DIAGNOSIS

Intracardiac Thrombosis
- Common, associated with atrial fibrillation and mitral valve disease
- Thrombus in the cardiac chambers can mimic myxoma
- Usually located adjacent to posterior and lateral atrial wall and appendage

Cardiac Metastasis
- May be larger than myxoma
- More often multiple
- More often high grade enhancement
- Often associated with pericardial effusion
- Look for other adjacent metastatic sites: Lung, mediastinum
- Most common primary sites: Lung, breast, melanoma

Cardiac Lipoma
- Often in interatrial septum
- Show fat density on CT and fat signal on MR

Primary Cardiac Malignancies
- Most often angiosarcoma, less common fibrosarcoma and liposarcoma
- Also may have associated pericardial effusion, adenopathy, lung metastases

Cardiac Lymphoma
- Generally have increased uptake on PET scanning
- Look for other areas of involvement: Lung, mediastinum
- Broad based attachment to septum - no stalk

Pericardial Metastases
- Often associated with pericardial effusion
- Often extend beyond the left atrial wall
- Most common primary sites: Lung, breast, melanoma

Pericardial Primary Tumors
- Solitary fibrous tumor
- Cysts

Cardiac Sarcoidosis
- Can rarely produce cardiac masses
- Usually have lung or mediastinal disease typical of sarcoidosis

Cardiac Wegener Granulomatosis
- Very rarely can produce cardiac masses
- Cavitary lung masses

Papillary Fibroelastoma
- Most common tumor of the valvular epithelium
- Solitary (rarely multiple) arising from aortic or mitral valve
- Most have a stalk
- May embolize and cause stroke

PATHOLOGY

General Features
- General path comments: Soft gelatinous or friable frond-like tumor, may be firm
- Genetics
  - Carney complex: Familial cardiac myxoma
    - Less than 10% of all myxomas
- Etiology: Unknown cell of origin, probably primitive mesenchymal cell
- Epidemiology: 90% sporadic
- Associated abnormalities
  - Tumor emboli can lead to intracranial aneurysms
  - Peripheral emboli can lead to ischemic changes
  - If obstructing mitral valve, left atrial enlargement and pulmonary venous congestion
  - If obstructing tricuspid valve, ascites, anasarca
  - Right atrial myxoma may cause pulmonary tumor emboli

Gross Pathologic & Surgical Features
- Hemorrhage, thrombus and hemosiderin present in 80%
- Calcification common in right sided myxomas (50%)

Microscopic Features
- Most commonly rings and syncytial chains of myxoma cells embedded in myxomatous matrix
- May contain hematopoietic, glandular, mesenchymal, and atopic endocrine elements; rarely thymic tissue

CLINICAL ISSUES

Presentation
- Most common signs/symptoms
  - Symptoms of valvular obstruction (40%)
    - Left atrium: Orthopnea, dyspnea
    - Right atrium: Peripheral edema, hepatic congestion, ascites
  - Constitutional (30%): Fatigue, weight loss, fever
  - Arrhythmias
  - Peripheral embolization (50% to brain causing stroke or mycotic aneurysms)
    - Myocardial infarction, from embolization to coronaries
    - In presence of valvular mitral stenosis, can protect from large tumor emboli
- Other signs/symptoms
  - About 70% express interleukin-6 (IL-6)
    - Can lead to symptoms similar to connective tissue disease
  - Elevated erythrocyte sedimentation rate (ESR)
  - May have auscultation findings
    - Resembling mitral valve disease
    - Tumor plop in about 15%
  - May have electrocardiographic abnormalities
    - Mainly signs of left atrial hypertrophy
    - Arrhythmias rarely
    - Transient heart blocks

Demographics
- Age
  - Mean age at presentation is 50
  - Range from 1 month to 81 years
- Gender: Approximately 60% female

Natural History & Prognosis
- Very slow growth
- Some may be managed conservatively in poor operative candidates
- May become infected, producing fever, weight loss and septic emboli
- 3 year survival over 95%

Treatment
- Surgical resection
  - Traditional approach is via median sternotomy
  - May require valve replacement
- May recur after removal in 5%
- Newer minimally invasive techniques promising

DIAGNOSTIC CHECKLIST

Image Interpretation Pearls
- Stalk connecting to atrial septum

SELECTED REFERENCES

1. Niarchos C et al: Ascites and other extracardiac manifestations associated with right atrial myxoma: a case report. Angiology. 56(3):357-60, 2005
2. Grebenc ML et al: Cardiac myxoma: imaging features in 83 patients. Radiographics. 22(3):673-89, 2002
3. Spuentrup E et al: Visualization of cardiac myxoma mobility with real-time spiral magnetic resonance imaging. Circulation. 104(19):E101-1, 2001
4. Araoz PA et al: CT and MR imaging of benign primary cardiac neoplasms with echocardiographic correlation. Radiographics. 20(5):1303-19, 2000

ATRIAL MYXOMA

IMAGE GALLERY

Variant

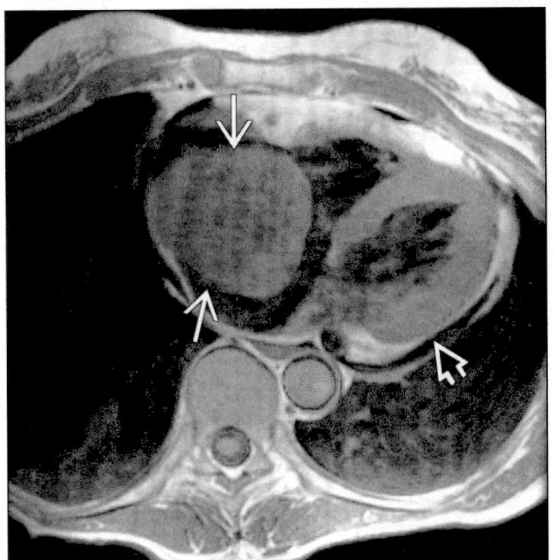

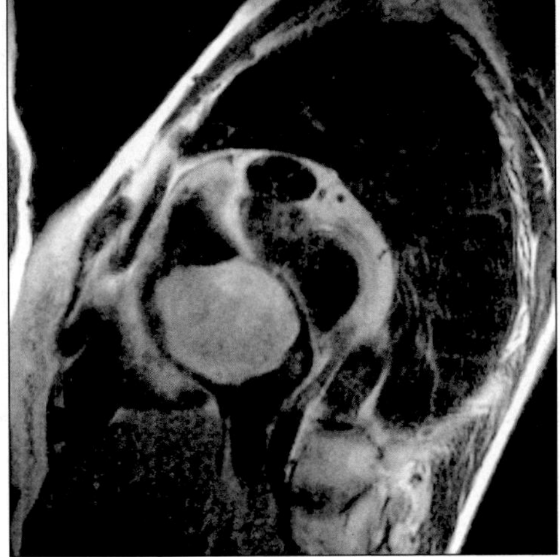

(Left) *Axial T1WI MR shows large, well-delineated, heterogeneous mass → filling most of RA. An attachment to the lateral atrial wall but not to the atrial septum is seen. Note: Small pericardial effusion ⇨.* ***(Right)*** *Coronal T2WI FSE MR shows a high signal intensity mass, consistent with, but not diagnostic of right atrial myxoma. Surgery revealed benign myxoma.*

Typical

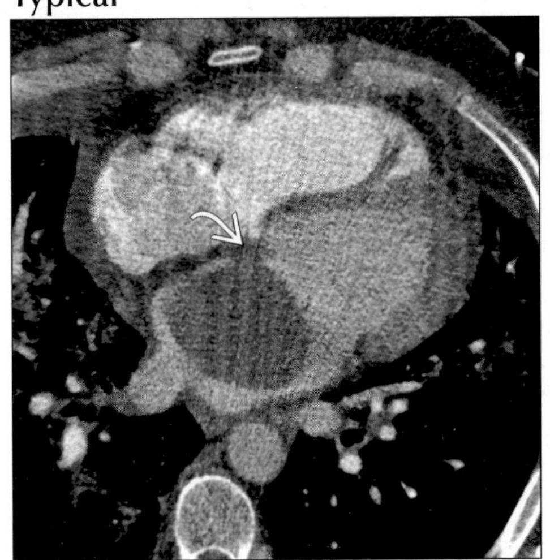

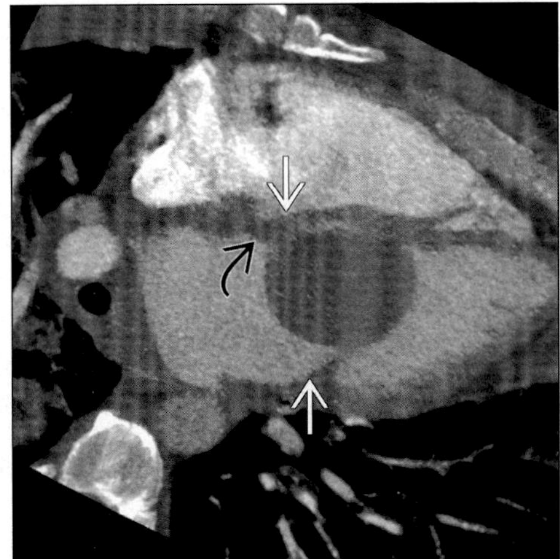

(Left) *Four chamber view coronary CTA in systole shows spheric smooth left atrial mass connected via small stalk ↷ to atrial septum. Note high level of image noise due to EKG tube modulation.* ***(Right)*** *Four chamber view coronary CTA in diastole shows better signal to noise ratio and prolapse of mass through mitral valve annulus →. Note stalk ↷.*

Typical

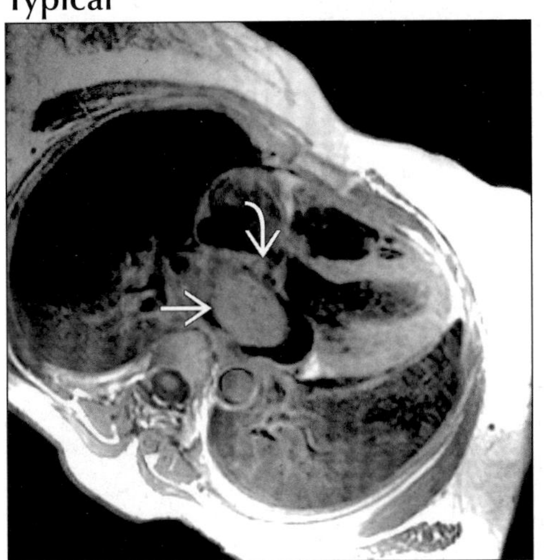

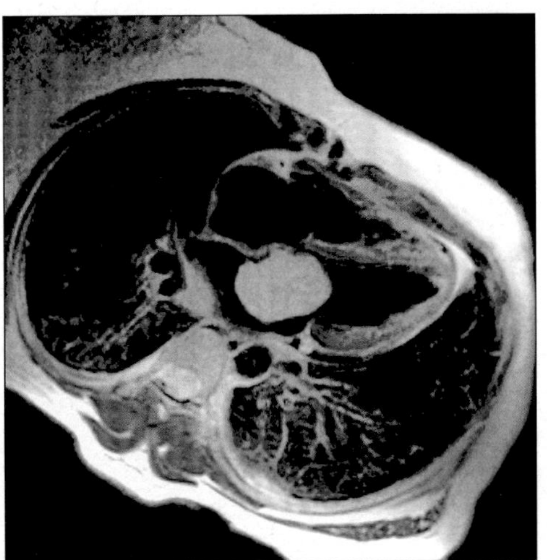

(Left) *Four chamber view T1WI MR shows large left atrial mass → isointense to left ventricular myocardium. One or two short thin stalks are identified ↷.* ***(Right)*** *Four chamber view T2WI MR shows mass now hyperintense compared to myocardium. Mass prolapses through mitral annulus.*

CARDIAC LIPOMA

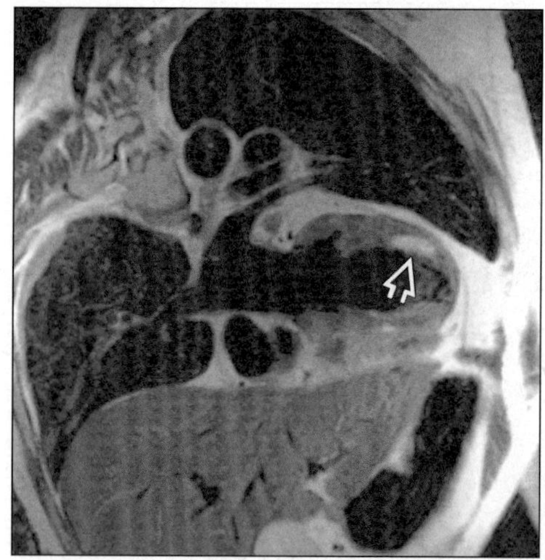

Paraseptal LV long axis black blood T1WI shows intramyocardial, well-defined oval, high signal intensity lesion ➔, with little if any mass effect. No gadolinium was administered.

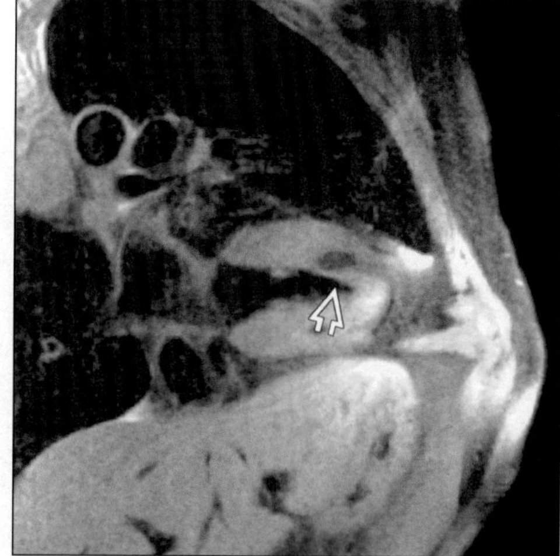

Paraseptal LV long axis black blood T1WI with fat-saturation in the same patient as previous image, shows signal dropout in the lesion ➔, indicating that it is composed completely of fat (lipoma).

TERMINOLOGY

Definitions

- Benign encapsulated cardiac mass consistent of mature adipocytes

IMAGING FINDINGS

General Features

- Best diagnostic clue
  - Follows fat density in all pulse sequences
  - Fat attenuation on CT
- Location
  - Common locations are atrial septum, right atrium (RA) and left ventricle (LV)
  - Most arise from endocardial surface and protrude into chamber lumen
  - May arise from epicardial fat and grow within pericardial space
  - Rarely intramyocardial
  - Rarely arising from valves
  - Rarely multiple lipomas
    - Multiple lipomas have been described in tuberous sclerosis
- Size
  - Variable ranging from few mm to > 15 cm
  - Usually large at time of diagnosis
- Morphology
  - Sessile or polypoid encapsulated mass with sharp demarcation
  - Fat density on CT, typical fat signal on MR

Radiographic Findings

- Radiography
  - Chest radiography findings
    - Usually normal
    - May demonstrate signs of obstruction of valve distal to lipoma if intracavitary
    - May present as mass continuous with pericardium
    - May have calcifications
    - May present as nonspecific cardiomegaly

CT Findings

- NECT
  - Fat density (< -50 HU) within otherwise water density or soft tissue density cardiac chambers/myocardium

DDx: Other Fat Containing Cardiac Lesions

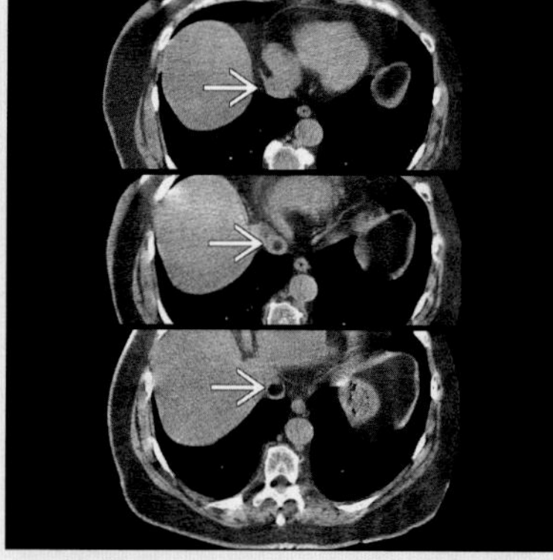

Fat Invagination into IVC

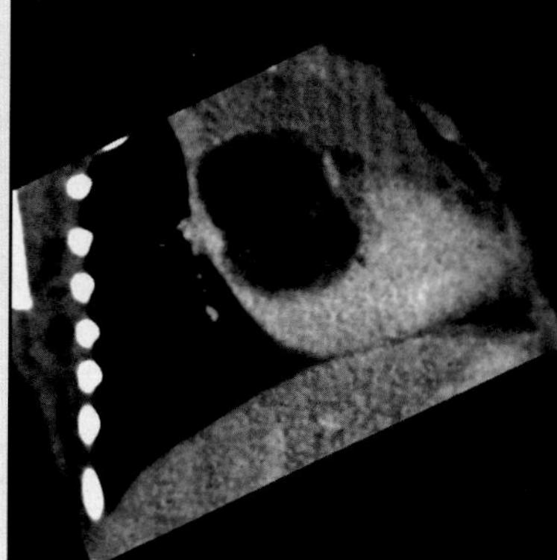

Cardiac Teratoma

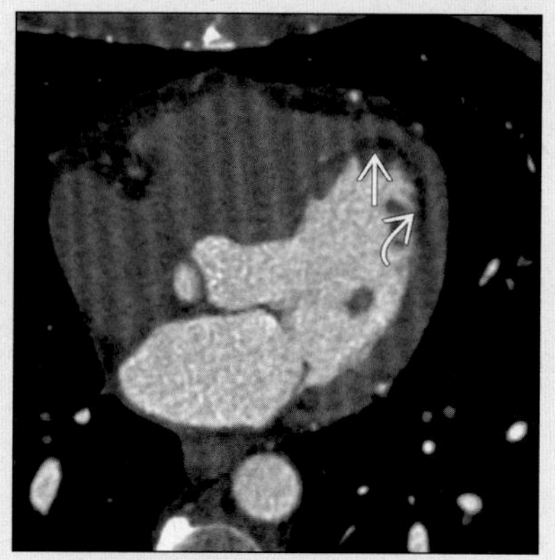

Fat 2° to Myocardial Infarct

CARDIAC LIPOMA

Key Facts

Terminology
- Benign encapsulated mass consistent of mature adipocytes

Imaging Findings
- Follows fat density in all pulse sequences
- Fat attenuation on CT
- Common locations are atrial septum, right atrium (RA) and left ventricle (LV)
- Most arise from endocardial surface and protrude into chamber lumen
- May arise from epicardial fat and grow within pericardial space
- May have thin nonenhancing septation
- Bright mass with dark capsule on T1WI
- T1 C+: No significant enhancement

Top Differential Diagnoses
- Atrial Myxoma
- Liposarcoma
- Metastatic Disease
- Lipomatous Hypertrophy of Intraatrial Septum

Pathology
- Second most common benign primary heart tumor
- True lipomas are encapsulated and contain neoplastic mature adipocytes

Clinical Issues
- May cause arrhythmias
- May cause progressive obstructive or compressive symptoms requiring surgery
- Recurrences post surgery rare

  - Dilatation of obstructed chambers/vasculature
- CECT
  - Fat density mass usually predominantly intraluminal or in epicardial space
    - Filling defect on contrast-enhanced CT
  - May rarely be purely within LV myocardium
  - No significant enhancement
  - No signs of invasion
  - May have thin nonenhancing septation

MR Findings
- T1WI
  - Bright mass with dark capsule on T1WI
  - May demonstrate few thin septations
  - Fat-saturation images demonstrate signal dropout of mass
- T2WI: Follows fat on T2WI
- PD/Intermediate: Follows fat intensity
- T1 C+: No significant enhancement
- MRA: Filling defect in cardiac chambers
- Lipomatous hypertrophy of atrial septum has bilobed appearance due to relative sparing of foramen ovale

Nuclear Medicine Findings
- PET
  - Usually no uptake
  - Lipomatous hypertrophy of interatrial septum however may be hot on FDG PET
    - This is due to presence of brown fat
    - Not a true neoplasm

Echocardiographic Findings
- Echocardiogram
  - Sensitive tool to demonstrate extent and effect on cardiac function
  - Echogenic intraluminal mass
  - Usually broad-based and not very mobile spheric or polypoid mass
  - TEE helpful in guiding transvenous biopsy

Angiographic Findings
- Conventional: Intraatrial or intraventricular filling defect

Imaging Recommendations
- Best imaging tool: MR or CT are usually diagnostic
- Protocol advice
  - Fat-saturation of T1WI helpful in characterizing fat content and visualizing capsule and potential non-fatty components of masses
    - If solid non-fatty components are present, consider alternative diagnoses (teratoma, liposarcoma, etc.)

DIFFERENTIAL DIAGNOSIS

Atrial Myxoma
- Most common benign primary tumor
- Typically left atrium
- Hypointense on T1

Cardiac or Pericardial Teratoma
- Rare tumors, usually present in infancy
- May contain large amount of fat
- May have mature tissues from all three germ cell layers
- May be complicated by cardiac compression and pericardial effusion

Other Primary Benign Tumors
- Usually readily distinguished by signal characteristics on MR

Liposarcoma
- Very rare
- May show invasion of neighboring structures
- May become symptomatic from obstructive symptoms
- Four pathological types: Well-differentiated, myxoid, round cell, pleomorphic

Other Malignant Tumors
- Metastatic disease
- Usually readily distinguished by signal characteristics on MR and HU range on CT

Thrombus
- Most commonly in atria

- Usually does not follow signal characteristics of epicardial fat on all sequences

Lipomatous Hypertrophy of Intraatrial Septum

- Not a true neoplasm
- No capsule present
- Consists of brown fat
- Dumbbell appearance of atrial septum due to sparing of fossa ovalis
- May demonstrate FDG uptake on PET scan

PATHOLOGY

General Features

- General path comments
  - True cardiac lipomas are rare
  - Second most common benign primary heart tumor
  - Usually single subendocardial, myocardial or subpericardial homogeneous circumscribed tumor
- Epidemiology
  - All ages, equal sex distribution
  - More common in overweight patients

Gross Pathologic & Surgical Features

- Most are spherical, sessile or polypoid masses of homogeneous yellow fat
- Usually 1-15 cm but may be up to 4000 g

Microscopic Features

- True lipomas are encapsulated and contain neoplastic mature adipocytes
- Lipomas do not contain brown fetal fat cells
  - Lipomatous hypertrophy of intraatrial septum is characterized by infiltration of mature adult type or fetal fat cells between myocardial fibers with absence of capsule

CLINICAL ISSUES

Presentation

- May be asymptomatic
- May cause arrhythmias
- Subepicardial tumors may cause compression symptoms
- Intraluminal subendocardial tumors may cause location specific symptoms, such as obstruction

Natural History & Prognosis

- Frequently incidentally noted on autopsy
- May cause progressive obstructive or compressive symptoms requiring surgery
- Generally good outcome
- Recurrences post surgery rare

Treatment

- No treatment necessary if asymptomatic
- Surgical resection if symptomatic

DIAGNOSTIC CHECKLIST

Consider

- Repeat T1WI with fat-saturation to prove fatty content

Image Interpretation Pearls

- If soft tissue component consider liposarcoma or teratoma as alternate diagnosis

SELECTED REFERENCES

1. Kosar F et al: A case of a large intrapericardial lipoma occupying pericardial space. J Card Surg. 22(5):427-9, 2007
2. Matsushita T et al: Aortic valve lipoma. Ann Thorac Surg. 83(6):2220-2, 2007
3. Taori K et al: Intrapericardial teratoma diagnosed on CT. J Thorac Imaging. 22(2):185-7, 2007
4. Ou P et al: Images in cardiovascular medicine. Cardiac teratoma in a newborn with right ventricular outflow tract obstruction. Circulation. 113(2):e17-8, 2006
5. Kato S et al: [Cardiac liposarcoma at the right ventricular outflow tract (RVOT) following lipomatous hypertrophy of the interatrial septum (LHIS); report of a case] Kyobu Geka. 57(2):143-6, 2004
6. Uemura S et al: Extensive primary cardiac liposarcoma with multiple functional complications. Heart. 90(8):e48, 2004
7. Frank H: Cardiac and Paracardiac Masses. In: Manning, WJ, Pennell DJ. Cardiovascular Magnetic Resonance. Churchill Livingstone, Philadelphia, 2002
8. Gaerte SC et al: Fat-containing lesions of the chest. Radiographics. 22 Spec No:S61-78, 2002
9. Colucci WS et al: Primary tumors of the heart. In: Braunwald E. Heart Disease: A Textbook of Cardiovascular Medicine. 6th ed. W.B. Saunders Company, Philadelphia, 2001
10. Grebenc ML et al: Primary cardiac and pericardial neoplasms: radiologic-pathologic correlation. Radiographics. 20(4):1073-103, 2000
11. Vander Salm TJ: Unusual primary tumors of the heart. Semin Thorac Cardiovasc Surg. 12(2):89-100, 2000
12. Beghetti M et al: Images in cardiovascular medicine. Intrapericardial teratoma. Circulation. 97(15):1523-4, 1998

CARDIAC LIPOMA

IMAGE GALLERY

Typical

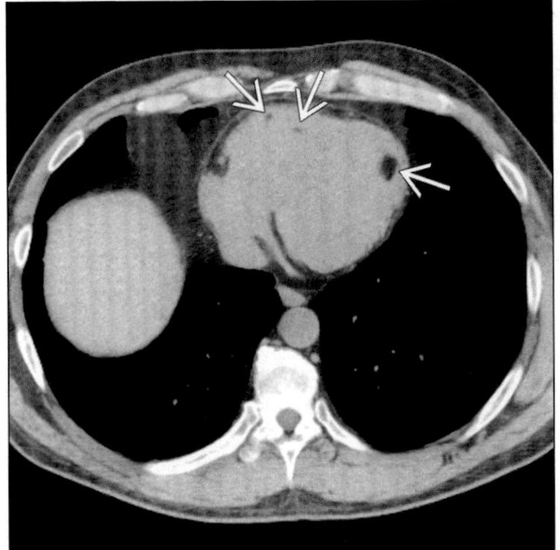

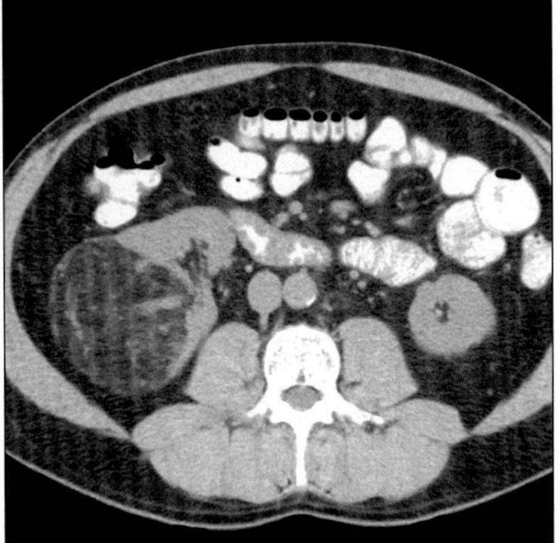

(Left) *Axial NECT shows multiple, intramyocardial, well-defined, rounded, low-attenuation lesions (~ -50 HU), indicating multiple cardiac lipomas →.* ***(Right)*** *Oblique NECT in the same patient as previous image, shows large right renal angiomyolipoma. This constellation of findings is consistent with tuberous sclerosis, which was a known diagnosis in this patient.*

Variant

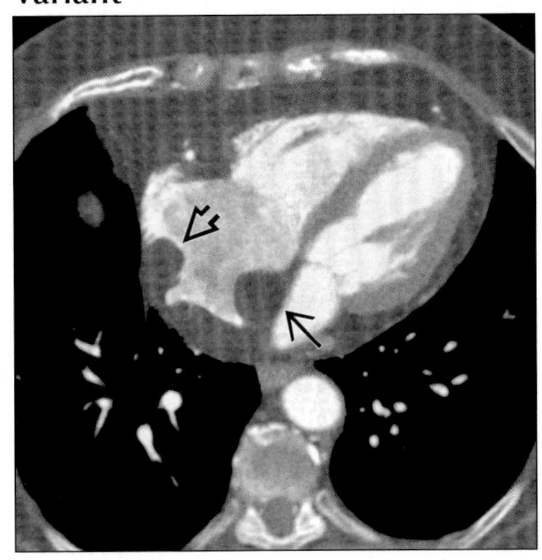

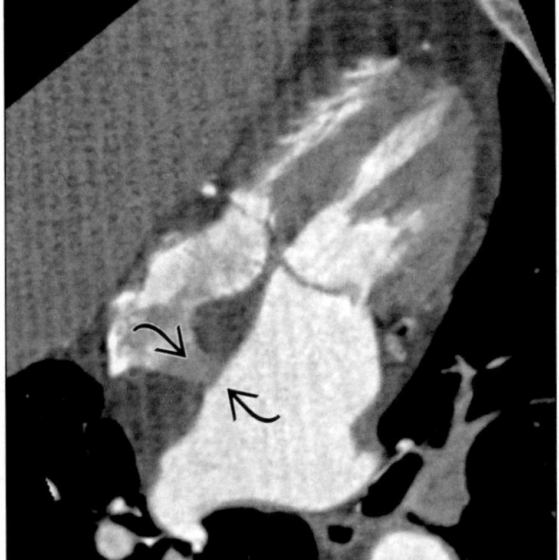

(Left) *Axial coronary CTA shows lipoma of the crista terminals →, which appeared as a right atrial mass on echocardiography. Note presence of lipomatous hypertrophy of the interatrial septum →.* ***(Right)*** *Four chamber view coronary CTA in the same patient as previous image, shows lipomatous hypertrophy with typical dumbbell appearance of interatrial septum due to sparing of the fossa ovalis →.*

Other

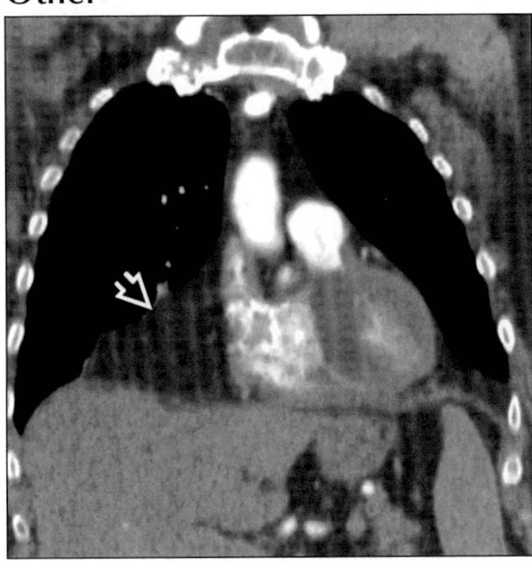

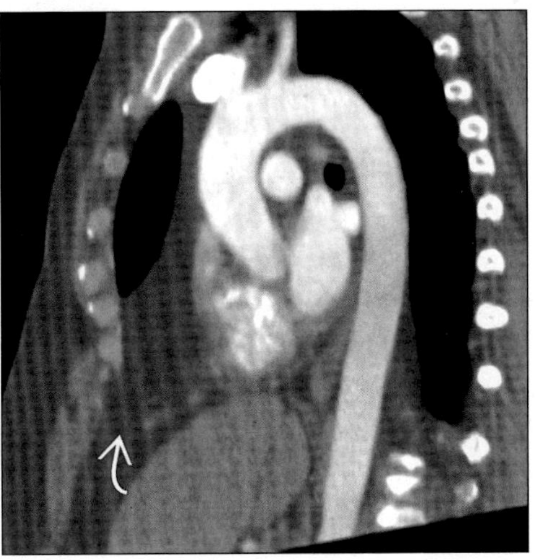

(Left) *Coronal CECT shows large fat-containing mass in right cardiophrenic angle →. The mass is actually extrapericardial and represents a Morgagni hernia.* ***(Right)*** *Oblique CECT in the same patient as previous image, shows a defect in the diaphragm → with extension of omental fat into the thoracic cavity (Morgagni hernia).*

VENTRICULAR THROMBUS

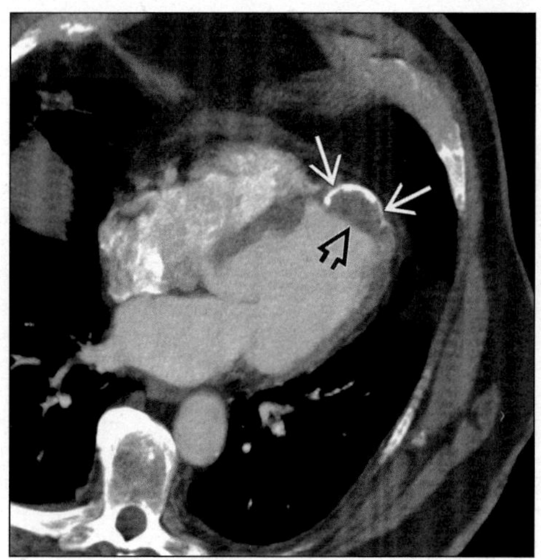

Axial CTA shows apical left ventricular LAD territory infarct with apical linear myocardial calcification ➡, and adjacent mural LV thrombus ⇨.

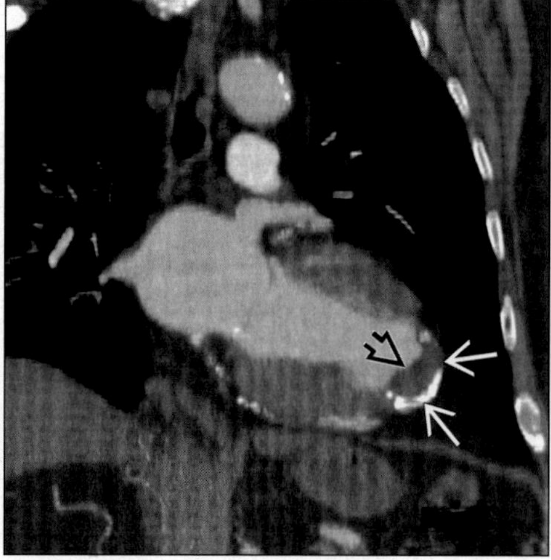

Long axis CTA in the same patient as previous image, shows mural thrombus ⇨ and small calcified apical LV aneurysm ➡.

TERMINOLOGY

Definitions

- Thrombus within ventricle typically due to flow disturbance, akinetic or dyskinetic wall due to prior infarct/aneurysm

IMAGING FINDINGS

General Features

- Best diagnostic clue
  - Intraluminal filling defect
  - Nonenhancing mural rim of tissue lining infarction
    - Underlying infarct may be evident from myocardial thinning, linear myocardial calcification, linear subendocardial fatty metaplasia, aneurysm, or wall-motion abnormality
- Location
  - Left atrium (LA) thrombus common in atrial fibrillation and mitral stenosis
  - Left ventricle (LV) mural thrombus in 40-60% of patients with anterior MI if no anticoagulant therapy
- Size: Variable
- Morphology
  - Broad based lining akinetic wall if due to LV infarct/aneurysm
  - May be ovoid or lobular intraluminal mass or filling defect
    - Often pedunculated connection to wall
    - Mobile

Radiographic Findings

- Radiography
  - Chest radiography finding
    - Only clue may show calcifications projected over an infarcted area
    - May demonstrate bulge from LV aneurysm

CT Findings

- NECT: May demonstrate calcification if old thrombus
- CECT
  - Filling defect and underlying signs of LV infarction
  - Mural thrombus may mimic normal thickness wall

DDx: Ventricular Thrombus

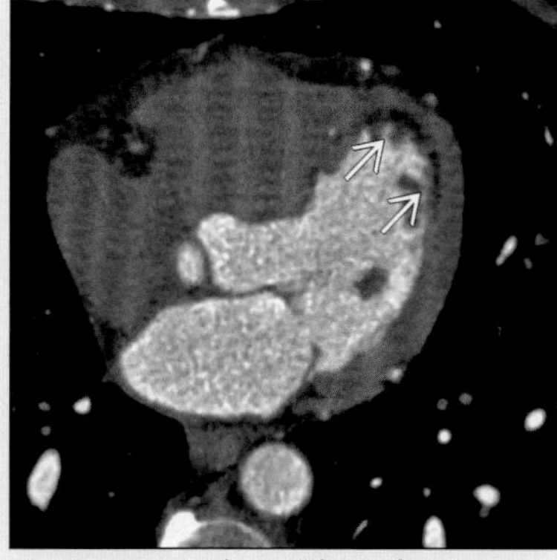

MI without Thrombus

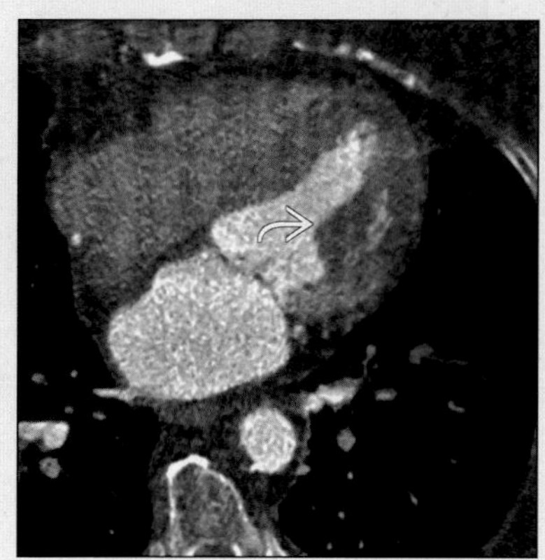

LVH Papillary Muscle

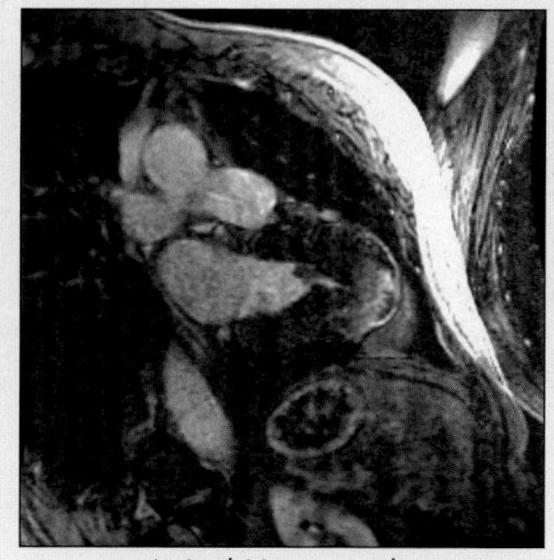

Apical Hypertrophy

VENTRICULAR THROMBUS

Key Facts

Imaging Findings

- Left atrium (LA) thrombus common in atrial fibrillation and mitral stenosis
- Left ventricle (LV) mural thrombus in 40-60% of patients with anterior MI if no anticoagulant therapy
- Criteria for increased risk of embolization
  - Increased mobility, protrusion into the ventricular chamber
- Mural thrombus may mimic normal wall
- Thrombus appears slightly lower in attenuation compared to remote normal myocardium
- Wall-motion abnormality in underlying myocardium
- Related imaging findings
  - Chronic infarct: Myocardial calcification, wall thinning, subendocardial fatty metaplasia, wall-motion abnormality, delayed hyper-enhancement on MR, aneurysm or pseudoaneurysm
  - Acute infarct: Normal thickness myocardium, akinesis, delayed hyper-enhancement and increased T2 signal on MR, subendocardial or transmural perfusion defects on MR or CT

Pathology

- Most frequent intracardiac mass

Clinical Issues

- 10% of mural LV thrombi result in systemic emboli
- Left chambers: Stroke, peripheral emboli
- Right chambers: Pulmonary emboli

  - Look for signs of infarction (calcium or fatty metaplasia)
  - Thrombus appears slightly lower in attenuation compared to remote normal myocardium
- Cardiac Gated CTA
  - Wall-motion abnormality in underlying myocardium
  - May demonstrate mobility of pedunculated thrombi
  - Underlying chronic infarction, aneurysm or pseudoaneurysm may be most obvious finding
    - Laminated mural thrombus may be subtle finding
  - Thrombus usually 35-50 HU whereas remote normal myocardium is 80-100 HU

MR Findings

- Increased signal on spin-echo sequences
  - Pitfall: Slow-flowing blood may also have increased signal on spin echo sequences
- Delayed contrast-enhanced spoiled gradient echo technique is highly sensitive for detecting intra-cardiac thrombus
- No enhancement of thrombus on first pass perfusion or delayed enhanced images
- May be difficult to differentiate from other atrial or ventricular masses
- Usually related findings from infarction
  - Subendocardial defect in coronary territory on first-pass perfusion imaging
  - Subendocardial or transmural delayed hyperenhancement
  - Myocardial thinning
  - Hypo-, a-, or dyskinesia
  - Aneurysm or pseudoaneurysm

Echocardiographic Findings

- Echocardiogram
  - Preferred technique
  - Ventricular thrombi usually anterior and apical
  - May be laminar and adherent to wall or pedunculated and mobile echogenic masses in areas of hypokinesis
  - Criteria for increased risk of embolization
    - Increased mobility, protrusion into the ventricular chamber
    - Visualization in multiple views
    - Contiguous zones of akinesis and hyperkinesis
  - Experimental use of antifibrinogen labeled echogenic immunoliposomes for thrombus specific enhancement of echogenicity

Angiographic Findings

- Conventional
  - Filling defect may be free floating (atrial thrombus ball)
  - May be negative in case thrombus is broadly adherent to wall
    - Only hint may be presence of wall-motion abnormality on ventriculography

Imaging Recommendations

- Best imaging tool: MR or CT

DIFFERENTIAL DIAGNOSIS

Benign Neoplasm

- Frequently intraluminal extension
- Contrast-enhancement excludes fresh thrombus
- Organized thrombus may demonstrate low grade enhancement

Primary or Secondary Malignancy

- Invasion of atrial or ventricular wall and contrast-enhancement exclude thrombus

Vegetation

- Will not resolve with anticoagulation

Pannus

- Typically related to prosthetic valve replacements

Apical Hypertrophic Cardiomyopathy

- MR or cardiac CT helpful for differentiating these

VENTRICULAR THROMBUS

LV Noncompaction or Prominent Normal Trabeculation

- May mimic mural thrombus

PATHOLOGY

General Features

- General path comments: Most frequent intracardiac mass
- Etiology
  - Right atrium (RA) thrombus
    - Low cardiac output state
    - Atrial fibrillation
    - Central catheters or pacemaker wires, transvenous ablation procedures
    - Embolic thrombus from deep venous thrombosis (DVT), or extension of tumor-thrombus from kidney, liver or adrenal glands
    - Rheumatic tricuspid stenosis, heart surgery, cardiomyopathy, extension of tumor-thrombus from kidney, liver or adrenal glands
    - Heart surgery
    - Cardiomyopathy
  - Right ventricle (RV) thrombus
    - Rare, same as RA thrombus
  - LA thrombus
    - Atrial fibrillation most common
    - Mitral stenosis
  - LV thrombus
    - Myocardial infarction (MI), LV aneurysm
  - Rarely LV thrombosis can be found as a sequela of chemotherapy
  - Rarely LV apical thrombus can be the sequela of Takotsubo cardiomyopathy (stress-induced transient "apical ballooning" akinesis)

Gross Pathologic & Surgical Features

- Freshly thrombosed blood at surface, may have organized thrombus in deep layers

Microscopic Features

- May be layered and adherent to myocardium
- Central layers: May be organized
  - Fibroblasts
  - Macrophages
- Superficial layers: Fibrin, platelets and red blood cells

CLINICAL ISSUES

Presentation

- Symptoms of underlying condition
  - Most frequently myocardial infarction
- May be asymptomatic until complication occurs
- Left chambers: Stroke, peripheral emboli
  - 10% of mural LV thrombi result in systemic emboli
- Right chambers: Pulmonary emboli

Demographics

- Age: Parallels that of myocardial infarction as the most common underlying cause

Natural History & Prognosis

- Mural thrombus formation within 48 h to 72 h post MI carries a poor prognosis from associated complications

Treatment

- Anticoagulation for 3-6 months with warfarin
- Aspirin may prevent further platelet deposition
- Percutaneous left atrial appendage transcatheter occlusion in high risk patients with atrial fibrillation to prevent stroke

DIAGNOSTIC CHECKLIST

Consider

- If a presumed thrombus does not resolve with anticoagulation, consider differential diagnoses

SELECTED REFERENCES

1. Korosoglou G et al: Prompt resolution of an apical left ventricular thrombus in a patient with takotsubo cardiomyopathy. Int J Cardiol. 116(3):e88-91, 2007
2. Morlese JF et al: Acute ventricular and aortic thrombosis post chemotherapy. Br J Radiol. 80(952):e75-7, 2007
3. Mueller J et al: Cardiac CT angiography after coronary bypass surgery: prevalence of incidental findings. AJR Am J Roentgenol. 189(2):414-9, 2007
4. Rustemli A et al: Evaluating cardiac sources of embolic stroke with MRI. Echocardiography. 24(3):301-8; discussion 308, 2007
5. Fieno DS et al: Cardiovascular magnetic resonance of primary tumors of the heart: A review. J Cardiovasc Magn Reson. 8(6):839-53, 2006
6. Peters PJ et al: The echocardiographic evaluation of intracardiac masses: a review. J Am Soc Echocardiogr. 19(2):230-40, 2006
7. White RD: MR and CT assessment for ischemic cardiac disease. J Magn Reson Imaging. 19(6):659-75, 2004
8. Mohiaddin RH et al: Valvular Heart Disease. In: Manning, WJ, Pennell DJ. Cardiovascular Magnetic Resonance. Churchill Livingstone, Philadelphia, 2002
9. Antman EM et al: Acute Myocardial Infarction. In: Braunwald E. Heart Disease: A Textbook of Cardiovascular Medicine. 6th ed. W.B. Saunders Company, Philadelphia, 2001
10. Dähnert WF: Radiology Review Manual 4th Ed., Lippincott Williams & Wilkins, Philadelphia. 316, 1999
11. Dinarevic S et al: Left ventricular pannus causing inflow obstruction late after mitral valve replacement for endocardial fibroelastosis. Pediatr Cardiol. 17(4):257-9, 1996

VENTRICULAR THROMBUS

IMAGE GALLERY

Typical

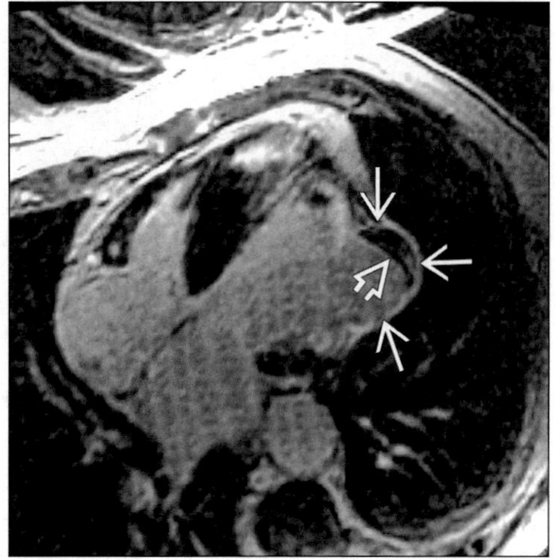

(Left) *LV short axis DE MR shows delayed hyper-enhancement in the RCA territory with pseudoaneurysm formation → and unenhanced mural thrombus → lining the pseudoaneurysm.* ***(Right)*** *Four chamber view DE MR in the same patient as previous image, shows hyper-enhanced wall (consistent of epicardium ± fibrosis, typically fused with pericardium) of pseudoaneurysm →, and unenhanced thrombus →.*

Variant

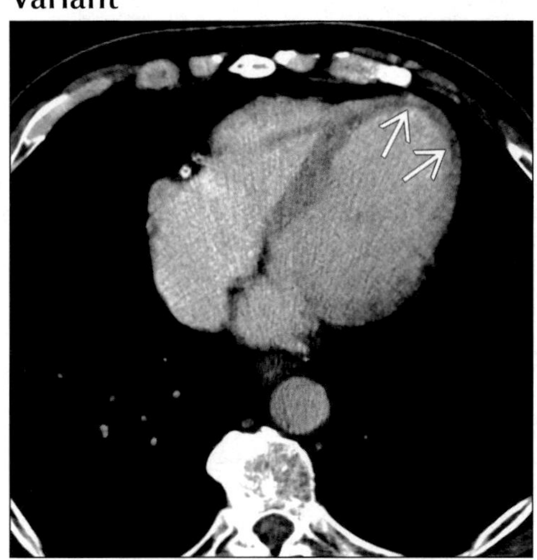

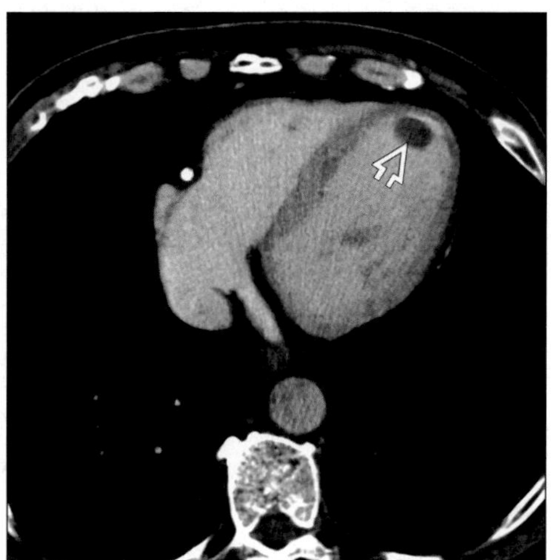

(Left) *Axial CECT shows thinning and fatty metaplasia of LV apex →, indicating remote myocardial infarction. No thrombus is seen on this level.* ***(Right)*** *Axial CECT in the same patient as previous image, shows oval thrombus in LV apex →, which has focal areas of attachment to the LV wall, but is not broadly mural based.*

Typical

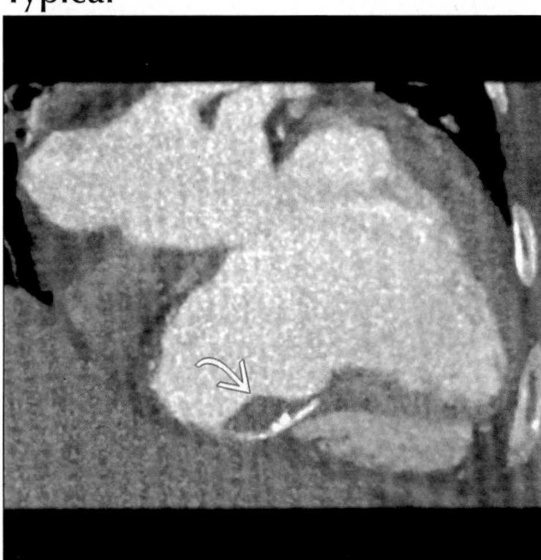

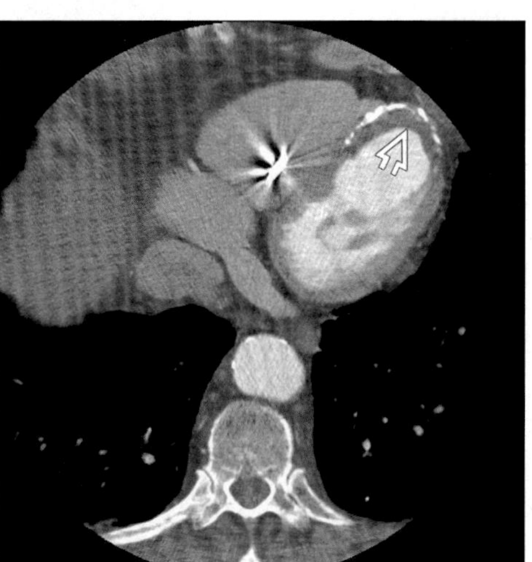

(Left) *Long axis cardiac CT shows basal inferior thin-walled aneurysm with a broad connection to the LV cavity and mural thrombus →. Note: Lower attenuation of thrombus compared to normal myocardium.* ***(Right)*** *Axial CTA shows apical LV aneurysm with thin calcified wall and broad-based, non-enhanced, mural thrombus →. Note: Mural thrombus can mimic normal myocardium, especially in absence of calcium.*

CARDIAC SARCOMA

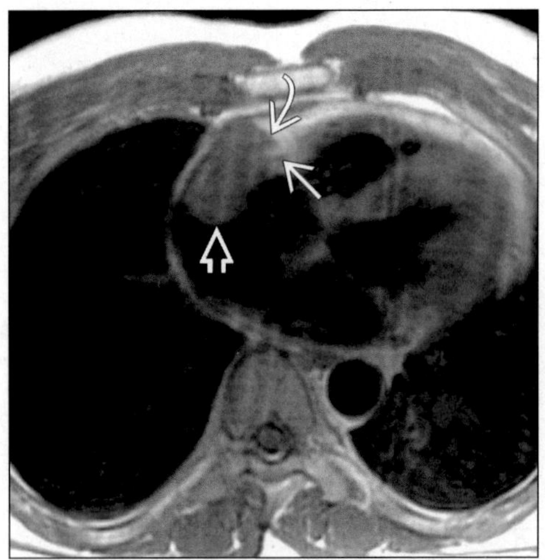

Axial T1WI MR image shows a right atrial mass that invades the epicardial fat ➡. Note: Tumor surrounded by epicardial fat ➡ of right atrio-ventricular groove; flow-void of RCA ➡.

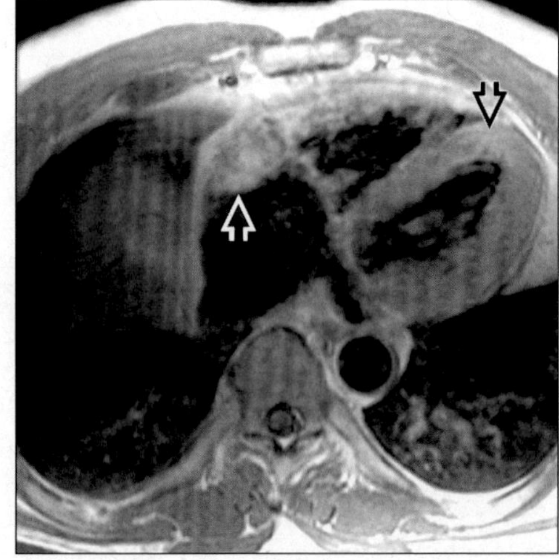

Axial T1WI MR with gadolinium shows the mass vividly enhancing ➡ compared to myocardium ➡. Invasion and enhancement indicate malignancy, the location suggests angiosarcoma. Biopsy revealed angiosarcoma.

TERMINOLOGY

Definitions

- Cardiac tumors that arise from one of the connective tissues (mesodermal cell origin) of the heart

IMAGING FINDINGS

General Features

- Location
  - Angiosarcoma, the most common primary malignant cardiac tumor, affects more frequently the right atrium (RA)
  - Malignant fibrous histiocytoma (MFH), osteosarcoma and leiomyosarcoma typically affect left atrium (LA)
  - Mesothelioma affects the visceral or parietal pericardium
- Invasive features are often present

Radiographic Findings

- Radiography
  - Cardiomegaly or focal cardiac mass
  - Other findings depend on location of mass and obstructive physiology
  - Secondary findings
    - Pleural and pericardial effusion
    - Atelectasis
    - Congestive heart failure (CHF)
    - Pulmonary venose hypertension (redistribution, Kerley B lines, edema)
    - Pleural effusion
    - Enlarged IVC and SVC

CT Findings

- NECT
  - Cardiomegaly, congested lungs or enlarged SVC/IVC
  - Fibrosarcoma demonstrates calcification in 25% of case
  - Disturbance of fat planes by invasion
  - Hemorrhagic pericardial effusion
- Broad-based tumor
- May extend into great vessels
- Invasion of myocardium, pericardium and mediastinal structures
- Positive contrast-enhancement, often heterogeneous

DDx: Angiosarcoma

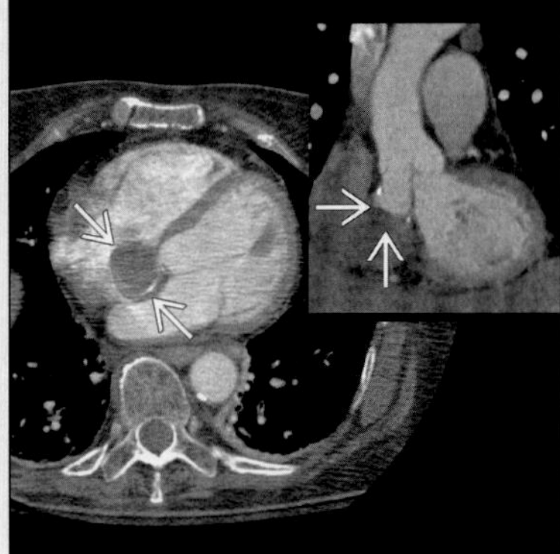

Sinus of Valsalva Aneurysm

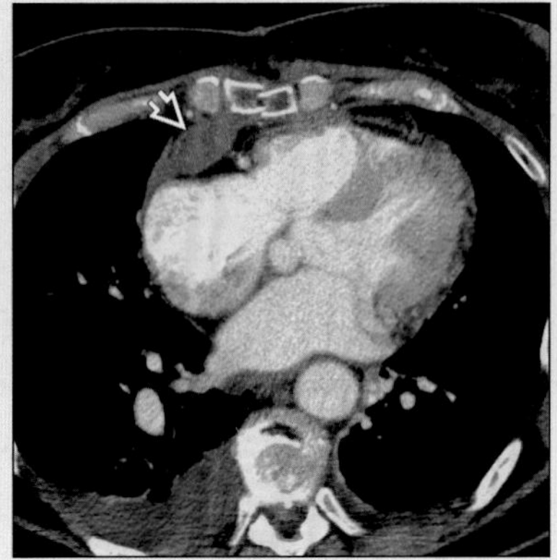

Loculated Effusion

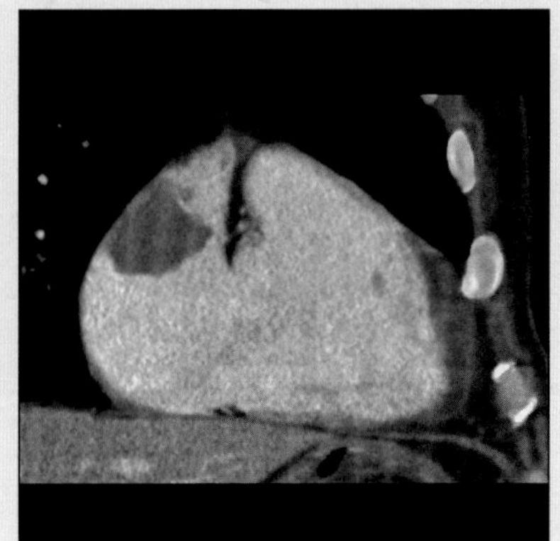

Right Atrial Thrombus

CARDIAC SARCOMA

Key Facts

Terminology

- Primary cardiac tumors that arise from from cardiac connective tissues (mesodermal cell origin)

Imaging Findings

- Angiosarcoma, the most common primary malignant cardiac tumor, affects more frequently the right atrium (RA)
- MFH, osteosarcoma and leiomyosarcoma typically affect left atrium (LA)
- Mesothelioma affects the visceral or parietal pericardium
- Heterogeneous, broad-based, large masses filling most of the affected chambers
- Valvular destruction and extracardiac extension frequent
- Central tumor necrosis
- Fibrosarcoma demonstrates characteristic calcification
- Positive contrast-enhancement, often heterogeneous
- Hemorrhagic pericardial effusion

Pathology

- Sarcomas are the second most common of all primary cardiac neoplasm after myxoma
- Spectrum including angiosarcoma (37%), undifferentiated sarcomas (24%), fibrosarcoma and malignant fibrous histiocytoma (MFH) (11-24%), rhabdomyosarcoma and leiomyosarcoma, osteosarcoma

Clinical Issues

- Nonspecific, depend on involved chambers

- ○ Degree of enhancement depends on vascularity of sarcoma
- Enhancing thickened pericardium
- Detection of pulmonary metastases
- Angiosarcoma typically right atrial enhancing tumors with low attenuation areas and pericardial extension
- May have central necrosis

MR Findings

- Heterogeneous, broad-based, large masses filling most of the affected chambers
- Central tumor necrosis
- Valvular destruction and extracardiac extension frequent
- Violation of fat planes
- Intermediate heterogeneous signal on T1WI, higher signal on T2WI
- Nodular or homogeneous pericardial thickening ± enhancement and hemorrhagic effusion
- Liposarcoma may demonstrate macroscopic fat
  - ○ Cases with little or no fat have been described

Echocardiographic Findings

- Echocardiogram
  - ○ Compression and distortion of anatomy by irregular echogenic mass
  - ○ Abnormal physiology depending on tumor location and extent
  - ○ TEE useful in detection and guidance of transvenous biopsy

DIFFERENTIAL DIAGNOSIS

Atrial Myxoma

- Most common benign primary tumor
- Typically left atrium with a stalk connecting it to atrial septum
- Hypointense on T1W1

Other Primary Benign Tumors

- Rhabdomyoma, lipoma, hemangioma, etc.
- No signs of invasion
- Lipoma has fibrous capsule and follows fat on all pulse sequences (including fat-saturated T1WI)
- Fibroma
  - ○ Increased incidence (~ 14%) in Gorlin syndrome (multiple nevoid basal cell skin carcinomas, cysts of the jaw, bifid ribs)
  - ○ Tumor calcification in 25% of cases
- Hemangioma may be part of Kasabach-Merritt syndrome (= hemangioma thrombocytopenia syndrome: Multiple hemangioendotheliomas, thrombocytopenia, consumptive coagulopathy)
  - ○ Vivid enhancement on CT
  - ○ Intermediate T1 signal intensity, hyperintense on T2WI
- Teratoma
  - ○ Chest x-ray may show formed teeth, other calcification, or a lipid/fluid level
  - ○ More commonly right-sided chambers
  - ○ May occur in pericardium
  - ○ Heterogeneous multiloculated complex cystic mass on echocardiography
  - ○ Contains tissues from all three germ cell layers (including teeth, hair, fat, bone, epithelium etc.)

Other Malignant Tumors

- Metastatic disease
- Lymphoma, pericardial mesothelioma

Thrombus

- Most commonly in atria or adjacent to infarcted myocardium
- No myocardial invasion

PATHOLOGY

General Features

- General path comments
  - ○ Sarcomas in general are the second most common primary cardiac neoplasm after myxoma
    - ▪ More frequent than true cardiac lipoma
  - ○ Malignant tumor of mesenchymal cell origin

- Spectrum including angiosarcoma (37%), undifferentiated sarcomas (24%), fibrosarcoma and malignant fibrous histiocytoma (MFH) (11-24%), rhabdomyosarcoma and leiomyosarcoma, osteosarcoma
- Very variable appearance
- Usually large heterogeneous invasive masses
- May replace myocardial walls
- Cardiac angiosarcoma
  - 80% lateral right atrial wall
  - May invade tricuspid valve, right ventricle, inferior and superior vena cava
- Rhabdomyosarcoma
  - Most common cardiac sarcoma in pediatric population, but may present at any age
  - No chamber predilection
- Mesothelioma
  - Tumor of the pericardium
  - Leads to constriction of chambers, rather than invading the myocardium
  - No link to asbestos exposure (unlike pleural mesothelioma)

- Etiology: Unknown
- Biopsies may be false negative, if tumor is covered with thrombus

Gross Pathologic & Surgical Features

- Cut surfaces typically firm and heterogeneous
- May be hemorrhagic and multilobular

Microscopic Features

- Variable appearance depending on cell type
- Microscopic features parallel the corresponding soft-tissue sarcoma
- May have areas of necrosis and hemorrhage
- MFH, leiomyosarcoma and osteosarcoma may have myxoid stroma similar to that of benign myxomas

CLINICAL ISSUES

Presentation

- Most common signs/symptoms
  - Nonspecific, depend on involved chambers
  - Dyspnea, chest pain, arrhythmia, peripheral edema
- Other signs/symptoms
  - Tamponade
  - Embolization
- Clinical Profile: Usually present after 3-6 month duration of symptoms

Demographics

- Age
  - Mean age at presentation 41 years
  - Extremely rare in infants and children
    - Rhabdomyosarcoma most common sarcoma in children
    - Sarcomas make up 75% of all malignant cardiac tumors in children and 95% of all primary malignancies (5% are lymphomas)
- Gender: No gender predilection

Natural History & Prognosis

- Rapidly progressive
- Extremely poor prognosis
  - Overwhelming majority are fatal
  - Typical survival 3-12 months (median survival = 6 months)
  - Survival over 4 years has been reported
  - Better prognosis if absence of metastasis, no central necrosis, low mitotic count

Treatment

- Aggressive surgery offers significant palliation and improves survival
- Local recurrence frequent
- Heart transplantation in rare cases
- Adjuvant radiation or chemotherapy does not prolong life but improves quality of life

DIAGNOSTIC CHECKLIST

Consider

- CT imaging of right atrial or ventricular tumors difficult due to mixing artifact (contrast from SVC with un-opacified blood from IVC)
- Delayed scans are crucial because RV and RA will be homogeneously opacified

SELECTED REFERENCES

1. JH Raaf et al: Cardiac Sarcoma. EMedicine (www.emedicine.com/med/topic282.htm), 2008
2. Murinello A et al: Cardiac angiosarcoma--a review. Rev Port Cardiol. 26(5):577-84, 2007
3. Uzun O et al: Cardiac tumours in children. Orphanet J Rare Dis. 2:11, 2007
4. Sakaguchi M et al: Cardiac angiosarcoma with right atrial perforation and cardiac tamponade. Ann Thorac Cardiovasc Surg. 12(2):145-8, 2006
5. Sparrow PJ et al: MR imaging of cardiac tumors. Radiographics. 25(5):1255-76, 2005
6. Frank H: Cardiac and Paracardiac Masses. In: Manning, WJ, Pennell DJ. Cardiovascular Magnetic Resonance. Churchill Livingstone, Philadelphia, 2002
7. Chiles C et al: Metastatic involvement of the heart and pericardium: CT and MR imaging. Radiographics. 21(2):439-49, 2001
8. Colucci WS et al: Primary tumors of the heart. In: Braunwald E. Heart Disease: A Textbook of Cardiovascular Medicine. 6th ed. W.B. Saunders Company, Philadelphia, 2001
9. Araoz PA et al: CT and MR imaging of benign primary cardiac neoplasms with echocardiographic correlation. Radiographics. 20(5):1303-19, 2000
10. Grebenc ML et al: Primary cardiac and pericardial neoplasms: radiologic-pathologic correlation. Radiographics. 20(4):1073-103; quiz 1110-1, 1112, 2000

CARDIAC SARCOMA

IMAGE GALLERY

Typical

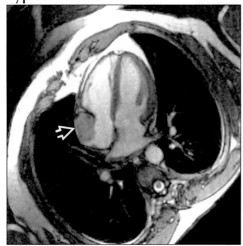

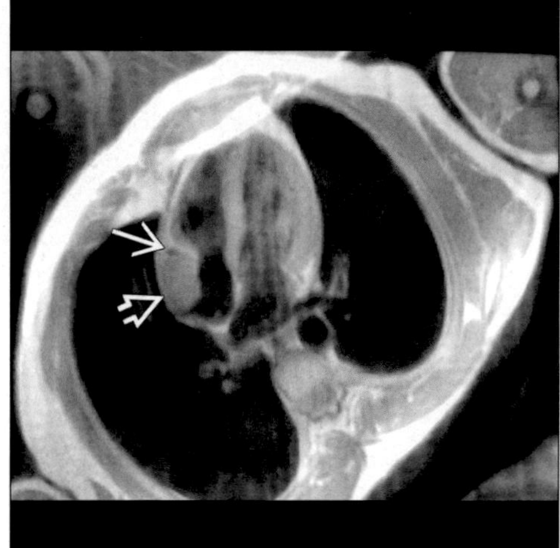

(Left) Four chamber view SSFP shows a broad-based mass along the lateral wall of the right atrium, and extending to the atrio-ventricular groove. *(Right)* Four chamber view T1WI FSE MR shows mass abutting and slightly displacing the flow void from the RCA. Biopsy revealed cardiac angiosarcoma.

Variant

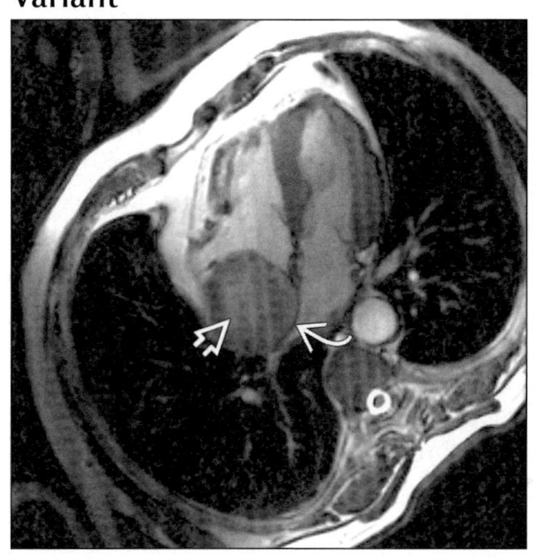

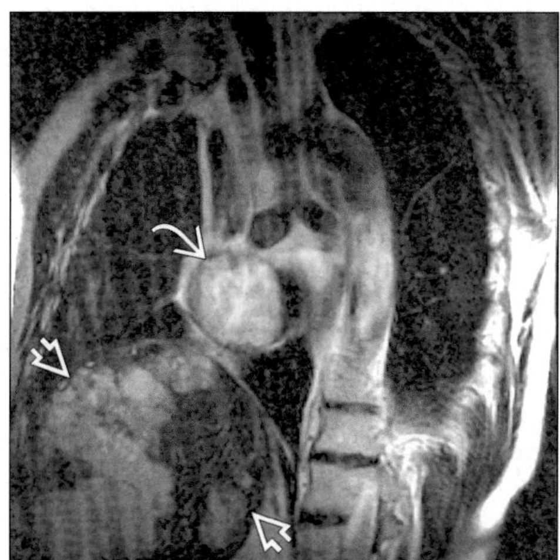

(Left) Four chamber view SSFP shows a large heterogeneous mass filling most of the right atrium and bowing the atrial septum towards the left. Note: Increased central signal due to high water content. *(Right)* Coronal oblique T2WI MR in the same patient as previous image shows biopsy proven extraskeletal myxoid chondrosarcoma metastatic to the liver and right atrium. Note: Increased T2 signal in metastases.

Typical

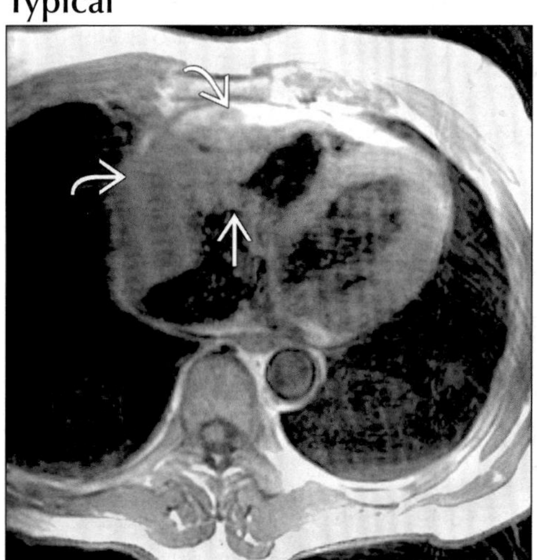

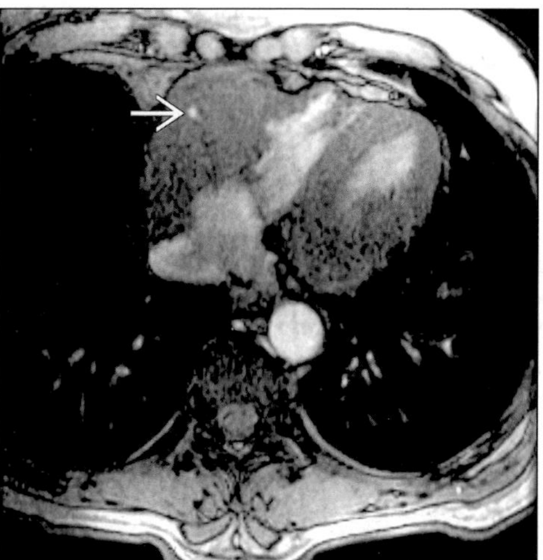

(Left) Axial T1WI MR SE shows typical appearance of a large primary cardiac angiosarcoma originating in the right atrium and invading the epicardial fat and pericardium, tricuspid valve, and RV. *(Right)* Axial SSFP shows high flow signal from the RCA, which is completely encased by the tumor.

CARDIAC METASTASES

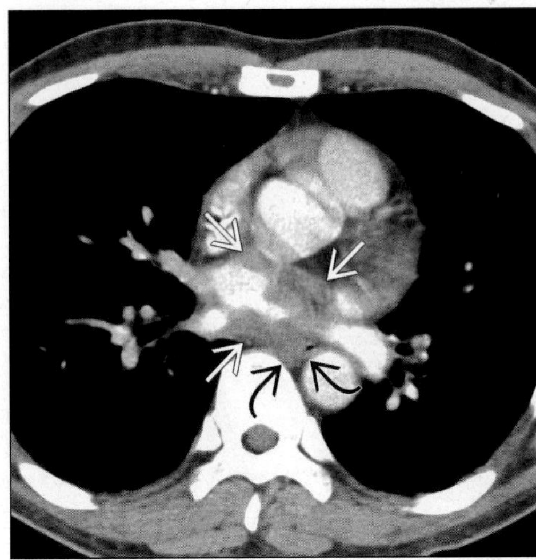

Axial CECT shows broad-based, enhancing mass ➡ in left atrium. Note: Loss of fat planes between aorta and vertebral bodies ⇨, suggesting extra cardiac growth.

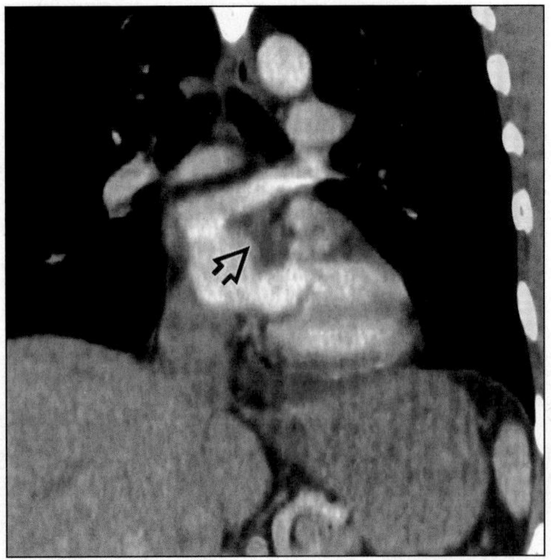

Coronal CECT shows same broad-based, lobular mass as previous image ⇨, at roof of left atrium between left superior pulmonary vein and atrial appendage ostia.

TERMINOLOGY

Definitions

- Deposit and growth of malignant tissue from remote primary tumor into myocardium, or other cardiac tissues
  - Commonly growth into cardiac chambers

IMAGING FINDINGS

General Features

- Best diagnostic clue: Cardiac mass in the presence of remote primary neoplasm or metastatic disease
- Location
  - Right atrium (RA) and right ventricle (RV) much more commonly affected than left atrium (LA) and left ventricle (LV)
  - Epicardium most commonly affected layer
- Size: Variable
- Very variable imaging features, may be clinically and radiographically occult

Radiographic Findings

- Radiography
  - Frequently normal
  - May mimic valvular heart disease
  - Cardiomegaly or specific chamber enlargement if obstruction occurs
  - Other metastases (lungs, bones)
  - Altered pulmonary vascularity
  - Secondary findings
    - Congestive heart failure (CHF)
    - Pleural and pericardial effusion
    - Atelectasis
  - Rarely focal cardiac mass
  - Rarely calcification (osteosarcoma metastasis)

CT Findings

- NECT
  - Usually normal, except if
    - Lung, bone, or mediastinal metastases are present
    - Massive cardiac involvement leading to chamber enlargement
    - Calcifications or fat are present (osteosarcoma or liposarcoma metastases)
- CTA

DDx: Cardiac Metastasis

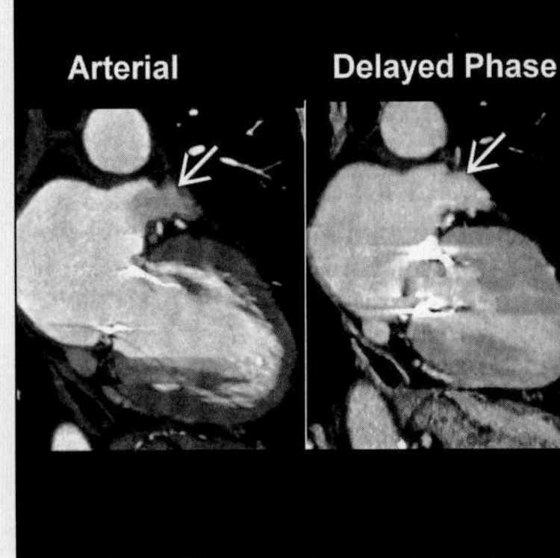

Pseudo-Mass

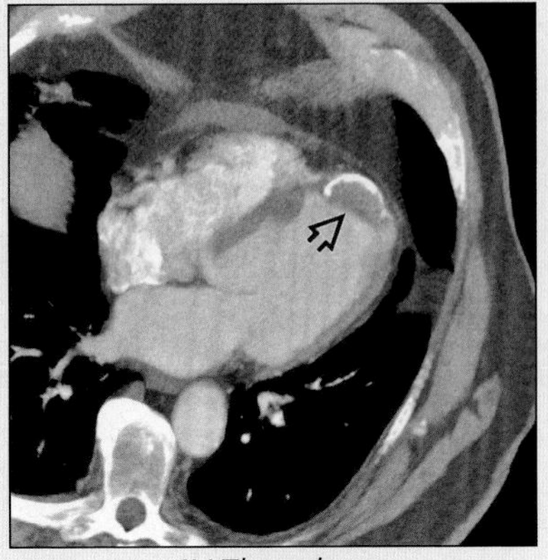

LV Thrombus

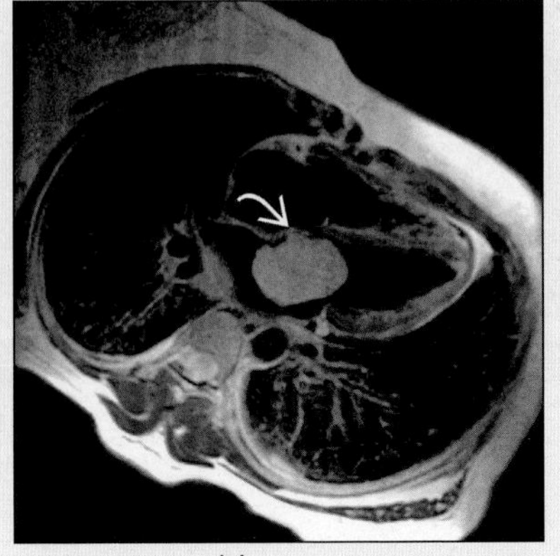

Myxoma

CARDIAC METASTASES

Key Facts

Terminology
- Deposit and growth of malignant tissue from remote primary tumor into myocardium, or other cardiac tissues

Imaging Findings
- Right atrium (RA) and right ventricle (RV) are much more commonly affected than left atrium (LA) and left ventricle (LV)
- Positive contrast-enhancement, depending on vascularity

Pathology
- Almost any cancer can metastasize to the heart
- 20-40 times more frequent than primary cardiac tumors
- Clinically silent cardiac metastases are commonly found on autopsy of cancer patients
  - Leukemias (46% of autopsies), melanoma (37%), thyroid cancer (30%), lung cancer (28%), sarcomas (26%), esophageal cancer (23%), renal cell cancer (22%), lymphoma (22%), breast (21%)
- But bronchogenic carcinoma is the primary tumor in 36% of all patients with cardiac metastases due to its high prevalence
- Leukemia & lymphoma are the primary malignancy in 20%
- Breast cancer is the primary tumor in 7%
- Esophageal cancer is the primary tumor in 6%
- Epicardium most often involved with metastases, even though all layers of the pericardium and myocardium may be affected

  - Very variable appearance
  - Invasion of myocardium, pericardium and mediastinal structures
  - Diffuse involvement or focal metastasis
  - Positive contrast-enhancement, depending on vascularity
  - Secondary findings
    - Pericardial effusion, often hemorrhagic
    - Pulmonary or osseous metastases
  - Direct invasion of lung cancer via pulmonary veins
  - Extension of renal or adrenal mass into RA via IVC
    - Inhomogeneous mixing of contrast opacified and non-opacified blood in the IVC may mimic tumor thrombus
    - In doubt, 2 min delayed scan or MR can confirm presence of IVC tumor

MR Findings
- Similar to CT
- Dark filling defects on white blood cine images
- High signal intensity filling defects on T1W black blood images
  - Slow flow may artificially cause high signal "pseudo filling defects"
- May reveal hemodynamic consequences of mass
  - Obstruction of RA inflow, pulmonary veins, RV or LV outflow tracts, or AV-valves
  - Valvular regurgitation due to tumor infiltration of leaflets
- Gadolinium enhancement more sensitive than CT for lower grade enhancing tumors
  - Use identical pulse sequence, slice orientation, shimming and tuning settings before and after Gd administration
    - Allows for comparable pre- and post-contrast images
- Best to image mass in 3 orthogonal planes ± specific cardiac planes
- Tissue characterization with fat-saturated images, T2WI, and T1WI pre- and post-contrast administration aids in assessment of composition of mass
  - Allow to differentiate lipoma from other neoplasms
  - Some primary cardiac tumors have typical MR properties (myxoma, fibroma, pericardial cysts, etc.) although these are often not reliable for differentiating benign from malignant

Echocardiographic Findings
- Echocardiogram
  - 25% no positive findings
  - Pericardial effusion (50%)
  - Mass or myocardial thickening evident in 40%
  - May demonstrate associated thrombus
  - Limited to the heart
    - May not detect associated metastatic disease in other organ systems, such as the lungs

DIFFERENTIAL DIAGNOSIS

Thrombus
- Most commonly in atria and adjacent to aneurysms
- No myocardial invasion

Atrial Myxoma
- Most common benign primary tumor
- Typically left atrium; intraluminal
- Hypointense on T1

Other Primary Benign Tumors
- Rhabdomyoma, hemangioma etc.
- Fibromas have a characteristically low signal on T2-weighted images

Other Malignant Tumors
- Primary malignant cardiac tumors
  - Lymphoma, sarcomas, pericardial mesothelioma etc.
- Direct invasion from neighboring cancers

Chronic Organized Pericardial Hematoma
- Demonstrate typical calcification pattern

Pericardial Infections
- May produce thickening and enhancement of pericardium that can mimic metastatic involvement

CARDIAC METASTASES

PATHOLOGY

General Features

- General path comments
  - Very variable appearance
  - Epicardium most often involved with metastases, even though all layers of the pericardium and myocardium may be affected
  - Usually large, heterogeneous, invasive masses
  - May replace myocardial walls
- Etiology
  - Four pathways of tumor spread to the heart are described
    - Hematogenic spread from primary tumor
    - Retrograde lymphatic extension
    - Direct contiguous extension into the heart
    - Transvenous extension
  - Almost any cancer can metastasize to the heart
  - Malignant melanoma and lymphoma have the highest propensity to metastasize to the heart
    - But bronchogenic carcinoma is the primary tumor in 36% of all patients with cardiac metastases due to its high prevalence
    - Leukemia & lymphoma are the primary malignancy in 20%
    - Breast cancer is the primary tumor in 7%
    - Esophageal cancer is the primary tumor in 6%
- Epidemiology
  - 20-40 times more frequent than primary cardiac tumors
  - 10% incidence in cancer patients
  - Up to 40% on autopsy series
  - Cardiac metastases are commonly found on autopsy of cancer patients
    - Leukemias (46% of autopsies), melanoma (37%), thyroid cancer (30%), lung cancer (28%), sarcomas (26%), esophageal cancer (23%), renal cell cancer (22%), lymphoma (22%), breast (21%)
- Associated abnormalities
  - Extracardiac metastases are typically present
  - Primary tumor may be evident on imaging study

Gross Pathologic & Surgical Features

- Frequently associated sanguineous pericardial effusion
- Multiple infiltrating masses in epicardium, myocardium and endocardium

Microscopic Features

- Variable appearance depending on cell type
- Microscopic features parallel the corresponding primary tumor
- Osteosarcoma metastases are unique in that they contain bone elements
  - Calcium may not be readily visible on MR (signal voids)
  - CT best modality for evaluating for osteosarcoma metastasis

CLINICAL ISSUES

Presentation

- Most common signs/symptoms: Frequently asymptomatic
- Other signs/symptoms
  - Tamponade from hemorrhagic effusion or compressing tumor mass
  - Shortness of breath
  - Cough, chest pain
  - Peripheral edema
  - Weight loss
  - Conduction disorders
  - Myocardial ischemia
  - Clinical symptoms are specific to other organ systems that also have metastatic involvement

Natural History & Prognosis

- Extremely poor

Treatment

- Chemotherapy for palliation
- Radiation therapy for palliation: May reduce pericardial effusion

DIAGNOSTIC CHECKLIST

Consider

- If MR or CT is ordered to clarify suspected masses on echocardiography, careful review of extracardiac structures is important
  - May reveal additional extracardiac masses that allow to establish the diagnosis of metastatic disease

SELECTED REFERENCES

1. Dodd JD et al: Cardiac septal aneurysm mimicking pseudomass: appearance on ECG-gated cardiac MRI and MDCT. AJR Am J Roentgenol. 188(6):W550-3, 2007
2. Garcia JR et al: Usefulness of 18-fluorodeoxyglucose positron emission tomography in the evaluation of tumor cardiac thrombus from renal cell carcinoma. Clin Transl Oncol. 8(2):124-8, 2006
3. Feys A et al: Cardiac metastasis from a stage IIIb cervix carcinoma. Acta Cardiol. 60(1):73-5, 2005
4. Kim JH et al: Non-small cell lung cancer initially presenting with intracardiac metastasis. Korean J Intern Med. 20(1):86-9, 2005
5. Tesolin M et al: Cardiac metastases from melanoma. Radiographics. 25(1):249-53, 2005
6. Wang ZJ et al: CT and MR imaging of pericardial disease. Radiographics. 23 Spec No:S167-80, 2003
7. Meng Q et al: Echocardiographic and pathological characteristics of cardiac metastasis in patients with lymphoma. Oncol Rep. 9(1):85-8, 2002
8. Chiles C et al: Metastatic involvement of the heart and pericardium: CT and MR imaging. Radiographics. 21(2):439-49, 2001
9. Chahinian AP et al: Tumors of the heart and great vessels in Holland*Frei. Cancer Medicine. 5th Ed., BC Becker, 2000
10. Shimotsu Y et al: Fluorine-18-fluorodeoxyglucose PET identification of cardiac metastasis arising from uterine cervical carcinoma. J Nucl Med. 39(12):2084-7, 1998

IMAGE GALLERY

Typical

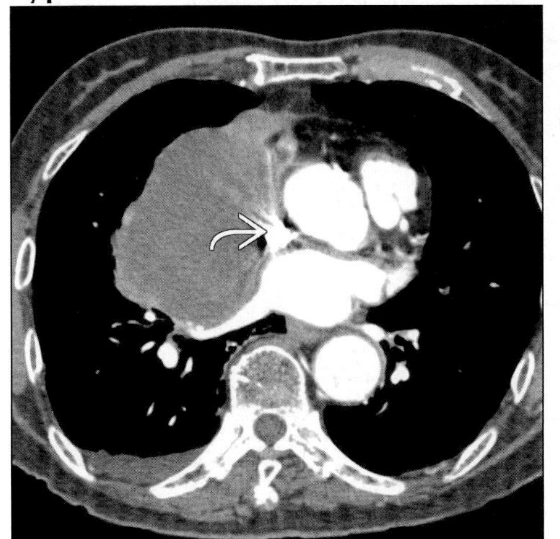

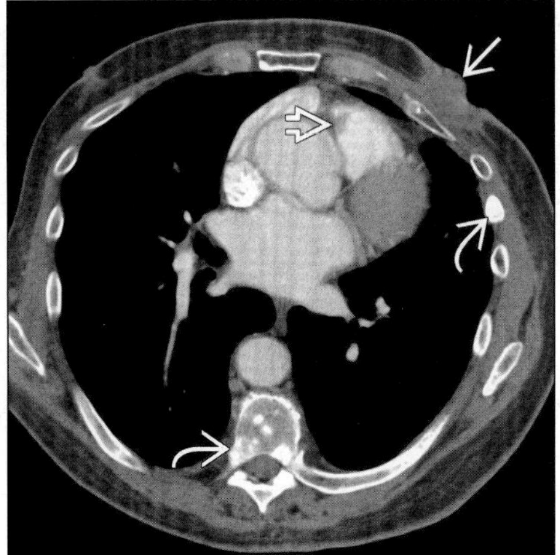

*(**Left**) Axial CECT shows large mass displacing SVC ➔, aorta and right-sided structures towards left. Squamous cell sarcoma metastasis to pericardium. (**Right**) Axial CECT in different patient with advanced metastatic disease shows skeletal ➔ and soft tissue metastasis ➔ as well as small metastatic deposits in the right ventricular outflow tract ➔.*

Typical

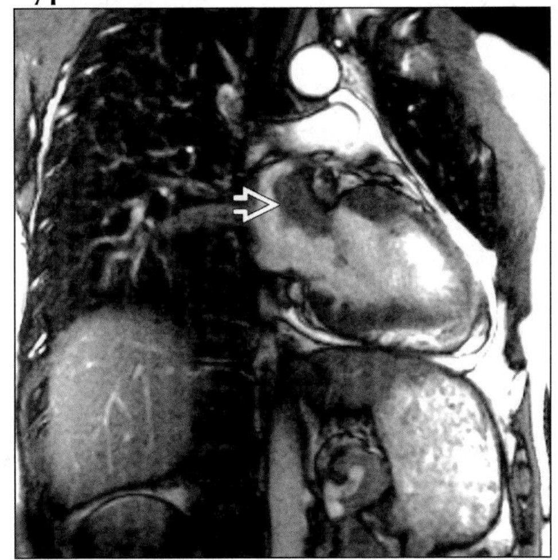

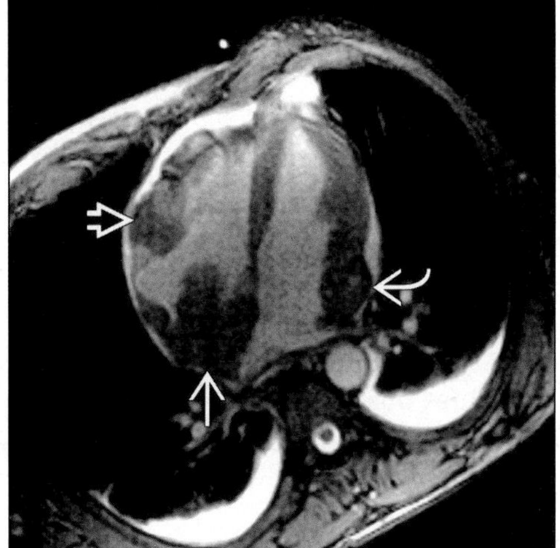

*(**Left**) Long axis horizontal SSFP shows broad based atrial mass ➔ invading base of mitral valve leaflet, representing spindle cell sarcoma metastasis. (**Right**) Four chamber view SSFP in patient with lymphoma shows pleural effusions and multiple lobulated masses in right atrium ➔, atrial septum and right ventricle ➔, and left atrioventricular groove ➔.*

Typical

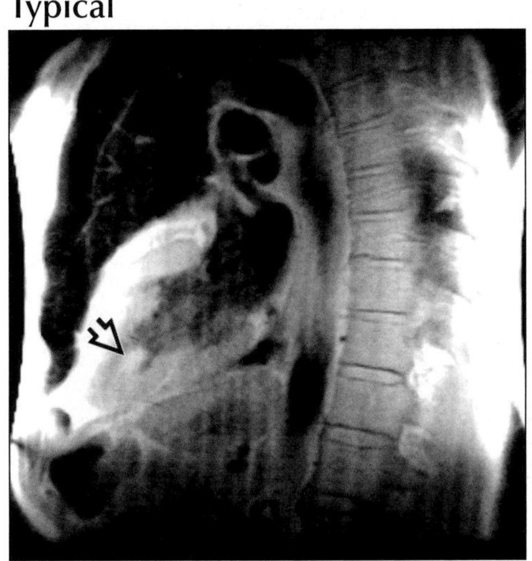

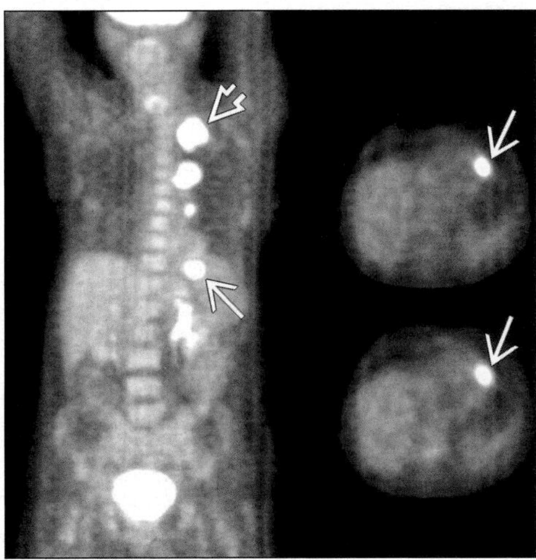

*(**Left**) Long axis T1WI MR black blood post gadolinium in patient with lung cancer shows subtle enhancing mass ➔ within LV cavity anterior to posterior-medial papillary muscle. (**Right**) Coronal and axial glucose starved FDG-PET shows lung ➔, hilar and left ventricular ➔ high uptake foci. Autopsy revealed non-small carcinoma with LV and other metastasis.*

PAPILLARY FIBROELASTOMA

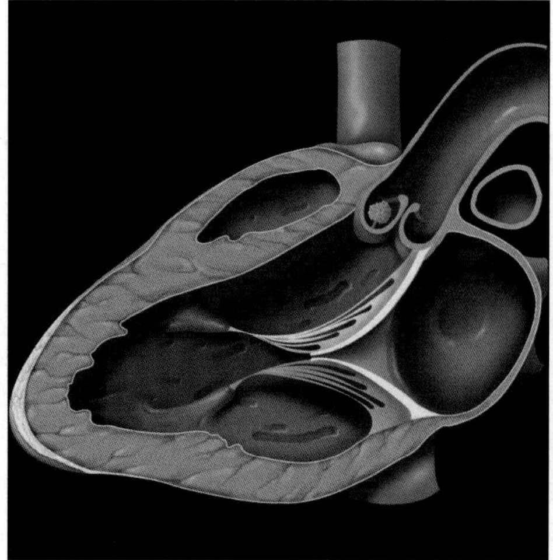

Three chamber view graphic shows a small mass with a thin stalk and multiple frond-like projections arising from the aortic side of the aortic valve.

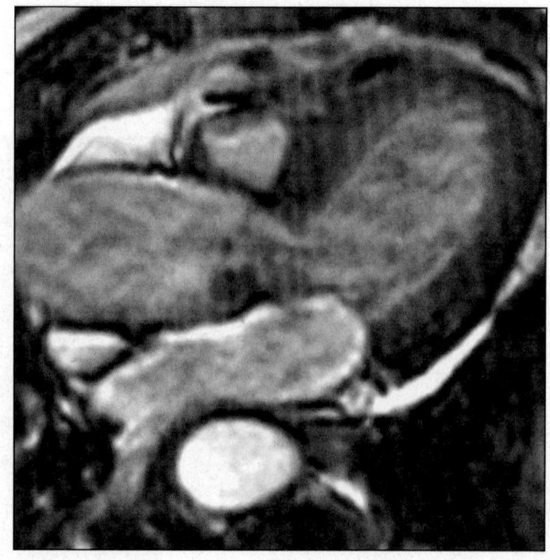

Three chamber view SSFP shows a subcentimeter, sharply marginated mass of intermediate signal intensity arising from the aortic side of an aortic valve leaflet.

TERMINOLOGY

Definitions

- Benign endocardial papillomas that predominantly affect the cardiac valves

IMAGING FINDINGS

General Features

- Best diagnostic clue
  - Pedunculated, valvular/paravalvular mass
  - Low signal intensity on T2-weighted images due to high fibrous content of the lesion
- Location
  - Tend to arise from heart valves in 90% of cases
    - Aortic valve (29%), mitral valve (25%), pulmonary valve (13%), tricuspid valve (17%)
  - Typically on the aortic side of the aortic valve and on the atrial side of the mitral valve
- Size: Median size is 8 mm, with a range of 2-28 mm; 99% of all tumors measure less than 20 mm
- Morphology
  - Round, oval or irregular in shape
  - "Speckled appearance" or "stippling" around the perimeter of the tumor has also been described

Imaging Recommendations

- Best imaging tool: Echocardiography has been the primary imaging modality in years past, although MR is rapidly becoming the gold standard for evaluation of cardiac masses
- Protocol advice: Lesions are best detected on bright blood SSFP sequences at MR due to their inherent low signal; tumors tend to be obscured by the blood pool on conventional spin-echo black blood images

DIFFERENTIAL DIAGNOSIS

Thrombus

- May be indistinguishable from fibroelastomas
- Thrombus results in higher incidence of valvular dysfunction than fibroelastomas

Atrial Myxoma

- More typically arise from the interatrial septum
- Generally larger than fibroelastomas

DDx: Papillary Fibroelastoma

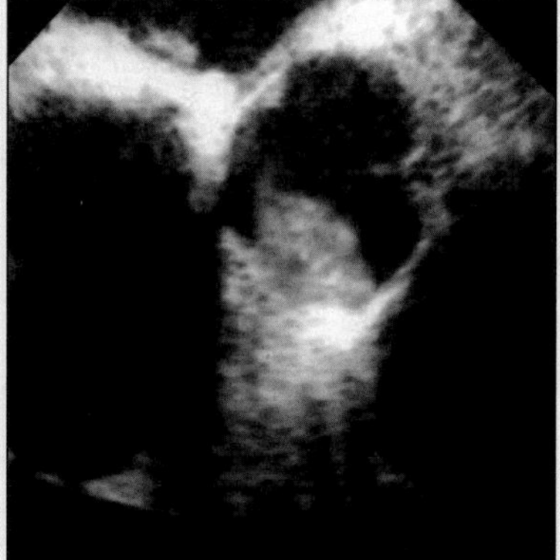

Aortic Valve Thrombus

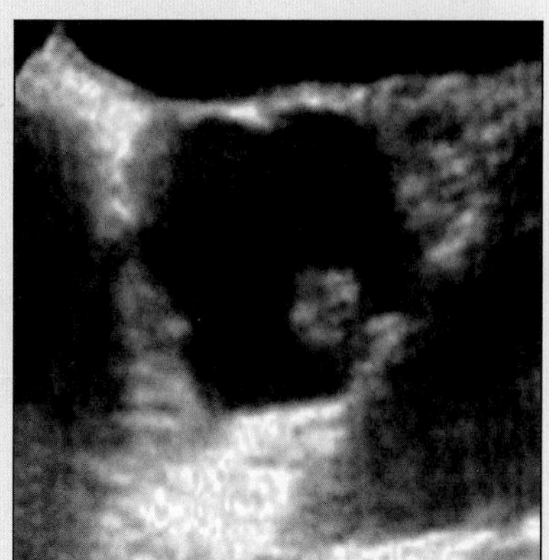

Aortic Valve Thrombus

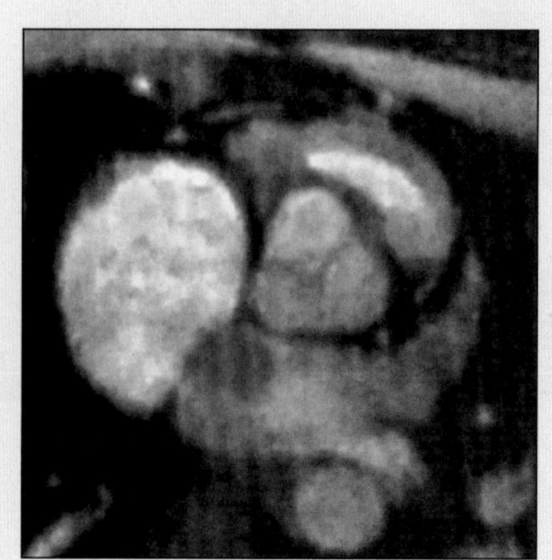

Left Atrial Myxoma

PAPILLARY FIBROELASTOMA

Key Facts

Imaging Findings

- Tend to arise from heart valves in 90% of cases
- Median size is 8 mm, with a range of 2-28 mm; 99% of all tumors measure less than 20 mm

Pathology

- 2nd most common benign primary cardiac neoplasm
- Accounts for roughly 75% of all cardiac valvular tumors

Clinical Issues

- Patients are generally symptomatic
  - Most lesions are incidentally discovered at autopsy, or while undergoing coronary surgery, echocardiography or cardiac catheterization
- Simple surgical excision with possible leaflet repair or valve replacement

PATHOLOGY

General Features

- Epidemiology
  - 2nd most common benign primary cardiac neoplasm
  - Accounts for roughly 75% of all cardiac valvular tumors
- Associated abnormalities
  - Rheumatic valvulitis, valvular fibrosis and/or calcification
  - Hypertropic cardiomyopathy
  - Aortic aneurysm
  - Congenital heart disease

Gross Pathologic & Surgical Features

- Gelatinous masses with a characteristic "sea anemone" appearance; these fronds are best seen by immersing the tumor in water

CLINICAL ISSUES

Presentation

- Most common signs/symptoms
  - Patients are generally asymptomatic
    - Most lesions are incidentally discovered at autopsy, or while undergoing coronary surgery, echocardiography or cardiac catheterization
- Other signs/symptoms
  - Patients may become symptomatic if tumor fragments or thrombus on the surface of the tumors result in an embolic event
    - Transient ischemic attacks or stroke from cerebrovascular occlusion
    - Dyspnea from pulmonary emboli
    - Myocardial infarction from coronary artery occlusion

Demographics

- Age: Mean age 60 years

Natural History & Prognosis

- Patients are generally asymptomatic with little incidence of valvular dysfunction; in the setting of thromboembolic events, lesions can be surgically excised with virtually no reported recurrence

Treatment

- Simple surgical excision with possible leaflet repair or valve replacement

SELECTED REFERENCES

1. Sun JP et al: Clinical and echocardiographic characteristics of papillary fibroelastomas: a retrospective and prospective study in 162 patients. Circulation. 103(22):2687-93, 2001
2. Grebenc ML et al: Primary cardiac and pericardial neoplasms: radiologic-pathologic correlation. Radiographics. 20(4):1073-103; quiz 1110-1, 1112, 2000
3. Edwards FH et al: Primary cardiac valve tumors. Ann Thorac Surg. 52(5):1127-31, 1991

IMAGE GALLERY

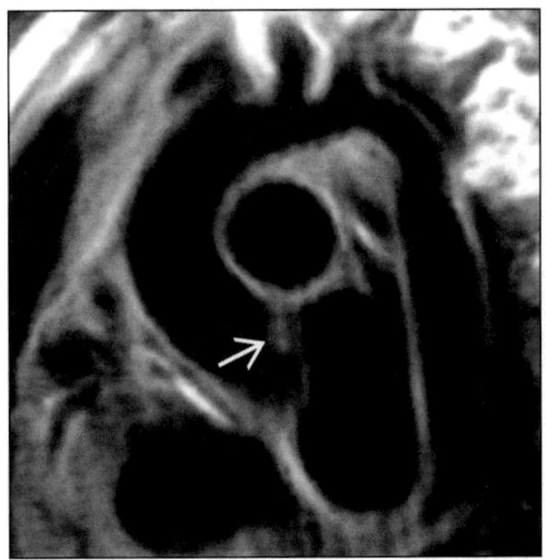

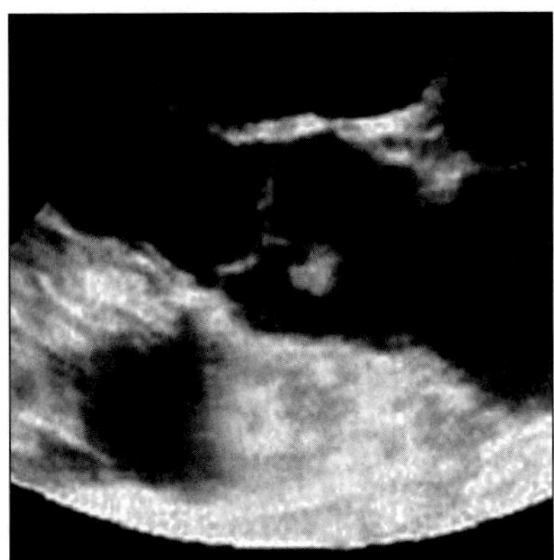

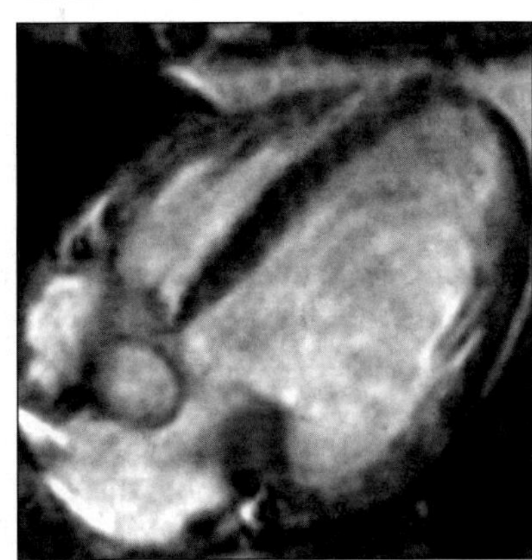

(Left) *LVOT T1WI FS MR shows a sharply marginated mass of intermediate signal intensity ➔ arising from an aortic valve leaflet consistent with a papillary fibroelastoma.* ***(Center)*** *Transthoracic echocardiogram shows a well-circumscribed, subcentimeter hyperechoic mass arising via a thin stalk from an aortic valve leaflet.* ***(Right)*** *Four chamber view SSFP shows an ill-defined hypointense mass arising from the atrial side of the posterior mitral valve leaflet. The mitral valve leaflet is partially obscured by the mass.*

FIBROMA

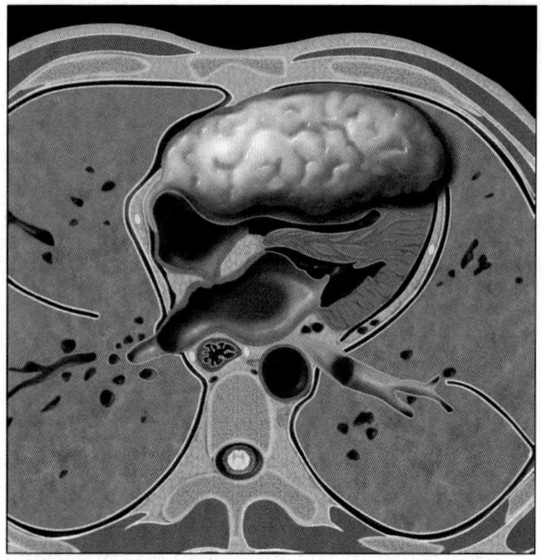

Axial graphic shows fibroma compressing both ventricles.

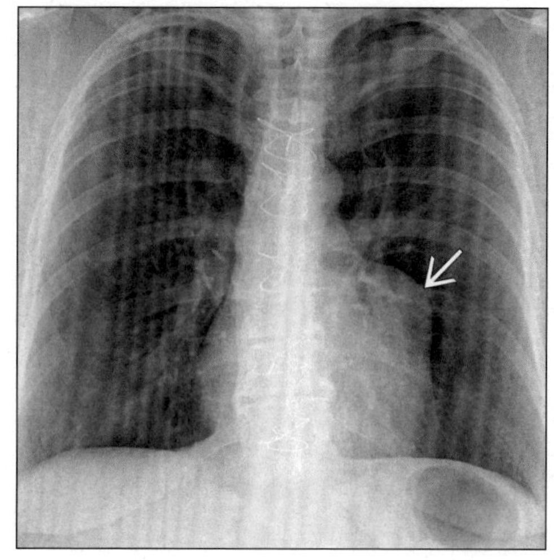

Coronal radiograph shows mass along superior left heart border ➔.

TERMINOLOGY

Abbreviations and Synonyms

- Fibrous hamartoma, fibroelastic hamartoma

Definitions

- Benign congenital cardiac neoplasm composed of fibroblasts and collagen

IMAGING FINDINGS

General Features

- Best diagnostic clue: Solitary myocardial mass
- Location: Almost always arise in septum or left ventricular free wall
- Size: Diameter range: 2-5 cm
- Morphology: Discrete or infiltrative mass, calcifications; no necrosis, hemorrhage, or cysts

Radiographic Findings

- Radiography: Cardiomegaly or focal bulge

CT Findings

- NECT: Homogeneous mass, can have calcification
- CECT: Heterogeneous enhancement

MR Findings

- T1WI: Isointense or hypointense
- T2WI: Homogeneously hypointense
- T1 C+ FS: Heterogeneous enhancement, poorly vascularized fibrous tissue may enhance poorly

Echocardiographic Findings

- Echocardiogram
  - Large, solid, noncontractile mass in myocardium
    - Calcification can be seen
    - May mimic focal hypertrophic cardiomyopathy

Imaging Recommendations

- Best imaging tool: Echocardiography

DIFFERENTIAL DIAGNOSIS

Metastatic Disease

- Multifocal masses with known primary neoplasm

Atrial Myxoma

- Endocardial mass attached to fossa ovalis

DDx: Other Cardiac Masses

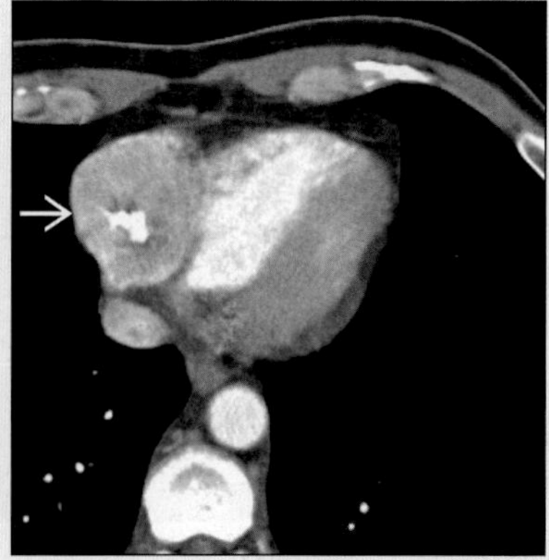

Paraganglioma

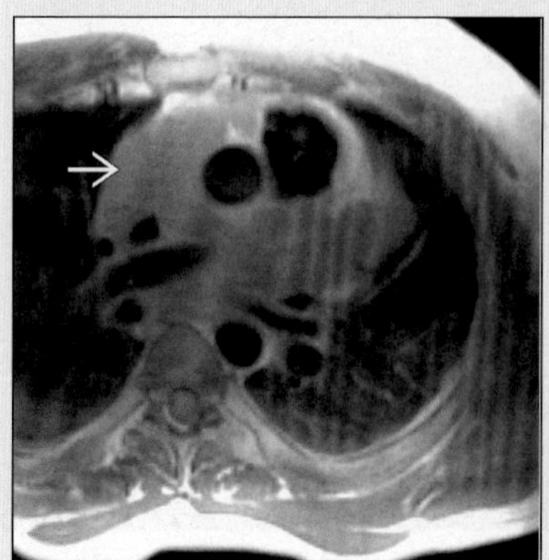

Angiosarcoma

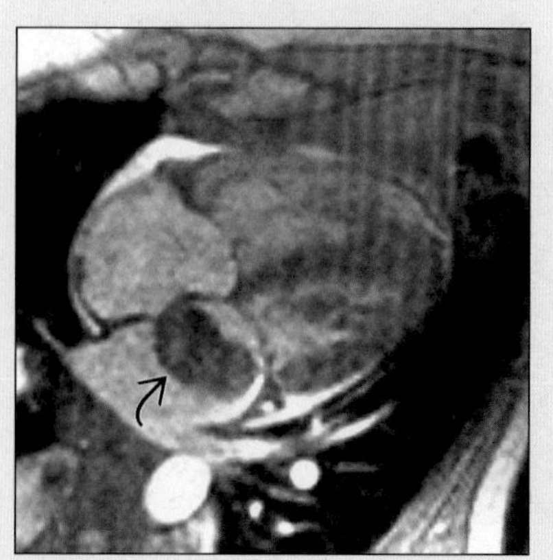

Atrial Myxoma

FIBROMA

Key Facts

Terminology
- Benign congenital cardiac neoplasm composed of fibroblasts and collagen

Imaging Findings
- Best diagnostic clue: Solitary myocardial mass
- Large, solid, noncontractile mass in myocardium

Top Differential Diagnoses
- Metastatic Disease

Pathology
- Infants: Fibroblast rich tumor with little collagen

Clinical Issues
- Most common signs/symptoms: Heart failure, arrhythmias, sudden death
- Can be dormant, regress
- Surgical excision is treatment of choice
- Controversial conservative approach if asymptomatic

Rhabdomyoma
- Ventricular masses in young patients
  - 50% have tuberous sclerosis

Hemangioma
- Endocardial or intramural masses
  - High signal on T2WI, enhance intensely

Paraganglioma
- Epicardial tumor at roof of left atrium
  - Central necrosis, calcification, high on T2WI

Angiosarcoma
- Large, heterogeneous, invasive right atrial masses with extensive pericardial involvement

PATHOLOGY

General Features
- Etiology: May be a hamartoma rather than neoplasm
- Epidemiology: About 100 reported cases in 30 years
- Associated abnormalities: Gorlin syndrome

Gross Pathologic & Surgical Features
- Large, firm, white, fibrous masses within ventricular myocardium with discrete or infiltrative margins
  - 50% calcify: No necrosis, hemorrhage, cystic change

Microscopic Features
- Infants: Fibroblast rich tumor with little collagen
- Adolescents and adults: Predominantly collagenous
- Occasional mitoses, elastic tissue

CLINICAL ISSUES

Presentation
- Most common signs/symptoms: Heart failure, arrhythmias, sudden death

Demographics
- Age: 85% children, 15% adolescents and adults

Natural History & Prognosis
- Can interfere with mechanical or electrical function
- Can be dormant, regress

Treatment
- Surgical excision is treatment of choice
- Controversial conservative approach if asymptomatic

SELECTED REFERENCES

1. Araoz PA: CT and MR imaging of benign primary cardiac neoplasms with echocardiographic correlation. RadioGraphics. 20:1303-19, 2000
2. Grebenc ML et al: Primary cardiac and pericardial neoplasms: radiologic-pathologic correlation. RadioGraphics. 20: 1073-1103, 2000
3. Burke AP et al: Cardiac fibroma: clinicopathologic correlates and surgical treatment. J Thorac Cardiovasc Surg. 108: 862-70, 1994

IMAGE GALLERY

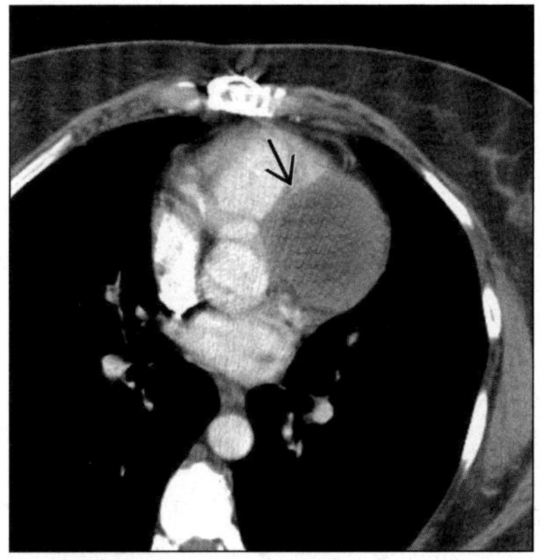
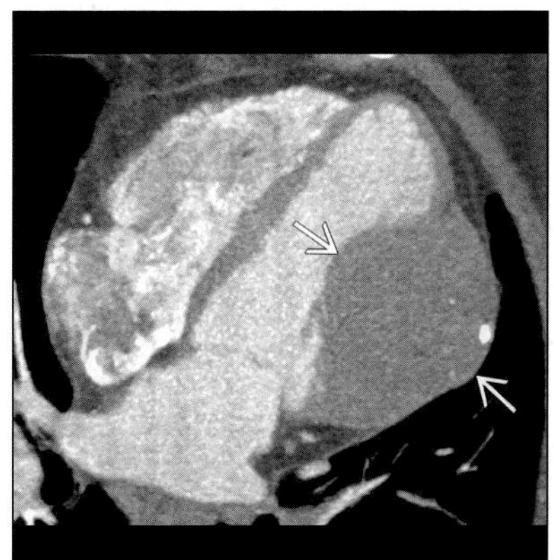
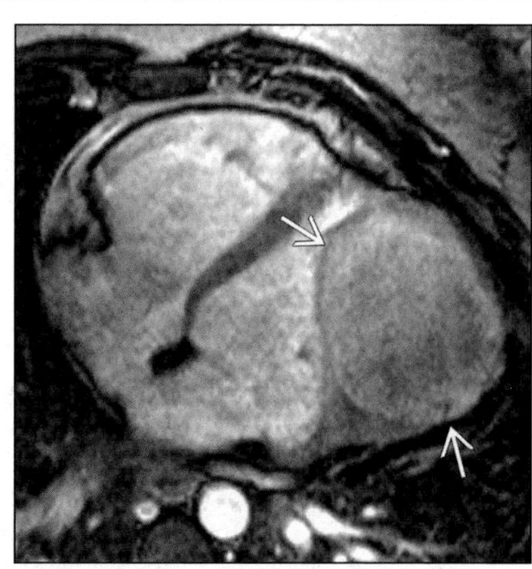

*(**Left**) Axial CECT shows a homogeneous intrapericardial well-marginated mass → arising from the left ventricular myocardium. (**Center**) Axial cardiac CT shows large posterolateral isodense myocardial mass ➔, with smooth margins, and small dense calcifications. Abutting but not invading through pericardium. (Courtesy C. White, MD). (**Right**) Axial SSFP shows a fibroma ➔ at the lateral wall of the left ventricle. (Courtesy C. White, MD).*

LIPOMATOUS HYPERTROPHY, INTERATRIAL SEPTUM

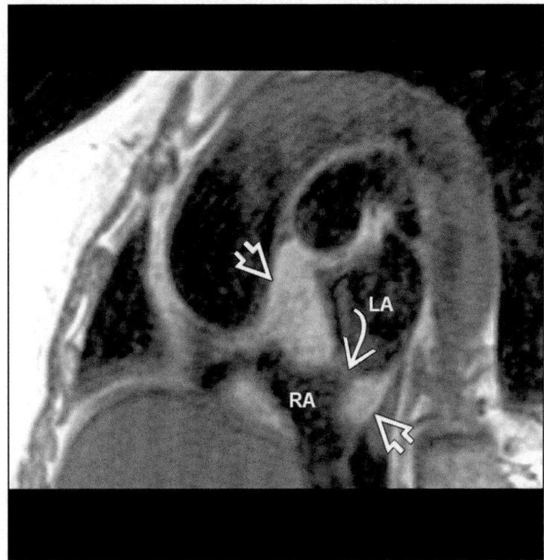

Oblique black blood SE MR shows high T1 signal tissue within atrial septum ➡ with sparing of fossa ovalis ➡, resulting in classic dumbbell appearance of LHIS.

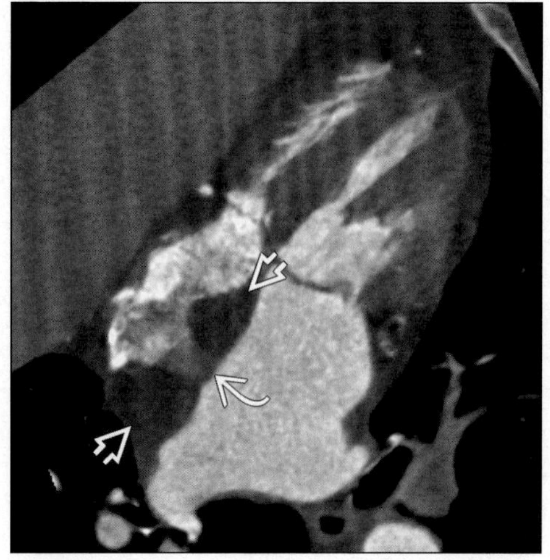

Four chamber view cardiac CT shows classic case of lipomatous hypertrophy of interatrial septum with low attenuation material within atrial septum ➡ and sparing of fossa ovalis ➡.

TERMINOLOGY

Abbreviations and Synonyms

- Lipomatous hypertrophy of the interatrial septum (LHIS)
- Lipomatous hypertrophy of the atrial septum (LHAS)
- Massive fatty deposits
- Lipomatous hamartoma
- Lipomatous hyperplasia

Definitions

- Deposition of excessive amounts of fat within the interatrial septum, first described in 1964 by Prior
- Not a true neoplasm

IMAGING FINDINGS

General Features

- Best diagnostic clue
  - Characteristic dumbbell-shaped lesion sparing the fossa ovalis
    - Though it need not have this shape to qualify
- Location
  - Within septum secundum
    - Spares fossa ovalis
- Size
  - Typically between 11 and 28 mm
  - Amounts of fatty deposit increases with age
- Morphology
  - Characteristically the area of most fatty deposition will be anterior or superior to the fossa ovalis
  - 80% will demonstrate dumbbell shape

Radiographic Findings

- Radiography: Chest radiograph is normal

CT Findings

- NECT
  - Low attenuation material posteriorly within otherwise water density heart
  - May also demonstrate increased mediastinal and epicardial fat
- CTA
  - Dumbbell-shaped, fat-density lesion that spares the fossa ovalis
  - May be contiguous with epicardial fat
  - Usually is an incidental diagnosis

DDx: Atrial Septal Masses

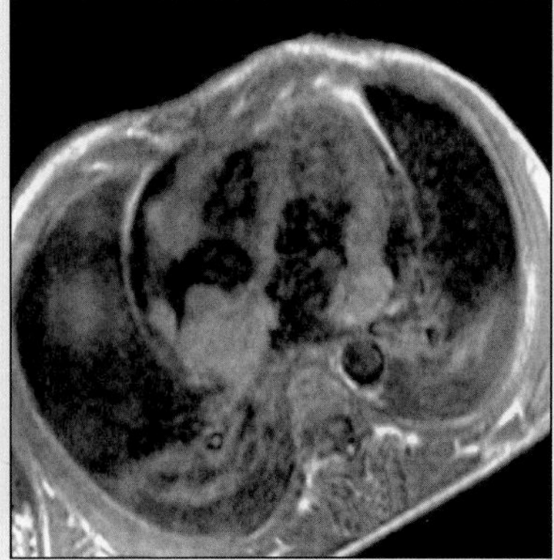

Lymphoma

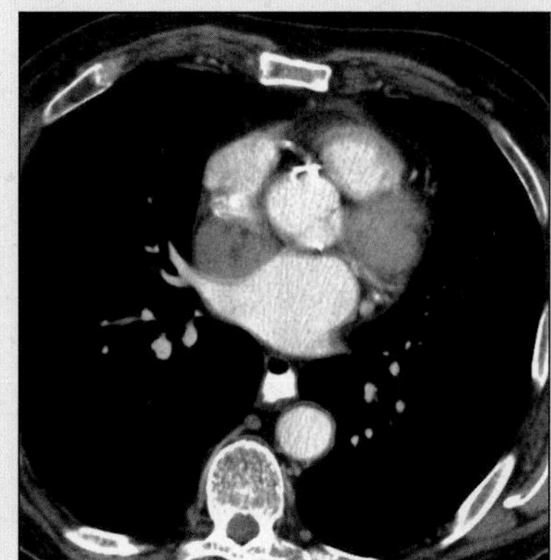

Melanoma

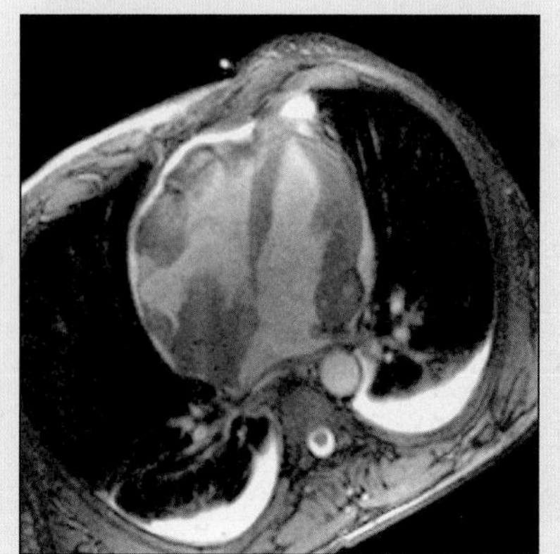

Metastatic Disease

LIPOMATOUS HYPERTROPHY, INTERATRIAL SEPTUM

Key Facts

Terminology
- LHIS; LHAS; massive fatty deposits; lipomatous hamartoma
- Not a true neoplasm
- Deposition of excessive amounts of fat within the interatrial septum

Imaging Findings
- Location of fat within septum secundum with sparing fossa ovalis
- Characteristic dumbbell-shaped fatty lesion
- Incidental finding that does not require additional imaging, unless findings are not unequivocal and exclusion of a neoplasm is required
- FDG PET shows focal increased FDG uptake
  - Positive correlation of SUV and thickness of LHIS on CT

Pathology
- No capsule present
- Proliferation of fat cells rather than hypertrophy
- Mature adipose tissue with cells resembling brown fat

Clinical Issues
- Prevalence increases with age
- Usually asymptomatic
- Reportedly associated with supraventricular arrhythmias and sudden death
- May occasionally present as obstructive right atrial mass and exertional dyspnea
- Rarely may cause obstructive symptoms that necessitate resection

  - Multiplanar reconstructions may be helpful to determine caval obstruction

MR Findings
- Characteristic bright T1 signal with loss of normal bright T1 signal on fat-suppressed sequences
- Classic dumbbell shape

Nuclear Medicine Findings
- PET
  - FDG PET shows focal increased FDG uptake
  - Standardized uptake value (SUV) of lipomatous hypertrophy of interatrial septum ~ 1.6-6.1 times greater than SUV of adjacent blood pool
  - Positive correlation of SUV and thickness of LHIS on CT
  - Image fusion with CT will confirm location during staging and may avoid pitfall of diagnosing metastatic disease

Echocardiographic Findings
- Echogenic lesion within interatrial septum
- Typically echo-dense globular shape with sparing of fossa ovalis
- Often incidental diagnosis that requires no further follow-up
  - Occasionally diagnosis is not unequivocal and further testing (such as MR) may be necessary to exclude cardiac mass

Imaging Recommendations
- Best imaging tool
  - Incidental finding that does not require imaging, unless one imaging modality is not unequivocal and exclusion of a mass is required
    - MR SE or FSE sequences
- Protocol advice: SE or FSE sequences without fat-saturation followed by otherwise identical sequence with fat-saturation

DIFFERENTIAL DIAGNOSIS

Lipoma
- Primary cardiac lipomas are rare
- True lipoma will have a fibrous capsule, lipomatous hypertrophy does not

Liposarcoma
- Rare
- Usually large, filling entire cavity
- Signs of malignancy (invasion of neighboring structures, mass effect, metastasis)

Teratoma
- Rare
- Demonstrates mass effect
- Not dumbbell-shaped
- May demonstrate fat or lipid collection but also various other tissues (soft tissue, hair, teeth, bone, etc.)

Myocardial Infarction
- Linear fat is within myocardium, but not within atrial septum

Arrhythmogenic Right Ventricular Dysplasia (ARVD)
- Fat typically within right ventricular myocardium
- Occasionally within LV myocardium, but virtually never within atrial septum

Myxoma
- Most common primary cardiac neoplasm
- May be adjacent to fossa ovalis but is usually connected to septum via a stalk and mobile
- Does not have features of fat on either CT or MR

Other Benign Tumors
- Rhabdomyoma, fibroma, mesothelioma
- Typically no fat density/signal characteristics

Thrombus
- May be adherent to the atrial wall

LIPOMATOUS HYPERTROPHY, INTERATRIAL SEPTUM

- Will not follow characteristics of fat on either CT or MR

Metastatic Disease

- Usually not fat density or signal characteristics
- Other cardiac or extracardiac metastatic deposits

PATHOLOGY

General Features

- Etiology: Hyperplasia rather than hypertrophy of local fat cells
- Associated abnormalities: Associated with large amount of epicardial fat and increased body mass index

Gross Pathologic & Surgical Features

- If resected will show features characteristic of mass-like fat deposits
  - Constrained by normal structures
- No capsule present

Microscopic Features

- Proliferation of fat cells rather than hypertrophy
- Mature adipose tissue with cells resembling brown fat
- Vacuolated cytoplasm and centrally-placed nuclei

CLINICAL ISSUES

Presentation

- Most common signs/symptoms: Most commonly asymptomatic
- Other signs/symptoms
  - Reportedly associated with supraventricular arrhythmias and sudden death
  - Syncope
  - May present as obstructive right atrial mass and exertional dyspnea

Demographics

- Age: Prevalence increases with age
- Gender: No gender predilection
- Prevalence reported from 1-8%
- More common in obese persons

Natural History & Prognosis

- Usually asymptomatic
- Rarely may cause obstructive symptoms that necessitate resection

Treatment

- Usually no treatment necessary
- Rarely resection of obstructive variants

DIAGNOSTIC CHECKLIST

Consider

- Add fat-saturated T1WI to regular T1WI if differentiating from cardiac masses or metastases, such as melanoma

Image Interpretation Pearls

- Fat density material in atrial septal location with sparing of fossa ovalis is diagnostic of LHIS

SELECTED REFERENCES

1. Pugliatti P et al: Lipomatous hypertrophy of the interatrial septum. Int J Cardiol. 2007
2. Tugcu A et al: Lipomatous Hypertrophy of the Interatrial Septum Presenting as an Obstructive Right Atrial Mass in a Patient with Exertional Dyspnea. J Am Soc Echocardiogr. 2007
3. Fan CM et al: Lipomatous hypertrophy of the interatrial septum: increased uptake on FDG PET. AJR Am J Roentgenol. 184(1):339-42, 2005
4. Kuester LB et al: Lipomatous hypertrophy of the interatrial septum: prevalence and features on fusion 18F fluorodeoxyglucose positron emission tomography/CT. Chest. 128(6):3888-93, 2005
5. Heyer CM et al: Lipomatous hypertrophy of the interatrial septum: a prospective study of incidence, imaging findings, and clinical symptoms. Chest. 124(6):2068-73, 2003
6. Iacovoni A et al: [Lipomatous hypertrophy of the interatrial septum: its assessment with TEE, CT and MRI] G Ital Cardiol. 28(11):1273-7, 1998
7. Meaney JF et al: CT appearance of lipomatous hypertrophy of the interatrial septum. AJR Am J Roentgenol. 168(4):1081-4, 1997
8. Burke AP et al: Lipomatous hypertrophy of the atrial septum presenting as a right atrial mass. Am J Surg Pathol. 20(6):678-85, 1996
9. Shirani J et al: Clinical, electrocardiographic and morphologic features of massive fatty deposits ("lipomatous hypertrophy") in the atrial septum. J Am Coll Cardiol. 22(1):226-38, 1993
10. Lund JT et al: Cardiac masses: assessment by MR imaging. AJR Am J Roentgenol. 152(3):469-73, 1989
11. Simons M et al: Lipomatous hypertrophy of the atrial septum: diagnosis by combined echocardiography and computerized tomography. Am J Cardiol. 54(3):465-6, 1984
12. Prior JT: Lipomatous hypertrophy of cardiac interatrial septum: a lesion resembling hibernoma, lipoblastomatosis and infiltrating lipoma. Arch Pathol. 78:11-5, 1964

LIPOMATOUS HYPERTROPHY, INTERATRIAL SEPTUM

IMAGE GALLERY

Variant

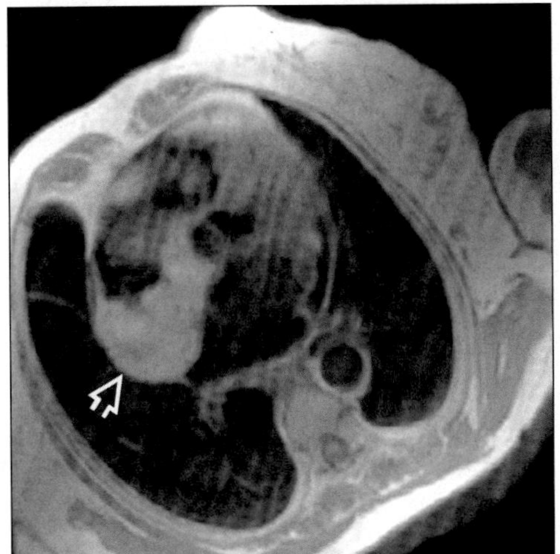

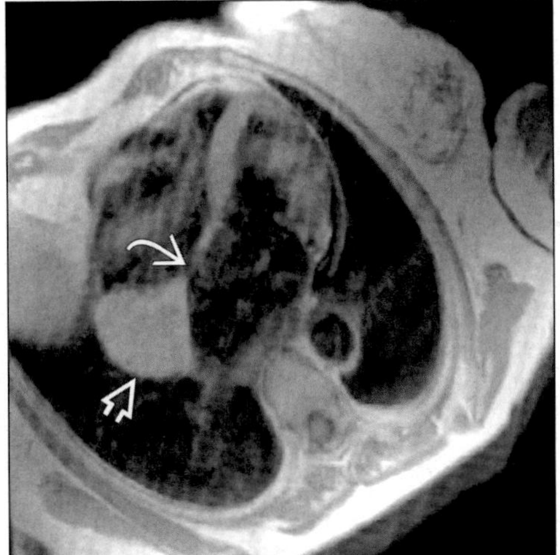

*(**Left**) Oblique black blood SE MR shows a large amount of high T1 signal tissue involving SVC (not shown) inflow and atrial septum, simulating a mass. (**Right**) Oblique black blood SE MR at lower level shows T1 bright tissue confined to atrial septum and sparing of fossa ovalis, suggesting lipomatous hypertrophy of septum.*

Typical

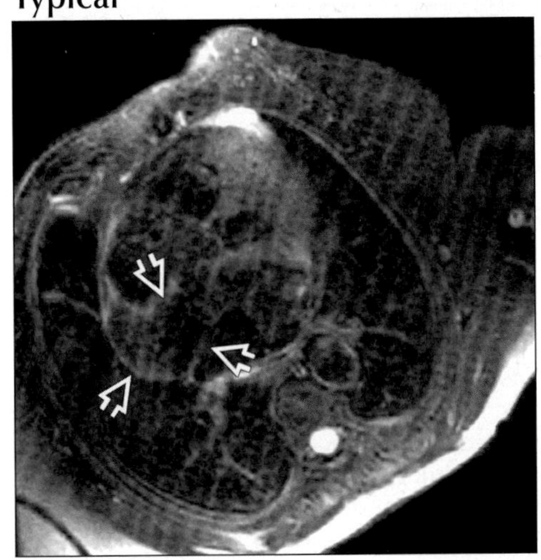

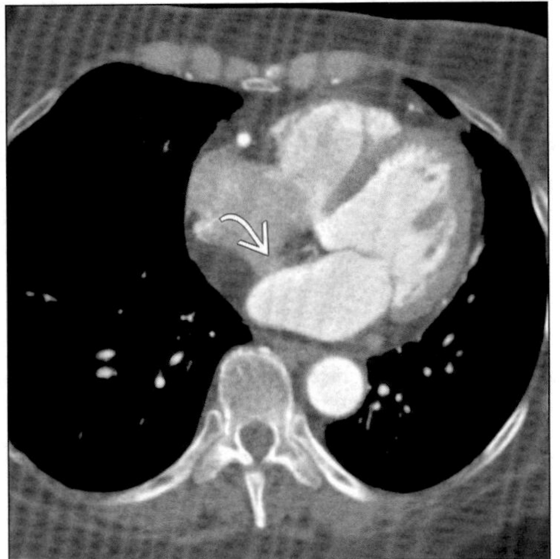

*(**Left**) Fat-suppressed black blood MR in same patient as previous two images shows complete signal dropout of the tissue proving fatty composition of the "mass". (**Right**) Axial CTA shows typical fatty infiltration of interatrial septum with dumbbell appearance due to sparing of fossa ovalis.*

Typical

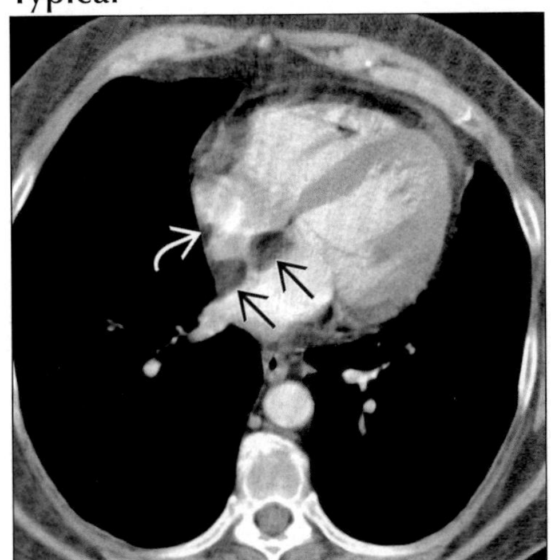

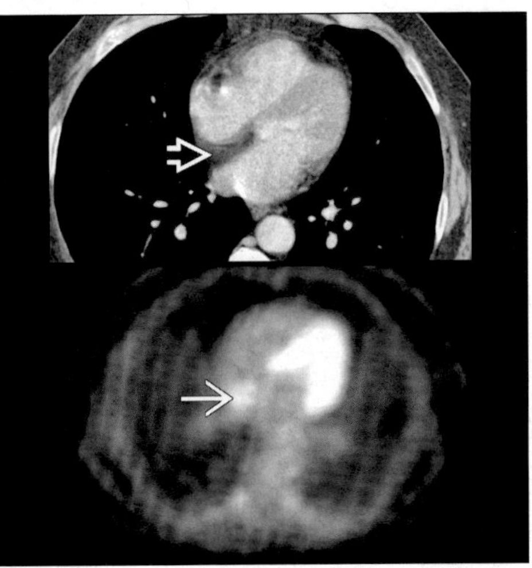

*(**Left**) Axial non-gated CTA shows lipomatous hypertrophy of interatrial septum and crista terminalis. The fossa ovalis membrane cannot be discerned due to motion artifact and borderline spatial resolution. (**Right**) Axial PET/CT shows lipomatous hypertrophy of interatrial septum on CT with corresponding increased FDG uptake on PET, which can mimic metastatic deposits if not recognized as LHIS.*

LYMPHOMA

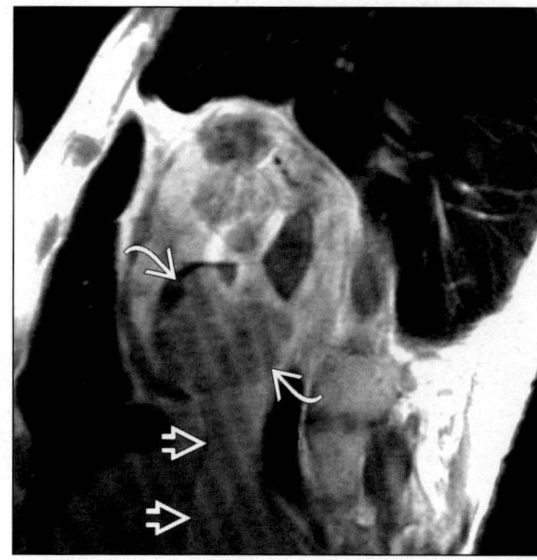

Short Axis T1WI MR black blood shows broadly attached large lobulated mass in RA obstructing the IVC inflow. Note: Bright signal in IVC despite black blood technique due to slow IVC flow.

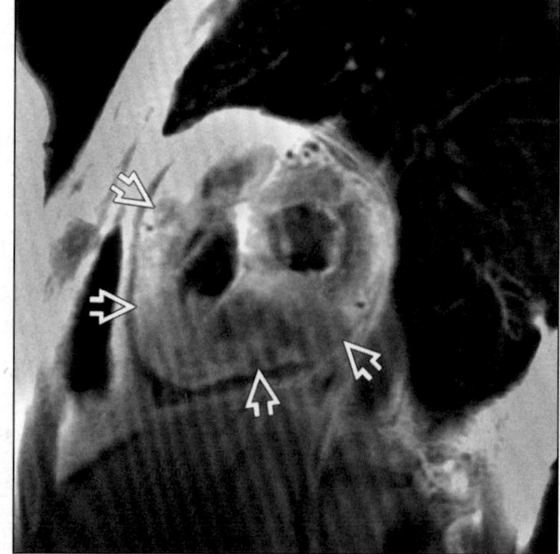

Short Axis T1WI MR black blood shows lobulated heterogeneously enhancing masses in RV and LV myocardium. A positive biopsy and no extracardiac lymphoma indicate primary cardiac lymphoma.

TERMINOLOGY

Abbreviations and Synonyms

- Primary cardiac lymphoma (PCL)
- Secondary cardiac lymphoma
- Malignant lymphoma of the heart

Definitions

- Primary cardiac lymphoma
  - Non-Hodgkin lymphoma involving only the heart or pericardium
  - Rare
  - More frequent in HIV/AIDS patients
- Secondary cardiac lymphoma
  - Cardiac involvement in patients with prior systemic lymphoma
  - Approximately one third of lymphoma patients develop secondary cardiac lymphoma (on pathology series)

IMAGING FINDINGS

General Features

- Best diagnostic clue: Enhancing, large, lobulated, intracavitary mass
- Location
  - Right atrium most frequently involved, followed by right ventricle, left ventricle and atrium, interatrial septum
  - Secondary lymphoma more commonly has pericardial involvement
  - May involve myocardium diffusely
    - Can mimic hypertrophic cardiomyopathy
  - Often predominantly intracavitary
    - Frequently nodular or lobulated
  - Epicardial involvement often demonstrates encasement of coronary arteries
  - Can involve exclusively pericardial space
  - Secondary cardiac lymphoma will have other non-cardiac foci
    - Check non cardiac structures
  - PCL reported to be more common in the right atrium

DDx: Cardiac Lymphoma

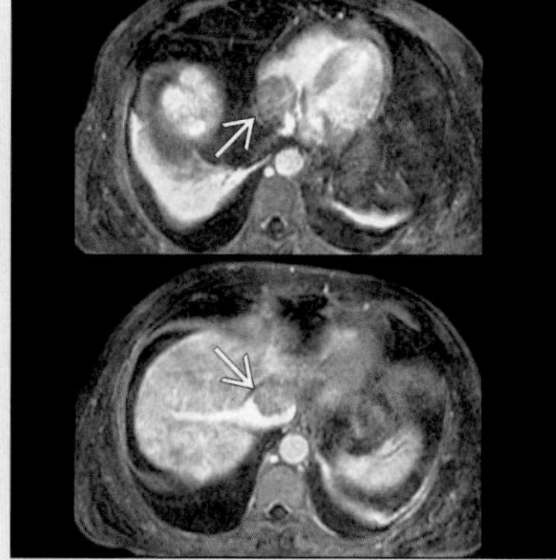

Angioinvasive Liver CA

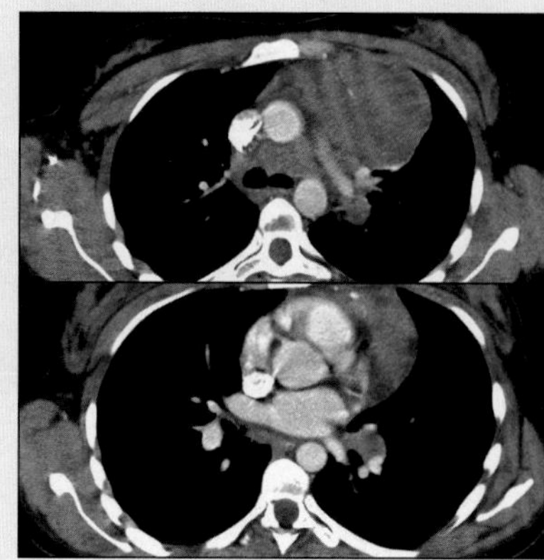

Mediastinal Lymphoma

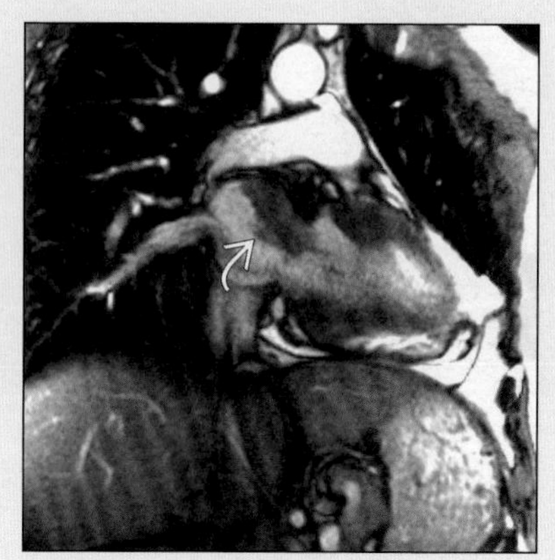

Sarcoma

LYMPHOMA

Key Facts

Terminology

- Primary cardiac lymphoma
  - Non-Hodgkin lymphoma involving only the heart or pericardium
  - Rare in general population, more frequent in HIV/AIDS patients
- Secondary cardiac lymphoma
  - Cardiac involvement in systemic lymphoma
- Approximately one third of lymphoma patients have cardiac involvement on post mortem examination

Imaging Findings

- Enhancing, large, lobulated, intracavitary mass
- May involve myocardium diffusely
  - Can mimic hypertrophic cardiomyopathy
- Epicardial involvement often demonstrates encasement of coronary arteries
- PCL reported to be more common in the right atrium
- Contrast-enhanced T1 weighted and delayed enhanced images may improve contrast between mass and non-affected myocardium

Clinical Issues

- Secondary lymphoma frequently not clinically apparent until patient dies of other complications
- Primary cardiac lymphoma 25-60 times more common in HIV/AIDS compared to general population

Diagnostic Checklist

- Imaging of abdomen and pelvis may reveal other lymphoma involvement and change diagnosis from primary to secondary cardiac lymphoma

- Size: Variable, but often large, filling most of affected cavity
- Morphology
  - Typically lobulated and intracavitary
  - May be diffusely infiltrating

Radiographic Findings

- Radiography
  - Signs of congestive heart failure (RV, LV, or biventricular failure, depending on involved structures)
  - May have cardiomegaly and pericardial effusion
  - May demonstrate other manifestations of lymphoma if secondary lymphoma

CT Findings

- Gated CT superior to non-gated CT
- Hypo- or iso-attenuating with respect to myocardium
- May miss diffuse myocardial infiltration without cavitary component
- Lobular mass with heterogeneous enhancement
- May demonstrate other manifestations of lymphoma, which then would indicate that cardiac involvement is secondary

MR Findings

- T1 and T2 weighted sequence may show diffusely infiltrating lymphoma as isointense, which makes it difficult to determine its extent
- T1 C+ MR and delayed enhanced imaging may improve contrast between brighter mass and non-affected darker or "nulled" myocardium
  - Usually heterogeneous enhancement
- Predominantly intraluminal masses are readily detected on white blood cine sequences
  - May demonstrate jets from flow obstruction
- May demonstrate encasement of coronary arteries
- May be used to monitor treatment success/remission and recurrence
- Chamber enlargement if obstructing physiology

Echocardiographic Findings

- Transthoracic echocardiography for initial evaluation of suspected cardiac mass
- Hypoechoic mass, pericardial effusion

Imaging Recommendations

- Best imaging tool: Cardiac gated MR
- Protocol advice
  - White blood cine images to assess for flow obstruction
  - T1 weighted spin echo sequences pre- and post-gadolinium (identical spatial locations) to assess for abnormal enhancement
  - Delayed enhancement imaging may improve contrast between unaffected and infiltrated myocardium

DIFFERENTIAL DIAGNOSIS

Other Primary Cardiac Tumors

- Myxoma
  - Most common primary cardiac tumor
  - Usually attached to atrial septum via stalk
  - Left atrium most common location
  - Low grade patchy enhancement
  - Bright on T2WI
- Sarcomas
  - Most common primary cardiac malignancy
  - Second most common of all (benign or malignant) primary cardiac tumors after myxoma
- Leiomyoma, rhabdomyoma, fibroma, hemangioma, lipoma, etc.

Metastatic Disease

- 40 times more common than all primary cardiac neoplasms

Non-Neoplastic Disorders

- Hypertrophic cardiomyopathy

LYMPHOMA

PATHOLOGY

General Features

- Etiology
  - Primary cardiac/pericardial involvement by a T cell phenotype has been described in post (non-cardiac) transplant patients
  - HIV/AIDS
    - Isolated cardiac tumors in HIV/AIDS are typically primary lymphoma
    - Primary cardiac non-Hodgkin lymphoma 25-60 times more common compared to general population
    - Secondary cardiac tumors often due to widespread Kaposi sarcoma
- Epidemiology
  - Primary cardiac lymphoma has an incidence of 0.06% in general population on pathology series
  - Only 1.3% of all primary cardiac tumors are PCL

Gross Pathologic & Surgical Features

- Multiple firm nodules, contiguous invasion of pericardium

CLINICAL ISSUES

Presentation

- Most common signs/symptoms: Dyspnea, systemic venous hypertension, chest pain, arrhythmias, right ventricular or bi-ventricular failure, syncope, pericardial effusion
- Other signs/symptoms
  - May mimic CHF
  - Rapid progression
  - May be occult until presenting with cardiac tamponade
  - Secondary lymphoma frequently occult in vivo and detected post mortem

Demographics

- Gender: No gender predilection

Natural History & Prognosis

- Secondary lymphoma frequently not clinically apparent until patient dies of other lymphoma related causes
- T-cell lymphomas invade the heart more frequently and are more aggressive than B-cell lymphomas
  - T-cell lymphomas are more likely to have cardiac manifestations
- Clinical outcome of PCL is variable
  - Early diagnosis and treatment may result in complete remission
  - Prognosis of HIV associated primary cardiac lymphoma is poor

Treatment

- Chemotherapy or combination of chemotherapy and radiation
- Autologous stem cell transplant has been described
- Pericardial drainage if tamponade
- Surgical treatment in some cases

DIAGNOSTIC CHECKLIST

Consider

- Rapidly progressive and treatment resistive congestive heart failure may be first presenting symptom

Image Interpretation Pearls

- Additional imaging of abdomen & pelvis may reveal other lymphomatous involvement & change the diagnosis from primary to secondary cardiac lymphoma

SELECTED REFERENCES

1. Mahesha V et al: Primary cardiac post-transplantation lymphoproliferative disorder--T cell type: a case report and review of the literature. J Clin Pathol. 60(4):447-8, 2007
2. Montiel V et al: Primary cardiac lymphoma and complete atrio-ventricular block: case report and review of the literature. Acta Cardiol. 62(1):55-8, 2007
3. Nascimento AF et al: Primary Cardiac Lymphoma: Clinical, Histologic, Immunophenotypic, and Genotypic Features of 5 Cases of a Rare Disorder. Am J Surg Pathol. 31(9):1344-1350, 2007
4. De Filippo M et al: Primary cardiac Burkett's type lymphoma: transthoracic echocardiography, multidetector computed tomography and magnetic resonance findings. Acta Radiol. 47(2):167-71, 2006
5. Chinen K et al: Cardiac involvement by malignant lymphoma: a clinicopathologic study of 25 autopsy cases based on the WHO classification. Ann Hematol. 84(8):498-505, 2005
6. Gulati G et al: Comparison of echo and MRI in the imaging evaluation of intracardiac masses. Cardiovasc Intervent Radiol. 27(5):459-69, 2004
7. Khan NU et al: Cardiac involvement in non-Hodgkin's lymphoma: with and without HIV infection. Int J Cardiovasc Imaging. 20(6):477-81, 2004
8. Kubo S et al: Primary cardiac lymphoma demonstrated by delayed contrast-enhanced magnetic resonance imaging. J Comput Assist Tomogr. 28(6):849-51, 2004
9. Rockwell L et al: Cardiac involvement in malignancies. Case 3. Primary cardiac lymphoma. J Clin Oncol. 22(13):2744-5, 2004
10. Daehnert W: Radiology Review Manual. Fifth Edition. Lippincott Williams & Wilkins, Philadelphia, 2003
11. Lam KY et al: Tumors of the heart. A 20-year experience with a review of 12,485 consecutive autopsies. Arch Pathol Lab Med. 117(10):1027-31, 1993
12. McDonnell PJ et al: Involvement of the heart by malignant lymphoma: a clinicopathologic study. Cancer. 49(5):944-51, 1982
13. Abbara S et al. Pericardial and Myocardial Disease. In: Miller SW: Cardiac Imaging - The Requisites. Elsevier Mosby, Philadelphia, PA, 2005 245-283

IMAGE GALLERY

Typical

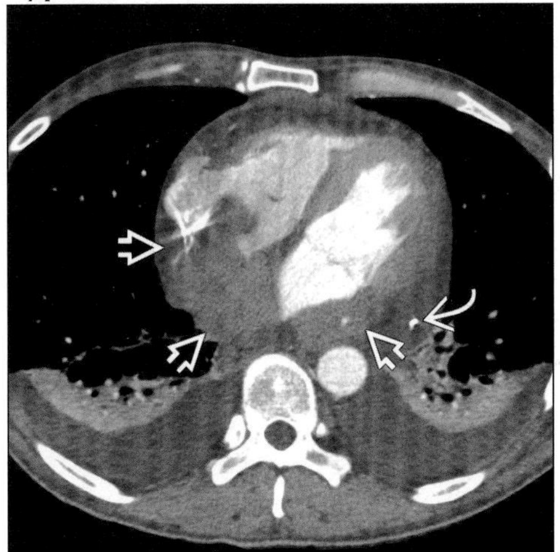

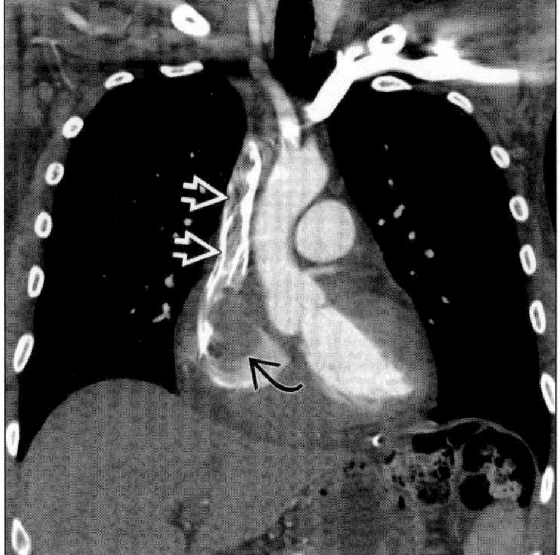

(Left) *Axial CECT shows large lobulated masses, broadly infiltrating the right and left atrial walls ➔. Note: Pericardial drain ➔ with small remaining amount of pericardial fluid; bilateral pleural effusions/atelectasis.* ***(Right)*** *Coronal CECT in the same patient as previous image shows large, lobular, intracavitary, right atrial component of lymphoma ➔ partially obstructing the SVC ➔ inflow.*

Typical

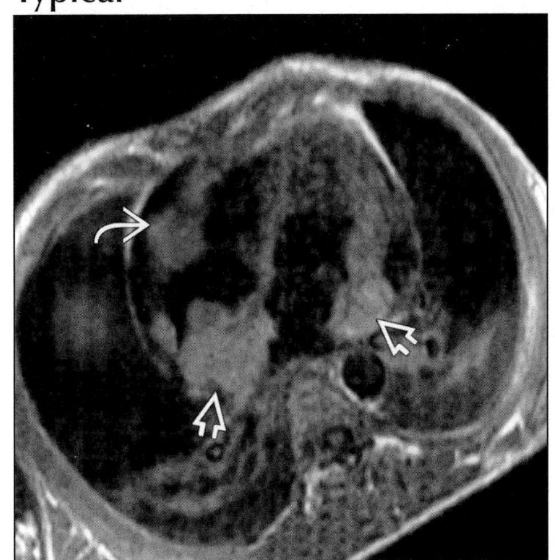

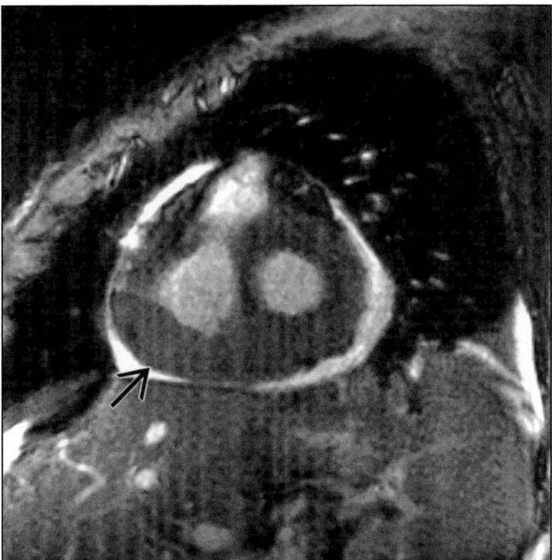

(Left) *Axial T1WI MR black blood SE after gadolinium administration in same patient as previous image shows heterogeneously enhancing masses involving both atria ➔ and the right ventricular anterior free-wall ➔.* ***(Right)*** *Short axis SSFP in a different patient shows lymphoma with markedly thickened RV diaphragmatic free-wall ➔, but without any discrete intracavitary component of mass. Note: Small pericardial effusion.*

Typical

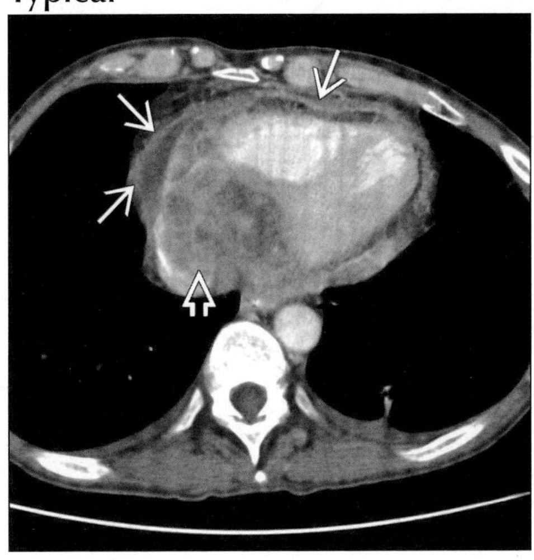

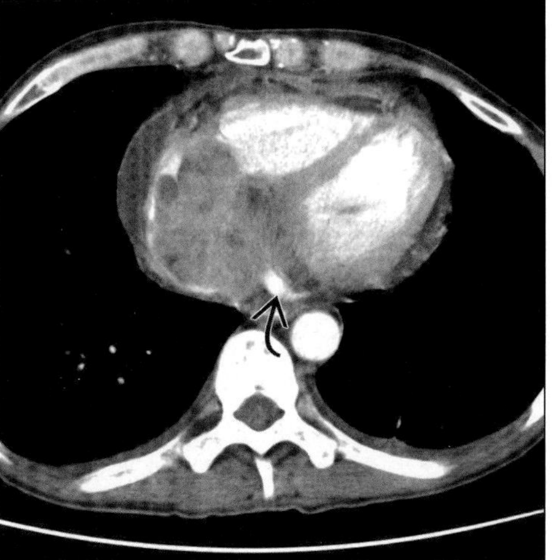

(Left) *Axial CECT shows large, right atrial, lobulated, heterogeneously enhancing mass ➔, and thickened and enhancing pericardium ➔ with small pericardial effusion.* ***(Right)*** *Axial CECT in the same patient as previous image, shows that mass fills most of the right atrium and obstructs the tricuspid valve. Note: Coronary sinus ➔ inflow obstruction. Patient is HIV+ and biopsy confirmed primary cardiac non-Hodgkin lymphoma.*

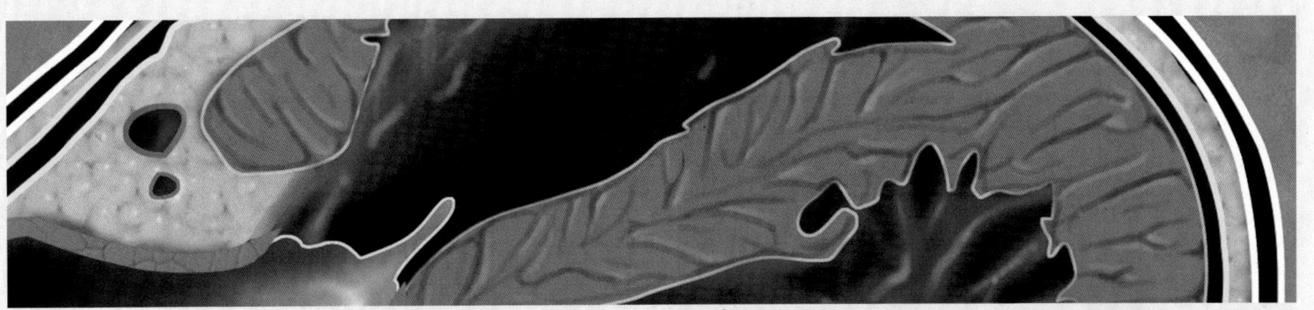

SECTION 5: Cardiomyopathy

HYPERTROPHIC CARDIOMYOPATHY

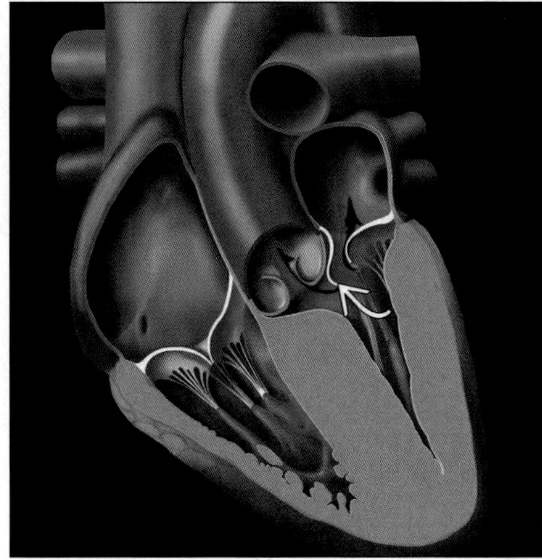

Graphic of five chamber systolic view shows concentric HCM. Note: Increased LVOT flow velocity (Venturi effect) and systolic anterior motion of anterior mitral valve leaflet, which causes mitral regurgitation.

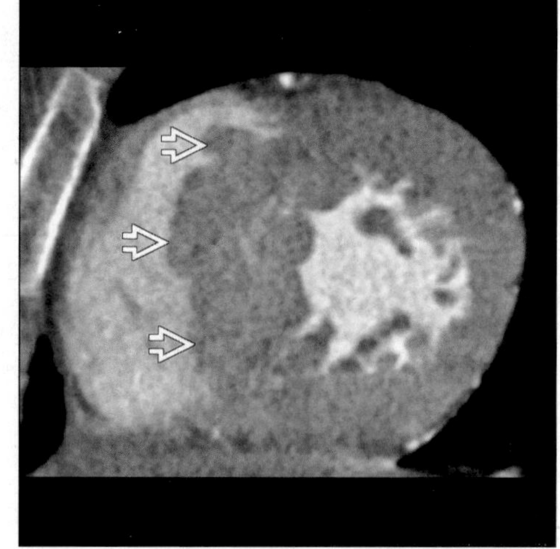

Short axis coronary CTA in diastole shows diffuse hypertrophy of the left ventricle with an asymmetric thickening (3 cm) involving the interventricular septum in a patient with HOCM.

TERMINOLOGY

Abbreviations and Synonyms

- Hypertrophic cardiomyopathy (HCM)

Definitions

- HCM is a genetic disease of the cardiac sarcomere
  - Increased left ventricular (LV) mass with resultant hypertrophy without an obvious etiology
  - Hypertrophy tends to be asymmetric involving basal septum but disorder can present with atypical patterns of hypertrophy such as mid-cavity or apical
  - When LV outflow tract obstruction is present the disease is referred to as hypertrophic obstructive cardiomyopathy (HOCM) or idiopathic hypertrophic subaortic stenosis (IHSS)

IMAGING FINDINGS

General Features

- Best diagnostic clue
  - Hallmark is myocardial hypertrophy which cannot be explained by another disease (i.e., hypertension, aortic stenosis)
    - Most common diagnostic criterion of HCM is LV wall thickness > 15 mm, although cases may exist with less hypertrophy
- Location
  - Degree and distribution of LV hypertrophy in HCM is variable
    - Most common location is basal septum hypertrophy with or without obstruction
    - Asymmetric septal hypertrophy (ASH) defined by a ratio of the wall thickness of the septum to a non-hypertrophied segment > 1.3
    - Rare cases exist of concentric hypertrophy, mid-cavity hypertrophy, and apical hypertrophy
- Morphology: Nondilated and hyperdynamic LV

Radiographic Findings

- Radiography
  - Variable findings
    - Cardiac silhouette may range from normal to markedly increased

DDx: Hypertrophic Cardiomyopathy

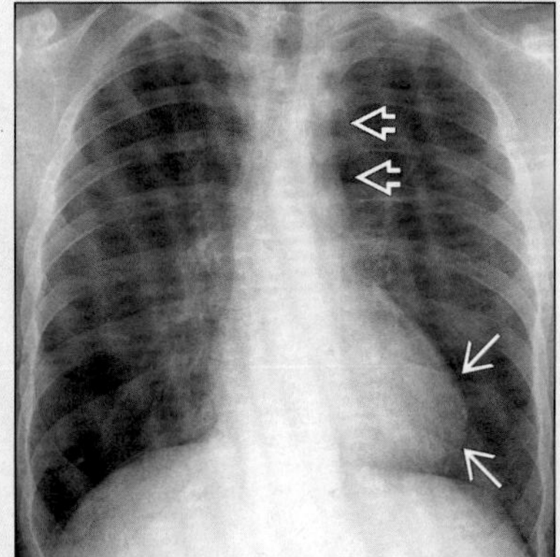

Aortic Coarctation

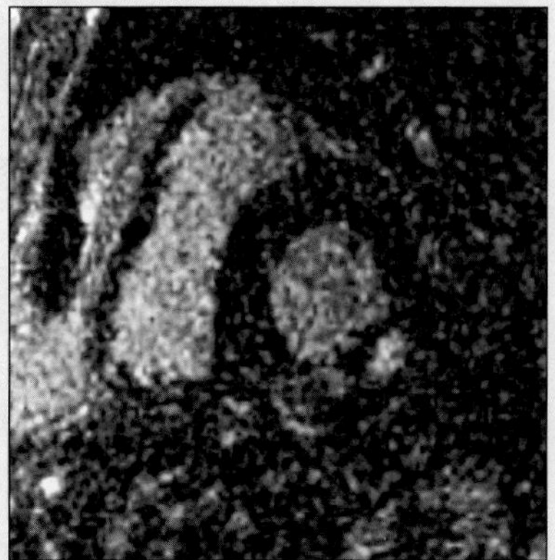

Sarcoid

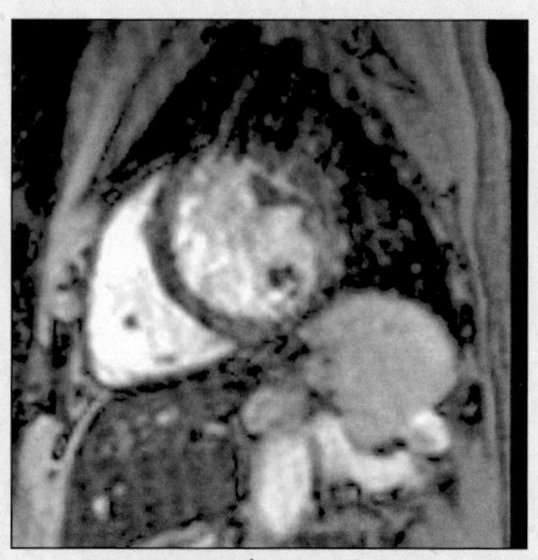

Hemochromatosis

HYPERTROPHIC CARDIOMYOPATHY

Key Facts

Terminology
- HCM is a genetic disease of the cardiac sarcomere
- Increased left ventricular (LV) mass with resultant hypertrophy without an obvious etiology

Imaging Findings
- Hallmark is myocardial hypertrophy which cannot be explained by another disease (i.e., hypertension, aortic stenosis)
- Most common diagnostic criterion of HCM is LV wall thickness > 15 mm, although cases may exist with less hypertrophy
- Most common location is basal septum hypertrophy with or without obstruction
- Morphology: Nondilated and hyperdynamic LV
- LV outflow tract (LVOT) obstruction with abnormal flow dynamics in some cases
- Mitral valve regurgitation and systolic anterior motion (SAM) of the mitral valve leaflet
- Echocardiography is diagnostic

Top Differential Diagnoses
- Aortic Stenosis
- Restrictive Cardiomyopathy
- Systemic Arterial Hypertension
- Aortic Coarctation

Pathology
- Autosomal dominant with incomplete penetrance and variable expressivity resulting in clinical heterogeneity among patients and family members

Clinical Issues
- Most common cause of sudden cardiac death (SCD) in both preadolescent and adolescent children

---

- Left atrial enlargement frequently (radiograph: Right retrocardial double density) is observed, especially when significant mitral regurgitation is present

MR Findings
- Quantification of left ventricular mass
  - LV hypertrophy can be asymmetric or symmetric and involve the basal, mid, apical and septal portions
- Delayed myocardial enhancement with gadolinium usually representing areas of increased fibrosis
  - Delayed enhancement can be diffuse or focal and involve any portion of LV wall
  - Delayed enhancement has been shown to be more common at junction of the RV wall and septum
  - Volume of delayed hyperenhancement on MR correlates with risk for sudden cardiac death
- LV outflow tract (LVOT) obstruction with abnormal flow dynamics in some cases
- Mitral valve regurgitation and systolic anterior motion (SAM) of the mitral valve leaflet

Nuclear Medicine Findings
- Radionuclide imaging with thallium or technetium may show reversible defects
  - Mostly in absence of coronary artery disease
  - Reversible defects on radionuclide scanning are more common in children and adolescents with a history of sudden death or syncope

Echocardiographic Findings
- Echocardiogram
  - Echocardiography is diagnostic
  - Two-dimensional echocardiography findings
    - Diagnostic for hypertropic cardiomyopathy
    - Color Doppler flow studies typically reveal mitral regurgitation from SAM of the anterior mitral valve leaflet
    - 2D images demonstrate septal thickening and SAM of anterior mitral valve leaflet

Imaging Recommendations
- Best imaging tool
  - Echocardiography
    - Widely available, first line modality
  - MR
    - Excellent tool in experienced hands
    - Less robust and less widely available when compared to echocardiography

DIFFERENTIAL DIAGNOSIS

Aortic Stenosis
- Morphology: Thickening, fusion and/or calcification of the aortic valve apparatus
- Extremely elevated peak systolic pressure gradient
- Severe aortic stenosis (AS) leads to concentric left ventricular hypertrophy
- Echocardiography is the most important technique for diagnosis and follow-up of patients with AS
- MR findings
  - Systolic flow void (jet) on cine exam arises at valve level (not LVOT) and extends into proximal aorta
  - Secondary left ventricular hypertrophy in severe AS

Restrictive Cardiomyopathy
- Replacement of cardiac tissue with scar tissue
  - Secondary to variant of systemic disorders such as amyloidosis, sarcoidosis, hemochromatosis, chemotherapy or radiation
  - Primary or idiopathic restrictive cardiomyopathy is uncommon
- Increased resistance to ventricular filling due to increased myocardial stiffness
- Leads to diastolic dysfunction
- Best diagnostic clue: Increased left ventricular thickness and mass with infiltration of myocardium
- Chest radiography findings
  - Demonstrate the typical appearance of congestive heart failure but without cardiomegaly
    - Pulmonary venous hypertension
    - LV dilatation may also be seen in some cases

Systemic Arterial Hypertension

- Leading cause of concentric left ventricular hypertrophy

Aortic Coarctation

- Narrowing of the aortic lumen with obstruction to blood flow
- Classic plain film appearance of rib notching and the figure "3" sign
  - Focal aortic narrowing, presence of collaterals
- Gated CT or MR may reveal bicuspid aortic valve ± ascending aortic aneurysm
- Phase-contrast MR can estimate of flow velocities and gradient

PATHOLOGY

General Features

- Genetics
  - Autosomal dominant with incomplete penetrance and variable expressivity resulting in clinical heterogeneity among patients and family members
    - Morphologic evidence of disease is found by echocardiography in approximately 25% of first-degree relatives of patients with HCM
- Etiology: Molecular basis for HCM is mutations in several genes encoding for structural components of thick and thin filaments
- Epidemiology
  - Prevalence is 1:500 in young healthy adults
  - HCM is reported in 0.5% of outpatient population referred for echocardiography
    - Overall prevalence of HCM is 0.16-0.29% of the population

Gross Pathologic & Surgical Features

- Macroscopically characterized by left ventricular hypertrophy, which may be asymmetrical or symmetrical
  - Both symmetric and asymmetric forms of HCM can have right ventricular involvement in up to 15% of cases
  - Any portion of LV can be affected by HCM (basal, mid-ventricular or apical)

Microscopic Features

- Pathologic hallmarks are myocyte hypertrophy and disarray together with expansion of the interstitial collagen compartment (fibrosis) resulting in gross disorganization of muscle bundles and changes in intramyocardial arteries and capillaries

Staging, Grading or Classification Criteria

- HCM can be separated into obstructive and non-obstructive types

CLINICAL ISSUES

Presentation

- Most common signs/symptoms
  - Most patients are asymptomatic
  - Other symptoms/signs include chest pain, palpitations, syncope (often during exercise), sudden cardiac death
- Other signs/symptoms: Congestive heart failure with orthopnea and paroxysmal nocturnal dyspnea
- Most common cause of sudden cardiac death (SCD) in both preadolescent and adolescent children
  - SCD usually caused by arrhythmias in the form of ventricular fibrillation (VF) or sustained ventricular tachycardia (VT)

Demographics

- Age: Can present at any age from infancy to adulthood
- Gender: No gender preference, however symptoms tend to be more severe and fatal in males

Natural History & Prognosis

- Can be a chronic illness requiring life-style restrictions or be the cause of sudden death
  - Risk of sudden death in children is has high as 6% per year
- Mode of death for patients with HCM depends on age
  - SCD is the most common mode of death in young, otherwise healthy individuals and athletes between age of 10 and 35 years
  - Heart failure and HCM-related stroke from atrial fibrillation is the most common cause of death in elderly

Treatment

- Beta blockers or calcium channel blockers to improve diastolic relaxation and reduce risk of arrhythmias
- Septal myomectomy or catheter based alcohol septal ablation for symptomatic relief in refractory cases
- Automatic intracardiac defibrillator in those patients at high risk for sudden cardiac death

SELECTED REFERENCES

1. Soler R et al: Magnetic resonance imaging of delayed enhancement in hypertrophic cardiomyopathy: relationship with left ventricular perfusion and contractile function. J Comput Assist Tomogr. 30(3):412-20, 2006
2. Hughes SE: The pathology of hypertrophic cardiomyopathy. Histopathology. 44(5):412-27, 2004
3. Moon JC et al: Toward clinical risk assessment in hypertrophic cardiomyopathy with gadolinium cardiovascular magnetic resonance. J Am Coll Cardiol. 41(9):1561-7, 2003
4. Braunwald E et al: Contemporary evaluation and management of hypertrophic cardiomyopathy. Circulation. 106(11):1312-6, 2002
5. Wilson JM et al: Magnetic resonance imaging of myocardial fibrosis in hypertrophic cardiomyopathy. Tex Heart Inst J. 29(3):176-80, 2002
6. Dong SJ et al: Left ventricular wall thickness and regional systolic function in patients with hypertrophic cardiomyopathy. A three-dimensional tagged magnetic resonance imaging study. Circulation. 90(3):1200-9, 1994
7. Casolo GC et al: Detection of apical hypertrophic cardiomyopathy by magnetic resonance imaging. Am Heart J. 117(2):468-72, 1989
8. Higgins CB et al: Magnetic resonance imaging in hypertrophic cardiomyopathy. Am J Cardiol. 55(9):1121-6, 1985

HYPERTROPHIC CARDIOMYOPATHY

IMAGE GALLERY

Typical

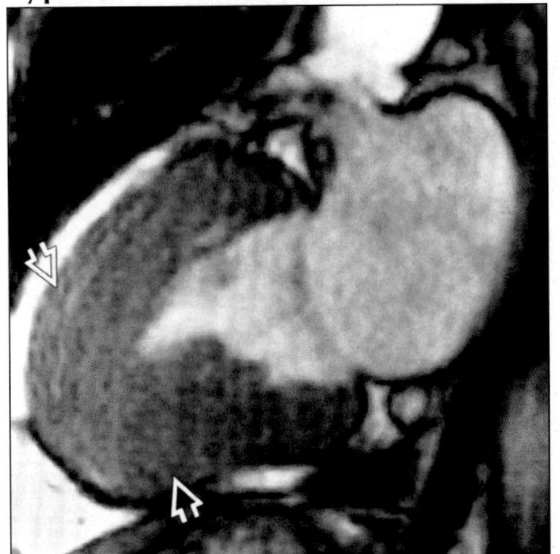

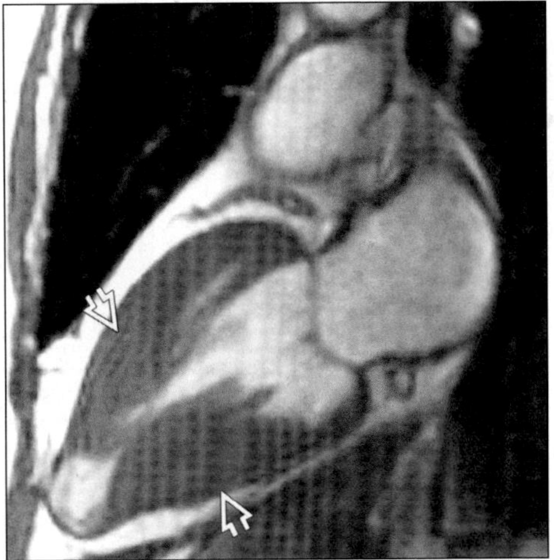

(Left) *SSFP paraseptal long axis shows apical variant of hypertrophic cardiomyopathy . Note, spade-shaped appearance of LV cavity.* ***(Right)*** *SSFP paraseptal long axis shows mid ventricular variant of hypertrophic cardiomyopathy .*

Typical

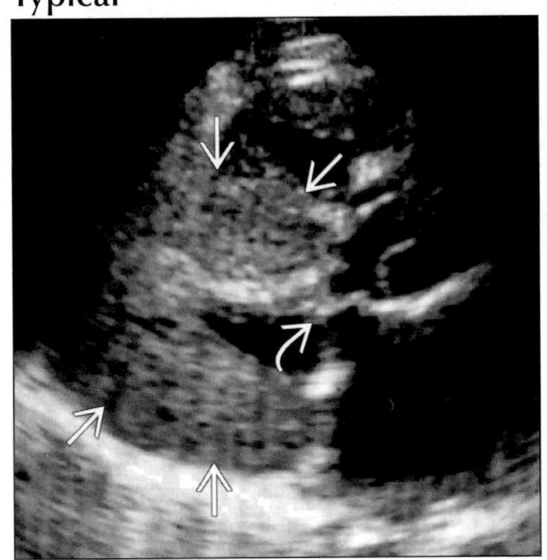

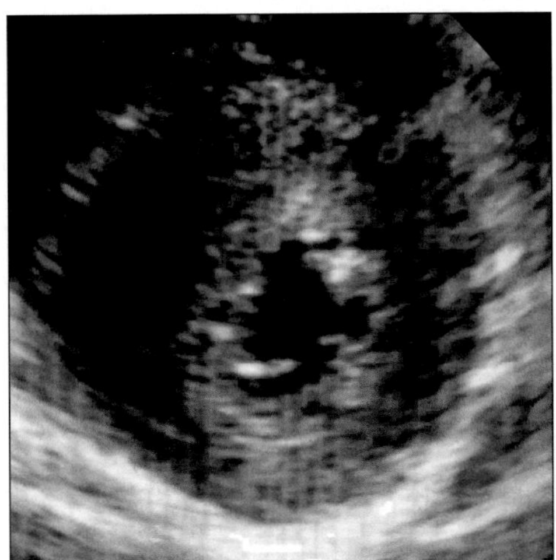

(Left) *Parasternal long axis echocardiogram shows hypertrophic cardiomyopathy with severe wall thickening and systolic cavity obliteration. Note systolic anterior motion (SAM) of the anterior mitral valve leaflet .* ***(Right)*** *LV short axis echocardiogram shows severe hypertrophic cardiomyopathy in the same patient as previous image.*

Typical

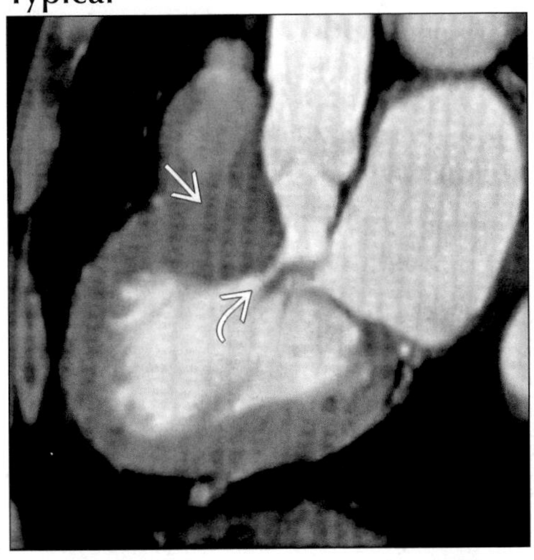

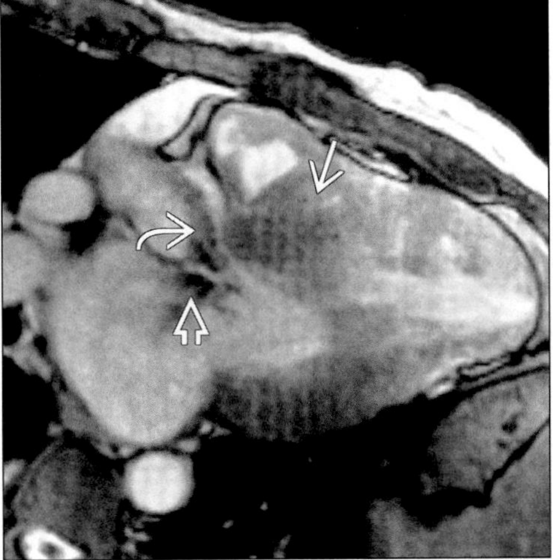

(Left) *Three chamber view coronary CTA shows hypertrophic obstructive cardiomyopathy with asymmetric septal hypertrophy . Note SAM of the anterior mitral valve leaflet and resultant malcoaptation of mitral valve (causing regurgitation).* ***(Right)*** *Three chamber view SSFP shows hypertrophic obstructive cardiomyopathy with basal septal hypertrophy . Note the mitral regurgitation jet and LVOT flow acceleration .*

DILATED CARDIOMYOPATHY

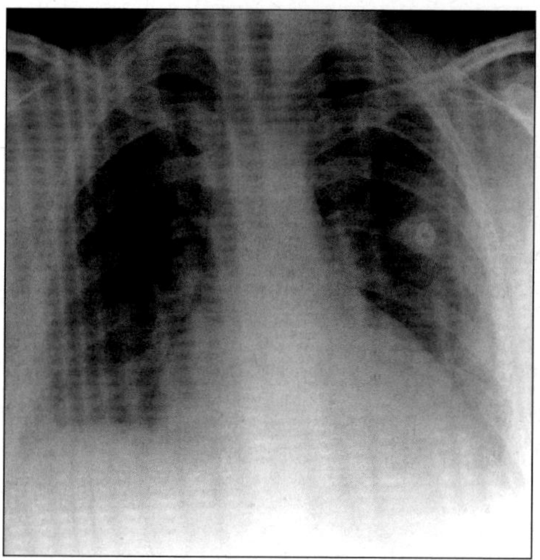

Posteroanterior radiograph shows enlarged cardiac silhouette consistent with dilated cardiomyopathy.

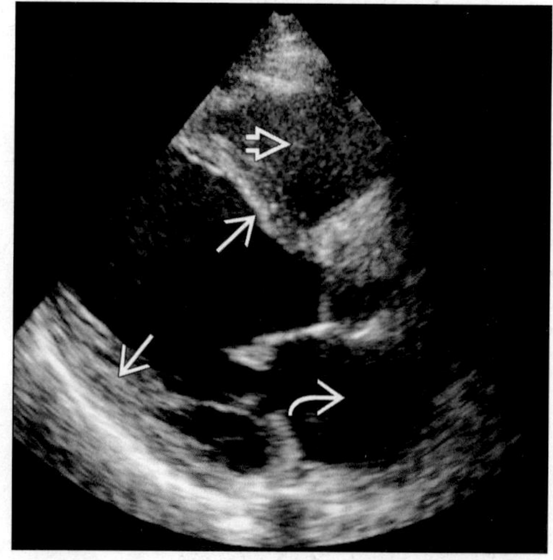

Parasternal long axis echocardiographic view shows dilated left ventricle at end diastole. Endocardial borders →. Left atrium ↷ and right ventricle ⇨.

TERMINOLOGY

Abbreviations and Synonyms

- Dilated Cardiomyopathy (DCM)

Definitions

- Left ventricular chamber dilation with systolic dysfunction with or without right ventricular dysfunction, LVEF < 40%
  - Systolic dysfunction (LVEF < 40%)
- Multiple etiologies: Final common end point of a variety of disease processes which cause myocardial damage
  - Idiopathic, familial, myocarditis, ischemic heart disease, infiltrative disease (amyloid, sarcoid), peripartum cardiomyopathy, hypertension, infectious, connective tissue disease, toxic (alcohol, cocaine), chemotherapy (doxorubicin), and metabolic (hypophosphatemia, hypocalcemia, uremia), endocrinopathies (thyroid dysfunction, pheochromocytoma, Cushing disease)

IMAGING FINDINGS

Radiographic Findings

- Radiography
  - Cardiomegaly with cardiac shadow > 50% of thorax width on posteroanterior view
  - Pleural effusions
  - Dilation of superior vena cava and azygous vein

CT Findings

- Cardiac CTA can exclude ischemic etiology as the presence if no atherosclerotic plaque is identified
  - Volume rendered multiphase data sets can accurately demonstrate increased LV chamber dimensions and LV volumes
    - Quantify ventricular volumes, mass, and ejection fraction (EF)

MR Findings

- MR Cine
  - Quantify ventricular volume, mass, and ejection fraction (EF)
    - Findings include ventricular dilation and decreased systolic function

DDx: Cardiomyopathies

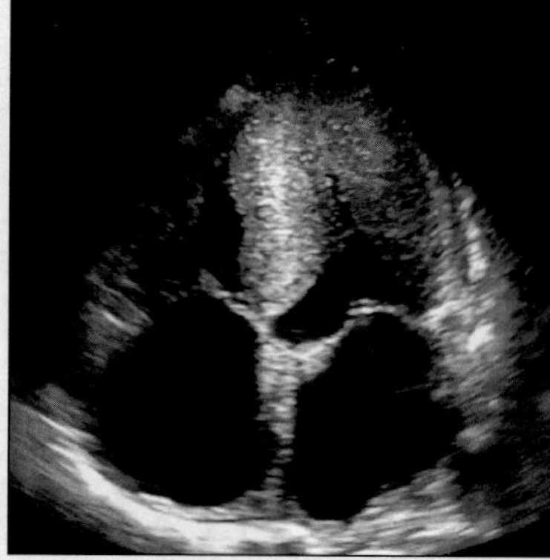

Restrictive Cardiomyopathy

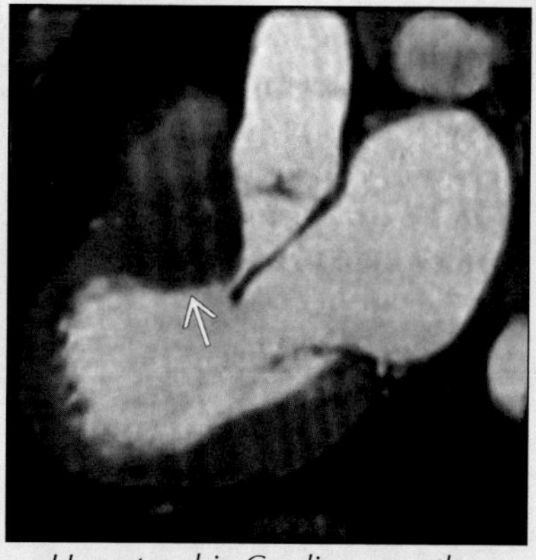

Hypertrophic Cardiomyopathy

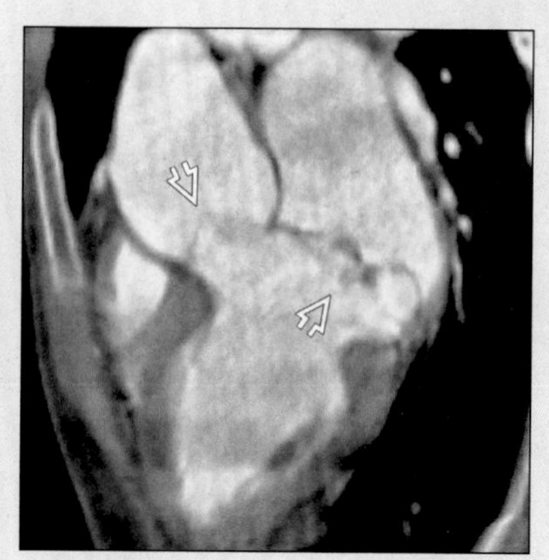

Aortic and Mitral Regurgitation

DILATED CARDIOMYOPATHY

Key Facts

Terminology
- Left ventricular chamber dilation with systolic dysfunction with or without right ventricular dysfunction, LVEF < 40%

Imaging Findings
- Cardiomegaly with cardiac shadow > 50% of thorax width on posteroanterior view
- Left ventricular or multichamber dilatation and severe contractile dysfunction of left ventricle with EF < 40%
- MR is most accurate method for assessing cardiac anatomy, left ventricular volumes, mass, and ejection fraction
- Echocardiography is most practical in the initial work-up of cardiomyopathy

Top Differential Diagnoses
- Restrictive Cardiomyopathy
- Hypertrophic Cardiomyopathy
- Valvular Heart Disease

Pathology
- Occult ischemic cardiomyopathy is most common dilated cardiomyopathy in United States
- Most patients present between the ages of 20 to 60 years old
- More prevalent and higher mortality in older individuals, African Americans and males

Clinical Issues
- Prognosis is related to severity of LV dysfunction
- Treat reversible causes

    - Tagging tracks deformation of myocardium throughout cardiac cycle and allows detailed evaluation of regional function
    - First pass perfusion is normal in cases of idiopathic dilated cardiomyopathy
    - Delayed contrast enhancement
        - Non-ischemic etiology demonstrates lack of delayed hyperenhancement or the presence of isolated intramyocardial mid-wall enhancement in a non-coronary distribution
        - Ischemic etiology demonstrates subendocardial or transmural hyperenhancement in a coronary distribution
        - Superior interstudy reproducibility for EF, LV volumes and mass when compared with echocardiography
- Can help to determine cause of dilated cardiomyopathy

Nuclear Medicine Findings
- PET: Can determine and quantify degree of myocardial perfusion and viability to distinguish idiopathic dilated cardiomyopathy from ischemic cardiomyopathy
- Radionuclide ventriculography
    - Assess myocardial perfusion and ventricular function

Echocardiographic Findings
- Echocardiogram
    - Left ventricular or multichamber dilatation and severe contractile dysfunction of left ventricle with EF < 40%
    - Global hypokinesis
        - Right ventricle may also be dilated and hypokinetic
    - Excellent for excluding valvular disease as the etiology
    - Can detect the presence of LV apical thrombus which is common in the setting of severe LV systolic dysfunction and/or apical wall motion abnormality
- Two-dimensional (2D) echocardiography
    - Measure ventricular wall thickness
    - Quantify LV volumes, mass, and ejection fraction
- Doppler echocardiography
    - Assess valvular function and hemodynamics
    - Comprehensive exam including conventional Doppler of mitral valve inflow and tissue Doppler of the LV myocardium can estimate cardiac filling pressures (i.e., pulmonary capillary wedge pressure)
        - Can use serial Doppler exam to assess response to therapy

Angiographic Findings
- Coronary angiography and left ventriculography
    - Utilized to exclude significant coronary artery disease as the etiology
    - Dilated left ventricle with reduced systolic function
    - Mural thrombi may occasionally be visualized at the apex
    - Normal coronary arteries are seen in idiopathic dilated cardiomyopathy

Imaging Recommendations
- Best imaging tool
    - MR is most accurate method for assessing cardiac anatomy, left ventricular volumes, mass, and ejection fraction
    - Echocardiography is most practical in the initial work-up of cardiomyopathy

DIFFERENTIAL DIAGNOSIS

Restrictive Cardiomyopathy
- Increased resistance to ventricular filling due to abnormal myocardial stiffness
- Biatrial enlargement with normal ventricular size
- Diastolic dysfunction
- Chest radiography findings of congestive heart failure without cardiomegaly

Hypertrophic Cardiomyopathy
- Genetic disease of the cardiac sarcomere
- Ventricular hypertrophy with increased LV mass without an obvious etiology

- Hypertrophy tends to be asymmetric involving the basal interventricular septum, but the disease may manifest with atypical patterns of hypertrophy such as mid cavity or apical

Valvular Heart Disease

- Chronic, severe mitral regurgitation and aortic regurgitation
  - Volume loaded left ventricle with increased volumes and decreased systolic function
  - Left ventricular dimensions are used as criteria to determine the timing of valve surgery
- End-stage aortic stenosis
  - Longstanding severe left ventricular pressure overload can cause a "burned out" dilated chamber
    - Results in low gradient (low output) aortic stenosis

PATHOLOGY

General Features

- Genetics
  - Familial dilated cardiomyopathy estimated to account for 25% of idiopathic cases
    - Mode of inheritance usually autosomal dominant although cases of autosomal recessive, X-linked, and mitochondrial inheritance have been described
  - Inherited syndromes
    - Dilated cardiomyopathy may be an important component of inherited disorders such as neuromuscular disease (i.e., muscular dystrophies, myotonic dystrophy)
- Etiology
  - Occult ischemic cardiomyopathy is most common dilated cardiomyopathy in United States
  - Idiopathic is the leading cause world wide
- Epidemiology
  - Most patients present between the ages of 20 to 60 years old
  - More prevalent and higher mortality in older individuals, African Americans and males

Gross Pathologic & Surgical Features

- Dilatation of all four chambers
- Intracavitary thrombi

Microscopic Features

- Interstitial and perivascular fibrosis

Staging, Grading or Classification Criteria

- New York Heart Association (NYHA) criteria is most often used to assess functional class of patients with heart failure - also has prognostic implications

CLINICAL ISSUES

Presentation

- Most common signs/symptoms: Biventricular failure with progressive and gradual dyspnea with exertion, impaired exercise capacity, orthopnea, paroxysmal nocturnal dyspnea, and peripheral edema
- Other signs/symptoms: Arrhythmia, angina, conduction disturbance, thromboembolic complications
- Clinical Profile: Obtain good history and laboratory tests to exclude lifestyle factors and other etiologies for potentially reversible causes of dilated cardiomyopathy

Demographics

- Age: Advancing age is reported as an independent risk factor for mortality
- Gender: Heart failure tends to be more common in men than in women
- Ethnicity: African Americans have almost a 3-fold increase in risk for developing dilated cardiomyopathy

Natural History & Prognosis

- Symptoms are progressive over months to years
- Prognosis is related to severity of LV dysfunction
- Outcome worse when the etiology is infiltrative, HIV infection, doxorubicin therapy, ischemic heart disease, and connective tissue disease

Treatment

- Treat reversible causes
- ACE inhibitors, hydralazine/nitrates, beta blockers, digoxin, diuretics
- Anticoagulation in subjects with lower LVEF to prevent thromboembolic complications
- Device therapy with ICD +/- biventricular pacing
- Cardiac transplantation

DIAGNOSTIC CHECKLIST

Consider

- Left ventricular or multichamber dilatation and severe contractile dysfunction of left ventricle with EF < 40%

SELECTED REFERENCES

1. Colletti PM: Cardiac imaging 2006. AJR Am J Roentgenol. 186(6 Suppl 2):S337-9, 2006
2. Rochitte CE et al: The emerging role of MRI in the diagnosis and management of cardiomyopathies. Curr Cardiol Rep. 8(1):44-52, 2006
3. Abbara S et al: Pericardial and Myocardial disease. In: Miller. Cardiac imaging The Requisites. 2nd Ed. Mosby. 270-2, 2005
4. Mestrioni L et al: Dilated Cardiomyopathies. In: Fuster V et al eds. Hurst's The Heart. 11th Ed. Mc Graw-Hill. 1889-907, 2004
5. Felker CM et al: Underlying causes and long-term survival in patients with initially unexplained cardiomyopathy. N Engl J Med. 342:1077-84, 2000
6. Cooke CE et al: Idiopathic Dilated Cardiomyopathy. N Engl J Med. 332:1384-6.1995
7. Dec GW et al: Idiopathic dilated cardiomyopathy. N Engl J Med. 331:1564-75, 1994

DILATED CARDIOMYOPATHY

IMAGE GALLERY

Typical

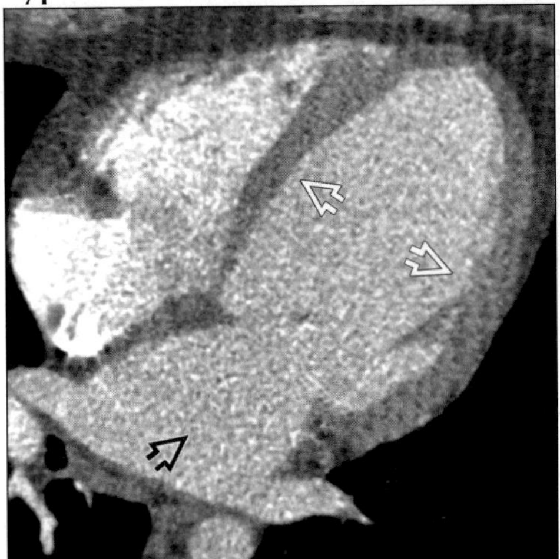

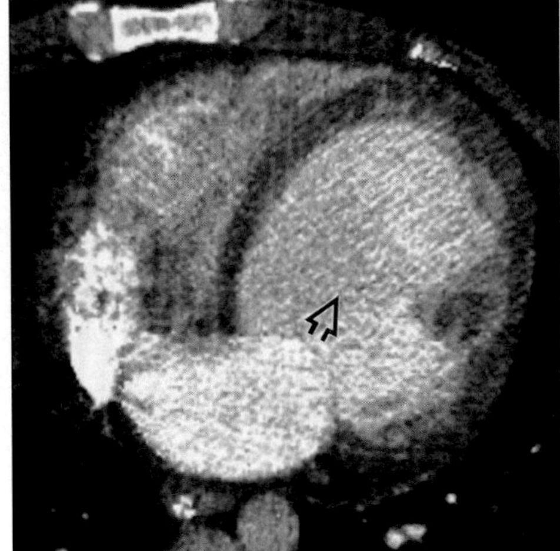

*(**Left**) Four chamber view CECT shows dilated cardiomyopathy →. No CT evidence of a myocardial infarction (thinning, fatty metaplasia, calcification) suggesting a non-ischemic etiology. Mild LA dilation →. (**Right**) Axial CECT shows globular left ventricular dilation → in a patient with tachycardia induced cardiomyopathy.*

Typical

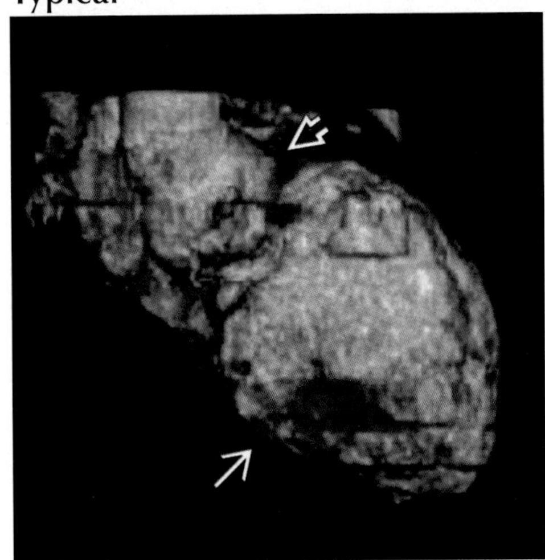

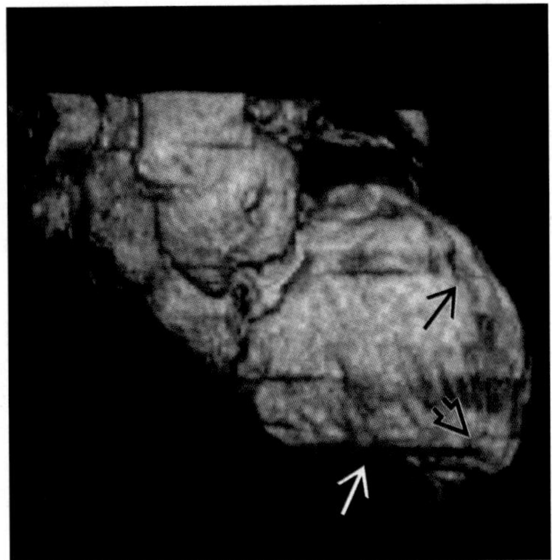

*(**Left**) 4D volume rendered CT ventriculogram at end diastole shows a globular enlarged heart in a patient with idiopathic dilated cardiomyopathy. Left ventricle →, aortic root →. (**Right**) 4D volume rendered CT ventriculogram in the same patient at end systole. Note severely reduced systolic function with minimal wall motion at the inferior wall →. The anterior wall → and apex → in this projection are akinetic.*

Typical

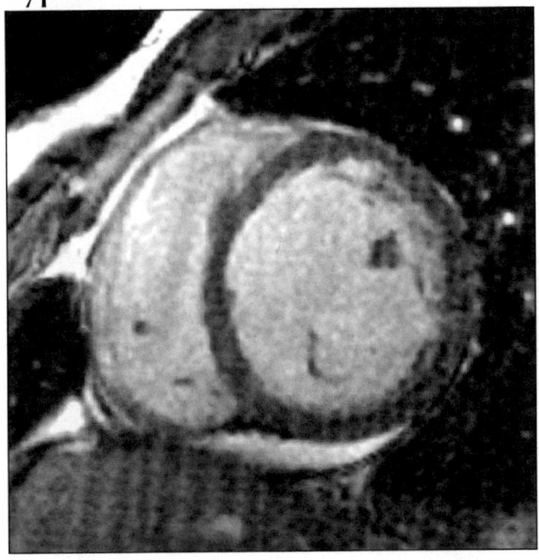

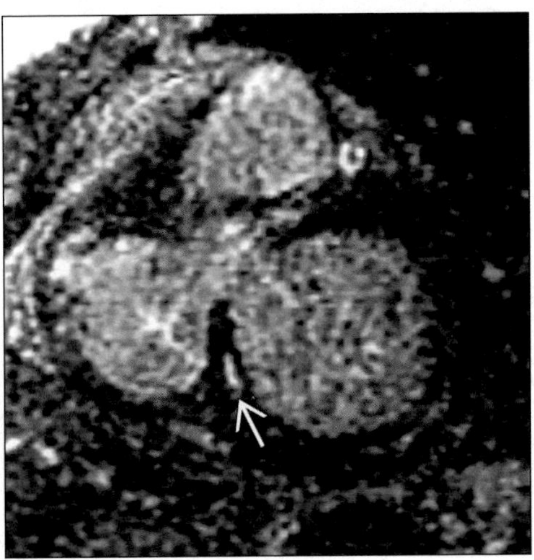

*(**Left**) Short axis SSFP shows marked dilatation of the left ventricle in a case of idiopathic dilated cardiomyopathy. (**Right**) Short axis 2D delayed enhanced MR in the same patient with idiopathic dilated cardiomyopathy shows an area of intramyocardial mid wall hyperenhancement consistent with scar/fibrosis →.*

RESTRICTIVE CARDIOMYOPATHY

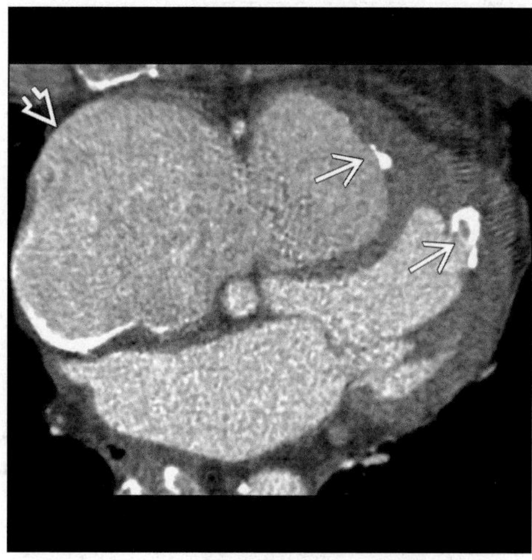

Axial cardiac CT shows severe right atrial enlargement ➡ in a sarcoid-induced restrictive cardiomyopathy patient. Note: Right and left ventricular apical obliteration and endocardial calcification ➡.

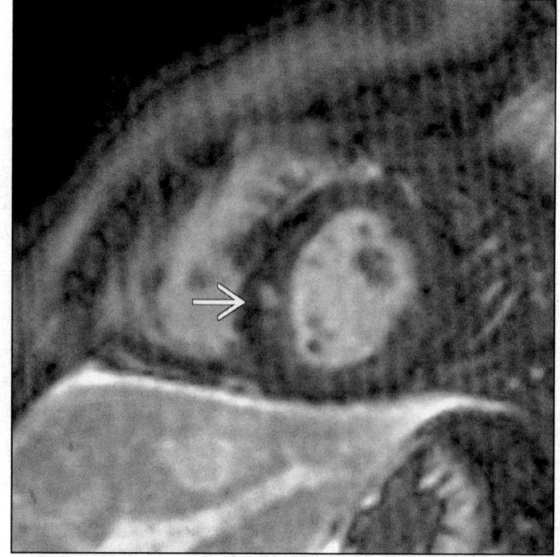

Short axis DE MR (inversion recovery) in a 3 y/o boy with glycogen storage disease. Note midwall septal delayed enhancement ➡. (Courtesy G. Reddy, MD).

TERMINOLOGY

Definitions

- Abnormal diastolic function and relatively well-preserved systolic function
  - Nondilated ventricle with normal wall thickness
  - Replacement of cardiac tissue with fibrosis
  - Restrictive physiology which causes increased ventricular filling pressures
  - Biatrial enlargement
- Primary or idiopathic restrictive cardiomyopathy is uncommon
  - Diagnosis of exclusion because restrictive physiology manifested in other systemic disorders such as amyloid, sarcoid, hemochromatosis

IMAGING FINDINGS

General Features

- Best diagnostic clue
  - Normal ventricular cavity size
  - Increased filling pressures on Doppler echo hemodynamics
- Location
  - Ventricles most commonly involved
    - Atria and conduction system may also be affected
- Size
  - Normal to slightly enlarged overall cardiac size
  - Secondary dilation of atria due to high LV filling pressures
- Morphology: Can be associated with increased cardiac mass

Radiographic Findings

- Radiography
  - CXR: Demonstrates typical appearance of congestive heart failure without cardiomegaly
    - Pulmonary venous hypertension
    - Left ventricle (LV) enlargement may also be seen in some cases
    - Biatrial enlargement
  - Not definitive in evaluation of restrictive cardiac diseases

CT Findings

- Multidetector contrast-enhanced CT angiography can accurately depict ventricular and atrial cavity sizes

DDx: Cardiomyopathies

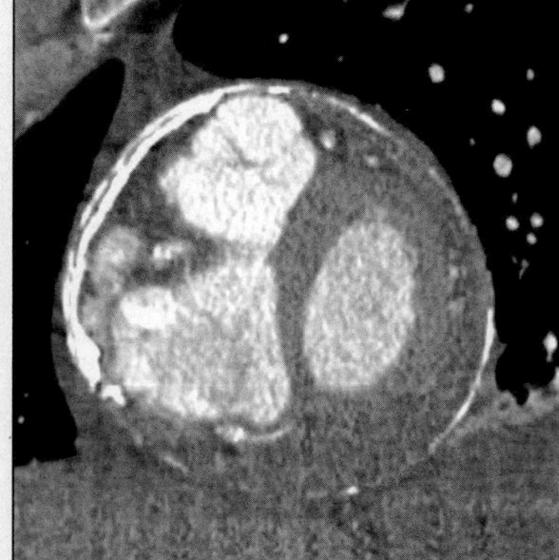

Constrictive Pericarditis

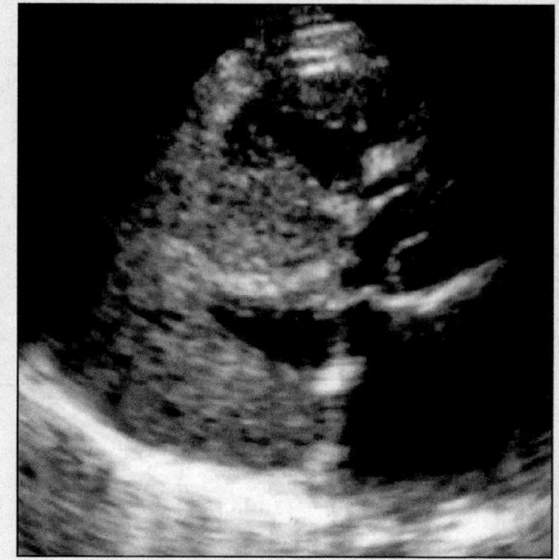

Hypertrophic Cardiomyopathy

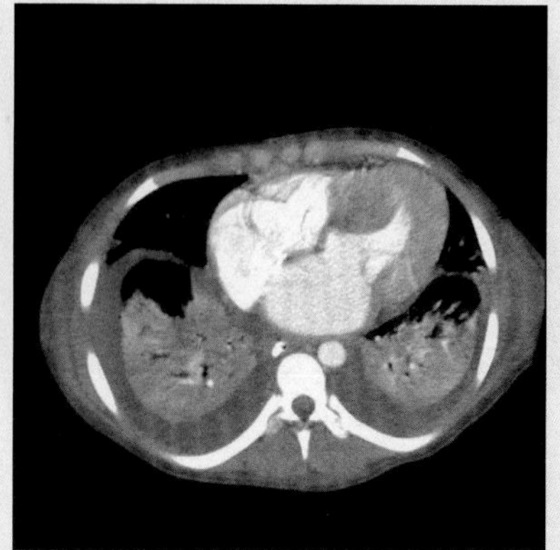

Left Ventricular Failure

RESTRICTIVE CARDIOMYOPATHY

Key Facts

Terminology
- Nondilated ventricle with normal wall thickness
- Replacement of cardiac tissue with fibrosis
- Restrictive physiology which causes increased ventricular filling pressures
- Biatrial enlargement

Imaging Findings
- CXR: Demonstrates typical appearance of congestive heart failure without cardiomegaly
- Most accurate imaging modality to assess ventricular morphology and function
- Abnormal delayed contrast-enhancement may be diagnostic such disorders as amyloid and sarcoid
- MR is best imaging tool
- Doppler echo parameters can identify restrictive filling pattern

Top Differential Diagnoses
- Constrictive Pericarditis
- Hypertropic Cardiomyopathy
- Hypertensive Heart Disease with Left Ventricular Hypertrophy

Pathology
- Primary idiopathic restrictive cardiomyopathy is uncommon and has no identifiable cause
- Familial restrictive cardiomyopathy is also a rare entity with autosomal dominant transmission

Clinical Issues
- Physical exam consistent with pulmonary and systemic congestion
- Goal of treatment is to control symptoms to improve the patient's quality of life

- Helpful in excluding the diagnosis of constriction pericarditis

MR Findings
- Most accurate imaging modality to assess ventricular morphology and function
  - Primary restrictive cardiomyopathies are associated with normal wall thickness, small ventricular cavity sizes, and normal systolic function
  - Time velocity curves demonstrate abnormal diastolic filling
- Abnormal delayed contrast-enhancement may be diagnostic such disorders as amyloid and sarcoid
- Normal pericardium (< 3 mm, absence of adhesions, no enhancement) excludes constrictive pericarditis
- May depict endocardial enhancement in case of endomyocardial fibrosis

Echocardiographic Findings
- Echocardiogram
  - Normal left ventricular cavity size
  - Biatrial enlargement
  - Normal systolic function
  - Abnormal diastolic function
    - Mitral inflow Doppler pattern assesses ventricular compliance and filling pressures by comparing early (E) and late (A) diastolic filling
    - Tissue Doppler pattern assesses myocardial motion during early (E') and late (A') diastolic filling

Imaging Recommendations
- Best imaging tool
  - MR is best imaging tool
    - Accurately depicts atrial and ventricular morphology
    - Delayed enhancement imaging identifies scar and fibrosis
    - Demonstrate early termination of left ventricular filling
    - High sensitivity, specificity, and predictive accuracy (88%, 100%, and 93%, respectively) in differentiating restrictive cardiomyopathy from constrictive pericarditis
  - Echocardiography alone is not definitive
    - Doppler echo parameters can identify restrictive filling pattern
- Protocol advice
  - SSFP cine images for ventricular morphology and function
  - Delayed enhancement imaging for fibrosis

DIFFERENTIAL DIAGNOSIS

Constrictive Pericarditis
- Evidence of pericardial thickening
  - Pericardial thickness > 4 mm on MR
  - Irregular appearance of pericardium with nodular thickening
  - Pericardial calcification identified on CT
  - Echocardiography findings
    - Pericardial thickening ± effusion
    - Respiratory phasic variations of ventricular filling pattern
- Pericardial adhesions
  - Taglines orthogonal to pericardium on cine imaging necessary
    - Break in tagline indicates normal pericardial sliding motion
    - Distortion or "pulling" of taglines indicates pericardial adhesion

Hypertropic Cardiomyopathy
- Asymmetric pattern of hypertrophy
- Evidence of dynamic left ventricular outflow tract obstruction
- Systolic function preserved, even late in disease

Hypertensive Heart Disease with Left Ventricular Hypertrophy
- Concentric left ventricular hypertrophy
- Spares right ventricular myocardium

RESTRICTIVE CARDIOMYOPATHY

PATHOLOGY

General Features

- General path comments
  - Primary idiopathic restrictive cardiomyopathy is uncommon and has no identifiable cause
  - Familial restrictive cardiomyopathy is also a rare entity with autosomal dominant transmission
  - Secondary restrictive cardiomyopathy is most common and includes the following diagnoses
    - Infiltration with amyloid, sarcoid, hemochromatosis, glycogen storage disorders
    - Chemotherapy or radiation
    - Hypereosinophilic syndrome
    - Endomyocardial fibrosis
  - Left ventricular scarring leads to impaired diastolic relaxation with reduced filling
  - Restrictive cardiomyopathy associated with
    - Elevated ventricular diastolic pressures
    - Low stroke volume with preserved systolic function

Gross Pathologic & Surgical Features

- Biatrial enlargement
- Increased left ventricular mass

Microscopic Features

- Diffuse infiltration of amyloid in amyloidosis
- Patchy infiltration of granulomas in sarcoidosis
- Extensive iron deposits in hemochromatosis
- Myocyte hypertrophy/fibrosis in endomyocardial fibrosis

CLINICAL ISSUES

Presentation

- Most common signs/symptoms: Gradually worsening shortness of breath and progressive exercise intolerance
- Other signs/symptoms
  - Orthopnea
  - Paroxysmal nocturnal dyspnea
- Clinical Profile
  - Physical exam consistent with pulmonary and systemic congestion
    - Pulmonary edema
    - Increased central venous pressure (jugular venous distension, peripheral edema, hepatomegaly)
  - Fatigue, weakness, anorexia

Demographics

- Age: Increased incidence in the elderly
- Gender: More common in women
- Ethnicity: Nonspecific

Natural History & Prognosis

- 70% of people with restrictive cardiomyopathy die within 5 years of disease symptomology

Treatment

- Goal of treatment is to control symptoms to improve the patient's quality of life
- Goal is to reduce symptoms by lowering elevated filling pressures without significantly reducing cardiac output
  - Low dose diuretics and nitrates for preload reduction
  - Beta blockers and/or calcium channel blockers to improve diastolic relaxation
- Medical treatment of underlying systemic disorder
  - Steroids for sarcoid; chemotherapy and stem cell transplant for amyloid, phlebotomy for hemochromatosis
- Pacemaker for patients with conduction abnormalities to properly time atrial contraction which improves ventricular filling
- ICD for refractory ventricular arrhythmias
- Cardiac transplantation in medical refractory cases

DIAGNOSTIC CHECKLIST

Image Interpretation Pearls

- MR for cardiac morphology and function
- Delayed enhancement imaging for fibrosis imaging
- Doppler echo for LV hemodynamics/filling pressures

SELECTED REFERENCES

1. Marijon E et al: Typical clinical aspect of endomyocardial fibrosis. Int J Cardiol. 112(2):259-60, 2006
2. Rochitte CE et al: The emerging role of MRI in the diagnosis and management of cardiomyopathies. Curr Cardiol Rep. 8(1):44-52, 2006
3. Cury RC et al: Images in cardiovascular medicine. Visualization of endomyocardial fibrosis by delayed-enhancement magnetic resonance imaging. Circulation. 111(9):e115-7, 2005
4. Chinnaiyan KM et al: Constrictive pericarditis versus restrictive cardiomyopathy: challenges in diagnosis and management. Cardiol Rev. 12(6):314-20, 2004
5. Wald DS et al: Restrictive cardiomyopathy in systemic amyloidosis. QJM. 96(5):380-2, 2003
6. Friedrich MG: Cardiovascular Magnetic Resonance in Cardiomyopathies. In: Cardiovascular Magnetic Resonance, Manning WJ, Pannell DJ (ed), Churchill-Livingstone, Philadelphia. 415-8, 2002
7. Ammash NM et al: Clinical profile and outcome of idiopathic restrictive cardiomyopathy. Circulation. 101(21):2490-6, 2000
8. Berensztein CS et al: Usefulness of echocardiography and doppler echocardiography in endomyocardial fibrosis. J Am Soc Echocardiogr. 13(5):385-92, 2000
9. Myers RB et al: Constrictive pericarditis: clinical and pathophysiologic characteristics. Am Heart J. 138(2 Pt 1):219-32, 1999
10. Angelini A et al: Morphologic spectrum of primary restrictive cardiomyopathy. Am J Cardiol. 80(8):1046-50, 1997
11. Kushwaha SS et al: Restrictive cardiomyopathy. N Engl J Med. 336(4):267-76, 1997
12. Leung DY et al: Restrictive Cardiomyopathy: Diagnosis and Prognostic Implications. In: The Practice of Clinical Echocardiography, Otto CN (ed), W.B. Saunders, Philadelphia. 473-94, 1997
13. Benotti JR et al: Clinical profile of restrictive cardiomyopathy. Circulation. 61(6):1206-12, 1980

IMAGE GALLERY

Typical

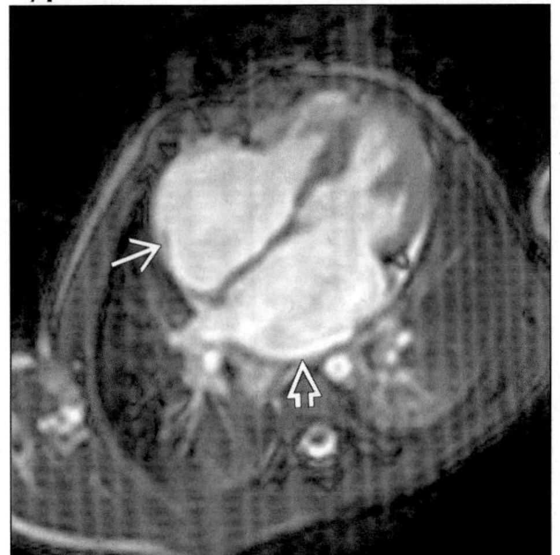

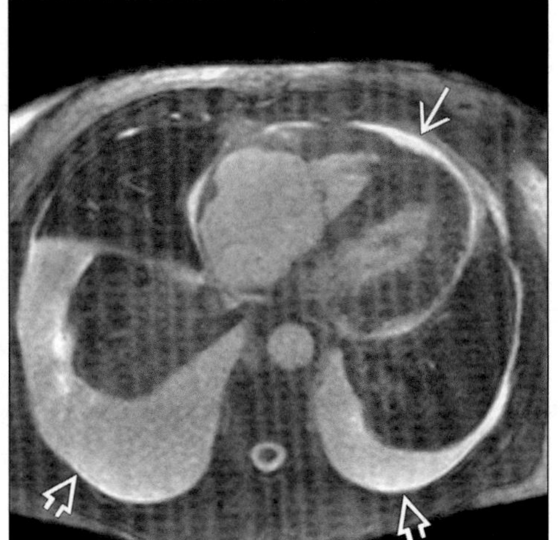

(Left) *Long axis SSFP corresponding to prior image shows 3 y/o boy with glycogen storage disease. Dilated LA ➡ and RA ➡. (Courtesy G. Reddy, MD).* ***(Right)*** *Axial SSFP shows enlarged right atrium, bilateral pleural effusions ➡ as well as a small pericardial effusion ➡ in a 39 y/o patient with restrictive cardiomyopathy. (Courtesy G. Reddy, MD).*

Typical

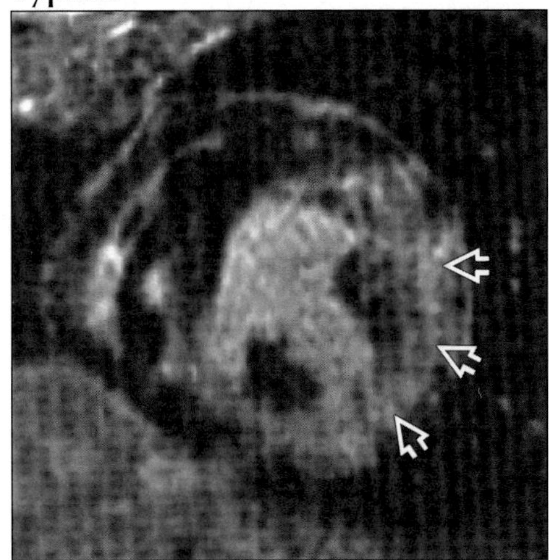

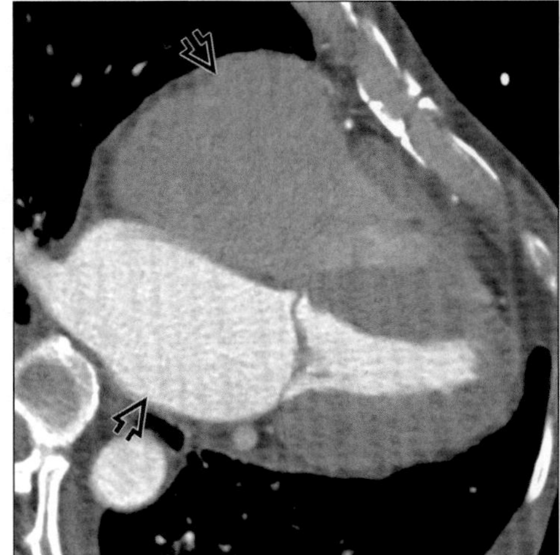

(Left) *LV short axis DE MR shows diffuse pattern of delayed hyperenhancement ➡ indicating massive fibrosis. This is not an ischemic pattern because the lesions neither follow coronary territories, nor are subendocardial based.* ***(Right)*** *Four chamber view coronary CTA shows marked biatrial enlargement ➡ in a 47 y/o patient with restrictive cardiomyopathy due to hemochromatosis. (Courtesy J. Kirsch, MD).*

Typical

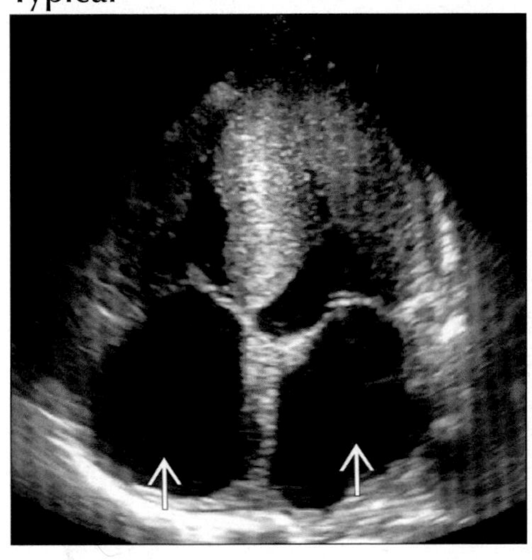

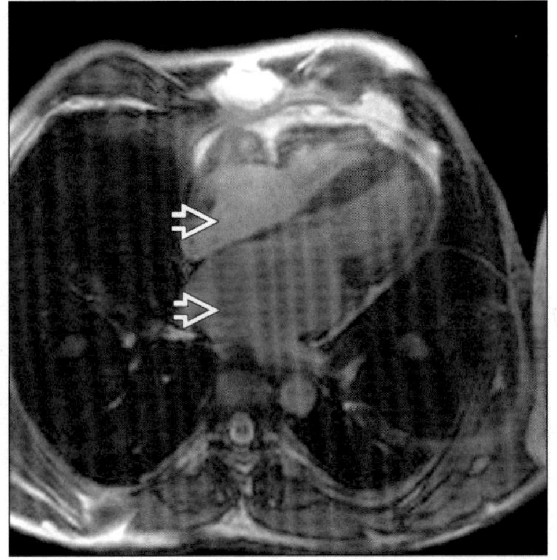

(Left) *Apical four chamber echocardiogram shows cardiomegaly and biatrial enlargement in a patient with amyloid ➡.* ***(Right)*** *Long axis SSFP shows cardiomegaly and biatrial prominence ➡ in a patient with restrictive cardiomyopathy due to sarcoidosis. (Courtesy J. Kirsch, MD).*

MYOCARDITIS

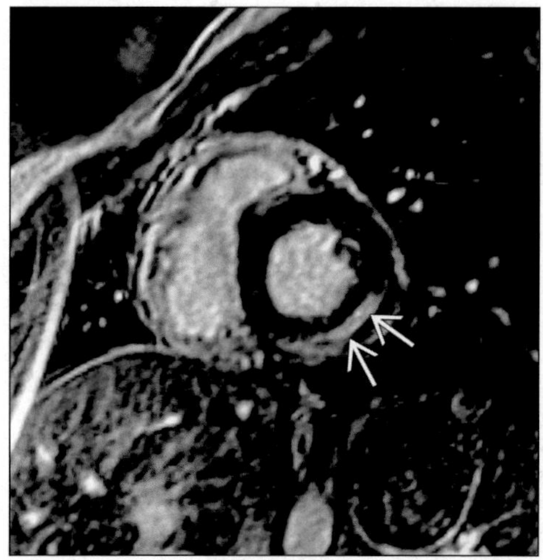

Short axis DE MR shows subepicardial delayed hyperenhancement ➔ in the inferolateral basal segment in a young patient with myocarditis. Note: Subendocardium is normal.

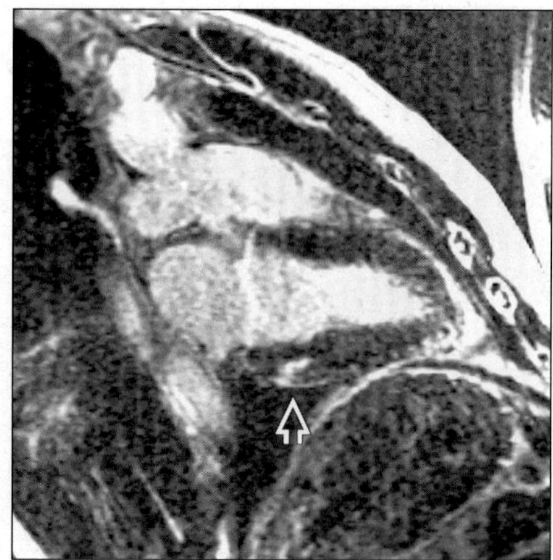

Three chamber view DE MR shows focal area of hyperenhancement in the basal subepicardial infero-lateral wall ➔ in a patient with acute myocarditis.

TERMINOLOGY

Definitions

- Inflammatory infiltrate of the myocardium with necrosis and/or degeneration of adjacent myocytes

IMAGING FINDINGS

General Features

- Best diagnostic clue: New dilated cardiomyopathy in an otherwise healthy person shortly after a viral syndrome
- Location
  - Generally diffuse global LV systolic dysfunction
    - Occasionally may be localized to the inferolateral wall

Radiographic Findings

- Radiography
  - Cardiomegaly often noted on PA chest radiograph
  - Pulmonary edema in cases of acute myocarditis

CT Findings

- NECT: Cardiomegaly
- Cardiac Gated CTA
  - Normal coronary arteries helps exclude ischemia as a possible etiology of new dilated cardiomyopathy
  - LV dilation and global hypokinesis on multiphase cine reconstructions
  - Accurately quantifies LV volumes, ejection fraction, and end-diastolic wall thickness
  - Preliminary research shows reasonable correlation of MDCT delayed enhancement with MR delayed enhancement for the detection of myocarditis

MR Findings

- T2WI: Myocardial segments with inflammation from **acute** myocarditis may show increased T2 signal due to edema
- T1 C+
  - Global relative gadolinium enhancement of myocardium compared to skeletal muscle
    - Calculate by dividing myocardial enhancement by the skeletal muscle enhancement
  - Global relative enhancement of more than 4.0 is diagnostic of myocarditis

DDx: Myocarditis

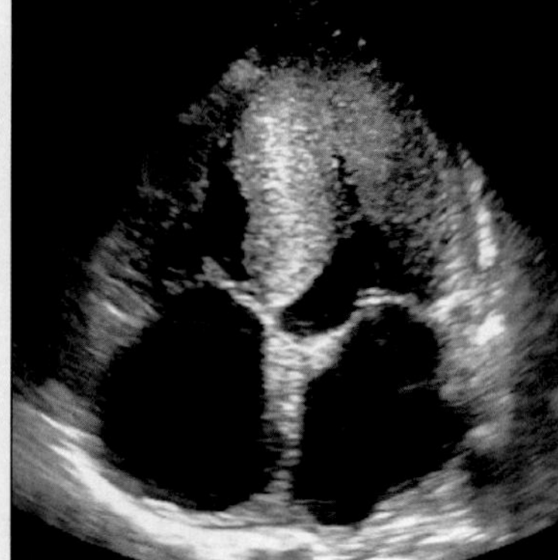

Restrictive Cardiomyopathy

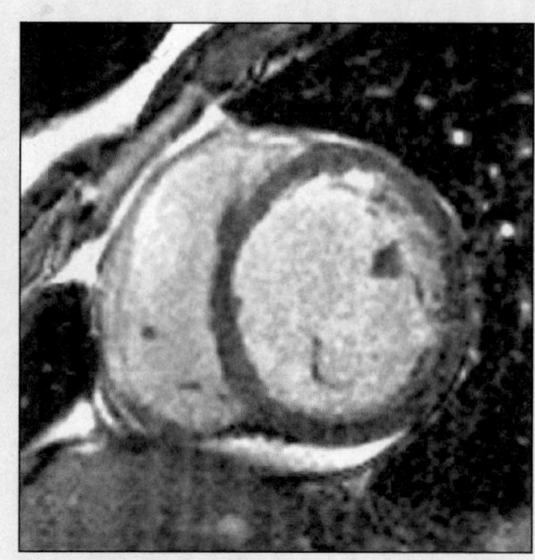

Idiopathic Dilated Cardiomyopathy

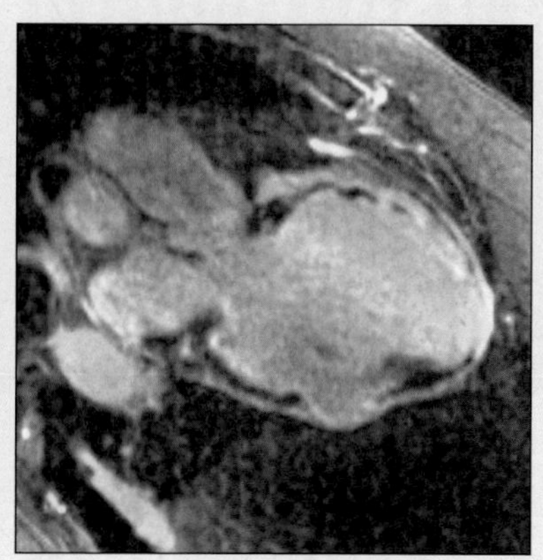

Ischemic Cardiomyopathy

MYOCARDITIS

Key Facts

Terminology
- Inflammatory infiltrate of the myocardium with necrosis and/or degeneration of adjacent myocytes

Imaging Findings
- New dilated cardiomyopathy in an otherwise healthy person shortly after a viral syndrome
- Echocardiography to exclude other causes of heart failure (valvular, amyloidosis, congenital) and to evaluate the degree of cardiac dysfunction (usually diffuse hypokinesis and diastolic dysfunction)
- Coronary CTA or invasive angiography useful to exclude obstructive coronary artery disease
- MR: **T2WI** for edema, **T1WI** pre- and post-contrast global relative enhancement, **delayed enhancement** for myocardial scar/fibrosis

Pathology
- Diagnosed by established histological, immunological, and immunochemical criteria

Clinical Issues
- Highly variable clinical presentation from subclinical to acute fulminant heart failure
- In developing countries viral causes is the most frequent
- True incidence of idiopathic or "viral" myocarditis is unknown
- Estimated that myocarditis is responsible for approximately 10% of unexplained dilated cardiomyopathy and heart failure

---

  - Normal relative myocardial enhancement ratio is < 2.5
- SSFP White Blood Cine
  - Quantify LV volumes, ejection fraction, and end diastolic wall thickness
  - Clearly demonstrates extent of LV systolic dysfunction
  - Excellent for assessing recovery of function
- Delayed Enhancement
  - Areas of hyperenhancement with the LV suggest myocardial inflammation
  - Typical pattern in the acute phase is affecting the subepicardial region in the infero-lateral wall
    - Contrast that to ischemic hyperenhancement which is always subendocardial
  - May be diffuse in cases of severe myocarditis
  - Can also demonstrate mid-wall hyperenhancement in a non-coronary distribution

Nuclear Medicine Findings
- Antimyosin scintigraphy can identify myocardial inflammation with high sensitivity (91-100%) and negative predictive power (93-100%), but
  - Low specificity (31-44%) and low positive predictive power (28-33%)
- Gallium scanning is used to reflect severe myocardial cellular infiltration and has a good negative predictive value, although specificity is low

Echocardiographic Findings
- Echocardiogram
  - Can quickly exclude other causes of new dilated cardiomyopathy and heart failure (i.e., ischemic or valvular)
  - Evaluate the degree of LV systolic dysfunction which has prognostic implications
  - Excellent modality for serial monitoring to assess recovery of function

Other Modality Findings
- Complete blood count - leukocytosis
- Elevated erythrocyte sedimentation rates
- Rheumatologic screening - to rule out systemic inflammatory diseases
- Elevated cardiac enzymes (creatine kinase or cardiac troponins)

Imaging Recommendations
- Best imaging tool: Cardiac MR
- Protocol advice: MRI: T2WI for edema, T1WI pre- and post-contrast for global relative enhancement, delayed enhancement for myocardial inflammation

DIFFERENTIAL DIAGNOSIS

Ischemic Cardiomyopathy
- Delayed-enhancement pattern is subendocardial (coronary distribution)

Nonischemic Dilated Cardiomyopathy
- Mid-wall hyperenhancement in the septum

Infiltrative Cardiomyopathy
- Patchy delayed-enhancement

PATHOLOGY

General Features
- General path comments
  - Diagnosed by established histological, immunological, and immunochemical criteria
  - Limited utility to endomyocardial biopsy and generally reserved for patient with major clinical manifestations
  - Clinicopathologic classification combining histology and clinical features may provide most prognostic information
    - Fulminant myocarditis: Acute illness after a distinct viral prodrome, multiple foci of active myocarditis by histology, and LV dysfunction
    - Acute myocarditis: Less distinct onset of viral illness with established LV dysfunction

- Chronic active myocarditis: Less distinct onset of illness associated with clinical/histologic relapses, and LV dysfunction
- Chronic persistent myocarditis: Less distinct onset of illness associated by persistent histologic changes often with foci of myocyte necrosis but without LV dysfunction
  - Myocardial damage has 2 main phases
    - Acute phase (first 2 weeks): Myocyte destruction is a direct consequence of the offending agent
    - Chronic phase: Continuing myocyte destruction is autoimmune in nature
- Etiology
  - Multiple etiologies exist however the majority of cases are classified as "idiopathic"
  - In developing countries viral causes are the most frequent
    - Coxsackie B is the most common viral pathogen related to myocarditis and dilated cardiomyopathy
    - Other newer emerging viruses include adenovirus, parvovirus B19, echovirus, Epstein-Barr virus
    - Other causes include autoimmune disorders (SLE, Wegener granulomatosis, giant cell arteritis, and Takayasu arteritis)
- Epidemiology
  - True incidence of idiopathic or "viral" myocarditis is unknown
  - Incidence and prevalence are difficult to study due to lack of an established noninvasive "gold standard"
  - Estimated that myocarditis is responsible for approximately 10% of unexplained dilated cardiomyopathy and heart failure

Microscopic Features

- Eosin methylene blue (EMB) should reveal the simultaneous findings of lymphocyte infiltration and myocyte necrosis

Staging, Grading or Classification Criteria

- WHO Marburg Classification (1996)
  - Cell types: Lymphocytic, eosinophilic, neutrophilic, giant cell, granulomatous, or mixed
  - Distribution: Focal (outside vessel lumen), confluent, diffuse, or reparative (in fibrotic areas)
  - Amount: None (grade 0), mild (grade 1), moderate (grade 2), or severe (grade 3)

CLINICAL ISSUES

Presentation

- Most common signs/symptoms
  - Highly variable clinical presentation from subclinical to acute fulminant heart failure
  - Majority of symptomatic cases of post-viral myocarditis present with a syndrome of heart failure and dilated cardiomyopathy
    - Fatigue and decreased exercise capacity are the initial manifestations
    - In fulminant cases biventricular failure and cardiogenic shock may result
- Other signs/symptoms
  - Chest pain is usually associated with accompanied pericarditis
    - May mimic myocardial ischemia on ECG
    - May be associated with fevers, sweats, chills, and dyspnea
  - Cardiogenic shock
    - Young patients with preceding febrile illness
    - Accompanied by classic ECG for myocarditis and elevation in cardiac enzymes
    - These patients need coronary angiogram to exclude significant epicardial coronary stenosis as the cause
    - Frequently require intra-aortic balloon pump or ventricular assist device as a bridge of transplant
  - Sudden cardiac death
    - Ventricular tachycardia and/or fibrillation may be the culprit in young patients who die suddenly in the absence of known heart disease

Natural History & Prognosis

- Majority of cases of acute myocarditis - many of which are not detected clinically - have a benign course
- Some patients develop heart failure, serious arrhythmias, disturbances of conduction, or even circulatory collapse
- 2/3 with mild symptoms recover completely without any residual cardiac dysfunction
- 1/3 subsequently develop dilated cardiomyopathy

Treatment

- Avoidance of exercise
- Electrocardiographic monitoring
- Antiarrhythmic drugs in selected patients
- Treatment of congestive heart failure
- Anticoagulation
- Nonsteroidal anti-inflammatory drugs are not effective and may actually enhance the myocarditis and increase mortality
- Immunosuppressive therapy is not recommended for myocarditis at this time
- Transplant in those cases of cardiogenic shock

SELECTED REFERENCES

1. Dambrin G et al: Diagnostic value of ECG-gated multidetector computed tomography in the early phase of suspected acute myocarditis. A preliminary comparative study with cardiac MRI. Eur Radiol. 17(2):331-8, 2007
2. Abdel-Aty H et al: Diagnostic performance of cardiovascular magnetic resonance in patients with suspected acute myocarditis: comparison of different approaches. J Am Coll Cardiol. 45(11):1815-22, 2005
3. Liu PP et al: Cardiovascular magnetic resonance for the diagnosis of acute myocarditis: prospects for detecting myocardial inflammation. J Am Coll Cardiol. 45(11):1823-5, 2005
4. Roditi GH et al: MRI changes in myocarditis--evaluation with spin echo, cine MR angiography and contrast enhanced spin echo imaging. Clin Radiol. 55(10):752-8, 2000
5. Friedrich MG et al: Contrast media-enhanced magnetic resonance imaging visualizes myocardial changes in the course of viral myocarditis. Circulation. 97(18):1802-9, 1998
6. Alpert JS et al: Update in cardiology. Ann Intern Med. 125(1):40-6, 1996

IMAGE GALLERY

Typical

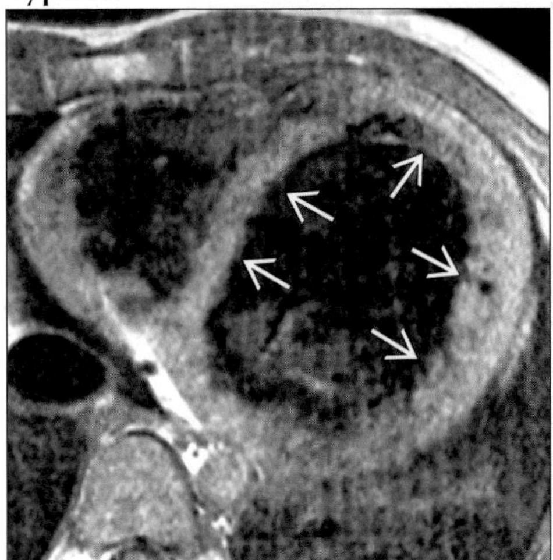

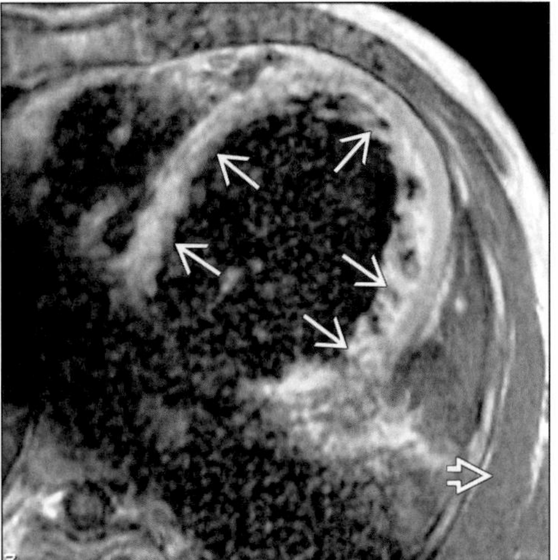

(Left) *Axial T1WI MR before gadolinium shows a dilated left ventricle. Note the global pattern of T1 signal within the myocardium ➡.* ***(Right)*** *Axial T1WI MR after gadolinium administration shows global increase in T1 signal from the myocardium ➡. Using skeletal muscle enhancement as a reference ⇨ a global relative enhancement ratio can be calculated. In this patient the ratio was > 4.0 which is positive for myocarditis.*

Typical

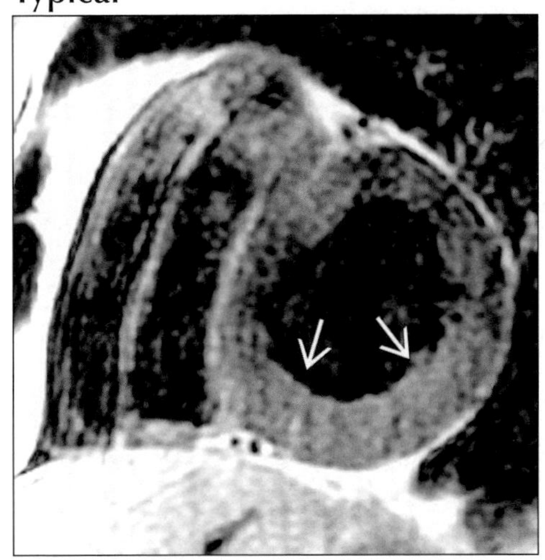

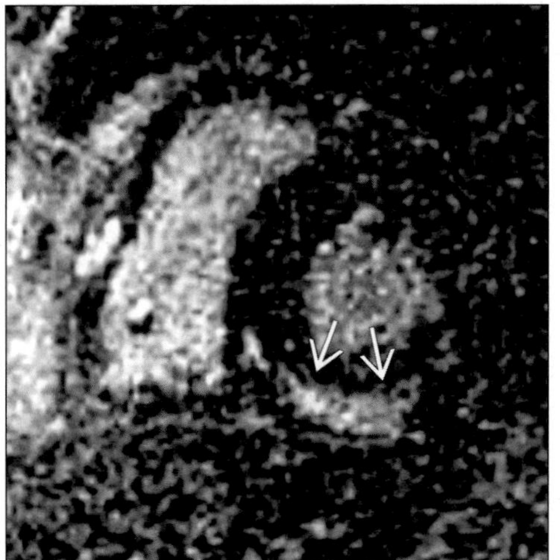

(Left) *Short axis T2WI MR shows increased signal in the inferior wall due to acute myocarditis with associated edema ➡.* ***(Right)*** *Short axis DE MR in the same patient as previous image, shows a corresponding area of hyperenhancement in the subepicardial wall suggesting myocardial inflammation ➡.*

Typical

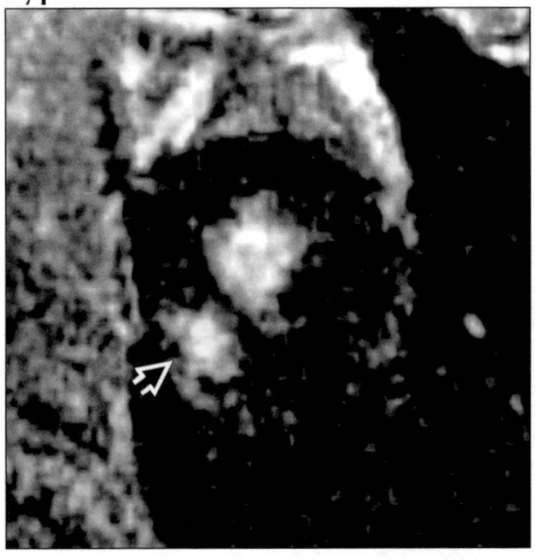

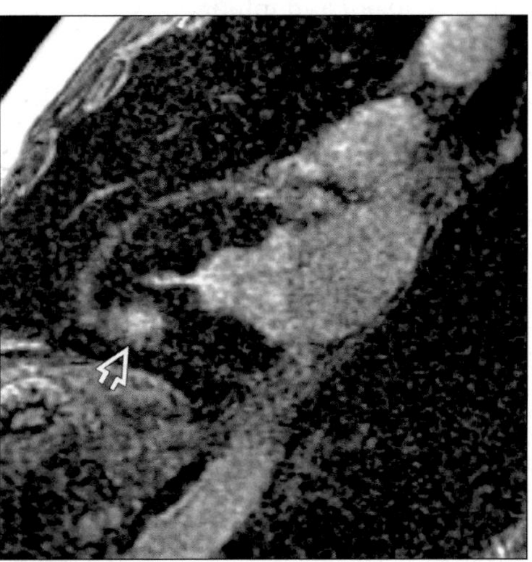

(Left) *Short axis DE MR in a patient with myocarditis shows mid-wall hyperenhancement ⇨ which is typical for this disease.* ***(Right)*** *Corresponding two chamber DE MRI shows the same area of inferior apical wall hyperenhancement ⇨.*

ARRHYTHMOGENIC RV DYSPLASIA

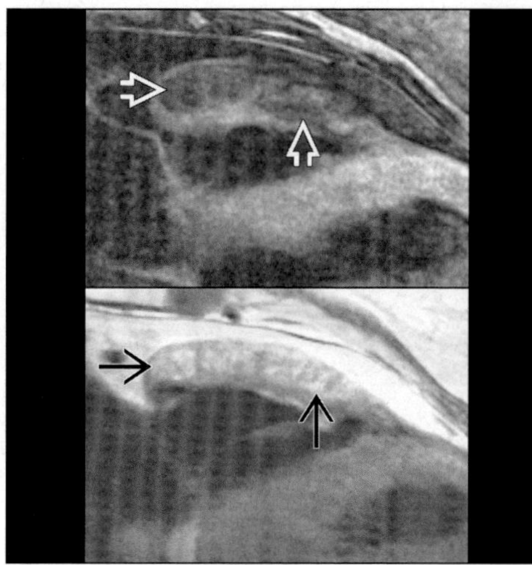

High resolution T1WI SE images (top) with and (bottom) without fat-saturation shows extensive bright tissue within RV myocardium ➔, with signal dropout ➔ on fat-saturation, indicating intramyocardial RV fat.

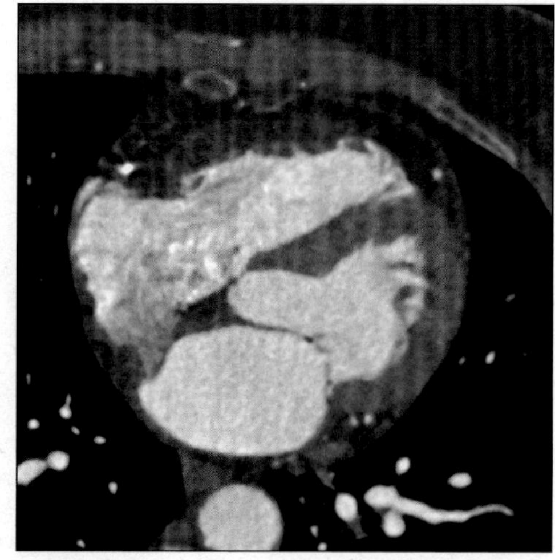

Axial coronary CTA in the same patient as previous image, shows large amount of low attenuation material (fat) within RV anterior freewall.

TERMINOLOGY

Abbreviations and Synonyms

- Arrhythmogenic right ventricular dysplasia (ARVD)
- Arrhythmogenic right ventricular cardiomyopathy (ARVC)
- RV dysplasia

Definitions

- Cardiomyopathy characterized by fibrofatty degeneration of right ventricle (RV) leading to spectrum of arrhythmias including sudden cardiac death (SCD)

IMAGING FINDINGS

General Features

- Best diagnostic clue
  - Diagnosis is made by using a set of major and minor criteria (task force criteria)
  - ARVD is considered present if either
    - Two major criteria are present, or
    - One major and two minor criteria are present, or
    - Four minor criteria are present
  - RV fatty infiltration detected by MR considered equivalent to a major criterium
    - By original task force criteria, only fat detected on pathology is considered a major criteria
  - RV global dilatation considered major criterium
  - RV aneurysm considered major criterium
  - Regional RV wall-motion abnormality considered minor criterium
  - Other criteria involve family history of SCD (major if pathology proven ARVD, minor if not), and EKG abnormalities
- Location: RV anterior free wall most commonly involved
- Size: Variable involvement
- Morphology: Patchy distribution: May lead to false negative biopsy
- Reduced right ventricular function
- Fatty infiltration of the myocardium
- Right ventricular dilatation, with wall thinning, localized aneurysms, and dyskinetic segments

Radiographic Findings

- Radiography

DDx: Arrhythmogenic RV Dysplasia

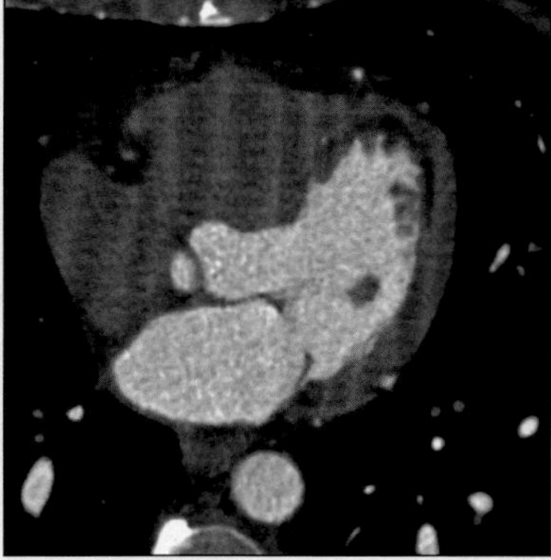

LV Fat from Remote MI

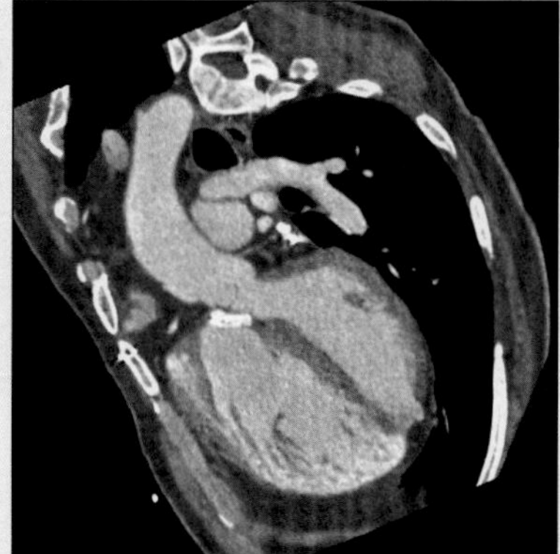

RVH due to VSD (Repaired)

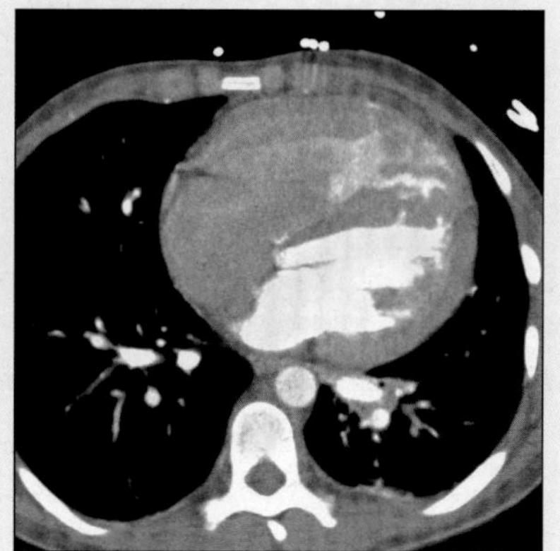

RVH due to PDA

ARRHYTHMOGENIC RV DYSPLASIA

Key Facts

Terminology
- Cardiomyopathy characterized by fibrofatty degeneration of right ventricle (RV) leading to spectrum of arrhythmias including sudden cardiac death (SCD)

Imaging Findings
- Diagnosis is made by using a set of major and minor criteria (task force criteria)
- Patchy distribution: May lead to false negative biopsy
- Dilated right ventricle
- RV aneurysms and thickened trabeculae
- FSE or SE techniques may reveal fatty infiltration of RV or LV myocardium
  - Repeating sequence with fat-saturation enhances accuracy
- Delayed enhancement imaging may demonstrate delayed hyperenhancement representing fibrosis
- MR excellent for RV volumes and morphology
- Detection of fat within RV by CT is of uncertain clinical significance and currently still under investigation

Pathology
- Fibrofatty infiltration of the myocardium with dysfunction and occasionally associated aneurysm

Clinical Issues
- Cause of syncope, serious ventricular arrhythmias and sudden death
- Should be considered in athletes of any age as the cause of syncope or cardiovascular collapse

---

- Chest radiography findings
  - Usually normal
  - May show evidence of right ventricular dilatation especially on lateral view

CT Findings
- NECT: RV dilatation
- CTA
  - Dilated right ventricle
  - Reduced systolic function
    - Essential to use fast techniques
  - Detection of fat within RV by CT is of uncertain clinical significance and currently still under investigation
  - May detect RV aneurysm

MR Findings
- SSFP White Blood Cine
  - In CINE mode, altered RV function and dyskinesis
  - RV aneurysms and thickened trabeculae
  - Typically no left ventricle (LV) involvement
- Black Blood SE
  - FSE or SE techniques may reveal fatty infiltration of RV or LV myocardium
    - Repeating sequence with fat-saturation enhances accuracy
  - Thinned right ventricular myocardium
  - May detect RV aneurysm
- Delayed Enhancement
  - May demonstrate delayed hyperenhancement representing fibrosis
    - Keep in mind that inversion times (TI) for RV is different from that of the LV

Echocardiographic Findings
- Echocardiogram
  - Hypokinetic and dilated right ventricle
    - Can range from mild to severe, decrease right ventricle (RV) ejection fraction
  - May detect RV aneurysm
  - Not useful fro demonstration of intramyocardial RV fat

Angiographic Findings
- Conventional
  - Right ventricular angiography findings
    - Best viewed with biplane 45 degree right and left anterior oblique
    - Infundibular aneurysms
    - Inferior dyskinesis
    - Thickened trabeculae

Imaging Recommendations
- Best imaging tool
  - MR excellent for RV volumes and morphology
  - Demonstration of RV intramyocardial fat is dependent on technique and interobserver variability is poor
- Protocol advice
  - If demonstration of fat is desired, maximize in-plane resolution and image in systole
    - FSE does not allow systolic imaging (except for investigational pulse sequences)

DIFFERENTIAL DIAGNOSIS

Right Ventricular Infarction
- Not commonly associated with localized aneurysm formation

Volume Overloaded Right Ventricle
- Ventricular or atrial septal defect

Normal Epicardial Fat
- Thinned myocardium may make differentiation of myocardial from epicardial fat difficult
- Normal hearts may have fat intermixed with myocardial fibers

PATHOLOGY

General Features
- General path comments
  - Fibrofatty infiltration of the myocardium

- Beginning in the subepicardium and extending endocardially
- Should have > 3% fibrous tissue and > 49% fat
- Involves predominantly RV inflow, apex, and infundibulum
- Can involve the LV in 40-76% of autopsy cases

- Etiology: Fibrofatty infiltration of the myocardium with dysfunction and occasionally associated aneurysm
- Familial/genetics
  - Typically autosomal dominant with incomplete penetrance
  - Several genes implicated
    - Altered gene associated with plakoglobin (inadequate cell-cell adhesion)
    - Cardiac ryanodine receptor defect: Calcium released from sarcoplasmic reticulum; may be responsible for adrenergically mediated arrhythmias
- Degenerative
  - Myocyte defect due to ultrastructural abnormality
    - Genetically determined atrophy
  - Inflammation
    - Possibly due to viral infection
  - Apoptosis

CLINICAL ISSUES

Presentation

- Most common signs/symptoms: Cause of syncope, serious ventricular arrhythmias and sudden death
- Clinical Profile: Should be considered in athletes of any age as the cause of syncope or cardiovascular collapse
- Ventricular arrhythmias: Ventricular tachycardia with left bundle branch block (LBBB) morphology
- Syncope
- Sudden death
  - 3-4% of sudden deaths in young athletes in the U.S.
  - Most common cause of sudden death in young athletes in Italy
- Heart failure
  - Isolated RV or biventricular
  - Look for typical EKG changes of arrhythmogenic right ventricular cardiomyopathy (ARVC) (see below)
- Diagnosis
  - Typical imaging findings
  - EKG
    - Epsilon waves: Small depolarization at the beginning of the ST segment
    - T-wave inversions in early V leads
  - Biopsy showing fibrofatty infiltration

Treatment

- Avoid vigorous athletics
- In the absence of arrhythmias, beta blocker therapy is appropriate
- Implantable cardioverter defibrillator (ICD)
  - In patients with a history of ventricular tachyarrhythmia (VT), cardiac arrest, or syncope
  - Antiarrhythmics may be needed for repeated discharges
    - Sotalol has shown some efficacy
    - Amiodarone not yet tested in a clinical study

SELECTED REFERENCES

1. Bomma C et al: Evolving role of multidetector computed tomography in evaluation of arrhythmogenic right ventricular dysplasia/cardiomyopathy. Am J Cardiol. 100(1):99-105, 2007
2. Wu YW et al: Structural and functional assessment of arrhythmogenic right ventricular dysplasia/cardiomyopathy by multi-slice computed tomography: comparison with cardiovascular magnetic resonance. Int J Cardiol. 115(3):e118-21, 2007
3. Tandri H et al: Magnetic resonance imaging of arrhythmogenic right ventricular dysplasia: sensitivity, specificity, and observer variability of fat detection versus functional analysis of the right ventricle. J Am Coll Cardiol. 48(11):2277-84, 2006
4. Tandri H et al: Normal reference values for the adult right ventricle by magnetic resonance imaging. Am J Cardiol. 98(12):1660-4, 2006
5. Abbara S et al: Value of fat suppression in the MRI evaluation of suspected arrhythmogenic right ventricular dysplasia. AJR Am J Roentgenol. 182(3):587-91, 2004
6. Castillo E et al: Arrhythmogenic right ventricular dysplasia: ex vivo and in vivo fat detection with black-blood MR imaging. Radiology. 232(1):38-48, 2004
7. Tandri H et al: Magnetic resonance and computed tomography imaging of arrhythmogenic right ventricular dysplasia. J Magn Reson Imaging. 19(6):848-58, 2004
8. Bluemke DA et al: MR Imaging of arrhythmogenic right ventricular cardiomyopathy: morphologic findings and interobserver reliability. Cardiology. 99(3):153-62, 2003
9. Tandri H et al: Magnetic resonance imaging findings in patients meeting task force criteria for arrhythmogenic right ventricular dysplasia. J Cardiovasc Electrophysiol. 14(5):476-82, 2003
10. Kayser HW et al: Diagnosis of arrhythmogenic right ventricular dysplasia: a review. Radiographics. 22(3):639-48; discussion 649-50, 2002
11. Gemayel C et al: Arrhythmogenic right ventricular cardiomyopathy. J Am Coll Cardiol. 38(7):1773-81, 2001
12. Corrado D et al: Arrhythmogenic right ventricular cardiomyopathy: diagnosis, prognosis, and treatment. Heart. 83(5):588-95, 2000
13. Burke AP et al: Arrhythmogenic right ventricular cardiomyopathy and fatty replacement of the right ventricular myocardium: are they different diseases? Circulation. 97(16):1571-80, 1998
14. Blake LM et al: MR features of arrhythmogenic right ventricular dysplasia. AJR Am J Roentgenol. 162(4):809-12, 1994

IMAGE GALLERY

Typical

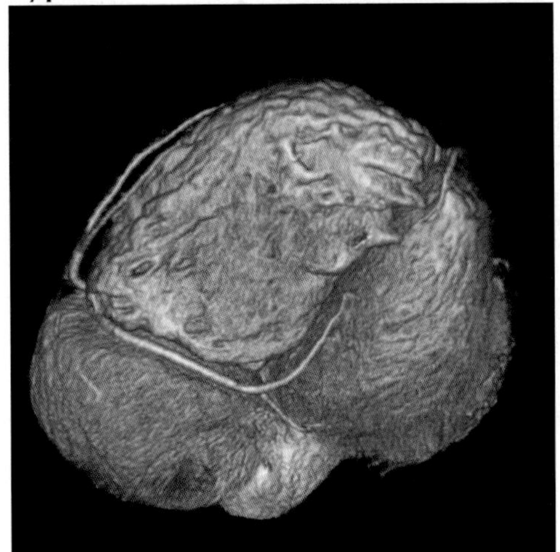

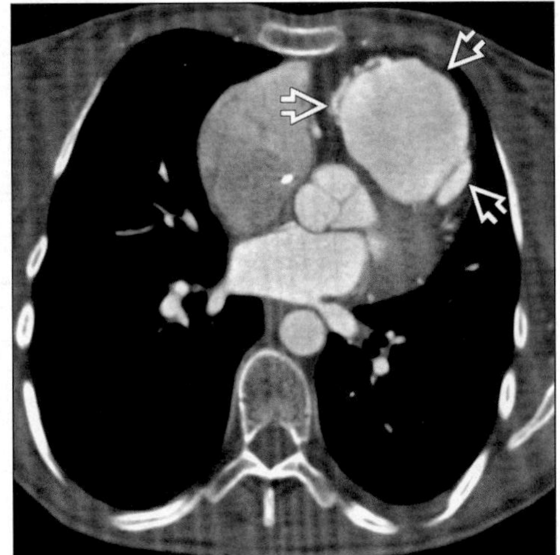

(Left) *Oblique coronary CTA shows markedly enlarged right ventricle in a patient that met task force criteria for ARVD.* ***(Right)*** *Axial coronary CTA shows markedly dilated right ventricular outflow tract (RVOT) ➡ in same patient as previous image.*

Typical

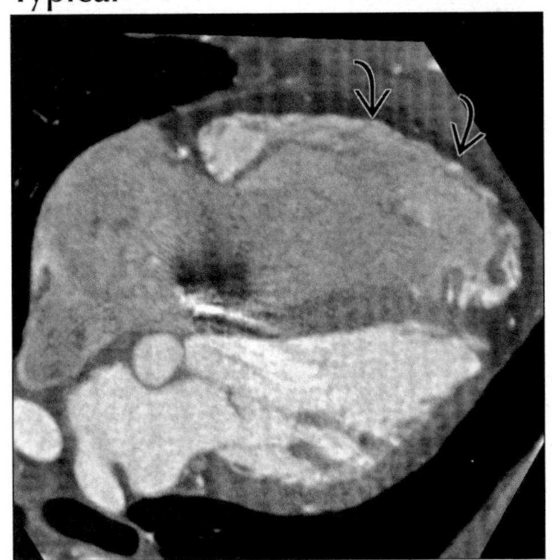

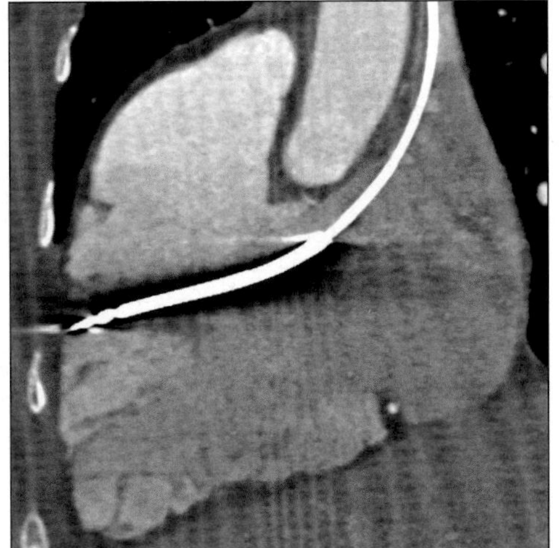

(Left) *Oblique cardiac CT shows globally dilated right ventricle with severely thinned and scalloped anterior free wall ➡ in a patient that met criteria for ARVD.* ***(Right)*** *RV long axis view of cardiac CTA in the same patient as previous image, shows markedly dilated RV with wall thinning and internal defibrillator lead in place.*

Typical

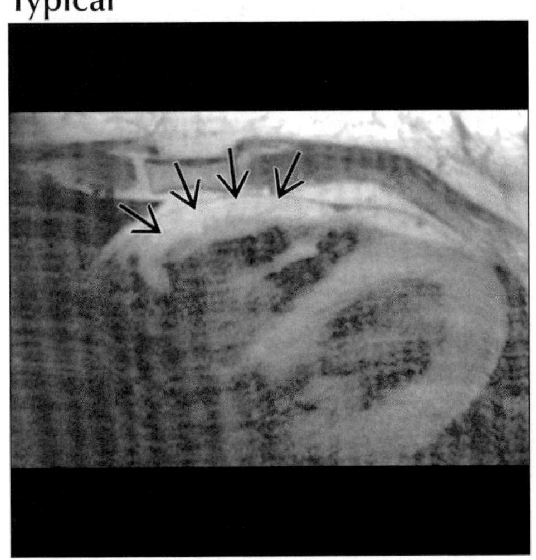

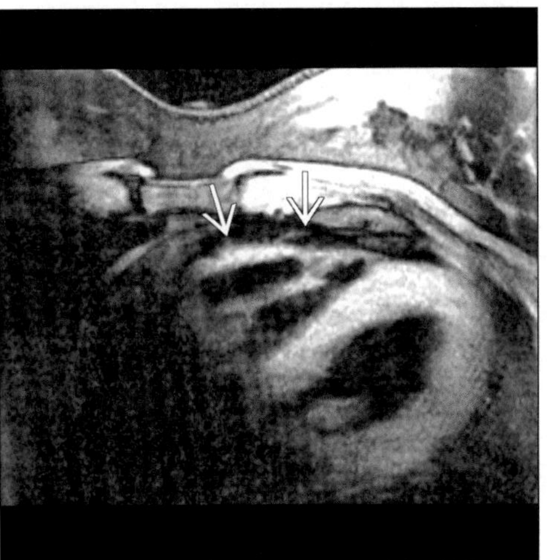

(Left) *High resolution systolic T1WI SE image shows extensive bright tissue encroaching into RV myocardium ➡ and interdigitating with normal myocardium.* ***(Right)*** *High resolution T1WI SE systolic image with fat-saturation shows signal dropout of the tissue confirming it is fat. Note: Normal myocardium appears as white fingerlike extensions within fat ➡.*

ENDOMYOCARDIAL FIBROSIS

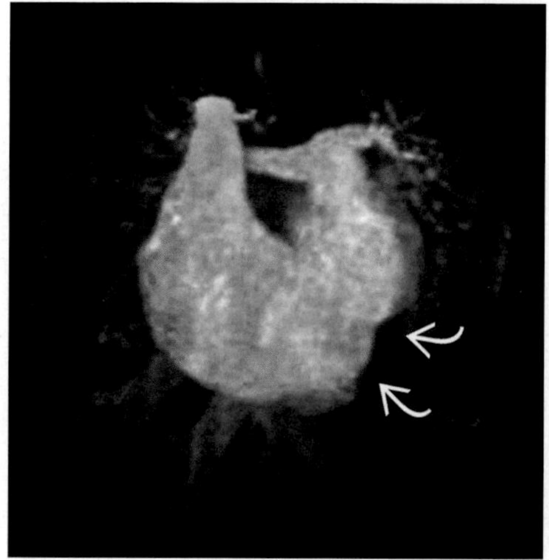

CE-MRA shows RV apical obliteration ➡, inflow and outflow tract dilatation associated with RA, hepatic veins and SVC enlargement characterizing right heart restrictive physiology.

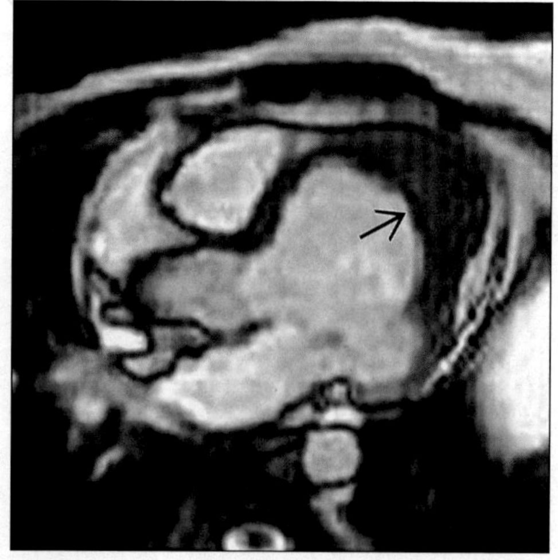

LVOT MR cine shows apical obliteration and LV dilatation, typical EMF findings. Note a dark spot in the endocardial surface of the apex ➡, which may indicate either fibrosis or thrombus.

TERMINOLOGY

Abbreviations and Synonyms

- Davies disease, restrictive obliterative cardiomyopathy, EMF, Löffler endocarditis

Definitions

- Idiopathic disorder in tropical regions characterized by development of restrictive cardiomyopathy
- EMF and Löffler endocarditis are thought to be different manifestations of same disease process, both associated with eosinophilia
  - Löffler endocarditis: Nontropical eosinophilic EMF
- Fibrosis of endocardial surface of heart leads to reduced compliance and, ultimately, restrictive physiology as endomyocardial surface becomes more generally involved
  - Endocardial fibrosis involves inflow tracts of right and left ventricles and may affect atrioventricular valves, leading to tricuspid and mitral regurgitation

IMAGING FINDINGS

General Features

- Best diagnostic clue
  - Ventricular apex obliteration by fibrous formation in the endomyocardium of a patient with heart failure
    - Detection of endomyocardial fibrosis by delayed-enhancement MR is the best noninvasive diagnostic tool
    - Eosinophilia usually present but not always
    - Associated signs of right/left heart failure or both, including systemic/pulmonary venous congestion, AV valve regurgitation and dilated atria
- Location: 45% biventricular, 40% right ventricle and 15% left ventricle
- Morphology
  - Generalized cardiomegaly is unusual because ventricles are not typically dilated
    - Atrial enlargement may modify cardiac silhouette
  - Echocardiography and cardiac MR can demonstrate dilated atria, normal-sized ventricles, regurgitant AV jets, venous congestion and effusions (restrictive heart physiology)

DDx: Endomyocardial Fibrosis

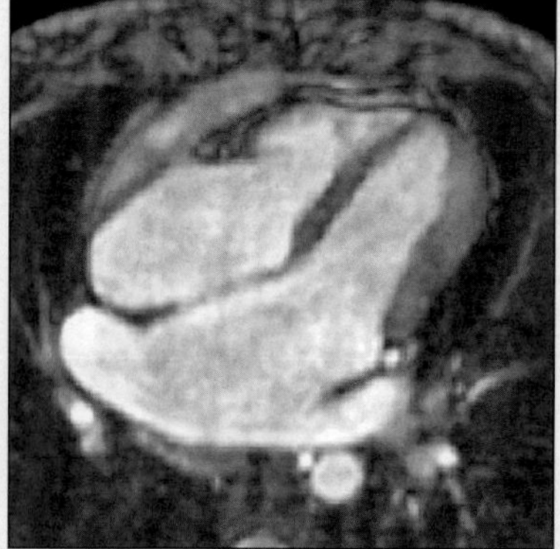

Constrictive Pericarditis

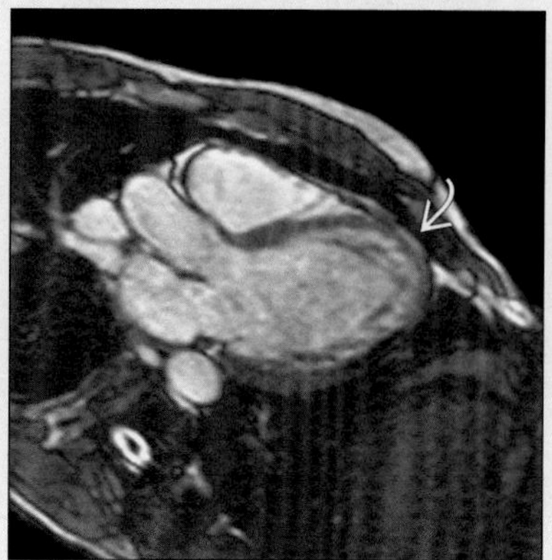

Noncompacted Myocardium

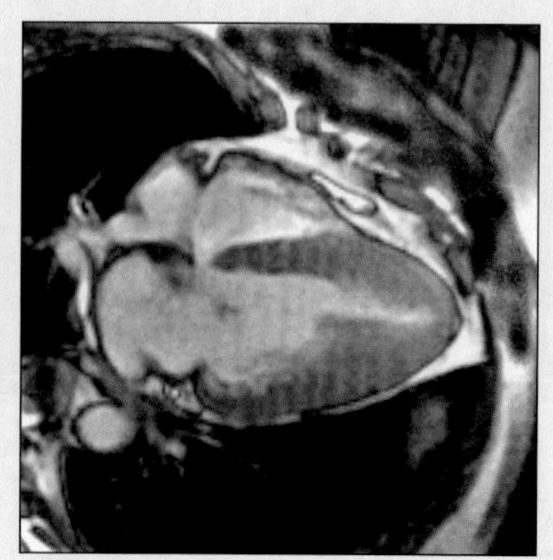

Apical Hypertrophic CMP

ENDOMYOCARDIAL FIBROSIS

Key Facts

Terminology

- EMF: Idiopathic disorder of tropical regions characterized by development of restrictive cardiomyopathy
- Endocardial fibrosis involves inflow tracts of right and left ventricles and may affect atrioventricular valves
  - Leading to tricuspid and mitral regurgitation

Imaging Findings

- Echocardiography: First line tool to detect restrictive physiology and obliterative changes, but limited potential for tissue characterization
- Cardiac MR: Best modality to confirm noninvasively typical EMF fibrosis pattern, clear depiction of thrombus and restrictive physiology
- Clear demonstration of heart morphology and restrictive physiology (dilated atria, regurgitation AV jets, obliterative changes and LV/RV function) on cine-MR
- Detects thrombus and inflammatory/fibrotic changes in endocardial surface, allowing highly accurate and histologically-correlated noninvasive tissue characterization
- Ventricular apex obliteration by fibrous formation in the endomyocardium of a patient with heart failure

Top Differential Diagnoses

- Constrictive Pericarditis
- Noncompaction of Myocardium
- Apical Hypertrophic Cardiomyopathy
- Rheumatic Heart Disease
- Ischemic Cardiomyopathy

Imaging Recommendations

- Best imaging tool
  - Echocardiography: First line tool to detect restrictive physiology and obliterative changes, but limited potential for tissue characterization
  - Cardiac MR: Best modality to confirm noninvasively typical EMF fibrosis pattern, clear depiction of thrombus and restrictive physiology
  - Coronary CTA: May be used selectively for exclusion of coronary artery disease and pericardial thickening
  - Cardiac cath: "Mushroom sign" describes the shape of the affected ventricle when the apex is obliterated completely by fibrosis
- Protocol advice
  - Delayed-enhancement and cine-SSFP images should always be part of the cardiac MR protocol
    - On DE images, low signal intracardiac lesion represents thrombus, hyperenhancement indicates inflammatory infiltration (early stage EMF) or fibrosis (late stage EMF)
    - Cine-SSFP images permit accurate morphologic and functional heart evaluation, as well as exclusion of pericardial thickening
- Chest radiography
  - Predominantly atrial enlargement, according to EMF type (RV, LV or biventricular)
  - Reduced pulmonary vessel markings in right-sided form and pulmonary congestion in left-sided involvement
  - Relatively normal-sized heart in a patient with signs/symptoms of severe heart failure
- Echocardiography
  - Findings include apical obliteration, thrombi adherent to endocardial surface, mitral and tricuspid regurgitation jets, small or normal-size ventricle(s) with severe atrial dilation
  - Restrictive filling pattern in Doppler waveforms of LV correlates with the functional status of the patient
  - In severe heart failure, pericardial effusion can be demonstrated and has prognostic significance
- Cardiac MR
  - Clear demonstration of heart morphology and restrictive physiology (dilated atria, regurgitation AV jets, obliterative changes and LV/RV function) on cine-MR
  - Small or normal-size ventricle(s) with severe atrial dilation
  - Detects thrombus and inflammatory/fibrotic changes in endocardial surface through delayed-hyperenhancement, allowing highly accurate and histologically-correlated noninvasive tissue characterization
  - Exclusion of constrictive pericarditis by normal-appearing pericardium (thickness lesser than 3 mm)
  - DE-images may demonstrate distinct hyperenhancement patterns usually consistent with other cardiomyopathies (hypertrophic CMP, ischemic CMP) and either focal or diffuse pericardial enhancement (CP)
- CE-3D MRA
  - Demonstrates typical angiographic pattern (mushroom sign) indicating apical obliteration of the involved ventricle
- Conventional angiography
  - Traditionally, DSA has been considered the standard tool when making the diagnosis of EMF
  - Coronary arteries are usually normal, hemodynamic findings consistent with restrictive cardiomyopathy (raised end-diastolic pressures in involved ventricle)
  - Left and right ventriculography exhibits distortion of chamber morphology by fibrosis and obliteration and variable degrees of mitral & tricuspid regurgitation

DIFFERENTIAL DIAGNOSIS

Constrictive Pericarditis

- Tubular appearance of ventricles on four-chamber view, and elliptical-shaped LV on short-axis view (diastolic phase)
- Pericardial thickening greater than 4-6 mm

- Focal or diffuse pericardial enhancement on CE-MR may indicate either inflammation or fibrosis, more frequently over right heart chambers and right atrioventricular groove
- Negative MR exam makes CP very unlikely

Noncompaction of Myocardium

- Characterized by persistent embryonic myocardial morphology - two-layered appearance of the ventricular myocardium (endocardial = noncompacted, epicardial = compacted)
- Noncompated/compacted thickness ratio > 2.3 (diagnostic)
- Noncompaction affects more frequently apex and infero-lateral segments of the left ventricle

Apical Hypertrophic Cardiomyopathy

- Apical obliteration is transient and typically occur only in systole, compared to the constant fashion during both systole and diastole in EMF
- On DE-MR images, hyperenhanced areas are located mainly in midwall myocardium and are patch in distribution, sparing the endocardial surface

Rheumatic Heart Disease

- Thickened AV valves leaflet (normal in EMF)
- Obliterative changes absent
- Evidence of previous group A streptococcal pharyngitis usually exist

Ischemic Cardiomyopathy

- Post-infarction thrombus formation may obliterate somewhat LV apex, then may mimic non-ischemic cardiomyopathies
- Thrombus-related myocardium usually very thin (lesser than 5 mm) and transmurally infarcted as can be observed on DE MR images (ischemic transmural hyperenhancement)
- Severe wall motion abnormality mostly in left anterior descending artery distribution

PATHOLOGY

General Features

- Etiology
  - Specific single etiology of EMF has not been established; potential causes include the following
  - Infectious
    - Parasites (e.g., helminths), Protozoans (e.g., toxoplasmosis, malaria)
  - Inflammatory
    - Eosinophilia (hypereosinophilic states)
  - Nutritional
    - General malnutrition, high-tuber diet and hypomagnesemia
- Epidemiology
  - Tropical EMF: 90% cases in tropical and subtropical regions of Africa, India and South America
  - EMF accounts for 22% of cases of heart failure in Nigerian children; EMF is most common type of restrictive cardiomyopathy in tropical countries

Gross Pathologic & Surgical Features

- Heart size is not usually enlarged, ventricular cavities obliterated by endocardial thickening and thrombosis

Microscopic Features

- Early phase (0-5 weeks): Eosinophilic infiltration of myocardium with necrosis of subendocardium, consistent with acute myocarditis
- Intermediate phase (after 10 months): Thrombus formation over initial lesions, with a decrement in amount of inflammatory activity
- Late phase (after years of activity): Fibrotic phase is reached, when endocardium is replaced by fibrosis

CLINICAL ISSUES

Presentation

- Most common signs/symptoms
  - RV involvement: Dyspnea, ascites, peripheral edema, hepatomegaly, distended neck veins
  - LV involvement: Dyspnea, S3 gallop and pulmonary edema
  - Most patients are admitted in class III or IV (NYHA)

Demographics

- Age: Older children (aged 5-15 y) and young adults
- Gender: Women of reproductive age and children are more commonly affected than men

Natural History & Prognosis

- Poor overall prognosis, 90% mortality rate at 2 years after the onset of symptoms

Treatment

- Endocardial decortication for class III or IV; recurrence occurs in 15% cases in post-operative period
- Successful surgery has a clear benefit on symptoms and seems to favorably affect survival as well
- Löffler endocarditis: Immune suppressant and cytotoxic medications with varying degrees of success

SELECTED REFERENCES

1. Syed IS et al: Cardiac magnetic resonance imaging of eosinophilic endomyocardial disease. Int J Cardiol. 2007
2. Macedo R et al: MRI to assess arrhythmia and cardiomyopathies. J Magn Reson Imaging. 24(6):1197-206, 2006
3. Cury RC et al: Images in cardiovascular medicine. Visualization of endomyocardial fibrosis by delayed-enhancement magnetic resonance imaging. Circulation. 111(9):e115-7, 2005
4. Hassan WM et al: Pitfalls in diagnosis and clinical, echocardiographic, and hemodynamic findings in endomyocardial fibrosis: a 25-year experience. Chest. 128(6):3985-92, 2005
5. Fernandes F et al: [Radiological findings in endomyocardial fibrosis] Arq Bras Cardiol. 68(4):269-72, 1997
6. Kushwaha SS et al: Restrictive cardiomyopathy. N Engl J Med. 336(4):267-76, 1997

ENDOMYOCARDIAL FIBROSIS

IMAGE GALLERY

Typical

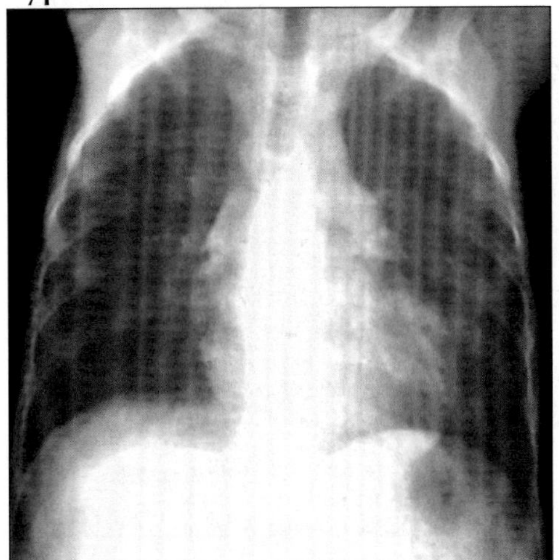

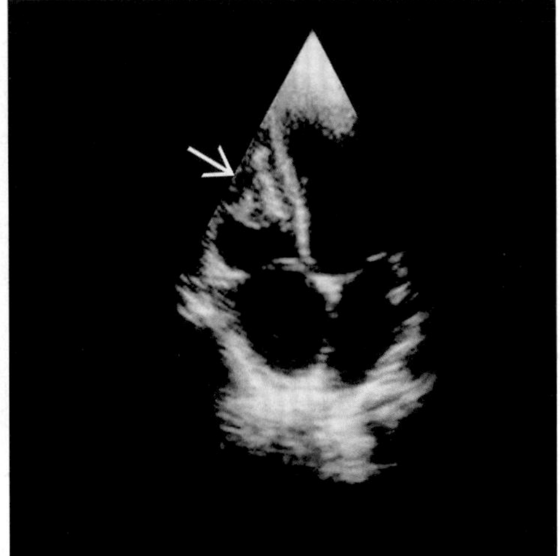

(Left) Posteroanterior radiograph shows RA enlargement, decreased pulmonary blood flow and mild cardiomegaly in a patient with right-sided EMF. CXR findings are usually nonspecific. *(Right)* Four chamber view echocardiogram shows an intraventricular mass-like lesion ➡ in RV and gross enlargement of right atrium in a patient with right-sided EMF and no evidence of disease on LV.

Typical

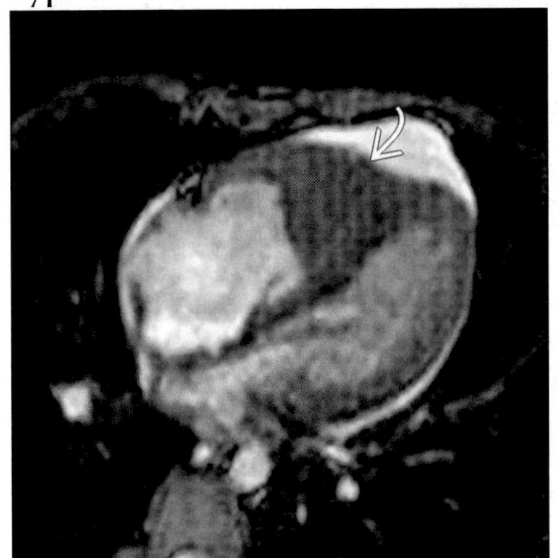

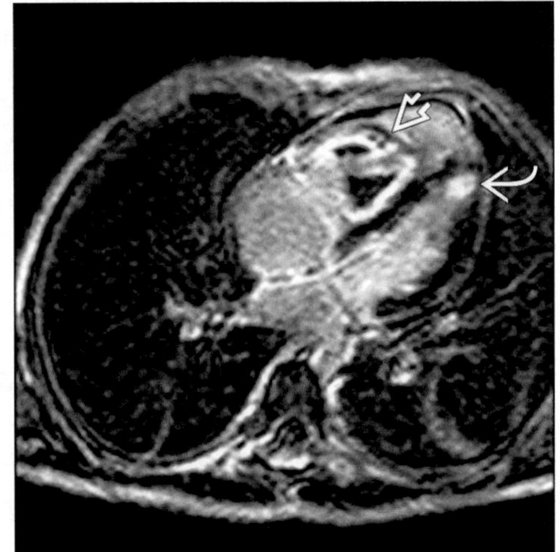

(Left) Four chamber view MR cine shows mid-apical obliteration of RV ➡, dilated RA and a small pericardial effusion. Mild LV apex involvement. *(Right)* Four chamber view DE MR shows RV endocavitary thrombus and endomyocardial hyperenhancement ➡ in a patient with eosinophilic leukemia (Löffler endocarditis). LV apex also involved ➡.

Typical

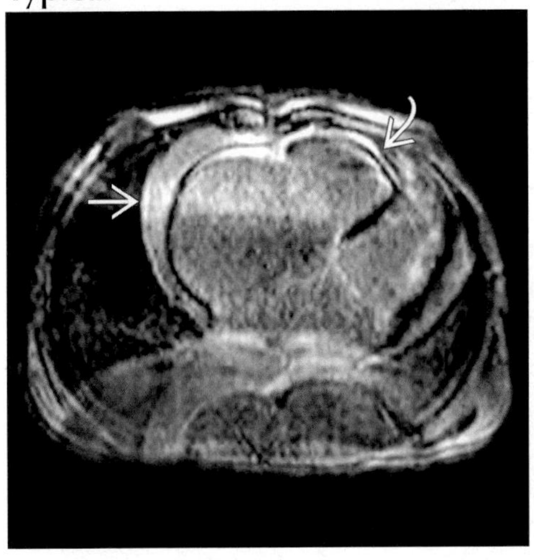

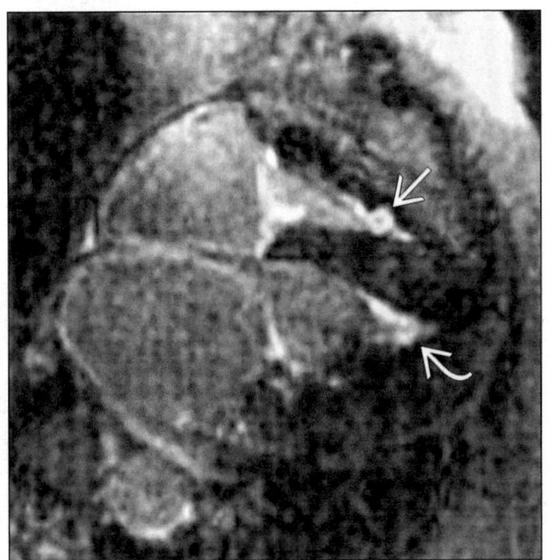

(Left) Four chamber view DE MR shows typical recurrent endocardial fibrosis on RV apex ➡ in a patient 2 years after surgical decortication. Note also moderate pericardial effusion ➡. *(Right)* Four chamber view DE MR detects small ventricles and dilated atria. Observe endomyocardial fibrosis on both RV and LV. Left ventricle ➡, right ventricle ➡.

HYPEREOSINOPHILIC SYNDROME

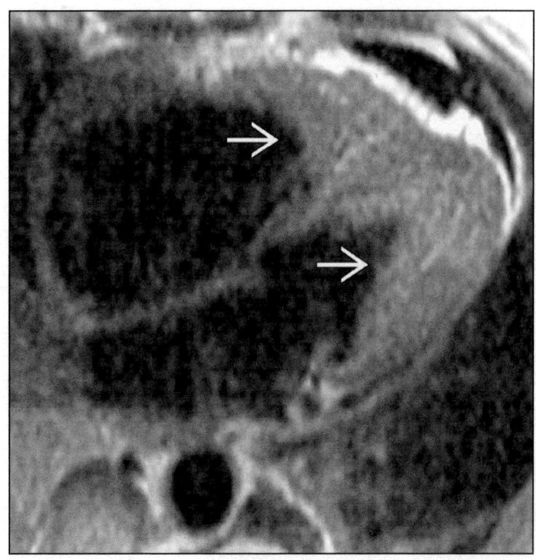

Four chamber view T1WI FSE MR shows bi-apical intraventricular thrombus ➔. Also note the myocardial thickening predominantly involving the left ventricular apex.

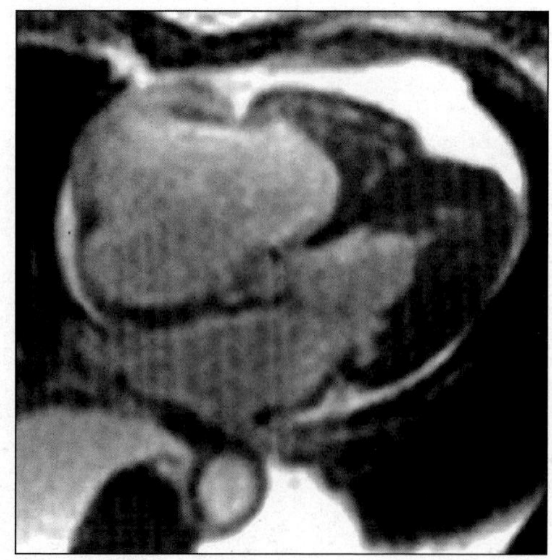

Four chamber view SSFP MR shows thrombus within the apices of both ventricles with thickening of the left ventricular myocardium. Bi-atrial enlargement is also visible.

TERMINOLOGY

Abbreviations and Synonyms

- Eosinophilic myocarditis
- Loeffler myocarditis
- Endomyocardial fibrosis
  - Similar pathophysiology to Loeffler endocarditis that may or may not be associated with hypereosinophilia

Definitions

- Prolonged hypereosinophilia (> 1500/mm^3) usually > six months duration which ultimately leads to the development of a restrictive cardiomyopathy

IMAGING FINDINGS

General Features

- Best diagnostic clue
  - MR findings often variable and nonspecific
    - Increased T2 signal in ventricular apices
    - Subendocardial late enhancement following gadolinium administration, particularly within apices
    - Regional areas of hypokinesis or akinesis in setting of endomyocardial fibrosis
    - Intraventricular thrombus, particularly in apices
    - Findings of restrictive cardiomyopathy can occur in later fibrotic stages of the disease, including diastolic dysfunction with bi-atrial enlargement
    - Enlarged atria, valvular regurgitation and tethered valves from fibrosed chordae tendinae

Imaging Recommendations

- Best imaging tool: Contrast-enhanced MR

DIFFERENTIAL DIAGNOSIS

Other Causes of Restrictive Cardiomyopathy

- Sarcoidosis
- Amyloidosis
- Hemochromatosis

DDx: Restrictive Cardiomyopathy

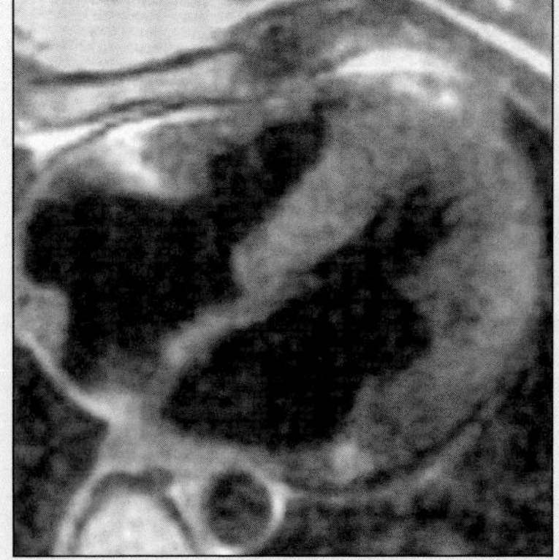

Amyloidosis

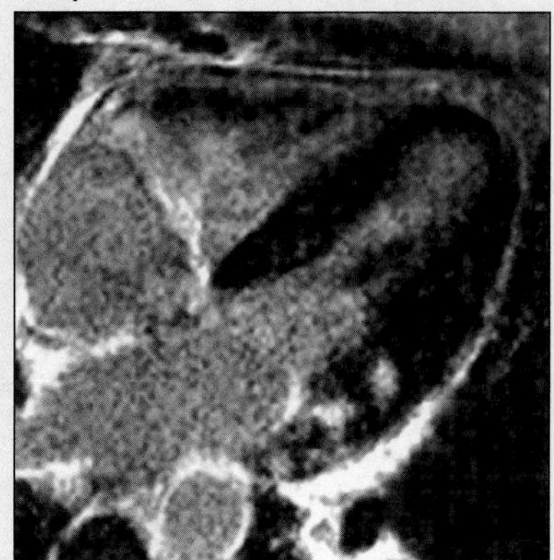

Sarcoidosis

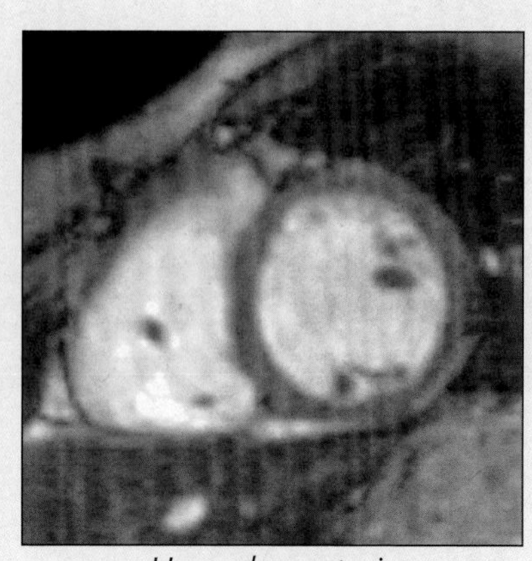

Hemochromatosis

HYPEREOSINOPHILIC SYNDROME

Key Facts

Terminology
- Eosinophilic myocarditis
- Prolonged hypereosinophilia (> 1500/mm^3) usually > six months duration which ultimately leads to the development of a restrictive cardiomyopathy

Imaging Findings
- Increased signal in the apices of both ventricles on T2 and STIR images
- Bi-atrial enlargement
- Subendocardial enhancement following gadolinium administration, particularly within the ventricular apices
- Regional areas of hypokinesis or akinesis in the setting of endomyocardial fibrosis
- Intraventricular thrombus, particularly in the ventricular apices

Top Differential Diagnoses
- Other Causes of Restrictive Cardiomyopathy

PATHOLOGY

General Features
- Genetics
  - Interstitial chromosomal deletion on chromosome band 4q12
    - Gene deletion leads to excess levels of tyrosine kinase which transforms hematopoietic stem cells into excess levels of eosinophils

Gross Pathologic & Surgical Features
- Increased stiffness of the ventricular walls, often with subsequent bi-atrial enlargement
- Reduction of the ventricular cavity volume by organized thrombus
- Pericardial effusions

CLINICAL ISSUES

Presentation
- Most common signs/symptoms: Biventricular congestive heart failure
- Other signs/symptoms: Fever, night sweats, weight loss, myalgias, dyspnea, non-productive cough and generalized fatigue

Demographics
- Gender: 85-90% male predominance

Natural History & Prognosis
- Three stages of disease progression
  - Acute necrotic stage
    - Infiltration of the endocardium and myocardium with eosinophils leading to microabscess formation within the myocardium
  - Thrombotic-necrotic stage
    - Formation of thrombi along damaged endocardium of ventricles & occasionally right atrium
  - Late fibrotic stage
    - Progressive scarring leading to entrapment of chordae tendinae resulting in mitral and/or tricuspid regurgitation

Treatment
- Low-dose imatinib (tyrosine kinase inhibitor), steroids and cytotoxic agents
- Conventional heart failure therapy, including digitalis and diuretics

SELECTED REFERENCES

1. Cury RC et al: Images in cardiovascular medicine. Visualization of endomyocardial fibrosis by delayed-enhancement magnetic resonance imaging. Circulation. 111(9):e115-7, 2005
2. Puvaneswary M et al: Idiopathic hypereosinophilic syndrome: magnetic resonance imaging findings in endomyocardial fibrosis. Australas Radiol. 45(4):524-7, 2001
3. Pitt M et al: Hypereosinophilic syndrome: endomyocardial fibrosis. Heart. 76(4):377-8, 1996

IMAGE GALLERY

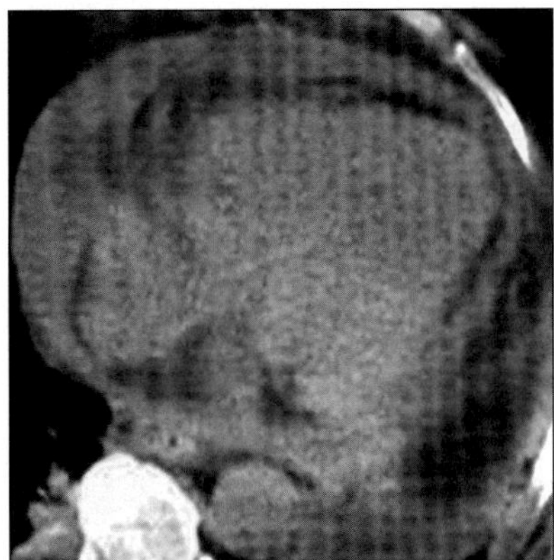

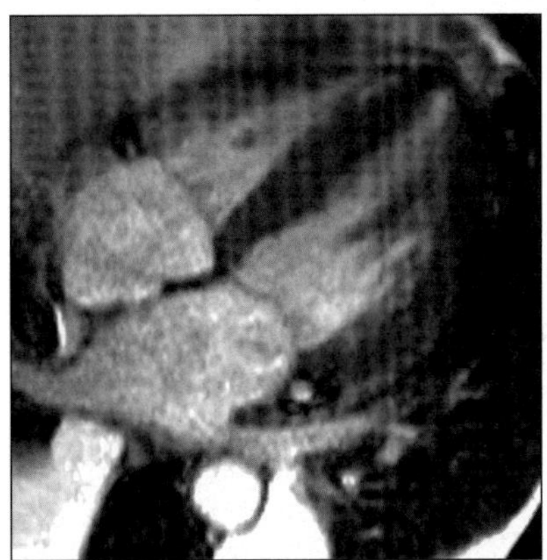

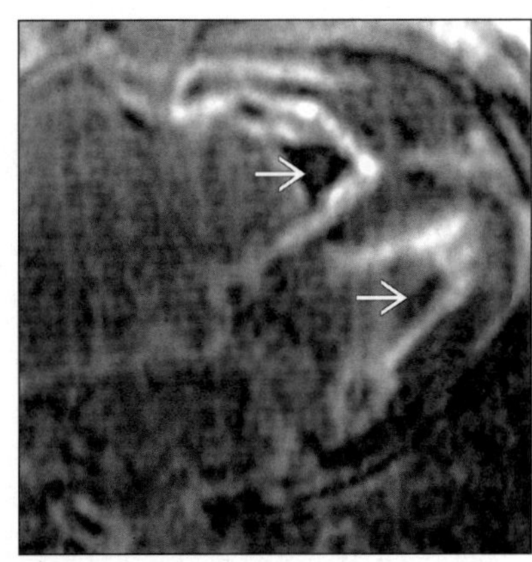

(Left) *Axial NECT shows mild atrial enlargement and a moderate pericardial effusion.* ***(Center)*** *Four chamber view SSFP MR shows mild bi-atrial enlargement. There is ventricular rigidity with global hypokinesis of the left ventricle, consistent with diastolic dysfunction.* ***(Right)*** *Four chamber view T1WI MR following contrast administration shows endocardial delayed hyperenhancement in a predominantly bi-apical distribution and adjacent nonenhancing ventricular thrombus* ➔.

CARDIAC SARCOIDOSIS

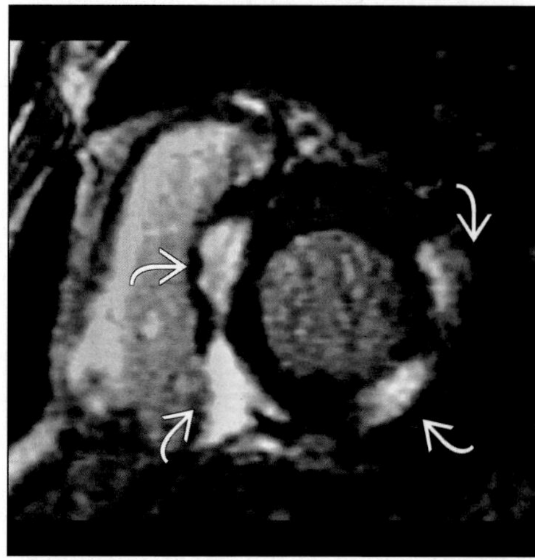

LV short axis DE MR shows patchy subepicardial delayed hyperenhancement in a patient with cardiac sarcoidosis ➔.

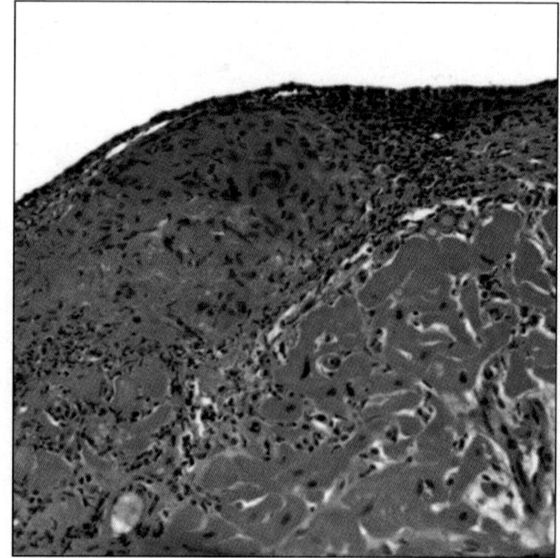

Endomyocardial biopsy shows extensive fibrosis with giant cells, compact non-caseating granulomas, and accompanying lymphocytic infiltrate, consistent with cardiac sarcoidosis.

TERMINOLOGY

Definitions

- Sarcoidosis is a systemic chronic granulomatous disease of unknown etiology that most commonly affects young adults
- Cardiac sarcoidosis is appearance of microscopic or macroscopic non-caseating granulomas in the pericardium, myocardium or endocardium that leads to sequelae

IMAGING FINDINGS

General Features

- Best diagnostic clue: Presence of hyperechogenic region on echocardiogram and delayed hyperenhancement on cardiac MR with corresponding wall motion abnormality in a non-ischemic pattern
- Location
  - Left ventricular free wall and papillary muscles are the most common locations for granulomas and scars, followed by the intraventricular septum
  - Myocardial sarcoid granulomas tend to be in the base of the heart
- Size: Granuloma formation may be microscopic or macroscopic

Radiographic Findings

- Chest radiographs may show mild to moderate cardiac enlargement along with other features of congestive heart failure such as pericardial effusion
- In the presence of concurrent pulmonary sarcoidosis, features such as hilar lymphadenopathy, interstitial lung disease and honeycombing may be seen

MR Findings

- T1WI FS
  - Depicts nodular pattern with peripherally increased signal intensity inside the myocardium on gadolinium enhanced images
  - Inflammatory changes can also appear on gadolinium-enhanced images as areas of focal increased signal intensity with or without myocardial wall thickening
- T2WI FS
  - Identifies myocardial edema due to inflammation in acute phase

DDx: Myocardial Disease

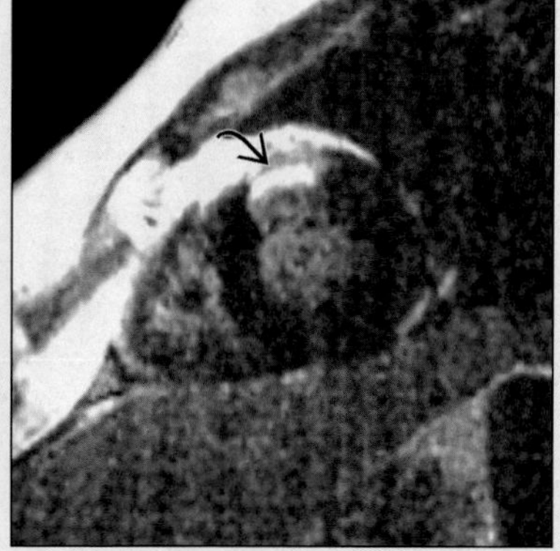

Myocardial Infarct

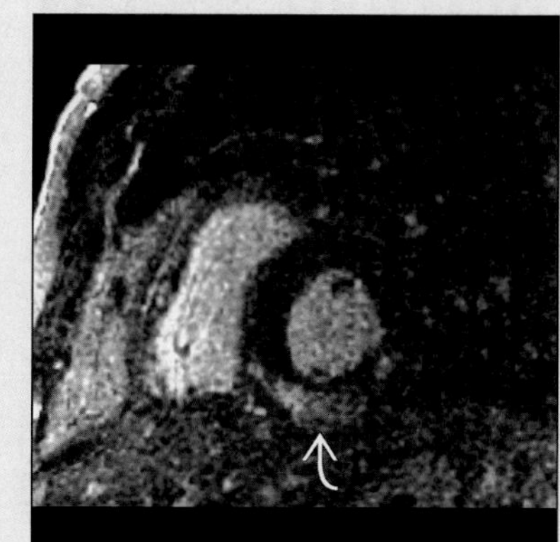

Acute Viral Myocarditis

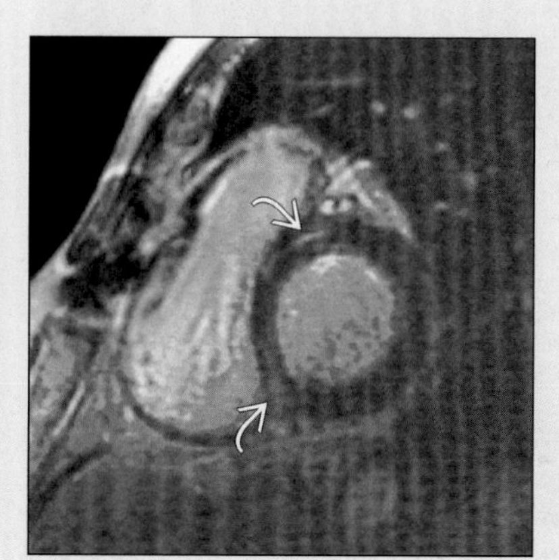

Non-Ischemic Cardiomyopathy

CARDIAC SARCOIDOSIS

Key Facts

Terminology
- Cardiac Sarcoidosis is appearance of microscopic or macroscopic non-caseating granulomas in the pericardium, myocardium or endocardium that leads to sequelae

Imaging Findings
- Granulomatous involvement of the myocardium with scar formation may appear hyperechogenic on echocardiogram
- Delayed enhancement cardiac MR may show areas of myocardial, epicardial or endocardial hyperenhancement in a non-ischemic pattern (not confined to coronary artery territories)
- Sequelae of the disease may include ventricular aneurysms, valvular regurgitation, mitral valve prolapse, LV dilatation or segmental or global LV hypokinesia and pericardial effusions

Top Differential Diagnoses
- Myocardial Infarction
- Arrhythmogenic Right Ventricular Dysplasia (ARVD)
- Myocarditis

Clinical Issues
- Majority of patients are asymptomatic
- Presentation depends on location and extent of granulomatous inflammation

---

  - Hyperintensity manifests mostly in the mid myocardium or epicardium
- MR Cine
  - Assessment of focal wall motion abnormalities in different coronary territories with possible involvement of the LV and RV
  - Occasionally, LV or RV wall aneurysms may be seen secondary to ventricular wall thinning
- Delayed Enhancement
  - Areas of delayed hyperenhancement correspond to myocardial inflammation, granulomatous and scar formation
  - Distribution of DE is mostly epicardial or mid-myocardial and along the RV border of the interventricular septum
  - Steroid therapy has been demonstrated to reduce the size of hyperenhancement on DE-MR
  - DE-MR can thus be used as a tool for judging response to treatment

Nuclear Medicine Findings
- Segmental defects are seen on scintigraphy with thallium-201and FDG-PET which correspond to areas of granulomatous replacement
- Defects decrease on exercise stress thallium, a phenomena known as reverse distribution; this helps differentiation from defects secondary to coronary artery disease

Echocardiographic Findings
- Granulomatous involvement of the myocardium with scar formation may appear hyperechogenic on echocardiogram
- There might be mild thickening of the myocardium initially leading to asymmetric hypertrophy
- As the disease progresses, this evolves into scarring that is seen as thinning of the myocardium, resulting in aneurysmal formation
- Sequelae of the disease may include ventricular aneurysms, valvular regurgitation, mitral valve prolapse, LV dilatation or segmental or global LV hypokinesia and pericardial effusions
- Microscopic granulomas may be missed, so the test cannot reliably establish or exclude the diagnosis

Angiographic Findings
- Used to exclude coronary artery disease as an etiological factor

Imaging Recommendations
- Best imaging tool
  - Cardiac MR
    - Delayed enhancement cardiac MR may show areas of myocardial, epicardial or endocardial hyperenhancement in a non-ischemic pattern (not confined to coronary artery territories)
    - Cine SSFP demonstrates focal areas of thinning and wall motion abnormality with aneurysmal formations
- Protocol advice: T1WI fast spin echo sequences before and after gadolinium administration, T2WI FSE, delayed imaging and cine MR with SSFP sequences are part of the comprehensive evaluation of patients with sarcoidosis

DIFFERENTIAL DIAGNOSIS

Myocardial Infarction
- Chest pain, shortness of breath, EKG abnormalities
- Abnormal cardiac biomarkers, associated with coronary artery disease on conventional or CT angiography
- Delayed enhancement MR shows hyperenhancement in an ischemic pattern with infarcts starting from the subendocardium
- Areas of hyperenhancement correspond to coronary artery territories

Arrhythmogenic Right Ventricular Dysplasia
- Usually presents with right ventricular distribution, which is somewhat rare in cardiac sarcoidosis
- FSE or SE techniques may show fatty infiltration of the RV

- Ventricular aneurysms and focal wall motion abnormalities may be seen

Myocarditis

- Inflammatory infiltrate of the myocardium with necrosis and/or degeneration of adjacent myocytes
- Pattern of delayed enhancement in acute cases is subepicardial predominantly in the basal infero-lateral wall

PATHOLOGY

General Features

- Genetics
  - Genetic factors may play a role
  - Positive association is reported with HLA-DQB1*0601
  - Disease is more common in monozygotic twins than dizygotic twins and there is familial clustering in 19% of affected African American families
- Etiology
  - Exaggerated immune response to a variety of antigens which cause CD4 cells accumulation and release of inflammatory cytokines leading to granuloma formation
  - Infectious and environmental agents have been implicated as potential antigens
- Associated abnormalities: Sarcoid infiltration of the myocardium might cause ventricular stiffness, or diminished systolic function

Gross Pathologic & Surgical Features

- Non-caseating epithelioid granulomas are seen
- Granulomas may involve the pericardium, myocardium or endocardium, the myocardium is most frequently involved

Microscopic Features

- Microscopic examination reveals T lymphocytes and mononuclear phagocytes, which are seen at sites of inflammation initially
- As the disease progresses, there is granuloma formation consisting of aggregated macrophages, epithelioid cells, and giant cells
- Dense band of fibroblasts, collagen and proteoglycans usually encase the aggregate of inflammatory cells

CLINICAL ISSUES

Presentation

- Most common signs/symptoms
  - Majority of patients are asymptomatic
  - Common presentations include
    - Conduction abnormalities: Ranging from benign first degree AV block to complete heart block
    - RBBB is more common than LBBB; sustained or non-sustained ventricular tachycardia is the second most common presentation
    - Supra ventricular arrhythmias are less common than ventricular ones
  - Clinical evidence of cardiac sarcoidosis is present in less than 5% of patients with sarcoidosis, but myocardial involvement can occur in up to 25%
- Other signs/symptoms
  - Mitral valve regurgitation is the most common valvular abnormality seen
  - CHF may also be seen; second most common cause of sarcoid-related mortality after sudden death due to conduction abnormalities
  - Isolated pericardial involvement is rare, as is cardiac tamponade and constrictive pericarditis due to cardiac sarcoidosis

Demographics

- Age: Sarcoidosis in general is seen mostly in young and middle aged adults
- Ethnicity
  - In the US, African Americans have a 3-4 fold greater risk of the disease compared to Caucasians
  - Higher incidence of concurrent involvement of the myocardium in certain races, e.g., Japanese (up to 50% of patients with sarcoidosis might have cardiac involvement)

Natural History & Prognosis

- Cardiac involvement of sarcoidosis is associated with a poorer prognosis compared to sarcoidosis that does not involve the heart
- It accounts for 13-25% of the deaths from sarcoidosis
- Mortality rate may exceed 40% at 5 years and 55% within 10 years

Treatment

- Corticosteroids
- Immunosuppressive therapy
- Anti-arrhythmic therapy
- Medical management of heart failure using standard therapies

SELECTED REFERENCES

1. Borchert B et al: Utility of endomyocardial biopsy guided by delayed enhancement areas on magnetic resonance imaging in the diagnosis of cardiac sarcoidosis. Clin Res Cardiol. 96(10):759-62, 2007
2. Doughan AR et al: Cardiac sarcoidosis. Heart. 92(2):282-8, 2006
3. Tadamura E et al: Images in cardiovascular medicine. Multimodality imaging of cardiac sarcoidosis before and after steroid therapy. Circulation. 113(20):e771-3, 2006
4. Smedema JP et al: The additional value of gadolinium-enhanced MRI to standard assessment for cardiac involvement in patients with pulmonary sarcoidosis. Chest. 128(3):1629-37, 2005
5. Tadamura E et al: Effectiveness of delayed enhanced MRI for identification of cardiac sarcoidosis: comparison with radionuclide imaging. AJR Am J Roentgenol. 185(1):110-5, 2005
6. Bargout R et al: Sarcoid heart disease: clinical course and treatment. Int J Cardiol. 97(2):173-82, 2004

CARDIAC SARCOIDOSIS

IMAGE GALLERY

Typical

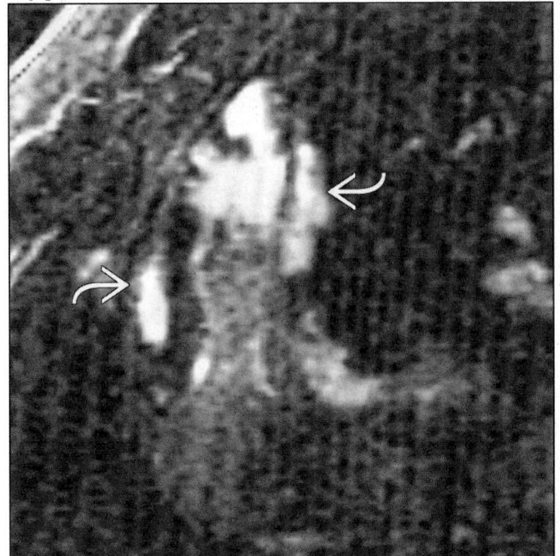

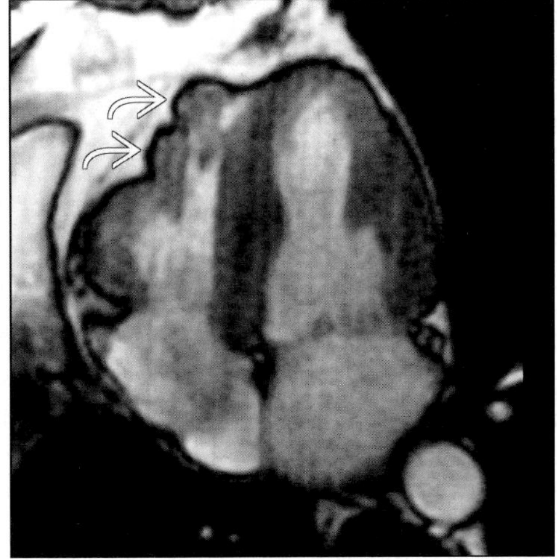

(Left) *Four chamber view DE MR shows multiple areas of subepicardial delayed enhancement ➔ corresponding to areas of granuloma formation in a patient with cardiac sarcoidosis.* ***(Right)*** *Four chamber view SSFP shows aneurysmal dilatation ➔ of the right ventricle in a patient with myocardial thinning due to cardiac sarcoidosis.*

Typical

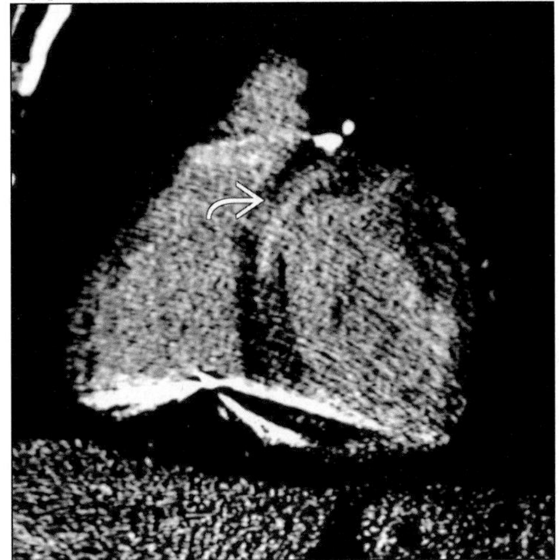

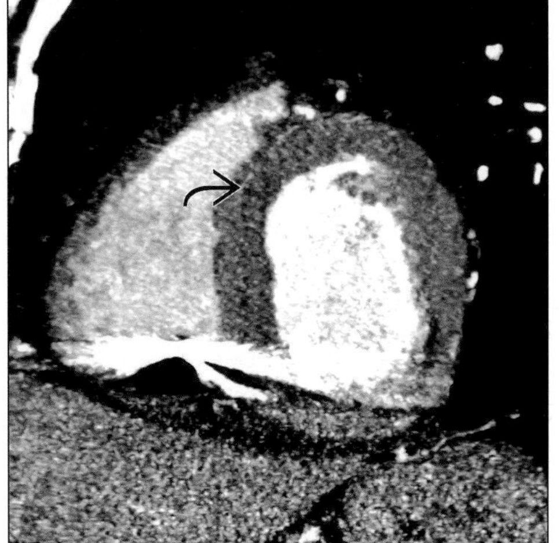

(Left) *LV short axis delayed enhancement cardiac CT shows hyperenhancement ➔ due to sarcoid granuloma in a young patient without coronary disease who could not undergo MR due to an implanted device.* ***(Right)*** *LV short axis cardiac CT of the same patient as previous image, shows normal myocardial perfusion of the corresponding segment ➔ by CT.*

Typical

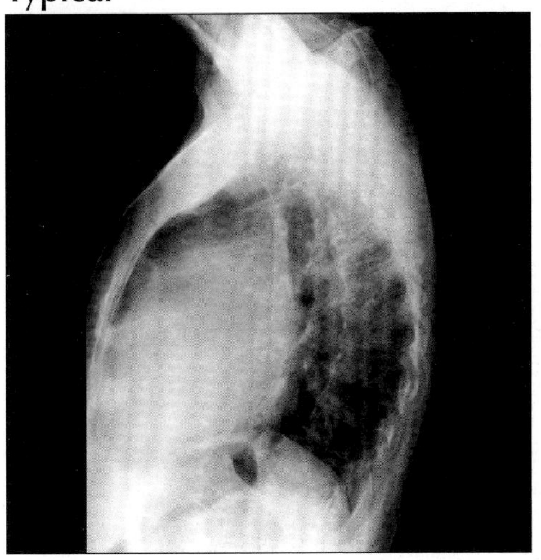

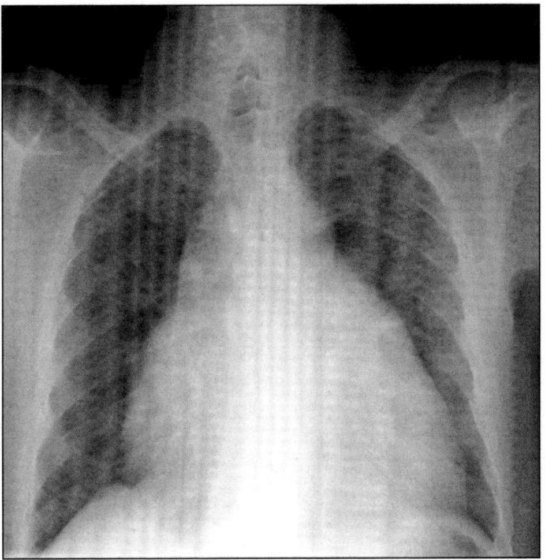

(Left) *Lateral radiograph shows prominent cardiomegaly in a patient with later stage of cardiac sarcoidosis.* ***(Right)*** *Posteroanterior radiograph shows cardiomegaly due to heart failure in a patient with cardiac sarcoidosis.*

CARDIAC AMYLOIDOSIS

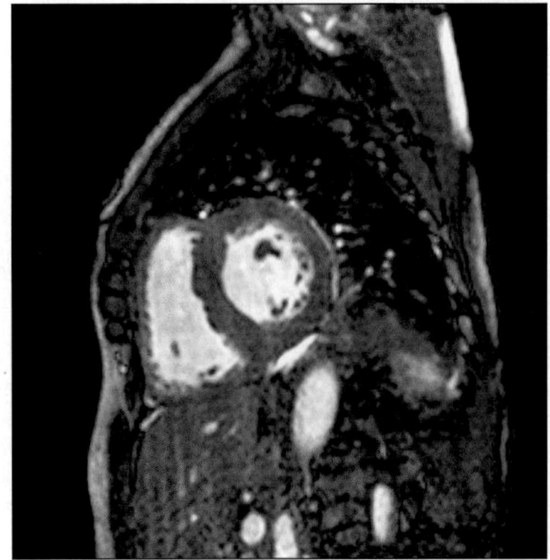

Short axis SSFP shows concentric left ventricular myocardial thickening in a patient with biopsy proven cardiac amyloidosis. (Courtesy A. Fuisz, MD).

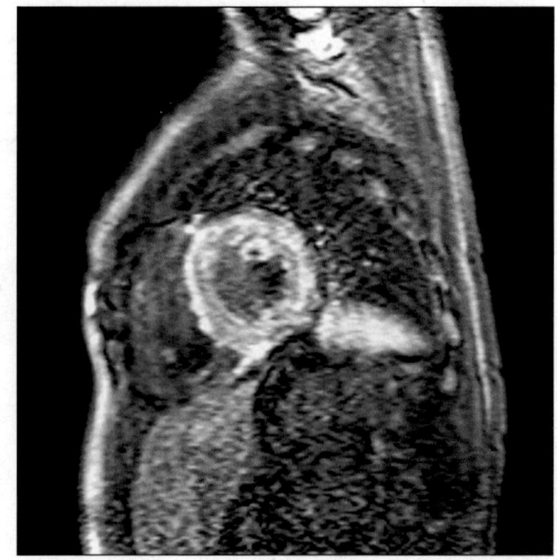

Short axis DE MR image of the same patient, shows myocardial delayed enhancement that is most prominent in the subendocardial region.

TERMINOLOGY

Abbreviations and Synonyms

- Stiff heart syndrome

Definitions

- Amyloidosis is a heterogeneous group of diseases characterized by extracellular deposits of insoluble fibrillar protein
- Cardiac amyloidosis may be primary, part of systemic amyloidosis or chronic systemic diseases

IMAGING FINDINGS

General Features

- Best diagnostic clue
  - Nonspecific
    - Concentric left ventricular (LV) hypertrophy
    - Enlarged atria
    - Pericardial and pleural effusions
- Location
  - Diffuse process that can involve nearly any portion of the heart
    - In addition to affecting ventricular wall thickness and atrial size, atrial septal thickening may be observed, also valvular thickening/regurgitation

MR Findings

- T1 C+
  - Diffuse heterogeneous enhancement (entire LV) of thickened subendocardial myocardium on delayed enhancement (DE) images
  - This distribution likely represents retention of gadolinium within areas of amyloid infiltration, rather than fibrotic myocardium
    - "Zebra" pattern: Biventricular subendocardial enhancement lending a striped appearance to the ventricular septum
  - Tagged cine sequence identifies areas of decreased myocardial contraction

Other Modality Findings

- Abnormal global or regional myocardial relaxation early in disease process, with restrictive pattern and increased filling pressures later
- Thickened ventricular walls with abnormal granular echotexture ("starry sky" appearance) on echocardiogram

DDx: Cardiomyopathies

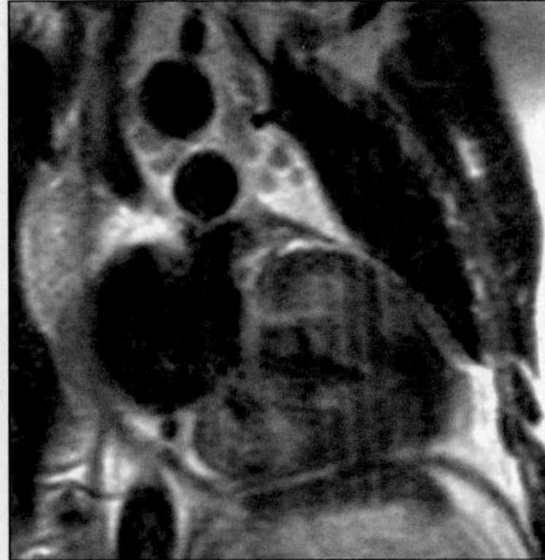

Sarcoidosis

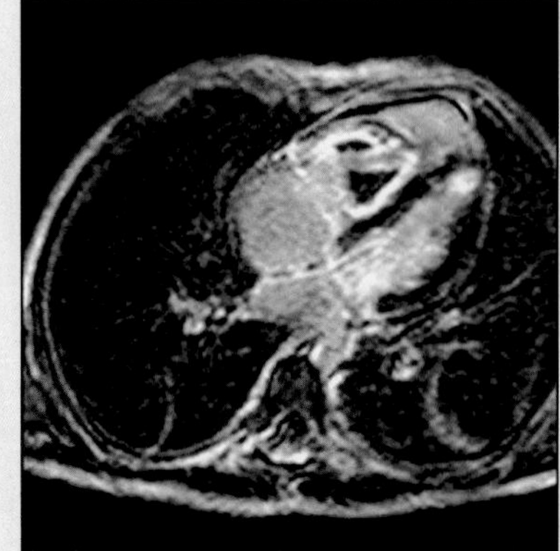

Löffler Endocarditis

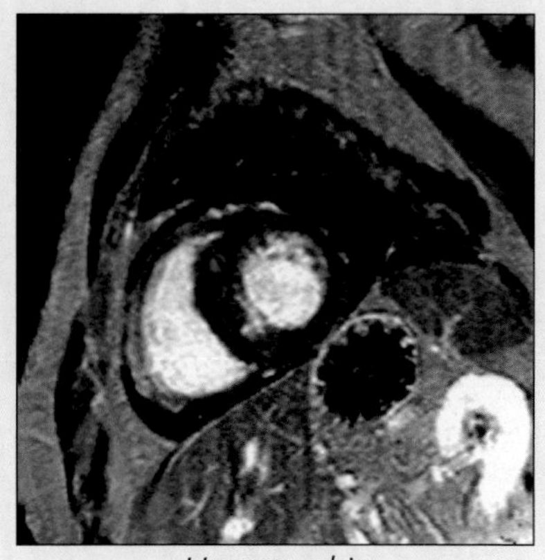

Hypertrophic

CARDIAC AMYLOIDOSIS

Key Facts

Terminology
- Amyloidosis is a heterogeneous group of diseases characterized by extracellular deposits of insoluble fibrillar protein

Imaging Findings
- Concentric left ventricular thickening
- Enlarged atria
- Pericardial and pleural effusions
- Amyloidosis is a diffuse process and can involve nearly any portion of the heart (valves, septum etc.)
- DE: Diffuse subendocardial delayed enhancement of entire LV and RV
  - Striped appearance of ventricular septum

Top Differential Diagnoses
- Hypertrophic Cardiomyopathy
- Hypertension
- Sarcoidosis
- Infiltrative Lymphoma

Pathology
- Cardiac amyloidosis is most commonly associated with AL type

Clinical Issues
- Many patients will have no symptoms, or minor symptoms
- Advanced cases may present with signs of symptoms of right heart failure, including increased jugular venous pressure, hepatomegaly, peripheral edema
- Left heart failure in absence of ischemic disease
- Atrial fibrillation, and other conduction abnormalities

Imaging Recommendations
- Best imaging tool: Echocardiography and MR
- Protocol advice
  - SSFP cine sequence to evaluate wall thickening
  - DE images to assess for diffuse subendocardial enhancement
    - Inversion times may be shorter than usual due to diffuse gadolinium retention in areas of infiltration
  - DE imaging < 8 min after contrast administration suggested to observe differential enhancement within myocardium, which later may equilibrate

DIFFERENTIAL DIAGNOSIS

Hypertrophic Cardiomyopathy
- Myocardial hypertrophy, often asymmetric
- Most patients are asymptomatic, leading cause of sudden death in children

Hypertension
- Concentric LV hypertrophy, impaired diastolic filling
- Aortic root dilation, increased vessel tortuosity

Sarcoidosis
- Infiltrating, noncaseating granulomas
- Affects conduction system and may lead to fatal arrhythmias
- Subcarinal and hilar adenopathy on chest radiography
- DE distribution does not follow ischemic pattern
- Increased T2 signal in regions of active disease

Infiltrative Lymphoma
- Right atrium and ventricle most commonly involved, but may involve all chambers
- Depending on location may cause dyspnea and arrhythmias

PATHOLOGY

General Features
- General path comments
  - Five types of amyloidosis
    - Immunoglobulin amyloidosis (AL type amyloidosis)
    - Secondary amyloidosis
    - Senile systemic amyloidosis (SSA)
    - Familial amyloidosis (hereditary amyloidosis)
    - Hemodialysis-associated amyloidosis
  - Immunoglobulin amyloid (AL)
    - Deposition of insoluble monoclonal immunoglobulin (Ig), light (L) chains, or L-chain fragments involving muscle, connective tissue, blood vessel wall, and peripheral nerves
    - Includes primary amyloidosis, multiple myeloma, and other plasma cell dyscrasias
    - 85% of newly diagnosed cases of amyloidosis
    - Cardiac amyloidosis is most often of AL type
  - Secondary amyloidosis
    - Reactive amyloid fibrils accumulate in response to systemic inflammation (rheumatoid arthritis, chronic infection, inflammatory bowel disease, etc.)
    - Can also affect multiple organ systems; however, renal involvement is pronounced
  - Senile systemic amyloidosis
    - Amyloid fibrils are derived from transthyretin; prevalence of 25% in patients > 80 years of age
    - Mainly involves atria, less frequently aorta or entire heart
  - Familial amyloidosis (hereditary amyloidosis)
    - Related to an autosomal dominant mutation, most commonly the transthyretin gene
  - Hemodialysis-associated amyloidosis
    - B2 microglobulin amyloid fibril subunit accumulates in bones, joints
- Genetics: Various mutations in the genes encoding the amyloid protein have been discovered
- Etiology

- Precipitation of amyloid protein can be elicited by a variety of genetic and physiologic factors
- Cardiovascular amyloidosis is most commonly associated with AL type

- Epidemiology
  - Variable depending on cause
    - Generally onset occurs between 50-80 years of age
- Associated abnormalities
  - Amyloidosis includes disorders caused by accumulation of abnormal protein within extracellular interstitium of various organs and tissues of the body
  - Accumulated amyloid can lead to the progressive malfunction of the affected organ

Gross Pathologic & Surgical Features

- Definitive diagnosis depends on results on histologic results from a biopsy
- Endomyocardial biopsy is the gold standard for diagnosis
- In cases where clinical, imaging, and ECG findings suggest cardiac amyloidosis amyloid protein may be obtained from extracardiac sites
  - Tongue, subcutaneous fat pad, bone marrow

Microscopic Features

- Histologic evaluation may include H&E staining, methyl violet, crystal violet, and thioflavin
  - All of which reveal characteristic infiltration pattern of amyloid surrounding blood vessels and myocardial fibers
- Congo red dye is a more specific stain for amyloid, with apple green birefringence noted under polarized light
- Specific protein types can be identified using immunoelectron microscopy, and staining for AK, ATTR, serum amyloid A, apolipoprotein A-1

CLINICAL ISSUES

Presentation

- Most common signs/symptoms
  - Many patients will have no symptoms, or minor symptoms
  - Advanced cases may present with signs of symptoms of right heart failure, including increased jugular venous pressure, hepatomegaly, peripheral edema
  - Left heart failure in absence of ischemic disease
  - Atrial fibrillation, and other conduction abnormalities
  - Diffuse low voltage QRS complexes
- Other signs/symptoms: Most common cardiovascular complications are congestive heart failure, typically due to restrictive cardiomyopathy and conduction system disturbances

Demographics

- Age
  - Usually occurs in patients 50–80 years old
  - Senile cardiac amyloidosis after age 60-70
- Gender: Usually males, except for isolated atrial amyloidosis, which is more common in females

Natural History & Prognosis

- Pathophysiology is typically a restrictive cardiomyopathy resulting from infiltration of myocardium by amyloid deposits
- This alters cellular metabolism, calcium transport, receptor regulation, cellular edema
- Amyloid-infiltrated myocardium is noncompliant, altering diastolic function, and occasionally systolic function
- Cardiac conduction abnormalities are also attributable to the amyloid infiltration
- Amyloid pulmonary vasculature resulting in pulmonary hypertension and cor pulmonale has been described
- Prognosis depends on underlying disease process; AL amyloidosis has poor prognosis (5% survive > 10 years)
  - Marked LV hypertrophy, CHF, and RV dilatation are poor prognostic features

Treatment

- Depends on underlying disease process
- ACE inhibitors, long acting nitrate, and other diuretics used carefully have shown varied efficacy
- Some medications (e.g., digoxin) should be used with great caution due to extracellular binding by amyloid fibrils
- Atrial fibrillation has been successfully treated with ibutilide and amiodarone; anticoagulation is required
- Pacemaker may be required to treat symptomatic bradycardia or other severe conduction abnormality
- Some benefit from chemotherapy or prednisone
- Some may benefit from a heart transplant (variable survival ~ 32-118 months)
  - Allograft amyloid deposits as early as 5 months post-transplant may be seen with AL amyloidosis

SELECTED REFERENCES

1. Van Geluwe F et al: Amyloidosis of the heart and respiratory system. Eur Radiol. 16(10):2358-65, 2006
2. vanden Driesen RI et al: MR findings in cardiac amyloidosis. AJR Am J Roentgenol. 186(6):1682-5, 2006
3. Hassan W et al: Amyloid heart disease. New frontiers and insights in pathophysiology, diagnosis, and management. Tex Heart Inst J. 32(2):178-84, 2005
4. Maceira AM et al: Cardiovascular magnetic resonance in cardiac amyloidosis. Circulation. 111(2):186-93, 2005
5. Ikeda S: Cardiac amyloidosis: heterogenous pathogenic backgrounds. Intern Med. 43(12):1107-14, 2004
6. Lekakis J et al: Myocardial adrenergic denervation in patients with primary (AL) amyloidosis. Amyloid. 10(2):117-20, 2003
7. Gertz MA et al: Primary systemic amyloidosis. Curr Treat Options Oncol. 3(3):261-71, 2002
8. Dubrey SW et al: Long term results of heart transplantation in patients with amyloid heart disease. Heart. 85(2):202-7, 2001
9. McCarthy RE 3rd et al: A review of the amyloidoses that infiltrate the heart. Clin Cardiol. 21(8):547-52, 1998
10. Skinner M et al: Treatment of 100 patients with primary amyloidosis: a randomized trial of melphalan, prednisone, and colchicine versus colchicine only. Am J Med. 100(3):290-8, 1996
11. Velusamy M et al: Primary cardiac amyloidosis. J Ark Med Soc. 91(8):398-9, 1995

IMAGE GALLERY

Typical

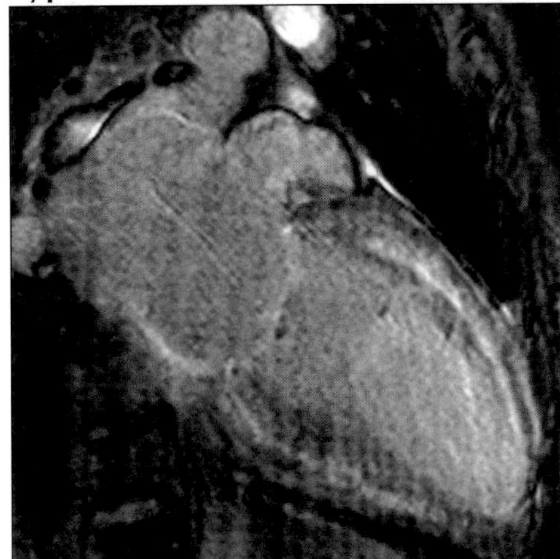

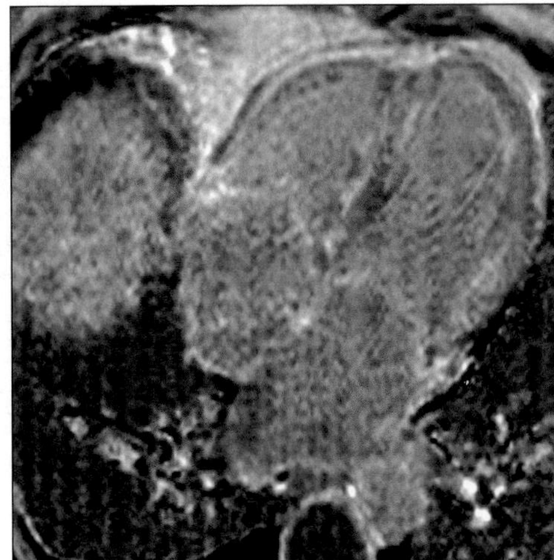

(Left) *Long axis vertical T1WI MR shows extensive subendocardial delayed enhancement in a 71 yo man with amyloidosis. (Courtesy S. Flamm, MD).* ***(Right)*** *Four chamber view T1WI MR shows diffuse subendocardial enhancement. (Courtesy S. Flamm, MD).*

Typical

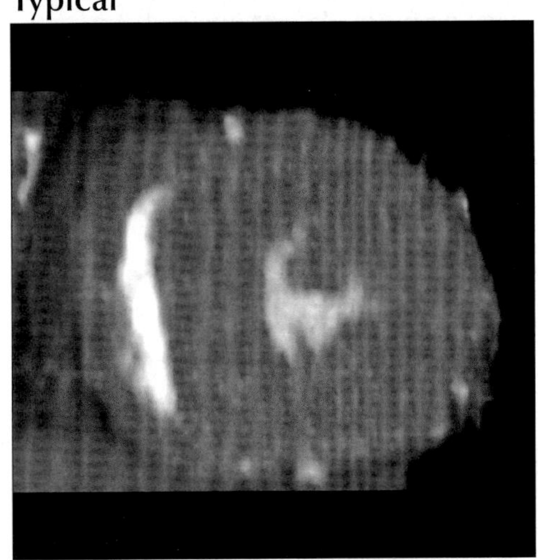

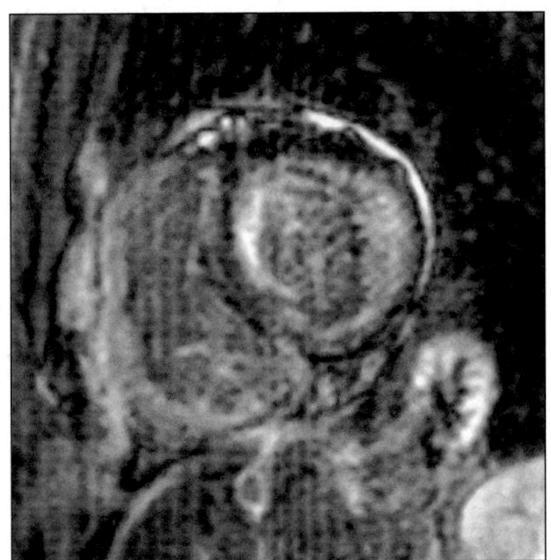

(Left) *Short axis CECT reveals concentric wall thickening of both ventricles in a 39 yo woman with amyloidosis.* ***(Right)*** *Short axis DE MR shows diffuse subendocardial enhancement in a 34 yo with amyloidosis. (Courtesy G. Reddy, MD).*

Typical

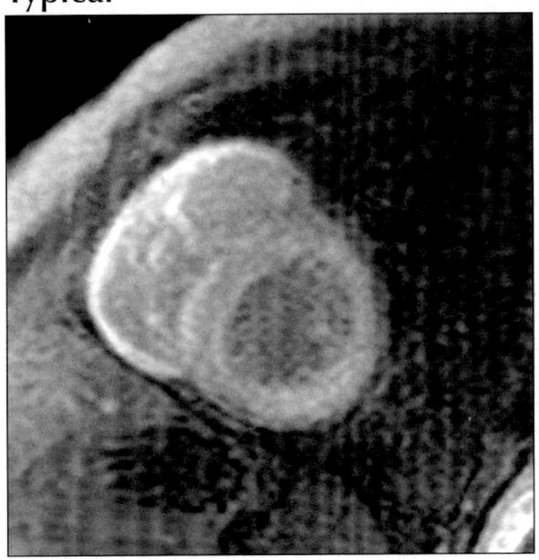

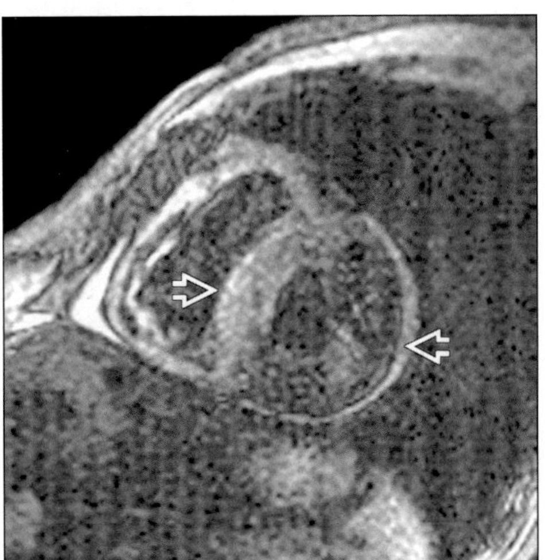

(Left) *Short axis T1WI MR shows concentric high signal in the walls of the ventricle in this 38 yo patient with longstanding amyloidosis. (Courtesy J. Kirsch, MD).* ***(Right)*** *Short axis T2WI MR corresponding to prior image shows concentric high signal in the walls of the ventricle ➪. (Courtesy J. Kirsch, MD).*

LV NON-COMPACTION

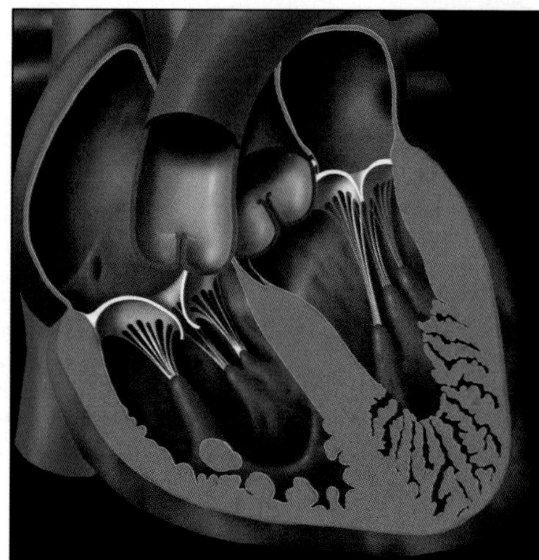

Coronal graphic shows extensive trabeculations within the left ventricle. There is predominant involvement of the LV apex with thinned underlying myocardium.

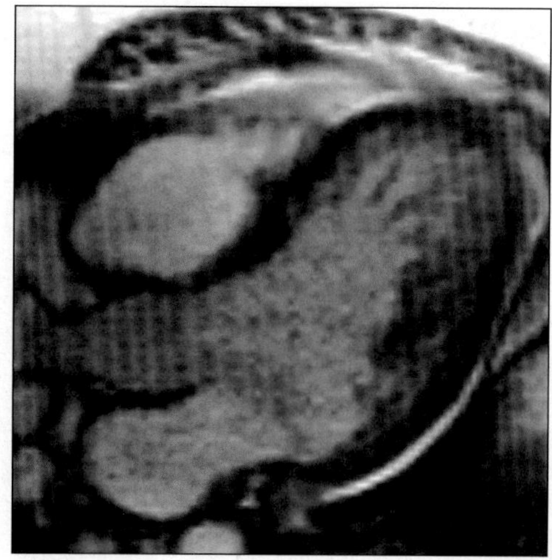

Three chamber view SSFP shows extensive trabeculations involving the lateral wall and apex of the left ventricle with a ratio of trabeculated to compact myocardium of more than 2.3 to 1.

TERMINOLOGY

Abbreviations and Synonyms

- LV non-compaction (LVNC)
- Spongy myocardium
- Left ventricular hypertrabeculation

Definitions

- An arrest in the normal process of myocardial compaction, resulting in persistence of multiple prominent ventricular trabeculations and deep intertrabecular recesses
    - LVNC is being increasingly recognized as a distinct cardiomyopathy with a specific underlying cause and prognosis

IMAGING FINDINGS

General Features

- Best diagnostic clue
    - > 2.3:1 ratio of non-compacted to compacted myocardium on MR
        - Measurements should be obtained at end-diastole
    - Subendocardial perfusion defects on contrast-enhanced MR can be seen
    - Delayed enhanced MR may demonstrate hyperenhancement corresponding to myocardial fibrosis
    - PET and thallium-201 scintigraphy may demonstrate transmural perfusion defects corresponding to areas of non-compacted myocardium
    - Plain film radiography has little role in the diagnosis of LVNC
        - Radiographic findings of congestive heart failure such as cardiomegaly and pulmonary edema can be seen in severely afflicted individuals
- Location
    - Predominantly involves mid to apical aspect of left ventricle
        - Sporadic right ventricular involvement up to 41% has been reported
- Morphology
    - 4 echocardiographic criteria have been proposed
        - Coexisting cardiac abnormalities are absent
        - A maximal end systolic ratio of non-compacted to compacted layers > 2:1 is diagnostic

DDx: Abnormal Thickening of the Left Ventricle

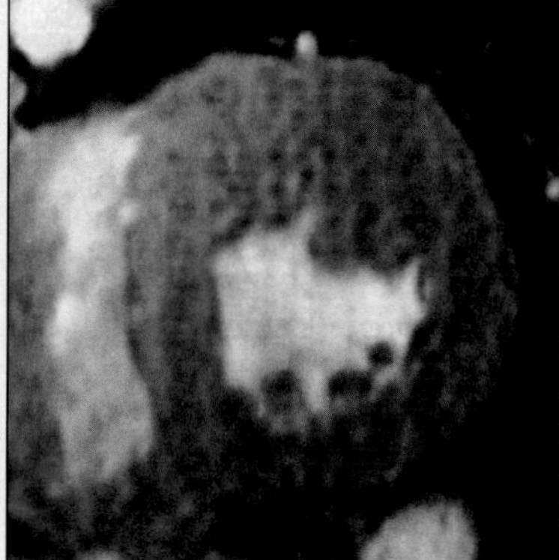

Hypertrophic Cardiomyopathy

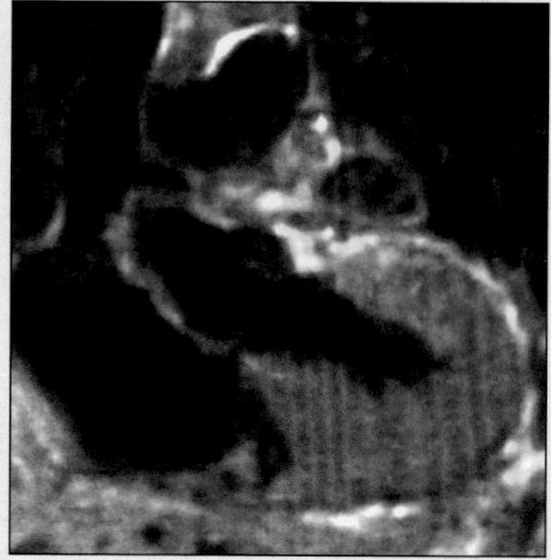

Hypertrophic Cardiomyopathy

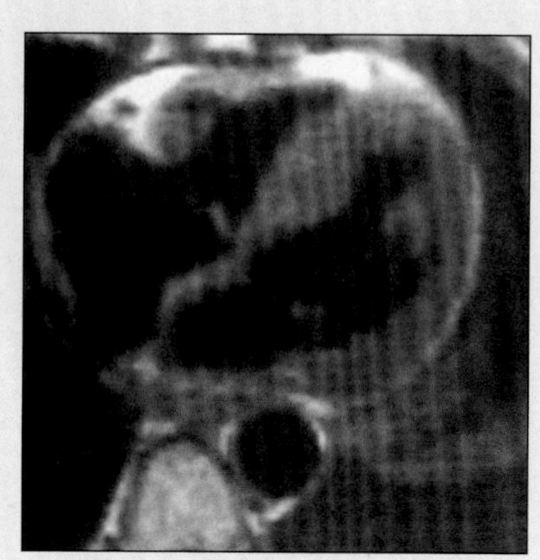

Hypertrophic Cardiomyopathy

LV NON-COMPACTION

Key Facts

Terminology
- Spongy myocardium
- An arrest in the normal process of myocardial compaction, resulting in persistence of multiple prominent ventricular trabeculations and deep intertrabecular recesses
- LVNC is being increasingly recognized as a distinct form of cardiomyopathy with a distinct underlying cause and prognosis

Imaging Findings
- > 2:1 Ratio of non-compacted to compacted myocardium by echo criteria
- Predominantly involves the mid to apical aspect of the left ventricle
- Echocardiography has been traditionally utilized
- Cardiac MR is playing an increasingly important role
  - > 2.3:1 ratio of non-compacted to compacted myocardium by MR criteria
  - May detect fibrosis on delayed enhanced imaging

Top Differential Diagnoses
- Hypertrophic Cardiomyopathy
- Left Ventricular Thrombus

Pathology
- An arrest in endomyocardial morphogenesis, which normally occurs between weeks 5 to 8 of fetal life

Clinical Issues
- Anticoagulation for the prevention of systemic embolism
- Beta-blockers for the treatment of ventricular arrhythmias and heart failure
- Cardioverter-defibrillator implantation

    - Predominant localization of the pathology was mid-lateral, apical and mid-inferior regions of the left ventricle
    - Color Doppler evidence of deep perfused intertrabecular recesses

Imaging Recommendations
- Best imaging tool
  - Echocardiography has been traditionally utilized
  - Cardiac MR is playing an increasingly important role, and will likely become the imaging modality of choice

DIFFERENTIAL DIAGNOSIS

Hypertrophic Cardiomyopathy
- Particularly the apical form

Left Ventricular Thrombus
- Usually adjacent to infarcted myocardium

PATHOLOGY

General Features
- Genetics
  - Both familial and sporadic forms of non-compaction have been described
  - Familial form
    - Familial recurrence was seen in 18% of the largest reported adult population with LVNC
    - Loose association with a mutation of the G4.5 gene
  - Sporadic form
    - Coexistent mitochondrial myopathies have yet to be fully validated
  - Equivocal association with Barth syndrome
    - Rare disorder linked to chromosome Xq28
    - Characterized by dilated cardiomyopathy, skeletal myopathy and neutropenia
- Etiology
  - An arrest in endomyocardial morphogenesis, which normally occurs between weeks 5 and 8 of fetal life
    - Normal compaction involves the transformation of large intertrabecular spaces into capillaries, as well as evolution of the coronary circulation
- Epidemiology
  - Median age at diagnosis is 7 years (1-22 years)
  - 0.014% prevalence for all patients referred for echocardiography
  - Slight male predominance according to largest reported series
- Associated abnormalities
  - Congenital cardiac anomalies
    - Obstruction of the right or left ventricular outflow tracts
    - Complex cyanotic congenital heart disease
    - Coronary artery anomalies
  - Biventricular non-compaction can occur with variable involvement of the right ventricle
    - Right ventricular involvement has been reported in up to 50% of patients in some series
  - Intraventricular thrombus formation due to slow blood movement within heavily trabeculated regions of the left ventricle
  - Ventricular and supra-ventricular arrhythmias
  - Subendocardial fibroelastosis

Gross Pathologic & Surgical Features
- Excessive trabeculation of the left ventricle which predominantly involves the apex and mid ventricle
  - May also involve the right ventricle to a lesser degree
- Areas of subendocardial ischemia have been demonstrated during postmortem evaluation of individuals with severe non-compaction

Microscopic Features
- Interstitial fibrosis of the endomyocardium commonly seen

LV NON-COMPACTION

CLINICAL ISSUES

Presentation

- Most common signs/symptoms
  - Clinical manifestations are highly variable depending on the severity of left ventricular involvement
    - Individuals with mild forms of LVNC may remain asymptomatic
  - Congestive heart failure
    - Both systolic and diastolic ventricular dysfunction have been described
    - Mean ejection fractions as low as 33% have been reported in some published series
    - Restrictive hemodynamics by cardiac catheterization may be present
  - Cardiac arrhythmias
    - Atrial fibrillation has been reported in up to 25% of individuals
    - Ventricular tachyarrhythmias have been reported in up to 50% of individuals
    - Sudden cardiac death has been reported in up to 50% of patients in larger case series
    - Paroxysmal supraventricular tachycardia and complete heart block have also been reported
    - Nonspecific resting ECG abnormalities have been frequently described, including inverted T waves, ST segment changes, axis shifts, intraventricular conduction abnormalities, and AV block
  - Thromboembolic events
    - Cerebrovascular accidents, transient ischemic attacks, pulmonary embolism and mesenteric infarction have all been described in patients with LVNC
    - Embolic events are thought to be related to the development of thrombi within prominent ventricular trabeculations due to sluggish blood flow
    - Atrial fibrillation and impaired systolic function have likewise been implicated in the development of system emboli
- Other signs/symptoms
  - Facial dysmorphisms amongst children have been rarely described
    - Prominent forehead
    - Low-set ears
    - Strabismus
    - High-arching palate
    - Micrognathia

Demographics

- Age: Congenital anomaly that is present at birth
- Gender: Slight male predilection

Natural History & Prognosis

- 60% of patients had either died or have undergone cardiac transplantation within 6 years of diagnosis in one large series

Treatment

- Anticoagulation for prevention of systemic embolism
- Beta-blockers for treatment of ventricular arrhythmias and heart failure
- Metabolic cocktail for individuals with underlying mitochondrial myopathies
  - Coenzyme Q10
  - Thiamine
  - Riboflavin
  - Carnitine
- Cardioverter-defibrillator implantation
- Orthotopic heart transplant

SELECTED REFERENCES

1. Dodd JD et al: Quantification of left ventricular noncompaction and trabecular delayed hyperenhancement with cardiac MRI: correlation with clinical severity. AJR Am J Roentgenol. 189(4):974-80, 2007
2. Jassal DS et al: Delayed enhancement cardiac MR imaging in noncompaction of left ventricular myocardium. J Cardiovasc Magn Reson. 8(3):489-91, 2006
3. Weiford BC et al: Noncompaction of the ventricular myocardium. Circulation. 109(24):2965-71, 2004
4. Pignatelli RH et al: Clinical characterization of left ventricular noncompaction in children: a relatively common form of cardiomyopathy. Circulation. 108(21):2672-8, 2003
5. McCrohon JA et al: Images in cardiovascular medicine. Isolated noncompaction of the myocardium: a rarity or missed diagnosis? Circulation. 106(6):e22-3, 2002
6. Rigopoulos A et al: Isolated left ventricular noncompaction: an unclassified cardiomyopathy with severe prognosis in adults. Cardiology. 98(1-2):25-32, 2002
7. Zambrano E et al: Isolated noncompaction of the ventricular myocardium: clinical and molecular aspects of a rare cardiomyopathy. Lab Invest. 82(2):117-22, 2002
8. Jenni R et al: Echocardiographic and pathoanatomical characteristics of isolated left ventricular non-compaction: a step towards classification as a distinct cardiomyopathy. Heart. 86(6):666-71, 2001
9. Oechslin EN et al: Long-term follow-up of 34 adults with isolated left ventricular noncompaction: a distinct cardiomyopathy with poor prognosis. J Am Coll Cardiol. 36(2):493-500, 2000
10. Ritter M et al: Isolated noncompaction of the myocardium in adults. Mayo Clin Proc. 72(1):26-31, 1997

IMAGE GALLERY

Typical

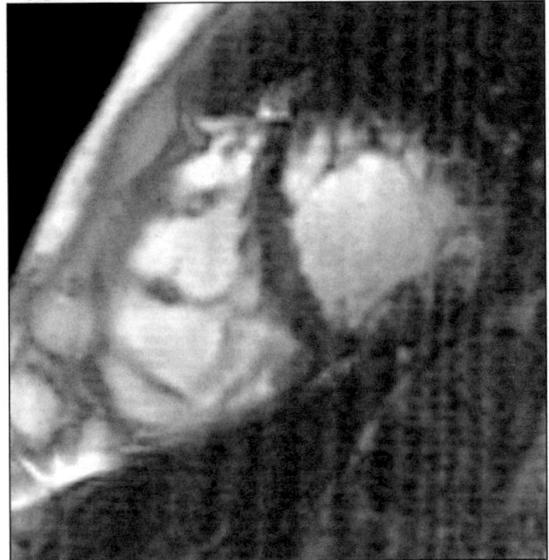

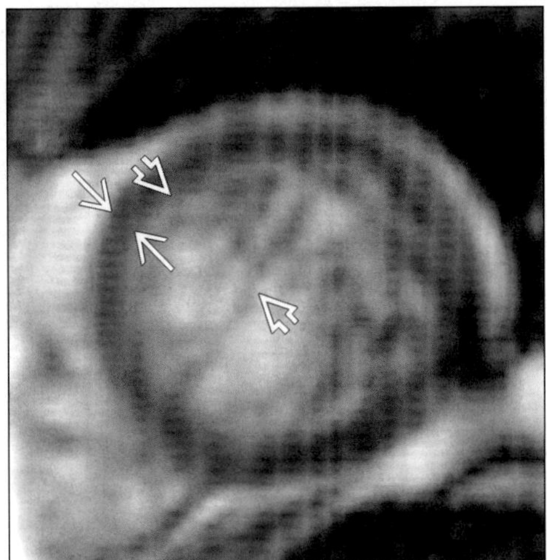

(Left) *LV short axis SSFP through the mid ventricle shows extensive trabeculations involving the anterior, lateral, and inferior walls. Extensive trabeculations of the right ventricle are also noted.* ***(Right)*** *LV short axis SSFP through the apical portion of the left ventricle in the same patient, shows extensive apical trabeculations. The ratio of trabeculated myocardium ➡ to compact myocardium ➡ by far exceeds the threshold of 2.3:1.*

Typical

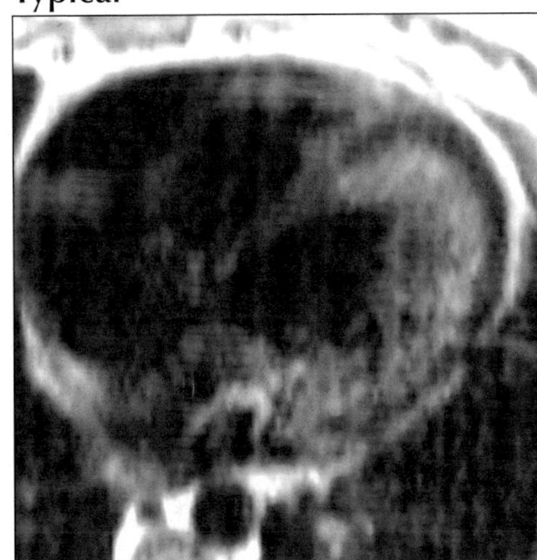

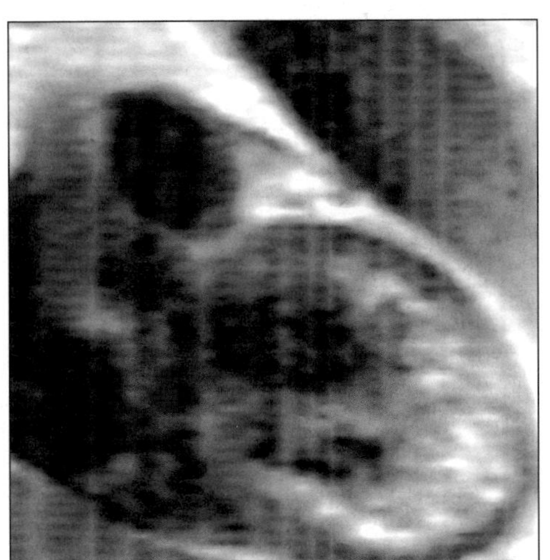

(Left) *Four chamber view FSE MR shows increased signal within the LV apex and lateral free wall, indicative of slow blood flow through regions with extensive left ventricular trabeculations.* ***(Right)*** *Long axis vertical FSE MR shows increased signal within the apex of the left ventricle, consistent with sluggish blood flow from extensive trabeculations.*

Variant

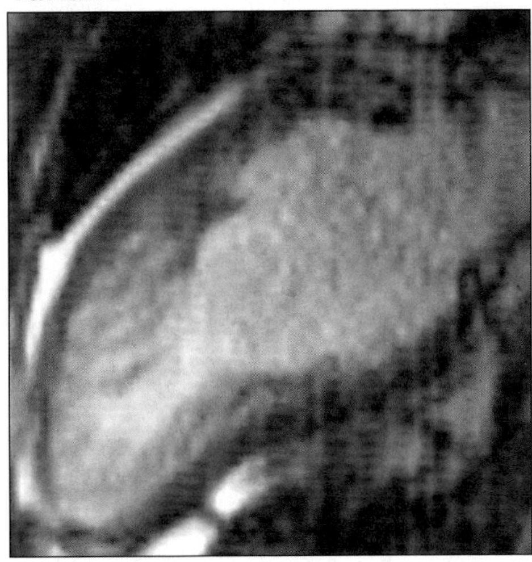

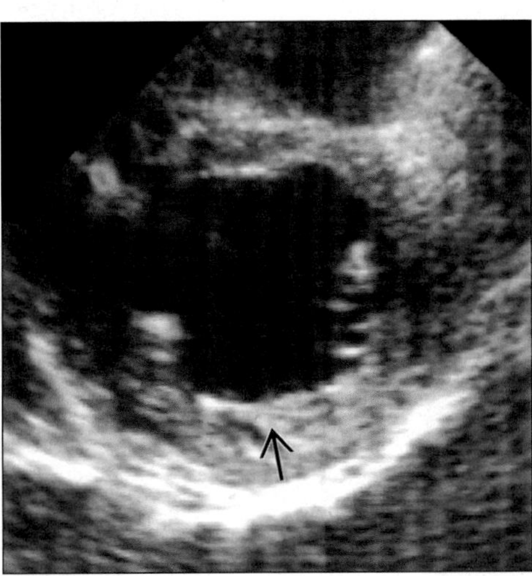

(Left) *Long axis vertical SSFP shows extensive circumferential trabeculations predominantly involving the apical portion of the anterior wall.* ***(Right)*** *LV short axis echocardiogram shows extensive trabeculations ➡ within the left ventricle that predominantly involve the inferior wall.*

CHAGAS DISEASE

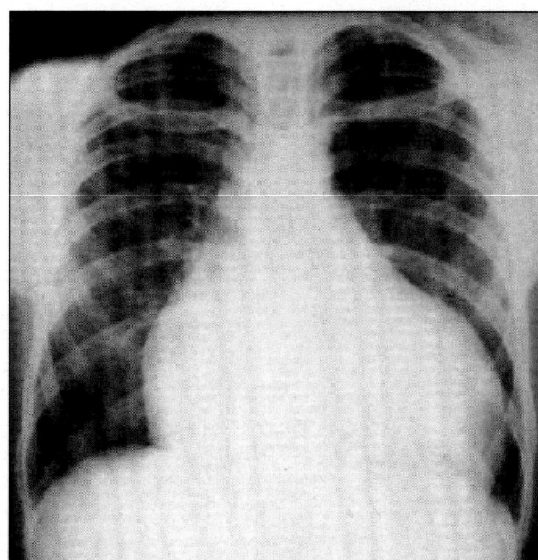

Posteroanterior radiograph shows global cardiomegaly and clear lung fields in a patient with chronic chagasic cardiomyopathy. No evidence of pulmonary congestion or pleural effusion.

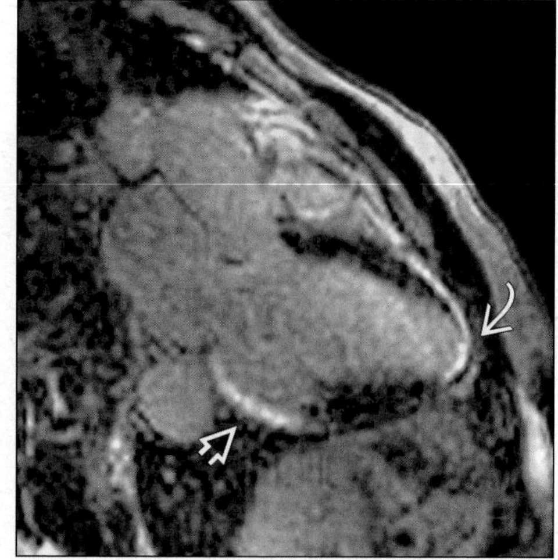

LVOT DE MR shows typically-located myocardial fibrosis on LV apex ➘ and inferolateral wall ➪ in a patient with several episodes of nonsustained VT on 24-hour Holter monitoring.

TERMINOLOGY

Abbreviations and Synonyms

- American trypanosomiasis; chagasic cardiomyopathy; Chagas heart disease

Definitions

- Chagas disease caused by a parasitic infection with Trypanosoma cruzi, transmitted through feces of infected bloodsucking insects in endemic areas of most Latin American countries

IMAGING FINDINGS

General Features

- Best diagnostic clue
  - Myocardial fibrosis on DE MR typically affecting apex and inferolateral regions of left ventricle in a heart failure patient from endemic region
  - Left ventricular wall becomes thinner, allowing the formation of an apical aneurysm, a feature of Chagas heart disease (the vortex lesion)
- Location: Apex, inferior and inferolateral segments of left ventricle
- Morphology
  - Asymptomatic stage (indeterminate phase): Normal-size ventricles and atria, normal heart function
  - Clinical stages: Varying degrees of global heart enlargement and systolic dysfunction

Imaging Recommendations

- Best imaging tool
  - DE MR may demonstrate predominantly midwall and subepicardial hyperenhancement areas encompassing multiple coronary territories (non-ischemic pattern)
  - Echocardiography, cine-MR & gated-CTA (advanced clinical phase) show global biventricular dysfunction with segmental akinesis and aneurysms, usually involving LV apex and infero-lateral walls
- Protocol advice
  - DE MR should be included in any cardiac MR protocol for cardiomyopathy evaluation
  - Delayed enhancement imaging patterns may aid in specific diagnosis for cardiomyopathies

DDx: Myocardial Disease

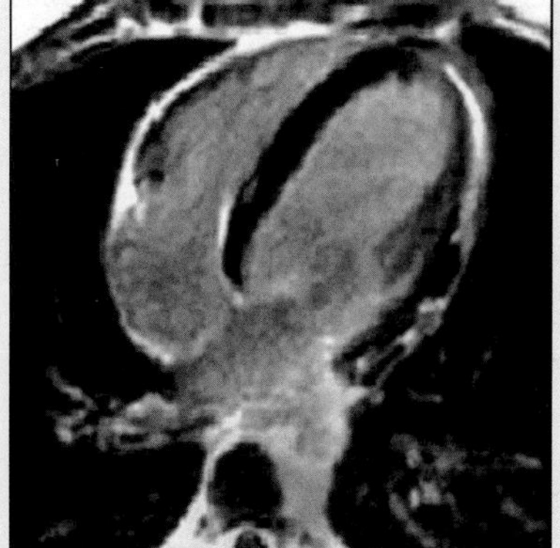

Acute Viral Myocarditis

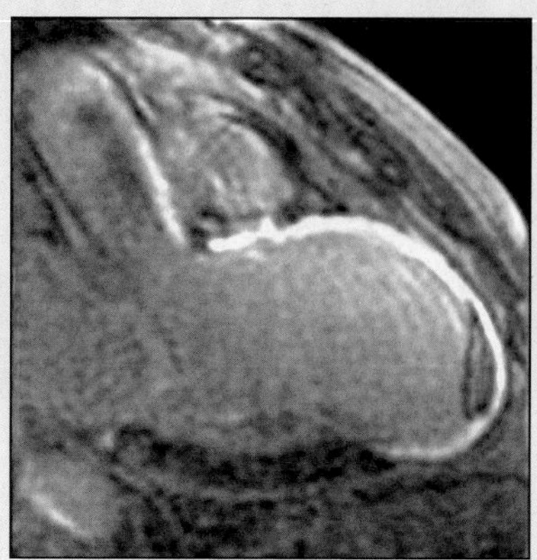

Ischemic LV Aneurysm/Thrombus

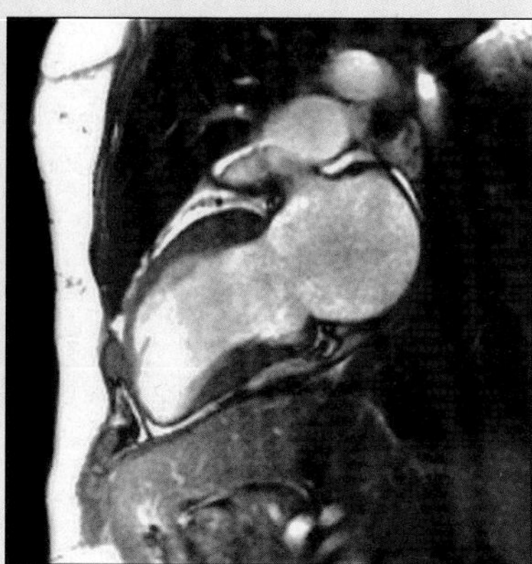

Takotsubo Cardiomyopathy

CHAGAS DISEASE

Key Facts

Terminology
- Chagas disease caused by a parasite T cruzi, transmitted through feces of infected bloodsucking insects in endemic areas

Imaging Findings
- Fibrosis on DE MR typically affects apex and inferolateral regions of LV myocardium
- Lesions are predominantly midwall and subepicardial encompassing multiple coronary territories (non-ischemic pattern), but a ischemic pattern may also be observed
- Thinner LV wall, allowing the formation of an apical aneurysm, a feature of Chagas heart disease (the vortex lesion)
- Increased LV volumes, segmental or global wall motion abnormalities and intracavitary thrombus

Top Differential Diagnoses
- Myocarditis
- Ischemic Cardiomyopathy
- Congenital Aneurysm
- Apical Hypertrophic Cardiomyopathy

Pathology
- In the USA, 100,000-675,000 immigrants from Latin America are infected with T cruzi
- Internationally, an estimated 18 million people are infected in 18 countries of Latin America

Clinical Issues
- Prognostic factors in Chagas disease
  - Impaired LV function, New York Heart Association Class III/IV, cardiomegaly and nonsustained ventricular tachycardia

---

- Chest radiography
  - Global heart enlargement
  - Congested lung fields
- Echocardiography
  - First line tool for morphologic and functional evaluation
  - Increased LV volumes
  - Segmental or global wall motion abnormalities
  - Apical aneurysm and intracavitary thrombus
- Cardiac MR
  - Location, extension, and severity of global and regional systolic dysfunction, most severe in apex and inferolateral wall
  - DE MR based myocardial fibrosis extension correlates with global and regional function measures and may detect subclinical Chagas heart disease (indeterminate form)
  - Prevalence of fibrosis on DE MR images: Indeterminate phase (20%), Chagas heart disease without ventricular tachycardia (85%) and with ventricular tachycardia (100%)
  - MR-defined fibrosis may present a non-ischemic pattern (midwall and subepicardial location in multiple coronary artery distributions)
  - But a ischemic pattern may also be noted (subendocardial and transmural involvement)
- Coronary CT angiography
  - May exclude significant coronary artery disease in selected Chagas patients with atypical chest pain
- Conventional angiography
  - Typical LV apical aneurysm (the vortex lesion)
  - Normal epicardial coronary arteries

DIFFERENTIAL DIAGNOSIS

Myocarditis
- Negative serologic tests for trypanosoma cruzi and geographic history absent
- Due to its indolent course, Chagas patients present at non-acute stages of disease for imaging evaluation, and T2WI are usually negative (chronic myocarditis)
- T2WI in viral myocarditis frequently show T2 signal abnormalities (edema); imaging evaluation occurs in acute stage of disease process
- Cine-MR and DE MR rarely demonstrate LV apical aneurysm in myocarditis

Ischemic Cardiomyopathy
- DE MR findings most frequently follow an ischemic pattern (subendocardial ⇒ transmural) located in a single coronary artery distribution
- Clinical history may reveal prior MI and multiple risk factors for coronary atherosclerosis
- Endocardial involvement is a hallmark for ischemic lesions

Congenital Aneurysm
- Imaging pattern may be indistinguishable of Chagas disease, in cases showing fibrotic apical and lateral aneurysms
- Negative serologic tests for trypanosoma cruzi and geographic history absent

Apical Hypertrophic Cardiomyopathy
- LV aneurysm wall in apical HCM represents very thin myocardium with or without delayed enhancement
- Normal Global LV function
- Asymmetric LV hypertrophy

Takotsubo Cardiomyopathy
- Type of non-ischemic cardiomyopathy in which there is a sudden temporary dysfunction of the myocardium
- Triggered by emotional stress

PATHOLOGY

General Features
- Etiology
  - Chagas disease is a protozoosis caused by the flagellate protozoa trypanosoma cruzi
  - Brazilian physician Carlos R.J. Chagas discovered American trypanosomiasis in 1909 in its parasite vector before describing all the epidemiological and clinical aspects of the infection

  - Insect vectors of Chagas disease belong to the Hemiptera order, Reduviidae family, and Triatominae subfamily (kissing bugs)
- Epidemiology
  - In the USA, according to estimates 100,000-675,000 immigrants from Latin America are infected with Trypanosoma cruzi
  - Internationally, an estimated 18 million people are infected in 18 countries of Latin America
  - 200,000 new cases each year
- Associated abnormalities
  - Megaesophagus and megacolon
  - Direct destruction due to intracellular parasitism leading to parasympathetic intramural denervation

Gross Pathologic & Surgical Features

- Cardiomegaly
- Ventricular wall thinning
- Thrombus
- LV aneurysm or multiple aneurysms

Microscopic Features

- Intracellular parasite multiplication ⇒ rupture of infected cells ⇒ inflammatory response ⇒ fibrosis
- Cellular lesions mainly affect the myocytes (myocytolysis) and the nervous cells (leading to an autonomic denervation)
- Arteriolar dilatation with organized thrombi and severe diffuse fibrosis in watershed myocardial regions (LV apex and inferior-basal LV wall)

CLINICAL ISSUES

Presentation

- Most common signs/symptoms
  - Chagas heart disease: Most frequent and serious manifestation
  - Typically leads to arrhythmias, cardiac failure, thromboembolic phenomena, and sudden death
    - Arrhythmia: Palpitations, dizziness, syncope, and Adams-Stokes syndrome
    - Atypical chest pain without evidence of coronary artery disease (15-20% of patients)
    - Heart failure: Dyspnea
    - Symptoms related to the clinical manifestations of thromboembolism, mainly in brain, lungs, and limbs

Demographics

- Age
  - Symptomatic acute phases mainly occur in newborns or young children
  - Chronic chagasic cardiomyopathy is generally detected in the third, fourth, or fifth decade of life
  - Patients develop cardiac and/or digestive dysfunction 10-30 years after the acute infection
- Gender: Chronic chagasic cardiomyopathy occurs earlier and is more severe in males than in females

Natural History & Prognosis

- Acute phase (1 week after initial infection), usually asymptomatic
  - Mortality in the acute phase, due to acute myocarditis and/or meningoencephalitis, fewer than 5% cases
- Chronic phase
  - Indeterminate form: No symptoms, normal EKG, normal radiological study of heart, esophagus, and colon
    - 50-70% of patients in the indeterminate phase never develop chronic lesions and remain asymptomatic
    - Prognosis for the chronic latent or indeterminate phase of infection is excellent
  - Clinical forms: Cardiac, digestive and mixed
    - In endemic areas, chagasic heart disease is the most common cause of cardiomyopathy and a leading cause of cardiovascular death among patients aged 30-50 years, 21,000 deaths annually
  - Independent prognostic factors in chronic Chagas disease
    - Impaired LV function
    - New York Heart Association Class III/IV
    - Cardiomegaly
    - Nonsustained ventricular tachycardia

Treatment

- Acute phase: Always requires treatment with benznidazole, cures 100% of children younger than 2 years and 60-70% of patients who are older and acutely infected
  - Corticosteroids are limited to severe illness with myocarditis or meningoencephalitis
- Chronic heart form
  - Diuretics, digitals and angiotensin-converting enzyme inhibitors ⇒ heart failure
  - Class III antiarrhythmic drugs (sotalol and amiodarone)
  - Anticoagulant treatment is justified in patients at risk for thromboembolic complications

SELECTED REFERENCES

1. Marcu CB et al: Chagas' heart disease diagnosed on MRI: the importance of patient "geographic" history. Int J Cardiol. 117(2):e58-60, 2007
2. Marin-Neto JA et al: Pathogenesis of chronic Chagas heart disease. Circulation. 115(9):1109-23, 2007
3. Rassi A Jr et al: Predictors of mortality in chronic Chagas disease: a systematic review of observational studies. Circulation. 115(9):1101-8, 2007
4. Mahrholdt H et al: Delayed enhancement cardiovascular magnetic resonance assessment of non-ischaemic cardiomyopathies. Eur Heart J. 26(15):1461-74, 2005
5. Rochitte CE et al: Myocardial delayed enhancement by magnetic resonance imaging in patients with Chagas' disease: a marker of disease severity. J Am Coll Cardiol. 46(8):1553-8, 2005
6. Sarabanda AV et al: Ventricular tachycardia in Chagas' disease: a comparison of clinical, angiographic, electrophysiologic and myocardial perfusion disturbances between patients presenting with either sustained or nonsustained forms. Int J Cardiol. 102(1):9-19, 2005

IMAGE GALLERY

Typical

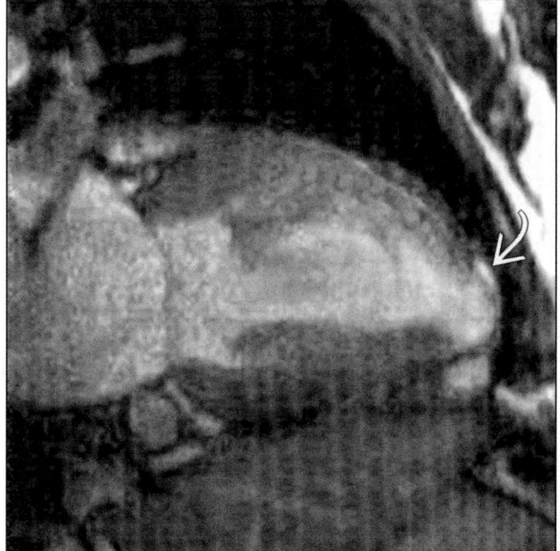

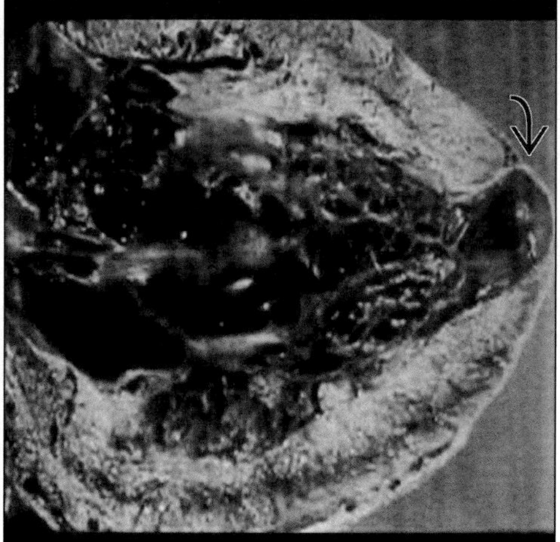

(Left) *Long axis MR cine shows typical LV apex aneurysm (vortex aneurysm). **(Right)** Long axis gross pathology shows typical vortex aneurysm .*

Typical

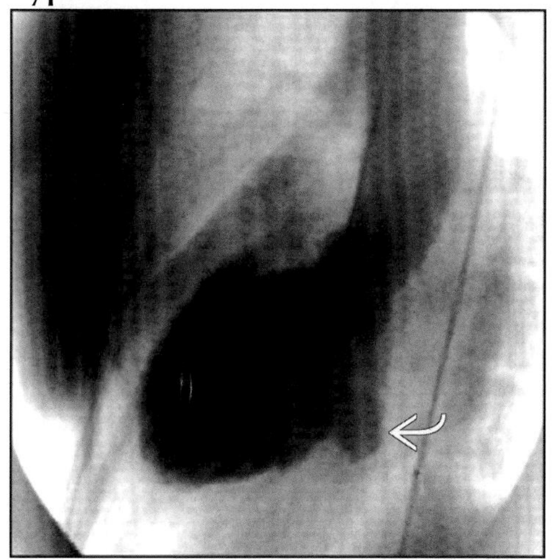

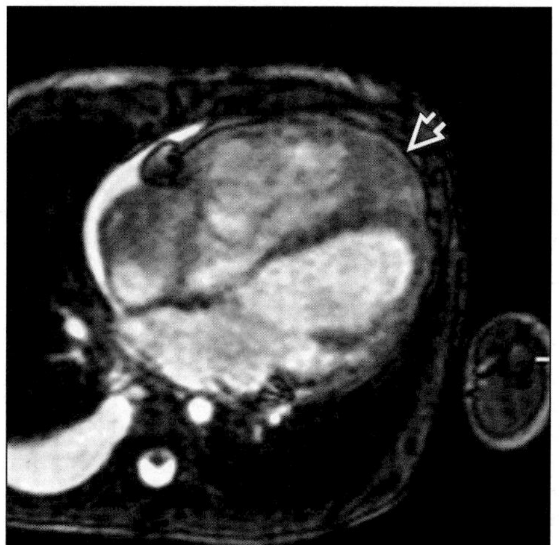

(Left) *Catheter angiography shows a diffusely dilated LV and a basal inferolateral aneurysm in a Chagas patient presenting with recurrent syncope. **(Right)** MR cine shows four-chamber enlargement, slow flow on RA and RV apex , pericardial and pleural effusion in a child with acute Chagas myocarditis.*

Typical

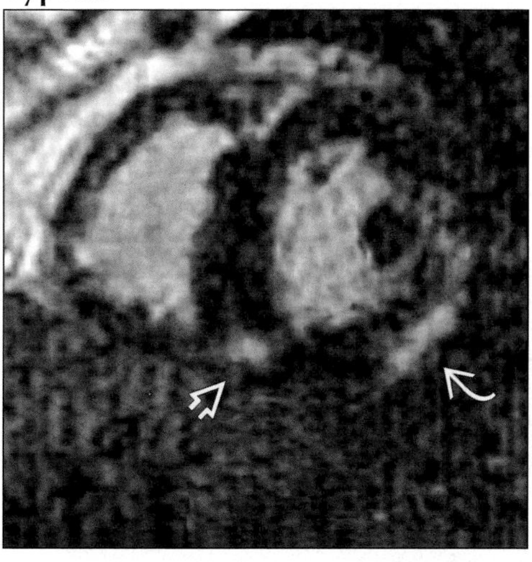

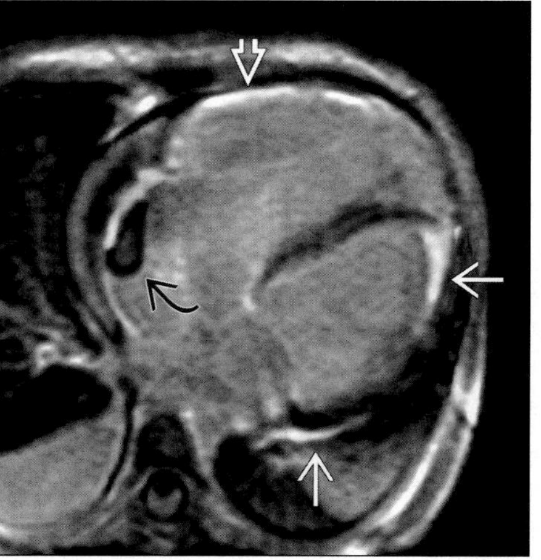

(Left) *Short axis DE MR shows midwall and subepicardial hyperenhanced areas , consistent with myocardial fibrosis, in a patient with the indeterminate form of Chagas heart disease. **(Right)** Four chamber view DE MR shows lesions on LV apex and inferolateral wall in a young child with acute Chagas myocarditis. Note: Extensive hyperenhancement in RV free wall , thrombus in the RA .*

HEMOCHROMATOSIS

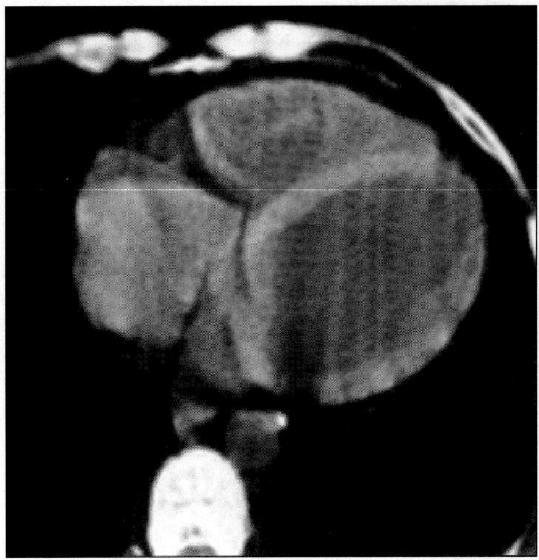

Axial NECT shows diffusely increased attenuation throughout the myocardium, indicative of excessive myocardial iron deposition.

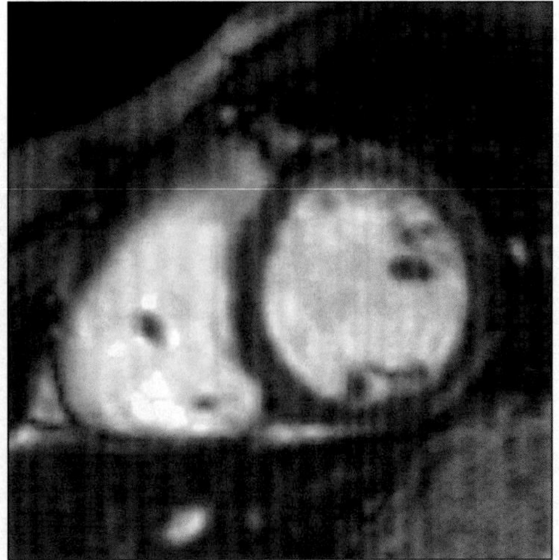

Short axis GRE shows diffusely decreased signal intensity throughout the left ventricular myocardium and liver, indicative of severe iron overload.

TERMINOLOGY

Abbreviations and Synonyms

- Hemosiderosis

Definitions

- Primary (hereditary or idiopathic) hemochromatosis
  - Autosomal recessive genetic disorder
  - Progressive increase in total body iron stores with abnormal multiorgan iron deposition
  - Liver is primary site of abnormal iron deposition, although abnormal iron deposition can likewise occur in the heart and pancreas

IMAGING FINDINGS

General Features

- Best diagnostic clue
  - Excess iron levels can be displayed qualitatively by MR by hypointense signal changes in affected organs on T2 or T2* weighted images
  - Echocardiography or MUGA scan can depict heart failure from iron overload in later stages of the disease, but provide no detail regarding the etiology of the disease
  - NECT: Global hyperdensity of myocardium
- Location: Diffuse involvement of the myocardium

Imaging Recommendations

- Best imaging tool
  - T2* MR imaging can be used to quantify myocardial iron levels
    - MR quantification is most clinically relevant in the setting of secondary hemochromatosis
    - T2* value of less than 20 is associated with heart failure

DIFFERENTIAL DIAGNOSIS

Transfusional Iron Overload

- Often termed hemosiderosis or secondary hemochromatosis
- Abnormal amounts of iron accumulate in the reticuloendothelial system of the liver, spleen and bone marrow, as well of the myocardium

DDx: Hemochromatosis

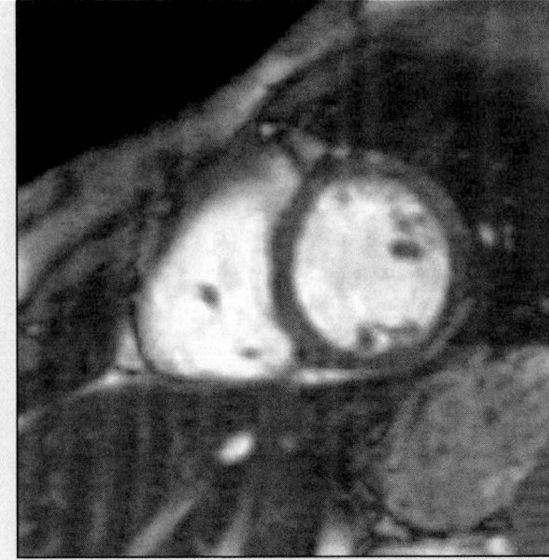

Transfusional Iron Overload

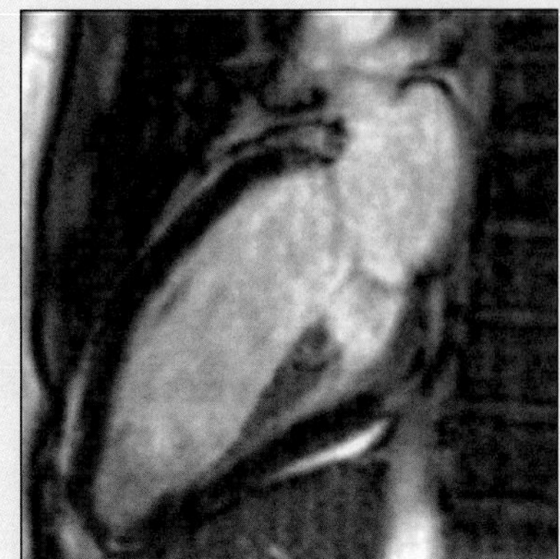

Thalassemia Major

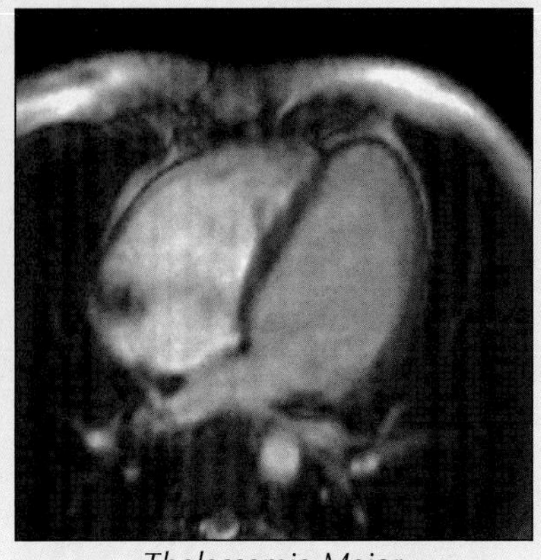

Thalassemia Major

HEMOCHROMATOSIS

Key Facts

Terminology

- Progressive increase in total body iron stores with abnormal multiorgan iron deposition
  - Primary (hereditary or idiopathic) hemochromatosis; autosomal recessive genetic disorder
  - Secondary hemochromatosis; sequela of multiple blood transfusions

Imaging Findings

- Signs of heart failure from iron overload in later stages of the disease
- Excess iron levels can be displayed qualitatively by MR by hypointense signal changes in affected organs on T2 or T2* weighted images
- T2* MR imaging can be used to quantify myocardial iron levels

- Cardiac imaging findings are indistinguishable from primary hemochromatosis

PATHOLOGY

General Features

- Genetics
  - Autosomal recessive disorder characterized by an abnormal HFE glycoprotein
    - Results in excessive cellular uptake by iron-based transferrin
- Etiology
  - Iron overload is most commonly due to multiple transfusions or abnormally elevated iron absorption
  - Excess unbound iron deposited in the myocardium is highly cardiotoxic
- Epidemiology
  - Primary form occurs predominantly in white populations of Northern European descent
  - M:F ratio is 1.8:1
- Associated abnormalities
  - Excessive liver deposition with development of cirrhosis, portal hypertension and hepatocellular carcinoma
  - Excessive pancreatic deposition can result in type 1 diabetes mellitus
  - Abnormal deposition in skin
  - Pituitary hypogonadism

CLINICAL ISSUES

Presentation

- Most common signs/symptoms: Congestive heart failure in the setting of significant cardiac involvement
- Other signs/symptoms
  - Polyarthralgia
  - Loss of libido, sexual impotence

Demographics

- Gender: M:F ratio is 1.8:1

Natural History & Prognosis

- Onset of heart failure from iron toxicity generally results in irreversible cardiac damage with a dismal prognosis

Treatment

- Iron chelation therapy

SELECTED REFERENCES

1. Anderson LJ et al: Cardiovascular T2-star (T2*) magnetic resonance for the early diagnosis of myocardial iron overload. Eur Heart J. 22(23):2171-9, 2001
2. Hershko C et al: Pathophysiology of iron overload. Ann N Y Acad Sci. 850:191-201, 1998
3. Pattynama PM et al: Evaluation of cardiac function with magnetic resonance imaging. Am Heart J. 128(3):595-607, 1994

IMAGE GALLERY

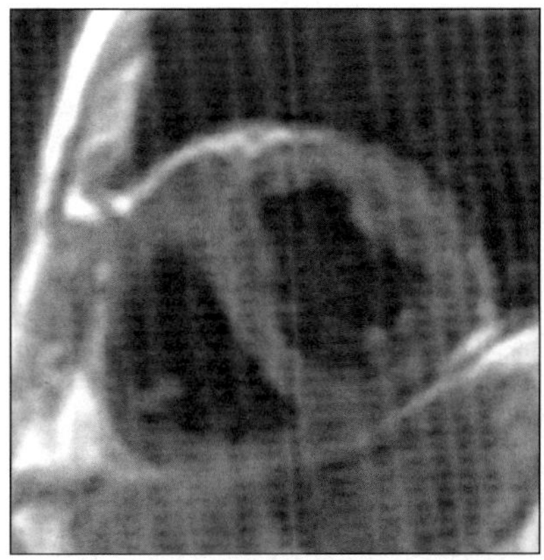
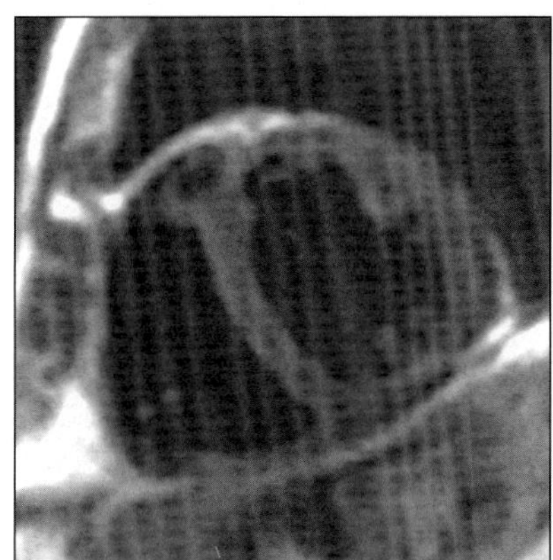
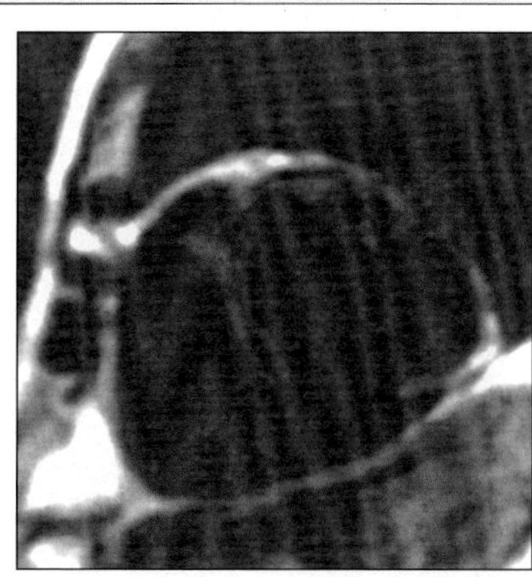

(Left) *Short axis GRE with a TE of 10 msec shows mildly hypointense myocardium and adjacent liver from iron deposition disease.* ***(Center)*** *Short axis GRE of the same patient with a TE of 30 msec shows moderately hypointense changes throughout the myocardium and liver.* ***(Right)*** *Short axis GRE of the same patient with a TE of 50 msec shows severe hypointense changes throughout the myocardium and liver. The progressively longer echo times results in greater T2* weighting.*

TAKOTSUBO CARDIOMYOPATHY

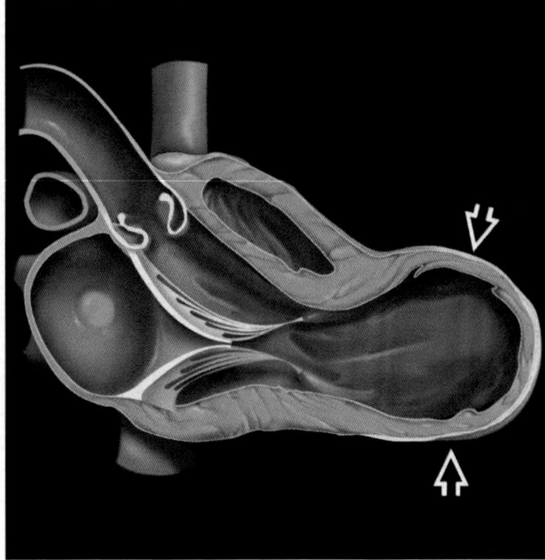

Three chamber view graphic shows wall thinning and dilatation (ballooning) of the left ventricular apex.

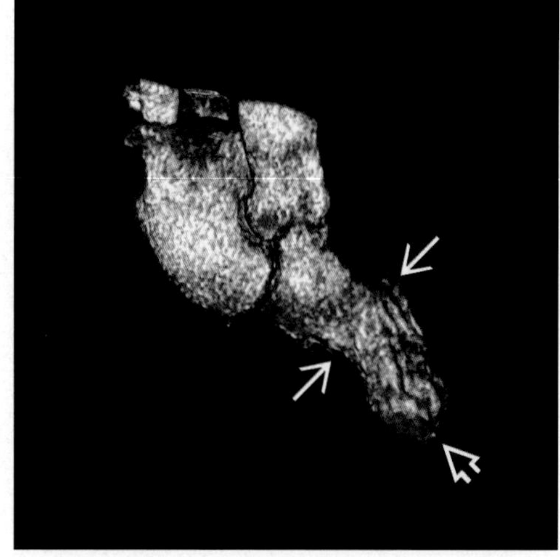

Cardiac CT 3D ventriculogram shows an akinetic LV apex with ballooning and preserved mid-ventricular contraction.

TERMINOLOGY

Abbreviations and Synonyms

- Transient left ventricular apical ballooning syndrome
- Stress-induced cardiomyopathy
- Ampulla cardiomyopathy
- Broken-heart syndrome

Definitions

- Sudden onset of transient akinesia or dyskinesia of apical (or less frequently mid portions) left ventricle without significant coronary artery stenosis
- Generally occurs following periods of severe emotional or physical stress
- Often accompanied by acute chest pain, reversible ST segment abnormalities, and elevation of cardiac biomarkers
- Degree of ECG changes and biomarker elevation do not correlate with the extent of akinesis

IMAGING FINDINGS

General Features

- Best diagnostic clue
  - Distinctive ballooning of mid to apical left ventricle (LV)
  - Normal or hyperkinetic left ventricular base
  - Left ventricle resembles Japanese octopus pot (tako: Octopus, tsubo: Pot) which has a narrow mouth and a large round base
- Location
  - Akinesis and ballooning are usually seen in the LV apex
  - Reports in literature of ballooning of mid-left ventricle in similar clinical setting
  - Distribution of dysfunctional myocardium does not correspond to perfusion territory of single epicardial coronary vessel

CT Findings

- Cardiac Gated CTA
  - Absence of significant (> 50%) stenosis in epicardial coronary arteries

DDx: Cardiomyopathy

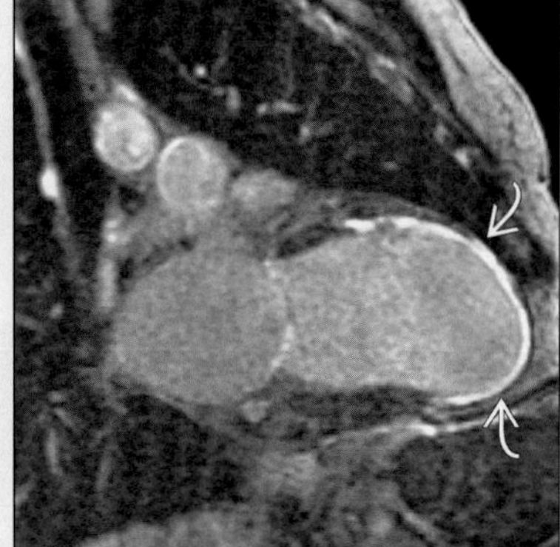

Antero-Apical LV Infarct

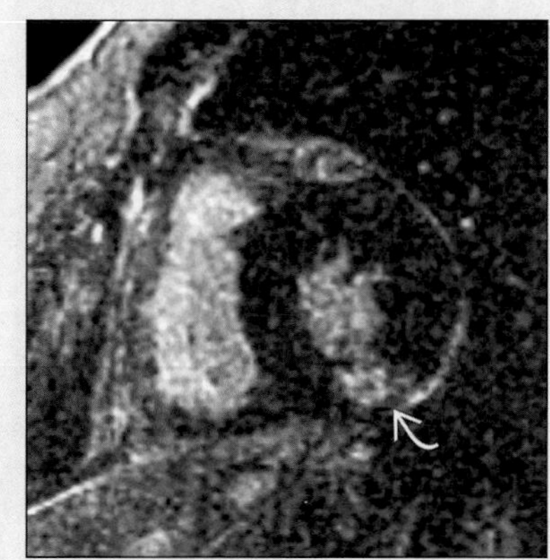

Acute Myocarditis

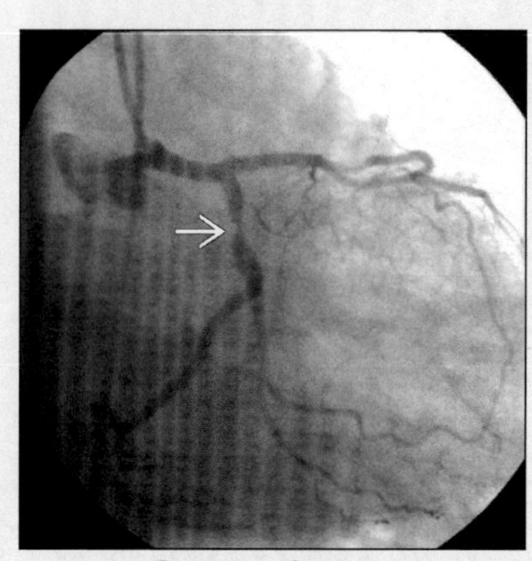

Coronary Stenosis

TAKOTSUBO CARDIOMYOPATHY

Key Facts

Terminology
- Sudden onset of transient akinesia or dyskinesia of the LV apex in absence of coronary artery stenosis

Imaging Findings
- Distinctive ballooning of the mid to apical left ventricle with normal or hyperkinetic basal LV
- Cardiac MR: Apical akinesis and ballooning without abnormal delayed hyperenhancement

Top Differential Diagnoses
- Acute Myocardial Infarction
- Acute Myocarditis
- Coronary Vasospasm

Pathology
- Most patients present after a period of severe emotional distress
- Primary abnormality is myocardial stunning rather than myocardial infarction

Clinical Issues
- Patients tend to be post-menopausal females
- Chest pain and dyspnea
  - Initial presentation closely resembles that of acute myocardial infarction or acute coronary syndrome
- Prompt and aggressive pharmacological and hemodynamic support can result in rapid reversal of the ventricular dysfunction

---

  - Functional assessment on multi-phase reconstructions shows classical ballooning of left ventricular apex during systole although basal segments of left ventricle contract normally

MR Findings
- T2WI FS: T2 hyperintensity in anterior-apical wall suggests myocardial edema
- MR Cine: Akinesis or dyskinesia of apical LV as well as dilation or ballooning is best seen in horizontal long axis and vertical long axis views
- Delayed Enhancement: Cases of apical ballooning syndrome are characterized by an absence of delayed hyperenhancement

Nuclear Medicine Findings
- Moderate to severe myocardial ischemia is seen in left ventricular apex during resting SPECT with technetium-99m
- Perfusion defect improves markedly after 3-5 days

Echocardiographic Findings
- Two-chamber and four-chamber views shows dilatation of left ventricular apex

Angiographic Findings
- Conventional
  - Syndrome resembles ischemic cardiomyopathy, however most patients have normal epicardial coronary arteries
  - Some individuals may have mild atherosclerotic disease without significant obstruction
  - Rarely multivessel epicardial spasm is evident, which may be spontaneous or induced by ergonovine or acetylcholine infusion
  - Left ventriculogram shows normal or hyperkinetic contraction of basal to mid-ventricle with dilatation of left ventricular apex

Imaging Recommendations
- Best imaging tool: Cardiac MR: Apical akinesis and ballooning with no evidence of delayed hyperenhancement
- Protocol advice
  - SSFP Cine images in horizontal long axis, vertical long axis and short axis views
  - De-MR is key to differentiate from acute myocardial infarct

DIFFERENTIAL DIAGNOSIS

Acute Myocardial Infarction
- Initial clinical presentation
  - Chest pain
  - Dyspnea
- Patients with acute myocardial infarction have evidence of significant atherosclerotic plaque in coronaries at catheterization
- Evidence of perfusion defects on
  - Nuclear perfusion studies
  - Cardiac MR
- Delayed enhancement MR shows subendocardial or transmural hyperenhancement in coronary territories

Acute Myocarditis
- Delayed enhancement MR shows subepicardial or mid-myocardial hyperenhancement
- Myocardial involvement is not confined to coronary artery territories

Coronary Vasospasm
- Prinzmetal angina
- Due to focal coronary artery vasospasm and may be associated with acute myocardial infarction (MI), serious ventricular arrhythmias, and sudden death
- Coronary vasoconstriction and dynamic coronary obstruction are also components of atherosclerotic coronary artery disease, which can present as stable and unstable angina pectoris

PATHOLOGY

General Features
- General path comments: Takotsubo cardiomyopathy was first described in Japan

TAKOTSUBO CARDIOMYOPATHY

- Etiology
  - Most patients present after period of severe emotional distress
    - May include unexpected death of a loved one, domestic abuse, catastrophic medical diagnosis or natural disasters
  - Physical stressors such as work, asthma attack, gastric endoscopy have also been reported to be associated with the initial presentation
  - It has been suggested that cause may be diffuse coronary microvascular dysfunction
    - Supported by presence of myocardial ischemia in absence of significant epicardial coronary artery disease
  - Other theories include
    - Catecholamine-mediated epicardial coronary spasm
    - Microvascular coronary spasm
    - Direct catecholamine-mediated myocyte injury

Gross Pathologic & Surgical Features

- Primary abnormality is myocardial stunning rather than myocardial infarction

Microscopic Features

- Endomyocardial biopsy shows no evidence of myocarditis

CLINICAL ISSUES

Presentation

- Most common signs/symptoms
  - Chest pain and dyspnea
  - Pain is preceded in some cases by emotional or physical stress, leading to the term stress-induced cardiomyopathy
  - ECG changes: ST-segment elevation and deep inverted T-waves in precordial leads with QT interval prolongation
    - Q-waves are present in 40% of patients
  - Slight elevation of cardiac biomarkers such as troponin I or T and CK-MB
    - However, degree of elevation of biomarkers does not correlate with extent of ventricular dysfunction
  - Initial presentation closely resembles that of acute myocardial infarction or acute coronary syndrome
- Other signs/symptoms: Patients may have more serious presentations such as cardiogenic shock or ventricular fibrillation

Demographics

- Age
  - Frequent in subjects older than 50 years
  - Patients tend to be post-menopausal females
- Gender: M:F = 1:6

Natural History & Prognosis

- Prognosis is generally favorable
- Most patients recover to normal left ventricular function and do not have recurrence
- Most common complication is heart failure with or without pulmonary edema
- May be risk of thrombus formation in the akinetic apex

Treatment

- Prompt and aggressive pharmacological and hemodynamic support can result in rapid reversal of ventricular dysfunction
- Some patients require intra-aortic balloon counterpulsation
  - Short-term anticoagulation may be required in case of apical thrombus formation

SELECTED REFERENCES

1. Arora S: Autonomic imbalance in patients with takotsubo cardiomyopathy: cause or association? QJM. 100(9):593-4; author reply 594-6, 2007
2. Celik T et al: Stress-induced (Takotsubo) cardiomyopathy: A transient disorder. Int J Cardiol. 2007
3. Cocco G et al: Stress-induced cardiomyopathy: A review. Eur J Intern Med. 18(5):369-79, 2007
4. Dorfman TA et al: An Unusual Manifestation of Takotsubo Cardiomyopathy. Clin Cardiol. 2007
5. Haghi D et al: Guidelines for diagnosis of takotsubo (ampulla) cardiomyopathy. Circ J. 71(10):1664; author reply 1665, 2007
6. Kawai S: Typical and atypical forms of takotsubo (ampulla) cardiomyopathy. Circ J. 71(10):1665, 2007
7. Kimura K et al: Images in cardiovascular medicine. Rapid formation of left ventricular giant thrombus with Takotsubo cardiomyopathy. Circulation. 115(23):e620-1, 2007
8. Matsuzaki M: Stress 'Takotsubo' cardiomyopathy: questions still remain. Nat Clin Pract Cardiovasc Med. 4(11):577, 2007
9. Nanda S et al: Takotsubo cardiomyopathy--a new variant and widening disease spectrum. Int J Cardiol. 120(2):e34-6, 2007
10. Pilgrim TM et al: Takotsubo cardiomyopathy or transient left ventricular apical ballooning syndrome: A systematic review. Int J Cardiol. 2007
11. Gianni M et al: Apical ballooning syndrome or takotsubo cardiomyopathy: a systematic review. Eur Heart J. 27(13):1523-9, 2006
12. Iqbal MB et al: Stress, emotion and the heart: tako-tsubo cardiomyopathy. Postgrad Med J. 82(974):e29, 2006
13. Bybee KA et al: Systematic review: transient left ventricular apical ballooning: a syndrome that mimics ST-segment elevation myocardial infarction. Ann Intern Med. 141(11):858-65, 2004

TAKOTSUBO CARDIOMYOPATHY

IMAGE GALLERY

Typical

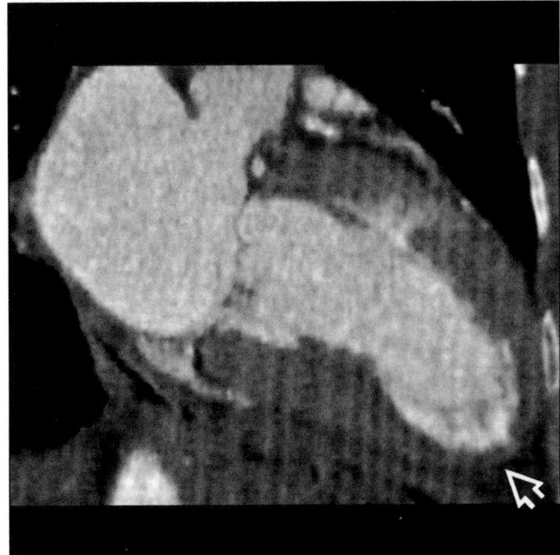

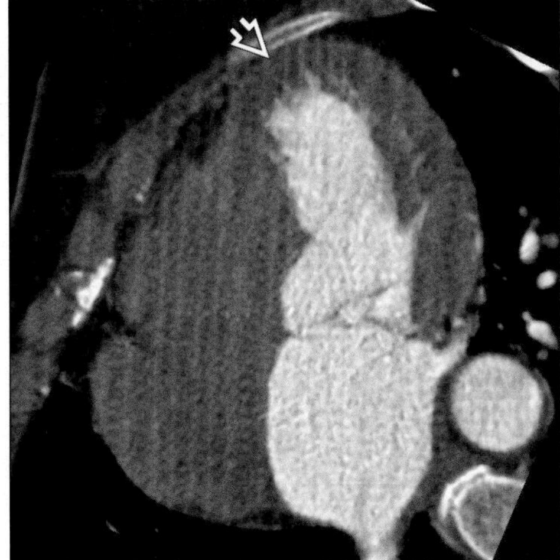

(Left) Long axis vertical cardiac CT shows myocardial thinning and dilatation ➡ of the left ventricular apex in a patient with Takotsubo cardiomyopathy. ***(Right)*** Long axis horizontal cardiac CT shows mild systolic LV apical thinning ➡ in a patient with transient apical ballooning syndrome. Functional cine images (not shown) revealed akinesis of this segment.

Variant

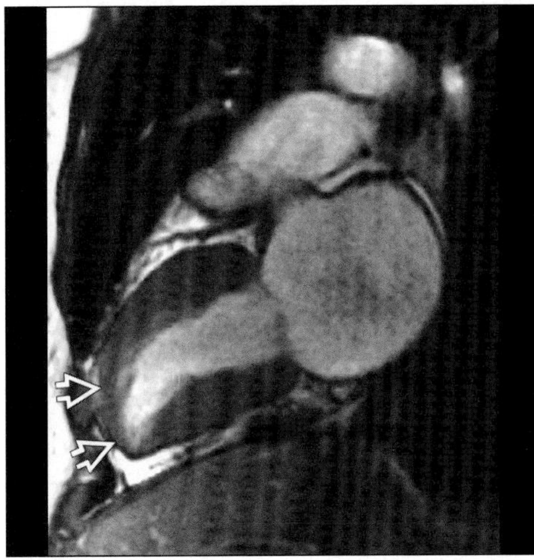

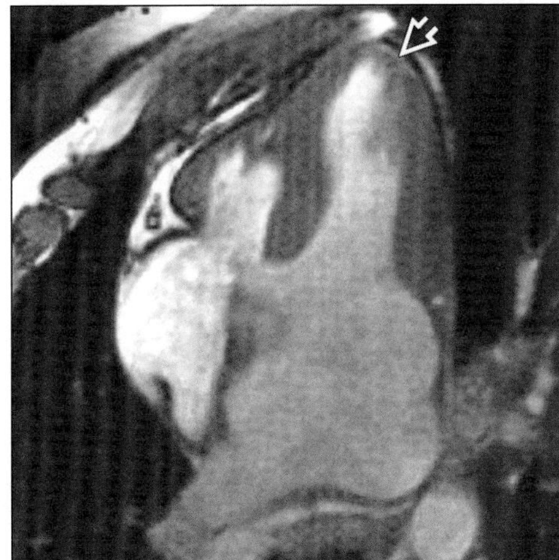

(Left) Long axis vertical SSFP shows subtle LV apical myocardial thinning ➡ and akinesia (on cines) of a patient with apical ballooning syndrome. ***(Right)*** Four chamber view SSFP in same patient as previous image shows LV apical akinesis and mild relative systolic myocardial thinning ➡. Coronary angiography was normal and LV function recovered, indicating Takotsubo cardiomyopathy.

Typical

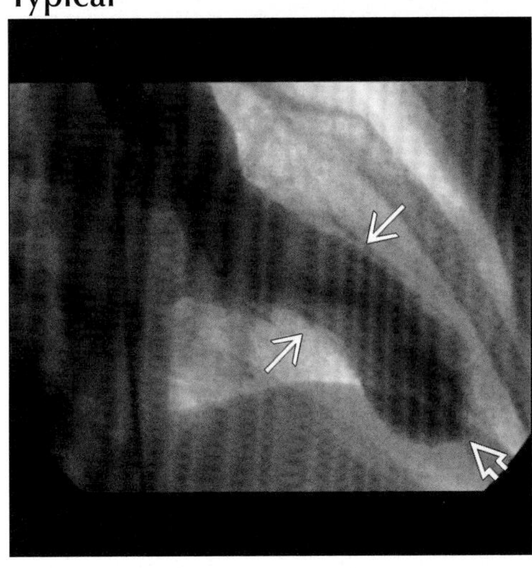

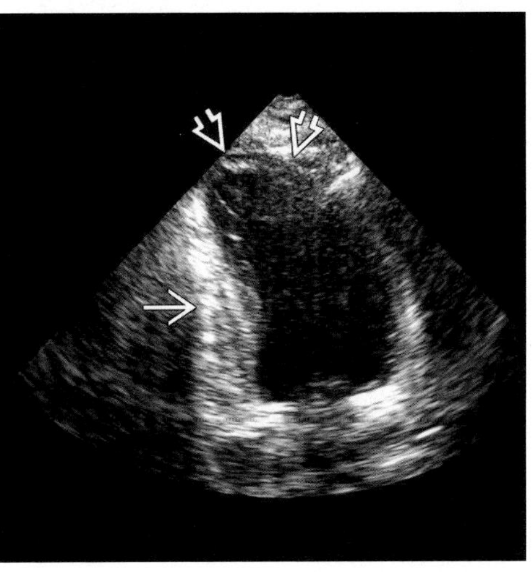

(Left) Right anterior oblique catheter angiography shows ballooning of the apex during systole. Area of normal contraction during systole ➔. Area of apical dilatation ➡. ***(Right)*** Conventional echocardiogram two-chamber view shows LV with relative ➔ thickening of the mid-ventricle and LV apical ballooning ➡.

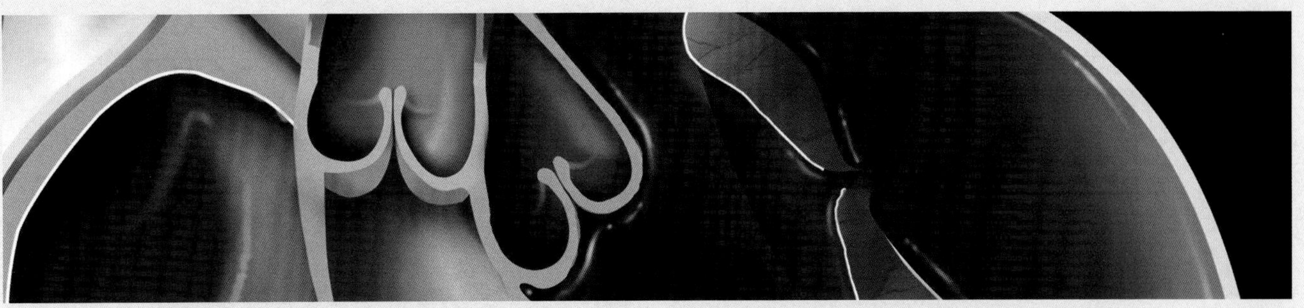

SECTION 6: Coronary Artery

Introduction and Overview

Coronary Artery

CORONARY ANATOMY

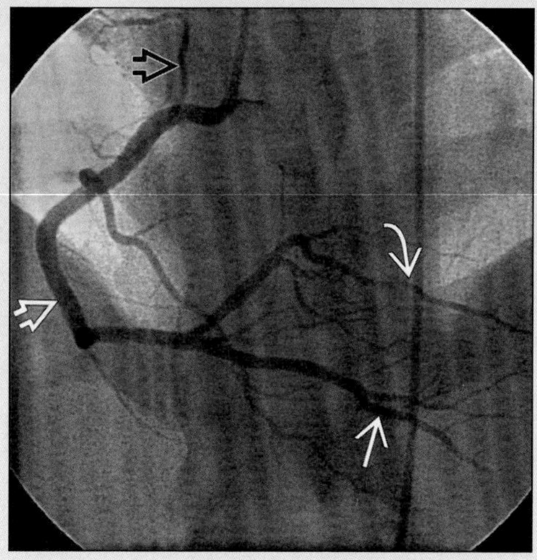

Oblique catheter angiography shows dominant RCA bifurcating into PDA and PLV. Note: Conus branch is first branch of RCA in cephalad direction.

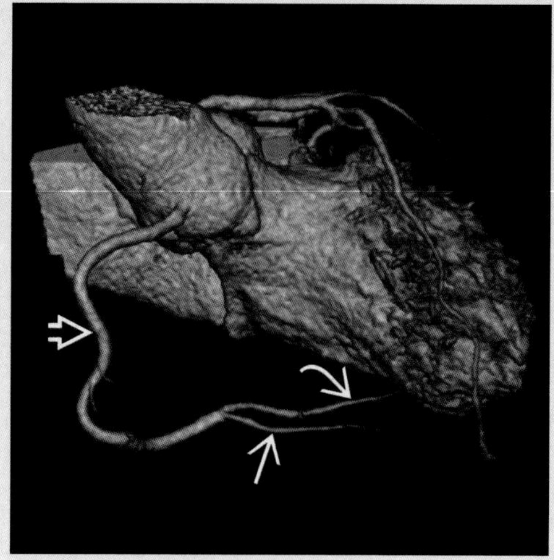

Oblique coronary CTA volume rendered image (VRT) shows dominant RCA bifurcating into PDA and PLV. Note that the RV is not seen with this VRT setting due to contrast wash-out of RV.

TERMINOLOGY

Abbreviations

- Coronary arteries and their branches
  - Left main (LM) coronary artery
  - Left anterior descending (LAD) coronary artery
  - Diagonal branches: D1, D2, D3 (1 proximal, 2 second, etc.)
  - Ramus intermedius (RI) or ramus
  - Left circumflex (LCX, CX) coronary artery
  - Obtuse marginal branch: OM1, OM2, OM3 (off LCX, 1 proximal)
  - Posterior lateral branch (PL, PLB)
  - Posterior left ventricular branch (PLV)
  - Posterior descending artery (PDA)
  - Right coronary artery (RCA)
  - Acute marginal branch (AM); branch off RCA
  - Sinoatrial node branch (SAN, SA node branch)
  - Atrioventricular node branch (AVN, AV node branch)
- Grafts
  - Left internal mammary artery (LIMA)
  - Right internal mammary artery (RIMA)
  - Saphenous vein graft (SVG)
  - Coronary artery bypass graft (CABG)

Synonyms

- Epicardial arteries

Definitions

- Coronary arteries are the vasa privata of the heart

Alternative International Nomenclature

- Ramus interventricularis anterior (RIVA) = LAD
- Ramus circumflexus (RCX) = LCX
- Ramus interventricularis posterior (RIVP, RIP) = PDA
- Ramus marginalis (RM, M) = OM
- Right posterolateral branch (RPL) - PLV from RCA
  - Ramus posterolateralis dexter (RPD) - PLV branch from RCA - careful not to confuse with
  - Right posterior descending artery (RPD) - PDA from RCA

IMAGING ANATOMY

General Anatomic Considerations

- Coronary arteries are often **divided into 15 or 17 segments** for standardized reporting
- Original 15 segment model was published via an AHA committee by W. Gerald Austen in 1975
  - Proximal RCA: RCA from ostium to 1/2 the distance to the acute margin of heart
  - Mid RCA: Continuation of above to the acute RV margin
  - Distal RCA: RCA from the acute margin to the origin of the PDA
  - PDA off RCA: Entire posterior descending branch
  - PLV off RCA: Only in 17 segment model, not originally included in 15 segment model
  - LM: From ostium to bifurcation into LAD and LCX (or trifurcation if ramus intermedius is present)
  - Proximal LAD: LAD proximal to and including origin of first septal perforator (or D1) branch
  - Mid LAD: LAD distal to origin of first septal branch (or D1) and extending to the origin of second diagonal branch (D2)
  - Distal (or apical) LAD: Terminal LAD distal to D2
  - First diagonal branch (D1): Entire branch from its origin off the LAD
  - Second diagonal (D2): Entire branch from its origin off the LAD
  - Ramus intermedius: (If present) in the 17 segment model, not originally included in 15 segment model
  - Proximal LCX: LCX from its origin off LM to origin of first obtuse marginal branch
  - Obtuse Marginal: Largest lateral branch of LCX
  - Distal LCX: From the origin of the OM branch on to crux of heart
  - Posterolateral branch
  - PDA: If present as branch of LCX

Anatomic Relationships

- Dominance is determined by the coronary artery that supplies the posterior descending artery (PDA) territory and inferior LV wall

CORONARY ANATOMY

Coronary Artery 17 Segment Model

- 1 Proximal RCA: RCA from ostium to 1/2 the distance to the acute margin of heart
- 2 Mid RCA: Continuation of above to the acute RV margin
- 3 Distal RCA: RCA from the acute margin to the origin of the PDA
- 4 PDA off RCA: Entire posterior descending branch
- 16 PLV off RCA: Not included in 15 segment model
- 5 LM: From ostium to bifurcation or trifurcation
- 6 Proximal LAD: LAD proximal to and including origin of first septal perforator (or D1) branch
- 7 Mid LAD: LAD distal to origin of first septal branch (or D1) and extending to the origin of second diagonal branch (D2)
- 8 Distal (or apical) LAD: Terminal LAD distal to D2
- 9 First diagonal branch (D1): Entire branch from its origin off the LAD
- 10 Second diagonal (D2): Entire branch from its origin off the LAD
- 17 Ramus intermedius: (If present) not included in 15 segment model
- 11 Proximal LCX: LCX from its origin off LM to origin of first obtuse marginal branch
- 12 Obtuse marginal: Largest lateral branch of LCX
- 13 Distal LCX: From the origin of the OM branch on to crux of heart
- 14 Posterolateral branch or obtuse marginal branch
- 15 PDA/distal LCX if present (left dominant system)

    - Approximately 85% of patients are right dominant (RCA provides PDA)
    - Remainder is split between left dominant (LCx provides PDA) or codominant (RCA and LCx provide PDA branches)
- RCA
    - Travels within the right atrioventricular groove
    - Provides small branches to the right atrium and anterior freewall and acute marginal branches to the right ventricle
    - RCA branches supply the sinus node in 60% of population
        - Most common alternative supply is via left circumflex (LCx) atrial branches
    - 1st branch of RCA is a conus branch in approximately 50% of patients
        - Alternative origin of the conus branch is via a separate ostium directly form the right sinus of Valsalva
        - Conus branch supplies the right ventricular outflow tract
    - Dominant RCA usually bifurcates at the crux of the heart into the PDA and PLV branches
    - PDA runs within the inferior (or posterior) interventricular groove and gives rise to septal perforators
    - PLV branch usually courses cephalad to curve above the great cardiac vein, before turning caudal and towards the inferior left ventricular
    - Atrioventricular (AV) nodal branch usually originates from the posterior left ventricular (PLV) branch of the RCA as it passes through the crux of the heart
- LM
    - Arises from left sinus of Valsalva
    - Variable length from virtually not present to approximately 2 centimeters
    - Typically bifurcates into LAD and LCX
        - Typically has no side branches
    - May trifurcate into LAD, LCX and a ramus intermedius
    - Most common site of stenosis is at the mid or distal portion
    - In the LM stenoses of > = 50% Are considered significant, compared to all other segments where 70% or greater is considered significant
- LCX
    - Arises from LM
    - Rarely may arise directly from left sinus of Valsalva, or as an anomalous origin from the right sinus or the RCA (most common coronary anomaly)
    - Runs around mitral valve annulus in the left atrio-ventricular (AV) groove
    - Gives rise to obtuse marginal branch
    - Non-dominant LCX often terminates as an OM branch
    - Native LCX distal to OM branches is often diminutive
    - If dominant will give rise to posterior left ventricular branch and PDA
- LAD
    - Often referred to RIVA, internationally
    - Originates from LM
    - Runs anteriorly within the anterior interventricular groove
    - Gives rise to septal perforator branches that penetrate the LV septum and to diagonal branches that run on the anterior wall of the LV
    - Often wraps around the apex and may form collaterals to the distal PDA if flow limiting obstructions are present

Normal Variants and Anomalies

- Coronary ostium typically arises from the peak convexity of the ipsilateral sinus of Valsalva; normal variants include
    - High ostium
        - May arise at or above sino-tubular junction
    - Commissural ostium
        - Ostium within 5 mm of the commissure (junction of adjacent sinuses)
- Separate ostia of LCX and LAD from left coronary sinus

CORONARY ANATOMY

Oblique catheter angiography shows LM, LAD, and LCX. Note large obtuse marginal branches off LCX, and presence of small ramus intermedius.

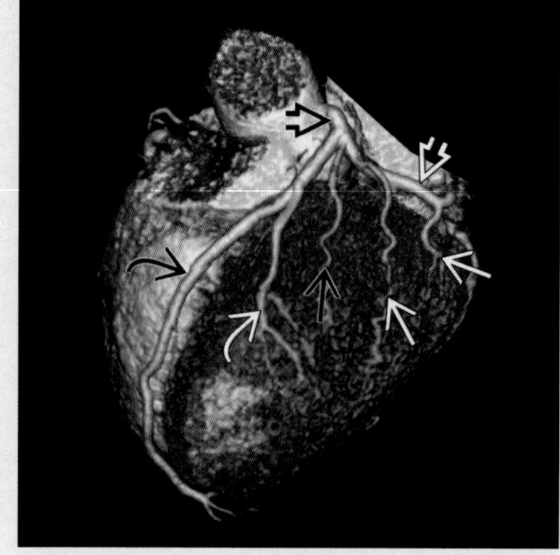

Oblique coronary CTA shows LM, LAD, diagonal branch and LCX. Note: Small obtuse marginal branches, and presence of small ramus intermedius.

- Anomalous origin of a coronary artery is defined by an origin from the opposite coronary sinus (LM, LAD or LCX from right sinus, or RCA from left sinus)
  - "Benign" variants of anomalous coronary arteries have course either retroaortic or pre pulmonic/anterior to the right ventricular outflow tract
  - "Malignant" variants have an interarterial course between aorta and pulmonary artery
    - Transseptal course is a variation of the "malignant" type where the abnormal vessel runs in the myocardium just below the interarterial space; this variant is considered less malignant compared to interarterial anomalies
  - Coronary artery origin from the non-coronary sinus is very rare
- Coronary-cameral fistulae are abnormal connections between a coronary artery and cardiac chamber
  - Vessels often enlarged and tortuous
  - May have aneurysmal dilatation just proximal to fistulous connection
    - Often large or giant aneurysm if fistula to coronary sinus
  - May be associated with flow reversal and steal phenomenon via collaterals if draining into low pressure system
  - Extreme form is Bland-White-Garland syndrome
    - Anomalous left coronary artery arising from the pulmonary artery (ALCAPA)
    - Less common is anomalous right coronary artery arising from the pulmonary artery (ARCAPA)

ANATOMY-BASED IMAGING ISSUES

Challenges

- LM and proximal LCX are often "hidden" underneath the left atrial appendage (LAA) on 3D cardiac CT
  - Manual or automated LAA segmentation may be necessary to allow viewing these coronary segments
  - Segmentation may mimic stenosis by inadvertently "resecting" portions of the coronary arteries
  - Multiplanar reformation with thin slices is best tool to visualize difficult areas

PATHOLOGY-BASED IMAGING ISSUES

Imaging Protocols

- Coronary CT angiography requires retrospective cardiac gating or prospective triggering
  - EKG-based tube current modulation is used to reduce radiation dose of retrospective gated acquisition
  - Optimal tube output is applied in mid to late diastole, and the tube current is ramped down during systole
- High flow rates of 5-7 cc/sec are required to achieve suitable contrast to noise ratios

Imaging Pitfalls

- Slab misregistration artifact at cardiac-gated MDCT may mimic coronary artery stenosis
  - Coronal or sagittal oblique images may be useful to differentiate artifact from a true stenosis
    - Slab line that extends beyond the confines of the coronary artery is indicative of slab artifact
    - Involvement of all visible coronary arteries (right and left-sided branches) at one axial slice level is highly suggestive of slab artifact

CORONARY ANATOMY

IMAGE GALLERY

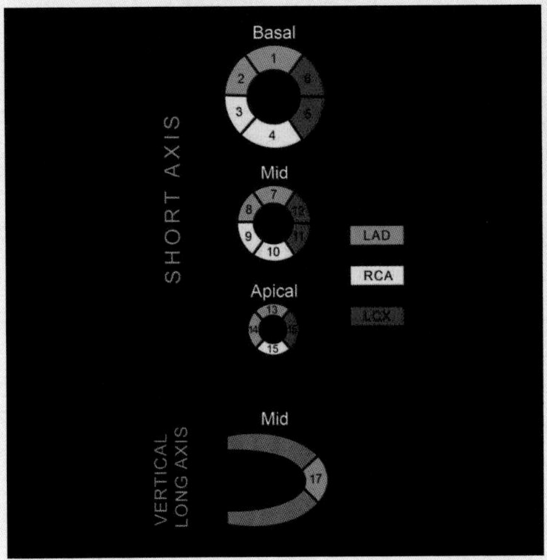

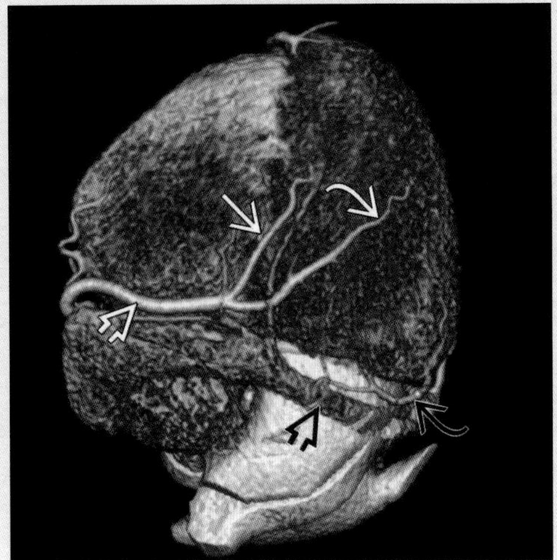

(Left) *Graphic shows 17 segment LV myocardial segment model with corresponding color coded coronary artery perfusion territories, assuming a right dominant system.* ***(Right)*** *Oblique coronary CTA volume rendered view of inferior cardiac surface shows right dominant system. Distal RCA bifurcates into PDA and PLV. Note: Coronary sinus, and distal LCX.*

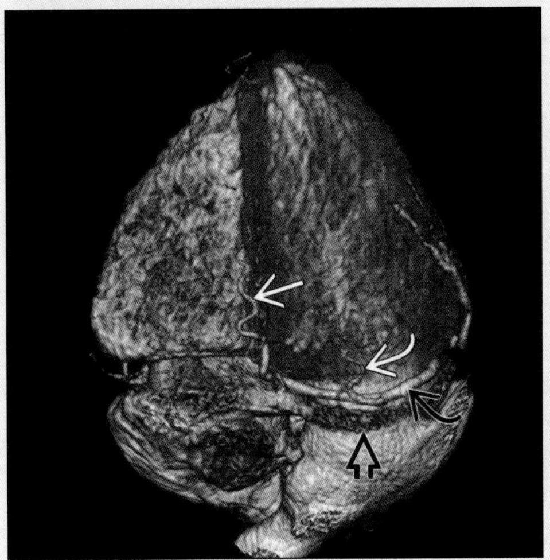

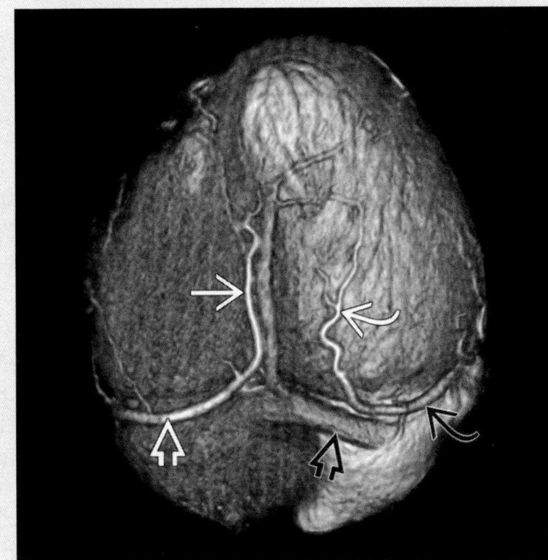

(Left) *Oblique coronary CTA volume rendered technique (VRT) view of inferior cardiac surface shows left dominant system. Distal LCX bifurcates into PLV and PDA. Note: Coronary sinus.* ***(Right)*** *Oblique coronary CTA VRT shows co-dominant system. Distal RCA terminates as a PDA. Distal LCX terminates as a large PLV. Note: Coronary sinus.*

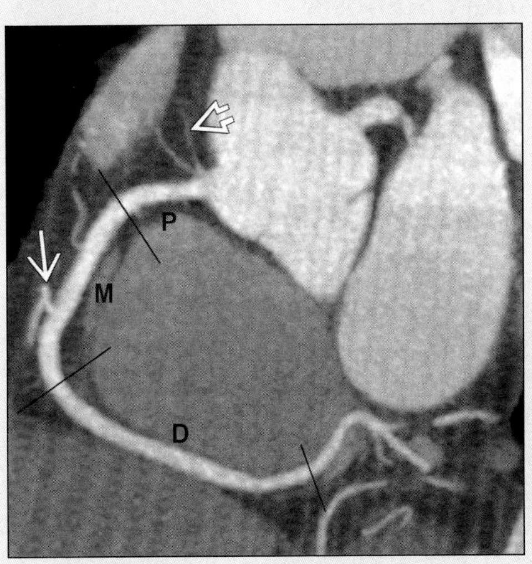

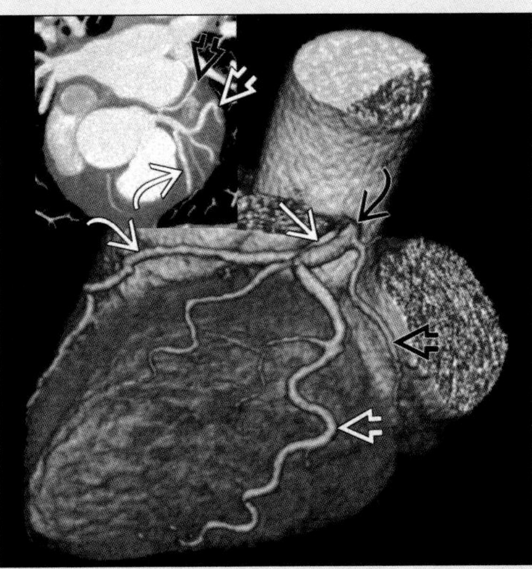

(Left) *Oblique coronary CTA shows proximal (P), mid (M), and distal (D) RCA. The PDA takeoff is not visible in this plane. Note: Acute marginal branch and split conus branch.* ***(Right)*** *Oblique coronary CTA shows LM, proximal LAD, mid LAD, very large first diagonal branch, and small LCX.*

ANOMALOUS LEFT CORONARY ARTERY, MALIGNANT

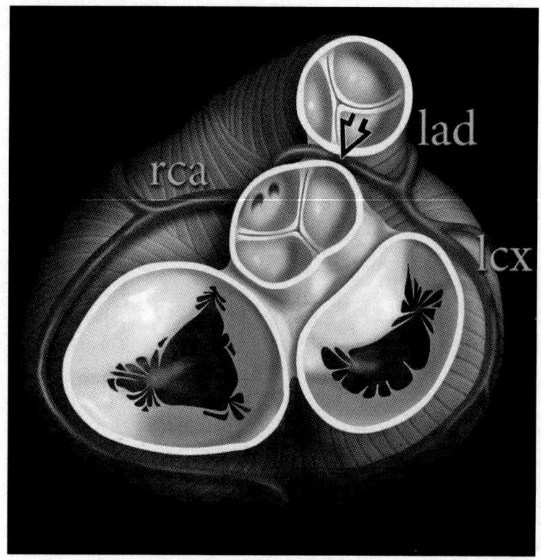

Graphic shows a malignant course of an anomalous left main coronary artery ➪ arising via a separate ostium from the right sinus of Valsalva. Note inter-arterial course ➪.

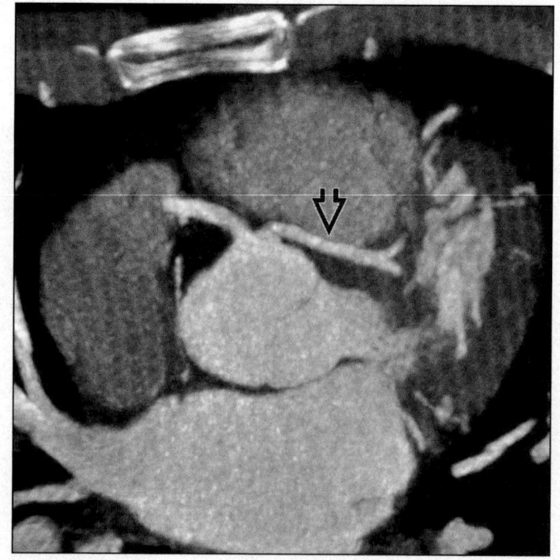

Axial coronary CTA shows an anomalous LM ➪ arising from the right sinus of Valsalva and passing between the right ventricular outflow tract and the aorta. Note: Intramyocardial course (considered protective).

TERMINOLOGY

Definitions

- Origin of the left coronary artery (LCA or left main [LM]) or LAD from the right sinus of Valsalva with an inter-arterial course causing risk for myocardial ischemia or sudden death
- Other "malignant" types of anomalies include
  - Origin of the left coronary artery from the pulmonary trunk
  - High-flow angiomas

IMAGING FINDINGS

General Features

- Best diagnostic clue: Left coronary artery arising from the right sinus of Valsalva or the RCA
- Location
  - Septal course: Through the ventricular septum beneath the right ventricular infundibulum
  - Inter-arterial course: Between the aorta and pulmonary artery
  - Anterior or posterior to the aorta, or mixed

CT Findings

- CTA: Contrast-enhanced CT is gold standard for diagnosing and characterizing anomalous coronary arteries

MR Findings

- MRA: Contrast-enhanced MRA shows excellent ability in non-invasive diagnosis of anomalous coronary arteries

Angiographic Findings

- Conventional: Multiple projection views are required for correctly diagnosing an inter-arterial course of the left coronary artery

DIFFERENTIAL DIAGNOSIS

Coronary Artery Stenosis

- Coronary stenosis due to atherosclerotic disease should be excluded in younger patients

DDx: Coronary Anomaly

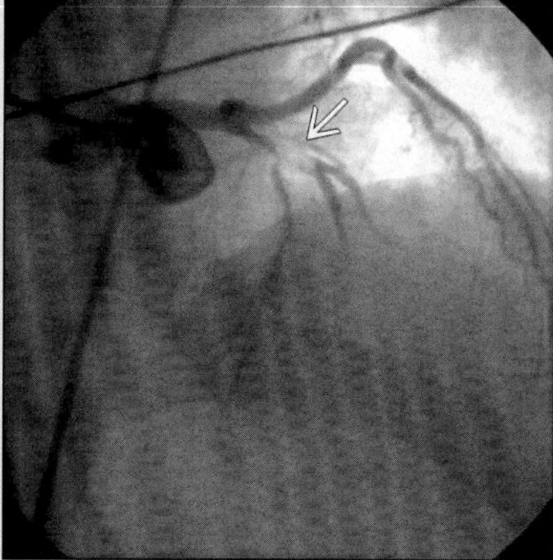

Atherosclerotic Stenosis

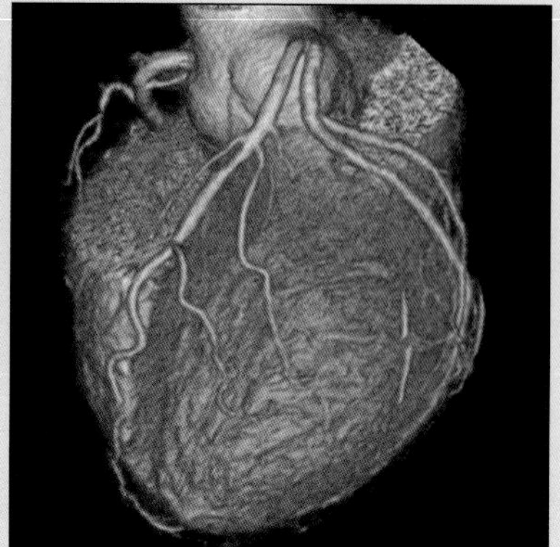

Separate LAD and LCX Ostia

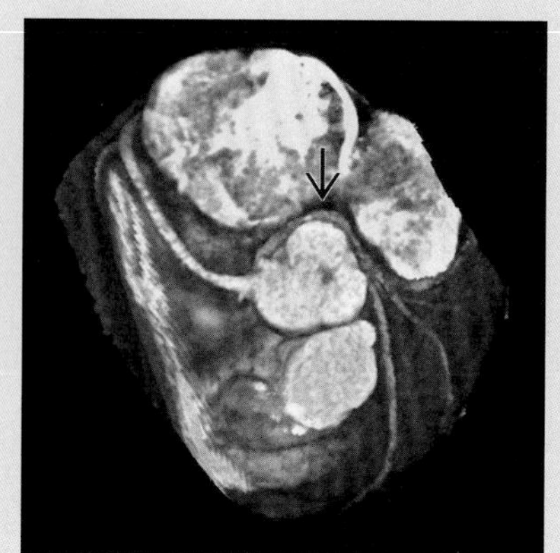

Retroaortic Course of LM

ANOMALOUS LEFT CORONARY ARTERY, MALIGNANT

Key Facts

Terminology

- Origin of LCA or LAD from right sinus of Valsalva or RCA with inter-arterial course causing myocardial ischemia or sudden death

Imaging Findings

- Contrast-enhanced CT is an excellent tool for diagnosing and tracing route of anomalous coronary artery
- Coronary MRA should be considered for young patients
- Invasive coronary angiography requires multiple projection views for a correct diagnosis

Clinical Issues

- Children and young adults with myocardia ischemia or sudden death
- Treatment: Coronary bypass or reimplantation of coronaries above the appropriate coronary sinus

Coronary Artery Aneurysm

- Kawasaki disease may present with the following: Rupture, thrombosis and stenosis

Benign Anomalous Coronary Artery

- LCA arising from the right side with anterior course to the pulmonary artery
- LCA or LCX with a retroaortic course
- LAD and LCX arising from the left sinus of Valsalva from separate ostia

PATHOLOGY

General Features

- General path comments
  - Normal histology and mechanism of sudden death not known
    - Squeezing between aorta and pulmonary artery, kinking or spasm
    - Acute angle of takeoff or slit-like origin
- Epidemiology: Malignant inter-arterial course of left coronary artery is found in approximately 1.3% of all coronary anomalies

Gross Pathologic & Surgical Features

- There are several anatomical features of symptomatic (malignant) left coronary arteries
  - Vessel lumen is slit-like at the point of origin
  - Initial vessel segment runs within the aortic wall
  - Vessel originates at an acute angle
  - Vessel follows an inter-arterial path

CLINICAL ISSUES

Presentation

- Most common signs/symptoms
  - Myocardial infarction or heart failure in an infant or young patient
  - Ventricular arrhythmias
- Other signs/symptoms: Complications due to compression of the left coronary artery commonly occur during or immediately after exercise

Demographics

- Age: Children and young adults with myocardia ischemia or sudden death

Treatment

- Coronary bypass or reimplantation of coronaries above appropriate coronary sinus
- Excellent prognosis with early treatment

SELECTED REFERENCES

1. Dodd JD et al: Congenital anomalies of coronary artery origin in adults: 64-MDCT appearance. AJR Am J Roentgenol. 188(2):W138-46, 2007
2. McConnell MV et al: Identification of anomalous coronary arteries and their anatomic course by magnetic resonance coronary angiography. Circulation. 92(11):3158-62, 1995

IMAGE GALLERY

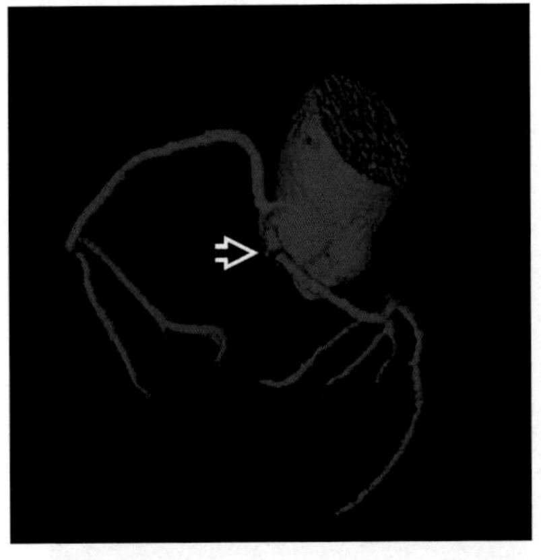

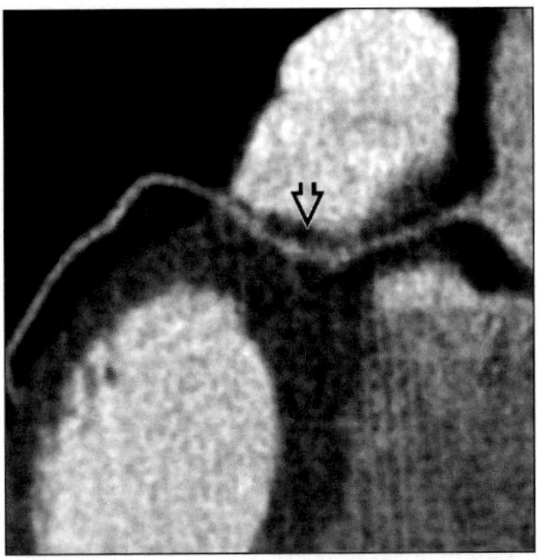

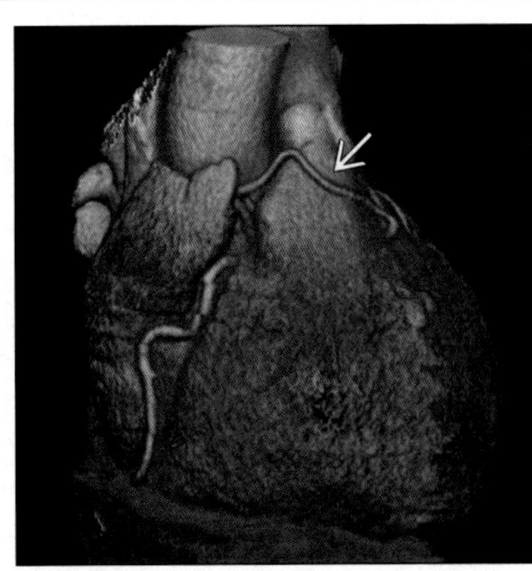

(Left) *Coronary CTA shows anomalous left coronary artery ➡ arising from the right sinus of Valsalva and coursing between the pulmonary artery (removed) and the aorta.* ***(Center)*** *Curved MPR coronary CTA shows an anomalous LAD arising from the right side and passing through the ventricular septum ⇨.* ***(Right)*** *3D coronary CTA shows LM coronary artery arising from the right side and passing anterior to the pulmonary outflow tract ➡ (benign type).*

ANOMALOUS LEFT CORONARY ARTERY, BENIGN

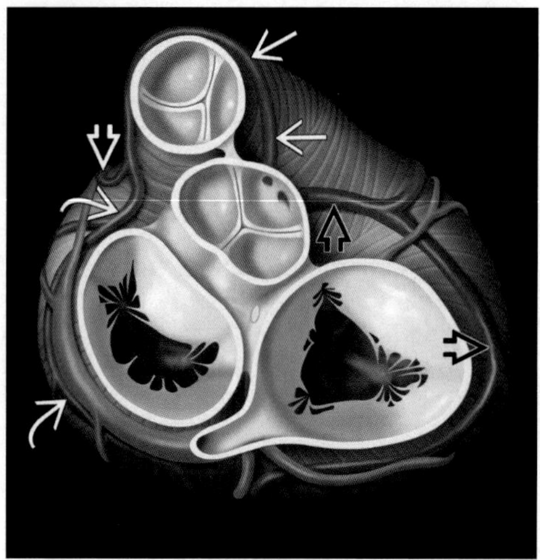

Graphic shows anomalous LM ➡ originating from right sinus of Valsalva separately from RCA ⇨. Note, LM courses anterior to RVOT and bifurcates into LAD ➡ and LCX ➡.

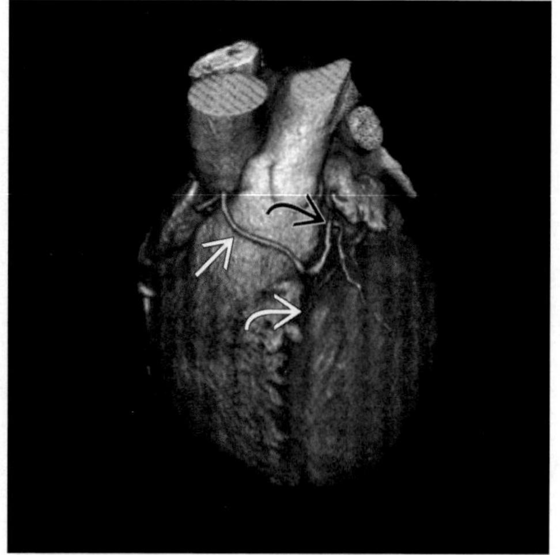

Oblique coronary CTA volume rendering shows anomalous LM ➡ coursing anterior to RVOT and giving rise to a very small LAD ➡ before traveling posteriorly to give rise to the LCX ⇨.

TERMINOLOGY

Abbreviations and Synonyms

- Anomalous left main coronary artery

Definitions

- Left main (LM) coronary artery arises from right sinus of Valsalva or from right coronary artery (RCA) and courses anterior to the right ventricular outflow tract (RVOT) to give rise to the left anterior descending (LAD) and left circumflex (LCX) coronary arteries

IMAGING FINDINGS

General Features

- Best diagnostic clue: Abnormal vessel anterior to RVOT and absence of a coronary ostium at left sinus of Valsalva
- Location
  - Typically has shared ostium with RCA at right sinus of Valsalva
  - LAD and LCX run in their normal respective locations, but LM bifurcation is shifted towards the LV apex compared to normals

CT Findings

- Cardiac Gated CTA
  - Gating of CTA is necessary to allow depiction of coronary ostia and course
  - Abnormal vessel arising from right sinus of Valsalva or RCA and coursing anterior to RVOT
  - Volume rendered 3D images can be helpful to evaluate spatial relationships

MR Findings

- MR/MRA useful for proximal coronary arteries
  - Preferred in children and young adults due to absence of radiation
  - May be useful in renal failure patients (non-contrast MRA)

Imaging Recommendations

- Best imaging tool
  - Cardiac MDCT
  - MR in children and young patients

DDx: Anomalous Left Main Coronary Artery, Malignant Variant

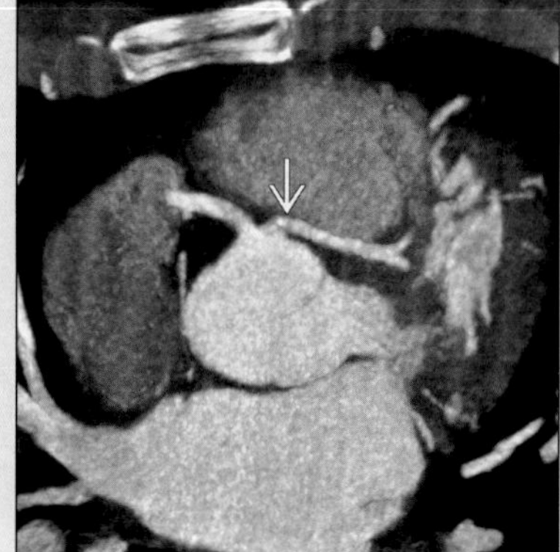

LM between PA & Ao

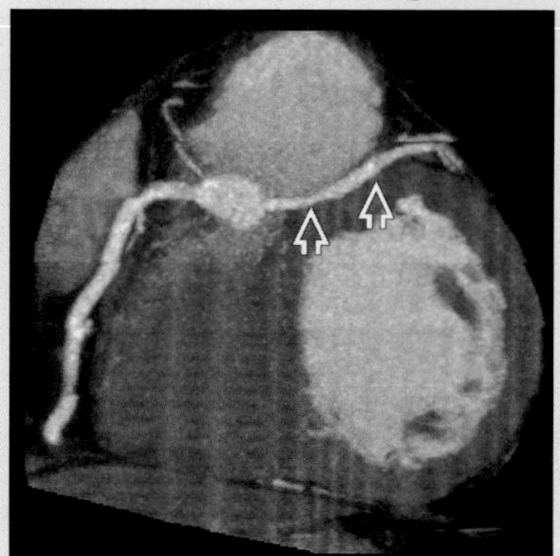

Intramyocardial LM

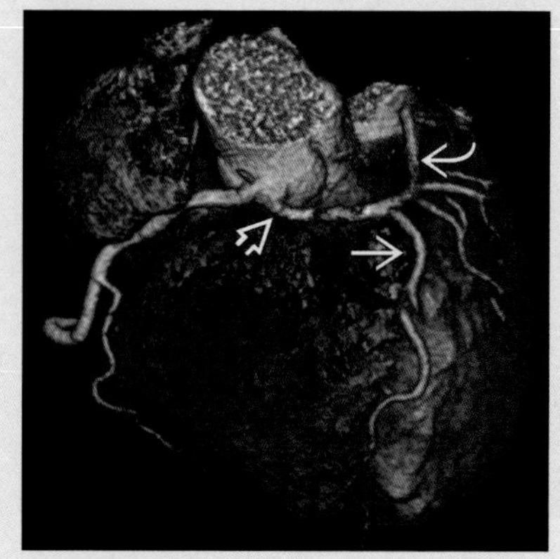

LAD & LCX from Anomalous LM

ANOMALOUS LEFT CORONARY ARTERY, BENIGN

Key Facts

Terminology
- Left main (LM) coronary artery arises from right sinus of Valsalva or from right coronary artery (RCA) and courses anterior to the right ventricular outflow tract (RVOT) to give rise to the left anterior descending (LAD) and left circumflex (LCX) coronary arteries

Imaging Findings
- Gating of CTA is necessary to allow depiction of coronary ostia and course

Pathology
- Epidemiology: Primary congenital anomalies of the coronary arteries have an incidence of 1-2% of general population

Clinical Issues
- Most common signs/symptoms: Usually asymptomatic
- Other signs/symptoms: Malignant variants may present with sudden cardiac death or arrhythmia

DIFFERENTIAL DIAGNOSIS

Malignant Variant of Anomalous LM
- Courses between PA and Aorta
- Sometimes has intramyocardial course, which is said to be relatively protective

Absent Left Main
- Split origin of LAD and LCX from left sinus of Valsalva
- Anomalous origin of LAD from the right sinus of Valsalva (benign or malignant) also has absent of LM
- Anomalous LCX also has absent LM

Coronary Artery Fistula
- May have a prominent conus branch as a feeder, which may mimic an anomalous LM

PATHOLOGY

General Features
- Epidemiology: Primary congenital anomalies of the coronary arteries have an incidence of 1-2% of general population

CLINICAL ISSUES

Presentation
- Most common signs/symptoms: Usually asymptomatic
- Other signs/symptoms: Malignant variants may present with sudden cardiac death or arrhythmia

Demographics
- Gender: No gender predisposition

Natural History & Prognosis
- Typically clinically silent
- Coronary artery abnormalities in general are second most common cause of sudden death in young athletes
  - Hypertrophic cardiomyopathy is first most common

DIAGNOSTIC CHECKLIST

Consider
- Check space between aorta and RVOT/PA to exclude malignant variant

Image Interpretation Pearls
- Left sinus of Valsalva without coronary artery ostium

SELECTED REFERENCES

1. Dodd JD et al: Congenital anomalies of coronary artery origin in adults: 64-MDCT appearance. AJR Am J Roentgenol. 188(2):W138-46, 2007
2. Datta J et al: Anomalous coronary arteries in adults: depiction at multi-detector row CT angiography. Radiology. 235(3):812-8, 2005
3. Liberthson RR: Sudden death from cardiac causes in children and young adults. N Engl J Med. 334(16):1039-44, 1996

IMAGE GALLERY

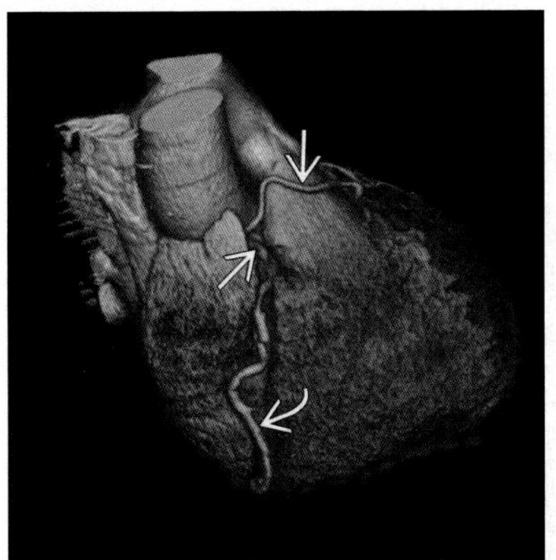

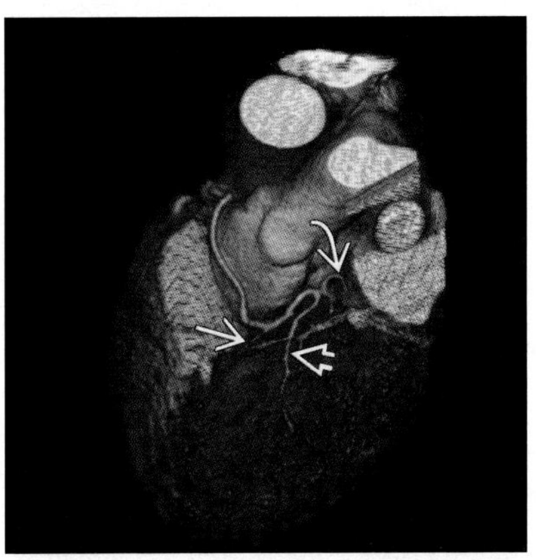

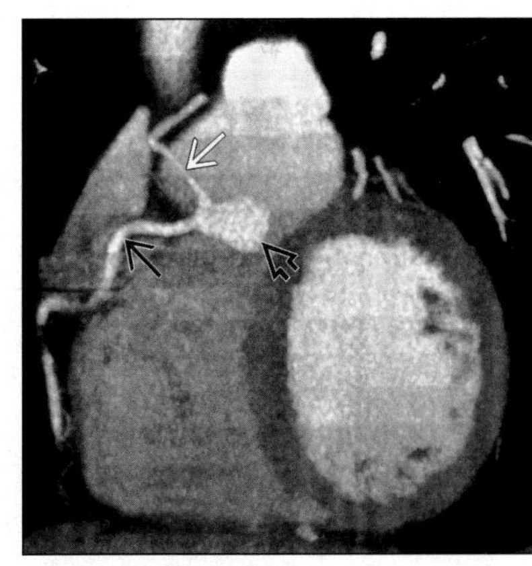

*(**Left**) Oblique coronary CTA volume rendering shows anomalous LM ➡ originating from the right and traveling anteriorly to RVOT. Note RCA ➡. (**Center**) Oblique coronary CTA volume rendering (same patient as previous image) shows anomalous left coronary artery giving rise to a minute LAD ➡, and then coursing posteriorly and giving rise to a larger diagonal branch ➡ followed by the LCX ➡. (**Right**) Oblique coronary CTA MIP image shows an anomalous LM ➡ originating from a common ostium with the RCA ⇨ from the right sinus of Valsalva ⇨.*

ANOMALOUS LCX

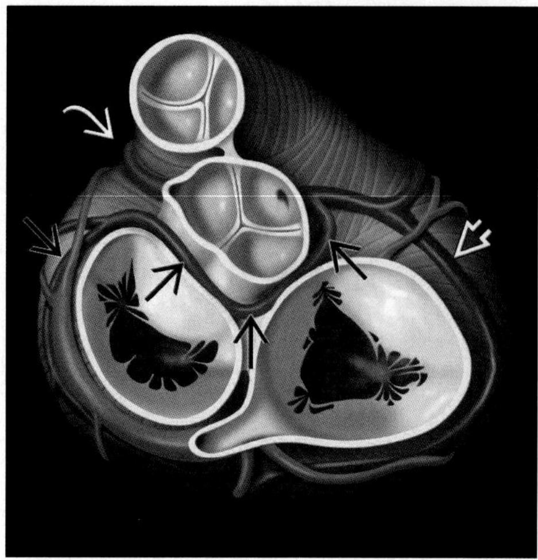

Oblique graphic shows anomalous LCX ➔ arising from right sinus of Valsalva and coursing behind non-coronary sinus of Valsalva. RCA ➔ and LAD ➔ are normal.

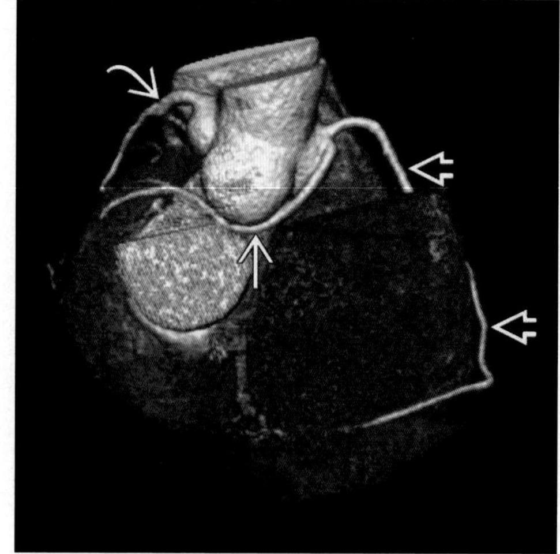

Posterior volume rendering of coronary CTA shows anomalous LCX ➔ arising from right sinus of Valsalva and coursing behind non-coronary sinus of Valsalva. RCA ➔ and LAD ➔ are normal.

TERMINOLOGY

Abbreviations and Synonyms

- Anomalous left circumflex (LCX) coronary artery

Definitions

- Left circumflex originates from right sinus of Valsalva and courses posterior and inferior to the non-coronary cusp towards the left
  - Left anterior descending (LAD) coronary artery originates directly from left sinus of Valsalva
  - No left main (LM) coronary artery segment is present

IMAGING FINDINGS

General Features

- Best diagnostic clue
  - Abnormal vessel between non-coronary cusp and roof of atria
  - No LCX branch off LM/LAD
  - Abnormal vessel arising from right sinus of Valsalva or RCA that courses posteriorly
- Location: Originates either from right coronary artery (RCA), a common ostium with RCA, or directly from the right sinus of Valsalva
- Size: Anomalous LCX is usually a smaller non-dominant vessel

CT Findings

- Cardiac Gated CTA
  - Considered gold standard as it demonstrates anomalous vessels at high spatial and contrast resolution and depicts relationship with surrounding structures
  - Anomalies with a course outside of the space between aorta and pulmonary artery are considered benign

Imaging Recommendations

- Best imaging tool
  - Cardiac gated MDCT is best imaging tool
  - Cardiac MR in young patients and other patients where radiation is to be avoided or minimized
- Protocol advice: Cardiac gating is necessary to eliminate aortic pulsation artifact

DDx: Anomalous Coronary Artery

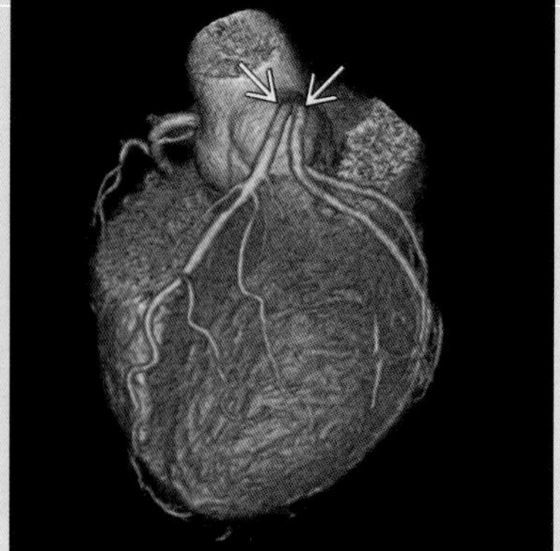

Separate LCX Ostium

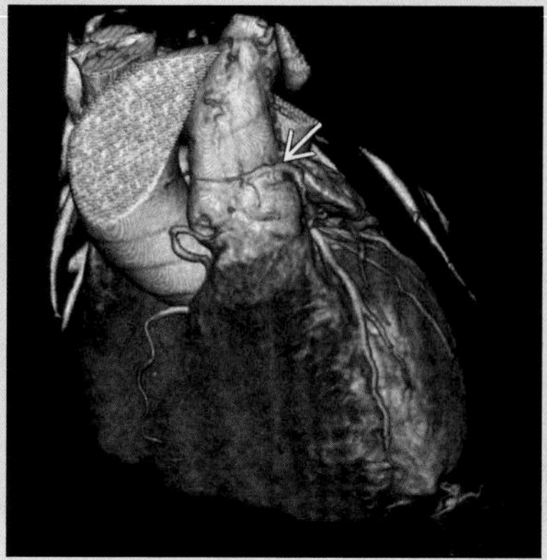

Coronary Fistula

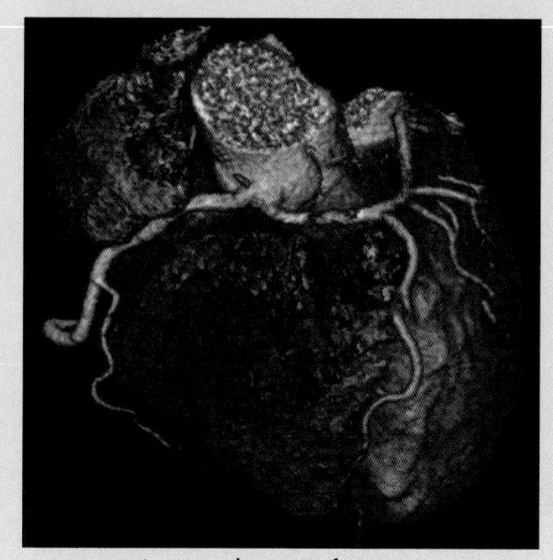

Anomalous Left Main

ANOMALOUS LCX

Key Facts

Terminology

- Left circumflex originates from right sinus of Valsalva and courses posterior and inferior to the non-coronary cusp towards the left
- Left anterior descending (LAD) coronary artery originates directly from left sinus of Valsalva
- No left main (LM) coronary artery segment is present

Imaging Findings

- Cardiac gated MDCT is best imaging tool
- Cardiac MR in young patients and other patients where radiation is to be avoided or minimized

Clinical Issues

- Age: Any
- Anomalous LCX is the most common variant of true coronary anomalies
- Usually benign incidental finding

DIFFERENTIAL DIAGNOSIS

Anomalous RCA, Benign Variant

- This variant also runs posterior and inferior to the non-coronary aortic sinus, but in opposite direction

Coronary Fistula

- Usually multiple tortuous and enlarged feeders

Sino-Atrial (SA) Node Branch

- Prominent SA nodal branch can be confused with anomalous LCX
- Best clue is identification of a normal LCX branch off the LM

PATHOLOGY

General Features

- Epidemiology: Primary congenital anomalies of the coronary arteries can be found in 1-2% of the general population

CLINICAL ISSUES

Presentation

- Most common signs/symptoms: Asymptomatic

Demographics

- Age: Any
- Gender: No sex predilection
- Anomalous LCX is the most common variant of true coronary anomalies

Natural History & Prognosis

- Usually benign incidental finding

Treatment

- No treatment necessary

DIAGNOSTIC CHECKLIST

Consider

- Volume rendered CTA images not useful unless atria are removed during segmentation

Image Interpretation Pearls

- Space between aortic non-coronary sinus and the atria does normally not contain any vessels
  - If a vessel in this space is detected it is pathognomonic for anomalous coronary artery and either represents anomalous LCX or anomalous RCA

SELECTED REFERENCES

1. Dodd JD et al: Congenital anomalies of coronary artery origin in adults: 64-MDCT appearance. AJR Am J Roentgenol. 188(2):W138-46, 2007
2. Datta J et al: Anomalous coronary arteries in adults: depiction at multi-detector row CT angiography. Radiology. 235(3):812-8, 2005

IMAGE GALLERY

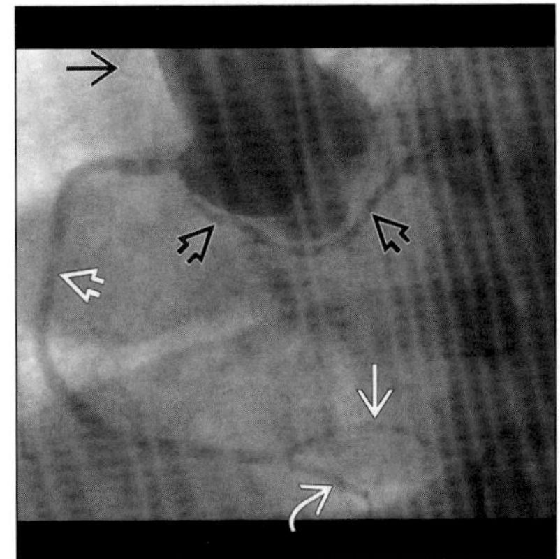

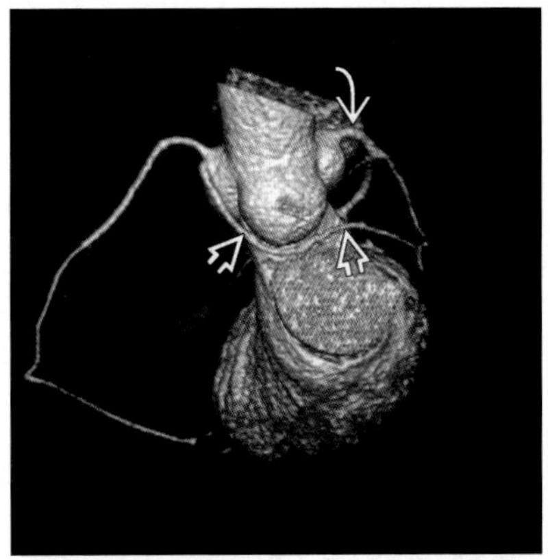

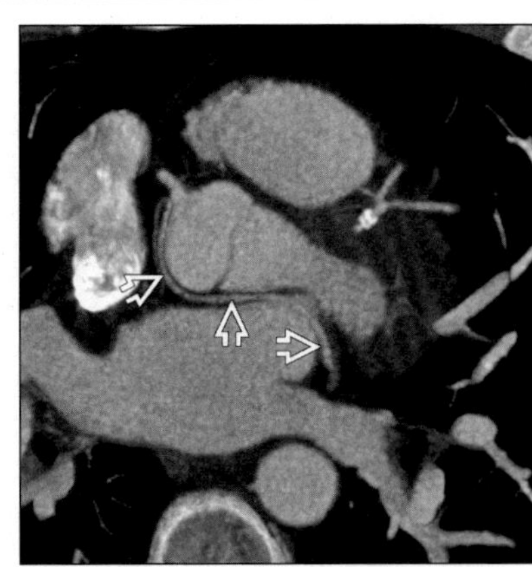

*(**Left**) Left anterior oblique invasive angiogram shows RCA ➡, conus branch ⇨, posterior left ventricular (PLV) branch ➡, posterior descending artery (PDA) ➡, and an anomalous LCX ⇨. (**Center**) Posterior view of volume rendered coronary CTA in the same patient as previous image, shows anomalous LCX ➡ as it courses posterior and inferior to the non coronary sinus. Note: LAD ➡ originates directly from left sinus. (**Right**) Oblique coronary CTA MIP image shows relationship of anomalous LCX ➡ to right and left atrium.*

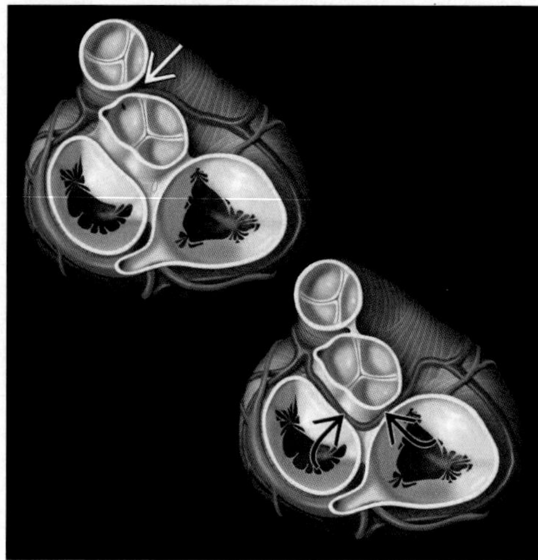

Posterior view graphics show relationship between anomalous RCA & aorta & pulmonary artery. Malignant variant: RCA between Ao and PA ➔, benign variant: RCA posterior to aorta ⇨.

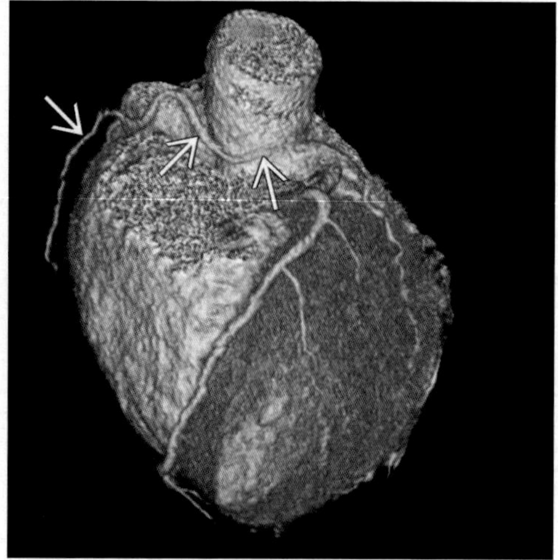

Anterior volume rendered coronary CTA shows anomalous origin of non-dominant RCA ➔ from left sinus of Valsalva. RCA courses between pulmonary artery (removed) & aorta ("malignant" course).

TERMINOLOGY

Definitions

- Malignant variant: Right coronary artery (RCA) originates from left sinus of Valsalva and courses between the aorta and the pulmonary artery
- Benign variant: RCA originates from left sinus of Valsalva and courses posterior and inferior to the aortic root

IMAGING FINDINGS

General Features

- Best diagnostic clue
  - Absence of coronary artery ostium at the right sinus of Valsalva (SOV), but present right coronary artery more distally
    - RCA has to be traced back to its abnormal origin to differentiate from ostial RCA occlusion
- Location
  - Origin of malignant anomalous RCA is variable
    - Typically arises from left coronary cusp between origin of LM and anterior commissure
    - May arise from left main (LM)
    - May arise superior to sino-tubular junction, either above left SOV or above junction of right and left SOV
    - Courses between anterior aspect of aortic root and posterior pulmonary artery wall
  - Benign variant is uncommon
    - Arises from left SOV and courses posterior and inferior to aortic root
- Morphology: May be oval in crossection which has been suggested to be a sign of compression, however this view is controversial

CT Findings

- Cardiac Gated CTA
  - Gating of CTA is necessary to allow depiction of coronary ostium and course of abnormal vessels
  - Volume rendered 3D images can be helpful to demonstrate spatial relationship of aortic root and anomalous vessel

Imaging Recommendations

- Best imaging tool
  - Cardiac MDCT
  - MR in children and young patients

DDx: RCA Anomaly

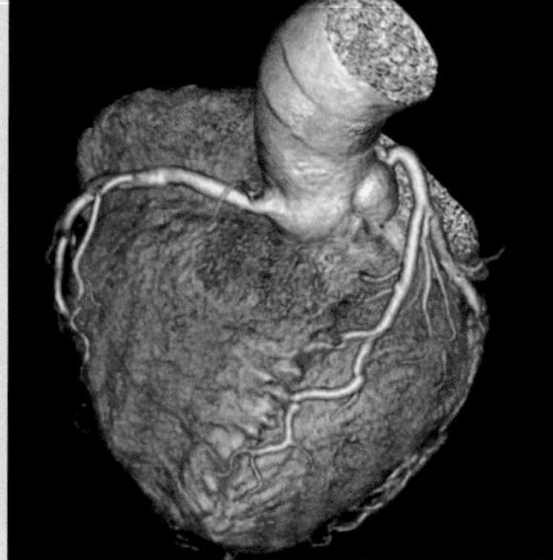

Normal RCA Origin

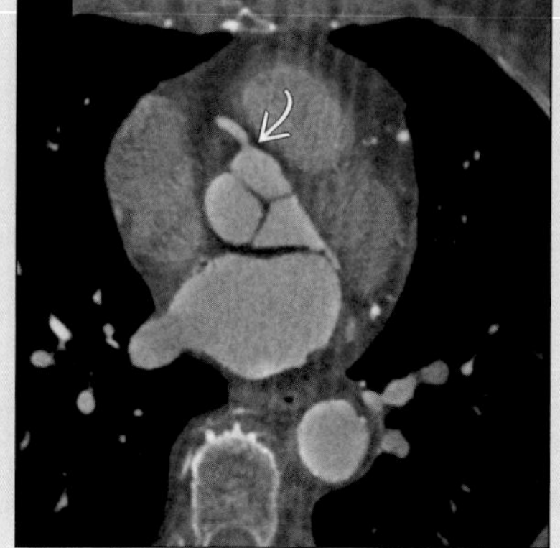

Normal RCA Origin

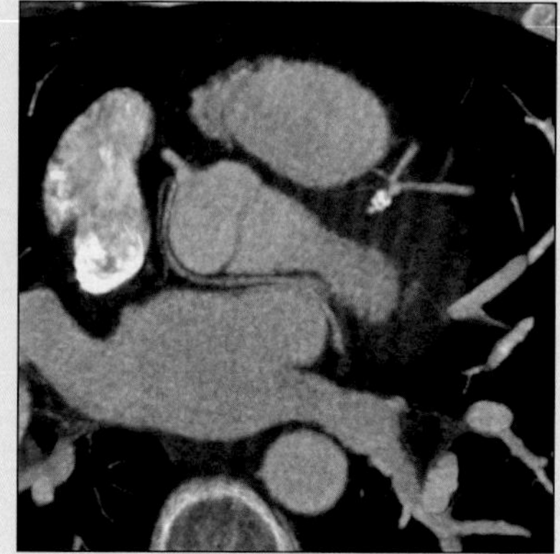

LCX Anomaly

ANOMALOUS ORIGIN RCA BENIGN/MALIGNANT

Key Facts

Terminology

- Malignant variant: Right coronary artery (RCA) originates from left sinus of Valsalva and courses between aorta and pulmonary artery
- Benign variant: RCA originates from left sinus of Valsalva and courses posterior and inferior to aortic root

Imaging Findings

- Absence of coronary artery ostium at the right sinus of Valsalva, but present right coronary artery more distally
- Benign variant is rare
- Malignant variant typically arises from left coronary cusp between origin of LM and anterior commissure
- May arise above sino-tubular junction, either above left or above junction of rt and lt sinus of Valsalva

DIFFERENTIAL DIAGNOSIS

Other Coronary Anomalies

- Anomalous left main may have similar intra arterial course compared to malignant anomalous RCA

Coronary Artery Fistula

- Abnormal vessels, but normal coronary ostium at sinus of Valsalva

PATHOLOGY

General Features

- Epidemiology: Primary congenital coronary anomalies have an incidence of 1-2%
- Associated abnormalities: Often isolated abnormality

Gross Pathologic & Surgical Features

- Slit-like ostium and intramural course of proximal "malignant" anomalous RCA is believed to have higher association with sudden cardiac death

CLINICAL ISSUES

Presentation

- Most common signs/symptoms: Often asymptomatic
- Other signs/symptoms: Malignant variants may present with sudden cardiac death or arrhythmia

Demographics

- Gender: No gender predisposition

Natural History & Prognosis

- Benign variant typically clinically silent
- Malignant coronary artery anomalies are second most common cause of sudden death in young athletes

DIAGNOSTIC CHECKLIST

Image Interpretation Pearls

- Right sinus of Valsalva without coronary artery ostium
- Abnormal vessel coursing behind (benign, uncommon) aortic root or between aorta and pulmonary artery (more common)

SELECTED REFERENCES

1. Dodd JD et al: Congenital anomalies of coronary artery origin in adults: 64-MDCT appearance. AJR Am J Roentgenol. 188(2):W138-46, 2007
2. Datta J et al: Anomalous coronary arteries in adults: depiction at multi-detector row CT angiography. Radiology. 235(3):812-8, 2005
3. Liberthson RR: Sudden death from cardiac causes in children and young adults. N Engl J Med. 334(16):1039-44, 1996

IMAGE GALLERY

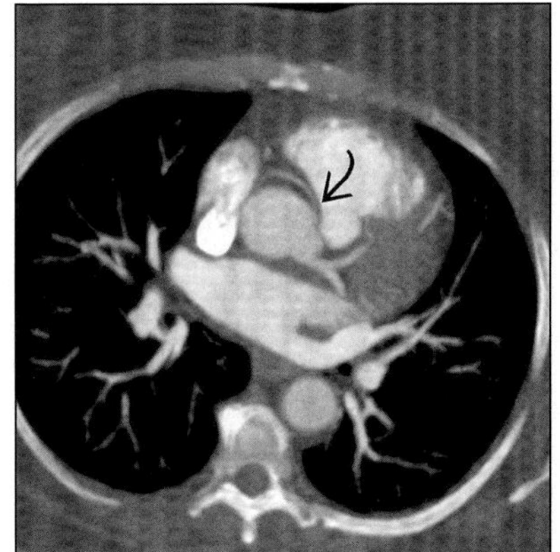

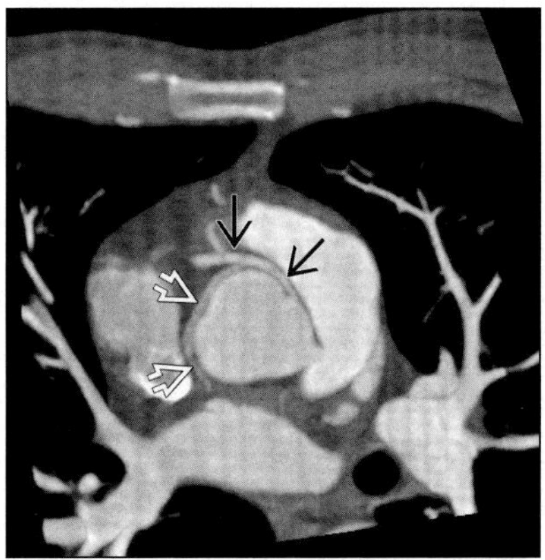

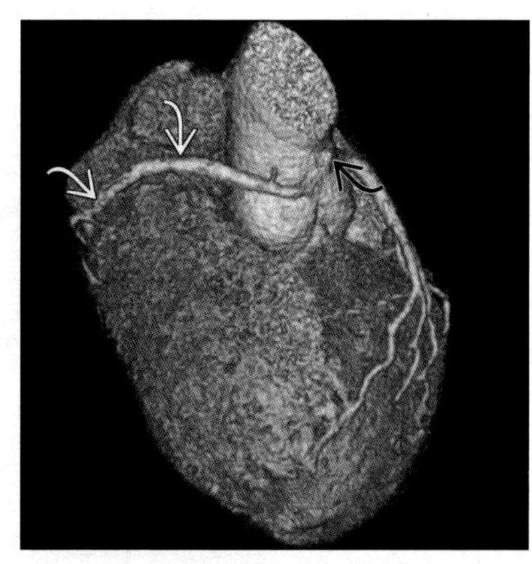

(Left) Oblique coronary CTA shows RCA originating from anterior edge of left sinus of Valsalva and coursing between the pulmonary artery and ascending aorta (malignant variant). Note: Narrowed ostium ➔. *(Center)* Oblique coronary CTA in a different patient shows anomalous RCA ➔ originating from left SOV & also taking a malignant course. Note: Sino-atrial nodal branch ➔. *(Right)* Oblique coronary CTA volume rendering shows malignant variant of RCA ➔ anomaly (dominant vessel). Note: RCA origin is above sino-tubular junction ➔.

BLAND-WHITE-GARLAND SYNDROME

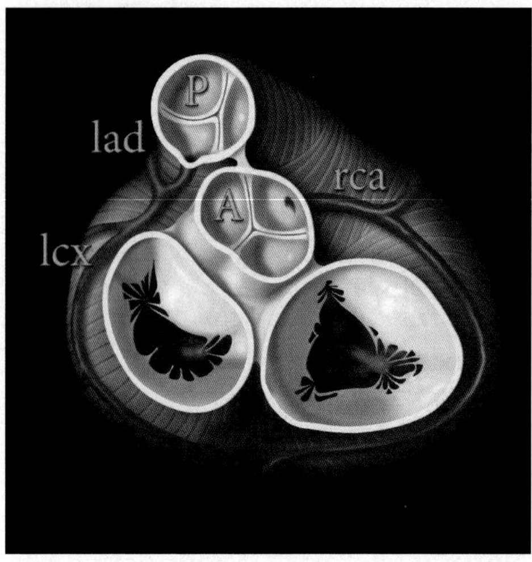

Graphic shows anomalous origin of the left coronary artery from the pulmonary artery.

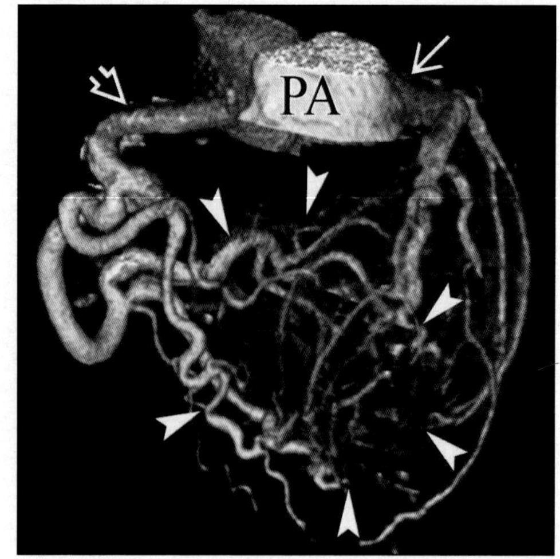

Coronary CTA 3-D image (cardiac chambers removed) shows anomalous LM origin ➡ from PA. Note multiple collateral vessels in LAD vascular territory (arrowheads) and dilated RCA ⇨. (Courtesy reference 3).

TERMINOLOGY

Abbreviations and Synonyms

- Anomalous left coronary artery from the pulmonary artery (ALCAPA)

Definitions

- Anomalous origin of a coronary artery from the pulmonary artery (PA)

IMAGING FINDINGS

General Features

- Best diagnostic clue: Left main coronary artery originates from the pulmonary artery
- Location: Left coronary artery originates from pulmonary artery then courses in its usual path down the anterior interventricular groove
- Size: Large left coronary artery, collaterals and right coronary artery with a left-to-right shunt

Imaging Recommendations

- Best imaging tool
  - Best non-invasive test: Coronary CTA
  - Cardiac MR a useful alternative
    - Does not currently have the spatial resolution of cardiac CTA
    - Does allow depiction of perfusion deficits
    - Delayed-enhanced gadolinium sequences allows detection of infarcted myocardium
  - Best invasive test: Coronary angiography

DIFFERENTIAL DIAGNOSIS

Other Coronary Artery Anomalies

- Anomalous vessels do not originate from PA

Coronary Fistula

- Normal origin of coronary artery, but abnormal branch vessels connecting to PA

DDx: Bland White Garland Syndrome

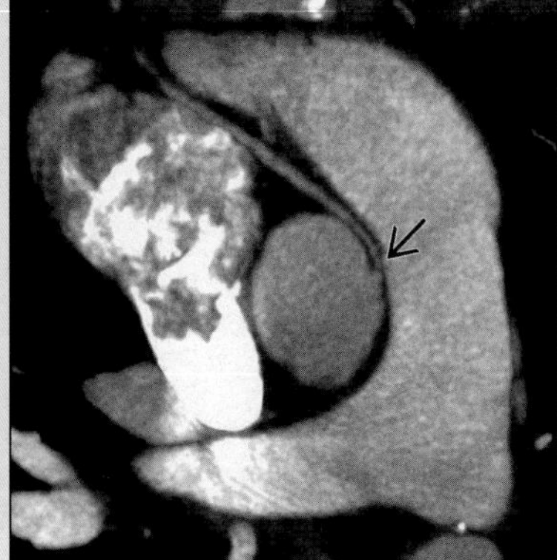

RCA from Left Coronary Sinus

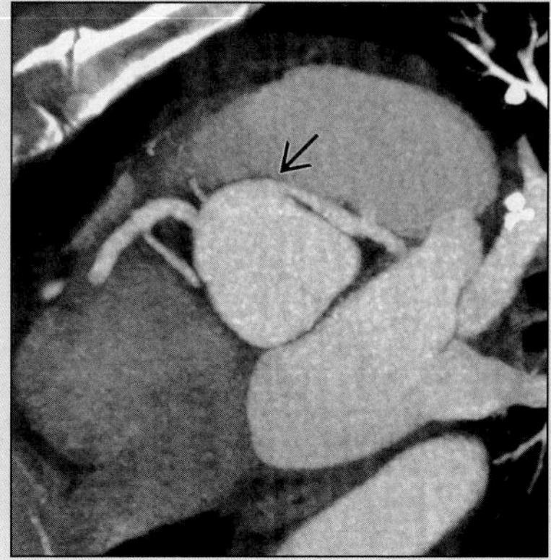

LM from Right Coronary Sinus

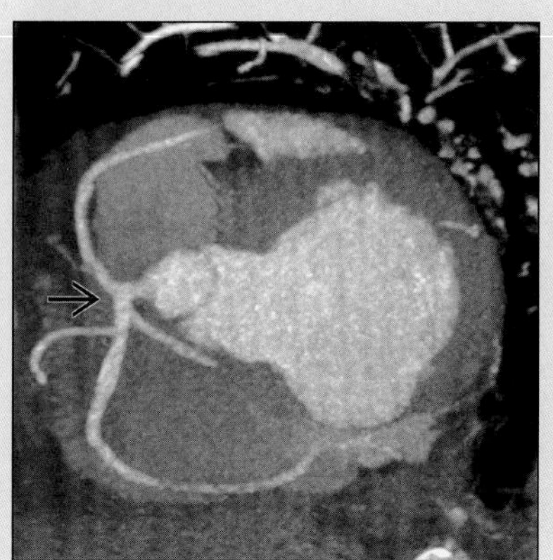

Single Coronary Artery

BLAND-WHITE-GARLAND SYNDROME

Key Facts

Terminology

- Anomalous origin of left coronary artery from the pulmonary artery

Imaging Findings

- Location: Left coronary artery originates from pulmonary artery then courses in its usual path down the anterior interventricular groove
- Size: Large left coronary artery, collaterals and right coronary artery with a left-to-right shunt
- Best non-invasive test: Coronary CTA

Clinical Issues

- 90% of patients present in infancy with heart failure
- Rare in adults; present with angina/myocardial infarction/heart failure
- Most commonly treated in infancy with direct re-implantation of anomalous coronary artery into aorta

PATHOLOGY

General Features

- Associated abnormalities: Coronary steal phenomenon, myocardial ischemia, myocardial infarction, congestive heart failure, mitral regurgitation

CLINICAL ISSUES

Presentation

- Most common signs/symptoms
  - Shortness of breath
  - Angina
  - Myocardial infarction

Demographics

- Age
  - 90% of patients present in infancy with heart failure
  - Rare in adults; present with angina/myocardial infarction/heart failure

Natural History & Prognosis

- Degree of survival into adulthood depends on degree of collateralization from the right coronary artery

Treatment

- Infants
  - Direct re-implantation of anomalous coronary artery into aorta
  - Intrapulmonary conduit from left coronary artery to the aorta
- Adults
  - Ligation of left coronary artery and bypass graft

DIAGNOSTIC CHECKLIST

Image Interpretation Pearls

- Absence of left main origin from left sinus of Valsalva differentiates ALCAPA from coronary fistula

SELECTED REFERENCES

1. Ichikawa M et al: Detection of Bland-White-Garland Syndrome by multislice computed tomography in an elderly patient. Int J Cardiol. 114(2):288-90, 2007
2. Choong CK et al: Bland-White-Garland syndrome in pregnancy: reoperation of ALCAPA with an internal thoracic radial artery "Y"-graft. Ann Thorac Surg. 81(4):1512-4, 2006
3. Kim SY et al: Coronary artery anomalies: classification and ECG-gated multi-detector row CT findings with angiographic correlation. Radiographics. 26(2):317-33; discussion 333-4, 2006
4. Mohrs OK et al: Assessment of nonviable myocardium due to Bland-White-Garland syndrome using contrast-enhanced MRI. J Cardiovasc Magn Reson. 6(4):941-4, 2004
5. Hansen A et al: Echocardiographic diagnosis of Bland-White-Garland syndrome. Heart. 85(2):152, 2001

IMAGE GALLERY

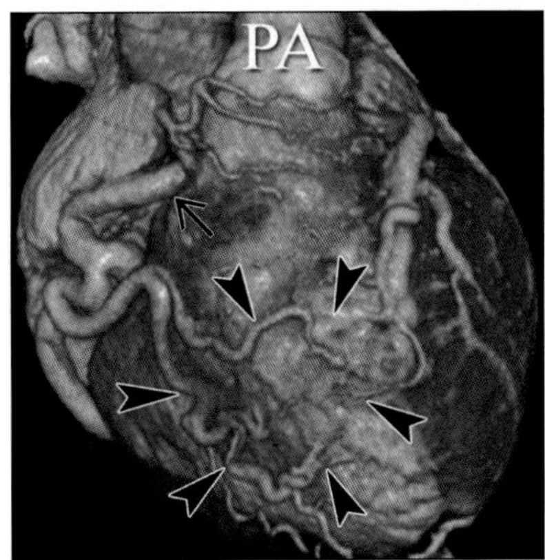

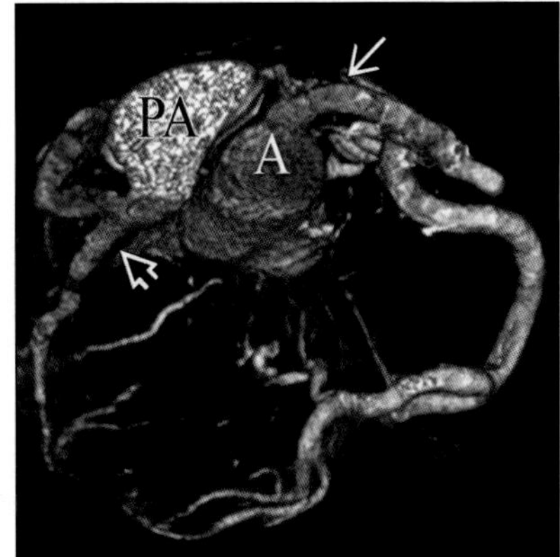

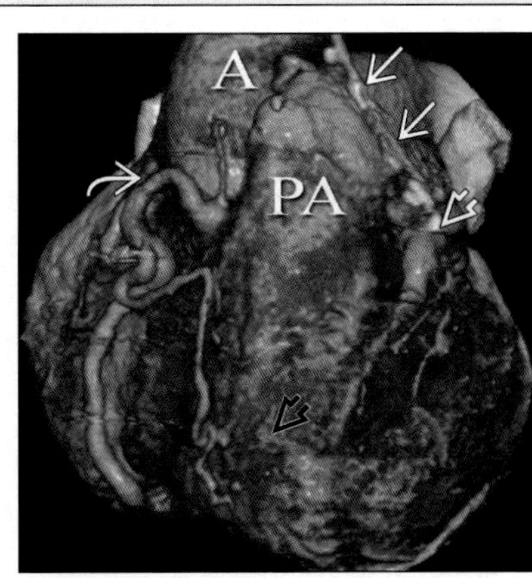

*(**Left**) Coronary CTA 3D image shows markedly dilated RCA → and multiple collateral vessels in LAD vascular territory (arrowheads). (**Center**) Coronary CTA 3D image shows anomalous origin of LM ➡ from PA. Note dilated RCA ➡ arising normally from aorta (A). (**Right**) Post-operative coronary CTA 3D image following ligation of LM os at PA & anastomosis between left internal mammary artery ➡ & LCA ➡. Note decrease in size of RCA ➡ & collaterals ⇨. (Courtesy reference 3).*

CORONARY EMBOLISM

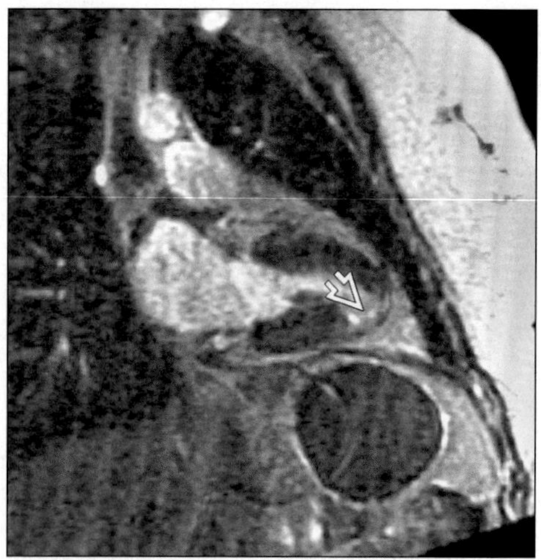

LV long axis delayed enhancement MR shows focal non-transmural subendocardial hyperenhancement ⇨ in inferior apical wall in patient with patent foramen ovale and clean coronaries by angiography.

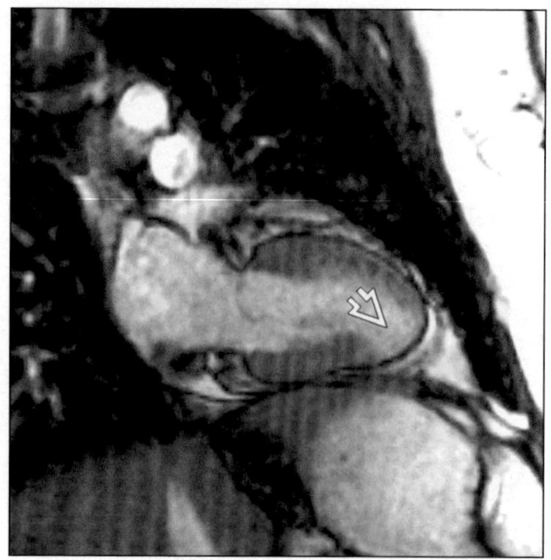

LV long axis SSFP MR of same patient as previous image shows transmural increased signal ⇨ indicating small acute infarct with corresponding edema.

TERMINOLOGY

Definitions

- Dislodged thrombus, tumor, cholesterol, air or fat obstructing coronary artery

IMAGING FINDINGS

General Features

- Best diagnostic clue
  - MR demonstrates focal subendocardial delayed hyper enhancement in presence of
    - Patent foramen ovale or atrial septal defect (ASD)
    - Left atrial appendage (LAA) thrombus
    - Left atrial (LA) myxoma or other mass

CT Findings

- Cardiac gated CTA
  - May show subtle subendocardial perfusion defect
  - Regional akinesis (stunning) but maintained global function
  - May demonstrate underlying pathology (myxoma, LAA thrombus, etc.)

MR Findings

- SSFP white blood cine
  - Focal wall motion abnormality with otherwise maintained global left ventricular (LV) function
- T2 weighted FSE
  - Edema adjacent to infarcted myocardium
- First pass perfusion
  - Focal subendocardial perfusion defect matching the delayed hyper enhancement
- Delayed enhancement
  - Focal area of delayed hyper enhancement based on the subendocardial myocardium

Angiographic Findings

- Invasive coronary angiography may demonstrate clean coronary arteries

Imaging Recommendations

- Best imaging tool: Cardiac MR is the best modality to suggest diagnosis
- Protocol advice: Include T1 pre and post-contrast images to exclude myocarditis

DDx: Delayed Enhancement Patterns in Coronary Artery Disease & Cardiomyopathy

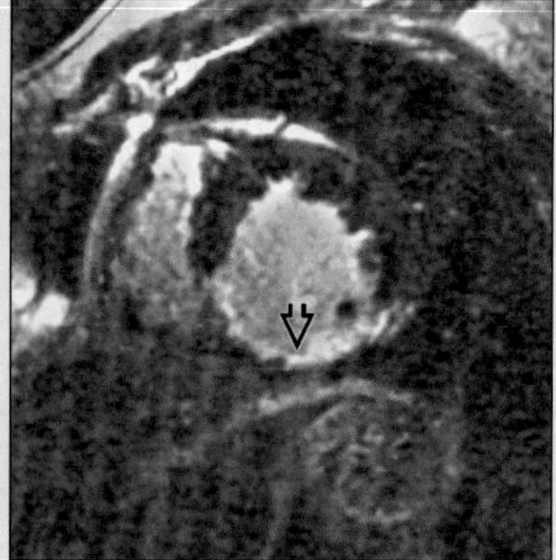

Chronic RCA Infarct

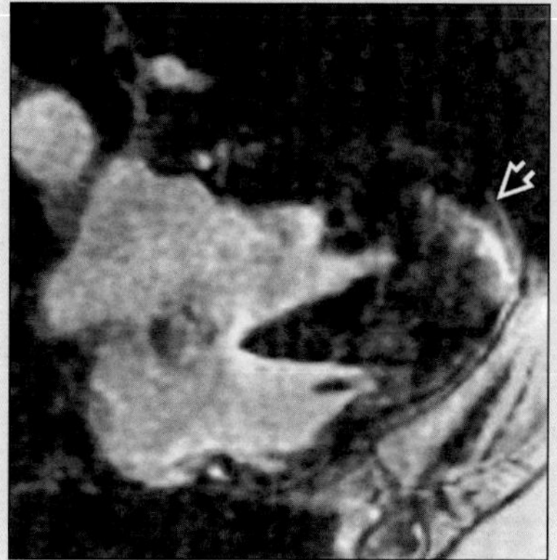

Apical Cardiomyopathy

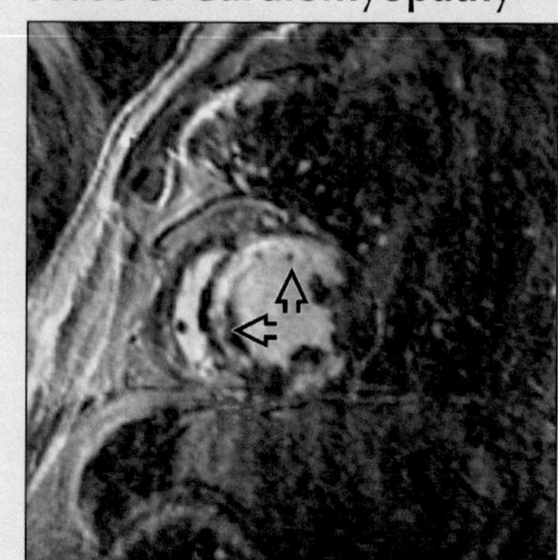

Acute LAD Infarct

CORONARY EMBOLISM

Key Facts

Terminology

- Dislodged thrombus, tumor, cholesterol, air or fat obstructing coronary artery

Imaging Findings

- MR demonstrates focal subendocardial delayed hyper enhancement in presence of
- Patent foramen ovale or atrial septal defect (ASD)
- Left atrial appendage (LAA) thrombus
- Left atrial (LA) myxoma or other mass
- Focal wall motion abnormality with otherwise maintained global left ventricular (LV) function
- Edema adjacent to infarcted myocardium
- Invasive coronary angiography may demonstrate clean coronary arteries

Top Differential Diagnoses

- Acute Myocardial Infarction due to Atherosclerotic Coronary Artery Disease
- Myocarditis

DIFFERENTIAL DIAGNOSIS

Acute Myocardial Infarction due to Atherosclerotic Coronary Artery Disease

- Associated coronary artery disease

Myocarditis

- Clean coronary arteries but elevated cardiac markers
- Linear mid-myocardial or sub epicardial hyper enhancement
- Increased relative global enhancement (myocardium vs. skeletal muscle)

PATHOLOGY

General Features

- Etiology
  - Dislodged thrombus from deep venous thrombosis or fat from long bone after fracture
  - Left atrial myxoma or other neoplasm
  - Plaque or cholesterol dislodged during coronary angioplasty
- Epidemiology: Rare
- Associated abnormalities: Deep venous thrombosis (DVT), left atrial appendix thrombus, LA myxoma or other tumor

Gross Pathologic & Surgical Features

- Usually small focal myocardial necrosis based on the subendocardial myocardium

CLINICAL ISSUES

Presentation

- Most common signs/symptoms
  - Usually atypical presentation due to small area of infarction
  - Chest pain, pain in chin, left arm or epigastrium
- Other signs/symptoms: Borderline elevated cardiac enzymes

Treatment

- Treat underlying cause
  - ASD closure device, resection of myxoma, treat DVT

DIAGNOSTIC CHECKLIST

Consider

- Coronary embolus is diagnosis of exclusion
  - Coronary artery disease with acute coronary syndrome and myocarditis need to be excluded

SELECTED REFERENCES

1. Duman D et al: Paradoxical mesentery embolism and silent myocardial infarction in primary antiphospholipid syndrome: a case report. Heart Surg Forum. 9(2):E592-4, 2006
2. Rana O et al: Images in clinical medicine. Cholesterol emboli after coronary angioplasty. N Engl J Med. 354(12):1294, 2006

IMAGE GALLERY

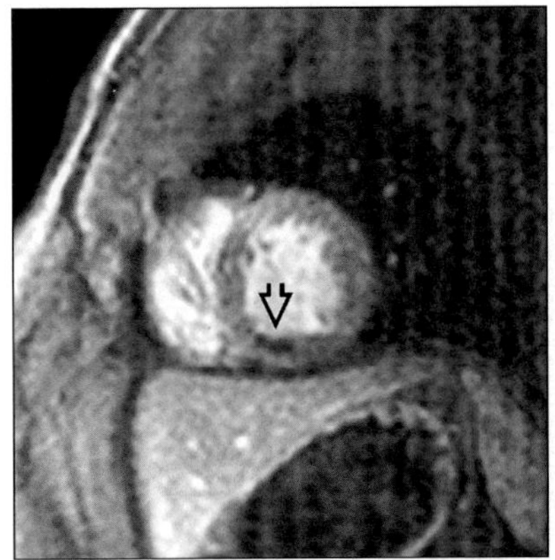
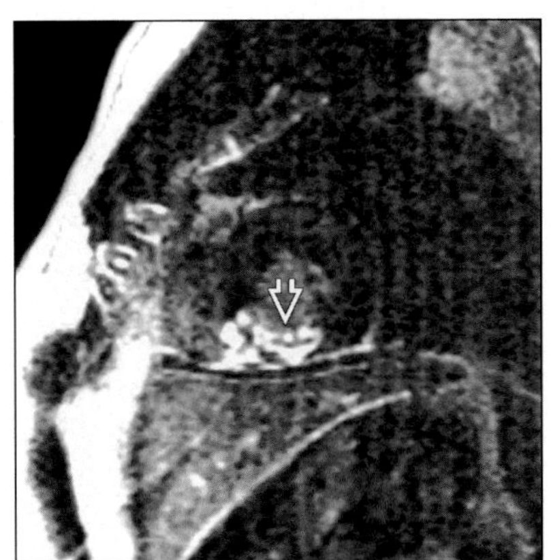
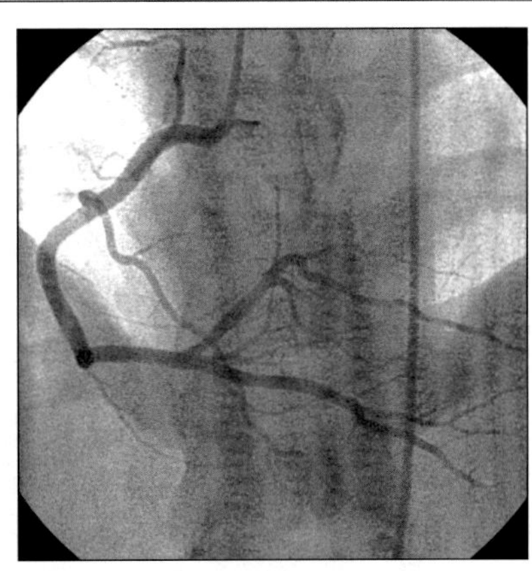

*(**Left**) LV short axis MR first pass perfusion image in patient with patent foramen ovale shows subendocardial perfusion defect ⇨ in inferior septal wall. (**Center**) LV short axis delayed enhanced image of same patient as previous image shows subendocardial based hyperenhancement with central dark area of microvascular obstruction ➡, indicating ischemic injury. (**Right**) Invasive coronary angiogram of dominant RCA shows no evidence of coronary artery disease suggesting embolus with interval resolution as etiology for ischemic myocardial injury.*

CORONARY ARTERY ANEURYSM

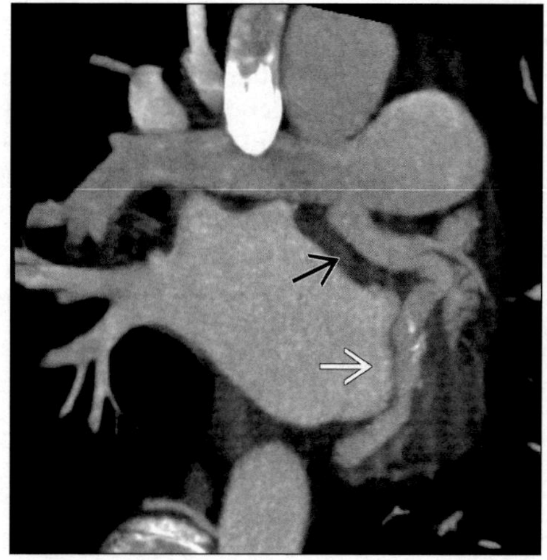

Oblique coronary CTA shows left main ➔ and left circumflex ➔ aneurysm in a 37 year old male with childhood history of Kawasaki disease.

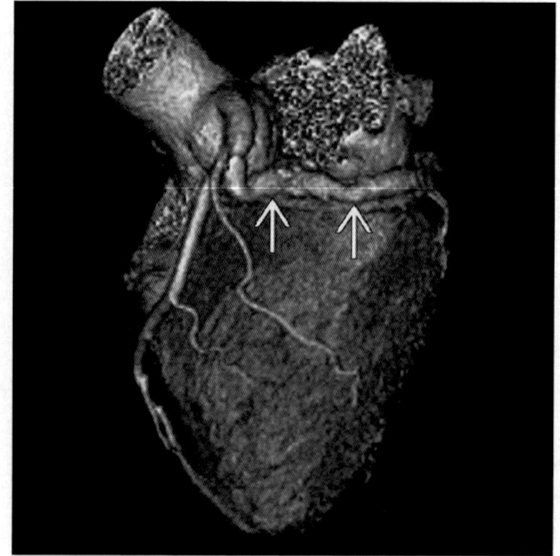

Left anterior oblique cardiac CT shows left circumflex coronary aneurysm ➔ in a volume rendered image also of the same patient as previous image.

TERMINOLOGY

Definitions

- Coronary artery diameter > 1.5 times normal adjacent segments

IMAGING FINDINGS

General Features

- Best diagnostic clue: Dilatation of coronary artery
- Morphology
  - Fusiform or saccular dilatation
    - Can be thrombosed or dissected

CT Findings

- Cardiac Gated CTA
  - Aneurysmal dilatation well-depicted
  - Calcification frequently present in atherosclerosis
  - Detects mural thrombus that may be occult on invasive angiography

MR Findings

- Can use coronary angiography sequence
  - Lumen dark on double IR FSE
  - Bright on GRE or b-SSFP unless thrombus
  - Difficult to detect calcification

Echocardiographic Findings

- Transthoracic and transesophageal echocardiogram
  - Aneurysm detection in proximal coronaries

Angiographic Findings

- Coronary angiography findings
  - Fusiform and saccular dilation of coronary arteries
  - Can underestimate size if mural thrombus is present

Imaging Recommendations

- Best imaging tool: Gated coronary CTA

DIFFERENTIAL DIAGNOSIS

Coronary Fistula

- Usually has dilated portion of fistula branch
- Coronary ectasia proximal to fistula if large shunt/steal

Pseudoaneurysms

- Post-trauma/surgery → ascending aorta common site

DDx: Other Aneurysms

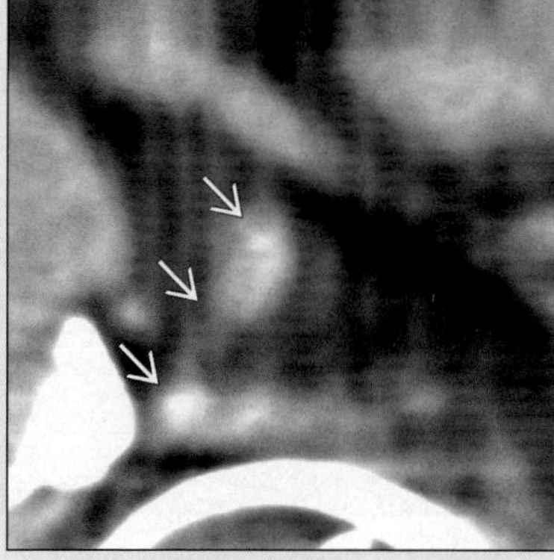

False Aneurysm

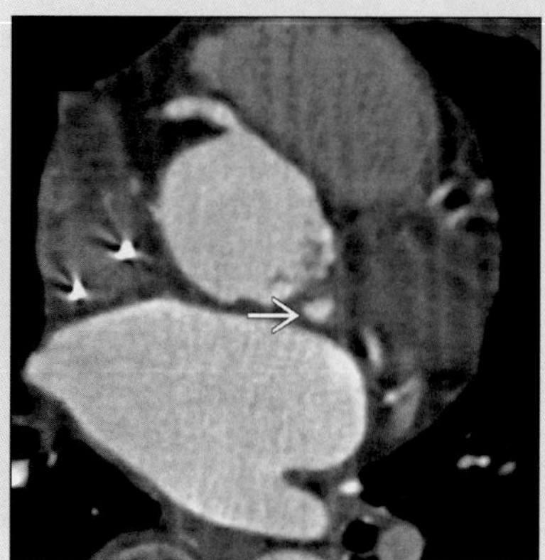

False Aneurysm

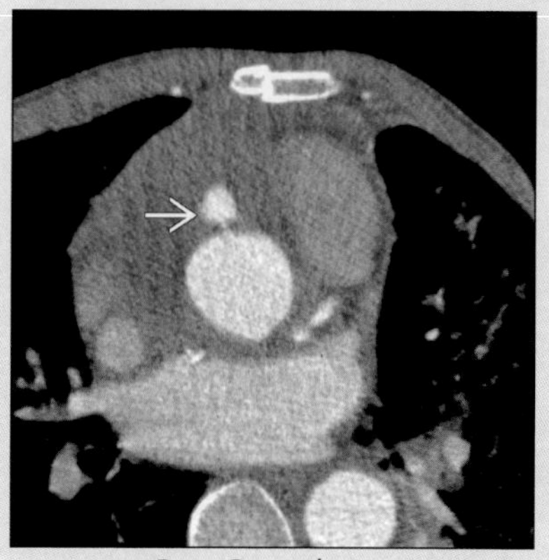

Post Cannulation

CORONARY ARTERY ANEURYSM

Key Facts

Terminology
- Coronary artery diameter > 1.5 times normal adjacent segments

Imaging Findings
- Best diagnostic clue: Dilatation of coronary artery
- Best imaging tool: Gated coronary CTA
  - Invasive angiography may underestimate luminal diameter if mural thrombus present

Pathology
- Atherosclerosis most common in USA
- Kawasaki disease most common worldwide
- Other: Congenital, trauma, procedural (angioplasty, stent, laser, atherectomy), mycotic emboli, dissection, connective tissue disease (SLE, Marfan, Behcet)

Clinical Issues
- Can be asymptomatic
- Can result in thrombosis and myocardial infarction

PATHOLOGY

General Features
- General path comments: Depends on etiology
- Etiology
  - Atherosclerosis most common in USA
  - Kawasaki disease most common worldwide
  - Other: Congenital, trauma, procedural (angioplasty, stent, laser, atherectomy), mycotic emboli, dissection, connective tissue disease (SLE, Marfan, Behcet)
- Epidemiology: 4.9% angiograms, 1.5% necropsy
- Associated abnormalities: Atherosclerosis

Gross Pathologic & Surgical Features
- Dilatation of coronary artery, may have thrombus

Microscopic Features
- In atherosclerosis, may demonstrate thinning or destruction of media

CLINICAL ISSUES

Presentation
- Most common signs/symptoms
  - Can be asymptomatic
  - Acute coronary syndrome, CHF that may be caused by aneurysm or concurrent disease
- Clinical Profile
  - Can result in thrombosis and myocardial infarction
  - Incidental finding on coronary angiography

Demographics
- Gender: Male predominant

Natural History & Prognosis
- Related to severity of concomitant obstructive disease in patients with atherosclerosis

Treatment
- Anticoagulants, antiplatelet therapy
- Bypass and exclusion of aneurysm
- Covered stent graph

DIAGNOSTIC CHECKLIST

Consider
- Angina or acute myocardial infarction in patient under 20 should prompt search for aneurysm

SELECTED REFERENCES

1. Murthy PA et al: MDCT of coronary artery aneurysms. AJR Am J Roentgenol. 184(3 Suppl):S19-20, 2005
2. Waller BF: Nonatherosclerotic coronary heart disease. In: Hurst JW, et al. (eds). The Heart, 11th ed. McGraw-Hill, New York. 1181, 2004
3. Glickel SZ et al: Coronary artery aneurysm. Ann Thorac Surg. 25(4):372-6, 1978

IMAGE GALLERY

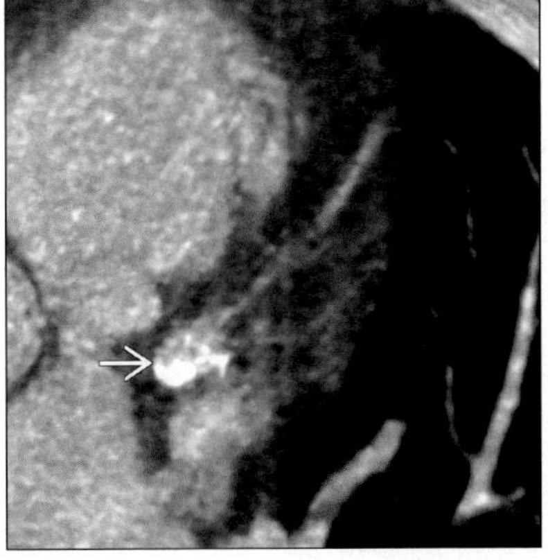

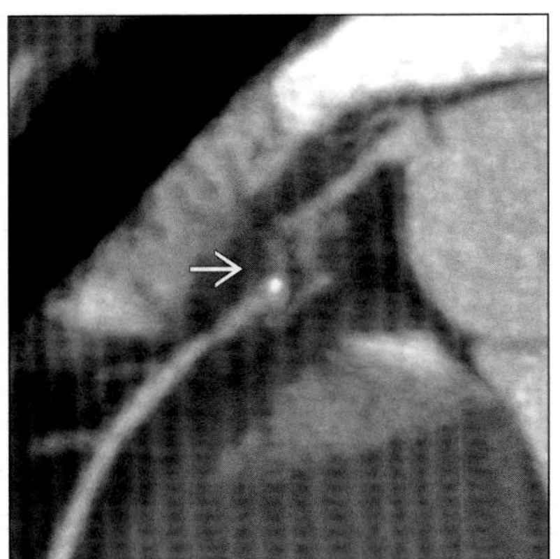

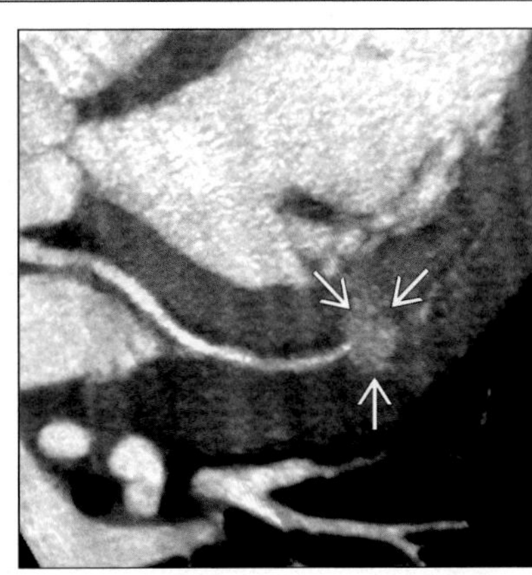

(Left) *Oblique coronary CTA shows partly calcified aneurysm in proximal LAD ➡. Adjacent coronary segments had stenotic lesions, indicating atherosclerosis as underlying disease.* ***(Center)*** *Oblique CECT shows recanalized thrombosed aneurysm in patient with Kawasaki disease ➡.* ***(Right)*** *Curved MPR coronary CTA shows left obtuse marginal coronary pseudoaneurysm ➡ following balloon angioplasty.*

CORONARY CALCIFICATION

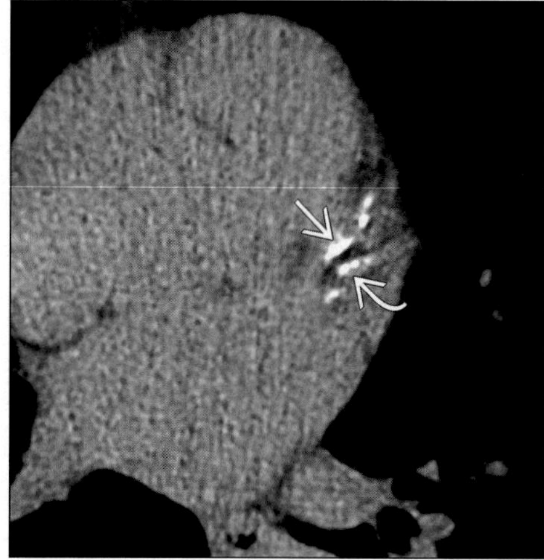

Axial gated nonenhanced cardiac CT obtained for coronary calcium scoring shows calcification in left anterior descending coronary artery ➡, and a diagonal branch ⮫.

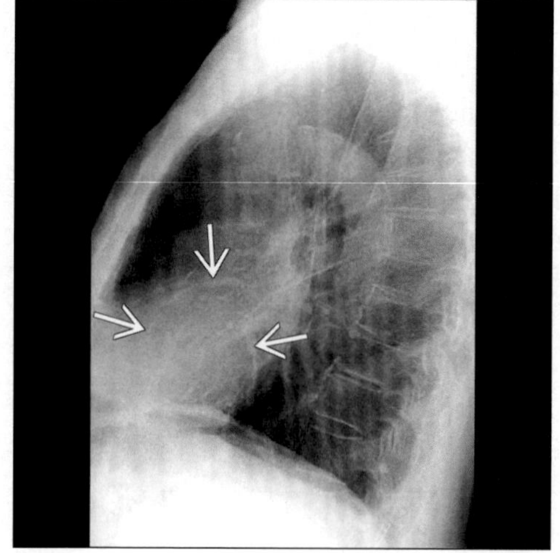

Lateral radiograph shows classic appearance of coronary calcifications ➡. Visibility of coronary calcium on radiographs indicates extensive coronary artery disease. (Courtesy H. Mann, MD).

TERMINOLOGY

Definitions

- Deposition of calcium hydroxyapatite in atherosclerotic plaque
- Quantitative software used to analyze non-contrast gated CT scan yields coronary artery calcium score (CACS)

IMAGING FINDINGS

General Features

- Best diagnostic clue: Identification of 3 or more contiguous pixels of increased attenuation (> 130 HU) in the wall of a coronary artery

Radiographic Findings

- Radiography: Low sensitivity

Fluoroscopic Findings

- Low sensitivity: Only 52% of calcific deposits seen on EBCT could be detected

CT Findings

- NECT
  - Calcium labeling threshold is 130 HU
  - Plaques have area of at least 3 contiguous pixels
  - Scoring predicated on use of 3 mm thick slices
  - Volume score is sum of area of calcific plaque
  - Agatston score weighs each plaque by a cofactor derived from peak plaque attenuation coefficient
    - Cofactor 1 for HU 131-200
    - Cofactor 2 for HU 201-300
    - Cofactor 3 for peak HU 301-400
    - Cofactor 4 for peak HU 401+
  - Risk stratification not significantly affected by scoring technique
  - Most studies use Agatston scoring
  - Volume scoring does not use cofactor and therefore is more reproducible
  - Can calculate calcium mass using phantom reference
- Electron beam CT (EBCT)
  - Temporal resolution up to 33 msec freezes coronary artery motion
  - Over 600 articles published validating use of EBCT

DDx: Other Calcifications

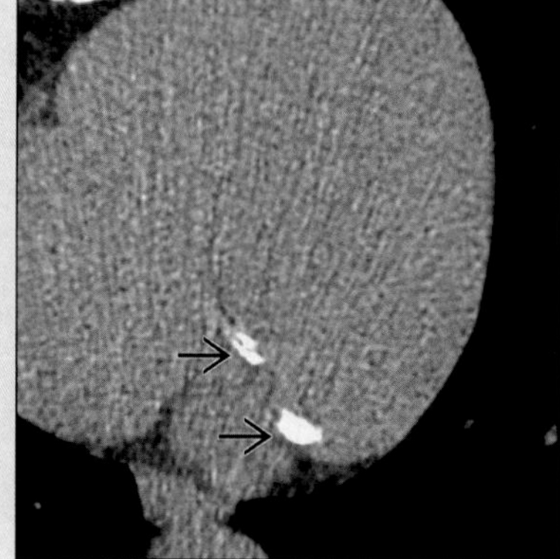

Mitral Annular Calcium

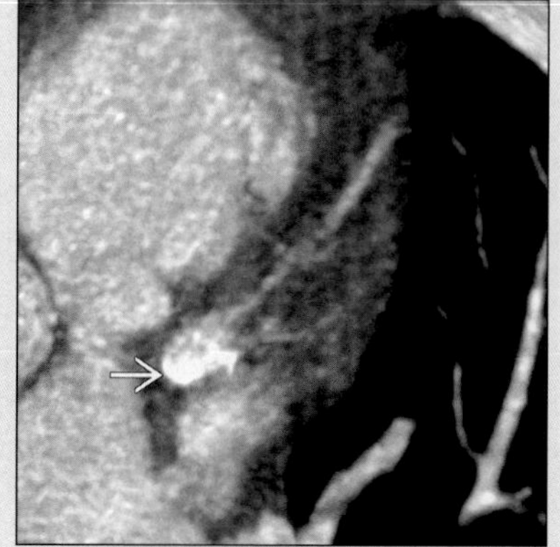

Calcified Aneurysm

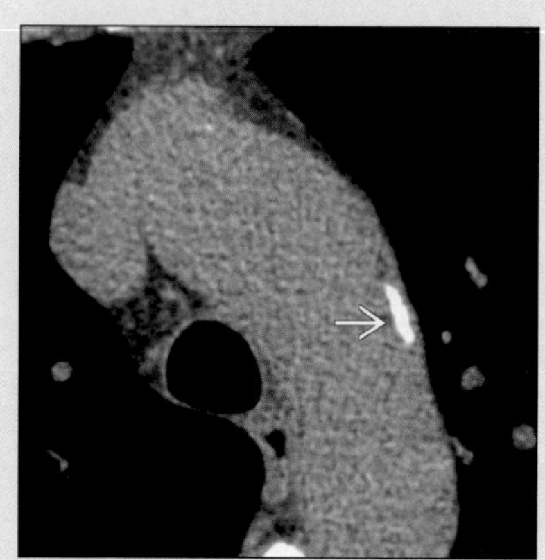

Aortic Calcium

CORONARY CALCIFICATION

Key Facts

Terminology

- Deposition of calcium hydroxyapatite in atherosclerotic plaque
- Quantitative software used to analyze non-contrast gated CT scan yields coronary artery calcium score (CACS)

Imaging Findings

- Best diagnostic clue: Identification of 3 or more contiguous pixels of increased attenuation (> 130 HU) in the wall of a coronary artery
- Volume score is sum of area of calcific plaque
- Agatston score weighs each plaque by a cofactor derived from peak plaque attenuation coefficient

Pathology

- Calcium is a frequent finding in atherosclerotic plaque
- Represents about 20% of total plaque burden
- Functions as a "marker" for plaque burden

Clinical Issues

- Part of risk assessment algorithms used to select candidates for cholesterol lowering drug therapy
- Meta-Analysis on prognostic value of CACS in ACCF/AHA consensus document yielded a 3-5 yr relative risk ratio (RR) of CHD of 4.3 (95% confidence interval = 3.5 to 5.2) for any measurable calcium

    - Low dose
    - Poor photon flux results in poor SNR
    - Limited access to scanners
- Multidetector row CT
    - Widespread availability
    - Good correlation with EBCT over large range of calcium values
    - Temporal resolution limited by mechanical speed of gantry rotation
    - Axial mode
        - Prospective gating
        - Low dose
    - Helical mode
        - Retrospective gating
        - Higher dose

Imaging Recommendations

- Best imaging tool: Multidetector row CT

DIFFERENTIAL DIAGNOSIS

Soft Atherosclerotic Plaque

- Not seen on non contrast-enhanced CT
- Can be present along with calcified plaques
- Presence of extensive calcified plaque can interfere with evaluation of coronary stenosis

Annular Calcification

- Corresponds to location of valve annulus

Calcification of an Infarct

- Calcification in myocardium

Calcification of Aortic Wall

- Must avoid aortic wall calcification in calculation of CACS

Pericardial Calcification

- Seen with constrictive pericarditis

PATHOLOGY

General Features

- General path comments
    - Calcium found at advanced stage of atherosclerotic plaque development
        - Calcium hydroxyapatite deposition a regulated process similar to osteogenesis
    - Calcified plaques are unlikely to rupture
    - Amount of calcified plaque is correlated with amount of "soft" vulnerable plaque
        - Calcified plaque represents about 20% of total plaque burden

Gross Pathologic & Surgical Features

- Positive correlation between amount of CAC and percent stenosis at same site
- Correlation nonlinear with large confidence limits

CLINICAL ISSUES

Presentation

- Clinical Profile
    - Part of risk assessment algorithms used to select candidates for cholesterol lowering drug therapy
    - Identify conditions that render risk assessment superfluous (established atherosclerotic cardiovascular disease)
    - Identify presence of major risk factors: Smoking, hypertension, low HDL cholesterol, family history of premature coronary artery disease
        - Family history includes myocardial infarction (MI), unstable angina, stable angina, coronary artery procedures, evidence of myocardial ischemia in a male first-degree relative < 55 yo or female first-degree relative < 65 yo
    - If 2 or more major risk factors are present, estimate 10 year likelihood for development of major coronary events

- Framingham Heart Study (FHS) risk for "hard" events (MI, death) can be calculated online (http://hin.nhbli.nih.gov/atpiii/calculator.asp)
- Other risk assessment algorithms are PROspective CArdiovascular Munster (PROCAM) and Systemic COronary Risk Evaluation (SCORE)

- National Cholesterol Education Program (NCEP) categories of 10 year absolute risk of hard event
  - High risk: CHD, CHD risk equivalents including 2+ major risk factors plus 10 year FHS risk for hard CHD greater than 20%
  - Moderately high risk: 2+ major risk factors plus 10 year FHS risk for hard CHD 10-20%
  - Moderate risk: 2+ major risk factors plus 10 year FHS risk for hard CHD less than 10%
  - Lower risk: 0 to 1 major risk factor (10 year FHS risk for hard CHD usually less than 10%)
- Predictive power of risk assessment tools measured by area under receiver-operating characteristic (ROC) curve
  - Central question in evaluating efficacy of CACS is whether it increases area under ROC curve compared to clinical risk factors alone
- Meta-Analysis on prognostic value of CACS in ACCF/AHA consensus document yielded a 3-5 yr relative risk ratio (RR) of CHD of 4.3 (95% confidence interval = 3.5 to 5.2) for any measurable calcium
  - CACS 1-112 had RR 1.9
  - CACS 100-400 had RR 4.3
  - CACS 400-999 had RR 7.2
  - CACS 1000+ had RR 10.8
- Bayes theorem should restrict use of CACS to FHS intermediate risk patients (10-20% risk of CHD over 10 years); for these patients, annual hard event rates
  - CACS 0-99 rate 0.4% per year
  - CACS 100-399 rate 1.3% per year
  - CACS 400 rate 2.4% per year
  - Therefore, FHS intermediate risk patient with CACS > 400 upgraded to high risk

- Coronary calcification in symptomatic patients
  - Presence of any calcium is sensitive but not specific for presence of obstructive coronary disease (greater than 50% luminal stenosis)
    - Similar performance to nuclear exercise testing, though no information about exercise tolerance
  - Can be used to distinguish ischemic cardiomyopathy from primary dilated cardiomyopathy
  - Helps triage of emergency department patients with chest pain
    - Small studies show sensitivities of 98-100% for identifying patients with acute MI with high negative predictive value

Demographics

- Age: Incidence increases from only a few percent in the second decade of life to nearly 100% by the 8th decade
- Gender
  - General incidence in women is similar to that in men who are a decade younger
  - Separation in prevalence with age is eliminated by age 70

Natural History & Prognosis

- Progression of CACS measured as percentage of baseline score
- Annual CACS progression 14-27% (average 24%)
- Need to factor in interscan variability when evaluating progression
  - Approximately 15%
  - Standard deviation 10%
- Rapid progression (> 15% per year) increases RR of MI
- Stable CACS associated with low risk of cardiovascular events
- Statins not proven to effect CACS progression

Treatment

- Progressively more aggressive lipid lowering regimes with increasing CAC scores

DIAGNOSTIC CHECKLIST

Consider

- Reconstructing full field of view images with 5 mm slice thickness to evaluate extracardiac structures
  - Lung nodules requiring follow-up in 2-5%

Image Interpretation Pearls

- Avoid measuring plaque in aortic wall near origins of right coronary artery and left main coronary artery

SELECTED REFERENCES

1. Greenland P et al: ACCF/AHA 2007 clinical expert consensus document on coronary artery calcium scoring by computed tomography in global cardiovascular risk assessment and in evaluation of patients with chest pain: a report of the American College of Cardiology Foundation Clinical Expert Consensus Task Force (ACCF/AHA Writing Committee to Update the 2000 Expert Consensus Document on Electron Beam Computed Tomography) developed in collaboration with the Society of Atherosclerosis Imaging and Prevention and the Society of Cardiovascular Computed Tomography. J Am Coll Cardiol. 49(3):378-402, 2007
2. Hecht HS et al: Coronary artery calcium scanning: Clinical paradigms for cardiac risk assessment and treatment. Am Heart J. 151(6):1139-46, 2006
3. Rumberger JA: Clinical use of coronary calcium scanning with computed tomography. Cardiol Clin. 21(4):535-47, 2003
4. O'Rourke RA et al: American College of Cardiology/American Heart Association Expert Consensus document on electron-beam computed tomography for the diagnosis and prognosis of coronary artery disease. Circulation. 102(1):126-40, 2000

CORONARY CALCIFICATION

IMAGE GALLERY

Typical

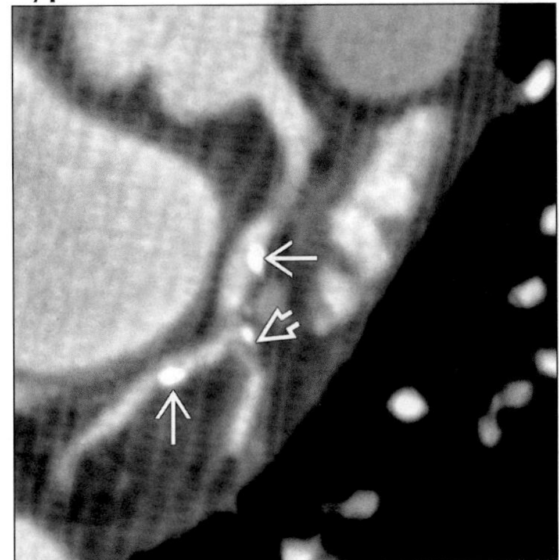

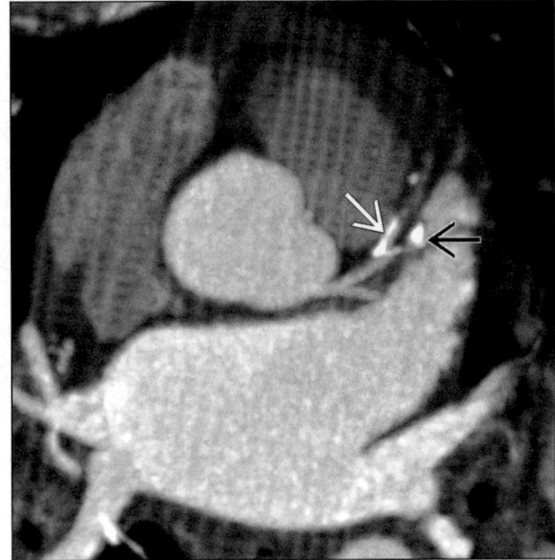

(Left) *Oblique CECT shows calcified plaque in left circumflex artery ➡. A mixed plaque (calcified and non-calcified components) at the ostium of the obtuse marginal branch ➡ is causing a stenosis.* ***(Right)*** *Axial coronary CTA maximum intensity projection image shows calcified plaque within the LAD ➡ and a diagonal branch →.*

Typical

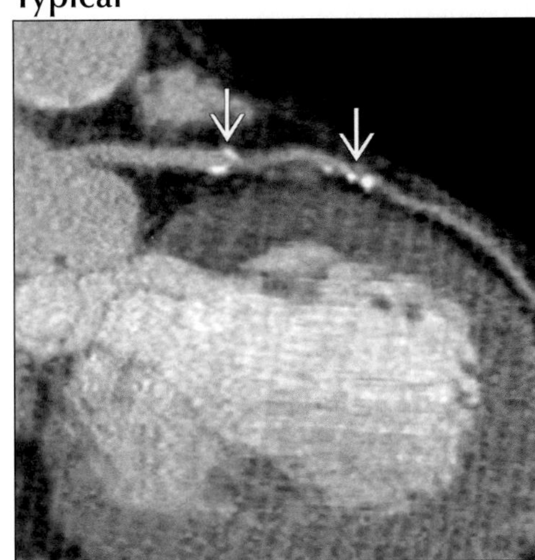

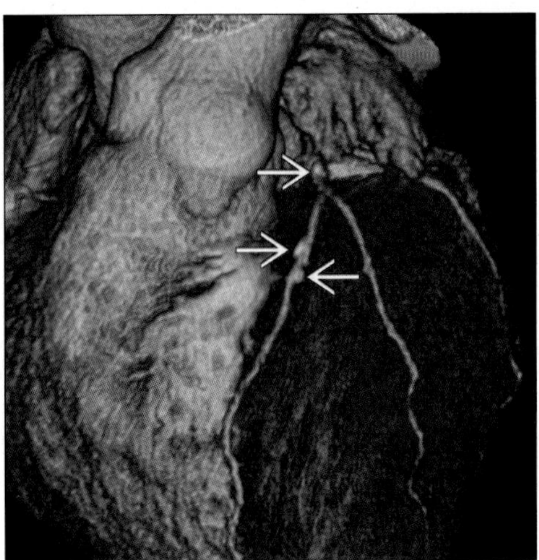

(Left) *Oblique CTA shows coronary artery calcification ➡ within LAD, making it difficult to judge the underlying lumen for significant stenosis.* ***(Right)*** *Coronal coronary CTA volume rendering image shows coronary calcium ➡ as bright thickened structures on the coronary arteries, and therefore preclude exclusion of stenoses on 3D imaging.*

Typical

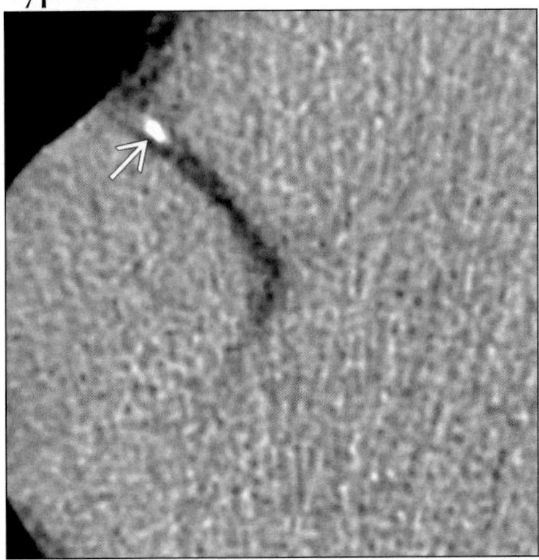

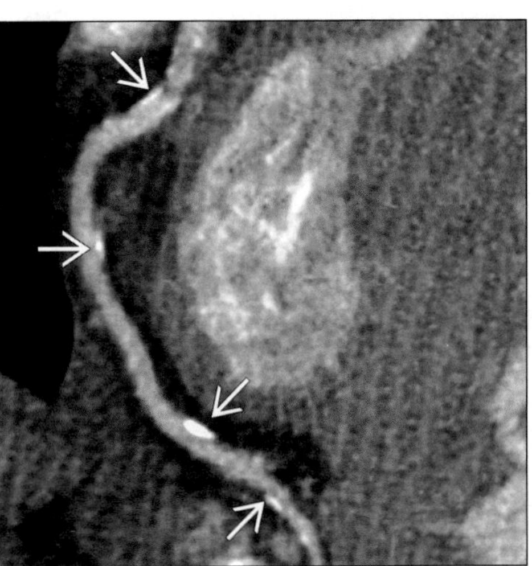

(Left) *Axial NECT shows calcium in the right atrioventricular groove ➡, indicating right coronary artery plaque.* ***(Right)*** *Curved MPR coronary CTA shows multiple calcified plaques ➡ within right coronary artery.*

CORONARY ATHEROSCLEROTIC PLAQUE

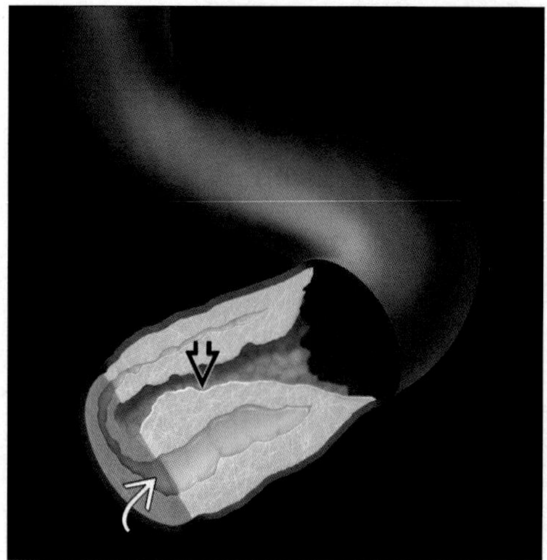

Graphic shows atheroma with relatively thick fibrous cap ⊳ and lipid rich core ➡ with significant stenosis. Vulnerable plaque are thin cap fibroatheromas with much thinner caps.

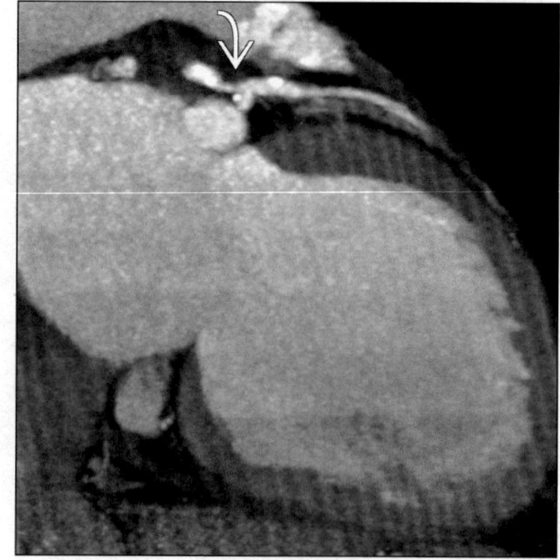

Coronary CTA two-chamber view shows atherosclerotic low density non-calcified potentially "vulnerable" plaque ➡ in the left main coronary artery (so-called widow maker).

TERMINOLOGY

Definitions

- Coronary atherosclerosis occurs when deposits of fatty substances, cholesterol, cellular waste products, calcium and other substances build up in the inner lining of a coronary artery
    - This build up is called coronary plaque

IMAGING FINDINGS

General Features

- Best diagnostic clue: Narrowing of coronary artery lumen
- Location: Occur in any part of coronary arterial tree
- Size
    - Controversial
        - Most consider low grade (minimal luminal narrowing) lesions with a lipid rich core and thin fibrous cap (vulnerable plaque) most prone to rupture
        - Usually do not cause significant luminal narrowing, but can be large due to positive remodeling
        - Ultimate event causing myocardial infarction is rupture of fibrous cap and subsequent luminal thrombosis
        - Some consider high grade lesions to have the highest individual risk of occlusion
- Morphology
    - Eight plaque types are based on five phases of atherosclerosis
        - A: Rupture-prone plaque with lipid rich core and thin fibrosus cap infiltrated by macrophages
        - B: Ruptured plaque with sub-occlusive thrombus and early organization
        - C: Erosion-prone plaque with proteoglycan matrix in a smooth muscle cell-rich plaque
        - D: Eroded plaque with sub-occlusive thrombus
        - E: Intraplaque hemorrhage secondary to leaking vasa vasorum
        - F: Calcific nodule protruding into the vessel lumen
        - G: Chronic stenotic plaque with severe calcification, old thrombus, eccentric lumen

DDx: Coronary Atherosclerosis

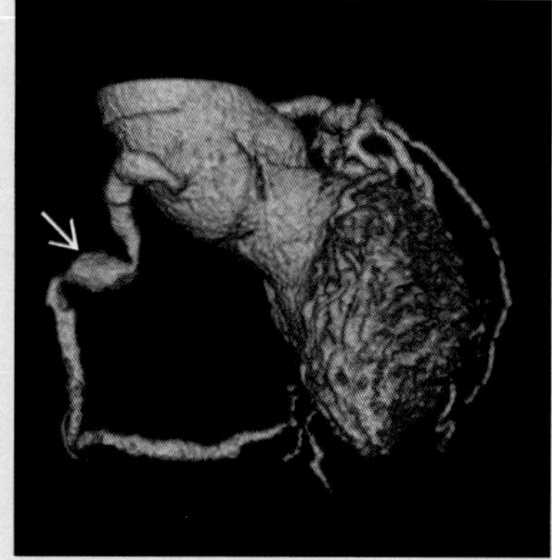

Kawasaki Disease

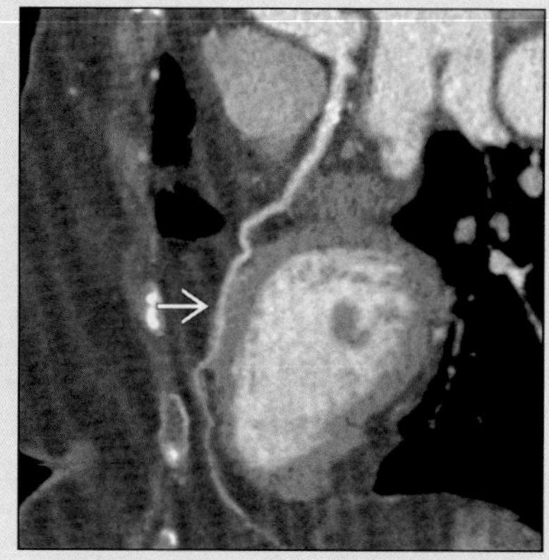

Myocardial Bridge

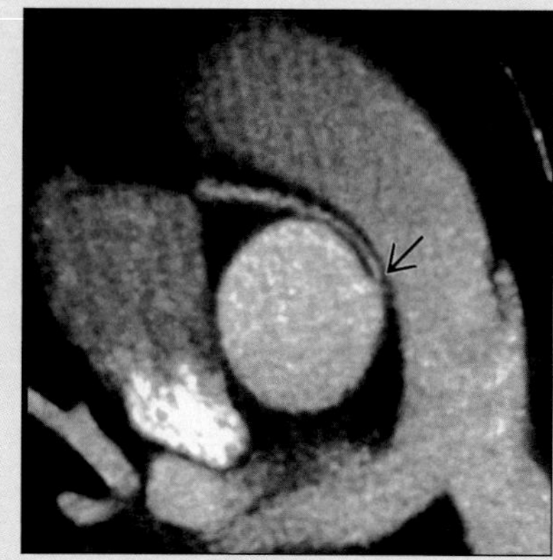

Anomalous Coronary Origin

CORONARY ATHEROSCLEROTIC PLAQUE

Key Facts

Terminology

- Coronary atherosclerosis occurs when deposits of fatty substances, cholesterol, cellular waste products, calcium and other substances build up in the inner lining of a coronary artery
- This build up is called coronary plaque

Imaging Findings

- Most consider low grade (minimal luminal narrowing) lesions with a lipid rich core and thin fibrous cap (vulnerable plaque) most prone to rupture
- Ultimate event causing myocardial infarction is rupture of fibrous cap and subsequent luminal thrombosis
- Eight plaque types are based on five phases of atherosclerosis
- CTA differentiates calcified and non-calcified plaque but not lipid rich and fibrous plaques
- Large potential, as invasive coronary angiography underestimates burden of soft plaque
- Coronary MR has potential for accurate plaque characterization
- Intravascular ultrasound (IVUS) can detect diseased segments in angiographic normal coronaries

Clinical Issues

- Atherosclerotic plaque develops over several years, usually without symptoms
- Plaque erosion and rupture with associated thrombus account for the bulk of acute infarcts
- HMG-CoA reductase inhibitors (statins) reduce coronary events in primary and secondary prevention trials

CT Findings

- NECT
  - Highly accurate in detection of coronary artery calcified plaque
    - Coronary calcified plaque is an independent predictor of subsequent hard myocardial events (myocardial infarction/death) in symptomatic and asymptomatic individuals
    - High sensitivity, low specificity, therefore is less useful for individual patient risk stratification
- CTA
  - CTA differentiates calcified and non-calcified plaque but not lipid rich and fibrous plaques
    - Large potential, as invasive coronary angiography underestimates burden of soft plaque
    - CTA shows considerable overlap in attenuation values between "vulnerable" lipid rich and stable fibrous plaque types

MR Findings

- Coronary MR has potential for accurate plaque characterization
  - Spin echo T2-weighted imaging
    - Intra-plaque lipid appears bright
    - Muscularis and external elastic lamina are dark
    - Adventitial fat (triglyceride rich) is bright
  - Multispectral imaging
    - T1WI, T2WI, TOF, PDWI techniques combined to identify components
    - Identify calcium, lipid and hemorrhage
- Resolution is limited, though methods are improving
  - Intravascular MR can improve resolution and signal to noise ratio

Echocardiographic Findings

- Echocardiogram
  - Transthoracic
    - Proximal coronary lesions occasionally detected
- Intravascular ultrasound (IVUS) can detect diseased segments in angiographic normal coronaries
  - Invasive technique done at the time of coronary catheterization
  - Normal intima not visible
  - Lesion extent: Lumen - external elastic lamina thickness
  - External elastic lamina; echo lucent border
  - Can differentiate calcific from soft plaque
  - Detect plaque rupture and erosion
  - Can guide therapy
    - Optimal deployment of stents; prevent incomplete apposition
    - Detect dissection; guide stent deployment
    - Plaque characterization still under development

Other Modality Findings

- Optical coherence tomography (OCT) findings
  - Intraluminal OCT catheter necessary
  - Examines interferogram generated by backscatter of coherent light source
  - High-resolution images; can measure on the scale of microns
  - Requires clear field: Saline or perfluorocarbon flush
  - Penetrates only 1-2 mm

Angiographic Findings

- Conventional
  - Soft plaque may not be evident on invasive angiography
  - May appear normal or with mild stenosis
  - Raised irregular lumen narrowing
  - Narrowing may be concentric or eccentric
- Angioscopy findings
  - Imaging catheter placed at the time of cardiac catheterization
  - Requires saline flush to clear blood from the field
  - Distinguish lesion type
    - Yellow surface: Lipid containing lesion with thin collagenous cap
    - White lesion: Thick fibrous caps, predominantly fibrous lesions
    - Yellow plaques are more likely to rupture

Imaging Recommendations

- Best imaging tool

- Traditional: Invasive coronary angiography for stenosis detection
- Contemporary: CTA in low and intermediate pre-test probability patients
  - CTA slightly limited in higher pre-test probability patients due to calcified plaques which may obscure coronary lumen

DIFFERENTIAL DIAGNOSIS

Coronary Artery Anomaly

- Origin of left or right coronary artery from contralateral sinus of Valsalva with passage between aorta and pulmonary trunk

Myocardial Bridge

- Intramyocardial course of coronary with systolic narrowing

Collagen Vascular Disease

- Systemic lupus erythematosus, scleroderma, polyarteritis nodosa

Inflammatory Vasculitis

- Kawasaki disease
- Takayasu arteritis

Thoracic Radiotherapy

- Particularly mediastinal radiotherapy for lymphoma

Post-Heart Transplant Coronary Fibrosis

- 64-slice cardiac CT provides moderate to excellent detection of post-transplant coronary vasculopathy

PATHOLOGY

General Features

- General path comments
  - Detection of plaque
    - Multiple stages of development: From fatty streaks to complex lesions with hemorrhage and calcification
  - Identification of vulnerable plaque
    - Thin fibrous cap
    - Large acellular lipid core
    - Inflammation in the cap and at the cap shoulders
    - Increased monocyte and macrophage content
    - Expression of matrix metalloproteinase (with collagenase activity)

CLINICAL ISSUES

Presentation

- Atherosclerotic plaque develops over several years, usually without symptoms
- Coronary arteries may appear normal on coronary angiography, yet still contain substantial plaque
  - Plaque erosion and rupture with associated thrombus account for the bulk of acute infarcts
  - Greater than 65% of infarcts are caused in vessels with < 70% stenosis
  - Coronaries may remodel to maintain lumen size while dilating to accommodate plaque burden (Glagov effect), revealing an apparently normal coronary artery on angiography (positive remodeling)

Treatment

- Lipid lowering medication can improve lumen diameter
  - In general a minor effect
- HMG-CoA reductase inhibitors (statins) reduce coronary events in primary and secondary prevention trials
  - Several proposed plaque stabilizing properties

DIAGNOSTIC CHECKLIST

Consider

- In patients presenting with anginal symptoms
- Coronary luminal narrowing with atherosclerotic plaque

SELECTED REFERENCES

1. Leber AW et al: Accuracy of 64-slice computed tomography to classify and quantify plaque volumes in the proximal coronary system: a comparative study using intravascular ultrasound. J Am Coll Cardiol. 47(3):672-7, 2006
2. Carr JJ et al: Calcified coronary artery plaque measurement with cardiac CT in population-based studies: standardized protocol of Multi-Ethnic Study of Atherosclerosis (MESA) and Coronary Artery Risk Development in Young Adults (CARDIA) study. Radiology. 234(1):35-43, 2005
3. Achenbach S et al: Assessment of coronary remodeling in stenotic and nonstenotic coronary atherosclerotic lesions by multidetector spiral computed tomography. J Am Coll Cardiol. 43(5):842-7, 2004
4. Leber AW et al: Accuracy of multidetector spiral computed tomography in identifying and differentiating the composition of coronary atherosclerotic plaques: a comparative study with intracoronary ultrasound. J Am Coll Cardiol. 43(7):1241-7, 2004
5. Fujii K et al: Intravascular ultrasound assessment of ulcerated ruptured plaques: a comparison of culprit and nonculprit lesions of patients with acute coronary syndromes and lesions in patients without acute coronary syndromes. Circulation. 108(20):2473-8, 2003
6. Naghavi M et al: From vulnerable plaque to vulnerable patient: a call for new definitions and risk assessment strategies: Part I. Circulation. 108(14):1664-72, 2003
7. Naghavi M et al: From vulnerable plaque to vulnerable patient: a call for new definitions and risk assessment strategies: Part II. Circulation. 108(15):1772-8, 2003
8. Yabushita H et al: Characterization of human atherosclerosis by optical coherence tomography. Circulation. 106(13):1640-5, 2002
9. Libby P: Current concepts of the pathogenesis of the acute coronary syndromes. Circulation. 104(3):365-72, 2001
10. Fayad ZA et al: Noninvasive in vivo human coronary artery lumen and wall imaging using black-blood magnetic resonance imaging. Circulation. 102(5):506-10, 2000
11. Virmani R et al: Lessons from sudden coronary death: a comprehensive morphological classification scheme for atherosclerotic lesions. Arterioscler Thromb Vasc Biol. 20(5):1262-75, 2000
12. Falk E et al: Coronary plaque disruption. Circulation. 92(3):657-71, 1995

CORONARY ATHEROSCLEROTIC PLAQUE

IMAGE GALLERY

Typical

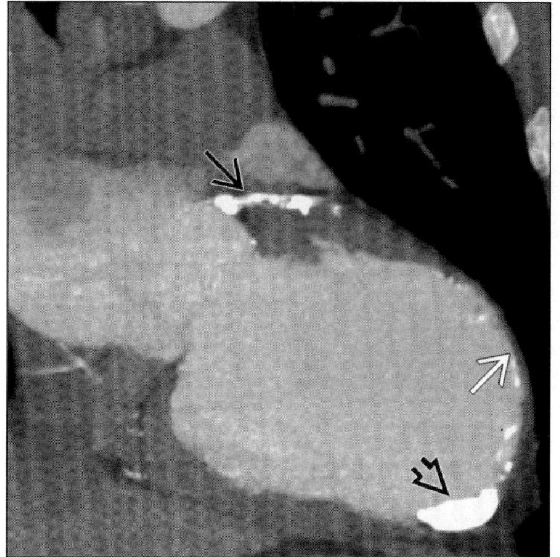

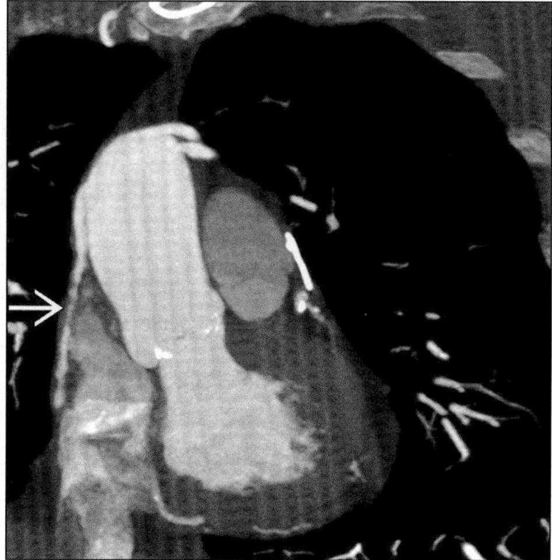

(Left) *Coronary CTA two-chamber view shows heavily calcified LAD ⇨. Marked anterior wall-wall thinning ➡ and calcified apical aneurysm ⇨ are consistent with chronic myocardial infarction in LAD territory.* ***(Right)*** *Oblique coronal coronary CTA shows atherosclerotic plaque in a vein graft ➡. 10-15% of vein grafts show stenoses 1 month post-operatively.*

Typical

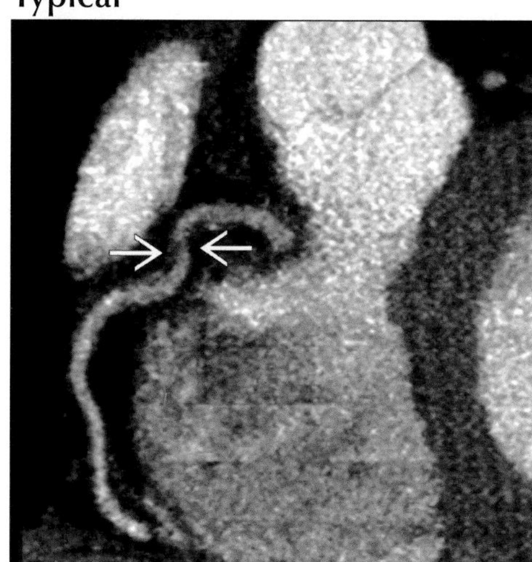

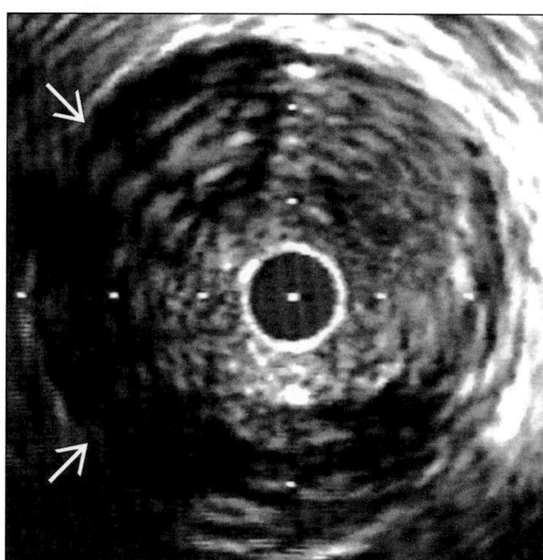

(Left) *Sagittal oblique coronary CTA MIP shows non-calcified plaque ➡ in the proximal right coronary causing significant luminal narrowing.* ***(Right)*** *Corresponding intravascular ultrasound axial view confirms hypoechogenicity ➡ consistent with a lipid-rich plaque.*

Typical

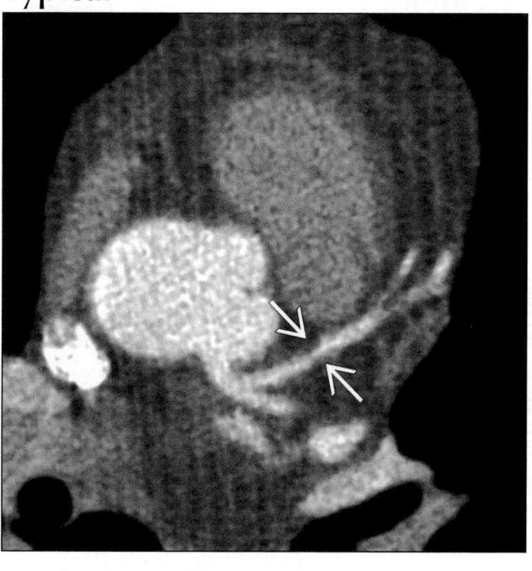

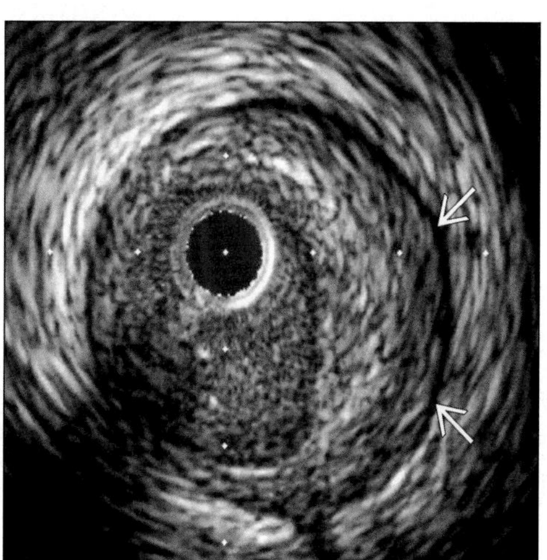

(Left) *Axial coronary CTA shows non-calcified plaque ➡ in the left anterior descending artery with significant luminal narrowing.* ***(Right)*** *Corresponding intravascular ultrasound axial view confirms hyperechogenicity consistent with fibrous plaque ➡.*

CORONARY THROMBOSIS

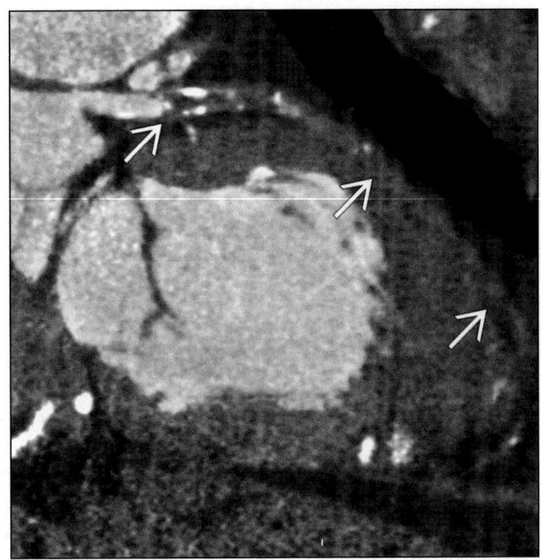

Coronary CTA in a 58 year old man with sudden onset acute chest pain shows acute thrombosis of the left anterior descending (LAD) coronary artery ➡.

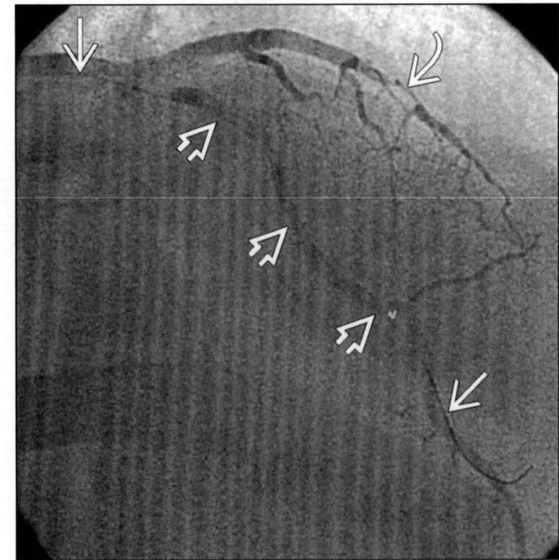

Corresponding coronary angiogram shows a guide wire ➡ has been passed down the LAD. Contrast outlines soft thrombus within the lumen ➡. Note the tight stenosis in the left circumflex artery ➡.

TERMINOLOGY

Definitions

- Obstruction/occlusion of a coronary artery by thrombus

IMAGING FINDINGS

General Features

- Best diagnostic clue: Abrupt cut-off of coronary lumen on coronary angiography

CT Findings

- CTA
  - Coronary CTA shows low density material within and usually completely occluding coronary lumen
    - Smooth abrupt cut-off of contrast material
    - Often an ↑ in diameter of the coronary artery

MR Findings

- MR 3D free-breathing navigator-gated sequences using fibrin-binding molecular MR contrast agents being developed which may aid in thrombus detection
  - Coronary in-stent thrombosis
  - Thrombus burden in patients with acute coronary syndromes

Echocardiographic Findings

- Echocardiogram
  - Ancillary findings
    - Reduced ejection fraction
    - Regional wall hypokinesis
    - Hyperkinesis of the contralateral wall

Ultrasonographic Findings

- Intravascular ultrasound shows characteristic hypoechogenic filling defect within coronary lumen

Other Modality Findings

- Optical coherence tomography
  - May allow differentiation between white and red thrombus

Angiographic Findings

- Conventional: Coronary angiography shows smooth round interface with contrast material; abrupt cut-off
- Fiberoptic angioscopy allows direct visualization of intraluminal thrombus

DDx: Coronary Artery Thrombosis

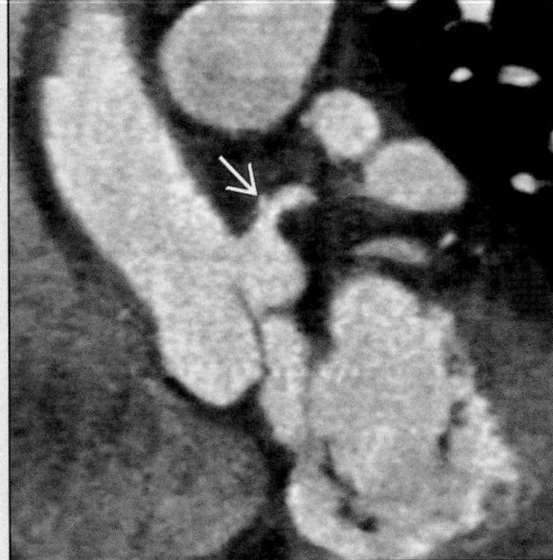

Coronary Dissection

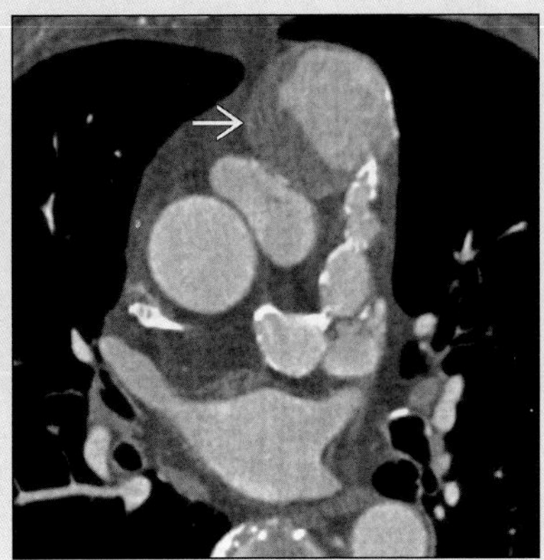

Kawasaki Disease

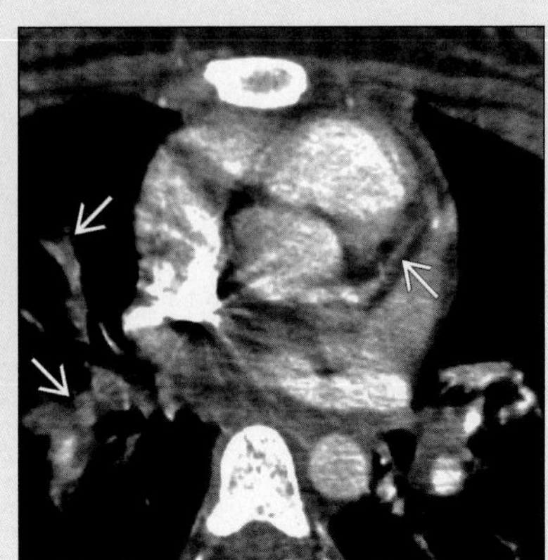

Takayasu Arteritis

CORONARY THROMBOSIS

Key Facts

Terminology
- Obstruction/occlusion of a coronary artery by thrombus

Imaging Findings
- Best diagnostic clue: Abrupt cut-off of coronary lumen on coronary angiography
- Coronary CTA shows low density material within and usually completely occluding coronary lumen
- MR 3D free-breathing navigator-gated sequences using fibrin-binding molecular MR contrast agents being developed which may aid in thrombus detection
- Intravascular ultrasound shows characteristic hypoechogenic filling defect within coronary lumen
- Conventional: Coronary angiography shows smooth round interface with contrast material; abrupt cut-off
- Fiberoptic angioscopy allows direct visualization of intraluminal thrombus

Pathology
- Etiology: Coronary atherosclerotic disease considered the underlying cause of acute coronary thrombosis in nearly all patients
- Initiating event is a "crack" or fissure, usually in the fibrous cap
- Exposes subendothelial matrix elements leading to thrombus formation

Clinical Issues
- Gender: Mortality rate among men and women is equal over their lifetimes
- Coronary artery thrombosis is considered primary cause of acute myocardial infarction

Imaging Recommendations
- Best imaging tool
  - Invasive
    - Coronary angiography
  - Non-invasive
    - Coronary CTA

DIFFERENTIAL DIAGNOSIS

Embolus
- Important for secondary prevention
  - May suggest hypercoagulable state

Vasculitis (Autoimmune)
- May lead to artery occlusion with or without thrombus
- More often part of a systemic disease
- Systemic lupus erythematous
- Rheumatoid arthritis

Coronary Dissection
- Can result from percutaneous intervention
  - With advancement of the guidewire
  - During expansion of a balloon catheter

Kawasaki Disease
- Long term complications include coronary aneurysms, stenosis and thrombosis

Takayasu Arteritis
- More commonly affects large vessels (aorta and great vessels) but can affect the coronary circulation

Cocaine
- Non-atherosclerotic cause of coronary artery thrombosis
  - Suspect in young patients diagnosed with myocardial infarction

PATHOLOGY

General Features
- General path comments
  - Generally white thrombus (platelet rich), with secondary areas of red thrombus formation (red cells, thrombin, fibrin)
  - Various stages of thrombus maturing will affect therapy
- Etiology: Coronary atherosclerotic disease considered the underlying cause of acute coronary thrombosis in nearly all patients

Gross Pathologic & Surgical Features
- Plaques that rupture tend to have
  - Thin fibrous cap
  - Lipid-rich core
  - Few smooth muscle cells
  - Large number of macrophages and monocytes

Microscopic Features
- Initiating event is a "crack" or fissure, usually in the fibrous cap
- Exposes subendothelial matrix elements leading to thrombus formation
  - Collagen
  - Lipid
  - Release of tissue activating factor

Staging, Grading or Classification Criteria
- Coronary artery thrombosis may be
  - Totally occlusive; acute myocardial infarction
    - Associated with stagnation of coronary artery blood flow
  - Mural; unstable angina
    - Not associated with stagnation of blood flow

CLINICAL ISSUES

Presentation
- Most common signs/symptoms
  - Acute, intense severe chest pain

        - Pain radiates usually to left arm
        - Often occurs in the early morning due to circadian rhythm of platelet and fibrinolytic activity
        - Impending sense of doom
    - Dyspnea
    - Indigestion common (especially inferior wall infarction)
    - Syncope (have a high suspicion for ventricular tachycardia as the cause)
- Other signs/symptoms
    - Signs include
        - Pallor
        - Irregular pulse (arrhythmia)
        - Hypotension
        - Elevated jugular venous pulse
- Clinical Profile
    - Risk factors include
        - Older age
        - Smoking
        - Hypercholesterolemia
        - Diabetes
        - Family history
        - Male gender/postmenopausal female gender
        - Hypertension

Demographics

- Gender: Mortality rate among men and women is equal over their lifetimes
- Ethnicity: Mortality from coronary artery thrombosis is lower in African-American men and women

Natural History & Prognosis

- Coronary artery thrombosis is considered primary cause of acute myocardial infarction

Treatment

- Oxygen
- Analgesia
    - Sublingual nitrates, Morphine
- Medical reperfusion
    - Earlier treatment is pivotal for improving outcome
    - Aspirin
    - Thrombolytics
        - Tissue plasminogen activator
        - Streptokinase
- Medical antiarrhythmics
    - Heparin
    - Beta-blockers
    - ACE (angiotensin converting enzyme) inhibitors
- Intra-aortic balloon counterpulsation pump (patients with Killip class IV or V)
- Left ventricular assist device
- Emergency transplantation (young patients)
- Elective coronary angiography and revascularization

DIAGNOSTIC CHECKLIST

Consider

- In patients presenting with acute myocardial infarction
- Most commonly result of ruptured "vulnerable" non-stenotic plaque

SELECTED REFERENCES

1. DeMaria AN et al: Imaging vulnerable plaque by ultrasound. J Am Coll Cardiol. 47(8 Suppl):C32-9, 2006
2. Iijima R et al: Comparison of coronary arterial finding by intravascular ultrasound in patients with "transient no-reflow" versus "reflow" during percutaneous coronary intervention in acute coronary syndrome. Am J Cardiol. 97(1):29-33, 2006
3. Sano K et al: Assessment of vulnerable plaques causing acute coronary syndrome using integrated backscatter intravascular ultrasound. J Am Coll Cardiol. 47(4):734-41, 2006
4. Baker WF Jr: Thrombolytic therapy: current clinical practice. Hematol Oncol Clin North Am. 19(1):147-81, vii, 2005
5. Libby P et al: Pathophysiology of coronary artery disease. Circulation. 111(25):3481-8, 2005
6. Tyczynski P et al: Intravascular ultrasound assessment of ruptured atherosclerotic plaques in left main coronary arteries. Am J Cardiol. 96(6):794-8, 2005
7. Botnar RM et al: In vivo magnetic resonance imaging of coronary thrombosis using a fibrin-binding molecular magnetic resonance contrast agent. Circulation. 110(11):1463-6, 2004
8. Porto I et al: Intravascular ultrasound to guide the management of intracoronary thrombus: a case report. Cardiovasc Ultrasound. 2(1):18, 2004
9. Golino P et al: Involvement of tissue factor pathway inhibitor in the coronary circulation of patients with acute coronary syndromes. Circulation. 108(23):2864-9, 2003
10. Gurbel PA et al: Onset and extent of platelet inhibition by clopidogrel loading in patients undergoing elective coronary stenting: the Plavix Reduction Of New Thrombus Occurrence (PRONTO) trial. Am Heart J. 145(2):239-47, 2003
11. Naghavi M et al: From vulnerable plaque to vulnerable patient: a call for new definitions and risk assessment strategies: Part I. Circulation. 108(14):1664-72, 2003
12. Naghavi M et al: From vulnerable plaque to vulnerable patient: a call for new definitions and risk assessment strategies: Part II. Circulation. 108(15):1772-8, 2003
13. Singh M et al: Treatment of saphenous vein bypass grafts with ultrasound thrombolysis: a randomized study (ATLAS). Circulation. 107(18):2331-6, 2003
14. Ramee SR et al: A randomized prospective multicenter study comparing intracoronary urokinase to rheolytic thrombectomy with the Possis Angiojet catheter for intracoronary thrombus: final results of the Vegas-2 trial. Circulation. 98:1-86, 1998
15. Boston DR et al: Management of intracoronary thrombosis complicating percutaneous transluminal coronary angioplasty. Clin Cardiol. 19(7):536-42, 1996
16. Kaplan BM et al: Prospective study of extraction atherectomy in patients with acute myocardial infarction. Am J Cardiol. 78(4):383-8, 1996
17. Gossage JR: Acute myocardial infarction. Reperfusion strategies. Chest. 106(6):1851-66, 1994
18. Badimon L et al: Thrombus formation on ruptured atherosclerotic plaques and rethrombosis on evolving thrombi. Circulation. 86(6 Suppl):III74-85, 1992
19. Brochier ML et al: Thrombosis and thrombolysis in unstable angina. Am J Cardiol. 68(7):105B-109B, 1991
20. Minor RL Jr et al: Cocaine-induced myocardial infarction in patients with normal coronary arteries. Ann Intern Med. 115(10):797-806, 1991
21. Rehr RB et al: Thrombosis in unstable angina: angiographic aspects. Cardiovasc Clin. 18(1):183-94, 1987

IMAGE GALLERY

Typical

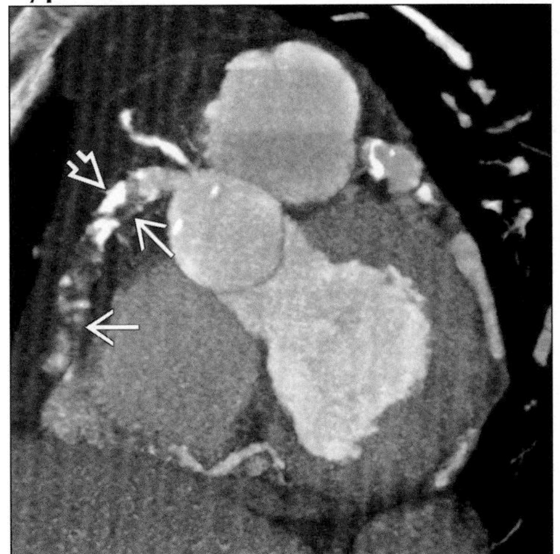

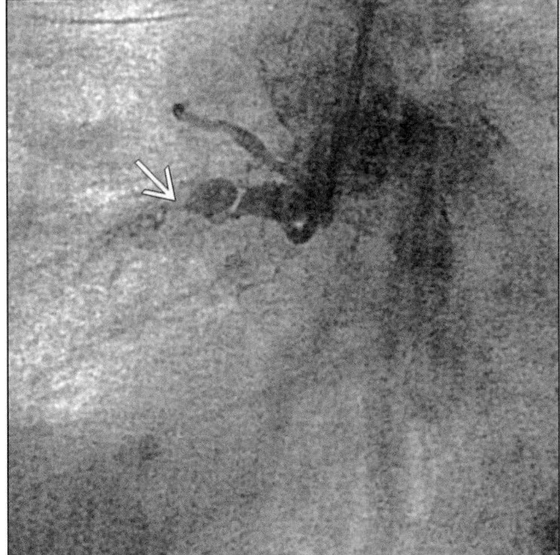

(Left) Coronary CTA in a 47 year old man with acute chest pain shows low density material ➡ consistent with thrombus in the RCA. Note also multiple calcified plaques ➡. *(Right)* Corresponding coronary angiogram shows abrupt cut-off of contrast in the RCA ➡ consistent with coronary thrombosis.

Typical

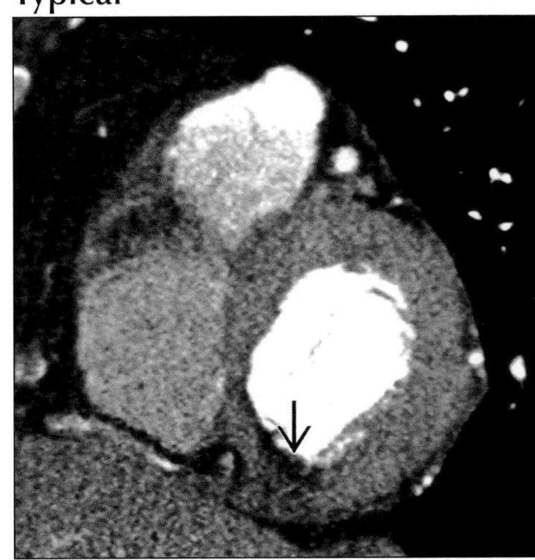

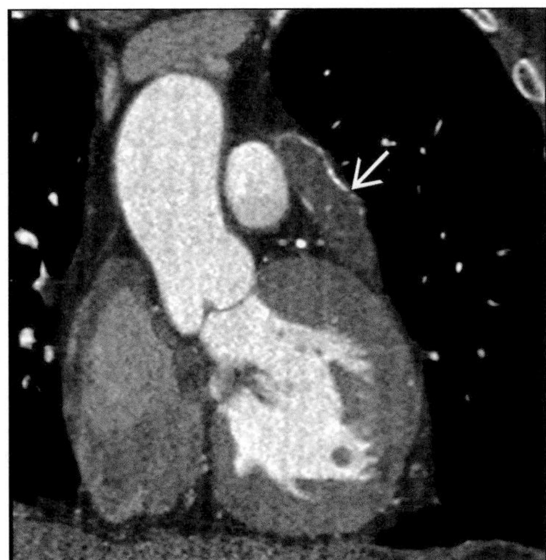

(Left) Corresponding CTA in short axis shows a subendocardial perfusion defect ➡ in the inferior segment RCA vascular territory. *(Right)* Coronary CTA in another patient post coronary artery bypass grafting (CABG) shows a thrombosed vein graft ➡. ~ 10% of grafts occlude during the first month post surgery.

Typical

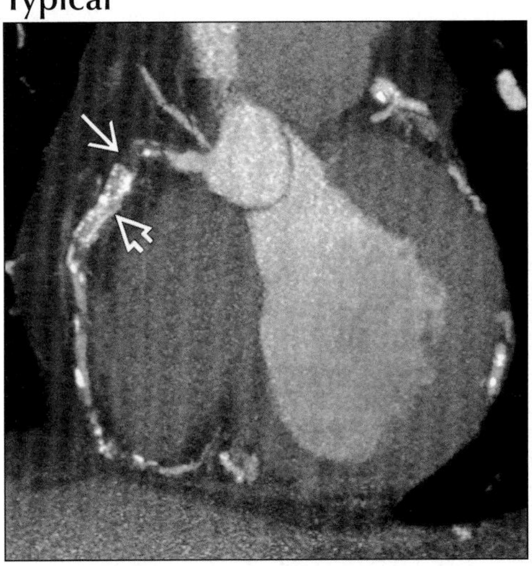

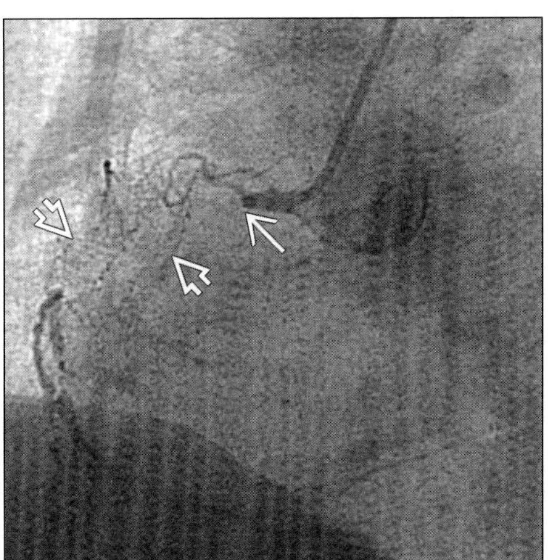

(Left) Coronary CTA in a 62 year old man post stent insertion shows complete thrombosis ➡ within the proximal RCA and the stent ➡. *(Right)* Corresponding coronary angiogram shows abrupt cut-off of contrast in the proximal RCA ➡. Extensive collaterals ➡ result in RCA reconstitution distally.

CORONARY ARTERY STENOSIS

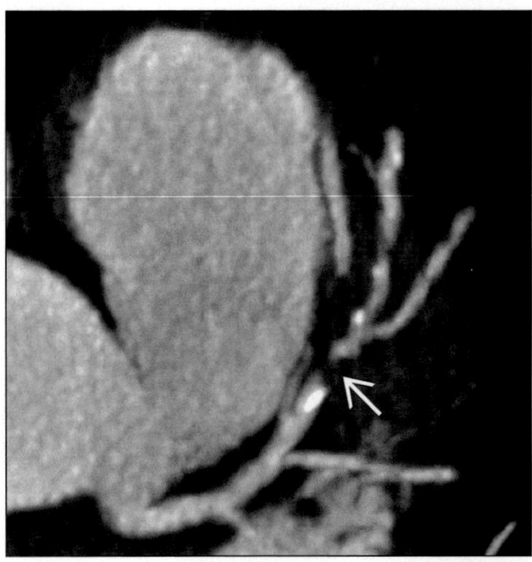

Coronary CTA shows a large non-calcified plaque ➔ in the mid left anterior descending coronary artery (LAD) resulting in a hemodynamically significant coronary stenosis.

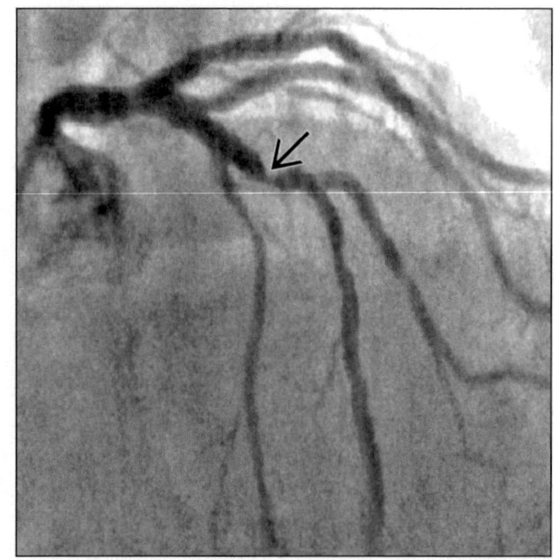

Corresponding coronary angiogram confirms the hemodynamically significant stenosis ➔ in the mid LAD.

TERMINOLOGY

Definitions

- Fixed obstructive coronary artery disease

IMAGING FINDINGS

General Features

- Coronary angiography is the clinical gold standard to detect and quantify coronary artery stenosis
  - Hemodynamically significant stenosis = 70% luminal narrowing except for LM = 50% luminal narrowing

Radiographic Findings

- Radiography
  - Chest radiography findings
    - Usually normal in the absence of acute ischemia & congestive heart failure

CT Findings

- NECT: Presence of coronary calcium is definitive for presence of coronary artery disease (CAD): Potential use as a screening tool in asymptomatic patients
- CTA
  - Requires high spatial, contrast and temporal resolution
    - Spatial: Submillimeter detector size 64-slice CT voxel size: 0.4 mm^3
    - Contrast: High iodine contrast concentration [370 mg/L iodine] and rapid injection rate [5-6 mL/s]
    - Temporal: Rapid gantry rotation (330-350 msec) + half scan reconstruction result in temporal resolution of 165 ms
    - Dual source scanners reduce temporal resolution to 83 ms
  - 64-slice CT sensitivity = 85-95%, specificity = 90-100% for detection of significant coronary artery stenosis
  - Can detect plaque "positive remodeling" that may go undetected with invasive angiography
  - Significant limitations remain (dual-source CT minimizes)

DDx: Coronary Stenosis (Acute Coronary Syndrome)

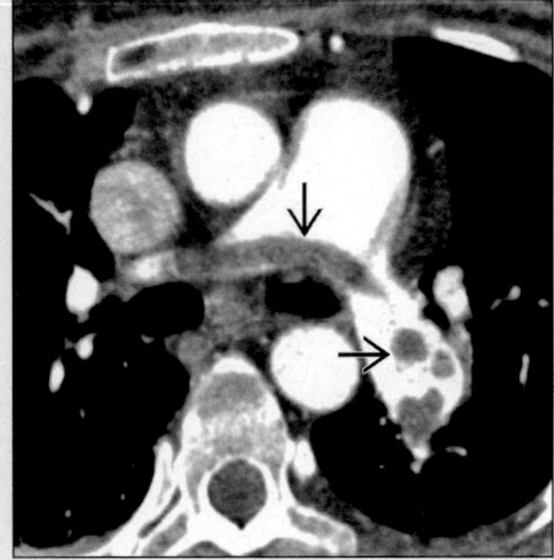

Pulmonary Embolism

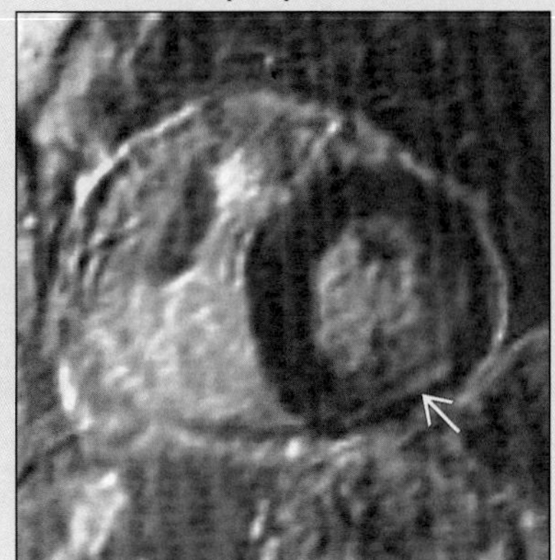

Acute Myocarditis

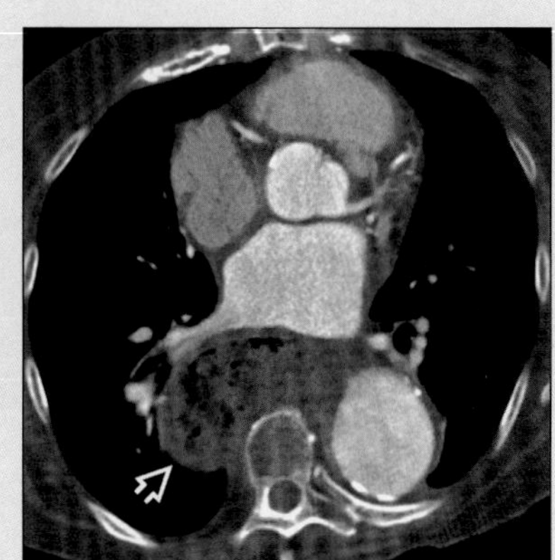

Hiatus Hernia/Reflux

CORONARY ARTERY STENOSIS

Key Facts

Terminology
- Fixed obstructive coronary artery disease

Imaging Findings
- Coronary angiography is the clinical gold standard to detect and quantify coronary artery stenosis
- Hemodynamically significant stenosis = 70% luminal narrowing except for LM = 50% luminal narrowing
- 64-slice CT sensitivity = 85-95%, specificity = 90-100% for detection of significant coronary artery stenosis
- Sophisticated cardiac MR sequences for coronary artery stenosis work-up
- IVUS is the gold standard for plaque characterization
- PET excellent for assessing perfusion, ischemia, and viability

Pathology
- Plaque components include collagenous cap, lipid core, smooth muscle cell proliferation and inflammatory cells
- Atherosclerotic plaque is the most common cause of stenosis

Clinical Issues
- Most common signs/symptoms: Chest, shoulder, neck or jaw pain that is reproducible with exertion
- Treatment is complex and driven by pretest probability of disease and the need for percutaneous coronary intervention (PCI)

        - Motion artifact (5-20% of coronary segments), large calcified plaques may cause blooming artifact across the coronary lumen, contraindications to contrast dye, radiation dose (6-13 mSv)

MR Findings
- Sophisticated cardiac MR sequences for coronary artery stenosis work-up
    - Global and regional wall motion abnormalities
        - Cine steady-state free-precession white blood sequences - high temporal/spatial/contrast resolution
        - Identified areas of wall motion abnormality in areas of ischemia
        - Reversible (stunned or hibernating myocardium) or irreversible (acute/chronic myocardial infarction)
    - Myocardial perfusion
        - Resting and stress perfusion using dobutamine/adenosine infusion
        - Abnormal myocardial perfusion reserve yields diagnostic accuracy of 87% for coronary artery stenosis
    - Myocardial viability
        - Low-dose dobutamine stress
        - Delayed enhancement with gadolinium using gradient echo inversion recovery sequences
        - Non-viable scar tissue appears as bright or "hyperenhanced" myocardium
    - Coronary arteries
        - New coronary angiography sequences available can generate 2 or 3-dimensional images
        - Breath-hold or respiratory navigator-gated techniques have led to improved image quality but not comparable to CT

Nuclear Medicine Findings
- PET
    - PET excellent for assessing perfusion, ischemia, and viability
        - FDG-glucose uptake in hypoperfused segments indicates viable hibernating myocardium
        - Limitations include cost, time requirement and limited availability
- Nuclear cardiology: Thallium or technetium imaging
    - Comparison of exercise (high-flow state) with rest (low-flow state)
    - Can use pharmacologic equivalent of exercise to uncover lesions by demonstrating differential perfusion in normal vs. diseased territories
        - Dobutamine and arbutamine increase cardiac work, oxygen myocardial consumption (MVO_2) and perfusion
        - Adenosine and dipyridamole augment coronary flow
    - Indicators of ischemic defect
        - Reduced tracer uptake, wall thinning, LV dilation in the stress image, increased lung uptake (slow transit time)
    - Care required in interpretation
        - Apical thinning, breast attenuation artifacts, motion artifacts and inadequate exercise

Echocardiographic Findings
- Echocardiogram
    - Baseline study usually normal
    - Stress echo most commonly performed with graded dobutamine stress and permits rapid acquisition of stress images in several planes
        - Positive test: Angina, serious arrhythmias, new wall motion abnormality, symptoms of heart failure, significant hypotension
        - Evaluate lack of increase in systolic function, or appearance of hypokinetic, akinetic, or dyskinetic segments
- Pulsed Doppler
    - Small intracoronary Doppler catheters allow measurement of selective coronary artery flow velocity across a lesion
    - By noting the increase in flow velocity following a strong coronary vasodilator (papaverine/adenosine) the coronary flow reserve (CFR) can be defined
    - CFR provides an index of the functional significance of coronary lesions rather than relying on purely angiographic morphological criteria

CORONARY ARTERY STENOSIS

Ultrasonographic Findings

- Intravascular ultrasound (IVUS)
  - Selective catheterization of coronary arteries with a motorized pullback catheter probe
  - Reflection of acoustic waves (spatial resolution 80-150 μm)
  - IVUS is the gold standard for plaque characterization
    - Hypoechoic plaque = lipid-rich plaque
    - Hyperechoic plaque = mixed plaque
    - Highly echogenic with acoustic shadow = calcified plaque

Other Modality Findings

- Exercise/pharmacological stress testing may induce angina
  - Ischemia at low workloads associated with poorer prognosis

Angiographic Findings

- Coronary angiography findings
  - High-resolution assessment (voxel size: 0.2 mm^3) of the number, location, character and severity of stenotic lesions
  - Provides information of the volume of myocardium likely subtended, presence of ruptured plaque, calcification and collaterals
- Left ventriculography
  - May demonstrate abnormal wall-motion in regions of stunned or infarcted myocardium

Imaging Recommendations

- Best imaging tool
  - Best non-invasive test for coronary artery stenosis currently: Coronary CTA
  - Best invasive test for coronary artery stenosis: Coronary catheterization with IVUS

DIFFERENTIAL DIAGNOSIS

Other Cardiac Disease

- Acute myocarditis, pericarditis, coronary spasm, aortic stenosis, hypertrophic cardiomyopathy, mitral valve prolapse, cocaine abuse, syndrome X

Non Cardiac Source of Symptoms

- Musculoskeletal diseases of the chest wall, shoulders
- Gastrointestinal diseases (hiatus hernia, acid reflux, cholecystitis, peptic ulcer)
- Vascular: Aortic dissection or pulmonary embolism

PATHOLOGY

General Features

- General path comments
  - Atherosclerosis
    - Plaque components include collagenous cap, lipid core, smooth muscle cell proliferation and inflammatory cells
    - Accumulation of modified lipid leads to endothelial cell activation
    - This triggers inflammatory cell migration and activation
    - This leads to smooth muscle cell recruitment and activation leading to fibrous cap formation
    - Plaque erosion/rupture, platelet aggregation and thrombosis
  - Non-atherosclerotic vascular disease
    - Lupus, Marfan, Behçet, Kawasaki disease, aneurysm and thrombosis
- Genetics
  - Mendelian disorders most dramatic examples of genetic contributions to atherosclerosis
  - Genetic factors may also influence atherosclerosis in more subtle ways and at many stages
    - For example: Cholesterol, hypertension, reduced high density lipoproteins
- Etiology: Atherosclerotic plaque is the most common cause of stenosis
- Epidemiology: Leading cause of mortality and morbidity in the developed world

CLINICAL ISSUES

Presentation

- Most common signs/symptoms: Chest, shoulder, neck or jaw pain that is reproducible with exertion
- Clinical Profile: Risk profiling is a critical part of evaluating patients suspected of significant coronary artery stenosis

Demographics

- Age: Likelihood of death or nonfatal ischemic event increases with age
- Ethnicity: African-Americans and Asian Indians have a higher risk of coronary artery disease and cardiovascular mortality

Treatment

- Treatment is complex and driven by pretest probability of disease and the need for percutaneous coronary intervention (PCI)
- Divide into symptom relief, coronary revascularization, secondary prevention

DIAGNOSTIC CHECKLIST

Consider

- Most common differential diagnosis are gastroesophageal reflux and musculoskeletal chest pain

SELECTED REFERENCES

1. Achenbach S: Computed tomography coronary angiography. J Am Coll Cardiol. 48(10):1919-28, 2006
2. Armstrong PW: Stable coronary syndromes. In Topol EJ (ed) Textbook of Cardiovascular Medicine. Lippincott-Raven, Philadelphia. 333-64, 1998

IMAGE GALLERY

Typical

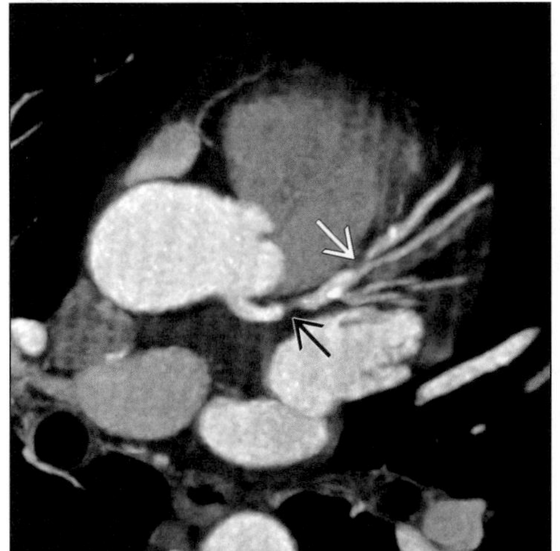

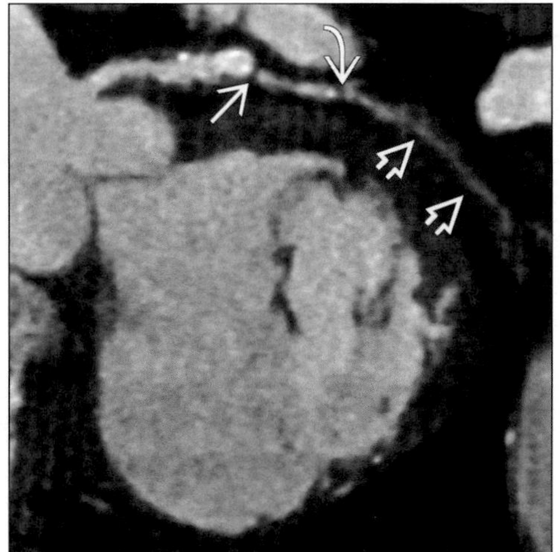

(Left) *Coronary CTA shows left main coronary stenosis (widow-maker). Note second coronary stenosis in mid segment LAD.* ***(Right)*** *Coronary CTA of the LCX shows two tight, ring-like stenosis, one at its origin and one in the proximal segment. Note diffuse circumferential mid and distal segment atherosclerotic plaque with extensive positive and negative remodeling.*

Typical

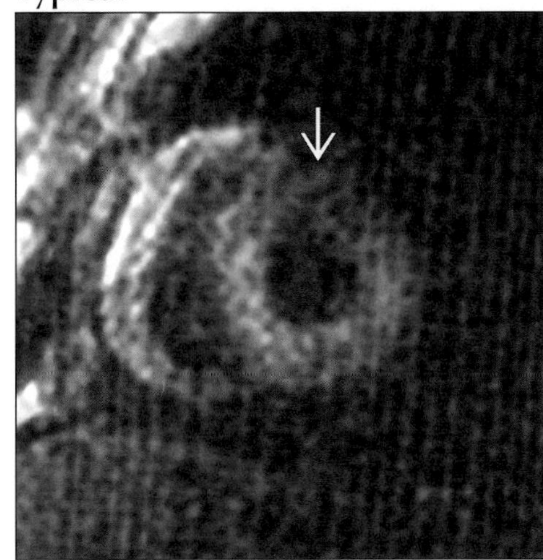

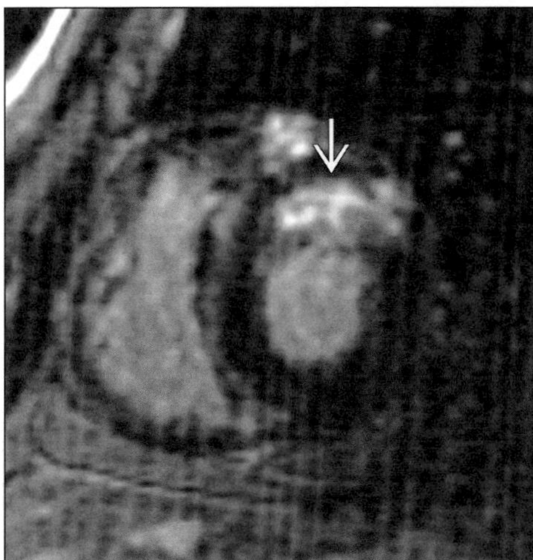

(Left) *1st pass perfusion hybrid gradient echo-planar MR shows perfusion defect in the anterior segment left ventricular myocardium corresponding in the LAD vascular territory.* ***(Right)*** *Corresponding inversion-recovery fast gradient-echo image 10 minutes post gadolinium shows delayed "hyperenhancement" of the anterior segment left ventricular myocardium consistent with myocardial infarction/scar.*

Typical

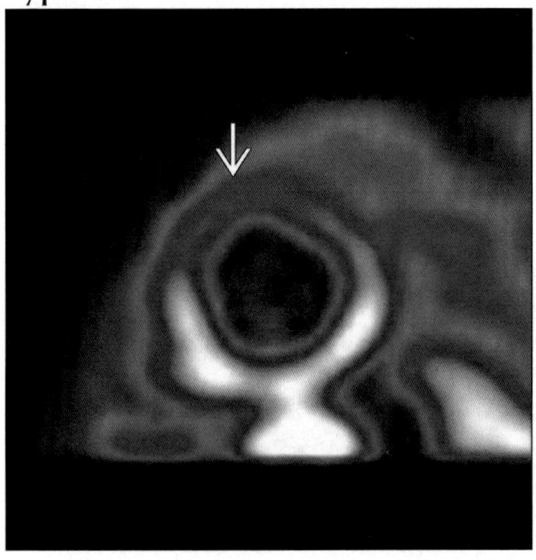

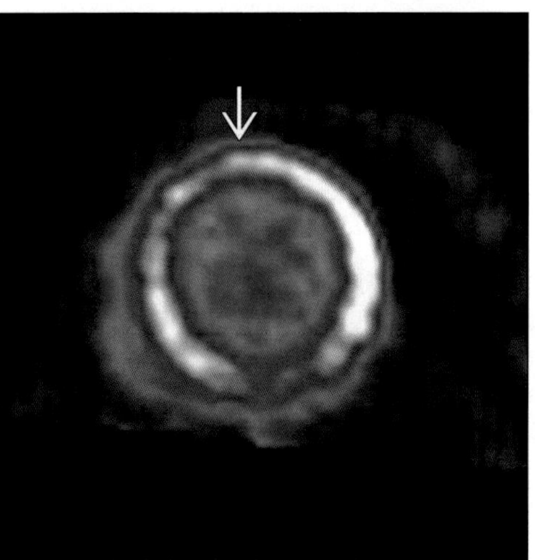

(Left) *Perfusion phase of a cardiac FDG PET scan in another patient shows perfusion defect in the anterior segment left ventricular myocardium.* ***(Right)*** *Corresponding FDG uptake phase shows good uptake within the anterior segment indicating viable but hibernating left ventricular myocardium.*

ISCHEMIA RCA STENOSIS

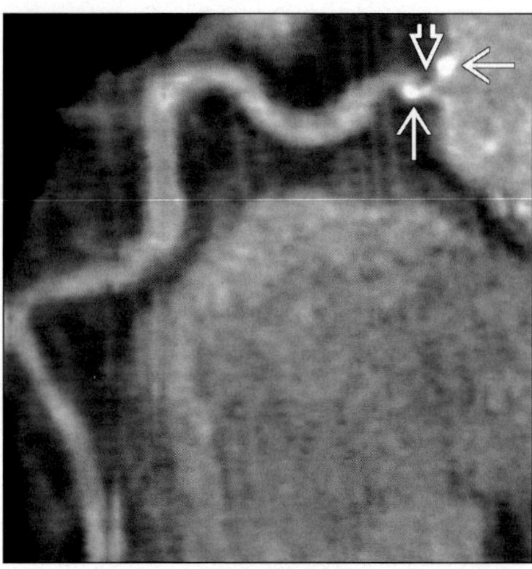

Curved MPR coronary CTA shows calcified ➡ and noncalcified ➡ plaque at the RCA ostium causing a significant stenosis.

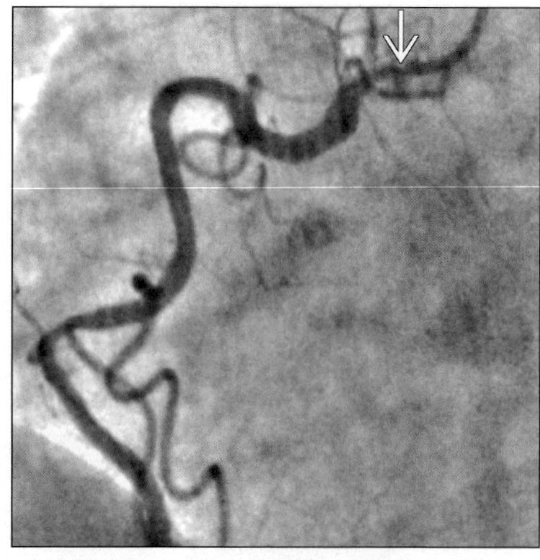

Corresponding invasive coronary angiogram confirms a significant stenosis ➡ at the RCA ostium.

TERMINOLOGY

Definitions

- Obstructive coronary disease in the right coronary artery (RCA)

IMAGING FINDINGS

General Features

- Location: RCA originates from right sinus slightly more caudal than left main coronary artery and supplies right ventricle/inferior aspect of left ventricle
- Morphology
  - RCA traverses the right atrioventricular groove
    - Provides small branches to right atrium and marginal branches to right ventricle
    - In ~ 60%, RCA atrial branches supply sinus node; otherwise, left circumflex (LCx) atrial branches serve this function
    - In ~ 50%, 1st branch of RCA is a conus branch, supplying right ventricular outflow tract; otherwise, conus branch originates from separate right sinus ostium
    - Dominance is defined as coronary artery supplying posterior descending artery (PDA); ~ 85% of patients are RCA dominant, remainder having either dominant LCx or codominant RCA and LCx
    - PDA of RCA (or LCx) courses along inferior interventricular groove, providing septal perforators, a feature that may aid in its identification and differentiation from posterolateral segment of RCA (or LCx), which gives off branches to posterior ventricle
    - In > 90%, artery to atrioventricular node originates from posterior left ventricular (PLV) branch of RCA as it passes through crux

Radiographic Findings

- Chest Radiography Findings
  - Usually normal in the absence of heart failure

Fluoroscopic Findings

- Coronary angiography is the gold standard to detect and quantify RCA stenosis

CT Findings

- CTA

DDx: Ischemia RCA Stenosis

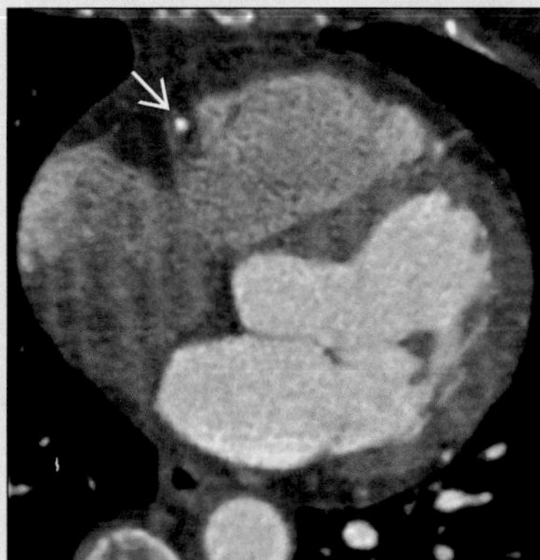

RCA Myocardial Bridge

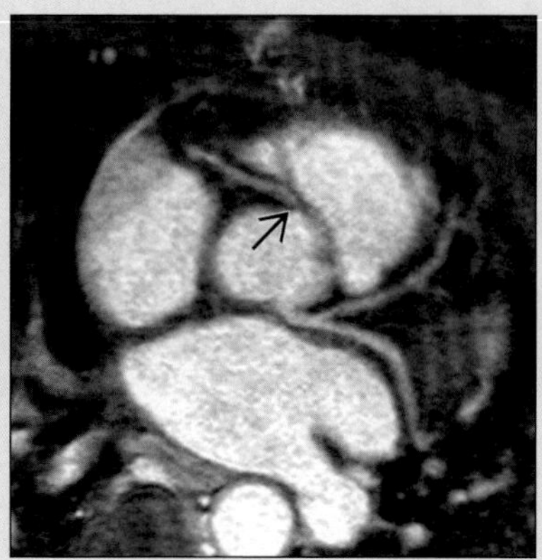

Right Coronary Anomaly

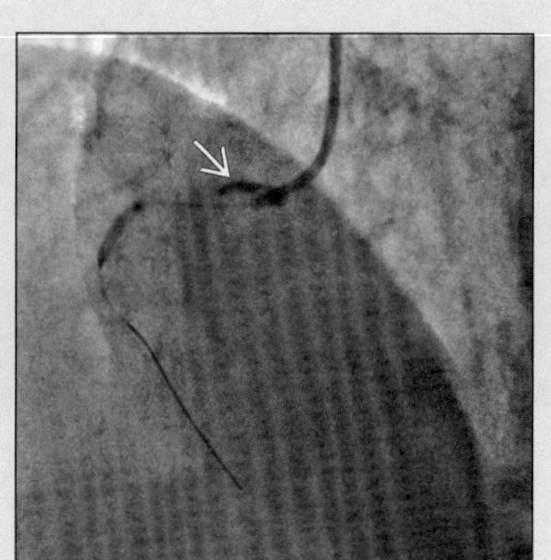

Right Coronary Dissection

ISCHEMIA RCA STENOSIS

Key Facts

Terminology
- Fixed obstructive coronary disease in the right coronary artery (RCA)

Imaging Findings
- Location: RCA originates from right sinus slightly more caudal than left main coronary artery and supplies right ventricle/inferior aspect of left ventricle
- Coronary angiography is the gold standard to detect and quantify RCA stenosis
- 64-slice CT sensitivity = 85-95% and specificity = 90-100% for detecting significant coronary artery stenosis
- Sophisticated cardiac MR sequences for RCA stenosis work-up
- Evaluate lack of increase in systolic function, or appearance of hypokinetic, akinetic, or dyskinetic segments in the inferior left ventricular wall
- PET: PET excellent for inferior left ventricular wall perfusion, ischemia, and viability (limitations: Cost, time, availability)
- Best non-invasive test: Coronary CTA

Clinical Issues
- Angina may be typical but GI symptoms more common
- ST segment depression in inferior ECG leads
- Treatment is complex and driven by pretest probability of disease and the likely need for definitive structural treatment

  - 64-slice CT sensitivity = 85-95% and specificity = 90-100% for detecting significant coronary artery stenosis

    - Genu of RCA may move rapidly during ventricular systole [systolic reconstruction phase (30%) often best for RCA analysis]

MR Findings
- Sophisticated cardiac MR sequences for RCA stenosis work-up
  - Cine steady state free-precession white blood sequences
    - Regional wall hypokinesis/akinesis/dyskinesis in the inferior/inferior-septal left ventricular wall
  - Myocardial perfusion
    - 1st pass perfusion shows perfusion defect in the inferior left ventricular wall
  - Myocardial viability
    - Delayed enhancement with gadolinium using gradient echo inversion recovery sequences
    - Non-viable myocardium appears as bright or "hyperenhanced" myocardium in the inferior left ventricular wall
  - Coronary arteries
    - New coronary angiography sequences are now available which can generate 2 or 3-dimensional images

Nuclear Medicine Findings
- PET: PET excellent for inferior left ventricular wall perfusion, ischemia, and viability (limitations: Cost, time, availability)
- Nuclear Cardiology Findings
  - Thallium or technetium imaging to detect reversible flow limited zones; reduced uptake, thinning
  - Must differentiate inferior myocardium from diaphragm and liver; exercise reduces splanchnic flow improving contrast
  - Including an analysis of right ventricle on thallium-201 stress scintigrams improves detection of proximal RCA lesions

Echocardiographic Findings
- Echocardiogram
  - Baseline study usually normal
  - Stress echo most commonly performed with graded dobutamine stress
    - Increases contractility and oxygen consumption
    - Evaluate lack of increase in systolic function, or appearance of hypokinetic, akinetic, or dyskinetic segments in the inferior left ventricular wall
- Pulsed Doppler: Coronary flow velocity reserve useful for non-invasive assessment of RCA stenosis (sensitivity 91%, specificity 88%)

Ultrasonographic Findings
- Pulsed Doppler
  - Small intracoronary Doppler catheters allow measurement of selective coronary artery flow velocity across a lesion
    - High-frequency sound waves are reflected from moving red blood cells and shift in sound frequency proportional to blood flow velocity
  - By noting increase in flow velocity following a strong coronary vasodilator (papaverine/adenosine), coronary flow reserve (CFR) can be defined
  - CFR provides index of functional significance of coronary lesions rather than relying on purely angiographic morphological criteria
- Intravascular Ultrasound
  - Selective catheterization of coronary arteries using a motorized pullback catheter probe
  - Reflection of acoustic waves (spatial resolution 80-150 μm)
  - Gold standard for plaque characterization
    - Hypoechoic plaque = lipid-rich plaque
    - Hyperechoic plaque = mixed plaque
    - Highly echogenic with acoustic shadow = calcified plaque

Angiographic Findings
- Conventional
  - Hemodynamically significant stenosis = 70% luminal narrowing

- Can evaluate collateral supply to ischemic territory
- Limitations
  - Severity of stenosis is generally estimated visually, but estimation is limited by the fact that interobserver variability may range from 30-60%
  - Diffuse disease may lead to underestimation of stenoses
- Left Ventriculography Findings
  - Reduced wall motion and thickening in the infero-posterior territory

Imaging Recommendations

- Best imaging tool
  - Best non-invasive test - coronary CTA
  - Best invasive test - coronary angiography

DIFFERENTIAL DIAGNOSIS

Cardiac Disease

- Acute myocarditis, coronary spasm, syndrome X, hypertrophic cardiomyopathy, cocaine abuse, mitral valve prolapse

Non-Cardiac Disease

- Musculoskeletal diseases of the chest wall, shoulders
- Gastrointestinal diseases (hiatus hernia, acid reflux, peptic ulcer disease, cholecystitis)
- Vascular: Aortic stenosis, aortic dissection, pulmonary embolism

PATHOLOGY

General Features

- General path comments: Vascular occlusion with inferior segment necrosis

Gross Pathologic & Surgical Features

- Myocardial thinning of the inferior segment

Microscopic Features

- Initiating event is a fissure in the diseased arterial wall plaque cap
  - Results in exposure of subendothelial matrix elements such as collagen, stimulating platelet activation and thrombus formation

CLINICAL ISSUES

Presentation

- Most common signs/symptoms
  - More difficult to diagnose because of inferior, posterior location of ischemia
  - Angina may be typical but GI symptoms more common
  - Rarely, abdominal discomfort above umbilicus
  - Frequently associated with nausea or vomiting
  - Can present with diaphragmatic irritation when ischemia is severe
- Other signs/symptoms: Hiccups
- ECG findings
  - ST segment depression in inferior ECG leads
  - RCA stenosis is an independent predictor of atrial fibrillation in pre-surgical and post CABG patients
- Sinus and AV node ischemic symptoms more common; bradycardia
- Bradyarrhythmias, sinus bradycardia, atrioventricular (AV) block

Treatment

- Treatment is complex and driven by pretest probability of disease and the likely need for definitive structural treatment
- Divide into symptom relief, coronary revascularization, secondary prevention
  - Symptom relief
    - Rapid-acting nitrate
    - Beta-blockers/calcium channel blockers
    - Long-acting nitrate
  - Coronary revascularization
    - Angioplasty has excellent 5-year survival for single ~ 93% and multivessel disease ~ 87%
    - Technically difficult in "shepard's crook" RCA (approximately 5% general population)
    - Coronary artery bypass graft (CABG)
    - Graft options include right internal mammary, radial, gastroepiploic artery or saphenous vein graft
  - Secondary prevention
    - Cardiac rehabilitation: Explanation, understanding, specific interventions (smoking cessation, diet, exercise), long-term adaptation
    - Antiplatelet therapy (aspirin or clopidogrel), lipid-lowering therapy (stains or fibrates), Beta-blockers, ACE inhibitors

SELECTED REFERENCES

1. Larose E et al: Right ventricular dysfunction assessed by cardiovascular magnetic resonance imaging predicts poor prognosis late after myocardial infarction. J Am Coll Cardiol. 49(8):855-62, 2007
2. Achenbach S: Computed tomography coronary angiography. J Am Coll Cardiol. 48(10):1919-28, 2006
3. Kumar A et al: Contrast-enhanced cardiovascular magnetic resonance imaging of right ventricular infarction. J Am Coll Cardiol. 48(10):1969-76, 2006
4. Somsen GA et al: Right ventricular ischaemia due to right coronary artery stenosis. Heart. 90(6):696, 2004
5. Ueno Y et al: Noninvasive assessment of significant right coronary artery stenosis based on coronary flow velocity reserve in the right coronary artery by transthoracic Doppler echocardiography. Echocardiography. 20(6):495-501, 2003
6. Mendes LA et al: Right coronary artery stenosis: an independent predictor of atrial fibrillation after coronary artery bypass surgery. J Am Coll Cardiol. 25(1):198-202, 1995
7. Gossman DE et al: Percutaneous transluminal angioplasty for shepherd's crook right coronary artery stenosis. Cathet Cardiovasc Diagn. 15(3):189-91, 1988
8. Gutman J et al: Enhanced detection of proximal right coronary artery stenosis with the additional analysis of right ventricular thallium-201 uptake in stress scintigrams. Am J Cardiol. 51(8):1256-60, 1983

IMAGE GALLERY

Typical

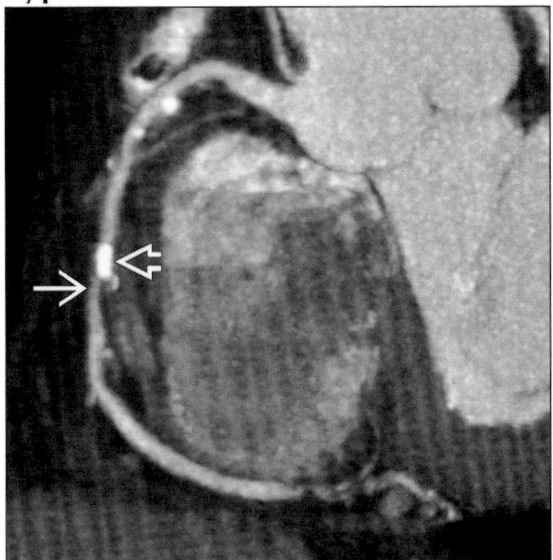

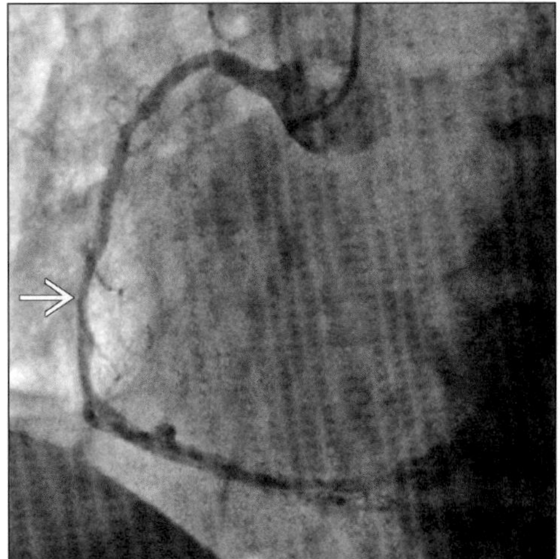

*(**Left**) Coronal oblique coronary CTA shows diffuse moderate to severe narrowing ➔ of the mid segment RCA distal to a large calcified plaque ➔. (**Right**) Corresponding invasive coronary angiogram confirms a moderate to severe stenosis ➔ of the mid segment RCA. Note how difficult it is to appreciate the extent and amount of RCA plaque burden compared with CTA.*

Typical

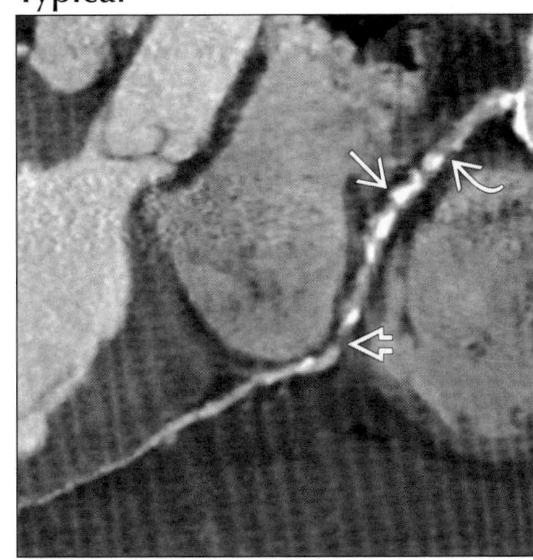

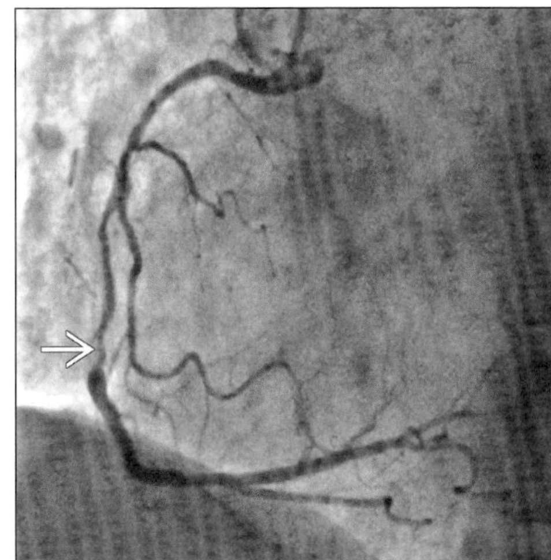

*(**Left**) Curved multiplanar reformat coronary CTA shows extensive calcified ➔ and noncalcified ➔ plaque in the proximal and mid segment RCA, and a tight stenosis ➔ in the distal portion of the mid segment. (**Right**) Corresponding invasive coronary angiogram confirms a significant stenosis ➔ in the mid segment RCA.*

Typical

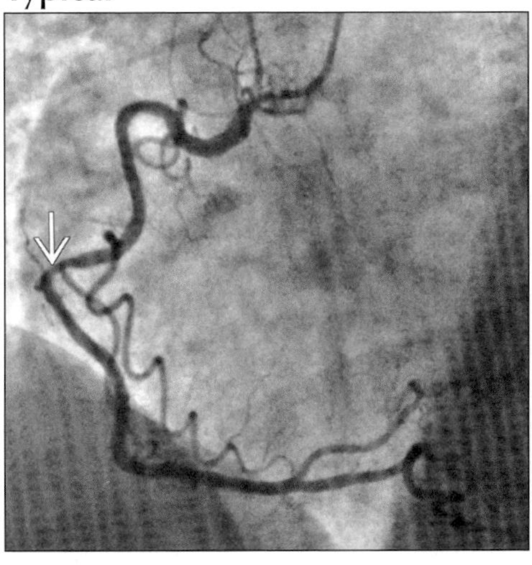

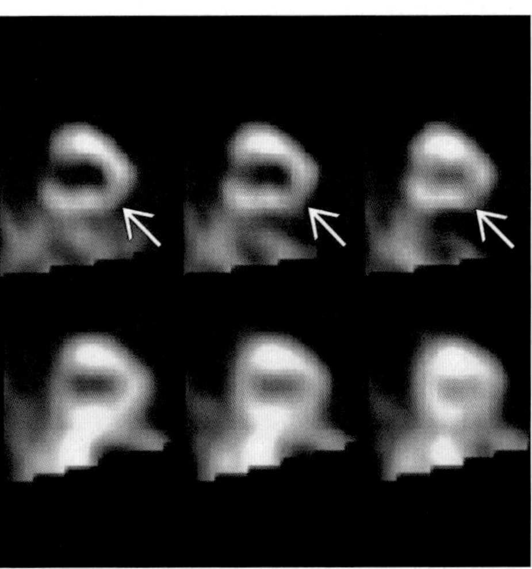

*(**Left**) Invasive coronary angiogram shows luminal narrowing ➔ of the mid segment RCA of uncertain hemodynamic significance. (**Right**) Corresponding SPECT scan shows a hypoperfusion defect in the inferior apical segment ➔ suggesting a hemodynamically significant RCA stenosis.*

LEFT MAIN CORONARY STENOSIS

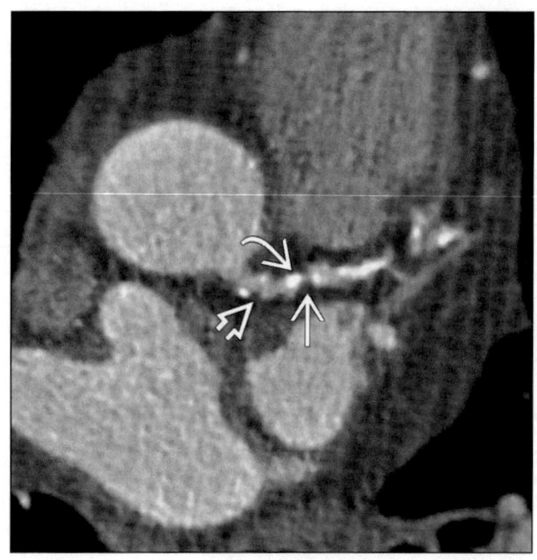

Axial coronary CTA shows significant stenosis in the distal portion of the LM. Note calcified and noncalcified plaque throughout the LM.

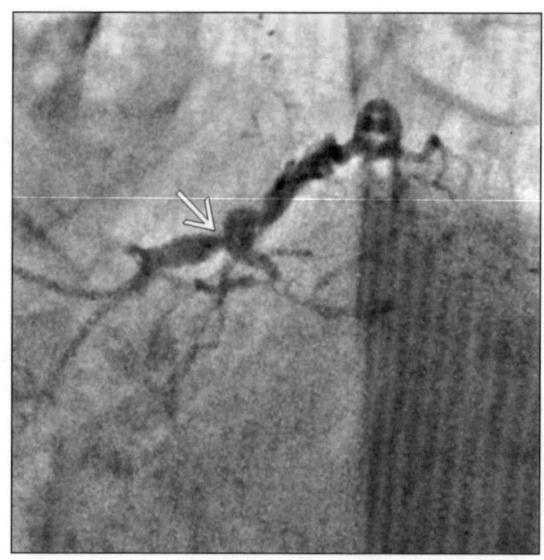

Corresponding invasive coronary angiogram confirms significant stenosis of the distal portion of the LM.

TERMINOLOGY

Definitions

- Left main (LM) coronary stenosis ≥ 50% luminal narrowing

IMAGING FINDINGS

General Features

- Best diagnostic clue
  - Stenosis ≥ 50% of the LM identified at
    - Invasive coronary angiography, cardiac coronary CT (CTA), cardiac coronary MR, intravascular ultrasound (IVUS)
- Location: Most common site of stenosis is at the mid or distal portion
- Size
  - Degree of stenosis is related to survival
    - LM stenosis between 50-70% = 3-year survival of 66%, LM stenosis > 70% = 3-year survival of 41%
- LM stenosis findings in stress testing
  - ST-depression > 2 mm
  - Downsloping ST-depression
  - Hypotension
  - ST-segment elevation strongly predictive of LM stenosis
  - Patients who stop at stage I or II Bruce protocol stage with ECG changes: 25% have LM stenosis
  - Patients who stop at stage III or IV Bruce protocol stage with ECG changes: < 1% have LM stenosis

Radiographic Findings

- Radiography
  - Chest radiography findings
    - Usually normal in the absence of heart failure

CT Findings

- CTA
  - Requires high spatial, temporal and contrast resolution
    - Sensitivity - 85-95% for the detection of significant coronary stenosis
    - Sensitivity - 95-99% for the detection of significant coronary stenosis
    - Very high negative predictive value
  - Coronary CTA allows considerable plaque characterization and has shown good agreement with IVUS

DDx: Left Main Coronary Stenosis

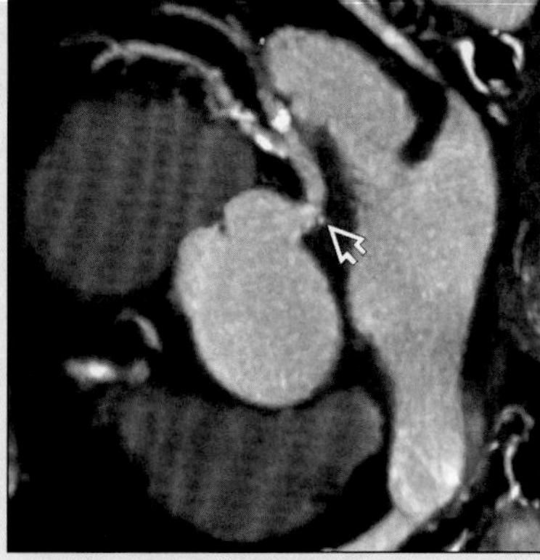

Coronary Dissection

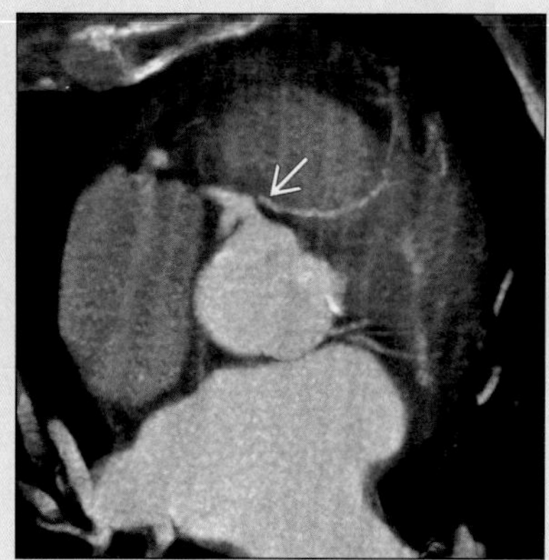

Coronary Anomaly

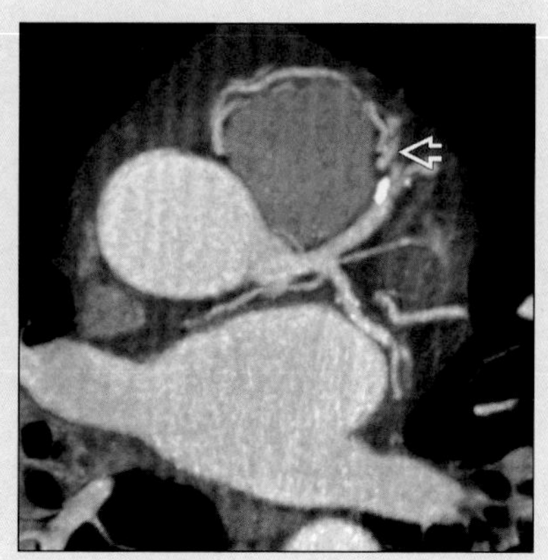

Coronary Fistula

LEFT MAIN CORONARY STENOSIS

Key Facts

Terminology

- Left main (LM) coronary stenosis ≥ 50%

Imaging Findings

- Most common site of stenosis is the mid or distal portion
- Degree of stenosis is related to survival
- Coronary angiography is considered the clinical gold-standard
- LM stenosis between 50-70% = 3-year survival of 66%
- LM stenosis > 70% = 3-year survival of 41%
- Coronary CTA allows considerable plaque characterization and has shown good agreement with IVUS
- Coronary CTA excellent diagnostic accuracy in detecting instent re-stenosis of LM stents
- High index of suspicion at angiography if ostial lesion suspected; sinus injection first is mandatory; careful advancement of catheter; limited number of shots

Clinical Issues

- Spectrum varies from asymptomatic to sudden death
- 80% of patients have concomitant lesions in other vessels
- Significant LM narrowing puts patient at high risk of subsequent hard cardiac event (infarction or death)
- Exact treatment is controversial but most agree that intervention is warranted and significantly affects prognosis

- Coronary CTA excellent diagnostic accuracy in detecting instent re-stenosis of LM stents
  - Lower diagnostic accuracy for bifurcation stents due to overlapping struts

MR Findings

- Whole heart MR
  - Images entire heart in one acquisition
  - Steady-state free precession sequence covering the entire heart
  - Prospective navigator gating and volume tracking
  - Does not have the spatial resolution of cardiac 64+ slice CTA
  - Useful non-invasive alternative in patients with contraindications to CT

Nuclear Medicine Findings

- PET: High sensitivity for detection of ischemic territory
- Nuclear cardiology findings
  - Thallium or technetium imaging to detect flow limited zones; large region of anteroapical and lateral reduced uptake, thinning
  - Left ventricle (LV) dilatation may appear during stress
  - LM stenosis appears as reduced uptake in the septum and anterior and lateral walls
  - Approx 60% of patients with LM stenosis have multiple thallium defects

Echocardiographic Findings

- Echocardiogram
  - Reduced wall motion and wall thickening
  - Chamber enlargement may be apparent

Ultrasonographic Findings

- Intravascular ultrasound (IVUS)
  - Permits detailed, high-quality, cross-sectional imaging of the LM in vivo
  - Excellent plaque characterization
  - Many patients with angiographically normal LM have abnormal IVUS studies
  - Absolute luminal area measurement helpful if no unaffected reference segment for % stenosis determination is present

Angiographic Findings

- Conventional
  - Coronary angiography is considered the clinical gold-standard
  - Care with image interpretation
    - Narrowing may be slit-like
    - Diffuse disease may be difficult to quantify
    - Ostial lesions may be missed if catheter is pushed past the lesion; may be hypotension and no reflux of contrast back into aorta
    - High index of suspicion at angiography if ostial lesion suspected; sinus injection first is mandatory; careful advancement of catheter; limited number of shots
    - Anteroposterior projection is the most useful
    - Glagov effect (vessel dilates in response to plaque formation)
  - Interobserver variability is considerable for LM stenosis

Imaging Recommendations

- Best imaging tool
  - Evolving topic: Clinical gold-standard is coronary angiography
  - Multidetector cardiac CTA is a rapidly evolving non-invasive alternative
  - IVUS if available

DIFFERENTIAL DIAGNOSIS

Other Causes of Acute Chest Pain

- Non-LM coronary artery stenosis
- Coronary anomaly
- Coronary artery aneurysm
- Coronary dissection

LEFT MAIN CORONARY STENOSIS

PATHOLOGY

General Features

- Etiology
  - Poorly understood
    - Atherosclerosis (principal cause)
    - Non-atherosclerotic considerations: Syphilis, giant cell arteritis, Takayasu arteritis, trauma (iatrogenic), anomalous take-off

CLINICAL ISSUES

Presentation

- Most common signs/symptoms
  - Clinical presentations have a low sensitivity and predictive value
  - Spectrum of symptoms varies from asymptomatic to sudden death
  - Unstable angina is the most common symptom, especially crescendo angina
- Clinical Profile
  - 80% of patients have concomitant lesions in other vessels
  - Prevalence
    - 9% in coronary artery bypass patients
    - 5% in patients with chronic angina
    - 7% of patients with acute myocardial infarction
    - Totally isolated LM stenosis is rare (< 0.5-1% of patients)
- Heart failure: Indicative of large region of ischemia
- ECG may show ST depression and T-wave inversion of all precordial leads

Demographics

- Gender: LM stenosis is more common in females (reason unknown)

Natural History & Prognosis

- Significant LM narrowing puts patient at high risk of subsequent hard cardiac event (infarction or death)
  - If no collateral flow 75% blood supply to LV may be removed

Treatment

- Exact treatment is controversial but most agree that intervention is warranted and significantly affects prognosis
- Coronary bypass surgery has been recommended over medical treatment
  - Many are now considering stent treatment for LM disease although this is an evolving topic
- Angioplasty without stenting associated with poor early and long-term results
- Rotational atherectomy (debulking) of the LM plaque advocated by some before stenting
- Stents: Evolving stent technology, bare metal versus drug-eluting
- American College of Cardiology Guidelines consider LM stenosis a class I indication for bypass surgery
  - Predictors of survival: Age, congestive heart failure, hypertension, stenosis percentage, coronary artery dominance

DIAGNOSTIC CHECKLIST

Consider

- In any patient presenting with crescendo angina

Image Interpretation Pearls

- Left main coronary stenosis ≥ 50% luminal narrowing
- Most common site of stenosis is at the mid or distal portion
- 80% of patients have concomitant lesions in other vessels

SELECTED REFERENCES

1. Sheiban I et al: Long-term clinical and angiographic outcomes of treatment of unprotected left main coronary artery stenosis with sirolimus-eluting stents. Am J Cardiol. 100(3):431-5, 2007
2. Suh WM et al: Utility of cardiac MRI in guiding revascularization therapy in unprotected left main stenosis: a case report. Cardiovasc Revasc Med. 8(3):209-12, 2007
3. Caussin C et al: Comparison of coronary minimal lumen area quantification by sixty-four-slice computed tomography versus intravascular ultrasound for intermediate stenosis. Am J Cardiol. 98(7):871-6, 2006
4. Caussin C et al: Comparison of coronary minimal lumen area quantification by sixty-four-slice computed tomography versus intravascular ultrasound for intermediate stenosis. Am J Cardiol. 98(7):871-6, 2006
5. Giannoglou GD et al: Prevalence of narrowing >or=50% of the left main coronary artery among 17,300 patients having coronary angiography. Am J Cardiol. 98(9):1202-5, 2006
6. Huang HW et al: Trends in percutaneous versus surgical revascularization of unprotected left main coronary stenosis in the drug-eluting stent era: a report from the American College of Cardiology-National Cardiovascular Data Registry (ACC-NCDR). Catheter Cardiovasc Interv. 68(6):867-72, 2006
7. Jönsson A et al: Left main coronary artery stenosis no longer a risk factor for early and late death after coronary artery bypass surgery--an experience covering three decades. Eur J Cardiothorac Surg. 30(2):311-7, 2006
8. Valgimigli M et al: Distal left main coronary disease is a major predictor of outcome in patients undergoing percutaneous intervention in the drug-eluting stent era: an integrated clinical and angiographic analysis based on the Rapamycin-Eluting Stent Evaluated At Rotterdam Cardiology Hospital (RESEARCH) and Taxus-Stent Evaluated At Rotterdam Cardiology Hospital (T-SEARCH) registries. J Am Coll Cardiol. 47(8):1530-7, 2006
9. Valgimigli M et al: Single-vessel versus bifurcation stenting for the treatment of distal left main coronary artery disease in the drug-eluting stenting era. Clinical and angiographic insights into the Rapamycin-Eluting Stent Evaluated at Rotterdam Cardiology Hospital (RESEARCH) and Taxus-Stent Evaluated at Rotterdam Cardiology Hospital (T-SEARCH) registries. Am Heart J. 152(5):896-902, 2006

LEFT MAIN CORONARY STENOSIS

IMAGE GALLERY

Typical

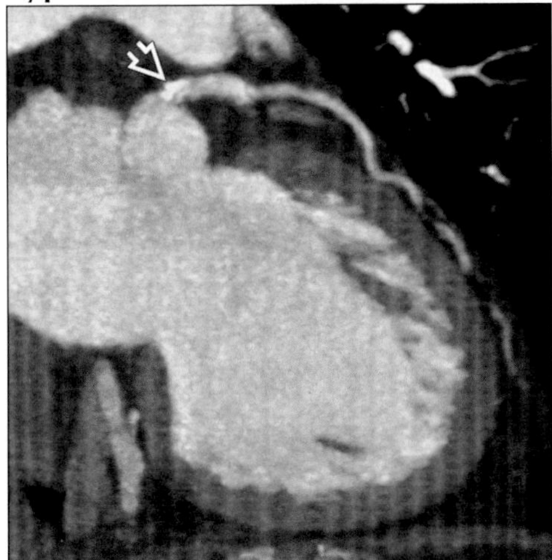

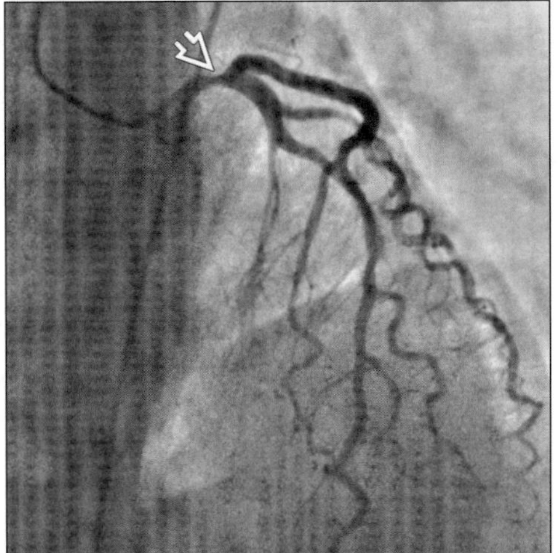

(Left) *Coronal oblique coronary CTA shows a calcified plaque* ➔ *at the LM ostium extending into its proximal portion, which makes stenosis evaluation difficult, but suggests a significant stenosis.* ***(Right)*** *Corresponding invasive coronary angiogram confirms a significant stenosis* ➔ *of the LM.*

Typical

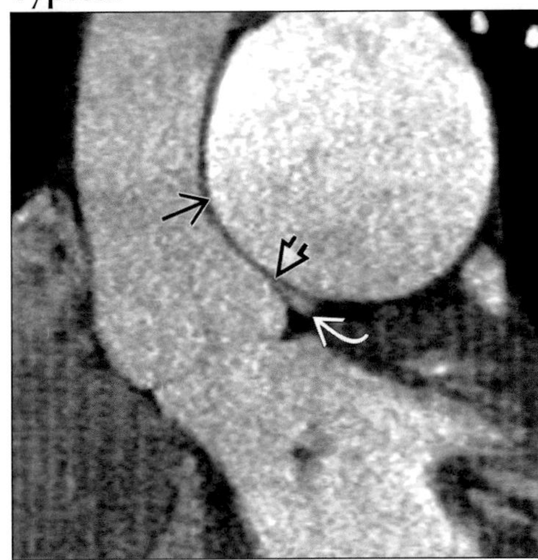

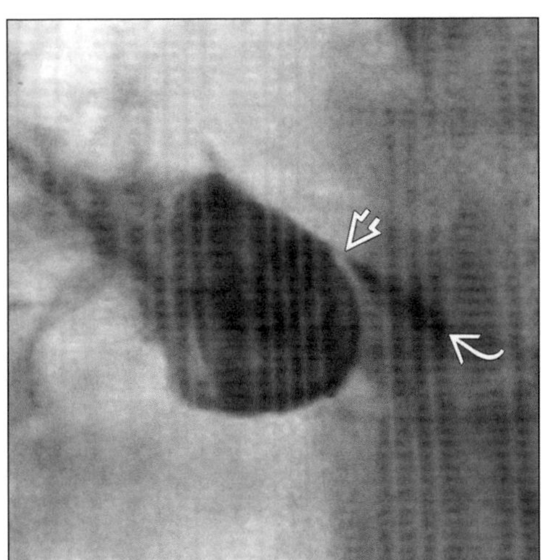

(Left) *Coronal oblique CTA shows massively enlarged main pulmonary artery* → *due to persistent patent ductus arteriosus. This is causing marked extrinsic ostial compression* ➔ *of the LM* ➦. ***(Right)*** *Corresponding invasive angiogram confirms ostial high grade stenosis* ➔ *of the LM* ➦ *from extrinsic compression.*

Typical

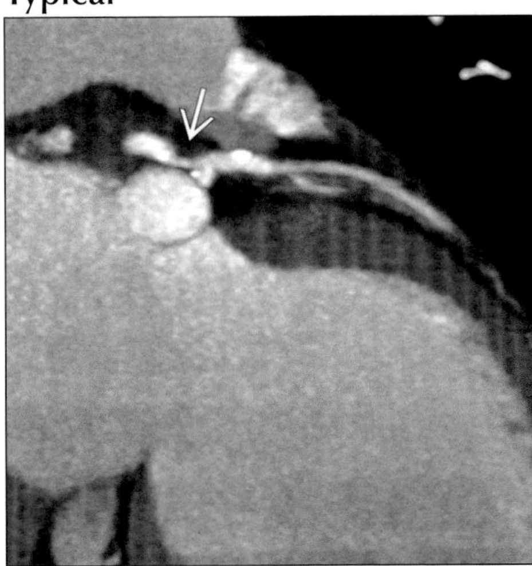

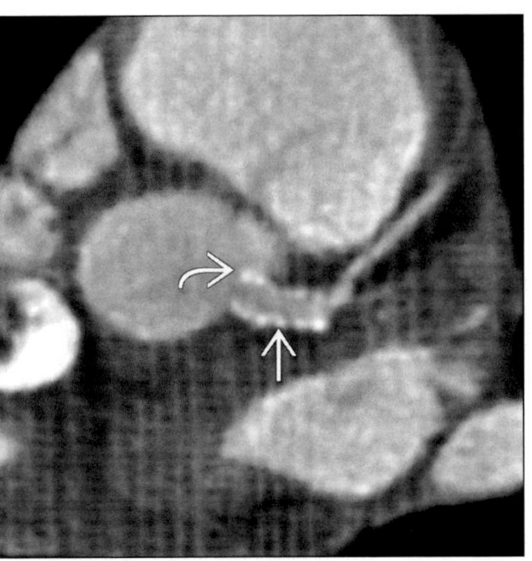

(Left) *Sagittal oblique coronary CTA shows a large non-calcified plaque* ➔ *causing hemodynamically significant stenosis of the LM. Patient declined surgery.* ***(Right)*** *Corresponding CTA post percutaneous coronary intervention shows a large, widely patent stent* ➔ *placed across the LM. Note struts* ➦ *jutting out into aortic lumen.*

CORONARY ARTERY DISSECTION

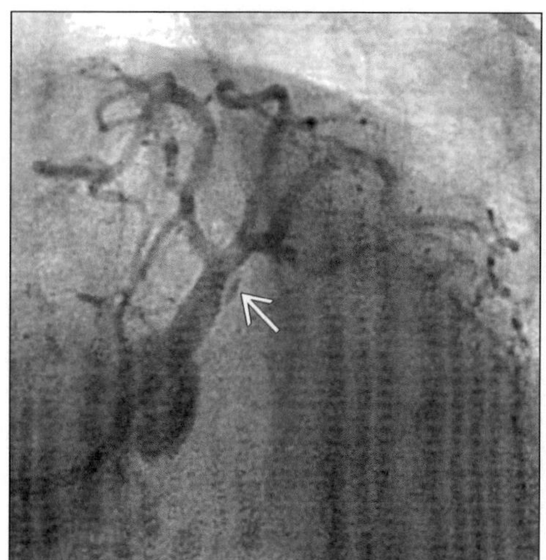

Coronary angiogram in 79 year old woman with chest pain demonstrates a coronary artery dissection following stent wire manipulation in left main coronary artery →.

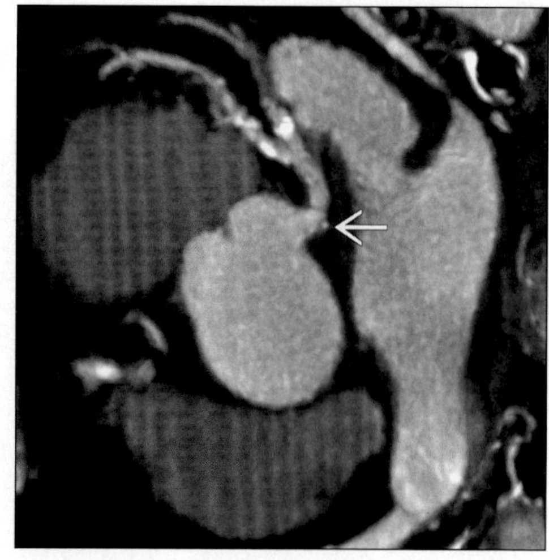

Corresponding coronary CTA shows tiny amount of contrast in coronary artery wall → corresponding to the invasive angiogram dissection.

TERMINOLOGY

Definitions

- Intimal tear of coronary artery wall with a false lumen between the adventitia and tunica media

IMAGING FINDINGS

General Features

- Best diagnostic clue: Contrast in the wall of a coronary vessel
- Location
  - Right coronary system more commonly affected in males
  - Left coronary system more commonly affected in females

CT Findings

- Cardiac Gated CTA
  - May show contrast within coronary artery wall outside true lumen
  - Thrombosed false lumen may be difficult to differentiate from non-calcified plaque
  - Misregistration artifact may mimic dissection
    - Reconstruction of different cardiac phases may result in a dataset where line is not persistent which proves its artificial nature
    - Artifact appears as unusually straight line (not anatomic) in X-Y plane between adjacent slabs
    - May extend beyond confines of vessel

Echocardiographic Findings

- Transesophageal
  - Linear echogenic flap
  - Color Doppler may allow differentiation of true and false lumen
- Intravascular ultrasound (IVUS)
  - IVUS can confirm presence of intimal flap and may aid placement of stent guidewire into the true lumen
  - Can demonstrate contrast (black echogenicity) or thrombus (grey echogenicity) within the false lumen

Angiographic Findings

- Conventional
  - Intimal flap may be apparent as linear filling defect in vessel lumen
    - Flap may be mobile or fixed

DDx: Coronary Artery Dissection

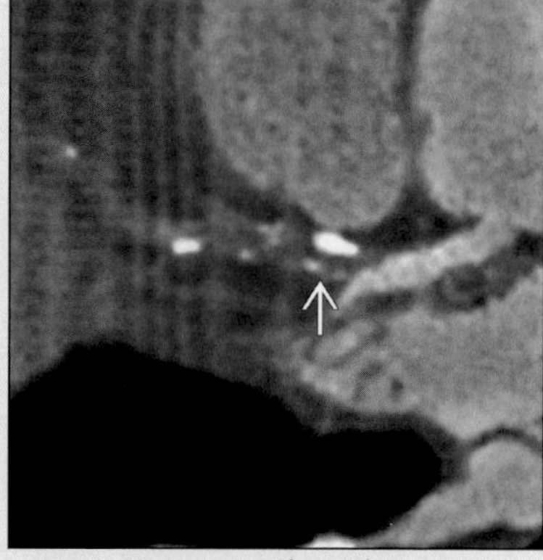

Coronary Thrombosis

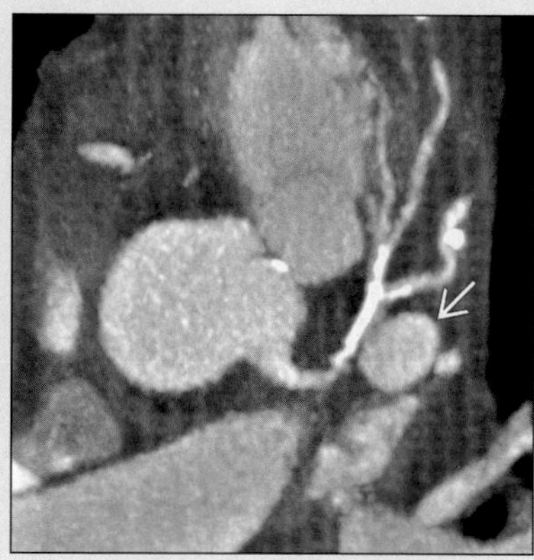

Coronary Aneurysm

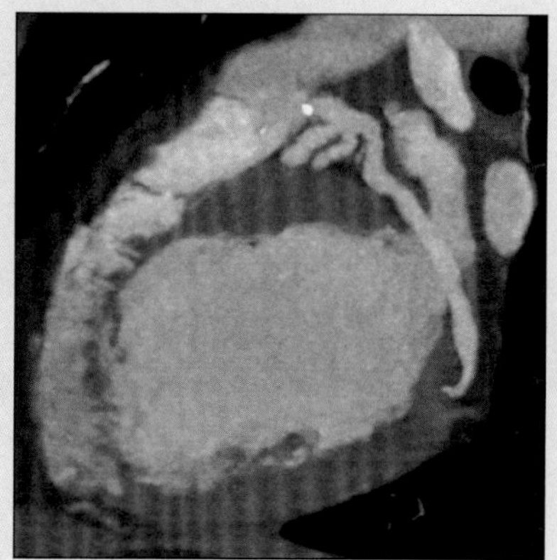

Kawasaki Disease

CORONARY ARTERY DISSECTION

Key Facts

Terminology
- Intimal tear of coronary artery wall with a false lumen between the adventitia and tunica media

Imaging Findings
- Best diagnostic clue: Contrast in the wall of a coronary vessel
- Right coronary system more commonly affected in males
- Left coronary system more commonly affected in females
- May show contrast within coronary artery wall outside true lumen
- Misregistration artifact may mimic dissection
- IVUS can confirm presence of intimal flap and may aid placement of stent guidewire into the true lumen
- Flap may be mobile or fixed

Pathology
- Subintimal disruption
- Small cystic spaces in the media of coronary vessels

Clinical Issues
- Age: Young patients with coronary dissection can present with heart failure and acute myocardial infarction
- Risk of acute occlusion varies depending on the degree of dissection
- Overall prognosis ill-defined
- Many small dissections will heal spontaneously
- Thrombolytics may exacerbate dissections
- Placement of stent will tack down dissection and is considered definitive therapy

  - Linear or spiral-shaped false lumen contrast staining
  - Spectrum from small benign to large occlusive flap

DIFFERENTIAL DIAGNOSIS

Thrombus
- Less often linear
- May be mobile, making flap differentiation difficult

Intraplaque Hemorrhage
- Not uncommon in complicated plaques, and as a result of plaque rupture
- May have similar clinical sequelae to dissection

Coronary Aneurysm
- Spindle shaped or saccular expansion of coronary artery wall without evidence of flap
- No intimal tear
- Dilatation involves all layers of vessel wall

Pseudoaneurysm
- Focal dilation of coronary artery with disruption of one or more layers of its walls

PATHOLOGY

General Features
- General path comments
  - Subintimal disruption
  - Thrombus formation can play an intimate role in stabilizing dissection
- Etiology
  - Spontaneous
  - Peri/post partum
  - Atherosclerosis
  - Coronary vasculitis
    - Kawasaki disease
    - Polyarteritis nodosa
    - Systemic lupus erythematosus
    - Giant cell arteritis
  - Coronary intervention
    - Cannulation of vessel
    - Advancing guidewire
    - Balloon angioplasty
    - Can be found in ~ 60% of post-procedure examinations
    - Directional atherectomy followed by balloon angioplasty
    - Edge dissection after stent deployment
  - Blunt chest trauma
  - Aortic dissection
- Epidemiology: Approximately 100 reported spontaneous cases

Microscopic Features
- Small cystic spaces in the media of coronary vessels
- Eosinophilic infiltrate in the adventitia - possible association?

CLINICAL ISSUES

Presentation
- Most common signs/symptoms
  - Asymptomatic
  - Recurrent angina
  - May cause acute myocardial infarction in young patients
  - Unexplained sudden heart failure in spontaneous dissection
  - Sudden death
- Asymptomatic in most procedural complications

Demographics
- Age: Young patients with coronary dissection can present with heart failure and acute myocardial infarction
- Gender: Equal gender distribution

Natural History & Prognosis
- Risk of acute occlusion varies depending on the degree of dissection
  - About 5-10% acutely occlude, usually in the first 12 hours after stopping heparin post-procedure

- Spiral and long (> 10 mm) dissections have worse outcomes
- Overall prognosis ill-defined

Treatment

- Many small dissections will heal spontaneously
- Thrombolytics may exacerbate dissections
- Antithrombotics and antiplatelet therapy (Gp IIb/IIIa) can reduce the risk of acute thrombosis and occlusion
- Placement of stent will tack down dissection and is considered definitive therapy
- Edge dissections associated with stent deployment do not require treatment

DIAGNOSTIC CHECKLIST

Consider

- In young patients presenting with acute myocardial infarction
- Intimal flap appears as linear filling defect in vessel lumen

SELECTED REFERENCES

1. Kurum T et al: Spontaneous coronary artery dissection after heavy lifting in a 25-year-old man with coronary risk factors. J Cardiovasc Med (Hagerstown). 7(1):68-70, 2006
2. Ohlmann P et al: Images in cardiovascular medicine. Spontaneous coronary dissection: computed tomography appearance and insights from intravascular ultrasound examination. Circulation. 113(10):e403-5, 2006
3. Tepe SM et al: MRI demonstration of acute myocardial infarction due to posttraumatic coronary artery dissection. Int J Cardiovasc Imaging. 22(1):97-100, 2006
4. van Gaal WJ 3rd et al: Treatment of spontaneous coronary dissection with drug-eluting stents--late clinical, angiographic and IVUS follow up. J Invasive Cardiol. 18(2):E93-4, 2006
5. Butler R et al: Spontaneous dissection of native coronary arteries. Heart. 91(2):223-4, 2005
6. Chai HT et al: Utilization of a double-wire technique to treat long extended spiral dissection of the right coronary artery. Evaluation of incidence and mechanisms. Int Heart J. 46(1):35-44, 2005
7. Gowda RM et al: Clinical perspectives of the primary spontaneous coronary artery dissection. Int J Cardiol. 105(3):334-6, 2005
8. Justice LT et al: Left main dissection and thrombosis in a young athlete. Cardiol Rev. 13(5):260-2, 2005
9. Thompson EA et al: Gender differences and predictors of mortality in spontaneous coronary artery dissection: a review of reported cases. J Invasive Cardiol. 17(1):59-61, 2005
10. Moukarbel GV et al: Spontaneous coronary artery dissection: management options in the stent era. J Invasive Cardiol. 16(6):333-5, 2004
11. Porto I et al: Intravascular ultrasound imaging in the diagnosis and treatment of spontaneous coronary dissection with drug-eluting stents. J Invasive Cardiol. 16(2):78-80, 2004
12. Rogers JH et al: Coronary artery dissection and perforation complicating percutaneous coronary intervention. J Invasive Cardiol. 16(9):493-9, 2004
13. Milano AD et al: Fate of coronary ostial anastomoses after the modified Bentall procedure. Ann Thorac Surg. 75(6):1797-801; discussion 1802, 2003
14. Roig S et al: Spontaneous coronary artery dissection causing acute coronary syndrome: an early diagnosis implies a good prognosis. Am J Emerg Med. 21(7):549-51, 2003
15. Sarmento-Leite R et al: Spontaneous coronary artery dissection: stent it or wait for healing? Heart. 89(2):164, 2003
16. Badmanaban B et al: Spontaneous coronary artery dissection presenting as cardiac tamponade. Ann Thorac Surg. 73(4):1324-6, 2002
17. Kamineni R et al: Spontaneous coronary artery dissection: report of two cases and a 50-year review of the literature. Cardiol Rev. 10(5):279-84, 2002
18. Maresta A et al: Spontaneous coronary dissection of all three coronary arteries: a case description with medium-term angiographic follow-up. Ital Heart J. 3(12):747-51, 2002
19. Lerakis S et al: Transesophageal echo detection of postpartum coronary artery dissection. J Am Soc Echocardiogr. 14(11):1132-3, 2001
20. Mulvany NJ et al: Isolated dissection of the coronary artery: a postmortem study of seven cases. Pathology. 33(3):307-11, 2001
21. Ichiba N et al: Images in cardiovascular medicine. Plaque rupture causing spontaneous coronary artery dissection in a patient with acute myocardial infarction. Circulation. 101(14):1754-5, 2000
22. Hobbs RE et al: Chronic coronary artery dissection presenting as heart failure. Circulation. 100(4):445, 1999
23. Knisely BL et al: Imaging of cardiac transplantation complications. Radiographics. 19(2):321-39; discussion 340-1, 1999
24. Cherng WJ et al: Diagnosis of coronary artery dissection following blunt chest trauma by transesophageal echocardiography. J Trauma. 39(4):772-4, 1995
25. Jakob M et al: Transoesophageal colour Doppler detection of coronary artery dissection. Lancet. 343(8912):1574-5, 1994
26. Carrozza JP Jr et al: Complications of directional coronary atherectomy: incidence, causes, and management. Am J Cardiol. 72(13):47E-54E, 1993
27. DeMaio SJ Jr et al: Clinical course and long-term prognosis of spontaneous coronary artery dissection. Am J Cardiol. 64(8):471-4, 1989
28. Thayer JO et al: Spontaneous coronary artery dissection. Ann Thorac Surg. 44(1):97-102, 1987
29. Sanborn TA et al: The mechanism of transluminal angioplasty: evidence for formation of aneurysms in experimental atherosclerosis. Circulation. 68(5):1136-40, 1983
30. Albertal M et al: Angiographic and clinical outcome of mild to moderate nonocclusive unstented coronary artery dissection and the influence on coronary flow velocity reserve. The Debate I Study Group.
31. Celik SK et al: Primary spontaneous coronary artery dissections in atherosclerotic patients. Report of nine cases with review of the pertinent literature.

CORONARY ARTERY DISSECTION

IMAGE GALLERY

Typical

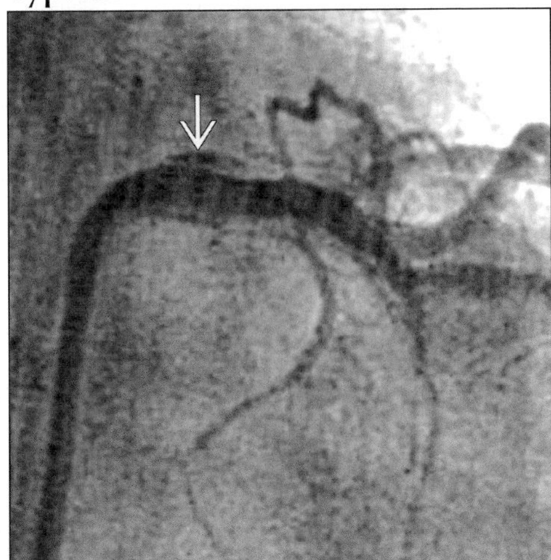

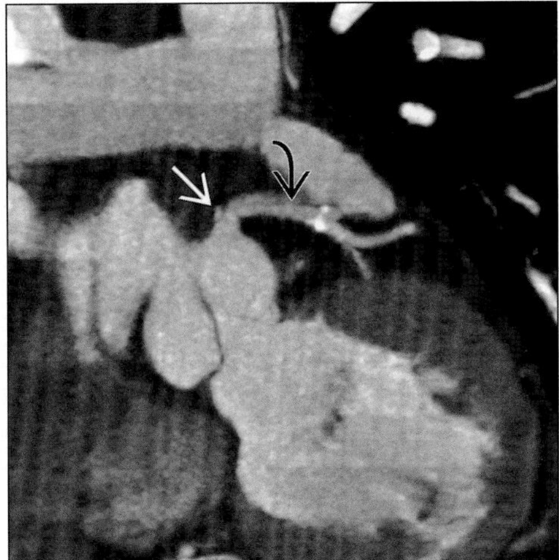

(Left) *Coronary angiogram demonstrates dissection of the left main coronary artery* ➡. ***(Right)*** *Corresponding coronary CTA shows contrast in wall of left main coronary artery* ➡ *corresponding to the dissection seen on the invasive angiogram. Note the linear "slab" artifact that can sometimes mimic dissection* ↷.

Typical

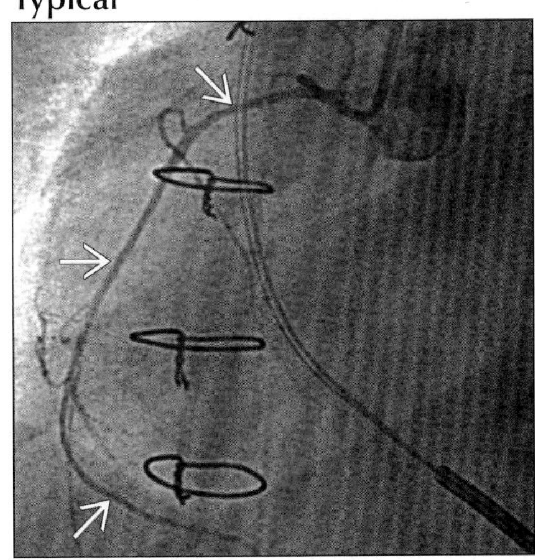

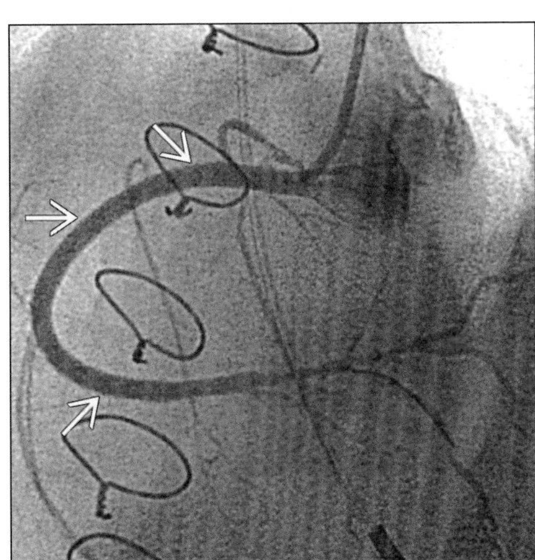

(Left) *Coronary angiogram in a 53 year old woman with sudden onset acute chest pain demonstrates spontaneous dissection of the entire right coronary artery* ➡. ***(Right)*** *Corresponding coronary angiogram post stenting of the entire right coronary artery demonstrates normal coronary lumen* ➡ *and widely patent stents.*

Typical

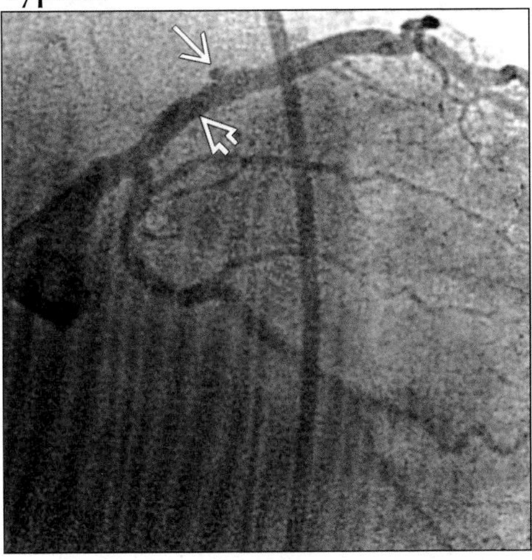

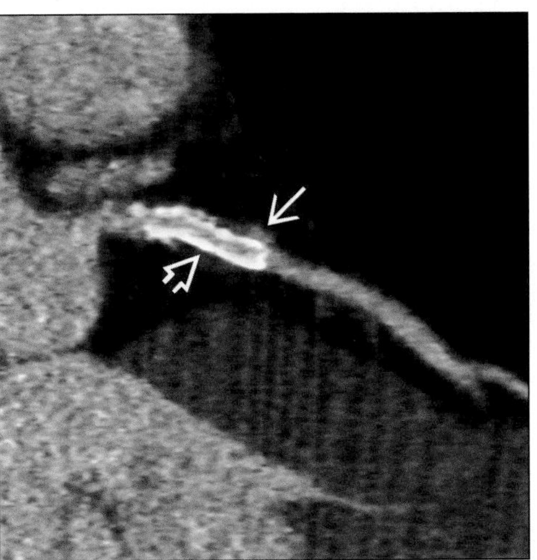

(Left) *Coronary angiogram shows a small coronary edge dissection* ➡ *secondary to stent insertion (obscured by contrast)* ⇨. ***(Right)*** *Corresponding coronary CTA shows a corresponding area of contrast in the wall of the coronary artery* ➡ *at the stent* ⇨ *edge consistent with a stent edge dissection.*

ACUTE MYOCARDIAL INFARCTION

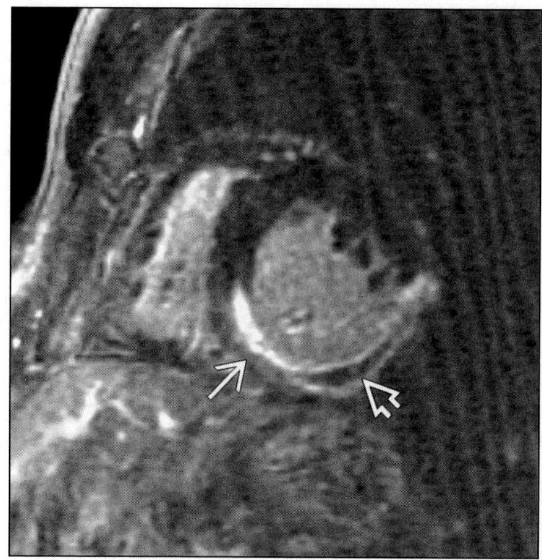

Short axis De-MRI shows large area of hyperenhancement ➡ in the inferior wall representing myocardial necrosis with central area of hypoenhancement ➡ (microvascular obstruction).

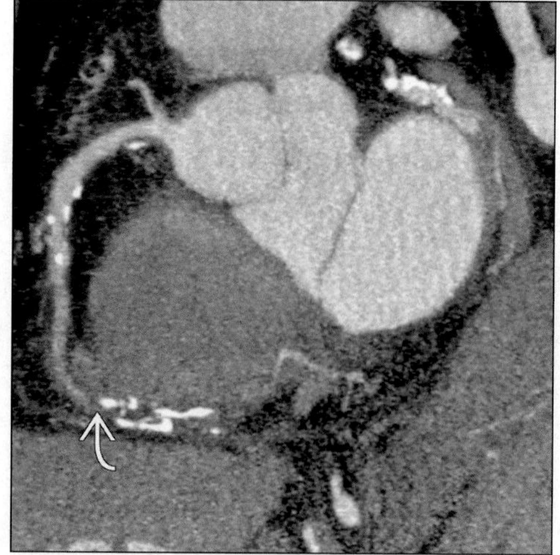

Oblique coronary CTA shows occlusion of the distal RCA ➡ with calcified and non-calcified plaque (thrombus) distal to the occlusion.

TERMINOLOGY

Abbreviations and Synonyms

- AMI, acute MI

Definitions

- Atherosclerotic plaque rupture followed by thrombosis and acute coronary occlusion leading to ischemic myocyte damage
  - Increased cardiac enzymes (troponin, CK and CK-MB) due to resulting cell integrity loss
- Myocardial infarction and unstable angina are considered acute coronary syndromes, while stable angina is a chronic condition
- AMI can be: ST elevation MI or non-ST elevation MI

IMAGING FINDINGS

General Features

- Best diagnostic clue: Coronary artery filling defect on invasive coronary angiogram
- General findings
  - Diminished perfusion and function of the affected area
  - Reduced regional contractility
    - Hypokinesis: Decreased systolic thickening
    - Akinesis: No contraction
    - Dyskinesis: Paradoxical motion
  - Increased cell membrane permeability
    - Increased uptake of extracellular agents
    - Leakage of intracellular proteins and enzymes
  - Altered regional metabolism

Radiographic Findings

- Radiography
  - Chest radiography findings
    - Abnormal findings are rare in the acute setting
    - Interstitial edema if heart failure ensues
    - Abnormal cardiac silhouette: Changes may result from acute valve dysfunction; regional aneurysm; cardiac rupture; pericardial tamponade
    - Sudden severe pulmonary edema in papillary muscle rupture → poor prognosis

CT Findings

- CTA

DDx: Acute Myocardial Infarction

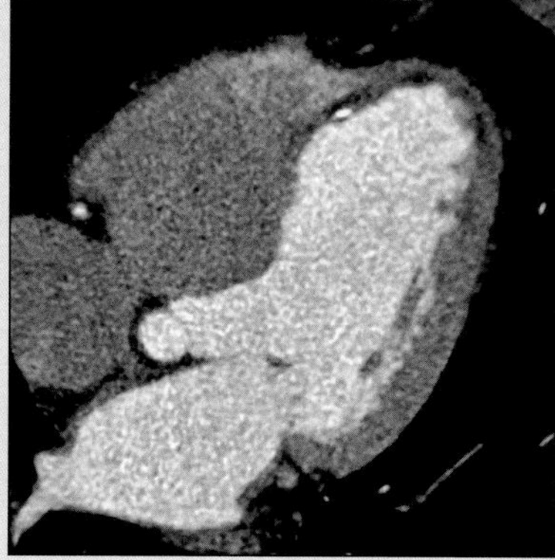

Chronic Infarct

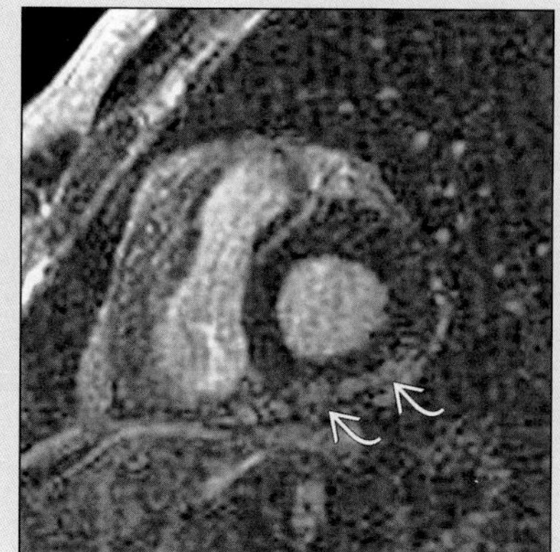

Acute Myocarditis

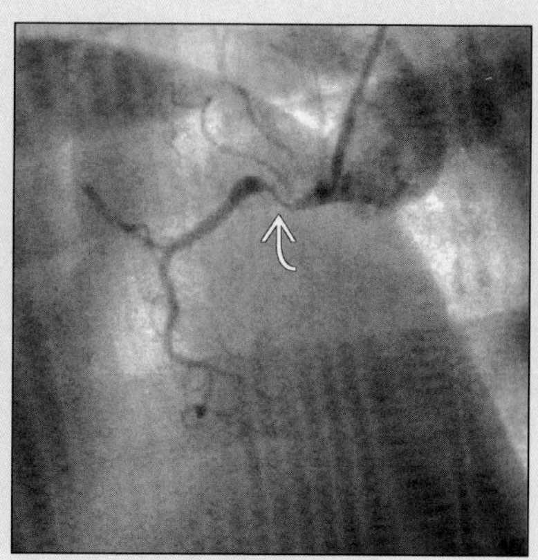

RCA Vasospasm

ACUTE MYOCARDIAL INFARCTION

Key Facts

Terminology
- Atherosclerotic plaque rupture followed by thrombosis and acute coronary occlusion leading to ischemic myocyte damage
- Myocardial infarction and unstable angina are considered acute coronary syndromes, while stable angina is a chronic condition

Imaging Findings
- CT evaluation of Hounsfield units (HU), LV thinning and presence of calcifications may differentiate chronic from acute MI
- T2WI: Affected area demonstrates increased signal intensity consistent with myocardial edema
- Reduced regional wall motion and systolic wall thickening
- Delayed-enhancement in the infarcted area due to myocardial necrosis (myocyte rupture → Gd enters cells)
- Central hypointense region surrounded by delayed-enhancement represents microvascular obstruction
- Reduced regional function: Hypokinesis, akinesis or dyskinesis

Clinical Issues
- Increased risk of ventricular arrhythmias and death
- Urgent treatment affects outcome (mortality and morbidity)
- Normal EKG does **not** exclude an acute infarct
- Imaging important to determine prognosis and to identify culprit coronary vessel
- Acute percutaneous intervention to restore flow

  - Coronary occlusion with non-calcified material (thrombus)
  - May demonstrate regional wall motion and perfusion deficit
  - CT evaluation of Hounsfield units (HU), LV thinning and presence of calcifications may differentiate chronic from acute MI
    - Negative HU indicate fatty metaplasia in chronic infarct

MR Findings
- T2WI: Affected area demonstrates increased signal intensity consistent with myocardial edema
- T1 C+: Infarcted area may demonstrate late enhancement after gadolinium
- MR Cine
  - Reduced regional wall motion and systolic wall thickening
  - Decreased ejection fraction, but could be preserved due to compensation from remote myocardium
  - May demonstrate mitral regurgitation, if inferior MI involving the postero-medial papillary muscle
- First-pass perfusion
  - Reduced wash-in of contrast agent on first-pass perfusion imaging (Perfusion deficit)
- Delayed-enhancement
  - Delayed-enhancement in the infarcted area due to myocardial necrosis (myocyte rupture → Gd enters cells)
  - Central hypointense region surrounded by delayed-enhancement represents microvascular obstruction
  - Microvascular obstruction indicates worse prognosis
  - Degree of transmurality of delayed-enhancement may predict LV functional recovery (> 75% transmurality in the acute setting = no recovery in 6 months)
- Gold standard for functional assessment; ejection fraction, LV end diastolic and end systolic volumes and LV mass
- Best modality to assess MI complications: True aneurysm, false aneurysm, ventricular septal rupture

Nuclear Medicine Findings
- Radionuclide angiography
  - Reduced overall ejection fraction
  - Regional myocardial dysfunction
  - Aneurysm formation; dyskinesis
- Cardiac scintigraphy
  - Fixed defect of reduced or absent tracer uptake (at stress and rest imaging)
  - Increased chamber size
  - No redistribution of thallium
  - No re-injection uptake of Tc99m perfusion tracer

Echocardiographic Findings
- Echocardiogram
  - Altered ventricular function
    - Decrease in ventricular ejection fraction, but function may be preserved
    - Reduced regional function: Hypokinesis, akinesis or dyskinesis
- Color Doppler: Mitral regurgitation (MR) with papillary muscle dysfunction

Angiographic Findings
- Conventional
  - Occluded coronary artery
  - Patent but tightly stenotic coronary artery, or plaque disruption
  - Minimal stenosis may reflect post-infarction lysis of a large thrombus
  - May show evidence of embolus
  - Ventriculography shows reduced regional wall motion and ejection fraction

Imaging Recommendations
- Best imaging tool: Cardiac catheterization → allows intervention

DIFFERENTIAL DIAGNOSIS

Old Infarction
- Wall motion abnormalities
- Persistent hyperenhancement on MR

- Absent tracer uptake on scintigraphy
- T2WI will not demonstrate peri infarct signal increase (no edema)
- Myocardial calcium, fatty metaplasia and aneurysm indicate remote infarct

Acute Myocarditis

- Typical presentation: Chest pain, increased cardiac enzymes and normal cardiac catheterization
- MR is fundamental for diagnosis
- Delayed-enhancement MR demonstrates hyperenhancement in the sub-epicardial region (typical location = infero-lateral basal epicardial wall)
- Wall motion abnormalities may be associated
- Cell membrane integrity compromised

Coronary Vasospasm

- Prinzmetal angina
- Syndrome of chest pain at rest secondary to myocardial ischemia associated with ST-segment elevation

Broken Heart Syndrome

- Also known as Takotsubo cardiomyopathy or stress induced cardiomyopathy
- Reversible left ventricular dysfunction with apical ballooning
- MR may add to the diagnosis demonstrating regional wall motion abnormality with no evidence of delayed-enhancement

Unstable Angina

- Syndrome that is intermediate between stable angina and myocardial infarction
- Accelerating or "crescendo" pattern of chest pain that lasts longer than in stable angina, occurs at rest or is less responsive to medication
- Cardiac enzymes are not elevated; significant stenosis by angiography or positive ischemic test

PATHOLOGY

General Features

- General path comments
  - Myocardial necrosis
  - Vascular occlusion
  - Most often combined with ischemic or post-ischemic non-infarcted myocardium
- Etiology: Plaque rupture with thrombus formation

CLINICAL ISSUES

Presentation

- Most common signs/symptoms
  - Chest pain; substernal, pressing, occasionally radiating to the left arm
  - Associated with dyspnea, nausea, palpitations, radiation to the jaw
  - Any diffuse pain above the umbilicus - not sharp or pleuritic
- Clinical Profile
  - Increased risk of ventricular arrhythmias and death
  - Urgent treatment affects outcome (mortality and morbidity)
  - Normal EKG does **not** exclude an acute infarct

Treatment

- Imaging important to determine prognosis and to identify culprit coronary vessel
- Medical therapy; thrombolysis in absence of contraindications if presenting within the first 12 hours after symptoms develop
- Acute percutaneous intervention to restore flow
  - Best done within the first 3 hours
  - Optimally done with stent implantation and antiplatelet therapy with Gp IIb/IIIa inhibitor
- Acute coronary bypass is available but rarely indicated in the absence of shock and availability of percutaneous intervention
- In hospital mortality is ~ 6% while overall mortality for AMI is ~ 20%

DIAGNOSTIC CHECKLIST

Consider

- EKG changes such as ST elevation and increased cardiac enzymes are diagnostic for acute MI and will lead to invasive angiogram
- Cardiac CT and MRI can be used in patients where the diagnosis of acute coronary syndrome is unclear

Image Interpretation Pearls

- Cardiac CT can assess not only coronary stenosis/occlusion, but also global and regional LV function and myocardial perfusion
- Cardiac MRI is best to detect myocardial infarct (delayed-enhancement) and further characterize acute vs. chronic (T2WI)

SELECTED REFERENCES

1. Nieman K et al: Differentiation of recent and chronic myocardial infarction by cardiac computed tomography. Am J Cardiol. 98(3):303-8, 2006
2. Gerber BL et al: Accuracy of contrast-enhanced magnetic resonance imaging in predicting improvement of regional myocardial function in patients after acute myocardial infarction. Circulation. 106(9):1083-9, 2002
3. Antman EM et al: Acute Myocardial Infarction In: Braunwald E. Heart Disease: A Textbook of Cardiovascular Medicine 6th ed W.B. Philadelphia, 2001
4. Kim RJ et al: Relationship of MRI delayed contrast enhancement to irreversible injury, infarct age, and contractile function. Circulation. 100(19):1992-2002, 1999
5. Ryan TL et al: ACC/AHA Guidelines for the Management of Patients With Acute Myocardial Infarction. Circulation 100:1016-30, 1999
6. Topol EJ et al: Acute Myocardial Infarction. In Topol EJ. Textbook of Cardiovascular Medicine 6th ed W.B. Lippincott Raven, Philadelphia, 395-436, 1998
7. Wu KC et al: Prognostic significance of microvascular obstruction by magnetic resonance imaging in patients with acute myocardial infarction. Circulation. 97(8):765-72, 1998
8. Choi KM et al: Transmural extent of acute myocardial infarction predicts long-term improvement in contractile function.

ACUTE MYOCARDIAL INFARCTION

IMAGE GALLERY

Typical

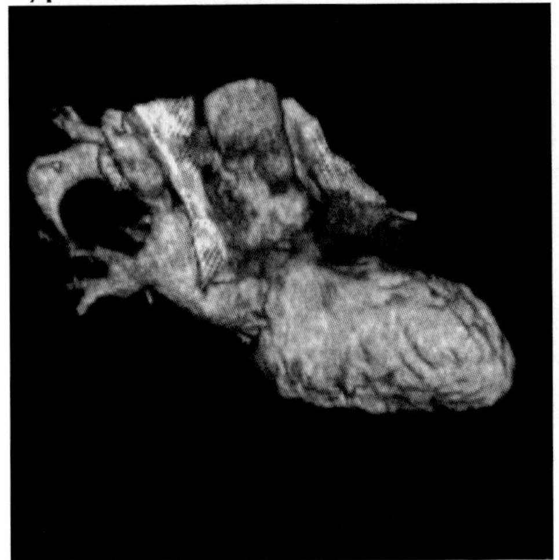

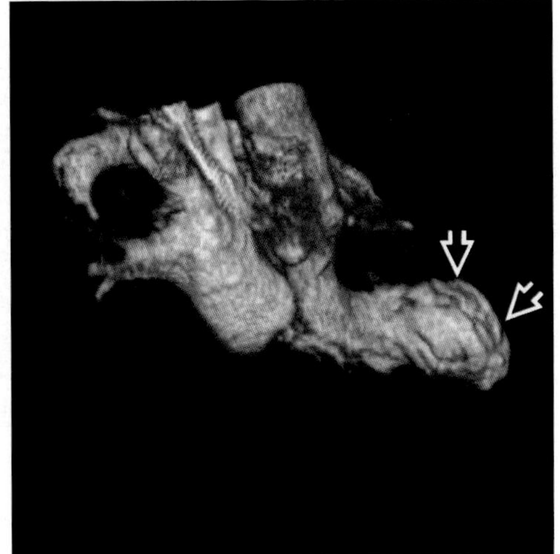

(Left) *Oblique cardiac CT 4D left ventriculogram shows normal left ventricular cavity in end-diastole.* ***(Right)*** *Oblique 4D left ventriculogram in end-systole (same patient as previous image) shows akinesis of left ventricular antero-apical wall → due to acute myocardial infarct in left anterior descending territory.*

Typical

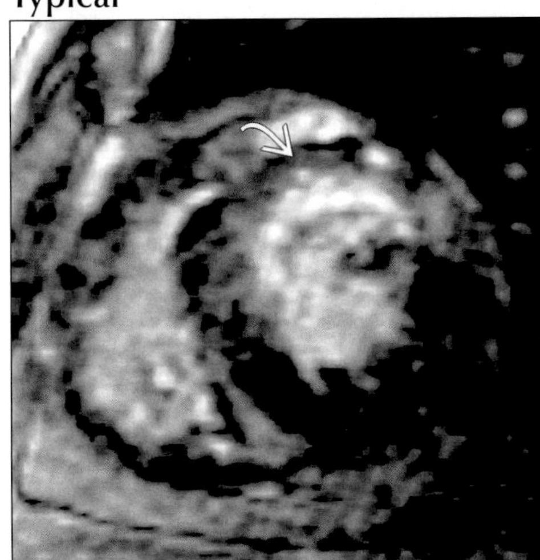

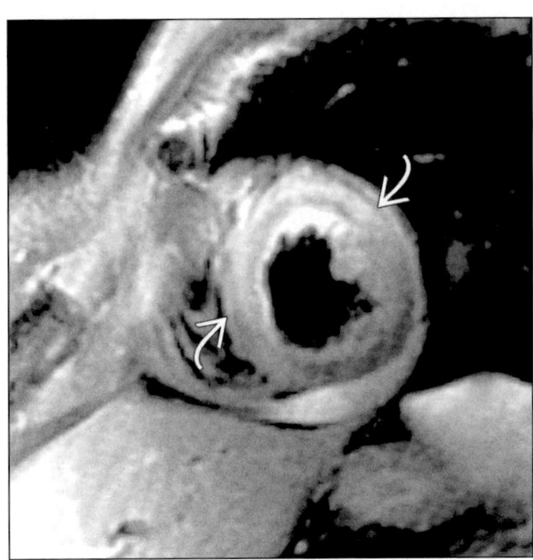

(Left) *Short axis Delayed-enhancement image shows hyperenhancement consistent with myocardial necrosis in the anterior & antero-septal walls → in setting of anterior AMI.* ***(Right)*** *Short axis T2WI FS MR shows area of hyperintensity in the anterior and antero-lateral walls → (8 to 1 o'clock) representing myocardial edema in the setting of anterior AMI.*

Typical

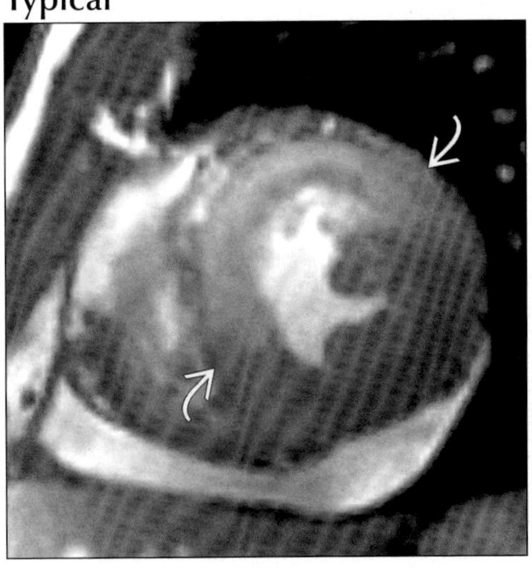

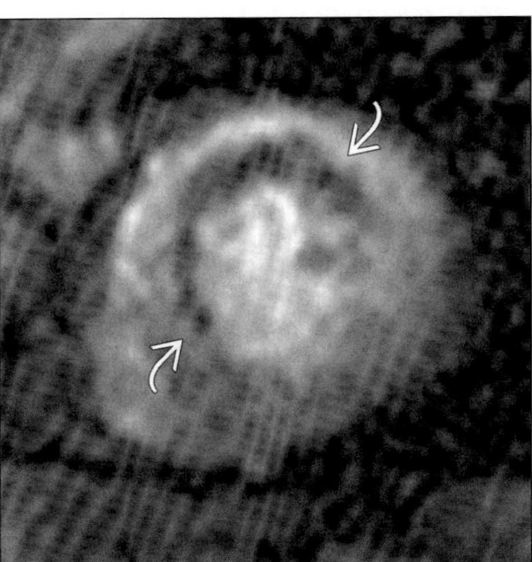

(Left) *Short axis MR cine in systole shows area of hypokinesis in anterior and antero-septal walls associated with increased myocardial signal → (edema) indicating AMI. Note: Pericardial effusion.* ***(Right)*** *Short axis first-pass perfusion MR image shows matching hypoperfusion in the anterior and antero-septal walls → suggesting microvascular obstruction.*

CHRONIC MYOCARDIAL INFARCTION

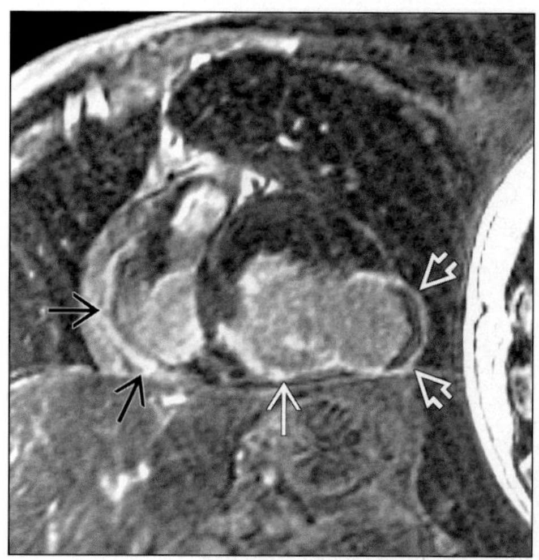

LV short axis DE MR shows hyperenhancement (infarct) of RV ➔, and LV inferior ➔, and infero-lateral walls, which has developed a large aneurysm ➔. Note unenhanced mural thrombus.

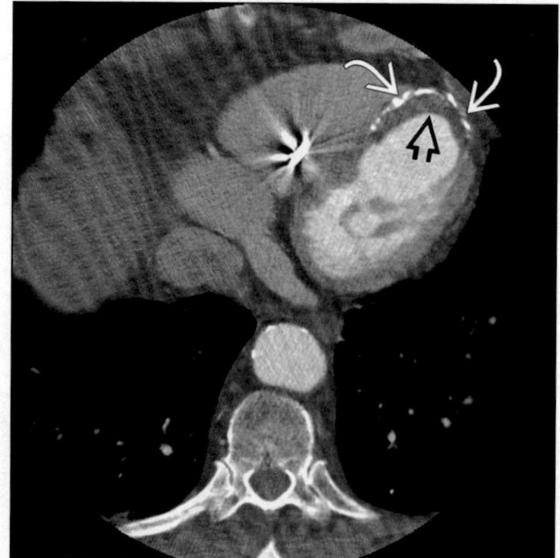

Axial CTA shows thinned and calcified myocardium ➔ and apical aneurysm. Note mural thrombus ➔ is hypodense (unenhanced) compared to remote normal myocardium.

TERMINOLOGY

Abbreviations and Synonyms

- Chronic myocardial infarction (MI), remote infarct

Definitions

- No exact definition of minimum amount of time after acute infarction
  - Though if the time after acute infarction is ≥ 8 weeks, it is generally accepted as chronic myocardial infarct
- Acute myocardial infarction: Myocardial cell death due to prolonged ischemia

IMAGING FINDINGS

General Features

- Best diagnostic clue
  - Linear myocardial calcification or subendocardial fatty metaplasia on CT are diagnostic of remote MI
  - Findings follow coronary vascular distribution
  - Myocardial thinning with akinesis, or dyskinesis
  - Myocardial aneurysm or pseudoaneurysm
  - Delayed hyperenhancement without increased T2 signal
- Location
  - Delayed enhancement or fatty metaplasia are subendocardial and may or may not be transmural
  - Usually confined to a coronary territory (or branch territory)
  - Delayed enhancement that is not subendocardial is non-ischemic in nature
- Size
  - Depends on location of culprit lesions(s)
    - The more proximal the culprit lesion, the larger the infarct territory
- General findings
  - Regional wall-motion abnormality
    - Hypokinesis: Decreased systolic thickening/contraction
    - Akinesis: No systolic thickening/contraction
    - Dyskinesis: No contraction and paradoxical motion
  - Regional myocardial thinning

DDx: Chronic Myocardial Infarction

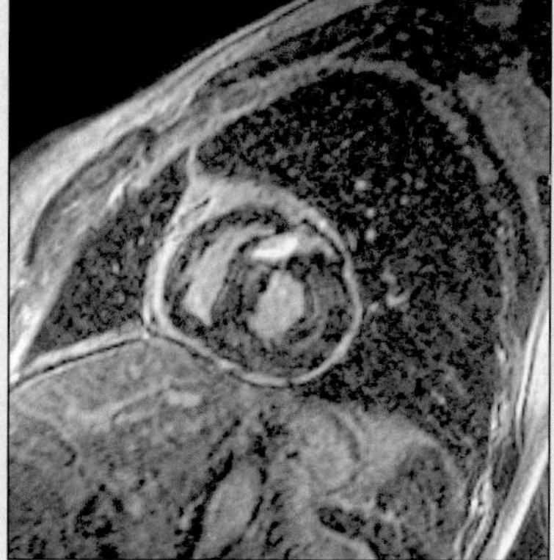

Non-Ischemic Myocardial Fibrosis

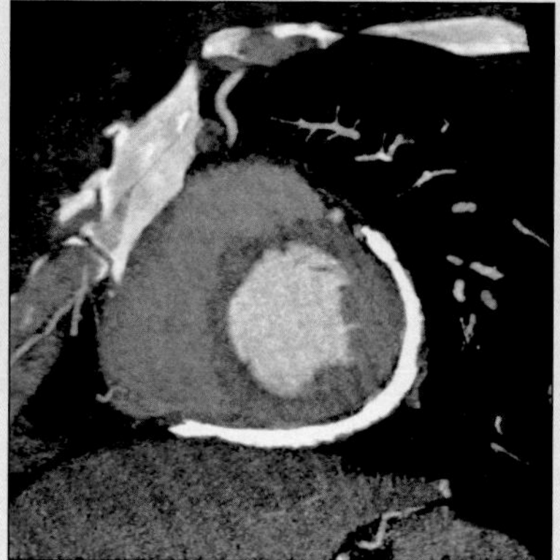

Pericardial Constriction

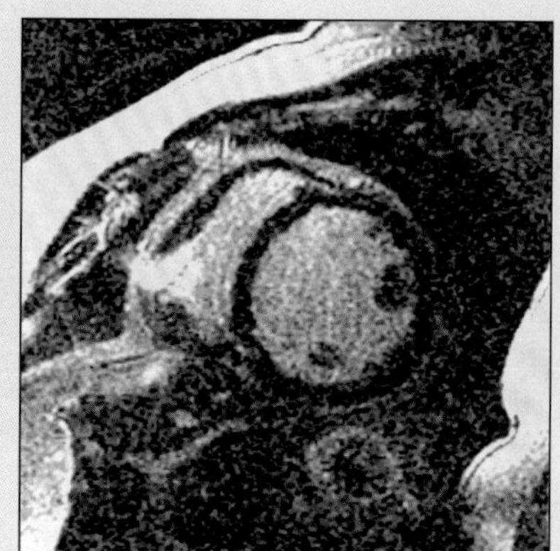

Non-Ischemic DCM

CHRONIC MYOCARDIAL INFARCTION

Key Facts

Terminology

- If the time after acute onset of the infarction is ≥ 8 weeks, it is generally accepted as chronic myocardial infarct
- Acute myocardial infarction: Myocardial cell death due to prolonged ischemia

Imaging Findings

- Linear myocardial calcification or subendocardial fatty metaplasia on CT are diagnostic of remote MI
- Myocardial thinning with akinesis, or dyskinesis
- Delayed hyperenhancement without increased T2 signal
- Presence of LV aneurysm or pseudoaneurysm
- Hypokinesis, akinesis or dyskinesis, depending on transmurality of the infarct

Clinical Issues

- May develop mitral regurgitation from remodeling and change of chordae tendineae geometry and resulting mitral valve malcoaptation

Diagnostic Checklist

- True aneurysm
  - Wide neck/base
  - Wall consists of endocardium, myocardium and epicardium ± mural thrombus
  - Low risk of rupture
- Pseudoaneurysm
  - Narrow base/neck
  - Wall consists of epi/pericardium ± thrombus
  - Higher risk of rupture

    - Degree of thinning ranges from few millimeters in remote transmural MI to near normal thickness myocardium in small subendocardial non-transmural MI

Radiographic Findings

- Radiography
  - Cardiomegaly
    - Enlarged LV from aneurysm, pseudoaneurysm, or dilated LV
    - Enlarged LA due to functional mitral valve regurgitation or increased filling pressures
  - Pulmonary venous hypertension secondary to mitral valve regurgitation or increased filling pressures
  - Myocardial calcifications indicate remote infarct
    - Must be differentiated from pericardial calcification in constrictive pericarditis

CT Findings

- NECT
  - Linear low attenuation (fat density, negative HU) within left ventricular myocardium
  - Linear calcification of myocardium
  - Enlarged LV
  - Secondary findings of sequela of chronic myocardial infarction
    - Enlarged left atrium
    - Pulmonary findings of pulmonary venous hypertension
- CTA
  - Linear calcification or fatty infiltration of subendocardial layers of LV myocardium on CT is diagnostic of remote MI
  - Typically, but not always myocardial thinning
  - LV aneurysm
- Cardiac Gated CTA
  - Functional images demonstrate hypokinesis, akinesis or dyskinesis, depending on the transmurality of the infarct
  - Very small remote infarcts may have normal wall thickness and normal wall motion
  - Obstructive coronary artery disease in the matching coronary territory

MR Findings

- T2WI
  - Absence of T2 prolongation (bright tissue) indicates absence of edema
    - Edema may be present in acute MI, but chronic MI may coexist
- MR Cine
  - Akinesis, hypokinesis or dyskinesis, depending on amount of remaining viable myocardium
  - Possible mural thrombus demonstrates absence of systolic thickening
- Delayed Enhancement
  - Delayed hyperenhancement must be based on subendocardial layer
    - Variable degree of transmurality depends on infarct size
  - Calcification will cause signal void within the delayed hyperenhancement
  - Most sensitive test for infarcted myocardium in vivo
  - Helps differentiate myocardium from mural thrombus
- First pass perfusion
  - Subendocardial perfusion defects in coronary territory
  - Helps delineate myocardium and mural thrombus

Nuclear Medicine Findings

- LV wall thinning with fixed defect
  - Akinesis in areas of fixed defects
- RV visualization plus high lung uptake are signs of severe LV dysfunction

Echocardiographic Findings

- Chronic LV remodeling
  - Infarcted segments wall is thinner and echo is more dense compared to non-infarcted segments
  - May demonstrate presence of aneurysm or pseudoaneurysm
- Functional mitral regurgitation
  - Abnormal coaptation secondary to tethering from LV dilatation/remodeling
- May detect mural thrombus

CHRONIC MYOCARDIAL INFARCTION

Angiographic Findings

- Coronary angiography may demonstrate signs of chronic coronary artery disease, not necessarily chronic MI
  - Severe coronary calcifications
  - Collaterals
- Left ventriculogram may demonstrate findings secondary to chronic MI
  - Dilated LV
  - Aneurysm
  - Mitral regurgitation

Imaging Recommendations

- Best imaging tool
  - Cardiac MR with delayed enhancement is highly sensitive and may depict smaller subendocardial defects
  - PET and SPECT demonstrate fixed defects but may miss smaller nontransmural infarcts
  - Linear calcification or fatty metaplasia detected on cardiac CT are diagnostic of remote MI
    - Absence of these findings does not necessarily exclude non-transmural chronic MI
- Protocol advice
  - MR viability protocol consists of function, T2 weighted fast spin echo, first pass perfusion, and delayed enhancement acquisitions
    - T2 weighted sequence may help differentiate acute from chronic MI

DIFFERENTIAL DIAGNOSIS

Acute MI

- Maintained myocardial thickness
- Increased T2 signal (edema)
- No fatty metaplasia, calcification or aneurysm

Non Ischemic Cardiomyopathies

- Nonischemic myocardial fibrosis or scar manifests in various patterns of delayed hyperenhancement
- Invariably sparing of subendocardium → allows for easy differentiation from ischemic infarct

Endocardial Fibroelastosis

- Delayed enhancement of endocardium
- Apical obliteration of ventricles, mitral and tricuspid regurgitation (distorted valve apparatus) with markedly enlarged atria, pericardial effusions

ARVD

- Fatty infiltration not subendocardial, usually in RV, occasionally in LV

Constrictive Pericarditis

- Calcifications of pericardium with sparing of myocardium

PATHOLOGY

Gross Pathologic & Surgical Features

- Thin plate of scar +/- aneurysm or pseudoaneurysm
- Mural thrombus commonly present

Microscopic Features

- Established scarring with collagen fibers

CLINICAL ISSUES

Natural History & Prognosis

- Left ventricular remodeling
  - LV dilatation
  - Increase in end-diastolic and end-systolic volumes are predictive of increased mortality
- May develop ischemic dilated cardiomyopathy (DCM)
- May develop mitral regurgitation from remodeling and change of chordae tendineae geometry and resulting mitral valve malcoaptation
- May develop aneurysm or pseudoaneurysms
  - Pseudo aneurysms uncommon at anterior apical walls
  - Commonly basal posterior and lateral walls

Treatment

- Medical treatment
- Surgical treatment includes
  - Coronary artery bypass grafts if viable myocardium exists
  - Dor procedure (named after Dr. Vincent Dor, who developed and frequently performed the procedure in the 1980s)
    - Resection of aneurysm with patch aneurysmorrhaphy
  - Linear aneurysmectomy
    - Aneurysm is resected and the edges are closed in a linear vertical fashion using two parallel layers of Teflon felt

DIAGNOSTIC CHECKLIST

Image Interpretation Pearls

- True aneurysm
  - Wide neck/base
  - Wall consists of endocardium, myocardium and epicardium ± mural thrombus
  - Low risk of rupture
- Pseudoaneurysm
  - Narrow base/neck
  - Wall consists of epi/pericardium ± thrombus
  - Higher risk of rupture

SELECTED REFERENCES

1. Saeed M et al: Discrimination of myocardial acute and chronic (scar) infarctions on delayed contrast enhanced magnetic resonance imaging with intravascular magnetic resonance contrast media. J Am Coll Cardiol. 48(10):1961-8, 2006
2. Kramer CM et al: Dissociation between changes in intramyocardial function and left ventricular volumes in the eight weeks after first anterior myocardial infarction. J Am Coll Cardiol. 30(7):1625-32, 1997
3. White HD et al: Left ventricular end-systolic volume as the major determinant of survival after recovery from myocardial infarction. Circulation. 76(1):44-51, 1987

CHRONIC MYOCARDIAL INFARCTION

IMAGE GALLERY

Typical

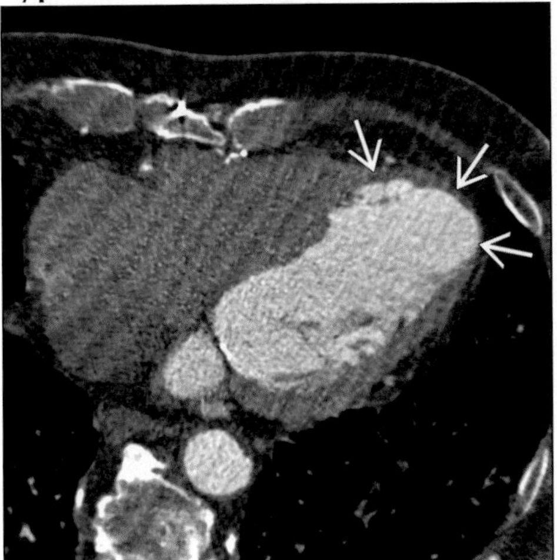

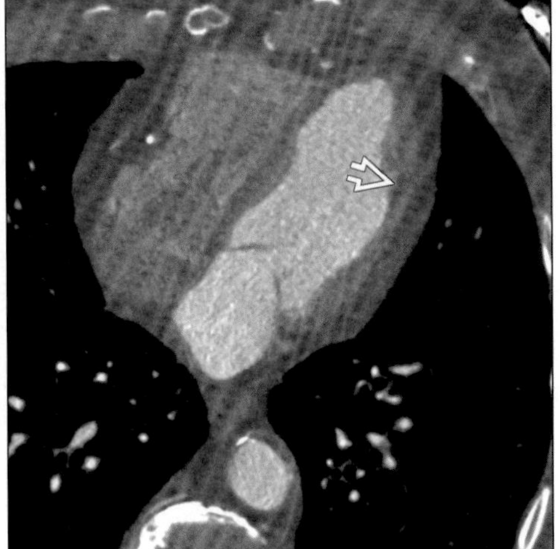

(Left) Axial cardiac CT shows marked thinning and aneurysmal dilatation of LV apex ➔, indicating remote transmural LAD territory myocardial infarction. *(Right)* Axial coronary CTA shows linear subendocardial fatty metaplasia ➔ but relatively preserved myocardial thickness indicating remote non-transmural infarct in diagonal branch or obtuse marginal branch territory.

Typical

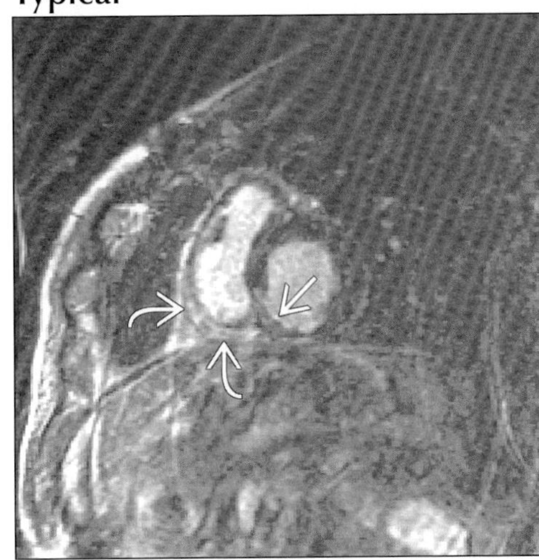

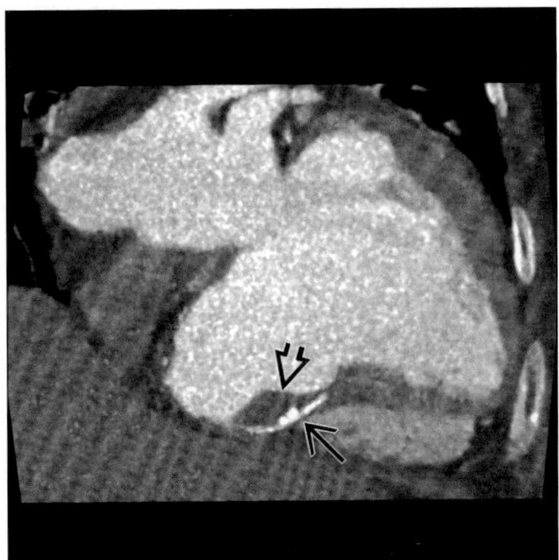

(Left) LV short axis DE MR in a patient with remote infarct and recent onset of arrhythmias shows RCA territory infarct with non-transmural delayed hyperenhancement ➔. Note: Transmural right ventricular infarct ➔. *(Right)* Long axis coronary CTA shows remote infarct with inferior-basal pseudoaneurysm. Note, mural calcification ➔ and mural thrombus ➔.

Typical

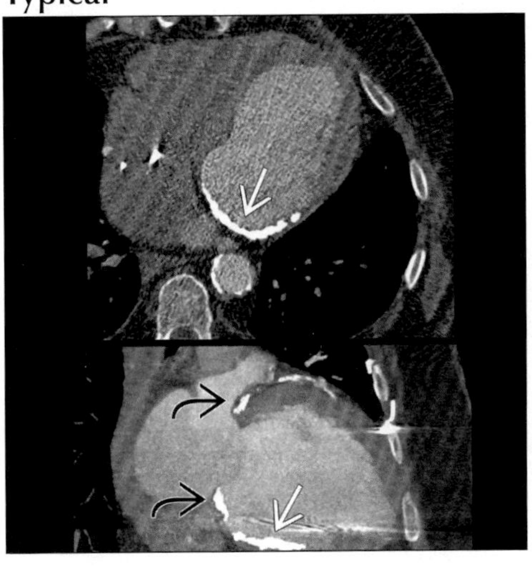

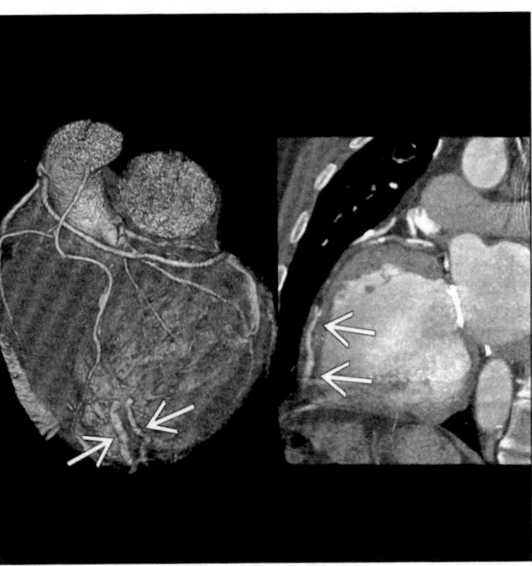

(Left) Oblique cardiac CT shows wall thinning and transmural calcification ➔ in the RCA territory, indicating remote transmural RCA territory infarct. Note: Unrelated mitral annular calcification ➔. *(Right)* Oblique cardiac CT images in a patient post CABG and LV aneurysmectomy shows two parallel layers of Teflon felt ➔ at resection site, indicating linear aneurysmectomy.

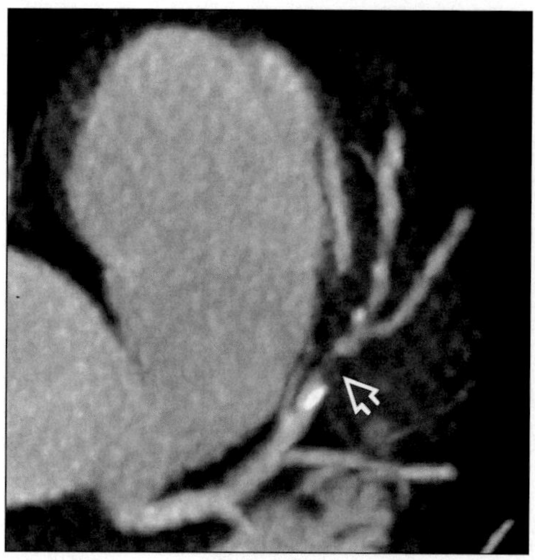

Coronary CTA shows large non-calcified plaque in the mid segment LAD ➡ causing a subtotal occlusion.

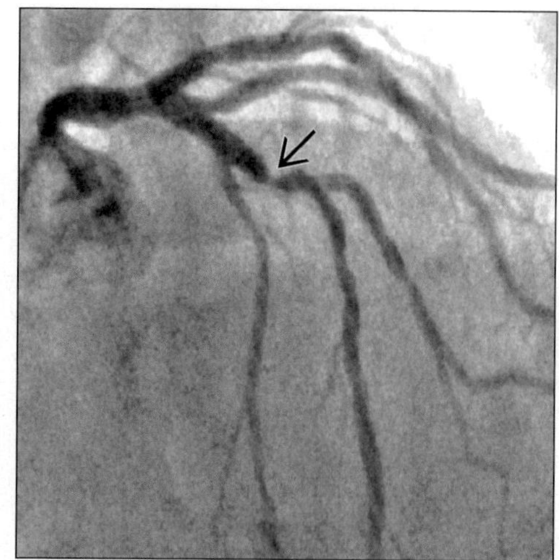

Corresponding invasive coronary angiogram confirms a subtotal occlusion in the mid segment LAD →.

TERMINOLOGY

Definitions

- Partial/total occlusion of the left anterior descending coronary artery (LAD)

IMAGING FINDINGS

General Features

- Best diagnostic clue: Partial/total occlusion of the left anterior descending coronary artery (LAD) on various imaging modalities (fluoroscopy, coronary CT, coronary MR)
- Location
  - Proximal LAD
    - Proximal to 1st septal perforator
    - Electrocardiographic (ECG) changes: ST ↑ V 1-6, I, aVL
  - Mid-LAD
    - Distal to 1st septal perforator, proximal to next large diagonal
    - ECG changes: ST ↑ V 1-6, I, aVL
  - Distal LAD
    - Distal to large diagonal
    - ECG changes: ST ↑ V 1-4, or ST ↑ I, aVL, V5-6
  - LAD diagonal branch "lateral" AMI
    - ECG changes: ST ↑ aVL, V5-6

Radiographic Findings

- Radiography
  - Chest Radiography Findings
    - Interstitial edema if heart failure ensues
    - Abnormal cardiac silhouette if anterior-apical aneurysm present

CT Findings

- CTA
  - Coronary CTA has a high sensitivity (85-95%), specificity (90-100%) and negative predictive value (95-100%) for the detection of hemodynamically significant stenosis
  - Thick multiplanar reformats (5 mm) may allow detection of myocardial hypoperfusion defect in anterior wall
  - Delayed scan (5 minutes after initial contrast bolus) may allow detection of myocardial infarction

DDx: Infarction LAD Distribution

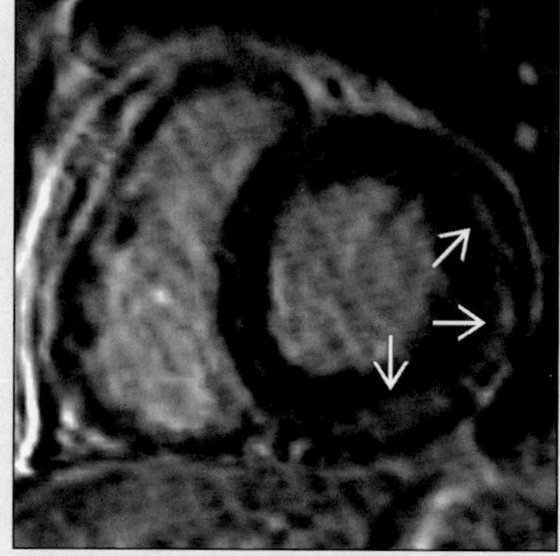

Acute Myocarditis

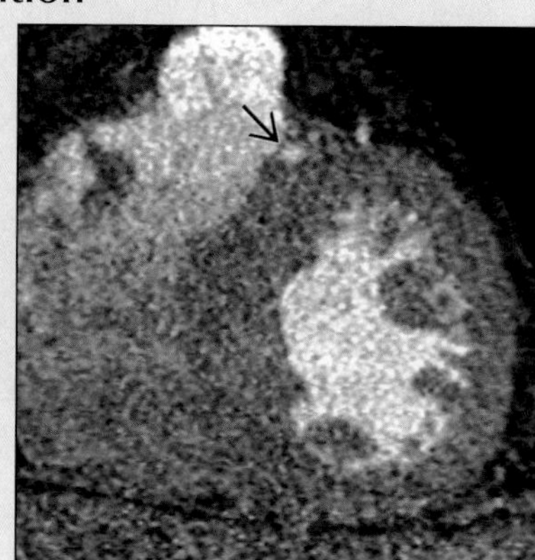

Myocardial Bridge (LAD)

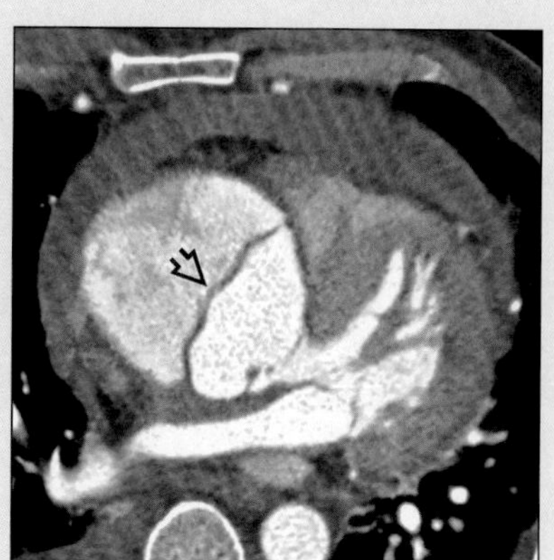

Acute Aortic Dissection

INFARCTION LAD DISTRIBUTION

Key Facts

Terminology
- Partial/total occlusion of the left anterior descending coronary artery (LAD)

Imaging Findings
- Coronary CTA has a high sensitivity (85-95%) and specificity (90-100%) for the detection of hemodynamically significant stenosis with very high negative predictive values
- Cardiac MR delayed enhancement can demonstrate presence, location and size of infarction
- Echo very useful bedside exam for complications of LAD infarction
- Invasive angiography remains the clinical gold-standard for detecting partial/total occluded LAD coronary artery
- PET is currently regarded as the gold-standard for myocardial viability assessment

Pathology
- Occlusive thrombus results in acute ST-segment elevation MI

Clinical Issues
- Classic LAD infarction causes severe, central, crushing chest pain
- Cardiogenic shock and arrhythmia are common complications in proximal LAD infarction
- LAD infarction has a higher rate of infarct expansion with potential for aneurysm and rupture
- LAD infarction has a higher rate of left ventricle (LV) thrombus

    - Newer techniques performing CTA immediately following percutaneous coronary intervention (avoids need for CTA contrast administration)

MR Findings
- Cardiac MR steady-state free precession sequence to assess LV global and regional wall motion
  - Standardized 17 segment AHA model utilized
- Acute infarction will cause increased signal intensity in the anterior segment on T2-weighted imaging
- 1st pass perfusion (stress followed by rest)
  - Hybrid gradient echo-planar sequence acquired during bolus of 0.1 mmol/kg gadolinium
  - Short axis stack (5-8 slices)
  - Repeat sequence 10 minutes later
- Cardiac MR delayed enhancement can demonstrate presence, location and size of infarction
  - Gradient-echo inversion recovery sequence
  - 7-10 mins after a bolus of 0.1 mmol/kg gadolinium
  - Vary inversion time to maximize nulling of normal myocardium
  - LAD infarction results in anterior segment hyperenhancement
  - Healthy viable myocardium appears black

Nuclear Medicine Findings
- PET
  - PET is currently regarded as the gold-standard for myocardial viability assessment
    - Validated for viability and subsequent prognosis
  - Qualitative assessment of regional myocardial blood flow
    - Most commonly used tracers are rubidium-82 and N-13 ammonia
    - Performed under rest and stress conditions
    - High diagnostic accuracy (sensitivity and specificity between 85-95%)
  - Quantitative assessment of regional myocardial blood flow
    - Tracer used is most commonly oxygen-15 water
  - Metabolic evaluation of myocardium
    - 5-fluoro deoxyglucose
    - Ischemia results in impaired fatty acid and increased glucose metabolism
  - Evolving technology includes hybrid PET/CT scanner
    - Allows superimposed imaging of coronary arteries with vascular territories & their metabolic activity
- Technetium-99m
  - Can demonstrate infarct size
  - Perfusion study can show viable myocardium
  - Sestamibi uptake dependent on perfusion, cell membrane integrity, mitochondrial function
  - Dysfunctional segments with > 50-60% uptake considered viable
  - Sensitivity/specificity for improvement post-revascularization = 81%/66%
- Thallium scan
  - Initial uptake determined by blood flow
  - Subsequent uptake dependent on cell membrane integrity/viability
  - Two protocols: Stress-redistribution-reinjection and rest-redistribution
    - Stress-redistribution-reinjection - can assess for stress-inducible ischemia and viability
    - Rest-redistribution - only assess viability
    - Dysfunctional but viable segments considered when tracer uptake increases > 10% or when activity > 50-60%
    - Sensitivity/specificity for improvement post-revascularization = 86%/59%

Echocardiographic Findings
- Echocardiogram
  - Standardized 17 segment AHA model utilized
  - Echo shows anterior segment akinesis acutely, anterior segment thinning chronically
    - Chronic infarction appears bright = fatty replacement
  - Normal echo makes proximal LAD infarction unlikely
    - LAD infarction results in regional wall motion abnormality of anterior segment
  - Echo very useful bedside exam for complications of LAD infarction

- LV thrombus, aneurysms/pseudoaneurysms, Dressler syndrome, post-infarction mitral regurgitation, papillary muscle rupture

Angiographic Findings

- Ventricular Angiography Findings
  - Reduced anterior-apical wall motion and EF
  - Reduced wall thickening, or dyskinesis
- Coronary Angiography Findings
  - Invasive angiography remains clinical gold-standard for detecting LAD stenosis/occlusion

DIFFERENTIAL DIAGNOSIS

Conditions with Overlapping Symptoms

- Acute aortic dissection, acute myocarditis, pneumonia, pancreatitis, reflux esophagitis, Takotsubo syndrome

PATHOLOGY

General Features

- General path comments
  - Vascular occlusion with anterior-apical necrosis
  - Myocardial thinning with LV thrombosis (40%)

Gross Pathologic & Surgical Features

- Initiating event in AMI LAD territory is a fissure in the diseased arterial wall
  - Loss of integrity of the plaque cap
- Results in exposure of subendothelial matrix elements such as collagen, stimulating platelet activation and thrombus formation
  - Release of tissue factor
- Occlusive thrombus results in acute ST-segment elevation MI
- If non-occlusive, results in unstable angina or non-ST elevation (non-transmural infarction)

CLINICAL ISSUES

Presentation

- Most common signs/symptoms
  - Classic LAD infarction causes severe, central, crushing chest pain, radiation to left arm
    - Impending sense of doom
  - Cardiogenic shock and arrhythmia are common complications in proximal LAD infarction
  - No conduction disturbance if lesion is mid or distal segment LAD
- Other signs/symptoms
  - Heaviness or burning, radiation to the jaw, neck, shoulder, back, or both arms
  - Indigestion/nausea/vomiting (suggestive of inferior wall MI)
  - Diaphoresis
  - Development of dyspnea is concerning, it indicates probable impending heart failure
  - Tachycardia worrisome (denotes large infarction)
  - Often accompanied by new left bundle branch block because of compromised flow to the His-Purkinje conduction tissue
- Clinical Profile: Risk factors: Smoking, cholesterol elevation, diabetes, hypertension, family history

Natural History & Prognosis

- LAD infarction has a higher rate of infarct expansion with potential for aneurysm and rupture
- LAD infarction has a higher rate of LV thrombus
- Significant number of LAD infarctions die before reaching hospital
- Mortality of in-patients with LAD infarction is declining (multifactorial)
  - More aggressive and better treatments: Smoking cessation, anti-cholesterol agents, diet, exercise, prophylactic aspirin

Treatment

- Thrombolysis
  - Absolute contraindications include: Acute intracranial hemorrhage, active bleeding, recent stroke, trauma or recent major surgery
  - Generally best results from thrombolysis are for LAD infarction
- Percutaneous intervention
  - Originally with balloon angioplasty
  - Stent insertion has now taken over
  - Considered by most to be the optimal reperfusion method if available in a timely manner
    - Danis Multicenter Randomized Study on Fibrinolytic Therapy versus Acute Coronary Angioplasty in Acute Myocardial Infarction (DANAMI-2) trial
- CABG (in unsuspected LM stenosis discovered on angiography)
- Analgesia: Morphine (2-4 mg IV), oxygen
- Aspirin (non-enteric)
  - International Studies of Infarct Survival (ISIS-2) trail
- Clopidogrel
  - Added benefit when combined with aspirin
  - CLARITY, CREDO and COMMIT trials
- Heparin IV (weight-adjusted dose)

SELECTED REFERENCES

1. Busk M et al: The Danish multicentre randomized study of fibrinolytic therapy vs. primary angioplasty in acute myocardial infarction (the DANAMI-2 trial): outcome after 3 years follow-up. Eur Heart J. 2007
2. Beinart SC et al: Long-term cost effectiveness of early and sustained dual oral antiplatelet therapy with clopidogrel given for up to one year after percutaneous coronary intervention results: from the Clopidogrel for the Reduction of Events During Observation (CREDO) trial. J Am Coll Cardiol. 46(5):761-9, 2005
3. Ryan TJ et al: 1999 update: ACC/AHA Guidelines for the Management of Patients With Acute Myocardial Infarction: Executive Summary and Recommendations: A report of the American College of Cardiology/American Heart Association Task Force on Practice Guidelines (Committee on Management of Acute Myocardial Infarction). Circulation. 100(9):1016-30, 1999
4. Topol EJ et al: Acute Myocardial Infarction. In: Topol EJ. Textbook of Cardiovascular Medicine. 6th ed. Philadelphia, W.B. Lippincott Raven. 395-436, 1998

INFARCTION LAD DISTRIBUTION

IMAGE GALLERY

Typical

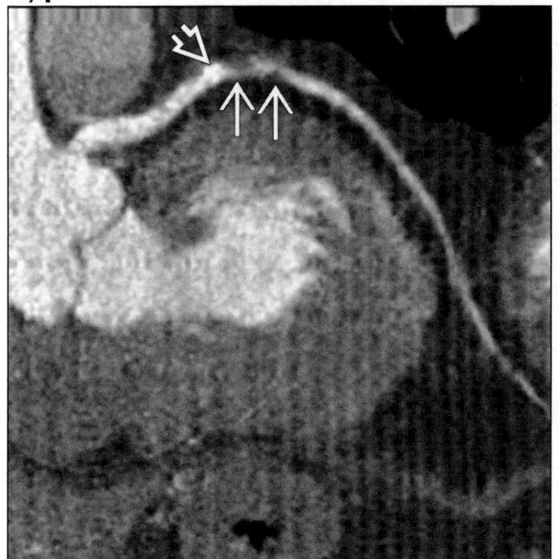

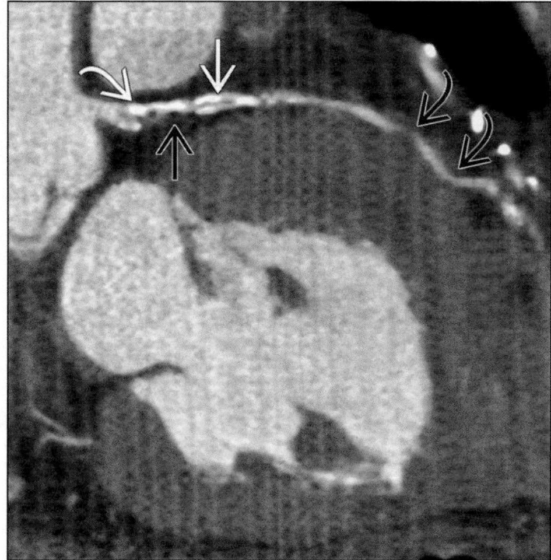

(Left) Curved multiplanar reformat coronary CTA shows two large non-calcified plaques ➡ causing significant stenosis of the LAD. Note calcified plaque proximal to stenosis ➡. ***(Right)*** Coronary CTA shows extensive calcified ➡ and noncalcified ➡ plaque in the proximal LAD extending into the distal LM ➡. Slab artifact mimics further stenosis in the mid segment ➡.

Typical

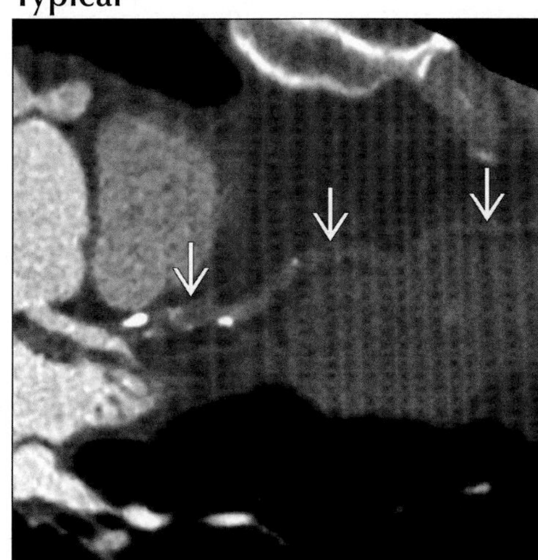

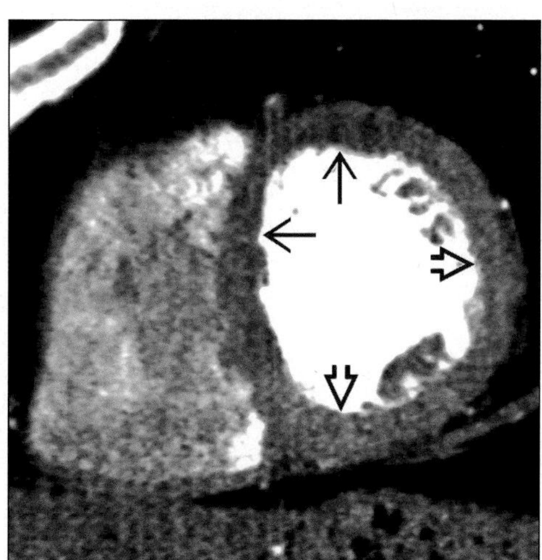

(Left) Curved multiplanar reformat of the LAD in a 39 year old man presenting with acute chest pain shows complete thrombosis of the LAD ➡. ***(Right)*** Corresponding short axis CTA image shows perfusion defect in the anterior and anteroseptal segments ➡ consistent with acute infarction. Compare to normally perfused myocardium ➡.

Typical

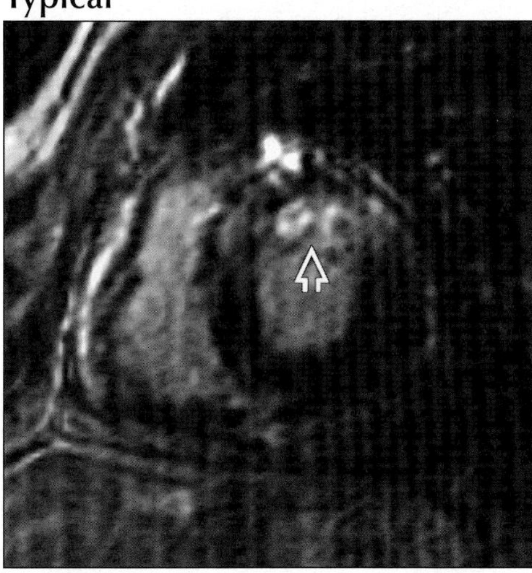

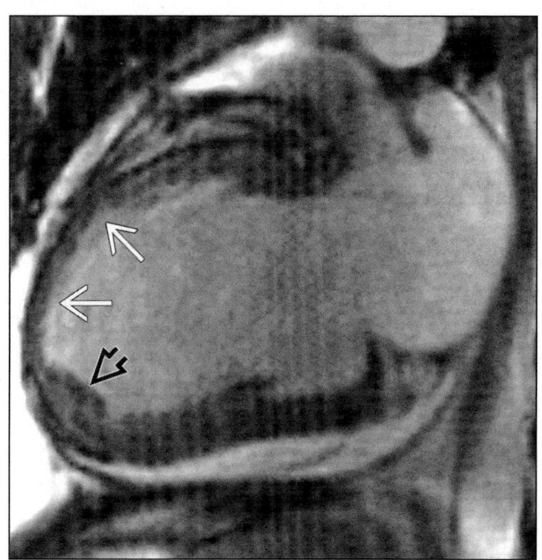

(Left) Delayed-enhanced cardiac MR in a 55-year-old man with acute chest pain shows anterior segment hyperenhancement ➡ consistent with AMI. Note subendocardial distribution (ischemia). ***(Right)*** Gradient-echo inversion recovery delayed enhanced MR two-chamber view shows hyperenhancement of the anterior wall ➡. Note acute LV apical thrombus ➡.

PAPILLARY MUSCLE RUPTURE

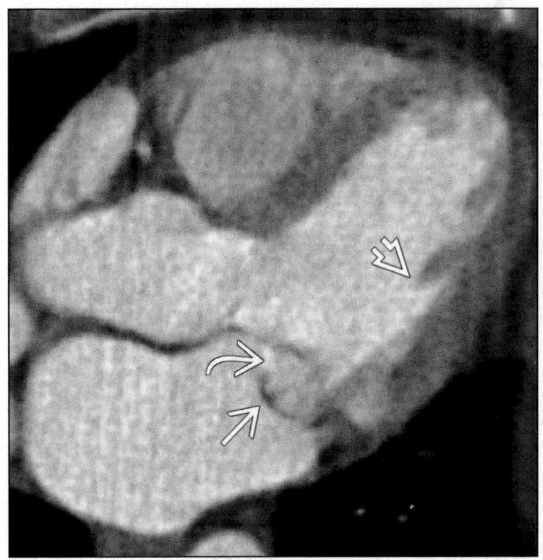

Three-chamber coronary CTA shows severe, posterior leaflet, mitral valve prolapse ➡ from an infarcted posterior papillary muscle ⇨. Note severe mitral regurgitant orifice ↷.

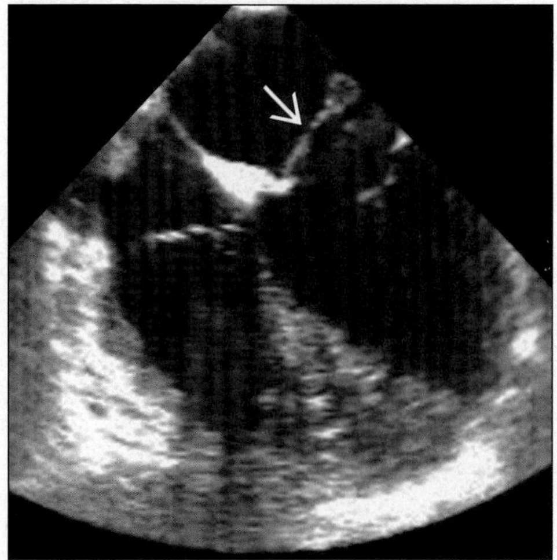

Four chamber view echocardiogram shows severe prolapse of anterior mitral leaflet ➡ into the left atrium secondary to acute papillary muscle rupture in the setting of acute myocardial infarction.

TERMINOLOGY

Definitions

- Partial or complete rupture of a papillary muscle (PM), most commonly in the setting of acute myocardial infarction (AMI)

IMAGING FINDINGS

General Features

- Best diagnostic clue: Flail of the chordae and/or PM into the left atrium along with severe mitral regurgitation on several imaging modalities
- Location: Posteromedial PM affected more commonly than the anterolateral PM
- Size: May be partial or complete
- Morphology
  - May affect one of the muscle heads, thus affecting several chordae
  - May affect trunk of the PM, thus affecting one half of the chordae
- Severe mitral regurgitation (MR) by multiple modalities
- Usually inferior ECG lead abnormalities

Radiographic Findings

- Radiography
  - Chest radiography findings
    - Heart failure
    - Pulmonary venous congestion with signs of pulmonary edema
    - Likely will not show evidence of left atrial enlargement in the acute setting
    - Specific CXR finding is right upper lobe edema, caused by mitral leaflet flail and jet of regurgitant blood directed into right superior pulmonary vein
  - Sudden onset of pulmonary edema within 2-9 days of MI

CT Findings

- CTA
  - Coronary arteries can be evaluated for significant coronary stenosis
  - Myocardial perfusion defect may be detected in acute myocardial infarction (MI)
  - Cine multiphasic reconstructions can show
    - Prolapse of chordae and mitral leaflet into left atrium

DDx: Papillary Muscle Rupture

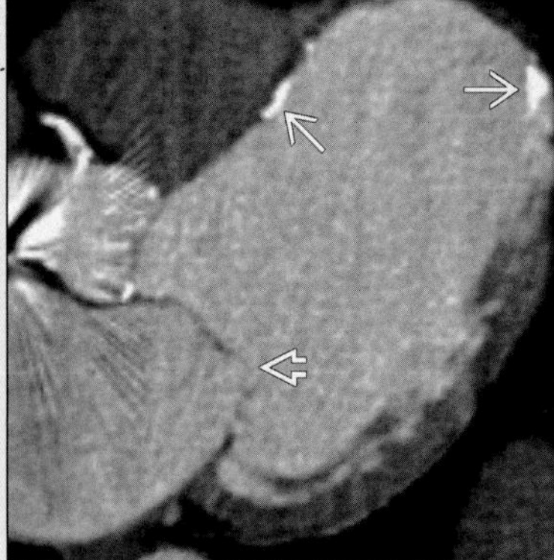

Ischemic Dilated Cardiomyopathy

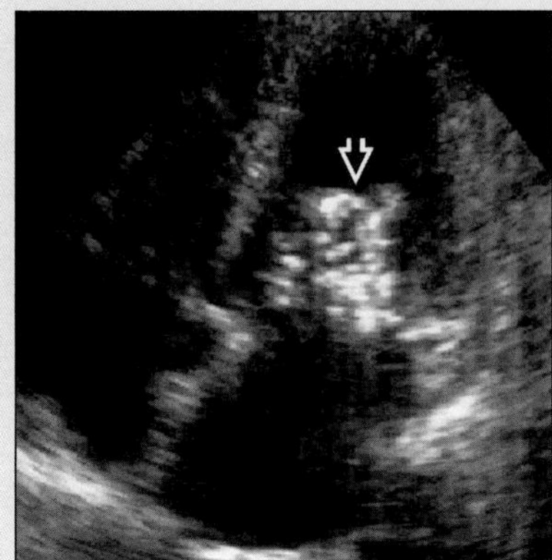

Infective Endocarditis

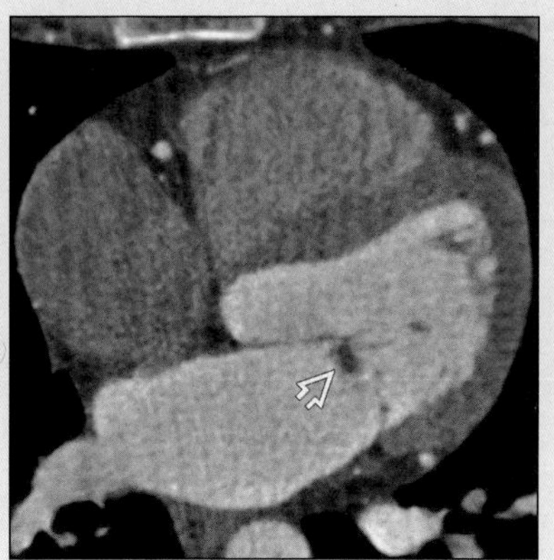

Papillary Fibroelastoma

PAPILLARY MUSCLE RUPTURE

Key Facts

Terminology

- Partial or complete rupture of a papillary muscle (PM), most commonly in the setting of acute myocardial infarction (AMI)

Imaging Findings

- Flail of the chordae and/or PM into the left atrium along with severe mitral regurgitation on several imaging modalities
- Posteromedial PM affected more commonly than the anterolateral PM
- Usually inferior ECG lead abnormalities
- Specific CXR finding is right upper lobe edema, caused by mitral leaflet flail and jet of regurgitant blood directed into right superior pulmonary vein
- TEE is superior to TTE in detecting PMR

Clinical Issues

- Acute hemodynamic collapse in setting of acute myocardial infarction (AMI)
- Severe mitral regurgitation: Detectable by several modalities
- Systolic murmur at the left lower sternal border, though may be very faint or absent
- Systolic function is better than anticipated, or hyperdynamic, in setting of hemodynamic compromise
- Once stabilized, early surgery is essential
- Most commonly presents 2-9 days post AMI with acute onset chest pain and shortness of breath

    - Global and regional left ventricular function abnormalities related to acute MI
  - Evolving technology, may not be suitable in the setting of acute PM rupture and AMI in which patients are unstable

MR Findings

- MR Cine
  - Can show
    - Prolapse of chordae and mitral leaflet into left atrium
    - Global and regional left ventricular function abnormalities related to acute MI
- Delayed Enhancement
  - Delayed hyperenhancement of affected PM
  - Can quantify extent of acute MI
- Flow void in LA representing regurgitation

Echocardiographic Findings

- Echocardiogram
  - Transthoracic and transesophageal echo (TEE)
    - Both can detect a flail mitral leaflet
    - Papillary muscle head in left atrium (LA) or left ventricle (LV)
    - Severe mitral regurgitation on Doppler exam: May be low-velocity broad-based flow
    - Better than expected systolic LV function is characteristic of papillary muscle rupture (PMR)
    - TEE shows leaflets especially well, and is ideally suited for patients on ventilators or in the operating room
    - TEE is superior to TTE in detecting PMR

Angiographic Findings

- Left ventriculography findings
  - Severe MR
  - Flail leaflet and papillary muscle head will frequently be apparent

Imaging Recommendations

- Best imaging tool: Transesophageal echocardiography if patient is stable

DIFFERENTIAL DIAGNOSIS

Cardiogenic Shock with Severe Reduction in Overall Systolic Function

- Prior myocardial infarction (MI) usually present
- Multivessel or left main coronary disease
- Evident from any modality that overall function is severely reduced

Ischemic Mitral Regurgitation

- Neighboring myocardium usually shows marked wall motion abnormality
- LV remodeling changes geometry of chordae tendinea leading to mitral valve malcoaptation
  - Lateral displacement of lateral wall changes angle of chordae (relative shortening) and results in incomplete systolic closure of posterior mitral valve leaflet
- No flail leaflet
- Lesser degree of regurgitation

Dilated Mitral Annulus

- More commonly associated with dilated LV

Chordal Rupture

- May have the same consequence as papillary muscle rupture and is difficult to distinguish
- May require TEE to distinguish from papillary muscle rupture
- Lesser degree of regurgitation is sometimes noted

Endocarditis

- Vegetation may appear as mobile structure attached to regurgitant valve
- Very different clinical setting, patient is usually septic
- Blood cultures are helpful in diagnosis

Ventricular Septal Rupture

- Post MI rupture of septum leading to ventricular septal defect (VSD)
- No mitral valve regurgitation

PAPILLARY MUSCLE RUPTURE

PATHOLOGY

General Features

- General path comments
  - More commonly involves posterior papillary muscle, resulting from single blood supply from posterior descending coronary artery
    - Anterior muscle is supplied by left anterior descending (LAD)
  - Rupture most often at the papillary muscle head
    - May be partial or complete
  - Typical necrosis apparent at site of rupture
  - Myocardial infarct size itself may not be large

CLINICAL ISSUES

Presentation

- Most common signs/symptoms: Most commonly presents 2-9 days post AMI with acute onset chest pain and shortness of breath
- Other signs/symptoms: Usually occurs 2-9 days after a first infarct
- Clinical Profile: PMR is always disabling and may be rapidly fatal
- Acute hemodynamic collapse in setting of acute myocardial infarction (AMI)
  - Potentially catastrophic and fatal
- Recurrent chest pain
- Sudden onset heart failure
- Severe mitral regurgitation: Detectable by several modalities
- Systolic murmur at the left lower sternal border, though may be very faint or absent
  - Absent murmur represents rapid equalization of pressure across the mitral valve
- Systolic function is better than anticipated, or hyperdynamic, in setting of hemodynamic compromise
- Thrombolytics may accelerate the course of rupture
- Associations
  - Prior MI
  - Extension of MI
  - Old age

Natural History & Prognosis

- Usually occurs at a first infarct

Treatment

- Stabilize patient with afterload reduction and diuretics
- Intraaortic balloon pump is frequently required
- Once stabilized, early surgery is essential
  - Coronary angiography may be helpful if the patient can be adequately stabilized
  - Mortality rate is < 10% for mitral valve replacement
  - 10 year survival rate is 90%

SELECTED REFERENCES

1. Masci PG et al: Images in cardiovascular medicine. Papillary muscle infarction after cardiopulmonary resuscitation. Circulation. 116(8):e308-9, 2007
2. Sanchez CE et al: Survival from combined left ventricular free wall rupture and papillary muscle rupture complicating acute myocardial infarction. J Am Soc Echocardiogr. 20(7):905, 2007
3. Kim TH et al: Images in cardiovascular medicine. Anterolateral papillary muscle rupture complicated by the obstruction of a single diagonal branch. Circulation. 112(16):e269-70, 2005
4. Marangelli V et al: Images in cardiovascular medicine. Three-dimensional imaging in rupture of papillary muscle after acute myocardial infarction. Circulation. 111(23):e385-7, 2005
5. Morishita S et al: A case of papillary muscle rupture caused by acute myocardial infarction. J Med. 32(5-6):301-9, 2001
6. Schwender FT: Papillary muscle calcification after inferoposterior myocardial infarction. Heart. 86(3):E8, 2001
7. McQuillan BM et al: Severe mitral regurgitation secondary to partial papillary muscle rupture following myocardial infarction. Rev Cardiovasc Med. 1(1):57-60, 2000
8. Nishimura RA et al: The case for an aggressive surgical approach to papillary muscle rupture following myocardial infarction: "From paradise lost to paradise regained". Heart. 83(6):611-3, 2000
9. Verma R et al: Images in clinical medicine. Rupture of papillary muscle during acute myocardial infarction. N Engl J Med. 341(4):247, 1999
10. Ha JW et al: Papillary muscle rupture during acute myocardial infarction. Clin Cardiol. 21(7):511-2, 1998
11. Park CW et al: Papillary muscle rupture complicating inferior myocardial infarction in a young woman with systemic lupus erythematosus and antiphospholipid syndrome. Nephrol Dial Transplant. 13(12):3202-4, 1998
12. Weiss SR et al: Isolated acute papillary muscle infarction in the absence of coronary artery disease resulting in cardiogenic shock and emergent mitral valve replacement. Cathet Cardiovasc Diagn. 43(2):185-9, 1998
13. Barbour DJ et al: Rupture of a left ventricular papillary muscle during acute myocardial infarction: analysis of 22 necropsy patients. J Am Coll Cardiol. 8(3):558-65, 1986
14. Killen DA et al: Surgical treatment of papillary muscle rupture. Ann Thorac Surg. 35(3):243-8, 1983
15. No authors listed: Case records of the Massachusetts General Hospital. Weekly clinicopathological exercises. Case 39-1982. Abrupt onset of dyspnea in a 59-year-old man. N Engl J Med. 307(14):873-80, 1982
16. Wei JY et al: Papillary muscle rupture in fatal acute myocardial infarction: a potentially treatable form of cardiogenic shock. Ann Intern Med. 90(2):149-52, 1979
17. Lie JT et al: Sudden appearance of a systolic murmur in acute myocardial infarction. Am Heart J. 90(4):507-12, 1975
18. Mary DA et al: Papillary muscle rupture following myocardial infarction. Thorax. 28(3):390-3, 1973
19. Heikkilä J: Electrocardiography in acute papillary muscle dysfunction and infarction: a clinicopathologic study. Chest. 57(6):510-7, 1970
20. De Busk RF et al: The clinical spectrum of papillary-muscle disease. N Engl J Med. 281(26):1458-67, 1969
21. Shelburne JC et al: A reappraisal of papillary muscle dysfunction; correlative clinical and angiographic study. Am J Med. 46(6):862-71, 1969
22. Christ G et al: Partial papillary muscle rupture complicating acute myocardial infarction. diagnosis by multiplane transoesophageal echocardiography.

PAPILLARY MUSCLE RUPTURE

IMAGE GALLERY

Typical

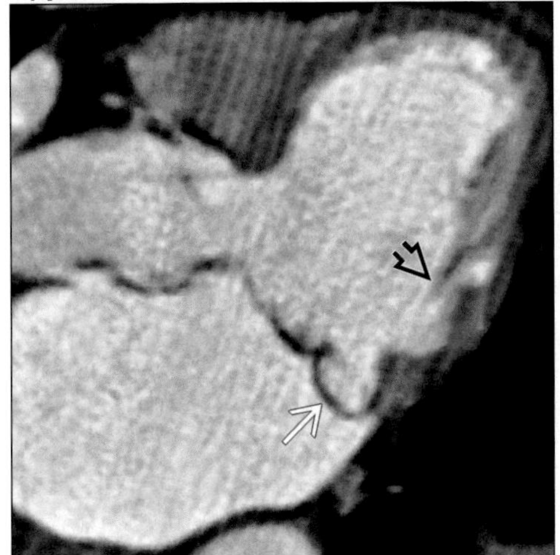

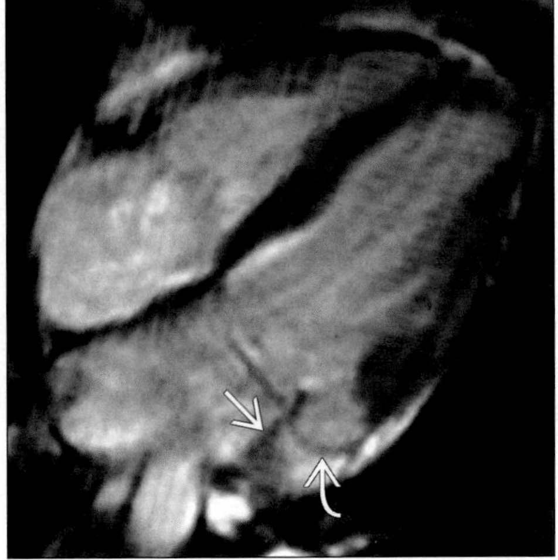

(Left) *Three-chamber coronary CTA shows marked posterior mitral leaflet prolapse ➡ secondary to papillary head rupture ⇨ in the setting of acute myocardial infarction.* ***(Right)*** *Four chamber view cardiac MR cine SSFP shows posterior mitral leaflet prolapse ↷ secondary to papillary muscle rupture. Note jet of blood ➡ into the left atrium representing mitral regurgitation.*

Typical

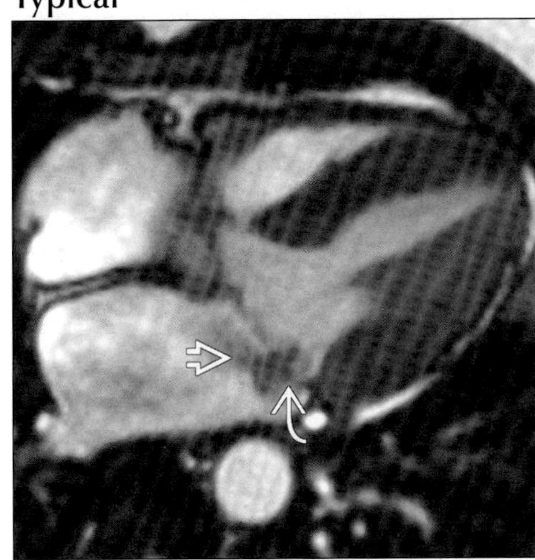

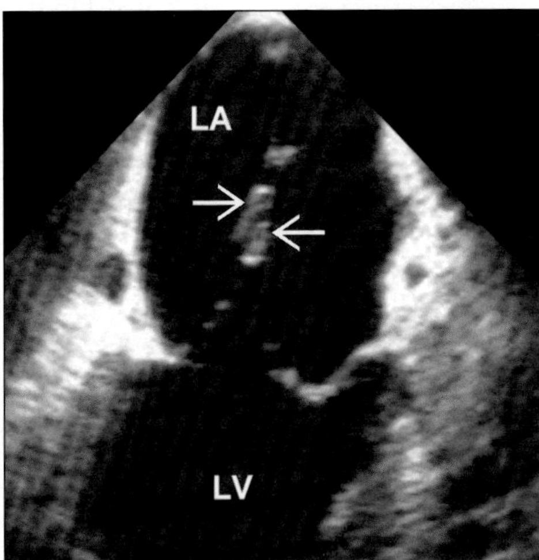

(Left) *Four chamber view cardiac MR cine SSFP shows posterior mitral leaflet prolapse ↷ secondary to ruptured chord from the papillary muscle head. Note jet of blood ⇨ into the left atrium (mitral regurgitation).* ***(Right)*** *Four chamber view echocardiogram shows complete, bi-leaflet, mitral leaflet flail ➡ into the left atrium from papillary muscle rupture in the setting of infective endocarditis.*

Typical

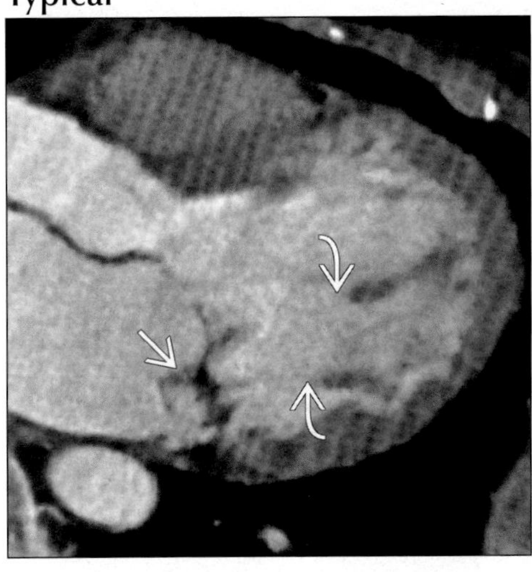

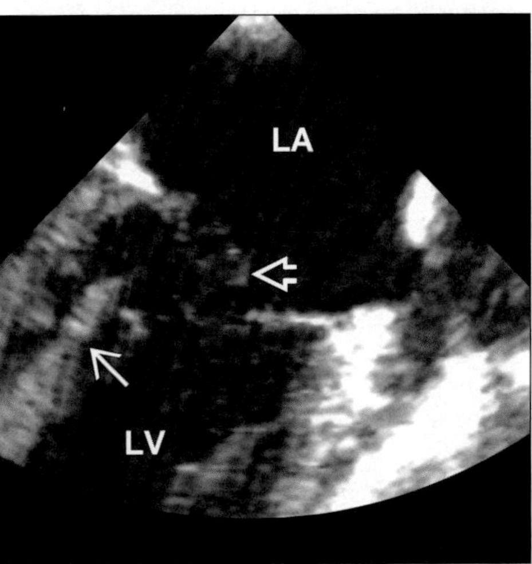

(Left) *Three-chamber coronary CTA shows prolapsed posterior mitral leaflet ➡ with complete chordae tendinea rupture ↷ from the papillary muscle heads in congenital mitral valve prolapse.* ***(Right)*** *Echo 4-chamber view shows papillary muscle infarction with rupture of the chordae ➡ and anterior mitral leaflet prolapse ⇨ into the left atrium.*

RIGHT VENTRICULAR INFARCTION

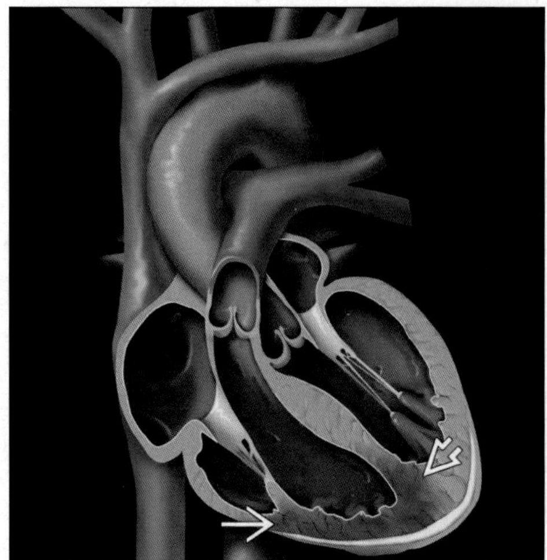

Graphic shows right ventricular infarction affecting the right ventricular free wall ➡. Note the involvement of the inferoseptal segment of the left ventricle ⇨.

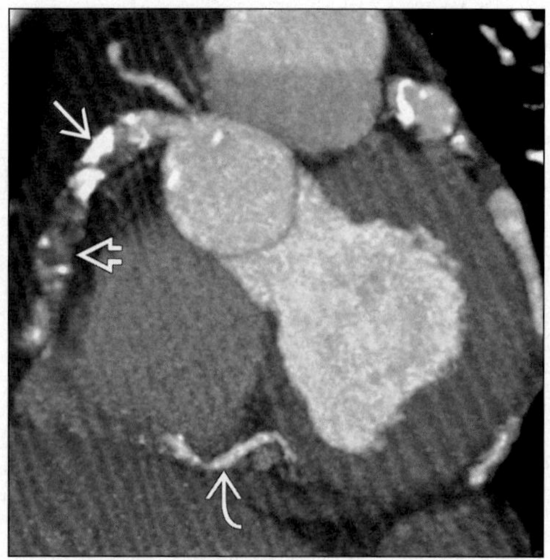

Coronal oblique coronary CTA shows extensive calcified and non-calcified plaque ➡ in the proximal segment and total occlusion ⇨ of the mid segment. Reconstitution distally through collaterals ↪.

TERMINOLOGY

Definitions

- Myocardial infarct of portions or all of the right ventricular (RV) free walls and RV septum
  - Subgroup of patients with inferior wall left ventricular (LV) infarction have concomitant right ventricular infarction also

IMAGING FINDINGS

General Features

- Best diagnostic clue
  - Occlusion of the right coronary artery (RCA) on imaging
  - Delayed hyperenhancement affecting RV inferior and anterior free walls
- Location: RV infarction usually involves inferior septum and inferior free wall rather than anterior free wall
- Size
  - The more proximal the culprit RCA lesion the larger is infarct size
  - More distal stenosis are counteracted by
    - Collateral coronary arterial supply
    - Thebesian vein supply
- Morphology
  - Posterior descending branch supplies inferior and posterior walls of right ventricle
  - Relative sparing of RV free wall due to extensive collateralization
- Electrocardiogram
  - ST-segment elevation in lead V4R, strong predictor of RV infarction

Radiographic Findings

- Chest Radiography
  - Hypotension in the absence of interstitial edema
  - Abnormal cardiac silhouette: Right ventricle (RV) enlargement

CT Findings

- CTA
  - Cardiac CTA sensitivity = 85-97% for detection of hemodynamically significant RCA stenosis
  - Allows detection of "positive remodeling" RCA plaque

DDx: Right Ventricular Infarction

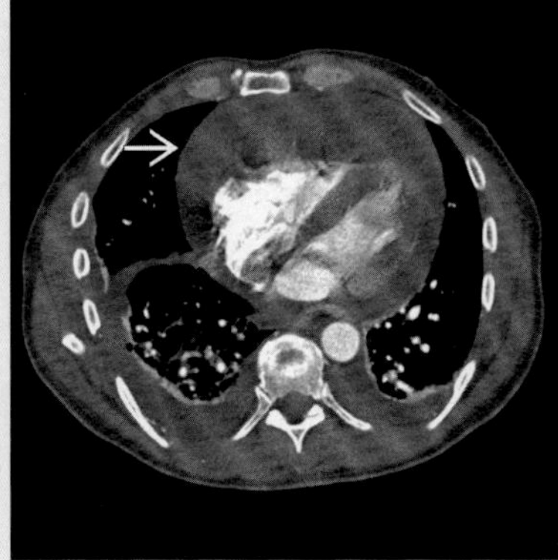

Acute Pericarditis

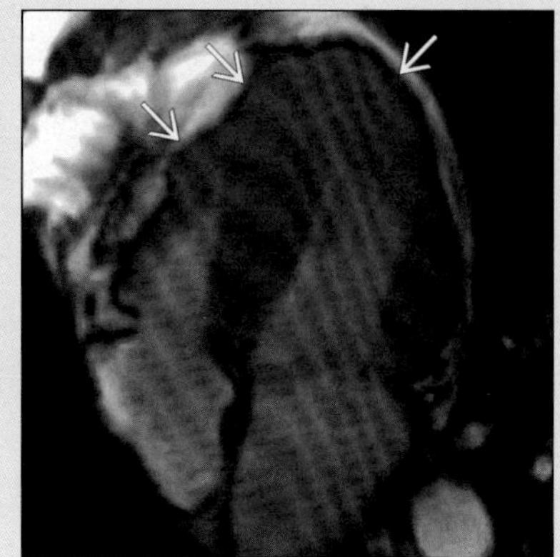

Hypertrophic Cardiomyopathy

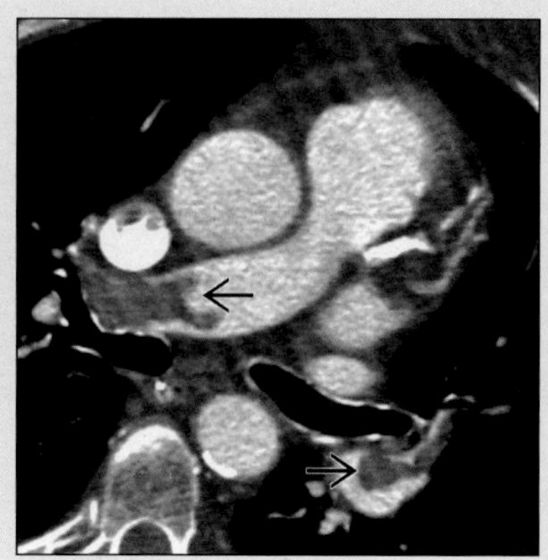

Pulmonary Embolism

RIGHT VENTRICULAR INFARCTION

Key Facts

Terminology
- Subgroup of patients with inferior wall left ventricular (LV) infarction have concomitant right ventricular (RV) infarction also

Imaging Findings
- RV infarction usually involves posterior septum and posterior wall rather than free wall due to better collateralization of free wall
- More proximal the culprit RCA lesion the larger the infarct size
- ST-segment elevation in lead V4R, strong predictor of RV infarction
- Delayed enhanced cardiac MR more sensitive and specific than ECG, physical examination or echocardiography
- Echocardiography sensitivity 82%, specificity 93% for RV infarction
- More than 90% are due to RCA occlusion

Pathology
- RV is less susceptible to infarction than LV due to collateralization

Clinical Issues
- Associated with reduced cardiac output, hypotension and pump failure
- Initial diagnosis dependent on ECG: Shows ST elevation in the right ventricular leads (V4R)
- Associated with increased mortality and morbidity
- Ventricular arrhythmias and atrioventricular (AV) conduction abnormalities
- Isolated RV infarction is very rare

  - Multiphasic cine reconstructions provide an accurate assessment of RV global/regional function and dilation
    - Ejection fraction and RV volumes can be quantified with volumetric, threshold-based software algorithms

MR Findings
- T1 C+: Reduced perfusion frequently not visible because of thin structure of the right ventricle
- Delayed Enhancement
  - Gradient-echo inversion recovery sequence shows infarcted myocardium as bright
    - Note: **Inversion time (TI)**, which has to be selected by the operator, **is different for the RV** compared to that for the LV
  - 7-10 minutes post gadolinium administration
  - Very low interobserver variability
  - Delayed enhanced cardiac MR more sensitive and specific than ECG, physical examination or echocardiography

Nuclear Medicine Findings
- Radionuclide Angiography Findings
  - Reduced RV ejection fraction
    - Regional myocardial dysfunction

Echocardiographic Findings
- Echocardiogram
  - 2D echocardiography
    - Altered ventricular function: Decrease in right ventricular ejection fraction
    - RV dilation
    - Reduced regional RV function
    - Paradoxical motion of interventricular septum
    - Myocardial performance index: Sum of isovolumic relaxation and contraction time/ejection fraction (MPI > 0.30 suggests RV infarction)
  - Doppler
    - Tricuspid regurgitation
    - Decrease in systolic velocity associated with worse prognosis
  - Echocardiography useful for excluding tamponade and pericarditis
  - Echocardiography sensitivity 82%, specificity 93% for RV infarction

Angiographic Findings
- Ventricular Angiography Findings
  - Reduced RV regional wall motion
  - Reduced RV ejection fraction
- Coronary Angiography Findings
  - More than 90% are due to RCA occlusion

Imaging Recommendations
- Best imaging tool: Delayed enhanced cardiac MR
- Protocol advice
  - Gradient-echo inversion recovery sequence, acquired 7-10 minutes post gadolinium administration
  - Select TI to achieve RV nulling (usually technologist aim to null LV myocardium, but TI for RV differs from that of LV)

DIFFERENTIAL DIAGNOSIS

Acute Pericarditis/Tamponade
- Silent cardiac exam; elevated jugular venous pressure

Hypertrophic Cardiomyopathy
- May involve RV myocardium (up to 33%)

Restrictive Cardiomyopathy
- Diastolic heart failure

Pulmonary Embolism
- May present with right heart failure

PATHOLOGY

General Features
- General path comments
  - RV is less susceptible to infarction than LV due to collateralization

- RV is a low pressure system
  - Highly dependent on diastolic pressure
- RV infarction results in marked increased diastolic pressures
- Can lead to LV dysfunction
  - Resultant drop in RV output
  - Raised right atrial pressures
- Increases in atrial natruretic peptide; detrimental to LV function

- Epidemiology
  - Isolated RV infarction is very rare and usual occurs in association with inferior LV infarction
    - Prevalence varies from 10-50%

CLINICAL ISSUES

Presentation

- Most common signs/symptoms
  - Classic triad
    - Distended neck veins
    - Normal lungs
    - Hypotension
- Other signs/symptoms: Right 3rd and 4th heart sounds
- Chest pain
- Hypotension
- Ventricular arrhythmias
- Associated with
  - Reduced cardiac output
  - Hypotension
  - Pump failure
- Initial diagnosis dependent on ECG
  - Shows ST elevation in the right ventricular leads (V3R, V4R)
- In RV infarction with unexplained hypoxia, always suspect right-to-left shunt at the atrial level

Natural History & Prognosis

- RV infarction is associated with increased mortality and morbidity
  - Ventricular arrhythmias and atrioventricular (AV) conduction abnormalities
- Isolated RV infarction is very rare
  - Usually in association with inferior wall LV infarction

Treatment

- Volume expansion is critical to medical treatment
- Acute reperfusion; percutaneous intervention or thrombolysis
- Acute reperfusion associated with rapid decrease in right atrial pressures
  - Important to decrease right atrial pressure because persistently elevated levels are associated with poorer outcomes

DIAGNOSTIC CHECKLIST

Consider

- In patients presenting with acute chest pain, right heart failure and hypotension

SELECTED REFERENCES

1. Jackson E et al: Ischaemic and non-ischaemic cardiomyopathies--cardiac MRI appearances with delayed enhancement. Clin Radiol. 62(5):395-403, 2007
2. Jenkins C et al: Reproducibility of right ventricular volumes and ejection fraction using real-time three-dimensional echocardiography: comparison with cardiac MRI. Chest. 131(6):1844-51, 2007
3. Kaandorp TA et al: Assessment of right ventricular infarction with contrast-enhanced magnetic resonance imaging. Coron Artery Dis. 18(1):39-43, 2007
4. Larose E et al: Right ventricular dysfunction assessed by cardiovascular magnetic resonance imaging predicts poor prognosis late after myocardial infarction. J Am Coll Cardiol. 49(8):855-62, 2007
5. Manka R et al: Silent inferior myocardial infarction with extensive right ventricular scarring. Int J Cardiol. 2007
6. Ibrahim T et al: Images in cardiovascular medicine. Assessment of isolated right ventricular myocardial infarction by magnetic resonance imaging. Circulation. 113(6):e78-9, 2006
7. Kumar A et al: Contrast-enhanced cardiovascular magnetic resonance imaging of right ventricular infarction. J Am Coll Cardiol. 48(10):1969-76, 2006
8. Kosuge M et al: Implications of the absence of ST-segment elevation in lead V4R in patients who have inferior wall acute myocardial infarction with right ventricular involvement. Clin Cardiol. 24(3):225-30, 2001
9. Mehta SR et al: Impact of right ventricular involvement on mortality and morbidity in patients with inferior myocardial infarction. J Am Coll Cardiol. 37(1):37-43, 2001
10. Haji SA et al: Right ventricular infarction--diagnosis and treatment. Clin Cardiol. 23(7):473-82, 2000
11. Menown IB et al: Early diagnosis of right ventricular or posterior infarction associated with inferior wall left ventricular acute myocardial infarction. Am J Cardiol. 85(8):934-8, 2000
12. Jugdutt BI: Right Ventricular Infarction: Contribution of Echocardiography to Diagnosis and Management. Echocardiography. 16(3):297-306, 1999
13. Bueno H et al: Combined effect of age and right ventricular involvement on acute inferior myocardial infarction prognosis. Circulation. 98(17):1714-20, 1998
14. Pu SY et al: Prediction of right ventricular infarction from standard surface ECG in patients with inferior myocardial infarction. Zhonghua Yi Xue Za Zhi (Taipei). 61(5):253-9, 1998
15. Zehender M et al: Right ventricular infarction as an independent predictor of prognosis after acute inferior myocardial infarction. N Engl J Med. 328(14):981-8, 1993
16. Bellamy GR et al: Value of two-dimensional echocardiography, electrocardiography, and clinical signs in detecting right ventricular infarction. Am Heart J. 112(2):304-9, 1986
17. Braat SH et al: Value of lead V4R for recognition of the infarct coronary artery in acute inferior myocardial infarction. Am J Cardiol. 53(11):1538-41, 1984
18. Garty I et al: The diagnosis and early complications of right ventricular infarction. Eur J Nucl Med. 9(10):453-60, 1984
19. Baigrie RS et al: The spectrum of right ventricular involvement in inferior wall myocardial infarction: a clinical, hemodynamic and noninvasive study. J Am Coll Cardiol. 1(6):1396-404, 1983
20. Candell-Riera J et al: Right ventricular infarction: relationships between ST segment elevation in V4R and hemodynamic, scintigraphic, and echocardiographic findings in patients with acute inferior myocardial infarction. Am Heart J. 101(3):281-7, 1981

IMAGE GALLERY

Typical

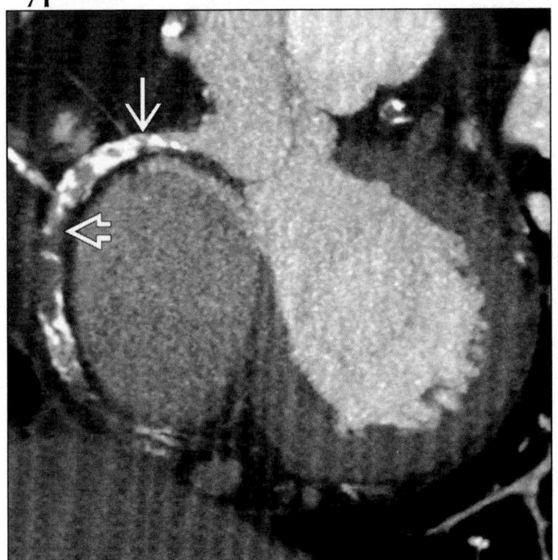

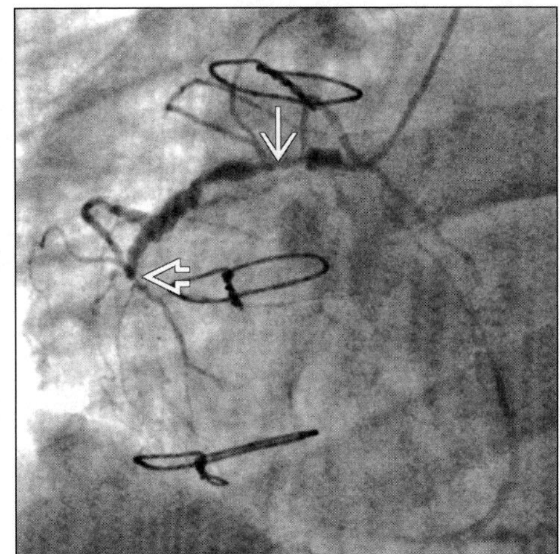

(Left) *Coronal oblique coronary CTA shows extensive plaque ➡ in the proximal segment and total occlusion ⇨ of the mid and distal segments.* ***(Right)*** *Corresponding invasive coronary angiogram confirms extensive plaque in the proximal segment ➡ and total occlusion ⇨ of the mid and distal segment RCA.*

Typical

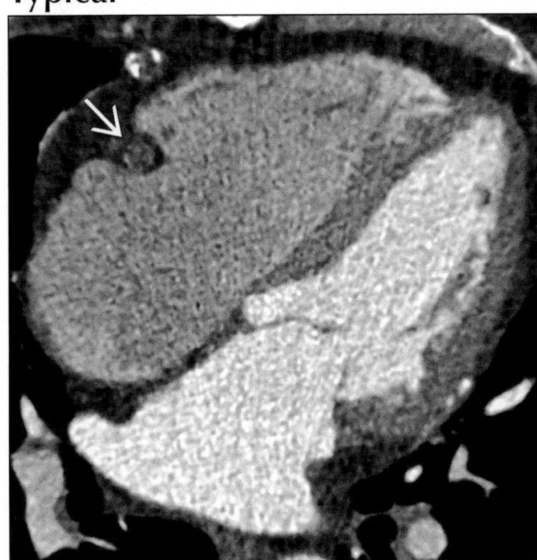

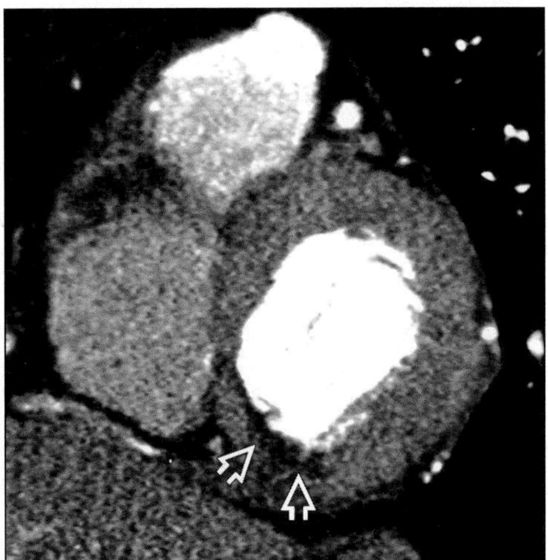

(Left) *Axial coronary CTA shows subtotal occlusion ➡ of the mid segment RCA.* ***(Right)*** *Corresponding short axis image shows inferior segment subendocardial perfusion defect ⇨ corresponding to RCA vascular territory myocardial infarction.*

Typical

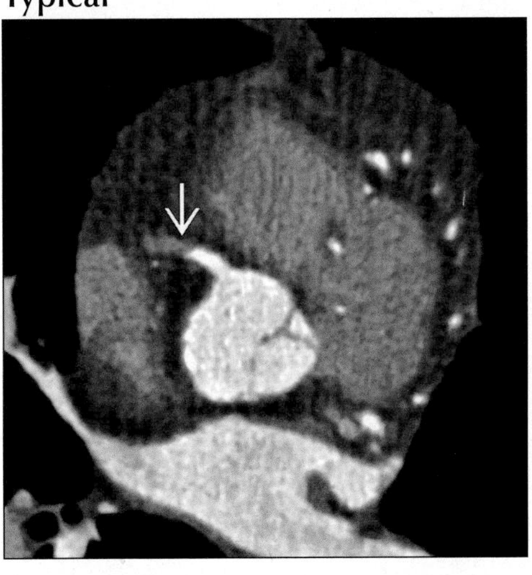

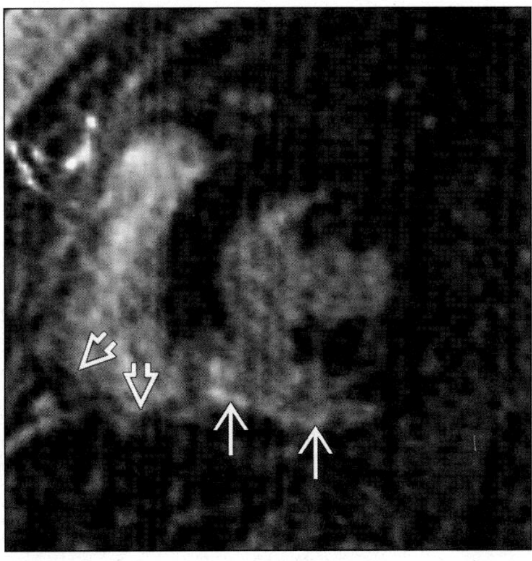

(Left) *Axial coronary CTA shows a total occlusion ➡ of the proximal segment RCA.* ***(Right)*** *Corresponding, delayed enhanced, inversion recovery, MR image shows inferior LV segment hyperenhancement ➡ consistent with inferior segment LV infarction. Note also RV inferior wall hyperenhancement ⇨ consistent with RV infarction.*

NON-ATHEROSCLEROSIS MI

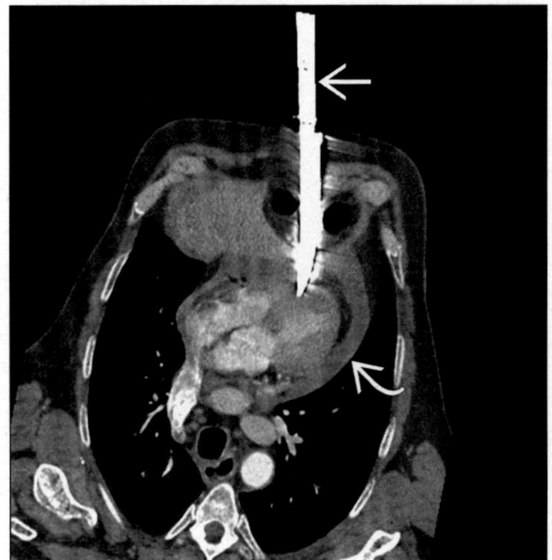

Coronary CTA (63 year old man) shows a knife injury to the heart. At surgery the knife tip had punctured the posterior descending coronary artery and right ventricle. Note hemopericardium.

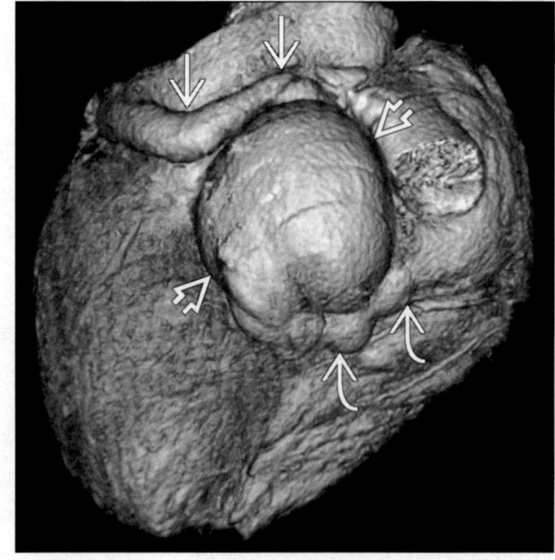

Coronary CTA 3D volumetric reformat (29 year old man with atypical chest pain) shows a giant coronary fistula. LCX becomes aneurysmal before draining into coronary sinus.

TERMINOLOGY

Definitions

- Myocardial infarction (MI) unrelated to coronary atherosclerosis

IMAGING FINDINGS

General Features

- Best diagnostic clue: Invasive angiography demonstrates normal appearing coronary arteries (2.8% prevalence)
- Location: EKG and enzymes similar to typical acute myocardial infarction (AMI)
- Morphology: Underlying cause often difficult to elucidate

Radiographic Findings

- Chest Radiography Findings
  - CXR: Acute pulmonary edema is a classic complication of cocaine abuse

CT Findings

- CTA
  - Coronary CTA has a high sensitivity (85-95%) and specificity (90-100%) for the detection of hemodynamically significant stenosis with very high negative predictive values
  - Thick multiplanar reformats (5 mm) may allow detection of hypoperfusion defect in anterior segment
  - Delayed scan (5 minutes after initial contrast bolus) may allow detection of myocardial infarction
    - Newer techniques performing CTA immediately following percutaneous coronary intervention (avoids need for CTA contrast administration)
  - CT of lung and mediastinum may provide clue to underlying etiology
    - Acute pulmonary edema: Increased ground-glass opacities and septal lines, classically seen in cocaine abuse
    - Cigarette smoking: Emphysema, respiratory bronchiolitis, Langerhans cell histiocytosis
    - Aortic wall abnormalities: Thickened in Takayasu arteritis

DDx: Non-Atherosclerosis MI

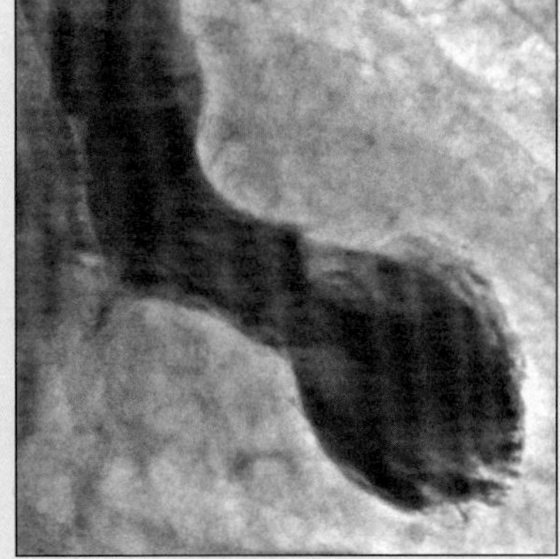

Takotsubo Cardiomyopathy

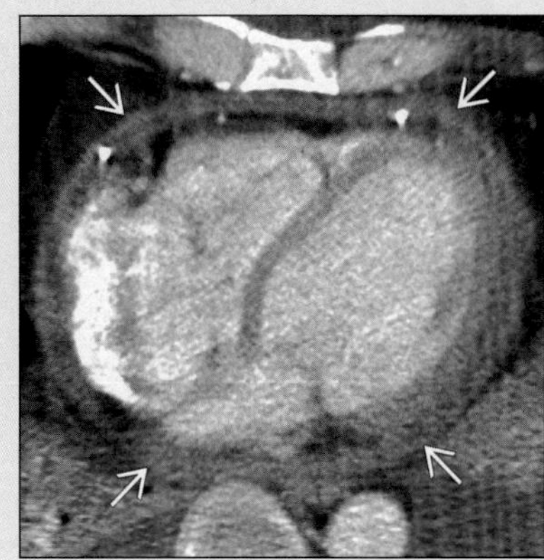

Acute Pericarditis

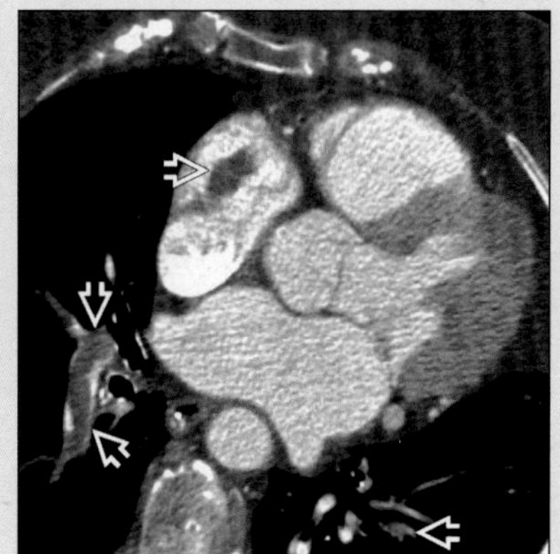

Acute Pulmonary Embolism

NON-ATHEROSCLEROSIS MI

Key Facts

Terminology
- Myocardial infarction unrelated to coronary atherosclerosis

Imaging Findings
- Invasive angiography demonstrates normal appearing coronary arteries (2.8% prevalence)
- EKG and enzymes similar to typical acute myocardial infarction (MI)
- Underlying cause often difficult to elucidate
- CXR: Acute pulmonary edema is a classic complication of cocaine abuse
- CT of lung and mediastinum may provide clue to underlying etiology

Pathology
- 6% of acute myocardial infarction (AMI) have normal coronary arteries at autopsy

Clinical Issues
- EKG and enzymes similar to typical acute myocardial infarction (MI)
- Younger patient population with less risk factors except for cigarette smoking
- Lower prevalence of atherosclerosis risk factors
- Mortality rate significantly lower than patients with atherosclerosis AMI who are high-risk or have LM disease
- Standard therapy for acute myocardial infarction

    - Radiation: Pulmonary fibrosis, fibrosing mediastinitis
    - Pulmonary parenchymal aneurysms: Polyarteritis nodosa
    - Pulmonary embolism in thrombotic states
    - Chest trauma: Pulmonary contusion, laceration, pneumothorax, fractured ribs

MR Findings
- Cardiac MR steady-state free precession sequence to assess LV global and regional wall motion
- Acute infarction will cause increased signal intensity in the anterior segment on T2-weighted imaging
- 1st pass perfusion (stress followed by rest)
- Cardiac MR delayed enhancement can demonstrate presence, location and size of infarction

Nuclear Medicine Findings
- PET: PET is currently regarded as the gold-standard for myocardial viability assessment

Echocardiographic Findings
- Echocardiogram
  - Echo shows anterior segment akinesis acutely, anterior segment thinning chronically
  - Echo very useful bedside exam for complications of infarction
    - LV thrombus

Angiographic Findings
- Coronary Angiography Findings
  - Normal appearing coronary arteries
  - It's now realized that many patients with apparently normal coronary angiograms have a significant coronary plaque burden with positive remodeling and that most myocardial infarctions arise from lesions causing < 50% luminal narrowing

DIFFERENTIAL DIAGNOSIS

Acute Aortic Dissection
- May dissect down and into the coronary artery ostia

Acute Myocarditis
- Prodromal flu-like symptoms

Pneumonia
- Chest pain, particularly with associated pleurisy

Pancreatitis
- Elevated amylase helps differentiate from cardiac

Reflux Esophagitis
- Exacerbated by lying down

Takotsubo Syndrome
- "Broken-heart" cardiomyopathy

PATHOLOGY

General Features
- General path comments: Pathology depends on underlying cause
- Etiology
  - Coronary vasospasm
    - Cocaine abuse
    - Ethanol abuse
    - Cigarette smoking
    - Endothelial dysfunction
    - Calcium channel withdrawl
  - Embolization
    - Very rare: Common sources include cardiac cavity and appendages, infective endocarditis, prosthetic valves
  - Inflammation/vasculitis
    - Takayasu arteritis usually affects large arteries, but is described
    - Syphilitic aortitis with ostial narrowing
    - Coxsackie virus B
    - Kawasaki disease
    - Radiation induced wall thickening
    - Polyarteritis nodosa, systemic lupus erythematosus (SLE), giant cell arteritis
  - Thrombosis/hypercoagulability
    - Factor VII activity

- Factor V leiden
- Protein C deficiency
- Hyperhomocystinuria
- Excessive estrogens
- Cigarette smoking
  - Spontaneous coronary dissection
    - Rare but well described entity occurring particularly in pregnant women
  - Myocardial bridge
    - Controversial; while many normal patients have a bridge and no associated ischemia, a small subgroup appear predisposed to ischemia in the vascular territory of the bridge
  - Chest trauma
  - Percutaneous coronary intervention
  - Re-instent stenosis
  - Anaphylaxis - wasp sting
- Epidemiology: 6% of acute myocardial infarction (AMI) have normal coronary arteries at autopsy

CLINICAL ISSUES

Presentation

- Most common signs/symptoms
  - Present with the classic clinical features of atherosclerosis AMI
    - Severe, central, crushing chest pain, radiation to left arm
- Other signs/symptoms: Heaviness or burning, radiation to the jaw, neck, shoulder, back, or both arms
- Clinical Profile
  - Lower prevalence of atherosclerosis risk factors
    - Hypertension
    - Hyperlipidemia
    - Diabetes
    - Congestive heart failure
    - Peripheral vascular disease
    - Malignancy
- No history of angina, no prodrome prior to AMI
- EKG and enzymes similar to typical AMI

Demographics

- Age: Younger patient population with less risk factors for atherosclerosis except for cigarette smoking

Natural History & Prognosis

- Mortality rate significantly lower than patients with atherosclerosis AMI who are high-risk or have LM disease

Treatment

- Standard therapy for AMI
- Greater survival than patients with AMI from atherosclerosis
- Percutaneous coronary intervention/surgery not generally used, except in coronary dissection

DIAGNOSTIC CHECKLIST

Consider

- In patients presenting with acute myocardial infarction with a normal coronary angiogram

SELECTED REFERENCES

1. Kardasz I et al: Myocardial infarction with normal coronary arteries: a conundrum with multiple aetiologies and variable prognosis: an update. J Intern Med. 261(4):330-48, 2007
2. Larsen AI et al: Characteristics and outcomes of patients with acute myocardial infarction and angiographically normal coronary arteries. Am J Cardiol. 95(2):261-3, 2005
3. Villines TC et al: Diffuse nonatherosclerotic coronary aneurysms: an unusual cause of sudden death in a young male and a literature review. Cardiol Rev. 13(6):309-11, 2005
4. Caussin C et al: Coronary plaque burden detected by multislice computed tomography after acute myocardial infarction with near-normal coronary arteries by angiography. Am J Cardiol. 92(7):849-52, 2003
5. Antman EM et al: Acute Myocardial Infarction In: Braundwald E. Heart Disease: A Textbook of Cardiovascular Medicine, 6th ed. Philadelphia, W.B. Saunders Company, 2001
6. Pinney SP et al: Myocardial infarction in patients with normal coronary arteries: proposed pathogenesis and predisposing risk factors. J Thromb Thrombolysis. 11(1):11-7, 2001
7. Tun A et al: Myocardial infarction with normal coronary arteries: the pathologic and clinical perspectives. Angiology. 52(5):299-304, 2001
8. Sztajzel J et al: Role of the vascular endothelium in patients with angina pectoris or acute myocardial infarction with normal coronary arteries. Postgrad Med J. 76(891):16-21, 2000
9. Alpert JS: Myocardial infarction with angiographically normal coronary arteries. Arch Intern Med. 154(3):265-9, 1994
10. Kutom AH et al: Myocardial infarction due to intracoronary thrombi without significant coronary artery disease in systemic lupus erythematosus. Chest. 100(2):571-2, 1991
11. Rajani RM et al: Acute myocardial infarction with normal coronary arteries in a case of polyarteritis nodosa: possible role of coronary artery spasm. Postgrad Med J. 67(783):78-80, 1991
12. Feit A et al: Bilateral coronary thrombosis in the absence of inducible coronary spasm, thrombocytosis, coagulation abnormalities, or angiographic evidence of coronary artery disease: previously undescribed method of myocardial infarction. Cathet Cardiovasc Diagn. 15(1):40-3, 1988
13. Zimmerman FH et al: Recurrent myocardial infarction associated with cocaine abuse in a young man with normal coronary arteries: evidence for coronary artery spasm culminating in thrombosis. J Am Coll Cardiol. 9(4):964-8, 1987
14. Diamond TH et al: Acute myocardial infarction with normal coronary arteries--viral myopericarditis and possible coronary vasospasm. A case report. S Afr Med J. 67(22):892-4, 1985
15. Gersh BJ et al: Coronary artery spasm and myocardial infarction in the absence of angiographically demonstrable obstructive coronary disease. Mayo Clin Proc. 56(11):700-8, 1981

IMAGE GALLERY

Typical

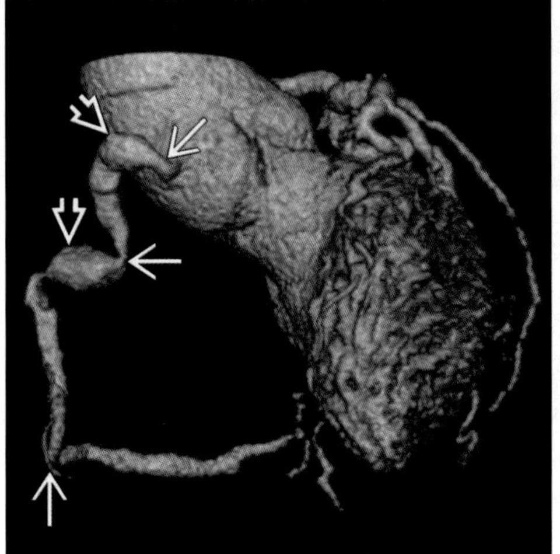

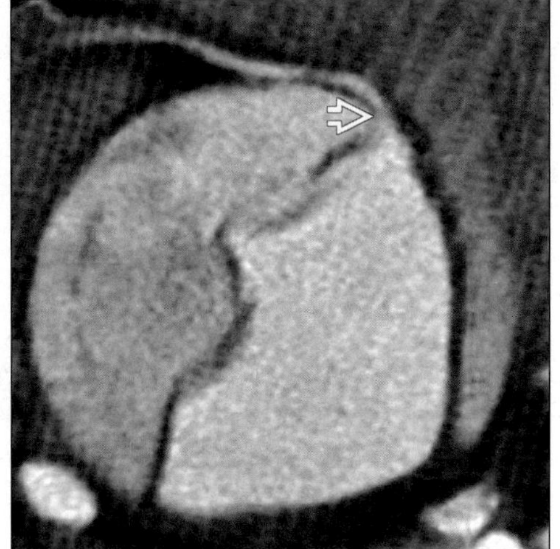

(Left) *Coronary CTA 3D volumetric reformat shows multiple RCA stenosis ⇒ and aneurysms ⇒ in a 23 year old man with known Kawasaki disease.* ***(Right)*** *Coronary CTA in a 38 year old bodybuilder shows acute aortic dissection involving the RCA ostium ⇒. The patient sustained an inferior segment AMI.*

Typical

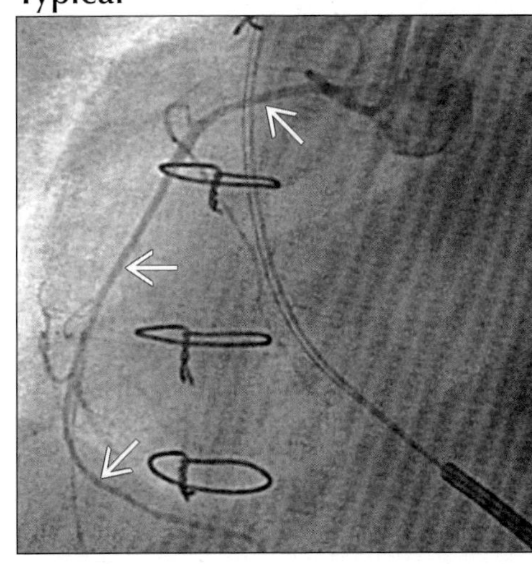

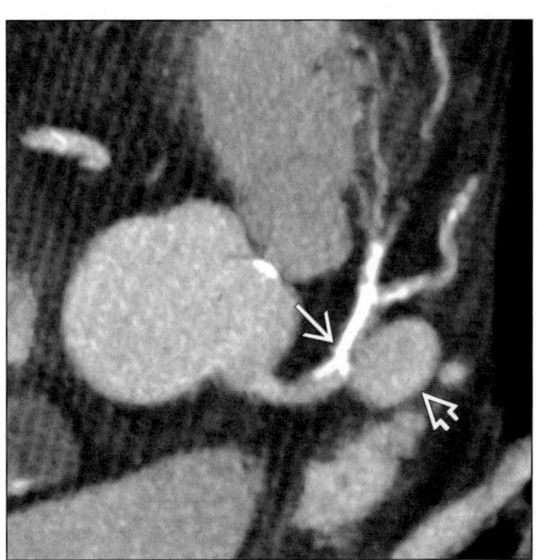

(Left) *Invasive coronary angiogram in a 33 year old woman shows spontaneous coronary dissection ⇒ of the entire RCA. The entire RCA was stented.* ***(Right)*** *Coronary CTA in a 52 year old man shows a focal aneurysm ⇒ arising from the lateral wall of the proximal LAD ⇒. Such aneurysms are prone to thrombosis and coronary occlusion.*

Typical

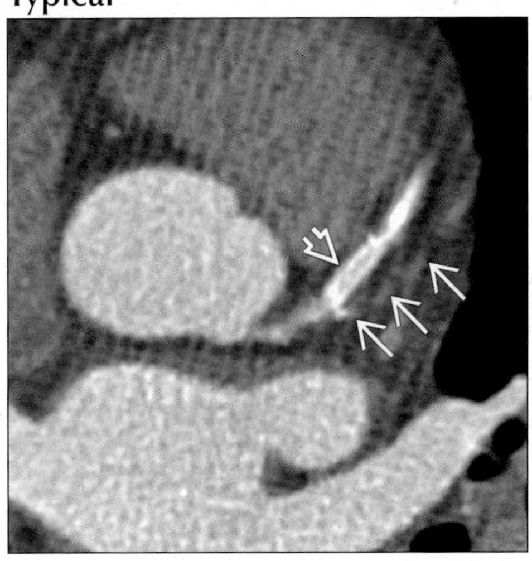

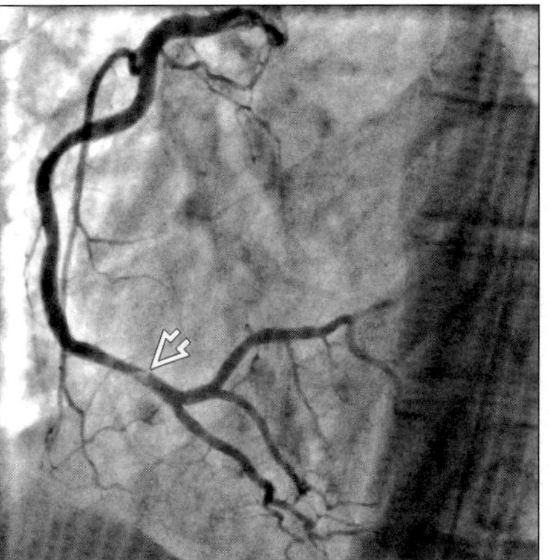

(Left) *Coronary CTA in a 56 year old man with a stented proximal LAD lesion ⇒ shows a "jailed" 1st diagonal branch ⇒ from the proximal stent placement. He sustained a small lateral AMI.* ***(Right)*** *Invasive coronary angiogram in a 32 year old cocaine user shows a filling defect ⇒, possibly embolic, in the distal segment of what is otherwise a normal right coronary artery.*

ISCHEMIC CARDIOMYOPATHY

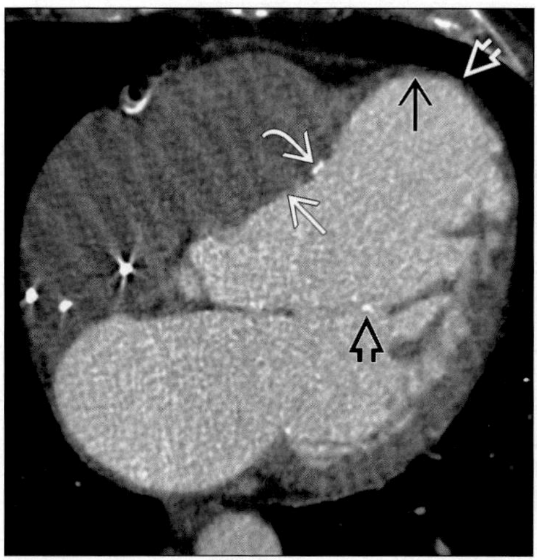

Coronary CTA shows a dilated LV with interventricular ➔ and apical ➔ wall thinning. Note the apical aneurysm formation ➔ as well as myocardial ➔ and chordae tendineae ➔ calcification.

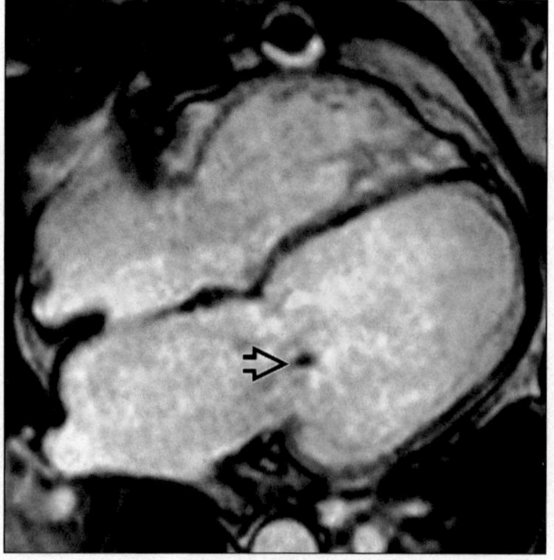

Cardiac MR steady state free precession 4-chamber image shows dilated LV and RV with circumferential wall thinning. Note the LV remodeling-related mitral regurgitation ➔.

TERMINOLOGY

Definitions

- Ischemic cardiomyopathy (ICM) may be defined as significantly impaired left ventricular dysfunction with left ventricular dilatation that results from coronary artery disease (CAD)

IMAGING FINDINGS

General Features

- Location: Usually diffuse LV involvement, usually three-vessel coronary disease
- Size: Depends on degree of coronary involvement
- Morphology: Ventricular wall thinning and fibrofatty involution
- Dilated hypokinetic left ventricle

Radiographic Findings

- Radiography
  - Enlarged cardiac silhouette, often globular shape
  - May reveal evidence of heart failure
    - Kerley B lines, interstitial edema and vascular redistribution to the upper lobes

CT Findings

- CTA
  - Coronary CTA has a high sensitivity (85-97%) & specificity (90-100%) for the detection of hemodynamically significant stenosis with very high negative predictive values
    - Delayed scan (5 minutes after initial contrast bolus) may allow detection of myocardial infarction
  - Cine multiplanar reformats allow assessment of global and regional function
    - Strong correlation with cardiac MR (gold standard)

MR Findings

- Cardiac MR steady-state free precession sequence to assess LV global and regional wall motion
  - Standardized 17 segment AHA model utilized
- 1st pass perfusion (stress followed by rest)
  - Vasodilation induced by dipyrimdole (0.56 mg/kg infused IV over 4 minutes)
  - Hybrid gradient echo-planar sequence acquired during bolus of 0.1 mmol/kg gadolinium

DDx: Ischemic Cardiomyopathy

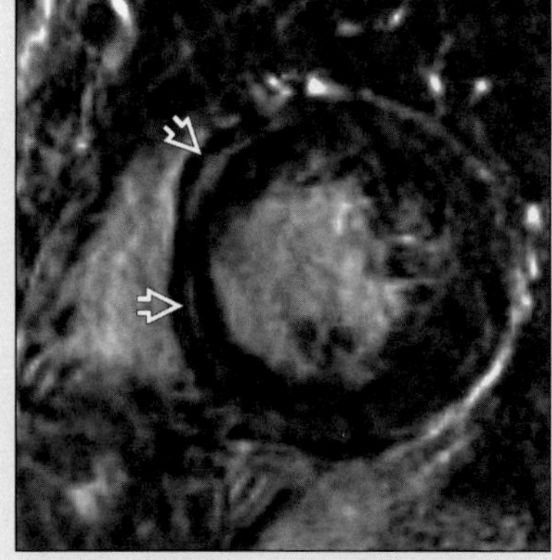

Chronic Myocarditis

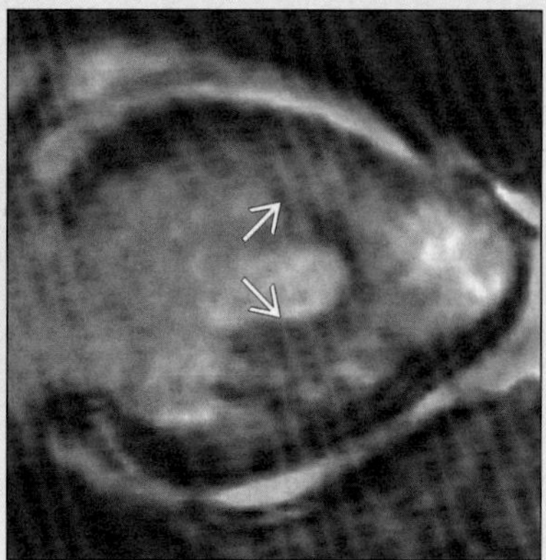

Non-Compaction Cardiomyopathy

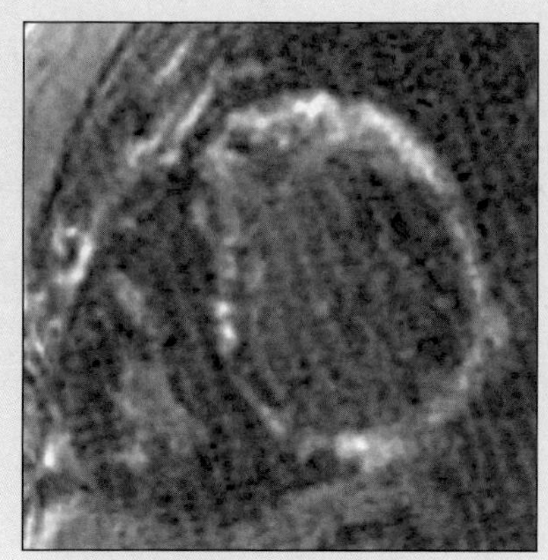

Cardiac Amyloidosis

ISCHEMIC CARDIOMYOPATHY

Key Facts

Terminology
- Ischemic cardiomyopathy (ICM) may be defined as significantly impaired left ventricular dysfunction (left ventricular ejection fraction 35-40%) that results from coronary artery disease (CAD)

Imaging Findings
- Ventricular wall thinning and fibrofatty involution
- Dilated hypokinetic left ventricle
- Controversial - currently PET is considered gold standard but evolving cardiac MR techniques also have high diagnostic accuracy
- Usually diffuse LV involvement, usually three-vessel coronary disease

Top Differential Diagnoses
- Myocarditis

Pathology
- After an acute thrombosis of a coronary artery, if the infarct is transmural, the ventricle undergoes a process of "remodeling"

Clinical Issues
- Angiographically diagnosed ischemic heart failure is associated with a shorter survival than nonischemic heart failure
- More extensive CAD is associated with a shorter survival
- Poor prognosis for 5-year survival; depends on
  - Ejection fraction
  - Functional status; poor class IV survival
  - Arrhythmias

  - Short axis stack (5-8 slices)
  - Repeat sequence 10 minutes later
- Cardiac MR delayed enhancement can demonstrate presence, location and size of infarction
  - Gradient-echo inversion recovery sequence
  - 7-10 minutes after a bolus of 0.1 mmol/kg gadolinium
  - Vary inversion time to maximize nulling of normal myocardium
  - Healthy viable myocardium appears black
  - Scar appears bright ("hyperenhanced")
  - Viability depends on degree of transmurality of scar
    - Rule of thumb: If 50% or less of wall thickness in any given segment is infarcted (white) then functional recovery after revascularization is likely (≥ 80% chance for recovery) → segment is considered "viable"

Nuclear Medicine Findings
- PET
  - PET has been regarded as the gold-standard for myocardial viability assessment, even though MR is considered superior by some
    - Validated for viability and subsequent prognosis
  - Qualitative assessment of regional myocardial blood flow
    - Most commonly used tracers are rubidium-82 and N-13 ammonia
    - Performed under rest and stress conditions
    - High diagnostic accuracy (sensitivity and specificity between 85-95%)
  - Quantitative assessment of regional myocardial blood flow
    - Most commonly used tracer is oxygen-15 Water
  - Metabolic evaluation of myocardium
    - Ischemia results in impaired fatty acid and increased glucose metabolism
    - Most commonly used tracer is 5-fluoxy deoxyglucose (FDG)
- Technetium-99m: Sestamibi uptake dependent on perfusion, cell membrane integrity, mitochondrial function
  - Dysfunctional segments with > 50-60% uptake considered viable
  - Sensitivity/specificity for improvement post-revascularization = 81%/66%
- Thallium scan
  - Initial uptake determined by blood flow
  - Subsequent uptake dependent on cell membrane integrity/viability
  - Two protocols: Stress-redistribution-reinjection and rest-redistribution
    - Stress-redistribution-reinjection: Assesses for stress-inducible ischemia and viability
    - Rest-redistribution: Assesses viability
    - Dysfunctional but viable segments considered when tracer uptake increases > 10% or when activity > 50-60%
    - Sensitivity/specificity for improvement in regional wall contractility post-revascularization = 86%/59%

Echocardiographic Findings
- Echocardiogram
  - Standardized 17 segment AHA model should be utilized
    - Echo shows segment akinesis acutely, segment thinning chronically
    - Chronic infarction appears bright = fatty replacement
  - Stress echo
    - Low-dose dobutamine (5-10 μg/kg/min)
    - Increased contractility in viable but dysfunctional myocardial segments (contractile reserve)
    - Sensitivity/specificity for improvement in regional wall contractility post-revascularization = 82%/79%

Angiographic Findings
- Coronary angiography usually reveals multiple stenoses and occlusions in several territories
- Ventricular angiography usually reveals reduced wall motion and ejection fraction, reduced wall thickening

Imaging Recommendations

- Best imaging tool: Controversial - currently PET is considered gold standard but cardiac MR evolving and may be superior

DIFFERENTIAL DIAGNOSIS

Idiopathic Dilated Cardiomyopathy

- Absent or insignificant coronary artery disease
- Diagnosis of exclusion

Chronic Myocarditis

- Wall thinning and LV dysfunction
- Usually post-viral infection (Coxsackie)

Arrhythmogenic Right Ventricular Dysplasia

- May effect LV in 15%

Restrictive Cardiomyopathy

- Often idiopathic
- Diastolic heart failure

Infiltrative Cardiomyopathy

- Often presents with diastolic heart failure
- Sarcoid, amyloid

PATHOLOGY

General Features

- General path comments
  - After acute coronary artery thrombosis with transmural infarct, the LV undergoes a process of "remodeling"
  - Occurs at a cellular and organ level
    - Cellular - destruction of connective tissue and slippage of myofibrils
    - Dilation in size and shape of ventricle
- Epidemiology: Approximately 70% of heart failure is caused by coronary artery disease

Staging, Grading or Classification Criteria

- Two subtypes of ICM
  - Transmural infarct: Ventricular remodeling, no viable myocardium, irreversible
  - Non-transmural: Hibernating myocardium
    - Reduced myocardial contraction due to chronic hypo-perfusion from CAD

CLINICAL ISSUES

Presentation

- Severe left ventricular (LV) dysfunction
  - Multivessel coronary artery disease
- Chest pain: Substernal, pressing, occasionally radiating to the left arm
  - Typical features of myocardial infarction may precede development of ischemic cardiomyopathy
  - May be preceded by silent infarcts
  - Symptoms of heart failure, depending on state of compensation
- Symptoms associated with arrhythmias: Atrial or ventricular

Natural History & Prognosis

- Angiographically diagnosed ischemic heart failure is associated with a shorter survival than nonischemic heart failure
- More extensive CAD is associated with a shorter survival

Treatment

- Poor prognosis for 5-year survival; depends on
  - Ejection fraction
  - Functional status; poor class IV survival
  - Arrhythmias
- Therapy for acute myocardial infarction (MI) can preserve tissue and alter progression of disease
- Medical therapy
  - Diuretics to reduce symptoms and allow patients to tolerate other medications; optimum medical management in euvolemic patients
  - Reduce activity of renin-angiotensin-aldosterone system
    - ACE inhibitors in patients without significant side effects
    - Angiotensin blockers (AT1 blockers); currently reserved for patients intolerant of ACE inhibitors
  - Beta blockers in all euvolemic patients without recent symptomatic heart failure or requirement for beta agonists
    - Conclusive data with carvedilol, metoprolol, and bisoprolol
    - Intolerance for heart failure decompensation or bradycardia
  - Digoxin: May reduce rate of hospitalization, no effect on mortality
  - Aspirin: Reduces risk of coronary thrombosis
  - Cholesterol lowering therapy: Statin therapy to reduce recurrent infarct
- Coronary revascularization (bypass surgery) can improve prognosis
  - Most reliable in patients with angina
  - Best data in patients with viable myocardium
  - Surgical risk is high; however, these patients derive the greatest benefit
- Implantable defibrillator
  - Latest data support implantation in patients with
    - Inducible or spontaneous arrhythmias
    - All patients with ejection fraction < 30% with ischemic etiology
- Transplantation
  - Intractable heart failure or arrhythmias
  - Benefit of revascularization expected to be minimal

SELECTED REFERENCES

1. Burch GE et al: Ischemic cardiomyopathy. Am Heart J. 79(3):291-2, 1970
2. Prognostic role of dobutamine stress echocardiography in myocardial viability: Curr Opin Cardiol. 2006 Sep;21(5):443-9. Review.

ISCHEMIC CARDIOMYOPATHY

IMAGE GALLERY

Typical

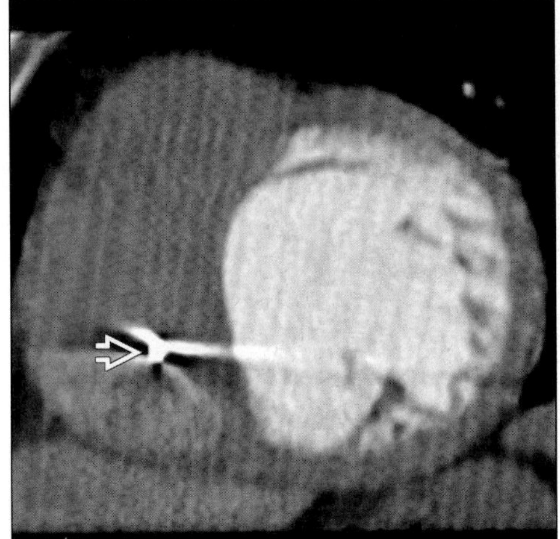

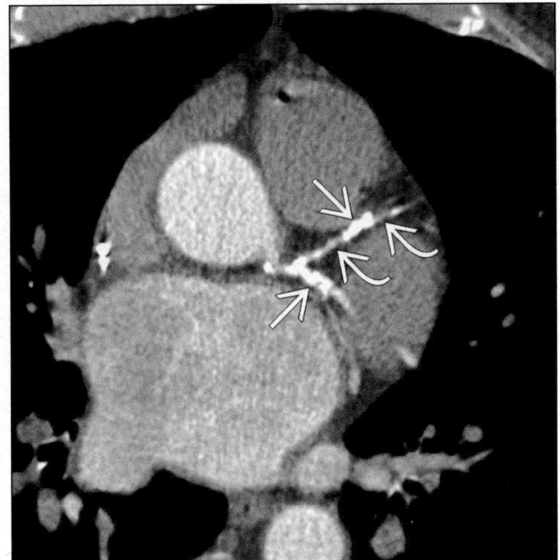

(Left) *Coronary CTA short axis view shows a dilated LV. Note the defibrillator wire in RV* → *due to recurrent arrhythmia (complication of ischemic cardiomyopathy).* ***(Right)*** *Corresponding coronary artery imaging shows an extensive calcified plaque* → *and multiple subtotal occlusions* ↪ *in the LM, LAD, and LCX. The RCA was also heavily diseased (not shown).*

Typical

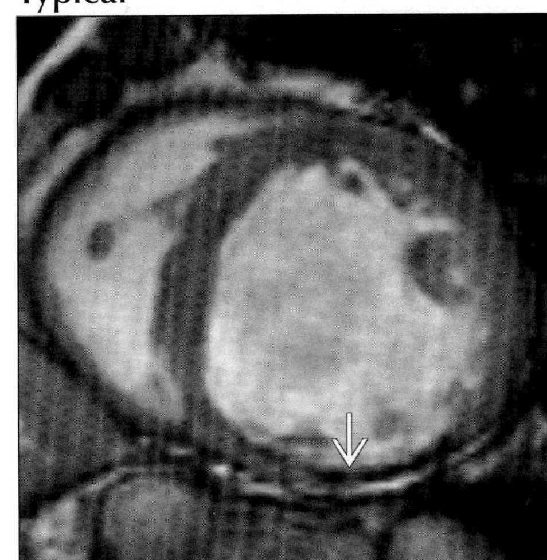

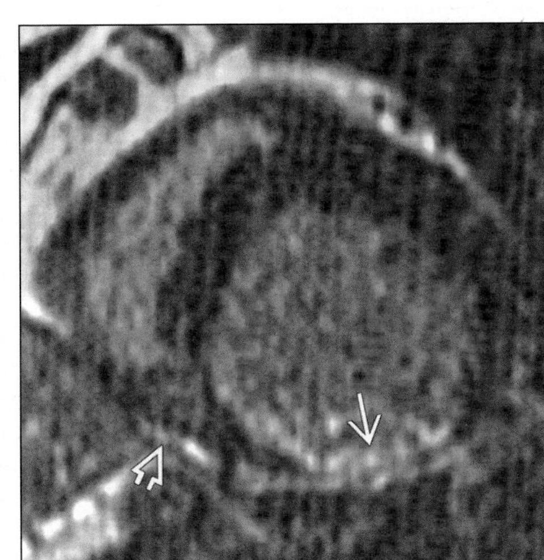

(Left) *Cardiac MR viability study: SSFP sequence shows poor global LV function, a dilated LV, and inferior segment wall thinning* → *consistent with RCA infarct. Query viability of remaining segments.* ***(Right)*** *Corresponding delayed enhancement image shows inferior segment transmural enhancement* → *confirming a RCA infarct. Entire remaining myocardium is black indicating viability. Note RCA infarct* →*.*

Typical

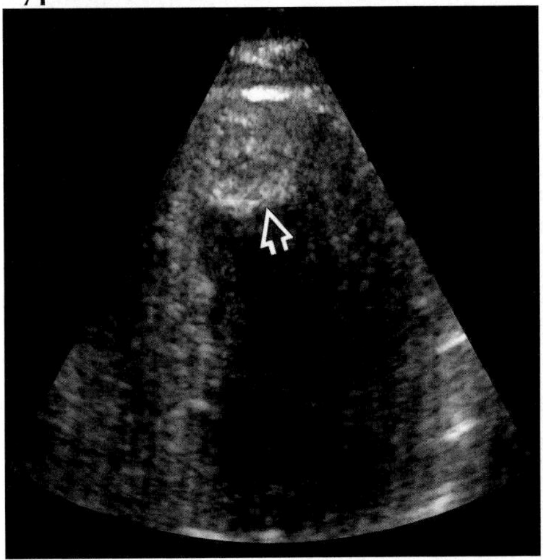

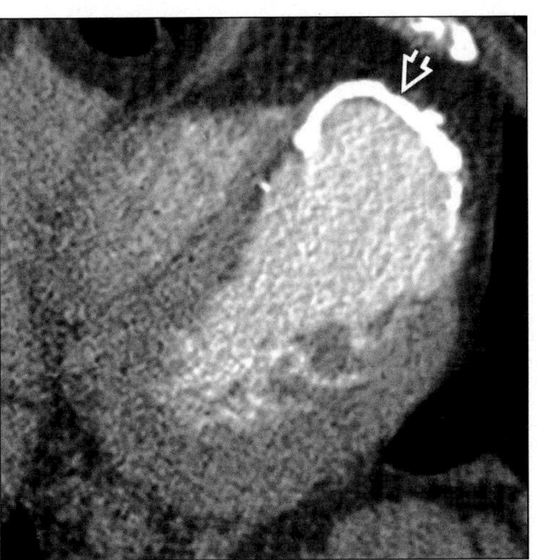

(Left) *Echocardiogram four-chamber view shows a dilated LV secondary to ischemic cardiomyopathy and an echogenic mass in the LV apex* → *consistent with an apical thrombus.* ***(Right)*** *Coronary CTA in a 72 year old man with ischemic cardiomyopathy shows a heavily calcified ventricular apical aneurysm* →*.*

NON-TRANSMURAL MYOCARDIAL INFARCTION

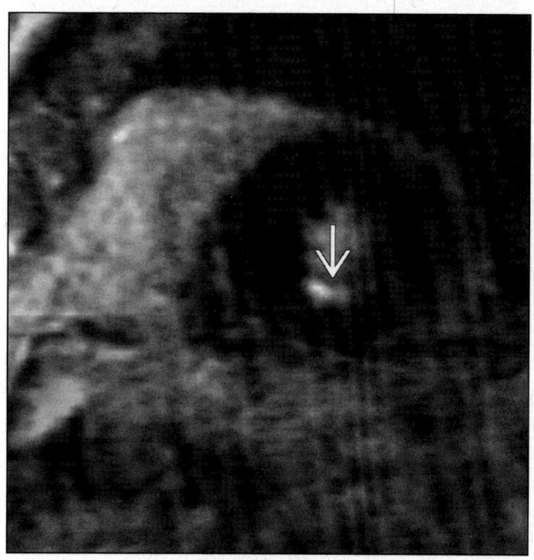

Short axis delayed enhancement MR shows a small focus of hyperenhancement ➔ in the subendocardial aspect of the inferior wall. Infarct spans less than 50% of transmurality (= viable myocardial segment).

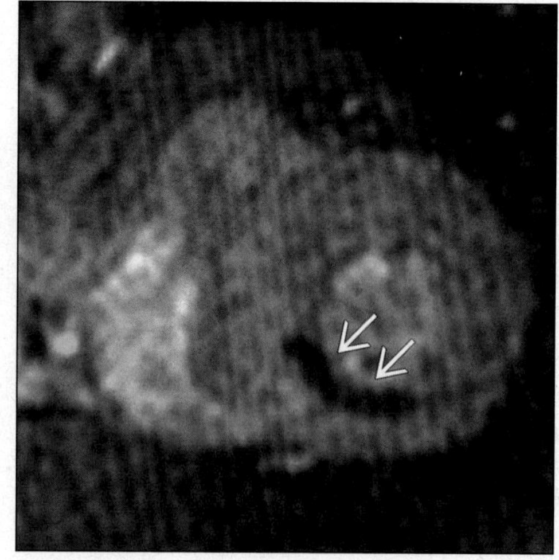

Short axis first-pass perfusion image shows subendocardial perfusion defect ➔ at rest consistent with myocardial infarct or critical stenosis.

TERMINOLOGY

Definitions

- Infarct affecting the subendocardial surface of the myocardium with less than 50% transmurality extension

IMAGING FINDINGS

General Features

- Morphology
  - Typically associated with non Q-wave infarction
  - Ischemic necrosis is limited to the subendocardial layers of the myocardium, extent is variable
- Most notable ECG change is a persistent ST segment depression
- Diminished perfusion and function in the affected area
  - Functional impairment is limited if minimal thickness involved
  - Function may be normal if infarct is remote and only small portion of transmurality affected

CT Findings

- CTA: Coronary CTA may demonstrate matching occlusion or high grade coronary stenosis
- Cardiac Gated CTA: Cine images may demonstrate regional wall motion abnormality
- Cardiac CT myocardial perfusion analysis reveals subendocardial hypoenhancement consistent with myocardial infarction (MI)
- CT perfusion underestimates infarct size as compared to delayed-enhancement MR
- Delayed-enhancement CT may be feasible, but with poor contrast-to-noise ratio when compared to MR
- Differentiation of acute vs. old MI by CT
  - HU values will be lower in old infarcts demonstrating negative numbers due to fatty metaplasia
  - LV thinning and calcifications may be present in old MI
  - LV remodeling with LV cavity dilation appears in large old infarcts

MR Findings

- T2WI

DDx: Subendocardial Myocardial Infarction

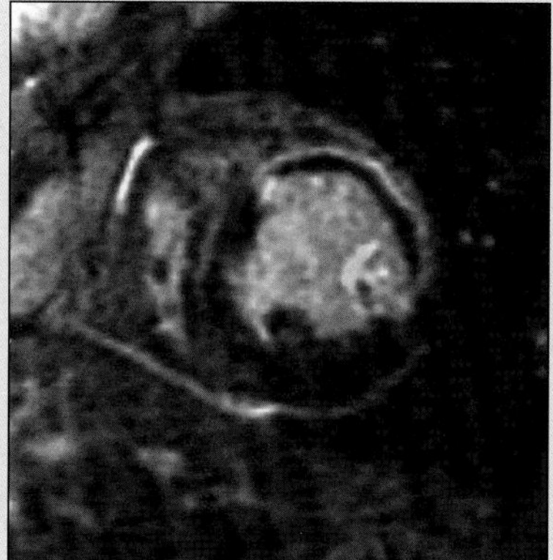

Transmural Myocardial Infarction

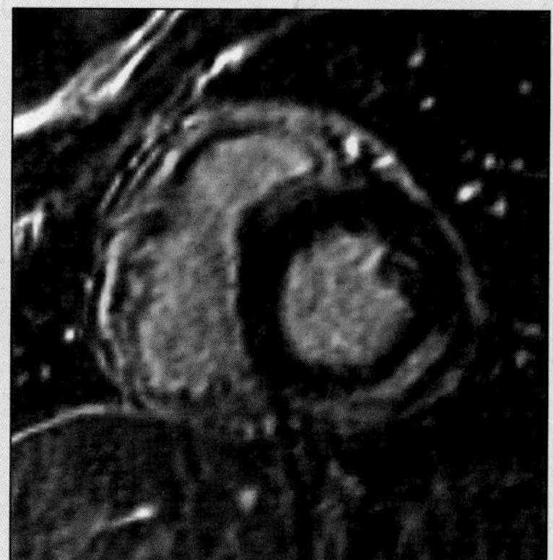

Myocarditis

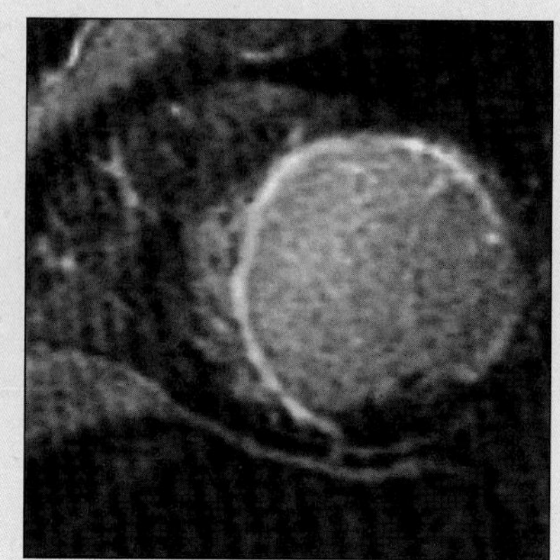

Chronic Myocardial Infarction

NON-TRANSMURAL MYOCARDIAL INFARCTION

Key Facts

Terminology
- Infarct affecting the subendocardial surface of the myocardium with less than 50% transmurality extension

Imaging Findings
- CTA: Coronary CTA may demonstrate matching occlusion or high grade coronary stenosis
- Cardiac CT myocardial perfusion analysis reveals subendocardial hypoenhancement consistent with myocardial infarction (MI)
- First-pass perfusion MR imaging shows perfusion defect due to reduced wash-in of gadolinium
- Delayed-enhancement MR shows hyperenhancement only in the inner border of LV myocardium
- Delayed-enhancement MR is the current gold standard for detection and quantification of non-transmural infarct
- Nuclear imaging will not detect 50% of subendocardial infarcts

Top Differential Diagnoses
- Myocarditis
- Transmural Myocardial Infarction

Pathology
- Result of early reperfusion before wavefront of infarction can extend transmurally

Clinical Issues
- Clinically determined by absence of Q wave on EKG, with serum marker of MI and appropriate clinical presentation

    - May show increased signal intensity representing myocardial edema if acute
    - Edema typically involves larger area than is infarcted
- Cine MR shows
    - Regional wall motion abnormality or reduced systolic thickening
- First-pass perfusion MR imaging shows perfusion defect due to reduced wash-in of gadolinium
- Delayed-enhancement MR shows hyperenhancement only in the inner border of LV myocardium

    - Delayed-enhancement MR is the current gold standard for detection and quantification of non-transmural infarct
    - High resolution images enable clear differentiation of transmural (100%) and nontransmural subendocardial infarcts
    - Myocardial viability depends on degree of transmurality
        - > 50% transmurality of delayed hyperenhancement → poor chance of functional recovery after revascularization = non-viable myocardium
        - < 50% delayed hyperenhancement → good chance of functional recovery after revascularization = viable myocardium
- Combination of stress-perfusion and delayed-enhancement MR may allow
    - Differentiation between inducible ischemia and infarcted myocardium
    - Detect peri-infarct ischemia

Nuclear Medicine Findings
- Radionuclide angiography finding
    - Reduced regional function
- Cardiac scintigraphy findings
    - Using perfusion marker, reduced tracer uptake demonstrated
        - Imaging may show thinning or partial thickness perfusion
        - However, usually apparent as wall thinning rather than dropout
    - Nuclear imaging will not detect 50% of subendocardial infarcts
        - Infarct detection may be compromised by partial volume effects

Echocardiographic Findings
- Echocardiogram
    - Reduced regional function
    - Not as sensitive as MR to detect subtle regional wall motion abnormalities

Angiographic Findings
- Coronary angiography findings
    - More commonly tightly stenosed coronary artery rather than occlusion
    - Tight stenoses which become occluded more likely to cause nontransmural infarct than mild stenoses which occlude
        - Chronic flow reduction may be a stimulus for collateral formation

DIFFERENTIAL DIAGNOSIS

Coronary Artery Stenosis
- Persistent ischemia may lead to myocardial necrosis and subendocardial infarct

Old Infarction
- Scintigraphy is a poor discriminating technique
- Persistent hyperenhancement on MR cannot discriminate old from new infarct
- T2WI will help to demonstrate increase in signal (edema) if acute
- Old infarct may demonstrate LV thinning (< 6 mm in end-diastole), fatty metaplasia or calcification

Myocarditis
- Patchy nature of disease may appear as nontransmural infarct
    - Serum markers and wall motion assessment will not adequately discriminate this diagnoses from infarction
    - Coronary angiography is essential to rule out MI
- Delayed-enhancement MR is the technique of choice to differentiate MI from myocarditis

- Acute myocarditis affects sub-epicardial rather than sub-endocardial region of LV

Transmural Myocardial Infarction

- Infarct extending throughout entire myocardial thickness
- Chronic infarct demonstrating more than 50% of delayed-hyperenhancement in transmural extension are unlikely to recover LV function
- Associated with worse prognosis and more complications

PATHOLOGY

General Features

- General path comments
  - Myocardial necrosis
    - Coagulation necrosis
    - Contraction band necrosis
    - Intramyocardial hemorrhage
  - Vascular occlusion
  - Result of early reperfusion before wavefront of infarction can extend transmurally

CLINICAL ISSUES

Presentation

- Chest pain; clinical picture of acute MI
- Clinically determined by absence of Q wave on EKG, with serum marker of MI and appropriate clinical presentation
  - Poor discrimination from transmural MI
- More commonly seen without ST elevation on presentation EKG
  - Natural history of MI not especially predictable on the basis of presenting EKG
- Confirmed by detection of markers in the serum
- Not uncommonly result of early reperfusion; prevent transmural extension
  - Thrombolysis
  - Percutaneous intervention
- May be associated with lethal arrhythmias, similar to transmural MI
- Wall thickening may be maintained
  - Result of varied orientation of myofibrils with wall thickness
  - Loss of oblique subendocardial fibers will not necessarily cause loss of normal thickening

Treatment

- Medical therapy; thrombolysis or early mechanical reperfusion can prevent progression to transmural infarct; salvage outer myocardial layers
  - Early reperfusion may prevent infarction altogether
- Acute percutaneous intervention to restore flow
  - Best done within the first 3 hours
  - Optimally done with stent implantation and antiplatelet therapy with Gp IIb/IIIa inhibitor
- Prognosis depends on extent of infarction and degree and location of coronary disease
- Nontransmural infarcts associated with
  - Better prognosis
  - Less infarct expansion
  - Decreased risk of cardiac rupture
  - Mural thrombosis
  - LV aneurysm

DIAGNOSTIC CHECKLIST

Consider

- Location, size and transmural extent of infarct
- De-MR is the best technique to assess non-transmural subendocardial infarcts

Image Interpretation Pearls

- Main differentials are transmural MI and myocarditis
- Combination of T2WI and De-MR help with
  - Differentiation of acute and chronic infarcts
  - Determination of area at risk in acute events

SELECTED REFERENCES

1. Ibrahim T et al: Diagnostic value of contrast-enhanced magnetic resonance imaging and single-photon emission computed tomography for detection of myocardial necrosis early after acute myocardial infarction. J Am Coll Cardiol. 49(2):208-16, 2007
2. Stork A et al: Value of T2-weighted, first-pass and delayed enhancement, and cine CMR to differentiate between acute and chronic myocardial infarction. Eur Radiol. 17(3):610-7, 2007
3. Cury RC et al: Diagnostic performance of stress perfusion and delayed-enhancement MR imaging in patients with coronary artery disease. Radiology. 240(1):39-45, 2006
4. Nieman K et al: Differentiation of recent and chronic myocardial infarction by cardiac computed tomography. Am J Cardiol. 98(3):303-8, 2006
5. Ibrahim T et al: Quantitative measurement of infarct size by contrast-enhanced magnetic resonance imaging early after acute myocardial infarction: comparison with single-photon emission tomography using Tc99m-sestamibi. J Am Coll Cardiol. 45(4):544-52, 2005
6. Abdel-Aty H et al: Delayed enhancement and T2-weighted cardiovascular magnetic resonance imaging differentiate acute from chronic myocardial infarction. Circulation. 109(20):2411-6, 2004
7. Mahrholdt H et al: Cardiovascular magnetic resonance assessment of human myocarditis: a comparison to histology and molecular pathology. Circulation. 109(10):1250-8, 2004
8. Wagner A et al: Contrast-enhanced MRI and routine single photon emission computed tomography (SPECT) perfusion imaging for detection of subendocardial myocardial infarcts: an imaging study. Lancet. 361(9355):374-9, 2003
9. Choi KM et al: Transmural extent of acute myocardial infarction predicts long-term improvement in contractile function. Circulation. 104(10):1101-7, 2001
10. Weissman HF et al: Effect of extent of transmurality on infarct expansion.Clin Res. 32:477A, 1984
11. Reimer KA et al: The "wavefront phenomenon" of myocardial ischemic cell death. II. Transmural progression of necrosis within the framework of ischemic bed size (myocardium at risk) and collateral flow. Lab Invest. 40(6):633-44, 1979

NON-TRANSMURAL MYOCARDIAL INFARCTION

IMAGE GALLERY

Typical

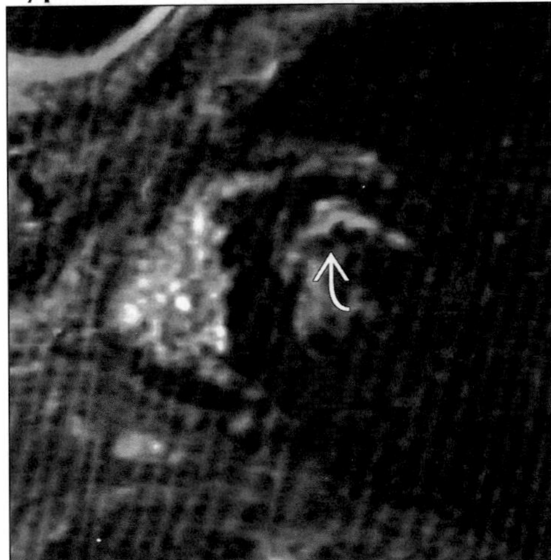

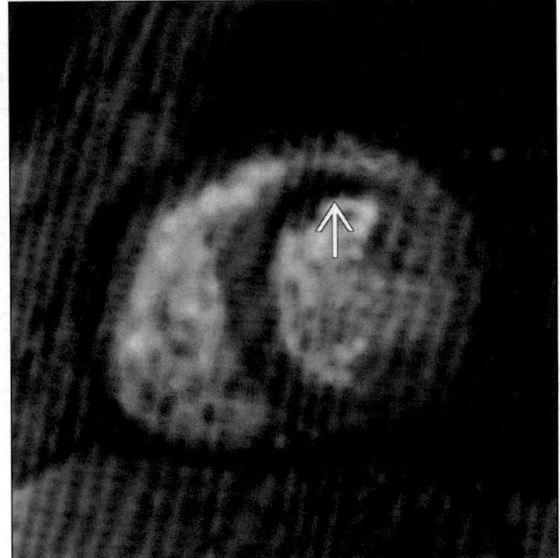

(Left) *Short axis delayed enhancement MR shows hyperenhancement ➔ in the subendocardial aspect of the anterior and antero-septal walls.* ***(Right)*** *Short axis First-pass perfusion MR shows subendocardial hypoperfusion in the anterior and antero-septal walls ➔.*

Typical

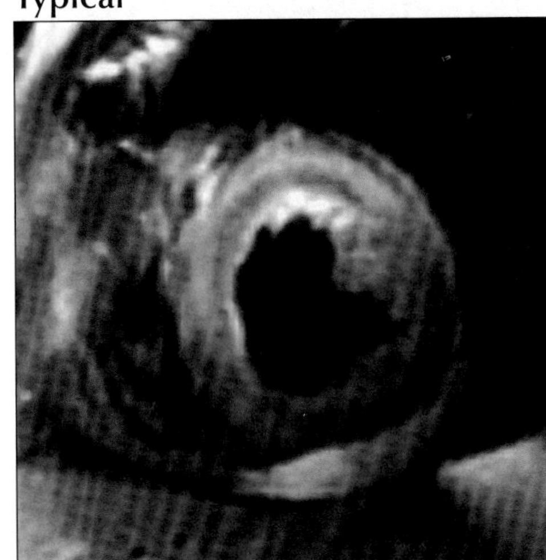

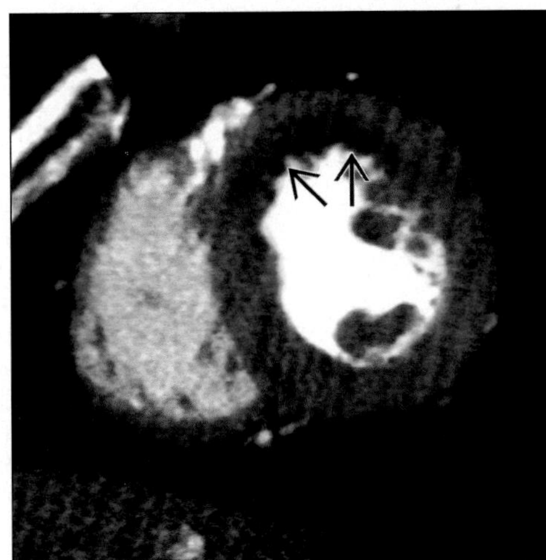

(Left) *Short axis T2WI FS MR shows increased signal in the anterior and antero-septal walls representing myocardial edema and potential area at risk.* ***(Right)*** *Short axis cardiac CT shows subendocardial hypoperfusion ➔ in the anterior and antero-septal walls.*

Typical

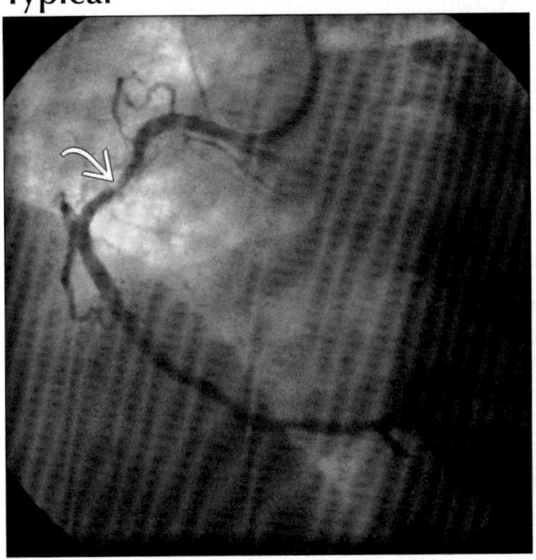

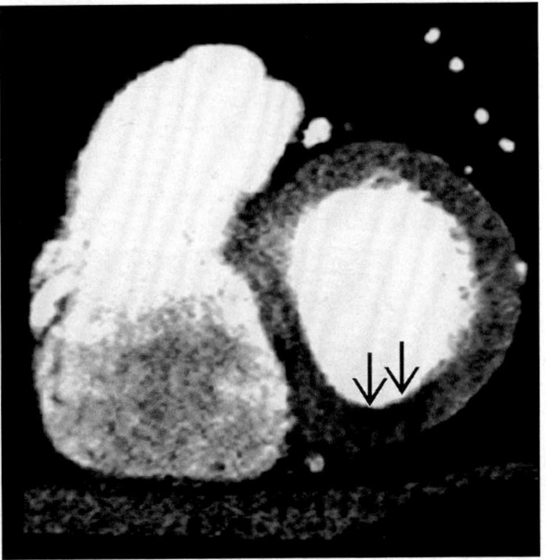

(Left) *LAO view of invasive cardiac catheterization shows high grade stenosis in the mid RCA ➔ in a patient with non-ST elevation MI.* ***(Right)*** *Short axis cardiac CT in the same patient as previous image, shows hypoperfusion ➔ of the inferior wall.*

POST INFARCTION LV ANEURYSM

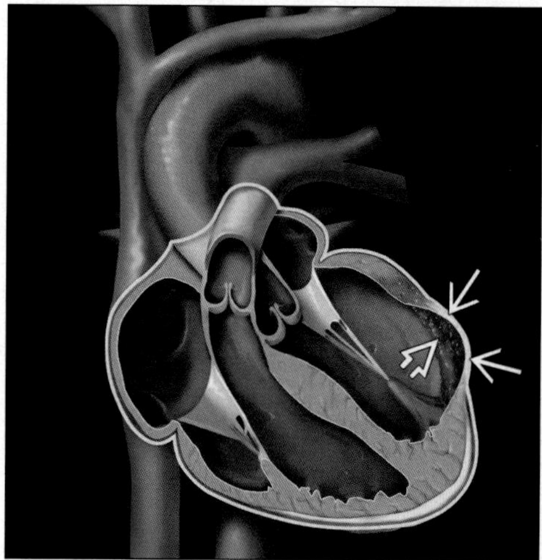

Graphic shows mid to apical anterolateral wall aneurysm ➡. Note thinning and fibrosis of the myocardium and outward bulge. Mural thrombus ➡ is layered against the aneurysm wall.

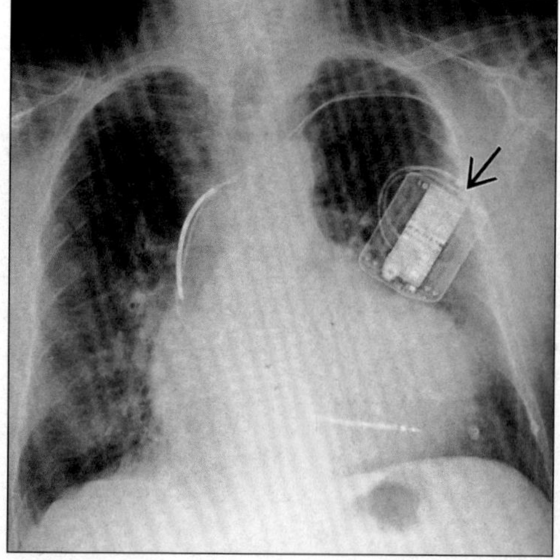

Posteroanterior radiograph shows cardiomegaly with an increased cardio-thoracic ratio in a patient s/p large anterior myocardial infarction and anteroapical aneurysm. Note implanted ICD ➡.

TERMINOLOGY

Definitions

- Akinetic or dyskinetic segment of well-demarcated thin, scarred, and fibrotic myocardium resulting from a healed transmural myocardial infarction (MI)

IMAGING FINDINGS

General Features

- Location
  - Anterior or apical aneurysms most common secondary to LAD territory infarctions
  - Inferior-basal or inferolateral true aneurysm are much less likely
    - Pseudoaneurysm are more common in these locations

Radiographic Findings

- Radiography
  - Enlarged cardiac silhouette
  - Occasionally can identify aneurysm as demarcated outpouching
  - Linear calcifications confined to LV
    - If linear calcification extend beyond LV → pericardial calcification/constriction

CT Findings

- NECT
  - Aneurysmal remodeling of LV and linear calcifications of infarcted myocardial wall (only in chronic MI)
    - Mural thrombus may calcify
  - Enlarged cardiac silhouette
- CECT
  - Thinned and scarred myocardium easily detected
  - Frequently accompanied with LV apical filling defect consistent with mural thrombus
- CTA
  - ECG gated arterial phase protocol
    - Significant coronary artery disease (> 70% stenosis) in vessel supplying aneurysmal segment
  - ECG gated multiphase (cine) reconstruction
    - Akinesis or dyskinesis apparent

MR Findings

- SSFP White Blood Cine

DDx: Post Infarction LV Aneurysm

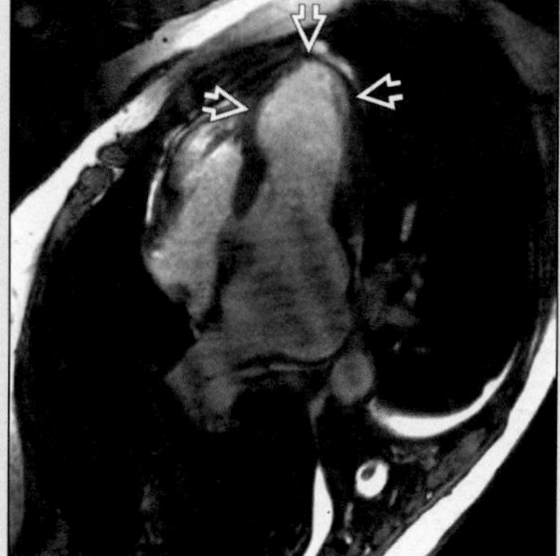

Takotsubo Cardiomyopathy

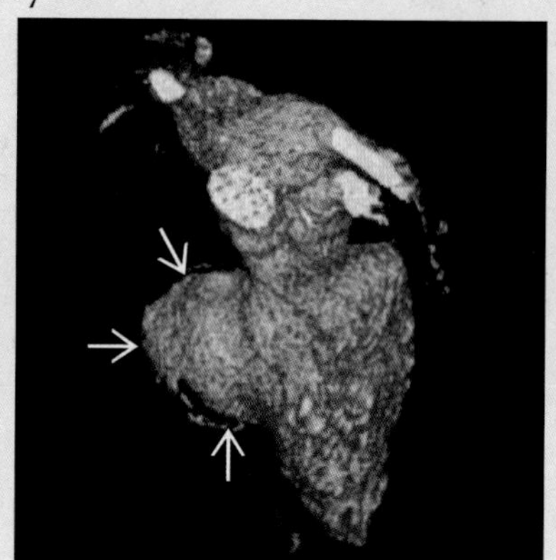

LV Pseudoaneurysm

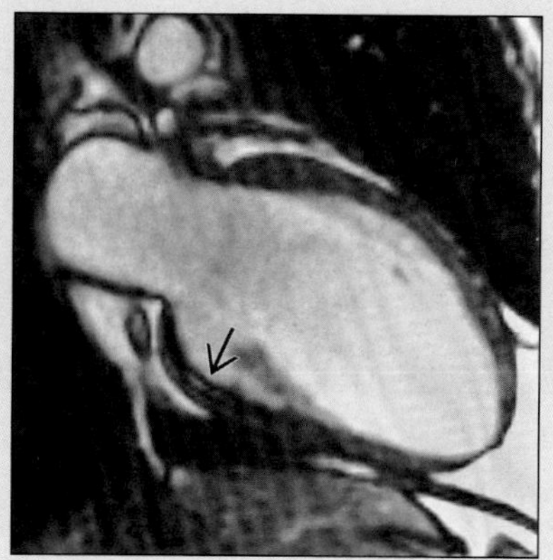

Inferior MI without Aneurysm

POST INFARCTION LV ANEURYSM

Key Facts

Terminology
- Akinetic or dyskinetic segment of well-demarcated thin, scarred, and fibrotic myocardium resulting from a healed transmural MI

Imaging Findings
- More common with left anterior descending (LAD) disease
- Aneurysmal segment will present as a transmural area of delayed hyperenhancement secondary to the scar/fibrosis
- Basal inferior or inferoposterior aneurysm are much less likely
- MR, echo and CT are excellent methods to identify aneurysm

Pathology
- Incidence is approximately 8-15% in patients who present with ST elevation MI
- Greater than 50% filled with organized clot

Clinical Issues
- Can lead to intractable heart failure
- Risk of systemic emboli and stroke
- Indicates poor prognosis: Mortality 6x higher than in patients without aneurysms
- History of MI is always present
- Frequently asymptomatic

Diagnostic Checklist
- LV aneurysms in all patients with transmural MI and LV dilation and systolic dysfunction

- LV aneurysm with wall thinning and associated wall motion abnormality
- Accurately quantifies LV volumes, mass, and wall thickness

- Delayed Enhancement
  - Transmural delayed hyperenhancement of aneurysm wall secondary to scar/fibrosis
    - Such segments are not viable and will not recover function if revascularized
  - May demonstrate underlying thrombus (nonenhanced area)
- First pass perfusion
  - Aneurysm wall will have a perfusion defect secondary to coronary artery occlusion
  - Thrombus can be detected as nonenhancing mural mass

Nuclear Medicine Findings
- Radionuclide scintigraphy findings
  - Fixed perfusion defect in the area affected
  - Detects wall motion abnormalities

Echocardiographic Findings
- Echocardiogram
  - Excellent method to identify aneurysm
  - Clear demonstration of akinesis or dyskinesis
  - Can demonstrate thrombus in the aneurysm
    - May require administration of LV contrast agents to increase sensitivity for detection of thrombus (filling defects)
  - Spontaneous echo contrast ("smoke") within the aneurysm suggests slow flow and increased likelihood for thrombus formation

Angiographic Findings
- Coronary angiogram
  - Coronary occlusion in vessel supplying infarcted territory and aneurysm
  - Typically absent collaterals
- Left ventriculogram
  - Detects wall motion abnormality in the aneurysmal segment
  - May detect apical filling defects
    - Can miss laminar mural thrombus

DIFFERENTIAL DIAGNOSIS

Pseudoaneurysm
- Narrow neck
- Typically basal inferior or lateral LV segments

Acute or Subendocardial MI
- Akinesis or hypokinesis without aneurysm

Takotsubo Cardiomyopathy
- Hallmarks are absence of coronary artery disease and recovery of wall-motion

PATHOLOGY

General Features
- General path comments
  - Transmural infarct
    - 70-85% located in the anterior and apical walls due to LAD occlusion and lack of collaterals
    - 10-15% involve the inferior-basal walls due to RCA occlusion
    - Lateral wall aneurysms are extremely rare
    - Uncommon in the setting of multivessel CAD with concomitant extensive collaterals
  - Size can vary but generally between 1-8 cm in diameter
- Epidemiology
  - Incidence is approximately 8-15% in patients who present with ST elevation MI
    - Recent improvements in revascularizations and post-MI medical therapy have minimized the development of LV aneurysms

Gross Pathologic & Surgical Features
- Frequently with evidence of pericarditis with dense, adherent pericardium

POST INFARCTION LV ANEURYSM

Microscopic Features

- Early phase demonstrates myocardial necrosis with inflammation
- Gradual replacement with scar tissue (fibrosis)
- Endocardial surface is smooth and nontrabeculated
- Border zone between the aneurysm and normal myocardium has patchy fibrosis and abnormal myocardial fiber arrangement
  - Potential for arrhythmogenic substrate
- Greater than 50% filled with organized clot
- Chronic aneurysm may demonstrate calcification

CLINICAL ISSUES

Presentation

- Most common signs/symptoms
  - History of MI is always present
  - Persistent ST elevation after myocardial infarction (MI); may be more representative of large infarct
  - Frequently asymptomatic
- Other signs/symptoms
  - Cardiac enlargement with diffuse dyskinetic apical impulse
  - Extra heart sounds (S3 and S4) from blood flow into a dilated, stiffened cavity
  - Often accompanied with ischemic mitral regurgitation due to altered ventricular geometry
- Clinical Profile
  - Heart failure and angina
    - Systolic bulging of the aneurysm "steals" part of the LV stroke volume
    - Leads to a reduction in cardiac output which further triggers adverse remodeling
    - Long term consequence is further LV dilation and increased filling pressures
  - Ventricular arrhythmias
    - Two mechanisms which drive ventricular arrhythmias and sudden cardiac death in patients with LV aneurysms
    - (1): Further myocardial ischemia leading to ventricular tachycardia or fibrillation
    - (2): Reentrant tachycardias from the "border zone"
  - Systemic embolization
    - > 50% patients have mural thrombus at the time of autopsy or surgery
  - Ventricular rupture
    - Mature LV aneurysms rarely rupture due to its dense fibrosis

Natural History & Prognosis

- Due to recent advances in revascularization the natural history of LV aneurysms is unclear
- Older literature suggests five year survival rates in patients with LV aneurysms to be 71%
- This is likely improved upon with modern day treatment of ST elevation MI
- Presence of aneurysm indicated poor prognosis
  - 6x higher mortality than in post infarction patients without aneurysms

Treatment

- Medical therapy
  - Afterload reduction with ACE-inhibitors can improve LV remodeling post-MI, limit infarct expansion, and lower blood pressure
  - Anti-ischemic medications
    - Beta blockers to control heart rate and lower blood pressure
  - Anticoagulation with warfarin
    - Empirically after a large anterior MI with significant LV dysfunction to reduce the likelihood of apical thrombus
    - If documented clot in aneurysm (echo, CT, or MR)
- Surgical therapy
  - Aneurysmectomy
    - ACC/AHA class IIa recommendation in patients with LV aneurysm with intractable ventricular arrhythmias and/or heart failure despite catheter-based or medical therapy
    - Must have sufficient functional myocardium remaining to warrant risk of surgery
    - Other possible indications included refractory angina and systemic embolization in those patient who cannot take warfarin
    - Coronary revascularization (CABG) is concurrently performed in most patients
- Catheter-based therapy
  - Endocardial mapping with endocardial resection/ablation can be performed to control intractable ventricular arrhythmias in "border zones"

DIAGNOSTIC CHECKLIST

Consider

- LV aneurysms in all patients with transmural MI and LV dilation and systolic dysfunction

SELECTED REFERENCES

1. Heatlie GL et al: LV aneurysm: comprehensive assessment of morphology, structure and thrombus using cardiovascular MR. Clin Radiol. 60(6):687-92, 2005
2. Konen E et al: True versus false left ventricular aneurysm: differentiation with MR imaging--initial experience. Radiology. 236(1):65-70, 2005
3. Antman EM et al: Acute Myocardial Infarction. In: Braundwald E. Heart Disease: A Textbook of Cardiovascular Medicine. 6th ed. W.B. Saunders Company. PA, 2001
4. HA JW et al: Left ventricular aneurysm after myocardial infarction. Clin Cardiol. 21(12):917, 1998
5. Buck T et al: Tomographic three-dimensional echocardiographic determination of chamber size and systolic function in patients with left ventricular aneurysm: comparison to magnetic resonance imaging, cineventriculography, and two-dimensional echocardiography. Circulation. 96(12):4286-97, 1997
6. Nicolosi AC et al: Quantitative analysis of regional systolic function with left ventricular aneurysm. Curr Surg. 45(5):387-9, 1988
7. Meizlish JL et al: Functional left ventricular aneurysm formation after acute anterior transmural myocardial infarction. Incidence, natural history, and prognostic implications. N Engl J Med. 311(16):1001-6, 1984
8. Faxon DP et al: Prognostic significance of angiographically documented left ventricular aneurysm from the Coronary Artery Surgery Study (CASS). Am J Cardiol. 50(1):157-64, 1982

POST INFARCTION LV ANEURYSM

IMAGE GALLERY

Typical

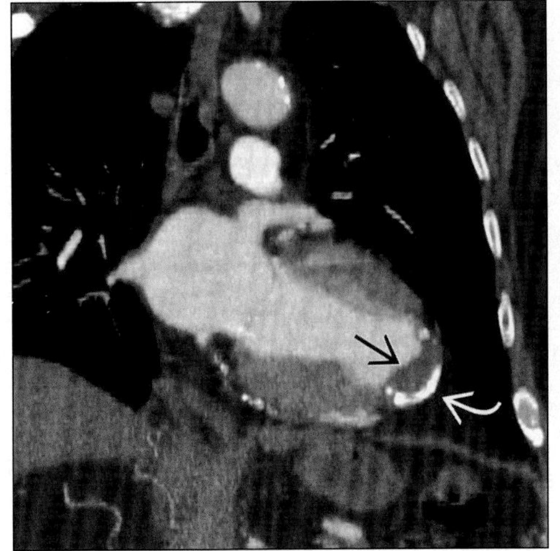

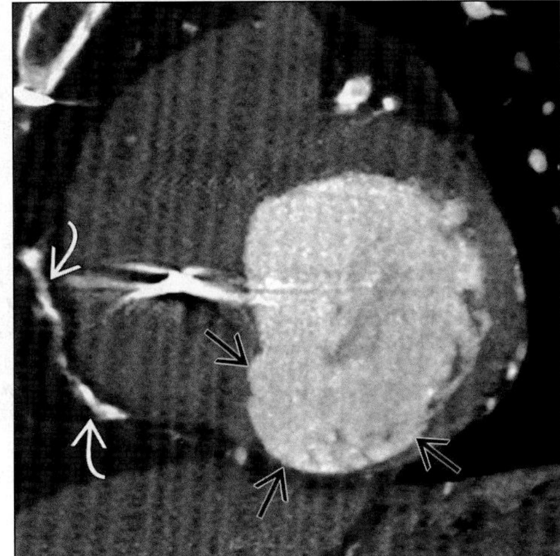

(Left) *Paraseptal two chamber cardiac CTA shows apical aneurysm and mural thrombus → (filling defect compared to the contrast-enhanced LV cavity). Note calcification ↗ of aneurysm wall.* ***(Right)*** *Short axis CTA in a different patient shows basal-mid inferoposterior aneurysm →. Note: Extensively calcified right coronary artery ↗, which was the culprit vessel.*

Typical

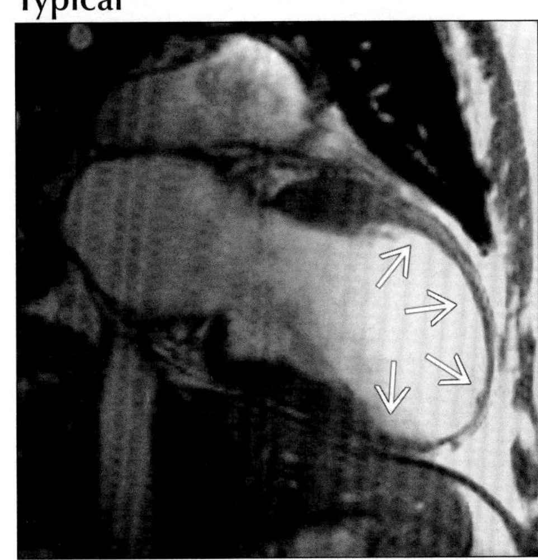

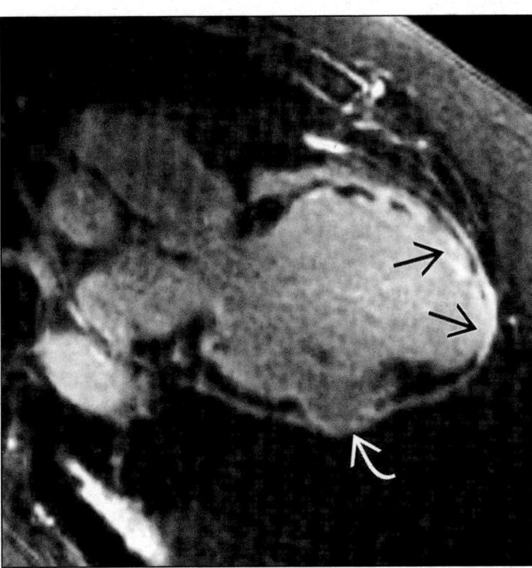

(Left) *Paraseptal two chamber SSFP shows large extensive anteroapical infarction with aneurysm. Note thinned myocardium which extends around the apex indicating large wrap around LAD ➔.* ***(Right)*** *Three chamber view DE MR in the same patient as previous image, shows transmural hyperenhancement in the anteroapex indicating lack of myocardial viability →. Note also another area of infarct ↗ laterally.*

Typical

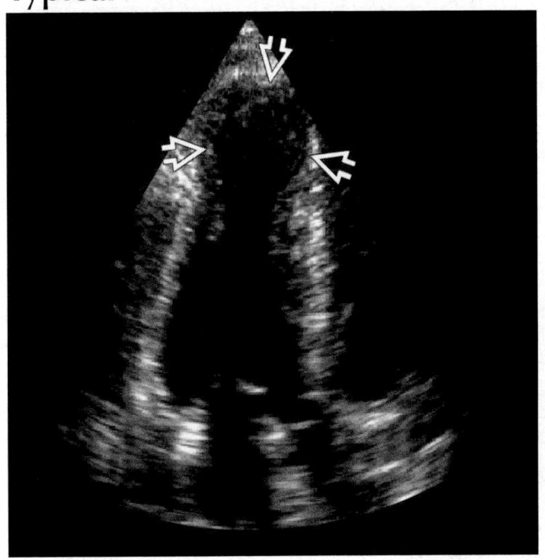

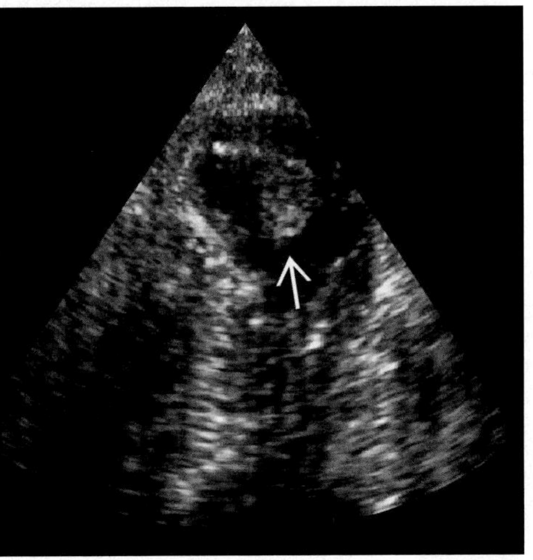

(Left) *Transthoracic echocardiogram apical three chamber view shows apical infarction with aneurysm in diastole. Note the outward bulge of the apex ➔.* ***(Right)*** *End systolic apical four chamber view in the same patient as previous image, shows echogenic material attached to the apex consistent with thrombus ➔. Apical dyskinesis was seen in cine images.*

POST INFARCTION LV PSEUDOANEURYSM

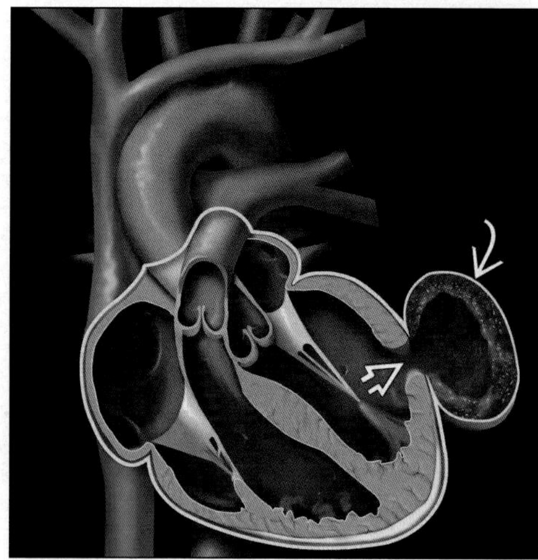

Graphic shows left ventricular pseudoaneurysm ➔ in the infero-lateral wall. Note that the neck ⇨ is substantially narrower than the pseudoaneurysm diameter.

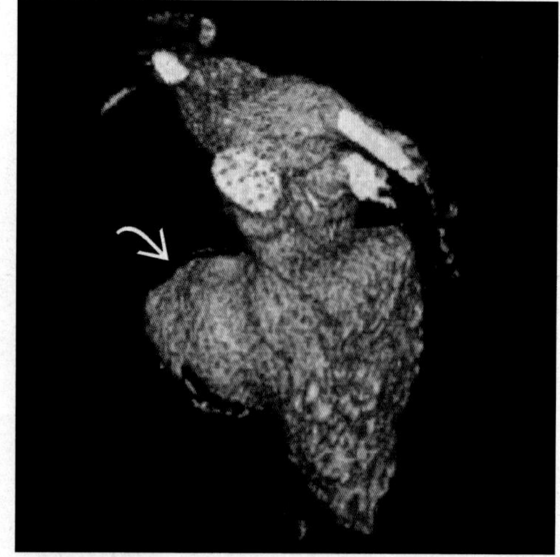

3D left ventriculogram of cardiac CT shows large pseudoaneurysm ➔ in the infero-septal wall.

TERMINOLOGY

Definitions

- Rupture contained by epicardium or scar tissue
- Unlike a true aneurysm, there is a tear of the endocardium and myocardium

IMAGING FINDINGS

CT Findings

- Cardiac Gated CTA
  - Neck narrower than aneurysm body
  - Can assess coronary arteries for stenosis/occlusion
  - Allows aneurysm measurements in any dimensions

MR Findings

- SSFP White Blood Cine: Most accurate for measuring dimensions of the pseudoaneurysm and its neck
- Delayed Enhancement
  - Delayed hyperenhancement of adjacent pericardium
  - Good technique to assess for residual thin layer of fibrotic myocardium
- First-pass perfusion
  - If performed in a long axis view of the LV can demonstrate flow of gadolinium into the pseudoaneurysm

Echocardiographic Findings

- Echocardiogram
  - Directly visualize connection between ventricular cavity and aneurysm
    - Abrupt change in ventricular wall contour
  - Similar to angiograms, echocardiogram demonstrates a narrow neck
    - Neck of pseudoaneurysm generally < 40% of maximal aneurysm diameter
    - True aneurysms are generally same size at neck and at maximal diameter
- Color Doppler
  - Hallmark Doppler finding is bidirectional flow into and out of pseudoaneurysm (to and fro murmur)
  - Since a true LV aneurysm is part of left ventricle there is no characteristic Doppler finding

Angiographic Findings

- Conventional
  - Left ventriculogram reveals a narrow orifice leading to a saccular aneurysm

DDx: LV Pseudoaneurysm

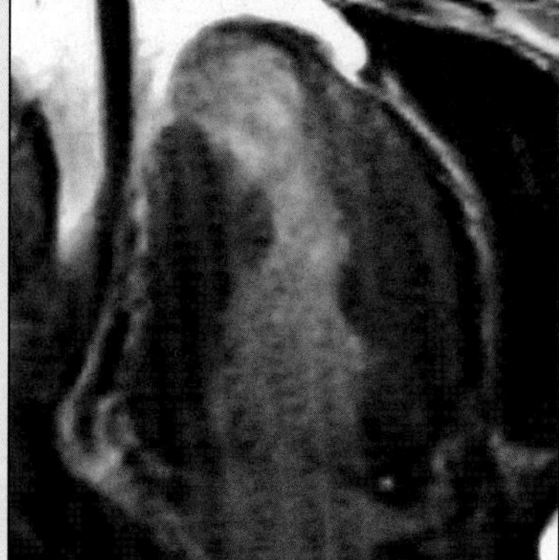

True Aneurysm with Thrombus

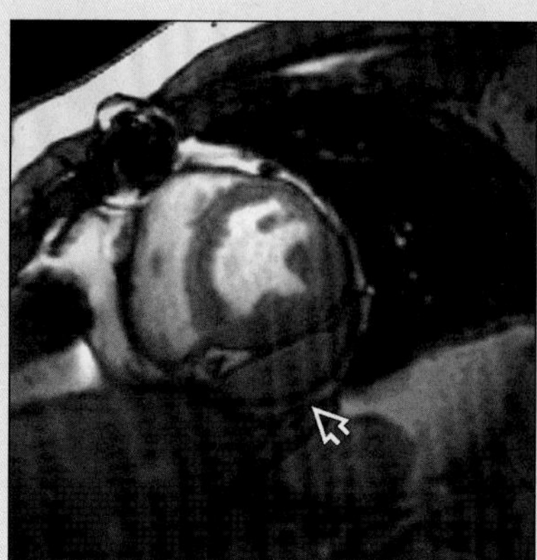

Hemopericardium

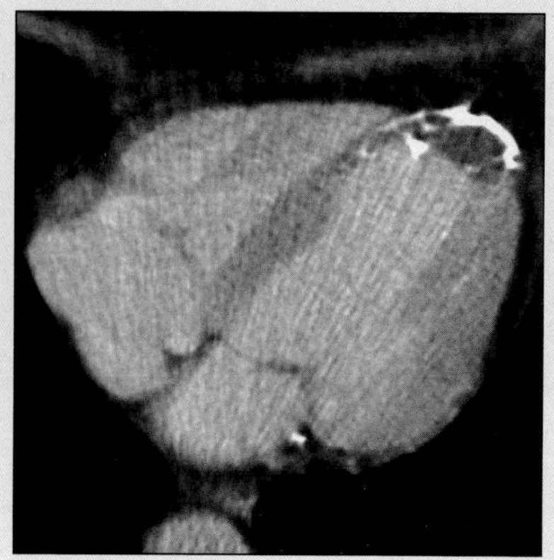

Apical Aneurysm with Thrombus

POST INFARCTION LV PSEUDOANEURYSM

Key Facts

Terminology
- Cardiac rupture contained by adherent pericardium or scar tissue

Imaging Findings
- Left ventriculogram or Cine images reveal a narrow orifice leading to a saccular aneurysm
- Cardiac MR cine imaging and CTA are the best technique to visualize the narrow aneurysm neck
- Delayed enhancement to assess if there is a residual thin layer of fibrotic infarcted myocardium
- Hallmark echocardiography Doppler finding is bidirectional flow into and out of the pseudoaneurysm

Clinical Issues
- To and fro murmur is often apparent
- Often accompanied by ST segment elevation on ECG
- Treatment: Prompt surgical intervention

 - Can result in a definitive diagnosis in > 85% of cases

Imaging Recommendations
- Best imaging tool: Cardiac MR
- Protocol advice: Cine, perfusion, and delayed enhancement

DIFFERENTIAL DIAGNOSIS

True Aneurysm
- All three layers of myocardium are intact and form aneurysm wall

PATHOLOGY

General Features
- Etiology
  - Most likely etiology is post myocardial infarction
    - Inferior wall infarctions lead to pseudoaneurysm twice as often as anterior infarcts
  - Cardiac surgery is the second most common cause for pseudoaneurysm
    - Most likely culprit surgeries are mitral valve replacement and aneurysmectomy
  - Trauma accounts for approximately 7% of cases

CLINICAL ISSUES

Presentation
- Most common signs/symptoms
  - Chest pain and dyspnea
  - To and fro murmur
  - Often accompanied by ST segment elevation on ECG
  - Small portion of patients remain asymptomatic
- Other signs/symptoms
  - Other complications include tamponade, heart failure, syncope, or arrhythmias
  - Much less likely (3%) is sudden cardiac death as the presenting manifestation

Natural History & Prognosis
- 30-45% of untreated pseudoaneurysms result in rupture

Treatment
- Prompt surgical intervention
  - Perioperative mortality is less than 10%

SELECTED REFERENCES

1. Komeda M et al: Surgical treatment of postinfarction false aneurysm of the left ventricle. J Thorac Cardiovasc Surg. 106(6):1189-91, 1993
2. Bolooki H: Surgical treatment of complications of acute myocardial infarction. JAMA. 263(9):1237-40, 1990
3. Dachman AH et al: Left ventricular pseudoaneurysm. Its recognition and significance. JAMA. 246(17):1951-3, 1981

IMAGE GALLERY

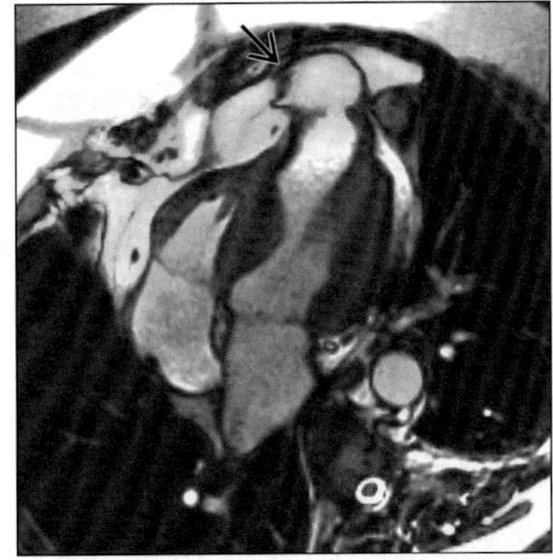

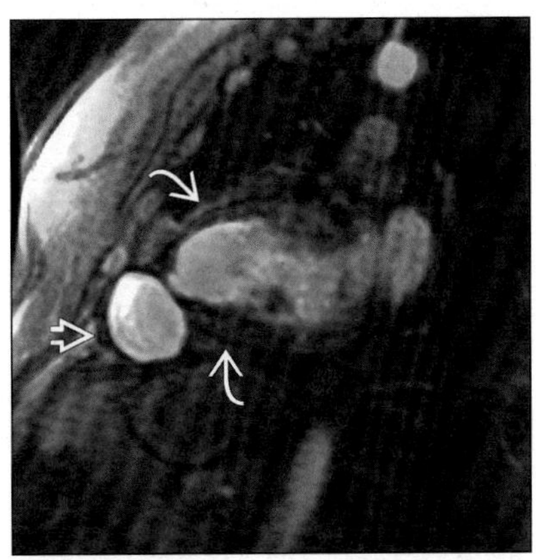

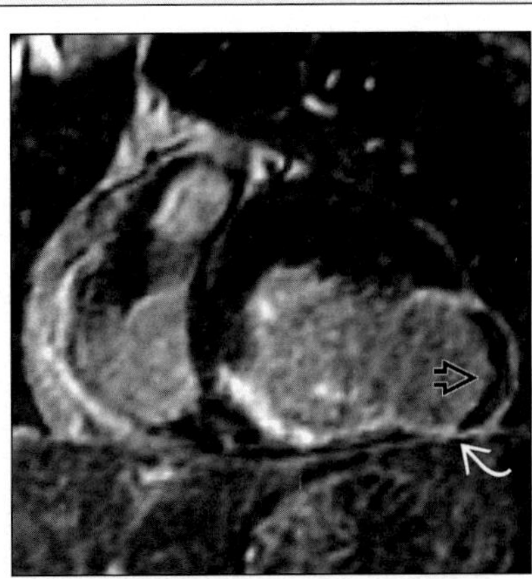

(Left) *Four chamber view MR cine shows a rare case of an LV-apical pseudoaneurysm ⇨ that is contained by the pericardium. This location rarely harbors pseudoaneurysms, but frequently is affected by true aneurysms.* ***(Center)*** *MR perfusion , two chamber view shows gadolinium filling the apical pseudoaneurysm ➡. There are also perfusion defects in the anterior and inferior ➡ apical walls.* ***(Right)*** *Short axis DE MR shows typical pseudoaneurysm in the infero-lateral wall with thin layer of delayed hyperenhancement ➡ as well as mural thrombus ⇨.*

POST INFARCTION MITRAL REGURGITATION

Cardiac MR 4-chamber image in a 52-year-old woman with chronic myocardial infarction shows a dilated LV and a dark jet of regurgitant blood through the mitral valve orifice →.

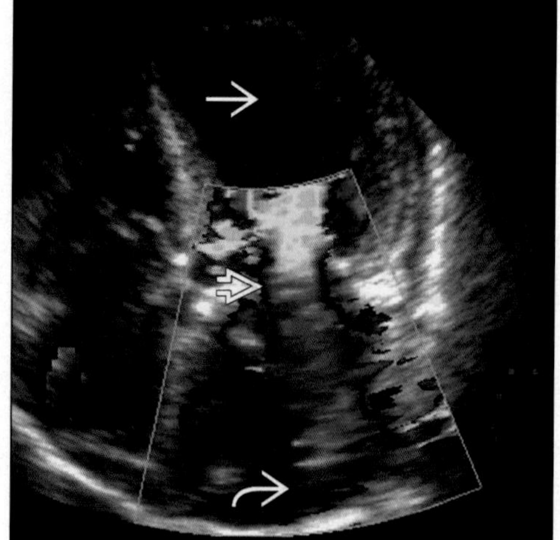

Echocardiogram 4-chamber view shows a dilated LV ➔ post infarction with severe mitral valve regurgitation ⇨ with the jet reaching the posterior wall of the dilated LA ↪.

TERMINOLOGY

Definitions

- Ischemic mitral regurgitation (IMR) is a frequent complication of myocardial infarction (MI) resulting from local and global ventricular remodeling

IMAGING FINDINGS

General Features

- Location: No definite relationship with infarct location

Imaging Recommendations

- Best imaging tool
  - Echocardiography is the clinical gold-standard
    - Echogenic papillary muscles, myocardial wall thinning and dilation
    - Chordal tethering results in leaflets being concave towards the atrium
    - Doppler (continuity equation or proximal isovelocity surface area)
    - Severe IMR is diagnosed when regurgitant volume > 30 mL, effective regurgitant orifice > 20 mm^2
  - Cardiac CT
    - Mitral regurgitant orifice area correlates well with echocardiography grading
- Cardiac MR
  - Steady-state-free-precession bright blood sequence shows mitral regurgitant jet
  - Cardiac MR delayed enhancement can demonstrate presence, location and size of infarction

DIFFERENTIAL DIAGNOSIS

Other Causes of Mitral Regurgitation

- Rheumatic heart disease
- Myxomatous degeneration, connective tissue disease
- Infective endocarditis
- Mitral valve prolapse, ruptured/elongated chordae tendinea, parachute mitral valve
- Dilated cardiomyopathy (annulus)

DDx: Post Infarction Mitral Regurgitation

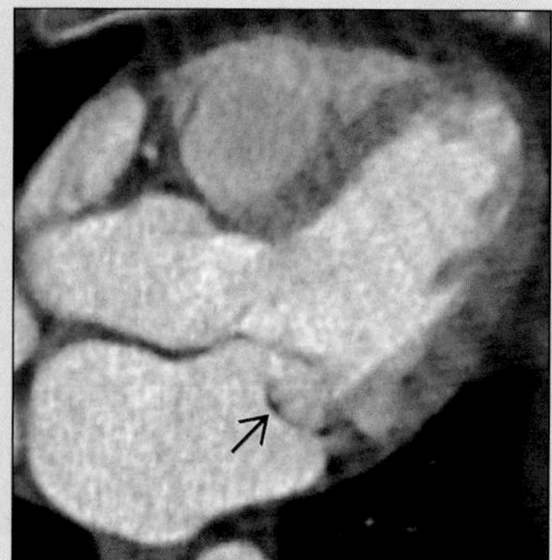

Mitral Valve Prolapse

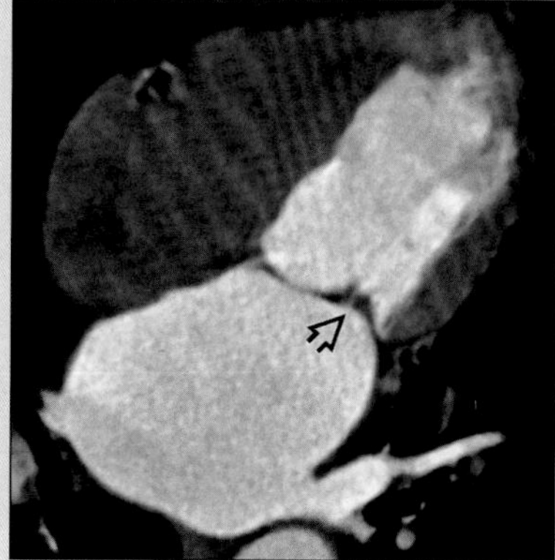

Rheumatic Heart Disease

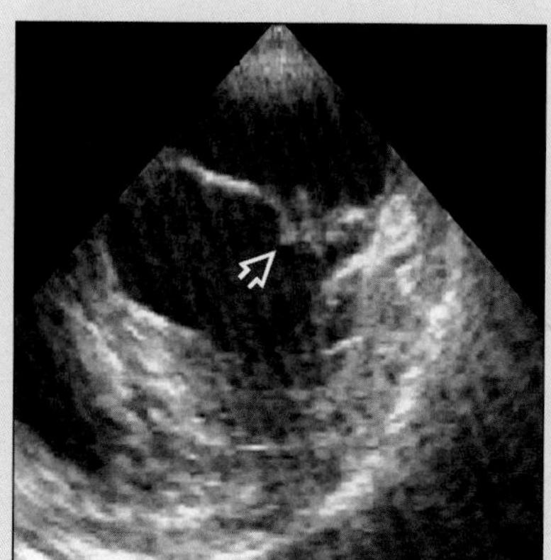

Infective Endocarditis

POST INFARCTION MITRAL REGURGITATION

Key Facts

Terminology

- Ischemic mitral regurgitation (IMR) is a frequent complication of myocardial infarction (MI) resulting from local and global ventricular remodeling

Imaging Findings

- Echocardiography is the clinical gold-standard investigation
- Cardiac MR delayed enhancement can demonstrate presence, location and size of infarction

Pathology

- Post infarction MR should be distinguished from structural valve abnormalities
- Ischemia causes papillary muscle displacement, mitral valve tethering and restriction of mitral leaflet movement resulting in malcoaptation

Clinical Issues

- MR in the setting of MI is associated with a poorer prognosis

PATHOLOGY

General Features

- Etiology
  - LV remodeling
    - Alteration in geometric relationship of annulus, valve leaflets, papillary muscles and myocardium
    - Ischemia causes papillary muscle displacement, mitral valve tethering and restriction of mitral leaflet movement resulting in malcoaptation
  - Papillary muscle rupture (usually presents abruptly with cardiogenic shock)
- Epidemiology
  - Angiographic prevalence studies: 1.6-19%
  - Echocardiographic prevalence studies: 8-74%

CLINICAL ISSUES

Presentation

- Most common signs/symptoms
  - Often asymptomatic, often underdiagnosed initially
  - Symptoms of heart failure eventually appear
    - Dyspnea, fatigue, raised jugular venous pulse, displaced apex beat, right ventricular heave

Demographics

- Age: Characteristically older, diabetes, hypertension

Natural History & Prognosis

- Post infarcted LV is less compliant and less able to increase contractility in response to the increased preload as a result of the MR
- Results in an increase in left atrium and ventricle, resultant pulmonary hypertension, and congestive heart failure
- Mitral regurgitation in the setting of MI is associated with a poorer prognosis
  - Regurgitant volume > 30 mL/beat; 5 year survival of 61%

Treatment

- Medical
  - Optimize blood pressure control, beta-blockers
- Resynchronization therapy
  - Improves LV function, reduces MR in certain patients
- Surgery
  - Consider in patients referred for coronary bypass surgery
  - Papillary muscle rupture
  - Annuloplasty in those with functional MR (annular dilation)

SELECTED REFERENCES

1. Otto CM: Clinical practice. Evaluation and management of chronic mitral regurgitation. N Engl J Med. 345(10):740-6, 2001

IMAGE GALLERY

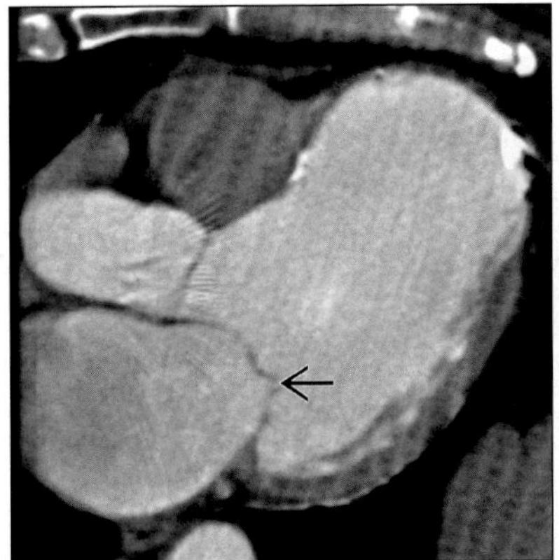

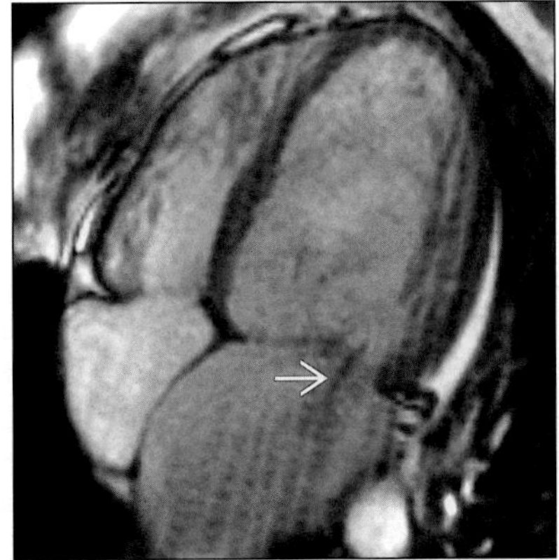

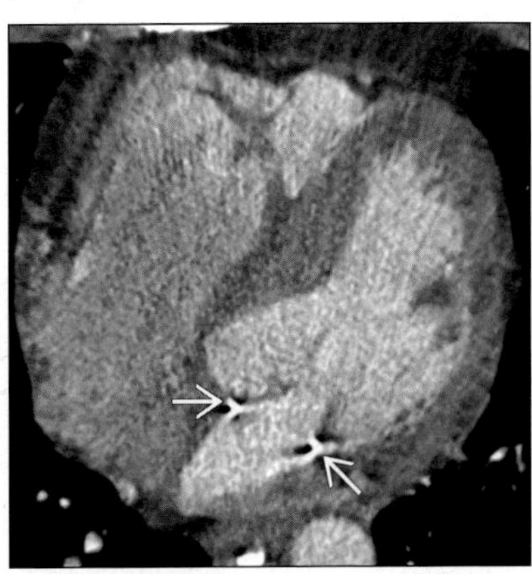

(Left) *CTA shows LV and mitral annular dilation with incomplete coaptation of mitral valve leaflets ⇨ consistent with moderate mitral regurgitation.* ***(Center)*** *Cardiac MR SSFP sequence shows LV and mitral annular dilation and a dark jet of blood ➡ passing through the mitral valve consistent with mitral regurgitation.* ***(Right)*** *CTA shows annular mitral ring ➡ in a patient post-mitral annuloplasty.*

LEFT VENTRICULAR FREE WALL RUPTURE

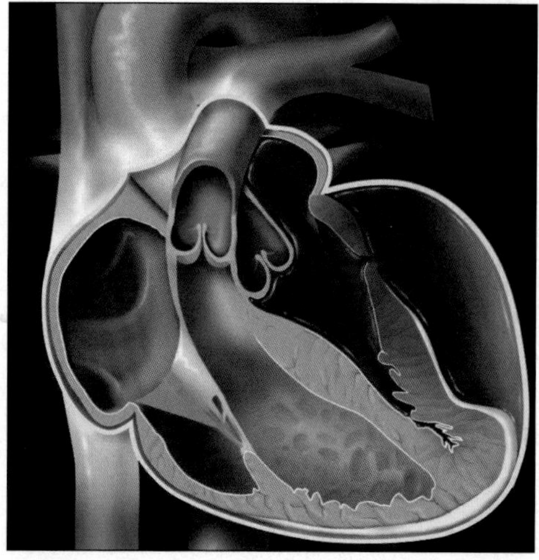

Graphic shows infarct with focal defect involving the lateral wall of the LV with adjacent pericardial hematoma with compression and deformity of the LV cavity.

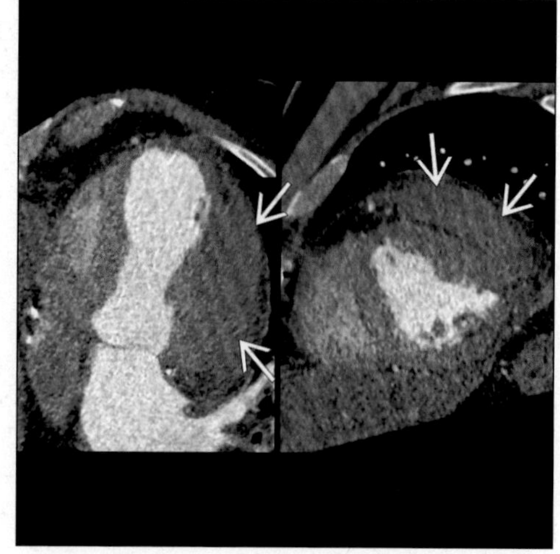

Oblique cardiac CT in a patient with circumflex thrombosis, transmural infarct and LV rupture shows large hematoma ➔ causing deformity of the left ventricle. (Courtesy W. Eicher, MD).

TERMINOLOGY

Abbreviations and Synonyms

- Left ventricular free wall rupture (LVFWR)

Definitions

- Left ventricular (LV) wall rupture with sudden hemodynamic deterioration
  - Usually seen in the setting of acute lateral wall myocardial infarction

IMAGING FINDINGS

General Features

- Best diagnostic clue: Sudden development of hemopericardium
- Location: Lateral aspect of left ventricle
- Size: Highly variable, depending on size of rupture

Radiographic Findings

- Radiography
  - Chest radiography findings
    - Flask-shaped heart, typical of pericardial effusion

MR Findings

- Complex pericardial collection
  - Heterogeneous fluid consistent with blood products of variable chronicity
- Cine images may demonstrate hypokineses or akinesis of free wall
- Delayed enhancement may demonstrate transmural hyperenhancement adjacent to hematoma

Echocardiographic Findings

- Echocardiogram
  - 2D echocardiography
    - Complex pericardial effusion
    - Tamponade physiology, diastolic right ventricle (RV) or right atrium (RA) collapse
- Color Doppler: May be able to demonstrate communication between LV and pericardium (or pseudoaneurysm), depending on size and extent of defect

Angiographic Findings

- Left ventricular angiography findings
  - Delineation of region of communication between LV and pericardial space

DDx: Left Ventricular Free Wall Rupture

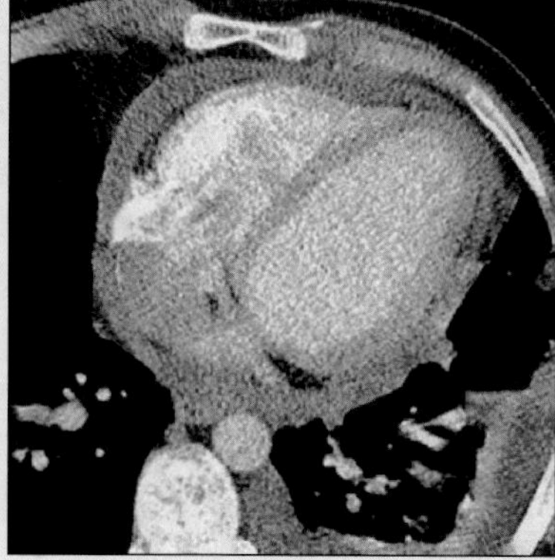

Hemopericardium

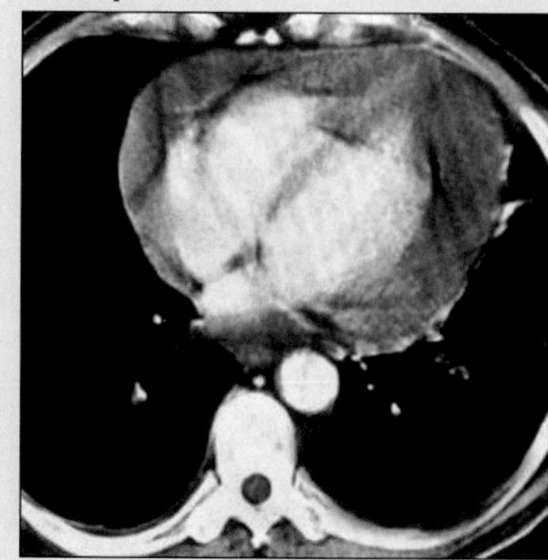

Hemopericardium

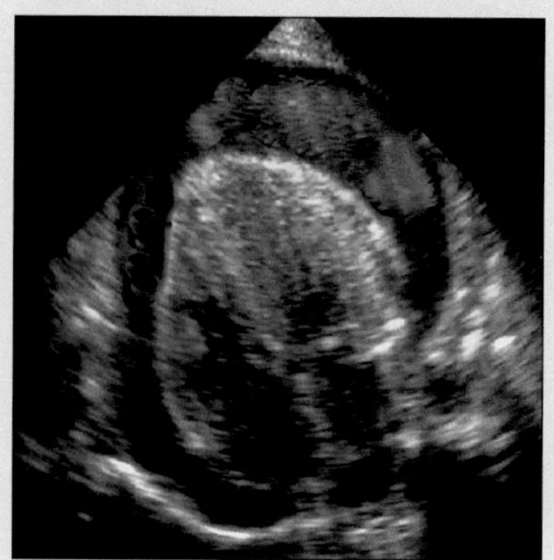

Pyogenic Pericardial Effusion

LEFT VENTRICULAR FREE WALL RUPTURE

Key Facts

Terminology

- Left ventricular (LV) wall rupture with sudden hemodynamic deterioration

Imaging Findings

- Best diagnostic clue: Sudden development of hemopericardium
- Delayed enhancement may demonstrate transmural hyperenhancement adjacent to hematoma

Top Differential Diagnoses

- Hemopericardium
- Exudative Pericardial Effusion

Clinical Issues

- Most common signs/symptoms: Tamponade physiology
- Early recognition is critical: Emergent surgical repair; high long-term survival if surgery is successful

DIFFERENTIAL DIAGNOSIS

Hemopericardium

- Trauma, neoplasm or ascending aortic rupture

Exudative Pericardial Effusion

- Infection or uremia

PATHOLOGY

General Features

- General path comments: Acute infarction of lateral wall
- Epidemiology: 6.2% in a recent study of 1,457 patients
- Associated abnormalities: Hemopericardium

Gross Pathologic & Surgical Features

- Contained ventricular rupture with blood and/or thrombus in the pericardial space

Staging, Grading or Classification Criteria

- 3 typical variants of rupture defect
  - Slit-like: Early infarct
    - Seen within the first 12 hours
    - Associated with delayed thrombolysis (> 14 hours after infarction)
  - Erosion at the borders of the infarct; extension of infarct, intermediate in timing
  - Expansion of the infarct; large infarction, late appearing

CLINICAL ISSUES

Presentation

- Most common signs/symptoms: Tamponade physiology
- Other signs/symptoms
  - Sudden or progressive hypotension
  - Sudden electromechanical dissociation
- Clinical Profile: Occurs early (< 24 hours), and late (4-7 days) post infarction

Demographics

- Age: Generally over 60 years (median age 65-70)
- Gender: No gender predilection

Natural History & Prognosis

- High mortality in the absence of prompt treatment

Treatment

- Early recognition is critical: Emergent surgical repair; high long-term survival if surgery is successful

SELECTED REFERENCES

1. Figueras J et al: Left ventricular free wall rupture: clinical presentation and management. Heart. 83(5):499-504, 2000
2. Becker RC et al: A composite view of cardiac rupture in the United States National Registry of Myocardial Infarction. J Am Coll Cardiol. 27(6):1321-6, 1996

IMAGE GALLERY

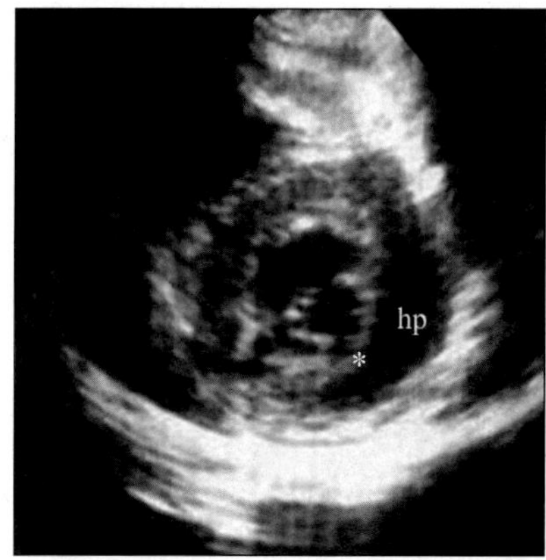

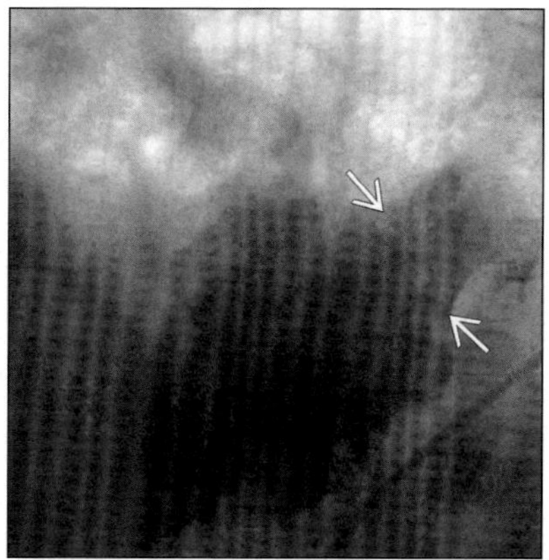

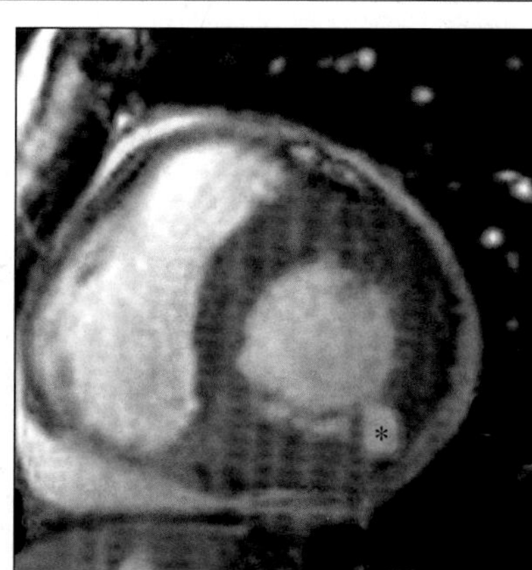

(Left) *Short axis echocardiogram shows irregularity of the LV free wall with a focal wall defect (*) and resultant hemopericardium (hp).* ***(Center)*** *Left ventriculogram shows contrast extending beyond the confines of the LV into the pericardial space →.* ***(Right)*** *Short axis SSFP MR shows near-transmural focal defect (*) within the posterior wall of the left ventricle, consistent with evolving free wall rupture.*

VENTRICULAR SEPTAL RUPTURE

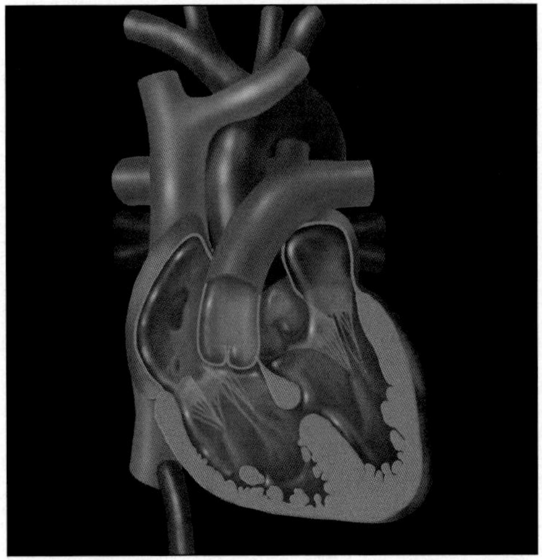

Graphic shows focal defect within the muscular portion of the ventricular septum.

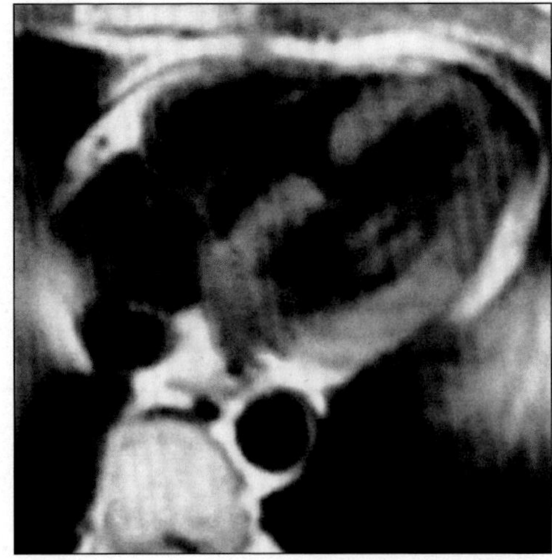

Four chamber view T1WI MR shows a focal defect within the mid-aspect of the muscular ventricular septum 6 weeks post LAD territory myocardial infarction.

TERMINOLOGY

Abbreviations and Synonyms

- Ventricular septal rupture (VSR) or acquired ventricular septal defect (VSD)

Definitions

- Abnormal communication between right and left ventricle
  - Generally following acute myocardial infarction (MI)

IMAGING FINDINGS

General Features

- Location
  - Anterior MI
    - Generally involves apical portion of septum
    - Usually simpler, discrete communication across the septum
  - Inferior MI
    - Generally involves inferoposterior septum
    - Tend to be more complex rupture with extensive hemorrhage and irregular, serpiginous tracts within areas of septal necrosis
- Size: Few mm to several cm
- Morphology
  - Defect in ventricular septum
  - Size of infarct in part determines prognosis

Radiographic Findings

- Radiography
  - Chest radiography findings
    - Right ventricular enlargement
    - Pulmonary congestion

CT Findings

- CTA: Gated study demonstrates focal defect involving the ventricular septum with areas of hypokinesis or akinesis adjacent to defect

MR Findings

- Multi-slice 2D gradient-echo
  - Excellent means of assessing dynamic 3D anatomy of defect
    - Peri-defect hypokinesis or akinesis on cine imaging

DDx: Congenital Ventricular Septal Defect

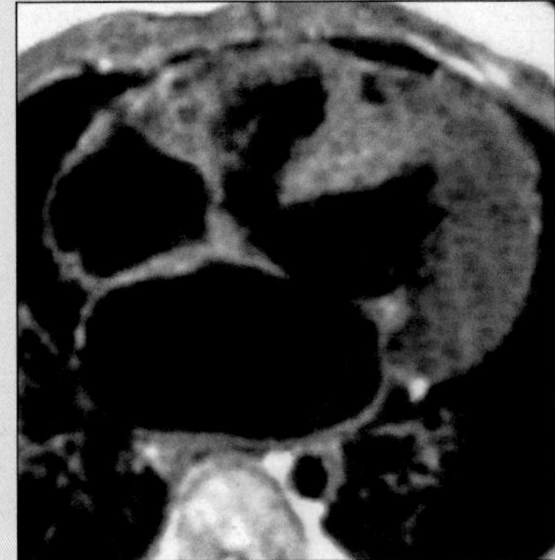

Perimembranous VSD

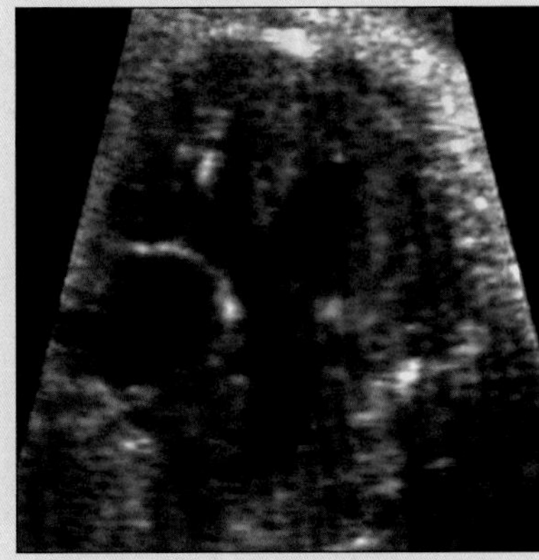

Inlet VSD Adjacent to AV Valves

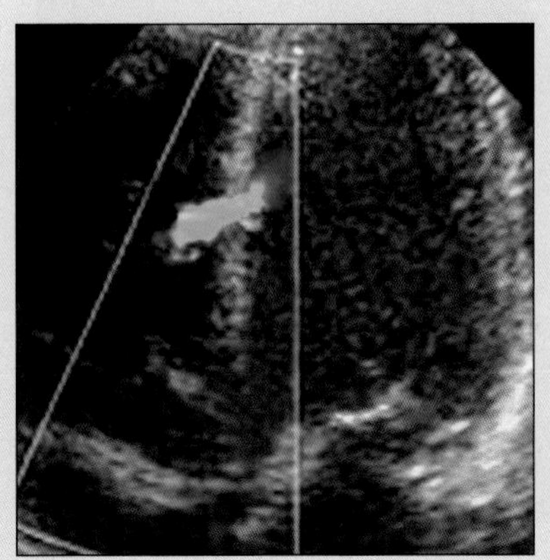

Muscular VSD with L-R Shunt

VENTRICULAR SEPTAL RUPTURE

Key Facts

Terminology
- Abnormal communication between rt & lt ventricle
  - Generally following acute myocardial infarction

Imaging Findings
- New VSD apparent on echo
- Best imaging tool: Doppler echocardiography
- Wall motion abnormalities usually correspond to infarction

Pathology
- Complication of anterior or inferior wall myocardial infarction
- Epidemiology: 1-2% incidence following acute myocardial infarction in prethrombolytic era

Clinical Issues
- Untreated symptomatic patients have a high mortality
- Requires prompt surgical treatment

  - Delayed post-gadolinium imaging often demonstrates transmural hyperenhancement surrounding septal defect

Echocardiographic Findings
- Echocardiogram
  - New VSD apparent on echo
  - Pattern of right ventricular (RV) overload
  - Wall motion abnormalities corresponding to infarction
- Color Doppler: Left to right shunt

Imaging Recommendations
- Best imaging tool: Doppler echocardiography

DIFFERENTIAL DIAGNOSIS

Congenital Ventricular Septal Defect
- Not preceded by myocardial infarct

PATHOLOGY

General Features
- General path comments
  - Necrosis of ventricular septum
    - Direct communication across septum, usually at ventricular apex for anterior infarction
- Etiology: Complication of anterior or inferior MI
- Epidemiology: 1-2% incidence following acute myocardial infarction in prethrombolytic era

CLINICAL ISSUES

Presentation
- Most common signs/symptoms
  - Recurrent chest pain after an infarction
  - Shortness of breath
  - Hypotension

Natural History & Prognosis
- Untreated symptomatic patients have a high mortality
- Higher mortality with inferior and/or right ventricular infarction when compared to an anterior infarction

Treatment
- Medical therapy to reduce afterload using intra-aortic balloon
- Requires prompt surgical treatment
  - Pericardial patch with or without infarct resection

SELECTED REFERENCES

1. Birnbaum Y et al: Ventricular septal rupture after acute myocardial infarction. N Engl J Med. 347(18):1426-32, 2002
2. Crenshaw BS et al: Risk factors, angiographic patterns, and outcomes in patients with ventricular septal defect complicating acute myocardial infarction. Circulation. 101:27-32, 2000

IMAGE GALLERY

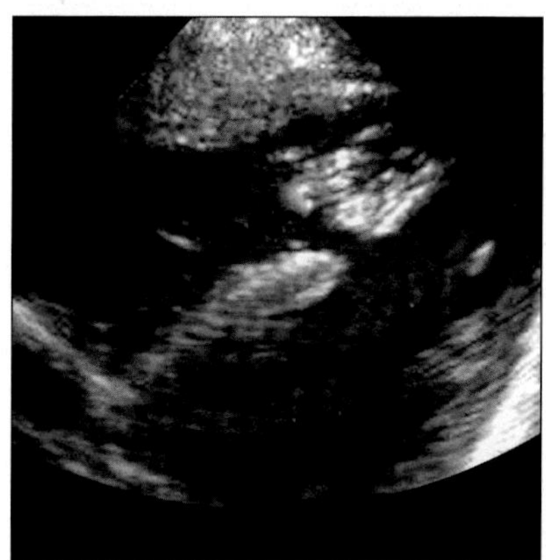

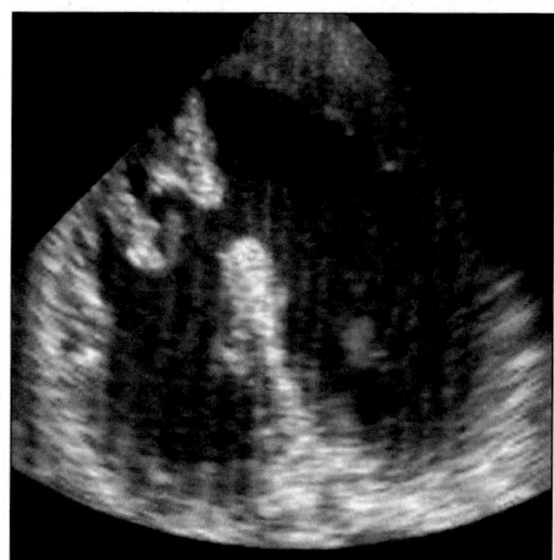

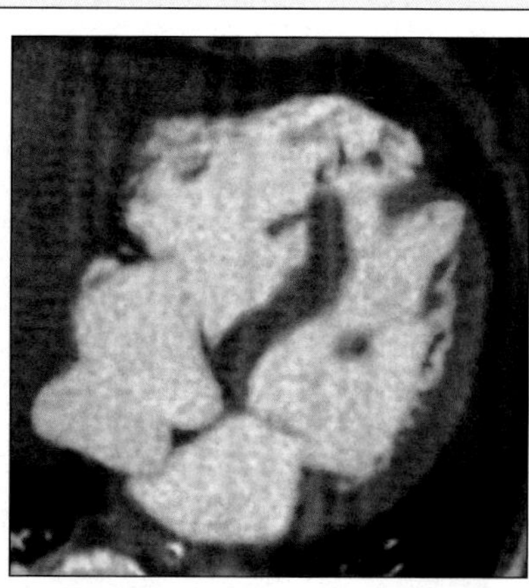

(Left) *Four chamber view echocardiogram shows focal defect within the muscular portion of the ventricular septum 2 weeks post LAD territory MI.* ***(Center)*** *Four chamber view echocardiogram shows large defect involving the apical portion of the muscular ventricular septum 3 weeks post LAD territory MI.* ***(Right)*** *Four chamber view CECT shows focal defect within the muscular portion of the ventricular septum near the apex following LAD territory MI.*

LEFT VENTRICULAR THROMBUS

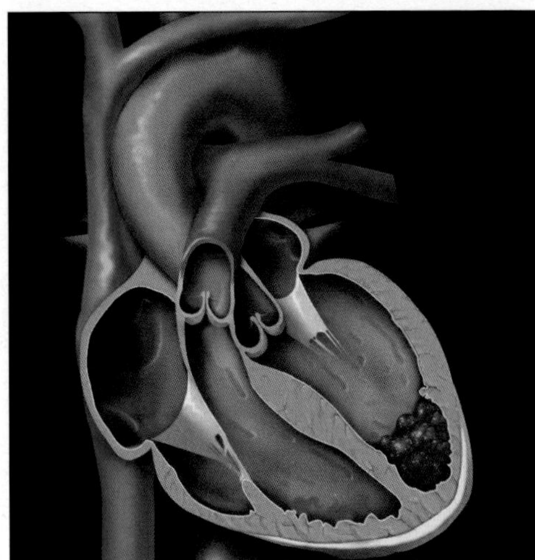

Graphic shows left ventricular apical infarct with decreased wall thickness and left ventricular thrombus.

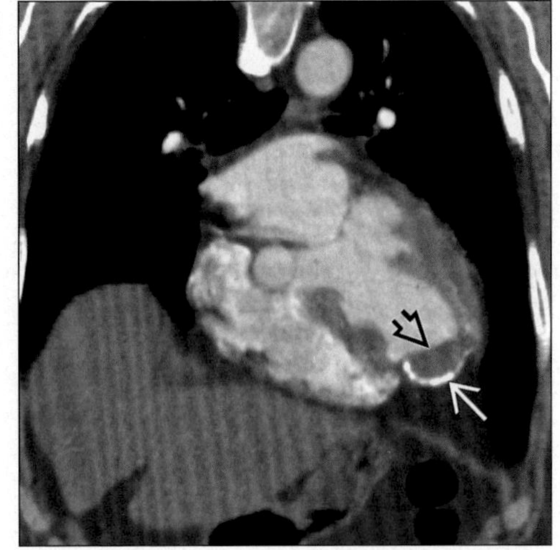

Coronal CECT shows left ventricular apical aneurysm with thin calcified wall →, and mural ventricular thrombus ⇨.

TERMINOLOGY

Abbreviations and Synonyms

- LV thrombus

IMAGING FINDINGS

General Features

- Found in the setting of reduced wall motion
  - Post MI, cardiomyopathy
- May have an irregular border
- Depending on the imaging modality, must be distinguished from the neighboring myocardium
- Size and shape of the thrombus can have prognostic significance

MR Findings

- With T2 weighted imaging can change from high intensity to low as thrombus matures
- First pass perfusion MR and delayed enhancement most sensitive for detection
- SSFP may demonstrate mobility of fresh thrombi

Echocardiographic Findings

- Echocardiogram
  - 2D echocardiography
    - 70-80% sensitivity, 90-95% specificity
    - More echodense than neighboring myocardium
    - Laminated or pedunculated, occasionally with fibrinous attachments
    - Associated wall motion abnormalities and aneurysms
    - Shaggy or mobile thrombi are more likely to embolize

Angiographic Findings

- Left ventricular angiography findings
  - Space-occupying lesion in area of reduced wall motion
  - Can demonstrate dye penetration in border zone between thrombus and myocardium

DIFFERENTIAL DIAGNOSIS

Papillary Muscles

- Move concordant with valve motion

DDx: LV Thrombus

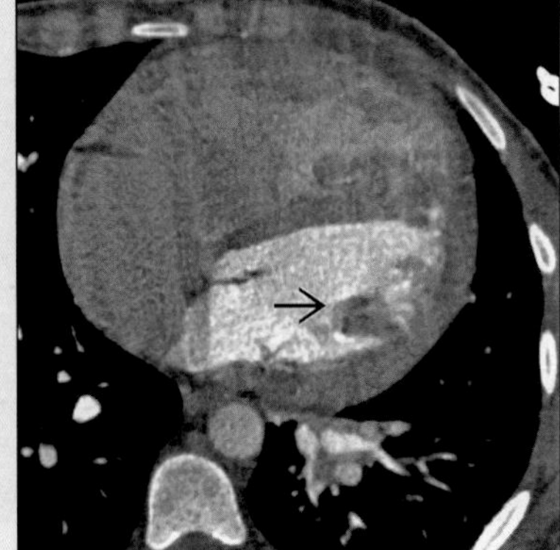

Papillary Muscle

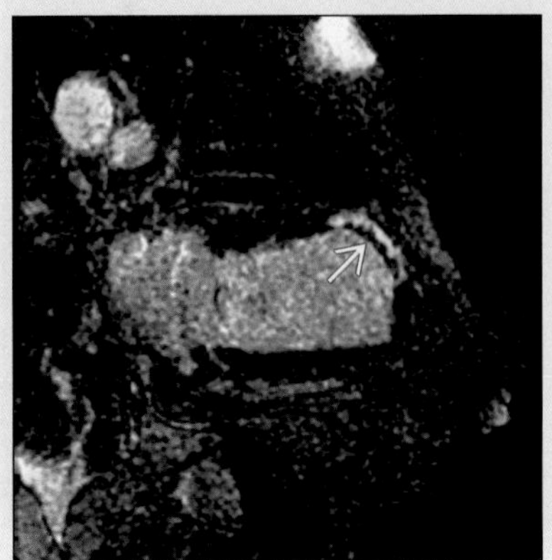

Non Reperfusion Infarct

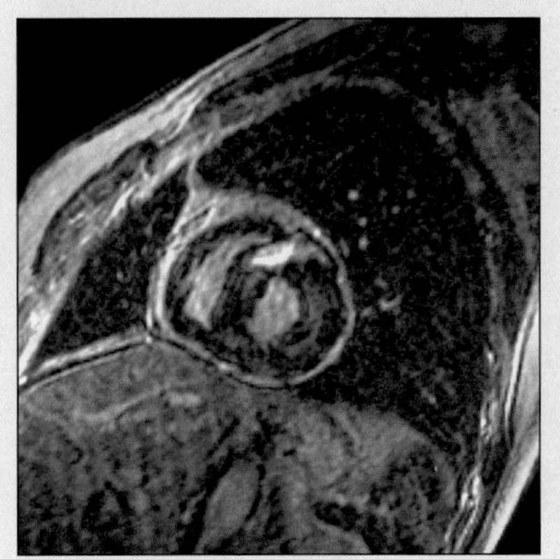

Hypertrophic Cardiomyopathy

LEFT VENTRICULAR THROMBUS

Key Facts

Imaging Findings

- Size and shape of the thrombus can have prognostic significance
- With T2 weighted imaging can change from high intensity to low as thrombus matures
- First pass perfusion MR and delayed enhancement most sensitive for detection
- SSFP may demonstrate mobility of fresh thrombi
- Shaggy or mobile thrombi are more likely to embolize

Pathology

- Associated abnormalities: MI, ventricular aneurysm, cardiomyopathy

Clinical Issues

- Frequent finding in anterior myocardial infarction (MI), and more commonly with dyskinetic segments
- Associated with blood stasis, increased coagulation, endothelial injury
- Risk for thromboembolism

Technical Artifacts

- Not persistent on multiple views
- Not associated with stasis

Cardiac Tumors

- May demonstrate enhancement

PATHOLOGY

General Features

- General path comments
  - Can be red or mixed red and white thrombus
  - Thrombus may form on surface of tumor complicating diagnosis
- Associated abnormalities: MI, ventricular aneurysm, cardiomyopathy

CLINICAL ISSUES

Presentation

- Clinical Profile
  - Recent MI or diagnosis of cardiomyopathy
  - Frequent finding in anterior myocardial infarction (MI), and more commonly with dyskinetic segments
  - Associated with blood stasis, increased coagulation, endothelial injury

Natural History & Prognosis

- Found in 30-40% with anterior MI, but < 5% with inferior MI
- 55-85% of thrombi were shown to resolve in a 3 year period without treatment
- Risk for thromboembolism

Treatment

- Warfarin anticoagulation
  - Observational studies suggest some benefit in prevention of thromboembolism
  - Current ACC/AHA recommendations do not support the use of prolonged anticoagulation in the absence of prospective studies

DIAGNOSTIC CHECKLIST

Consider

- Prescribe first pass perfusion and delayed enhanced MR in image plane that best demonstrates thrombus

SELECTED REFERENCES

1. Kontny F et al: Left ventricular thrombus formation and resolution in acute myocardial infarction. Int J Cardiol. 66(2):169-74, 1998
2. Weintraub WS et al: Decision analysis concerning the application of echocardiography to the diagnosis and treatment of mural thrombi after anterior wall acute myocardial infarction. Am J Cardiol. 64(12):708-16, 1989

IMAGE GALLERY

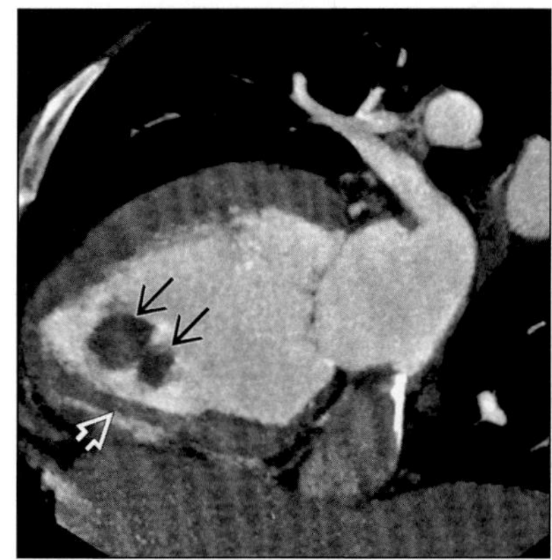

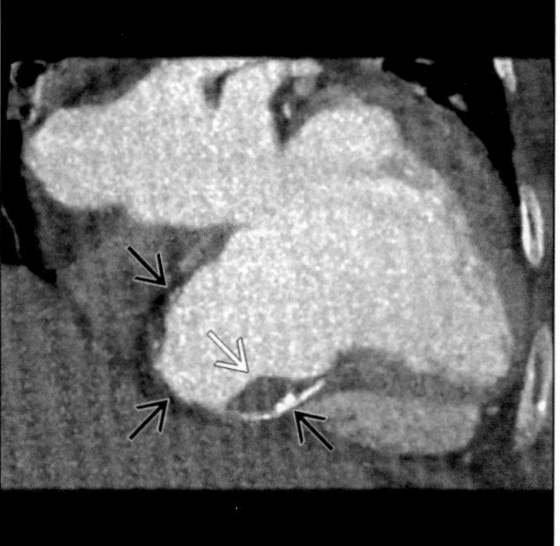

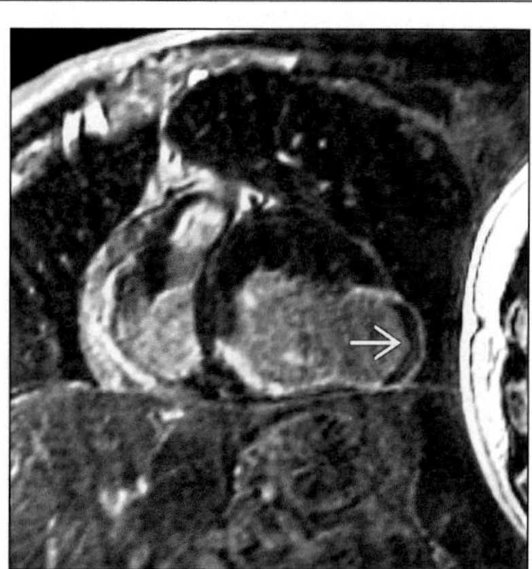

*(**Left**) Long axis coronary CTA shows two left ventricular filling defects → (mobile on function) in a patient with old inferior & acute anterior-apical infarct. Note thin inferior wall ➡. (**Center**) Long axis coronary CTA shows chronic posterior-lateral infarct resulting in aneurysm →, lined w/mural thrombus ➡. Note aneurysm wall calcification. (**Right**) LV short axis delayed enhanced MR in same patient shows extensive abnormal hyperenhancement & thinning (remote infarct) in RV, & inferior & lateral walls of LV. The aneurysm is lined with thrombus ➡.*

POST ANGIOPLASTY RESTENOSIS

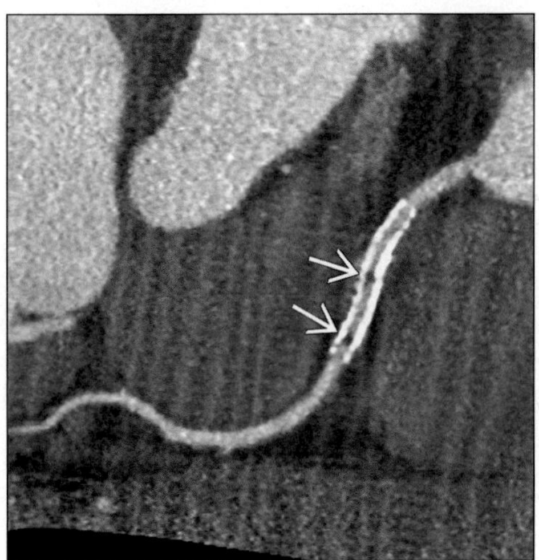

Coronary CTA in a patient who presented with recurrent angina following stenting to the RCA shows two filling defects ➔ within the stent suspicious for instent re-stenosis.

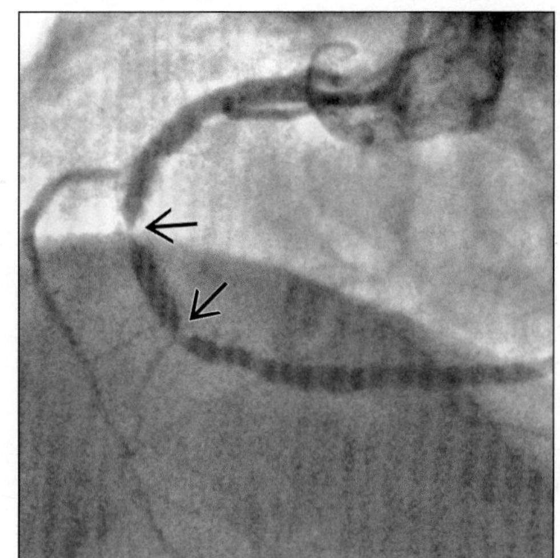

Corresponding invasive angiogram confirms two high-grade lesions ➔ within the stent confirming instent re-stenosis. (Courtesy S. Achenbach, MD).

TERMINOLOGY

Definitions

- Recurrent luminal narrowing of a coronary artery following angioplasty to alleviate a prior obstruction

IMAGING FINDINGS

General Features

- Size: Lumen diameter/area after treatment is a major predictor of restenosis
- Morphology
  - Varied characteristics of stenotic lesion
    - Concentric or eccentric
    - Smooth or rough

CT Findings

- CTA
  - Rate of assessable stents by coronary CT is low, but in evaluable stents diagnostic accuracy is high
    - Generally, about 60% of stents are evaluable with coronary CT
    - Evaluable stents: Diagnostic sensitivity 86%, specificity 98%
    - Higher for left main stents: Diagnostic sensitivity 100%, specificity 91%

Angiographic Findings

- Catheterization Findings
  - Diffuse or focal lesion development
  - May show evidence of dissection

DIFFERENTIAL DIAGNOSIS

Coronary Artery Stenosis

- New coronary stenosis on a non previously treated segment
- Incompletely stented lesion

Stent Thrombosis

- Stent occlusion

Post Angioplasty Dissection

- Intimal tear → contrast on both sides of intimal flap

DDx: Post Angioplasty Restenosis

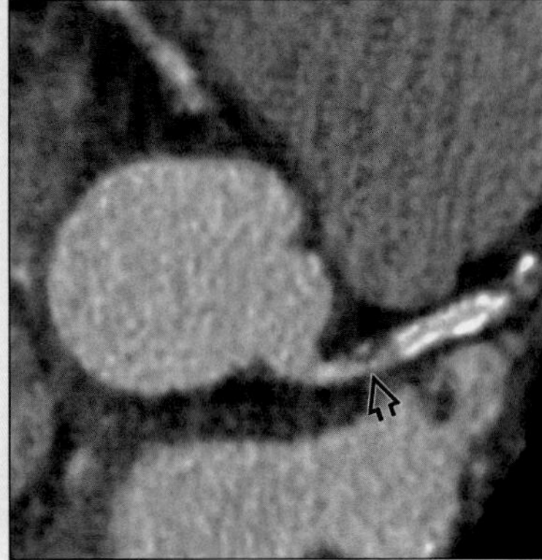

Incomplete Stenting

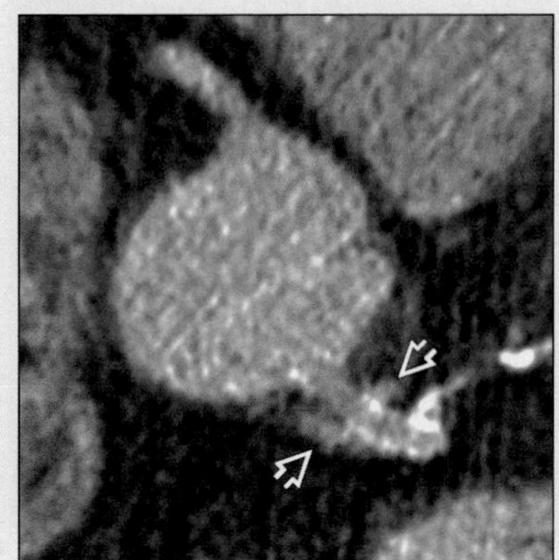

Stent Dissection

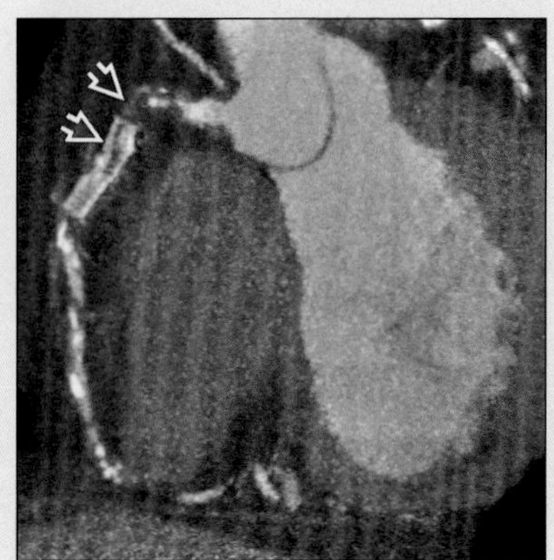

Stent Thrombosis

POST ANGIOPLASTY RESTENOSIS

Key Facts

Terminology
- Recurrent luminal narrowing of a coronary artery following angioplasty to alleviate a prior obstruction

Imaging Findings
- Rate of assessable stents by coronary CT is low, but in evaluable stents diagnostic accuracy is high
- Generally, about 60% of stents are evaluable with coronary CT

Pathology
- Post angioplasty lumen size: Prognostic indicator of clinical restenosis

Clinical Issues
- Can re-present with typical ischemic symptoms
- Greater incidence after treatment of total occlusion, small vessels, long lesions, thrombus, complicated dissections

PATHOLOGY

General Features
- General path comments
  - Elastic recoil
  - Reduction in area delimited by external and internal elastic laminae
  - Neointimal growth may play a lesser role than initially assumed
- Etiology
  - Balloon angioplasty is associated with vascular injury or dissection
  - Healing frequently results in tissue ingrowth and restenosis
- Epidemiology: Typically occurs within 6 months of the procedure

CLINICAL ISSUES

Presentation
- Most often asymptomatic restenosis
- Estimated 30-50% restenosis rate, lower with drug eluting stents
- Can re-present with typical ischemic symptoms
  - Recurrent angina
  - Acute myocardial infarction (MI)
  - Sudden onset heart failure
- Greater incidence after treatment of total occlusion, small vessels, long lesions, thrombus, complicated dissections
- Worse outcome in diabetics, heart failure, old age, smokers
- Prevention
  - Aspirin (indefinitely)
  - Gp IIb/IIIa inhibitor periprocedure
  - Careful balloon sizing
  - Avoidance of overexpansion
  - Stent placement reduced restenosis by 30-50%

Treatment
- Repeat balloon angioplasty
- Stent placement
  - Preferred treatment in vessels > 2.5 mm
- Rotational atherectomy
- Coronary bypass for severe stenoses not amenable to percutaneous treatment, or patients with multivessel disease

DIAGNOSTIC CHECKLIST

Image Interpretation Pearls
- On coronary CTA, filling defects in evaluable stents are suspicious for instent re-stenosis

SELECTED REFERENCES

1. Rixe J et al: Assessment of coronary artery stent restenosis by 64-slice multi-detector computed tomography. Eur Heart J. 27(21):2567-72, 2006
2. Bittl JA: Advances in coronary angioplasty. N Engl J Med. 335(17):1290-302, 1996

IMAGE GALLERY

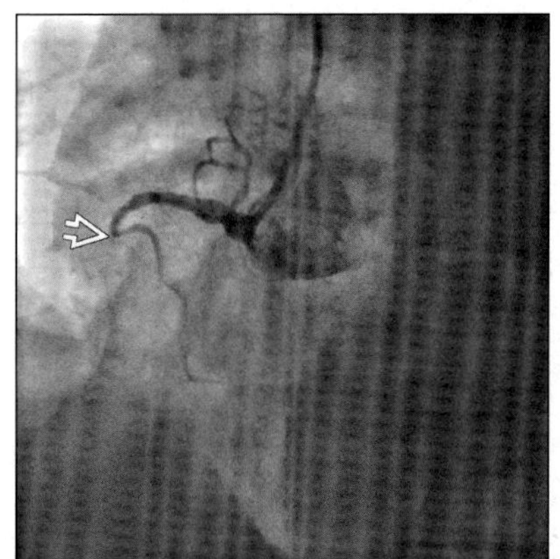

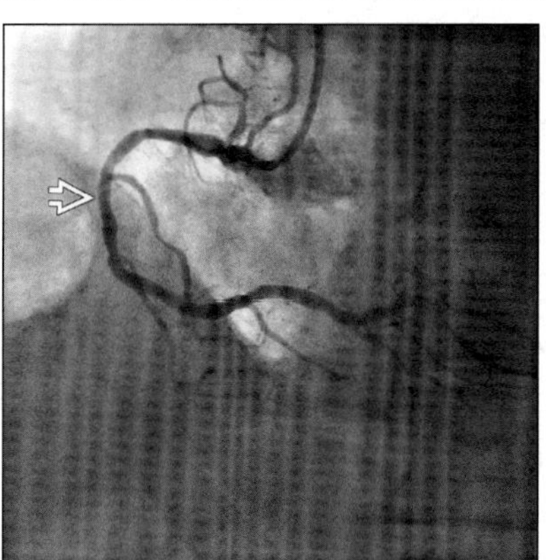

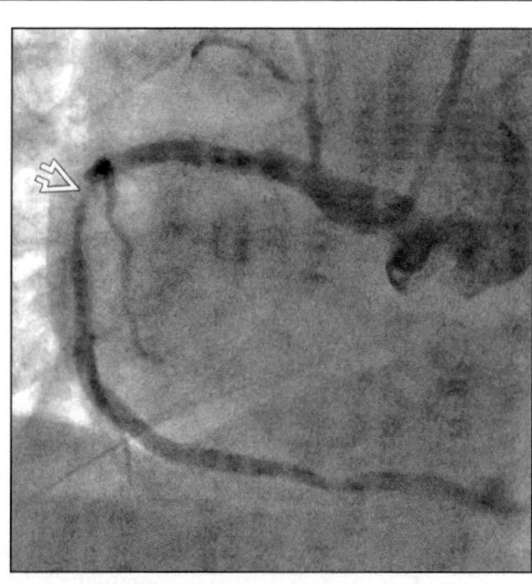

(Left) *Invasive coronary angiogram shows a total occlusion of the proximal RCA ⇨.* ***(Center)*** *The patient underwent percutaneous coronary intervention. Post angioplasty angiogram demonstrates a widely patent RCA lumen ⇨.* ***(Right)*** *Six months later the corresponding angiogram demonstrates marked luminal narrowing ⇨ consistent with post angioplasty restenosis. (Courtesy S. Achenbach, MD).*

POST-STENT RESTENOSIS

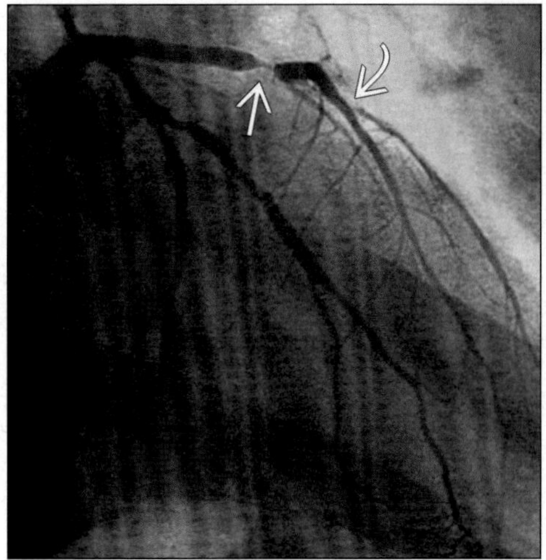

Catheter angiography shows an LAD stenosis ➔ proximal to the previously placed stent. A second stenosis is seen at the distal edge of the stent ➔.

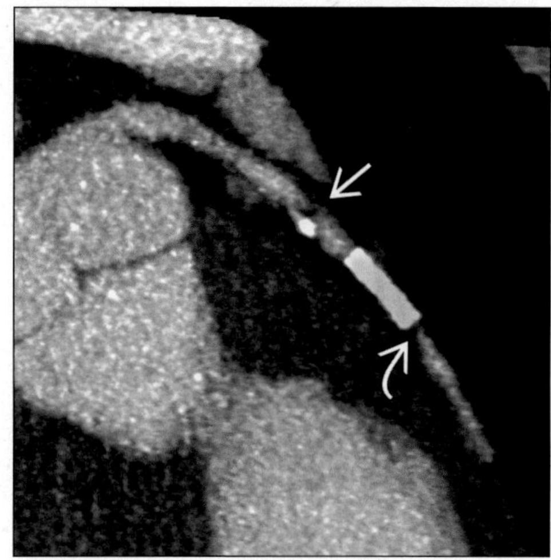

Multiplanar reformat of the LAD on cardiac CTA in the same patient shows the stenosis proximal to the stent ➔ and a second lesion at the distal stent edge ➔.

TERMINOLOGY

Abbreviations and Synonyms

- In-stent restenosis (ISR)

Definitions

- More than 50% stenosis inside or at the edges of a stent
- Target lesion or target vessel revascularization beyond 30 days, death, or MI in the target vessel territory

IMAGING FINDINGS

General Features

- Location: May appear anywhere along the stent, including the edges

CT Findings

- CTA
  - Gated cardiac CTA is an emerging tool for assessing stent patency
  - Prone to artifacts from the metal struts of the stent
    - Blooming artifact make the stent wall appear bigger which reduces the ability to assess the lumen
    - Extent of this artifact depends on the material and design of the stent
    - Beam hardening artifacts cause hypodense areas adjacent to the stent struts that can mimic in-stent restenosis
  - Post-processing techniques with sharper reconstruction filters will increase diagnostic accuracy
  - Stent size is one of the most important determinants of CT assessibility
    - Stents that are 3.0 mm or larger more likely assessable for in-stent restenosis than smaller ones
    - Since the left main is a larger caliber vessel and is protected from motion artifact, MDCT may have its biggest application in excluding restenosis after left main stenting

MR Findings

- MRA
  - Metallic stents cause susceptibility and radiofrequency artifacts on MRA

DDx: In-Stent Restenosis

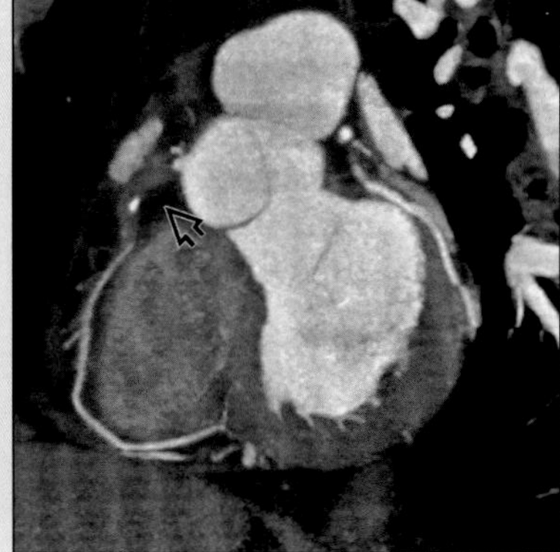

Native RCA Occlusion

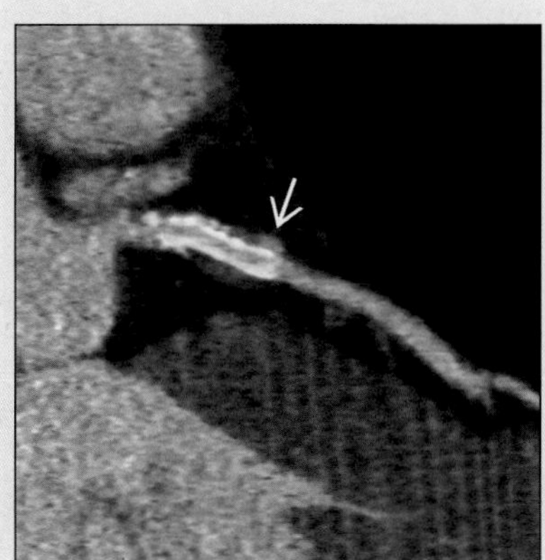

Coronary Stent Aneurysm

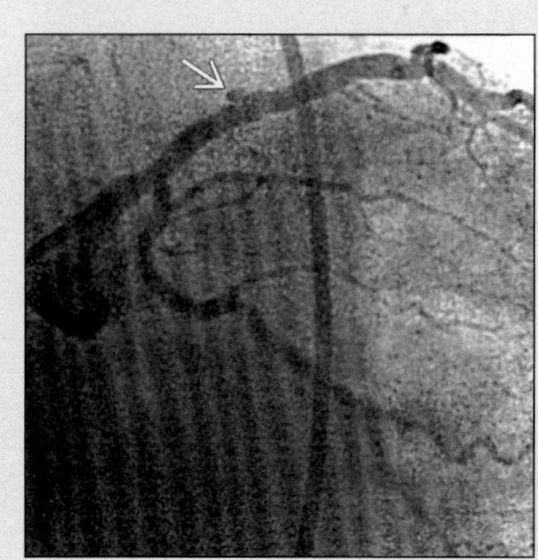

Angiogram of Same Stent Aneurysm

POST-STENT RESTENOSIS

Key Facts

Terminology

- In-stent restenosis (ISR)

Imaging Findings

- May appear anywhere along the stent, including the edges
- Metallic stents cause susceptibility and radiofrequency artifacts on MRA
- Invasive angiography: Gold standard for detecting post-stent restenosis
- Coronary CTA: Emerging tool for assessing stent patency
- Coronary CTA can assess restenosis in-stents larger than 3 mm
- IVUS: Aid in treatment post-stenting to check for adequate deployment
- IVUS: May be helpful at further characterizing the lesion and quantifying the degree of stenosis

Top Differential Diagnoses

- Coronary Artery Stenosis in a Non-Culprit Vessel
- Acute Stent Thrombosis
- Post-Stent Aneurysm

Pathology

- Neointimal proliferation from arterial damage
- Neointimal tissue peaks during first six months, after that there may be no further reduction in-stent diameter or even regression

Clinical Issues

- AMI is more likely to result for acute stent thrombosis within 30 days of the procedure
- Angiographic restenosis precedes clinical restenosis

    - Causes local signal void
  - There are emerging prototype stents of a dedicated MR alloy to minimize artifacts
    - These are still investigational in animal models

Angiographic Findings

- Conventional
  - Quantitative coronary angiography is the gold standard for detecting in-stent restenosis
  - In those stents treated with radiation, the appearance of a restenosis at the stent edges is termed "candy wrapper lesions"
  - Can distinguish acute or subacute stent thrombosis from in-stent restenosis
  - Intravascular ultrasound may be useful adjunct
    - May be helpful at further characterizing the lesion and quantifying the degree of stenosis
    - Aid in treatment post-stenting to check for adequate deployment and malapposition
  - Positive remodeling and decreased neointima proliferation are among the causes for late stent malapposition

DIFFERENTIAL DIAGNOSIS

Coronary Artery Stenosis in a Non-Culprit Vessel

- New coronary stenosis on a non previously stented segment

Acute Stent Thrombosis

- Defined as occurring within 24 hours after the intervention
- Subacute: Between 1 and 30 days after intervention
- Late: After 30 days of intervention

Post-Stent Aneurysm

- Coronary aneurysm after stent implantation is a rare complication
- Aneurysm could result from inflammation due to hypersensitivity reaction to the metal, the polymer or the drug (in drug-eluting stents)

PATHOLOGY

General Features

- General path comments
  - Neointimal proliferation from arterial damage
    - Generally a diffuse process but may be focal
  - Macrophage accumulation with cellular proliferation
    - Less of a thrombotic response than after conventional balloon angioplasty
  - Neointimal tissue peaks during the first six months after which time there may be no further reduction in-stent diameter or even regression
- Etiology
  - There are multiple predictors of in-stent restenosis
    - Longer total stent length
    - Smaller reference lumen diameter
    - Smaller final minimal lumen diameter (MLD) by angiography
    - Smaller stent lumen cross-sectional area (CSA) by IVUS
- Epidemiology
  - At one year, target lesion or target vessel revascularization is performed 12-14% of cases in the era of bare metal stents
    - Factors which influence restenosis include stent type, length, diameter, and post-deployment minimal luminal diameter
    - Small vessels, long lesions, and bifurcation lesions have much higher rates of restenosis
  - Newer drug eluting stents markedly reduce the incidence of in-stent restenosis and the rate of target vessel revascularization by approximately 75%
    - Trade off with drug eluting stents are high rates of acute stent thrombosis and longer duration of post-PCI antiplatelet therapy

Microscopic Features

- Pathophysiology of in-stent restenosis is multifactorial and comprises
  - Inflammation
  - Smooth muscle cell migration and proliferation

- Extracellular matrix formation
- All mediated by distinct molecular pathways

Staging, Grading or Classification Criteria

- Four described patterns of in-stent restenosis
  - Pattern I is a focal (< 10 mm length) lesion within the stent
  - Pattern II is a diffuse (> 10 mm length) lesion within the stent
  - Pattern III is a stenosis (> 10 mm length) extending outside the stent
  - Pattern IV is a totally occluded stent

CLINICAL ISSUES

Presentation

- Most common signs/symptoms
  - Angiographic restenosis precedes clinical symptoms
  - Recurrent angina is most likely symptom and develops within 6-12 months
    - After 1 year, recurrent angina is more likely due to progression of non-culprit lesions
- Other signs/symptoms
  - Acute myocardial infarction is unlikely to result from restenosis
  - This presentation is more likely to result from acute stent thrombosis within 30 days of the procedure
    - Mechanism is different from restenosis

Treatment

- Prevention
  - Post-PCI antiplatelet therapy with aspirin and clopidogrel
  - Periprocedural GP 2b/3a antagonists
  - Adequate stent deployment and contact with endothelium
- Repeat percutaneous coronary intervention
  - Repeat stenting now the preferred approach for treating restenosis as opposed to conventional balloon angioplasty
  - IVUS guidance helpful to evaluate the restenotic stent as well as peri-stent areas
- Intracoronary radiotherapy (or brachytherapy)
  - Adjunctive treatment with both beta and gamma radiation with restenosis of bare metal stents
  - Reduce the chance of subsequent recurrence by 40-50%
- Specialized revascularization devices
  - Rotational or directional atherectomy
  - Cutting balloon angioplasty
  - Laser angioplasty
  - No long term studies document the actual benefit of these devices
- Bypass surgery
  - For patients that are not candidates for repeat percutaneous coronary intervention and meet the established ACC/AHA guidelines for the use of CABG in patients with angina
  - Benefit of CABG is much lower rate of repeat revascularization

DIAGNOSTIC CHECKLIST

Consider

- Coronary CTA for vessels larger than 3 mm in diameter, such as the left main coronary artery
- Invasive angiography and IVUS are the reference standards for diagnosis and planning intervention

Image Interpretation Pearls

- Main artifacts caused by stent by CTA: Blooming artifact and beam hardening artifact

SELECTED REFERENCES

1. Sheth T et al: Coronary stent assessability by 64 slice multi-detector computed tomography. Catheter Cardiovasc Interv. 69(7):933-8, 2007
2. Van Mieghem CA et al: Multislice spiral computed tomography for the evaluation of stent patency after left main coronary artery stenting: a comparison with conventional coronary angiography and intravascular ultrasound. Circulation. 114(7):645-53, 2006
3. Spuentrup E et al: Artifact-free coronary magnetic resonance angiography and coronary vessel wall imaging in the presence of a new, metallic, coronary magnetic resonance imaging stent. Circulation. 111(8):1019-26, 2005
4. Cutlip DE et al: Beyond restenosis: five-year clinical outcomes from second-generation coronary stent trials. Circulation. 110(10):1226-30, 2004
5. Cutlip DE et al: Clinical restenosis after coronary stenting: perspectives from multicenter clinical trials. J Am Coll Cardiol. 40(12):2082-9, 2002
6. Mehran R et al: Treatment of focal in-stent restenosis with balloon angioplasty alone versus stenting: Short- and long-term results. Am Heart J. 141(4):610-4, 2001
7. Goldberg SL et al: Rotational atherectomy or balloon angioplasty in the treatment of intra-stent restenosis: BARASTER multicenter registry. Catheter Cardiovasc Interv. 51(4):407-13, 2000
8. Hoffmann R et al: Coronary in-stent restenosis - predictors, treatment and prevention. Eur Heart J. 21(21):1739-49, 2000
9. Mehran R et al: Angiographic patterns of in-stent restenosis: classification and implications for long-term outcome. Circulation. 100(18):1872-8, 1999
10. Kasaoka S et al: Angiographic and intravascular ultrasound predictors of in-stent restenosis. J Am Coll Cardiol. 32(6):1630-5, 1998
11. Kornowski R et al: In-stent restenosis: contributions of inflammatory responses and arterial injury to neointimal hyperplasia. J Am Coll Cardiol. 31(1):224-30, 1998
12. Kearney M et al: Histopathology of in-stent restenosis in patients with peripheral artery disease. Circulation. 95(8):1998-2002, 1997
13. Teirstein PS et al: Catheter-based radiotherapy to inhibit restenosis after coronary stenting. N Engl J Med. 336(24):1697-703, 1997
14. Hoffmann R et al: Patterns and mechanisms of in-stent restenosis. A serial intravascular ultrasound study. Circulation. 94(6):1247-54, 1996

POST-STENT RESTENOSIS

IMAGE GALLERY

Typical

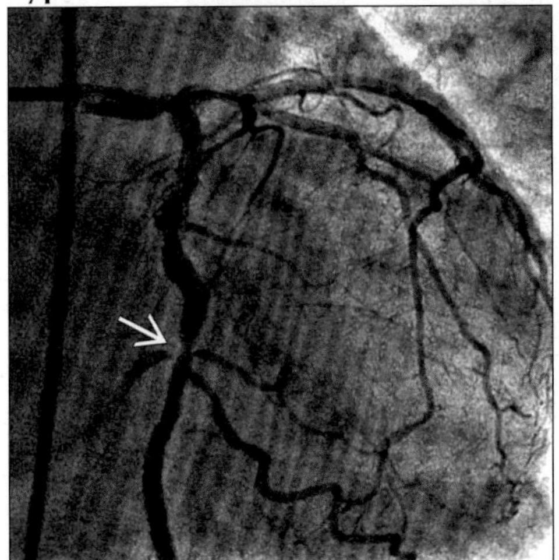

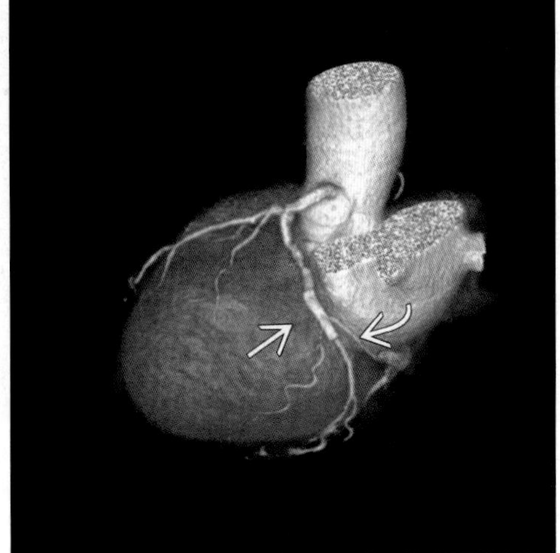

(Left) *Coronary angiogram shows a focal area of restenosis at the edge of a left circumflex stent* ➡. ***(Right)*** *Cardiac gated CTA volume rendered image shows the left circumflex stent in the same patient* ➡. *The area of restenosis at the edge of the stent cannot be assessed on this image* ➡.

Typical

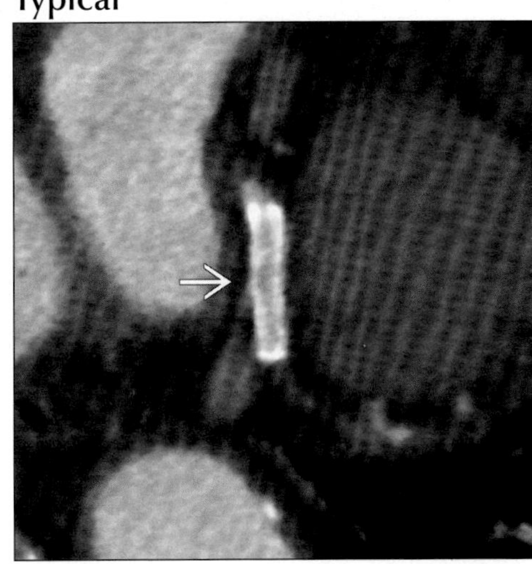

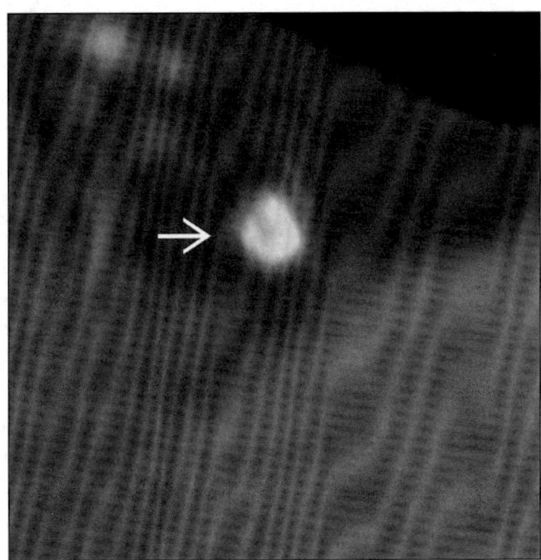

(Left) *Cardiac gated CTA multiple planar reformat of the left circumflex stent* ➡ *does not reveal the area of restenosis. Stents are prone to blooming artifact on CT.* ***(Right)*** *Cardiac gated CTA short axis image of the same LCX stent* ➡ *nicely demonstrates the blooming artifact, where the stent wall appears bigger which reduces the ability to assess the lumen.*

Typical

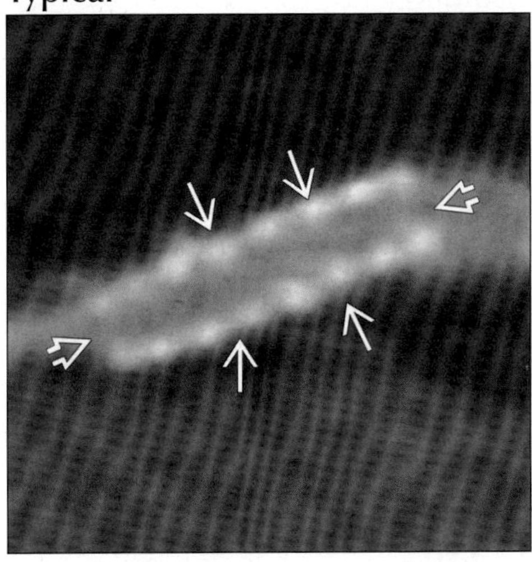

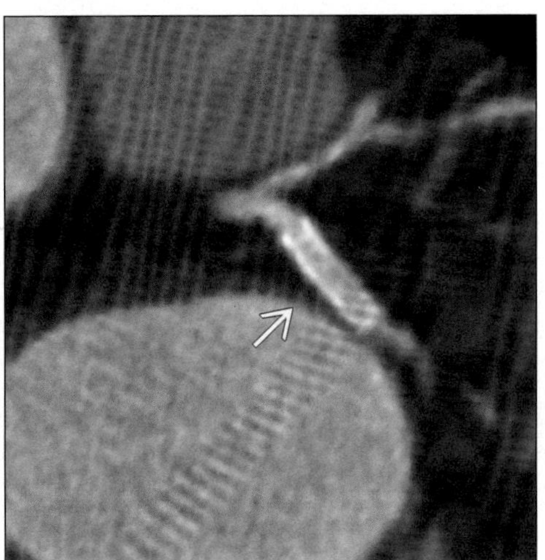

(Left) *Cardiac gated CTA multiple planar reformat of a larger caliber LAD stent nicely shows the vessel lumen* ➡ *and the stent struts* ➡. ***(Right)*** *Cardiac gated CTA multiplanar reformat of a LCX stent* ➡ *does not clearly demonstrate the struts or vessel lumen as in the previous case. This highlights the variability of CTA in-stent evaluation.*

POST CABG THROMBOSIS

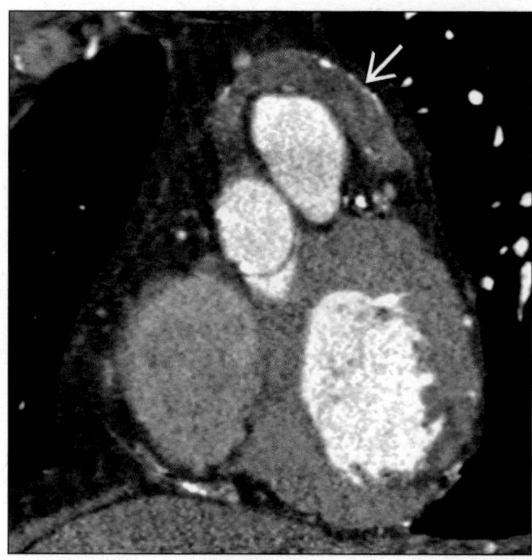

Coronary CTA in a 68 year old man with recurrent angina shows a thrombosed, occluded and expanded saphenous vein graft ➡ to an obtuse marginal branch.

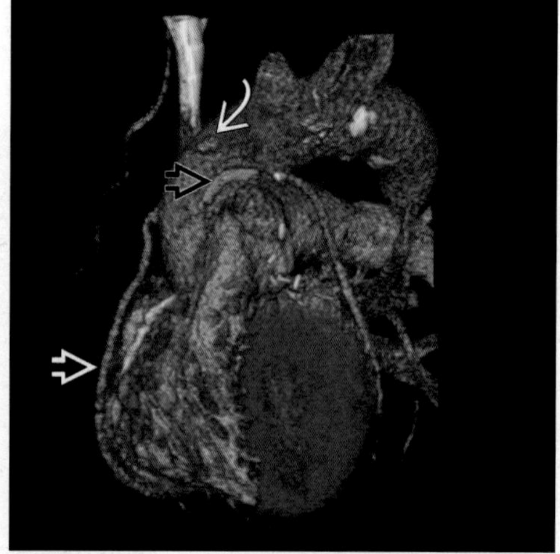

Oblique 3D coronary CTA in 64 yr old man with recurrent angina shows occluded vein graft ➡. Note the stent ➡ in a 2nd vein graft to a diagonal branch, and a patent vein graft ➡ to distal right coronary artery.

TERMINOLOGY

Definitions

- Acute saphenous vein graft failure due to subtotal/total occlusive thrombosis

IMAGING FINDINGS

General Features

- Best diagnostic clue
  - Acute subtotal/total occlusion of a saphenous vein graft by thrombus
    - Coronary angiography (traditional gold-standard but invasive)
- Location: Aorto-coronary reversed saphenous vein grafts
- Morphology
  - Low density material within graft lumen
    - May also demonstrate graft expansion

Radiographic Findings

- Radiography: Chest radiograph may reveal severe acute pulmonary edema (cardiogenic shock)

CT Findings

- NECT: May demonstrate slightly increased HU within occluded graft lumen
- CTA
  - Retrospective ECG gating and segmental reconstruction algorithm allow for high quality images of venous bypass graft occlusions
  - May demonstrate complete absence of luminal contrast in total occlusion with low density luminal material (thrombus)
  - May demonstrate crescentic rim of contrast in subtotal occlusion
  - May demonstrate expansion of vein graft
  - Smooth broad-based area of contrast outpouching at aortic anastomosis may be best clue
    - Aortic cannulation sites can mimic outpouching at occluded graft anastomosis
  - Functional imaging may demonstrate matching wall motion abnormality

MR Findings

- MRA

DDx: Post CABG Thrombosis

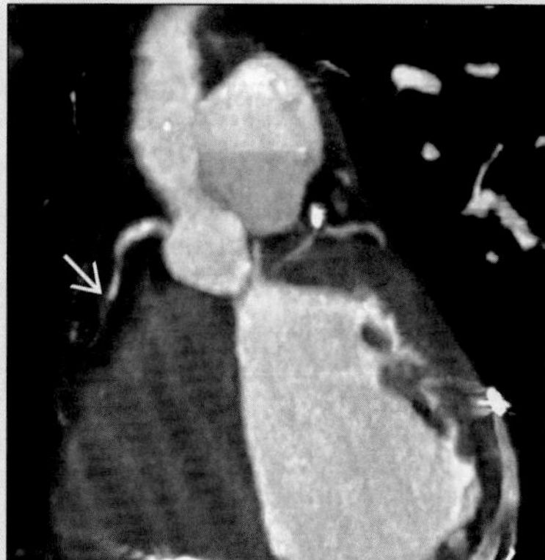

Native Coronary Stenosis/Occlusion

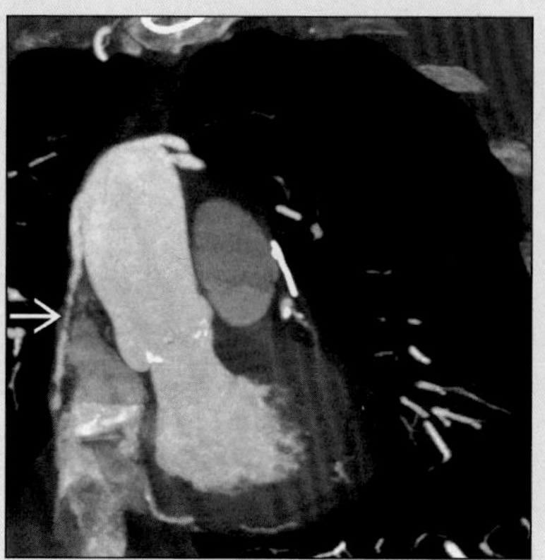

Graft Atherosclerosis

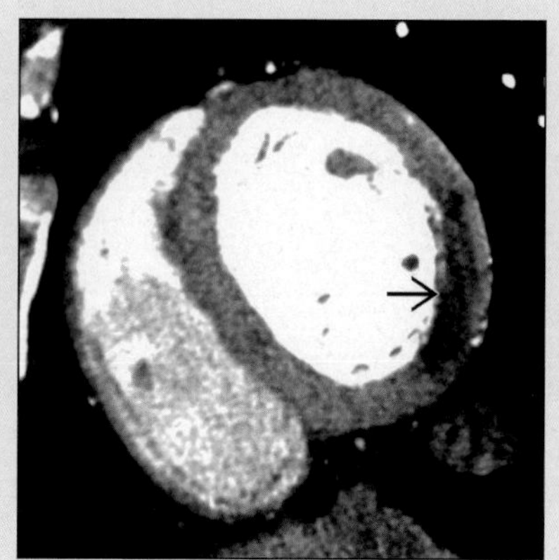

Perioperative Myocardial Infarction

POST CABG THROMBOSIS

Key Facts

Terminology

- Acute saphenous vein graft failure due to subtotal/total occlusive thrombosis

Imaging Findings

- Acute subtotal/total occlusion of a saphenous vein graft by thrombus
- Retrospective ECG gating and segmental reconstruction algorithm allow for high quality images of venous bypass graft occlusions
- Coronary angiography (traditional gold-standard but invasive)

Pathology

- Atherosclerosis is diffuse and concentric
- Lesions are friable and fragile
- Fibrous cap is absent or weak and thin

Clinical Issues

- Recurrent angina commonest presentation
- Myocardial infarction
- Arrhythmias
- Sudden death
- Prevention better than cure: Intensify medical therapy post-operatively
- ~ 10% of CABG occlude during the first month post surgery
- Balloon angioplasty: Unsatisfactory restenosis rate of at least 45%
- Directional atherectomy: Long term re-stenosis rate similar to angioplasty
- Stents: Best percutaneous option - re-stenosis rate = 16% at 6 months
- Re-operation, but significant disadvantages

- 3D gadolinium-enhanced MR techniques are more sensitive than 2D gradient echo or spin echo techniques for detecting graft occlusion
    - Sensitivity = 85%, specificity = 94%
- Respiratory navigating markedly improves image quality
- Occluded grafts are absent; correlation with operative notes crucial
    - May demonstrate small smooth outpouching of contrast at aortic anastomosis

Nuclear Medicine Findings

- Nuclear cardiology findings
    - Thallium or technetium imaging
        - Reduced tracer uptake in ischemic segments

Angiographic Findings

- Catheterization findings
    - Demonstrates graft occlusion
    - Abnormal wall motion on ventriculogram

Imaging Recommendations

- Best imaging tool
    - Coronary angiography (traditional gold-standard but invasive)
        - Many patients will need percutaneous transluminal coronary intervention
    - Cardiac CT (non-invasive)

DIFFERENTIAL DIAGNOSIS

Coronary Artery Stenosis

- New stenosis on native coronary arteries

CABG Atherosclerosis

- Within the 1st post-operative year is due to perianastomotic stenosis (within the 1st post-operative year is due to perianastomotic stenosis [especially at three-months], graft stenosis or occlusion especially at three-months), graft stenosis or occlusion
- After the 1st year post-operatively is due to stenosis in grafts and native coronary arteries

Perioperative Infarction

- Especially in left main stenosis and triple vessel disease

PATHOLOGY

General Features

- General path comments
    - Loss of endothelium with accumulation of fibrin
    - Adherence of platelets and white blood cells
    - Thrombus occluding vessel lumen especially at sites of anastomosis
- Etiology
    - Endothelial injury
        - Direct physical trauma during surgery
        - Leukocyte response
        - Ischemia of wall after loss of vasa vasorum
        - Risk factors such as smoking, high low density lipoprotein cholesterol
    - Low saphenous vein graft flow
        - Small luminal size of recipient artery
        - Diseased native artery distal to anastomosis
        - Bypass of subcritical lesion (< 70% stenosis)
    - Local atheroma development within the vein graft
    - Sequential "jump" grafts
    - Technical factors
        - Distal anastomosis errors
        - Insufficient/excessive graft length
        - Mismatched size of graft to recipient artery
        - Angle of graft to aorta < 90° can lead to "kinking"
    - Resistance to antiplatelet agents

Gross Pathologic & Surgical Features

- Atherosclerosis is diffuse and concentric
- Lesions are friable and fragile
- Prone to atherosclerotic embolism, particularly during re-operation

Microscopic Features

- Fibrous cap is absent or weak and thin
    - Foam cells and lipid debris exposed to bloodstream

POST CABG THROMBOSIS

- Infiltrate of inflammatory cells and lipid-laden multinucleate giant cells

CLINICAL ISSUES

Presentation

- Most common signs/symptoms
  - Recurrent angina commonest presentation
  - Myocardial infarction
  - New/worsening heart failure
  - Arrhythmias
  - Sudden death
- Range from no symptoms to recurrent angina and infarction
- Prevention
  - Prevention better than cure: Intensify medical therapy post-operatively
    - Aspirin
    - Dipyrimadole
    - Ticlopidine

Natural History & Prognosis

- ~ 10% of CABG occlude during the first month post surgery

Treatment

- Graft vasospasm minimized at surgery by bathing in
  - Topical {alpha}-adrenergic antagonist solutions (phenoxybenzamine)
  - Calcium channel blockers
- Balloon angioplasty: Unsatisfactory restenosis rate of at least 45%
  - Short focal lesions in the distal portion of graft respond best
- Directional atherectomy: Long term re-stenosis rate similar to angioplasty
  - Better initial gain in luminal diameter compared to angioplasty
    - Complicated by non-Q-wave infarction from distal embolism
- Stents: Best percutaneous option - re-stenosis rate = 16% at 6 months
  - Initial success rate = 98%
  - Newer drug-eluting stents may improve patency rates
- Re-operation, but significant disadvantages
  - More costly
  - Two-three times morbidity and mortality compared to initial procedure
  - Recurrent angina more common

DIAGNOSTIC CHECKLIST

Consider

- In patients re-presenting with angina post CABG
- Obstruction/occlusion in grafts or native vessels

SELECTED REFERENCES

1. Ropers D et al: Diagnostic Accuracy of Noninvasive Coronary Angiography in Patients After Bypass Surgery Using 64-Slice Spiral Computed Tomography With 330-ms Gantry Rotation. Circulation, 2006
2. Frazier AA et al: Coronary artery bypass grafts: assessment with multidetector CT in the early and late postoperative settings. Radiographics. 25(4):881-96, 2005
3. Serna DL et al: Antifibrinolytic agents in cardiac surgery: current controversies. Semin Thorac Cardiovasc Surg. 17(1):52-8, 2005
4. Yilmaz MB et al: Late saphenous vein graft occlusion in patients with coronary bypass: possible role of aspirin resistance. Thromb Res. 115(1-2):25-9, 2005
5. Poston R et al: Virchow triad, but not use of an aortic connector device, predicts early graft failure after off-pump coronary bypass. Heart Surg Forum. 7(5):E428-33, 2004
6. Enzweiler CN et al: Diameter changes of occluded venous coronary artery bypass grafts in electron beam tomography: preliminary findings. Eur J Cardiothorac Surg. 23(3):347-53, 2003
7. Singh M et al: Treatment of saphenous vein bypass grafts with ultrasound thrombolysis: a randomized study (ATLAS). Circulation. 107(18):2331-6, 2003
8. Stone GW et al: Prospective, randomized evaluation of thrombectomy prior to percutaneous intervention in diseased saphenous vein grafts and thrombus-containing coronary arteries. J Am Coll Cardiol. 42(11):2007-13, 2003
9. Shuhaiber JH et al: Mechanisms and future directions for prevention of vein graft failure in coronary bypass surgery. Eur J Cardiothorac Surg. 22(3):387-96, 2002
10. Saltman AE et al: Immediate vein graft thrombectomy for acute occlusion after coronary artery bypass grafting. Ann Thorac Surg. 67(6):1775-6, 1999
11. Motwani JG et al: Aortocoronary saphenous vein graft disease: pathogenesis, predisposition, and prevention. Circulation. 97(9):916-31, 1998
12. Mehta D et al: Towards the prevention of vein graft failure. Int J Cardiol. 62 Suppl 1:S55-63, 1997
13. No authors listed: The effect of aggressive lowering of low-density lipoprotein cholesterol levels and low-dose anticoagulation on obstructive changes in saphenous-vein coronary-artery bypass grafts. The Post Coronary Artery Bypass Graft Trial Investigators. N Engl J Med. 336(3):153-62, 1997
14. De Paulis R et al: Early coronary artery bypass graft thrombosis in a patient with protein S deficiency. Eur J Cardiothorac Surg. 10(6):470-2, 1996
15. Fitzgibbon GM et al: Coronary bypass graft fate and patient outcome: angiographic follow-up of 5,065 grafts related to survival and reoperation in 1,388 patients during 25 years. J Am Coll Cardiol. 28(3):616-26, 1996
16. Mak KH et al: Subacute stent thrombosis: evolving issues and current concepts. J Am Coll Cardiol. 27(2):494-503, 1996
17. Eeckhout E et al: Complications and follow-up after intracoronary stenting: critical analysis of a 6-year single-center experience. Am Heart J. 127(2):262-72, 1994
18. Comess K et al: Intracoronary ultrasound imaging of graft thrombosis. N Engl J Med. 327(23):1691-2, 1992
19. Grondin CM et al: Coronary artery bypass grafting with saphenous vein. Circulation. 79(6 Pt 2):I24-9, 1989
20. Walts AE et al: Thrombosed, ruptured atheromatous plaques in saphenous vein coronary artery bypass grafts: ten years' experience. Am Heart J. 114(4 Pt 1):718-23, 1987
21. Holmes DR Jr et al: Streptokinase for vein graft thrombosis--a caveat. Circulation. 63(3):729, 1981

IMAGE GALLERY

Typical

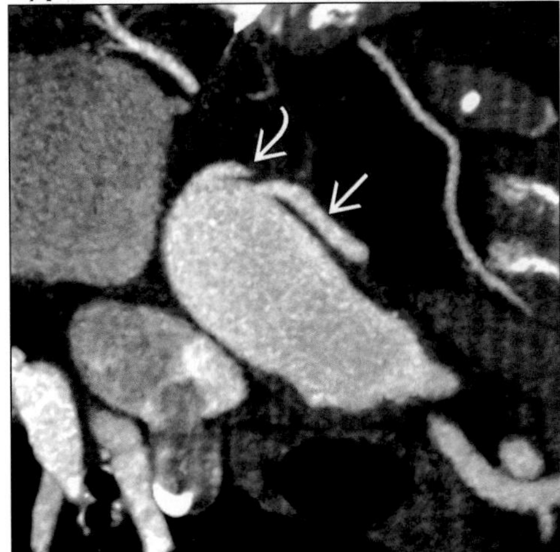

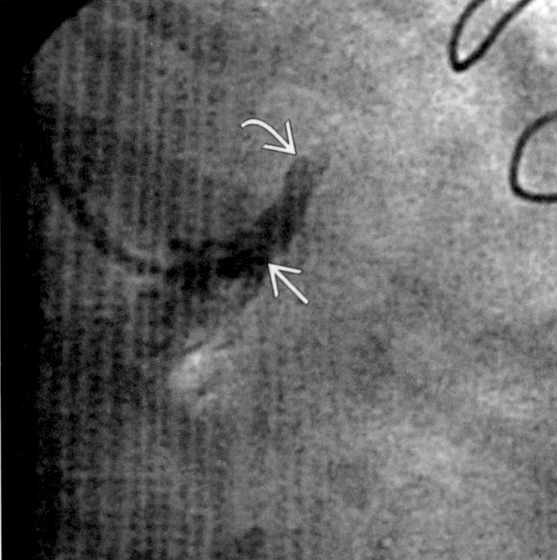

(Left) *Coronary CTA in a 68 year old man with recurrent angina shows one patent ➔ and one thrombosed saphenous vein graft ➔.* ***(Right)*** *Corresponding coronary angiogram shows catheter tip in saphenous vein graft ➔ and abrupt cut-off of contrast in the proximal portion of the graft ➔.*

Typical

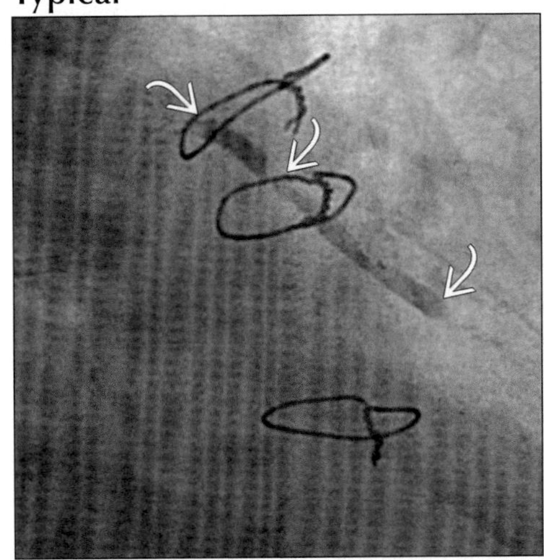

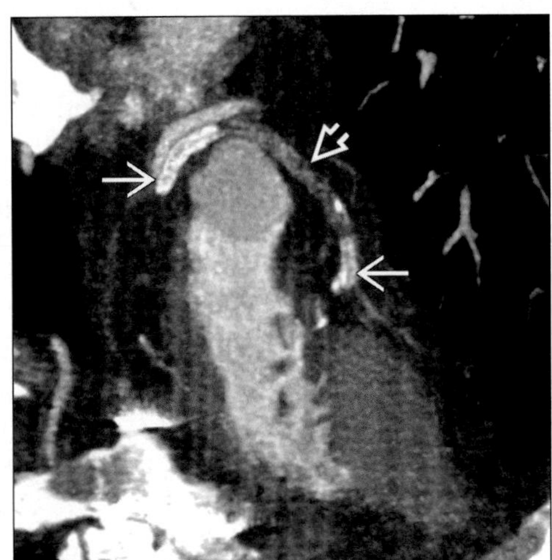

(Left) *Oblique coronary angiogram in a 66 year old man with recurrent angina shows subtotal occlusions ➔ of the proximal and mid portions of a saphenous vein graft.* ***(Right)*** *Corresponding coronary CTA shows two stents ➔ placed across the proximal and mid graft stenosis. Both stents and graft are now completely occluded with thrombus ➔.*

Typical

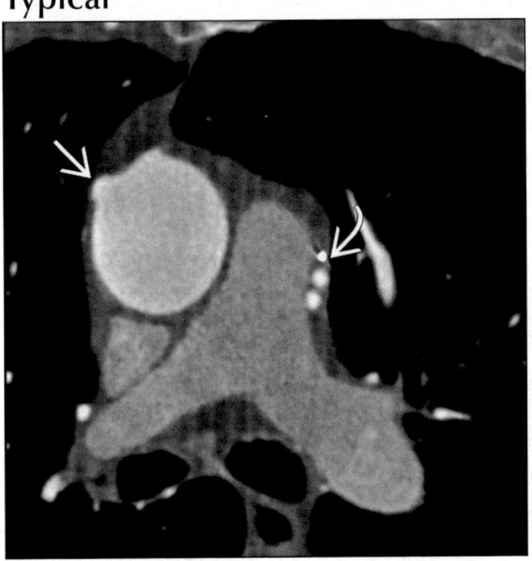

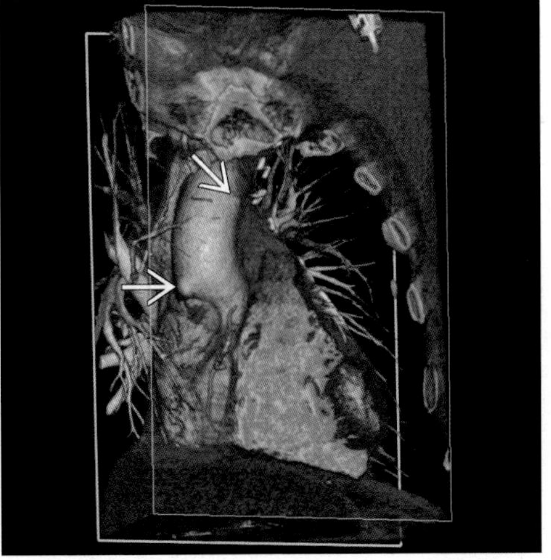

(Left) *Coronary CTA in a 72 year old man with recurrent angina shows a thrombosed, occluded graft ➔. Such outpouchings at the ascending aortic wall are typical of vein graft occlusions on CT. Note clips ➔ from patent LIMA graft.* ***(Right)*** *Coronary CTA 3D reformats can be useful in illustrating thrombosed, occluded saphenous vein grafts ➔.*

POST CABG ATHEROSCLEROSIS

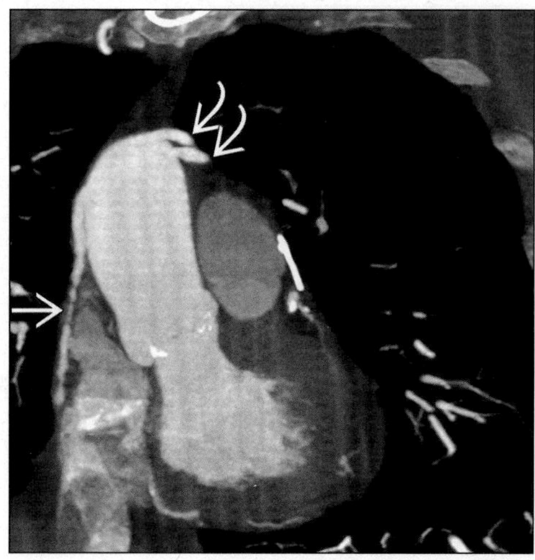

Coronary CTA shows severe atherosclerosis ➡ in venous graft to distal right coronary artery. Note two additional, patent venous grafts ⮫.

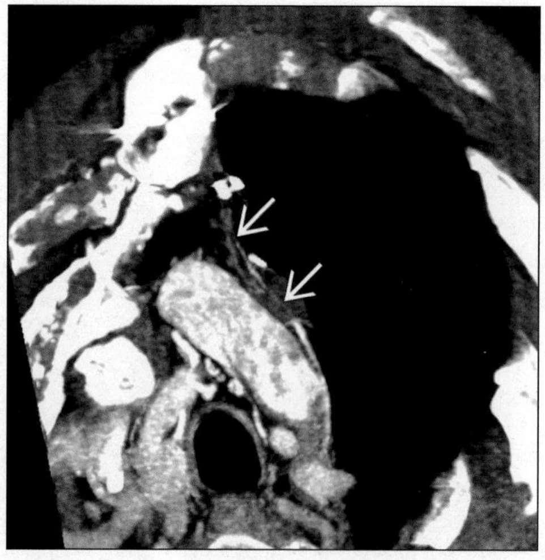

Coronary CTA shows severe atherosclerotic narrowing ➡ in the proximal portions of a left internal mammary artery graft.

TERMINOLOGY

Definitions

- Post-operative atherosclerotic disease of bypass grafts or native coronary arteries

IMAGING FINDINGS

General Features

- Best diagnostic clue: Stenosis or occlusion of graft or native coronary artery on coronary angiography or cardiac CT
- Location
  - Recurrent angina
    - Within a few hours to days post-operatively is due to venous graft thrombosis
    - Within the 1st post-operative year is usually due to perianastomotic stenosis (especially at three-months), graft stenosis or occlusion
    - After the 1st year post-operatively is usually due to stenosis in grafts and native coronary arteries

CT Findings

- CTA
  - Retrospective ECG gating image reconstruction algorithm allow high quality images of arterial and venous bypass grafts
    - Sensitivity = 100%, specificity = 98%
    - Accuracy for native coronary arteries decreased due to advanced disease and high prevalence of coronary calcium

MR Findings

- MRA
  - 3D gadolinium enhanced techniques are more sensitive than 2D gradient echo or spin echo techniques
    - Sensitivity = 85%, specificity = 94%
    - Respiratory navigating markedly improves image quality but takes more time
  - Phase-contrast velocity encoding of graft blood flow enables estimation of coronary flow reserve
    - Coronary flow reserve is useful for identifying hemodynamically significant stenosis and influencing need for intervention
- MR Cine

DDx: Post CABG Atherosclerosis

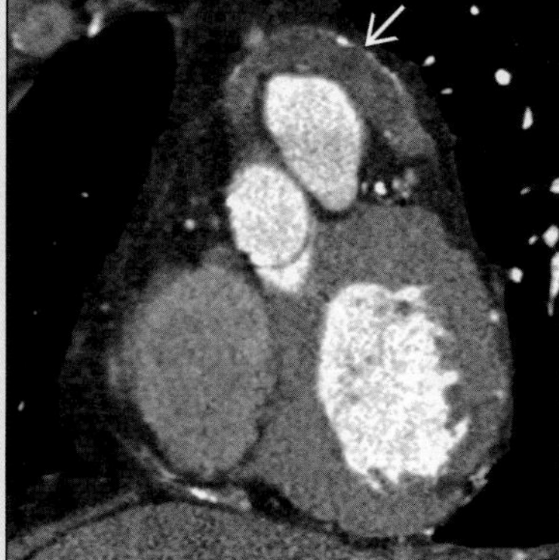

Thrombosed Vein Graft

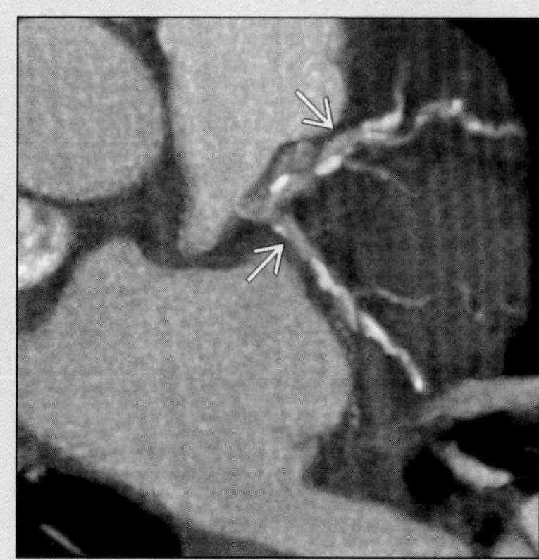

Native Coronary Thrombosis

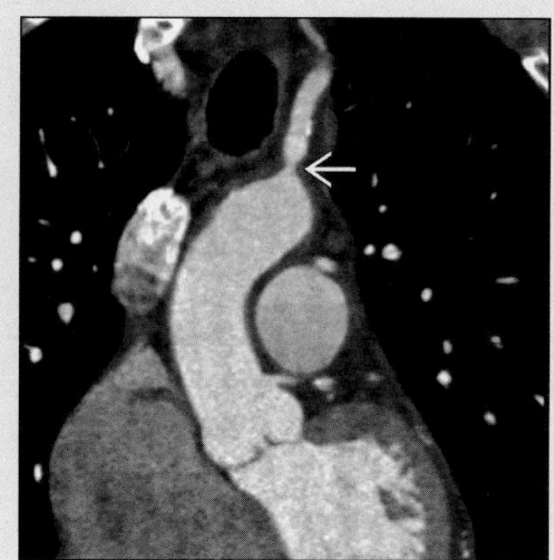

Subclavian Stenosis

POST CABG ATHEROSCLEROSIS

Key Facts

Terminology
- Significant post-operative atherosclerotic disease of bypass grafts or native coronary arteries

Imaging Findings
- Best diagnostic clue: Stenosis or occlusion of graft or native coronary artery on coronary angiography (traditional gold-standard but invasive) or cardiac CT (non-invasive)

Top Differential Diagnoses
- Graft Thrombosis

Pathology
- Neointimal hyperplasia of grafts
- Progression of atherosclerosis common in native coronary arteries proximal to grafts
- Due to lower blood flow through the native coronary proximal segments

Clinical Issues
- Angina recurs in 15-20% of patients during the first year post-op with an additional ~ 4% per year
- By 5th post-operative year 50% of patients have recurrent angina
- Saphenous vein grafts are most common to stenose/occlude
- Intensify risk factor modification especially aggressive lipid-lowering and antiplatelet therapies
- Percutaneous transluminal coronary intervention for graft stenosis
- Percutaneous transluminal coronary intervention for native coronary artery stenosis

- ○ Global and regional ventricular function can be assessed with steady state free-precession sequences
  - ▪ Good left ventricular function post-operatively is associated with better long term clinical outcome
- Delayed Enhancement: Amount of infarcted tissue depicted by delayed enhancement MR post-operatively correlates well with elevated biomarkers and long term clinical outcome

Nuclear Medicine Findings
- PET
  - High sensitivity and moderate specificity for predicting improvement in function post-operatively
    - Improvement most strongly predicted when 3 or more dysfunctional myocardial segments have a relative FDG uptake > 45% of normal myocardium
- Stress technetium or sestamibi imaging
  - Reduced tracer uptake in ischemic areas corresponding to areas of decreased perfusion/infarction

Echocardiographic Findings
- Echocardiogram
  - Transthoracic Doppler echo has a high accuracy for detecting left internal mammary artery (LIMA) graft stenosis but
    - Up to 10% of LIMA's are not visualized; other techniques may provide more complete evaluation

Angiographic Findings
- Catheterization findings
  - Demonstrates degree of luminal stenosis or occlusion
  - Abnormal wall motion on ventriculogram

Imaging Recommendations
- Best imaging tool
  - Coronary angiography
  - Cardiac CT

DIFFERENTIAL DIAGNOSIS

Graft Thrombosis
- May be in absence of graft atherosclerotic disease

Subclavian Artery Stenosis Proximal to Left Internal Mammary Artery (LIMA) Origin
- May have same effect as LIMA stenosis

PATHOLOGY

General Features
- General path comments
  - Neointimal hyperplasia of grafts
  - Proliferation of smooth muscle cells and extracellular matrix
  - Proliferation throughout the length of the graft with focal areas of stenosis
  - Even mild atherosclerotic stenosis in vein grafts leads to significant increased risk of ischemic events
- Etiology
  - Incomplete surgical revascularization with persistent distal coronary disease
  - Inadequate amount of conduit
  - Inadequate conduit lumen; especially LIMA
  - Intramyocardial location of target coronary vessel
  - Graft anastomosis to wrong coronary artery or to a vein
  - LIMA with extensive subclavian artery atherosclerosis
- Associated abnormalities
  - Progression of atherosclerosis common in native coronary arteries proximal to grafts
    - Due to lower blood flow through the native coronary proximal segments
    - Important when re-operation is considered
    - Can cause proximal side-branch ischemia

CLINICAL ISSUES

Presentation

- Most common signs/symptoms
  - Angina recurs in 15-20% of patients during the first year post-op with an additional ~ 4% per year
    - Accelerated form of atherosclerosis

Natural History & Prognosis

- By 5th post-operative year 50% of patients have recurrent angina
- Approximately 25% of patients require re-operation in 10 years; re-operation compared to initial operation
  - More costly
  - 2-3 times more likely to be complicated by death or myocardial infarction
  - Less effective in relieving angina
- Saphenous vein grafts are most common to stenose/occlude
  - 7% by 9 days, 10-15% by the first month

Treatment

- Intensify risk factor modification especially aggressive lipid-lowering and antiplatelet therapies
- Percutaneous transluminal coronary intervention for graft stenosis
  - Angioplasty
  - Drug-eluting stent
  - Directional atherectomy
  - Laser angioplasty
- Percutaneous transluminal coronary intervention for native coronary artery stenosis
  - Left main coronary stenting may be lifesaving in the presence of acute graft thrombosis
  - Approach via IVC or graft

DIAGNOSTIC CHECKLIST

Consider

- Post CABG atherosclerosis in patients with recurrence of angina postoperatively in
  - Grafts
  - Native coronary arteries

SELECTED REFERENCES

1. Anders K et al: Coronary artery bypass graft (CABG) patency: assessment with high-resolution submillimeter 16-slice multidetector-row computed tomography (MDCT) versus coronary angiography. Eur J Radiol. 57(3):336-44, 2006
2. Pache G et al: Initial experience with 64-slice cardiac CT: non-invasive visualization of coronary artery bypass grafts. Eur Heart J. 27(8):976-80, 2006
3. Chiurlia E et al: Follow-up of coronary artery bypass graft patency by multislice computed tomography. Am J Cardiol. 95(9):1094-7, 2005
4. Frazier AA et al: Coronary artery bypass grafts: assessment with multidetector CT in the early and late postoperative settings. Radiographics. 25(4):881-96, 2005
5. Gasparovic H et al: Three dimensional computed tomographic imaging in planning the surgical approach for redo cardiac surgery after coronary revascularization. Eur J Cardiothorac Surg. 28(2):244-9, 2005
6. Ohnesorge BM et al: CT for imaging coronary artery disease: defining the paradigm for its application. Int J Cardiovasc Imaging. 21(1):85-104, 2005
7. Salm LP et al: Comprehensive assessment of patients after coronary artery bypass grafting by 16-detector-row computed tomography. Am Heart J. 150(4):775-81, 2005
8. Stauder NI et al: Assessment of minimally invasive direct coronary artery bypass grafting of the left internal thoracic artery by means of magnetic resonance imaging. J Thorac Cardiovasc Surg. 129(3):607-14, 2005
9. Stein PD et al: Usefulness of 4-, 8-, and 16-slice computed tomography for detection of graft occlusion or patency after coronary artery bypass grafting. Am J Cardiol. 96(12):1669-73, 2005
10. Kavanagh EC et al: CT of a ruptured vein graft pseudoaneurysm: an unusual cause of superior vena cava obstruction. AJR Am J Roentgenol. 183(5):1239-40, 2004
11. Marano R et al: Non-invasive assessment of coronary artery bypass graft with retrospectively ECG-gated four-row multi-detector spiral computed tomography. Eur Radiol. 14(8):1353-62, 2004
12. Salm LP et al: Blood flow in coronary artery bypass vein grafts: volume versus velocity at cardiovascular MR imaging. Radiology. 232(3):915-20, 2004
13. Schlosser T et al: Noninvasive visualization of coronary artery bypass grafts using 16-detector row computed tomography. J Am Coll Cardiol. 44(6):1224-9, 2004
14. Willmann JK et al: Coronary artery bypass grafts: ECG-gated multi-detector row CT angiography--influence of image reconstruction interval on graft visibility. Radiology. 232(2):568-77, 2004
15. Bunce NH et al: Coronary artery bypass graft patency: assessment with true ast imaging with steady-state precession versus gadolinium-enhanced MR angiography. Radiology. 227(2):440-6, 2003
16. Langerak SE et al: Value of magnetic resonance imaging for the noninvasive detection of stenosis in coronary artery bypass grafts and recipient coronary arteries. Circulation. 107(11):1502-8, 2003
17. Bedaux WL et al: Assessment of coronary artery bypass graft disease using cardiovascular magnetic resonance determination of flow reserve. J Am Coll Cardiol. 40(10):1848-55, 2002
18. Hoogwerf BJ et al: A summary of the findings from the Post-CABG trial. Minerva Cardioangiol. 50(4):291-9, 2002
19. Ascione R et al: Clinical and angiographic outcome of different surgical strategies of bilateral internal mammary artery grafting. Ann Thorac Surg. 72(3):959-65, 2001
20. Gerber BL et al: Positron emission tomography using(18)F-fluoro-deoxyglucose and euglycaemic hyperinsulinaemic glucose clamp: optimal criteria for the prediction of recovery of post-ischaemic left ventricular dysfunction. Results from the European Community Concerted Action Multicenter study on use of(18)F-fluoro-deoxyglucose Positron Emission Tomography for the Detection of Myocardial Viability. Eur Heart J. 22(18):1691-701, 2001
21. Popma JJ et al: Lipid-lowering therapy after coronary revascularization. Am J Cardiol. 86(4B):18H-28H, 2000
22. Motwani JG et al: Aortocoronary saphenous vein graft disease: pathogenesis, predisposition, and prevention. Circulation. 97(9):916-31, 1998
23. Salm LP et al: Functional significance of stenoses in coronary artery bypass grafts. Evaluation by single-photon emission computed tomography perfusion imaging, cardiovascular magnetic resonance, and angiography.

POST CABG ATHEROSCLEROSIS

IMAGE GALLERY

Typical

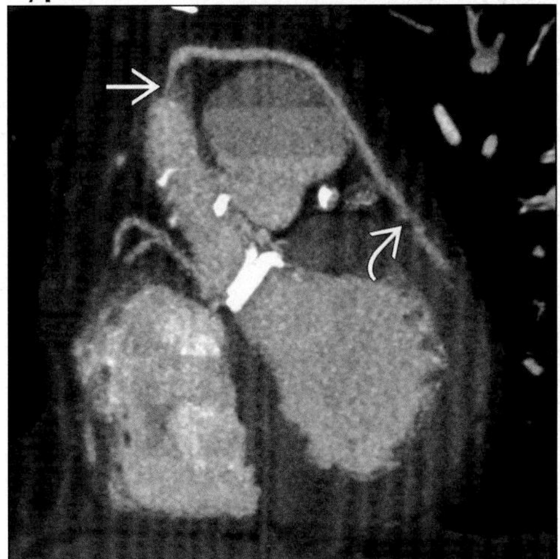

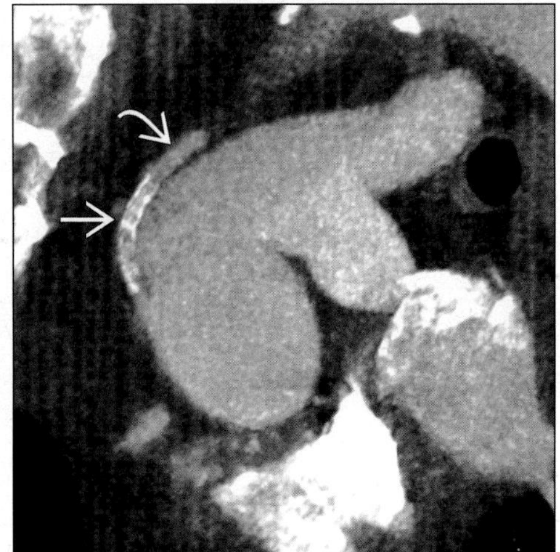

(Left) *Coronal coronary CTA shows severe ostial and mid segment stenosis of saphenous vein bypass graft to 1st obtuse marginal branch.* ***(Right)*** *Coronary CTA in a 67 year old man shows a stent in the proximal portion of a patent but atherosclerotic saphenous vein graft.*

Typical

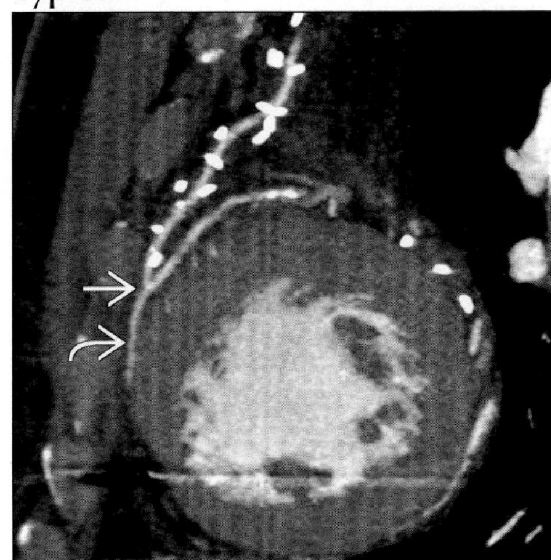

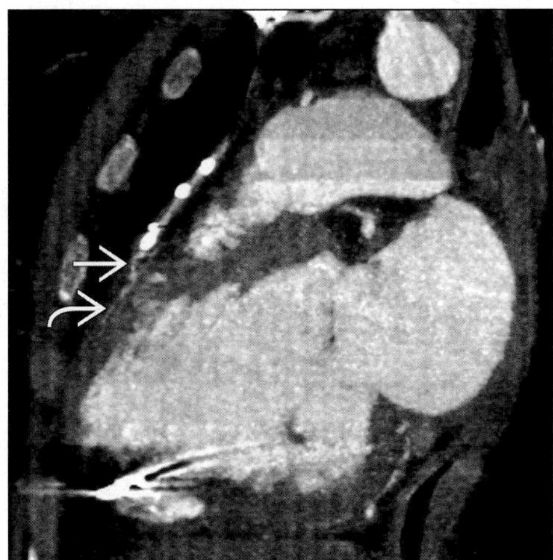

(Left) *Coronary CTA shows clean anastomosis of LIMA graft to distal left anterior descending artery. Good distal vessel run-off.* ***(Right)*** *In contrast, coronary CTA in another patient with recurrent angina shows stenosis at site of distal anastomosis of LIMA graft to distal left anterior descending artery, with poor distal vessel run-off.*

Typical

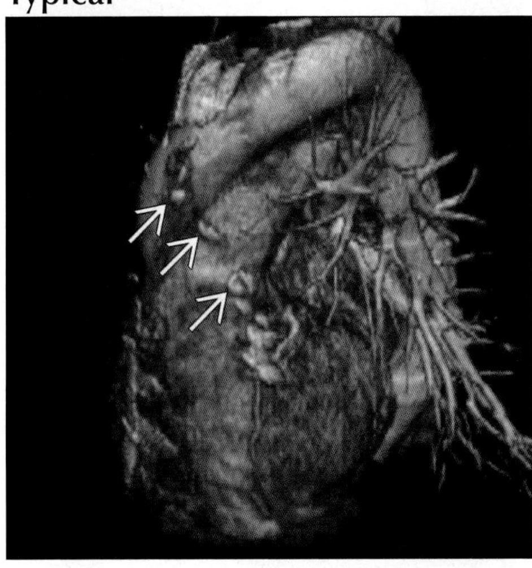

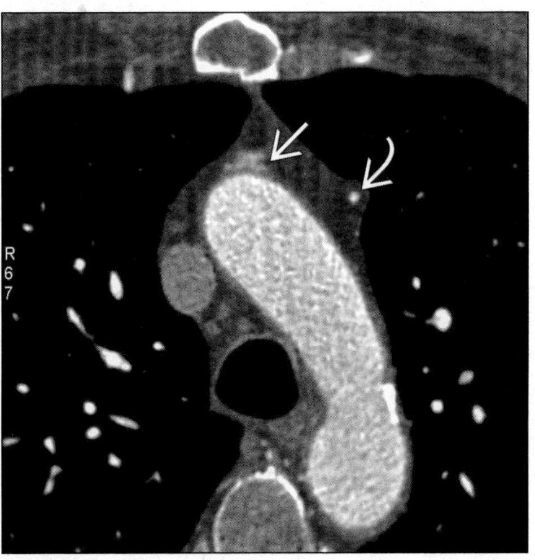

(Left) *Coronary CTA 3D reformats are useful in identifying suspected graft occlusions. The path of an occluded LIMA graft may be identified from the surgical clips.* ***(Right)*** *Coronary CTA occasionally on coronary CTA surgical pledglet material may be seen and may mimic graft atherosclerosis or occlusion. Note patent LIMA graft.*

MYOCARDIAL BRIDGE

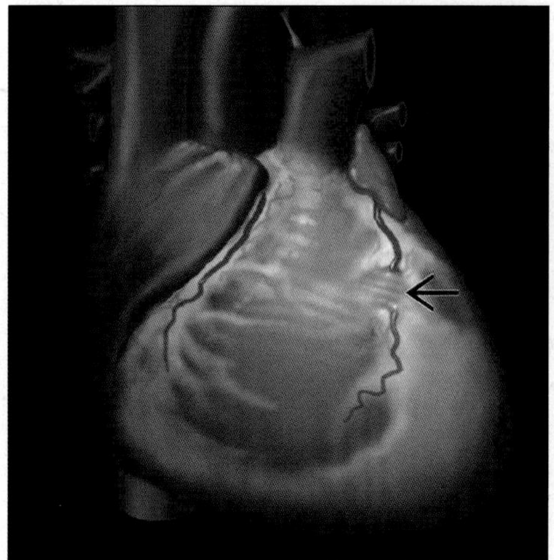

3-dimensional graphic illustration shows a short myocardial bridge ⇨ in the mid portion of the mid LAD.

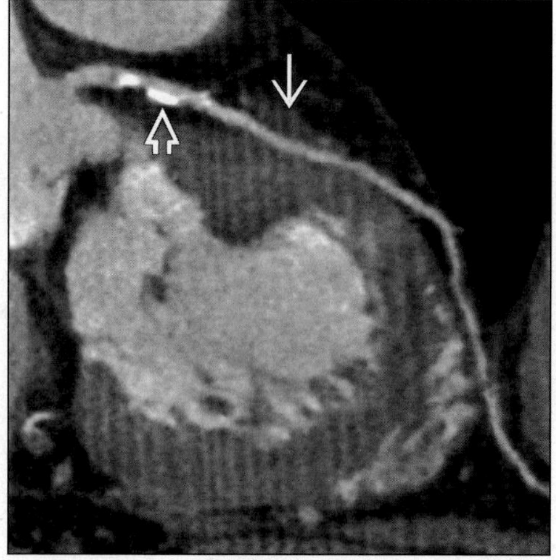

Coronary CTA shows mid left anterior descending artery myocardial bridge ➡. Note calcified plaque ⇨ proximal to the bridge but no atherosclerosis within bridge.

TERMINOLOGY

Definitions

- Congenital coronary anatomic variant in which a segment of epicardial coronary artery takes an intramyocardial course

IMAGING FINDINGS

General Features

- Best diagnostic clue: Coronary artery dives into and is covered by a "bridge" of myocardium
- Location: Most common = mid segment of left anterior descending coronary artery, left circumflex artery (~ 40%), right coronary artery (~ 20%)
- Morphology
  - Most patients have single bridge
    - Two and rarely three bridges are reported
    - May be superficial or deep

Imaging Recommendations

- Best imaging tool
  - Cardiac CT
    - Epicardial coronary dives into myocardium and resurfaces distally into epicardial fat
  - Intracoronary ultrasound shows a highly specific echolucent half-moon sign

DIFFERENTIAL DIAGNOSIS

Hypertrophic Cardiomyopathy

- Asymmetric myocardial hypertrophy may mimic a bridge

Cardiac Tumor

- May invade epicardial fat to engulf coronary arteries

Coronary Anomaly

- Classically a left main arising from the RCA and passing between the great vessels may bridge

PATHOLOGY

General Features

- Etiology
  - Cause of ischemia currently uncertain

DDx: Myocardial Bridge

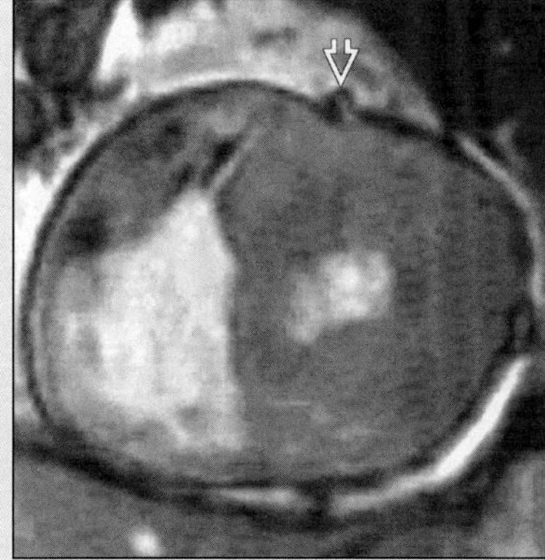

Hypertrophic Cardiomyopathy

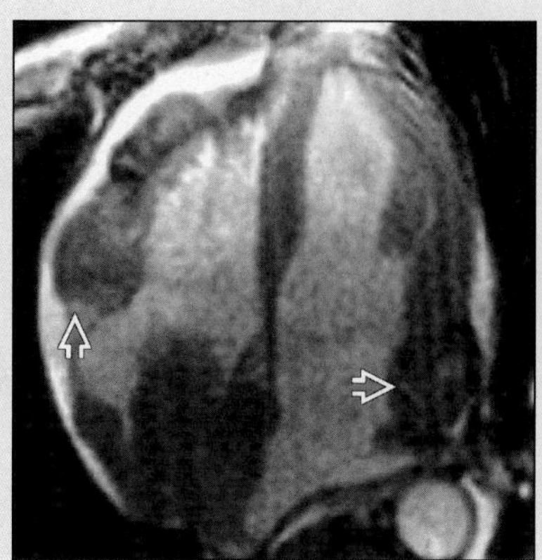

Cardiac Tumor

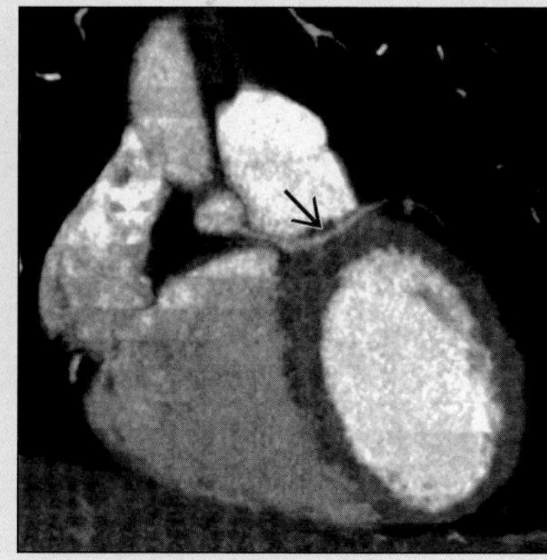

Coronary Anomaly

MYOCARDIAL BRIDGE

Key Facts

Terminology
- Congenital coronary anatomic variant in which a segment of epicardial coronary artery takes an intramyocardial course

Imaging Findings
- Location: Most common = mid segment of left anterior descending coronary artery, left circumflex artery (~ 40%), right coronary artery (~ 20%)
- Most patients have single bridge

Pathology
- Cause of ischemia currently uncertain

Clinical Issues
- Most patients asymptomatic; small subgroup develop ischemia

Diagnostic Checklist
- On cardiac CT, use multiplanar reformats to depict bridge

    - 85% of coronary blood flow is in diastole
    - Vessel compression occurs during systole
    - Leads to proximal segment wall shear stress which predisposes proximal segment to atherosclerosis
- Epidemiology
  - Prevalence of 1.5-16% in angiography studies (an underestimate)
    - Autopsy studies = up to 80%

Gross Pathologic & Surgical Features
- Intima of the tunneled segment is thin

Microscopic Features
- Synthetic smooth muscle cells are absent
- Such phenotypic morphology correlates with a low incidence of subsequent atherosclerosis in the tunneled segment
- Appears to lead to upstream shear wall stress in the proximal coronary segment, predisposing to atherosclerosis development upstream from the bridge

CLINICAL ISSUES

Presentation
- Most common signs/symptoms
  - Most patients asymptomatic; small subgroup develop ischemia
    - Angina, spasm, ST-segment depression during exercise, ventricular septal rupture, arrhythmias, myocardial stunning, sudden death

Demographics
- Age: Symptoms, if any, usually begin in third decade
- Gender: No gender predilection
- Myocardial bridging more common in young patients with hypertrophic cardiomyopathy

Natural History & Prognosis
- Most patients are asymptomatic
  - Small subgroup develop ischemia

Treatment
- Medical
  - Beta-blockers and calcium channel blockers
- Percutaneous coronary intervention - stenting
- Coronary artery bypass graft
- Septal myomectomy
- Septal alcohol ablation

DIAGNOSTIC CHECKLIST

Image Interpretation Pearls
- On cardiac CT, long and short axis multi planar reformations very useful

SELECTED REFERENCES

1. Goitein O et al: Myocardial bridging: noninvasive diagnosis with multidetector CT. J Comput Assist Tomogr. 29(2):238-40, 2005

IMAGE GALLERY

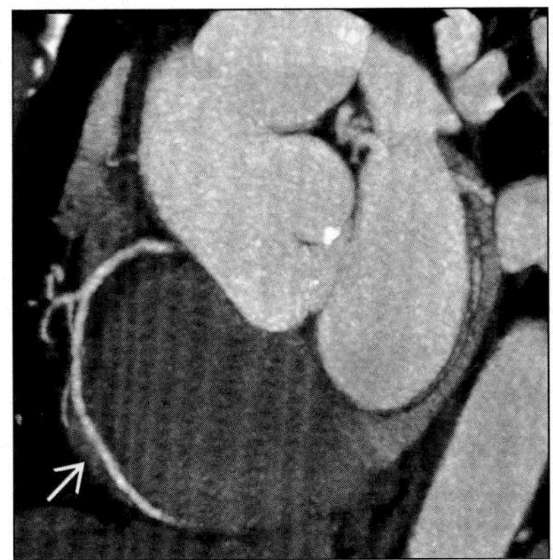
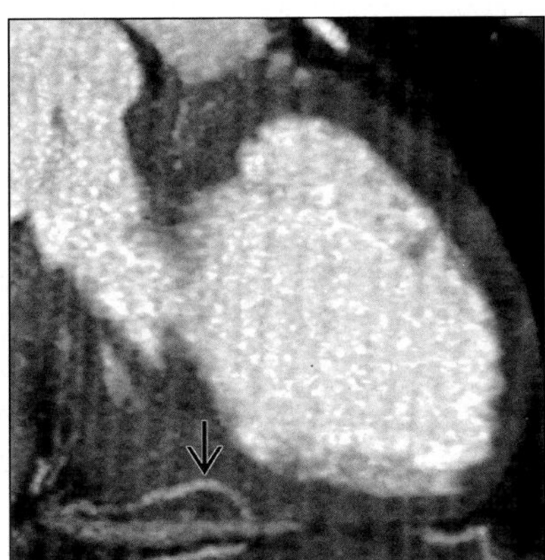
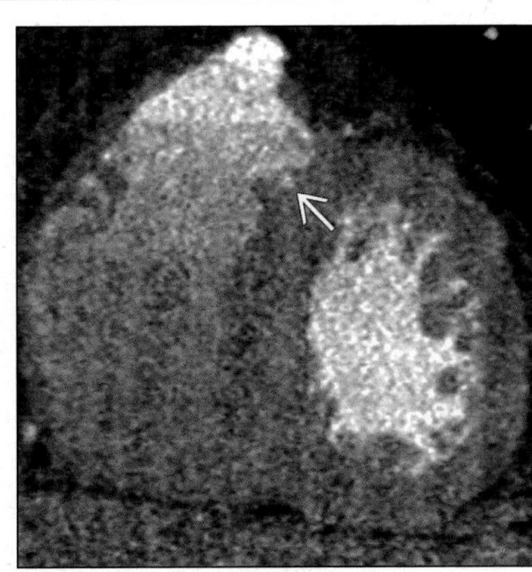

(Left) *Oblique coronary CTA shows a right coronary artery bridge ➔ which are much less common then left coronary artery bridges and usually occur in the mid segment.* ***(Center)*** *Coronary CTA shows a very uncommon posterior descending artery bridge ➔.* ***(Right)*** *Coronary CTA short axis view shows a deep myocardial mid segment LAD bridge ➔.*

CORONARY FISTULA

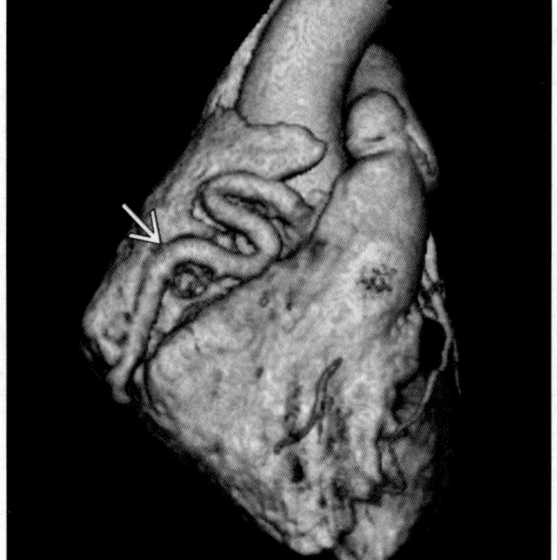

Anterior volume rendered view of a gated coronary CTA shows an enlarged and tortuous RCA ➡ in a patient with an incidental coronary fistula to the coronary sinus.

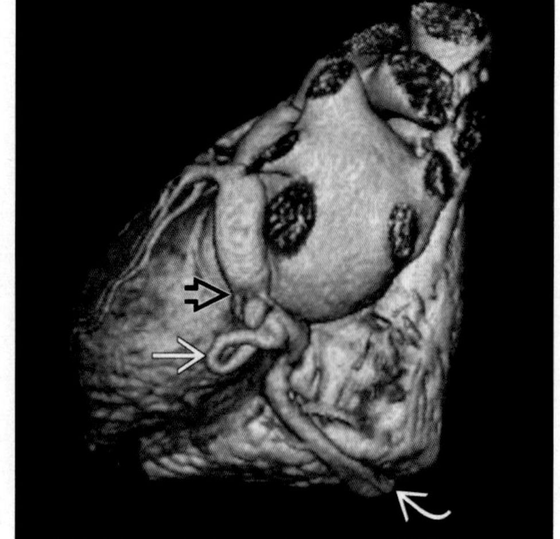

Inferior-posterior volume rendered view of gated coronary CTA in the same patient as previous shows enlarged distal RCA ➡ and its PLV branch ➡, which is very tortuous and connects to coronary sinus ⇨.

TERMINOLOGY

Abbreviations and Synonyms

- Coronary artery fistula
- Coronary cameral fistula
  - Abnormal direct connection between coronary artery and any cardiac chamber
- Coronary arteriovenous fistula (AV-fistula, AVF, CAVF)
  - Connection between coronary artery and pulmonary artery or coronary sinus or its tributaries

Definitions

- Abnormal connection between coronary artery branch and cardiac or vascular chambers without normal transition through capillary bed of the myocardium
  - May connect to pulmonary artery, coronary sinus, atria, or ventricles
- Usually congenital malformation, even though, rarely iatrogenic fistulas after biopsy, or traumatic fistulas may develop
- CAVFs are a differentiated from anomalous coronary artery origin from the pulmonary artery (Bland-White-Garland syndrome, ALCAPA, ARCAPA)
  - Main difference is that the abnormal vessel arises from the pulmonary artery, and no separate ostium from the aorta is identified

IMAGING FINDINGS

General Features

- Best diagnostic clue
  - Large tortuous vessels with abnormal connection to cardiac chamber, pulmonary artery or coronary venous system
    - Normal origins of coronary arteries from respective sinus of Valsalva
- Location
  - Connects a high pressure system (coronary artery) with low pressure system
    - Pulmonary artery
    - Right atrium
    - Right ventricle
    - Tricuspid annulus
    - Creat cardiac vein
    - Coronary sinus

DDx: Coronary Fistula

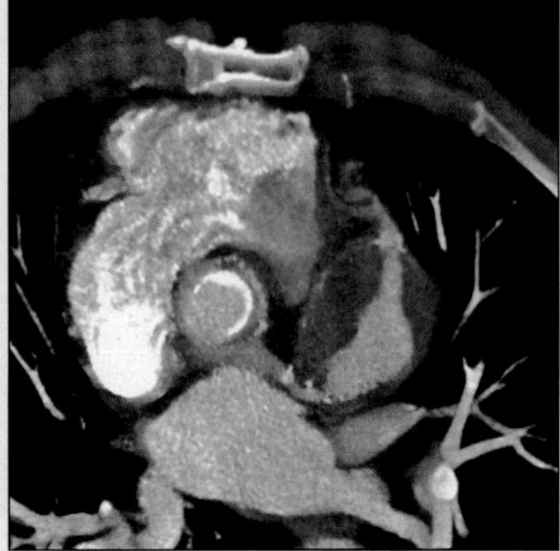

Coronary Aneurysm

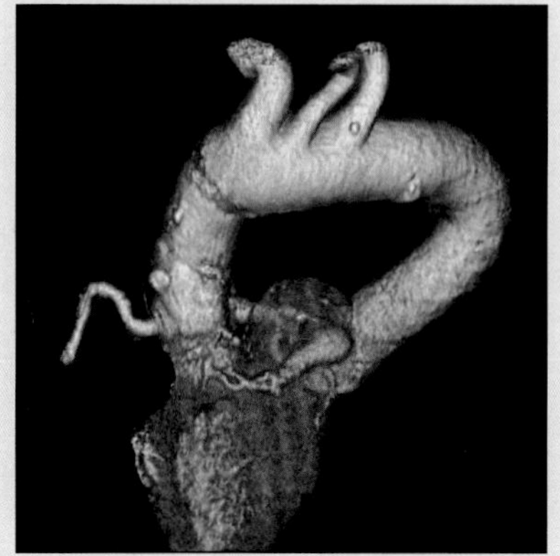

Coronary Aneurysm

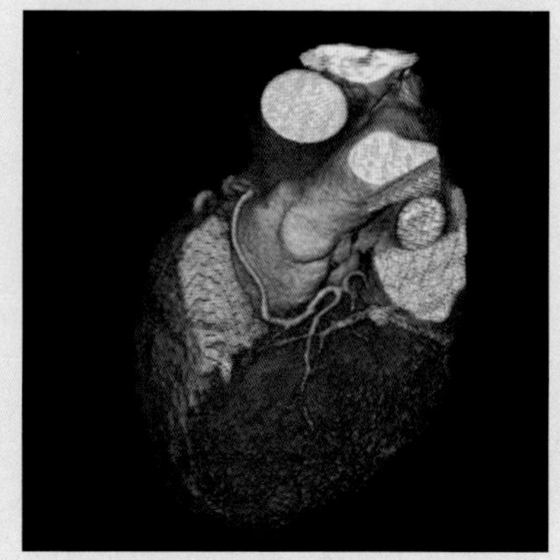

Anomalous Left Coronary Artery

CORONARY FISTULA

Key Facts

Terminology
- Coronary cameral fistula
  - Abnormal direct connection between coronary artery and any cardiac chamber
- Coronary arteriovenous fistula (AV-fistula, AVF, CAVF)
  - Connection between coronary artery and pulmonary artery or coronary sinus or its tributaries
- Usually congenital malformation, even though, rarely iatrogenic fistulas after biopsy, or traumatic fistulas may develop
- CAVFs are a differentiated from anomalous coronary artery origin from the pulmonary artery (Bland-White-Garland syndrome, ALCAPA, ARCAPA)

Imaging Findings
- Cardiac gated CT is excellent test to delineate number, size and anatomic course of feeding vessels

Top Differential Diagnoses
- Bland-White-Garland syndrome
  - Anomalous coronary artery origin from the pulmonary artery
  - Myocardial infarcts in infancy common

Pathology
- In larger angiographic series incidence of coronary artery fistula detected during diagnostic coronary angiography is 0.1%

Clinical Issues
- Treatment necessary only in larger fistulae

  - Feeders originate from right coronary arterial system in 55%, left coronary system in 35%, and both systems or other arteries in 10%
  - Within epicardial fat
    - May have feeders from bronchial or mediastinal arteries entering the epicardial fat space via the space between pericardial reflection and great vessel wall

Radiographic Findings
- Radiography
  - Usually normal
  - Rarely chamber enlargement

CT Findings
- Cardiac gated CT is excellent test to delineate number, size and anatomic course of feeding vessels
- Tortuous epicardial arterially enhancing vessels
  - Often multiple feeders identified
- Occasionally markedly enlarged and tortuous coronary arteries
- Drainage site is often identified
  - Jet of arterial density contrast into receiving chamber (lower HU) or coronary sinus may be appreciated
- Often aneurysmal dilatation immediately proximal to drainage site
- Rarely enlarged cardiac chambers from left to right shunting

MR Findings
- Findings similar to CT
  - CT superior in defining smaller feeders due to isovolumetric sub-millimeter spacial resolution and true volumetric imaging
- May detect late complications
  - Delayed enhanced imaging highly sensitive for non-transmural myocardial infarction

Echocardiographic Findings
- Enlarged feeding coronary artery
- Fistula drainage site demonstrates systolic and diastolic continuous turbulent flow pattern

Angiographic Findings
- Delineates size and detailed anatomy of fistulous vessels
- May potentially miss feeders that arise from unexpected locations
- Enables transcatheter coil embolization

Imaging Recommendations
- Best imaging tool: Cardiac gated CTA
- Protocol advice
  - Ensure field of view selection in z-dimension includes entire pulmonary artery
    - Avoid incomplete visualization of fistula
    - Typically cardiac CT start at mid pulmonary arterial level

DIFFERENTIAL DIAGNOSIS

Bland-White-Garland Syndrome
- Anomalous coronary artery origin from the pulmonary artery
  - Most commonly left coronary artery origin from pulmonary artery
- Large left to right shunt and steal phenomenon
- Often symptomatic in infancy
- Myocardial infarcts in infancy common
- May present in infancy with dyspnea and syncopes during feeding

Coronary Aneurysm
- No abnormal drainage into low pressure chamber
- No presence of "multiple feeders"

Anomalous Coronary Artery
- Abnormal origin of coronaries from sinus of Valsalva
- No abnormal "feeders"

PATHOLOGY

General Features
- Etiology

- Usually congenital malformation
    - Persistence of embryonic intertrabecular spaces and sinusoids
- May be iatrogenic (RV biopsy, pericardiocentesis, after septal myectomy, etc.) or due to other trauma
- May be complication of mycotic aneurysm

- Epidemiology
    - In larger angiographic series incidence of coronary artery fistula detected during diagnostic coronary angiography is 0.1%
        - Newer MDCT based detection of fistulas suggests higher incidence of smaller fistulas, but to date there are no published larger series

CLINICAL ISSUES

Presentation

- Most common signs/symptoms
    - Often asymptomatic if smaller fistula without significant steal
    - Depending on size of fistulas there is association with
        - Arrhythmias
        - Dyspnea
        - Congestive heart failure
        - Endocarditis
        - Angina pectoris if significant steal phenomenon
        - Myocardial infarction
- Other signs/symptoms
    - In pediatric population often presents as cardiac murmur
        - Lower to mid-left sternal border
        - Loud, superficial and continuous murmur
        - Maximal intensity of murmur relates to shunt entry site

Natural History & Prognosis

- Generally good, especially in smaller and moderate size fistula
    - Myocardial blood flow typically not compromised
- Rarely serious complications
    - Myocardial infarction
    - Pulmonary hypertension
    - Congestive heart failure
    - Tamponade due to rupture of coronary artery fistula is reported
- Rarely spontaneous closure

Treatment

- Treatment necessary only in larger fistulae
- Surgical ligation
    - Carries risk of myocardial infarction
- Catheter based interventions

DIAGNOSTIC CHECKLIST

Consider

- 3D volume rendered images helpful in delineating anatomy and identifying feeders
- If coronary fistula is suspected, ensure that scan range is extended superiorly to include aortic arch
    - Otherwise pulmonary fistula may be only partially visualized
    - Occasionally feeders from aortic arch can be present

SELECTED REFERENCES

1. Cowles RA et al: Bland-White-Garland syndrome of anomalous left coronary artery arising from the pulmonary artery (ALCAPA): a historical review. Pediatr Radiol. 37(9):890-895, 2007
2. Gulati GS et al: Utility of multislice computed tomography in the diagnosis of a right coronary artery fistula to the right atrium. J Postgrad Med. 53(3):191-2, 2007
3. Iwasawa Y et al: Cardiac tamponade due to rupture of coronary artery fistulas with a giant aneurysm containing a free floating ball thrombus: a case report. J Cardiol. 50(1):71-6, 2007
4. Kharouf R et al: Transcatheter closure of coronary artery fistula complicated by myocardial infarction. J Invasive Cardiol. 19(5):E146-9, 2007
5. Latson LA: Coronary artery fistulas: how to manage them. Catheter Cardiovasc Interv. 70(1):110-6, 2007
6. Oncel D et al: An Aneurysmal Left Circumflex Artery-to-Right Atrium Fistula in a Patient with Ischemic Symptoms: Accurate Diagnosis with Dual-Source CT Angiography. Cardiovasc Intervent Radiol. 2007
7. Gowda RM et al: Coronary artery fistulas: clinical and therapeutic considerations. Int J Cardiol. 107(1):7-10, 2006
8. Luo L et al: Coronary artery fistulae. Am J Med Sci. 332(2):79-84, 2006
9. Takahashi Y et al: Successful surgical treatment of a mycotic right coronary artery aneurysm complicated by a fistula to the right atrium. Jpn J Thorac Cardiovasc Surg. 53(12):661-4, 2005
10. Friedman WF et al: Diseases of the Heart, Pericardium and Pulmonary Vascular Bed. In: Braunwald E, Zipes DP, Libby P. Heart Disease 6th Ed. WB Saunders Company, Philadelphia. 1505-91, 2001
11. Vavuranakis M et al: Coronary artery fistulas in adults: incidence, angiographic characteristics, natural history. Cathet Cardiovasc Diagn. 35(2):116-20, 1995
12. Sarkis A et al: [Left coronaro-ventricular fistula after septal myectomy] Arch Mal Coeur Vaiss. 85(4):457-60, 1992

CORONARY FISTULA

IMAGE GALLERY

Typical

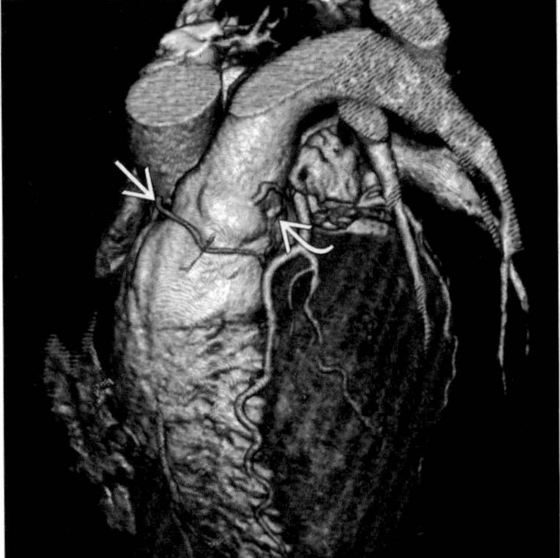

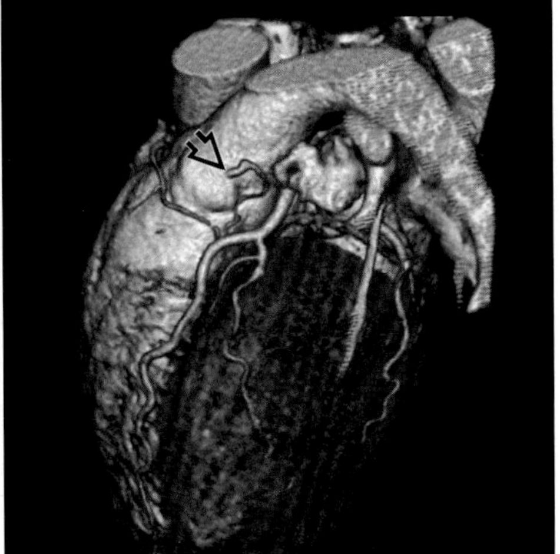

(Left) *Oblique volume rendered view of a gated coronary CTA shows multiple small tortuous RCA → and LAD fistula feeders → running at the surface of the pulmonary trunk.* ***(Right)*** *Left lateral oblique volume rendered coronary CTA in the same patient as previous image shows the fistulous connection to pulmonary trunk →.*

Typical

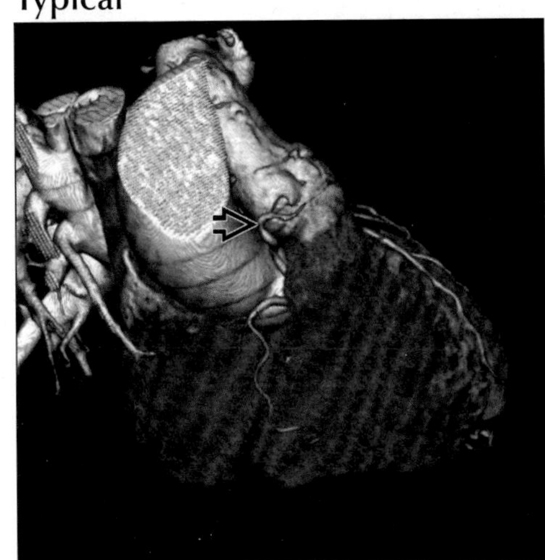

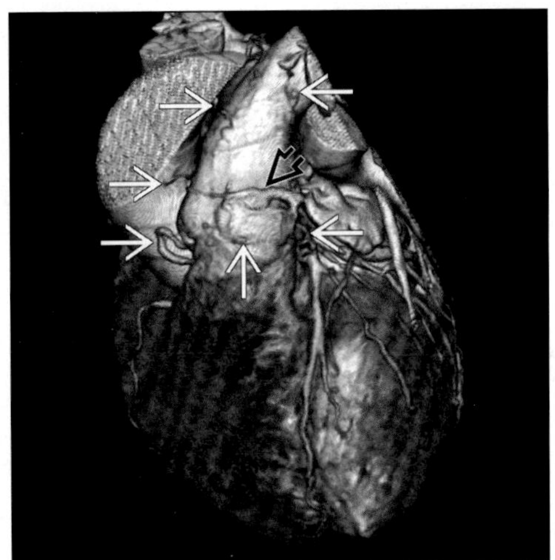

(Left) *Right lateral oblique volume rendered coronary CTA shows an enlarged conus branch →, giving rise to fistula feeders.* ***(Right)*** *Oblique volume rendered coronary CTA in the same patient as previous image shows multiple additional feeders → including extra-cardiac vessels from the mediastinum and aorta. Note: Site of fistulous connection →.*

Variant

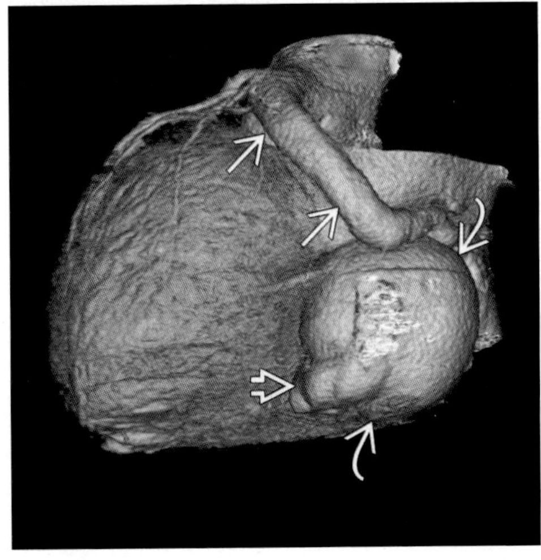

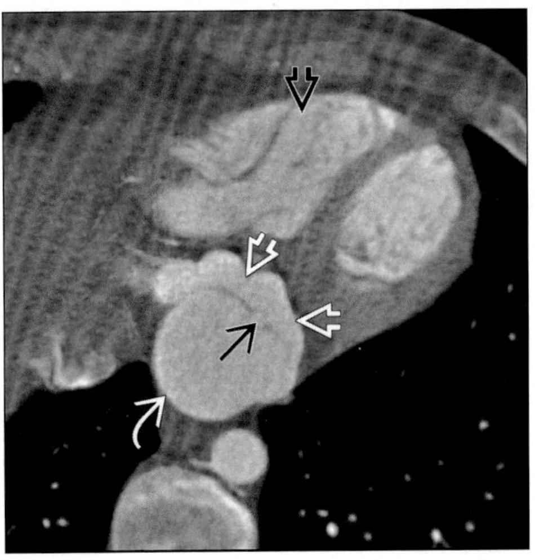

(Left) *Oblique coronary CTA shows a markedly enlarged LCX → with distal aneurysm → due to LCX to coronary sinus (CS) fistula. Note: Distal CS demonstrates arterial enhancement →.* ***(Right)*** *Oblique coronary CTA shows an enlarged, contrast-filled CS →, and a distal LCX aneurysm →. Note: Fistulous connection of aneurysm to CS →, and unusually homogeneous enhancement of RV → due to contrast shunting.*

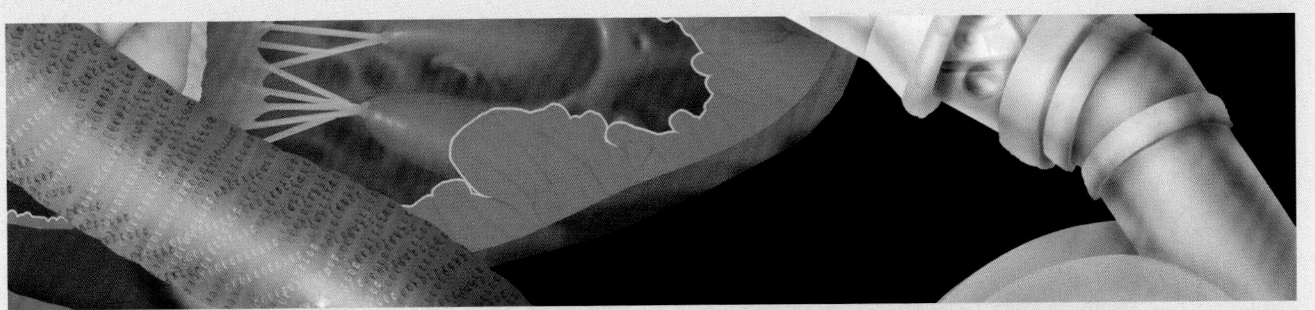

SECTION 7: Heart Failure

RIGHT HEART FAILURE

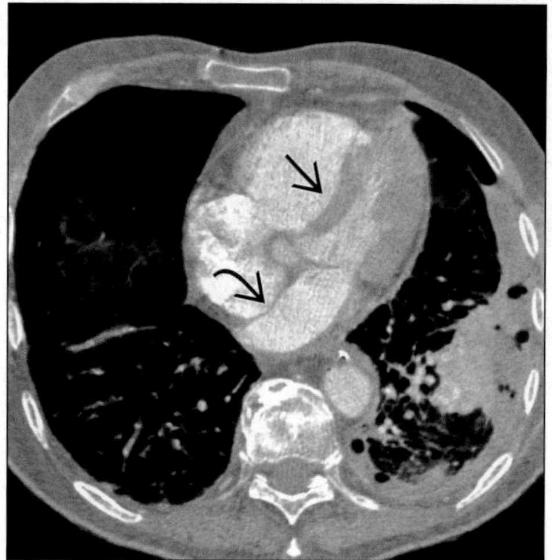

Axial CECT shows dilated right atrium and ventricle with bowing of ventricular ➔ and atrial ➔ septa towards the left. Note chronic lung disease.

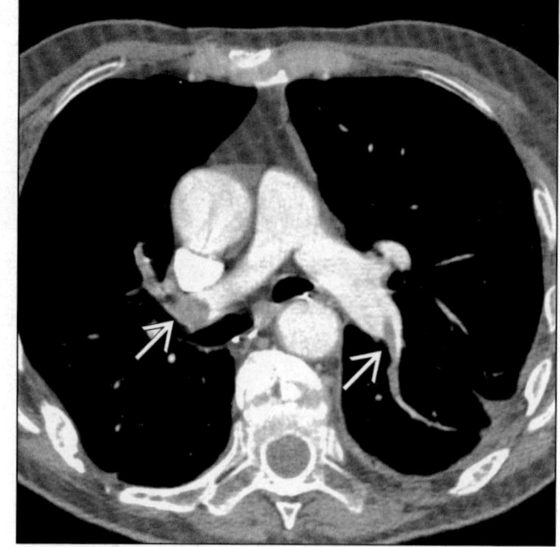

Axial CECT in same patient as previous image, shows extensive pulmonary embolism ➔ which has caused acute right ventricular failure.

TERMINOLOGY

Definitions

- Cor pulmonale = right ventricular (RV) failure due to pulmonary disease

IMAGING FINDINGS

Radiographic Findings

- Radiography: Chest radiograph classically demonstrates right-sided cardiomegaly and elevated central venous volume (large azygous vein)

CT Findings

- Dilated RV, right atrium (RA) and systemic veins
- Contrast refluxing into enlarged hepatic veins
- Cardiac-gated CT may demonstrate decreased RV function

MR Findings

- MR superior to echocardiography for assessing RV function
- Decreased ejection fraction from systolic dysfunction or decreased compliance from diastolic dysfunction
- Short-axis cine-white blood (SSFP) imaging optimal for assessing RV mass and thickness
- Normal RV functional parameters
  - RV end-diastolic volume 138 ± 40 mL
  - RV end-systolic volume 54 ± 21 mL
  - RV free wall mass 46 ± 11 gm (26 ± 5 gm/m²)
  - RV ejection fraction (%) = 61 ± 7
  - RV stroke volume = 84 ± 24 mL (46 ± 8 mL/m²)
- Right atrial pressure estimated by size of IVC
  - Small (< 1.5 cm) → 0-5 mmHg
  - Normal (1.5-2.5 cm) → 5-15 mmHg
  - Dilated (> 2.5 cm) → 15-20 mmHg
  - Dilated + enlarged hepatic veins → > 20 mmHg

Echocardiographic Findings

- Echocardiogram
  - RV function often difficult to assess on echo due to limited acoustic window
  - RV systolic dysfunction
  - Decreased RV outflow tract acceleration time
  - Tricuspid regurgitation, pulmonary regurgitation
  - Dilated inferior vena cava (IVC) and hepatic veins

DDx: Right Ventricular Failure

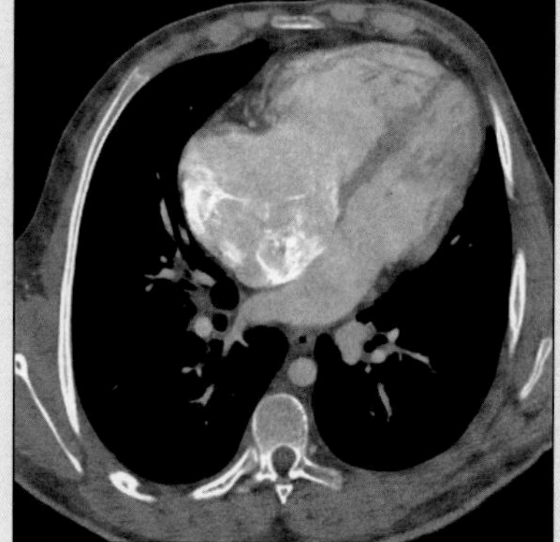

Ebstein Anomaly

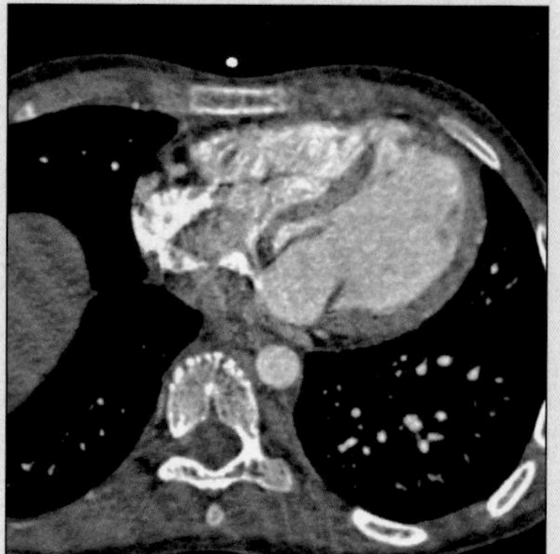

Ventricular Septal Defect

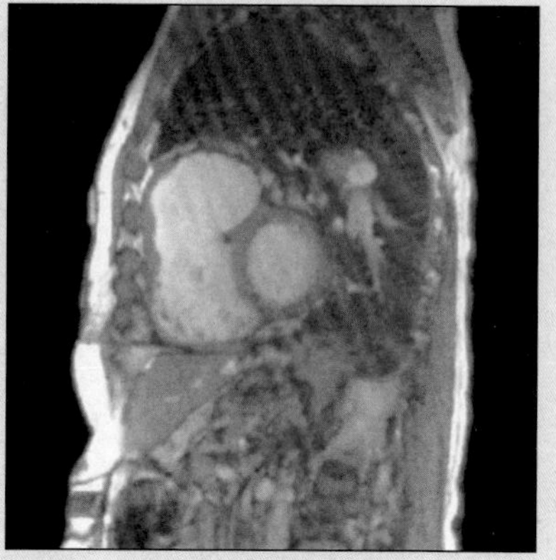

Tetralogy of Fallot

RIGHT HEART FAILURE

Key Facts

Terminology

- Cor pulmonale = right ventricular (RV) failure due to pulmonary disease

Imaging Findings

- Chest radiograph classically demonstrates right-sided cardiomegaly and elevated central venous volume (large azygous vein)
- Cardiac-gated CT may demonstrate decreased RV function
- MR superior to echocardiography for assessing RV function

Pathology

- Most common cause is left heart failure

Clinical Issues

- Associated with lower extremity edema, ascites, weight gain

DIFFERENTIAL DIAGNOSIS

Non-Cardiogenic Edema

- Endstage liver disease with ascites and pleural effusions, renal disease

Isolated Left Heart Failure

- Typically pulmonary symptoms predominate

PATHOLOGY

General Features

- General path comments: Typically pattern is left ventricular failure resulting in RV failure from chronic overload
- Etiology
  - Most common cause is left heart failure
  - Pulmonic or tricuspid valve disease
  - Shunts
- Epidemiology
  - Very common result of left heart failure
  - Major source of morbidity and mortality

Gross Pathologic & Surgical Features

- Often dilated/hypertrophied right ventricle
- May see hypertrophied right atrium

Staging, Grading or Classification Criteria

- Class I: No limitation during ordinary activity
- Class II: Slight limitation by shortness of breath ± fatigue during moderate exertion
- Class III: Symptoms with minimal exertion that interfere with normal daily activity
- Class IV: Inability to carry out physical activity; patients typically have marked neurohumoral activation, muscle wasting, and reduced oxygen consumption

CLINICAL ISSUES

Presentation

- Most common signs/symptoms: Associated with lower extremity edema, ascites, weight gain
- Likely concomitant pulmonary symptoms

Natural History & Prognosis

- Depends on New York Heart Association class
- Often difficult to treat due to volume overload

Treatment

- Diuretics, Inotropics agents, ACE inhibitors, Beta blockers
- Treat underlying coronary disease

SELECTED REFERENCES

1. Braunwald E et al: Heart Disease: A Textbook of Cardiovascular Medicine. 6th Ed. W.B. Saunders Co., Philadelphia, 1751-83, 2001
2. Goldman L et al: Cecil Textbook of Medicine. 21st Ed. W.B. Saunders Co., Philadelphia, 207-26, 2000

IMAGE GALLERY

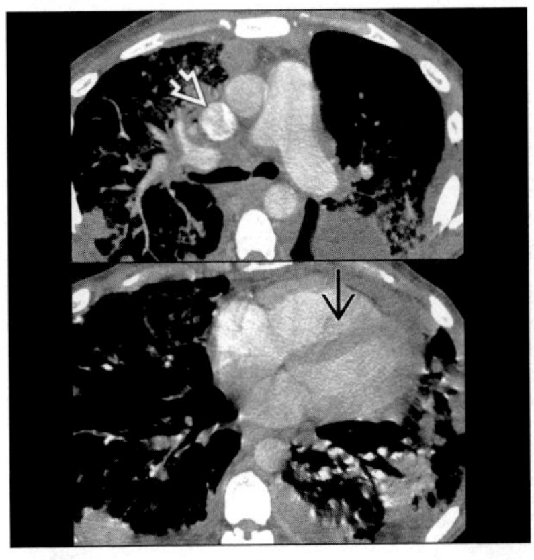

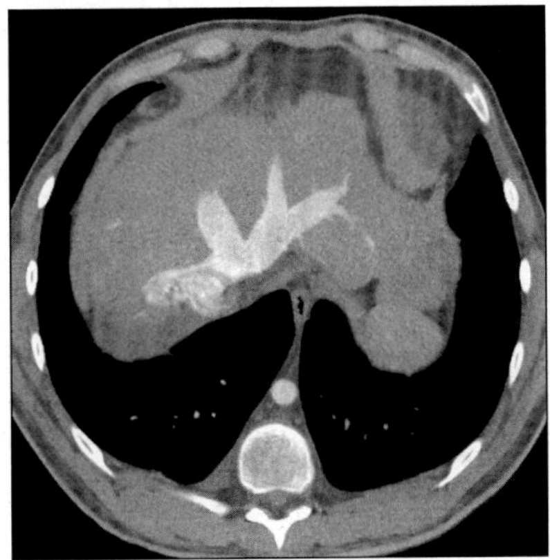

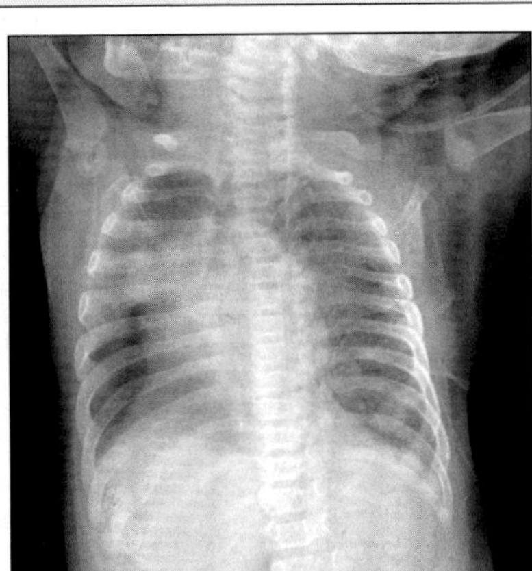

(Left) *Axial CECT shows enlarged superior vena cava ⯈ and flattening of the ventricular septum ⇒ in a patient with chronic lung disease (lymphoma) with secondary cor pulmonale.* ***(Center)*** *Axial CECT shows enlarged hepatic veins with reflux of contrast due to chronic right ventricular failure.* ***(Right)*** *Anteroposterior radiograph shows infant with chronic lung disease and enlarged right heart border due to cor pulmonale.*

LEFT HEART FAILURE

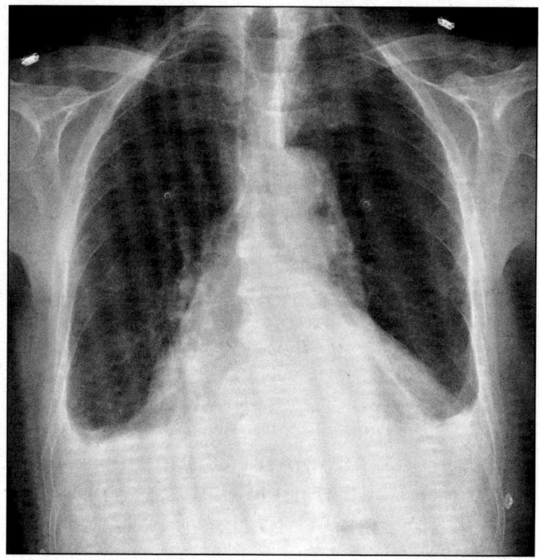

Posteroanterior radiograph shows cardiomegaly, pleural effusions, peribronchial cuffing and mild interstitial edema in patient undergoing treatment for LV failure.

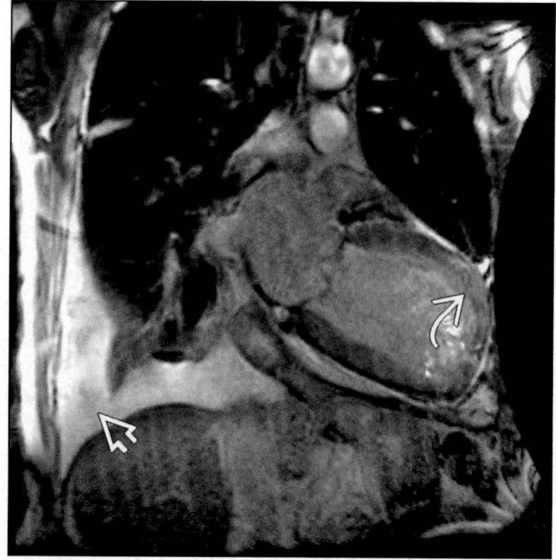

Long axis SSFP in same patient shows dilated LA and LV cavity with increased myocardial signal ➚ in anterior wall suggesting edema. Note pleural effusion ➾. (Corresponding delayed enhanced MR, next image).

TERMINOLOGY

Abbreviations and Synonyms

- Congestive heart failure (CHF), heart failure (HF)
- Left ventricular failure (LV failure)
- Cardiac failure
  - Often used synonymously with left heart failure, but LV failure should be differentiated from biventricular failure and right ventricular failure

Definitions

- Physiologic state where left ventricle is unable to pump at rate necessary to meet oxygen consumption needs of end organ tissue
- Systolic dysfunction refers to a decrease in myocardial contractility
- With pure diastolic heart failure, left ventricular end-systolic volume and stroke volume are preserved; there is, however, an abnormal decrease in left ventricular diastolic distensibility

IMAGING FINDINGS

General Features

- Best diagnostic clue: Cardiomegaly with pulmonary venous hypertension (Kerley lines, redistribution, pulmonary edema, effusion)

Radiographic Findings

- Radiography
  - Chest radiograph demonstrates enlarged cardiac silhouette with pulmonary edema and possibly pleural effusions
  - Increased pulmonary artery to bronchus ratio
  - Peribronchial cuffing
  - Pulmonary venous redistribution (larger apical veins, smaller basal veins) (pulmonary venous pressure = 18-23 mmHg)
  - Kerley B lines (pulmonary venous pressure = 20-25 mmHg)
  - Alveolar edema with "butterfly" or "batwing" distribution ± effusions (pulmonary venous pressure > 25 mmHg)
  - Edema shifts with patient positioning

DDx: Left Heart Failure

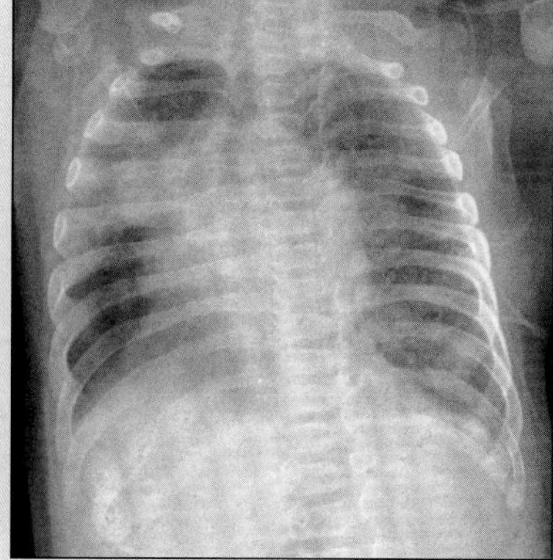

Cor Pulmonale

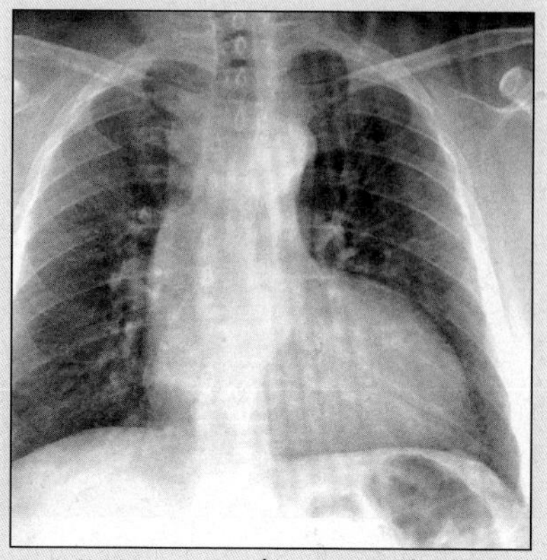

LV Hypertrophy w/o Failure

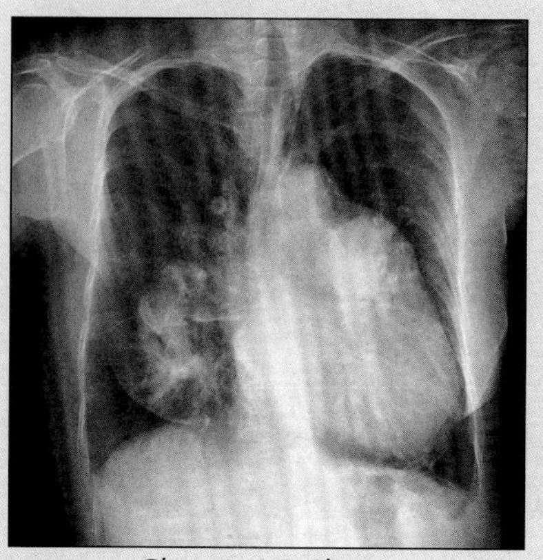

Chronic L-R Shunt

LEFT HEART FAILURE

Key Facts

Terminology

- Physiologic state where left ventricle is unable to pump at rate necessary to meet oxygen consumption needs of end organ tissue
- Systolic dysfunction refers to a decrease in myocardial contractility
- With pure diastolic heart failure, left ventricular end-systolic volume and stroke volume are preserved; there is, however, an abnormal decrease in left ventricular diastolic distensibility

Imaging Findings

- Chest radiograph demonstrates enlarged cardiac silhouette with pulmonary edema and possibly pleural effusions
- Pulmonary venous redistribution (larger apical veins, smaller basal veins) (pulmonary venous pressure = 18-23 mmHg)
- Kerley B lines (pulmonary venous pressure = 20-25 mmHg)
- Alveolar edema with "butterfly" or "batwing" distribution ± effusions (pulmonary venous pressure > 25 mmHg)
- Edema shifts with patient positioning
- Azygos, SVC and IVC distention if biventricular or RV failure
- Thickening of interlobular septa
- Bronchovascular bundle thickening

  - Cardiopulmonary ratio = transverse diameter of cardiac silhouette divided by transverse diameter of inner ribcage at level of diaphragms
  - Azygos, SVC and IVC distention if biventricular or RV failure

CT Findings

- NECT: Enlarged hilar nodes (mildly)
- HRCT
  - Thickening of interlobular septa
  - Bronchovascular bundle thickening
  - Ground glass or airspace opacities, most prominent in dependent portions of lungs
- Cardiac Gated CTA
  - May demonstrate underlying cardiac cause of failure
    - Myocardial infarction (thinning, calcification, fatty metaplasia, subendocardial perfusion defects)
    - LV dilatation
    - Mitral valve disorders
    - Shunts
    - Coronary artery disease

MR Findings

- Functional findings similar to echocardiography, but MR more precise in quantifying myocardial functional parameters (i.e., stroke volume, ejection fraction)
- Delayed contrast-enhanced MR may also be used to identify viable and non-viable myocardial tissue
- Viability on MR may be used to predict response to beta-blocker therapy and revascularization
- May demonstrate and characterize nonischemic causes of LV failure
  - Dilated or hypertrophic cardiomyopathies
  - Takatsubo disease
  - Myocarditis
  - Infiltrative cardiomyopathies
  - Masses

Nuclear Medicine Findings

- Radionuclide ventriculography alternative diagnostic test to evaluate LV function per ACC/AHA Chronic Heart Failure Evaluation and Management Guidelines

Echocardiographic Findings

- Echocardiogram
  - Echocardiography coupled with Doppler flow studies is most useful diagnostic test in evaluation of HF patients (per American College of Cardiology/ American Heart Association (ACC/AHA) Chronic Heart Failure Evaluation and Management Guidelines)
    - Determine LV function
    - Abnormalities of pericardium, myocardium, and valves
  - Findings variable depending on etiology
  - Decreased ejection fraction with systolic dysfunction
  - Decreased compliance with diastolic dysfunction

DIFFERENTIAL DIAGNOSIS

Etiology of Left Heart Failure

- Ischemic
- Restrictive
- Constrictive
- Infiltrative disease

Pneumonia

- Atypical pneumonia may have diffuse air space disease/interstitial markings on chest radiograph

Pericardial Effusion

- Enlarged cardiac silhouette on chest radiograph

PATHOLOGY

General Features

- Genetics: Some component of inheritance for dilated cardiomyopathy and idiopathic hypertrophic subaortic stenosis (IHSS) leading to left heart failure
- Etiology
  - Three major determinants of the left ventricular forward stroke volume/performance are the preload, myocardial contractility, and the afterload

  - Left atrium appears to adapt to left ventricular dysfunction in patients with CHF
  - Causes of CHF include
    - Myocardial ischemia or infarction
    - Arrhythmias
    - Systemic infection
    - Myocarditis
    - Nonischemic cardiomyopathies
    - Congenital AV fistula
    - Congenital heart disease
    - Papillary muscle rupture pericardial effusion
    - High output states: Anemia, pregnancy, valvular heart disease
- Epidemiology: One of the leading causes of death in the United States

Gross Pathologic & Surgical Features

- Often areas of infarcted myocardium in systolic dysfunction
- Myocyte hypertrophy vs. chamber enlargement

Microscopic Features

- Infarcted areas of myocardium in ischemic heart failure
- Infiltrating diseases in restrictive cardiomyopathy

Staging, Grading or Classification Criteria

- New York Heart Association (NYHA) Classification
  - Class I: No limitation during ordinary activity
  - Class II: Comfortable at rest; slight limitation by shortness of breath, palpitation, dyspnea, or angina during ordinary physical activity
  - Class III: Comfortable at rest; symptoms with minimal exertion that interfere with normal daily activity
  - Class IV: Inability to carry out any physical activity; these patients typically have marked neurohumoral activation, muscle wasting, and reduced peak oxygen consumption
- Framingham classification requires 2 major criteria or 1 major and 2 minor criteria for diagnosis of CHF
- Major criteria
  - Cardiomegaly on radiograph
  - Pulmonary edema
  - Jugular vein distention
  - Hepatojugular reflux
  - Rales
  - Nocturnal dyspnea
  - S3 gallop
  - Elevated central venous pressure > 16 cm H2O
  - Circulation time of 25 seconds
  - Weight loss with treatment (> = 4.5 kg/5 treatment days)
- Minor criteria
  - Pleural effusion
  - Bilateral ankle edema
  - Dyspnea with ordinary activity
  - Hepatomegaly
  - Decreased vital capacity
  - Tachycardia (> = 120 bpm)
  - Nocturnal cough

CLINICAL ISSUES

Presentation

- Most common signs/symptoms
  - Dyspnea on exertion
  - Shortness of breath
  - Jugular vein distention
  - Pulmonary rales
  - Cough
  - Orthopnea
  - Tachycardia
- Other signs/symptoms
  - Nocturia
  - Fatigue
  - Cerebral symptoms: Confusion, memory loss
  - Ascites
  - Edema
  - Pleural effusions

Demographics

- Age
  - Can affect any age
  - Frequency parallels that of underlying etiology
- Gender: M = F

Natural History & Prognosis

- Depending on NYHA class
- Depends on NYHA class
- Prognosis worsens with increasing NYHA class

Treatment

- Diuretics
- Inotropics agents
- ACE inhibitors
- Beta blockers
- Treat underlying coronary disease

DIAGNOSTIC CHECKLIST

Consider

- Pulmonary venous redistribution and azygos vein diameter may not be evaluable on non-upright radiographs

Image Interpretation Pearls

- RV or biventricular failure can be differentiated from LV failure by presence (RV failure) or absence (at least no severe RV failure) of distended systemic veins (IVC,SVC,azygos vein) on radiograph, CT, or MR

SELECTED REFERENCES

1. Braunwald E et al: Heart Disease: A Textbook of Cardiovascular Medicine. 6th Ed. W.B. Saunders Co., 1751-83, 2001
2. Goldman L et al: Cecil Textbook of Medicine. 21st Ed. W.B. Saunders Co., 207-26, 2000
3. American College of Cardiology/American Heart Association Chronic Heart Failure Evaluation and Management Guidelines: Relevance to the Geriatric Practice Journal of the American Geriatrics Society 51 (1), 123-126.

IMAGE GALLERY

Typical

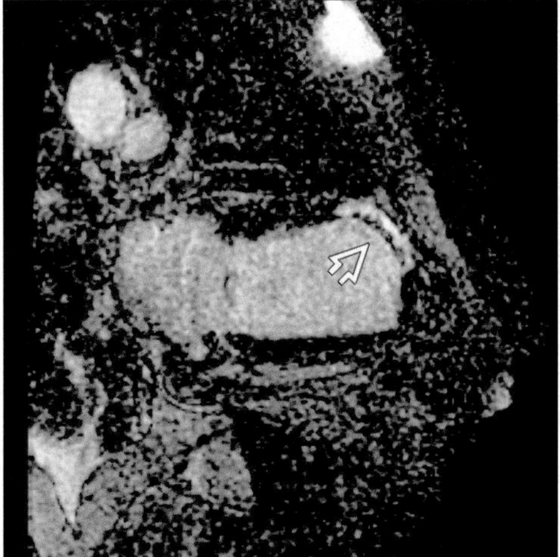

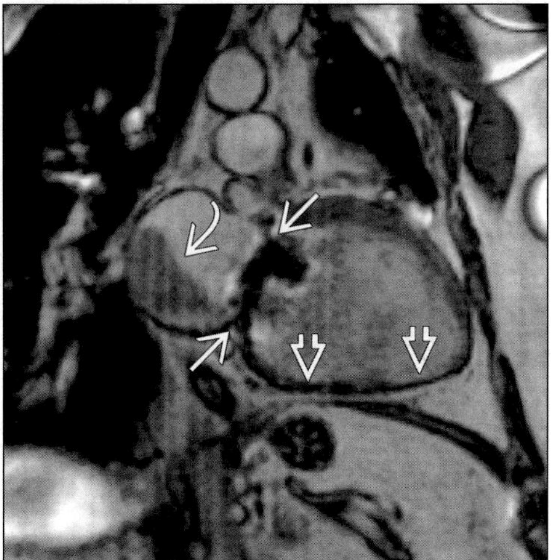

(Left) *Long axis vertical delayed enhanced MR in same patient as previous image shows area of abnormal hyperenhancement with some non-reperfusion* ⇨*, confirming acute myocardial infarction as underlying cause for LV failure.* ***(Right)*** *Long axis SSFP shows dilated RA and RV, mitral valve prosthesis* ➡*, RA thrombus* ↪*, and LV inferior wall thinning due to MI* ⇨ *(same patient as next two radiographs).*

Typical

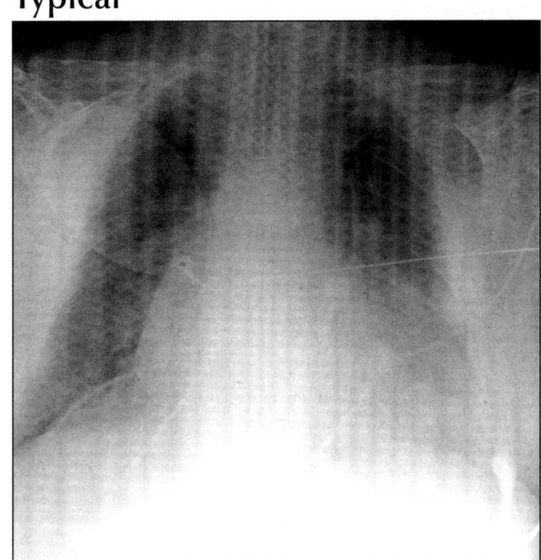

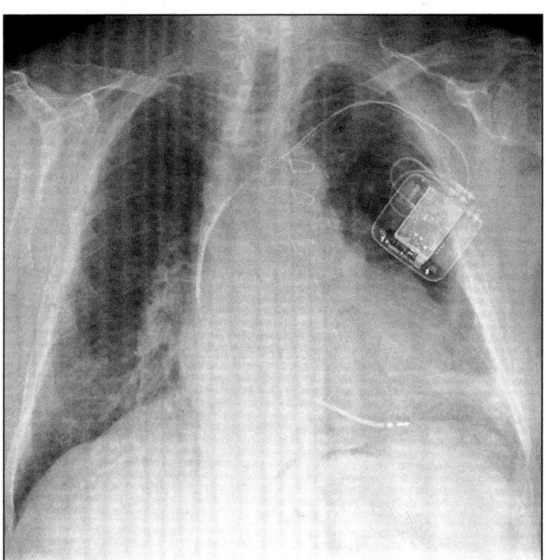

(Left) *Anteroposterior radiograph shows cardiomegaly, PVH and small effusion due to acute arrhythmia in a patient with remote MI. Note percutaneous pacemaker pads.* ***(Right)*** *Anteroposterior radiograph after thrombolysis and treatment of arrhythmia and ICD placement shows ongoing cardiomegaly, but decreased PVH and effusions. Significant clinical interval improvement.*

Typical

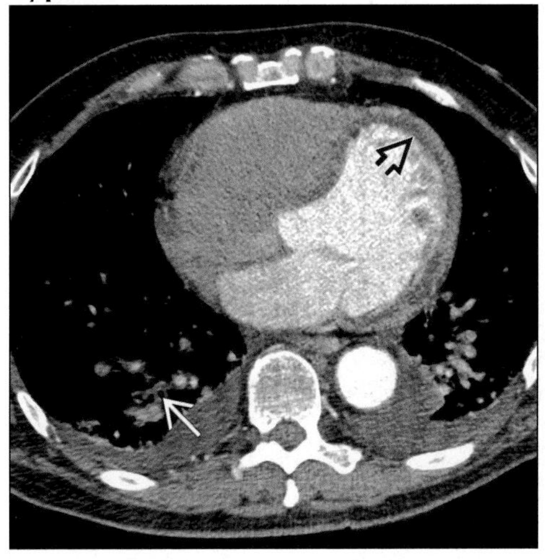

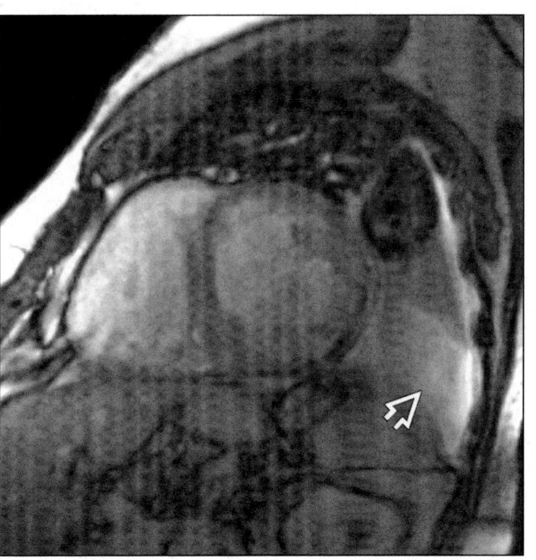

(Left) *Axial CECT shows bilateral pleural effusions, interstitial edema with bronchial cuffing* ➡ *and dilated LV with subendocardial rest perfusion defect* ⇨ *in a patient with LV failure due to ischemic cardiomyopathy.* ***(Right)*** *LV short axis SSFP systolic frame in the same patient as previous image shows left ventricular failure due to ischemic dilated cardiomyopathy with markedly enlarged end systolic volume. Note pleural effusion* ⇨.

HEART TRANSPLANT

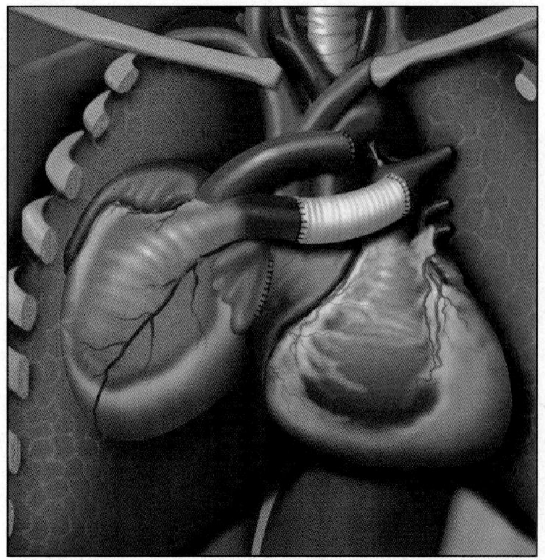

Graphic shows heterotopic heart transplant where the native RV provides the majority of right-side cardiac output and the donor LV provides the bulk of the left side cardiac output.

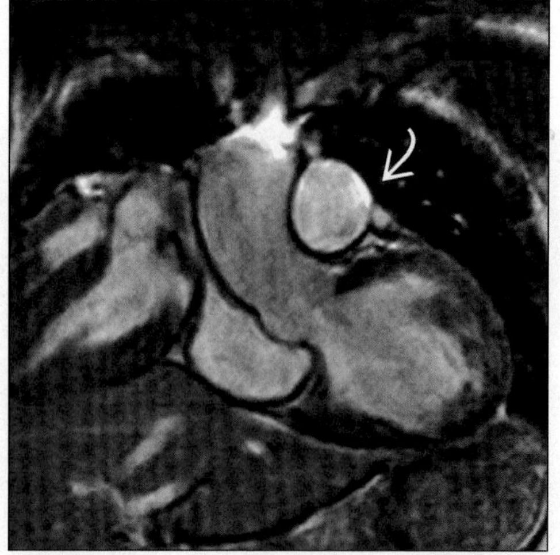

Coronal cardiac MR cine shows heterotopic heart transplant with native heart demonstrating dilated LV and MPA ➔ and transplanted heart on the right with preserved systolic function.

TERMINOLOGY

Definitions

- Most effective therapy for treatment of end-stage congestive heart failure
- Most common complications of cardiac transplantation
  - Infection
  - Rejection
  - Accelerated coronary artery atherosclerosis
  - Posttransplantation lymphoproliferative disease

IMAGING FINDINGS

General Features

- Best diagnostic clue
  - Cardiac allograft can be placed in an orthotopic or heterotopic position
  - Orthotopic heart transplant is the most common procedure
    - Recipient's heart is removed through a median sternotomy
    - Donor heart joined to receipt's atria, aorta and pulmonary artery
  - Heterotopic heart transplant is performed more rarely
    - Used for patients with severe pulmonary arterial hypertension

Imaging Recommendations

- Best imaging tool
  - Cardiac MR is best modality to identify transplant rejection, LV and RV failure
  - Coronary CTA and IVUS are best modalities to directly visualize accelerated coronary atherosclerosis
  - Serial echocardiograms are used to assess left and right ventricular function
  - Increased cardiac uptake on Gallium-67 scintigraphic in patients with moderate to severe transplant rejection
- Protocol advice
  - Delayed-enhancement and T2WI should always be part of the cardiac MR protocol

DDx: Complications of Heart Transplant

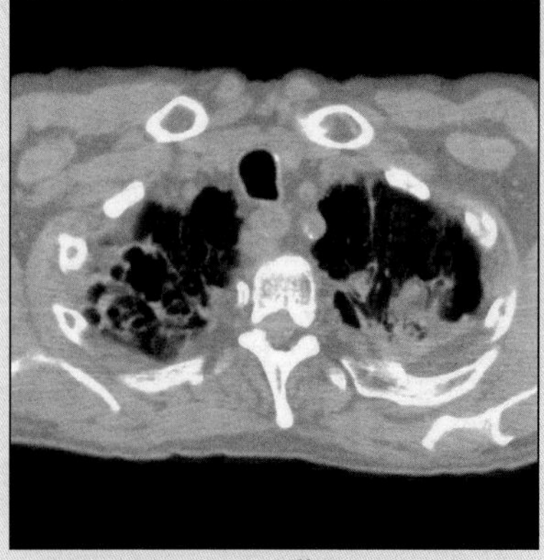

Aspergillosis

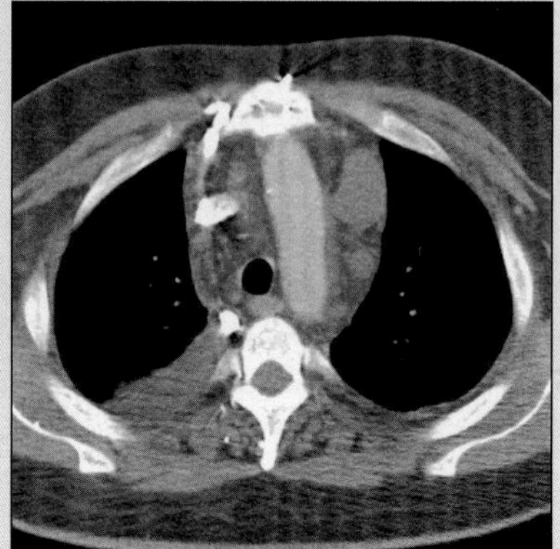

Lymphoma

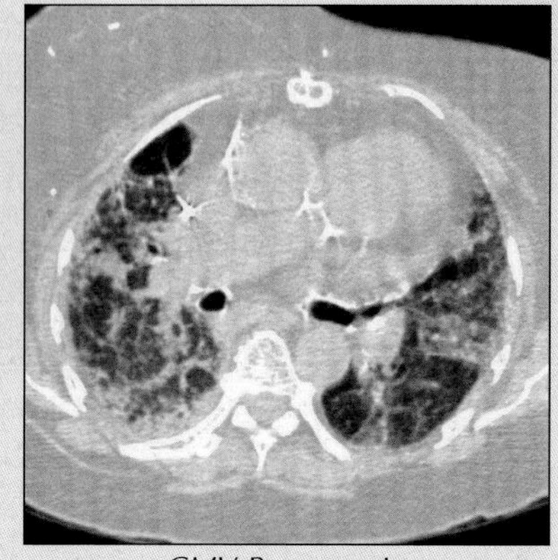

CMV Pneumonia

HEART TRANSPLANT

Key Facts

Terminology
- Most effective therapy for treatment of end-stage congestive heart failure

Imaging Findings
- Cardiac allograft can be placed in an orthotopic or heterotopic position
- Orthotopic heart transplant is the most common procedure
- Cardiac MR is best modality to identify transplant rejection, LV and RV failure
- Coronary CTA and IVUS are best modalities to directly visualize accelerated coronary atherosclerosis
- Delayed-enhancement and T2WI should always be part of the cardiac MR protocol

Top Differential Diagnoses
- Later infections are commonly caused by viruses (CMV) and opportunistic fungi (Pneumocystis, Candida, and Aspergillus)
- Rejection usually occurs between 2 weeks and 3 months after transplantation
- Pathophysiology of transplant vasculopathy: Concentric (not eccentric, like traditional CAD) hyperplasia with intimal proliferation of the vessels
- Incidence of any malignancy is 35% by 10 years

Clinical Issues
- Graft failure and infectious disease are leading causes of death in the first year after surgery
- Major complications in late post-operative stage: Coronary artery disease and neoplastic disease

        - Hyperenhancement in delayed images represent myocardial necrosis (rejection if early stage and transplant vasculopathy if subendocardial and late stage)
        - T2WI can demonstrate T2 prolongation in the myocardium consistent with myocardial edema
- Chest radiography
    - Enlarged cardiac silhouette
    - Pericardial effusions
    - Double right atria contour (overlap of donor and recipient right atria)
    - Pneumomediastinum; pneumothorax; pneumopericardium
    - Subcutaneous emphysema
    - Mediastinal fluid collections
- Computed tomography
    - High and redundant MPA
    - Space between SVC and ascending aorta and space between aorta and MPA
    - Aortic and MPA anastomosis
    - Atrial waist due to anastomosis of the right and left donor and recipient atria
    - Vertical atrioventricular groove

DIFFERENTIAL DIAGNOSIS

Infection
- First month of transplantation: Pseudomonas aeruginosa, Staphylococcus aureus, Enterococci, and Enterobacteriaceae
- Later infections are commonly caused by viruses (CMV) and opportunistic fungi (Pneumocystis, Candida, and Aspergillus)
- Aspergillus infection: Isolated pulmonary nodular disease, upper lobe predilection and associated with cavitations
- Mediastinitis: Mediastinal fluid collections, air inclusions and focal contrast-enhancement

Allograft Rejection
- Lymphocytic infiltration of the myocardium with myocyte necrosis
- Rejection usually occurs between 2 weeks and 3 months after transplantation
- Most cases of acute cellular rejection are diagnosed by endomyocardial biopsy when the patient is asymptomatic
- Symptoms are manifestations of LV dysfunction such as dyspnea, paroxysmal nocturnal dyspnea, orthopnea, palpitations, and syncope

Transplant Vasculopathy
- Incidence is approximately 9% at one year, 32% at five years and 46% at eight years
- High mortality rate: 3.8% in one year and 13% more than one year
- Pathophysiology of transplant vasculopathy: Concentric (not eccentric, like traditional CAD) hyperplasia with intimal proliferation of the vessels
- Diffuse process, starts with small, distal vessels and spreads to all coronary arteries
- Exacerbation of vascular disease with hyperlipidemia, hypertension, diabetes, and steroid use
- Diagnosis is difficult because heart transplantation patients have denervation of hearts and rarely present with chest pain
- Due to lack of symptoms, cardiac catheterization with IVUS are performed on an annual basis to monitor for coronary allograft vasculopathy
- 64-slice MDCT provides moderate to good test characteristics for the detection of transplant vasculopathy when compared to IVUS as the reference standard

Neoplastic Disease
- Incidence of any malignancy is 35% by 10 years
- Most common tumors
    - Skin cancer: Squamous cell/basal cell cancers/melanomas
    - Non-Hodgkin and Hodgkin lymphoma
    - Kaposi sarcoma
    - In situ carcinomas of the uterine cervix
    - Anogenital cancers

HEART TRANSPLANT

PATHOLOGY

General Features

- Etiology
  - Disease processes that require transplantation
    - Non-ischemic cardiomyopathy - 46%
    - Ischemic cardiomyopathy: 42%
    - Valvular disease: 3%
    - Adult congenital heart disease: 2%
    - Miscellaneous causes: 7%
- Epidemiology
  - Over 2,000 cardiac transplants are performed in the United States each year
  - First successful heart transplantation was performed in 1967
  - Over 73,000 cardiac transplantations have been performed worldwide

CLINICAL ISSUES

Presentation

- Most common signs/symptoms
  - Early disease is defined when it occurs less than one year after surgery
    - Graft failure and infectious disease are leading causes of death in the first year after surgery
    - Infectious disease accounts for almost 33% of the deaths in the first year
    - Acute rejection accounts for 12% of deaths
  - Major complications in late post-operative stage: Coronary artery disease and neoplastic disease

Natural History & Prognosis

- One-year survival of heart transplant recipients is over 80% with the 10-year survival rate approaching 50%
- Graft half-life for a combined group of adult and pediatric heart recipients is currently 9.9 years
- Improvement in early survival statistics due to
  - Establishing recipient selection criteria
  - Use of endomyocardial biopsy to diagnose rejection
  - Improvements in immunosuppression techniques

Treatment

- Re-transplantation occurs in 2% of cases

DIAGNOSTIC CHECKLIST

Consider

- First detect features of orthotopic or heterotopic transplantation
- Orthotopic transplantation shows enlarged atria due to anastomosis of donor heart with the receipt's atria
- Assess for complications
  - Impaired LV function (echo, MR and cardiac-gated CT)
  - Atherosclerotic plaque and coronary stenosis: Coronary angiogram; coronary CTA and IVUS
  - Rejection (cardiac MR): Hyperenhancement in delayed images and hyperintensity in T2WI suggest myocardial necrosis/edema
  - Chest X-ray and CT: Lung and mediastinal infections and tumors

SELECTED REFERENCES

1. Gregory SA et al: Comparison of sixty-four-slice multidetector computed tomographic coronary angiography to coronary angiography with intravascular ultrasound for the detection of transplant vasculopathy. Am J Cardiol. 98(7):877-84, 2006
2. Trulock EP et al: Registry of the International Society for Heart and Lung Transplantation: twenty-third official adult lung and heart-lung transplantation report--2006. J Heart Lung Transplant. 25(8):880-92, 2006
3. Nikolaou K et al: Morphological and functional magnetic resonance imaging after heterotopic heart transplantation. Ann Thorac Surg. 78(3):1064-6, 2004
4. Almenar L et al: Utility of cardiac magnetic resonance imaging for the diagnosis of heart transplant rejection. Transplant Proc. 35(5):1962-4, 2003
5. Farzaneh-Far A: Electron-beam computed tomography in the assessment of coronary artery disease after heart transplantation. Circulation. 103(10):E60, 2001
6. Marie PY et al: Detection and prediction of acute heart transplant rejection with the myocardial T2 determination provided by a black-blood magnetic resonance imaging sequence. J Am Coll Cardiol. 37(3):825-31, 2001
7. Rinaldi M et al: Neoplastic disease after heart transplantation: single center experience. Eur J Cardiothorac Surg. 19(5):696-701, 2001
8. Aranda JM Jr et al: Cardiac transplant vasculopathy. Chest. 118(6):1792-800, 2000
9. Bellenger NG et al: Left ventricular function and mass after orthotopic heart transplantation: a comparison of cardiovascular magnetic resonance with echocardiography. J Heart Lung Transplant. 19(5):444-52, 2000
10. Knollmann FD et al: CT of heart transplant recipients: spectrum of disease. Radiographics. 20(6):1637-48, 2000
11. Knisely BL et al: Imaging of cardiac transplantation complications. Radiographics. 19(2):321-39; discussion 340-1, 1999
12. Haramati LB et al: Lung nodules and masses after cardiac transplantation. Radiology. 188(2):491-7, 1993
13. Henry DA et al: Orthotopic cardiac transplantation: evaluation with CT. Radiology. 170(2):343-50, 1989
14. Adey CK et al: Heterotopic heart transplantation: a radiographic review. Radiographics. 7(1):151-60, 1987
15. Aherne T et al: Magnetic resonance imaging of cardiac transplants: the evaluation of rejection of cardiac allografts with and without immunosuppression. Circulation. 74(1):145-56, 1986

HEART TRANSPLANT

IMAGE GALLERY

Typical

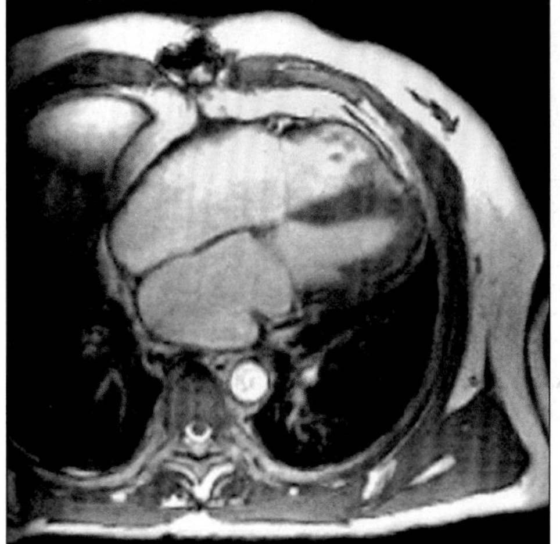

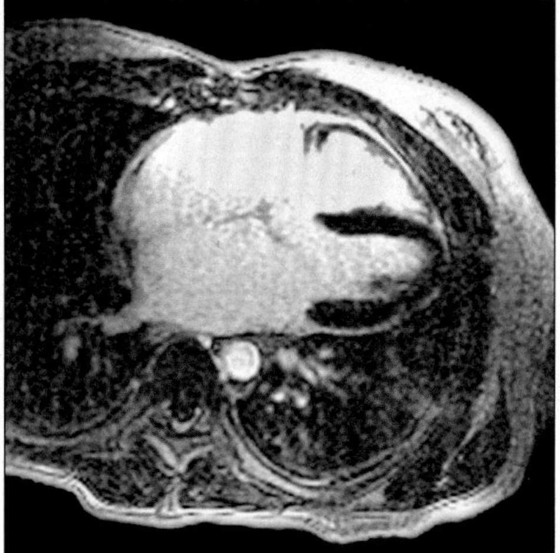

(Left) *Four chamber view cine cardiac MR shows orthotopic heart transplant with dilated appearance of both atria due to anastomosis between the transplanted and native atria.* ***(Right)*** *Four chamber view delayed-enhancement cardiac MR shows no evidence of hyperenhancement in the LV myocardium excluding the possibilities of rejection and severe transplant vasculopathy.*

Typical

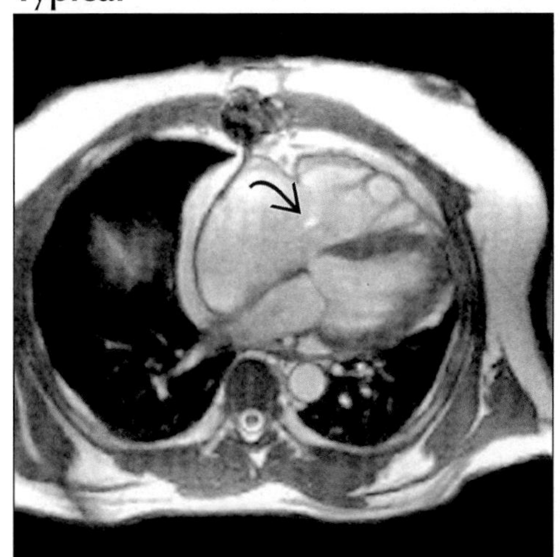

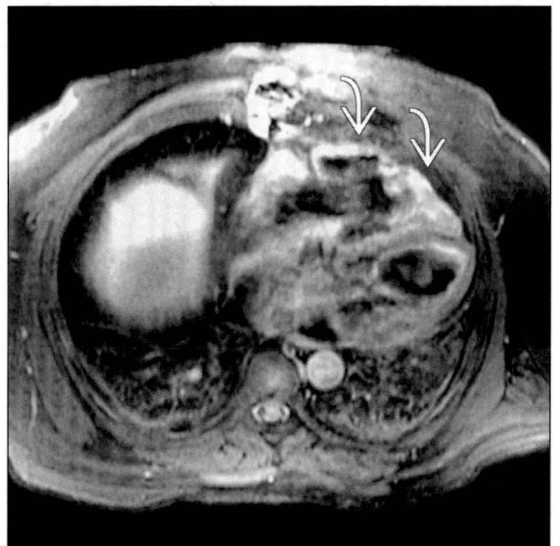

(Left) *Four chamber view cine cardiac MR shows dilated right atrium and ventricle with decreased function and evidence of tricuspid regurgitation →.* ***(Right)*** *Axial T2WI FS MR in the same patient as previous image, shows increased signal →, in the RV free wall suggesting edema and transplant rejection.*

Typical

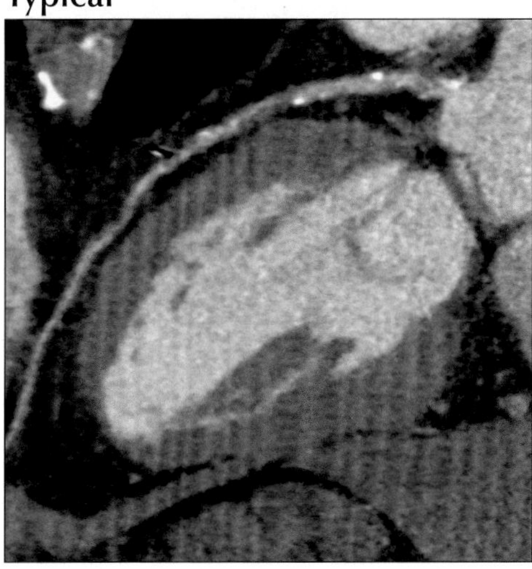

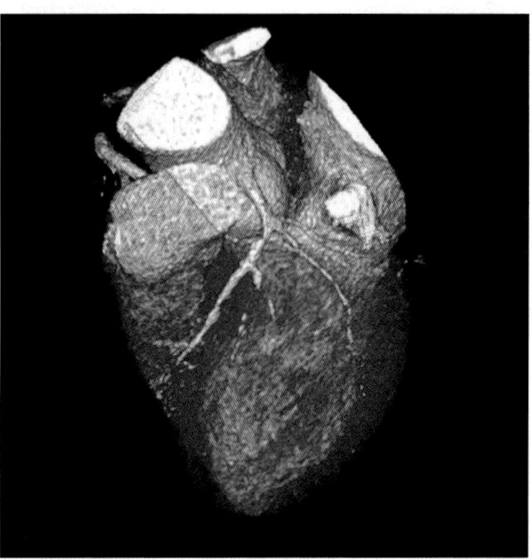

(Left) *Curved MPR coronary CTA shows moderate amount of calcified and non-calcified plaques in the LAD leading to at least moderate stenosis in a patient 3-years after heart transplant.* ***(Right)*** *Coronary CTA 3D volume rendering image shows areas of luminal narrowing in the LAD and diagonal branches in a patient 3 years after heart transplant.*

LV ASSISTANCE DEVICES

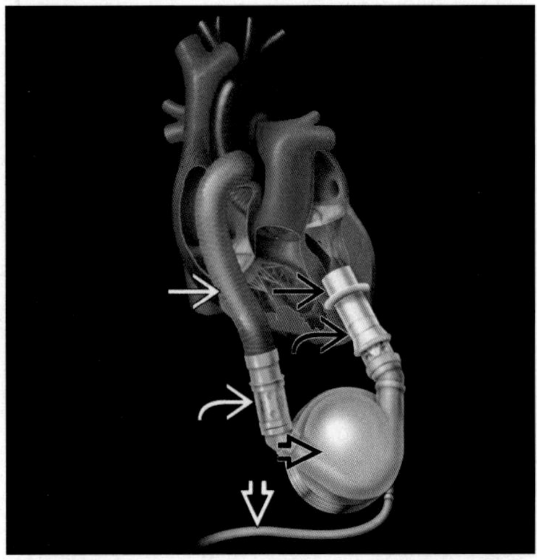

Coronal graphic shows pulsatile pump, sewing ring and cuff, inflow valved conduit, outflow valved conduit, outflow graft, and driveline.

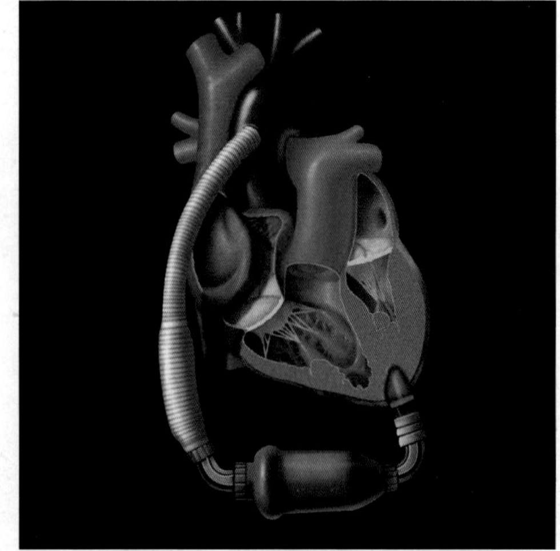

Coronal graphic shows second generation non-pulsatile continuous flow pump.

TERMINOLOGY

Abbreviations

- Left ventricular assistance device (LVAD)
- Right ventricular assist device (RVAD)

Definitions

- Battery-operated implanted mechanical pump device to augment cardiac output for failing ventricle
- FDA approval of first left ventricular assist device to bridge to transplant was in 1994

PRE-PROCEDURE

Indications

- Bridge to cardiac transplant
  - Effective hemodynamic support
  - Maintains or improves other organ function
- "Destination" therapy
  - For permanent use in patients not considered for transplant

Contraindications

- Device cannot be implanted in some very short or very thin patients

Getting Started

- Types
  - Extracorporeal nonpulsatile
  - Extracorporeal pulsatile
  - Implantable pulsatile
  - Total artificial heart

PROCEDURE

Patient Position/Location

- Best procedure approach
  - Preperitoneal pocket is preferred placement site
    - Improved control of bleeding
    - Easier management of pocket infections
    - Prevents development of intraabdominal adhesions
  - Intraabdominal position reserved for smaller patients

Components

- Pump
  - Surgically implanted in abdomen
- Inflow conduit
  - Conducts blood from left ventricular apex to pump
- Outflow conduit
  - Conducts blood from pump to ascending aorta
- Internal valves
  - Ensures unidirectional flow
- External power source
  - Pneumatic
    - Patient confined to hospital
  - Electrical
    - Portable battery packs can let patients live at home
  - Power leads pass through skin to pump
- External controller
  - System function settings
  - System status

Devices

- 1st generation pulsatile pumps simulate cardiac cycle
  - HeartMate Implantable
  - Novacor Implantable
  - Thoratec Extracorporeal Biventricular
- 2nd generation non-pulsatile continuous flow pumps

LV ASSISTANCE DEVICES

Key Facts

Terminology
- Implanted mechanical device to augment cardiac output for failing ventricle

Pre-procedure
- "Destination" therapy

Procedure
- 1st generation pulsatile pumps simulate cardiac cycle
- 2nd generation non-pulsatile continuous flow pumps

Post-procedure
- Typically a bridge to cardiac transplant
- Reverse remodeling while on LVAD has been described

Common Problems & Complications
- Thromboembolic
- Pleural complications
- Pericardial bleeding
- Abdominal complications

- Smaller and easier to implant
- Quieter
  - DeBakey VAD
- Artificial hearts
  - Significant complications limit use
    - CardioWest
    - AbioCor

Imaging Findings
- Radiographic
  - Can visualize radiopaque structures
  - Dacron conduits are not visible
- CT
  - Can visualize conduits as well as more radiodense components

POST-PROCEDURE

Expected Outcome
- Typically a bridge to cardiac transplant
- Reverse remodeling while on LVAD has been described
  - May reverse a number of adaptive cardiac changes at cellular/molecular level
  - May restore basic cardiac function in some patients

PROBLEMS & COMPLICATIONS

Complications
- Most feared complication(s)
  - Thromboembolic
    - Pulmonary infarction
    - Cerebral infarction
  - Pleural complications
    - Pneumothorax
    - Hemothorax presumptive diagnosis if sudden accumulation of large amount of pleural fluid
  - Pericardial bleeding
    - Hemopericardium
    - Focal accumulations of blood around inflow or outflow cannulas may be an expected post-operative finding
  - Abdominal complications
    - Hemoperitoneum
    - Abscess
    - Obstruction
  - Device failure

SELECTED REFERENCES

1. Wohlschlaeger J et al: Reverse remodeling following insertion of left ventricular assist devices (LVAD): a review of the morphological and molecular changes. Cardiovasc Res. 68(3):376-86, 2005
2. Goldstein DJ et al: Implantable left ventricular assist devices. N Engl J Med. 339(21):1522-33, 1998
3. Knisely BL et al: Imaging of ventricular assist devices and their complications. AJR Am J Roentgenol. 169(2):385-91, 1997

IMAGE GALLERY

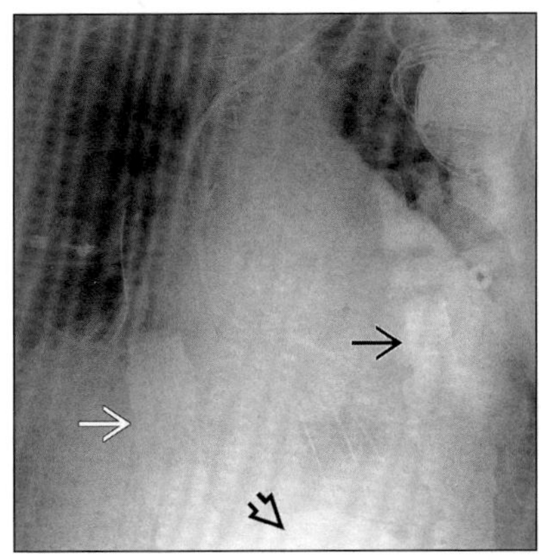

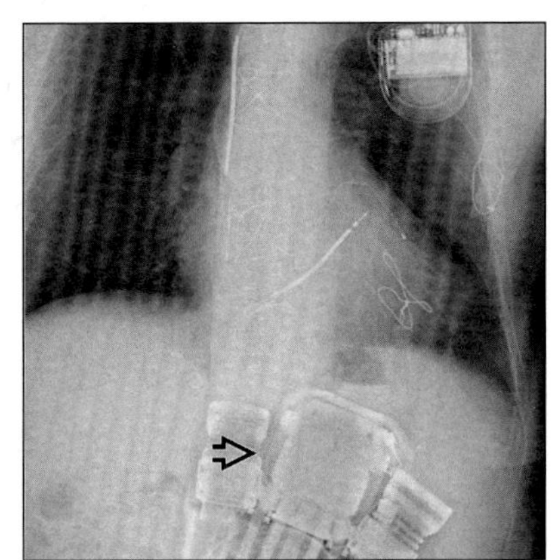

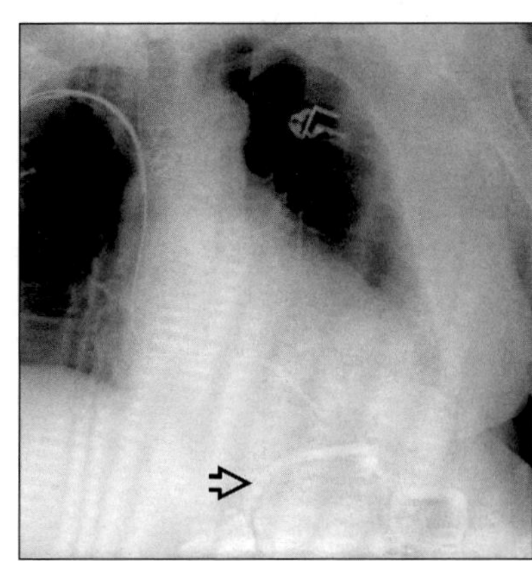

(Left) *Coronal radiograph shows a HeartMate device ⇨. Inflow cannula → arises in left ventricle. The outflow cannula is radiolucent Dacron and arises from outflow valved conduit ➡.* ***(Center)*** *Coronal radiograph shows a Novacor device ⇨. Inflow and outflow cannulas are nonradiopaque.* ***(Right)*** *Coronal radiograph shows a Novacor device ⇨.*

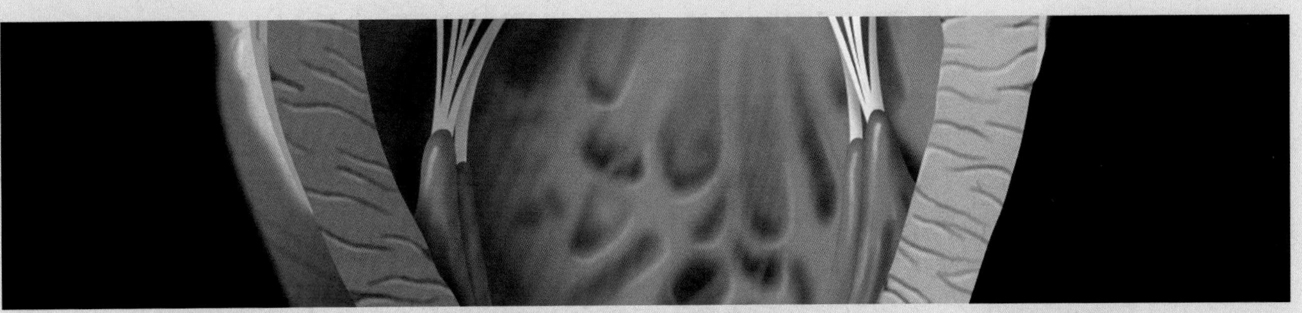

SECTION 8: Hypertension

LEFT VENTRICULAR HYPERTROPHY

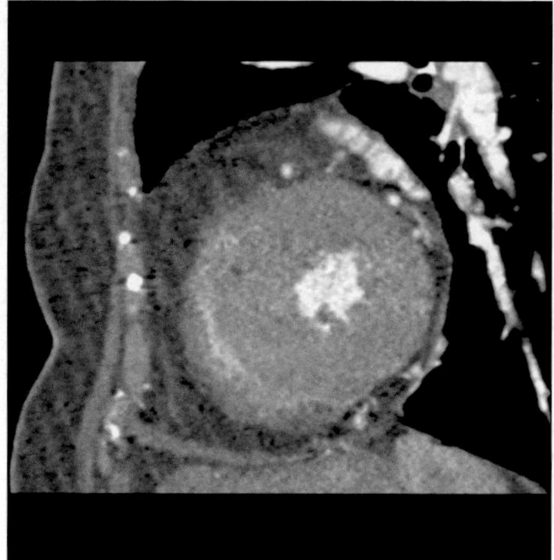

Short axis coronary CTA in mid-diastole shows concentric LV hypertrophy in patient with severe aortic valve stenosis.

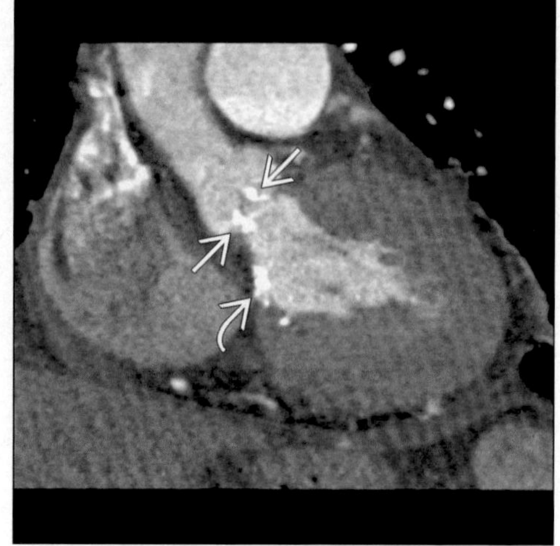

LVOT shows concentric LV hypertrophy and calcification of stenotic aortic valve ➡ and mitral annulus ↪.

TERMINOLOGY

Abbreviations and Synonyms

- Left ventricular (LV) hypertrophy (LVH)

Definitions

- Increase in left ventricular mass

IMAGING FINDINGS

General Features

- Best diagnostic clue
  - Equally distributed increase in ventricular wall thickness with normal ventricular chamber dimensions
  - LV thickening measured at end-diastole
  - LV thickness exceeding 1.1 cm indicates hypertrophy

MR Findings

- Cine-gradient echo or steady state free precession imaging
- MR is the method of choice for quantifying LV mass
- LV mass
  - Males 148 ± 26 gm (76 ± 13 gm/m^2)
  - Females 108 ± 21 gm (66 ± 11 gm/m^2)
- Normal end-diastolic wall thickness = 0.7-1.1 cm
  - Mild LVH = 1.2-1.4 cm
  - Moderate LVH = 1.5-1.9 cm
  - Severe LVH ≥ 2 cm
- Relative wall thickness
  - Eccentric hypertrophy < 0.30
  - Normal 0.3-0.45
  - Concentric hypertrophy > 0.45

Other Modality Findings

- Echocardiography
  - Mainstay for evaluating left ventricular function
  - Same findings as described for MR

DIFFERENTIAL DIAGNOSIS

Hypertrophic Cardiomyopathy

- Often asymmetric hypertrophy
- Absence of hypertension
- Dynamic outflow obstruction on echo/MR/gated CT
- Abnormal diastolic function

DDx: Left Ventricular Hypertrophy

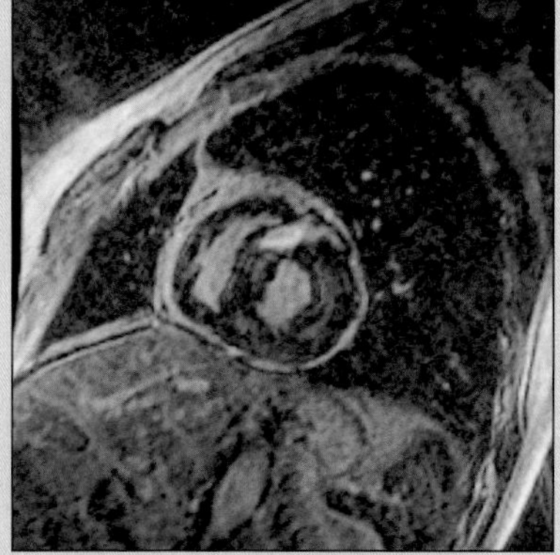

Hypertrophic Cardiomyopathy

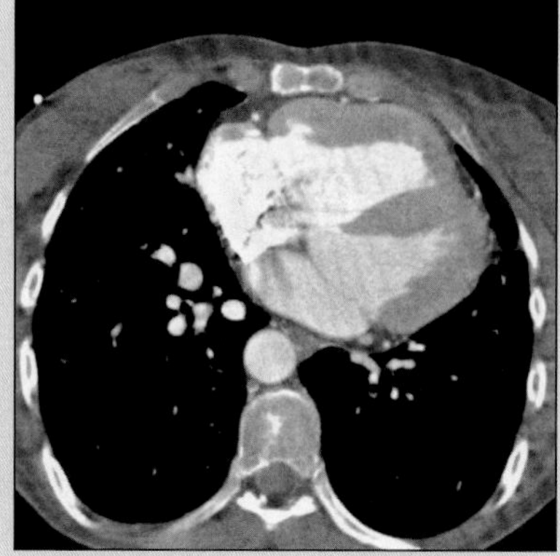

Right Ventricular Hypertrophy

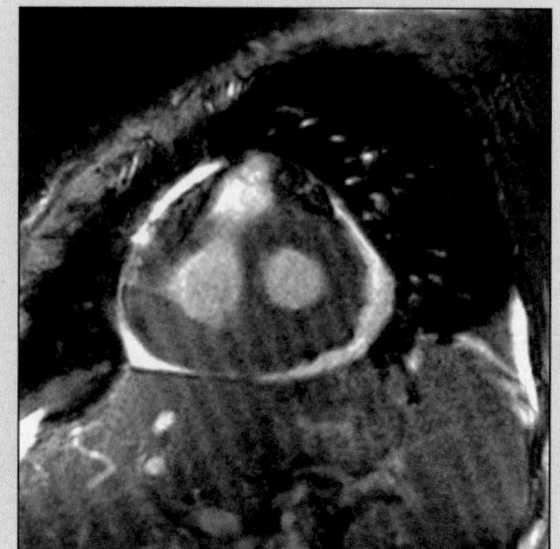

Metastatic Disease

LEFT VENTRICULAR HYPERTROPHY

Key Facts

Terminology
- Increase in left ventricular mass

Imaging Findings
- Equally distributed increase in ventricular wall thickness with normal ventricular chamber dimensions
- LV thickening measured at end-diastole
- LV thickness exceeding 1.1 cm indicates hypertrophy
- MR is the method of choice for quantifying LV mass
- Normal end-diastolic wall thickness = 0.7-1.1 cm

Pathology
- Systemic hypertension most common cause of left ventricular hypertrophy
- Less common causes include valvular stenosis or regurgitation

Restrictive Cardiomyopathy
- Absence of hypertension
- Right ventricular hypertrophy often present
- Abnormal diastolic function

PATHOLOGY

General Features
- Etiology
  - Systemic hypertension most common cause of left ventricular hypertrophy
  - Less common causes include valvular stenosis or regurgitation
- Epidemiology
  - 62 million persons in the US have systemic hypertension
  - 40% of African-American males over age 50 have systemic hypertension

Gross Pathologic & Surgical Features
- Characterization of hypertrophy
  - Concentric hypertrophy
    - Uniform increase in ventricular wall thickness
    - Normal ventricular chamber dimension
    - Increased ventricular mass
  - Eccentric hypertrophy
    - Increased ventricular dimensions
    - Normal wall thickness
    - Low or normal relative wall thickness
    - Increased ventricular mass
    - Seen in patients with valvular regurgitation
  - Asymmetric hypertrophy
    - Nonuniform increase in wall thickness
    - Associated with hypertrophic cardiomyopathy

CLINICAL ISSUES

Presentation
- Clinical Profile
  - Hypertension (systolic BP > 140 mmHg, diastolic BP > 90 mmHg)
  - Left ventricular hypertrophy on EKG

Natural History & Prognosis
- LVH in patients with systemic hypertension is significant risk factor for future morbid events

Treatment
- Treat underlying cause
- Medical therapy for hypertension
- Surgical therapy for valvular disease as indicated

SELECTED REFERENCES

1. Otto CM: Cardiomyopathies, hypertensive and pulmonary heart disease. In: Textbook of Clinical Echocardiography, 2nd ed. WB Saunders, Philadelphia, 183-203, 2000
2. Devereux RB et al: Left ventricular hypertrophy and hypertension. Clin Exp Hypertens. 15(6):1025-32, 1993

IMAGE GALLERY

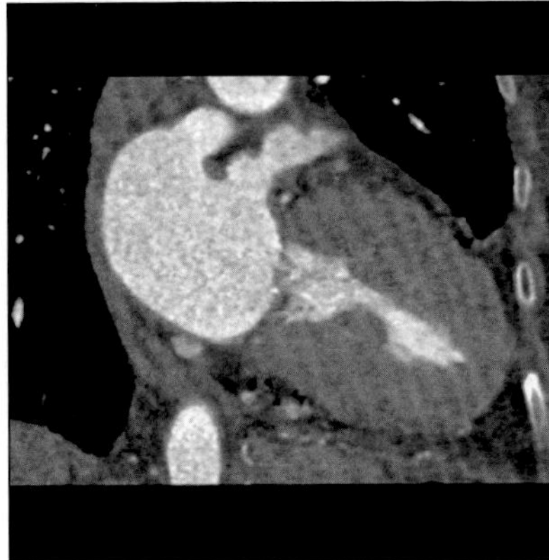

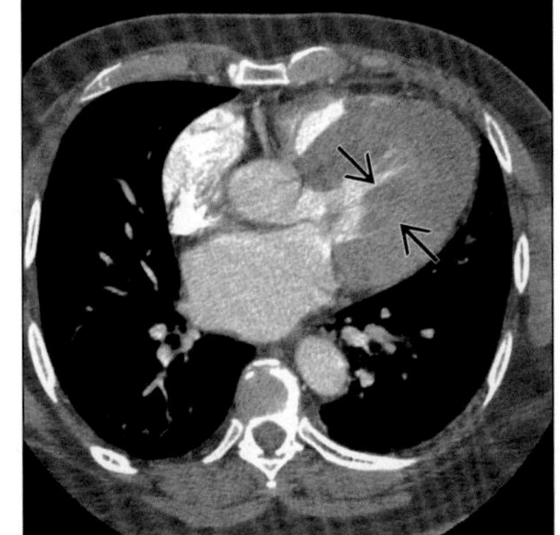

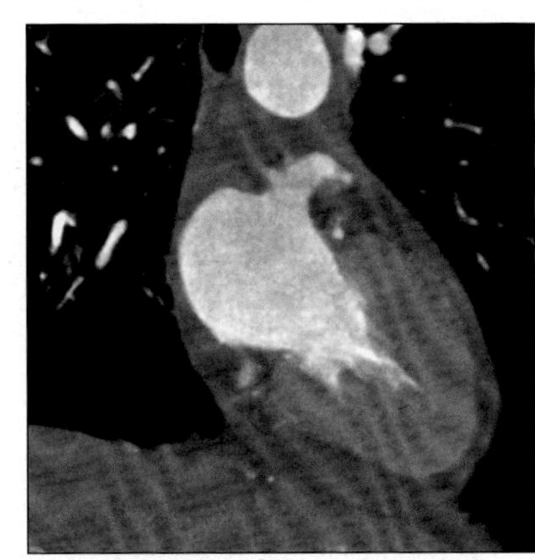

__(Left)__ Long axis coronary CTA shows concentric hypertrophy of LV myocardium and diminished LV cavity size and dilated left atrium in a patient with chronic systemic hypertension. __(Center)__ Axial coronary CTA in the same patient, shows symmetric hypertrophy of LV myocardium and hypertrophy of papillary muscles ⇒ without LV dilatation. Note: Mildly dilated left atrium. __(Right)__ Long axis coronary CTA in different patient shows concentric left ventricular hypertrophy and systolic near obliteration of LV cavity in patient with aortic stenosis (not shown).

RIGHT VENTRICULAR HYPERTROPHY

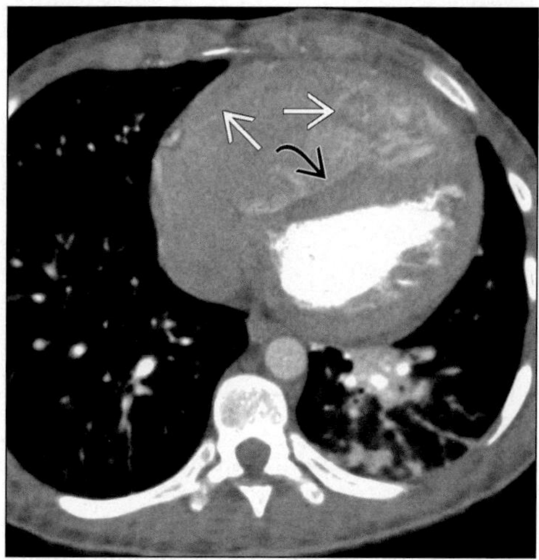

Axial cardiac CT shows RV myocardial and trabecular hypertrophy ➡ with flattening of the ventricular septum ⇨ and ventricular dilatation due to chronic shunt.

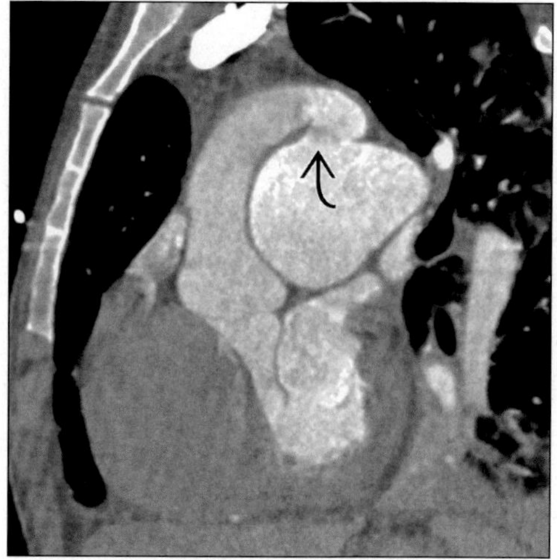

Oblique cardiac CT in same patient as previous image, shows large pulmonary artery with connection ⇨ to normal sized aorta indicating persistent ductus arteriosus as the underlying cause of RVH.

TERMINOLOGY

Abbreviations and Synonyms

- Right ventricle (RV) hypertrophy (RVH)

Definitions

- Increased right ventricular myocardial mass and wall thickness

IMAGING FINDINGS

General Features

- Best diagnostic clue: Right ventricular free wall thickness > 7 mm as assessed on MR, the best method for evaluating the RV

CT Findings

- Cardiac Gated CTA: Allows end diastolic wall thickness and functional RV assessment

MR Findings

- Short-access cine-gradient echo imaging optimal method for assessing right ventricular mass and thickness (now SSFP: True FISP, FIESTA, balanced FE)
- Temporal resolution should be 25-40 msec in order to accurately assess systole and diastole time points
- Normal RV functional parameters
  - RV end-diastolic volume 138 ± 40 mL
  - RV end-systolic volume 54 ± 21 mL
  - RV free wall mass 46 ± 11 gm (26 ± 5 gm/m^2)
  - RV ejection fraction (%) = 61 ± 7
  - RV stroke volume = 84 ± 24 mL (46 ± 8 ml/m^2)

DIFFERENTIAL DIAGNOSIS

RVH Due to Pulmonary Hypertension

- RV mass exceeds 60 gm
- Pulmonary artery (PA) pressure estimated as (P right atrium) + 4 V^2
  - V is peak velocity of regurgitant tricuspid valve jet
  - Right atrial pressure (P right atrium) estimated by size of inferior vena cava IVC
    - Small (< 1.5 cm) 0-5 mmHg
    - Normal (1.5-2.5 cm) 5-15 mmHg
    - Dilated (> 2.5 cm) 15-20 mmHg
    - Dilated, enlarged hepatic veins > 20 mmHg

DDx: Right Ventricular Hypertrophy

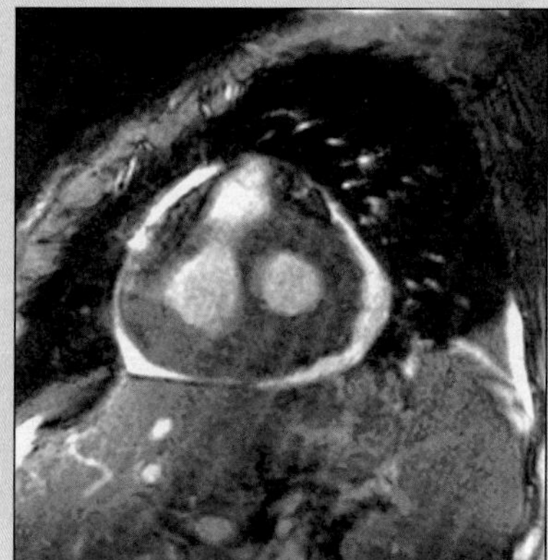

Cardiac Lymphoma

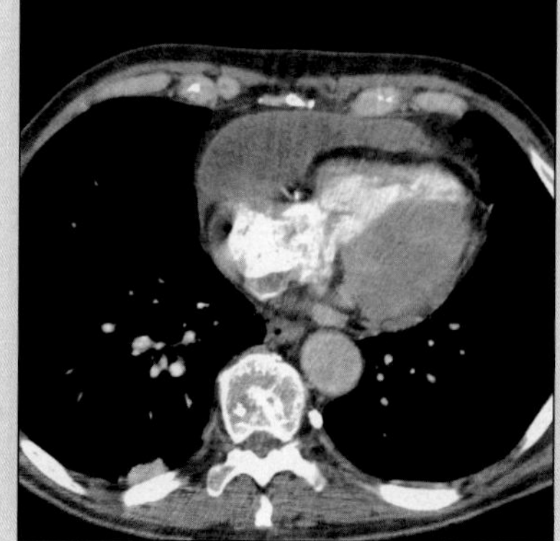

Loculated Effusion

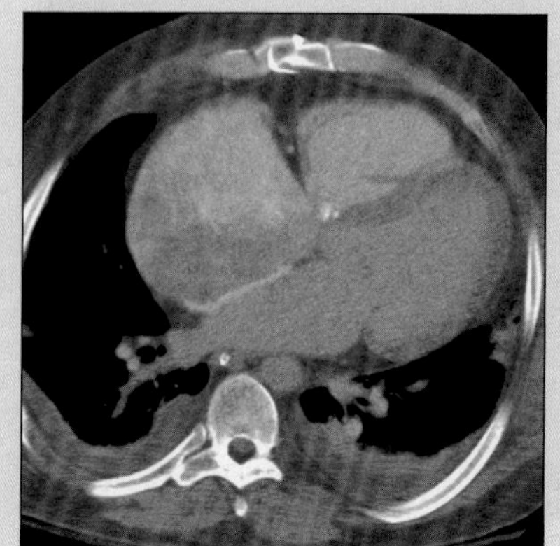

Right Atrium Enlargement

RIGHT VENTRICULAR HYPERTROPHY

Key Facts

Terminology
- Right ventricle (RV) hypertrophy (RVH)
- Increased right ventricular myocardial mass and wall thickness

Imaging Findings
- Best diagnostic clue: Right ventricular free wall thickness > 7 mm as assessed on MR, the best method for evaluating the RV
- Cardiac Gated CTA: Allows end diastolic wall thickness and functional RV assessment

Pathology
- Normal RV free wall mass = 26 ± 5 gm/m²
- Normal RV free wall thickness < 6 mm
- RVH occurs as a result of pulmonary arterial hypertension

Congenital Heart Disease
- Right ventricular hypertrophy a common manifestation of congenital heart disease
- Tetralogy of Fallot
- Transposition of great vessels

PATHOLOGY

General Features
- General path comments
  - Normal RV free wall mass = 26 ± 5 gm/m²
  - Normal RV free wall thickness < 6 mm
- Etiology
  - RVH occurs as a result of pulmonary arterial hypertension
    - Congenital heart disease
    - Primary pulmonary hypertension (etiology unknown)
    - Secondary pulmonary hypertension: Acquired heart disease, especially left ventricular dysfunction; valvular heart disease; chronic pulmonary edema (PE); pulmonary disease; chronic obstructive pulmonary disease (COPD); chronic interstitial lung disease; chronic bronchitis

CLINICAL ISSUES

Presentation
- Exertional dyspnea
- Chest pain
- Cor pulmonale
- Cyanosis
- Right axis deviation on EKG

Treatment
- Medical treatment
  - Treat underlying cause of secondary pulmonary hypertension
  - Pulmonary vasodilators
- Surgical treatment
  - Valve replacement
  - IVC filter for recurrent pulmonary emboli
  - Transplantation

SELECTED REFERENCES

1. Lorenz CH: Right ventricular anatomy and function in health and disease. In: Cardiovascular Magnetic Resonance, Manning WJ, Pannell DJ, Churchill-Livingstone, Philadelphia. 283-92, 2002
2. Otto CM: Echocardiographic evaluation of left and right ventricular systolic function. In: Textbook of Clinical Echocardiography, 2nd ed. WB Saunders, Philadelphia. 120-3, 2000

IMAGE GALLERY

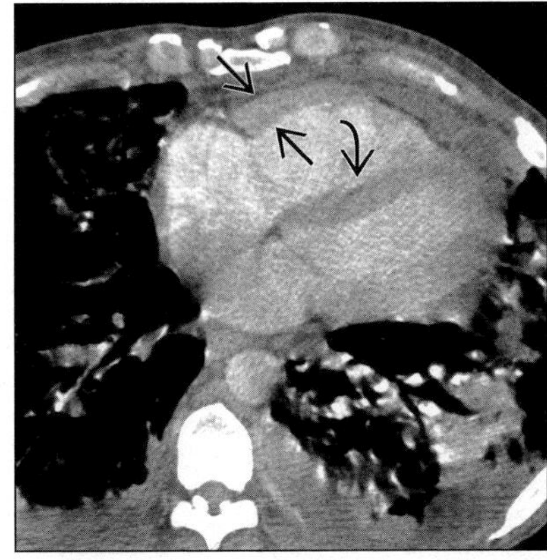
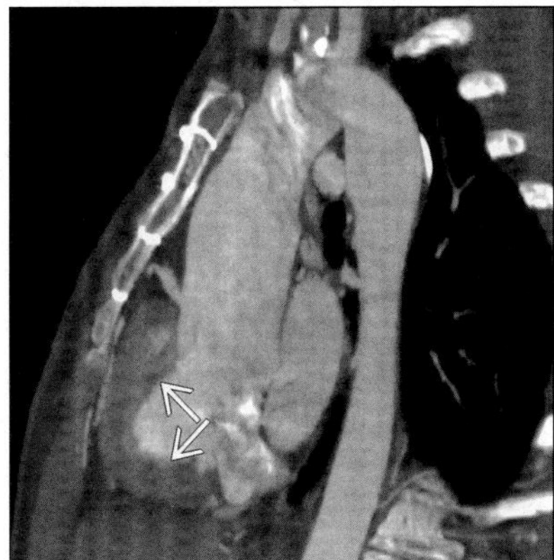
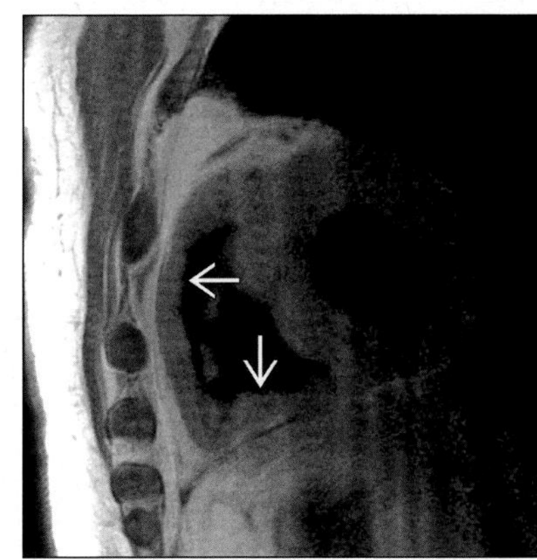

(Left) *Axial CECT shows cor pulmonale with RV hypertrophy ➔ and septal flattening ➔ due to chronic lung disease.* ***(Center)*** *Oblique cardiac CT in patient with tetralogy of Fallot shows aorta overriding a VSD. Marked RV hypertrophy ➔ without dilatation.* ***(Right)*** *Short axis T1WI FS MR shows concentric RV myocardial thickening ➔ of unknown cause. Cine images (not shown) demonstrated segmental wall motion abnormalities.*

PULMONARY ARTERIAL HYPERTENSION

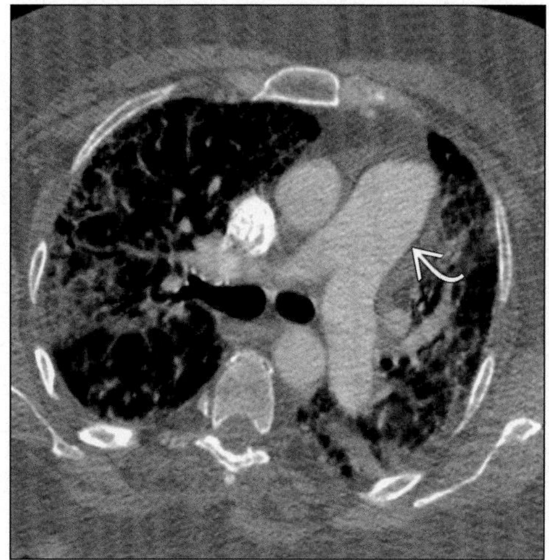

Axial CECT shows enlarged central pulmonary artery ➡ with rapid tapering (pruning) in patient with pulmonary arterial hypertension due to chronic obstructive pulmonary disease (COPD).

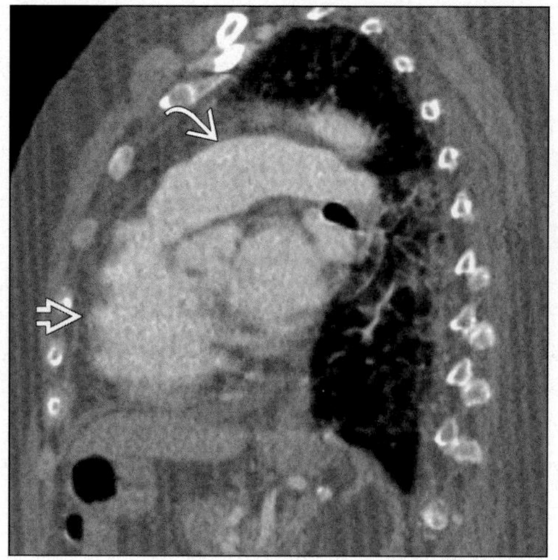

Oblique CECT shows enlarged right ventricle ➡ with filling of the retrosternal clear space and large pulmonary artery ➡ in patient with COPD, indicating cor pulmonale.

TERMINOLOGY

Abbreviations and Synonyms

- Pulmonary arterial hypertension (PAH)

Definitions

- Elevated mean pulmonary artery pressure > 25 mmHg at rest (> 30 mmHg during exercise)
- Classified as pre- or post-capillary

IMAGING FINDINGS

General Features

- Best diagnostic clue
  - Convex pulmonary artery (PA) segment on AP radiograph
    - Mild convex pulmonary artery segment may be normal in young adults up to the 3rd decade of life
  - Dilatation of central pulmonary arteries with rapid tapering (pruning)
  - Right ventricular (RV) hypertrophy

Radiographic Findings

- Radiography
  - Pre-capillary hypertension
    - Dilatation central pulmonary arteries with rapid pruning of peripheral pulmonary arteries
    - Normal sized heart early or cardiomegaly with right ventricular hypertrophy
    - Intimal calcification with severe long-standing hypertension
  - Associated findings with secondary disease: Emphysema, bronchiectasis, honeycombing
  - Post-capillary hypertension: Pulmonary veno-occlusive disease (PVOD)
    - Normal size left atrium
    - Edema, septal thickening and small pleural effusions
  - Post-capillary hypertension: Left atrial obstruction
    - Hemosiderosis: Nodular interstitial thickening with calcified nodules

CT Findings

- HRCT
  - Mosaic perfusion pattern common in pulmonary hypertension

DDx: Eisenmenger Syndrome

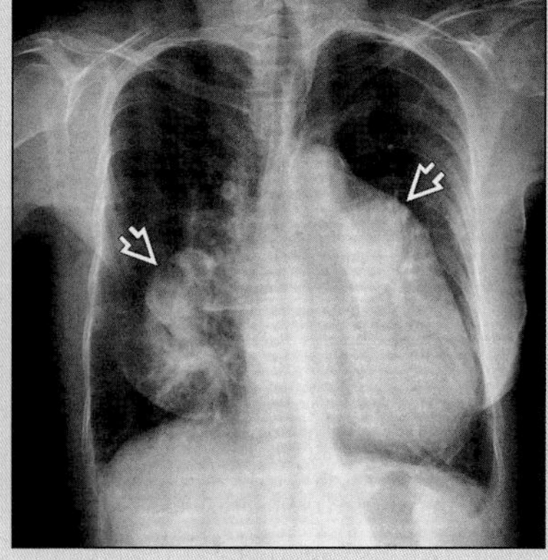

Large PA

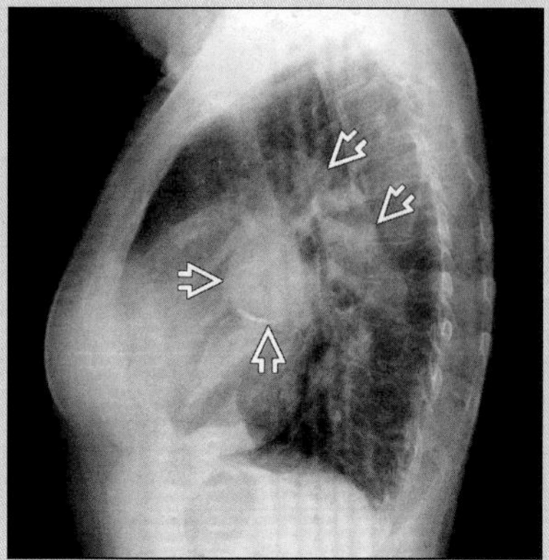

Right and Left PA

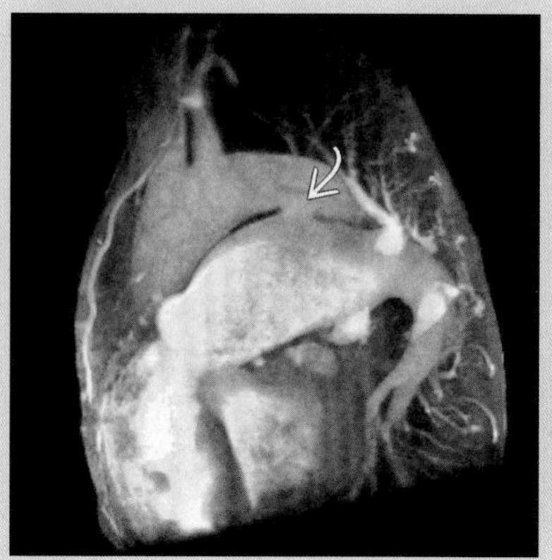

Persistent Ductus

PULMONARY ARTERIAL HYPERTENSION

Key Facts

Terminology
- Elevated mean pulmonary artery pressure > 25 mmHg at rest (> 30 mmHg during exercise)

Imaging Findings
- Convex pulmonary artery (PA) segment on AP radiograph
- Dilatation of central pulmonary arteries with rapid tapering (pruning)
- Right ventricular (RV) hypertrophy
- Intimal calcification with severe long-standing hypertension
- Normal main pulmonary artery smaller diameter than adjacent ascending aorta

Top Differential Diagnoses
- Adenopathy
- Idiopathic Dilatation
- Pulmonary Artery Stenosis

Pathology
- PAH secondary to parenchymal lung disease: Cor pulmonale
- Prevalence in men: 10% above age 35 and 25% above age 65
- 1% with acute pulmonary emboli will develop chronic thromboemboli

Clinical Issues
- No cure, 30% respond to medical therapy

Diagnostic Checklist
- Septal thickening may represent post-capillary hypertension, important to recognize before prostaglandin therapy

    - Geographic ground-glass attenuation represents normal or hyperperfused lung
    - Vessels in hypoattenuated lung have decreased caliber due to either vascular obstruction or hypoxic vasoconstriction
    - Geographic ground-glass opacities less well-defined than that seen with small airways disease
  - Post-capillary hypertension: Additional findings beyond pre-capillary hypertension
    - Central and gravity dependent ground-glass opacities, septal thickening
    - Centrilobular nodules
    - Pleural and pericardial effusions
    - Mediastinal adenopathy
  - Centrilobular nodules may also represent cholesterol granulomas which are seen in up to 25% of patients with pulmonary hypertension
- CTA
  - Normal transverse diameter of main pulmonary artery < 29 mm
    - Measured at bifurcation, perpendicular to long axis
  - Normal main pulmonary artery smaller diameter than adjacent ascending aorta
  - Normal cross-section artery-to-bronchus ratio ≤ 1
  - Good correlation between size of central pulmonary arteries and mean pulmonary artery pressure
  - Acute right ventricular dysfunction
    - Usually secondary to acute pulmonary embolus
    - Right ventricular dilatation (cavity wider than left ventricular cavity)
    - Convex deviation of interventricular septum towards the left ventricular cavity
  - Peripheral lobular or wedge-shaped opacities in those who develop pulmonary infarcts
    - Chronic thromboembolism and tumor emboli
  - Pericardial thickening or effusion common

MR Findings
- Less sensitive and specific than CT
- More difficult in dyspneic patients

Nuclear Medicine Findings
- Ventilation-perfusion
  - Usually low probability scans except in patients with chronic thromboemboli which has a high probability pattern
  - Need to reduce the number of particles to avoid risk of acute right heart failure from occlusion of capillary bed

Angiographic Findings
- Contrast injection has increased risk of complications, primarily used for pressure measurements

Imaging Recommendations
- Best imaging tool: CT useful to exclude chronic pulmonary embolism as a cause of hypertension and to look for PVOD prior to institution of prostaglandin therapy

DIFFERENTIAL DIAGNOSIS

Adenopathy
- Hilum more lobulated may have abnormal mediastinal contours from adenopathy
- Typical examples: Sarcoidosis, lymphoma

Idiopathic Dilatation
- Young women, unilateral enlargement main and left pulmonary artery, no pressure gradient

Pulmonary Artery Stenosis
- Unilateral enlargement main and left pulmonary artery, left upper lobe vessels larger than mirror image right upper lobe vessels (due to jet effect of flow across pulmonic valve)

PULMONARY ARTERIAL HYPERTENSION

PATHOLOGY

General Features

- General path comments: Hemodynamic vascular changes due to elevated pressure from either pre- or post-capillary obstruction
- Etiology
  - May be divided into primary PAH or secondary PAH
    - Primary PAH has no known cause and is rare: Diagnosis of exclusion
  - PAH secondary to parenchymal lung disease: Cor pulmonale
  - Pre-capillary
    - Congenital left to right shunt, (e.g., atrial septal defect)
    - Chronic thromboemboli
    - Tumor embolism: Hepatoma, gastric carcinoma, renal cell, right atrial sarcoma, breast, intravascular lymphomatosis
    - Infection: Schistosomiasis, AIDS
    - IV drug abuse: Talcosis
    - Portal hypertension (2%)
    - Primary pulmonary hypertension (PPH)
    - Lung disease: End stage interstitial lung disease or chronic emphysema
  - Post-capillary
    - PVOD
    - Mediastinal fibrosis (affecting pulmonary veins)
    - Left atrial obstruction: Mitral stenosis; left ventricular (LV) dysfunction, myxoma
- Epidemiology
  - Prevalence in men: 10% above age 35 and 25% above age 65
  - PPH: Women 3rd decade
  - 1% with acute pulmonary emboli will develop chronic thromboemboli
  - Pulmonary veno-occlusive disease, 1/3rd children
  - Schistosomiasis most common cause worldwide
- Associated abnormalities
  - RV dilatation and tricuspid regurgitation
    - Tricuspid regurgitation (TR) due to stretching of the tricuspid anulus and resulting malcoaptation of leaflets
  - Secondary systemic venous hypertension
    - Dilated azygos vein on frontal radiograph
    - Dilated inferior vena cava (IVC) on lateral radiograph

Microscopic Features

- Necrotizing arteritis and capillary plexiform lesion in PPH and left-to-right shunts
- Capillary hemangiomatosis in PVOD
- Pulmonary vein intimal fibrosis, recanalized thrombi and webs in PVOD
- Centrilobular cholesterol granulomas in 25% of those with pulmonary hypertension

CLINICAL ISSUES

Presentation

- Most common signs/symptoms
  - Nonspecific symptoms: Dyspnea, easy fatigue, chest pain
  - Raynaud phenomenon
- Other signs/symptoms: Pulmonary veno-occlusive disease often preceded by flu-like illness
- Swan-Ganz catheterization: Normal resting mean pulmonary artery pressure < 20 mmHg
  - Pre-capillary
    - Elevated mean pulmonary artery pressure and increased resistance
    - Normal pulmonary capillary wedge pressure (PCWP)
  - Post-capillary
    - Elevated mean pulmonary artery pressure and increased resistance
    - Elevated PCWP (may be normal, PVOD patchy in distribution)

Demographics

- Gender: Primary hypertension (women 3:1)
- Ethnicity: Schistosomiasis endemic in Middle East, Africa, and Caribbean

Natural History & Prognosis

- Poor, 5 year survival for untreated primary pulmonary hypertension
- 5 year survival for chronic thromboembolic hypertension 30%
- End stage complications: Right heart failure, pulmonary artery dissection, pulmonary artery thrombosis

Treatment

- No cure, 30% respond to medical therapy
- Oxygen of little benefit
- Anticoagulation for thromboemboli: Consider inferior cava filter and thromboendarterectomy
- Calcium channel blockers (potential lethal rebound if discontinued)
- Prostaglandin I2 (epoprostenol) for primary hypertension
  - May cause acute pulmonary edema and right heart failure in those with post-capillary hypertension
- Lung with or without heart transplant

DIAGNOSTIC CHECKLIST

Image Interpretation Pearls

- Septal thickening may represent post-capillary hypertension, important to recognize before prostaglandin therapy

SELECTED REFERENCES

1. Frazier AA et al: From the archives of the AFIP: Pulmonary vasculature: Hypertension and infarction. Radiographics. 20:491-524; quiz 530-491, 532, 2000
2. Sherrick AD et al: Mosaic pattern of lung attenuation on CT scans: Frequency among patients with pulmonary artery hypertension of different causes. AJR. 169:79-82, 1997

PULMONARY ARTERIAL HYPERTENSION

IMAGE GALLERY

Typical

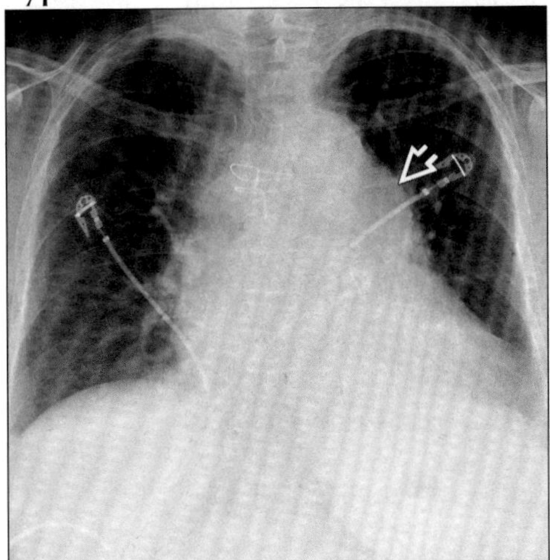

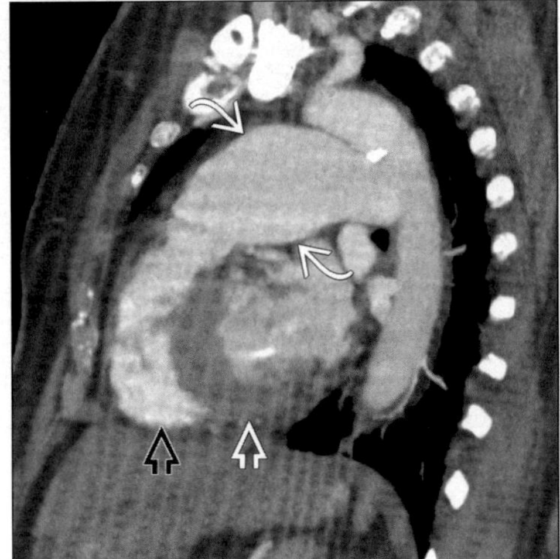

(Left) *PA radiograph shows convex pulmonary artery segment ➔ and very large central pulmonary arteries with rapid tapering (pruning) indicating PAH. Underlying etiology is chronic pulmonary embolism (PE).* ***(Right)*** *Oblique CECT in same patient as previous image shows markedly enlarged main pulmonary artery ➔. Note RV ➔ and LV ➔.*

Typical

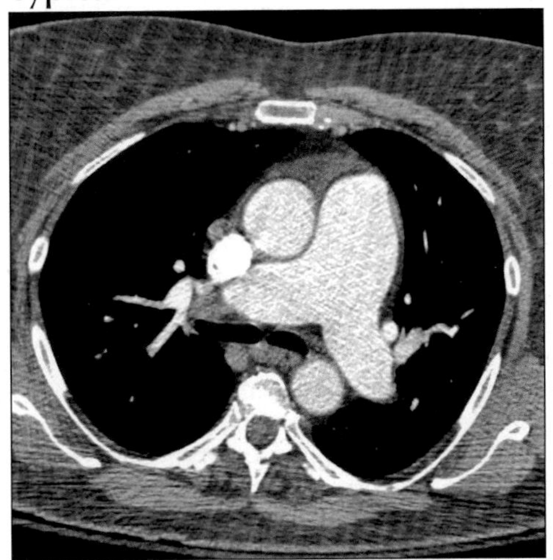

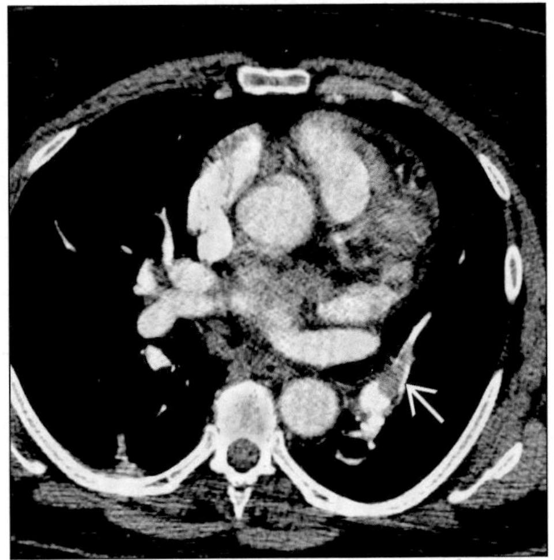

(Left) *Axial CECT in patient with chronic PE shows large central pulmonary arteries indicating secondary pulmonary arterial hypertension (precapillary).* ***(Right)*** *Axial CECT a few cuts lower than previous image shows pulmonary artery filling defect ➔ indicating acute PE.*

Typical

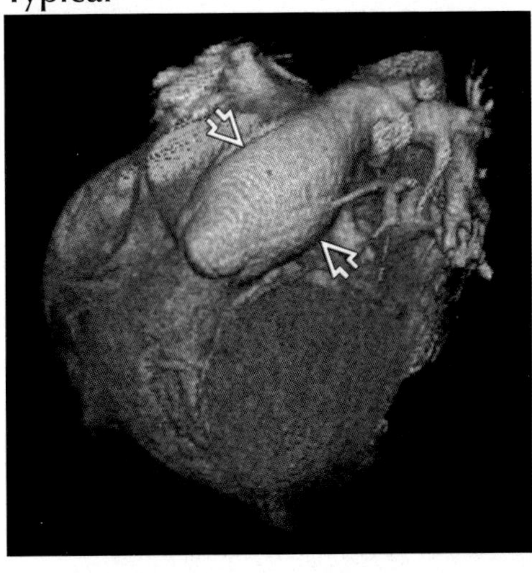

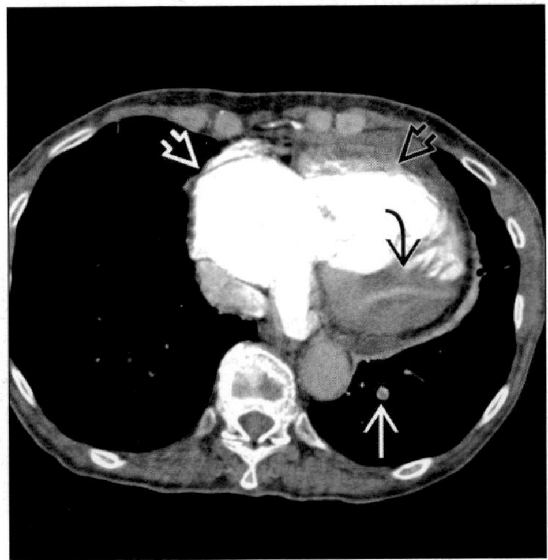

(Left) *Oblique coronary CTA volume rendered 3D image shows enlarged main pulmonary artery ➔ in a patient with primary pulmonary arterial hypertension.* ***(Right)*** *Axial CECT shows markedly enlarged right atrium ➔ and ventricle ➔, flattened ventricular septum ➔, and enlarged central pulmonary arteries (not shown) secondary to chronic PE ➔.*

BRANCH PULMONARY STENOSIS

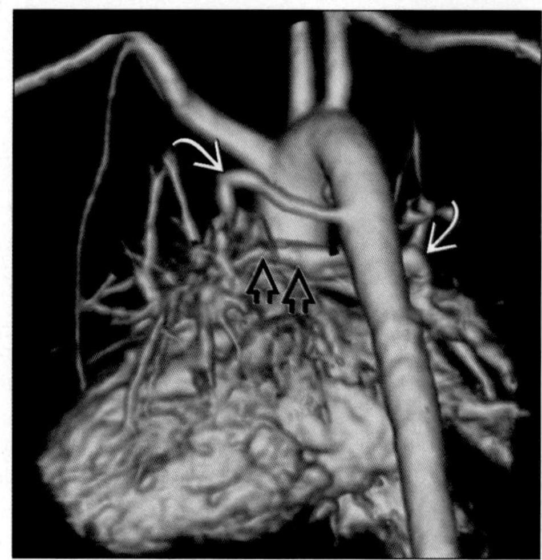

Oblique CECT volume rendering in tetralogy patient shows small stenosed native pulmonary arteries ⇨. Note multiple aorto pulmonary collateral arteries (MAPCA) ➡.

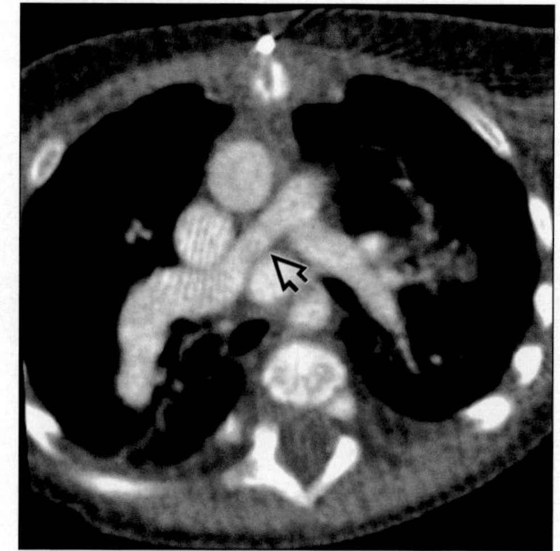

Oblique CECT shows smooth narrowing of right pulmonary artery ⇨ at insertion site of Blalock Taussig shunt (not shown). Note: Post-stenotic dilatation.

TERMINOLOGY

Definitions

- Stenosis of pulmonary artery (PA) and/or branches

IMAGING FINDINGS

General Features

- Best diagnostic clue
  - Focal web-like or long-segment tubular narrowing of pulmonary artery
  - Evidence for collateral aorto-pulmonary circulation to lung in chronic pulmonary artery stenosis

Radiographic Findings

- Radiography
  - Usually normal size heart with normal vascularity
    - Rarely decreased vascularity in severe stenosis
  - Post-stenotic dilatation may occasionally be evident, especially on left side
  - Right heart enlargement with filling of retrosternal space in chronic severe pulmonary artery stenosis

CT Findings

- NECT
  - May see calcification in setting of fibrosing mediastinitis
  - Right heart enlargement in chronic severe obstruction and resultant right ventricular (RV) failure
- CTA
  - Best test for evaluation of potential underlying mediastinal lesions causing extrinsic compression
  - Focal or tubular narrowing of pulmonary arteries
    - If extrinsic compression often also narrowing of corresponding pulmonary veins
  - Best test to depict aorto-pulmonary collaterals
  - Gated CTA may demonstrate associated congenital abnormalities

MR Findings

- T1WI: Useful for evaluating soft tissue anatomy of mediastinum or lesions surrounding stenosed pulmonary arteries
- T2WI: Useful for characterizing lesions creating extrinsic compression of pulmonary arteries
- MRA

DDx: Branch Pulmonary Stenosis

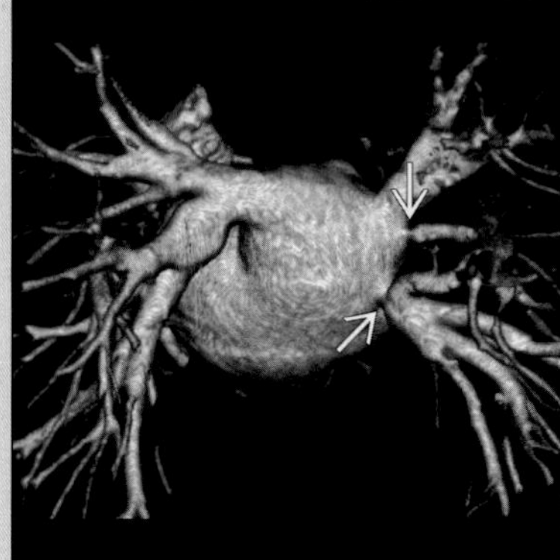

Pulmonary Vein Stenosis

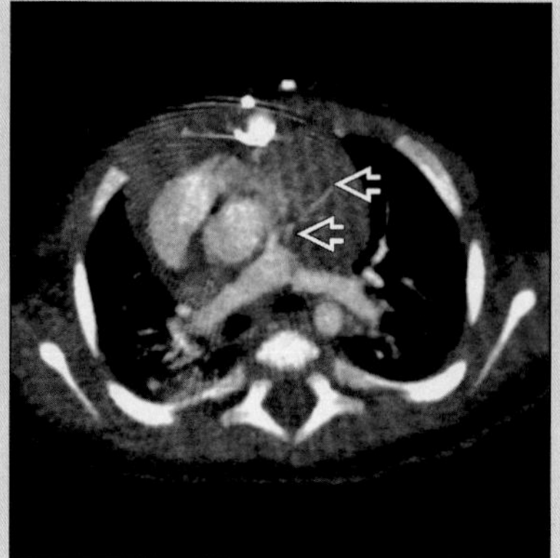

Pulmonary Atresia

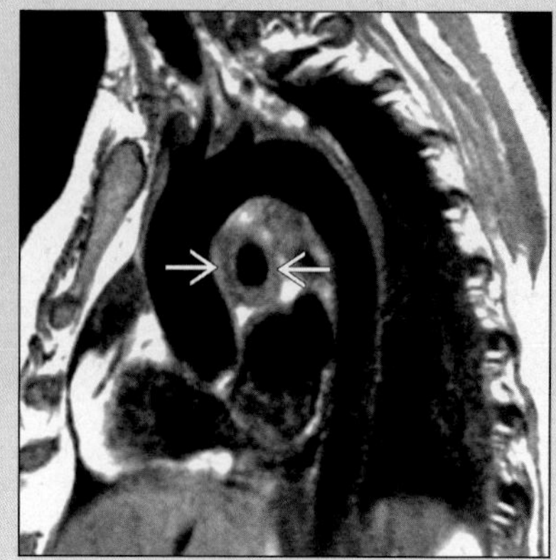

Takayasu Arteritis

BRANCH PULMONARY STENOSIS

Key Facts

Terminology
- Stenosis of pulmonary artery (PA) and/or branches

Imaging Findings
- Focal web-like or long-segment tubular narrowing of pulmonary artery
- Evidence for collateral aorto-pulmonary circulation to lung in chronic pulmonary artery stenosis
- Usually normal size heart with normal vascularity
- Post-stenotic dilatation may occasionally be evident, especially on left side
- Right heart enlargement with filling of retrosternal space in chronic severe pulmonary artery stenosis
- Echocardiography has limited usefulness due to limited acoustic window for evaluating branch pulmonary stenosis

Pathology
- Common anatomic component of complex cyanotic congenital heart disease
- Common long-term complication of congenital heart disease

Clinical Issues
- Surgical revascularization for proximal pulmonary artery stenosis/atresia associated with congenital heart disease
- Percutaneous balloon angioplasty ± stent in select cases

  - Focal or diffuse stenosis involving pulmonary artery
  - Focal or diffuse stenosis of pulmonary veins
  - Evidence for aorto-pulmonary collateral circulation in chronic pulmonary artery stenosis
  - Contrast-enhanced 3D MRA technique shown to be as accurate as conventional arteriography for detecting pulmonary stenoses and aorto-pulmonary collaterals
  - Phase-contrast velocity measurement important to characterize the hemodynamic significance of pulmonary stenosis
    - Peak systolic velocities exceeding 1.5 mm/sec imply hemodynamically significant stenosis
    - Cine-gradient-echo imaging may be helpful for characterizing associated congenital heart abnormalities
  - Noncontrast MRA of limited value

Echocardiographic Findings
- Echocardiogram
  - Echocardiography has limited usefulness due to limited acoustic window for evaluating branch pulmonary stenosis
  - May demonstrate associated cardiac abnormalities
    - Atrial septal defect
    - Pulmonic valve stenosis
- Pulsed Doppler
  - Parasternal and subcostal views most accurately determine PA flow velocities across valve and main PA stenoses
  - Peripheral stenoses not directly visualized

Angiographic Findings
- Conventional
  - Pressure gradient within pulmonary arterial system is diagnostic
  - Defines location, length, number and severity of stenotic segments
  - Balloon angioplasty in select cases only
    - Proximal well localized severe stenoses
    - May have stent placed

Imaging Recommendations
- Best imaging tool: CTA or MRA
- Routine spin echo and cine MR followed by contrast-enhanced 3D MRA

DIFFERENTIAL DIAGNOSIS

Isolated Pulmonary Stenosis
- Unusual cause of pulmonary stenosis

Pulmonary Stenosis Associated with Congenital Heart Disease
- Tetralogy of Fallot
- Pulmonary atresia
- Post-Fontan pulmonary palliation

Adult-Acquired Pulmonary Stenosis
- Chronic pulmonary embolism
- Vasculitis
  - Takayasu arteritis
    - Young to middle-aged women
    - Pulmonary arteries affected in > 50% of cases
    - Usually bilateral and multifocal
    - Predilection for upper lobe branches
  - Connective tissue disorders
    - Scleroderma
    - Rheumatoid arthritis
    - Systemic lupus erythematosus
  - Behçet disease
  - Wegener granulomatosis
  - Allergic angiitis and granulomatosis

Pulmonary Vein Stenosis
- Patients post-radiofrequency ablation of ectopic atrial foci
- Patients following re-anastomosis of anomalous pulmonary vein

BRANCH PULMONARY STENOSIS

PATHOLOGY

General Features

- Etiology
  - Most common cause is abnormal pulmonary circulation in congenital heart disease
    - Common anatomic component of complex cyanotic congenital heart disease
    - Common long-term complication of congenital heart disease
  - Stenosis may be acquired, especially in presence of pulmonary revascularization procedures (Fontan, Blalock-Taussig shunt)

Gross Pathologic & Surgical Features

- Narrowing of pulmonary artery or branches
- Thickening of pulmonary arterial wall
- Aorto-pulmonary collateral circulation through bronchial arteries

Microscopic Features

- Inflammation of vessel wall in setting of vasculitis

Staging, Grading or Classification Criteria

- Pulmonary arterial obstruction may be divided into four types
  - Type 1: Isolated stenosis of pulmonary trunk or main left or main right PA
  - Type 2: Stenosis at truncal bifurcation and extending into main PAs
  - Type 3: Multiple peripheral branch stenoses
  - Type 4: Combination of main and peripheral stenoses

CLINICAL ISSUES

Presentation

- Cyanotic congenital heart disease
- Features of systemic vasculitis
- Presentation of pulmonary vein stenosis related to venous hypertension
  - Pleural effusions
  - Pulmonary edema, unilateral or asymmetric

Natural History & Prognosis

- Branch pulmonary stenosis is a serious and long-term complication of congenital heart disease
- Prognosis is poor

Treatment

- Surgical revascularization for proximal pulmonary artery stenosis/atresia associated with congenital heart disease
- Percutaneous balloon angioplasty ± stent in select cases

DIAGNOSTIC CHECKLIST

Consider

- Check newborns for associated congenital malformations associated with intrauterine rubella infection
  - Atrial septal defect, pulmonic valve stenosis, persistent ductus arteriosus
- If peripheral pulmonary stenosis in conjunction with supravalvular aortic stenosis consider familial form or Williams syndrome

SELECTED REFERENCES

1. Seto T et al: [A case of the multiple peripheral pulmonary artery branch stenosis] Nihon Kokyuki Gakkai Zasshi. 43(12):755-60, 2005
2. Horstkotte D et al: [Congenital heart disease and acquired valvular lesions in pregnancy] Herz. 28(3):227-39, 2003
3. Geva T et al: Gadolinium-enhanced 3-dimensional magnetic resonance angiography of pulmonary blood supply in patients with complex pulmonary stenosis or atresia: comparison with x-ray angiography. Circulation. 106(4):473-8, 2002
4. Bacha EA et al: Comprehensive management of branch pulmonary artery stenosis. J Interv Cardiol. 14(3):367-75, 2001
5. Friedman WF et al: Congenital Heart Disease in Infancy and Childhood. In: Heart Disease - A Textbook of Cardiovascular Medicine. Vol 2. 1505-91, 2001
6. Dicle O et al: Multiple coarctation of the pulmonary artery. Eur J Radiol. 36(3):147-9, 2000
7. Shah R et al: Case 2. Congenital multiple peripheral pulmonary artery stenosis (Pulmonary branch stenosis or supravalvular pulmonary stenosis). AJR Am J Roentgenol. 175(3):854; 856-7, 2000
8. Kreutzer J et al: Isolated peripheral pulmonary artery stenoses in the adult. Circulation. 93(7):1417-23, 1996
9. Miyamura H et al: Spontaneous regression of peripheral pulmonary artery stenosis in Williams syndrome. Jpn Circ J. 60(5):311-4, 1996
10. Bletry O et al: [Severe pulmonary artery involvement of Takayasu arteritis. 3 cases and review of the literature] Arch Mal Coeur Vaiss. 84(6):817-22, 1991
11. Busch U et al: [Peripheral pulmonary stenosis: initial manifestation of a malignant teratoma] Z Kardiol. 77(9):613-6, 1988
12. Damuth TE et al: Major pulmonary artery stenosis causing pulmonary hypertension in sarcoidosis. Chest. 78(6):888-91, 1980
13. Carambas CR et al: Congenital pulmonary artery branch stenosis: association with renal artery stenosis. Chest. 75(3):402-4, 1979
14. Cohn LH et al: Surgical treatment of congenital unilateral pulmonary arterial stenosis with contralateral pulmonary hypertension. Am J Cardiol. 38(2):257-60, 1976

BRANCH PULMONARY STENOSIS

IMAGE GALLERY

Typical

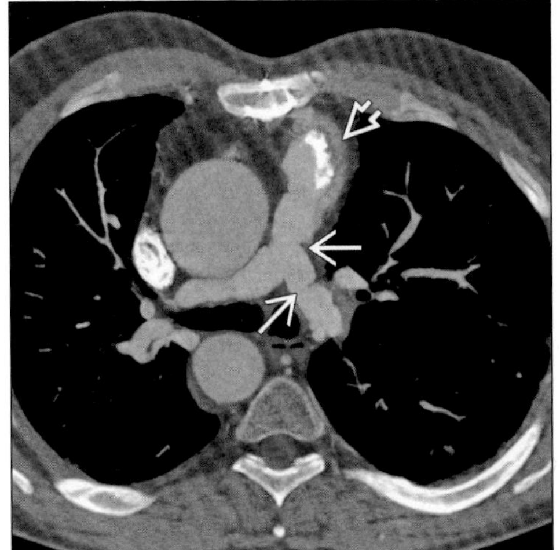

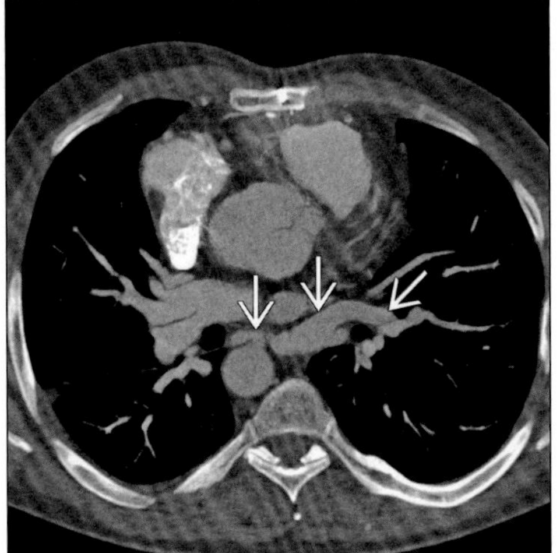

*(**Left**) Axial CECT in patient with tetralogy shows multiple web-like pulmonary artery stenoses ➔. Note: Patch repair of right ventricular outflow tract obstruction ➔ and right aortic arch. (**Right**) Oblique CECT in same patient as previous image shows large aorto-pulmonary collateral artery ➔ to left lung that has developed due to the hemodynamic pulmonary flow obstruction.*

Typical

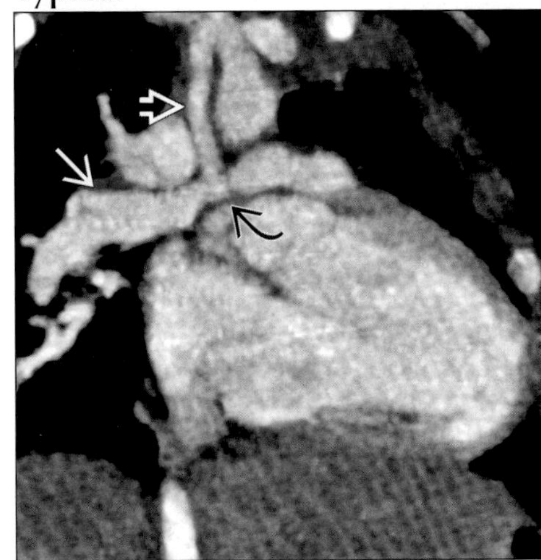

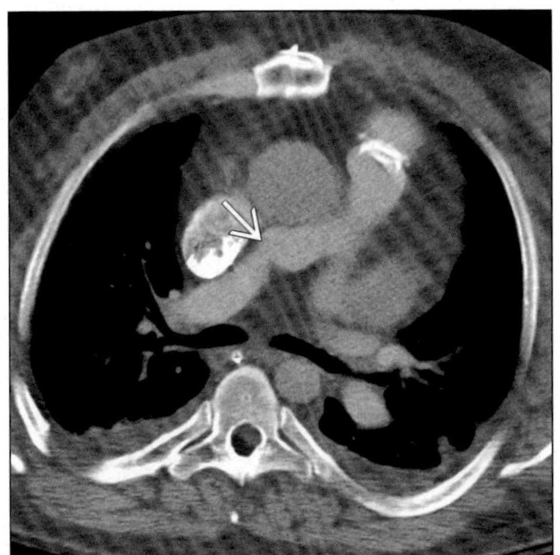

*(**Left**) Oblique CECT shows Blalock Taussig shunt ➔ connecting to right pulmonary artery. Note: Smooth perianastomotic stenosis ➔ with distal dilatation ➔. (**Right**) Oblique CECT in patient with tetralogy of Fallot shows deformity and mild pulmonary artery stenosis ➔ due to previous Waterston shunt palliation. Note: Prosthetic pulmonary artery valve.*

Typical

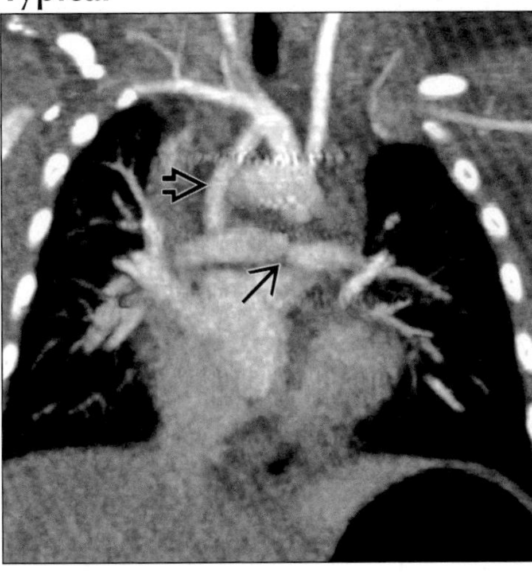

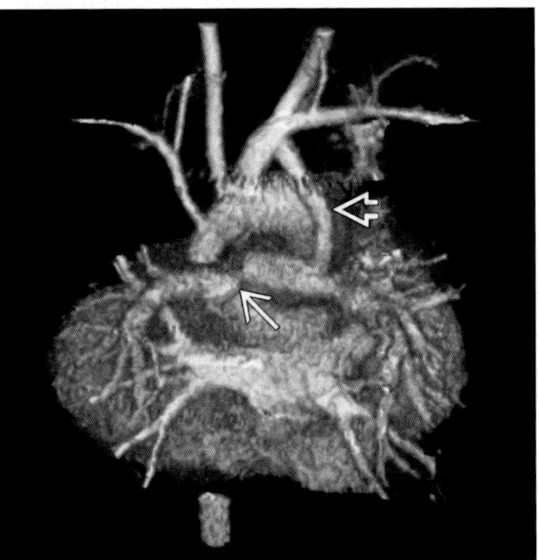

*(**Left**) Coronal CECT in patient with single ventricle and pulmonary atresia shows right Blalock Taussig (BT) shunt ➔ and web-like stenosis of left pulmonary artery ➔. (**Right**) Posterior volume rendering of CTA shows central pulmonary stenosis ➔. Note: BT shunt ➔.*

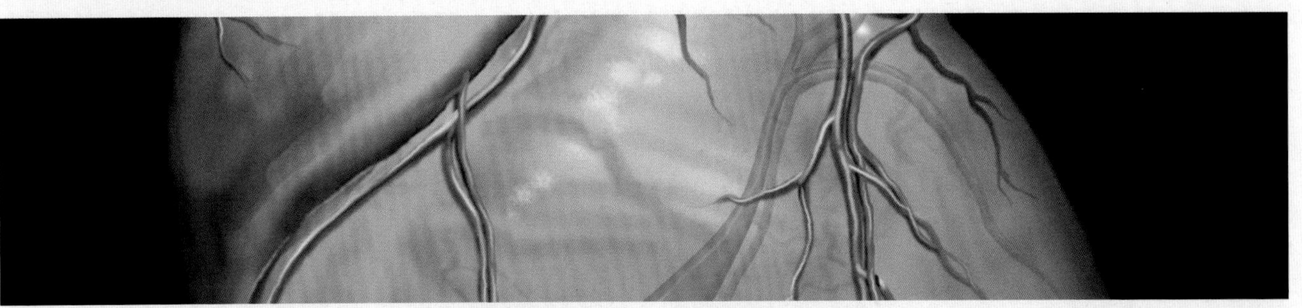

SECTION 9: Electrophysiology

PULMONARY VEIN MAPPING

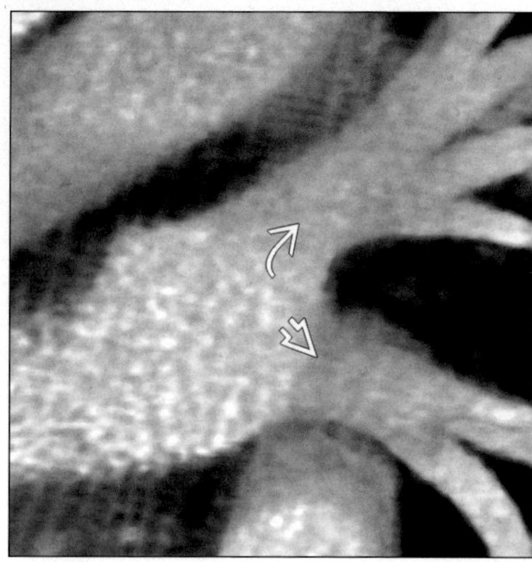

Oblique CTA shows left upper lobe pulmonary vein ➦ and left lower lobe pulmonary vein ➯.

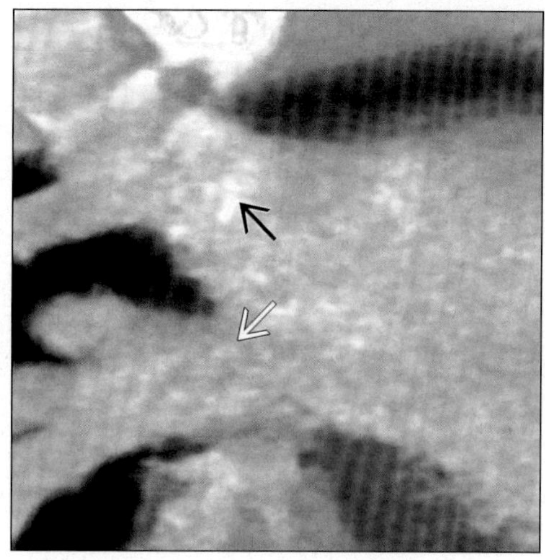

Oblique CTA shows right upper lobe pulmonary vein ➔ and right lower lobe pulmonary vein ➡.

TERMINOLOGY

Definitions

- Imaging of left atrium (LA) and pulmonary veins (PV) to help guide electrophysiological (EP) ablation procedure
- PVs return oxygenated blood from the lungs to the LA and may contain ectopic electrical foci that cause atrial fibrillation

IMAGING FINDINGS

General Features

- Location
  - Modal anatomy has paired upper and lower PVs bilaterally (56%)
  - Supernumerary pulmonary veins occur when there is overincorporation of primitive pulmonary venous structures by the developing LA (29%)
    - Usually on the right side
    - More common variant is separate drainage of right middle lobe
    - Less common is separate drainage of superior segment of right middle lobe
    - Can be separate drainage of lingula
    - May present challenge to performance of ostial ablations
  - Common pulmonary trunk occurs if under incorporation of primitive pulmonary veins (17%)
    - Usually on the left side
- Size
  - Maximal ostial diameters
    - Left superior PV = 18.0 ± 2.9 mm
    - Right superior PV = 18.4 ± 2.9 mm
    - Left inferior PV = 15.4 ± 2.2 mm
    - Right inferior PV = 15.5 ± 2.8 mm
    - 25% of patients have PV ostia < 10 mm which may not accommodate circumferential mapping catheters and increases risk of PV stenosis following radiofrequency catheter ablation (RFCA)
    - 14% of patients have PV ostia > 25 mm resulting in unstable positioning and/or inadequate contact of the circumferential mapping catheter
  - Average intrapatient variability in PV diameter was 7.9 ± 4.2 mm
    - Greater than 10% variation in 31% of patients

DDx: Variant Anatomy

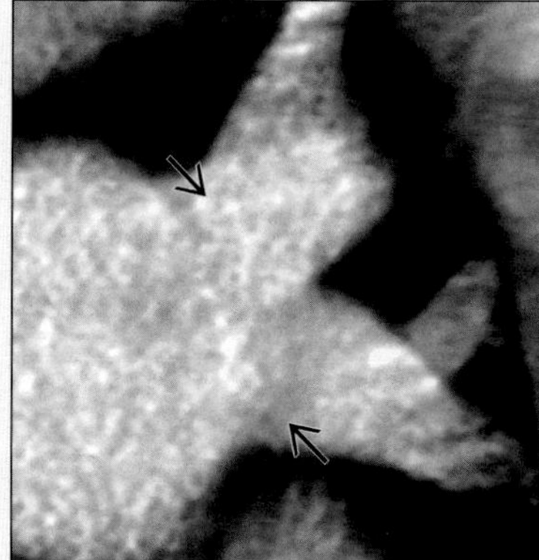

Conjoined LPV

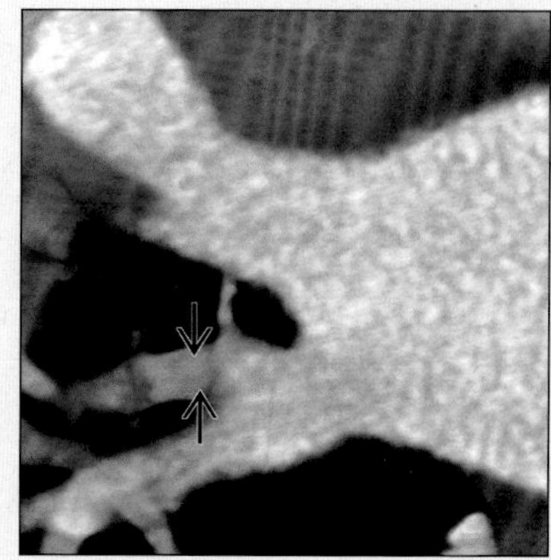

Ostial Branch RPV

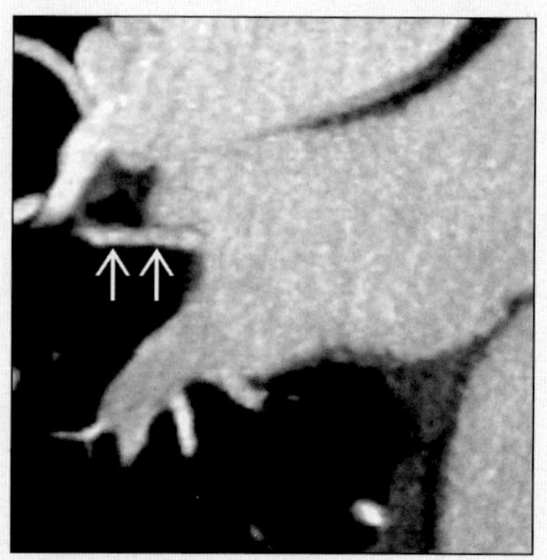

Supernumerary Vein

PULMONARY VEIN MAPPING

Key Facts

Terminology

- Pulmonary veins (PV) return oxygenated blood from the lungs to the left atrium (LA) and may contain ectopic electrical foci that cause atrial fibrillation

Imaging Findings

- Modal anatomy has paired upper and lower PVs bilaterally (56%)
- Supernumerary pulmonary veins occur when there is overincorporation of primitive pulmonary venous structures by the developing LA (29%)
- Can be separate drainage of lingula
- Common pulmonary trunk occurs when there is underincorporation of primitive pulmonary veins (17%)
- PV anatomy can be readily identified
- Reformatted images obtained to measure PV ostial diameters

    - Necessitates use of more than one circumferential mapping catheter during RFCA
- Morphology
  - Majority of PV ostia are oval
  - PVs can be straight or funnel-shaped
    - Straight PVs have only a gradual decrease in diameter from proximal (ostial) to distal
    - Funnel-shaped PV have a decrease in diameter by 60% over a length of 10 mm
    - 47% of patients have at least one funnel-shaped PV
    - Can interfere with stable placement of RFCA catheters
  - 41% of patients have branches within first 5 mm of PV (ostial branches)
    - An early branch may be prone to stenosis after an ostial RFCA
  - Angulation in both transverse and coronal planes may affect ease with which ostia are accessed

CT Findings

- CTA
  - May be used for fusion with electroanatomic map during procedure
  - PV anatomy can be readily identified
  - Reformatted images obtained to measure PV ostial diameters
- Cardiac Gated CTA: Can be used to assess diameters of PV during different phases of cardiac cycle

MR Findings

- MRA
  - PV anatomy readily identified without ionizing radiation
  - PV ostial diameters derived from reformatted images
- MR Cine
  - Phase contrast images can determine velocity profiles of PVs
  - May be useful as baseline if patient is to undergo RFCA which can be complicated by PV stenosis

Echocardiographic Findings

- Can be limited to superior pulmonary veins

Imaging Recommendations

- Best imaging tool: CTA
- Protocol advice: Use bolus timing software to scan during peak enhancement of LA

DIAGNOSTIC CHECKLIST

Consider

- PV anatomy impacts preprocedural planning of RFCA

Image Interpretation Pearls

- LA clot is a relative contraindication to RFCA

SELECTED REFERENCES

1. Mansour M et al: Assessment of pulmonary vein anatomic variability by magnetic resonance imaging: implications for catheter ablation techniques for atrial fibrillation. J Cardiovasc Electrophysiol. 15(4):387-93, 2004

IMAGE GALLERY

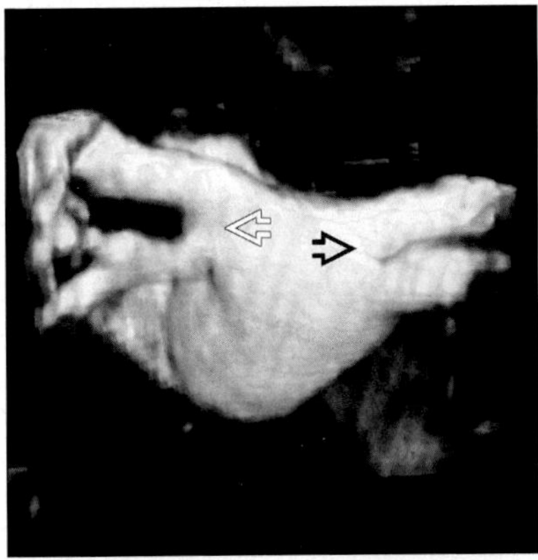

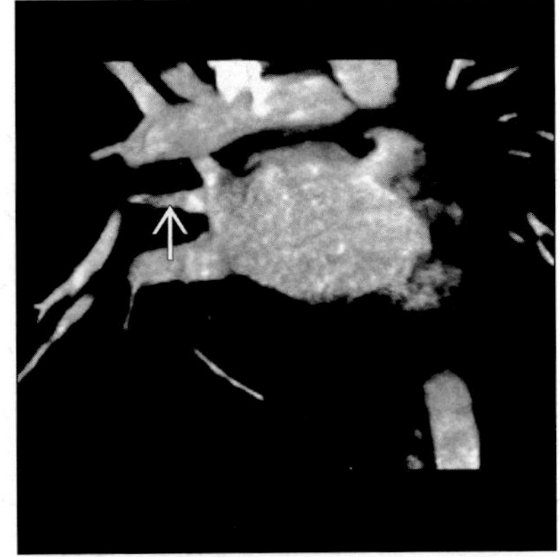

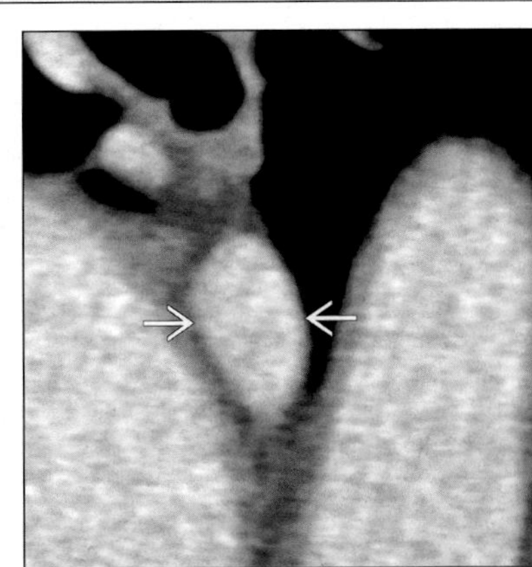

(Left) *Coronal shows normal modal anatomy depicted by contrast-enhanced MR with two veins on the left ⇨ and two on the right ➡.* ***(Center)*** *Coronal CECT shows ostial branch at right upper pulmonary vein ➡.* ***(Right)*** *Oblique CECT shows left inferior pulmonary vein ostium in cross-section ➡. Anteroposterior and cranio-caudal measurements can be obtained with this projection. Note: Oval shape is normal.*

PULMONARY VEIN STENOSIS

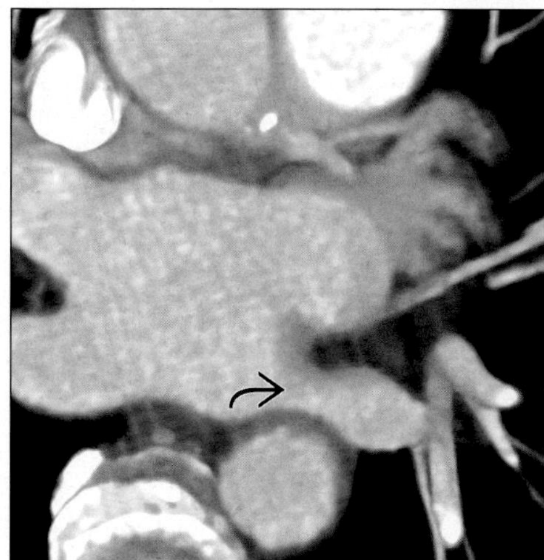

Oblique CTA shows stenosis at ostium of left inferior pulmonary vein ➚. Note: Normal mild concavity of PV may mimic stenosis, comparison with pre-treatment study most helpful.

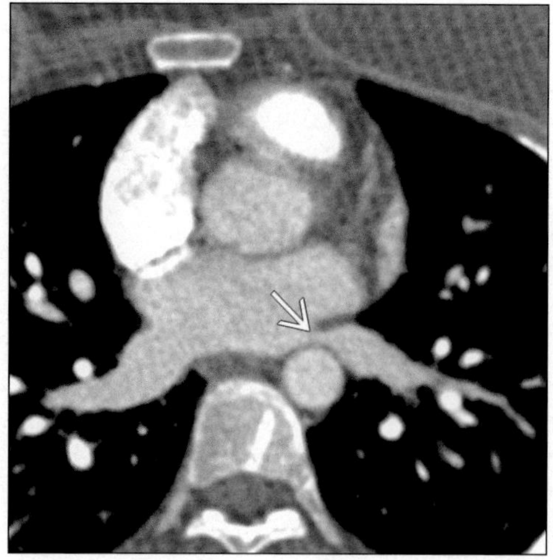

Axial CECT shows stenotic ostium of left inferior pulmonary vein ➡ after radiofrequency ablation.

TERMINOLOGY

Definitions

- Narrowed pulmonary vein (PV) after radio frequency catheter ablation (RFCA) for atrial fibrillation

IMAGING FINDINGS

General Features

- Best diagnostic clue: Direct visualization of narrowing on cross-sectional imaging modality
- Location: Any of the treated PVs
- Size: Mild diameter stenosis < 50%, severe > 70%

Radiographic Findings

- Radiography: Edema in lung drained by stenotic PV

CT Findings

- CECT
  - Direct visualization of PV stenosis with CT
    - Pitfall: Normal oval shape may mimic stenosis; comparison with pre-treatment images helpful
  - Delayed contrast-enhancement of affected veins and corresponding pulmonary arteries

MR Findings

- MRA
  - Direct visualization of PV stenosis
  - Can use 2D Cine PC to measure velocity

Echocardiographic Findings

- Echocardiogram
  - TEE may show increased PV velocity, turbulent flow at junction of PV & left atrium (LA), stenosis
    - Often limited to superior PVs

Angiographic Findings

- Conventional: Pulmonary angiography may reveal pruning of peripheral arteries, delayed transit of contrast through lungs to LA & PV stenosis itself

Imaging Recommendations

- Best imaging tool: CT
- Protocol advice: Bolus timing to LA

DDx: Pulmonary Vein Stenosis Progressing to Thrombosis

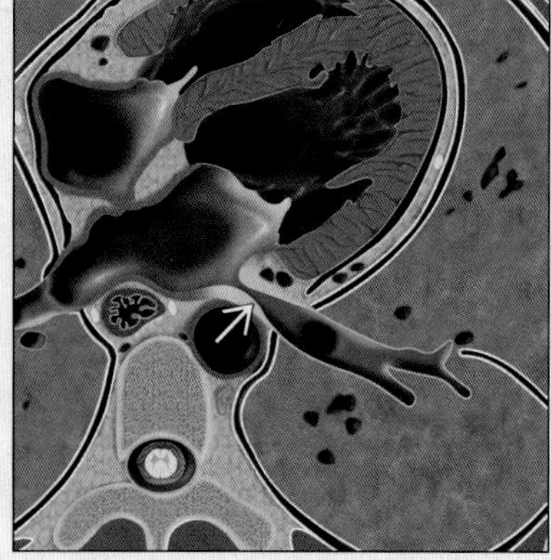

Stenosis from RFCA

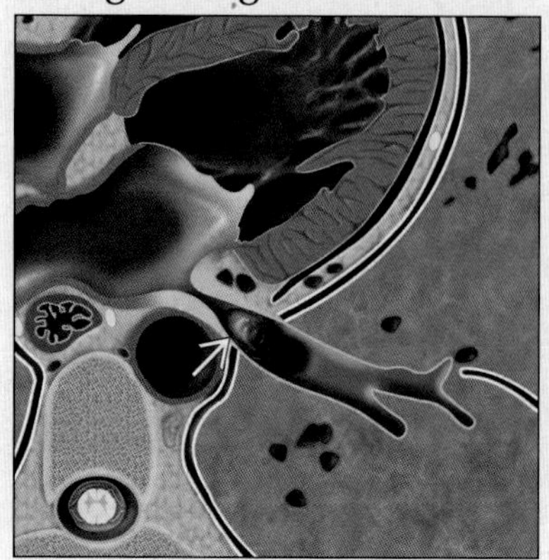

Secondary Thrombosis

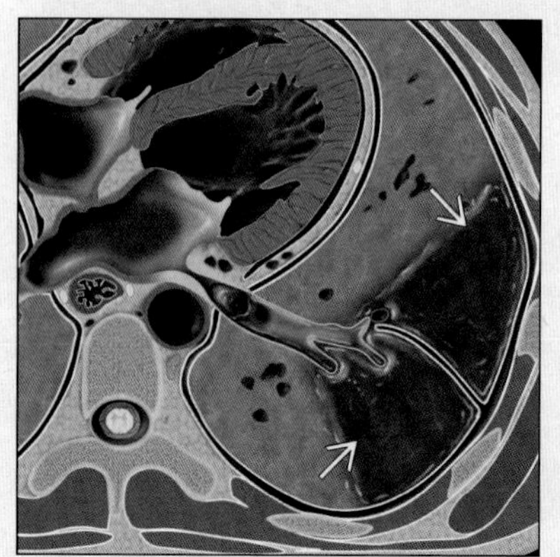

Focal Edema

PULMONARY VEIN STENOSIS

Key Facts

Terminology

- Narrowed pulmonary vein (PV) after radio frequency catheter ablation (RFCA) for atrial fibrillation

Imaging Findings

- Radiography: Edema in lung drained by stenotic PV
- Direct visualization of PV stenosis with CT
- Pitfall: Normal oval shape may mimic stenosis; comparison with pre-treatment images helpful
- Delayed contrast-enhancement of affected veins and corresponding pulmonary arteries
- Conventional: Pulmonary angiography may reveal pruning of peripheral arteries, delayed transit of contrast through lungs to LA & PV stenosis itself
- Bolus timing to LA

Pathology

- Risk factors include RFCA inside the PVs rather than around the ostia, use of excessive power

DIFFERENTIAL DIAGNOSIS

Pulmonary Vein Thrombosis

- Visualization of thrombus in lumen of PV

PATHOLOGY

General Features

- Etiology
  - Risk factors include RFCA inside the PVs rather than around the ostia, use of excessive power
  - RFCA may induce swelling (early) and fibrosis (late)
- Epidemiology
  - Incidence from 3% to 42% depending on technique, imaging technique, definition of stenosis
  - Rate falling because of RFCA delivered around ostia rather than within PVs

CLINICAL ISSUES

Presentation

- Most common signs/symptoms
  - Frequently asymptomatic
  - Dyspnea, cough, hemoptysis, pleuritic pain

Natural History & Prognosis

- If stenosis occurs post RFCA, about 10% progress and about 10% regress

Treatment

- Symptomatic patients or asymptomatic patients with severe stenosis can be treated with balloon angioplasty and stent deployment
- Rationale for treating asymptomatic patient is unknown risk of pulmonary hypertension, risk of progression to complete occlusion
- About half restenose prompting further intervention

DIAGNOSTIC CHECKLIST

Consider

- Preprocedural imaging helps size catheters

SELECTED REFERENCES

1. Mansour M et al: Assessment of pulmonary vein anatomic variability by magnetic resonance imaging: implications for catheter ablation techniques for atrial fibrillation. J Cardiovasc Electrophysiol. 15(4):387-93, 2004
2. Ghaye B et al: Percutaneous ablation for atrial fibrillation: the role of cross-sectional imaging. Radiographics. 23 Spec No:S19-33; discussion S48-50, 2003
3. Saad EB et al: Pulmonary vein stenosis after catheter ablation of atrial fibrillation: emergence of a new clinical syndrome. Ann Intern Med. 138(8):634-8, 2003
4. Saad EB et al: Pulmonary vein stenosis after radiofrequency ablation of atrial fibrillation: functional characterization, evolution, and influence of the ablation strategy. Circulation. 108(25):3102-7, 2003

IMAGE GALLERY

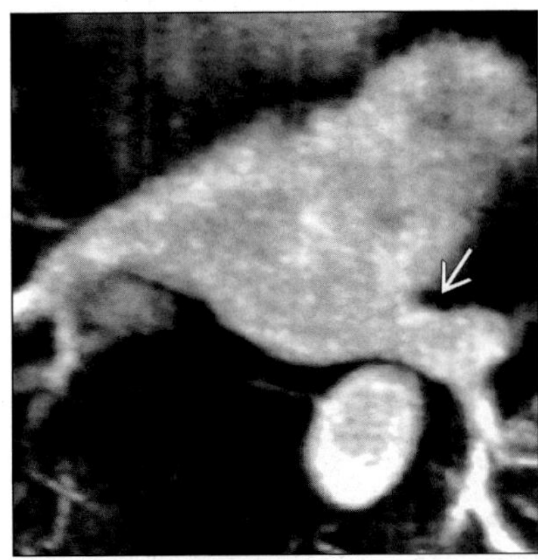

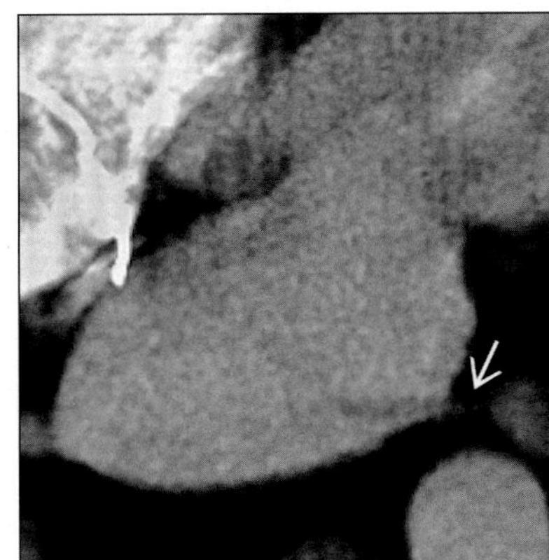

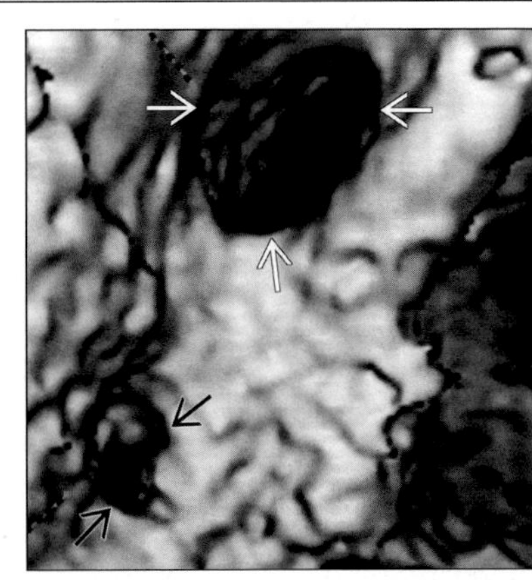

(Left) *Oblique MR angiogram shows normal left inferior pulmonary vein ➡ in a 57 year old male prior to pulmonary vein ablation for atrial fibrillation.* ***(Center)*** *Oblique cardiac CT in same patient as previous image, shows severe stenosis of left inferior pulmonary vein ➡ after radiofrequency ablation.* ***(Right)*** *Endoluminal view of the left-sided pulmonary veins in same patient as previous image, shows the severity of the left inferior pulmonary vein stenosis ⇨ compared to the left superior pulmonary vein ➡.*

PACEMAKERS/ICDS

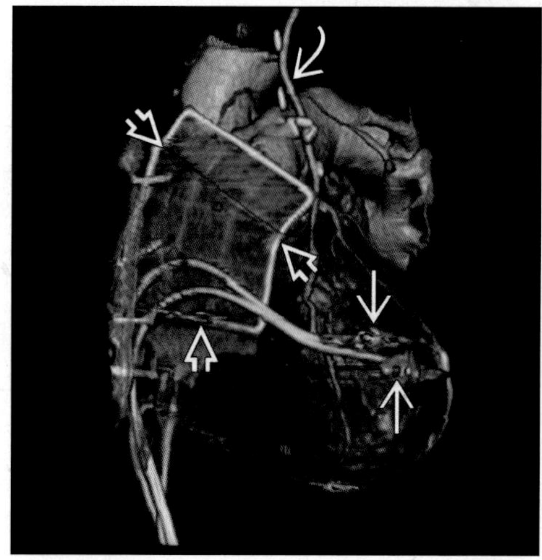

Oblique cardiac CT shows epicardial defibrillator patches and screw-in epicardial leads in left ventricular myocardium . Note, left internal mammary artery bypass graft .

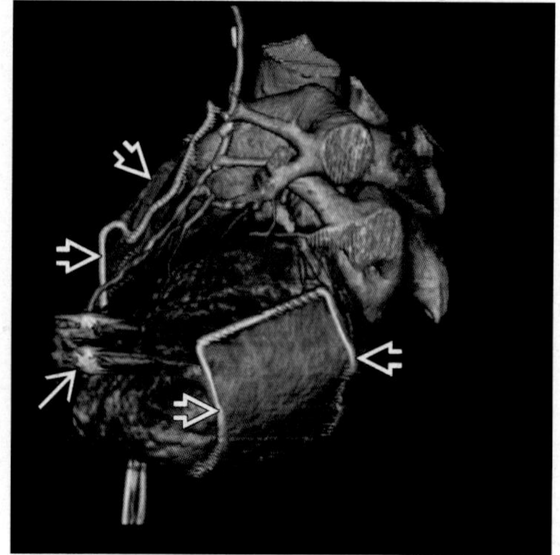

Posterior lateral view volume rendered cardiac CT shows defibrillator patches and tips of screw-in epicardial leads . Note, leads descend anteriorly towards devices in abdominal wall.

TERMINOLOGY

Abbreviations and Synonyms

- Implantable cardioverter defibrillator (ICD)
- Automatic implantable cardioverter-defibrillator (AICD)
- Permanent pacing device

Definitions

- Pacemakers are permanently implanted, battery-operated electronic devices, connected to the heart by pacing wires that use electrical impulses to regulate cardiac rate or rhythm
  - Substitute for a natural pacemaker (sinus node)
- ICDs are permanently implanted battery-operated electronic device that administer electric shocks via intracardiac or epicardial leads to the heart to restore normal cardiac rhythm if defined rapid ventricular arrhythmias are sensed

IMAGING FINDINGS

General Features

- Best diagnostic clue
  - Presence of epicardial, coronary sinus or right atrial and ventricular leads
  - Presence of Pacemaker or ICD generator
- Location
  - Usually right or left pectoral pocket containing device generator
  - Older devices and epicardial pacing or defibrillator devices in abdominal wall tissue
  - Temporary leads may have leads exit at right internal jugular vein and connect to extracorporal device
  - Leads typically ascend into superior vena cava (SVC) and right or left innominate and subclavian veins
  - Older leads may descend in subcutaneous tissue towards abdomen
  - Epicardial leads typically perforate pericardium anteriorly and descend towards abdomen within connective tissue
  - Lead tip locations
    - Right atrium - commonly atrial appendage

DDx: Pacemakers/ICDs

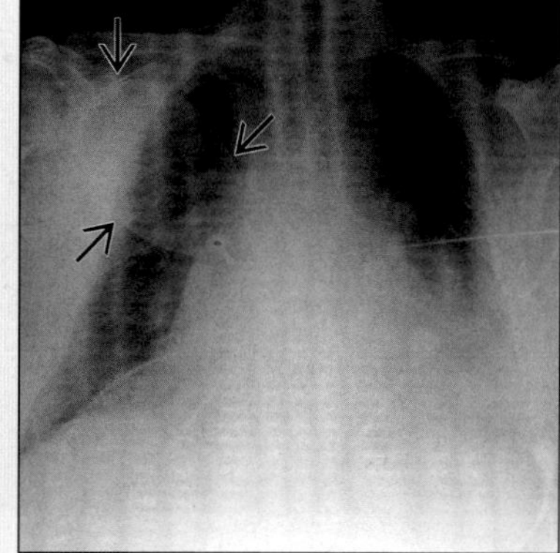

External Defibrillator

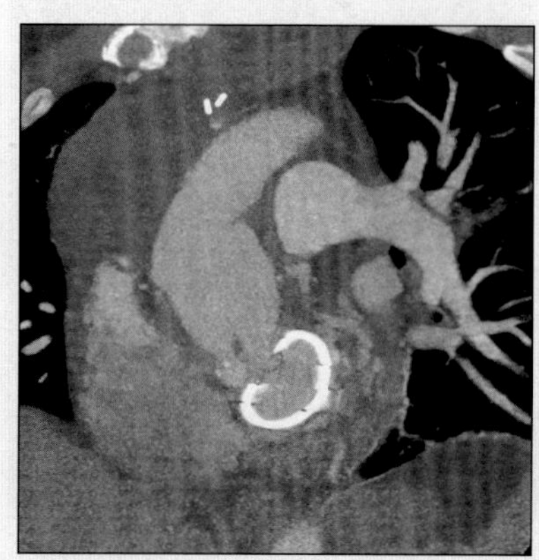

Open Annuloplasty Ring

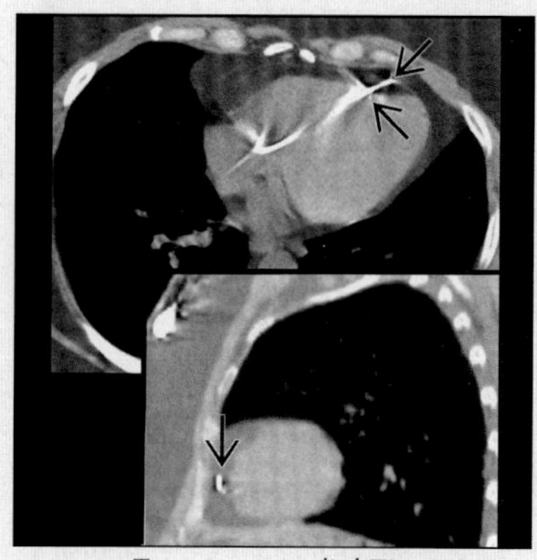

Transmyocardial Tip

PACEMAKERS/ICDS

Key Facts

Terminology

- Pacemakers are permanently implanted, battery-operated electronic devices, connected to the heart by pacing wires that use electrical impulses to regulate cardiac rate or rhythm
- Substitute for a natural pacemaker (sinus node)
- ICDs are permanently implanted battery-operated electronic device that administer electric shocks via intracardiac or epicardial leads to the heart to restore normal cardiac rhythm if defined rapid ventricular arrhythmias are sensed

Imaging Findings

- Radiograph may demonstrate lead fractures, tip dislodgement and device migration
- Fluoroscopy may be helpful in confirming lead fractures with only little fragment displacement
- **CT may demonstrate complication from device placement including**
- Hemothorax
- Pneumothorax or pneumopericardium
- Chamber or coronary sinus rupture with hemopericardium ± tamponade
- Ultrasound with Doppler sonography useful to detect venous thrombosis
- Best imaging tool: PA and lateral radiograph
- Protocol advice: Fluoroscopy may confirm suspected lead fracture

Diagnostic Checklist

- Beam hardening artifact may mimic right ventricular perforation by lead tip

---

    - Right ventricle near apex
    - Left ventricle either via coronary sinus in great cardiac vein or its tributaries (transvenous leads), or via pericardium within epicardial myocardium (epicardial leads)
- Size
  - Lead size varies 1-3 mm
    - ICD leads are generally thicker and have two separate thickened areas with a spring coil appearance which deliver the electrical shocks when triggered
- Morphology
  - Single chamber pacing
    - → One lead in RA
  - Dual chamber pacing
    - → Two leads, one in RA one in RV
  - Biventricular pacing
    - → RA and RV leads and one lead via coronary sinus in great cardiac vein or tributary
  - Epicardial pacing
    - → Two screw-in leads in left ventricular myocardium
    - Device location = abdominal wall
  - Epicardial defibrillator
    - → Two patches over anterior right ventricle and posterior lateral left ventricle
    - Device location = abdominal wall
  - ICD
    - → One multifunctional lead with defibrillator electrodes at SVC and RV level, sensing electrode at lead tip
    - ± Coronary sinus lead and right atrial lead if also biventricularly paced

Radiographic Findings

- Radiograph may demonstrate lead fractures, tip dislodgement and device migration

Fluoroscopic Findings

- Fluoroscopy may be helpful in confirming lead fractures with only little fragment displacement
  - Typically between first rib and clavicle
- Upper extremity maneuvers may be useful in displacing fragments better visualize and confirm fractures

CT Findings

- CECT
  - **CT may demonstrate complication from device placement including**
    - Hemothorax
    - Pneumothorax or pneumopericardium
    - Chamber or coronary sinus rupture with hemopericardium ± tamponade
    - Device infection

Ultrasonographic Findings

- Ultrasound with Doppler sonography useful to detect venous thrombosis
- Useful to evaluate device infection or seroma formation
  - Interrogation of tissue behind generator may be limited by immobile device and acoustic shadowing

Imaging Recommendations

- Best imaging tool: PA and lateral radiograph
- Protocol advice: Fluoroscopy may confirm suspected lead fracture

DIFFERENTIAL DIAGNOSIS

Deep Brain Stimulator

- Treatment of Parkinson disease
- Leads travel towards cranium
- May be multiple devices

Vagal Nerve Stimulator

- Leads terminate in neck near carotid arteries

Spinal Cord Stimulators

- One or two leads with multiple electrodes (4-6)
- Leads in epidural space of lower thoracic and upper lumbar spine

Other Pacemakers and Stimulators

- Diaphragmatic Pacemaker
- Gastric stimulator
- Bladder Pacemaker

PATHOLOGY

General Features

- ACC/AHA guidelines for ICD therapy include as class I indications
  - Cardiac arrest due to ventricular fibrillation (VF) or tachycardia (VT) not due to transient cause
  - Spontaneous sustained VT
  - Syncope with inducible VT or VF in electrophysiological (EP) study
  - Nonsustained VT in setting of ischemic heart disease and inducible VF or VT in EP study
- Other indications for ICD treatment include VT while awaiting transplant, familial conditions such as hypertrophic cardiomyopathy or long QT syndrome, and others
- Indications for permanent pacing therapy include among others
  - Acquired atrioventricular (AV) block with bradycardia, arrhythmia, asystole > 3 sec, or after surgery or ablation procedures
  - Bi- or trifascicular AV blocks
  - Sinus node dysfunction with bradycardia ± symptoms
  - Hypertrophic or dilated cardiomyopathies with sinus node dysfunction
  - Neuro cardiogenic syncopes

Gross Pathologic & Surgical Features

- Intraoperative placement of epicardial leads should consider phrenic nerve course to avoid phrenic stimulation
- Coronary sinus lead preferred over epicardial location for biventricular pacing
- Implantation of epicardial leads still necessary if
  - No suitable coronary vein identified
  - Coronary sinus placement failed
- Screw-in leads are the leads of choice in epicardial pacing
  - Development of epicardial fibrosis often leads to increases in pacing thresholds
- Epicardial leads may lead to post-operative pericardial adhesions
- Video-assisted thoracic surgical placement available but carries risks related to single lung ventilation
- Epicardial defibrillator patches more commonly used in the past
  - May migrate or cause excessive fibrosis or fluid collections

CLINICAL ISSUES

Presentation

- Complications
  - Cardiac perforation or coronary sinus transsection
  - Pneumothorax and/or pneumopericardium
  - Dislodgement of leads
  - Hemothorax, pleural effusions
  - Infection of pacer generator or ICD and/or leads
  - Stimulation of the diaphragm via phrenic nerve
  - Device migration
- Old leads frequently left in place when device and leads are replaced

Treatment

- In heart failure patients, a resynchronization-defibrillator combination device coupled with optimal medical therapy reduces all-cause mortality by 43%

DIAGNOSTIC CHECKLIST

Consider

- Carefully follow course of leads as fractures may be nondisplaced and subtle
- Compare lead position to initial post placement radiograph to exclude lead migration

Image Interpretation Pearls

- Beam hardening artifact may mimic right ventricular perforation by lead tip
  - Absence of pericardial fluid in absence of clinical symptoms suggests absence of free perforation

SELECTED REFERENCES

1. Chen HY: Delayed isolated hemothorax caused by temporary pacemaker: a case report. Int J Cardiol. 114(3):e109-10, 2007
2. Levin G et al: Noncardiac implantable pacemakers and stimulators: current role and radiographic appearance. AJR Am J Roentgenol. 188(4):984-91, 2007
3. Martinek M et al: Pneumopericardium followed by pericardial effusion after thoracic trauma and pacemaker implantation. Herz. 31(6):592-3, 2006
4. Ellery SM et al: Complications of biventricular pacing. Eur. Heart J. Suppl. 6(suppl_D):D117-21, 2004
5. Kuhlkamp V: Initial experience with an implantable cardioverter-defibrillator incorporating cardiac resynchronization therapy. J. Am. Coll. Cardiol. 39(5):790-7, 2002
6. Ho WJ et al: Right pneumothorax resulting from an endocardial screw-in atrial lead. Chest. 116(4):1133-4, 1999

IMAGE GALLERY

Typical

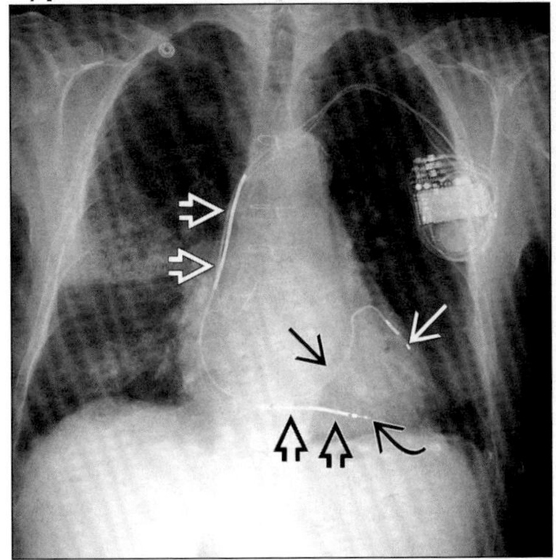

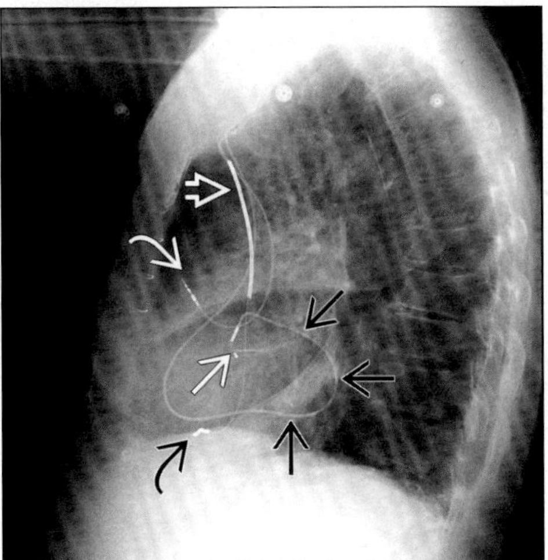

(Left) Posteroanterior radiograph shows ICD with defibrillator coils in SVC → and RV →, and sensing tip → in RV apex. A biventricular pacing lead traverses the coronary sinus → with tip in diagonal vein →. **(Right)** Lateral radiograph shows ICD lead with coil in SVC → and tip in RV apex →, right atrial appendage lead →, and pacing lead in coronary sinus → with tip in diagonal vein →.

Variant

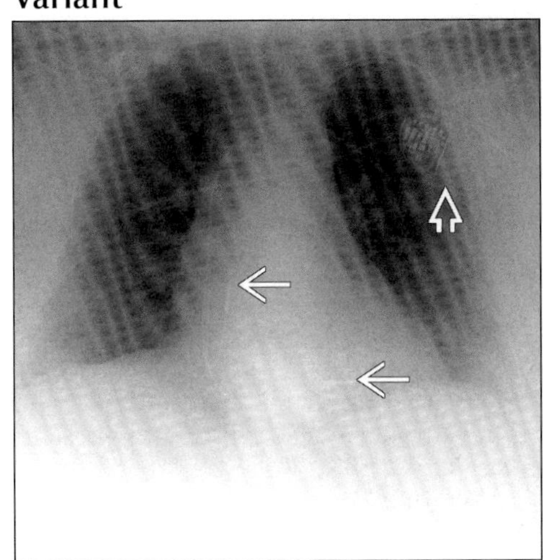

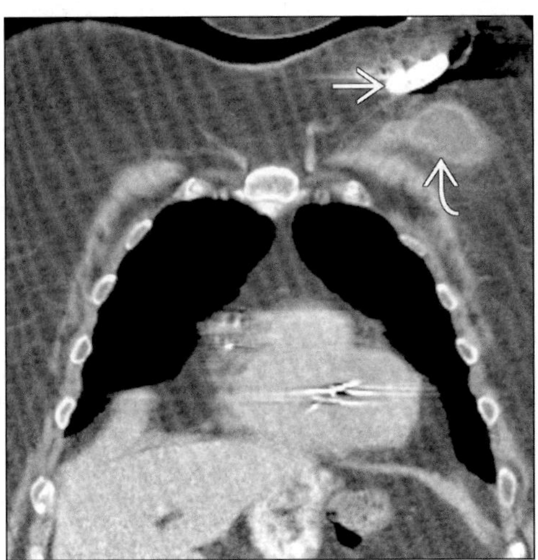

(Left) Anteroposterior radiograph shows left subclavian dual-lead pacemaker → with lead tips → projected over the right ventricle and left atrium. (Courtesy M Holbert, MD). **(Right)** Coronal CECT in same patient, shows a subcutaneous fluid collection → with enhancing thick rim adjacent to pacemaker generator → indicating abscess. (Courtesy M. Holbert, MD).

Typical

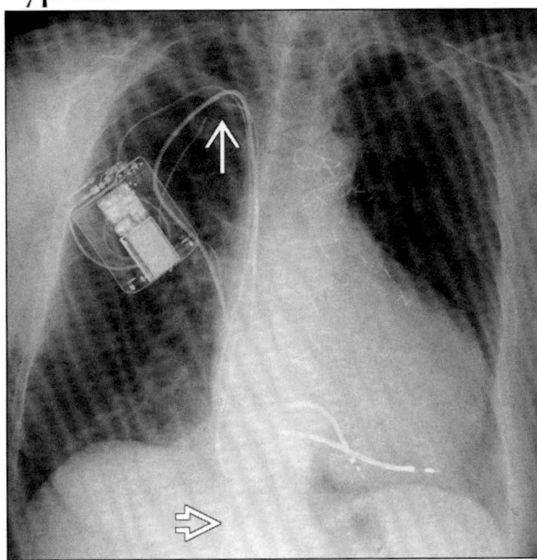

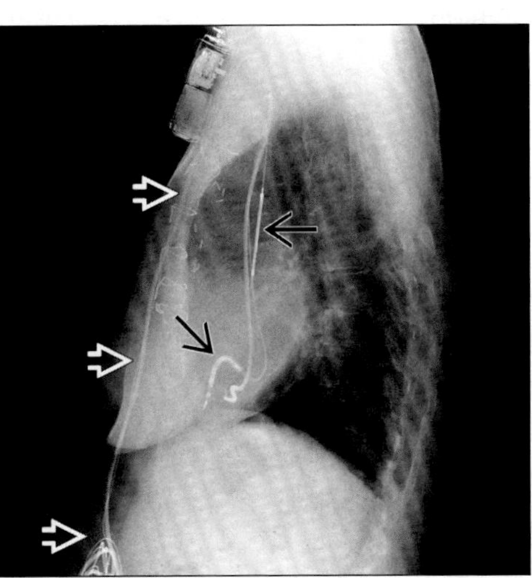

(Left) Anteroposterior radiograph shows fractured pacer wire →. Note, original pacer unit was in abdominal wall and original wires left in situ (subcutaneous course from subclavian vein to abdomen →). **(Right)** Lateral radiograph shows subcutaneous course of original wires →. Note that the new device is an ICD as evident by coil spring appearance of lead →.

CORONARY VEIN MAPPING

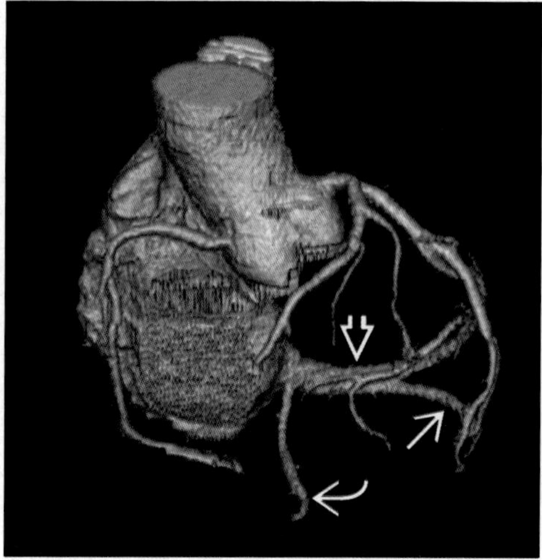

Anterior view cardiac CT volume rendering shows coronary arterial tree and coronary venous system. Note: Coronary sinus ➡, middle cardiac vein ➡, and marginal vein ➡.

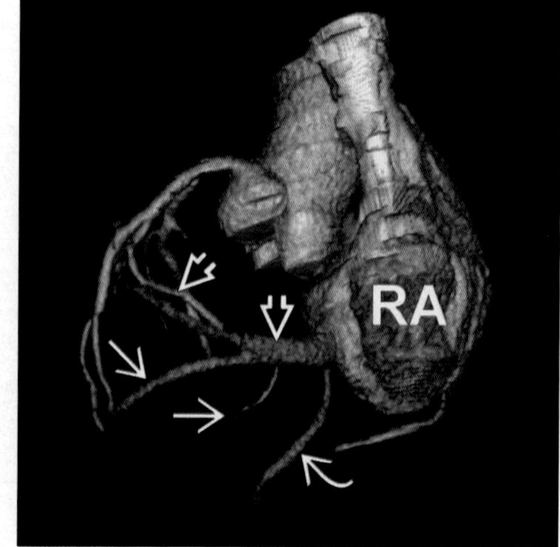

Posterior 3D cardiac CT shows coronary sinus ➡ and great cardiac vein paralleling left circumflex coronary artery ➡, marginal and posterior vein of left ventricle ➡, and middle cardiac vein ➡. RA = right atrium.

TERMINOLOGY

Abbreviations and Synonyms

- CT cardiac venography

Definitions

- Cardiac gated CT angiogram with contrast injection protocol tailored to optimize coronary venous enhancement

IMAGING FINDINGS

General Features

- Location
  - Cardiac veins are located within epicardial fat and drain into right atrium
    - Coronary sinus and great cardiac vein travel in left atrioventricular groove
    - Middle cardiac vein and anterior interventricular vein travel in the posterior and anterior interventricular grooves
    - Diagonal, marginal and posterior left ventricular tributaries are located on the anterior, lateral and inferior left ventricular surfaces
- Morphology
  - Cardiac venous anatomy is very variable
    - Coronary sinus consistently present (~ 100%)
    - Middle cardiac vein or "posterior interventricular vein" consistently present
    - Posterior vein of left ventricle (PVLV) variable 80-90%
    - Great cardiac vein consistently present
    - Marginal vein or lateral vein 70-90% often multiple
    - Anterior interventricular vein consistently present
    - Small cardiac veins ~ 10%
    - Anterior cardiac veins ~ 40%

Imaging Recommendations

- Best imaging tool
  - CTA best noninvasive imaging test
  - Invasive retrograde angiography prior to biventricular pacer placement
    - Rotational angiography promising new tool
- Protocol advice

DDx: Right Coronary Artery to Coronary Sinus Fistula

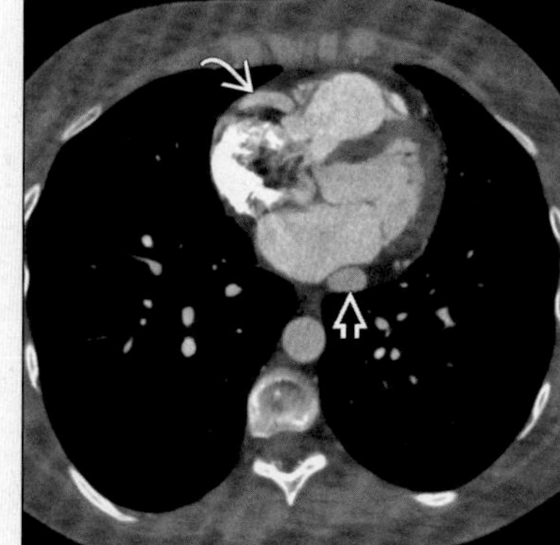

Enlarged Great Cardiac Vein

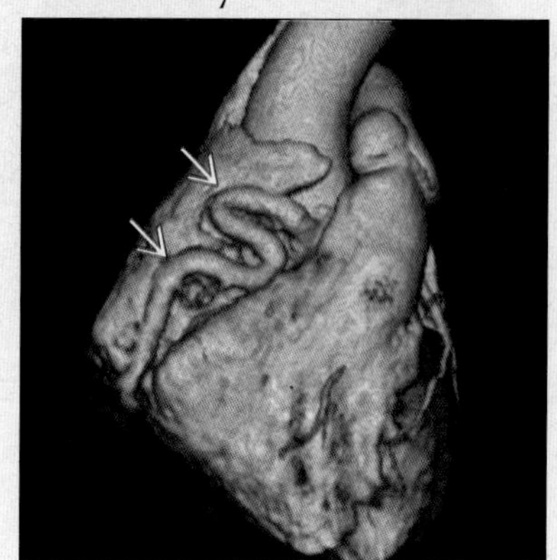

Dilated RCA

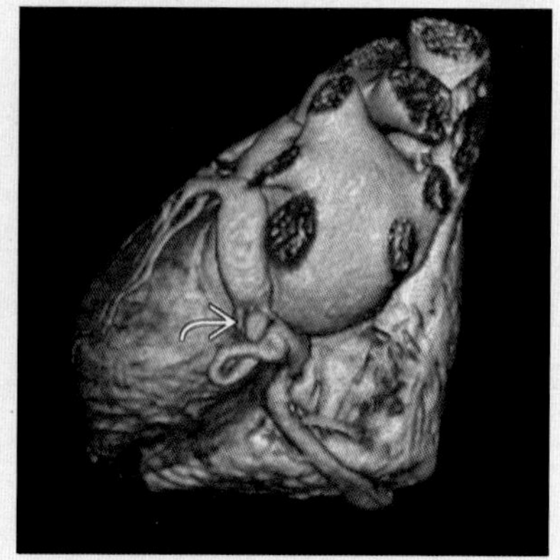

Fistula Site

CORONARY VEIN MAPPING

Key Facts

Terminology

- Cardiac gated CT angiogram with contrast injection protocol tailored to optimize coronary venous enhancement

Imaging Findings

- Cardiac veins are located within epicardial fat and drain into right atrium
- Coronary sinus and great cardiac vein travel in left atrioventricular groove
- Middle cardiac vein and anterior interventricular vein travel in the posterior and anterior interventricular grooves

Diagnostic Checklist

- CT allows evaluation for presence of suitable veins for coronary sinus lead placement
- Alternatively CT may be used for coronary arterial and venous anatomy delineation prior to surgical epicardial pacemaker lead placement

---

- Coronary CT protocol needs to be adjusted to allow for capturing coronary venous phase
  - Best venous enhancement approximately 8 seconds after initial arterial enhancement

DIFFERENTIAL DIAGNOSIS

Coronary Artery to Coronary Vein Fistula

- Abnormal connection between epicardial artery and veins
- Usually dilated and tortuous arteries and coronary sinus

Unroofed Coronary Sinus

- Abnormal connection between coronary sinus and right atrium
- Causes left to right shunt (left atrium into CS into RA)
- Rarest type of atrial septal defects (ASD)

DIAGNOSTIC CHECKLIST

Consider

- CT allows evaluation for presence of suitable veins for coronary sinus lead placement
- Alternatively CT may be used for coronary arterial and venous anatomy delineation prior to surgical epicardial pacemaker lead placement
  - Helps guide placement and avoid vascular injury
- May be used to guide complex electrophysiology procedures, such as trans-coronary venous or trans pericardial catheter ablation of ventricular fibrillation foci within myocardium

Image Interpretation Pearls

- Consider adding ~ 8 seconds to delay time for optimal venous enhancement
  - Also requires increasing contrast volume by 8 seconds multiplied with injection rate in milliliter

SELECTED REFERENCES

1. Abbara S et al: Noninvasive evaluation of cardiac veins with 16-MDCT angiography. AJR Am J Roentgenol. 185(4):1001-6, 2005
2. Jongbloed MR et al: Noninvasive visualization of the cardiac venous system using multislice computed tomography. J Am Coll Cardiol. 45(5):749-53, 2005
3. Muhlenbruch G et al: Imaging of the cardiac venous system: comparison of MDCT and conventional angiography. AJR Am J Roentgenol. 185(5):1252-7, 2005
4. Gerber TC et al: Evaluation of the coronary venous system using electron beam computed tomography. Int J Cardiovasc Imaging. 17(1):65-75, 2001
5. Schaffler GJ et al: Imaging the coronary venous drainage system using electron-beam CT. Surg Radiol Anat. 22(1):35-9, 2000

IMAGE GALLERY

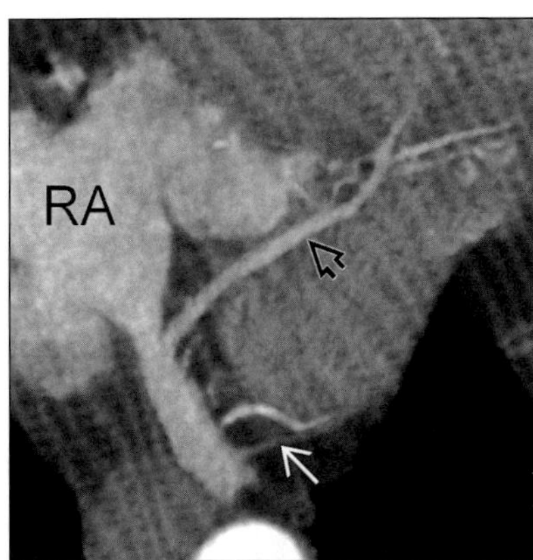

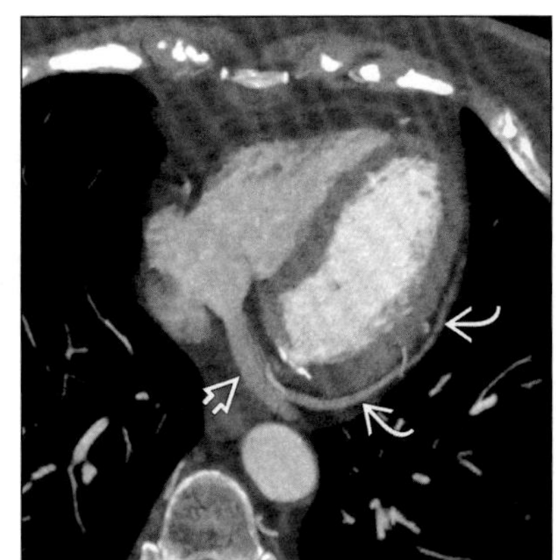

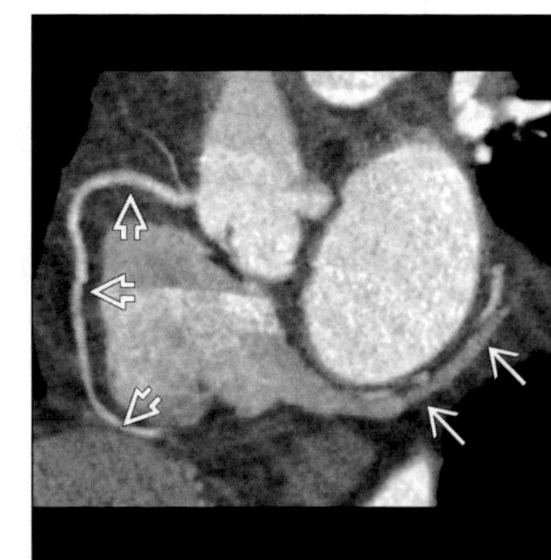

(Left) *Axial cardiac CT shows middle cardiac vein ⇨ entering coronary sinus close to its connection to the right atrium. Note: Very small PVLV ➡ paralleling posterior left ventricular (PLV) artery.* ***(Center)*** *Oblique cardiac CT MIP image shows large marginal vein ➡ in posterior lateral left ventricular epicardial fat and draining into coronary sinus ⇨.* ***(Right)*** *Atrioventricular (AV) valve plane cardiac CT shows right coronary artery ⇨ descending in right AV-groove and coronary sinus and great cardiac vein ➡ ascending in left AV-groove.*

LEFT ATRIAL THROMBUS

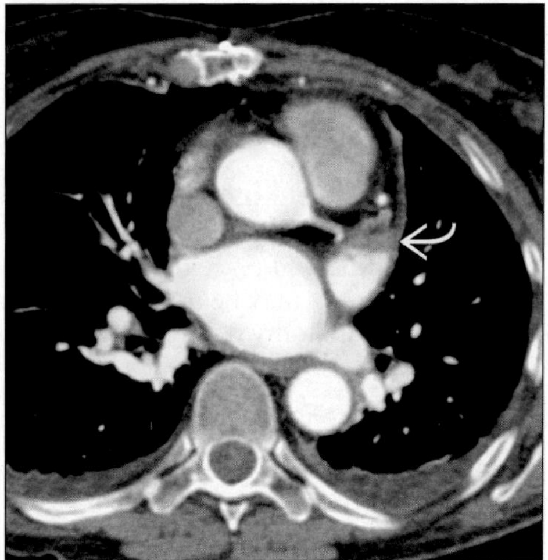

Axial coronary CTA shows mural non-enhancing LAA filling defect ➡ with well-defined borders, suggesting presence of thrombus.

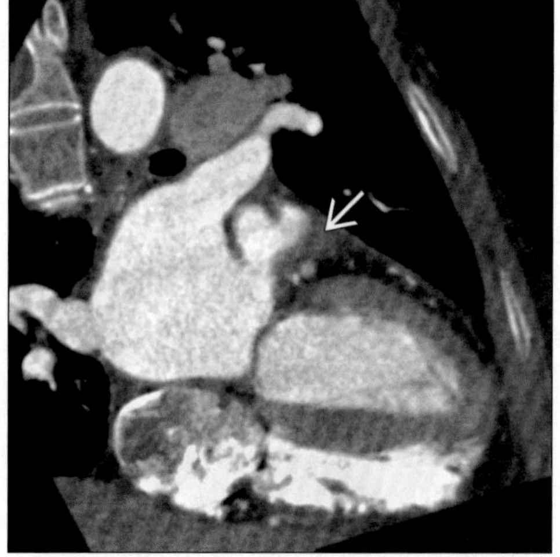

Oblique coronary CTA in same patient shows same filling defect occupying tip of LAA ➡. Trans esophageal echocardiography confirmed presence of LAA thrombus.

TERMINOLOGY

Abbreviations and Synonyms

- LA thrombus
- LAA thrombus

Definitions

- Thrombus formation in left atrial appendage or occasionally in body of left atrium
  - Usually due to atrial fibrillation or mitral valve stenosis

IMAGING FINDINGS

General Features

- Best diagnostic clue
  - Filling defect within left atrial appendage
    - Persistent on delayed contrast-enhanced scan
- Location
  - Thrombus usually forms in left atrial appendage (LAA)
  - Occasionally in body of left atrium (LA)
- Size: Variable
- Morphology
  - Chronic broad-based thrombus may develop neovascularization which will lead to low grade enhancement on contrast MR
    - May present diagnostic challenge when differentiating chronic thrombus from malignancy

Radiographic Findings

- Usually no signs on PA radiograph
- May demonstrate convexity of left atrial appendix segment of left heart border
- May demonstrate signs of underlying condition
  - Mitral valve stenosis
    - Pulmonary venous hypertension (Kerley B lines, pulmonary vein redistribution, pulmonary edema)
    - Right retrocardiac double density (enlarged LA)
    - Splaying of carina (enlarged LA)
    - Convex LAA segment
    - Convex PA segment if secondary pulmonary arterial hypertension (chronic mitral stenosis only)

CT Findings

- CTA

DDx: Left Atrial Appendage Thrombus

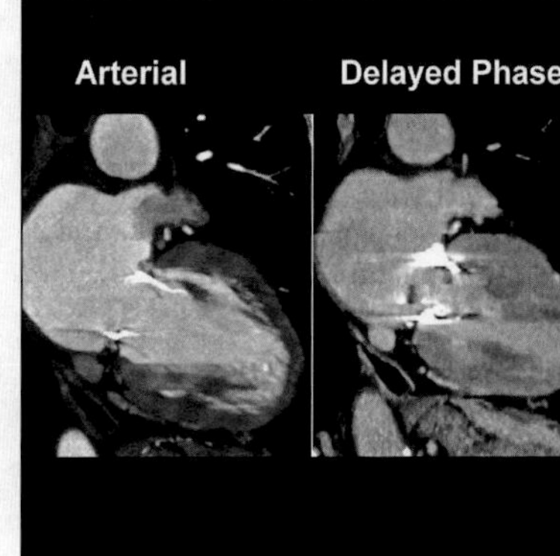

Smoke (Slow Mixing)

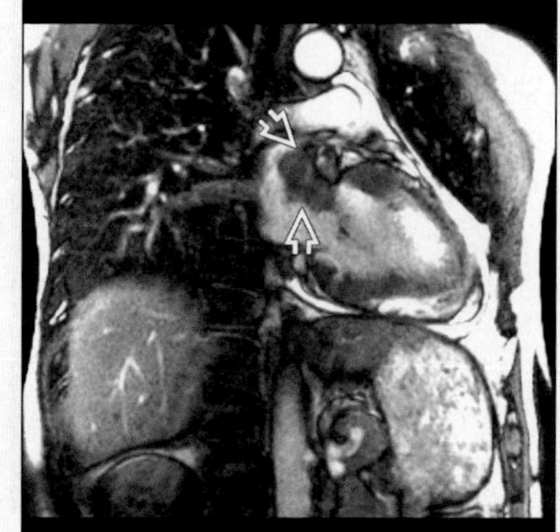

Spindle Cell Sarcoma

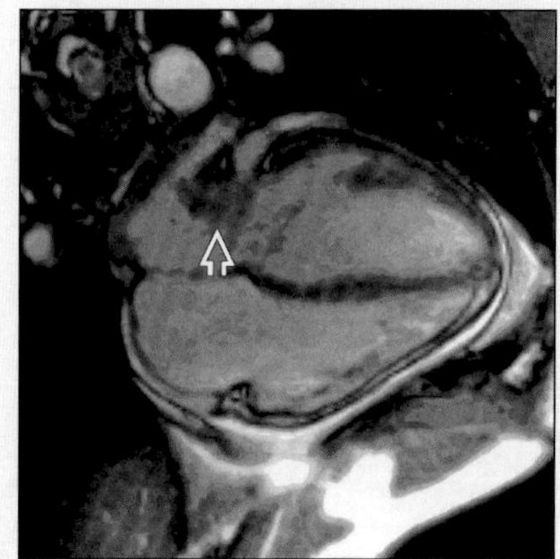

Left Atrial Sarcoma

LEFT ATRIAL THROMBUS

Key Facts

Terminology

- Thrombus formation in left atrial appendage or occasionally in body of left atrium
- Usually due to atrial fibrillation or mitral valve stenosis

Imaging Findings

- Chronic broad-based thrombus may develop neovascularization which will lead to low grade enhancement on contrast MR
- May present diagnostic challenge when differentiating chronic thrombus from malignancy
- TEE considered gold standard for excluding LAA thrombi
- Spontaneous echo contrast (SEC) or "smoke" and other artifacts may hamper identification or exclusion of LAA thrombus

Clinical Issues

- Recurrence common if underlying cause not treated
- Anticoagulant therapy (warfarin) substantially reduces embolic event risk in atrial fibrillation from LAA thrombus

Diagnostic Checklist

- One minute delayed gated scan to follow CTA or CTV if filling defect noted on initial images
- Slow mixing of opacified and non-opacified blood across neck of LAA may mimic thrombus on arterial phase gated CT
- Delayed scan allows for more complete mixing
- If filling defect persists → thrombus present
- If LAA fills with contrast → slow flow artifact (equivalent of smoke on TEE)

  - Thoracic CTA may incidentally demonstrate LAA thrombus
    - Thin cut reconstructions and delayed scans most helpful in demonstrating persistent filling defect
    - Pitfall: Motion or pulsation artifact
- Cardiac Gated CTA
  - Lower HU suggestive of thrombus
  - Sharper interface between filling defect and contrast opacified lumen suggestive of thrombus
  - HU > 80 more likely represent slow mixing
  - Delayed scans allow for differentiation of slow mixing and real LAA thrombus
  - When differentiating thrombus from malignancy CTA enhancement less helpful than MR enhancement
  - Cardiac CTA useful for anatomic metrics and exclusion of thrombus prior to percutaneous occlusion device implantation
    - Follow-up scan to confirm proper device placement and exclude residual perfusion
  - Cardiac CTA used for anatomic guidance of pulmonary vein radiofrequency (or cryo-) ablation to treat atrial fibrillation
    - Fusion of electroanatomic maps with CTA datasets possible
    - Mid expiration CT imaging preferred when fusion is performed as electroanatomic mapping is performed during free breathing

MR Findings

- Gadolinium-enhanced MR inferior to TEE for detection of left atrial appendage thrombus
- SSFP imaging in multiple planes helpful for outlining thrombus especially if in body of LV
- T1WI SE without and with gadolinium best test for assessing enhancement of the mass
- First pass perfusion and delayed enhanced acquisitions may also demonstrate absence of enhancement of large LA (body) or LV thrombi
- MR may be used for atrial appendage occlusion device placement planning
- MR used for pulmonary vein ablation/isolation procedures

Echocardiographic Findings

- Echocardiogram
  - TEE considered gold standard for excluding LAA thrombi
    - Spontaneous echo contrast (SEC) or "smoke" and other artifacts may hamper identification or exclusion of LAA thrombus
  - Visualization of left atrial appendage thrombus may be improved with the use of a thrombus-targeting ultrasonographic contrast agent (MRX-408A1)

Imaging Recommendations

- Best imaging tool
  - TEE
  - Cardiac CT with delayed phase scan is a promising tool
- Protocol advice: CTA delayed scan reduces false positive findings from slow mixing

DIFFERENTIAL DIAGNOSIS

Pseudo Thrombus (CTA)

- Low-attenuation within LAA due to slow mixing of contrast containing blood with non opacified blood
- More common in atrial fibrillation and poor LAA ejection fraction

Tumors

- Myxoma
- Metastasis
- Primary malignancy

Surgical Exclusion of LAA

- Performed after valve surgery to prevent LAA thrombosis

PATHOLOGY

General Features

- Etiology
  - Atrial fibrillation

  - Mitral valve disease of any cause
  - Left atrial thrombus formation on atrial septal defect (ASD) occluder systems have been reported
- Associated abnormalities
  - Often source of neurologic events or large artery occlusion
    - Cardiac (left atrial or ventricular) thrombus has to be excluded in the absence of otherwise identifiable source of embolic (cryptogenic) stroke or TIA
    - If negative, patent foramen ovale (PFO) and deep vein thrombosis (DVT) need to be excluded
    - Lower extremity ultrasound and pelvic MR venography are used to exclude DVT in patients with PFO and cryptogenic stroke

CLINICAL ISSUES

Presentation

- Most common signs/symptoms
  - Asymptomatic
  - Cryptogenic stroke
  - Other embolic events
- Other signs/symptoms
  - Symptoms from underlying disease
    - Atrial fibrillation
    - Mitral valve disease
  - In rheumatic mitral stenosis
    - Presence of coarse F-waves on EKG is associated with left atrial appendage dysfunction
    - Presence indicates higher thromboembolic risk

Demographics

- Age: Age range parallels that of underlying conditions
- Gender: M = F

Natural History & Prognosis

- May persist without complication
- May embolize to brain causing TIA or stroke
- May resolve spontaneously
- Recurrence common if underlying cause not treated

Treatment

- Anticoagulant therapy (warfarin) substantially reduces embolic event risk in atrial fibrillation from LAA thrombus
  - However carries bleeding risk
- Other drugs may have clinical roles in select cases
  - Ximelagatran
  - Antiplatelet therapy ± low-dose warfarin, etc.
- Surgical: Maze procedure and similar operations
- Catheter-based radiofrequency ablation (pulmonary vein isolation)
  - Prevention of thrombus formation
- Left atrial appendage obliteration
  - Surgical or catheter based occlusion device

DIAGNOSTIC CHECKLIST

Consider

- One minute delayed gated scan to follow CTA or CTV if filling defect noted on initial images
  - Slow mixing of opacified and non-opacified blood across neck of LAA may mimic thrombus on arterial phase gated CT
  - Delayed scan allows for more complete mixing
  - If filling defect persists → thrombus present
  - If LAA fills with contrast → slow flow artifact (equivalent of smoke on TEE)

SELECTED REFERENCES

1. Hesse B et al: Images in cardiovascular medicine. A left atrial appendage thrombus mimicking atrial myxoma. Circulation. 113(11):e456-7, 2006
2. Mohrs OK et al: Percutaneous left atrial appendage transcatheter occlusion (PLAATO): planning and follow-up using contrast-enhanced MRI. AJR Am J Roentgenol. 186(2):361-4, 2006
3. Mohrs OK et al: Thrombus detection in the left atrial appendage using contrast-enhanced MRI: a pilot study. AJR Am J Roentgenol. 186(1):198-205, 2006
4. Parekh A et al: Images in cardiovascular medicine. The case of a disappearing left atrial appendage thrombus: direct visualization of left atrial thrombus migration, captured by echocardiography, in a patient with atrial fibrillation, resulting in a stroke. Circulation. 114(13):e513-4, 2006
5. Blackshear JL et al: Stroke prevention in atrial fibrillation: warfarin faces its challengers. Curr Cardiol Rep. 7(1):16-22, 2005
6. Mutlu B et al: Fibrillatory wave amplitude as a marker of left atrial and left atrial appendage function, and a predictor of thromboembolic risk in patients with rheumatic mitral stenosis. Int J Cardiol. 91(2-3):179-86, 2003
7. Nakai T et al: Percutaneous left atrial appendage occlusion (PLAATO) for preventing cardioembolism: first experience in canine model. Circulation. 105(18):2217-22, 2002
8. von der Recke G et al: Transesophageal contrast echocardiography distinguishes a left atrial appendage thrombus from spontaneous echo contrast. Echocardiography. 19(4):343-4, 2002
9. von der Recke G et al: Use of transesophageal contrast echocardiography for excluding left atrial appendage thrombi in patients with atrial fibrillation before cardioversion. J Am Soc Echocardiogr. 15(10 Pt 2):1256-61, 2002
10. Sim EK et al: Co-existing left atrial thrombus and myxoma in mitral stenosis--a diagnostic challenge. Singapore Med J. 40(1):46-7, 1999
11. J Am Soc Echocardiogr: the use of a thrombus-targeting ultrasonographic contrast agent (MRX-408A1): In vivo experimental echocardiographic studies.

LEFT ATRIAL THROMBUS

IMAGE GALLERY

Variant

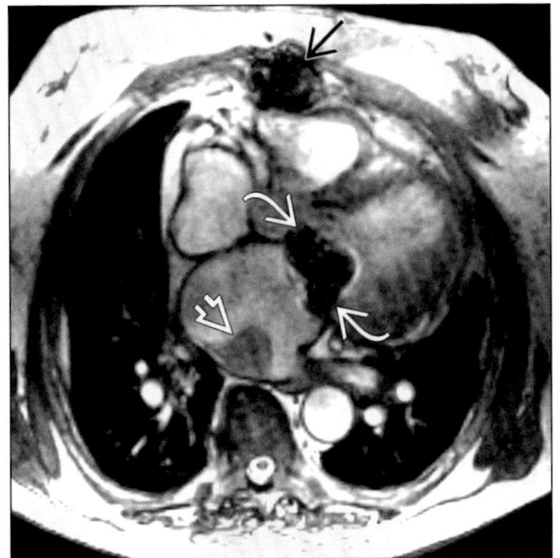

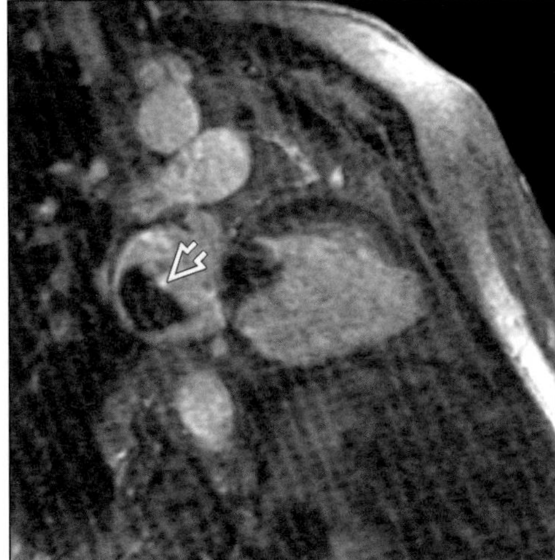

*(**Left**) Axial SSFP shows a broad-based mass arising from the posterior wall of the left atrium. Note: Artifacts from mitral valve replacement and sternotomy wires. (**Right**) Long axis delayed enhanced MR shows the same mass (thrombus) unenhanced and with contrast between most of the atrial wall and mass.*

Other

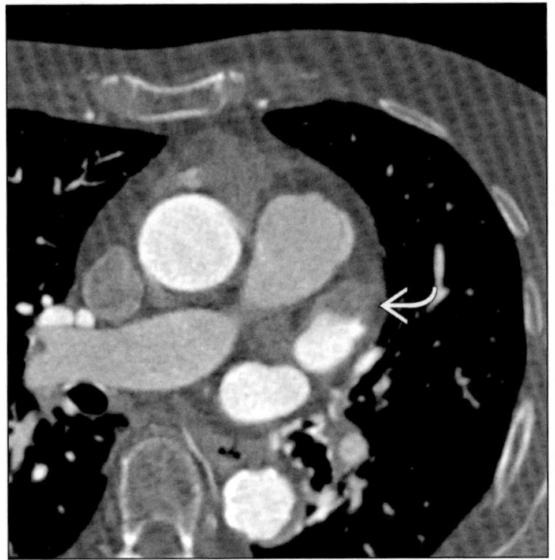

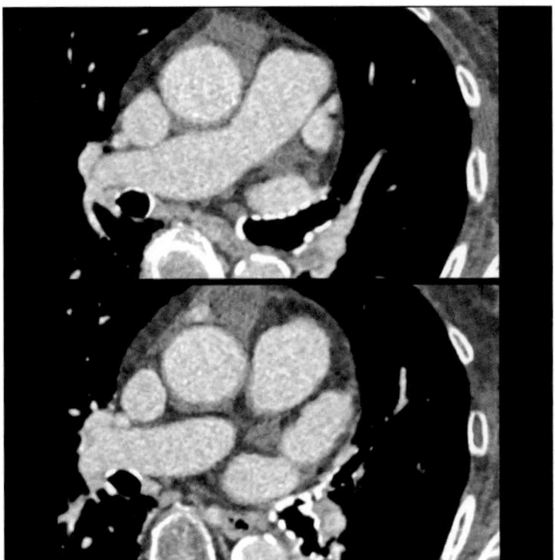

*(**Left**) Axial cardiac CT shows a relatively well-defined filling defect in LAA (falsely) suggesting possible LAA thrombus. (**Right**) Axial cardiac CT delayed scan in the same patient shows complete contrast filling of LAA, indicating absence of thrombus. This case illustrates the value of delayed scans to confirm presence/absence of LAA thrombus.*

Typical

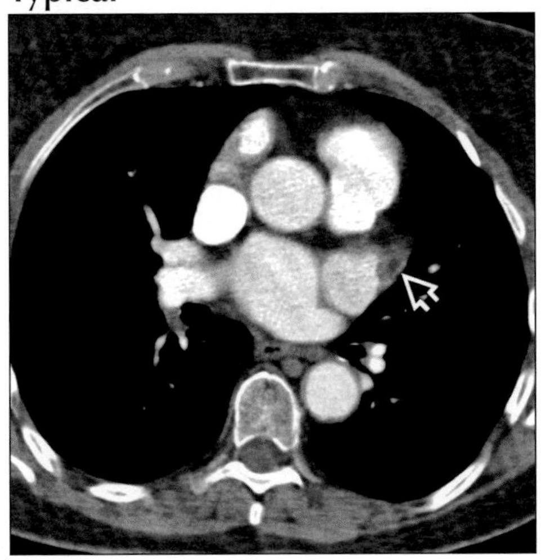

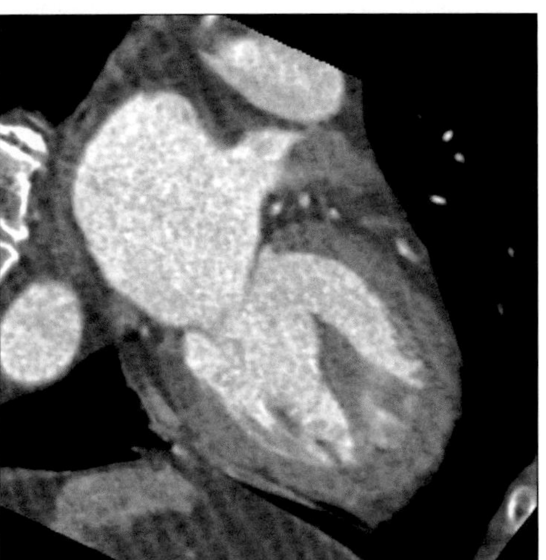

*(**Left**) Axial non-gated CECT shows well-defined filling defect in the left atrial appendage, suggesting presence of thrombus. (**Right**) Oblique cardiac CT shows large, low HU filling defect with sharp demarcation suggesting LAA thrombus. Presence of thrombus confirmed by TEE.*

PART II

Vascular

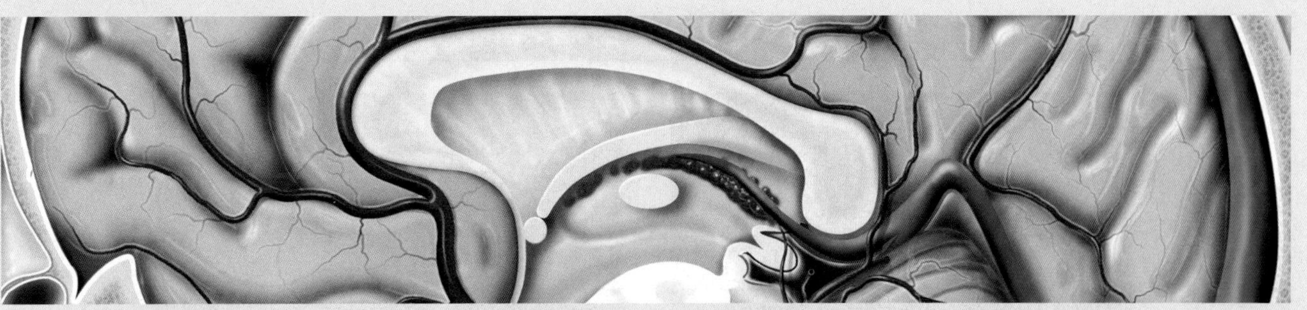

SECTION 1: Brain

Introduction and Overview

Brain

BRAIN VASCULATURE

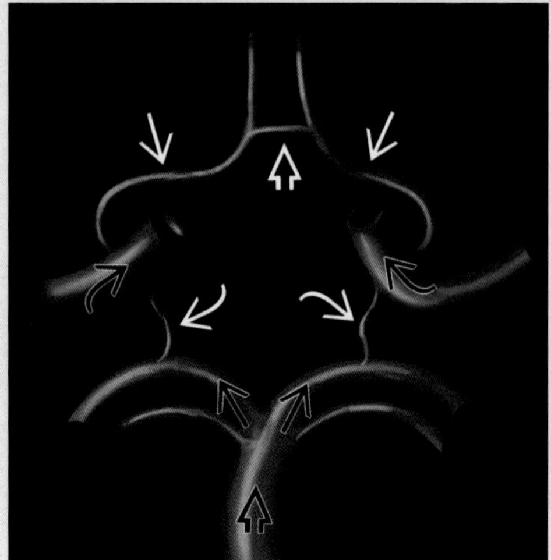

Graphic of the COW as seen from below shows ICAs, ACAs, ACoA, BA, PCAs, and PCoAs. This COW has all components intact, the less common configuration.

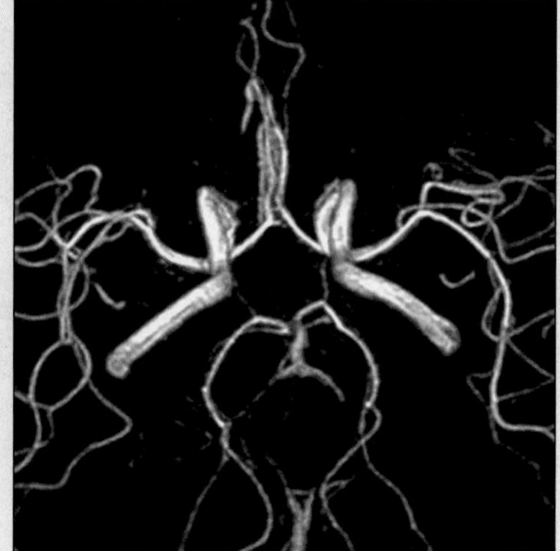

3D TOF MRA of the brain vasculature, superior-inferior MIP image with shaded-surface display technique, shows all components of a completely intact COW, a so-called "balanced" COW.

TERMINOLOGY

Abbreviations

- Circle of Willis (COW)
- External carotid (ECA), internal carotid (ICA), vertebral (VA), basilar arteries (BA)
- Anterior (ACA), middle (MCA), posterior cerebral arteries (PCA)
- Superior (SCA), anterior inferior (AICA), posterior inferior cerebellar arteries (PICA)
- Anterior (ACoA), posterior communicating arteries (PCoA)
- Superior sagittal (SSS), inferior sagittal (ISS), straight (SS), transverse (TS), sigmoid (SigS), cavernous sinuses (CS)
- Superficial middle cerebral vein (SMCV), veins of Trolard (V of T) and Labbé (V of L)
- Internal cerebral veins (ICV), basal veins of Rosenthal (BVR), vein of Galen (V of G), internal jugular vein (IJV)

IMAGING ANATOMY

Anatomic Relationships

- COW
  - Components
    - Terminal ICAs: Divide into ACAs/MCAs
    - Horizontal (A1) ACAs
    - ACoA; PCoA (branch of supraclinoid ICA)
    - BA: Formed from the union of distal VAs, terminates into PCAs
    - Precommunicating (P1) PCAs
  - COW surrounds suprasellar cistern, lies below hypothalamus/3rd ventricle
  - A1s normally pass above CNs 2, 3
  - Normal variants common (60% of COWs have one or more hypoplastic/absent segments)
    - Hypoplastic (10%) or absent (1-2%) A1
    - Duplicated/fenestrated ACoA; absent ACoA 5%
    - Hypoplastic/absent PCoA in one-third of cases
    - PCoA "infundibulum" (funnel-shaped junctional dilatation of PCoA origin from ICA) in 5-15%
    - "Fetal" PCA origin from ICA (PCoA large, P1 PCA hypoplastic) 20-30%
  - Anomalies (persistent carotid-basilar anastomoses)
    - Persistent trigeminal artery (PTA): 0.1-0.5% of cases; originates from pre-cavernous ICA, passes through or around sella, anastomoses with distal BA in the midline; vascular anomalies, aneurysms may be associated
    - All others (otic, hypoglossal, proatlantal intersegmental arteries) very rare
- ACA
  - A1 (horizontal) segment: From ACA origin to ACoA junction
    - Perforating branches: Medial lenticulostriate arteries, recurrent artery of Heubner (can also arise from A2)
  - A2 (vertical) segment: From ACoA junction to corpus callosum genu; orbital, frontal arteries
  - A3 (major cortical) branches: Bifurcation near corpus callosum genu into pericallosal, callosomarginal arteries
  - Vascular territory: Anteromedial basal ganglia (caudate head), ventromedial frontal lobes, medial 2/3rd of hemispheres, brain convexity
  - Variations: Hypoplastic A1 common (distal ACA territory supplied by ACoA collateral flow via contralateral ICA/ACA)
  - Anomalies: Infraoptic A1, azygous ACA (single ACA supplies both medial hemispheres) rare, azygous ACA has increased association with aneurysms and holoprosencephaly
- MCA
  - M1 (horizontal) segment: From MCA origin to bi-/trifurcation ("genu")
    - Perforating branches: Lateral lenticulostriate arteries
  - M2 (insular) segment: Over insula, divides into 6-8 major branches
  - M3 (sylvian) segment: From insula through lateral cerebral fissure

BRAIN VASCULATURE

Cerebral Vascular Pathologic Entities

Congenital Abnormalities
- Vessel aplasia/hypoplasia (moyamoya)
- Idiopathic progressive arteriopathy of childhood
- Sickle cell disease
- Phakomatoses (NF1, TS, VHL, Sturge-Weber)
- Connective tissue disorders (Marfan, Ehlers-Danlos)

Vasculopathies
- Atherosclerosis
- Primary angiitis of the CNS
- Vasculitides (SLE, antiphospholipid syndromes)
- Vasomotor disorders (PRES, eclampsia)
- Infectious processes (vasculitis, HIV, septic emboli)
- Oncotic lesions (intravascular lymphoma)
- Radiation vasculopathy
- Migraine

Cerebral Microvascular Disease
- Arteriolosclerosis/small vessel disease
- Hypertensive angiopathy/microbleeds
- Amyloid angiopathy
- CADASIL/CARASIL

Hemorrhagic Conditions
- Trauma
- Hypertensive hemorrhage
- Ischemic infarct hemorrhagic transformation
- Amyloid angiopathy
- Venous thrombosis
- Vascular malformations (AVM, CM, A-V fistula)
- Aneurysm
- Vascular neoplasms
- Superficial siderosis

- M4 (cortical) branches: Ramifications over lateral frontal/parietal/temporal lobes
- Vascular territory: Midlateral basal ganglia (putamen, globus pallidus), insula, most of lateral hemisphere surface
- Variations
  - "Early" branching MCA
  - "Accessory" M1 segment
- Anomalies: True "duplicated" M1, absent/hypoplastic M1, etc., rare

- PCA
  - P1 (horizontal or precommunicating) segment: BA to PCoA junction
    - Perforating branches: Thalamoperforating arteries
  - P2 (ambient) segment: Curves around midbrain
    - Posterolateral, posteromedial choroidal arteries
  - P3 (cortical) branches: Splenial artery (anastomoses with pericallosal artery), anterior/posterior inferior temporal, calcarine, parietooccipital arteries
  - Vascular territory: Posterior basal ganglia (thalami), midbrain, posterior 1/3 of medial hemisphere, occipital lobe, most of inferolateral temporal lobe
  - Variations: Hypoplastic P1 common ("fetal" PCA origin from ICA via PCoA)
  - Anomalies: Rare; with PTA, PCAs may arise from anterior (carotid) circulation via large PTA
- Cerebellar arteries
  - SCA: From distal BA, supplies superior cerebellum
  - AICA: From mid BA, supplies anterolateral mid cerebellum
  - PICA: From distal VA, supplies inferior cerebellum (and lateral medulla)
- Brainstem arteries
  - VA perforators: Supplies medulla
  - BA perforators: Supplies pons and midbrain
  - Anomalies: Fenestrated BA, aneurysms associated
- Major dural venous sinuses and drainage patterns
  - SSS
    - > 95% single midline channel from crista galli to sinus confluence (torcular Herophili)
    - Variations: Absent anterior segment (uncommon)
    - SSS + cortical veins (including Trolard) + falx tributaries drain upper hemispheres, subcortical WM
  - ISS
    - Small midline channel in inferior falx cerebri
    - Joins V of G to form SS
  - SS
    - Courses posteroinferiorly from falcotentorial apex to sinus confluence
    - 85% single midline channel from V of G to sinus confluence
    - Variations: 15% double or triple parallel channels
    - Anomalies: Absent SS (rare; usually seen in V of G malformations with persistent embryonic falcine sinus)
    - SS + V of G, ICV, BVR drain basal ganglia, thalami, deep WM
  - TS
    - Runs from sinus confluence laterally within tentorial attachment to calvarium
    - 75% right > left TS
    - Variations: Up to one-third have hypoplastic/absent TS segment (should not be mistaken for occlusion)
    - TS + cortical veins (including Labbé) + tentorial tributaries drain most of occipital/posterior temporal lobes
  - SigS
    - Located between TS and jugular bulb/IJV
    - Significant asymmetry in size of SigSs, jugular bulbs, IJVs common
  - CS
    - Multiseptated trabeculated venous channels on either side of sphenoid body
    - Lateral dural wall thick, easily recognized; inner wall very thin, difficult to delineate
    - Contains ICA, CN 6 within CS; CNs 3, 4, 5 (1st, 2nd divisions) in lateral dural wall
    - Communicates with orbit, clival and pterygoid (deep face) plexuses, SMCV, superior/inferior petrosal sinuses (which join with TS/SigS)

BRAIN VASCULATURE

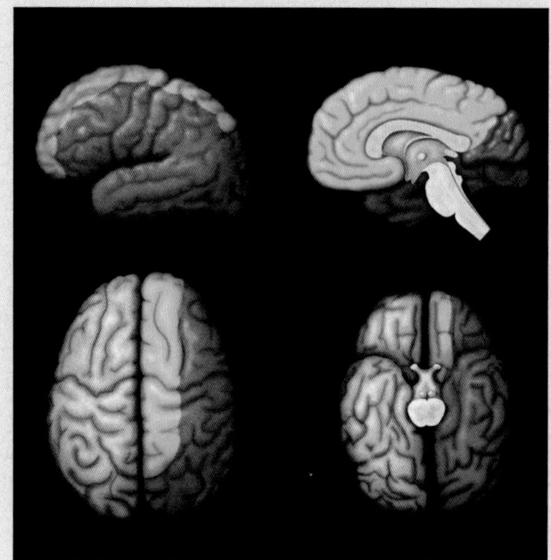

Graphic shows usual distribution of major supratentorial arterial territories. Green = ACA. Red = MCA. Purple = PCA. Superficial (cortical) "watershed zone" = confluence of territories.

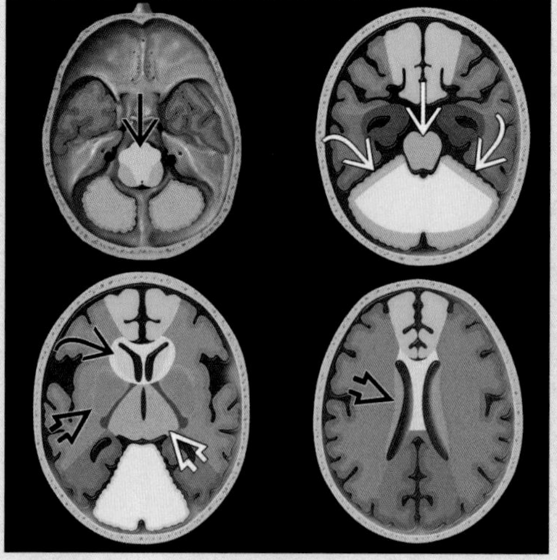

Graphic shows deep supply. Tan = PICA. ➔ = AICA. Yellow = SCA. VA ➔ and BA ➔ perforator territory. Medial ➔/lateral ➔ lenticulostriate and thalamoperforator ➔ territory.

    - Drains medial temporal lobes, basal brain structures
  - V of G
    - Formed from bilateral ICV and BVR
    - Also drains tributaries from the posterior fossa such as precentral cerebellar vein
  - Major superficial cortical veins (variations common; exist in reciprocal size relationship)
    - SMCV drains brain around sylvian fissure
    - V of T: Superior anastomotic vein between SMCV, SSS; drains superior hemispheric region
    - V of L: Inferior anastomotic vein between SMCV, transverse sinus; drains lateral hemispheric region
  - Major deep veins
    - ICV + subependymal, deep medullary veins (normally always present)
    - BVR + deep middle cerebral veins (variable)

ANATOMY-BASED IMAGING ISSUES

Imaging Pitfalls

- Arterial vascular territories quite variable (minimum to maximum areas of supply)
- Variations in COW common
  - Beware: "Absent" PCA on vertebral angiogram may be due to fetal origin (check ICA injection!)
  - Flow direction within COW can be assessed by phase-contrast MRA
- TS variations with hypoplastic/absent segment(s) are common and may mimic occlusion
- "Filling defects" within TS, SigS may be giant arachnoid granulations (round/ovoid > long/linear, CSF signal characteristics)
- Jugular bulbs, IJVs may be very asymmetric in size; slow/turbulent flow may mimic thrombosis/mass

Other Imaging Issues

- Both intra-, extracranial circulations must be evaluated in patients with unexplained nontraumatic intracranial hemorrhage, patients who may become candidates for ECA-ICA bypass, etc.
- Assessing entire COW very important in evaluating patients with aneurysmal subarachnoid hemorrhage both for aneurysms and potential for collateral flow

CLINICAL IMPLICATIONS

Clinical Importance

- COW variations are the rule, not exception; hypoplastic/absent segments limit potential collateral flow in case of major vessel occlusion
- Vascular "watershed": Confluence of ACA/MCA/PCA territories
  - Hypotensive infarcts commonly affect cortical watershed, basal ganglia
  - "Rosary-like" lesions along deep watershed common in severe carotid stenosis
- Venous occlusions represent < 1% of all "strokes" and have variable clinical presentation, are often overlooked on imaging studies

CUSTOM DIFFERENTIAL DIAGNOSIS

"Stroke" in Children, Young Adults

- Congenital heart disease with emboli
- Vascular malformation with hemorrhage
- Arterial dissection
- Vasculitis, drug abuse
- Idiopathic progressive arteriopathy of childhood
- Mitochondrial encephalopathies
- Blood dyscrasia, clotting disorder

"Stroke" in Middle-Aged, Older Adults

- Arterial thromboembolism, atherosclerosis
- Hypertensive intracranial hemorrhage
- Cerebral amyloid disease
- Aneurysmal, nonaneurysmal subarachnoid hemorrhage; vascular malformation
- Dural sinus/cerebral venous occlusion
- Neoplasm (primary or metastatic)
- Drugs
- Coagulopathy

IMAGE GALLERY

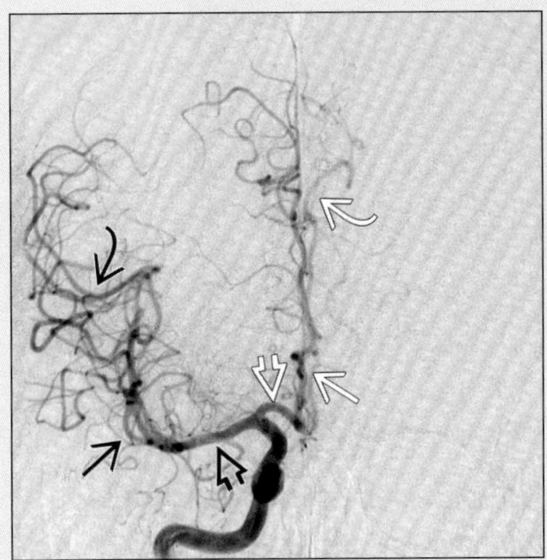

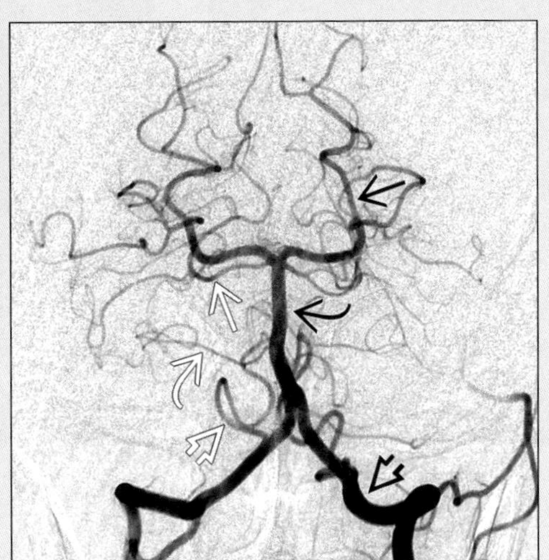

(Left) Anteroposterior DSA of the right ICA, arterial phase, shows normal cerebral anterior circulation vascular anatomy: MCA M1, M2, M3; ACA A1, A2, A3. **(Right)** Anteroposterior DSA left VA injection, arterial phase, shows normal cerebral posterior circulation vascular anatomy: VA, BA, PCA, PICA, AICA, SCA.

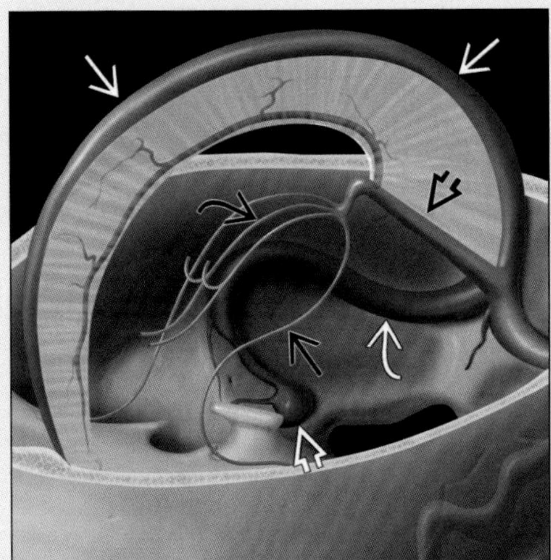

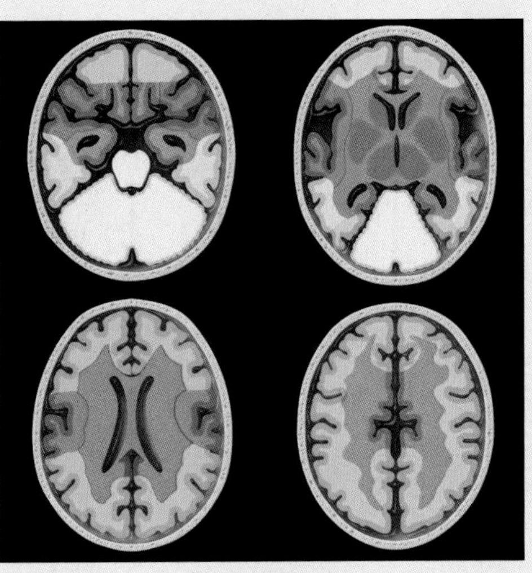

(Left) Graphic shows cerebral venous anatomy: SSS, TS, SigS, ICV, BVR, SS. Confluence of ICVs and BVRs = V of G. **(Right)** Axial graphic shows cerebral venous drainage territories. Green = SSS, V of T, cortical veins. Yellow = TS, V of L. Purple = CS, SMCV. Red = deep medullary veins, ICVs, BVRs, V of G, SS.

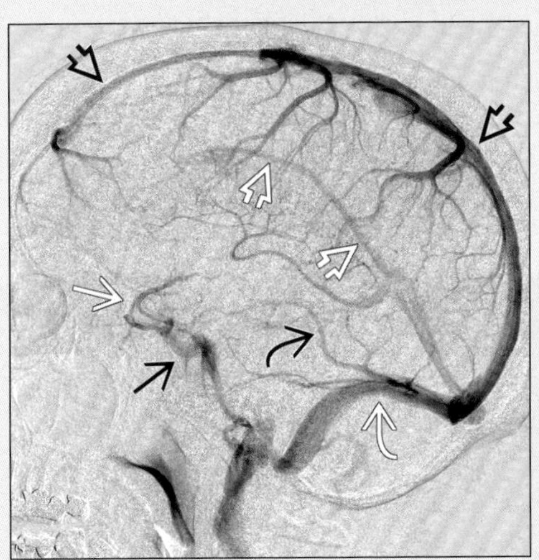

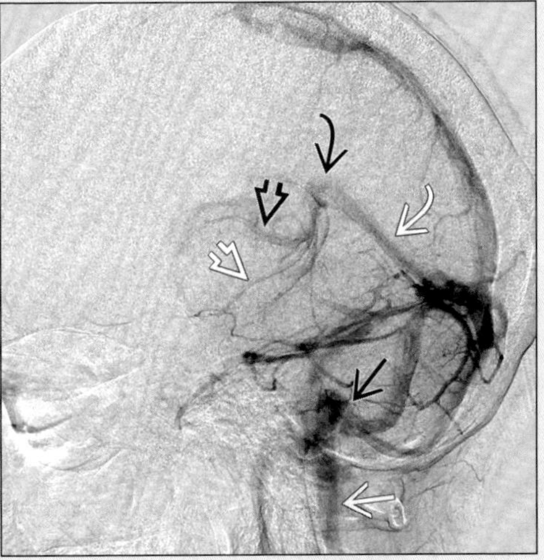

(Left) Lateral DSA of right ICA injection, venous phase, shows normal cerebral venous anatomy: SSS, ISS, V of L, TS, SMCV, CS. Co-dominant V of T drain into SSS. **(Right)** Lateral DSA of left VA injection, venous phase, shows normal cerebral deep venous anatomy: ICV, BVR, V of G, SS, SigS, IJV.

STURGE-WEBER SYNDROME

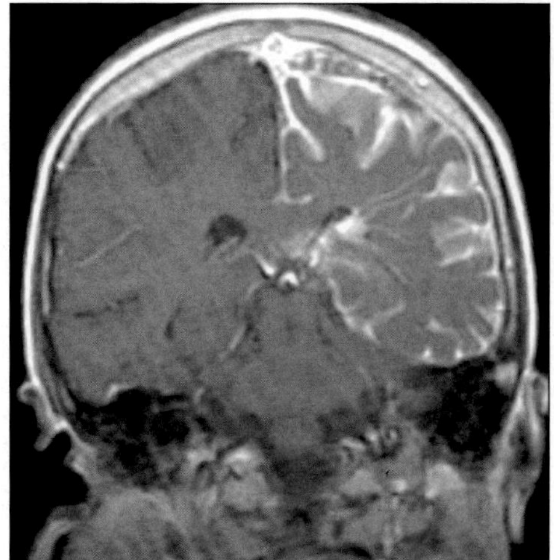

Coronal T1WI MR with intravenous gadolinium shows diffuse leptomeningeal enhancement of the left cerebral hemisphere and an enlarged enhancing left choroid plexus.

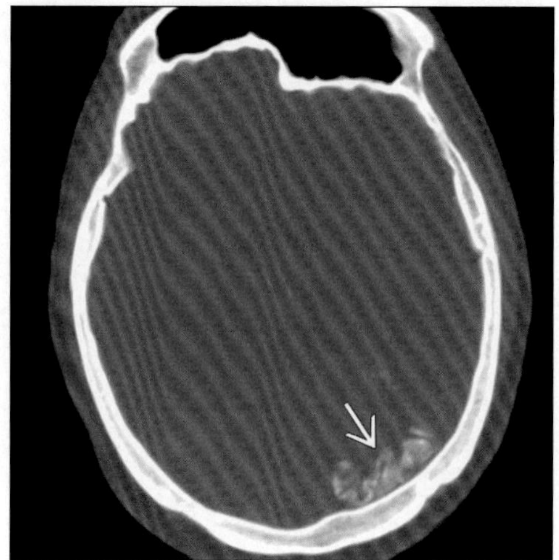

Axial NECT with bone windowing shows gyriform calcification in the left parietal lobe ➔ and an enlarged left frontal sinus.

TERMINOLOGY

Abbreviations and Synonyms

- Sturge-Weber syndrome (SWS); Sturge-Weber-Dimitri; encephalotrigeminal angiomatosis

Definitions

- Usually a sporadic congenital (but not inherited) malformation in which fetal cortical veins fail to develop normally
  - One of the neurocutaneous syndromes (phakomatoses)

IMAGING FINDINGS

General Features

- Best diagnostic clue: Cortical Ca++, atrophy, and enlarged ipsilateral choroid plexus
- Location
  - Pial angiomatosis unilateral 80%, bilateral 20%
  - Occipital > parietal > frontal/temporal lobes > diencephalon/midbrain > cerebellum
- Size: Small focal or bilateral multi-lobar involvement
- Morphology: Gyriform cortical Ca++
- Imaging features are sequelae of progressive venous occlusion and chronic venous ischemia

Radiographic Findings

- Radiography: Tram-track calcification

CT Findings

- NECT
  - Gyral/subcortical white matter (WM) Ca++
    - Ca++ not in leptomeningeal angioma
    - Progressive, generally posterior to anterior (2-20 yrs)
  - Late
    - Atrophy
    - Hyperpneumatization of paranasal sinuses
    - Thick diploe
- CECT
  - Serpentine leptomeningeal enhancement
  - Ipsilateral choroid plexus enlargement almost universal
    - Choroidal fissure if frontal involvement
    - Glomus in trigone if posterior involvement (most common)

DDx: Sturge-Weber

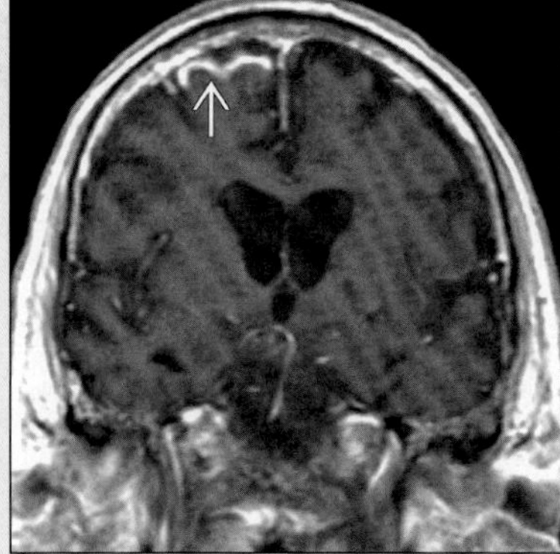

Meningitis

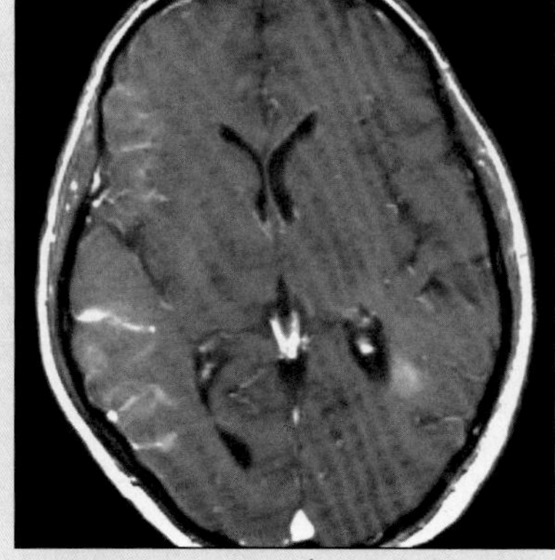

Leptomeningeal Metastases

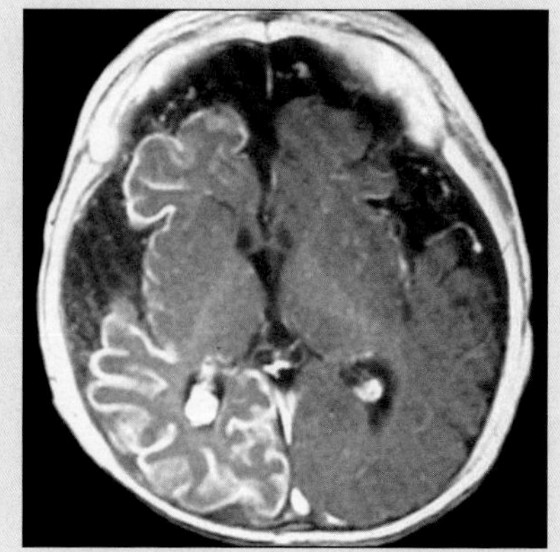

Klippel-Trenaunay-Weber

STURGE-WEBER SYNDROME

Key Facts

Terminology

- Sturge-Weber syndrome (SWS); Sturge-Weber-Dimitri; encephalotrigeminal angiomatosis
- Usually a sporadic congenital (but not inherited) malformation in which fetal cortical veins fail to develop normally
- One of the neurocutaneous syndromes (phakomatoses)

Imaging Findings

- Best diagnostic clue: Cortical Ca++, atrophy, and enlarged ipsilateral choroid plexus
- Pial angiomatosis unilateral 80%, bilateral 20%
- Imaging features are sequelae of progressive venous occlusion and chronic venous ischemia
- Gyral/subcortical white matter (WM) Ca++
- Atrophy
- Hyperpneumatization of paranasal sinuses
- Early: Serpentine leptomeningeal enhancement, pial angiomatosis of subarachnoid space
- Late: "Burnt-out" ⇒ ↓ pial enhancement, ↑ cortical/subcortical Ca++; atrophy
- Engorged, enhancing choroid plexus
- Best imaging tool: Enhanced MR

Top Differential Diagnoses

- Other Vascular Phakomatoses (Neurocutaneous Syndromes)
- Celiac Disease
- Meningitis, Leptomeningeal Metastases, Leukemia

Clinical Issues

- Clinical Profile: "Port-wine stain", seizures, hemiparesis

MR Findings

- T1WI
  - Atrophy over time
  - ↑ WM volume subjacent to pial angiomatosis (early); atrophy of WM and GM (late)
- T2WI
  - Early: Transient hyperperfusion ⇒ "accelerated" myelin maturation
  - Late: ↑ Signal in region of gliosis & ↓ cortical signal in regions of calcification
- FLAIR
  - Late: Gliosis in involved lobes
  - FLAIR C+: Improved visualization of leptomeningeal enhancement
- T2* GRE: Tram-track gyral calcifications
- DWI: Restricted diffusion in acute ischemia
- T1 C+
  - Early: Serpentine leptomeningeal enhancement, pial angiomatosis of subarachnoid space
  - Late: "Burnt-out" ⇒ ↓ pial enhancement, ↑ cortical/subcortical Ca++; atrophy
  - Engorged, enhancing choroid plexus
  - Orbital enhancement > 50%, best seen with T1 C+ fat-saturation
    - Choroidal angioma, periorbital soft tissues, bony orbit and frontal bone
- MRA: Rare high-flow arteriovenous malformations
- MRV
  - Progressive sinovenous occlusion
    - Lack of superficial cortical veins
    - ↓ Flow transverse sinuses/jugular veins
    - ↑↑ Prominence deep collateral (medullary/subependymal) veins
- MRS: ↑ Choline; ↓ NAA in affected areas

Nuclear Medicine Findings

- PET: Progressive hypoperfusion; progressive glucose hypometabolism
- Bone Scan
  - Hypertrophied ipsilateral skull vault, diploic involvement
  - Intracranial dystrophic gyral calcification
- SPECT: Transient hyperperfusion (early); hypoperfusion (late)
  - Pattern inconsistent, may be smaller or larger than abnormality detected on CT/MR

Ultrasonographic Findings

- Pulsed Doppler: ↓ Middle cerebral artery velocity

Angiographic Findings

- Conventional
  - Pial blush, rare arteriovenous malformation
  - Findings mostly venous: Paucity of normal cortical veins, extensive medullary and deep collaterals

Imaging Recommendations

- Best imaging tool: Enhanced MR
- Protocol advice
  - NECT to evaluate for calcification (may be more extensive than recognized on MR)
  - MR with contrast (assess extent, uni-/bilaterality, orbital involvement)
    - FLAIR + contrast improves conspicuity of leptomeningeal angiomatosis

DIFFERENTIAL DIAGNOSIS

Other Vascular Phakomatoses (Neurocutaneous Syndromes)

- Blue-rubber-bleb nevus syndrome
  - Multiple, small, cutaneous, venous malformations plus intracranial developmental venous anomalies
- Wyburn-Mason syndrome
  - Facial vascular nevus; visual pathway and/or brain arteriovenous malformation (AVM)
- Klippel-Trenaunay-Weber syndrome
  - Osseous/soft tissue hypertrophy, extremity vascular malformations
  - May be combined with some features of SWS
- PHACES
  - Posterior fossa malformations, hemangiomas, arterial anomalies, coarctation of the aorta, cardiac and eye anomalies, sternal clefts

STURGE-WEBER SYNDROME

- Meningioangiomatosis
  - Ca++ common; variable leptomeningeal enhancement
  - May invade brain through Virchow-Robin perivascular spaces
  - Atrophy usually absent

Celiac Disease

- Bilateral occipital Ca++; no angiomatous involvement of brain/face

Leptomeningeal Enhancement

- Meningitis, leptomeningeal metastases, leukemia

PATHOLOGY

General Features

- General path comments
  - Cutaneous nevus flammeus CN V1 & V2; ± visceral angiomatosis
  - Embryology
    - 4-8 week stage: Embryonic cortical veins fail to coalesce & develop ⇒ persistence of primordial vessels
    - Visual cortex adjacent to optic vesicle and upper fetal face
- Genetics
  - Usually sporadic: Probable somatic mutation or cutaneous mosaicism
    - Fibronectin (found in SWS port-wine-derived fibroblasts and SWS surgical brain samples) regulates angiogenesis and vasculogenesis
  - Very rarely familial, but occasionally with other vascular phakomatosis
- Etiology: Persistent fetal vasculature ⇒ deep venous occlusion/stasis ⇒ anoxic cortex
- Epidemiology: Rare: 1:50,000
- Associated abnormalities: 50% have extracranial port-wine stains (torso or extremities), so evaluate for other vascular phakomatoses

Gross Pathologic & Surgical Features

- Meningeal hypervascularity & angiomatosis
- Subjacent cortical & subcortical Ca++

Microscopic Features

- Pial angioma = multiple thin-walled vessels in enlarged sulci
- Cortical atrophy, Ca++
- Occasional underlying cortical dysplasia

Staging, Grading or Classification Criteria

- Roach Scale
  - Type I: Leptomeningeal plus facial; ± glaucoma
  - Type II: Facial only; ± glaucoma
  - Type III: Leptomeningeal only

CLINICAL ISSUES

Presentation

- Most common signs/symptoms
  - CN V1 facial nevus flammeus ("port-wine stain") 98%; (± V2, V3)
    - Need to look at mucous membranes for occult lesions
  - Eye findings especially with upper and lower lid nevus flammeus
    - Choroidal angioma 70% ⇒ ↑ intraocular pressure/congenital glaucoma ⇒ buphthalmos
    - Retinal telangiectatic vessels; scleral angioma; iris heterochromia
  - Seizures 90%; hemiparesis 30-66%
  - Stroke-like episodes; neurological deficit 65%; migraines
- Clinical Profile: "Port-wine stain", seizures, hemiparesis

Demographics

- Age
  - Facial lesion visible at birth
    - Pial angiomatosis may be occult if no facial lesion and no seizures to prompt imaging
  - Seizures develop first year of life
    - Infantile spasms ⇒ tonic/clonic, myoclonic
- Gender: M = F
- Ethnicity: No ethnic predilection

Natural History & Prognosis

- ↑ Extent of lobar involvement and atrophy ⇒ ↑ likelihood seizures
- If seizures ⇒ developmental delay 43%, emotional/behavioral problems 85%, special education 70%, employability 46%
- Progressive hemiparesis 30%, homonymous hemianopsia 2%

Treatment

- Treat seizures; resection affected lobes (hemisphere) may be required
- Laser skin lesions (cosmetic)
- Medical and surgical management of glaucoma

DIAGNOSTIC CHECKLIST

Consider

- In "Sturge-Weber-like" syndromes, look for extracranial manifestations

Image Interpretation Pearls

- Choroid plexus nearly always enlarged on involved side
  - May be only finding in first 6 months of life
  - If both sides enlarged, look for bilateral involvement

SELECTED REFERENCES

1. Comi AM: Advances in Sturge-Weber syndrome. Curr Opin Neurol. 19(2):124-8, 2006
2. Thomas-Sohl KA et al: Sturge-Weber syndrome: a review. Pediatr Neurol. 30(5):303-10, 2004
3. Comi AM et al: Increased fibronectin expression in SWS fibroblasts and brain tissue. Pediatr Res. 53(5):762-9, 2003
4. Lin DD et al: Early characteristics of Sturge-Weber syndrome shown by perfusion MRI and proton MRS imaging. AJNR. 24(9):1912-5, 2003
5. Pfund Z et al: Quantitative analysis of gray- & white-matter volumes and glucose metabolism in Sturge-Weber syndrome. J Child Neurol. 18(2):119-26, 2003

STURGE-WEBER SYNDROME

IMAGE GALLERY

Typical

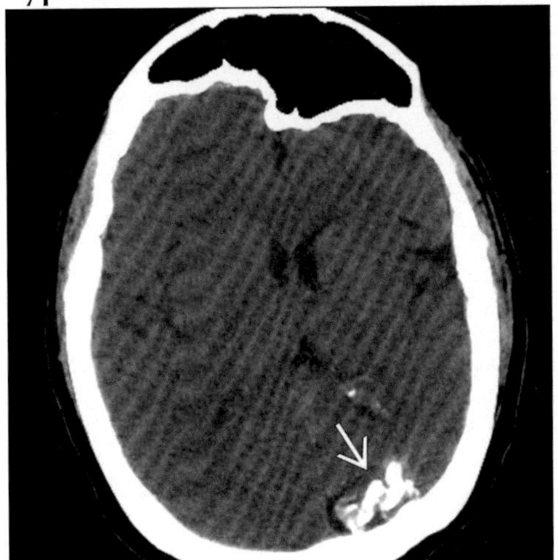

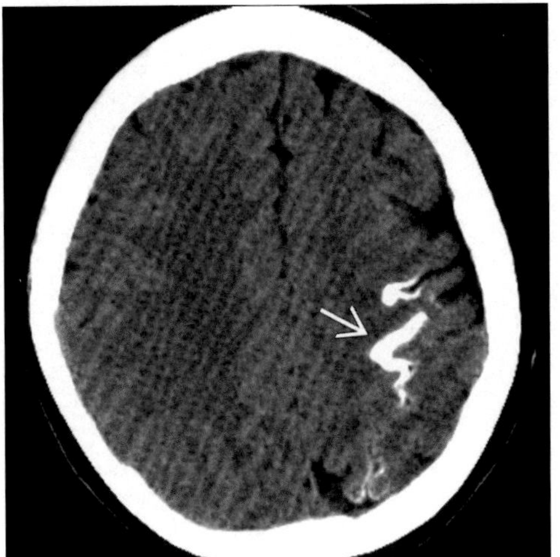

(Left) *Axial NECT shows gyriform calcification in the left occipital lobe ➡ associated with atrophy of the left cerebral hemisphere and an enlarged, hyperpneumatized left frontal sinus.* ***(Right)*** *Axial NECT shows gyriform calcification in the left frontal and parietal lobes ➡ in association with atrophy of the left cerebral hemisphere.*

Typical

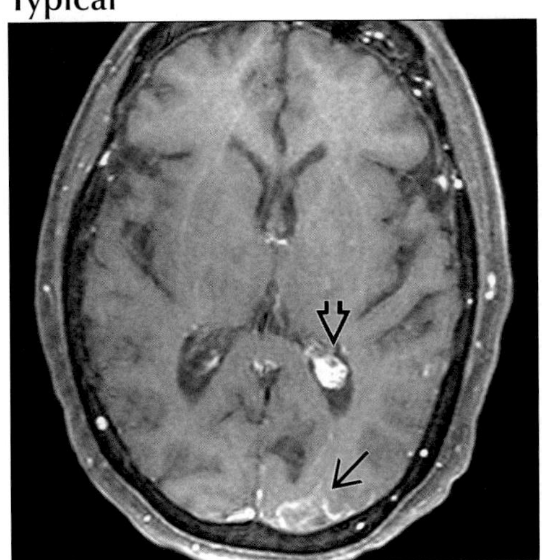

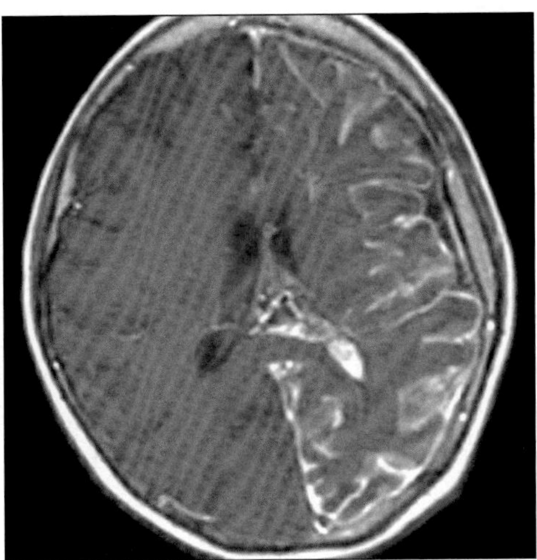

(Left) *Axial T1WI FS MR with intravenous gadolinium shows cortical gyriform enhancement in the left occipital lobe ➡ and asymmetric increased enhancement of an enlarged left choroid plexus ⇨.* ***(Right)*** *Axial T1WI MR with intravenous gadolinium shows diffuse leptomeningeal enhancement of the left cerebral hemisphere in addition to asymmetric enhancement of an enlarged left choroid plexus.*

Typical

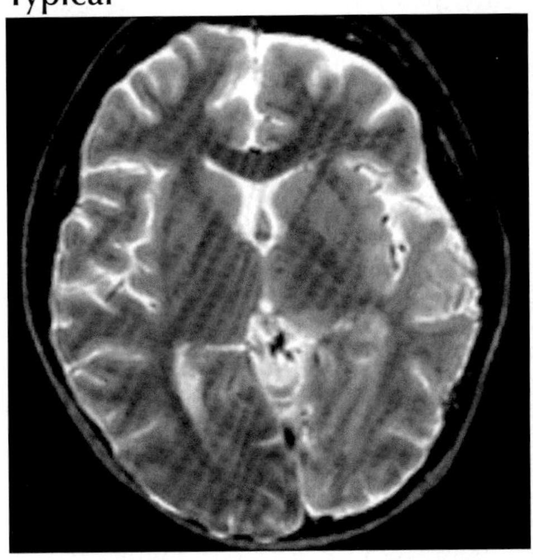

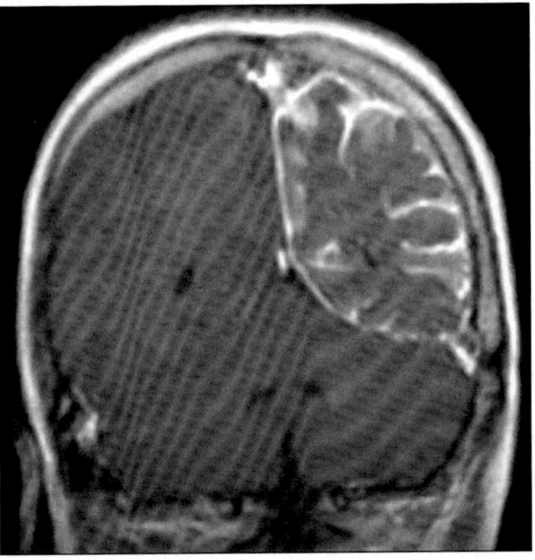

(Left) *Axial T2WI MR shows diffuse atrophy of the left cerebral hemisphere.* ***(Right)*** *Coronal T1WI MR with intravenous gadolinium shows diffuse leptomeningeal enhancement of the left cerebral hemisphere. Note ipsilateral thickening of the skull vault. Cortical calcifications are more difficult to visualize on MR compared with CT.*

VON HIPPEL LINDAU DISEASE

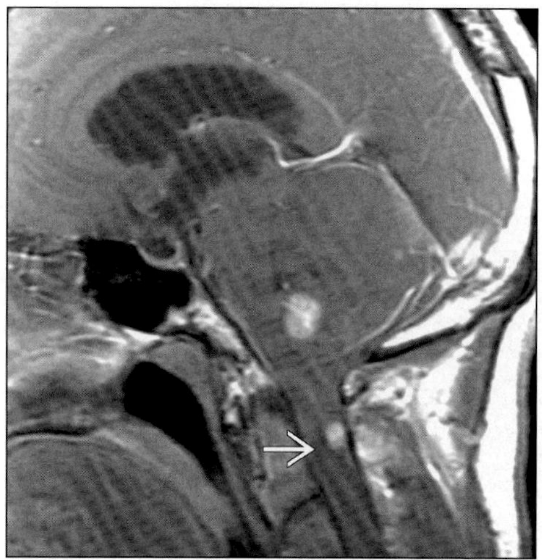

Sagittal T1WI MR with intravenous gadolinium shows two enhancing nodules. The nodule in the upper cervical spinal cord is associated with a small cyst ➔.

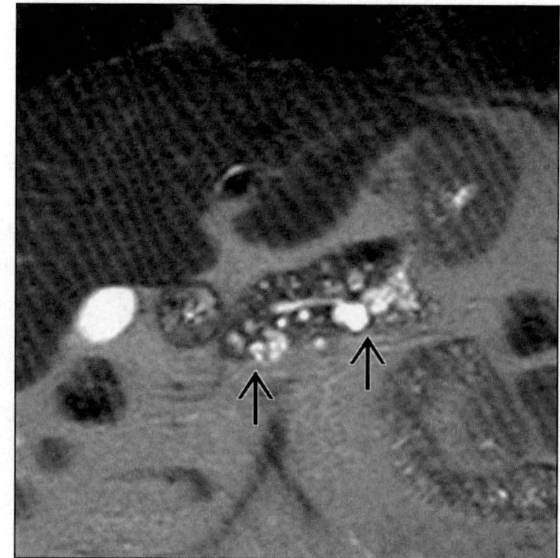

Coronal T2WI MR shows multiple pancreatic cysts ➔ and mild dilatation of the pancreatic duct.

TERMINOLOGY

Abbreviations and Synonyms

- von Hippel Lindau (VHL) syndrome

Definitions

- Autosomal dominant familial tumor syndrome with hemangioblastomas (HGBLs), clear cell renal carcinoma (RCC), cystadenomas, pheochromocytomas, islet cell tumors
  - Affects six different organ systems, including eye, ear, CNS
  - Involved tissues often have multiple lesions
  - Lesions = benign cysts, vascular tumors, carcinomas

IMAGING FINDINGS

General Features

- Best diagnostic clue: 2 or more CNS HGBLs or 1 HGBL + 1 visceral tumor characteristic of VHL
- Location
  - HGBLs in VHL
    - Typically multiple
    - 50% in spinal cord (posterior half)
    - 35-40% cerebellum
    - 10% brainstem (posterior medulla)
    - 1% supratentorial (along optic pathways, in cerebral hemispheres)
  - Ocular angiomas
    - Found in 75% of VHL gene carriers
    - Cause retinal detachment, hemorrhage
- Size: HGBLs vary from tiny to very large lesions with even larger associated cysts
- Morphology: Symptomatic HGBLs more often cystic than solid

CT Findings

- NECT
  - 2/3 of HGBLs have well-delineated cerebellar cyst + nodule
    - Nodule typically abuts pial surface
    - 1/3 solid, without cyst
    - ± Obstructive hydrocephalus due to compression of 4th ventricle
  - Endolymphatic sac (ELS) tumors
    - Lytic destructive lesions in the inner ear → hearing loss

DDx: Von Hippel Lindau Disease

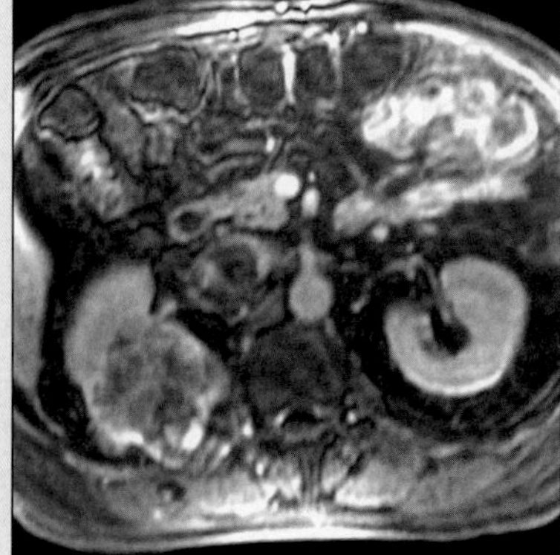

Solitary Clear Cell Renal Carcinoma

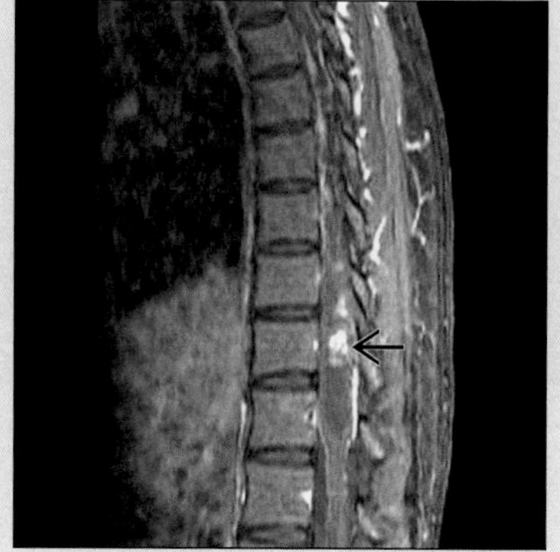

Pilocytic Astrocytoma

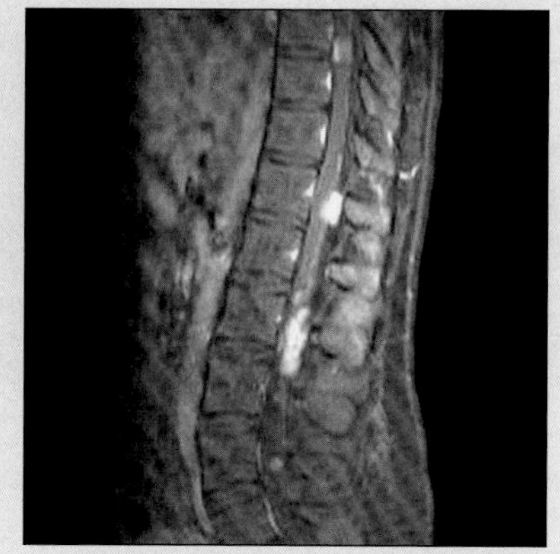

Hypervascular Metastases

VON HIPPEL LINDAU DISEASE

Key Facts

Terminology
- Autosomal dominant familial tumor syndrome with hemangioblastomas (HGBLs), clear cell renal carcinoma (RCC), cystadenomas, pheochromocytomas, islet cell tumors

Imaging Findings
- Best diagnostic clue: 2 or more CNS HGBLs or 1 HGBL + 1 visceral tumor characteristic of VHL
- T2WI: HGBL: Hyperintense cyst, often associated with edema when in the spinal cord
- Tumor nodule enhances strongly
- Associated cyst wall usually non-neoplastic, does not enhance
- Best imaging tool: MR without & with contrast for CNS lesions

Top Differential Diagnoses
- Vascular Metastasis
- Solitary Hemangioblastoma
- Pilocytic Astrocytoma
- Disseminated HGBLs without VHL
- Multiple AVMs in Vascular Neurocutaneous Syndromes

Pathology
- Etiology: Both alleles of VHL tumor suppressor gene on chromosome 3 inactivated

Clinical Issues
- Earliest symptom in VHL often visual

Diagnostic Checklist
- Solitary HGBL in a young patient may indicate VHL

- CECT
  - HGBL: Intense enhancement of tumor nodule = classic
    - Homogeneous enhancement of solid tumor or irregular peripheral enhancement less common
  - RCC: Enhancing renal mass

MR Findings
- T1WI
  - HGBL: Mixed iso ⇒ hypointense nodule, ± "flow voids"
    - Associated cyst slightly hyperintense to CSF
  - ELS tumor: May contain high signal due to proteinaceous fluid ± hemorrhage
- T2WI: HGBL: Hyperintense cyst, often associated with edema when in the spinal cord
- FLAIR
  - Cyst typically hyperintense due to proteinaceous content or prior hemorrhage
  - Variable high signal edema around lesion
- T2* GRE: Low signal "blooming" if blood products present, flow voids
- T1 C+
  - Tumor nodule enhances strongly
  - Associated cyst wall usually non-neoplastic, does not enhance
  - May detect tiny asymptomatic enhancing nodules
  - Enhancing renal masses and adrenal masses
  - ELS tumor: Intense enhancement

Ultrasonographic Findings
- Grayscale Ultrasound
  - Simple anechoic epididymal cysts, renal cysts, pancreatic cysts, hepatic cysts
  - Epididymal papillary cystadenoma
    - Solid with a non-shadowing echogenic focus
  - Solid renal mass: RCC

Angiographic Findings
- Conventional
  - DSA shows intensely vascular mass, prolonged stain
  - Arteriovenous (AV) shunting is common ± venous lakes

Imaging Recommendations
- Best imaging tool: MR without & with contrast for CNS lesions
- Protocol advice: Scan entire spine
- NIH recommendations for patients with family Hx of VHL
  - Contrast-enhanced MR of brain/spinal cord from age 11 y, every 2 years
  - US of abdomen from 11 y, yearly
  - Abdominal CT from 20 y, yearly or every other year
  - MR of temporal bone if hearing loss, tinnitus/vertigo

DIFFERENTIAL DIAGNOSIS

Vascular Metastasis
- Usually solid, not cyst + nodule
- Parenchymal edema is typically extensive (unusual in cerebellar HGBL)
- Some tumors (e.g., renal clear cell carcinoma) can resemble hemangioblastoma histopathologically
- Rare: RCC metastasis to an HGBL reported

Solitary Hemangioblastoma
- 25-40% of HGBLs occur in VHL
- No family history, other tumors or cysts
- No VHL gene alterations

Pilocytic Astrocytoma
- Common in cerebellum, brainstem
- Different age (usually younger than VHL patients)
- No family history, lacks retinal angioma/hemorrhages
- Tumor nodule often lacks large flow voids (more characteristic of HGBL)

Disseminated HGBLs without VHL
- Rare; occurrence recently reported
- Multiple sites of subarachnoid dissemination 1-8 yrs after initial complete resection of solitary HGBL
- Somatic deletion of one copy of the VHL gene in tumors (derived from single clone)

VON HIPPEL LINDAU DISEASE

Multiple AVMs in Vascular Neurocutaneous Syndromes

- E.g., HHT, Wyburn-Mason
- Small AVMs may resemble HGBL at angiography

PATHOLOGY

General Features

- General path comments
  - VHL characterized by development of
    - Capillary hemangioblastomas of CNS & retina
    - Cysts, renal clear cell carcinoma
    - Pheochromocytoma
    - Pancreatic cysts, islet cell tumors
    - ELS tumors
    - Epididymal cysts, cystadenomas
- Genetics
  - Autosomal dominant inheritance with high penetrance, variable expression
  - Germline mutations of VHL tumor suppressor gene
    - Chromosome 3p25-26, different mutations scattered throughout gene
    - Inactivating mutations (nonsense mutations/deletions) predispose to VHL type 1
    - Missense mutations predispose to VHL types 2A, 2B
- Etiology: Both alleles of VHL tumor suppressor gene on chromosome 3 inactivated
- Epidemiology: 1 in 35-50,000

Gross Pathologic & Surgical Features

- HGBL seen as well-circumscribed, very vascular, reddish nodule
  - 75% at least partially cystic, contain amber-colored fluid
- Rare: Leptomeningeal hemangioblastomatosis

Microscopic Features

- Two components in HGBL
  - Rich capillary network and large vacuolated stromal cells with clear cytoplasm

Staging, Grading or Classification Criteria

- Capillary hemangioblastoma = WHO grade I

CLINICAL ISSUES

Presentation

- Most common signs/symptoms
  - VHL is clinically very heterogeneous; phenotypic penetrance = 97% at 65 y
  - Retinal angiomas
    - Earliest symptom in VHL often visual
    - Retinal detachment, vitreous hemorrhages
  - Cerebellar HGBLs
    - H/A (obstructive hydrocephalus)
    - Nearly 75% of symptom-producing tumors have associated cyst
  - Spinal cord HGBLs
    - Progressive myelopathy
    - 95% associated syrinx
- Other signs/symptoms: HGBLs can produce erythropoietin and result in polycythemia
- Clinical Profile
  - Phenotypes based on absence or presence of pheochromocytoma
    - Type 1 = without pheochromocytoma
    - Type 2A = pheochromocytoma without renal cell carcinoma
    - Type 2B = pheochromocytoma with renal cell carcinoma
    - Type 2C = pheochromocytoma only
  - Diagnosis of VHL
    - Family history of VHL + single HGBL, RCC, pheochromocytoma, or possibly multiple pancreatic cysts
    - If no family history of VHL then need 2 or more HGBLs or 1 HGBL + 1 visceral tumor seen in VHL

Demographics

- Age
  - VHL presents in young adults
    - Retinal angioma: Mean age = 25 y
    - Cerebellar: Mean age = 30 y
  - Mean age of presentation with other VHL-associated tumors
    - Pheochromocytoma (30 y)
    - RCC (33 y)
- Gender: M = F

Natural History & Prognosis

- RCC develops in up to 70% of patients
  - Eventual cause of death in 15-50%
- HGBLs often have periods of tumor growth (usually associated with ↑ cyst size) separated by periods of arrested growth
- On average, new lesion develops every 2 yrs in VHL

Treatment

- Ophthalmoscopy yearly from infancy
- Physical/neurological examination annually from age 2 years
- Surgical resection of symptomatic cerebellar/spinal hemangioblastoma
  - Preoperative embolization of tumor significantly reduces intraoperative hemorrhage
- Stereotactic radiosurgery may control smaller lesions
- Laser treatment of retinal angiomata

DIAGNOSTIC CHECKLIST

Consider

- Look for ELS tumors in VHL patients with dysequilibrium, hearing loss or aural fullness
- MR for screening of both CNS and abdomen to reduce long term radiation exposure in young patients

Image Interpretation Pearls

- Solitary HGBL in a young patient may indicate VHL

SELECTED REFERENCES

1. Lin DD et al: Neuroimaging of phakomatoses. Semin Pediatr Neurol. 13(1):48-62, 2006

IMAGE GALLERY

Typical

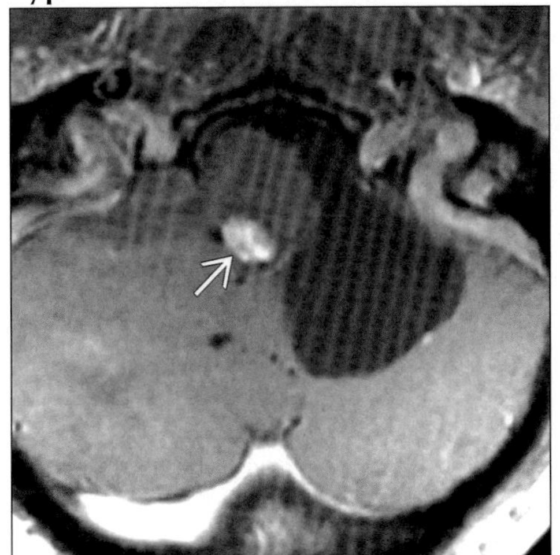

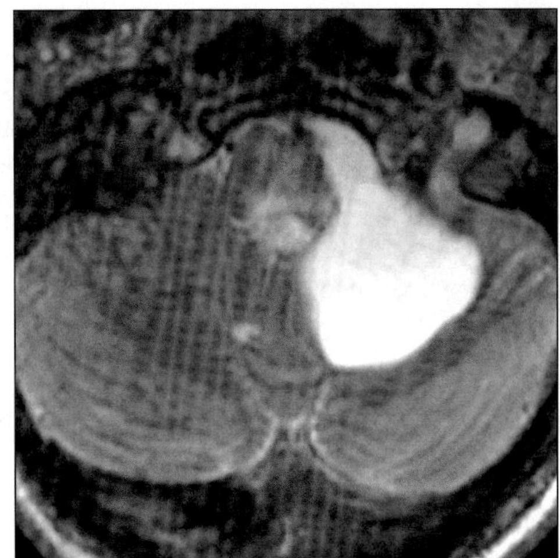

(Left) *Axial T1WI MR with intravenous gadolinium shows a lobulated cyst within the left cerebellar hemisphere with mild mass effect and an enhancing nodule ➡.* ***(Right)*** *Axial T2WI MR shows a cystic mass in the posterior fossa with mass effect on the medulla and cerebellar hemisphere.*

Typical

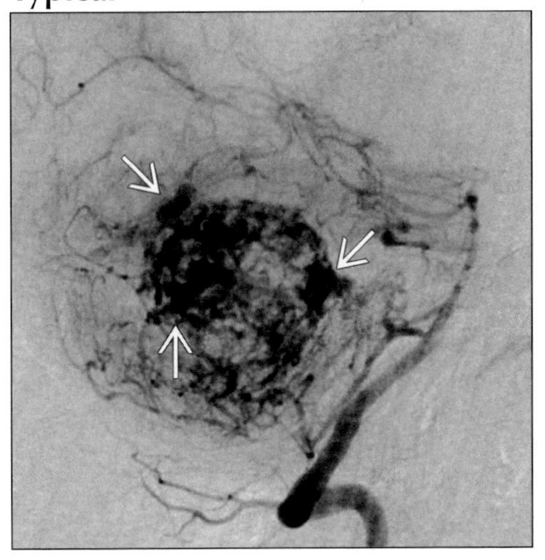

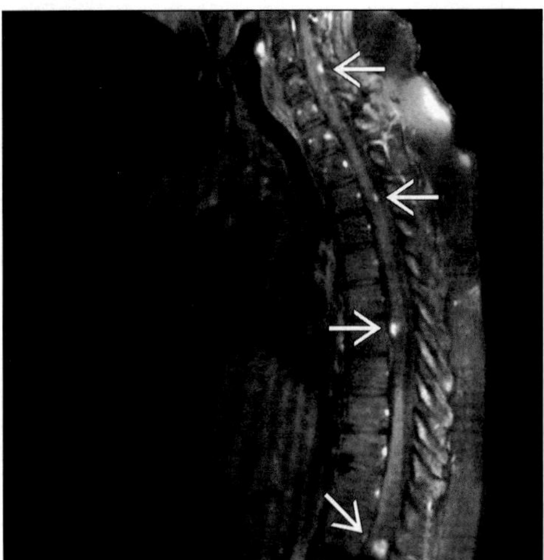

(Left) *Lateral vertebral artery DSA shows a vascular cerebellar mass with AV shunting into numerous peripherally located venous lakes ➡. The patient had no prior history of VHL. Preoperative embolization was performed to reduce blood loss during resection. Histopathologically proven HGBL.* ***(Right)*** *Sagittal T1WI FS MR in the same patient shows multiple spinal HGBLs ➡. Abdominal CT revealed multiple pancreatic and renal cysts (not shown).*

Typical

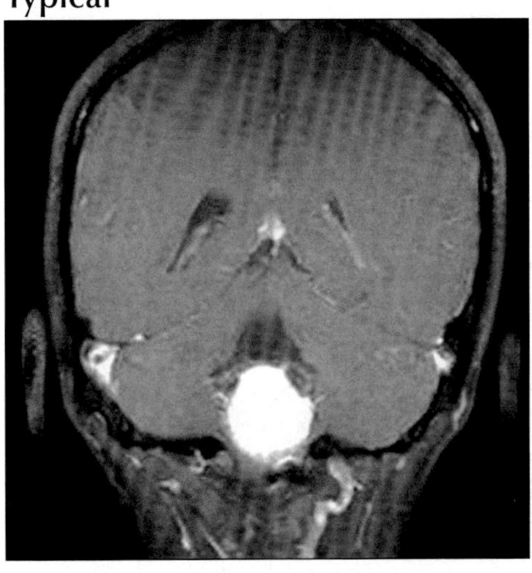

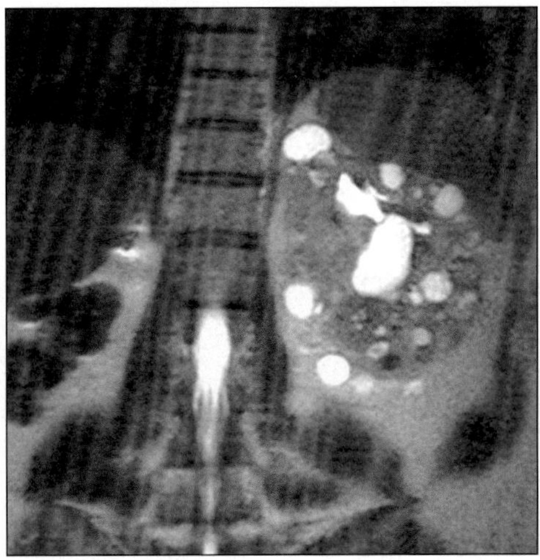

(Left) *Coronal T1WI FS MR with intravenous gadolinium shows a large enhancing mass in the roof of the fourth ventricle.* ***(Right)*** *Coronal T2WI MR shows multiple cysts in the left kidney. In patients with known or suspected VHL, a careful search for RCC and pancreatic cysts should be made. Gd-enhanced MR is sensitive for detection of spinal and intracranial HGBLs as well as ELS tumors. Early detection of the latter may prevent hearing loss.*

HEMANGIOBLASTOMA, BRAIN

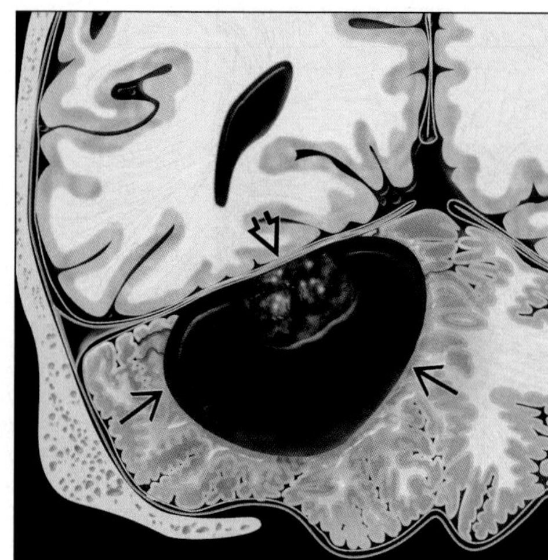

Coronal graphic depicts a classic cerebellar hemangioblastoma, seen here as a largely cystic mass ➔ with a very vascular tumor nodule that is abutting the pia ⇨.

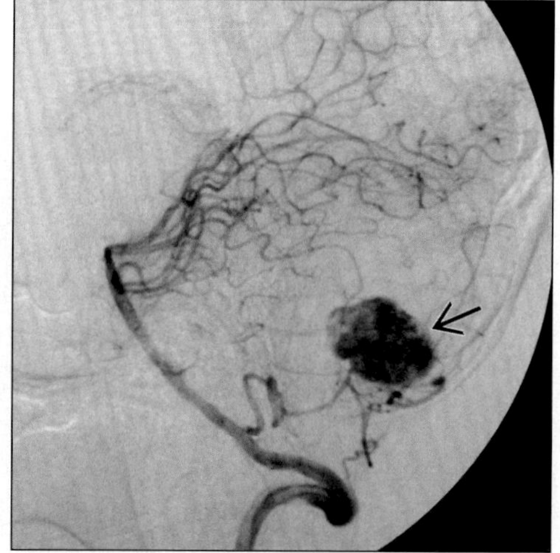

Lateral DSA of a right vertebral artery injection shows an enhancing tumor nodule ➔ supplied by the PICA with surrounding avascular region due to the cystic component of hemangioblastoma.

TERMINOLOGY

Abbreviations and Synonyms

- Hemangioblastoma (HGBL)
- Capillary hemangioblastoma

Definitions

- Vascular neoplasm of uncertain origin
- HGBL currently classified as meningeal tumor of uncertain histogenesis (WHO, 2000)

IMAGING FINDINGS

General Features

- Best diagnostic clue: Adult with intra-axial posterior fossa mass with cyst, enhancing mural nodule abutting pia
- Location
  - 90-95% posterior fossa
    - 80% cerebellar hemispheres
    - 15% vermis, 5% other: Medulla, 4th ventricle
  - 5-10% supratentorial: Around optic pathways, hemispheres; usually in von Hippel Lindau (VHL) syndrome
- Size: Varies from tiny to several cms
- Morphology
  - 60% cyst + "mural" nodule
  - 40% solid

CT Findings

- NECT: Low density cyst + isodense nodule
- CECT
  - Common
    - Nodule enhances intensely, relatively uniformly
    - Cyst wall usually doesn't enhance
  - Less common: Solid tumor
  - Rare: Ring-enhancing mass
- CTA: May demonstrate arterial feeders

MR Findings

- T1WI
  - Nodule isointense with brain ± "flow voids"
  - Cyst slightly hyperintense compared to CSF
- T2WI
  - Both nodule, cyst are hyperintense
  - Prominent "flow voids" in some cases

DDx: Hemangioblastoma

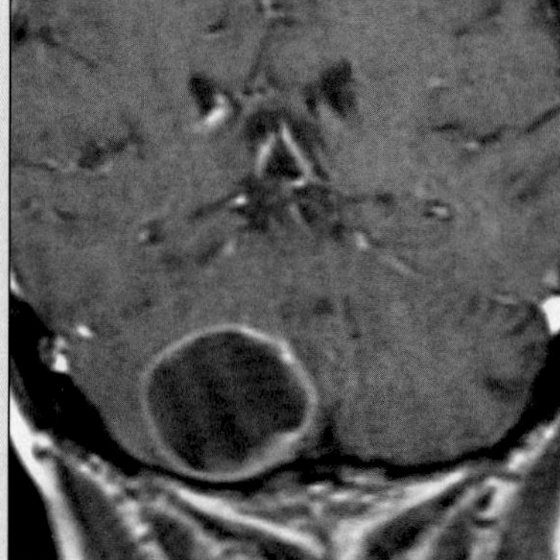

Breast Cancer Metastasis

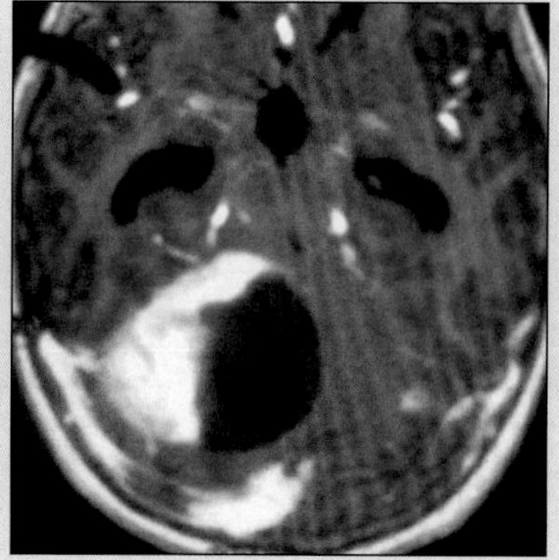

Juvenile Pilocytic Astrocytoma

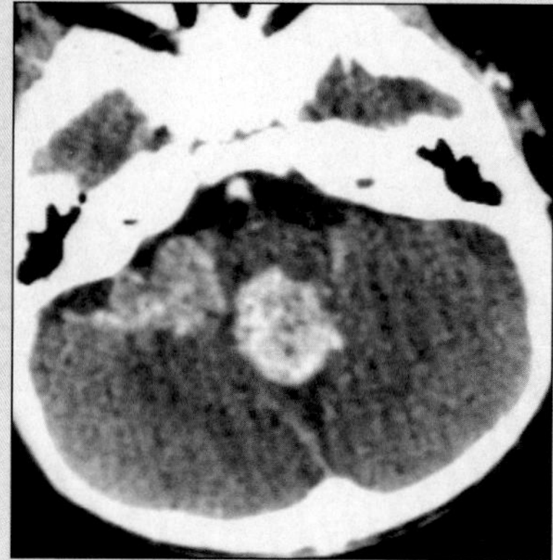

Ependymoma

HEMANGIOBLASTOMA, BRAIN

Key Facts

Terminology
- HGBL currently classified as meningeal tumor of uncertain histogenesis (WHO, 2000)

Imaging Findings
- Best diagnostic clue: Adult with intra-axial posterior fossa mass with cyst, enhancing mural nodule abutting pia
- 90-95% posterior fossa
- Size: Varies from tiny to several cms
- 60% cyst + "mural" nodule
- 40% solid

Top Differential Diagnoses
- Metastasis
- Astrocytoma
- Vascular Neurocutaneous Syndrome
- Cavernous Malformation (CM)
- Ependymoma

Pathology
- VHL phenotypes (based on presence, absence of pheochromocytoma and renal cell carcinoma)
- 1-2% of primary intracranial tumors
- 7-10% of posterior fossa tumors
- Associated abnormalities: Secondary polycythemia (may elaborate upregulated erythropoietin)
- WHO grade I

Diagnostic Checklist
- Screen entire neuraxis for other HGBLs
- Most common posterior fossa intra-axial mass in middle-aged/older adult = metastasis, not HGBL!

- PD/Intermediate: Hyperintense
- FLAIR: Both cyst, nodule hyperintense
- T2* GRE: May "bloom" if short T2 blood products present
- DWI: Cyst slightly or markedly low signal
- T1 C+
  - Common: Nodule enhances strongly, intensely
  - Less common: Solid tumor enhancement
  - Rare: Enhancement of cyst wall

Nuclear Medicine Findings
- Thallium-201 SPECT shows fast washout

Angiographic Findings
- Conventional
  - Large avascular mass (cyst)
  - Highly vascular nodule
    - Prolonged blush
    - ± AV shunting (early draining vein)
  - Rarely performed as diagnosis established with MR and pre-operative embolization not generally used
  - Can detect the rare aneurysm on feeding vessel

Imaging Recommendations
- Best imaging tool: Contrast-enhanced MR (sensitivity >> CT for small HGBLs)
- Protocol advice
  - Begin MR screening of patients from VHL families after age 10 y
    - Also screen complete spine to detect possible additional lesions

DIFFERENTIAL DIAGNOSIS

Metastasis
- Multiple > single
- Solid or necrotic > cystic
- May be very vascular
  - Vascular mets such as renal cell carcinoma (RCC) do not express inhibin A or GLUT1; HGBL does

Astrocytoma
- Juvenile pilocytic astrocytoma (JPA)
  - Usually in children
  - Tumor nodule often lacks flow voids
  - Tumor nodule usually does not abut pial surface
- Glioblastoma
  - Similar age range as HGBL
  - Posterior fossa uncommon location
  - Central necrosis with enhancing rim of tumor > cyst with mural nodule

Vascular Neurocutaneous Syndrome
- Hereditary hemorrhagic telangiectasia (HHT), Wyburn-Mason
- Multiple intracranial AVMs may mimic HGBLs

Cavernous Malformation (CM)
- Gross intratumoral hemorrhage rare in HGBL
- Complete hemosiderin rim typical in CMs

Ependymoma
- Younger patients; extrudes through ventricle foramina

PATHOLOGY

General Features
- General path comments
  - VHL phenotypes (based on presence, absence of pheochromocytoma and renal cell carcinoma)
    - Type 1 = without pheochromocytoma
    - Type 2A = with pheochromocytoma, RCC
    - Type 2B = with pheochromocytoma, without RCC
- Genetics
  - Familial HGBL (VHL disease)
    - Autosomal dominant
    - Chromosome 3p mutation
    - Suppressor gene product (VHL protein) causes neoplastic transformation
    - Multiple HGBLs are the rule (cerebellar + supratentorial or spinal HGBLs)
    - VEGF highly expressed in stromal cells
    - Other VHL gene mutations common
    - Other markers (visceral cysts, renal clear cell carcinoma, retinal angiomas), + family history

HEMANGIOBLASTOMA, BRAIN

- Etiology: Precise histogenesis unknown
- Epidemiology
  - VHL 1:36-40,000
  - Less than half (25-40%) HGBLs associated with VHL
  - 1-2% of primary intracranial tumors
    - 7-10% of posterior fossa tumors
  - 3-13% of spinal cord tumors
- Associated abnormalities: Secondary polycythemia (may elaborate upregulated erythropoietin)

Gross Pathologic & Surgical Features

- Red or yellowish well-circumscribed, unencapsulated highly vascular mass that abuts leptomeninges
- ± Cyst with yellow-brown fluid

Microscopic Features

- Nodule
  - Large vacuolated stromal cells
    - Neoplastic component
    - Lipid-containing vacuoles ("clear cell" morphology)
  - Immunohistochemistry
    - Negative for cytokeratin, EMA
    - Positive for inhibin A, GLUT1
    - Overexpress VEGF protein
  - Rich capillary network
  - Absence of endothelial tight junctions
    - May be the cause of associated cyst formation
- Cyst wall
  - Usually compressed brain (not neoplasm)
  - Variable intratumoral hemorrhage

Staging, Grading or Classification Criteria

- WHO grade I
- Low MIB-1 index (mean 0.8%)
- No difference between sporadic, VHL-associated HGBLs

CLINICAL ISSUES

Presentation

- Most common signs/symptoms
  - Sporadic HGBL
    - Headache (85%), dysequilibrium, dizziness
  - Familial
    - Retinal HGBL: Ocular hemorrhage often first manifestation of VHL
    - Other: Sx due to RCC, polycythemia, endolymphatic sac tumor

Demographics

- Age
  - Sporadic HGBL
    - Peak 40-60 y
    - Rare in children
  - Familial
    - VHL-associated HGBLs occur at younger age but are rare < 15 y
    - Retinal HGBL: Mean onset 25 y
- Gender: Slight male predominance

Natural History & Prognosis

- Usually benign tumor with slow growth pattern
  - Symptoms usually associated with cyst expansion (may occur rapidly)
  - Rare: Leptomeningeal tumor dissemination
- Two-thirds with one VHL-associated HGBL develop additional lesions
  - Average = one new lesion every 2 years
  - Require periodic screening, lifelong follow-up
  - Periods of intermixed growth, relative quiescence
  - Median life expectancy in VHL = 49 years

Treatment

- En bloc surgical resection (piecemeal may result in catastrophic hemorrhage)
  - 85% 10 year survival rate
  - 15-20% recurrence rate
- Pre-operative embolization
  - Sometimes used if large tumor nodule present
  - Partial (not complete) embolization does not reduce operative complications or morbidity
- Gamma knife surgery effective for smaller lesions

DIAGNOSTIC CHECKLIST

Consider

- Screen entire neuraxis for other HGBLs

Image Interpretation Pearls

- Most common posterior fossa intra-axial mass in middle-aged/older adult = metastasis, not HGBL!
- Most common posterior fossa primary brain tumor in middle-aged/older adult = HMGB!

SELECTED REFERENCES

1. Cornelius JF et al: Hemorrhage after particle embolization of hemangioblastomas: comparison of outcomes in spinal and cerebellar lesions. J Neurosurg. 106(6):994-8, 2007
2. Ammerman JM et al: Long-term natural history of hemangioblastomas in patients with von Hippel-Lindau disease: implications for treatment. J Neurosurg. 105(2):248-55, 2006
3. Chen Y et al: Absence of tight junctions between microvascular endothelial cells in human cerebellar hemangioblastomas. Neurosurgery. 59(3):660-70; discussion 660-70, 2006
4. Priesemann M et al: Benefits of screening in von Hippel-Lindau disease--comparison of morbidity associated with initial tumours in affected parents and children. Horm Res. 66(1):1-5, 2006
5. Tago M et al: Gamma knife surgery for hemangioblastomas. J Neurosurg. 102 Suppl:171-4, 2005
6. Hoang MP et al: Inhibin alpha distinguishes hemangioblastoma from clear cell renal cell carcinoma. Am J Surg Pathol. 27(8):1152-6, 2003
7. Kondo T et al: Diagnostic value of 201Tl-single-photon emission computerized tomography studies in cases of posterior fossa hemangioblastomas. J Neurosurg. 95(2):292-7, 2001
8. Wang C et al: Surgical management of medullary hemangioblastoma. Report of 47 cases. Surg Neurol. 56(4):218-26; discussion 226-7, 2001
9. Miyagami M et al: Clinicopathological study of vascular endothelial growth factor (VEGF), p53, and proliferative potential in familial von Hippel-Lindau disease and sporadic hemangioblastomas. Brain Tumor Pathol. 17(3):111-20, 2000

IMAGE GALLERY

Typical

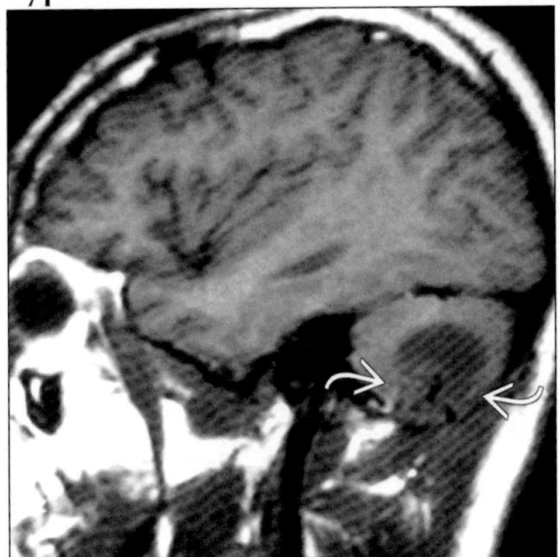

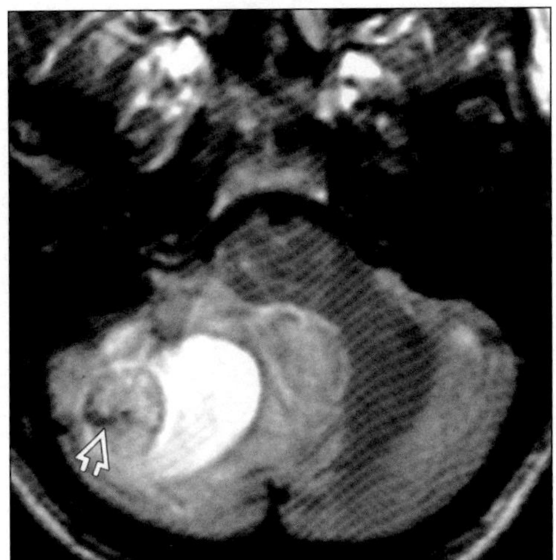

*(**Left**) Sagittal T1WI MR shows a mass in the cerebellum with a nodular soft tissue component inferiorly ➡ and a cystic component superiorly. Note the flow voids in the solid portion of the tumor. (**Right**) Axial PD MR image in the same patient as previous image, shows slightly hyperintense nodule and markedly hyperintense cyst. Flow voids ➡ in the nodule again evident from the very vascular hemangioblastoma.*

Typical

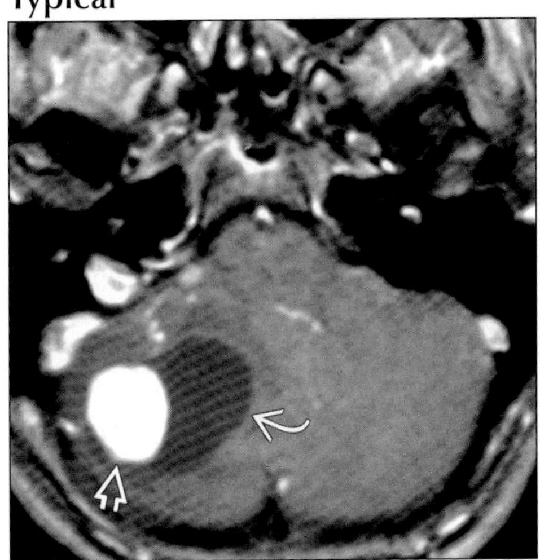

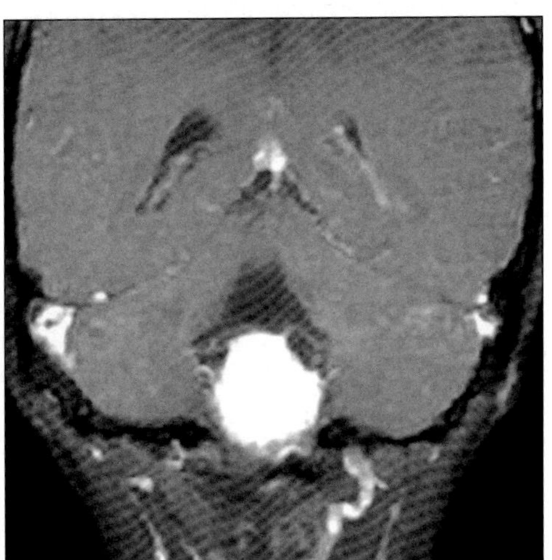

*(**Left**) Axial T1WI MR post-contrast depicts a classic solitary hemangioblastoma. There is an avidly enhancing nodule ➡ with an adjacent non-enhancing cyst ➡ in the right cerebellar hemisphere. (**Right**) Coronal T1WI FS MR post-contrast demonstrates a solidly enhancing mass (without a cyst) in the cerebellar vermis. This is a somewhat less common appearance and location of hemangioblastoma.*

Variant

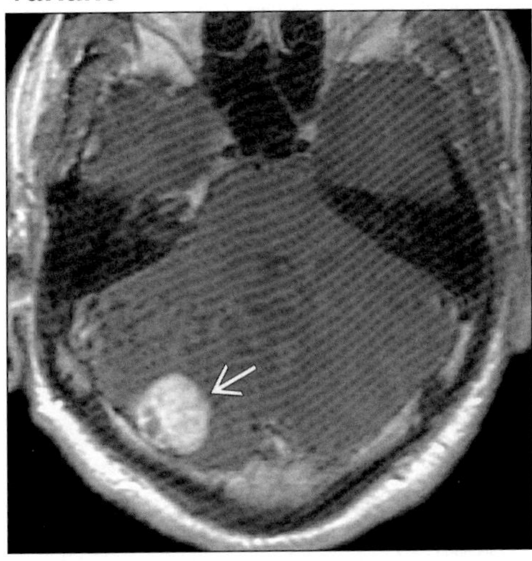

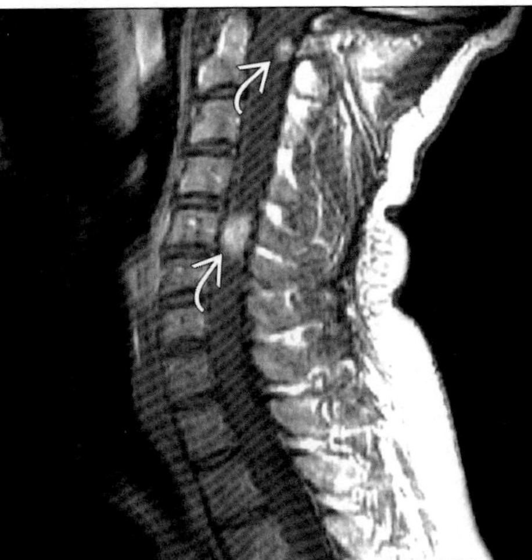

*(**Left**) Axial T1WI MR post-contrast shows a right cerebellar markedly enhancing mass ➡ abutting the pia with no significant associated large cystic component. (**Right**) Sagittal T1WI MR post-contrast in the same patient as previous image, shows additional enhancing lesions on the surface of the cervical spinal cord ➡. Patient with VHL and multiple hemangioblastomas.*

ARTERIOVENOUS MALFORMATION, BRAIN

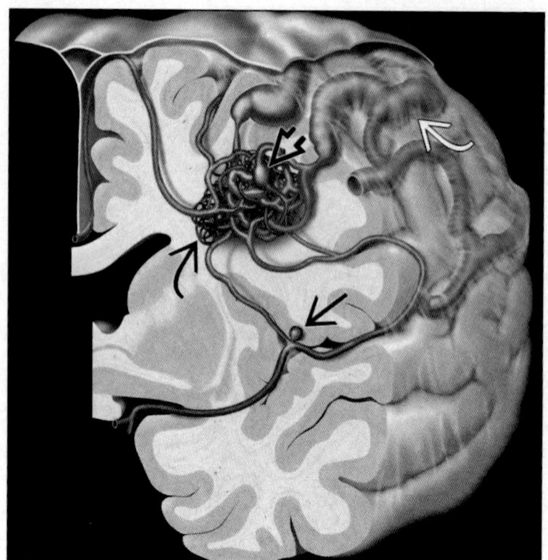

Coronal graphic shows a classic cerebral AVM. Note nidus ➔ with intranidal aneurysm ➔, enlarged feeding arteries with a "pedicle" aneurysm ➔, and draining venous varices ➔.

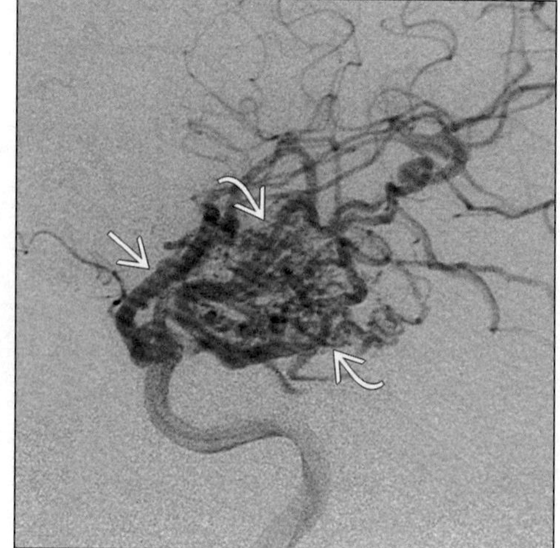

Lateral DSA of a selective ICA injection shows markedly enlarged arteries ➔ feeding a deep cerebral large AVM nidus ➔.

TERMINOLOGY

Abbreviations and Synonyms

- Arteriovenous malformation (AVM)

Definitions

- Vascular malformation with arteriovenous shunting, no intervening capillary bed

IMAGING FINDINGS

General Features

- Best diagnostic clue: "Bag of black worms" (flow voids) on MR with minimal/no mass effect
- Location
  - May occur anywhere in brain, spinal cord
  - 85% supratentorial; 15% posterior fossa
  - 98% solitary, sporadic
  - Rare: Multiple AVMs (usually syndromic)
- Size
  - Varies from microscopic to giant
  - Most symptomatic AVMs are 3-6 cm
- Morphology: Tightly packed mass of enlarged vascular channels

CT Findings

- NECT
  - May be normal with very small AVM
    - Iso/hyperdense serpentine vessels
    - Ca++ in 25-30%
    - Usually no significant mass effect even in larger lesions
    - Variable hemorrhage
- CECT: Strong enhancement of tubular vascular structures
- CTA: Enlarged arteries, draining veins, and intervening vascular nidus usually depicted well

MR Findings

- T1WI
  - Signal varies with flow rate, direction, presence/age of hemorrhage
  - Classic: Tightly packed mass looks like "honeycomb" of "flow voids"
- T2WI
  - Multiple tightly clustered low signal "flow voids"

DDx: Arteriovenous Malformation

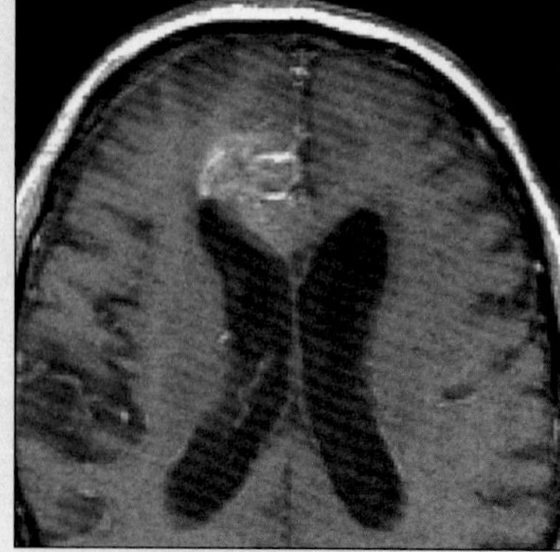

Glioblastoma

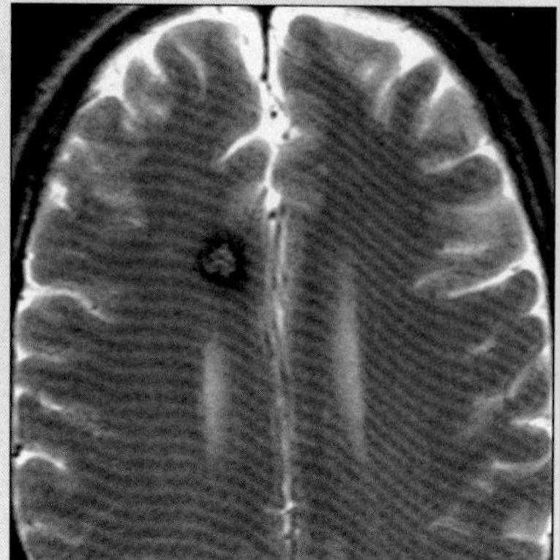

Cavernous Malformation

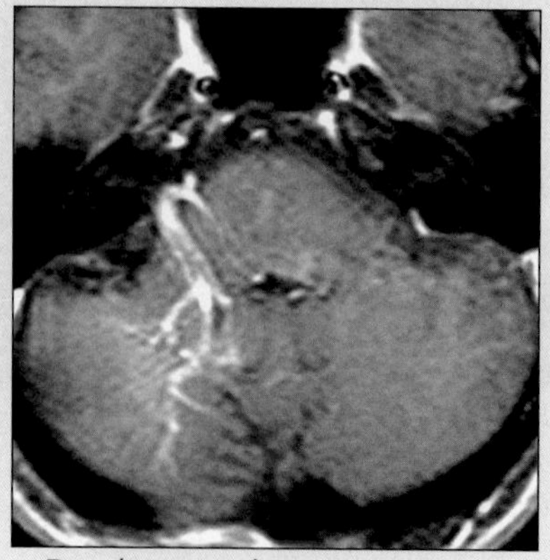

Developmental Venous Anomaly

ARTERIOVENOUS MALFORMATION, BRAIN

Key Facts

Terminology
- Vascular malformation with arteriovenous shunting, no intervening capillary bed

Imaging Findings
- Best diagnostic clue: "Bag of black worms" (flow voids) on MR with minimal/no mass effect
- 85% supratentorial; 15% posterior fossa
- 98% solitary, sporadic
- Ca++ in 25-30%
- Signal varies with flow rate, direction, presence/age of hemorrhage
- Classic: Tightly packed mass looks like "honeycomb" of "flow voids"
- Best imaging tool: DSA with superselective catherization

Top Differential Diagnoses
- Patent AVM vs. Glioblastoma with AV Shunting

Pathology
- General path comments: AVMs have dysregulated angiogenesis, undergo continued vascular remodeling
- Sporadic AVMs have multiple up-, down-regulated genes
- Multiple AVMs in HHT 1 (endoglin gene mutation)
- Cerebrofacial arteriovenous metameric syndromes (CAMS) have orbit/maxillofacial + intracranial AVMs
- Most common symptomatic cerebral vascular malformation (CVM)

Clinical Issues
- Headache with hemorrhage 50%
- Age: Peak presentation = 20-40 y (25% by age 15)

- Variable ages of hemorrhagic components can lead to mixed signal pattern
- Little/no brain within nidus (some gliotic, high signal tissue may be present)
- FLAIR: "Flow voids" ± surrounding high signal (gliosis)
- T2* GRE: May show some hypointense "blooming" if short T2 hemorrhagic products present
- DWI: Usually normal; vascular "steal" may cause ischemia in adjacent brain
- T1 C+: Strong enhancement of vascular elements
- MRA
  - Helpful for gross depiction of flow, post-embo/XRT
  - Does not depict detailed angioarchitecture
- MRV: May be useful for delineating presence/direction of venous drainage

Angiographic Findings
- Conventional
  - Delineates internal angioarchitecture (superselective best)
  - Depicts three components of AVMs
    - Enlarged arteries
    - Nidus of tightly packed vessels
    - Draining veins (AV shunting with early appearance of contrast in enlarged veins)
  - 27-32% of AVMs have "dual" arterial supply (pial, dural)
    - Dural supply to AVMs occurs through leptomeningeal anastomoses or transdural anastomoses (TDAs) with normal cortical arteries
    - Essential to examine ICA, ECA, vertebral circulations completely!
    - Frequency of TDAs increases with AVM volume, patient age
    - Identification of TDAs affects treatment decision (embolization, surgery)

Imaging Recommendations
- Best imaging tool: DSA with superselective catheterization
- Protocol advice: Standard contrast MR (include contrast-enhanced 3D MRA, GRE sequences)

DIFFERENTIAL DIAGNOSIS

Patent AVM vs. Glioblastoma with AV Shunting
- GBM enhances, has mass effect
- Some parenchyma between vessels

Thrombosed ("Cryptic") AVM Versus
- Cavernous malformation
- Developmental venous anomaly
- Calcified neoplasm
  - Oligodendroglioma, astrocytoma, metastasis

PATHOLOGY

General Features
- General path comments: AVMs have dysregulated angiogenesis, undergo continued vascular remodeling
- Genetics
  - Sporadic AVMs have multiple up-, down-regulated genes
    - Homeobox genes such as Hox D3 and B3 involved in angiogenesis may malfunction
  - Syndromic AVMs (2% of cases)
    - Multiple AVMs in HHT 1 (endoglin gene mutation)
    - Cerebrofacial arteriovenous metameric syndromes (CAMS) have orbit/maxillofacial + intracranial AVMs
- Etiology
  - Dysregulated angiogenesis
    - Vascular endothelial growth factors (VEGFs), receptors mediate endothelial proliferation, migration
    - Cytokine receptors mediate vascular maturation, remodeling
- Epidemiology
  - Most common symptomatic cerebral vascular malformation (CVM)
  - Prevalence of sporadic AVMs = .04-.52%
- Associated abnormalities

ARTERIOVENOUS MALFORMATION, BRAIN

- Flow-related aneurysm on feeding artery 10-15%
- Intranidal "aneurysm" > 50%
- Vascular "steal" may cause ischemia in adjacent brain
  - PET studies may show hemodynamic impairment

Gross Pathologic & Surgical Features

- Wedge-shaped, compact mass of tangled vessels

Microscopic Features

- Wide phenotypic spectrum
  - Feeding arteries usually enlarged but mature (may have some wall thickening)
  - Enlarged draining veins (may have associated varix, stenosis)
  - Nidus
    - Conglomeration of numerous AV shunts ("micro AVFs")
    - Thin-walled dysplastic vessels (no capillary bed)
    - Disorganized collagen, variable muscularization
    - Lack subendothelial support
    - Loss of normal contractile properties
    - No normal brain (may have some gliosis)
  - Perinidal capillary network (PDCN)
    - Nidus surrounded by dilated capillaries in brain tissue 1-7 mm outside nidus border
    - Vessels in PDCN 10-25x larger than normal capillaries
    - PDCN connects both to nidus, feeding arteries/draining veins, surrounding narrowed brain vessels
    - May be cause of recurrence of surgically resected AVMs

Staging, Grading or Classification Criteria

- Spetzler-Martin scale
  - Size
    - Small (< 3 cm) = 1
    - Medium (3-6 cm) = 2
    - Large (> 6 cm) = 3
  - Location
    - In "noneloquent" area = 0
    - If involves eloquent brain = 1
  - Venous drainage
    - Superficial only = 0
    - Deep = 1
  - Score from sum above correlates with ↑ surgical risk
- Craniofacial arteriovenous metameric syndromes (CAMS)
  - CAMS 1 = prosencephalic metameric AVMs (hypothalamus/hypophysis, nose)
  - CAMS 2 = lateral prosencephalic group (occipital lobe, thalamus, maxilla)
  - CAMS 3 = rhombencephalic group (cerebellum, pons, mandible)

CLINICAL ISSUES

Presentation

- Most common signs/symptoms
  - Headache with hemorrhage 50%
  - Seizure 25%
  - Focal neurologic deficit 20-25%
- Clinical Profile: Young adult with spontaneous (nontraumatic) ICH

Demographics

- Age: Peak presentation = 20-40 y (25% by age 15)
- Gender: M = F
- Ethnicity: Occurs in all ethnic groups

Natural History & Prognosis

- All brain AVMs are potentially hazardous
  - Risk of first hemorrhage is lifelong, rises with age (2-4%/year, cumulative)
  - Vast majority will become symptomatic during patient's lifetime
- Spontaneous obliteration rare (< 1% of cases)
  - 75% have small lesion (< 3 cm), single draining vein
  - 75% have "spontaneous" ICH

Treatment

- Endovascular embolization (liquid agents best), stereotactic radiosurgery, microvascular surgery

DIAGNOSTIC CHECKLIST

Consider

- MR of a vascular-appearing lesion that has brain parenchyma in-between "flow voids" may be a vascular neoplasm, not AVM

Image Interpretation Pearls

- Look carefully for pedicle, intranidal aneurysms
- A partially or completely thrombosed AVM may have little/no nidus, enlarged arteries at angiography
  - Look for subtle "early draining veins", they may be the only clue to the diagnosis!

SELECTED REFERENCES

1. Linfante I et al: Brain aneurysms and arteriovenous malformations: advancements and emerging treatments in endovascular embolization. Stroke. 38(4):1411-7, 2007
2. Richling B et al: Therapy of brain arteriovenous malformations: multimodality treatment from a balanced standpoint. Neurosurgery. 59(5 Suppl 3):S148-57; discussion S3-13, 2006
3. Sato S et al: Perinidal dilated capillary network in cerebral arteriovenous malformation. Neurosurgery 54:163-70, 2004
4. Berg J et al: Hereditary haemorrhagic telangiectasia: a questionnaire based study to delineate the different phenotypes caused by endoglin and ALK1 mutations. J Med Genet. 40(8):585-90, 2003
5. Shenkar R et al: Differential gene expression in human cerebrovascular malformations. Neurosurgery. 52(2):465-77; discussion 477-8, 2003
6. Suzuki M et al: Contrast-enhanced MRA for investigation of cerebral arteriovenous malformations. Neuroradiol. 45: 231-5, 2003
7. Battacharya JJ et al: Wyburn-Mason or Bonnet-Dechaume-Blanc as cerebrofacial arteriovenous metameric syndromes (CAMS): a new concept and classification. Interv Neuroradiol. 7:5-17, 2001
8. Vikkula M et al: Molecular genetics of vascular malformations. Matrix Biol. 20(5-6):327-35, 2001
9. Warren DJ et al: Cerebral arteriovenous malformations: comparison of novel MRA techniques and conventional catheter angiography. Neurosurgery. 48:973-83, 2001

IMAGE GALLERY

Typical

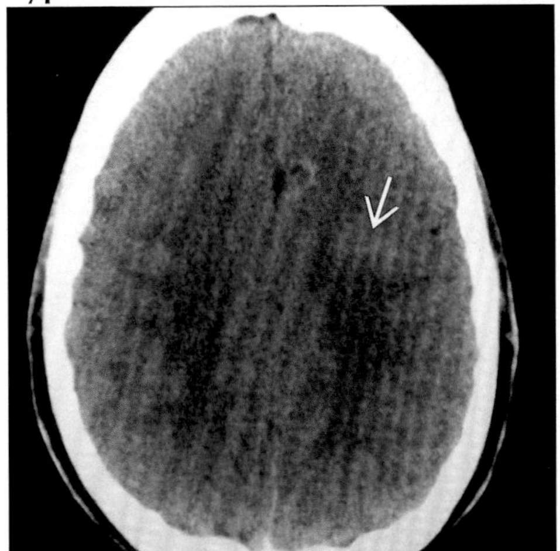

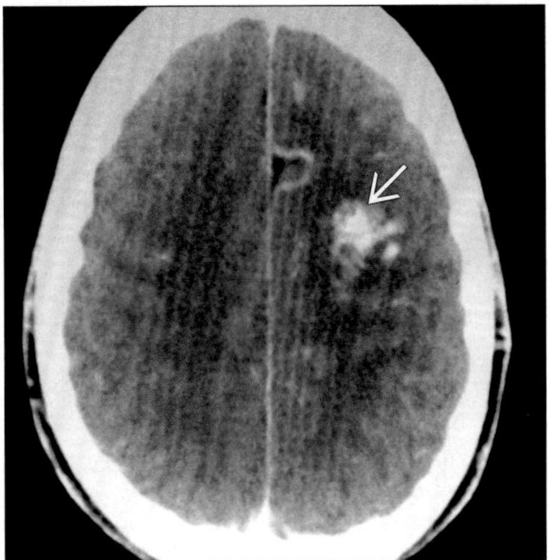

*(**Left**) Axial NECT shows subtle focus of calcification in the left frontal lobe ➡. There is no evidence of mass effect within the brain parenchyma. (**Right**) Axial CECT in the same case as previous image, shows enlarged enhancing arteries, nidus, and veins ➡ in the left frontal lobe parenchyma due to arteriovenous malformation.*

Typical

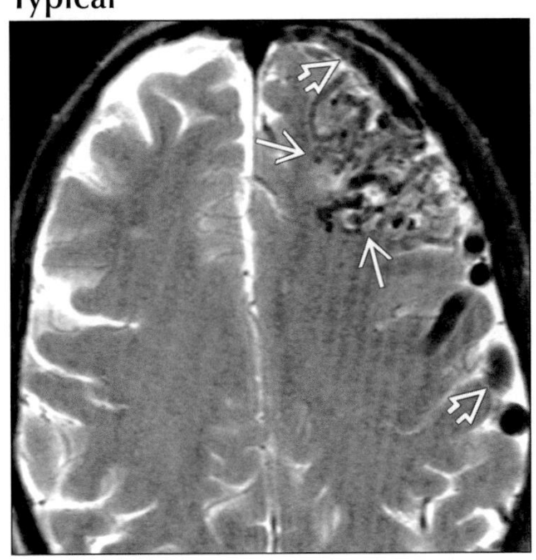

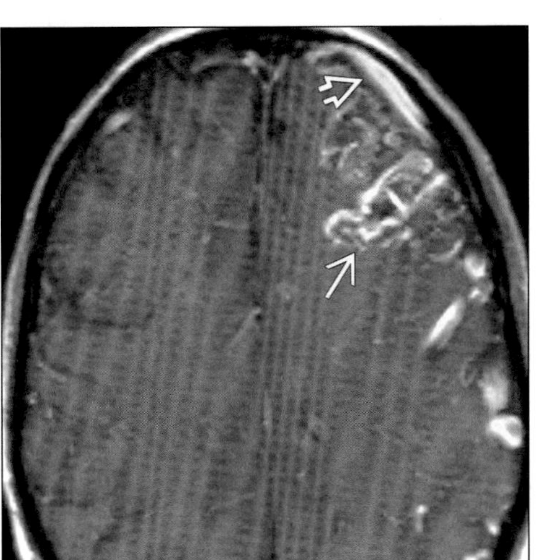

*(**Left**) Axial T2WI MR shows a large conglomeration of flow voids in the left frontal lobe characteristic of an AVM nidus ➡. Note very large superficial cortical draining veins ➡. (**Right**) Axial T1WI MR post-contrast in the same case as previous image shows abnormal curvilinear enhancement in the left frontal lobe representing the AVM nidus ➡ and associated enlarged draining veins ➡.*

Typical

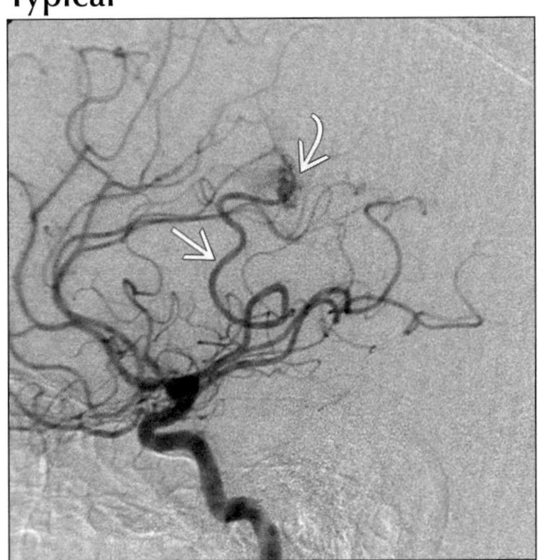

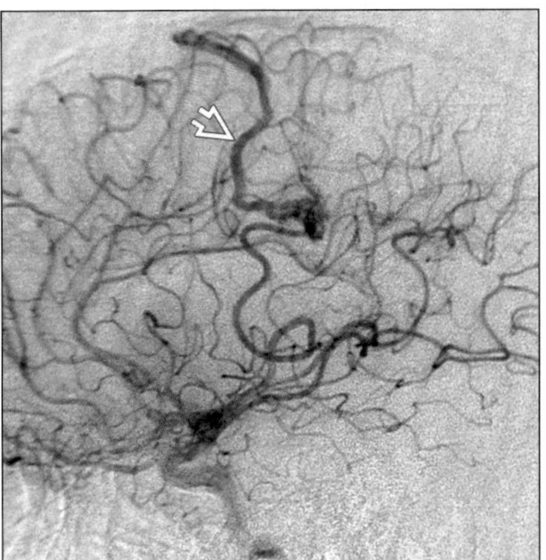

*(**Left**) Lateral DSA early arterial phase shows a small AVM nidus ➡ fed mainly from a slightly enlarged branch of the middle cerebral artery ➡. (**Right**) Lateral DSA late arterial phase in the same case as previous image, shows early draining superficial cortical vein ➡.*

DURAL AV SHUNTS, BRAIN

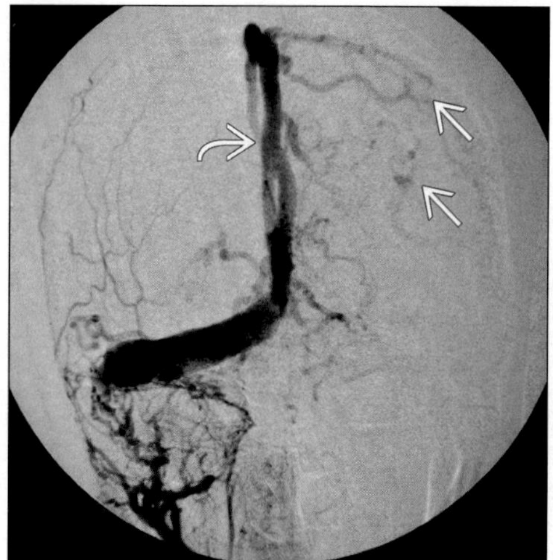

AP right ECA DSA shows a DAVF of the right transverse sinus. Note occlusion of both transverse-sigmoid sinuses and retrograde flow into the superior sagittal sinus ➔ and cortical veins ➔.

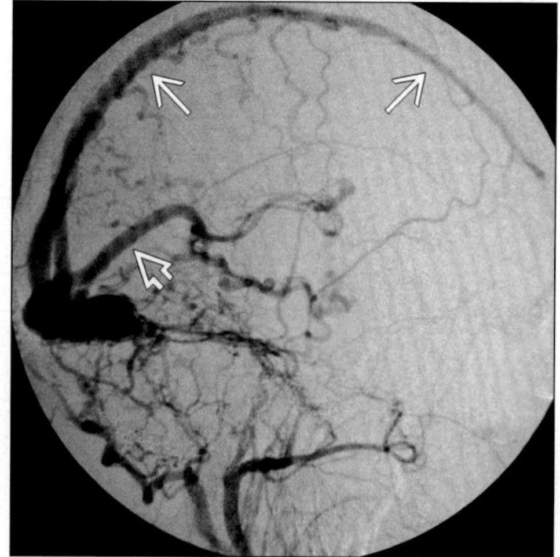

Lateral ECA DSA shows numerous feeding arteries and retrograde venous drainage into the straight ➔ and superior sagittal ➔ sinuses with reflux into the deep and superficial cerebral veins respectively.

TERMINOLOGY

Definitions

- Dural AV shunt; dural AV fistula (DAVF); dural AV malformation (DAVM)
- DAVF: Multiple AV shunts associated with a dural venous sinus (DVS) which is frequently stenotic or thrombosed

IMAGING FINDINGS

General Features

- Best diagnostic clue
  - Serpentine vessels on CTA/MRA without intraparenchymal AVM nidus
  - Enlarged foramen spinosum on bone window NECT from enlarged middle meningeal artery (MMA)
  - Dural venous sinus (DVS) stenosis ± occlusion is common
- Location
  - AV shunt typically located within the wall of a DVS (not within brain parenchyma as in pial AVMs)
  - Common sites: Transverse sinus (TS) ± sigmoid sinus (SS), cavernous sinus (CS), superior sagittal sinus (SSS), superior petrosal sinus (SPS)
  - Any DVS can be involved
- Adult-type DAVF
  - Multiple high-flow AV shunts into a single ± adjacent DVS which is frequently stenotic or occluded
- Infantile DAVF (rare)
  - Often multiple high-flow shunts involving different dural sinuses

Radiographic Findings

- Radiography: Enlarged groove(s) for MMA on lateral skull film

CT Findings

- NECT
  - Often normal
  - May see intraparenchymal hemorrhage (IPH) ± subarachnoid hemorrhage (SAH) which is atypical in location for aneurysm rupture
  - Look for enlarged foramen spinosum as MMA often supplies DAVFs

DDx: Intracranial Arteriovenous Shunts

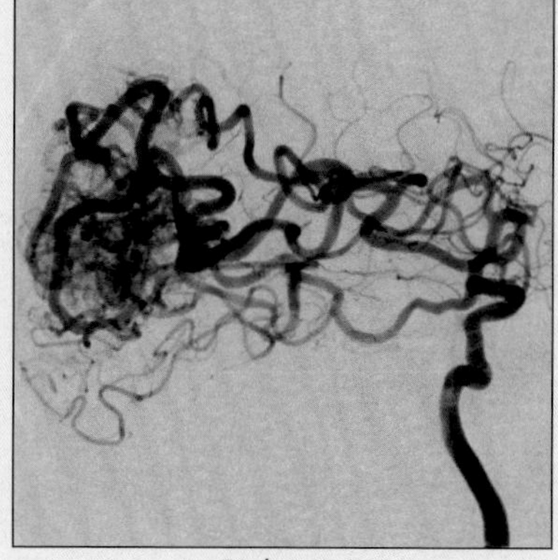

Pial AVM

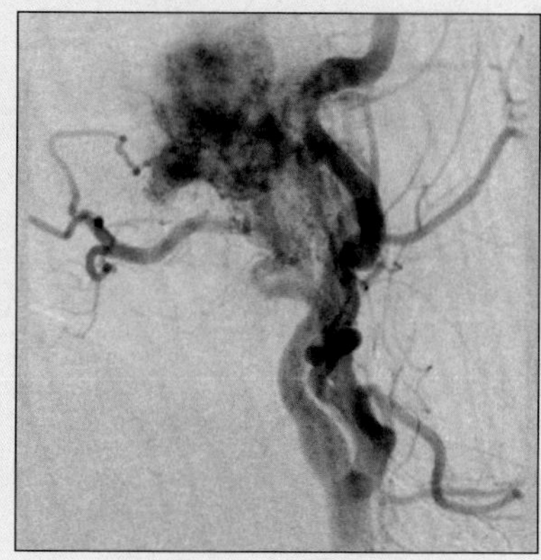

Glomus Jugulare

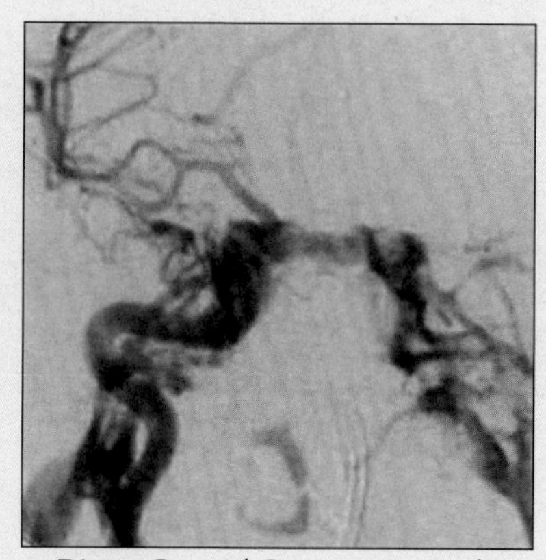

Direct Carotid Cavernous Fistula

DURAL AV SHUNTS, BRAIN

Key Facts

Terminology

- DAVF: Multiple AV shunts associated with a dural venous sinus (DVS) which is frequently stenotic or thrombosed

Imaging Findings

- Serpentine vessels on CTA/MRA without intraparenchymal AVM nidus
- Common sites: Transverse sinus (TS) ± sigmoid sinus (SS), cavernous sinus (CS), superior sagittal sinus (SSS), superior petrosal sinus (SPS)
- May see intraparenchymal hemorrhage (IPH) ± subarachnoid hemorrhage (SAH) which is atypical in location for aneurysm rupture
- TOF MRA may show enlarged feeding arteries ± draining vein(s)

Top Differential Diagnoses

- Pial AVM
- Vascular Neoplasm
- Direct Carotid Cavernous Fistula

Pathology

- 10-15% of all cerebrovascular malformations with AV shunting
- Grading scale based on venous drainage pattern + related to risk of ICH

Clinical Issues

- Bruit, pulsatile tinnitus, headache, focal neurological deficit from ICH
- Peak incidence in 5th decade of life
- Transvenous occlusion of recipient sinus/pouch with coils/liquid embolics may be curative

---

  - May see cerebral edema due to venous hypertension ± venous infarction
- CECT
  - May be normal with small shunts
  - May see serpentine feeders, enlarged, tortuous draining vein(s), DVS thrombosis or occlusion
  - Enlarged superior ophthalmic veins due to retrograde venous drainage, especially with CS DAVF (indirect carotid cavernous fistula)
  - Infantile DAVF may be associated with markedly dilated dural sinuses
- CTA
  - May be useful for static depiction of angioarchitecture
  - Look for enlarged ECA branches, serpentine vessels adjacent to recipient dural venous sinus

MR Findings

- T2WI: Thrombosed or stenotic dural venous sinus contains numerous flow voids from "micro" fistulae ("crack-like" vessels)
- FLAIR: Most sensitive for detection of associated SAH or parenchymal edema
- MRA
  - TOF MRA may show enlarged feeding arteries ± draining vein(s)
  - May be negative with small or slow-flow shunts or yield incomplete depiction of high-flow lesions
  - Time resolved contrast augmented MRA useful for gross depiction of angioarchitecture and dynamics
- MRV: May see occluded or stenotic dural sinus, enlarged cortical veins

Angiographic Findings

- Conventional
  - DSA shows dominant arterial supply via dural arteries; parasitization of pial arterial supply is common with large DAVFs
  - Feeding arteries usually ECA branches
    - MMA nourishes much of dura mater; commonest feeder to DAVFs
    - Occipital artery commonly contributes to TS/SS DAVFs
  - Dural branches from cavernous ICA: Meningohypophyseal trunk (MHT) and inferolateral trunk (ILT) may supply DAVF
    - MHT has two dural branches: (1) Marginal tentorial artery of Bernasconi & Cassinari, (2) basal tentorial artery
    - Ophthalmic artery gives rise to ethmoidal arteries, artery of falx cerebri, MMA (1%) that may supply DAVF
  - Vertebral artery may contribute to DAVF via muscular branches, posterior meningeal artery, artery of the falx cerebelli, arteries of Davidoff & Schechter
  - Flow-related aneurysms uncommon
  - Recipient dural sinus often thrombosed or stenotic
  - Tortuous engorged pial veins ("pseudophlebitic pattern") due to cortical venous reflux correlates with ↑ ICH risk

Imaging Recommendations

- Best imaging tool: 6 vessel catheter angiography required for definitive exclusion of intracranial DAVF + determination of angioarchitecture + treatment planning
- Screening MR, contrast augmented MRA
- DSA with rapid acquisitions (> 6 F/s) + ↑ contrast volume injected due to rapid flow

DIFFERENTIAL DIAGNOSIS

Pial AVM

- Contains a true nidus: Tangle of abnormal vessels
  - May have intranidal aneurysm → ↑ risk of ICH
- Dominant supply is from pial arteries, not dural as in DAVF
- Flow-related aneurysms common

Vascular Neoplasm

- Vascular skull base tumors (e.g., glomus jugulare) supplied by enlarged ECA branches
- AV shunting on DSA commonly seen but usually slower cf. DAVF and preceded by tumor blush

DURAL AV SHUNTS, BRAIN

- Mass lesion identified on CT/MR with strong enhancement after contrast administration ± erosion of skull base

Direct Carotid Cavernous Fistula

- High-flow AV shunt between cavernous ICA and CS
- Usually secondary to traumatic tear of ICA or ruptured cavernous ICA aneurysm
- No ECA contribution to shunt

PATHOLOGY

General Features

- General path comments
  - Absence of a true nidus (cf. pial AVM)
  - Cluster of numerous "micro" AV shunts inside dural sinus wall
- Etiology
  - Most DAVF are acquired, express active angiogenesis
    - May be idiopathic
    - Can occur in response to trauma, venous occlusion, or venous hypertension
  - Pathological activation of neoangiogenesis
    - Proliferating capillaries within granulation tissue in dural sinus obliterated by organized thrombi
    - Budding/proliferation of microvascular network in inner dura connects to plexus of thin-walled venous channels
    - High bFGF, VEGF expression in DAVFs
- Epidemiology: 10-15% of all cerebrovascular malformations with AV shunting

Gross Pathologic & Surgical Features

- Multiple enlarged dural feeders converge on dural sinus
- Venous hypertension with development of cortical venous reflux and high-flow venopathy is characterized by ectasias, varices, stenoses → ↑ risk of ICH

Staging, Grading or Classification Criteria

- Grading scale based on venous drainage pattern, correlates with risk of ICH
  - Grade 1: Draining into a dural venous sinus with antegrade flow
  - Grade 2: Drainage into a dural venous sinus with (a) retrograde flow within sinus; (b) reflux/retrograde flow into cortical veins; (a+b) retrograde flow in dural sinus and cortical vein(s)
  - Grade 3: Direct drainage into cortical vein(s) without ectasia
  - Grade 4: Direct drainage into cortical vein(s) with venous ectasia
  - Grade 5: Perimedullary venous drainage

CLINICAL ISSUES

Presentation

- Common
  - Bruit, pulsatile tinnitus
  - Headache, focal neurological deficit from ICH
  - CS DAVF: Exophthalmos, ophthalmoplegia, decreased visual acuity
- Uncommon
  - Progressive dementia
  - Cranial neuropathy
- Rare
  - Life-threatening congestive heart failure; usually neonates, infants

Demographics

- Age: Peak incidence in 5th decade of life
- Gender: M < F

Natural History & Prognosis

- May be clinically silent with low risk of ICH, discovered incidentally on DSA
- May be aggressive with rapid progression to venous hypertension and ICH
- SPS DAVF and ethmoidal DAVF (supplied by ethmoidal branches of ophthalmic artery) typically have high risk of ICH
- Spontaneous closure rare

Treatment

- Endovascular
  - Transvenous occlusion of recipient sinus/pouch with coils/liquid embolics may be curative
  - Transarterial embolization of feeders
    - ↓ Flow through shunt; may use particulate emboli, liquid embolics, EtOH
    - Usually performed on pre-operative basis or for palliation (e.g., pulsatile tinnitus)
- Surgical resection
  - Skeletonization of sinus
  - Drainage of parenchymal hematoma if significant mass effect
- Stereotactic radiosurgery
  - Success rate is inversely proportional to size/extent of DAVF
  - May require 2-3 years for complete obliteration, therefore more suitable for DAVFs with low ICH risk

DIAGNOSTIC CHECKLIST

Consider

- DAVF in pts with SAH blood pattern that is atypical for aneurysm rupture
- Definitive diagnosis or exclusion with DSA

Image Interpretation Pearls

- CTA/MRA shows serpiginous vessels without a visible nidus
- DSA confirms supply predominantly by dural arteries rather than pial arteries

SELECTED REFERENCES

1. Ng PP et al: Endovascular strategies for carotid cavernous and intracerebral dural arteriovenous fistulas. Neurosurg Focus. 15(4):ECP1, 2003
2. Ng PP et al: Endovascular treatment for dural arteriovenous fistulae of the superior petrosal sinus. Neurosurgery. 53(1):25-32; discussion 32-3, 2003

IMAGE GALLERY

Variant

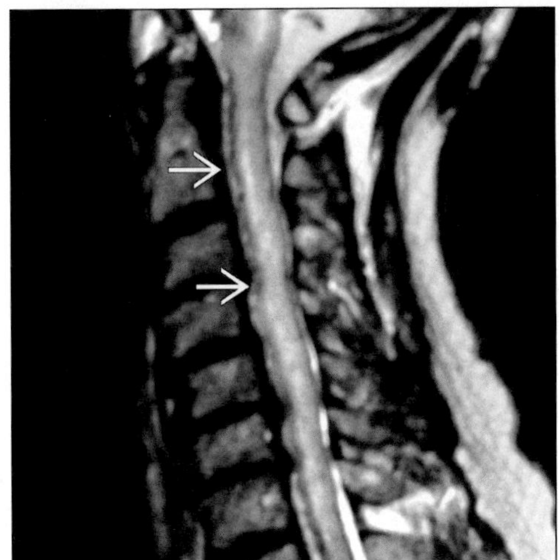

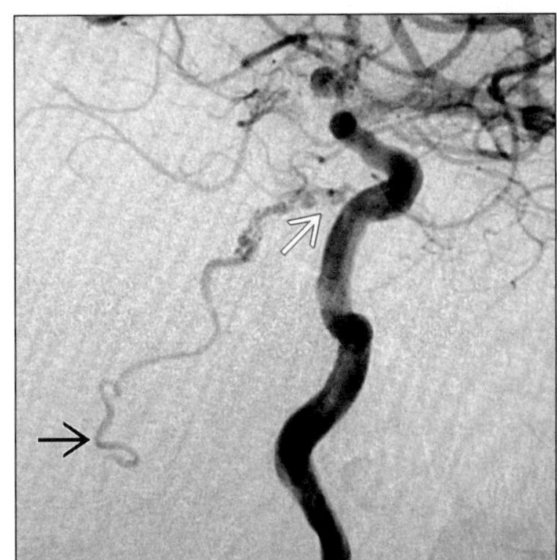

(Left) *Sagittal T2WI MR shows cord edema and flow voids anterior to the spinal cord ➡ in a patient with progressive upper extremity weakness and paresthesias.* ***(Right)*** *ICA DSA shows an enlarged MHT ➡ arising from the cavernous ICA supplying a DAVF of the superior petrosal sinus which is occluded. Perimedullary venous drainage ➡ resulted in venous hypertension and cord edema. Grade V DAVF.*

Typical

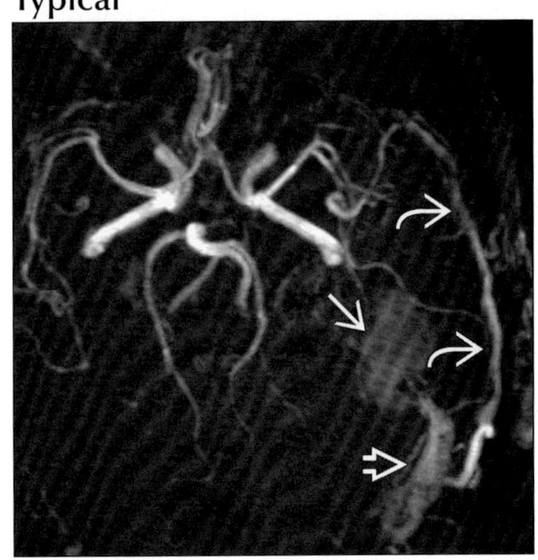

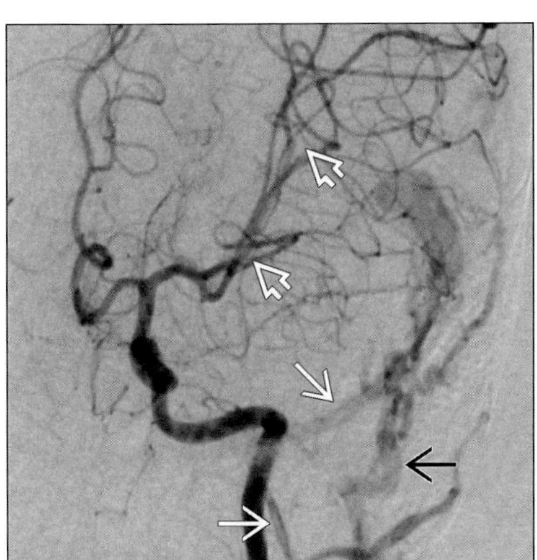

(Left) *TOF MRA shows an enlarged MMA ➡ supplying a DAVF of the left transverse-sigmoid sinus junction ➡. Note high signal from subacute intraparenchymal hematoma ➡.* ***(Right)*** *AP left carotid DSA shows enlarged middle meningeal ➡ and occipital ➡ arteries supplying the DAVF. There is mass effect on the middle cerebral artery with medial displacement of the Sylvian triangle ➡ from an underlying hematoma.*

Variant

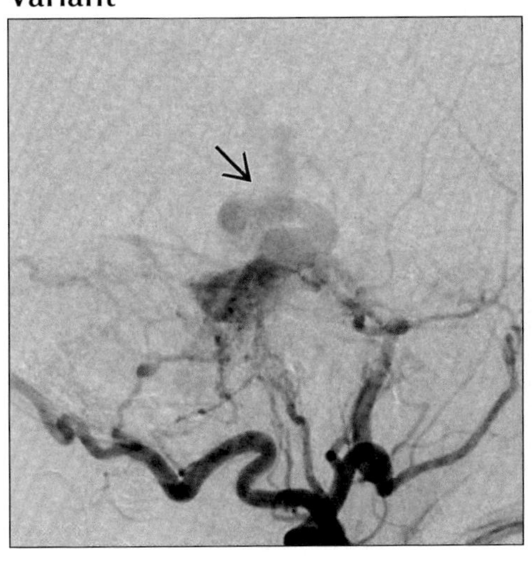

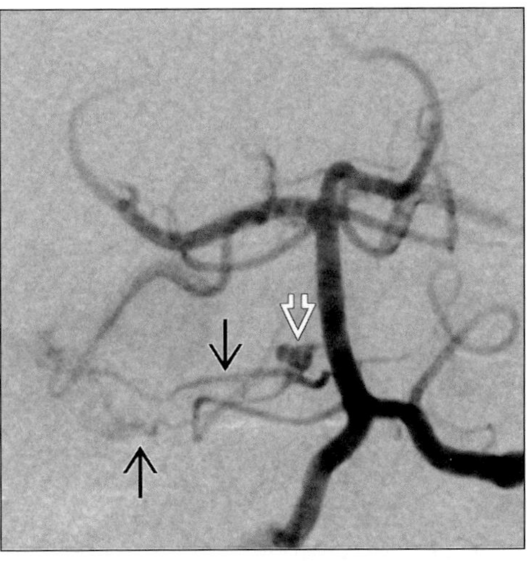

(Left) *Lateral right ECA DSA shows tentorial DAVF draining into lateral mesencephalic vein ➡ supplied by numerous occipital, middle meningeal & ascending pharyngeal artery feeders.* ***(Right)*** *Anteroposterior left vertebral artery DSA (same patient as previous image) shows supply to DAVF by branches of right AICA ➡ with a flow-related aneurysm proximally ➡. Flow-related aneurysms are uncommonly associated with DAVFs compared with pial AVMs.*

CAROTID CAVERNOUS FISTULA

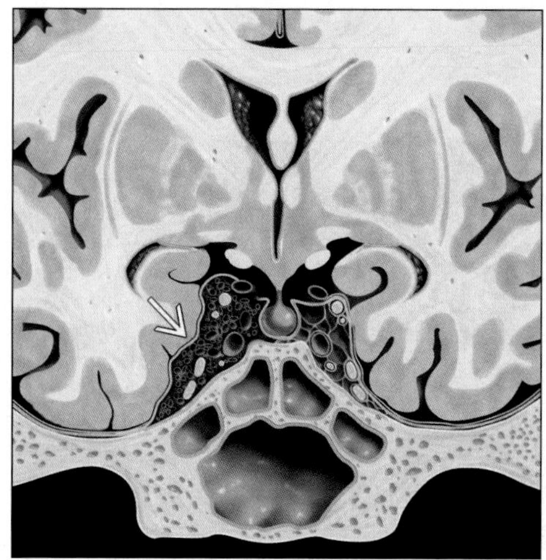

Coronal graphic of an indirect CCF shows engorgement of the right CS ➡ which contains a myriad of small arterial feeders and venous drainage channels.

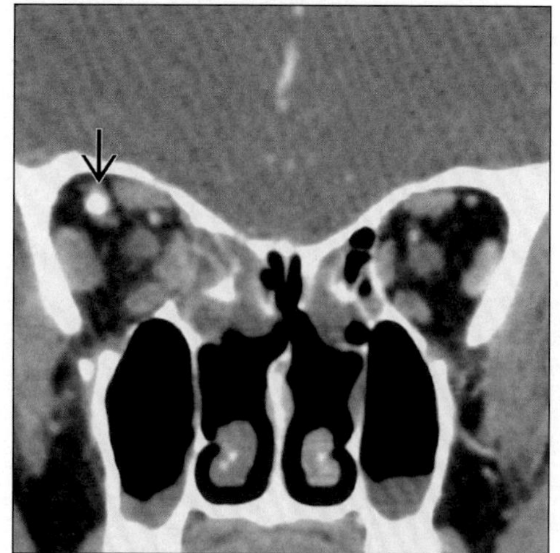

Coronal CTA shows dilatation of the right SOV ➡, enlargement of the extraocular muscles, and stranding of the intraconal fat in a patient with an indirect CCF.

TERMINOLOGY

Definitions

- Carotid cavernous fistula (CCF): Arteriovenous (AV) shunt between internal carotid artery (ICA) ± external carotid artery (ECA) and cavernous sinus (CS)
- Direct CCF: High-flow, single hole fistula between ICA and CS
- Indirect CCF: Dural AV fistula (DAVF) of CS, typically supplied by numerous ECA ± cavernous ICA branches

IMAGING FINDINGS

General Features

- Best diagnostic clue: Dilated superior ophthalmic vein (SOV) ± proptosis
- Location
  - AV shunt is between carotid circulation and CS
    - Direct CCF: Single, relatively large, high-flow communication between cavernous ICA and CS
    - Indirect CCF: Typically numerous small AV shunts from ECA ± cavernous ICA → CS ± circular (intercavernous) sinus
  - Bilateral CCFs uncommon; can occur with both types
- Classic imaging appearance
  - MR/CT: Proptosis (unilateral > bilateral), tortuosity and dilatation of SOV(s), enlarged CS

CT Findings

- NECT
  - Exophthalmos, intra ± peri-orbital edema, enlarged extraocular muscles, dilated SOV
  - Skull base fracture involving body of sphenoid bone, foramen lacerum and carotid canal best visualized with fine cuts on bone algorithm
    - Traumatic direct CCF more likely if present
- CTA
  - Dilated, strongly enhancing SOV
    - SOV may be stenotic or occluded anteriorly in longstanding CCFs due to high-flow venopathy
  - Enlarged CS
    - May see cavernous ICA aneurysm as etiology of direct CCF

MR Findings

- Dilatation of SOV

DDx: Proptosis and Extraocular Muscle Enlargement

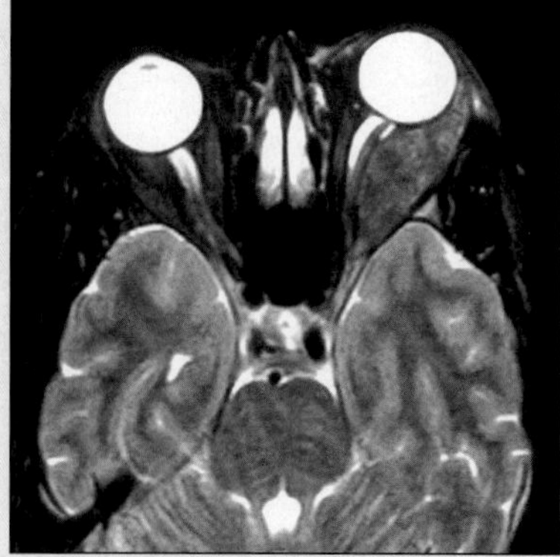

Orbital Pseudotumor

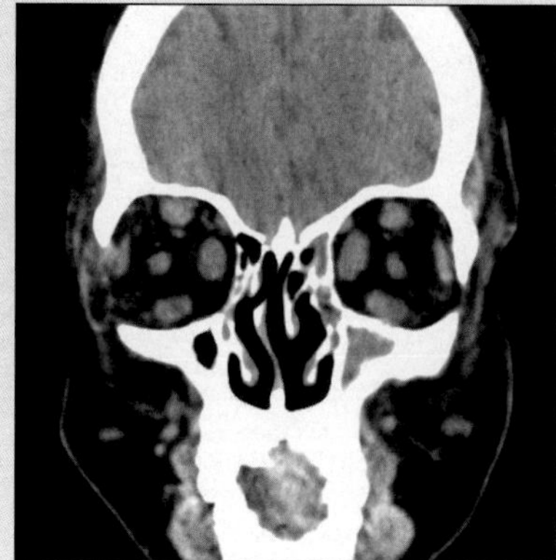

Thyroid Ophthalmopathy

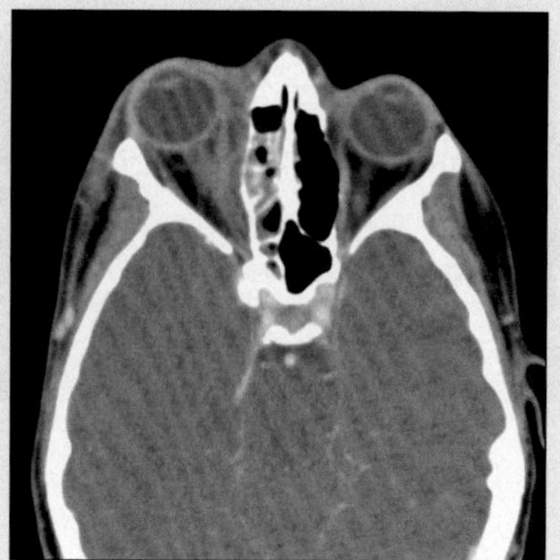

Subperiosteal Abscess

CAROTID CAVERNOUS FISTULA

Key Facts

Terminology
- Carotid cavernous fistula (CCF): Arteriovenous (AV) shunt between internal carotid artery (ICA) ± external carotid artery (ECA) and cavernous sinus (CS)
- Direct CCF: High-flow, single hole fistula between ICA and CS
- Indirect CCF: Dural AV fistula (DAVF) of CS, typically supplied by numerous ECA ± cavernous ICA branches

Imaging Findings
- Best diagnostic clue: Dilated superior ophthalmic vein (SOV) ± proptosis
- Size:
- MR/CT: Proptosis (unilateral > bilateral), tortuosity and dilatation of SOV(s), enlarged CS
- Exophthalmos, intra ± peri-orbital edema, enlarged extraocular muscles, dilated SOV
- DSA: Most sensitive and specific

Clinical Issues
- Most common signs/symptoms: Diplopia/ophthalmoplegia due to CN3, 4 or 6 palsies
- Chemosis, proptosis, bruit/pulsatile tinnitus, headache, retro-orbital pain, decreased visual acuity
- Indirect CCF most common in post-menopausal females
- Vision at risk due to raised intra-ocular pressure (IOP) and compromised retinal perfusion pressure resulting in retinal ischemia

Diagnostic Checklist
- Tolosa-Hunt syndrome presents with painful ophthalmoplegia (like CCF) but bruit/pulsatile tinnitus absent, SOV not enlarged

- Exophthalmos with enlargement of extraocular muscles
- Enlarged CS
  - Usually unilateral, occasionally bilateral (often asymmetric)
  - T2WI: Tiny flow voids representing arterial feeders may be visible adjacent to CS (indirect CCFs)
  - Cerebral edema ± intracranial hemorrhage (ICH) if cortical venous drainage present (rare)
- TOF MRA appearance can establish diagnosis: Visualization of CS, inferior petrosal sinus (IPS), SOV
- Time-resolved Gd-MRA depicts arterial shunting into sinus, early appearance of SOV

Ultrasonographic Findings
- Color Doppler
  - Shows flow reversal (intra- to extracranial) in enlarged SOV
  - Useful as rapid, bedside screening tool

Angiographic Findings
- Conventional
  - Definitive for diagnosis and treatment
  - Retrograde flow into SOV, angular and facial veins
    - SOV dilatation may be bilateral with large circular sinus, especially when ipsilateral IPS is stenotic or occluded
  - Direct CCF is a high-flow AV shunt
    - DSA with fast frame rate (> 6 fps) useful in determining exact site of fistula for endovascular repair
    - Proximal extent of fistula may be shown using ipsilateral compression of the common carotid artery (CCA) during CCA angiography (Mehringer maneuver)
    - Distal extent of fistula may be shown using ipsilateral CCA compression during vertebral artery angiography (Huber maneuver)
  - Indirect CCF is a DAVF of the CS
    - ECA feeders include: Ascending pharyngeal artery, distal internal maxillary artery, accessory meningeal artery, middle meningeal artery
    - ICA feeders include: Meningohypophyseal trunk, inferolateral trunk (arise from cavernous ICA segment)
  - IPS ± SOV may be stenotic or occluded in long-standing fistulas
    - IPS stenosis or occlusion increases venous outflow through SOV → exacerbates ophthalmoplegia
  - Venous egress may also include superior petrosal sinus, pterygoid, clival and pharyngeal venous plexi, cortical cerebral veins

Imaging Recommendations
- Best imaging tool
  - DSA: Most sensitive and specific
    - Best assessment of shunt location, direct vs. indirect CCF morphology, arterial feeders, venous drainage, planning for endovascular approach
- Screening Doppler U/S
- MR/CT: Dilated SOV ± proptosis is highly suggestive of underlying CCF
- Absence of dilated SOV does not exclude the diagnosis and should not preclude DSA

DIFFERENTIAL DIAGNOSIS

Thyroid Ophthalmopathy
- Most common cause of proptosis in adults
- 70% show clinical and biochemical evidence of hyperthyroidism
- Course of thyroid eye disease independent of hyperthyroidism
- Orbit findings bilateral in 80%
- Asymmetric involvement of extraocular muscles with inferior and medial rectus most common

Orbital Pseudotumor
- Idiopathic inflammatory condition of orbit
- Tolosa-Hunt syndrome: Variant with dominant involvement of CS ± superior orbital fissure; presents as painful ophthalmoplegia
- Most common intraorbital mass in adults
- Steroid responsive

CAROTID CAVERNOUS FISTULA

Cavernous Sinus Thrombosis

- Previously a life-threatening condition due to spread of facial, paranasal sinus & dental infections intracranially
  - Ophthalmoplegia, high fever, malaise, progressing to coma was typical
  - Now rare with effective antimicrobial therapy
- Increased density of CS on NECT
- Filling defects within or non-enhancement of CS on CECT or Gd-enhanced MR
- Enlarged cavernous sinus and SOV on routine MR

PATHOLOGY

General Features

- General path comments
  - Normal flow direction in SOV and CS is anterior → posterior
  - Presence of AV shunt results in retrograde (posterior → anterior) arterialized flow through CS and SOV (valveless) → orbital venous hypertension → edema, chemosis, proptosis, retinal ischemia
- Etiology
  - Direct CCF
    - Traumatic tear of cavernous ICA (sheared from its dural attachments to the foramen lacerum and anterior clinoid process)
    - Rupture of intracavernous ICA aneurysm
    - Iatrogenic (e.g., transsphenoidal pituitary resection)
    - Spontaneous (Marfan syndrome, Ehlers-Danlos syndrome, fibromuscular dysplasia, other collagen vascular diseases)
  - Indirect CCF
    - Mostly idiopathic
    - Others: Trauma, hypercoagulable states with CS thrombosis

Staging, Grading or Classification Criteria

- Barrow classification according to arterial supply
  - A = direct CCF
  - B = indirect CCF, supplied by ICA only
  - C = indirect CCF, supplied by ECA only
  - D = indirect CCF, supplied by ICA and ECA

CLINICAL ISSUES

Presentation

- Most common signs/symptoms: Diplopia/ophthalmoplegia due to CN3, 4 or 6 palsies
- Other signs/symptoms
  - Chemosis, proptosis, bruit/pulsatile tinnitus, headache, retro-orbital pain, decreased visual acuity
  - Large AV shunts (direct CCFs) may compromise antegrade ICA flow beyond fistula resulting in cerebral ischemia if circle of Willis collaterals inadequate
  - Cortical venous drainage may result in venous tortuosity, varices, stenoses → ↑ risk of ICH

Demographics

- Gender
  - Indirect CCF most common in post-menopausal females
  - Direct CCF most common in young males (increased incidence of trauma)

Natural History & Prognosis

- Vision at risk due to raised intra-ocular pressure (IOP) and compromised retinal perfusion pressure resulting in retinal ischemia
- Worsening ophthalmoplegia/diplopia, proptosis with corneal ulceration
- Risk of cerebral edema + ICH if cortical venous drainage present

Treatment

- Direct CCF
  - Acutely raised IOP: Acetazolamide, beta-blockers, lateral canthotomy as temporizing measures to save vision
  - Endovascular therapy with transarterial detachable balloon occlusion of fistula; alternatives include transvenous (TV) embolization with coils, ICA sacrifice, covered stent
- Indirect CCF
  - Carotid compression maneuver curative in up to 30% of low-flow fistulas; may be helpful for residual fistula post-embolization
  - Endovascular treatment with TV coil embolization usually curative
    - May have temporary exacerbation of ophthalmoplegia with CS thrombosis following embolization
    - May access CS via IPS or anterior facial vein & angular vein
    - Surgical exposure of SOV for direct cannulation can be used if endovascular access not possible
  - Transarterial embolization with particulate embolic agents (e.g., PVA) occasionally required as adjunct or for palliation if TV access not achievable
  - Anecdotal reports of successful endovascular treatment utilizing liquid embolics, covered stents

DIAGNOSTIC CHECKLIST

Consider

- Tolosa-Hunt syndrome presents with painful ophthalmoplegia (like CCF) but bruit/pulsatile tinnitus absent, SOV not enlarged

Image Interpretation Pearls

- Dilated SOV ± proptosis on CT or MR is highly suggestive of an underlying CCF
- DSA required for definitive diagnosis or exclusion

SELECTED REFERENCES

1. Ng PP et al: Endovascular strategies for carotid cavernous and intracerebral dural arteriovenous fistulas. Neurosurg Focus. 15(4):ECP1, 2003

CAROTID CAVERNOUS FISTULA

IMAGE GALLERY

Typical

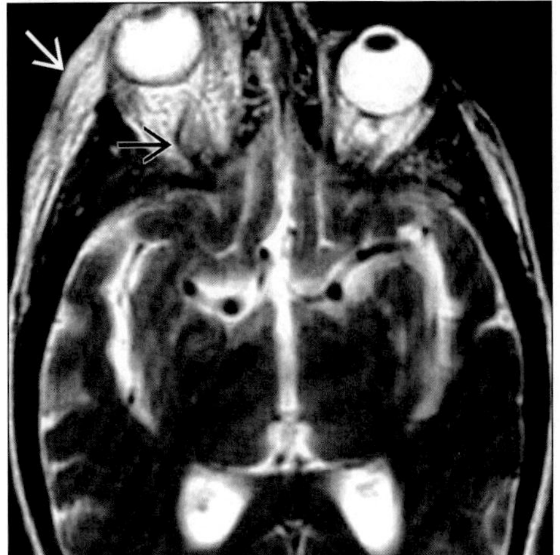

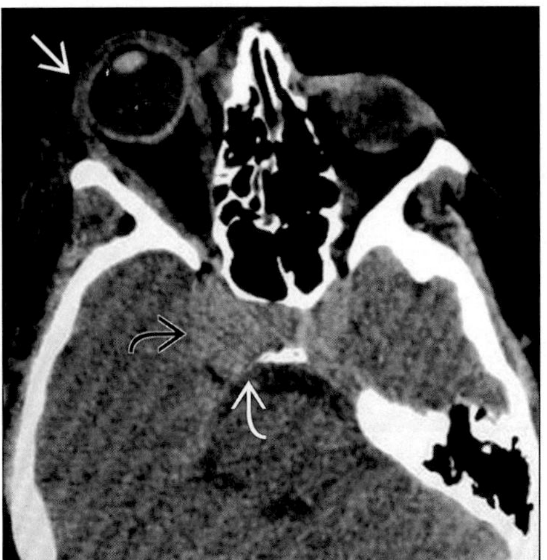

(Left) *Axial T2WI MR shows right-sided proptosis, dilatation of the SOV → as well as peri- and intra-orbital edema ➔ in a patient with direct CCF.* ***(Right)*** *Axial NECT shows marked proptosis ➔ in conjunction with periorbital edema in the same patient with direct CCF due to rupture of a cavernous ICA aneurysm. Note expansion of the right cavernous sinus ↗ and erosion of the dorsum sella ↗ by the aneurysm.*

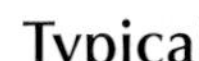

Typical

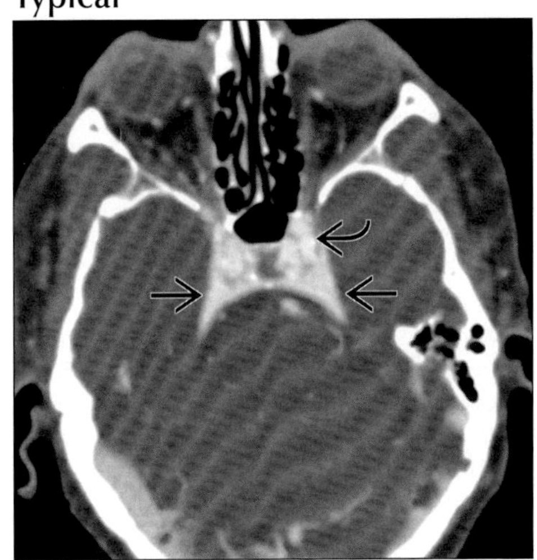

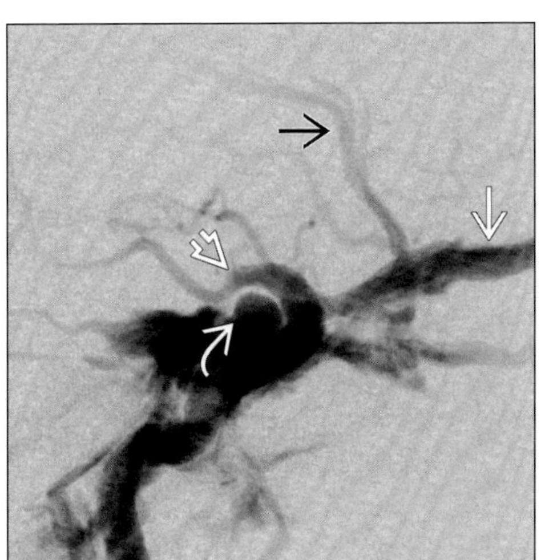

(Left) *Axial CTA shows engorgement of the cavernous sinuses bilaterally → and prominent vasculature within the anterior part of the left CS ↗.* ***(Right)*** *Lateral left ICA DSA shows a direct CCF due to rupture of a cavernous ICA aneurysm ↗. Note apparent truncation of the ICA beyond the posterior communicating artery ➔ due to preferential flow into the fistula. There is retrograde flow into a dilated SOV ➔ as well as cortical veins →.*

Typical

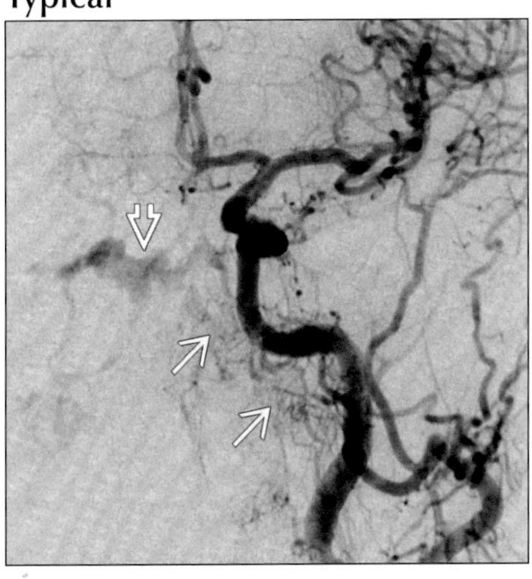

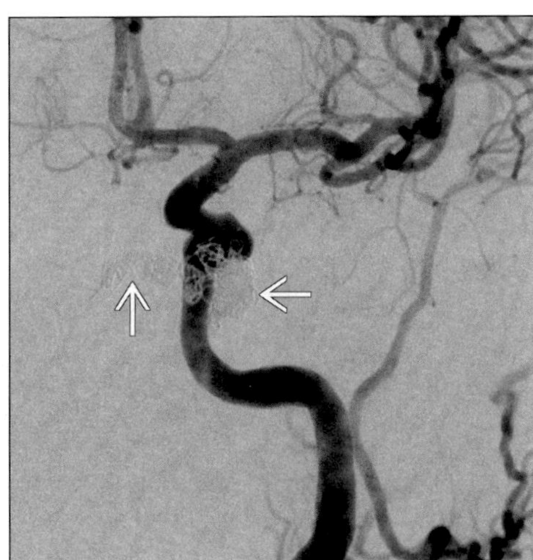

(Left) *Anteroposterior left CCA DSA shows an indirect CCF supplied mainly by small feeders arising from the ECA ➔. There is venous outflow via the circular sinus ➔ into the right CS. This venous drainage pathway may cause retrograde flow in the contralateral SOV.* ***(Right)*** *Left CCA DSA after transvenous coil embolization shows no residual arteriovenous shunting. Note coil mass within the left CS and circular sinus ➔.*

DEVELOPMENTAL VENOUS ANOMALY

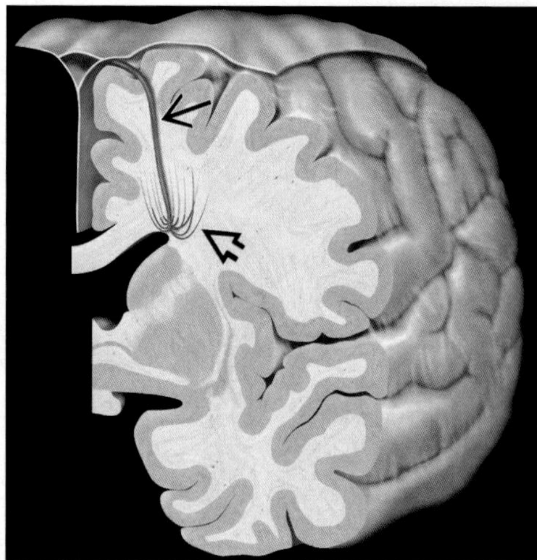

Coronal oblique graphic shows a classic DVA with the umbrella-like "Medusa head" of enlarged medullary white matter veins ⇨ and dilated transcortical collector vein → that drains into the SSS.

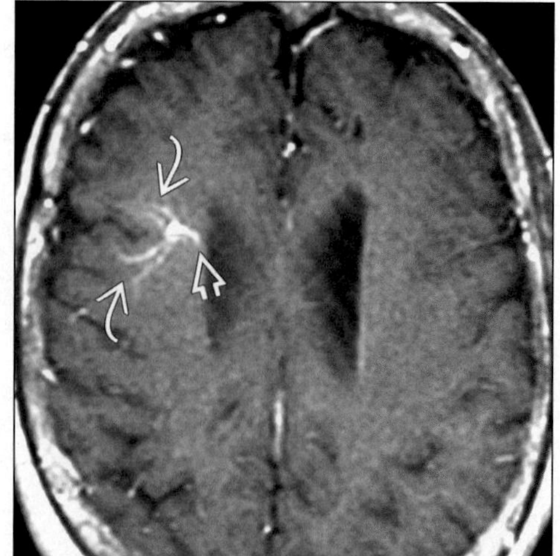

Axial T1WI MR shows enhancing, dilated, deep white matter medullary veins ➡ draining into a single collecting venous trunk ➡, typical of developmental venous anomaly.

TERMINOLOGY

Abbreviations and Synonyms

- Developmental venous anomaly (DVA); venous angioma

Definitions

- Congenital cerebral vascular anomaly with angiogenically mature venous elements
- May represent anatomic variant of otherwise normal venous drainage

IMAGING FINDINGS

General Features

- Best diagnostic clue: "Medusa head" (dilated medullary white matter veins) draining into solitary major venous trunk
- Location
  - Periventricular white matter: Main venous trunk drains into deep venous system
    - Usually into the thalamostriate/ependymal vein in the lateral aspect of the lateral ventricle
    - Near frontal horn = most common site
    - Other: Adjacent to fourth ventricle
  - Subcortical white matter: Main venous trunk drains into the dural venous sinuses
    - Supratentorial: Usually into the superficial sagittal sinus
    - Infratentorial: Usually into the transverse sinus
- Size: Varies (may be extensive) but usually < 2-3 cm
- Morphology
  - Umbrella-like collection of enlarged medullary (white matter) veins
  - Large "collector" vein drains into dural sinus or deep ependymal vein
  - Usually solitary
    - Can be multiple in blue rubber-bleb nevus syndrome

CT Findings

- NECT
  - Usually normal
  - Occasional: Ca++ if associated with cavernous malformation (CM)
  - Rare: Acute parenchymal hemorrhage (if draining vein spontaneously thromboses)

DDx: Developmental Venous Anomaly

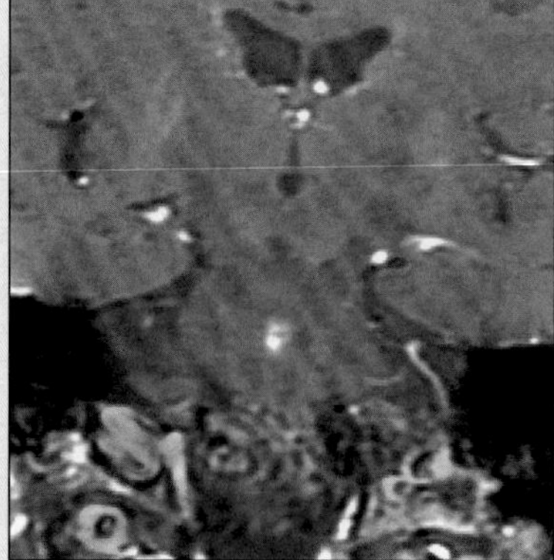

Capillary Telangiectasia

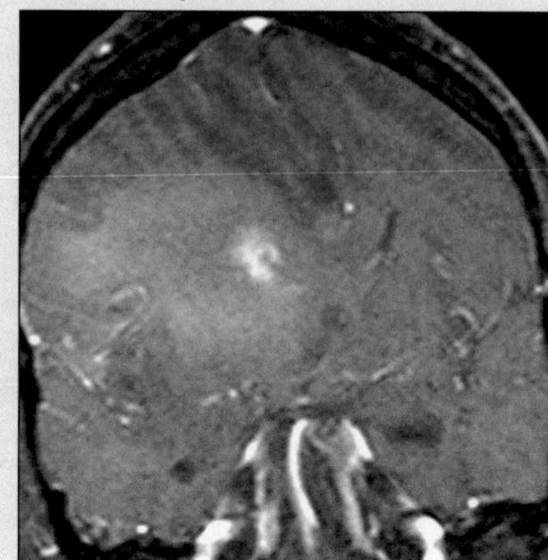

Glioblastoma

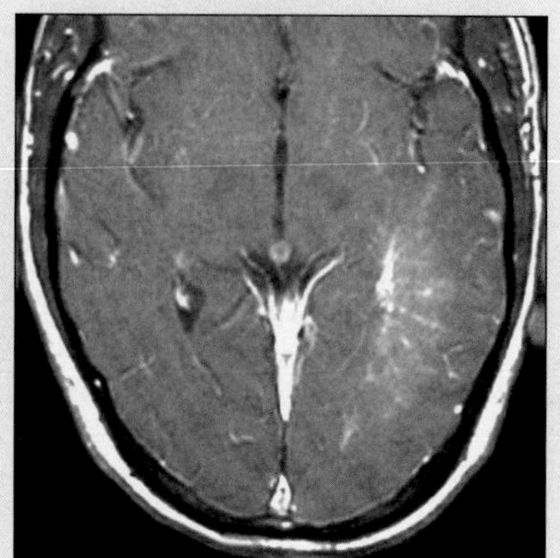

Dural Sinus Occlusion

DEVELOPMENTAL VENOUS ANOMALY

Key Facts

Terminology
- Congenital cerebral vascular anomaly with angiogenically mature venous elements

Imaging Findings
- Best diagnostic clue: "Medusa head" (dilated medullary white matter veins) draining into solitary major venous trunk
- Collector vein drains into dural sinus/ependymal vein
- Protocol advice: Include T2* sequence to look for hemorrhage, mixed CM

Top Differential Diagnoses
- AVM, Cavernous Malformation, Capillary Telangiectasia
- Vascular Neoplasm
- Dural Sinus Occlusion (with Venous Stasis, Collateral Drainage)
- Sturge-Weber Syndrome

Pathology
- Mutations in chromosome 9p
- Most common cerebral vascular malformation at autopsy
- 15-20% occur with co-existing CM
- Radially oriented dilated medullary veins
- Venous radicals are separated by normal brain

Clinical Issues
- Usually asymptomatic
- Stenosis or thrombosis of draining vein increases hemorrhage risk

---

- CECT
  - Numerous linear or dot-like enhancing foci
    - Well-circumscribed round/ovoid enhancing areas on sequential sections
    - Converge on single enlarged tubular draining vein
    - Occasionally seen as linear structure if oriented tangential in a single slice

MR Findings
- T1WI
  - Can be normal if DVA is small
  - Variable signal depending on size, flow
    - "Flow void" appearance possible
  - Hemorrhage may occur if associated with CM or with draining vein thromboses
- T2WI
  - ± "Flow void"
  - ± Blood products
- FLAIR: Usually normal; may show hyperintense region if venous ischemia or hemorrhage present
- T2* GRE
  - Hypointensity may bloom if co-existing CM present with short T2 hemorrhagic products
  - Hypointense blooming may also occur from intravascular conversion of oxyhemoglobin to deoxyhemoglobin due to slow flow
- DWI
  - Usually normal
  - Rare: Acute venous infarct seen as hyperintense area of restricted diffusion
- T1 C+
  - Strong enhancement
    - Stellate, tubular vessels converge on collector vein
    - Collector vein drains into dural sinus/ependymal vein
- MRA
  - Arterial phase usually normal
  - Contrast-enhanced MRA may demonstrate slow-flow DVA
- MRV: Delineates "Medusa head" and drainage pattern
- MRS: Normal; deoxyhemoglobin or short T2 hemorrhagic products may result in peak broadening

Angiographic Findings
- Conventional
  - DSA
    - Arterial phase normal in > 95% of cases
    - Capillary phase usually normal (rare: Prominent "blush" ± A-V shunt)
    - Venous phase: "Medusa head" and large collector vein
    - 5% atypical (transitional form of venous-arteriovenous malformation with enlarged feeders, A-V shunting)

Imaging Recommendations
- Best imaging tool: T1 C+ MR plus MRV
- Protocol advice: Include T2* sequence to look for hemorrhage, mixed CM

DIFFERENTIAL DIAGNOSIS

Other Vascular Malformations
- AVM, cavernous malformation, capillary telangiectasia
- Hemorrhage possible with AVM, CM

Vascular Neoplasm
- Enlarged medullary veins
- Mass effect, usually enhances

Dural Sinus Occlusion (with Venous Stasis, Collateral Drainage)
- Sinus thrombosis
- Medullary veins enlarge as collateral drainage

Sturge-Weber Syndrome
- May develop strikingly enlarged medullary, subependymal, choroid plexus veins
- Co-existing facial angioma

Venous Varix (Isolated)
- Occurs but is rare without associated DVA

DEVELOPMENTAL VENOUS ANOMALY

Demyelinating Disease

- Rare: Active, aggressive demyelination may have prominent medullary veins (or even associated DVA)

PATHOLOGY

General Features

- General path comments
  - Embryology
    - Arrested medullary vein development at time when normal arterial development nearly complete
    - Developmental arrest results in persistence of large primitive embryonic deep white matter veins
- Genetics
  - Mutations in chromosome 9p
    - Encodes for surface cell receptors
    - Tie-2 mutation results in missense activation
    - Segregates pedigrees with skin, oral and GI mucosa, brain venous malformations
  - Approximately 50% inherited as autosomal dominant
- Etiology
  - Does not express growth factors
  - May represent extreme anatomic variant of otherwise normal venous drainage
  - Expresses structural proteins of mature angiogenesis
- Epidemiology
  - Most common cerebral vascular malformation at autopsy
  - 60% of cerebral vascular malformations
  - 2.5-9% prevalence on contrast-enhanced MR scans
- Associated abnormalities
  - 15-20% occur with co-existing CM
  - Blue rubber-bleb nevus syndrome
  - Sinus pericranii
  - Sulcation-gyration disorders (may cause epilepsy)
  - Cervicofacial venous or lymphatic malformation

Gross Pathologic & Surgical Features

- Radially oriented dilated medullary veins
- Venous radicals are separated by normal brain
- Enlarged transcortical or subependymal draining vein

Microscopic Features

- Dilated thin-walled vessels diffusely distributed in normal white matter (no gliosis)
- Occasional: Thickened, hyalinized vessel walls
- 20% have mixed histology (CM most common), may hemorrhage

CLINICAL ISSUES

Presentation

- Most common signs/symptoms
  - Usually asymptomatic
  - Uncommon
    - Headache (if associated with CM)
    - Seizure (if associated with CM or cortical dysplasia)
    - Hemorrhage with focal neurologic deficit (if associated with CM)
- Clinical Profile: Asymptomatic patient with DVA found incidentally on MR

Demographics

- Age: All ages
- Gender: M = F
- Ethnicity: None known

Natural History & Prognosis

- Hemorrhage risk 0.15% per lesion/per year
  - Stenosis or thrombosis of draining vein increases hemorrhage risk
  - Co-existing CM increases hemorrhage risk

Treatment

- Solitary VA: None (attempt at removal may cause venous infarction of intervening normal brain)
- Histologically mixed VA: Determined by co-existing lesion

DIAGNOSTIC CHECKLIST

Consider

- DVAs contain (and provide main venous drainage for) intervening normal brain!

Image Interpretation Pearls

- Without contrast-enhanced MR, incidental DVAs may be missed
- T2* GRE useful to show the possible associated more concerning CM

SELECTED REFERENCES

1. Vieira Santos A et al: Spontaneous isolated non-haemorrhagic thrombosis in a child with development venous anomaly: case report and review of the literature. Childs Nerv Syst. 22(12):1631-3, 2006
2. Campeau NG et al: De novo development of a lesion with the appearance of a cavernous malformation adjacent to an existing developmental venous anomaly. AJNR Am J Neuroradiol. 26(1):156-9, 2005
3. Gabikian P et al: Developmental venous anomalies and sinus pericranii in the blue rubber-bleb nevus syndrome. J Neurosurg. 99:409-11, 2003
4. Wurm G et al: Recurrent cryptic vascular malformation associated with a developmental venous anomaly. Br J Neurosurg. 17(2):188-95, 2003
5. Desai K et al: Developmental deep venous system anomaly associated with congenital malformation of the brain. Pediatr Neurosurg. 36(1):37-9, 2002
6. Agazzi S et al: Developmental venous anomaly with an arteriovenous shunt and a thrombotic complication. Case report. J Neurosurg. 94(3):533-7, 2001
7. Kilic T et al: Expression of structural proteins and angiogenic factors in cerebrovascular anomalies. Neurosurg. 46:1179-92, 2000
8. Komiyama M et al: Venous angiomas with arteriovenous shunts. Neurosurg. 44:1328-35, 1999
9. Naff NJ et al: A longitudinal study of patients with venous malformations. Neurol. 50:1709-14, 1998

DEVELOPMENTAL VENOUS ANOMALY

IMAGE GALLERY

Typical

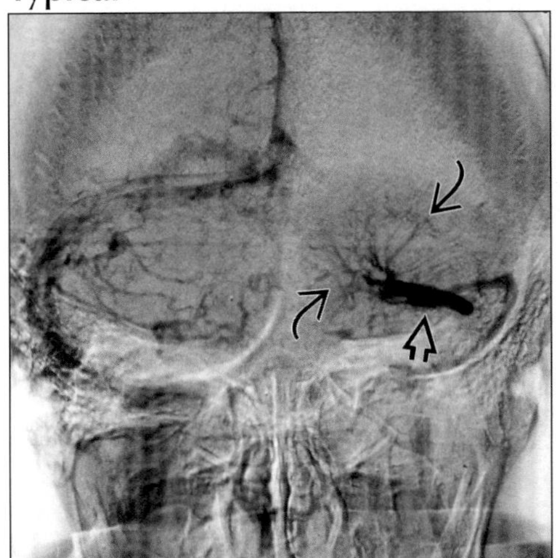

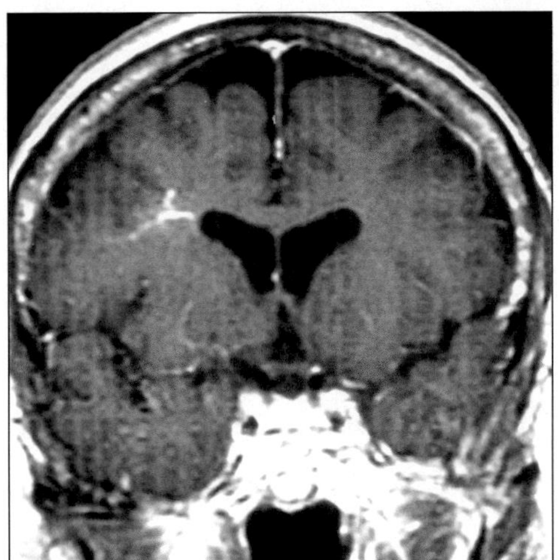

(Left) *Anteroposterior catheter angiography venous phase shows the classic "Medusa head" and large draining venous trunk of a typical DVA. The arterial and capillary phases were normal.* ***(Right)*** *Coronal T1WI MR shows enlarged, enhancing right frontal lobe draining veins coalescing into a main collector vein. Note the collector vein drains into the ependymal vein of the lateral ventricle.*

Typical

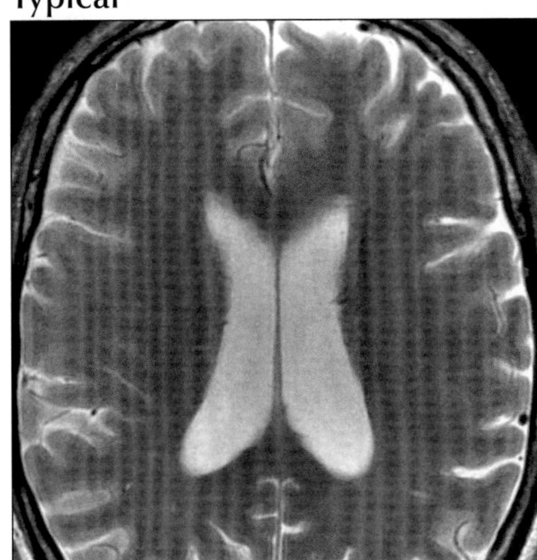

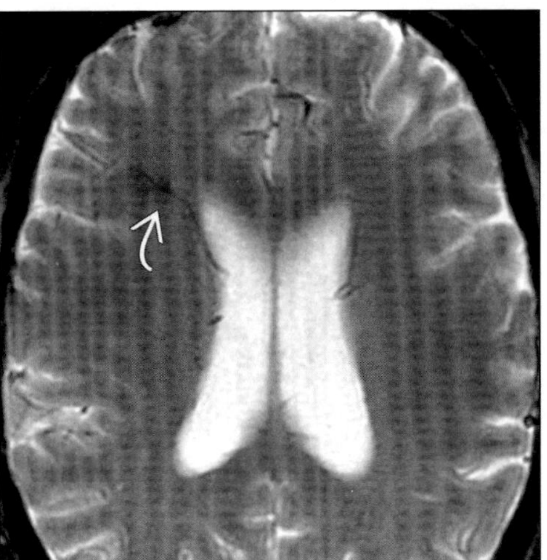

(Left) *Axial T2WI MR FSE shows a questionable dilated venous flow void in the right frontal lobe deep white matter.* ***(Right)*** *Axial T2WI MR GRE in the same case as previous image, more clearly shows the right frontal DVA. This is due to magnetic susceptibility blooming of the normal deoxyhemoglobin within the venous system.*

Typical

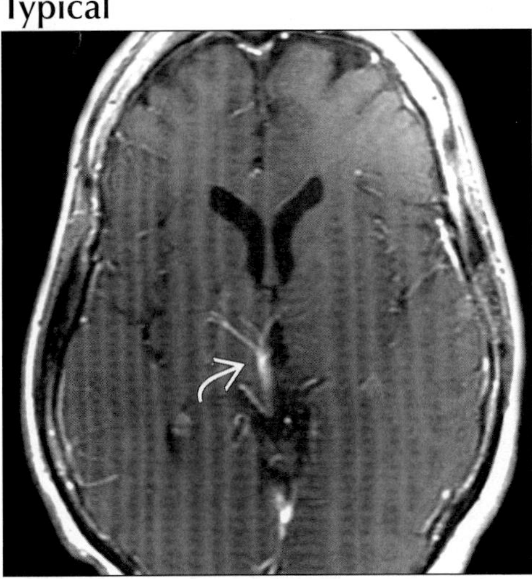

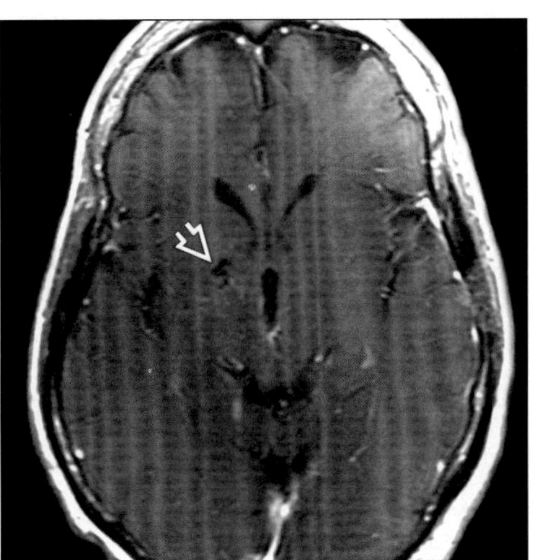

(Left) *Axial T1WI MR post-contrast shows an enhancing right thalamic DVA draining into the deep venous system.* ***(Right)*** *Axial T1WI MR post-contrast in the same case as previous image, shows a focus of chronic blood products from an adjacent cavernous malformation. These associated lesions can lead to hemorrhage.*

CAVERNOUS MALFORMATION

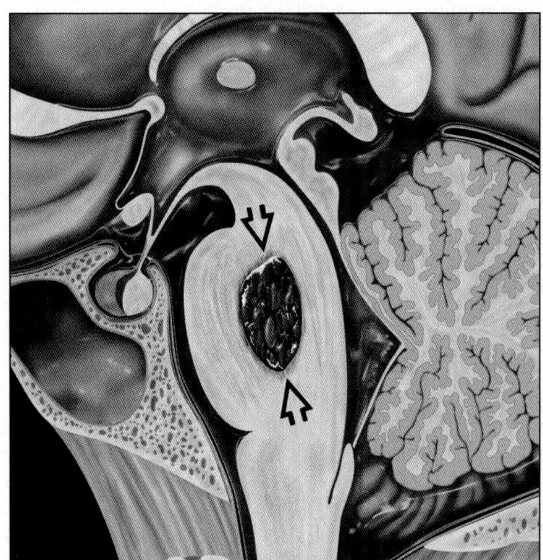

Sagittal graphic shows cavernous malformation (CM) of the pons with multiple locules of blood in different stages of degradation as well as Ca++. Hemosiderin rim surrounds the lesion ⇨.

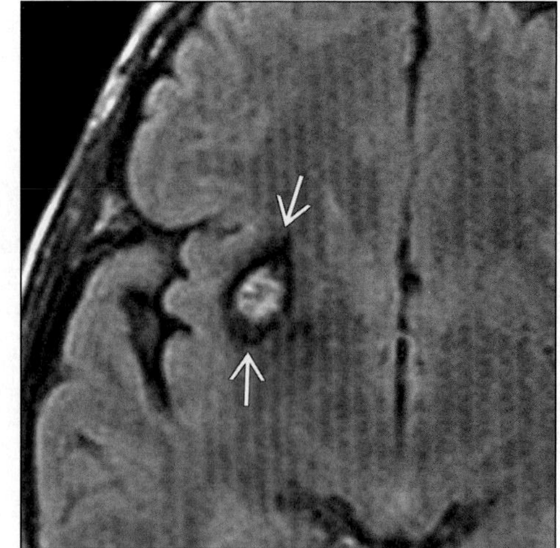

Axial T2WI MR FLAIR shows typical "popcorn" appearance of mixed signal intensity blood products centrally and complete low signal hemosiderin rim characteristic of CM ➡.

TERMINOLOGY

Abbreviations and Synonyms

- Cavernous malformation (CM); "cavernoma"
- Cavernous angioma obsolete incorrect term

Definitions

- Benign vascular hamartoma with masses of closely apposed immature blood "caverns", intralesional hemorrhages, no normal intervening neural tissue

IMAGING FINDINGS

General Features

- Best diagnostic clue: "Popcorn" mixed signal appearance with complete hypointense hemosiderin rim on T2WI MR
- Location
    - Occurs throughout CNS
    - Brain CMs common; spinal cord rare
- Size
    - CMs vary from microscopic to giant (> 6 cm)
    - Majority are between 0.5-3 cm
- Morphology
    - Discrete, lobulated mass of interwoven vascular channels
    - Locules of variable size contain blood products at different stages of evolution
    - Complete hemosiderin rim commonly surrounds lesion

CT Findings

- NECT
    - Negative in 30-50%
    - Well-delineated round/ovoid hyperdense lesion, usually < 3 cm
        - 40-60% Ca++
    - Surrounding brain usually appears normal
- CECT: Little/no enhancement unless mixed with other lesion (e.g., DVA)
- CTA: Usually negative

MR Findings

- T1WI
    - Variable, depending on hemorrhage/stage
        - Common: "Popcorn" appearance of mixed hyper-, hypointense blood-containing "locules"
- T2WI

DDx: Cavernous Malformation

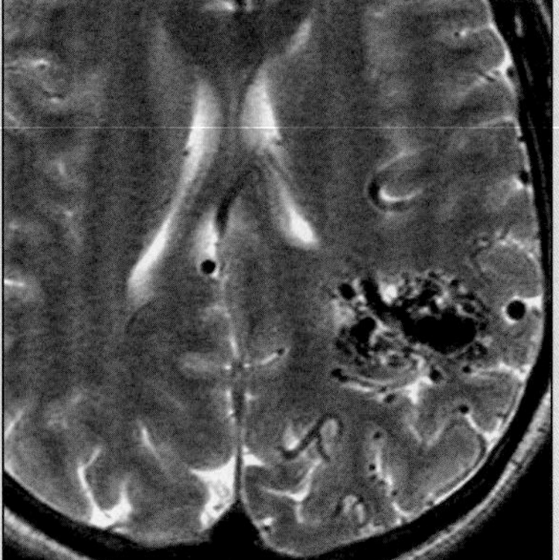

Arteriovenous Malformation

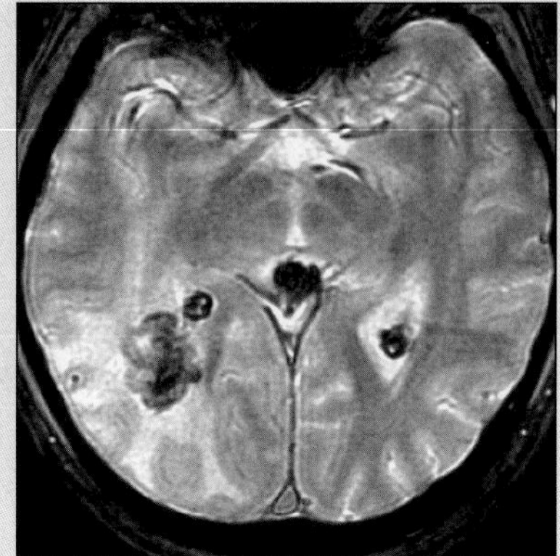

Hemorrhagic Metastasis

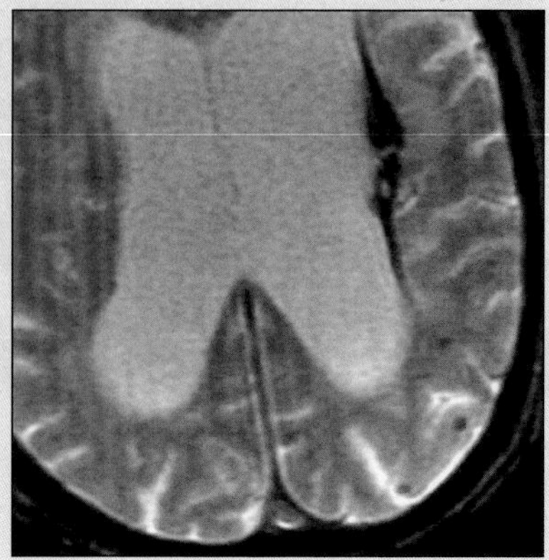

Hypertensive Hemorrhages

CAVERNOUS MALFORMATION

Key Facts

Terminology
- Benign vascular hamartoma with masses of closely apposed immature blood "caverns", intralesional hemorrhages, no normal intervening neural tissue

Imaging Findings
- Mixed signal core, complete hypointense hemosiderin rim
- Locules of blood with fluid-fluid levels
- Prominent susceptibility effect (hypointense "blooming") of short T2 blood products

Top Differential Diagnoses
- AVM ("flow voids" ± hemorrhage)
- Hemorrhagic neoplasm (incomplete hemosiderin rim, disordered evolution of blood products, enhancement)
- Hypertensive microbleeds (longstanding HTN)

Pathology
- Multiple (familial) CM syndrome is autosomal dominant, variable penetrance
- CMs are angiogenically immature lesions with endothelial proliferation, increased neoangiogenesis
- 75% occur as solitary, sporadic lesion

Clinical Issues
- Seizure 50%
- Clinical Profile: Familial CM = young adult Hispanic-American with repeated spontaneous intracranial hemorrhages
- Broad range of dynamic behavior (may progress, enlarge, regress)

  - Reticulated "popcorn-like" lesion most typical
    - Mixed signal core, complete hypointense hemosiderin rim
    - Locules of blood with fluid-fluid levels
  - Less common: Surrounding high signal edema from acute hemorrhage
- FLAIR: May show surrounding edema in acute lesions
- T2* GRE
  - Prominent susceptibility effect (hypointense "blooming") of short T2 blood products
  - Numerous punctate hypointense foci ("black dots") possible
  - Susceptibility-weighted imaging (SWI) even more sensitive
- DWI: Usually normal
- T1 C+: Minimal or no enhancement (may show associated vascular lesion)
- MRA
  - Normal (unless mixed malformation present)
  - Large acute hemorrhage may obscure more typical features of CM
  - Intrinsic high T1 signal may "shine-through" and mimic other vascular lesions

Angiographic Findings
- Conventional
  - DSA
    - DSA usually normal ("angiographically occult vascular malformation")
    - Slow intralesional flow without AV shunting
    - Avascular mass effect if large or acute hemorrhage
    - ± Associated other malformation (e.g., DVA)
    - Rare: Venous pooling, contrast "blush"

Imaging Recommendations
- Best imaging tool: MR (use T2* sequence; standard T1-, T2WI may be negative in small lesions!)
- Protocol advice
  - Use T2* GRE sequence with long TE
  - Include T1 C+ to look for associated anomalies (i.e., DVA)

DIFFERENTIAL DIAGNOSIS

"Popcorn" Lesion
- AVM ("flow voids" ± hemorrhage)
- Hemorrhagic neoplasm (incomplete hemosiderin rim, disordered evolution of blood products, enhancement)
- Calcified neoplasm (e.g., oligodendroglioma; usually shows some enhancement)

Multiple "Black Dots"
- Old trauma (DAI, contusions)
- Hypertensive microbleeds (longstanding HTN)
- Amyloid angiopathy (elderly, demented, white matter disease)
- Capillary telangiectasia (faint brush-like enhancement)

PATHOLOGY

General Features
- General path comments: Discrete collection of endothelial-lined, hemorrhage-filled caverns without intervening normal brain
- Genetics
  - Three separate loci implicated (CCM1, CCM2, CCM3 genes)
  - Multiple (familial) CM syndrome is autosomal dominant, variable penetrance
    - Mutation in chromosomes 3,7q (KRIT1 mutation at CCM1 locus)
    - Nonsense, frame-shift or splice-site mutations consistent with two-hit model for CM
    - Mutations encode a truncated KRIT1 protein
    - KRIT1 interacts with endothelial cell microtubules; loss of function leads to inability of endothelial cells to mature, form capillaries
  - Sporadic CM
    - No KRIT1 mutation
- Etiology
  - CMs are angiogenically immature lesions with endothelial proliferation, increased neoangiogenesis
  - VEGF, βFGF, TGFα expressed

CAVERNOUS MALFORMATION

  - Receptors (e.g., Flk-1) upregulated
- Epidemiology
  - Approximate prevalence 0.5%
  - 75% occur as solitary, sporadic lesion
  - 10-30% multiple, familial
- Associated abnormalities
  - DVA
  - Superficial siderosis
  - Cutaneous abnormalities
    - Cafe au lait spots
    - Hyperkeratotic capillary-venous malformations ("cherry angiomas")

Gross Pathologic & Surgical Features

- Discrete, lobulated, bluish-purple ("mulberry-like") nodule
- Pseudocapsule of gliotic, hemosiderin-stained brain

Microscopic Features

- Thin-walled endothelial-lined spaces
- Large gaps at endothelial cell junctions
- Embedded in collagenous matrix
- Hemorrhage in different stages of evolution
- ± Ca++
- Does not contain normal brain
- May be histologically mixed (DVA most common)

Staging, Grading or Classification Criteria

- Zabramski classification of CMs
  - Type 1 = subacute hemorrhage (hyperintense on T1WI; hyper- or hypointense on T2WI)
  - Type 2 = mixed signal intensity on T1-, T2WI with degrading hemorrhage of various ages (classic "popcorn" lesion)
  - Type 3 = chronic hemorrhage (hypointense on T1-, T2WI)
  - Type 4 = punctate microhemorrhages ("black dots"), poorly seen except on GRE sequences

CLINICAL ISSUES

Presentation

- Most common signs/symptoms
  - Seizure 50%
  - Neurologic deficit 25% (may be progressive)
  - 20% asymptomatic
- Clinical Profile: Familial CM = young adult Hispanic-American with repeated spontaneous intracranial hemorrhages

Demographics

- Age
  - Peak presentation = 40-60 y but may present in childhood
  - Familial CMs tend to present earlier than sporadic lesions
- Gender: M = F
- Ethnicity
  - Multiple (familial) CM syndrome in Hispanic Americans of Mexican descent
    - Founder mutation in KRIT1 (Q445X)
    - Positive family history = 90% chance of mutation resulting in CM
  - CMs may occur in any ethnic population

Natural History & Prognosis

- Broad range of dynamic behavior (may progress, enlarge, regress)
- De novo lesions may develop
- Propensity for growth via repeated intralesional hemorrhages
  - Sporadic = 0.25-0.7% per year
  - Risk factor for future hemorrhage = previous hemorrhage
  - Rehemorrhage rate high initially, decreases after 2-3 years
- Familial CMs at especially high risk for hemorrhage, forming new lesions
  - 1% per lesion per year

Treatment

- Total removal via microsurgical resection
  - Caution: If mixed DVA, venous drainage must be preserved
- Stereotaxic XRT limited effectiveness

DIAGNOSTIC CHECKLIST

Consider

- In patients with spontaneous ICH, do a T2* scan to look for additional lesions
- Atypical appearance of CM in setting of recent hemorrhage requires F/U imaging to confirm diagnosis

Image Interpretation Pearls

- CM should not be confused with cavernous hemangioma (true vasoproliferative neoplasm)
- "Giant" CMs can mimic neoplasm

SELECTED REFERENCES

1. Battistini S et al: Clinical, magnetic resonance imaging, and genetic study of 5 Italian families with cerebral cavernous malformation. Arch Neurol. 64(6):843-8, 2007
2. Baumann CR et al: Seizure outcome after resection of supratentorial cavernous malformations: a study of 168 patients. Epilepsia. 48(3):559-63, 2007
3. Gault J et al: Spectrum of genotype and clinical manifestations in cerebral cavernous malformations. Neurosurgery. 59(6):1278-84; discussion 1284-5, 2006
4. Tu J et al: Ultrastructural characteristics of hemorrhagic, nonhemorrhagic, and recurrent cavernous malformations. J Neurosurg. 103(5):903-9, 2005
5. Mathiesen T et al: Deep and brainstem cavernomas: a consecutive 8-year series. J Neurosurg. 99(1):31-7, 2003
6. Musunuru K et al: Widespread central nervous system cavernous malformations associated with cafe-au-lait skin lesions. Case report. J Neurosurg. 99(2):412-5, 2003
7. Reich P et al: Molecular genetic investigations in the CCM1 gene in sporadic cerebral cavernomas. Neurology. 60(7):1135-8, 2003
8. Rivera PP et al: Intracranial cavernous malformations. Neuroimaging Clin N Am. 13(1):27-40, 2003
9. Cave-Riant F et al: Spectrum and expression analysis of KRIT1 mutations in 121 consecutive and unrelated patients with Cerebral Cavernous Malformations. Eur J Hum Genet. 10(11):733-40, 2002

CAVERNOUS MALFORMATION

IMAGE GALLERY

Typical

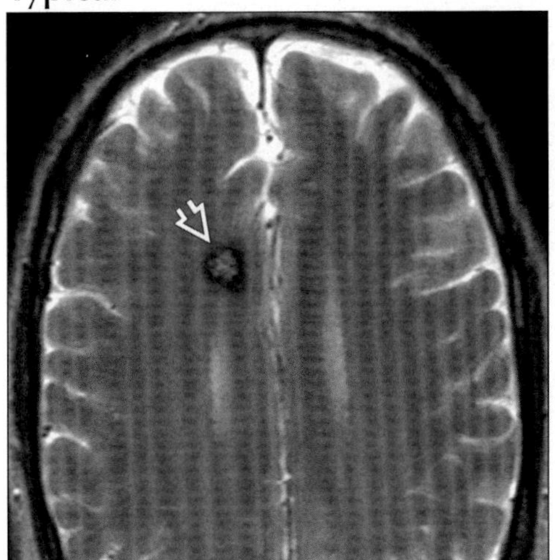

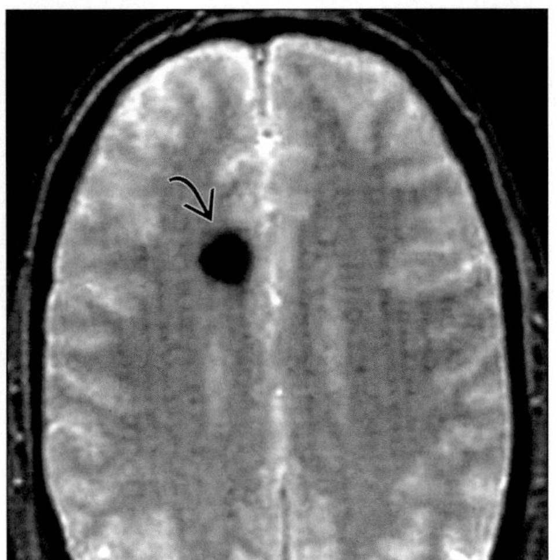

(Left) *Axial T2WI MR shows a classic cavernous malformation with central locules of different stages of blood degradation products encased by a complete low signal hemosiderin rim* ➢. ***(Right)*** *Axial T2WI MR GRE in the same case as previous image, shows obvious "blooming"* ➚ *of the right frontal lobe lesion due to the magnetic susceptibility of the various blood degradation products.*

Typical

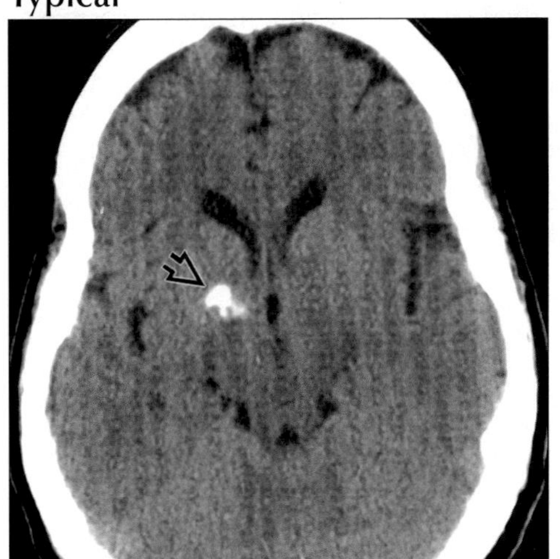

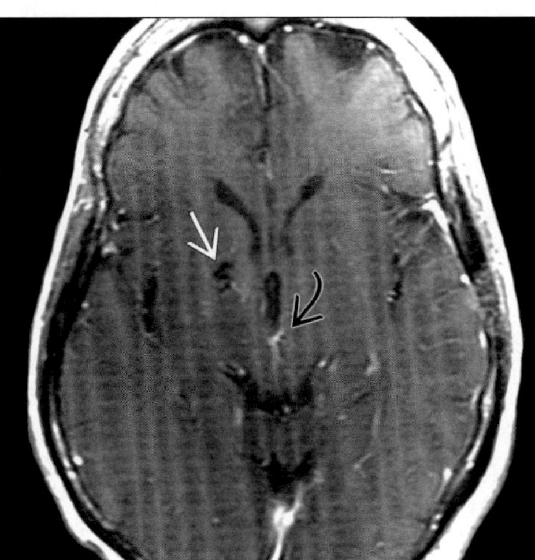

(Left) *Axial NECT of a CM shows dense focus of calcification centered in the right internal capsule* ➢ *without significant mass effect or surrounding edema.* ***(Right)*** *Axial T1WI MR post-contrast in the same case as previous image, shows no significant enhancement* ➔ *typical of CM. Note the adjacent developmental venous anomaly* ➚ *draining the bilateral thalami.*

Variant

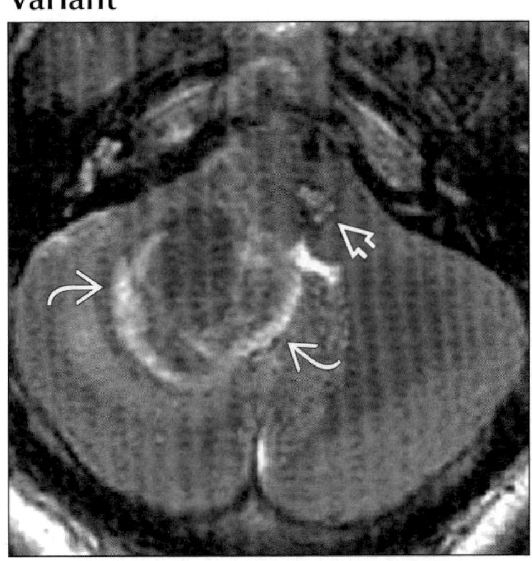

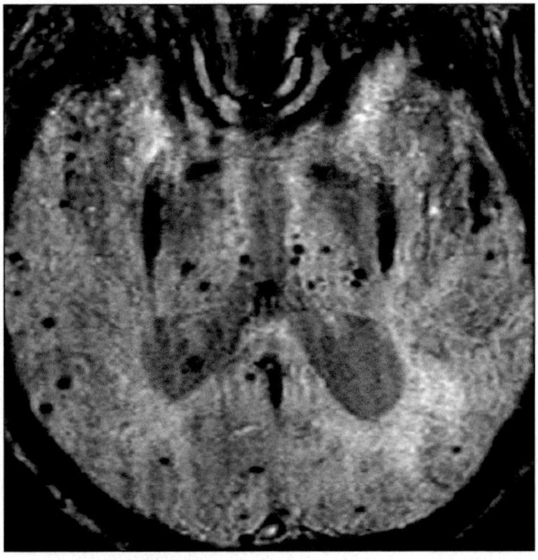

(Left) *Axial T2WI MR shows a large mixed signal acute/subacute hematoma with surrounding edema in the right cerebellar hemisphere* ➚ *due to hemorrhagic CM. Note additional CM in the pons* ➢. ***(Right)*** *Axial T2* MR SWI shows multifocal punctate hypointensities characteristic of type 4 CMs. SWI depicts these lesions much more readily than other MR sequences (Courtesy M. Haacke, PhD).*

CAPILLARY TELANGIECTASIA

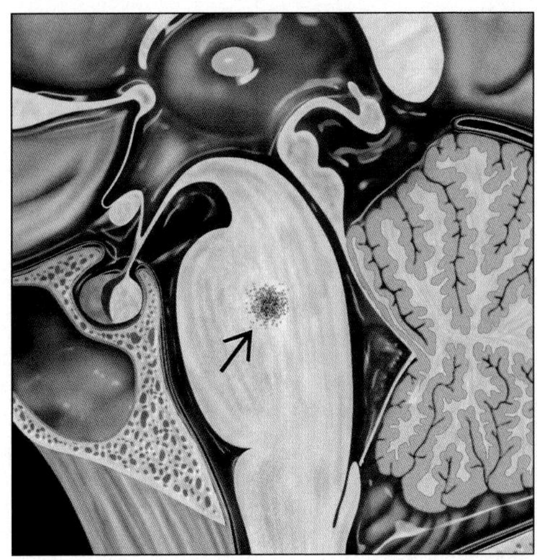

Sagittal graphic shows pontine capillary telangiectasia ⇒. Note enlarged stippled-appearing thin-walled capillaries with normal intervening brain parenchyma between the dilated vessels.

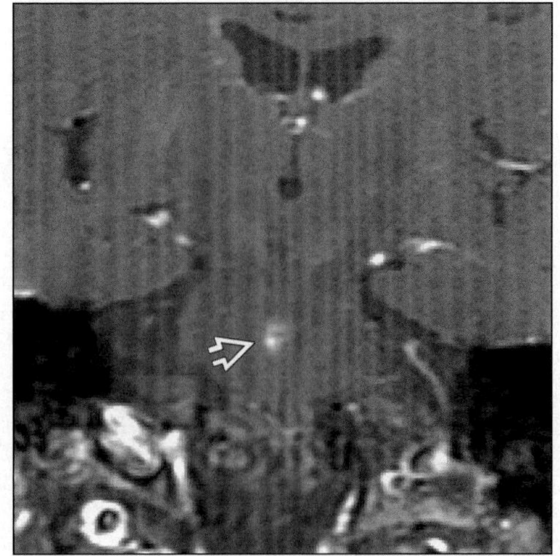

Coronal T1WI MR post-contrast shows faint brush-like focus of enhancement in the pons ⇨, the typical location and appearance of capillary telangiectasia.

TERMINOLOGY

Abbreviations and Synonyms

- Brain capillary telangiectasia (BCT)

Definitions

- Cluster of thin-walled ectatic capillaries interspersed with normal brain parenchyma

IMAGING FINDINGS

General Features

- Best diagnostic clue
  - Hypointense lesion on T2* GRE MR
  - Faint "brush-like" enhancement
- Location
  - Midbrain, pons, medulla, spinal cord most common
  - One-third found elsewhere (subcortical WM, etc.)
- Size
  - Few mm to 2 cm, usually < 1 cm
  - Rare reports of very large lesions
- Morphology
  - Small, poorly-demarcated lesion; no mass effect or edema
  - Macroscopic hemorrhage, calcifications, draining vein rare
    - If present, suggests a "mixed" or "transitional" capillary malformation

CT Findings

- NECT: Usually normal (occasionally may have Ca++ if "mixed malformation")
- CECT: May see mild punctate enhancement

MR Findings

- T1WI: Usually normal, may see very mild hypointense focus
- T2WI: 50% normal; 50% stippled foci of mild hyperintensity
- FLAIR: Usually normal; may show small foci of hyperintensity
- T2* GRE
  - Lesion moderately but not profoundly hypointense
    - Slow to stagnant blood flow results in oxy- to deoxyhemoglobin conversion
  - Less common: Multifocal BCTs ("gray dots")

DDx: Capillary Telangiectasia

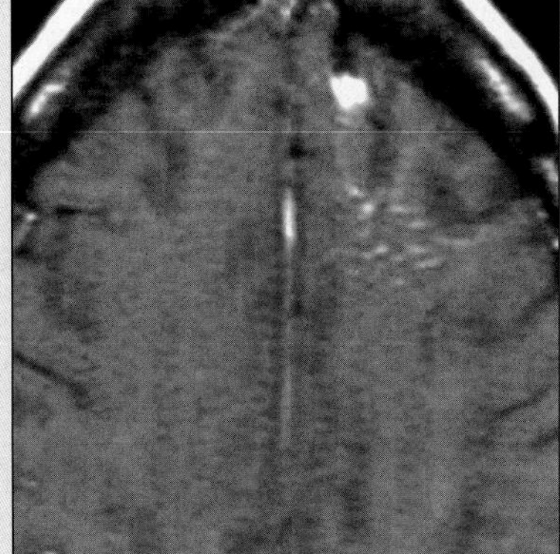

Developmental Venous Anomaly

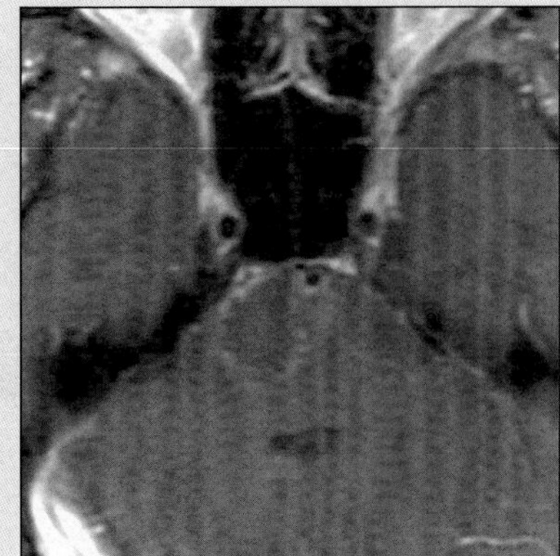

Brainstem Glioma

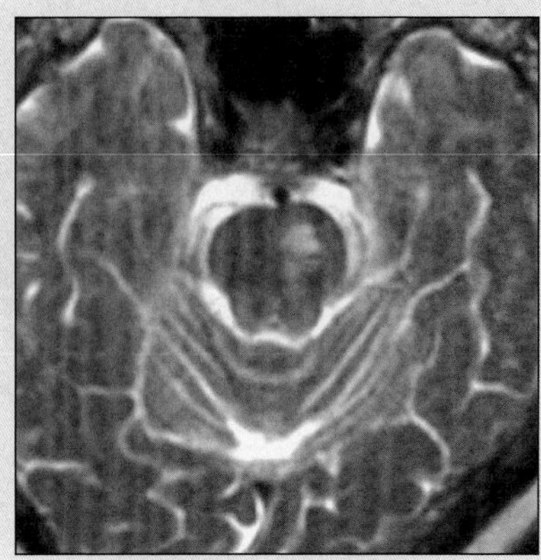

Brainstem Lacunar Infarct

CAPILLARY TELANGIECTASIA

Key Facts

Terminology
- Cluster of thin-walled ectatic capillaries interspersed with normal brain parenchyma

Imaging Findings
- Hypointense lesion on T2* GRE MR
- Faint "brush-like" enhancement
- Midbrain, pons, medulla, spinal cord most common
- Few mm to 2 cm, usually < 1 cm
- Slow to stagnant blood flow results in oxy- to deoxyhemoglobin conversion
- Best imaging tool: MR with T2*, T1 C+ sequences

Top Differential Diagnoses
- Developmental Venous Anomaly (DVA)
- Cavernous Malformation
- Arteriovenous Malformation
- Neoplasm

Pathology
- Epidemiology: 15-20% of all intracranial vascular malformations

Clinical Issues
- Asymptomatic, discovered incidentally
- Rare: Headache, vertigo, tinnitus, diplopia
- Any age but 30-40 y most common
- Clinically benign, quiescent unless histologically mixed with other vascular malformation
- No treatment necessary (normal intervening brain parenchyma)

Diagnostic Checklist
- Enhancing small pontine lesion that becomes moderately hypointense on T2* is usually a BCT

  - Susceptibility-weighted imaging (SWI) may be even more sensitive to detect small lesions
- DWI: Usually normal
- T1 C+
  - Faint stippled or speckled "brush-like" enhancement
  - May show punctate, linear/branching vessels, collecting vein (if mixed with DVA)

Angiographic Findings
- Conventional
  - Usually normal
  - Faint vascular "stain" or draining vein if mixed with DVA

Imaging Recommendations
- Best imaging tool: MR with T2*, T1 C+ sequences
- Protocol advice: Consider SWI for problematic lesions

DIFFERENTIAL DIAGNOSIS

Developmental Venous Anomaly (DVA)
- "Medusa-head" branching veins
- Large central draining venous trunk
- Can be mixed with BCT

Cavernous Malformation
- Blood locules with fluid-fluid levels
- Complete hemosiderin rim
- Can be mixed with BCTs, cause hemorrhage

Arteriovenous Malformation
- Nidus of flow voids, enlarged feeding and draining vessels
- Mixed signal of blood products if hemorrhaged
- Surrounding edema if recent hemorrhage

Neoplasm
- Strong > faint enhancement
- Mass effect
- Pons/cerebellum rare locations
- Unlikely to show deoxyhemoglobin blooming on GRE
  - If hemorrhagic neoplasm, usually subacute to chronic blood products (mixed signal changes on T1 as well as T2 and GRE)

Demyelinating Disease (Multiple Sclerosis)
- Usually multiple foci of periventricular and subcortical T2 hyperintensities
  - Classically oriented perpendicular to the ependyma
- Can enhance if hyperacute lesion (usually within 6 weeks)
  - Typically incomplete ring enhancement

Lacunar Ischemic Infarction
- More intense T2 high signal
- Restricted diffusion on DWI
- Can enhance if late acute to subacute stage

PATHOLOGY

General Features
- General path comments: Usually found incidentally at autopsy or imaging
- Genetics: None known
- Etiology
  - Sporadic BCTs: Unknown
  - May develop as complication of radiation (20% of children after cranial irradiation)
- Epidemiology: 15-20% of all intracranial vascular malformations
- Associated abnormalities
  - Osler-Weber-Rendu disease (hereditary hemorrhagic telangiectasia)
    - BCTs rare (AVMs more common)

Gross Pathologic & Surgical Features
- Rarely identified unless unusually large (greater than 2 cm reported) or hemorrhage (from other vascular malformation) present

Microscopic Features
- Cluster of thin-walled, dilated but otherwise histologically normal capillaries
- Normal brain in-between vascular channels

CAPILLARY TELANGIECTASIA

- No mass effect
- Uncomplicated BCTs have no gliosis, hemorrhage, Ca++, or hemosiderin-laden macrophages

CLINICAL ISSUES

Presentation

- Most common signs/symptoms
  - Asymptomatic, discovered incidentally
  - Rare: Headache, vertigo, tinnitus, diplopia
    - If symptomatic, usually larger lesion (greater than 2 cm) or mixed malformation
- Other signs/symptoms
  - Transient or intermittent course mimicking TIA or inflammatory process
    - Symptoms can be exacerbated by menstrual period or pregnancy
    - May be due to stimulation of hormone/steroid receptors on endothelial cells
- Clinical Profile: Asymptomatic middle-aged patient with a poorly-delineated brainstem lesion seen incidentally on T1 C+ MR scan

Demographics

- Age
  - Any age but 30-40 y most common
  - Few reports in children (as young as 15 months of age)
- Gender: No known preference

Natural History & Prognosis

- Clinically benign, quiescent unless histologically mixed with other vascular malformation
  - Mixed malformations can lead to subarachnoid or intraparenchymal hemorrhage
- Very rare reports of aggressive course with isolated BCT alone

Treatment

- No treatment necessary (normal intervening brain parenchyma)
- Rarely surgery or XRT for symptomatic lesion
  - Treatment directed at the associated mixed vascular lesion

DIAGNOSTIC CHECKLIST

Image Interpretation Pearls

- Enhancing small pontine lesion that becomes moderately hypointense on T2* is usually a BCT
- T2* "blooming" may help differentiate from a small enhancing neoplasm

SELECTED REFERENCES

1. Yoshida Y et al: Capillary telangiectasia of the brain stem diagnosed by susceptibility-weighted imaging. J Comput Assist Tomogr. 30(6):980-2, 2006
2. Koike S et al: Asymptomatic radiation-induced telangiectasia in children after cranial irradiation: frequency latency, and dose relation. Radiology. 203:93-9, 2004
3. Tang SC et al: Diffuse capillary telangiectasia of the brain manifested as a slowly progressive course. Cerebrovasc Dis. 15(1-2):140-2, 2003
4. Castillo M et al: MR imaging and histologic features of capillary telangiectasia of the basal ganglia. AJNR Am J Neuroradiol. 22(8):1553-5, 2001
5. Clatterbuck RE et al: The juxtaposition of a capillary telangiectasia, cavernous malformation, and developmental venous anomaly in the brainstem of a single patient: case report. Neurosurgery. 49(5):1246-50, 2001
6. Scaglione C et al: Symptomatic unruptured capillary telangiectasia of the brain stem: report of three cases and review of the literature. J Neurol Neurosurg Psychiatry. 71(3):390-3, 2001
7. Auffray-Calvier E et al: [Capillary telangiectasis, angiographically occult vascular malformations. MRI symptomatology apropos of 7 cases] J Neuroradiol. 26(4):257-61, 1999
8. Huddle DC et al: Clinically aggressive diffuse capillary telangiectasia of the brain stem: a clinical radiologic-pathologic case study. AJNR Am J Neuroradiol. 20(9):1674-7, 1999
9. Chang SD et al: Mixed arteriovenous malformation and capillary telangiectasia: a rare subset of mixed vascular malformations. Case report. J Neurosurg. 86(4):699-703, 1997
10. Lee RR et al: Brain capillary telangiectasia: MR imaging appearance and clinicohistopathologic findings. Radiology. 205(3):797-805, 1997
11. Barr RM et al: Slow-flow vascular malformations of the pons: capillary telangiectasias? AJNR Am J Neuroradiol. 17(1):71-8, 1996
12. McCormick PW et al: Cerebellar hemorrhage associated with capillary telangiectasia and venous angioma: a case report. Surg Neurol. 39(6):451-7, 1993

CAPILLARY TELANGIECTASIA

IMAGE GALLERY

Typical

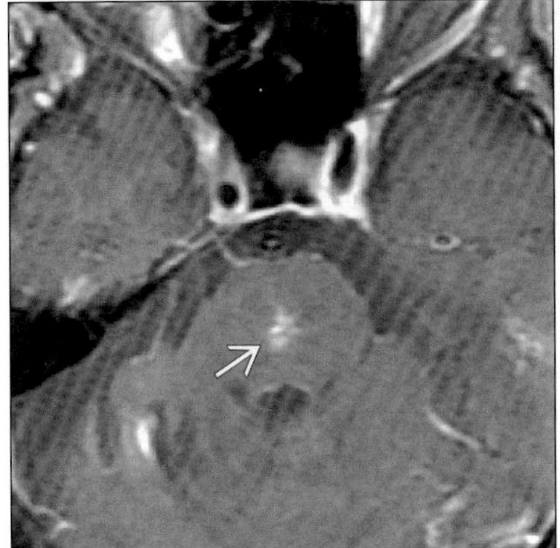

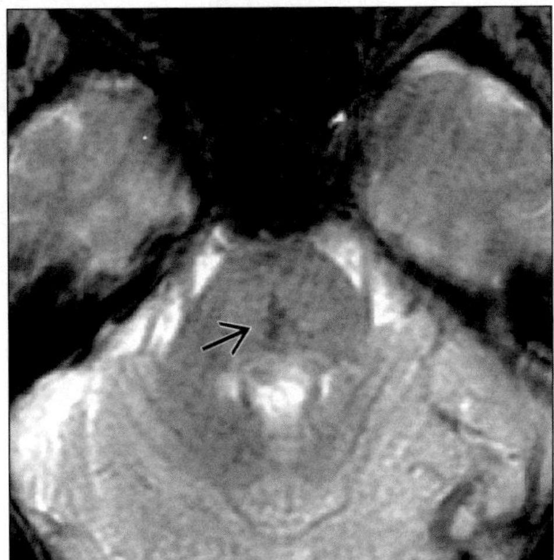

(Left) Axial T1WI MR following contrast administration depicts stippled faint enhancement in the central pons ➡ without mass effect suggestive of capillary telangiectasia. *(Right)* Axial T2WI MR GRE in the same case shows moderate lesion hypointensity ➡ due to susceptibility effect of deoxyhemoglobin confirming capillary telangiectasia.

Typical

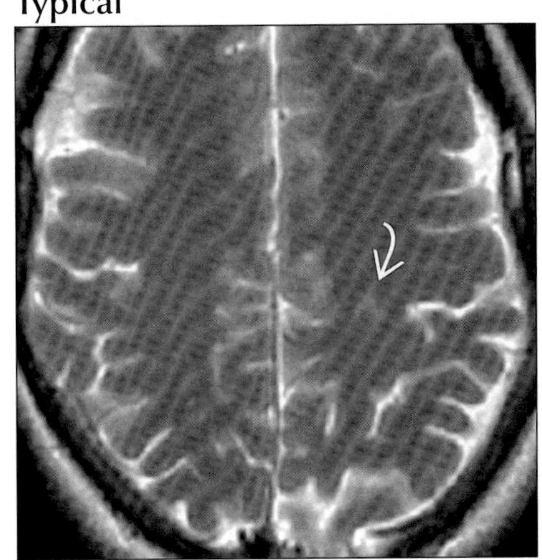

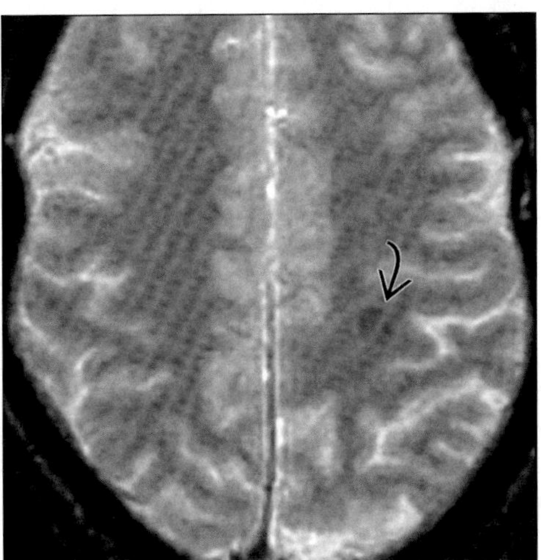

(Left) Axial T2WI MR FSE shows ill-defined faint focus of hyperintensity ➡ in the left posterior frontal lobe centrum semiovale white matter. The lesion also showed stippled enhancement. *(Right)* Axial T2WI MR GRE in the same case depicts lesion hypointensity ➡ verifying the presumed etiology of capillary telangiectasia. Note normal interspersed brain parenchyma.

Variant

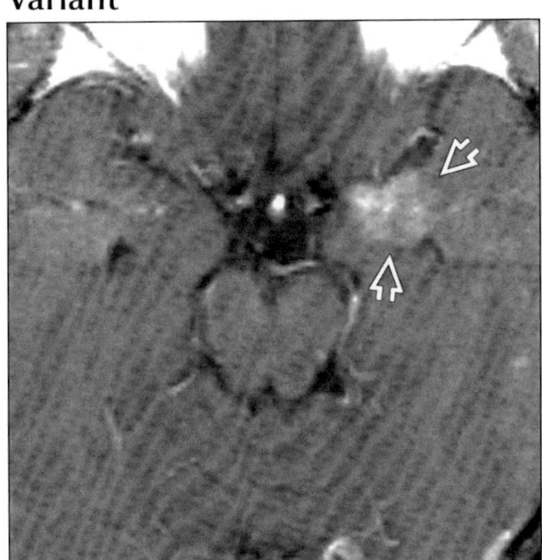

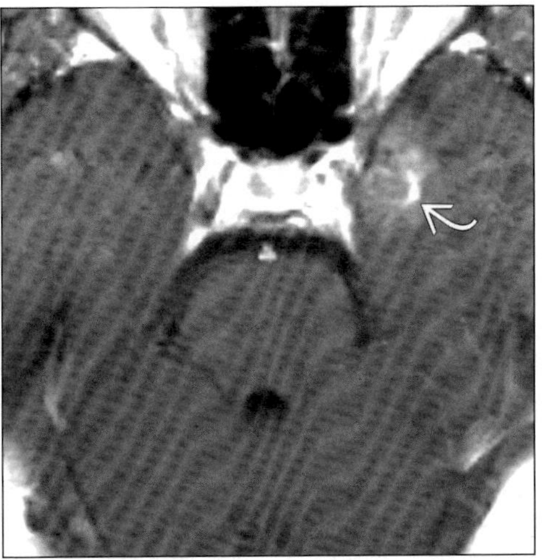

(Left) Axial T1WI MR post-contrast shows relatively large region of faint brush-like enhancement of the medial anterior left temporal lobe ➡ from capillary telangiectasia. *(Right)* Axial T1WI MR post-contrast of adjacent slice in the same case as previous image, identifies radially oriented vessels converging on a single venous trunk ➡ compatible with a DVA in this mixed malformation.

VEIN OF GALEN MALFORMATION

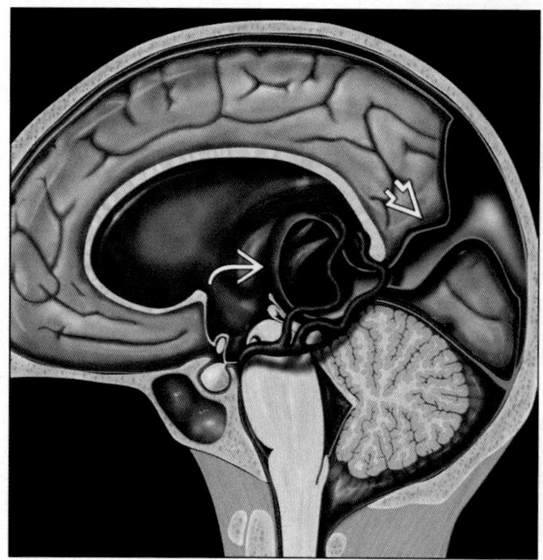

Sagittal graphic of a patient with a mural type VGAM depicting collicular and posterior choroidal artery feeders emptying into a dilated MPV ➔. Note persistent falcine sinus ➔.

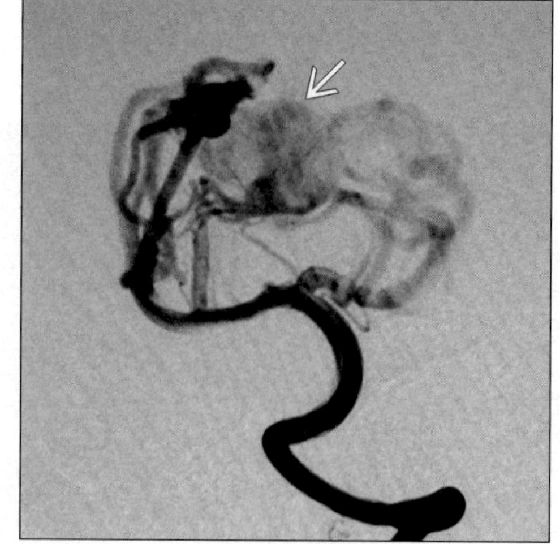

Early arterial phase of a left vertebral artery DSA shows large AV shunts from the posterior cerebral arteries draining into a dilated MPV ➔.

TERMINOLOGY

Definitions

- Vein of Galen malformation (VGAM): Arteriovenous fistula (AVF) resulting in aneurysmal dilatation of the "vein of Galen"
- VGAM is misnomer; malformation actually involves the median prosencephalic vein (MPV) of Markowski which becomes "aneurysmal"/dilated

IMAGING FINDINGS

General Features

- Best diagnostic clue
  - Dilated arteries with AV shunting into large midline venous pouch (MPV) in neonate/infant, often with associated dysplasia of dural venous sinuses (DVS)
  - Persistent falcine sinus
- Location: Quadrigeminal plate cistern, cistern of velum interpositum
- Size: Variable size, number, complexity of shunts depending on type, with commensurate dilatation of MPV
- Morphology
  - Myriad of complex shunts of various sizes from pericallosal arteries and posterior cerebral arteries (PCAs) + anterior choroidal artery (AChA) in "choroidal" type VGAM
  - Fewer shunts from PCAs, collicular arteries in "mural" type VGAM

Radiographic Findings

- Radiography
  - Cardiomegaly, wide mediastinum, edema on chest X-ray
  - Calcification of MPV wall ± cerebral cortex (dystrophic Ca++ from chronic venous ischemia) are late findings

CT Findings

- NECT
  - Venous pouch mildly hyperdense to brain
  - May show
    - MPV wall Ca++ (older children, thrombosed "aneurysm"/dilated MPV)
    - Hydrocephalus
    - Parenchymal ischemia (low attenuation), Ca++, atrophy

DDx: Pediatric Arteriovenous Shunts

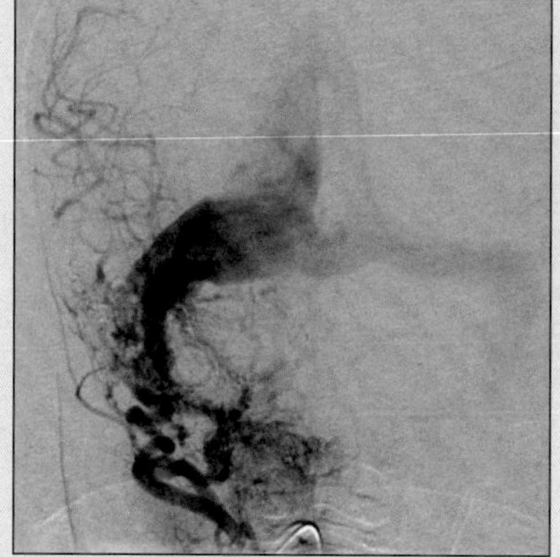

Dural AV Fistula

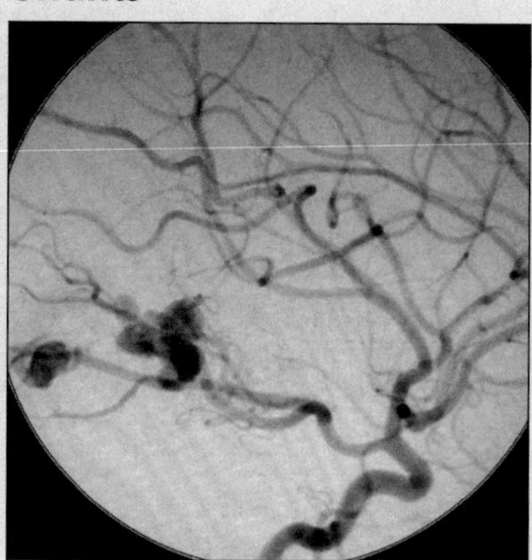

Pial AV Fistula

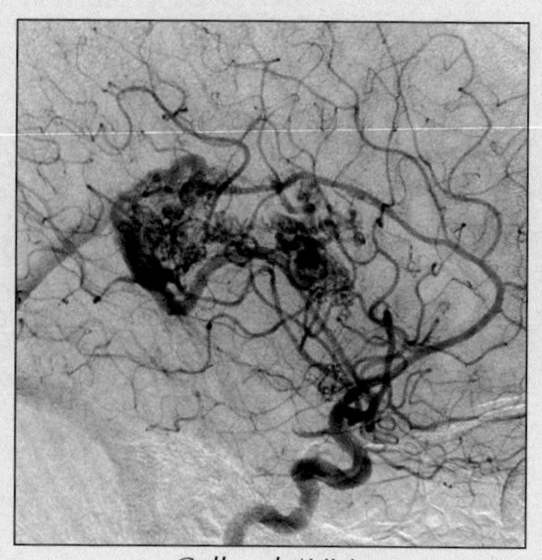

Callosal AVM

VEIN OF GALEN MALFORMATION

Key Facts

Terminology

- Vein of Galen malformation (VGAM): Arteriovenous fistula (AVF) resulting in aneurysmal dilatation of the "vein of Galen"
- VGAM is misnomer; malformation actually involves the median prosencephalic vein (MPV) of Markowski which becomes "aneurysmal"/dilated

Imaging Findings

- Antenatal US/MR: VGAM identified in 3rd trimester
- Dilated arteries with AV shunting into large midline venous pouch (MPV) in neonate/infant
- Choroidal type: Multiple feeders from pericallosal, choroidal, and thalamoperforating arteries
- Mural type: Few feeders from uni- or bilateral collicular or posterior choroidal arteries
- Persistent falcine sinus
- Hydrocephalus
- Cardiomegaly, wide mediastinum, edema on chest X-ray

Pathology

- AVF of MPV occurs during 6th-11th weeks gestation
- < 1% cerebral vascular malformations at any age

Clinical Issues

- Choroidal type: Neonates
    - Death from intractable CHF and multi-system failure without treatment
- Mural type: Infants/children
    - Progressive developmental delay; irreversible if chronic cerebral venous hypertension is unabated
- Delay transcatheter embolization (TCE) until 6 months or later if possible

---

        - Intraventricular hemorrhage (IVH) is rare
- CECT: Strong enhancement of feeding arteries and enlarged midline venous structures
- CTA: Multiplanar reformats (MPRs) provide excellent pre-angiographic delineation of VGAM

MR Findings

- T1WI
    - Arterial feeders: Flow voids
    - MPV: Flow void or mixed intensity due to fast or turbulent flow
    - Hyperintense foci within pouch: Thrombus
    - Hyperintense foci within brain: Ca++, hemorrhage (rare)
- T2WI
    - Arterial feeders: Flow voids
    - MPV: Flow void or mixed intensity due to fast or turbulent flow
    - Ischemic foci poorly seen due to unmyelinated infant brain
- DWI: Restriction in areas of acute ischemia/infarction
- MRA: Delineates arterial feeders and draining MPV

Ultrasonographic Findings

- Grayscale Ultrasound: MPV mildly echogenic midline mass
- Color Doppler: Arterial feeders; arterialized, turbulent flow within MPV
- Antenatal US/MR: VGAM identified in 3rd trimester
    - Cardiac dilatation, hydrops fetalis → poor prognosis

Angiographic Findings

- Conventional
    - "Choroidal" or "mural" classification based on angioarchitecture of VGAM
        - Choroidal: Multiple feeders from pericallosal, choroidal, and thalamoperforating arteries
        - Mural: Few feeders from uni- or bilateral collicular or posterior choroidal arteries
        - May see "limbic arterial ring": Persistent arterial bridge between anterior cerebral artery and AChA or PCA
    - Frequent DVS anomalies
        - Embryonic falcine sinus drains MPV in 50%, associated with absent or hypoplastic straight sinus
        - Variable absence and stenoses other sinuses

Imaging Recommendations

- Best imaging tool
    - Initial evaluation
        - Antenatal US/MR or postnatal US
        - MRI/MRA for better definition vascular anatomy, status of brain/ventricles; also for F/U
    - Catheter angiogram ideally performed in conjunction with first embolization at 6 months of age or later if clinically stable
- Protocol advice
    - Thin sagittal images define anatomy and relationship of VGAM to cerebral aqueduct
    - MRA C+ often superior to MRA C-; additional MRV usually not necessary

DIFFERENTIAL DIAGNOSIS

Childhood Dural Arteriovenous Fistula (DAVF)

- Neonatal presentation similar to VGAM
- Multifocal, large, fast-flow fistulas common

Arteriovenous Malformation (AVM)

- Congenital web of arteriovenous connections (nidus) without intervening capillary network
- May result in vein of Galen aneurysmal dilatation (VGAD)

Complex Developmental Venous Anomaly (DVA)

- Dilatation of several superficial or deep veins draining normal brain parenchyma
- No nidus or AV shunting

Pial AV Fistula

- Direct, high-flow connection between ≥ 1 pial artery and a single draining vein ± varix

VEIN OF GALEN MALFORMATION

- May be multiple in Rendu-Osler-Weber or Klippel-Trenaunay-Weber syndromes

PATHOLOGY

General Features

- General path comments
  - Embryology: Normal development
    - 7th-8th week: Choroid plexus drains via single temporary midline vein (MPV)
    - 10th week: Internal cerebral veins annex drainage of choroid plexus ⇒ regression MPV
- Etiology
  - VGAM
    - AVF of MPV occurs during 6th-11th weeks gestation
    - ↑ Flow through VGAM prevents involution of normally transient fetal venous drainage pattern
  - DVS occlusions/stenoses
    - Primary atresia vs occlusion 2° to turbulent flow
  - Cerebral ischemia/atrophy
    - Arterial "steal" and/or chronic venous HTN
  - Hydrocephalus (HC)
    - ↓ CSF resorption 2° to elevated DVS pressure (CSF resorption in neonates is via transependymal flow into medullary veins as arachnoid granulations not yet mature)
    - CSF resorption dependent on pressure gradient between ventricles and medullary veins but in VGAM ↑ DVS pressure transmitted to medullary veins → ↓ pressure gradient for CSF resorption → HC
    - Cerebral aqueduct obstruction secondary to compression by dilated MPV may contribute
- Epidemiology
  - Rare
    - < 1% cerebral vascular malformations at any age
    - Up to 30% of all pediatric vascular malformations
  - Most common extracardiac cause of high-output CHF in newborn period

Gross Pathologic & Surgical Features

- Dilated arterial feeders and midline venous pouch
- DVS anomalies
- Malformations of structures adjacent to MPV
  - Pineal gland, tela choroidea of 3rd ventricle

Staging, Grading or Classification Criteria

- "Choroidal" or "mural" classification based on angioarchitecture of VGAM (Lasjaunias et al)
  - Choroidal: Multiple feeders from pericallosal, choroidal, and thalamoperforating arteries
  - Mural: Few feeders from uni- or bilateral collicular or posterior choroidal arteries

CLINICAL ISSUES

Presentation

- Most common signs/symptoms: CHF, hydrocephalus
- Clinical Profile
  - Neonate: CHF, cranial bruit (choroidal VGAM)
  - Infant: Hydrocephalus (macrocranium), ± mild CHF (mural VGAM)
  - Older infant/child: Developmental delay, hydrocephalus, seizure, headache

Demographics

- Age: Neonatal > infant presentation; rare adult presentation
- Gender: M:F = 2:1

Natural History & Prognosis

- Choroidal type: Neonates
  - Increasing head circumference, delayed developmental milestones
  - Death from intractable CHF and multi-system failure without treatment
- Mural type: Infants/children
  - Progressive developmental delay; irreversible if chronic cerebral venous hypertension is unabated
  - Spontaneous thrombosis of slow flow VGAM rare

Treatment

- Choroidal VGAM (neonatal presentation)
  - Medical therapy for CHF until 6 months of age
    - Failure of therapy warrants earlier neurointervention
  - Delay transcatheter embolization (TCE) until 6 months or later if possible
    - Arterial embolization effective and safer than venous approach which is associated with ↑ risk IVH
- Mural VGAM (infant presentation)
  - TCE can be performed later (slower flow VGAM)
  - TCE technically easier (fewer arterial feeders)
- Treatment for hydrocephalus controversial
  - Shunt placement associated with complications
  - Shunt placement reserved for refractory hydrocephalus after all TCEs performed
- Aim of endovascular therapy is to permit normal neurological development, which does not necessitate complete angiographic cure of VGAM

DIAGNOSTIC CHECKLIST

Consider

- Delay catheter angiography + initial embolization until 6 months of age if clinically stable

Image Interpretation Pearls

- Imaging appearance diagnostic in the appropriate clinical setting
  - Look for dilated midline MPV, falcine sinus, HC

SELECTED REFERENCES

1. Lasjaunias PL et al: The management of vein of Galen aneurysmal malformations. Neurosurgery. 59(5 Suppl 3):S184-94; discussion S3-13, 2006
2. Gailloud P et al: Diagnosis and management of vein of galen aneurysmal malformations. J Perinatol. 25(8):542-51, 2005
3. Halbach VV et al: Endovascular treatment of mural-type vein of Galen malformations. J Neurosurg. 89(1):74-80, 1998

VEIN OF GALEN MALFORMATION

IMAGE GALLERY

Typical

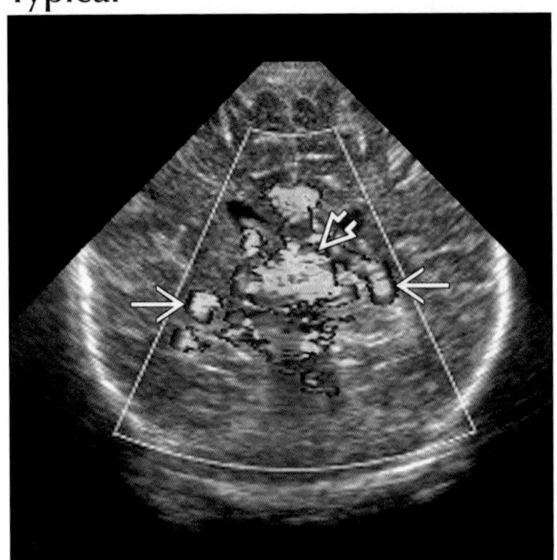

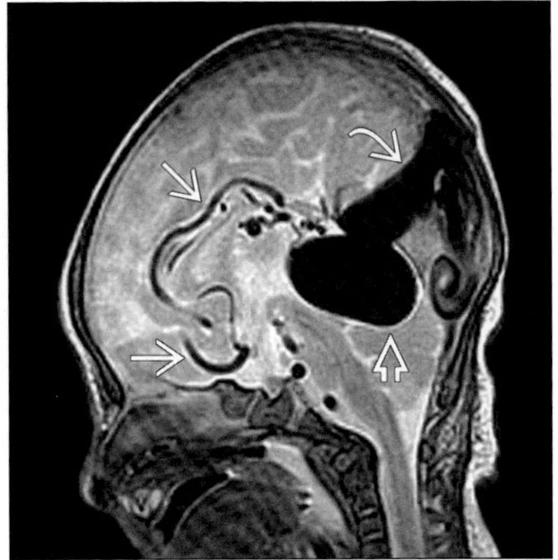

(Left) Coronal color Doppler ultrasound in a neonate with VGAM shows large arterial feeders bilaterally ➔ that drain into a dilated, midline MPV ➔. **(Right)** Sagittal T2WI MR shows enlarged pericallosal arteries ➔ that drain into a dilated MPV ➔. The straight sinus is absent and venous egress is via a persistent falcine sinus ➔.

Typical

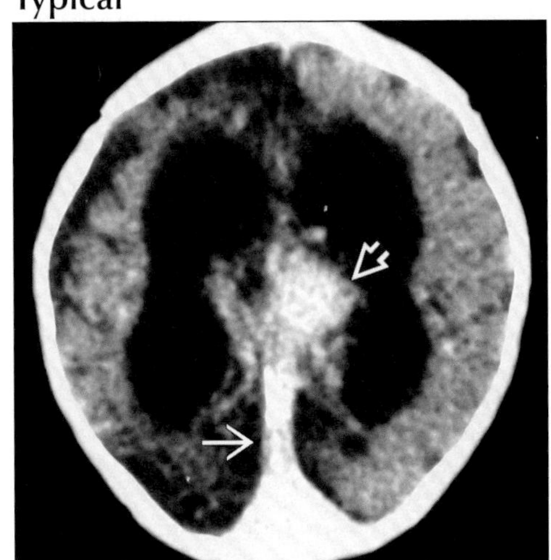

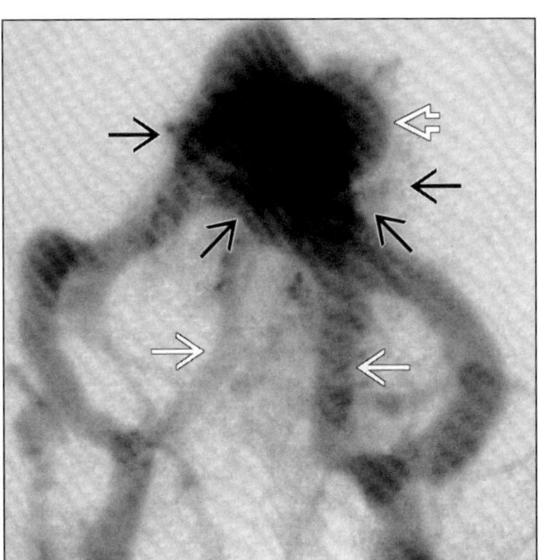

(Left) Axial CECT in a developmentally delayed infant with VGAM shows hydrocephalus and encephalomalacia due to long-standing venous hypertension. Note dilated MPV ➔ and falcine sinus ➔. **(Right)** Posteroanterior venous phase DSA shows a dilated MPV ➔ and adjacent superior sagittal sinus. Note also the occipital sinuses bilaterally ➔. Numerous small arterial feeders enter the MPV ➔.

Typical

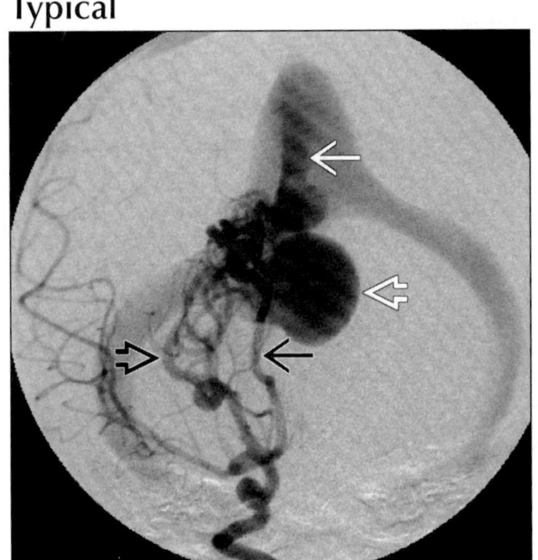

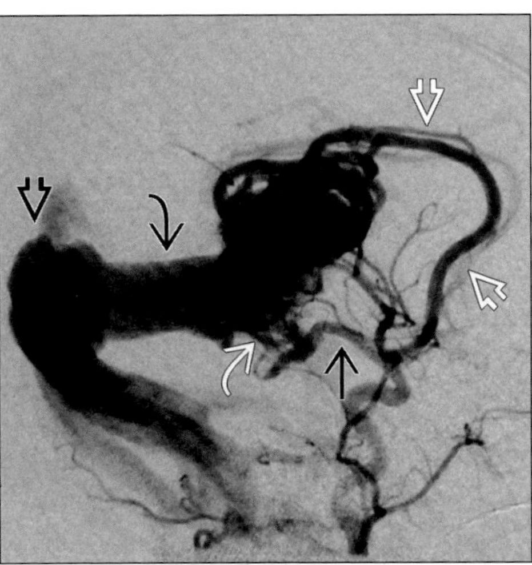

(Left) AP right ICA DSA in a 3 week old with heart failure shows a choroidal type VGAM supplied by anterior ➔ and posterior ➔ cerebral artery branches. Note MPV ➔ and falcine sinus ➔. **(Right)** Lateral carotid DSA shows a choroidal VGAM supplied by hypertrophied anterior cerebral arteries ➔ as well as posterior choroidal and thalamoperforating arteries ➔ via the PCoA ➔. A large falcine sinus ➔ and dilated torcular Herophili ➔ are present.

ACUTE ISCHEMIC STROKE

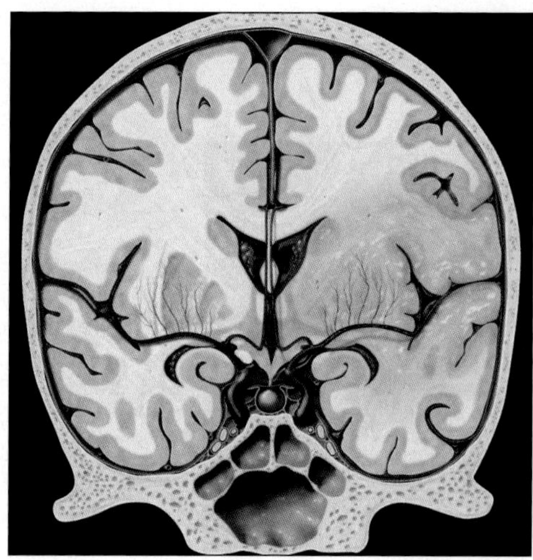

Coronal graphic illustrates left MCA M1 embolus. This proximal occlusion results in complete MCA territory infarction, including the deep gray nuclei perfused by lenticulostriate arteries.

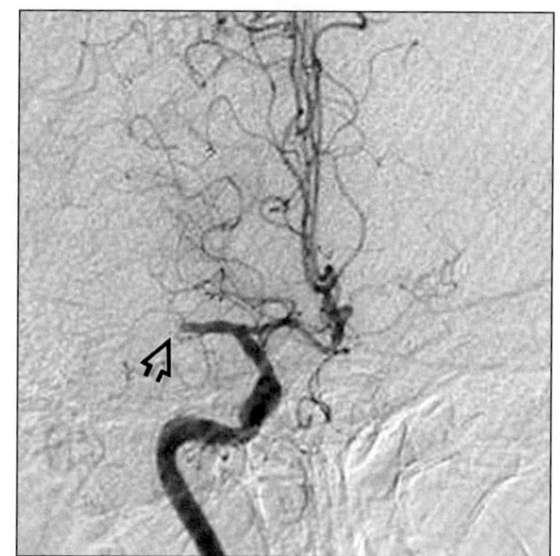

Anteroposterior DSA shows abrupt truncation ➪ of the M1 segment of the right middle cerebral artery compatible with thrombosis/embolus with resultant acute cerebral ischemia.

TERMINOLOGY

Abbreviations and Synonyms

- Stroke = lay term for sudden onset neurologic symptoms; many etiologies
- Cerebrovascular accident (CVA), acute cerebral ischemia/infarction

Definitions

- Interrupted blood flow to brain resulting in cerebral ischemia/infarction with variable neurologic deficit

IMAGING FINDINGS

General Features

- Best diagnostic clue: MR diffusion restriction with correlating ADC map
- Location: One or more vascular territories; vascular border-zones ("watershed")
- Size: Dependent on degree of compromise, collateral circulation
- Morphology
  - Cortical gray matter infarct: Usually wedge-shaped
  - Deep white matter infarct: Variable distribution

CT Findings

- NECT
  - Hyperdense vessel: Acute intravascular thrombus
    - Hyperdense MCA M1 segment (35-50%)
    - "Dot sign" = occluded MCA branches in sylvian fissure (16-17%)
  - Loss of gray-white matter distinction in first 3 hrs seen in 50-70%
    - Loss of insular "ribbon", obscuration of deep nuclei
  - Parenchymal hypodensity
    - If > 1/3 MCA territory initially, large lesion later
    - Temporary transition to isodensity (up to 54%) at 2-3 weeks post-onset = CT "fogging"
  - Gyral swelling, sulcal effacement 12-24 hrs
  - Hemorrhagic transformation possible
    - Delayed onset (24-48 hrs) is most typical
    - Usually due to reperfusion following lysis of vascular occlusion
- CECT
  - Enhancing cortical vessels = slow flow or collateralization acutely, absent vessels = occlusion

DDx: Acute Ischemic Stroke

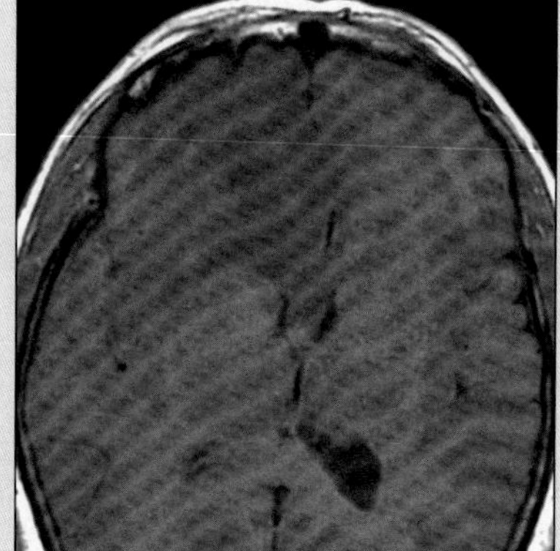

Astrocytoma

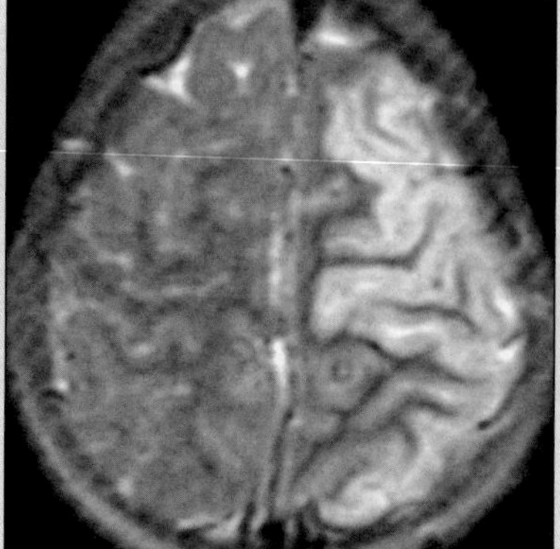

Cerebritis

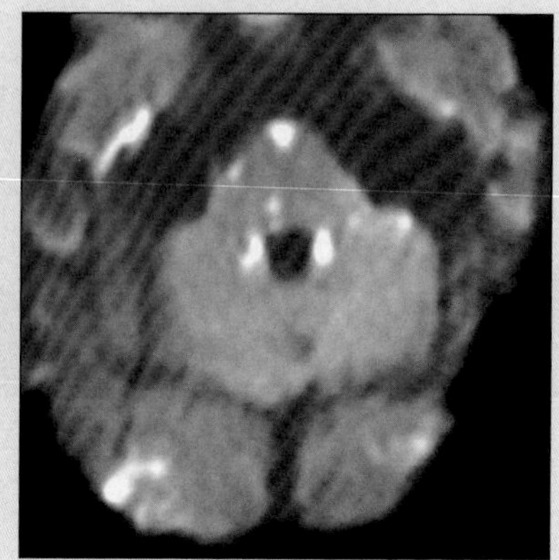

Contusion and DAI

ACUTE ISCHEMIC STROKE

Key Facts

Terminology

- Interrupted blood flow to brain resulting in cerebral ischemia/infarction with variable neurologic deficit

Imaging Findings

- Best diagnostic clue: MR diffusion restriction with correlating ADC map
- Location: One or more vascular territories; vascular border-zones ("watershed")
- Cortical gray matter infarct: Usually wedge-shaped
- Deep white matter infarct: Variable distribution
- DWI improves hyperacute stroke detection to 95% (conventional MR sequences positive in 70-80%)
- DWI/PWI "mismatch" = "penumbra" or "at risk" tissue
- MR with FLAIR, GRE, DWI, MRA, PWI
- NECT, perfusion CT, CTA
- DSA with thrombolysis in selected patients

Top Differential Diagnoses

- Hyperdense Vessel Mimics
- Other Intra-Parenchymal Brain Lesions

Pathology

- Second most common worldwide cause of death
- Number one cause of US morbidity

Clinical Issues

- Focal acute neurologic deficit
- Clinical diagnosis inaccurate in 15-20% of "strokes"
- "Time is brain": At present, IV rTPA window < 3 hrs; IA rTPA window < 6 hrs (reduces risk of hemorrhage)

Diagnostic Checklist

- DWI positive for acute infarct only if ADC correlates

  - Triphasic perfusion CT: Assess infarcted core vs. ischemic but viable penumbra to identify patients who will benefit most from revascularization
    - Determines cerebral blood volume (CBV) and/or flow (CBF), mean transit time (MTT)
    - ↓ CBV = infarcted core, ↑ MTT = ischemic penumbra
  - Cortical/gyral enhancement after 48-72 hrs
- CTA: Identifies occlusions, stenoses, collaterals

MR Findings

- T1WI: Early cortical swelling & hypointensity, loss of gray-white borders
- T2WI
  - Early cortical swelling, hyperintensity in affected distribution
  - May normalize 2-3 weeks post-onset = MR "fogging"
- PD/Intermediate: Loss of flow voids = slow flow vs. occlusion
- FLAIR
  - May be positive (hyperintense) when other sequences normal (as early as 3-6 hrs)
  - MR intra-arterial signal on FLAIR = early specific sign of major vessel occlusion
- T2* GRE
  - Sensitive for detection of acute "petechial" blood products
  - Shows thrombosed vessel as arterial "blooming" from clot susceptibility
- DWI
  - Hyperintense restriction from "cytotoxic" edema
    - DWI improves hyperacute stroke detection to 95% (conventional MR sequences positive in 70-80%)
    - Usually correlates to "infarct core"; some diffusion abnormalities reversible
    - May have reduced sensitivity in brainstem and medulla in first 24 hours
    - High signal may persist (after 10 days, T2 effect predominates over low ADC = "T2 shine-through")
  - Corresponding low signal on ADC maps
    - Confirms true restricted diffusion
    - May normalize after tissue reperfusion
    - Note: Hyperintensity on ADC map (T2 "shine-through") differentiates diffusion restriction mimics
  - Distinguishes cytotoxic from vasogenic edema in complicated cases
- T1 C+
  - Variable enhancement patterns evolve over time
    - Immediate: Intravascular enhancement (stasis from slow antegrade or retrograde collateral flow)
    - Early: Meningeal enhancement (pial collateral flow appears in first 24-48 hrs, then resolves over 3-4 days)
    - Late acute: Parenchymal enhancement (appears after 24-48 hrs, can persist for weeks/months)
- MRA: Demonstrates major vessel occlusions, stenoses, collateral status
- MRS
  - Elevated lactate, decreased NAA
    - At intermediate TE (135 or 144) lactate doublet inverts
- Perfusion MR
  - Bolus-tracking T2* Gadolinium perfusion imaging (PWI)
    - Non-quantitative; depicts relative perfusion maps (rCBV, rCBF, rMTT)
  - DWI/PWI "mismatch" = "penumbra" or "at risk" tissue
    - Found in 75-80% of cases
    - rCBF most accurate, rMTT most sensitive (to detect region of penumbra)

Nuclear Medicine Findings

- SPECT: Voxel-based maps reflect viable neurons, potentially salvageable tissue

Angiographic Findings

- Conventional
  - Vessel occlusion (cutoff, tapered, tram track, meniscus)
  - Slow antegrade flow, retrograde collateral flow
- Interventional: rTPA, GPIIb/IIIa inhibitors, mechanical thrombolysis

ACUTE ISCHEMIC STROKE

- Fibrinolytic therapy: Selected acute nonhemorrhagic ischemia within a 6 hr window (traditional approach)
- Mechanical thrombectomy or physiologic information (CBV, CBF, MTT) may widen window
- Significantly improves clinical outcomes

Imaging Recommendations

- Best imaging tool: MR + DWI, T2*
- Protocol advice
  - MR with FLAIR, GRE, DWI, MRA, PWI
  - NECT, perfusion CT, CTA
  - DSA with thrombolysis in selected patients

DIFFERENTIAL DIAGNOSIS

Hyperdense Vessel Mimics

- High hematocrit; calcification in vessel wall
- Low density brain → vessels appear hyperdense

Other Intra-Parenchymal Brain Lesions

- Infiltrating neoplasm (e.g., astrocytoma)
- Cerebritis, encephalitis
- Other inflammatory processes (e.g., acute MS)
- Cerebral contusion/DAI
- Evolving encephalomalacia

PATHOLOGY

General Features

- Etiology
  - Many causes of acute cerebral ischemia (thrombotic vs. embolic, dissection, vasculitis, hypoperfusion)
  - Early: Critical disturbance in CBF
    - Severely ischemic core has CBF < 6-8 mL/100 g/min (normal ~ 60 mL/100 g/min)
    - Causes oxygen depletion, energy failure, terminal depolarization, ion homeostasis failure
    - Represents bulk of final infarct → cytotoxic edema, cell death
  - Later: Evolution from ischemia to infarction depends on many factors (e.g., BP fluctuations, embolic fragmentation, hyperglycemia, reperfusion)
  - Ischemic "penumbra" CBF between 10-20 mL/100 g/min
    - Theoretically salvageable tissue
    - Target of thrombolysis, neuroprotective agents
- Epidemiology
  - Second most common worldwide cause of death
  - Number one cause of US morbidity
  - Newly-identified risk factors: C-reactive protein, homocysteine
- Associated abnormalities: Cardiac disease, prothrombotic states

Gross Pathologic & Surgical Features

- Acute thrombosis of major vessel
- Pale, swollen brain; GM/WM boundaries "smudged"

Microscopic Features

- After 4 hrs: Eosinophilic neurons with pyknotic nuclei
- 15-24 hrs: Neutrophils invade, necrotic nuclei look like "eosinophilic ghosts"
- 2-3 days: Blood-derived phagocytes
- 1 week: Reactive astrocytosis, ↑ capillary density
- End result: Fluid-filled cavity lined by astrocytes

CLINICAL ISSUES

Presentation

- Focal acute neurologic deficit
  - Varies with vascular distribution
  - Weakness, aphasia, decreased mental status

Demographics

- Usually older adults, no gender predilection
- Children, young adults → consider underlying disease; sickle cell, moyamoya, NF1, cardiac, drugs

Natural History & Prognosis

- Clinical diagnosis inaccurate in 15-20% of "strokes"
  - Seizure (Todd paralysis), migraine, inflammatory diseases
- "Malignant" MCA infarct (coma, death)
  - Up to 10% of all CVA patients
  - Fatal brain swelling with increased ICP

Treatment

- Generally unfavorable outcome without treatment
- "Time is brain": At present, IV rTPA window < 3 hrs; IA rTPA window < 6 hrs (reduces risk of hemorrhage)
- Patient selection = most important factor in outcome
  - Symptom onset < 6 hrs
  - CT shows no parenchymal hemorrhage
  - < 1/3 MCA territory CT hypodensity

DIAGNOSTIC CHECKLIST

Image Interpretation Pearls

- Perform DWI on all brain MRs; time cost < 1 min
- DWI positive for acute infarct only if ADC correlates

SELECTED REFERENCES

1. Parsons MW et al: Identification of the penumbra and infarct core on hyperacute noncontrast and perfusion CT. Neurology. 68(10):730-6, 2007
2. Wessels T et al: Contribution of diffusion-weighted imaging in determination of stroke etiology. AJNR Am J Neuroradiol. 27(1):35-9, 2006
3. Abou-Chebl A et al: Multimodal therapy for the treatment of severe ischemic stroke combining GPIIb/IIIa antagonists and angioplasty after failure of thrombolysis. Stroke. 36(10):2286-8, 2005
4. Kim EY et al: Prediction of hemorrhagic transformation in acute ischemic stroke: role of diffusion-weighted imaging and early parenchymal enhancement. AJNR Am J Neuroradiol. 26(5):1050-5, 2005
5. Seitz RJ et al: Initial ischemic event: perfusion-weighted MR imaging and apparent diffusion coefficient for stroke evolution. Radiology. 237(3):1020-8, 2005
6. Diaz J et al: Cerebral ischemia: new risk factors. Cerebrovasc Dis. 17 Suppl 1:43-50, 2004
7. Fiehler J et al: Predictors of apparent diffusion coefficient normalization in stroke patients. Stroke. 35(2):514-9, 2004

ACUTE ISCHEMIC STROKE

IMAGE GALLERY

Typical

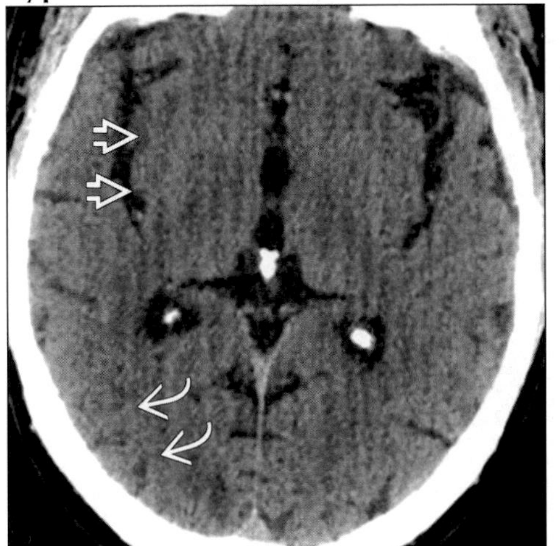

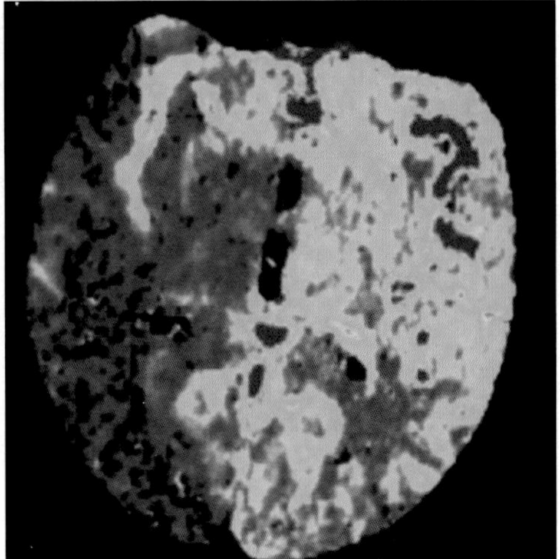

*(**Left**) Axial NECT shows very subtle loss of the right "insular ribbon" ⇨ and minimal effacement of right temporal sulci ↪. These findings are nearly undetectable on screening CT alone. (**Right**) Axial CECT perfusion image, cerebral blood flow map, in the same case as previous image, clearly shows large right MCA territory of ischemic but potentially salvagable brain tissue. (Courtesy A. Cianfoni, MD).*

Typical

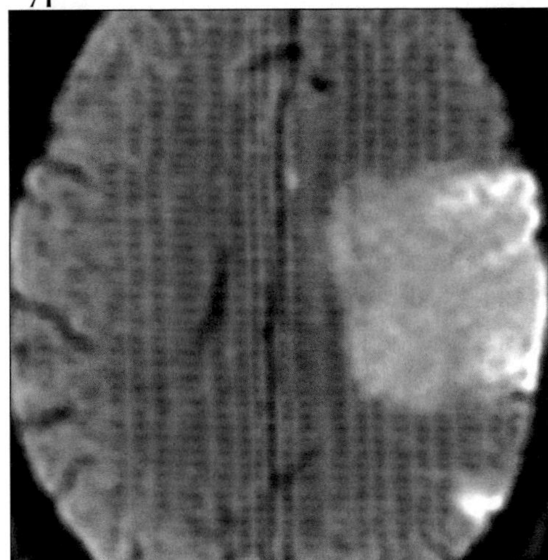

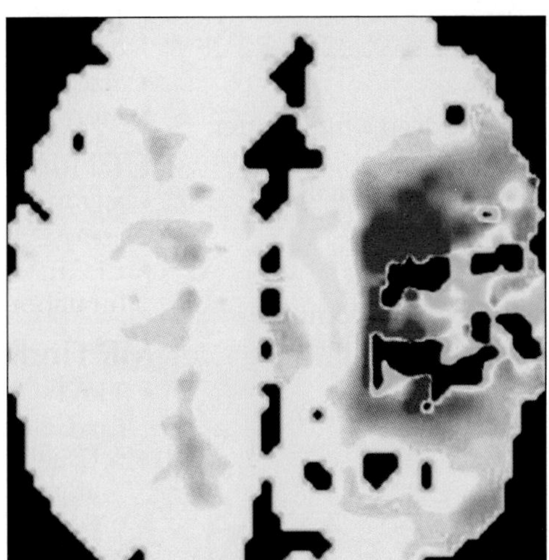

*(**Left**) Axial MR DWI shows left posterior frontal and parietal regions of infarction. Corresponding ADC image hypointensity confirmed true restricted diffusion (not shown). (**Right**) Axial MR PWI, mean transit time map, in the same patient as previous image, shows similar region of abnormality signifying no significant salvageable ischemic penumbra. (Courtesy A. Cianfoni, MD).*

Typical

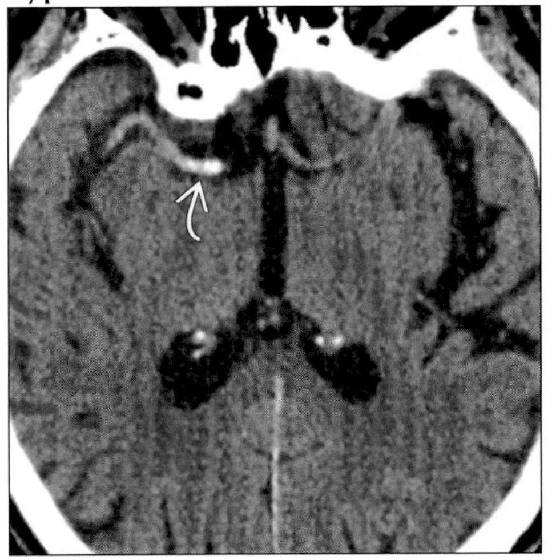

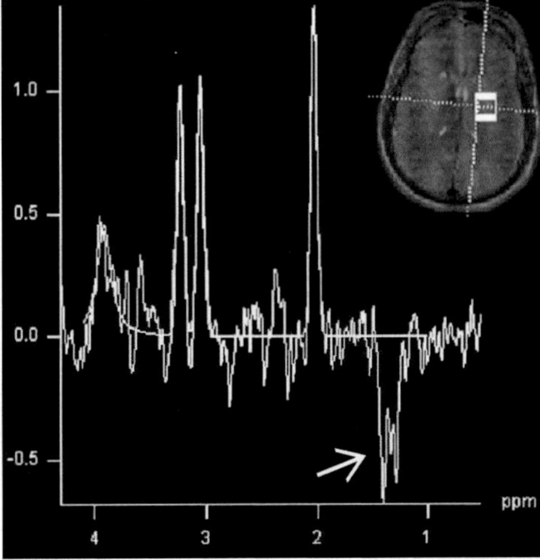

*(**Left**) Axial NECT demonstrates a hyperdense right MCA ↪ due to thrombus occluding the vessel. Note differing lower attenuation of the left-sided vessels confirming a true finding. (**Right**) MR spectroscopy, TE 144, of left lentiform nucleus in a patient with anoxic injury depicts inverted doublet peak centered at 1.3 ppm (lactate metabolite) → indicative of acute ischemia.*

SMALL VESSEL ISCHEMIA

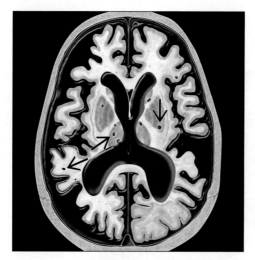

Axial graphic shows diffuse atrophy, left occipital cortical infarct and multiple foci of deep white matter/basal ganglia lacunar infarcts →, typical in small vessel ischemic disease.

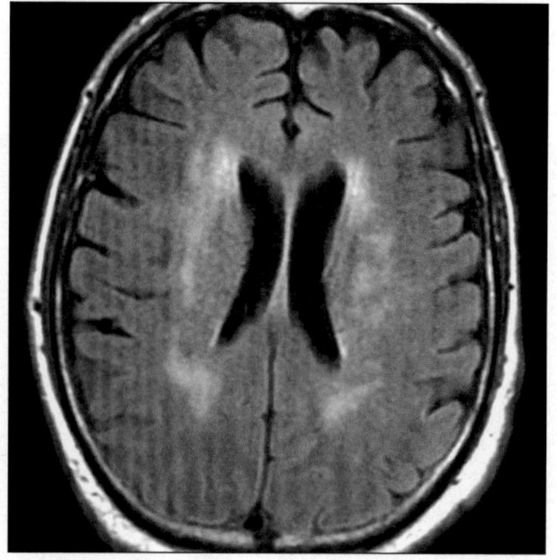

Axial T2WI MR FLAIR shows ill-defined patchy and confluent areas of deep white matter hyperintensity in the bilateral corona radiata consistent with chronic small vessel ischemic disease.

TERMINOLOGY

Abbreviations and Synonyms

- Arteriolosclerosis, microangiopathy, deep white matter (WM) ischemia
- Imaging correlate = leukoariosis or periventricular leukoencephalopathy

Definitions

- Sclerosis of small-sized arteries (arterioles), common from chronic hypertension and/or diabetes mellitus, often leading to dementia
- Ischemic myelin loss in deep WM and brainstem to frank subcortical infarction

IMAGING FINDINGS

General Features

- Best diagnostic clue
  - WM rarefaction on CT; patchy/confluent hyperintensity on PD/T2WI/FLAIR
  - Small, well-circumscribed foci of encephalomalacia (lacunar infarcts) in deep WM, basal ganglia & pons
- Location: Periventricular white matter (PVWM) and deep WM, basal ganglia, brainstem
- Size: Varies, progress with age
- Morphology: Focal, patchy or confluent

CT Findings

- NECT: Multifocal/confluent ill-defined hypodense areas ≥ 5 mm
- CECT: No enhancement unless acute/subacute infarction

MR Findings

- T1WI
  - ± Generalized atrophy (large ventricles, sulci)
  - Usually negative with PVWM disease (myelin pallor) alone
  - Focal hypointensities in PVWM and basal ganglia/pons with lacunar infarction
- T2WI
  - Ill-defined hyperintensities ≥ 5 mm = PVWM disease
  - Focal well-defined hyperintensities 3-15 mm = chronic lacunar infarcts
- FLAIR

DDx: Small Vessel Ischemia

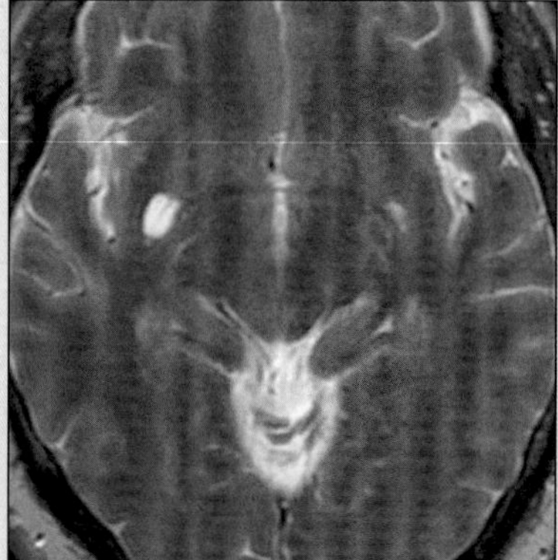

Dilated Perivascular Spaces

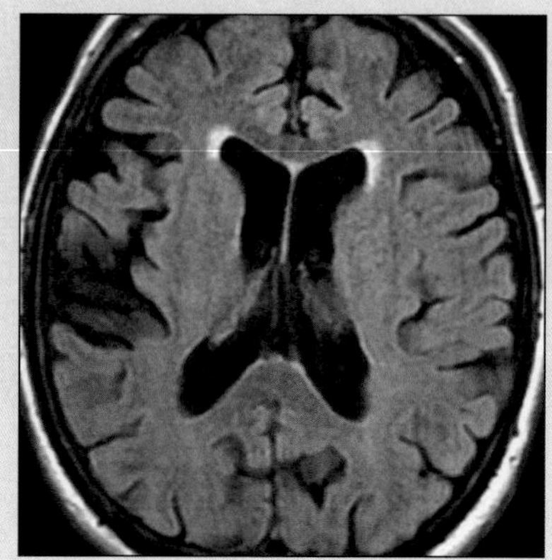

Ependymitis Granularis

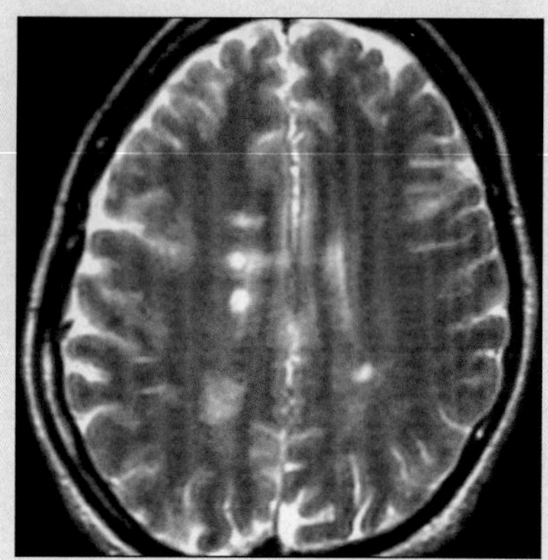

Multiple Sclerosis

SMALL VESSEL ISCHEMIA

Key Facts

Terminology
- Arteriolosclerosis, microangiopathy, deep white matter (WM) ischemia

Imaging Findings
- WM rarefaction on CT; patchy/confluent hyperintensity on PD/T2WI/FLAIR
- Small, well-circumscribed foci of encephalomalacia (lacunar infarcts) in deep WM, basal ganglia and pons
- Hyperintensities usually oriented parallel to ependyma
- T2* GRE: ± Multifocal "black dots" on T2* (overlap with chronic hypertension, amyloid)

Top Differential Diagnoses
- Perivascular (Virchow-Robin) Spaces
- Ependymitis Granularis
- Demyelinating Disease

Pathology
- Hypertensive occlusive disease of small penetrating arteries
- Embolic, atheromatous or thrombotic lesions in long single penetrating end arterioles supplying deep cerebral structures

Clinical Issues
- From normal to focal neurologic deficit; minimal cognitive impairment to demented
- Clinical profile: Older patient with cerebrovascular risk factors (hypertension, age, hypercholesterolemia, diabetes, etc.)

Diagnostic Checklist
- Use FLAIR, GRE sequences in all elderly patients

- Most conspicuous sequence for PVWM hyperintensities
  - Hyperintensities usually oriented parallel to ependyma
- Chronic lacunar infarcts hypointense centrally (CSF) with hyperintense gliotic rim
- T2* GRE: ± Multifocal "black dots" on T2* (overlap with chronic hypertension, amyloid)
- DWI: No associated restriction unless acute (lacunar) infarct present
- T1 C+: Nonenhancing unless acute/subacute infarction
- MRS: Reduced N-acetyl aspartate (NAA), ↓ NAA/Cr ratio (marker of neuronal/axonal disruption)
- DTI: Reduced fractional anisotropy (FA) and increased mean diffusivity (MD)
  - Consistent with axonal loss or dysfunction
  - Correlates with degree of cognitive impairment
- PWI: Can see ↓ cerebral blood flow (rCBF)

Angiographic Findings
- Conventional: Small and larger vessel arterial stenoses commonly associated

Imaging Recommendations
- Best imaging tool: NECT screen; MR (esp. if acutely symptomatic)
- Protocol advice: MR with FLAIR, DWI + GRE

DIFFERENTIAL DIAGNOSIS

Perivascular (Virchow-Robin) Spaces
- Variable size, well-delineated
- Most common near anterior commissure, cerebral WM
- Signal, attenuation identical to CSF
- Usually no peripheral high signal on FLAIR but can be seen esp. with larger foci

Ependymitis Granularis
- Younger patients, ≥ 40 years of age
- T2 hyperintensity parallel to ependyma usually near frontal horns, frontal horn "caps"
- Represents increased water content in less tightly integrated periventricular white matter
- Asymptomatic

Demyelinating Disease
- Usually young adult patients
- MS > ADEM
- Usually ovoid, periventricular T2 hyperintensities
- Oriented perpendicular to ependyma
- Callososeptal interface involved (rare with ASVD)

PATHOLOGY

General Features
- General path comments
  - "Microangiopathy-related cerebral damage" = PVWM hyperintensities, lacunar infarcts
  - PVWM hyperintensities on imaging does not always have pathologic correlate
  - Significance of white matter myelin pallor controversial; findings nonspecific, likely due to several types of arteriopathy
    - Arteriolosclerosis
    - Chronic hypertension and/or diabetes mellitus
    - Cerebral amyloid angiopathy
    - Cerebral autosomal dominant arteriopathy with subcortical infarct and leukoencephalopathy (CADASIL)
  - Clinical + radiographic picture overlaps with multi-infarct and/or vascular dementia and subcortical arteriosclerotic encephalopathy = Binswanger disease
- Genetics
  - General risk factors for peripheral/cerebral vascular diseases
    - APOE ϵ4 alleles
    - Angiotensinogen gene promoter
  - CADASIL
    - Notch3 mutations (chromosome 19)
- Etiology
  - Hypertensive occlusive disease of small penetrating arteries

SMALL VESSEL ISCHEMIA

- Embolic, atheromatous or thrombotic lesions in long single penetrating end arterioles supplying deep cerebral structures
- Epidemiology
  - Strong association with systemic hypertension
  - Lacunar infarcts account for 15-20% of all strokes
  - Most common stroke subtype associated with vascular dementia
    - Vascular dementia (VaD) third most common cause of dementia (after Alzheimer disease, Lewy body disease)

Gross Pathologic & Surgical Features

- Prominent sulci and ventricles common
- Periventricular WM spongiosis
- Multifocal lacunes often present

Microscopic Features

- PVWM hyperintensities have spectrum of histopathologic correlates
  - Degenerated myelin (myelin "pallor")
  - Axonal loss, increased intra/extracellular fluid
  - Gliosis, spongiosis
  - Arteriolosclerosis, small vessel occlusions
  - Dilated perivascular spaces
- Lacunar infarction
  - Neuronal/axonal loss
  - Ischemic necrosis and cavitation
  - Surrounding gliosis along margin of infarction
  - Hypertensive hyalinization of supplying arterioles
  - Pigmented macrophages occasionally seen, suggesting possible hemorrhagic component

Staging, Grading or Classification Criteria

- European Task Force on Age-Related White Matter Changes (ARWMC) rating scale for MR and CT (for ill-defined lesions ≥ 5 mm)
  - White matter lesions
    - 0 = no lesions (including symmetrical caps, bands)
    - 1 = focal lesions
    - 2 = beginning confluence of lesions
    - 3 = diffuse involvement, with or without U-fibers
  - Basal ganglia lesions
    - 0 = no lesions
    - 1 = 1 focal lesion (≥ 5 mm)
    - 2 = > 1 focal lesion
    - 3 = confluent lesions

CLINICAL ISSUES

Presentation

- Most common signs/symptoms
  - Broad range
    - From normal to focal neurologic deficit; minimal cognitive impairment to demented
- Clinical Profile: Older patient with cerebrovascular risk factors (hypertension, age, hypercholesterolemia, diabetes, obesity, smoking, etc.)

Demographics

- Age
  - PVWM hyperintensities almost universal after 65 y
  - Lacunar infarcts in 1/3 of asymptomatic patients > 65 y
- Gender: M = F

Natural History & Prognosis

- Increased risk of developing cognitive decline and dementia, pseudobulbar palsy, motor deficits
- Presence of multiple lacunar infarcts prognostic indicator of level of recovery as well as ongoing incidence of recurrence

Treatment

- Modification of known cerebrovascular risk factors
- Identification of possible embolic source

DIAGNOSTIC CHECKLIST

Consider

- Use FLAIR, GRE sequences in all elderly patients

SELECTED REFERENCES

1. Enzinger C et al: Progression of cerebral white matter lesions -- clinical and radiological considerations. J Neurol Sci. 257(1-2):5-10, 2007
2. Schmidt R et al: Progression of leukoaraiosis and cognition. Stroke. 38(9):2619-25, 2007
3. Matsusue E et al: White matter changes in elderly people: MR-pathologic correlations. Magn Reson Med Sci. 5(2):99-104, 2006
4. Nitkunan A et al: Correlations between MRS and DTI in cerebral small vessel disease. NMR Biomed. 19(5):610-6, 2006
5. Tajitsu K et al: [The correlation between lacunes and microbleeds on magnetic resonance imaging in consecutive 180 patients] No Shinkei Geka. 34(5):483-9, 2006
6. Wong A et al: Hyperhomocysteinemia is associated with volumetric white matter change in patients with small vessel disease. J Neurol. 253(4):441-7, 2006
7. Seifert T et al: Acute small subcortical infarctions on diffusion weighted MRI: clinical presentation and aetiology. J Neurol Neurosurg Psychiatry. 76(11):1520-4, 2005
8. Arboix A et al: New concepts in lacunar stroke etiology: the constellation of small-vessel arterial disease. Cerebrovasc Dis. 17 Suppl 1:58-62, 2004
9. Arima K et al: Cerebral arterial pathology of CADASIL and CARASIL (Maeda syndrome). Neuropathology. 23(4):327-34, 2003
10. Schmidt R et al: Risk factors and progression of small vessel disease-related cerebral abnormalities. J Neural Transm Suppl. (62):47-52, 2002
11. Marti-Fabregas J et al: Blood pressure variability and leukoaraiosis amount in cerebral small-vessel disease. Acta Neurol Scand. 104(6):358-63, 2001
12. Schmidt H et al: Angiotensinogen gene promoter haplotype and microangiopathy-related cerebral damage: results of the Austrian Stroke Prevention Study. Stroke. 32(2):405-12, 2001
13. Hirono N et al: Effect of the apolipoprotein E epsilon4 allele on white matter hyperintensities in dementia. Stroke. 31(6):1263-8, 2000
14. Scheltens P et al: White matter changes on CT and MRI: an overview of visual rating scales. European Task Force on Age-Related White Matter Changes. Eur Neurol. 39(2):80-9, 1998

SMALL VESSEL ISCHEMIA

IMAGE GALLERY

Typical

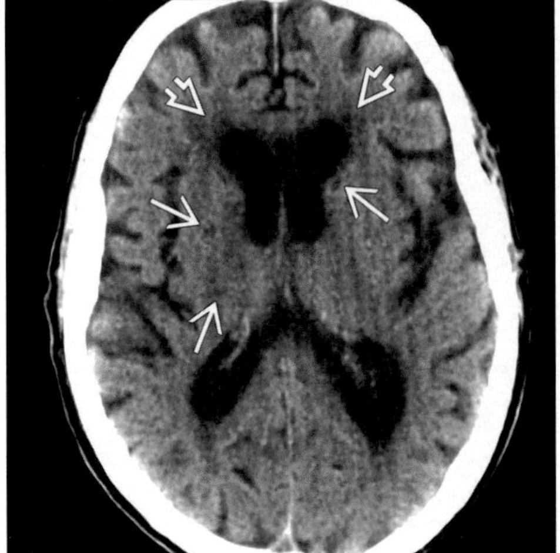

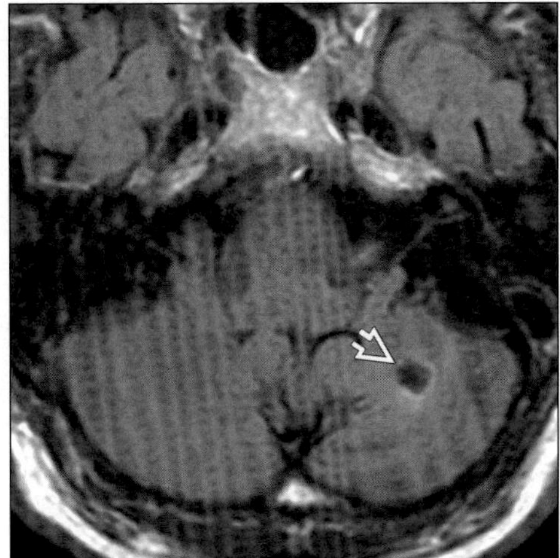

(Left) *Axial NECT demonstrates atrophy, diffuse periventricular hypodensity ➔ and multiple focal deep gray and white matter lacunar infarcts ➔ from small vessel ischemia.* ***(Right)*** *Axial T2WI MR FLAIR shows focal hypointense encephalomalacia (CSF signal) centrally with surrounding hyperintense gliosis deep in the left cerebellum ➔ from chronic lacunar infarction.*

Typical

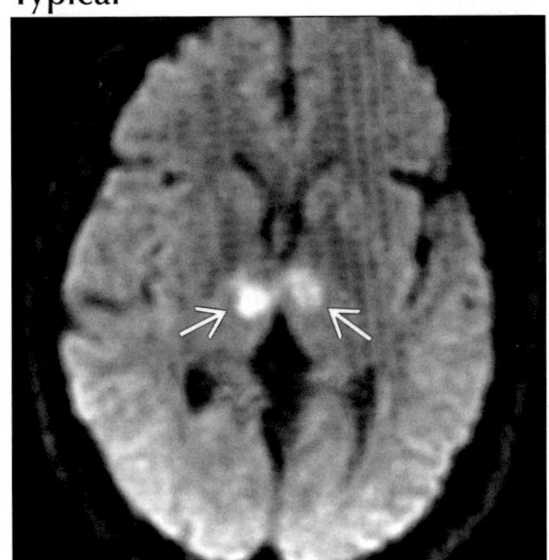

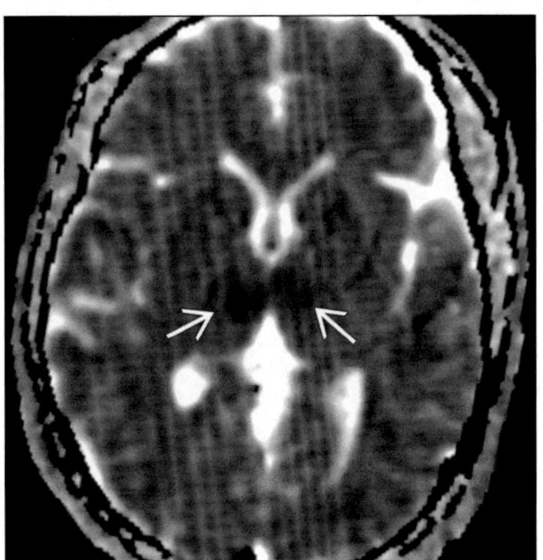

(Left) *Axial MR DWI shows foci of hyperintensity in the bilateral thalamic nuclei ➔ from occlusion of the "artery of Percheron" a small thalamoperforator from the posterior cerebral artery.* ***(Right)*** *Axial ADC map DWI in the same patient as previous image, depicts hypointensity in bilateral thalamic nuclei ➔ confirming suspected acute deep gray matter lacunar infarction from small vessel ischemic disease.*

Variant

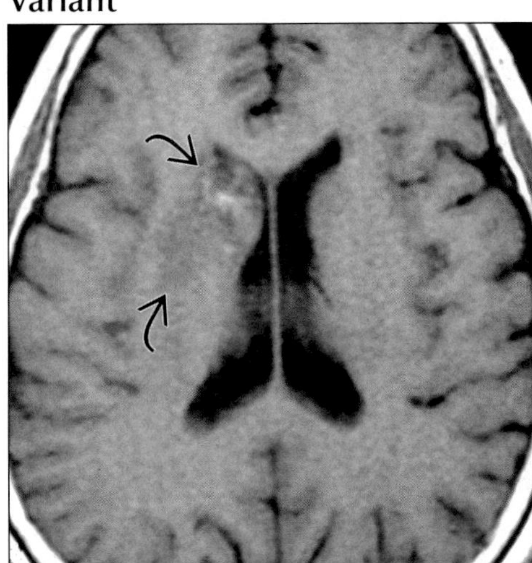

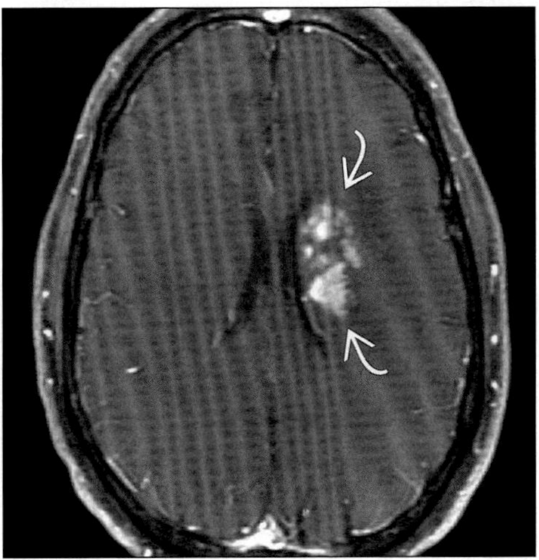

(Left) *Axial T1WI MR shows focus of hypointensity with punctate hyperintensity ➔ in the right caudate nucleus and adjacent deep white matter from subacute hemorrhagic lacunar infarction.* ***(Right)*** *Axial T1WI MR post-contrast demonstrates multifocal patchy enhancement ➔ in the left caudate nucleus and corona radiata deep white matter from subacute small vessel infarction.*

PEDIATRIC/YOUNG ADULT STROKE

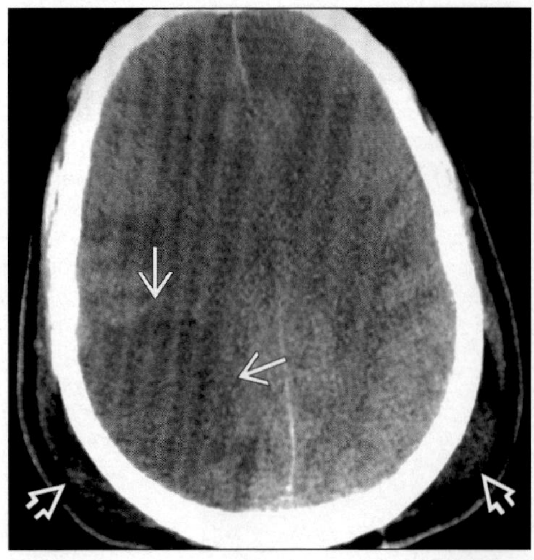

Axial NECT shows wedge-shaped (MCA territory) hypodensity in right frontoparietal lobe ➡ due to cerebral infarction following traumatic injury. Note scalp soft tissue swelling ➡.

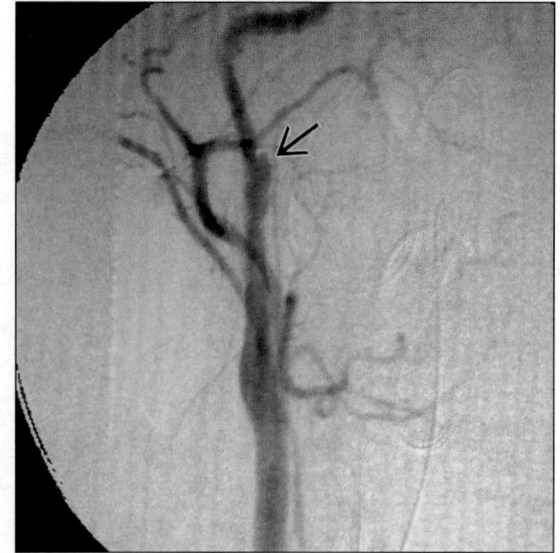

Anteroposterior DSA of right common carotid artery injection in the same patient as previous image, shows medial outpouching of the midcervical right ICA ➡ from post-traumatic pseudoaneurysm formation.

TERMINOLOGY

Abbreviations and Synonyms

- Cerebral ischemia/infarct, cerebrovascular accident (CVA), hypoxic-ischemic encephalopathy (HIE)

Definitions

- Acute alteration of neurologic function due to loss of vascular integrity with resultant parenchymal damage

IMAGING FINDINGS

General Features

- Best diagnostic clue: Edema, restricted diffusion (acutely) in affected territory
- Location
  - Neonatal: HIE: Periventricular white matter (WM) = pre-term; subcortical watershed WM = full-term; basal ganglia (BG) = either pre-term or full-term (indicates severe profound insult)
  - Child: Any part of brain can be affected; middle cerebral artery (MCA) territory most common
- Morphology
  - Ischemic stroke caused by arterial occlusion often conforms to specific arterial territory
  - Venous infarct territories often less well-delineated

CT Findings

- NECT
  - Decreased attenuation of affected region
    - Often wedge-shaped; arterial territory
    - Diffuse ischemic injury can result in "reversal sign", with gray matter (GM) diffusely decreased in attenuation relative to WM
    - Decreased periventricular/subcortical WM density, loss of distinction of BG/internal capsule (IC) in HIE
  - Insular ribbon sign ⇒ loss of distinction of insular cortex with adjacent WM
  - Hyperdense MCA sign ⇒ increased density of thrombosed MCA
  - Venous occlusion: Hyperdense dural sinus ⇒ "delta" sign
  - Hemorrhage identification
    - Petechial cortical hemorrhage; usually incidental
    - WM or deep nuclear hemorrhage often mass-like ⇒ "reperfusion" hematoma within infarcted tissue

DDx: Pediatric/Young Adult Stroke

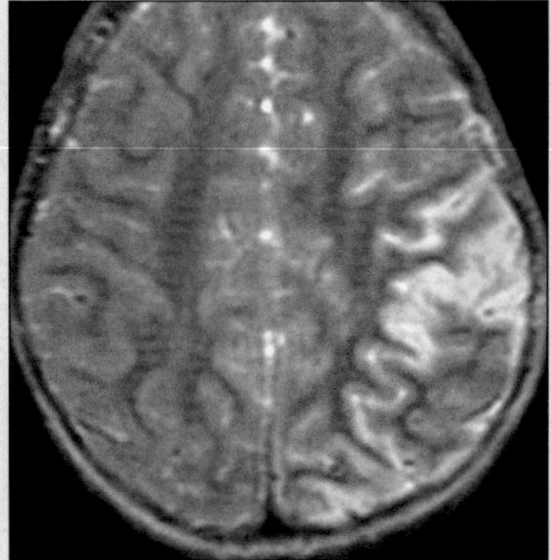

Cerebritis

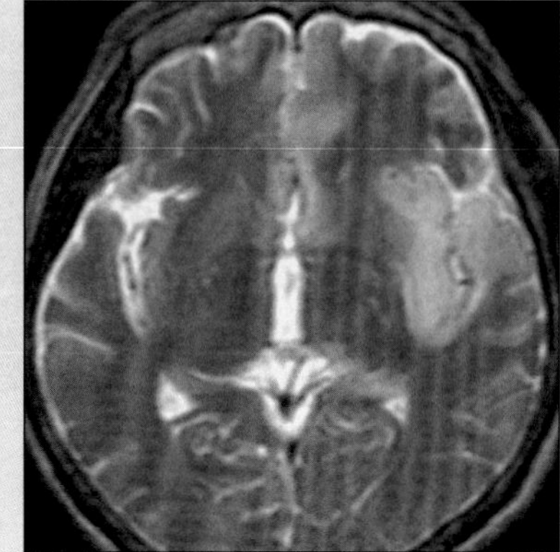

Herpes Encephalitis

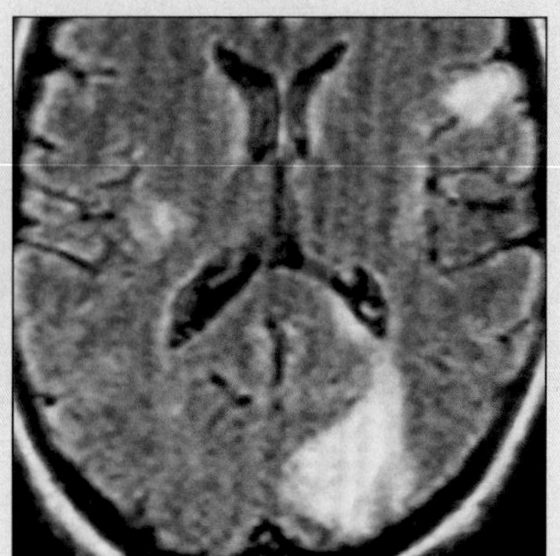

ADEM

PEDIATRIC/YOUNG ADULT STROKE

Key Facts

Terminology

- Acute alteration of neurologic function due to loss of vascular integrity with resultant parenchymal damage

Imaging Findings

- Ischemic stroke caused by arterial occlusion often conforms to specific arterial territory
- Venous infarct territories often less well-delineated
- T1WI: Best for HIE: Hyperintense signal in BG compared to IC (normally BG hypointense compared to myelinated IC)
- T2WI: Hyperintense edema evident in affected territory after 4-6 hours of arterial occlusion
- DWI: Restricted diffusion can be seen within 30 minutes of arterial occlusion
- MRA: Can demonstrate arterial narrowing and dilation in arteritides
- MRV: Can demonstrate focal venous occlusion
- MRS: ↑ Lactate hallmark of ischemia/infarct

Top Differential Diagnoses

- Inflammatory Processes
- Congenital Abnormalities
- Traumatic Injury

Pathology

- No underlying cause is discovered in > 33% of cases
- Incidence 2-3/100,000 per year in US

Clinical Issues

- Under-recognized as significant source of morbidity in pediatric population
- Children with stroke typically present in delayed fashion (> 24 hours)
- Capacity for recovery much greater than in adults

- CECT
  - Gyral enhancement of infarcted territory typically occurs after 4-7 days
  - Enhancement of venous sinus wall around nonenhancing clot ⇒ "empty delta" sign
- CTA
  - Invaluable for demonstrating focal vascular abnormalities in acute setting
  - May identify intimal flap in acutely dissected vessel

MR Findings

- T1WI
  - Gyral swelling and hypointensity in affected territory
  - Loss of normal vascular flow void
    - Entry slice artifact can cause false positive!
  - Best for HIE: Hyperintense signal in BG compared to IC (normally BG hypointense compared to myelinated IC)
  - May see hyperintense cortical ribbon from laminar necrosis
- T1WI FS
  - Axial head/neck images allows identification of crescent of mural hematoma in dissected vessel
    - Use in combination with MRA (2D or 3D)
- T2WI
  - Hyperintense edema evident in affected territory after 4-6 hours of arterial occlusion
  - Hypointense if hemorrhage, laminar necrosis
- FLAIR
  - More sensitive than T2WI for ischemia-induced parenchymal cytotoxic edema
  - Also shows loss of normal arterial flow voids
    - "Climbing ivy" ⇒ bright vessels in sulci distal to arterial occlusion due to slow flow
  - Excellent for detection of venous thrombosis
    - Iso/hyperintense thrombus compared to hypointense flowing blood in sinus
- DWI
  - Most sensitive imaging sequence for ischemic injury
  - Restricted diffusion can be seen within 30 minutes of arterial occlusion
  - Apparent diffusion coefficient (ADC) mapping essential to avoid false positive from "T2 shine through"
- T1 C+
  - Can provide earliest sign of proximal arterial occlusion ⇒ enhancement of arteries in territory distal to occlusion, classically in moyamoya
    - Collateral flow to distal vascular bed is slower
  - Beware! Contrast effect increased on 3T and GRE acquisitions ⇒ normal arteries/veins may show enhancement
- MRA
  - Sensitive in detection of arterial occlusion and stenosis in large and medium-sized cerebral vessels
  - Can demonstrate arterial narrowing and dilation in arteritides
- MRV: Can demonstrate focal venous occlusion
- MRS: ↑ Lactate hallmark of ischemia/infarct
- MR perfusion
  - Can provide valuable information regarding region at risk in setting of acute stroke
    - Ischemic penumbra ⇒ region with diminished perfusion not yet infarcted (perfusion-diffusion mismatch)
    - May define brain salvageable with acute stroke therapy

Nuclear Medicine Findings

- PET and SPECT can be used to investigate normal development, effect of therapy and subclinical pathology
  - Salvageable regions at risk (ischemic penumbra)
  - Effects of synangiosis surgery in moyamoya

Ultrasonographic Findings

- Grayscale Ultrasound
  - Affected territory hyperechoic in acute/subacute stage
  - HIE: Increased echogenicity periventricular WM
- Color Doppler
  - Direct Doppler evaluation ideal for surveillance of vascular occlusion in neonate with open sutures

PEDIATRIC/YOUNG ADULT STROKE

  - Transcranial Doppler evaluation of circle of Willis through temporal squamosa
    - Increased velocities can predict vessel stenoses
    - Used as screening tool in sickle cell anemia

Angiographic Findings

- Catheter angiography rarely necessary in acute evaluation of childhood stroke
  - Justified if contemplating endovascular therapy
  - Best modality for detailed evaluation of primary arteriopathies

Imaging Recommendations

- Best imaging tool: MR with DWI, MRA and MRV
- Protocol advice: Contrast can help in assessing timing of injury and in performing perfusion imaging

DIFFERENTIAL DIAGNOSIS

Inflammatory Processes

- Cerebritis
- Encephalitis
  - Viral ⇒ e.g., herpetic encephalitis
  - Autoimmune ⇒ e.g., ADEM

Congenital Abnormalities

- Tuberous sclerosis (cortical/subcortical tubers)

Traumatic Injury

- Cerebral contusion, diffuse axonal injury

Neoplastic Lesions

- Astrocytoma, ganglioglioma/neuroblastoma (verses mass-like ± hemorrhagic infarct)

PATHOLOGY

General Features

- General path comments: Anterior circulation > posterior, left > right
- Etiology
  - No underlying cause is discovered in > 33% of cases
  - Arterial etiologies
    - Arteriopathies: Vasculitis (radiation, infectious, autoimmune or drug-induced), connective tissue disorders (Marfan, Ehlers-Danlos, homocystinuria), CADASIL/CARASIL
    - Emboli ⇒ cardiac (congenital heart disease, R-L shunt, valve anomaly)
    - Aneurysms, vascular malformations
    - Cervical dissections ⇒ vertebral > carotid, penetrating trauma, birth trauma
  - Hypoperfusion
    - Cardiopulmonary collapse
  - Metabolic encephalopathies
    - Mitochondrial encephalopathies, organic acidurias, progeria
  - Venous occlusion
    - High association with sepsis or adjacent infection (mastoiditis), oral contraceptives
  - Coagulopathies
    - Factor deficiencies, lupus anticoagulant, protein C/protein S abnormality, polycythemia
- Epidemiology
  - Incidence 2-3/100,000 per year in US
    - Mortality 0.6/100,000
- Associated abnormalities: Cardiac disease (25-50%), sickle cell (200-400x increased risk), trauma, NF1, Down syndrome

CLINICAL ISSUES

Presentation

- Most common signs/symptoms
  - Under-recognized as significant source of morbidity in pediatric population
  - Children with stroke typically present in delayed fashion (> 24 hours)
    - Poor recognition/understanding of symptoms by child, caregiver, physician
- Other signs/symptoms
  - Seizure ⇒ deficit often attributed to post-ictal state (Jacksonian paralysis)
  - Poor feeding, developmental delay, speech difficulties, gait abnormality
  - Focal deficit often masked by lethargy, coma, irritability
  - Preceding transient events occur in 25%

Demographics

- Age: Incidence/mortality greatest < 1 year

Natural History & Prognosis

- Capacity for recovery much greater than in adults
  - Fewer concomitant risk factors
  - Greater capacity for compensatory mechanisms, collateral recruitment

Treatment

- No randomized trials of therapies
  - Clinical window of opportunity/benefit much narrower than in adults
- Aspirin is mainstay of chronic therapy for fixed vascular lesions and vasculopathies
- Immunosuppression for autoimmune etiologies
- Transfusion therapy for at-risk children with sickle cell

DIAGNOSTIC CHECKLIST

Image Interpretation Pearls

- Basically same imaging signs as in adults
- Have low threshold for use of CTA/MRA, MRS

SELECTED REFERENCES

1. Seidman C et al: Pediatric stroke: current developments. Curr Opin Pediatr. 19(6):657-62, 2007
2. Danchaivijitr N et al: Evolution of cerebral arteriopathies in childhood arterial ischemic stroke. Ann Neurol. 59(4):620-6, 2006
3. Boardman JP et al: Magnetic resonance image correlates of hemiparesis after neonatal and childhood middle cerebral artery stroke. Pediatrics. 115(2):321-6, 2005
4. Carvalho KS et al: Arterial strokes in children. Neurol Clin. 20(4):1079-100, vii, 2002

IMAGE GALLERY

Typical

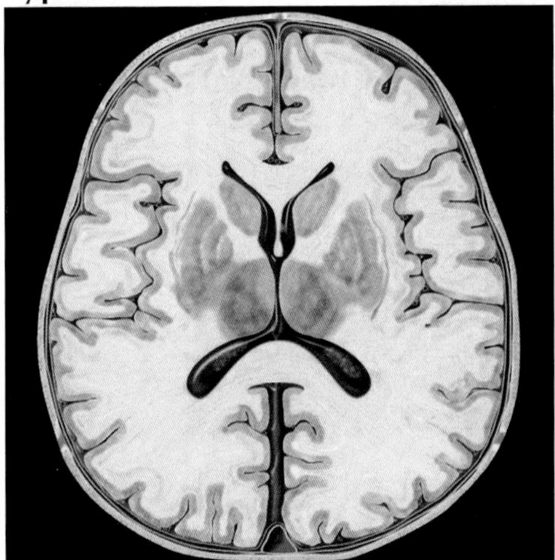

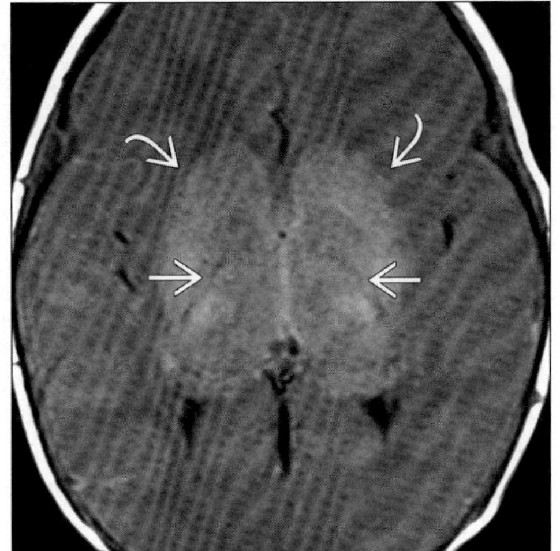

(Left) *Axial graphic shows deep pattern of HIE injury with edema of the lateral thalami and posterior putamina in profound, acute hypoxic ischemia of the newborn.* ***(Right)*** *Axial T1WI MR shows markedly abnormal increased signal in all the basal ganglia ➔ in this neonate with HIE. Note the abnormal relatively low signal of the internal capsules ➔.*

Typical

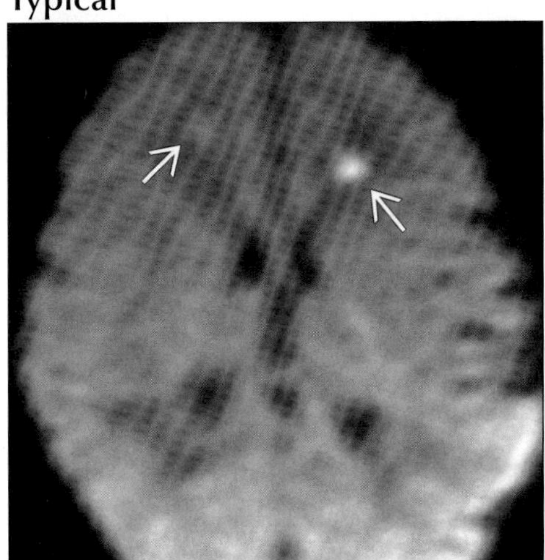

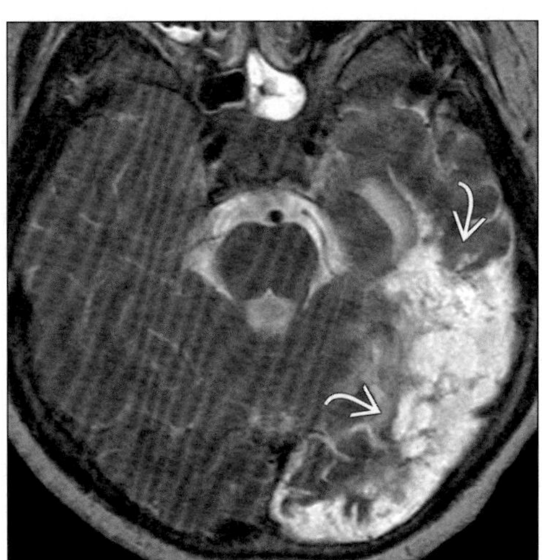

(Left) *Axial DWI MR demonstrates foci of restricted diffusion in the left greater than right bifrontal "watershed" white matter ➔ due to cerebral infarction from neonatal (full-term) asphyxia.* ***(Right)*** *Axial T2WI MR shows left temporal-occipital encephalomalacia ➔ from prior cerebral ischemic stroke in this patient with Down syndrome.*

Typical

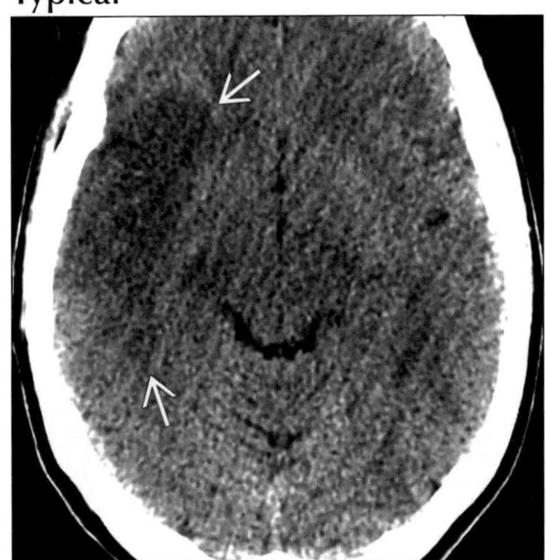

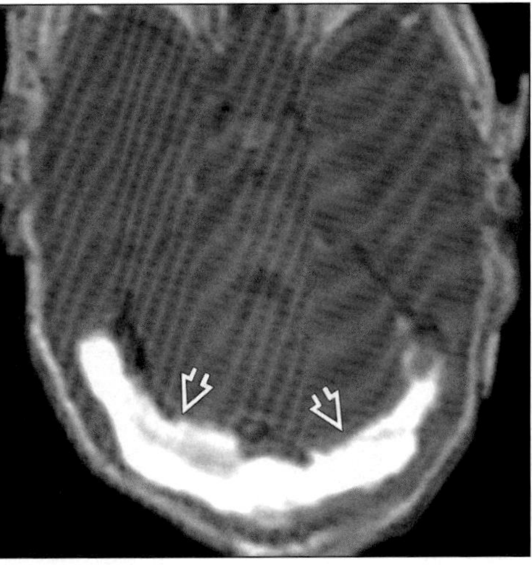

(Left) *Axial NECT depicts low-attenuation in the right frontotemporal lobe ➔ from acute cerebral ischemia in this patient with congenital hypoplastic/aplastic anemia (Diamond-Blackfan syndrome).* ***(Right)*** *Axial T1WI MR demonstrates diffuse high signal in enlarged bilateral transverse sinuses ➔ compatible with methemoglobin from dural sinus thrombosis in this 11 day old premature infant.*

CEREBRAL VENOUS SINUS THROMBOSIS

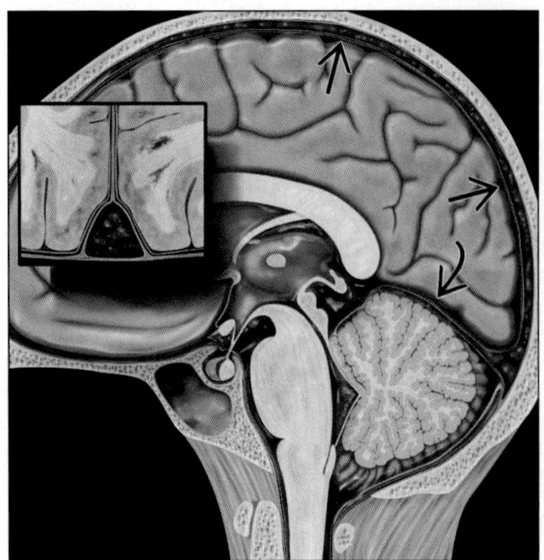

Sagittal graphic shows thrombosis of the superior sagittal sinus (SSS) ➔ and straight sinus ➔. Inset: Axial view of occluded SSS and associated parenchymal hemorrhagic infarcts.

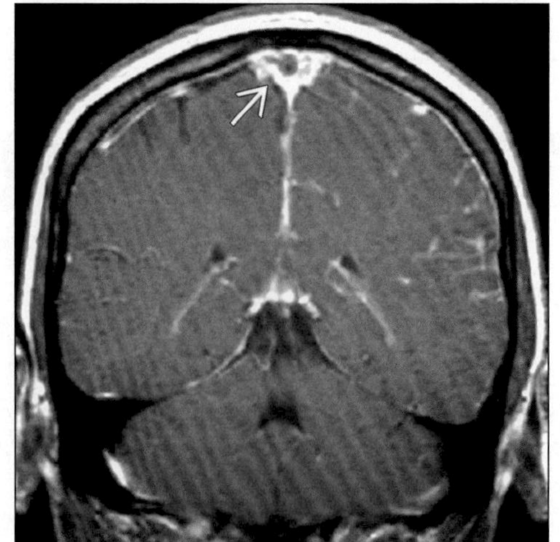

Coronal T1WI MR post-contrast shows an "empty delta" sign ➔ in the superior sagittal sinus due to central thrombus with surrounding enhancing dura and collateral venous channels.

TERMINOLOGY

Abbreviations and Synonyms

- Dural sinus thrombosis (DST); cerebral vein thrombosis (CVT)

Definitions

- Thrombotic occlusion of intracranial dural sinuses

IMAGING FINDINGS

General Features

- Best diagnostic clue
  - "Empty delta" sign on CECT, contrast-enhanced MR
  - Early imaging findings often subtle
- Location: Thrombus in dural sinus ± adjacent cortical vein(s)
- Size: Varies from small to extensive
- Morphology: Variable; usually linear, cigar-shaped

CT Findings

- NECT
  - Hyperdense dural sinus > cortical vein ("cord sign")
  - Venous infarct in 50%
    - Cortical/subcortical petechial hemorrhages, edema
    - If straight sinus/internal cerebral veins occlude, thalami/basal ganglia hypodense
- CECT
  - "Empty delta" sign in 25-30% of cases
    - Enhancing dura surrounds nonenhancing thrombus
  - "Shaggy," irregular veins (collateral channels)
- CTA: CT venogram (CTV) shows thrombus as filling defect(s) in dural sinus

MR Findings

- T1WI
  - Acute thrombus T1 isointense
  - Subacute thrombus becomes hyperintense
    - Most conspicuous sequence if clot subacute
- T2WI
  - Clot initially hypointense
    - Caution: If thrombus is hypointense, can mimic normal sinus "flow void" on T2WI
  - If venous infarct, mass effect with mixed blood/edema (hypo-/hyperintense signal) in adjacent parenchyma

DDx: Cerebral Venous Sinus Thrombosis

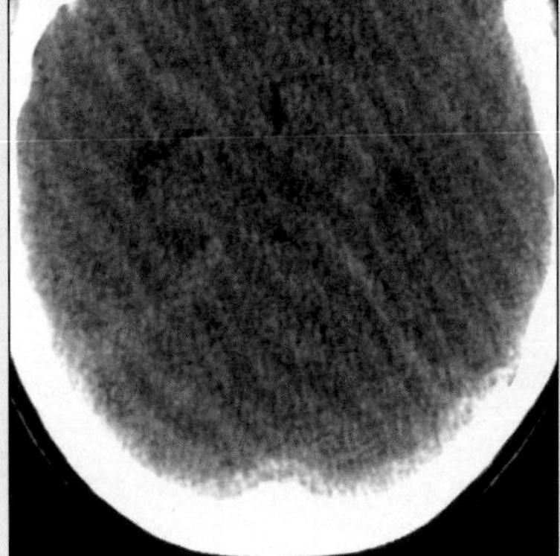

Diffuse Cerebral Edema

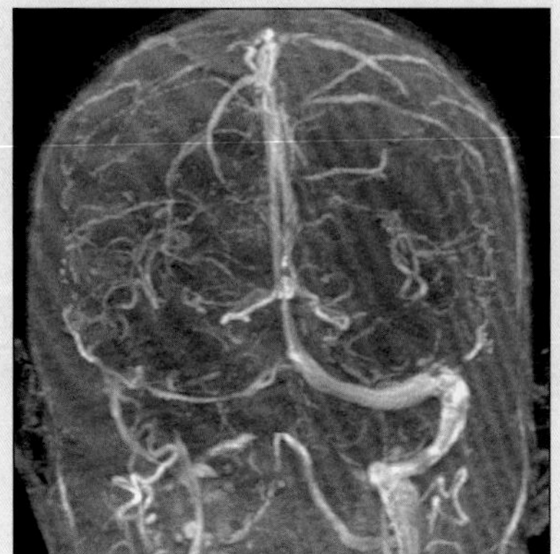

Hypoplastic Transverse Sinus

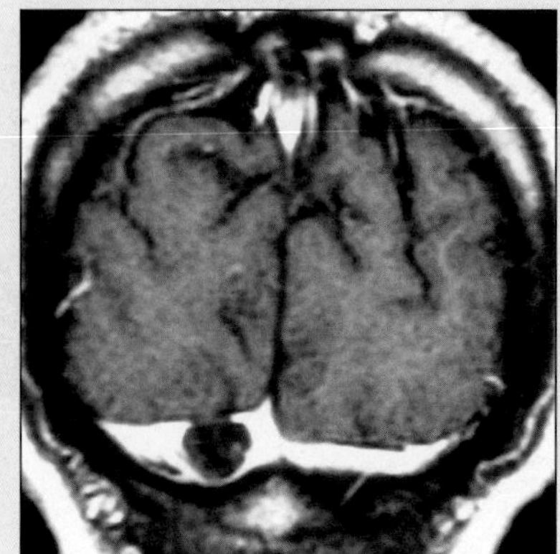

Arachnoid Granulation

CEREBRAL VENOUS SINUS THROMBOSIS

Key Facts

Terminology
- Thrombotic occlusion of intracranial dural sinuses

Imaging Findings
- Hyperdense dural sinus > cortical vein ("cord sign")
- Cortical/subcortical petechial hemorrhages, edema
- "Empty delta" sign in 25-30% of cases
- Acute thrombus T1 isointense
- Subacute thrombus becomes hyperintense
- Loss of normal venous sinus flow voids
- Absence of flow in occluded sinus on 2D TOF MRV
- PC MRV not limited by T1 hyperintense thrombus (does not misrepresent patency as can TOF MRV)

Top Differential Diagnoses
- Hypodense Brain (Normal Venous Sinuses)
- Anatomic Variant (Hypoplastic/Absent Dural Sinus)
- "Giant" Arachnoid Granulation

Pathology
- Resistance to activated protein C (typically due to factor V Leiden mutation) = most common cause of sporadic CVT
- Wide spectrum of predisposing causes (> 100 identified)
- Epidemiology: 1% of acute "strokes"

Clinical Issues
- Headache, vomiting, seizure ± neurologic deficit
- Extremely variable (from asymptomatic to coma, death)
- Heparin ± rtPA
- Endovascular thrombolysis, chemical or mechanical

 - Subacute thrombus appears hyperintense
 - Chronically occluded, fibrotic sinus eventually appears isointense
- PD/Intermediate
 - Loss of normal venous sinus flow voids
 - More sensitive sequence than T2WI
- FLAIR: Venous infarcts hyperintense
- T2* GRE
 - Acute thrombus hypointense, short T2 blood products "bloom"
 - Petechial and/or parenchymal hemorrhages hypointense
- DWI
 - Findings in parenchyma variable, heterogeneous
   - May restrict early, normalize later
   - Distinguishes cytotoxic from vasogenic edema
   - Parenchymal abnormalities more frequently reversible (30% resolve) than in arterial occlusions (< 1% resolve)
- T1 C+
 - Peripheral enhancement around acute clot
 - Chronic sinus thrombosis can enhance due to organizing fibrous tissue
- MRV
 - Absence of flow in occluded sinus on 2D TOF MRV
   - "Frayed" or "shaggy" appearance of venous sinus
   - Abnormal collateral channels (e.g., enlarged medullary veins)
 - Note: T1 hyperintense (subacute) clot can masquerade as flow on TOF MRV, evaluate standard sequences and source images to exclude artifacts
 - Contrast-enhanced MRV (CE-MRV) better demonstrates thrombus, small vein detail, and collaterals; much faster than 2D TOF
 - PC MRV not limited by T1 hyperintense thrombus (does not misrepresent patency as can TOF MRV)
- MRS: Helpful to differentiate venous infarct from tumor

Angiographic Findings
- Occlusion of involved sinus
- Slow flow in adjacent patent cortical veins
- Collateral venous drainage develops

Imaging Recommendations
- Best imaging tool
 - NECT, CECT scans ± CTV as initial screening
 - MR (include T2*, DWI, T1 C+), MRV
- Protocol advice
 - If CT scan negative, MR with MRV
 - If MRV equivocal, DSA

DIFFERENTIAL DIAGNOSIS

Hypodense Brain (Normal Venous Sinuses)
- Blood in normal vessels appears slightly hyperdense on NECT scans
 - Diffuse cerebral edema
 - Common artifact in newborns (combination of unmyelinated low density brain, physiologic polycythemia)

Anatomic Variant
- Congenital hypoplastic/absent sinus (transverse sinus flow gaps 31%, usually nondominant sinus)
 - Right transverse sinus dominant 59%, left dominant in 25%, codominant in 16%
- "High-splitting" tentorium
- Fat in sinus

"Giant" Arachnoid Granulation
- Round/ovoid filling defect (clot typically long, linear)
- CSF density/signal intensity
- Arachnoid granulations normal in 24% of CECT, 13% of MR
 - Transverse sinus most common location by imaging, L > R
 - Superior sagittal sinus most common location on histopathology (not well seen by imaging)

False "Empty Delta" Sign
- Subdural hematoma, subdural empyema

Neoplasm
- Venous infarct can enhance, mimic neoplasm
- Intravascular lymphomatosis (rare)

CEREBRAL VENOUS SINUS THROMBOSIS

PATHOLOGY

General Features

- Genetics
  - Inherited predisposing conditions
    - Resistance to activated protein C (typically due to factor V Leiden mutation) = most common cause of sporadic CVT
    - Protein S deficiency
    - Prothrombin (factor II) gene mutation (G20210A)
    - Antithrombin III deficiency
- Etiology
  - No cause identified in 20-25% of cases
  - Wide spectrum of predisposing causes (> 100 identified)
    - Trauma, infection, inflammation
    - Pregnancy, oral contraceptives
    - Metabolic (dehydration, thyrotoxicosis, cirrhosis, hyperhomocysteinemia, etc.)
    - Hematological (coagulopathy)
    - Collagen-vascular disorders (e.g., antiphospholipid antibody syndrome)
    - Vasculitis (e.g., Behçet)
    - Drugs (androgens, ecstasy)
  - Most common pattern: Thrombus initially forms in dural sinus
    - Clot propagates into cortical veins
    - Venous drainage obstructed, venous pressure elevated
    - Blood-brain barrier breakdown with vasogenic edema, hemorrhage
    - Venous infarct with cytotoxic edema ensues
- Epidemiology: 1% of acute "strokes"
- Associated abnormalities
  - Dural arteriovenous fistula (dAVF): Venous occlusive disease may be underlying etiologic factor
  - Ulcerative colitis
  - May have thromboses elsewhere: Pulmonary embolism, lower extremity DVT

Gross Pathologic & Surgical Features

- Sinus occluded, distended by acute clot
- Thrombus in adjacent cortical veins
- Adjacent cortex edematous, usually with petechial hemorrhage

Microscopic Features

- Thrombosis of veins, proliferative fibrous tissue in chronic thromboses

Staging, Grading or Classification Criteria

- Venous ischemia
  - Type 1: No abnormality
  - Type 2: High signal on T2WI/FLAIR; no enhancement
  - Type 3: High signal on T2WI/FLAIR; enhancement present
  - Type 4: Hemorrhage or venous infarction

CLINICAL ISSUES

Presentation

- Most common signs/symptoms
  - Headache, vomiting, seizure ± neurologic deficit
  - Clinical diagnosis often elusive

Demographics

- Age: All ages
- Gender: M < F

Natural History & Prognosis

- Extremely variable (from asymptomatic to coma, death)
  - Up to 50% of cases progress to venous infarction
  - Can be fatal if severe brain swelling, herniation

Treatment

- Heparin ± rtPA
- Endovascular thrombolysis, chemical or mechanical

DIAGNOSTIC CHECKLIST

Consider

- DSA in patients with suspected chronic DST
- Could a venous "filling defect" be a prominent arachnoid granulation?

Image Interpretation Pearls

- Review MRV source images
- Transverse sinus common site for hypoplastic segment variations that can mimic occlusion

SELECTED REFERENCES

1. Ferro JM et al: Interobserver agreement in the magnetic resonance location of cerebral vein and dural sinus thrombosis. Eur J Neurol. 14(3):353-6, 2007
2. Klingebiel R et al: Comparative evaluation of 2D time-of-flight and 3D elliptic centric contrast-enhanced MR venography in patients with presumptive cerebral venous and sinus thrombosis. Eur J Neurol. 14(2):139-43, 2007
3. Linn J et al: Diagnostic value of multidetector-row CT angiography in the evaluation of thrombosis of the cerebral venous sinuses. AJNR Am J Neuroradiol. 28(5):946-52, 2007
4. Chaudhary MY et al: Dural sinus thrombosis: frequency and imaging diagnosis. J Coll Physicians Surg Pak. 16(6):400-3, 2006
5. Sheerani M et al: Oral contraceptives and cerebral venous thrombosis: case report and a brief review of literature. J Pak Med Assoc. 56(11):559-61, 2006
6. Ferro JM et al: Delay in hospital admission of patients with cerebral vein and dural sinus thrombosis. Cerebrovasc Dis. 19(3):152-6, 2005
7. Curtin KR et al: Rheolytic catheter thrombectomy, balloon angioplasty, and direct recombinant tissue plasminogen activator thrombolysis of dural sinus thrombosis with preexisting hemorrhagic infarctions. AJNR Am J Neuroradiol. 25(10):1807-11, 2004
8. Ferro JM et al: Prognosis of cerebral vein and dural sinus thrombosis. Stroke. 35(3):664-70, 2004
9. Hinman JM et al: Hypointense thrombus on T2-weighted MR imaging: a potential pitfall in the diagnosis of dural sinus thrombosis. Eur J Radiol. 41(2):147-52, 2002
10. Kawaguchi T et al: Classification of venous ischaemia with MRI. J Clin Neurosci. 8 Suppl 1:82-8, 2001
11. Provenzale JM et al: Dural sinus thrombosis: findings on CT and MR imaging and diagnostic pitfalls. AJR Am J Roentgenol. 170(3):777-83, 1998

CEREBRAL VENOUS SINUS THROMBOSIS

IMAGE GALLERY

Typical

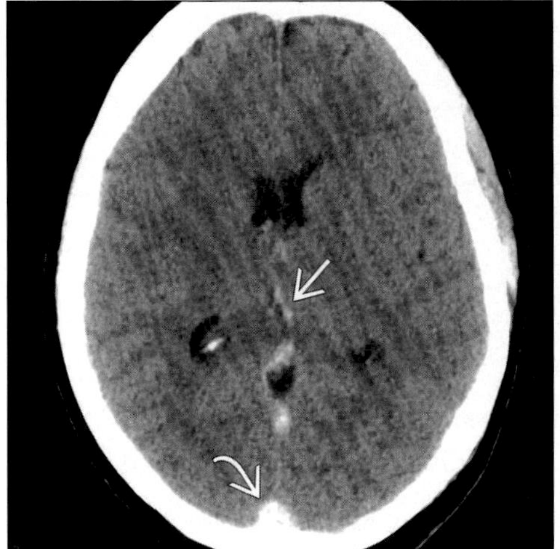

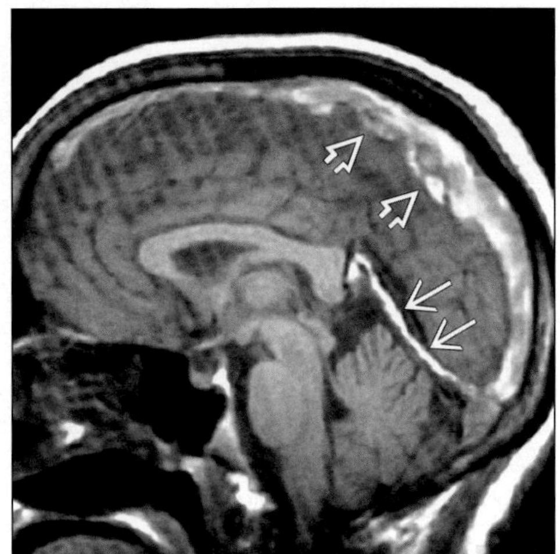

(Left) Axial NECT shows high density in the internal cerebral veins (deep venous system) ➡ and superior sagittal sinus (superficial venous system) ➡ from acute cerebral venous thrombosis. *(Right)* Sagittal T1WI MR demonstrates high signal and expansion of the superior sagittal sinus ➡ from subacute venous sinus thrombosis. There is also clot in the straight sinus ➡.

Typical

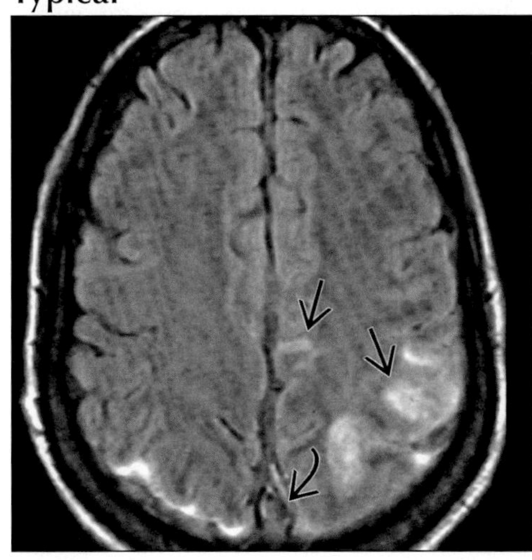

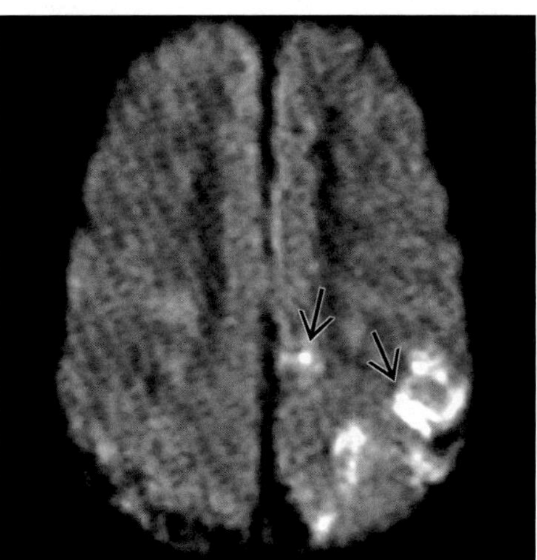

(Left) Axial T2WI MR FLAIR shows gyriform left frontoparietal cortical and adjacent subcortical hyperintensity ➡. There is also lack of normal "flow void" in the superior sagittal sinus ➡. *(Right)* Axial DWI MR in the same patient as previous image, depicts corresponding left frontoparietal regions of restricted diffusion ➡ secondary to acute cerebral venous infarction from the dural sinus thrombosis.

Typical

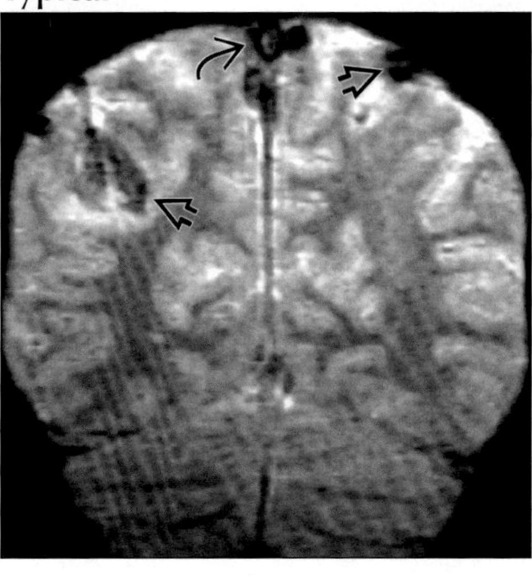

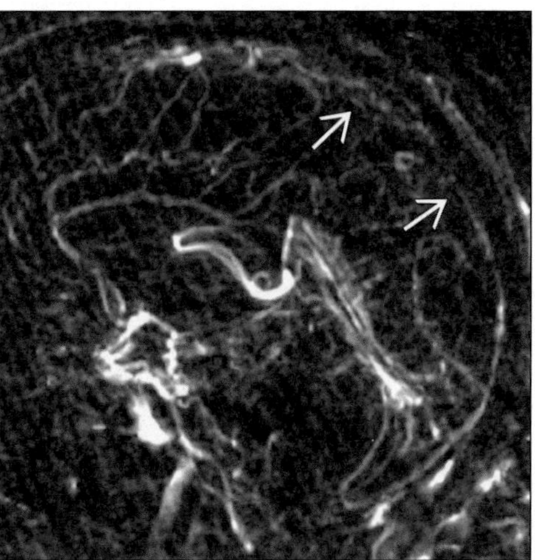

(Left) Coronal T2WI MR GRE shows multiple bilateral foci of hypointense "blooming" ➡ due to parenchymal hemorrhagic venous infarction. There is also "blooming" of clot in the dural sinus ➡. *(Right)* Sagittal 2D TOF MRV MIP image demonstrates lack of flow related enhancement in the superior sagittal sinus ➡ indicating venous occlusion from acute cerebral dural sinus thrombosis.

MIGRAINE

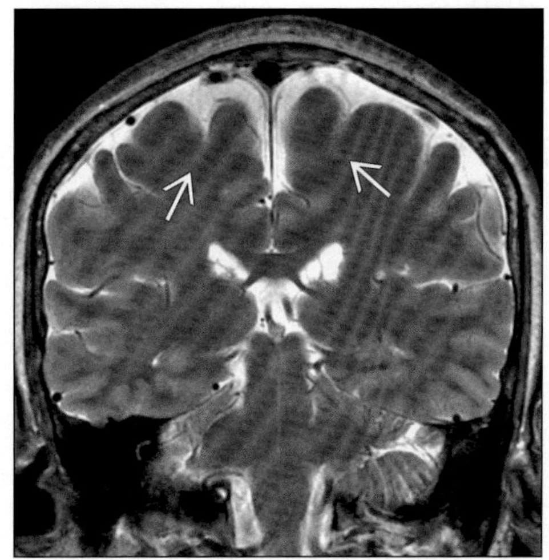

Coronal T2WI MR shows small punctate foci of increased signal intensity in the bilateral centrum semiovale ➡ in this patient with chronic recurrent severe throbbing headaches.

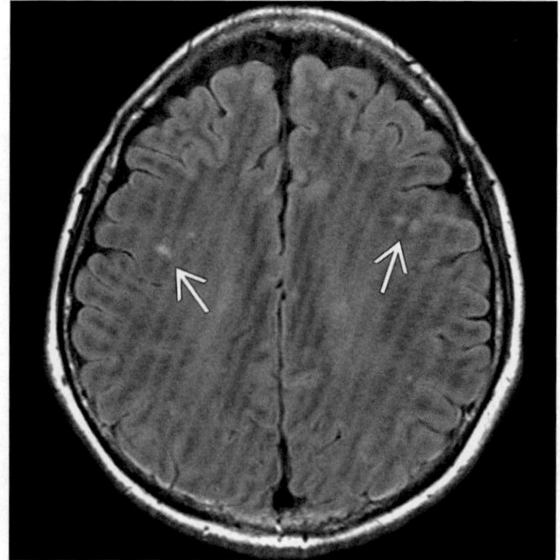

Axial T2WI MR FLAIR (same patient as previous image) more easily demonstrates bilateral centrum semiovale foci of increased signal intensity ➡ secondary to presumed migraine-induced chronic ischemia.

TERMINOLOGY

Abbreviations and Synonyms

- "Vascular headache"

Definitions

- Recurring severe headache occasionally preceded by scintillating scotomata

IMAGING FINDINGS

General Features

- Best diagnostic clue: Punctate deep white matter lesions on T2WI
- Location: Commonly identified in the corona radiata and centrum semiovale
- Size: Usually few millimeters in length
- Morphology: Punctate: Rounded, oval

CT Findings

- NECT: Generally none, may see punctate hypodensities
- CECT: Generally none, rare associated infarction will enhance in the late acute to subacute stage

MR Findings

- T1WI
  - Generally none, may see punctate hypointensities
  - Rarely supratentorial cortical or deep white matter infarcts, cerebellar infarcts
- T2WI
  - Punctate hyperintensities in deep white matter; commonly corona radiata and centrum semiovale, occasionally in the brainstem and cerebellum
    - Due to gliosis from presumed small vessel hypoperfusion/ischemia
  - Supratentorial cortical or deep white matter infarcts (usually posterior circulation territory), cerebellar infarcts may be rarely seen
- FLAIR
  - Punctate hyperintensities in deep white matter
  - Lesions more obvious than on other sequences
  - Differentiates abnormal lesions (high signal) from CSF spaces (low signal)
- DWI
  - Can be positive in complicated migraine

DDx: Migraine

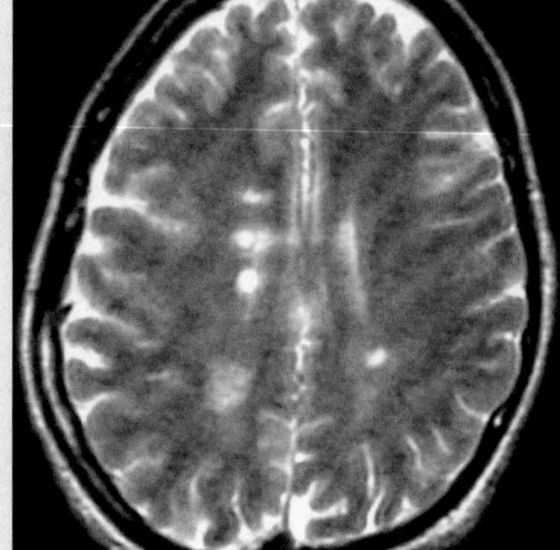

Multiple Sclerosis

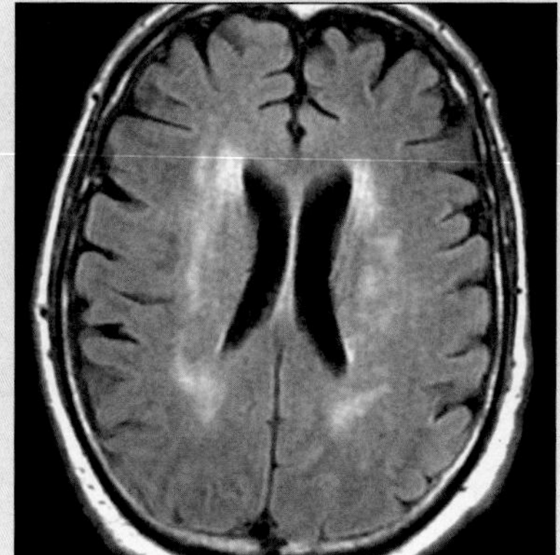

Small Vessel Ischemic Disease

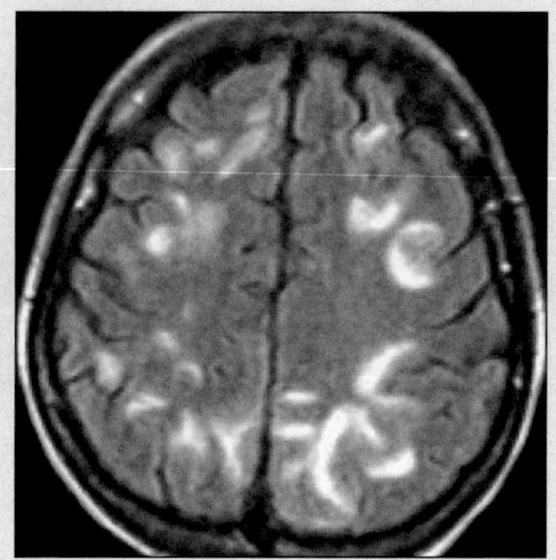

Vasculitis

MIGRAINE

Key Facts

Terminology

- "Vascular headache"
- Recurring severe headache occasionally preceded by scintillating scotomata

Imaging Findings

- Punctate deep white matter lesions on T2WI
- Supratentorial cortical or deep white matter infarcts (usually posterior circulation territory), cerebellar infarcts may be rarely seen
- Restricted diffusion when hemiplegic or hemisensory symptoms are (or have recently been) present
- MR perfusion imaging can demonstrate hypoperfusion, typically in occipital lobes during acute attack
- Rarely may show cerebrovascular foci of narrowing due to vasospasm

Top Differential Diagnoses

- Demyelinating Disease (Multiple Sclerosis)
- Deep White Matter Ischemia
- Vasculitis

Pathology

- Recent data suggest probable effect on trigeminal somatosensory and modulatory pain systems including the spinal trigeminal nucleus and thalamus
- Affects 10-15% of population
- Gliosis in deep white matter from presumed small vessel hypoperfusion/ischemia

Clinical Issues

- Throbbing head pain with sensitivity to light, sound and head movement

---

  - Restricted diffusion when hemiplegic or hemisensory symptoms are (or have recently been) present
  - Can spontaneously resolve unlike most typical ischemic lesions
  - DTI: ↓ Fractional anisotropy (FA) in thalamocortical tract (all migraineurs), ↓ FA in ventral trigeminothalamic tract (migraineurs with aura), ↓ FA in ventrolateral periaqueductal gray matter (migraineurs without aura)
- T1 C+: Cortical and subcortical enhancement of associated rare late acute to subacute infarct
- MRA: Rarely may show cerebrovascular foci of narrowing due to vasospasm
- MRS: May see decreased NAA and elevated lactate in the occipital lobes in migraineurs with visual aura
- MR perfusion imaging can demonstrate hypoperfusion, typically in occipital lobes during acute attack

Nuclear Medicine Findings

- PET
  - Abnormal activation in the brainstem identified
  - May be the cause of resultant trigeminovascular reflex

Imaging Recommendations

- Best imaging tool: MR with T2, FLAIR, DWI

DIFFERENTIAL DIAGNOSIS

Demyelinating Disease (Multiple Sclerosis)

- Clinically not associated with headaches but rather relapsing/remitting neurologic sx
- White matter lesions commonly oriented perpendicular to ependyma

Deep White Matter Ischemia

- Typically older patients or those with hypertension, diabetes, or hyperlipidemia

Vasculitis

- Cortical and deep white matter infarcts with occasional hemorrhage

Gliosis

- Any focal prior injury to the brain such as trauma, infection, etc.

PATHOLOGY

General Features

- General path comments
  - Classically thought to be primarily due to vasoconstriction of calcarine artery (leading to scintillating scotomata) followed by vasodilatation (leading to headache)
    - New hypotheses suggest initial abnormal brainstem activation
- Genetics
  - Rare autosomal dominant familial hemiplegic migraine
    - Patients present with hemiplegia that can last for days or weeks
    - Dysphagia and dysarthria in 50%
    - Hemihypesthesia in nearly 100%
    - Related to the CACNA1A (Ca++ channel), ATP1A2 (Na+/K+ ATPase), SCN1A (Na+ channel) genes
- Etiology
  - Recent data suggest probable effect on trigeminal somatosensory and modulatory pain systems including the spinal trigeminal nucleus and thalamus
  - Probably caused by impaired central neural inhibitory mechanisms in brainstem neurons (possibly in the midbrain dorsal raphe)
    - Neuronal dysfunction of excitation followed by spreading depression
    - Phase of vasoconstriction and vasodilatation
    - Secretion of vasoactive peptides at the terminations of the trigeminal nerve
- Epidemiology: Affects 10-15% of population

MIGRAINE

- Associated abnormalities
  - Rarely can produce supratentorial cortical/deep white matter or cerebellar infarcts
    - More common in migraineurs with aura
    - Can occur either during the episode of migraine or between attacks
    - Usually clinically silent

Microscopic Features

- Gliosis in deep white matter from presumed small vessel hypoperfusion/ischemia

CLINICAL ISSUES

Presentation

- Most common signs/symptoms
  - Throbbing head pain with sensitivity to light, sound and head movement
  - Lateralized headache in 60%
- Other signs/symptoms
  - Nausea, vomiting, scalp tenderness common
  - Transient vertigo, ataxia, dysarthria, tinnitus, diplopia, sensorial clouding and blindness possible
- "Common" migraine: 80% of cases
  - Unilateral, throbbing, severe headache
- "Classic" migraine: 10-20% of cases
  - Headache preceded by aura of sensory, motor, or visual ("scintillating scotomata") symptoms lasting 30 minutes or less
    - Most commonly visual premonitory symptoms due to occipital lobe neuronal dysfunction
- "Complicated" migraine
  - Neurologic deficits last longer than 30 minutes (or permanent)
- "Ophthalmic" migraine: Scintillating scotomata without headache or neurologic deficits (common)

Demographics

- Gender: M < F

Natural History & Prognosis

- Variable; usually very painful
- Chronic and recurrent
- Rarely neurologic deficit from infarction

Treatment

- Relief by darkness and sleep
- Analgesics, e.g., aspirin, acetaminophen, ± caffeine; ibuprofen; naproxen
- Ergot derivatives, e.g., dihydroergotamine mesylate
- Serotonin receptor agonists, e.g., sumatriptan

DIAGNOSTIC CHECKLIST

Consider

- In a patient with a history of severe headache, cerebral aneurysm must always be excluded! Evaluate vascular flow voids on T2WI or perform MRA

Image Interpretation Pearls

- While punctate deep white matter T2 hyperintensities are a nonspecific finding (and can be seen in many etiologies of ischemia, demyelination and gliosis), migraine should always be considered especially in non-elderly patients with a history of headache
- MR FLAIR imaging best differentiates focal white matter abnormal lesions (high signal) from CSF spaces (low signal)
- In patients with headache and focal neurologic symptoms, MR imaging with DWI should be performed to exclude infarction from complicated migraine

SELECTED REFERENCES

1. DaSilva AF et al: Interictal alterations of the trigeminal somatosensory pathway and periaqueductal gray matter in migraine. Neuroreport. 18(4):301-5, 2007
2. Goadsby PJ: Recent advances in understanding migraine mechanisms, molecules and therapeutics. Trends Mol Med. 13(1):39-44, 2007
3. Leone M et al: Functional neuroimaging and headache pathophysiology: new findings and new prospects. Neurol Sci. 28 Suppl 2:S108-13, 2007
4. Liang Y et al: Migrainous infarction with appearance of laminar necrosis on MRI. Clin Neurol Neurosurg. 109(7):592-6, 2007
5. Marshall N et al: MRA captures vasospasm in fatal migrainous infarction. Headache. 47(2):280-3, 2007
6. Rozen TD: Vanishing cerebellar infarcts in a migraine patient. Cephalalgia. 27(6):557-60, 2007
7. Toth M et al: [The prevalence of white matter abnormalities on magnetic resonance images in migraine] Ideggyogy Sz. 60(5-6):239-44, 2007
8. Bono G et al: Complications of migraine: migrainous infarction. Clin Exp Hypertens. 28(3-4):233-42, 2006
9. Borsook D et al: Functional imaging of the trigeminal system: applications to migraine pathophysiology. Headache. 46 Suppl 1:S32-8, 2006
10. Kruit MC et al: Brain stem and cerebellar hyperintense lesions in migraine. Stroke. 37(4):1109-12, 2006
11. May A: A review of diagnostic and functional imaging in headache. J Headache Pain. 7(4):174-84, 2006
12. Resnick S et al: Migraine with aura associated with reversible MRI abnormalities. Neurology. 66(6):946-7, 2006
13. Afridi SK et al: A positron emission tomographic study in spontaneous migraine. Arch Neurol. 62(8):1270-5, 2005
14. Kruit MC et al: Infarcts in the posterior circulation territory in migraine. The population-based MRI CAMERA study. Brain. 128(Pt 9):2068-77, 2005
15. Kruit MC et al: MRI findings in migraine. Rev Neurol (Paris). 161(6-7):661-5, 2005
16. Bussone G: Pathophysiology of migraine. Neurol Sci. 25 Suppl 3:S239-41, 2004
17. Swartz RH et al: Migraine is associated with magnetic resonance imaging white matter abnormalities: a meta-analysis. Arch Neurol. 61(9):1366-8, 2004
18. Gonzalez-Alegre P et al: Prolonged cortical electrical depression and diffuse vasospasm without ischemia in a case of severe hemiplegic migraine during pregnancy. Headache. 43(1):72-5, 2003
19. Osborn RE et al: MR imaging of the brain in patients with migraine headaches. AJNR Am J Neuroradiol. 12(3):521-4, 1991

MIGRAINE

IMAGE GALLERY

Typical

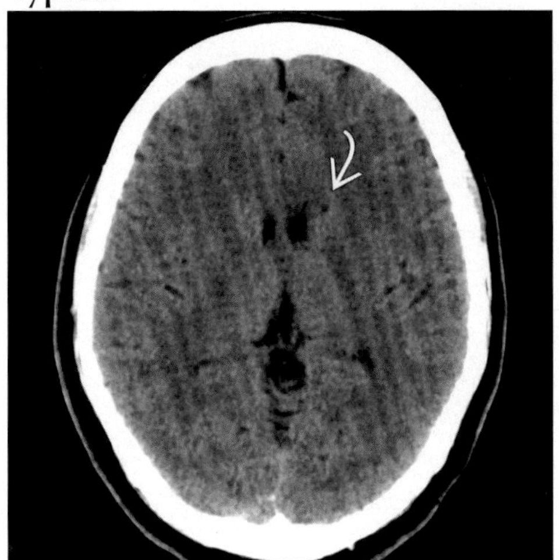

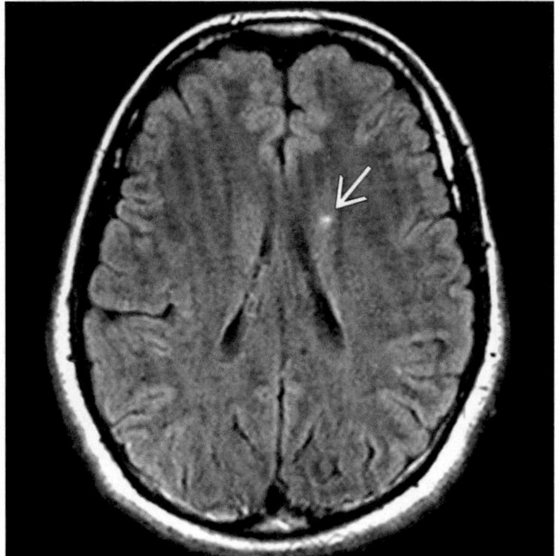

*(**Left**) Axial NECT shows a punctate focus of hypodensity adjacent to the left caudate ➔ in this patient with chronic headaches. This may represent a lesion or normal perivascular space. (**Right**) Axial T2WI MR FLAIR in the same patient as previous image confirms a small focus of gliosis ➔, a non-specific but abnormal finding, most compatible with the history of migraine in this young patient.*

Typical

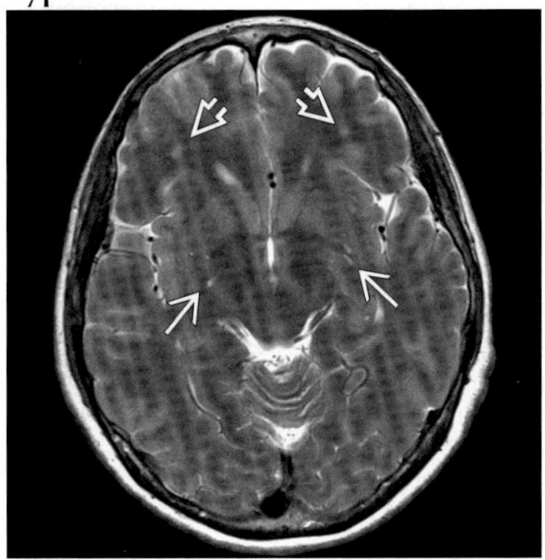

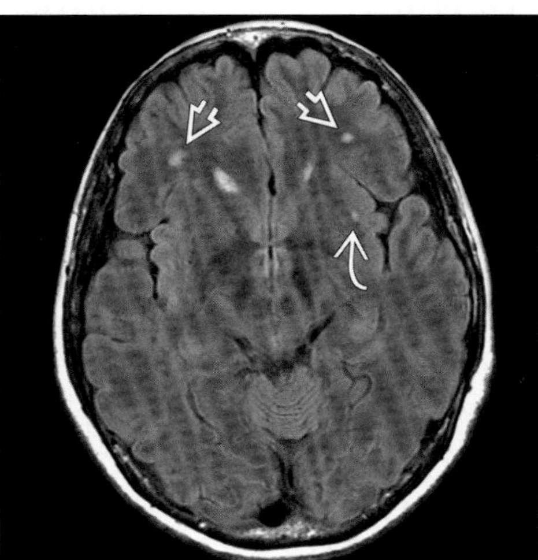

*(**Left**) Axial T2WI MR shows multiple punctate foci of hyperintensity in the bilateral frontal white matter ➔. Additional high intensity foci are seen adjacent to the anterior commissure ➔. (**Right**) Axial T2WI MR FLAIR in the same patient as previous image confirms migrainous lesions in bifrontal white matter ➔, and differentiates left subinsular lesion ➔ from the remaining CSF perivascular spaces.*

Variant

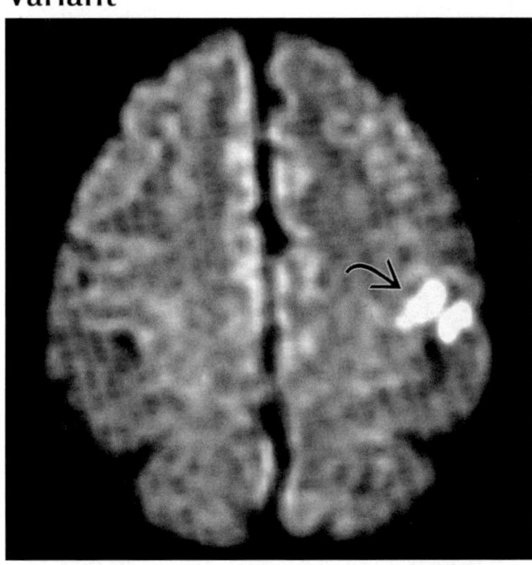

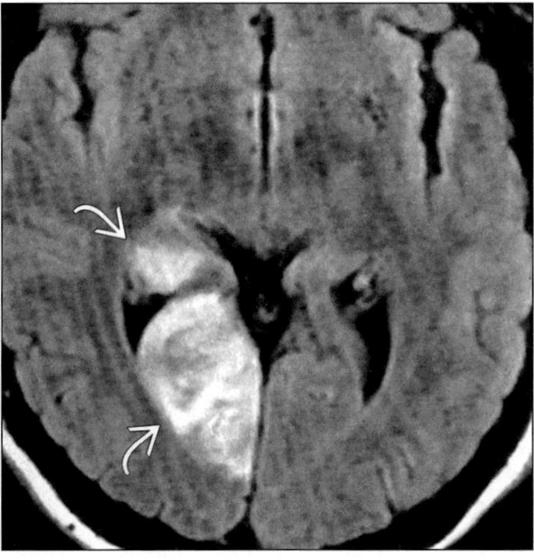

*(**Left**) Axial DWI MR shows restricted diffusion ➔ in a patient with acute aphasia during a migraine. While these lesions can resolve, this likely represents infarction from complicated migraine. (**Right**) Axial T2WI MR FLAIR shows high signal in the right occipital and medial temporal lobes ➔, PCA distribution, due to infarction from complicated migraine. (Courtesy M. Brant-Zawadzki, MD).*

SICKLE CELL ANEMIA

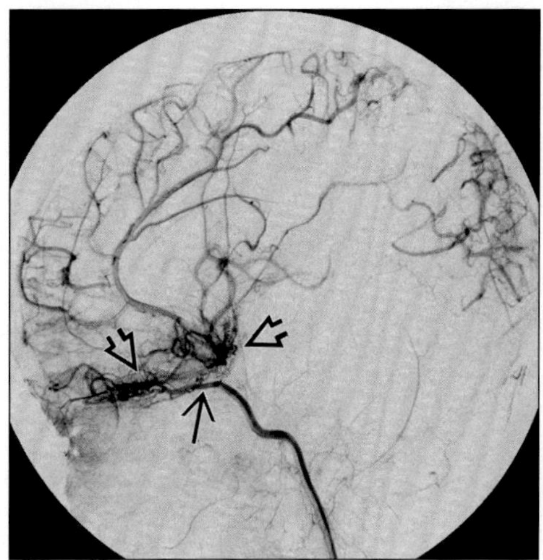

Lateral DSA shows marked stenosis of the distal internal carotid artery ⇒ with multiple hypertrophied surrounding collateral vessels ⇨. Moyamoya pattern from sickle cell anemia.

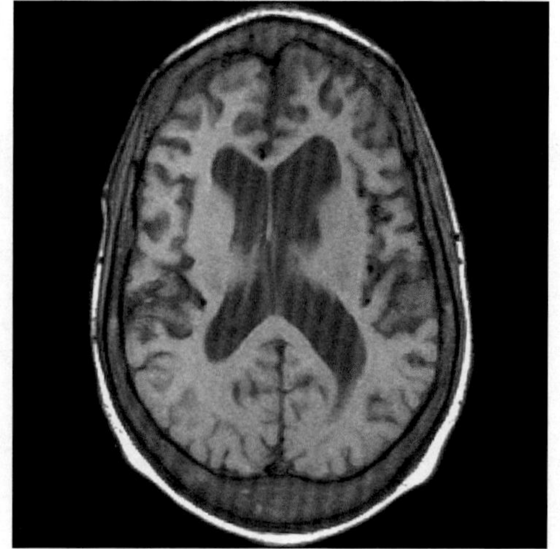

Axial T1WI MR shows diffuse atrophy of the cerebral parenchyma and widening of the calvarium with intrinsic isointense signal from hematopoietic marrow secondary to sickle cell anemia.

TERMINOLOGY

Abbreviations and Synonyms

- Sickle cell disease (SCD)

Definitions

- Abnormality in hemoglobin (Hgb) → change in shape ("sickling") → increased "stickiness" of erythrocytes (RBCs) → capillary occlusions, ischemia, infarctions, premature RBC destruction (hemolytic anemia)

IMAGING FINDINGS

General Features

- Best diagnostic clue
  - Narrowing of the distal ICAs, proximal ACAs/MCAs with cerebral infarction
    - Moyamoya pattern (hypertrophied lenticulostriate collaterals)
- Location: Stenoses: Distal ICAs, proximal cerebral vessels; ischemia: Supratentorial cortex, deep white matter
- Use MR to document previous as well as new ischemic events
- Caveat: Cognitive impairment does not correlate with imaging findings

Radiographic Findings

- Radiography
  - Thick skull with expanded diploic space
  - Opacified paranasal sinuses

CT Findings

- NECT
  - Calvarial thickening
  - Focal encephalomalacia due to cortical infarction
  - Adult sickle cell moyamoya: Intraventricular bleed may be initial presentation
- CECT: Punctate enhancement in basal ganglia due to moyamoya collaterals
- CTA: Stenosis of distal ICA, proximal circle of Willis (COW) vessels

MR Findings

- T1WI
  - Hemorrhagic infarcts may be seen

DDx: Sickle Cell Anemia

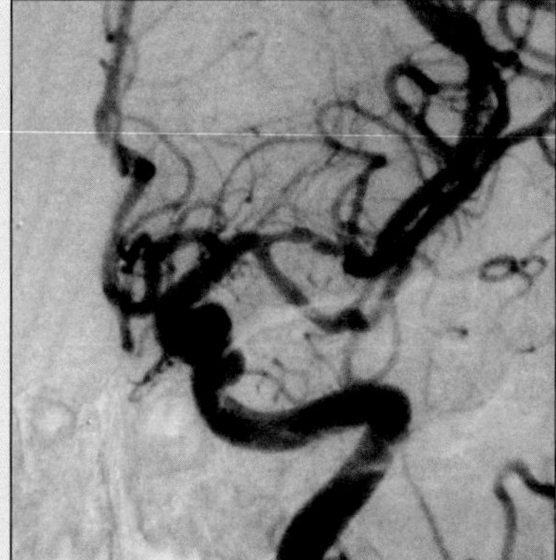

Vasculitis

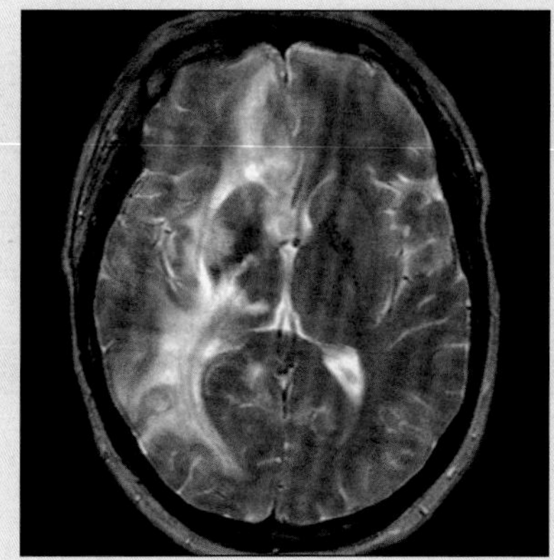

Primary Arteritis of the CNS

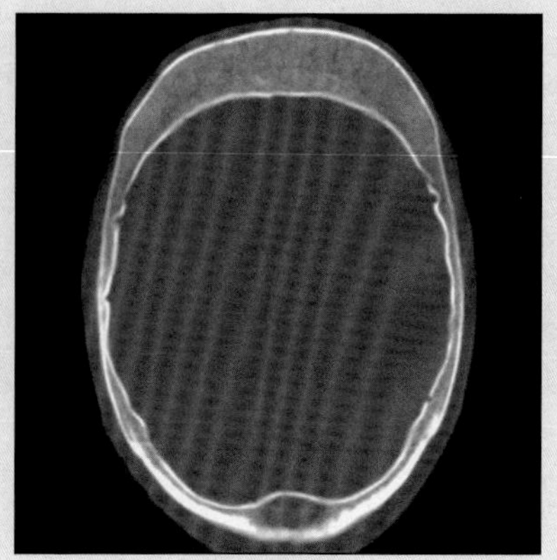

Thalassemia

SICKLE CELL ANEMIA

Key Facts

Terminology
- Abnormality in hemoglobin (Hgb) → change in shape ("sickling") → increased "stickiness" of erythrocytes (RBCs) → capillary occlusions, ischemia, infarctions, premature RBC destruction (hemolytic anemia)

Imaging Findings
- Hemorrhagic infarcts may be seen
- T2WI: Cortical, deep white matter infarcts (often in distal watershed ACA/MCA territory)
- Stenosis of distal ICA, proximal COW
- Thick skull with expanded diploic space

Top Differential Diagnoses
- Vasculitis/Arteritis
- Connective Tissue Disorders
- Arteriopathy

Pathology
- Hgb S becomes "stiff" (erythrocytes are sickle-shaped) when deoxygenated
- Primary cause of stroke in African-American children
- Stroke incidence decreased if Hgb S kept to less than 30% by transfusion (but need initial ischemic event to initiate therapy)

Clinical Issues
- Age: Infarctions are generally first seen in children about 10 years of age
- Hgb S found in 10% of African-Americans

Diagnostic Checklist
- African-American child with cerebral infarction: Always consider SCD!

  - Punctate flow voids in basal ganglia correspond to moyamoya collaterals
  - Abnormal signal intensity in bone marrow which may be expanded
- T2WI: Cortical, deep white matter infarcts (often in distal watershed ACA/MCA territory)
- FLAIR: Multifocal hyperintensities ± ivy sign of moyamoya (bright sulci from slow flow collaterals)
- DWI: Focal hyperintensities due to acute infarctions
- T1 C+: Vascular enhancement from stasis and leptomeningeal collaterals in territory with proximal stenosis
- MRA
  - Stenosis of distal ICA, proximal COW
    - Caveat: Turbulent dephasing due to anemia, rapid flow can mimic stenosis on "bright blood" MRA
    - Suggestion: Use lowest possible TE for bright blood MRA or use black blood MRA if stenosis suspected
  - MRA source images: Multiple dots in basal ganglia due to moyamoya collaterals
  - Aneurysms in atypical locations
- MRS: ↑ Lactate, ↓ NAA, ↓ Cho, ↓ Cr in areas of infarction (lactate seen only in acute/subacute infarctions)
- Perfusion studies: ↓ rCBF, ↓ rCBV, ↑ TTP, ↑ MTT

Nuclear Medicine Findings
- PET: Focal areas of low brain perfusion

Ultrasonographic Findings
- Transcranial Doppler: Excellent screening modality
  - Hyperdynamic flow in cerebral arteries secondary to proximal stenosis
  - 10% annual risk of stroke if abnormal ICA or MCA velocities!

Angiographic Findings
- Conventional
  - Stenosis of distal ICA, proximal COW; fusiform aneurysms; moyamoya collaterals; EC-IC collaterals
    - Hydrate, transfuse before catheter study
    - Risk of stroke higher than in other populations
  - Moyamoya may be associated with persistent primitive carotid-basilar arterial communications

Imaging Recommendations
- Best imaging tool: MR with DWI, MRA; ± DSA
- Protocol advice
  - MR to differentiate acute from previous infarcts
  - MRA to exclude distal ICA, COW stenosis and moyamoya collaterals

DIFFERENTIAL DIAGNOSIS

Vasculitis/Arteritis
- Infectious, autoimmune, idiopathic or substance abuse etiologies
- Classic imaging findings: Cortical and deep white matter infarcts, parenchymal hemorrhage

Connective Tissue Disorders
- Marfan, Ehlers-Danlos, homocystinuria
- Progressive arterial narrowing and occlusion

Arteriopathy
- NF1, Down syndrome, radiation-induced vasculopathy
- Can show vascular moyamoya pattern

Dissection
- Smooth tapering of vascular lumen
- T1 hyperintense crescent = thrombus

Arterial Vasospasm
- Temporal relationship to subarachnoid hemorrhage
- Drug-related (sympathomimetics)

Thick Skull with Expanded Diploe
- Other chronic anemias (thalassemia)

PATHOLOGY

General Features
- General path comments

SICKLE CELL ANEMIA

- Initial endothelial injury from abnormal adherence of sickled RBCs
- Subsequently internal elastic lamina fragmentation and degeneration of muscularis result in large vessel vasculopathy and aneurysm formation
  - May be reversed with transfusion
- Genetics
  - Homozygous for Hgb S
  - Mutation in β-globin: Glutamic acid ⇒ valine
- Etiology
  - Heterozygous Hgb S affords increased resistance to malaria (hence prevalence)
  - Homozygous SS leads to sickling and vascular occlusion ("crisis")
  - Hgb S becomes "stiff" (erythrocytes are sickle-shaped) when deoxygenated
    - RBCs lose pliability required to traverse capillaries
    - RBCs have "sticky" membrane
    - Result: Microvascular occlusion, cell destruction (hemolysis)
- Epidemiology
  - Primary cause of stroke in African-American children
    - Stroke incidence decreased if Hgb S kept to less than 30% by transfusion (but need initial ischemic event to initiate therapy)
  - 11% suffer cerebral infarction by age 20 years, 24% by age 45 years
  - Incidence of cerebral lesions in sickle cell trait: 10-19%
- Associated abnormalities
  - Anemia, reticulocytosis, granulocytosis
  - Susceptibility to pneumococci (due to malfunctioning spleen)
  - Occasionally causes pseudotumor cerebri (idiopathic intracranial hypertension without evidence for other etiology such as venous sinus occlusion, etc.)

Gross Pathologic & Surgical Features

- Bone, brain, renal and splenic infarcts; hepatomegaly

Microscopic Features

- Severe anemia with sickled cells on smear
- Vascular occlusions due to masses of sickled RBCs

CLINICAL ISSUES

Presentation

- Most common signs/symptoms
  - Vasoocclusive crisis with infarctions involving
    - Spleen, brain, bone marrow, kidney, lung
  - Formation of gallstones, priapism, neuropathy, skin ulcers
- Clinical Profile
  - Stroke in African-American children
    - 17-26% of all patients with SCD
    - 75% are ischemic, 25% are hemorrhage
- Bone infarcts, avascular necrosis during crisis
- Osteomyelitis, especially Salmonella
- Gross hematuria from renal papillary necrosis
- Splenic infarction from exposure to high altitude
- Infections common, especially pneumococcus after splenic infarction

Demographics

- Age: Infarctions are generally first seen in children about 10 years of age
- Gender: No predilection
- Ethnicity
  - Hgb S found in 10% of African-Americans
    - SCD found primarily in African-Americans and their decendents

Natural History & Prognosis

- Unrelenting, severe hemolytic anemia beginning at a few months of age after Hgb S replaces Hgb F (fetal)
  - Cognitive dysfunction occurs even in absence of cerebral infarctions
- Repeated ischemic events leading to strokes with worsening motor and intellectual deficits
- Poor for homozygous SCD without transfusions
- Usually live to adulthood albeit with complications

Treatment

- Repeated transfusions to keep Hgb S less than 30% decreases both incidence of stroke and intimal hyperplasia in COW vessels
- Folic acid for anemia
- Hydroxyurea improves hematologic parameters (can lower TCD velocities), may be an alternative to chronic transfusions
- Hydration and oxygenation during crises

DIAGNOSTIC CHECKLIST

Image Interpretation Pearls

- African-American child with cerebral infarction: Always consider SCD!

SELECTED REFERENCES

1. Zimmerman SA et al: Hydroxyurea therapy lowers transcranial Doppler flow velocities in children with sickle cell anemia. Blood. 110(3):1043-7, 2007
2. Debaun MR et al: Etiology of strokes in children with sickle cell anemia. Ment Retard Dev Disabil Res Rev. 12(3):192-9, 2006
3. Adams RJ: TCD in sickle cell disease: an important and useful test. Pediatr Radiol. 35(3):229-34, 2005
4. Zimmerman RA: MRI/MRA evaluation of sickle cell disease of the brain. Pediatr Radiol. 35(3):249-57, 2005
5. Gebreyohanns M et al: Sickle cell disease: primary stroke prevention. CNS Spectr. 9(6):445-9, 2004
6. Henry M et al: Pseudotumor cerebri in children with sickle cell disease: a case series. Pediatrics. 113(3 Pt 1):e265-9, 2004
7. Oguz KK et al: Sickle cell disease: continuous arterial spin-labeling perfusion MR imaging in children. Radiology. 227(2):567-74, 2003
8. Steen RG et al: Cognitive impairment in children with hemoglobin SS sickle cell disease: relationship to MR imaging findings and hematocrit. AJNR Am J Neuroradiol. 24(3):382-9, 2003
9. Steen RG et al: Prospective brain imaging evaluation of children with sickle cell trait: initial observations. Radiology. 228(1):208-15, 2003
10. Oyesiku NM et al: Intracranial aneurysms in sickle-cell anemia: clinical features and pathogenesis. J Neurosurg. 75(3):356-63, 1991

SICKLE CELL ANEMIA

IMAGE GALLERY

Typical

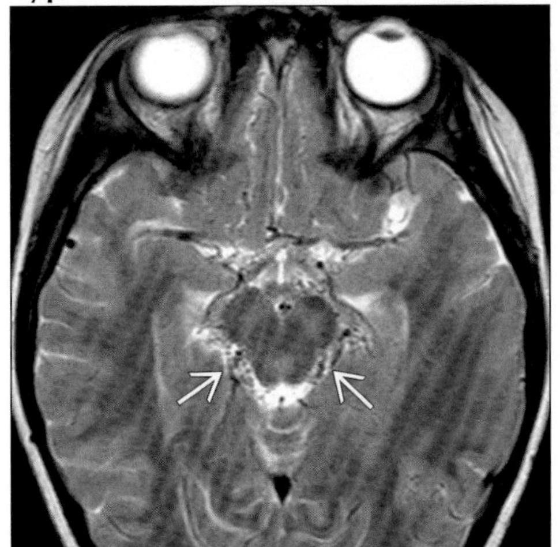

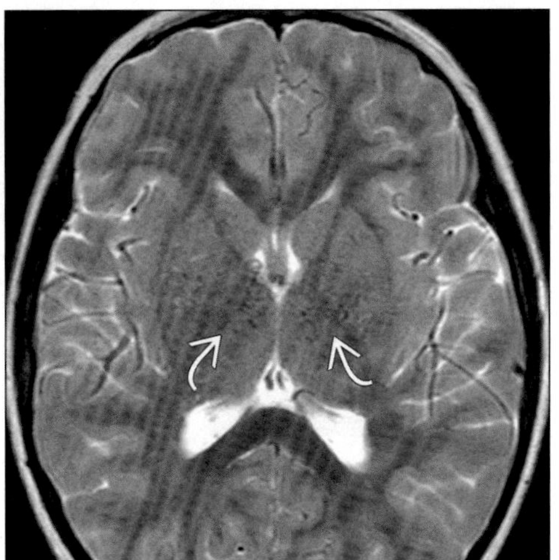

*(**Left**) Axial T2WI MR demonstrates multiple serpiginous flow voids ➔ in the basal cisterns surrounding the midbrain from collateral vessels due to moyamoya from sickle cell disease. (**Right**) Axial T2WI MR in the same patient more superior slice depicts multiple punctate flow voids ➔ in bilateral basal ganglia from hypertrophied collateral lenticulostriate moyamoya arteries.*

Typical

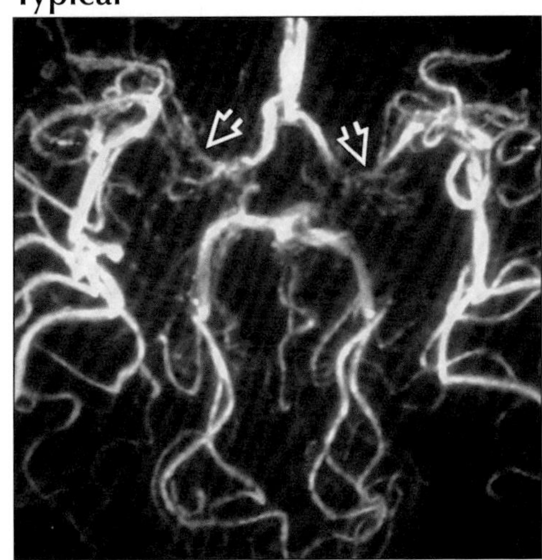

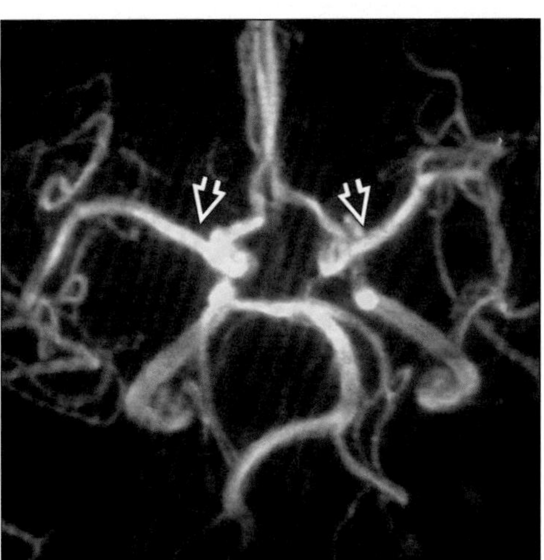

*(**Left**) Superior-inferior 3D TOF MRA shows severe narrowing of the bilateral proximal middle cerebral arteries ➔ in this 2 year old patient with sickle cell anemia. (**Right**) Superior-inferior 3D TOF MRA in the same patient 16 months later demonstrates resolution of the arterial narrowing ➔ following transfusion therapy.*

Typical

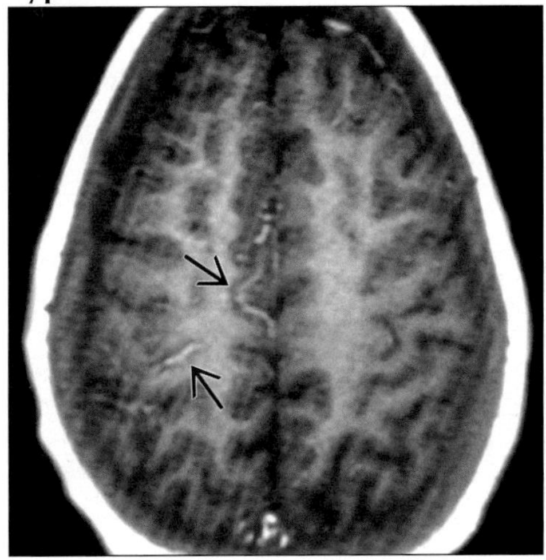

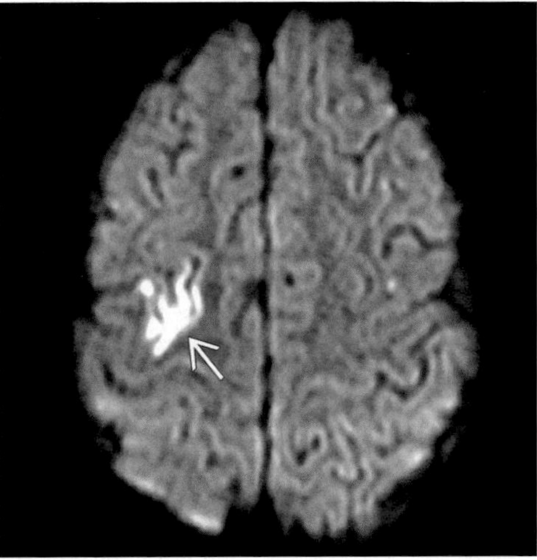

*(**Left**) Axial T1WI MR post-contrast in a patient with left hand weakness shows vascular enhancement overlying the right posterior frontal lobe ➔ from stagnant flow due to sickle cell disease. (**Right**) Axial DWI MR in a different patient with sickle cell anemia shows restricted diffusion ➔ in the cortex and subcortical white matter of posterior right frontal lobe from acute infarction.*

VASCULITIS, INTRACRANIAL

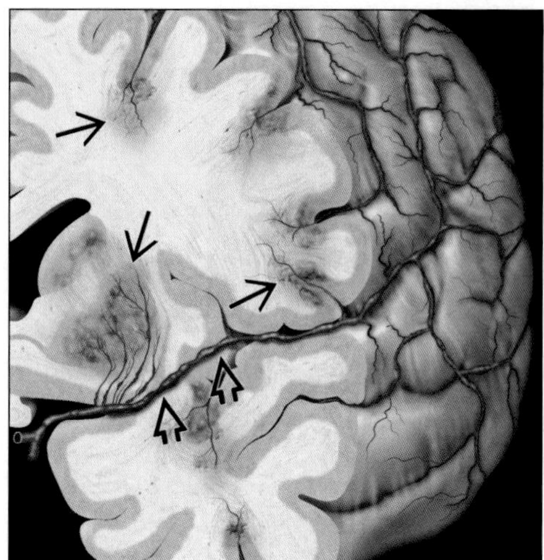

Coronal oblique graphic shows vessel wall irregularity ⇨ due to vasculitis with resultant foci of edema and scattered hemorrhages → in basal ganglia and gray-white matter junctions.

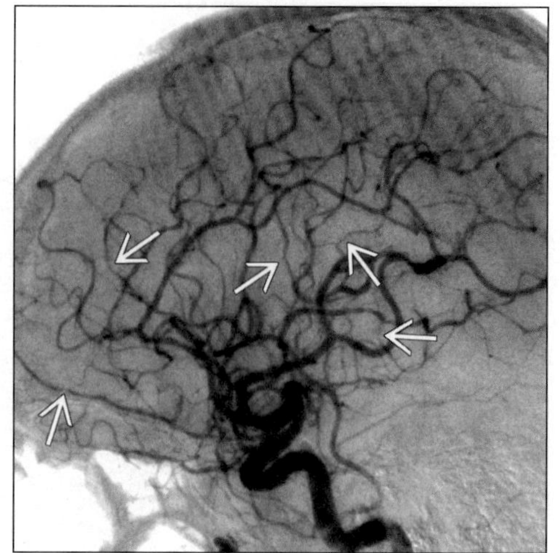

Lateral DSA left common carotid artery injection demonstrates a subtle but classic example of multiple foci of irregular vessel narrowing in the distal vasculature ➔ due to vasculitis.

TERMINOLOGY

Abbreviations and Synonyms

- Inflammatory vasculopathy (more general term indicating any vascular pathology)
- Arteritis (specifies arterial inflammation)
- Angiitis (inflammation of either arteries or veins)

Definitions

- Heterogeneous group of CNS disorders characterized by inflammation and necrosis of blood vessel walls
- Involves either arteries or veins

IMAGING FINDINGS

General Features

- Best diagnostic clue
  - Irregularities, stenoses and vascular occlusions in a pattern atypical for atherosclerotic disease
  - Imaging workup can be normal; need clinical/laboratory correlation
- Location: Arteries and veins are affected; occurs in intracranial vessels of any size
- Size: Degree of vessel narrowing may range from normal/minimally stenotic to occluded
- Morphology
  - Classic appearance: Multifocal areas of stenoses (smooth/irregular) alternating with dilated segments
  - Variety of angiographic appearances depending on etiology including vascular irregularities, stenoses, aneurysms and occlusions

CT Findings

- NECT
  - Relatively insensitive; may be normal
  - May see secondary signs such as ischemia/infarction: Multifocal low density areas in basal ganglia, subcortical white matter
  - May see hemorrhage
- CECT: May see patchy areas of enhancement

MR Findings

- T1WI: Can be normal early; ± multifocal cortical/subcortical hypointensities
- T2WI: Multifocal WM hyperintensities, cortical/subcortical infarcts (infarcts commonly hemorrhagic)
- FLAIR: Subcortical, basal ganglia hyperintensities

DDx: Vasculitis, Intracranial

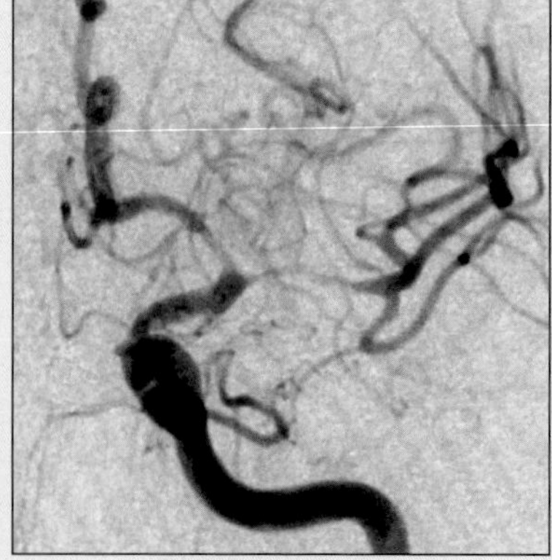

Left MCA/ACA ASVD

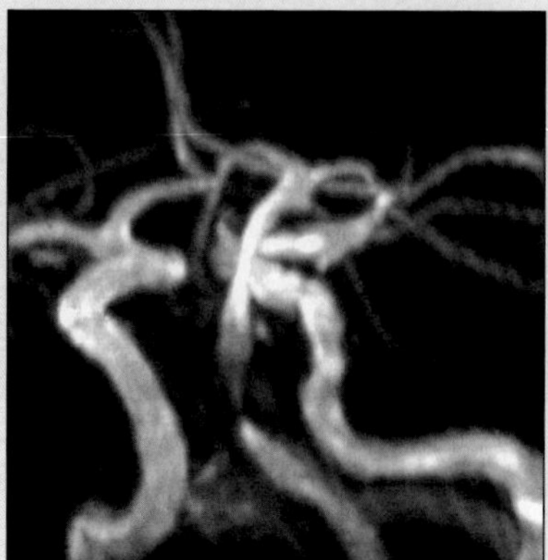

LICA/Basilar ASVD

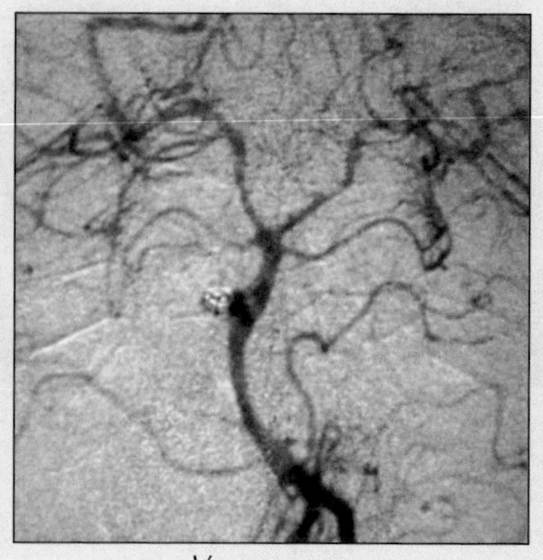

Vasospasm

VASCULITIS, INTRACRANIAL

Key Facts

Terminology
- Inflammatory vasculopathy (more general term indicating any vascular pathology)
- Heterogeneous group of CNS disorders characterized by inflammation and necrosis of blood vessel walls

Imaging Findings
- Irregularities, stenoses and vascular occlusions in a pattern atypical for atherosclerotic disease
- Location: Arteries and veins are affected; occurs in intracranial vessels of any size
- Multifocal WM hyperintensities, cortical/subcortical infarcts (infarcts commonly hemorrhagic)
- T1 C+: May see patchy areas of enhancement

Top Differential Diagnoses
- Intracranial Atherosclerotic Vascular Disease
- Arterial Vasospasm

Pathology
- Pattern of vessel wall inflammation, necrosis common to all vasculitides
- Primary or secondary; caused by broad spectrum of infectious, inflammatory agents, drugs, etc.

Clinical Issues
- Stroke related to manifestations of vascular involvement (stenosis, occlusion, aneurysm)
- Varies depending upon etiology; typically progressive if untreated
- Most patients with CNS vasculitis should be treated aggressively with a combination of steroids or other immunosuppressive medications

- T2* GRE: May show short T2 hemorrhagic "blooming"
- DWI
  - Can see restricted diffusion (acute infarction)
  - Increase in ADC values noted in "normal" brain
- T1 C+: May see patchy areas of enhancement
- MRA
  - May see some classic angiographic signs if larger vessels involved/vascular occlusion; may be normal
  - 3T MRA more sensitive to detect lesions

Ultrasonographic Findings
- Pulsed Doppler
  - TCD may be used to monitor cerebral blood flow velocities if large arteries are involved
  - If positive, can be used to evaluate therapy response

Angiographic Findings
- Conventional
  - Alternating stenosis and dilatation ("beading") primarily involving 2nd, 3rd order branches
  - Less common: Long segment stenoses, pseudoaneurysms

Imaging Recommendations
- Best imaging tool
  - DSA is cornerstone diagnostic procedure
  - Rarely MR imaging findings may be negative in the setting of CNS vasculitis confirmed on angiography
- Protocol advice
  - DSA if lab studies positive, MR/MRA negative
  - CTA/MRA useful screening; spatial resolution may be insufficient for subtle disease in distal vasculature

DIFFERENTIAL DIAGNOSIS

Intracranial Atherosclerotic Vascular Disease
- Advanced patient age
- Typical distribution (carotid siphon, proximal intracranial vessels); extracranial disease as well

Arterial Vasospasm
- Temporal relationship to subarachnoid hemorrhage
- Involves proximal vasculature

PATHOLOGY

General Features
- General path comments
  - Pattern of vessel wall inflammation, necrosis common to all vasculitides
  - Primary or secondary; caused by broad spectrum of infectious, inflammatory agents, drugs, etc.
- Etiology
  - Bacterial meningitis
    - Infarction due to vascular involvement in 25%
    - H. Influenzae most common; esp. children
  - Tuberculous meningitis
    - Vessels at the skull base commonly involved, i.e., supraclinoid ICA and M1 occlusions and stenoses
  - Mycotic arteritis (aspergillus, cocci, etc.)
    - Actinomyces; invades vessel walls leading to hemorrhage
    - Narrowing of the basal cerebral or cortical vessels
  - Viral arteritis
    - Herpes simplex most common in North America
    - HIV-associated vasculitis increasing, esp. children
  - Syphilis arteritis
    - Two forms: Syphilitic meningitis and gummatous vasculitis
    - Diffuse vasculitis of cortical arteries and veins
    - Gummatous vasculitis usually affects proximal MCA branches
  - Polyarteritis nodosa
    - Most common systemic vasculitis to involve the CNS (though late)
    - Microaneurysms due to necrosis of the internal elastic lamina in 75%
  - Cell mediated arteritides
    - Giant cell arteritis (granulomatous infiltration of the arterial walls)
    - Takayasu (primarily involves aorta, great vessels)
    - Temporal arteritis (systemic; involves temporal, other extracranial arteries)
  - Wegener
    - May cause intracerebral and meningeal granulomas or vasculitis

VASCULITIS, INTRACRANIAL

- CNS involved in 15-30% due to direct invasion from nose/sinuses
- Chronic systemic arteritis involving lungs, kidneys and sinuses
- Sarcoid (CNS involvement in 3-5% of cases)
  - Can extend along perivascular spaces, involve penetrating arteries
  - Meningitis, vasculitis involving vessels at the base of the brain
- Granulomatous angiitis (PACNS)
  - Primary angiitis isolated to the CNS (idiopathic)
  - Manifest as multiple intracranial stenoses
- Collagen vascular disease (SLE, rheumatoid, scleroderma)
  - SLE: Most common to involve the CNS
  - Vasculitis relatively uncommon (variable findings; small vessel irregularities/stenoses/occlusions up to fusiform aneurysms)
  - CVA seen in 50% due to cardiac disease or coagulopathy
- Drug abuse vasculitis
  - Drug can injure vessels directly or secondarily (usually hypersensitivity to contaminants)
  - Associated with both legitimate and illegal "street" drugs including amphetamines, cocaine, heroin, phenylpropanolamine and ergots
- Radiation
  - Acute arteritis; transient white matter edema
  - Chronic changes more severe with vessel obliteration and brain necrosis, leukomalacia, calcifying microangiopathy and atrophy
  - Effects compounded with concomitant chemotherapy
- Moyamoya disease
  - Sometimes referred to as "idiopathic progressive arteriopathy of childhood"
  - Moyamoya is an angiographic pattern, not a specific disease; may be acquired or inherited
  - Any progressive occlusion of the supraclinoid ICAs may develop moyamoya pattern
  - Pattern has been reported with neurofibromatosis, atherosclerosis, radiation therapy
  - Prognosis depends upon the rapidity and extent of the vascular occlusions as well as the development of effective collaterals
- Epidemiology: CNS vasculitis occurs in a variety of clinical settings, some of which exhibit a distinct age preference; others a tissue tropism
- Associated abnormalities: May have many, particularly with vasculitis secondary to systemic disease

Gross Pathologic & Surgical Features

- Characterized by ischemic lesions and small petechial hemorrhages
- Vessels of any size can be involved
- May see venulitis with parenchymal hemorrhages

Microscopic Features

- Inflammation and necrosis of blood vessel walls

Staging, Grading or Classification Criteria

- Several different classification systems have been proposed
  - Can be primary intracranial or secondary to a systemic disease
  - Can be divided into true vasculitis (angiitis) and noninflammatory vasculopathy
  - Can be divided into those due to immune complex deposition vs. cell-mediated disorders
  - Can be infectious or noninfectious

CLINICAL ISSUES

Presentation

- Most common signs/symptoms
  - Stroke related to manifestations of vascular involvement (stenosis, occlusion, aneurysm)
  - Patients presenting with symptoms suggestive of vasculitis require brain neuroimaging, lumbar puncture, and angiography, but only biopsy allows a definite diagnosis

Demographics

- Age: Variable from childhood to adulthood
- Gender: Depends upon the type of vasculitis; generally no gender predilection

Natural History & Prognosis

- Varies depending upon etiology; typically progressive if untreated

Treatment

- Most patients with CNS vasculitis should be treated aggressively with a combination of steroids or other immunosuppressive medications

DIAGNOSTIC CHECKLIST

Consider

- Diagnosis is frequently made on the basis of clinical presentation, brain MR, and cerebral angiography without pathologic confirmation
- Despite the high sensitivity of MR imaging for CNS vasculitis, angiography may still be required to render an accurate diagnosis

SELECTED REFERENCES

1. Kuker W: Cerebral vasculitis: imaging signs revisited. Neuroradiology. 49(6):471-9, 2007
2. White ML et al: Analysis of central nervous system vasculitis with diffusion-weighted imaging and apparent diffusion coefficient mapping of the normal-appearing brain. AJNR Am J Neuroradiol. 28(5):933-7, 2007
3. Benseler SM: Central nervous system vasculitis in children. Curr Rheumatol Rep. 8(6):442-9, 2006
4. Markl M et al: High resolution 3T MRI for the assessment of cervical and superficial cranial arteries in giant cell arteritis. J Magn Reson Imaging. 24(2):423-7, 2006
5. Mazlumzadeh M et al: Treatment of giant cell arteritis using induction therapy with high-dose glucocorticoids: a double-blind, placebo-controlled, randomized prospective clinical trial. Arthritis Rheum. 54(10):3310-8, 2006
6. Schmidt WA: Takayasu and temporal arteritis. Front Neurol Neurosci. 21:96-104, 2006
7. Carolei A et al: Central nervous system vasculitis. Neurol Sci. 24 Suppl 1:S8-S10, 2003

IMAGE GALLERY

Typical

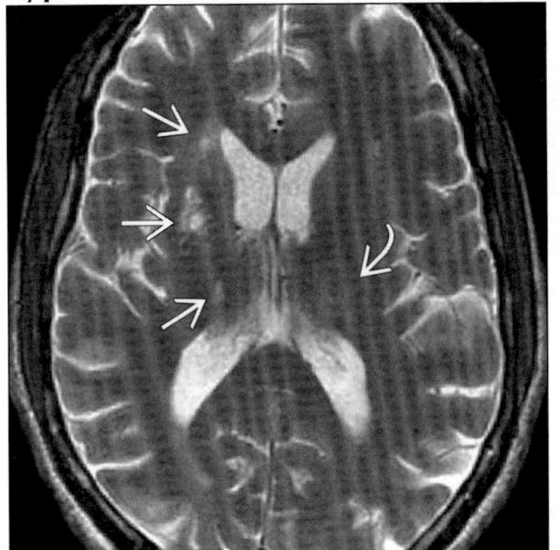

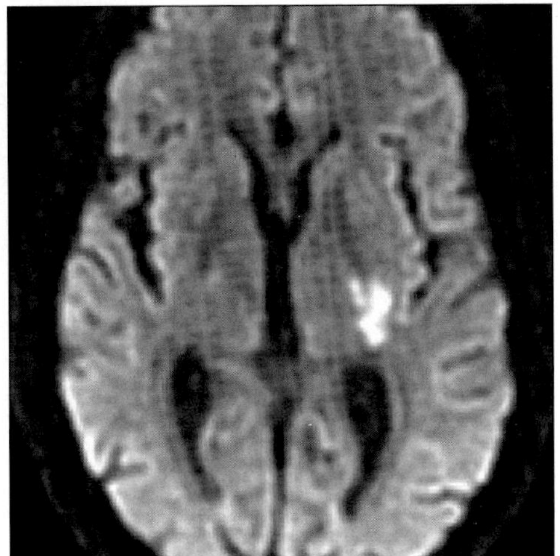

*(**Left**) Axial T2WI MR shows foci of marked hyperintensity in right caudate, lentiform, and thalamic nuclei ➡ from old lacunar infarcts. There is a vague hyperintensity in the left thalamus ➡. **(Right)** Axial DWI MR in the same patient as previous image, shows restricted diffusion in the left thalamus and left posterior internal capsule confirming suspected acute lacunar infarct. Patient with HIV vasculitis.*

Typical

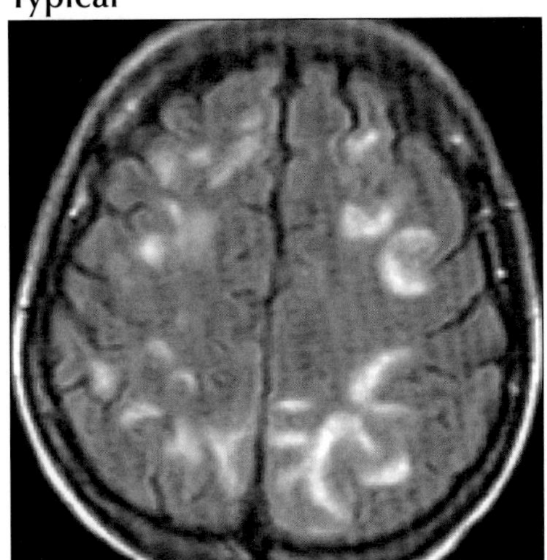

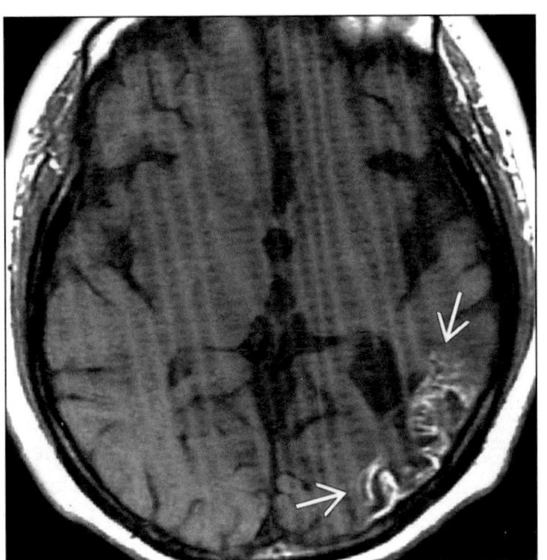

*(**Left**) Axial FLAIR MR image shows diffuse subcortical hyperintense foci from severe chronic ischemic disease in this patient with vasculitis due to systemic lupus erythematosus. **(Right)** Axial T1WI MR in a different patient with SLE vasculitis depicts frank infarction ➡ of the left posterior temporal and occipital lobes with associated chronic hemorrhage/laminar necrosis.*

Typical

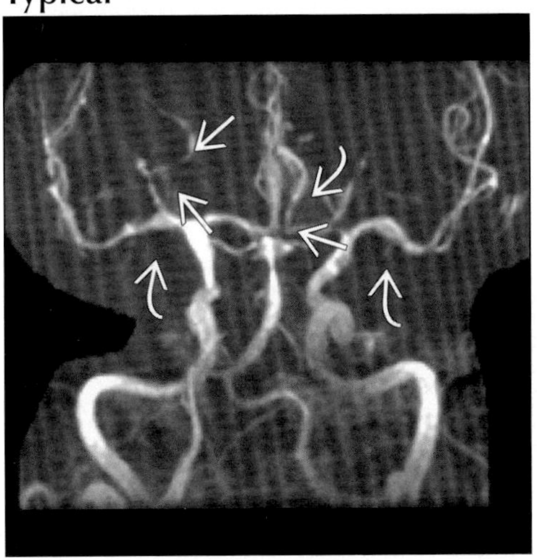

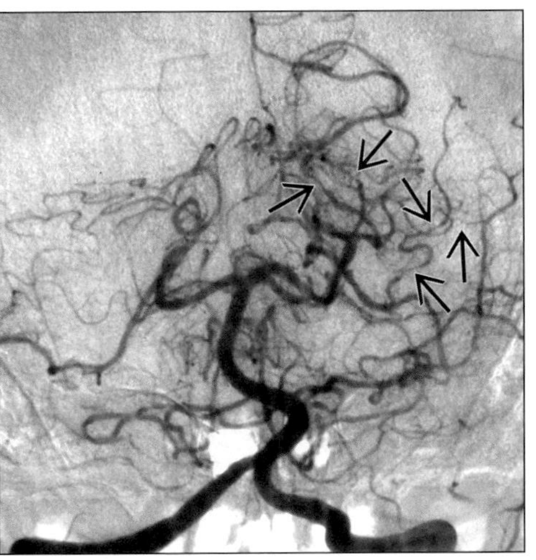

*(**Left**) Anteroposterior TOF MRA MIP image shows multifocal areas of alternating vessel constriction ➡ and dilatation ➡ in this HIV positive patient with severe vasculitis. **(Right)** Anteroposterior DSA of the vertebrobasilar circulation depicts multiple foci of severe narrowing ➡ consistent with vasculitis in this patient with a history of intravenous drug abuse.*

MOYAMOYA

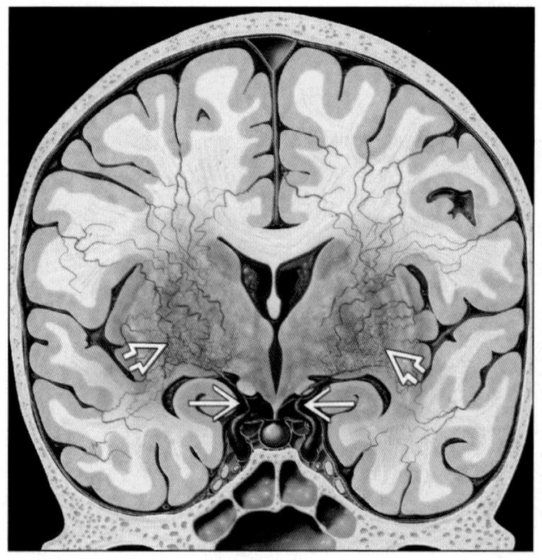

Coronal graphic shows severe tapering of both distal internal carotid arteries ➡ and markedly enlarged lenticulostriate arteries ⇨, the "puff of smoke" moyamoya pattern.

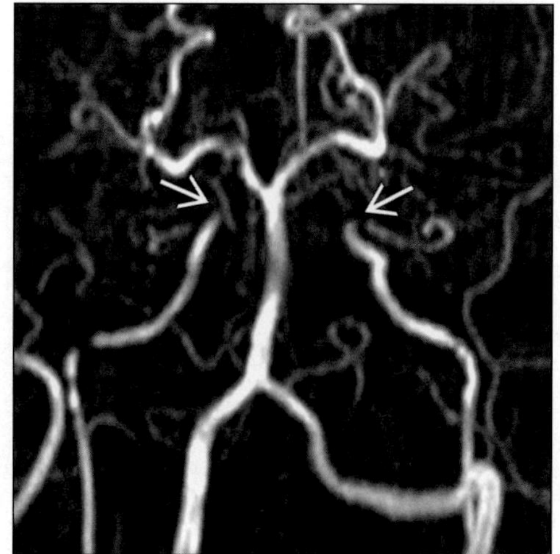

Anteroposterior 3D TOF MRA MIP image shows complete lack of flow related signal in the distal internal carotid arteries ➡ due to vessel occlusion, a classic moyamoya appearance.

TERMINOLOGY

Abbreviations and Synonyms

- Idiopathic progressive arteriopathy of childhood; spontaneous occlusion of the circle of Willis (COW)

Definitions

- Progressive narrowing of distal ICA & proximal COW vessels with secondary collateralization
- Moyamoya collateralization may occur with **any** progressive vascular occlusion (inherited or acquired)

IMAGING FINDINGS

General Features

- Best diagnostic clue: Multiple punctate dots (CECT) & flow-voids (MR) in basal ganglia (BG)
- Location: COW; anterior > > posterior circulation
- Size: Large vessel occlusion
- Morphology: "Puff or spiral of smoke" (moyamoya in Japanese) = cloud-like lenticulostriate & thalamoperforator collaterals on angiography

CT Findings

- NECT
  - Children: 50-60% show anterior > posterior atrophy
  - Adults: Hemorrhage (esp. intraventricular)
- CECT: Enhancing dots (big lenticulostriates) in BG & abnormal "net-like" vessels at base of brain
- CTA: Abnormal COW & "net-like" collaterals
- Xe-133 CT: ↓ Cerebral reserve with acetazolamide challenge

MR Findings

- T1WI: Multiple dot-like flow voids in BG
- T2WI
  - Hyperintense cortical, white matter, & small vessel infarcts
  - Collateral vessels = "net-like" cisternal filling defects
- FLAIR
  - Bright sulci = leptomeningeal "ivy sign"
    - Slow-flowing engorged pial vessels, thickened arachnoid membranes
- T2* GRE: Hemosiderin blooming if prior hemorrhage
- DWI: Positive in acute stroke; **very** useful in "acute on chronic" disease
- T1 C+

DDx: Moyamoya

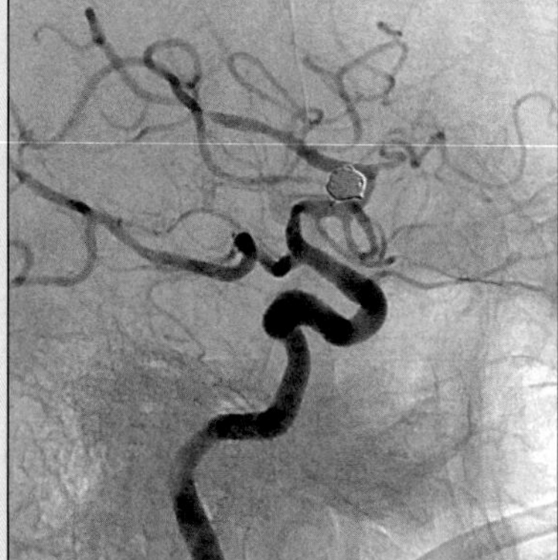

SAH Vasospasm

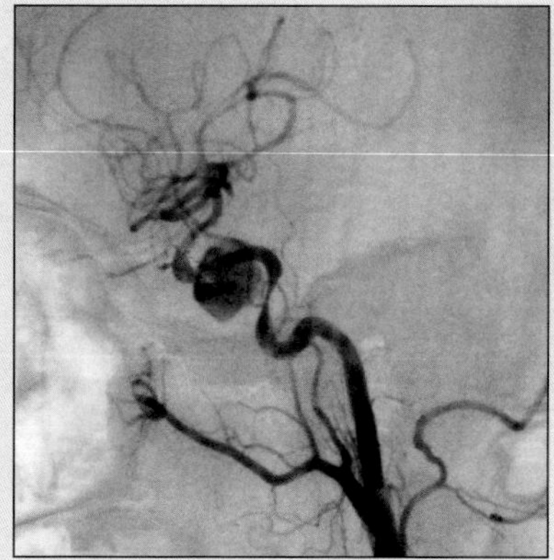

ICA Dissection/Pseudoaneurysm

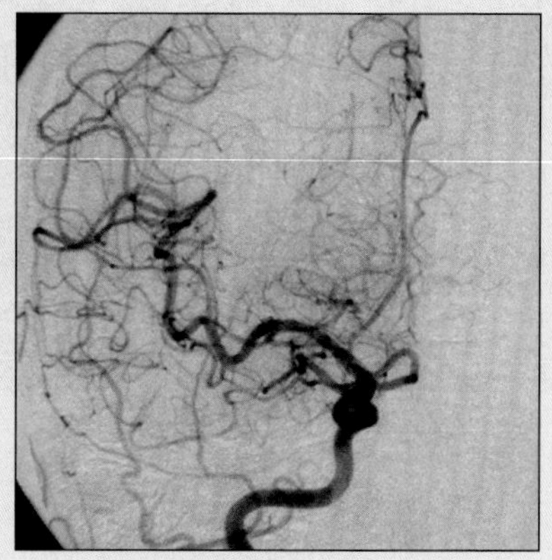

ACA Tumor Encasement

MOYAMOYA

Key Facts

Terminology

- Idiopathic progressive arteriopathy of childhood; spontaneous occlusion of the circle of Willis (COW)
- Progressive narrowing of distal ICA & proximal COW vessels with secondary collateralization
- Moyamoya collateralization may occur with **any** progressive vascular occlusion (inherited or acquired)

Imaging Findings

- Best diagnostic clue: Multiple punctate dots (CECT) & flow-voids (MR) in basal ganglia (BG)
- Morphology: "Puff or spiral of smoke" (moyamoya in Japanese) = cloud-like lenticulostriate & thalamoperforator collaterals on angiography
- Bright sulci = leptomeningeal "ivy sign"
- DWI: Positive in acute stroke; **very** useful in "acute on chronic" disease
- Catheter angiography: Predominantly (not exclusively) anterior circulation
- Dilatation & branch extension of anterior choroidal artery predicts adult hemorrhagic events

Pathology

- Many etiologies: Idiopathic, genetic, inflammatory, congenital mesenchymal defects, premature aging syndromes, prothrombotic states

Clinical Issues

- Initially described in Japanese children as a specific entity

Diagnostic Checklist

- Moyamoya outside of Asia: Need to seek etiology
- Moyamoya in children typically presents with cerebral ischemia vs. hemorrhage in adults

---

 - Lenticulostriate collaterals ⇒ enhancing "dots" in BG & "net-like" thin vessels in cisterns
 - Leptomeningeal enhancement (contrast-enhanced "ivy sign"); ↓ after "effective bypass surgery"
- MRA: Narrowed distal ICA & proximal COW vessels, ± patent synangiosis; note: Turbulent dephasing from rapid flow can mimic stenoses on "bright blood" MRA ⇒ use lowest possible TE to minimize artifact
- MRV: Some vasculopathies leading to moyamoya may also involve veins
- MRS
 - Lactate in acutely infarcted tissue
 - NAA/Cr & Cho/Cr ratios in frontal white matter improve after revascularization
- Perfusion-weighted imaging (PWI): ↓ Perfusion deep hemispheric white matter, relative ↑ perfusion posterior circulation
 - PWI may be abnormal when MR still normal
 - Relative cerebral blood volume (rCBV) & time to peak (TTP) correlate with stage/severity of disease

Nuclear Medicine Findings

- PET: ↓ Hemodynamic reserve capacity
- SPECT 123I-Iomazenil: Neuronal density preserved if asymptomatic, ↓ if symptomatic

Ultrasonographic Findings

- Grayscale Ultrasound: Reduction of ICA lumen size
- Pulsed Doppler
 - Doppler spectral waveforms in ICA show no flow (occluded) or high resistance (stenotic) flow pattern
 - ↑ End-diastolic flow velocity & ↓ vascular resistance in ECA collaterals
- Color Doppler: Aliasing suggests stenoses
- Power Doppler: Contrast improves visualization of slow flow stenotic vessels & collaterals

Angiographic Findings

- Conventional
 - Catheter angiography: Predominantly (not exclusively) anterior circulation
   - Narrow proximal COW & ICA (earliest)
   - Lenticulostriate & thalamoperforator collaterals (intermediate)
   - Transdural & transosseous ECA-ICA collaterals (late)
 - Dilatation & branch extension of anterior choroidal artery predicts adult hemorrhagic events

Imaging Recommendations

- Best imaging tool: MR/MRA
- Protocol advice
 - MRA: COW
 - DWI: Seek "acute on chronic" ischemia
 - MR: FLAIR & T1 C+ illustrate "ivy sign" (reversible if patent bypass)
 - Contrast material improves visualization of synangiosis & collaterals
 - Catheter angiography defines anatomy of occlusions pre-bypass

DIFFERENTIAL DIAGNOSIS

"Ivy Sign"

- Leptomeningeal metastases, subarachnoid hemorrhage (SAH), meningitis; also seen with high inspired oxygen

Punctate Foci in Basal Ganglia

- Cribriform lacunar state: No enhancement

Severely Attenuated ICA or Circle of Willis

- SAH vasospasm, meningitis/vasculitis, dissection, tumor encasement, congenital hypoplasia

PATHOLOGY

General Features

- General path comments
 - Nearly endless list of etiologies reported
 - Results from any slowly progressive intracranial vascular occlusion
- Genetics
 - Inherited (primary) moyamoya

MOYAMOYA

- Several gene loci: Chr 3p26-p24.2 & 17q25 (amongst others)
  - Disorders with ↑ association secondary moyamoya
    - Down syndrome, tuberous sclerosis, sickle cell disease, connective tissue disease, progeria
    - Midline anomalies (morning glory syndrome); syndromes w/aneurysms, cardiac & ocular defects
    - NF1, irradiation & suprasellar tumor a disastrous combination
    - Inflammatory: CNS angiitis (of childhood), basal meningitis (TB), leptospirosis, radiation angiopathy, local infection (tonsillitis/otitis), atherosclerosis
    - Vasculopathies & prothrombotic states: Kawasaki, anticardiolipin antibody, Factor V Leiden, polyarteritis nodosa, Behcet, SLE
- Etiology: Many: Idiopathic, genetic, inflammatory, congenital mesenchymal defects, premature aging syndromes, prothrombotic states
- Epidemiology
  - 10% of cases are familial
  - 1:100,000 in Japan
- Associated abnormalities: Dependent upon primary etiology

Gross Pathologic & Surgical Features

- Increased perforating (early) & ECA-ICA (late) collaterals in atrophic brain
- Intracranial hemorrhage (adults)
- Increased saccular aneurysms (esp. basilar in adults)

Microscopic Features

- Intimal thickening & hyperplasia
- Excessive infolding & thickening of internal elastic lamina
- Increased periventricular pseudoaneurysms (cause of hemorrhage)

Staging, Grading or Classification Criteria

- Staging criteria (Suzuki)
  - Stage I: Narrowing of ICA bifurcation
  - Stage II: ACA, MCA, PCA dilated
  - Stage III: Maximal basal moyamoya collaterals; small ACA/MCA
  - Stage IV: Fewer collaterals (vessels); small PCA
  - Stage V: Further reduction in collaterals; absent ACA, MCA, PCA
  - Stage VI: Extensive pial collaterals from external carotid branches

CLINICAL ISSUES

Presentation

- Most common signs/symptoms
  - In childhood: TIAs, alternating hemiplegia (exacerbated by crying), headache, occasionally just developmental delay & poor feeding
  - In adulthood: SAH & intraventricular hemorrhage
- Clinical Profile
  - Children more likely to have TIAs & to progress, adults more likely to infarct (but slower progression)
  - Children more likely to have ipsilateral anterior **plus** posterior circulation involvement

Demographics

- Age: Bimodal age peaks: 6 yrs > 35 yrs
- Gender: M:F = 1:1.8
- Ethnicity
  - Initially described in Japanese children as a specific entity
  - Remains most frequent cause of stroke in Asian children

Natural History & Prognosis

- Progressive narrowing, collateralization & ischemia
- Prognosis depends on etiology, ability to form collaterals, age/stage at diagnosis
- Pediatric cases usually advance to stage V within 10 yrs onset
  - Infantile moyamoya progresses faster
- Hemorrhagic moyamoya has poorer outcome

Treatment

- Anticoagulation; correct/control prothrombotic states & inflammatory etiologies
- Hypertransfusion regimens for sickle cell related moyamoya
- Encephalo-duro-arterio-synangiosis (EDAS), a method of indirect bypass
  - 5 yr risk of ipsilateral stroke post EDAS 15%
- Perivascular sympathectomy or superior cervical ganglionectomy; percutaneous angioplasty (adult)

DIAGNOSTIC CHECKLIST

Consider

- Moyamoya outside of Asia: Need to seek etiology

Image Interpretation Pearls

- Asymmetric atrophy found on childhood CT, look for abnormal vascular pattern
- Moyamoya in children typically presents with cerebral ischemia vs. hemorrhage in adults

SELECTED REFERENCES

1. Kuroda S et al: Radiological findings, clinical course, and outcome in asymptomatic moyamoya disease: results of multicenter survey in Japan. Stroke. 38(5):1430-5, 2007
2. Takagi Y et al: Histological features of middle cerebral arteries from patients treated for Moyamoya disease. Neurol Med Chir (Tokyo). 47(1):1-4, 2007
3. Hallemeier CL et al: Clinical features and outcome in North American adults with moyamoya phenomenon. Stroke. 37(6):1490-6, 2006
4. Ruan LT et al: Color and power Doppler sonography of extracranial and intracranial arteries in Moyamoya disease. J Clin Ultrasound. 34(2):60-9, 2006
5. Scott RM et al: Long-term outcome in children with moyamoya syndrome after cranial revascularization by pial synangiosis. J Neurosurg. 100:142-9, 2004
6. Morioka M et al: Angiographic dilatation and branch extension of the anterior choroidal and posterior communicating arteries are predictors of hemorrhage in adult moyamoya patients. Stroke. 34(1):90-5, 2003
7. Yoon HK et al: "Ivy sign" in childhood moyamoya disease: depiction on FLAIR and contrast-enhanced T1-weighted MR images. Radiology. 223(2):384-9, 2002

MOYAMOYA

IMAGE GALLERY

Typical

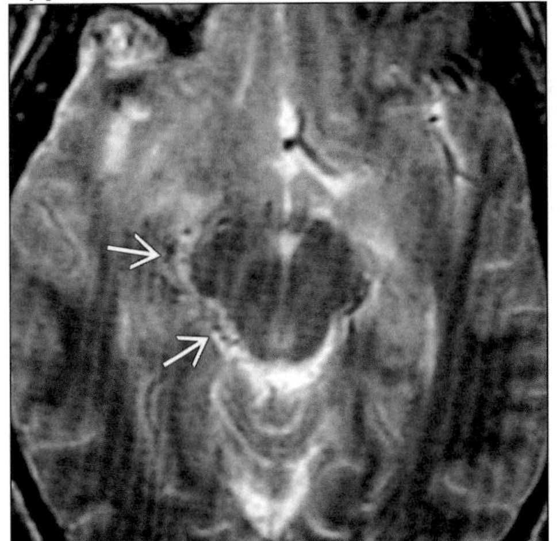

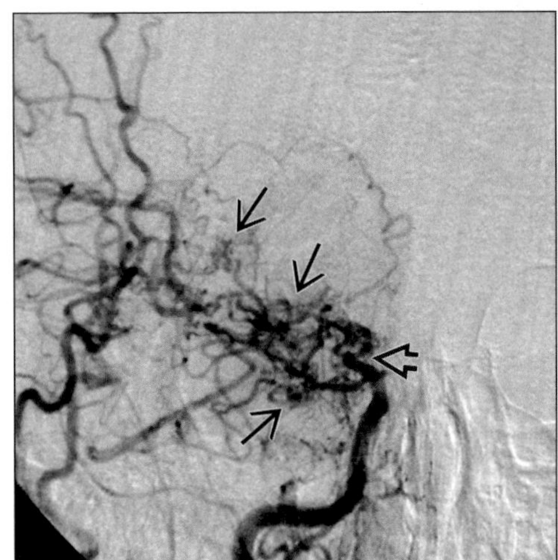

(Left) *Axial T2WI MR shows curvilinear "net-like" flow voids ➡ in the right ambient (lateral perimesencephalic) cistern from collateral moyamoya vessels.* ***(Right)*** *Anteroposterior DSA in the same patient as previous image, shows abrupt termination of the right ICA ⇨ with hypertrophied collateral moyamoya vessels ➡ producing the typical "puff of smoke" pattern.*

Typical

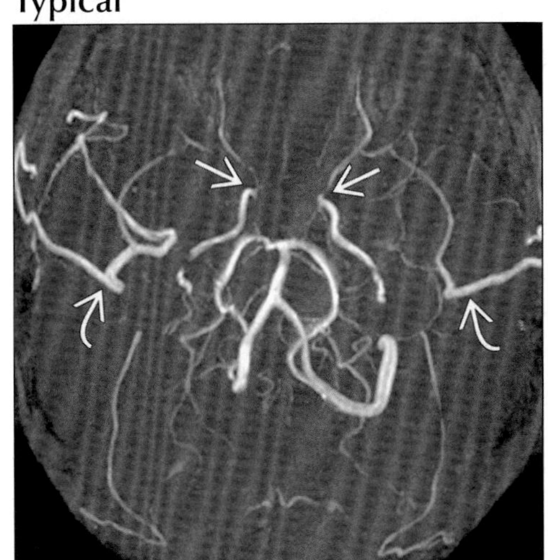

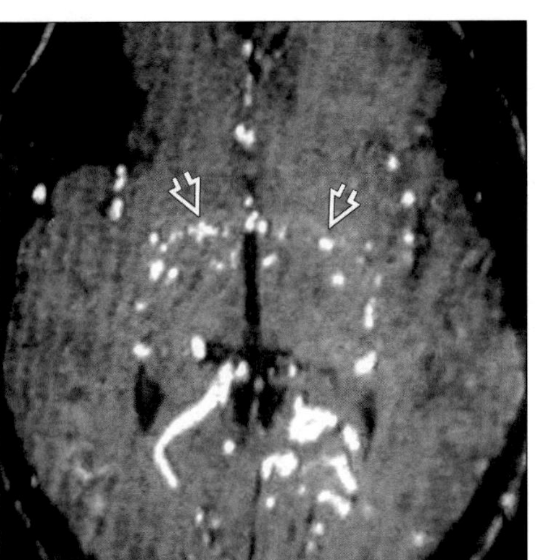

(Left) *Axial collapsed 3D TOF MRA MIP image shows complete occlusion of the distal internal carotid arteries ➡ with hypertrophy of the external carotid artery branches ➡ from moyamoya.* ***(Right)*** *Axial TOF MRA source image in a different patient depicts multiple punctate dilated vessels ⇨ in the lentiform nuclei from hypertrophied moyamoya lenticulostriate collateral vasculature.*

Typical

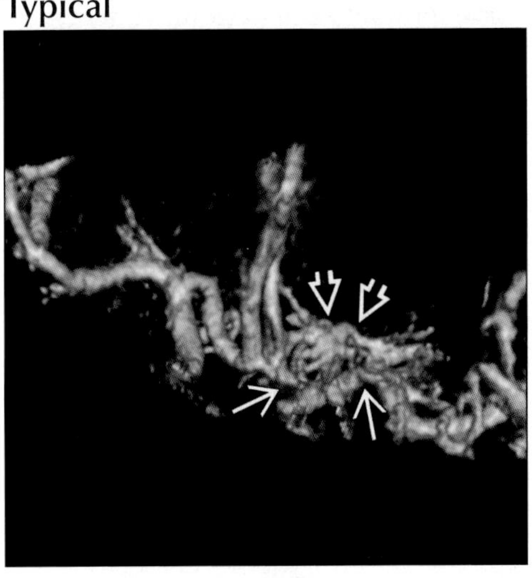

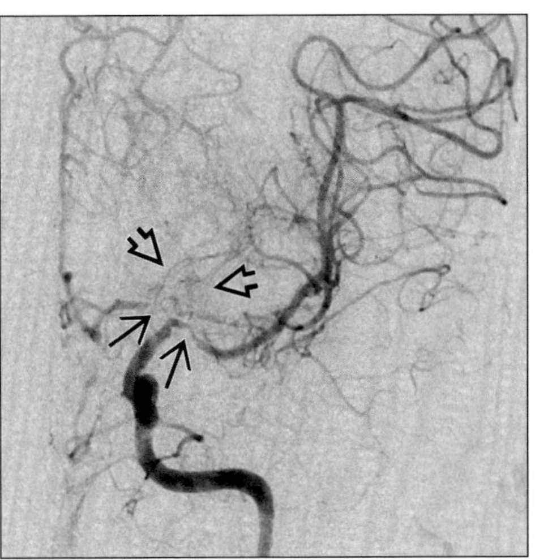

(Left) *Anteroposterior CECT angiogram demonstrates narrowing of the proximal left MCA and ACA ➡ with associated mass of collateral vasculature ⇨ in this 45 year old Japanese patient with TIA.* ***(Right)*** *Anteroposterior DSA in the same patient as previous image, confirms severe focal narrowing in proximal left MCA and ACA ➡ as well as hypertrophy of the lenticulostriates ⇨ in this patient with moyamoya.*

ATHEROSCLEROSIS, EXTRACRANIAL

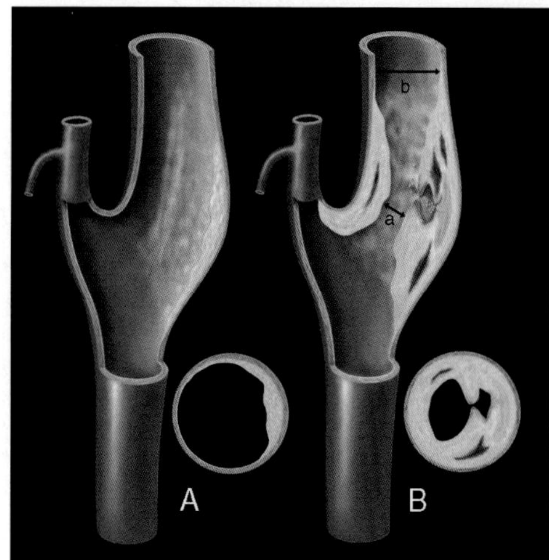

Graphic of ASVD. (A) Mild: "Fatty streaks"; slight intimal thickening. (B) Severe: Intraplaque hemorrhage, ulceration, platelet aggregation. NASCET calculation: % stenosis = (b-a) / (bx100).

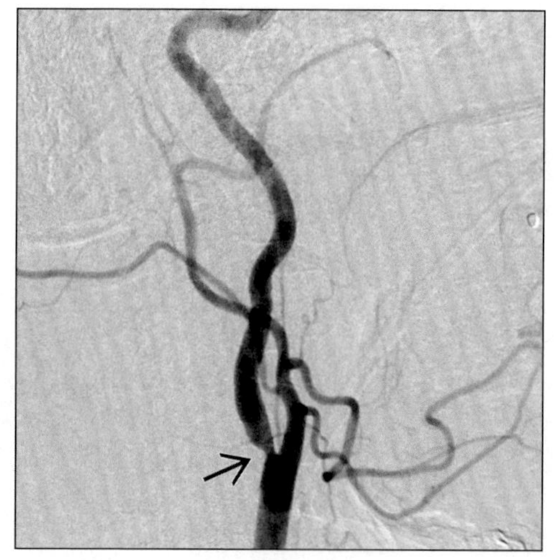

Lateral oblique DSA, common carotid artery injection, shows classic example of atherosclerotic stenosis ⇒ at the origin of the internal carotid artery.

TERMINOLOGY

Abbreviations and Synonyms

- Atherosclerotic vascular disease (ASVD)

Definitions

- Pathologic degenerative process resulting from deposition of plasma lipids in arterial walls

IMAGING FINDINGS

General Features

- Best diagnostic clue
  - Smooth or irregular narrowing of arterial lumen
  - Calcium deposition in arterial walls
- Location: Proximal internal carotid (ICA) and vertebral (VA) arteries most common sites in head and neck
- Size
  - Vessels affected are large, medium and small arteries and arterioles
  - Plaque ranges from microscopic lipid deposition to fatty streaks to eccentric luminal filling defects
    - Vary from 0.3-1.5 cm in diameter
  - "Fatty streaks" may coalesce to form larger masses
- Morphology
  - Begins initially as smooth, slight eccentric thickening of the vessel intima
  - Progresses to more focal and prominent eccentric thickening (subintimal macrocyte and smooth muscle cell deposition)
  - Subintimal hemorrhage from "new vessels" further narrows the lumen
  - Rupture of fibrous cap and intima can occur, resulting in the "ulcerated plaque"

CT Findings

- NECT
  - Identify calcification in vessel walls
  - Large plaques may show low density foci (lipid)
- CECT
  - Opacifies the vessel lumen, differentiate plaque from patent lumen
  - Identify ectasia, tortuosity and fusiform vessel dilatation
- CTA
  - Further enables visualization and accurate estimation of degree of stenosis

DDx: Atherosclerosis, Extracranial

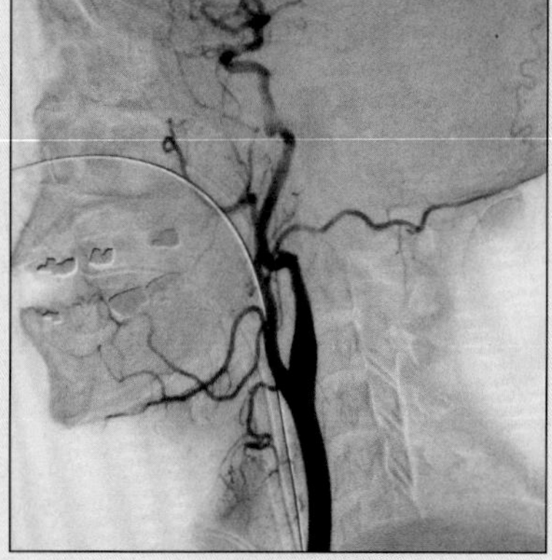

ICA Dissection

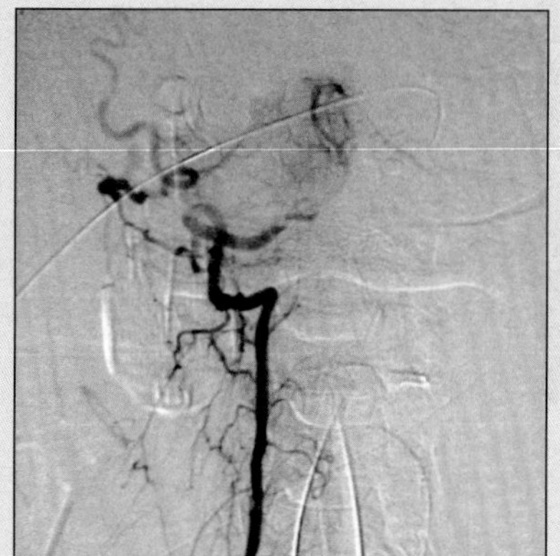

Vertebral Artery Dissection

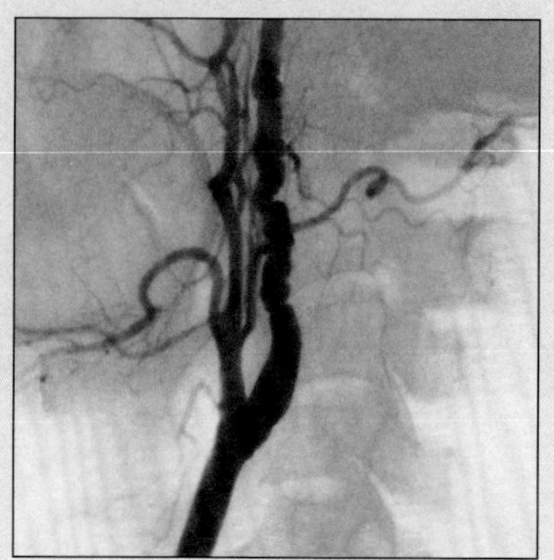

ICA Fibromuscular Dysplasia

ATHEROSCLEROSIS, EXTRACRANIAL

Key Facts

Terminology
- Pathologic degenerative process resulting from deposition of plasma lipids in arterial walls

Imaging Findings
- Smooth or irregular narrowing of arterial lumen
- Proximal internal carotid (ICA) and vertebral (VA) arteries most common sites in head and neck
- Plaque surface irregularity associated with increased risk of stroke at all degrees of stenosis
- Ultrasound as initial screening procedure
- CTA/MRA
- Late phase angiogram important in setting of high grade stenosis or suspected occlusion to identify "string-sign" and rule out "pseudo-occlusion"

Top Differential Diagnoses
- Dissection
- Fibromuscular Dysplasia (FMD)
- Vasospasm

Pathology
- Leading cause of morbidity and mortality in West
- Three main hypotheses have been proposed: Lipid hypothesis, injury hypothesis, and "unifying theory"
- NASCET method: % stenosis = (normal lumen - minimal residual lumen) / (normal lumen x 100)

Clinical Issues
- Variable; asymptomatic, carotid bruit, TIA, stroke
- Endarterectomy if carotid stenosis ≥ 70% (NASCET)
- Percutaneous carotid stenting (± distal protection): Becoming treatment of choice

        - Reconstruct/reformat multiplanar images

MR Findings
- T1WI
    - Wall thickening and luminal narrowing
    - Absence of "flow-void" may occur if vessel occluded or severely stenotic
    - Can detect lipid, calcium, hemorrhage in plaque
- T2WI
    - Useful to further characterize plaque components
    - Evaluate fibrous cap (> 100 μm stable, < 100 μm vulnerable)
- MRA
    - Degree of stenosis visualized
    - Signal loss may occur if high-grade (i.e., > 95%) stenosis
    - Contrast-enhanced MRA provides more accurate assessment than unenhanced MRA or MOTSA
        - Minimizes saturation effects: Improved estimation of degree of stenosis
        - Maximizes longitudinal field of view: Visualization of aortic arch to skull base vasculature

Nuclear Medicine Findings
- (111) In-platelet scintigraphy may be used to detect thrombotic complications in carotid plaques

Ultrasonographic Findings
- Grayscale imaging allows visualization of hypo- (non-calcified) or hyper- (calcified) echoic plaque
- Hypoechoic plaques are independent risk factors for stroke; strong correlation with ↑ lipoprotein(a)
- Doppler imaging measures flow velocity; peak systolic velocity best parameter for quantifying stenosis
- Spectral analysis allows evaluation of waveform; morphologic changes with increasing stenosis
- Color Doppler may detect high grade occlusions more reliably than conventional Doppler

Angiographic Findings
- Conventional
    - Identifies degree of stenosis, morphology of plaque, tandem stenoses, potential collateral pathways as well as coexisting pathology (i.e., aneurysm)
    - Plaque surface irregularity associated with increased risk of stroke at all degrees of stenosis
    - Tandem lesions (distal stenoses) present in approximately 2% of patients with significant cervical ICA lesions
        - Hemodynamic effect of tandem stenoses is additive if both lesions are severe enough to reduce flow separately
    - Late phase angiogram important in setting of high grade stenosis or suspected occlusion to identify "string-sign" and rule out "pseudo-occlusion"

Imaging Recommendations
- Best imaging tool: CTA or MRA
- Protocol advice
    - Ultrasound as initial screening procedure
    - CTA/MRA
    - Consider DSA in equivocal cases

DIFFERENTIAL DIAGNOSIS

Dissection
- Typically spares carotid bulb; no calcification
- Seen in young-middle age groups
- Smoother, longer narrowing

Fibromuscular Dysplasia (FMD)
- "String of beads" > > segment stenosis

Vasospasm
- Usually iatrogenic (catheter-induced), transient

Extrinsic Compression (Rare)
- Tumor encasement, hematoma, infectious process

PATHOLOGY

General Features
- General path comments

ATHEROSCLEROSIS, EXTRACRANIAL

- Complex, multifactorial process, pathogenesis of which remains controversial
- Probably no single cause, no single initiating event, and no exclusive pathogenetic mechanism
- Irregular plaque surface = increased stroke risk; collateral circulation = lower stroke risk
- Significant ICA narrowing in 20-30% of carotid territory strokes (vs. 5-10% general population)

- Genetics
  - Probably multigenic
  - Many polymorphisms identified
- Etiology
  - Three main hypotheses have been proposed: Lipid hypothesis, injury hypothesis, and "unifying theory"
    - Lipid hypothesis: Relates ASVD to high plasma LDL levels causing LDL-cholesterol deposits in the arterial intima
    - Injury hypothesis: ASVD is initiated by focal endothelial damage that initiates platelet aggregation and plaque formation
    - Unifying theory: Suggests that endothelial injury is accompanied by increased permeability to macromolecules such as LDL
  - Other factors include diet, genetics, mechanical stress (e.g., wall shear, anatomic variations), inflammation, hyperhomocysteinemia
- Epidemiology
  - Leading cause of morbidity and mortality in West
  - Ischemic stroke = up to 40% of deaths in elderly
  - Cerebral infarctions occur in > 70% of patients with carotid occlusion
  - 90% of large, recent infarcts caused by emboli
  - Strong epidemiological and experimental evidence that increased dietary lipid (especially cholesterol, saturated fats) correlates with development of atherosclerotic lesions

Gross Pathologic & Surgical Features

- Two well-accepted lesions described: Atheromatous plaque and fatty streak
  - Atheromatous plaque: Most important lesion, being principal cause of arterial narrowing in adults
  - Fatty streak: Important precursor; present universally in children, even in first year of life
- Intimal "fatty streaks" are earliest macroscopically visible lesions
- Plaques are whitish-yellow, protrude intraluminally and vary in size

Microscopic Features

- Fibroatheromatous plaques are basic lesion of ASVD; and develop following lipid deposition
- Plaques contain cells (monocytes/macrophages, leukocytes, smooth muscle); connective tissue; intra/extracellular lipid deposits
- Necrotic core of lipid material, cholesterol, cellular debris, lipid-laden foam cells and fibrin form deep within plaque
- Neovascularization occurs; may lead to vessel rupture causing intraplaque hemorrhage and ulceration
- Atheromatous plaque itself may also rupture (fibrous cap weakens and fractures); may lead to emboli

Staging, Grading or Classification Criteria

- Methods for calculating degree of stenosis vary; NASCET, ACAS, ECST AND VACSG
- NASCET method: % Stenosis = (normal lumen - minimal residual lumen) / (normal lumen x 100)
- Mild < 50%; moderate 50-69%; severe 70-99%

CLINICAL ISSUES

Presentation

- Most common signs/symptoms: Variable; asymptomatic, carotid bruit, TIA, stroke
- Clinical Profile: Patient with typical risk factors for stroke: Smoking, HTN, diabetes, obesity, hypercholesterolemia, advanced age

Demographics

- Age: Usually middle aged to elderly
- Gender: Male > female
- Ethnicity: African-American with highest risk of ASVD

Natural History & Prognosis

- Progressive, significant stenosis may cause decreased cerebral perfusion

Treatment

- Endarterectomy if carotid stenosis ≥ 70% (NASCET)
- Symptomatic moderate stenosis (50-69%) also benefits from endarterectomy (NASCET)
- Asymptomatic patients may also benefit from treatment even with stenosis of only 60% (ACAS)
- Percutaneous carotid stenting (± distal protection): Becoming treatment of choice

DIAGNOSTIC CHECKLIST

Consider

- For calculation of degree of stenosis, at least two DSA projections required to profile plaque adequately
- For pre-op patients undergoing CEA/stenting, adequacy of collateral circulation becomes critical; consider cerebral CTA/MRA or DSA
- Pseudo-occlusion (very high grade stenosis) may not be noted on CTA/MRA and seen only on late phase angiogram; CEA/stenting still an option if ICA patent!

SELECTED REFERENCES

1. Saam T et al: The vulnerable, or high-risk, atherosclerotic plaque: noninvasive MR imaging for characterization and assessment. Radiology. 244(1):64-77, 2007
2. Miralles M et al: Quantification and characterization of carotid calcium with multi-detector CT-angiography. Eur J Vasc Endovasc Surg. 32(5):561-7, 2006
3. Gaitini D et al: Diagnosing carotid stenosis by Doppler sonography: state of the art. J Ultrasound Med. 24(8):1127-36, 2005
4. Fayad ZA et al: Magnetic resonance imaging and computed tomography in assessment of atherosclerotic plaque. Curr Atheroscler Rep. 6(3):232-42, 2004
5. Binaghi S et al: Three-dimensional computed tomography angiography and magnetic resonance angiography of carotid bifurcation stenosis. Eur Neurol. 46(1):25-34, 2001

IMAGE GALLERY

Typical

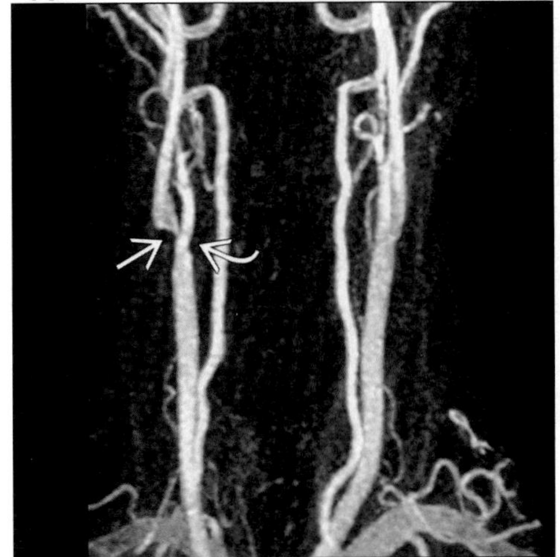

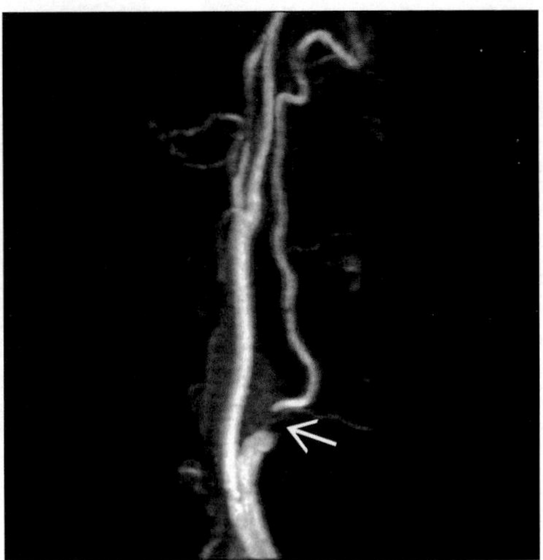

(Left) *Anteroposterior 3D TOF post-contrast MRA MIP image shows moderate stenosis at the origin of the right ICA and mild atherosclerotic plaque at the right CCA-ECA junction.* ***(Right)*** *Lateral oblique 3D TOF post-contrast MRA MIP image shows severe stenosis at the origin of right vertebral artery. MRA permits 360° rotation to adequately visualize the entire vessel.*

Typical

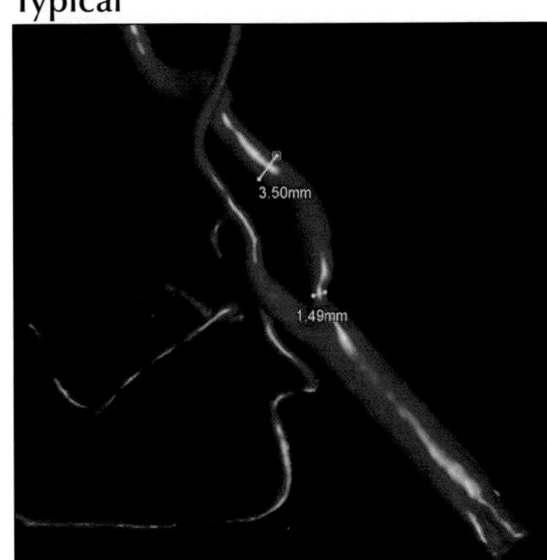

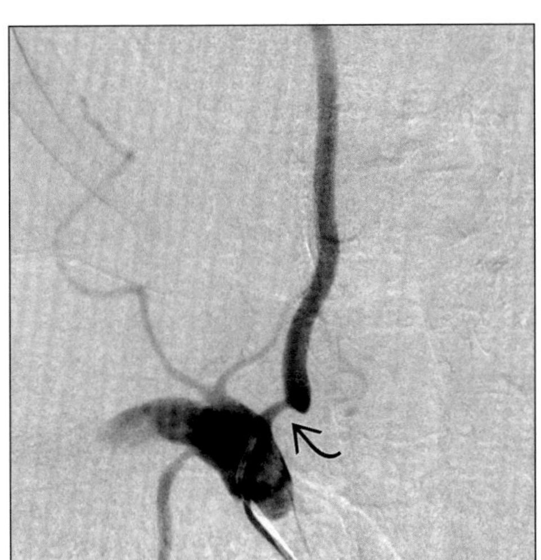

(Left) *3D rotational DSA image shows narrowing at the origin of the ICA. NASCET criteria % stenosis = (3.50 - 1.49) / (3.50 x 100) = 57% diameter stenosis which is moderate in degree.* ***(Right)*** *Anteroposterior DSA of a right subclavian artery injection shows moderate stenosis at the origin of the right vertebral artery from atherosclerosis.*

Typical

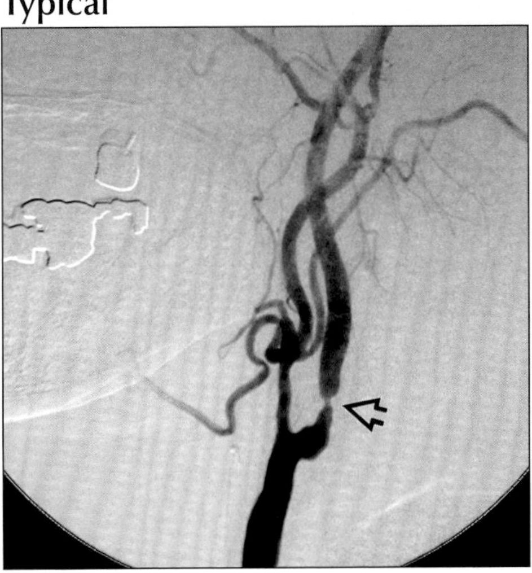

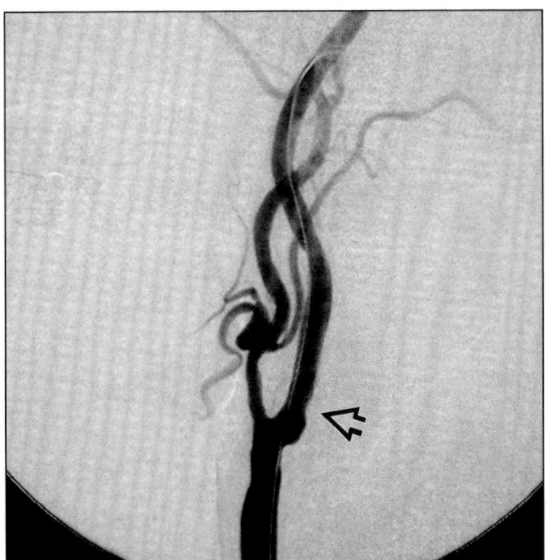

(Left) *Lateral oblique DSA, common carotid artery injection, depicts severe atherosclerotic stenosis of the post-bulbar proximal internal carotid artery.* ***(Right)*** *Lateral oblique DSA in the same case, CCA injection following placement of an ICA stent, demonstrates an excellent angiographic result with marked improvement of ICA lumen diameter.*

ATHEROSCLEROSIS, INTRACRANIAL

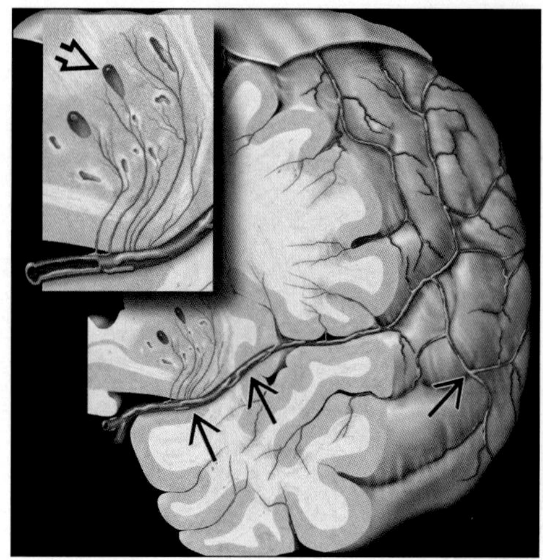

Coronal oblique graphic shows atherosclerotic plaques ⇒ in the left MCA. Inset also demonstrates disease extent into the small penetrating vessels and resultant lacunar infarction ⇨.

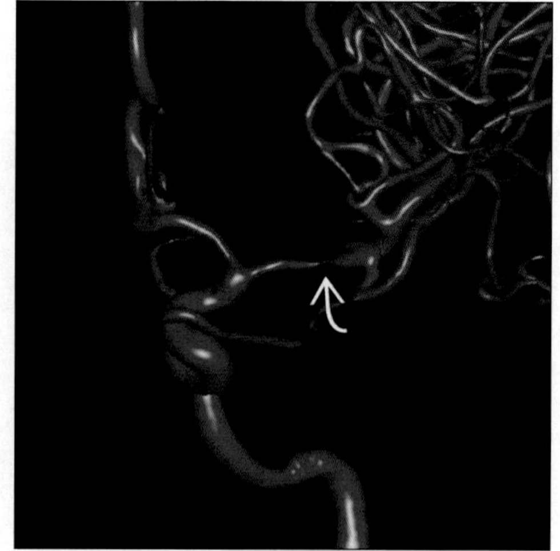

Anteroposterior rotational 3D DSA shows focal narrowing of the M1 segment of the left middle cerebral artery ➔ from intracranial atherosclerosis.

TERMINOLOGY

Abbreviations and Synonyms

- Intracranial arterial stenosis

Definitions

- Focal narrowing of intracranial arterial lumen

IMAGING FINDINGS

General Features

- Best diagnostic clue: Stenotic intracranial artery on CTA, MRA or conventional angiogram
- Location
  - Usually involves distal internal carotid (ICA) or basilar artery (BA)
  - Less common sites
    - Circle of Willis (COW)
    - Middle cerebral artery stenosis rare (2% of cases) but high stroke death risk
- Size: Variable, usually focal
- Morphology: Variable; usually eccentric, irregular ± ulceration

CT Findings

- NECT: Mural calcifications may be present
- CTA
  - Thin-section acquisition and 3D reconstruction/reformatted post-processed images improves detection/evaluation of narrowed lumen
  - Calcifications in vessel wall may reduce specificity

MR Findings

- T1WI
  - Decreased/absent flow void in expected position of artery (slow flow or occlusion)
  - Also seen with slow flow from upstream (extracranial) stenosis or vessel dissection
- T2WI
  - Decreased flow void in expected position of artery (slow flow or occlusion)
  - Propensity for deep white matter borderzone and deep gray/white matter lacunar infarcts
- FLAIR: Slow flow or occlusion may appear hyperintense ("bright dot sign")
- MRA
  - Focal stenosis, ectasia or irregularity on 3D time of flight (TOF) or contrast-enhanced MRA (CE-MRA)

DDx: Atherosclerosis, Intracranial

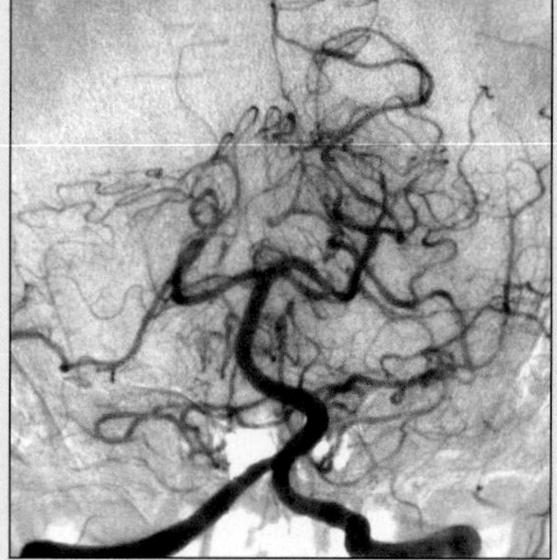

Vasculitis

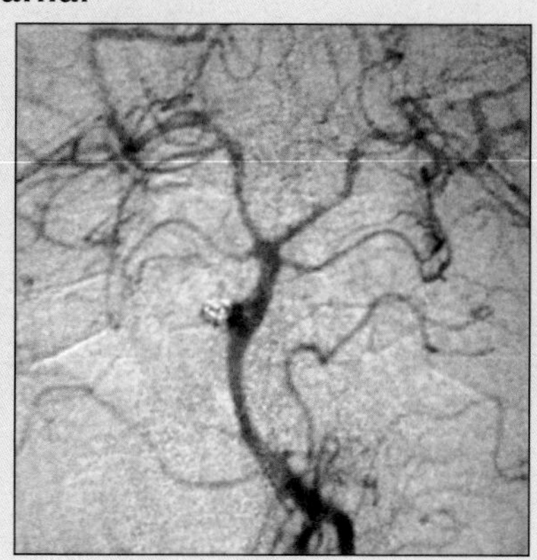

Vasospasm

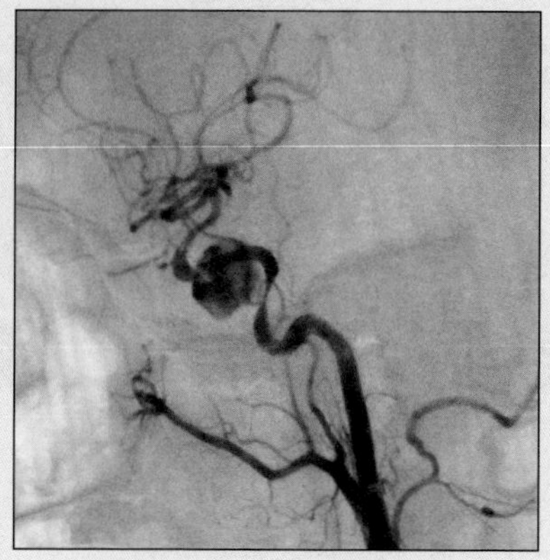

ICA Dissection/Pseudoaneurysm

ATHEROSCLEROSIS, INTRACRANIAL

Key Facts

Terminology

- Focal narrowing of intracranial arterial lumen

Imaging Findings

- Usually involves distal internal carotid (ICA) or basilar (BA) artery
- Less common location: Circle of Willis (COW)
- Focal stenosis, luminal irregularities, thrombosis, occlusion
- Less common: Ectasia and elongation, serpentine fusiform aneurysms
- CTA or MRA excellent screening modality; followed by DSA if equivocal

Top Differential Diagnoses

- Vasculitis/Arteritis
- Vasospasm
- Moyamoya
- Dissection

Pathology

- Atherosclerosis is a systemic, multifactorial disease
- Third most common cause of thromboembolic stroke, after carotid and cardiac sources
- Ischemic symptoms depend on collaterals
- Arterial irregularity from disrupted endothelium may form thrombogenic surface

Clinical Issues

- Most common signs/symptoms: Transient ischemic attack; due to emboli, severe stenosis, progressive occlusion
- Progressive disease unless treated aggressively
- Angioplasty and/or stenting in some cases

        - Caveat: 3D TOF MRA tends to overestimate stenosis due to spin saturation (poor evaluation of slow flow and in-plane flow)
        - CE-MRA less affected by spin saturation and much faster imaging sequence
        - Combined with CTA, sensitivity and specificity approach DSA
    - 3T MRA improves spatial resolution; comparable to DSA
- Perfusion-weighted imaging (PWI): ↓ Perfusion esp. deep hemispheric white matter

Ultrasonographic Findings

- Trans-Cranial Doppler (TCD): Increased velocities

Angiographic Findings

- Conventional
    - DSA: Focal stenosis, luminal irregularities, thrombosis, occlusion
        - Less common: Ectasia and elongation, serpentine fusiform aneurysms
    - DSA most sensitive and specific test; goals include
        - Grade extracranial stenosis, criteria standardized by NASCET (North American Symptomatic Carotid Endarterectomy Trial)
        - Identify "tandem" lesions
        - Assess collateral status
        - Potential assessment of plaque ulceration
        - Potential intervention (angioplasty ± stenting)

Imaging Recommendations

- Best imaging tool: DSA remains gold standard
- Protocol advice: CTA or MRA excellent screening modality; followed by DSA if equivocal

DIFFERENTIAL DIAGNOSIS

Vasculitis/Arteritis

- Usually involves smaller (tertiary) branches
- More likely associated with hemorrhage
- Can be primary or secondary
- Often associated with systemic disease
- Elevated ESR, autoimmune parameters

Vasospasm

- Subarachnoid hemorrhage related, maximal 7 days post-bleed
- Drug-related (sympathomimetics)

Moyamoya

- Usually involve distal ICA and proximal COW with relative sparing of basilar artery
- Frequently bilateral

Dissection

- Smooth tapering
- T1 hyperintense crescent = thrombus, best seen with fat-saturation imaging
- Younger patients
- Can have minimal or no history of trauma

Non-Occlusive Thrombus or Embolus

- Appearance of rounded, central non-opacification with peripheral enhancing rim on contrast study

PATHOLOGY

General Features

- General path comments
    - Atherosclerosis is a systemic, multifactorial disease
    - Intracranial atherosclerosis associated with atherosclerosis of carotids, coronaries, aorta, renal arteries, iliofemoral system
    - Anatomy
        - Most often involves regions of arterial curvature or bifurcations, e.g., distal ICA and BA
        - May involve distal arterioles leading to vasculitis pattern of alternating stenosis and dilatation
- Etiology
    - Probably multiple etiologies; main three are
        - Lipid hypothesis: High plasma LDL leads to LDL-cholesterol deposition in intima
        - Response to injury hypothesis: Focal endothelial change or intimal injury leads to platelet aggregation and plaque formation

ATHEROSCLEROSIS, INTRACRANIAL

    - Unifying hypothesis: Endothelial injury leads to increased permeability of LDL: Plaques grow by thrombus formation on plaque surface and transendothelial leakage of plasma lipids
- Epidemiology
  - Third most common cause of thromboembolic stroke, after carotid and cardiac sources
  - Most common cause of intracranial vascular stenosis in adults

Gross Pathologic & Surgical Features

- Earliest macroscopic finding: Intimal fatty streaks
- Fibrous atheromatous plaques contain
  - Smooth muscle cells, monocytes, other leukocytes
  - Connective tissue: Collagen, elastic fibers, proteoglycans
  - Intra- and extracellular lipid deposits
  - New capillaries at plaque periphery (angiogenesis)
    - Leads to intraplaque hemorrhage and ulceration
    - Hemorrhage leads to dystrophic ferrocalcinosis (seen as calcification on CT, as iron on MR)
- Arterial narrowing due to plaque
  - Ischemic symptoms depend on collaterals
    - Slow occlusion leads to more collaterals, fewer symptoms
    - Rapid occlusion (from thrombosis or emboli) does not permit time for collaterals to develop, infarct likely
- Arterial irregularity from disrupted endothelium may form thrombogenic surface leading to thrombosis or emboli

Microscopic Features

- Earliest findings
  - Lipid deposition, cellular reaction in intima
- Later findings and determinants of stability in atherosclerotic plaques (MR holds promise for characterization of intraplaque composition)
  - Lipid core
  - Fibrous cap (thicker cap is more stable and less likely to rupture)
  - Inflammatory changes
  - Calcification
  - Intraplaque hemorrhage

Staging, Grading or Classification Criteria

- NASCET criteria (used in cervical disease), greater than 70% stenosis considered flow-limiting and likely to benefit from angioplasty, stenting or surgery

CLINICAL ISSUES

Presentation

- Most common signs/symptoms: Transient ischemic attack; due to emboli, severe stenosis, progressive occlusion
- Plaque rupture usually leads to stroke
- Vascular stenosis leads to stuttering ischemia from intermittent thrombosis

Demographics

- Age: Older age groups
- Gender: M = F
- More common in Western countries

Natural History & Prognosis

- Progressive disease unless treated aggressively
- Poor prognosis without treatment, better prognosis with treatment

Treatment

- Low saturated fat and cholesterol diet; exercise
- Cholesterol lowering drugs, EtOH (in moderation)
- Plaque stabilization ("statin" drugs) may decrease stroke
- Angioplasty and/or stenting in some cases
  - Drug-eluting stents appear to have less restenosis
- Rarely extracranial to intracranial surgical bypass

DIAGNOSTIC CHECKLIST

Consider

- CTA and/or MRA as excellent screening tool
- DSA gold standard, allows potential intervention

Image Interpretation Pearls

- Status of collaterals important; patients with developed collaterals tolerate stenosis/occlusion better

SELECTED REFERENCES

1. Feldmann E et al: The Stroke Outcomes and Neuroimaging of Intracranial Atherosclerosis (SONIA) trial. Neurology. 68(24):2099-106, 2007
2. Jovin TG et al: Management of symptomatic intracranial atherosclerotic disease. Curr Cardiol Rep. 9(1):32-40, 2007
3. Kang DW et al: Early recurrent ischemic lesions on diffusion-weighted imaging in symptomatic intracranial atherosclerosis. Arch Neurol. 64(1):50-4, 2007
4. Chen XY et al: Diagnostic accuracy of MRI for middle cerebral artery stenosis: a postmortem study. J Neuroimaging. 16(4):318-22, 2006
5. Knopman DS: Dementia and cerebrovascular disease. Mayo Clin Proc. 81(2):223-30, 2006
6. Abou-Chebl A et al: Drug-eluting stents for the treatment of intracranial atherosclerosis: initial experience and midterm angiographic follow-up. Stroke. 36(12):e165-8, 2005
7. Lee DK et al: Lesion patterns and stroke mechanism in atherosclerotic middle cerebral artery disease: early diffusion-weighted imaging study. Stroke. 36(12):2583-8, 2005
8. Qureshi AI et al: Clinical and angiographic results of dilatation procedures for symptomatic intracranial atherosclerotic disease. J Neuroimaging. 15(3):240-9, 2005
9. Suwanwela NC et al: Risk factors for atherosclerosis of cervicocerebral arteries. Neuroepidemiology. 22:37-40, 2003
10. Hirai T et al: Prospective evaluation of suspected stenoocclusive disease of the intracranial artery. AJNR Am J Neuroradiol. 23:93-101, 2002
11. Lernfelt B et al: Cerebral atherosclerosis as predictor of stroke and mortality in representative elderly population. Stroke. 33:224-9, 2002
12. Summers PE et al: MR Angiography in cerebrovascular disease. Clin Radiol. 56:437-56, 2001
13. Nakayama Y et al: Diagnostic value of perfusion MRI in classifying stroke. Keio J Med. 49 Suppl 1:A51-4, 2000
14. Consigny PM: Pathogenesis of atherosclerosis. AJR Am J Roentgenol. 164: 553-8, 1995

ATHEROSCLEROSIS, INTRACRANIAL

IMAGE GALLERY

Typical

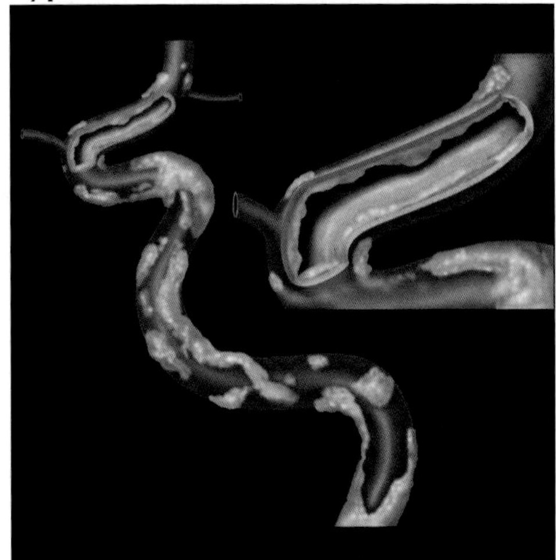

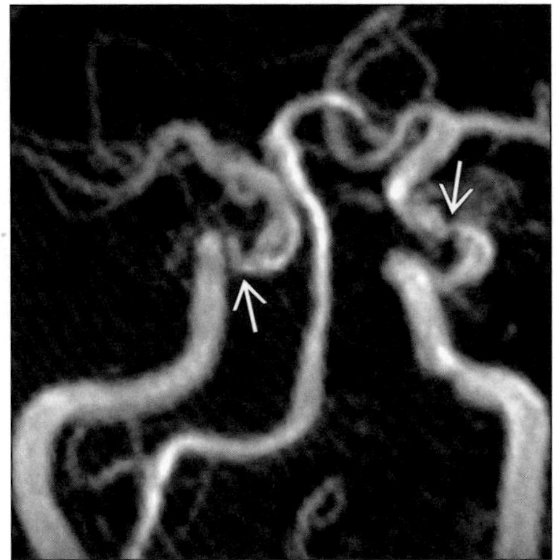

(Left) *Lateral graphic shows internal carotid artery atherosclerotic plaques causing irregularity along the vessel wall and luminal narrowing, particularly at the carotid siphon (inset).* ***(Right)*** *Anteroposterior 3D TOF MRA MIP image shows multiple foci of flow related signal attenuation especially in the cavernous internal carotid arteries from atherosclerotic arterial stenosis.*

Typical

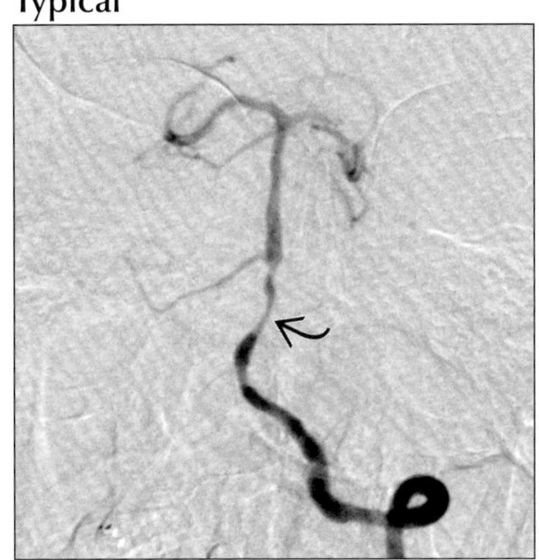

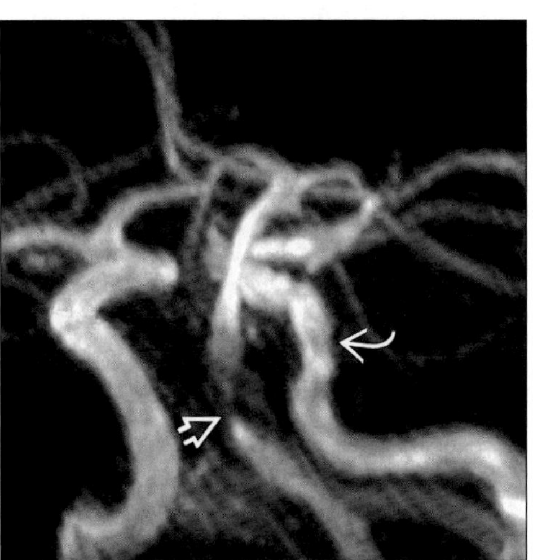

(Left) *Anteroposterior DSA of a left vertebral artery injection shows significant stenosis of the proximal basilar artery, a common location for atherosclerotic disease.* ***(Right)*** *Anteroposterior oblique 3D TOF MRA MIP image in a different patient also depicts severe atherosclerotic stenosis of the proximal basilar artery as well as mild left ICA disease.*

Typical

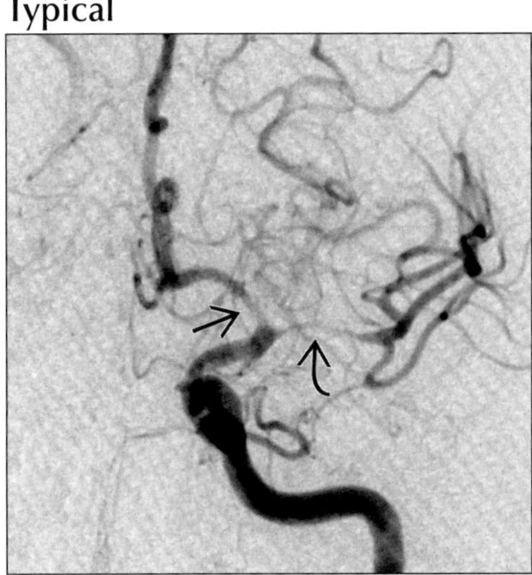

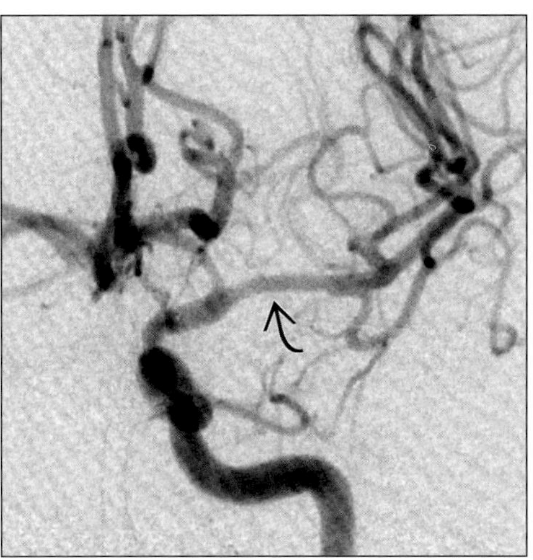

(Left) *Anteroposterior DSA of a left ICA injection demonstrates severe stenosis of the proximal middle cerebral and mild-moderate stenosis of the proximal anterior cerebral arteries.* ***(Right)*** *Anteroposterior DSA of the left ICA in the same patient as previous image, following left MCA angioplasty and stenting shows an excellent angiographic result with markedly improved luminal diameter.*

EC-IC BYPASS

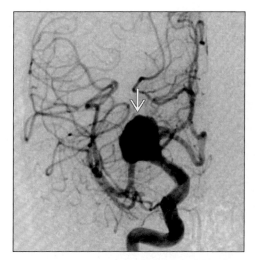

Posteroanterior right ICA DSA shows a wide-necked aneurysm of the carotid terminus ➔ incorporating the origins of the M1 and A1 segments. This was not suitable for surgical clipping or coil embolization.

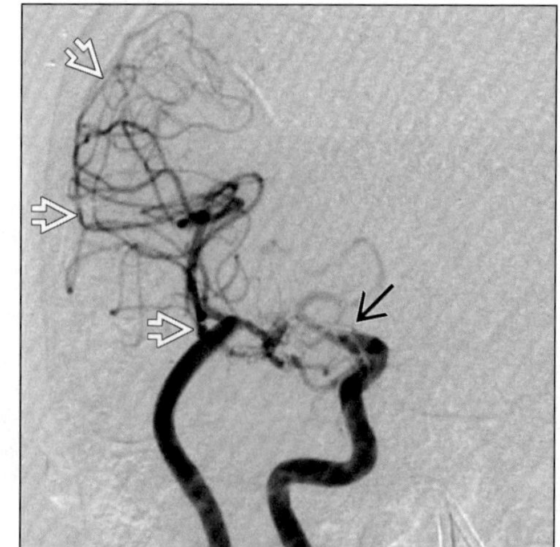

Posteroanterior right CCA DSA S/P saphenous vein bypass (same patient as previous) shows filling of MCA cortical branches via bypass graft ➔. Supraclinoid ICA was ligated above anterior choroidal artery ➔.

TERMINOLOGY

Definitions

- Arterial bypass between extracranial (EC) circulation to intracranial (IC) circulation
- Used for cerebral blood flow augmentation to prevent ischemic stroke

IMAGING FINDINGS

General Features

- Best diagnostic clue
  - Absent flow void/enhancement in native bypassed vessel on MR or CTA
  - Craniotomy defect on skull XR, CT
- Size: Small caliber ECA branch bypass vs. large caliber saphenous vein graft
- Morphology: Vein graft will have valves along its course (vein is reversed to permit cranial flow)

CT Findings

- NECT
  - Look for adverse features
    - Immediate post-op: Extra-axial hematoma, brain edema from surgical retraction
    - New ischemia due to graft occlusion or thromboemboli
    - Thrombosed graft may appear as hyperdense cord
- CECT: Absent enhancement of native vessel being bypassed, enhancement of bypass graft
- CTA
  - Patent graft enhances with arterial phase imaging
  - STA-MCA bypass
    - STA enters skull via burr hole adjacent to craniotomy defect
    - STA enlarges due to increased flow to supply IC circulation
  - Saphenous vein EC-IC bypass
    - Large caliber vessel coursing superficial to native cervical ICA, joins intracranial ICA or MCA
    - Native ICA non-enhancing or gracile
    - Valves along course of saphenous vein appear as focal dilatations
  - Morphology of anastomosis site(s) difficult to assess due to artifact from adjacent metallic surgical clips

DDx: Native Collateral Pathways

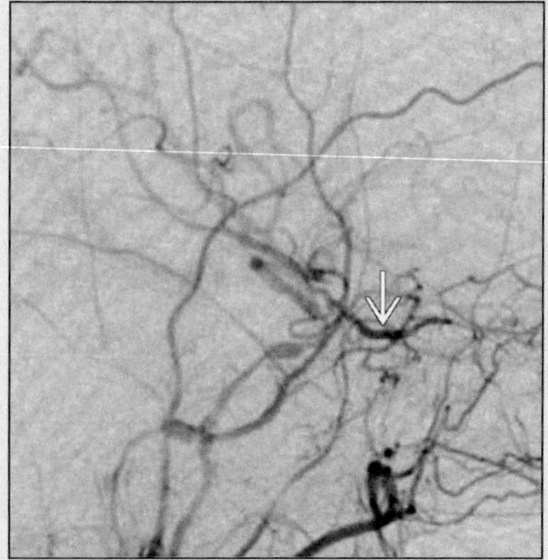

Ophthalmic Artery to ICA

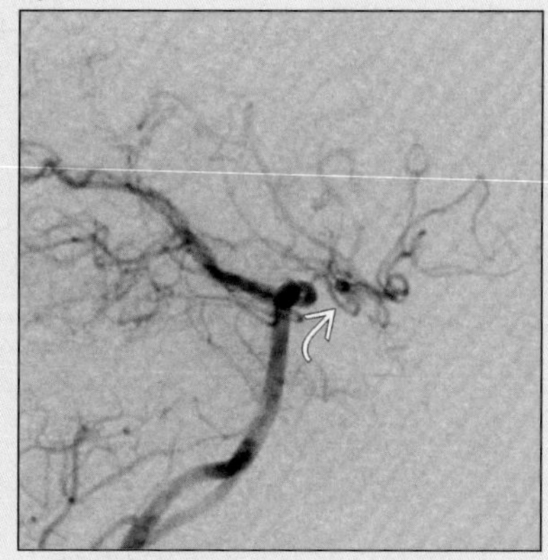

Posterior Communicating Artery

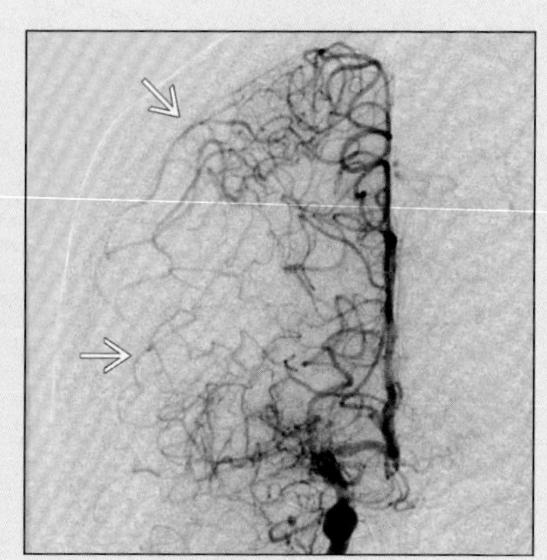

Leptomeningeal from ACA, PCA

EC-IC BYPASS

Key Facts

Terminology
- Arterial bypass between extracranial (EC) circulation to intracranial (IC) circulation
- Used for cerebral blood flow augmentation to prevent ischemic stroke

Imaging Findings
- Small caliber ECA branch bypass vs. large caliber saphenous vein graft
- CECT: Absent enhancement of native vessel being bypassed, enhancement of bypass graft
- MRA: Not routinely used to assess graft patency due to limited resolution ± susceptibility artifact from surgical clips
- DSA: Gold-standard for assessment of bypass graft patency and morphology of anastomosis site(s)
  - Must visualize entire course of graft

Pathology
- Direct: End-end or end-side anastomosis between an EC and IC artery
  - STA-MCA vs. reversed vein graft
- Indirect: Induced revascularization pathways from EC circulation to brain surface
  - Types: EMS, EDAS, omentum transposition

Clinical Issues
- EC-IC bypass may be considered in those with abnormal perfusion imaging, especially if lack of cerebrovascular reserve with Diamox challenge

Diagnostic Checklist
- Consider intracranial stent placement as alternative to EC-IC bypass in select cases

MR Findings
- T1WI: Absent flow void ± intravascular hyperintensity seen with slow flow or occlusion/thrombosis of native bypassed vessel
- MRA
  - Not routinely used to assess graft patency due to limited resolution ± susceptibility from surgical clips
  - 2D TOF superior to 3D techniques in differentiating slow flow from occlusion
- Perfusion MR/CT
  - Pre-operative work-up
    - Measure parameters: Cerebral blood flow (CBF), cerebral blood volume (CBV), mean transit time (MTT), time to peak (TTP)
    - Cerebral ischemia: ↓ CBF, ↑ TTP, ↑ MTT; CBV may ↑ if good collaterals or ↓ if collaterals poor
    - Diamox challenge: Diamox (acetazolamide): Intracranial vasodilator which results in vasodilatation and ↑ flow to ischemic areas unless maximal vasodilation from autoregulatory mechanisms has already occurred → candidate for EC-IC bypass

Ultrasonographic Findings
- Color Doppler
  - Intra-operative Doppler useful to determine patency of graft at time of surgery
  - STA-MCA bypass: Normal high resistance waveform of ECA branches changes to low-resistance waveform

Other Modality Findings
- F-18 FDG PET and/or HMPAO SPECT may reveal ischemia; may be done in conjunction with Diamox challenge to assess cerebrovascular reserve

Angiographic Findings
- Conventional
  - Gold-standard for assessment of bypass graft patency and morphology of anastomosis site(s)
  - CCA injection used to assess anterior circulation bypass
    - Avoids iatrogenic spasm of ECA or venous graft/injury to proximal venous anastomosis
  - STA-MCA bypass
    - STA enters skull via burr hole
    - Typically end to side anastomosis to MCA branch at M3/M4 junction
    - Patent bypass should show antegrade and retrograde filling of the MCA branches
  - Saphenous vein-ICA bypass
    - Saphenous vein is grafted onto CCA or ICA proximally and enters skull via craniectomy to a distal anastomosis with ICA/MCA
    - Native ICA is often ligated at origin at time of bypass
    - Venous graft has valves seen as undulations along its course; valves are oriented to permit cranially directed flow
  - Look for adverse features
    - Must visualize entire course of graft from CCA bifurcation to intracranial anastomosis
    - Need to exclude stenosis at anastomosis site(s) due to surgical technique vs. vasospasm
    - Vasospasm typically affects a longer vessel segment, smoother morphology ± affects adjacent intracranial vessels cf. focal true anastomotic stenosis
    - Vasospasm should respond to vasodilators (e.g., verapamil or nitroglycerin) cf. true anastomotic stenosis

Imaging Recommendations
- Best imaging tool
  - Pre-op assessment to include CT/MR perfusion to identify suitable candidates for EC-IC bypass (those with limited or no cerebrovascular reserve after Diamox challenge)
  - Post-op assessment of graft patency and anastomotic stenoses with DSA
- Long-term follow-up of graft patency can be monitored with CTA
- May assess graft function with perfusion CT/MR (compare to pre-operative baseline)

EC-IC BYPASS

DIFFERENTIAL DIAGNOSIS

Native Collateral Pathways

- Circle of Willis (COW) is complete in < 30% of people
  - ACoA, PCoA collateral supply to ischemic hemisphere
- ECA to ICA collaterals: Internal maxillary artery → cavernous ICA, MMA → ophthalmic → ICA
- Leptomeningeal collaterals: cortical branches of MCA, ACA, PCA supplies adjacent vascular territory

PATHOLOGY

General Features

- General path comments
  - Native ICA/MCA stenosis or occlusion is commonest need for EC-IC bypass
    - Underlying etiology usually atherosclerosis; dissection or vasculitis also possible
  - Bypass also required in patients with cervical/skull base tumors unable to tolerate carotid sacrifice, fusiform or complex intracranial aneurysms when parent vessel reconstruction not possible
  - Collateral pathways
    - MCA lesion: Leptomeningeal collaterals from ACA, PCA
    - ICA lesion: Anterior communicating artery (ACoA), posterior communicating artery (PCoA), ECA to ICA via ophthalmic artery, cavernous ICA branches
    - May provide sufficient perfusion to negate need for EC-IC bypass: Balloon test occlusion can be performed prior to ICA sacrifice for aneurysm or skull base tumor
    - Limited collaterals in context of ICA stenosis/occlusion with isolated hemisphere (absent ACoA & PCoA)
  - When collaterals insufficient to meet cerebral demand, hemodynamic failure ensues
  - Hemodynamic failure may cause postural ischemia at first and ultimately watershed infarction

Staging, Grading or Classification Criteria

- Direct: End-end or end-side anastomosis between an EC and IC artery
  - Low flow: Surgical anastomosis between external carotid artery (ECA) branch and an intracranial vessel
    - Commonest type: Superficial temporal artery (STA) to middle cerebral artery (MCA)
    - Others: Occipital artery to posterior cerebral artery (PCA) or posterior inferior cerebellar artery (PICA) or MCA
  - High flow: Reversed venous graft between ECA or common carotid artery (CCA) and supraclinoid ICA most commonly
- Indirect: Induced revascularization pathways from EC circulation to brain surface
  - Types: Encephalo-myo-synangiosis (EMS), encephalo-duro-arterio-synangiosis (EDAS), omentum transplantation
  - EMS: Temporalis muscle flap applied to brain surface
  - EDAS: STA is mobilized and laid onto brain surface after incising the dura and arachnoid
  - Omentum transposition: May use transposition flap or vascularized free flap with anastomoses to STA and superficial temporal vein
  - Typically used for Moya-moya disease or variant

CLINICAL ISSUES

Presentation

- Most common signs/symptoms
  - MCA or ICA stenosis/occlusion
    - Hemiparesis, hemianesthesia, language deficits (dominant hemisphere involvement), visual field cuts possible with involvement of Meyer loop or visual cortex in context of fetal PCA
  - Giant fusiform aneurysm: Mass effect, thromboembolic events, subarachnoid hemorrhage
  - Bypass graft failure: Hemodynamic/postural cerebral ischemia or stroke

Demographics

- Age
  - Atherosclerosis: Older patients
  - Moya-moya and other vasculitides: Younger patients

Natural History & Prognosis

- High risk of ipsilateral stroke within 1-year in patients with proven lack of cerebrovascular reserve with Diamox imaging

Treatment

- Chronic ICA occlusion is not amenable to carotid artery stenting or endarterectomy
  - Medical treatment with permissive hypertension to maximize collateral flow
- High grade MCA stenosis maybe amenable to balloon angioplasty ± stent placement
  - Medical treatment with anticoagulants and antiplatelet agents
- EC-IC bypass may be considered in those with abnormal perfusion imaging, especially if lack of cerebrovascular reserve with Diamox challenge

DIAGNOSTIC CHECKLIST

Consider

- Intracranial stent placement as alternative to EC-IC bypass in select cases

Image Interpretation Pearls

- DSA best for assessment of graft patency, anastomotic stenoses, post-operative vasospasm

SELECTED REFERENCES

1. Guthikonda M et al: Future of extracranial-intracranial bypass. Neurol Res. 24 Suppl 1:S80-3, 2002
2. No authors listed: Failure of extracranial-intracranial arterial bypass to reduce the risk of ischemic stroke. Results of an international randomized trial. The EC/IC Bypass Study Group. N Engl J Med. 313(19):1191-200, 1985

EC-IC BYPASS

IMAGE GALLERY

Typical

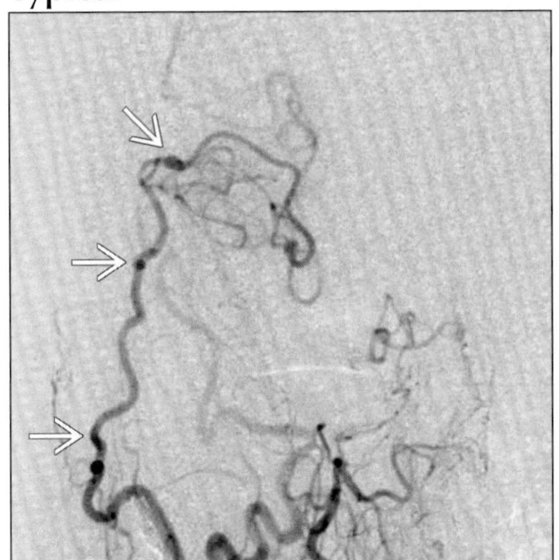

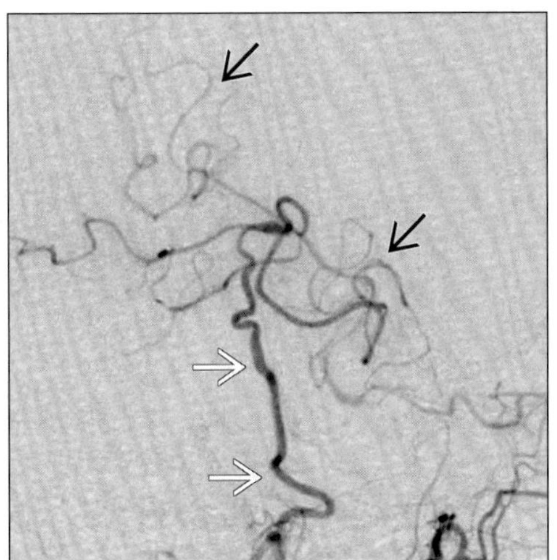

(Left) *Posteroanterior right CCA DSA in a patient with ICA occlusion treated with STA-MCA bypass shows a mildly enlarged STA* → *entering the skull via a burr hole to anastomose with a cortical branch of the MCA.* ***(Right)*** *Lateral DSA projection in the same patient as previous image, shows prominent STA* → *filling the territory of the inferior division MCA* →.

Typical

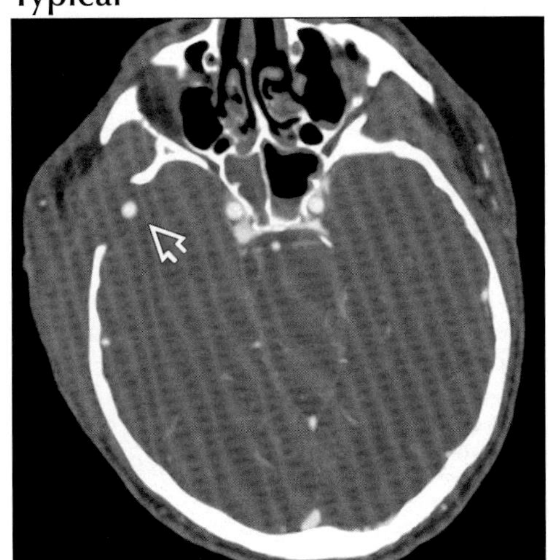

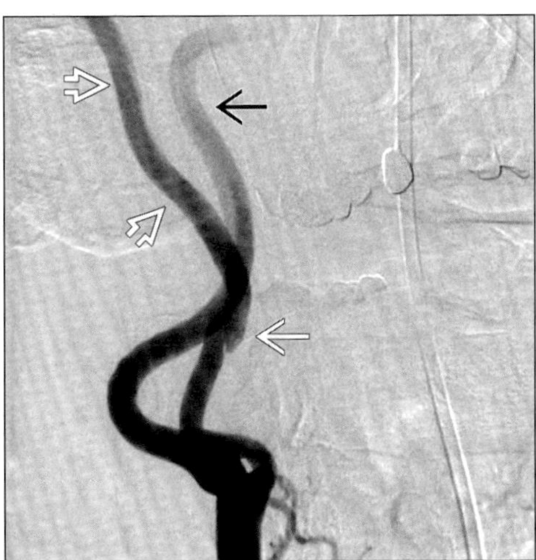

(Left) *Axial CTA S/P high-flow venous bypass graft shows the enhancing graft running along a craniectomy defect* → *before entering the skull. Note overlying scalp soft tissue swelling.* ***(Right)*** *Oblique right CCA DSA of the proximal graft anastomosis shows an end-to-end anastomosis between the saphenous vein and ECA. Note venous valve* → *which is oriented to permit superiorly directed flow. The graft* → *fills faster than the native ICA* →.

Typical

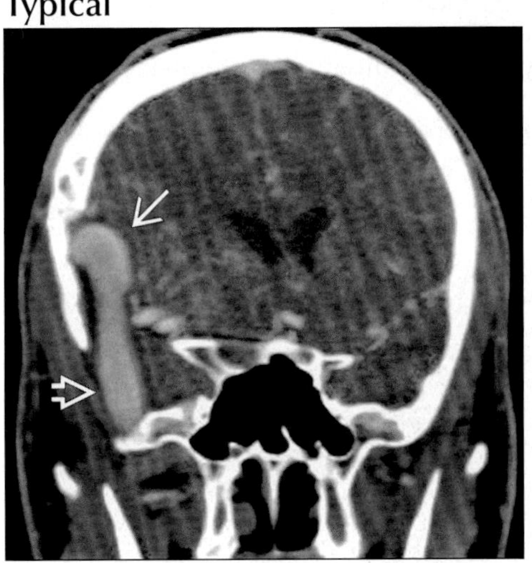

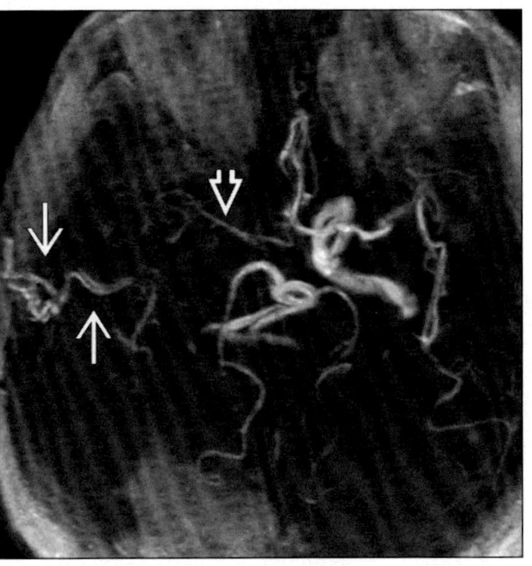

(Left) *Coronal CTA shows a large venous bypass graft* → *entering the skull via a small craniectomy* →*. The patient had a large fusiform aneurysm of his ICA that could not be treated with preservation of the ICA.* ***(Right)*** *Axial MIP image from a TOF MRA in a patient with STA-MCA bypass shows the STA entering the skull to anastomose with a branch* → *of the MCA. Note right ICA occlusion and attenuated MCA* → *from decreased antegrade flow.*

RADIATION VASCULOPATHY, CNS

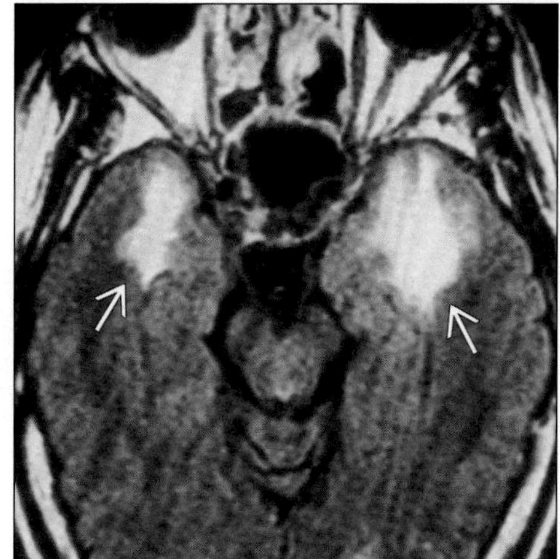

Axial T2WI MR FLAIR shows bilateral anterior temporal lobe white matter hyperintense signal ➡ in this 61 year old male who received prior radiation treatment for nasopharyngeal carcinoma.

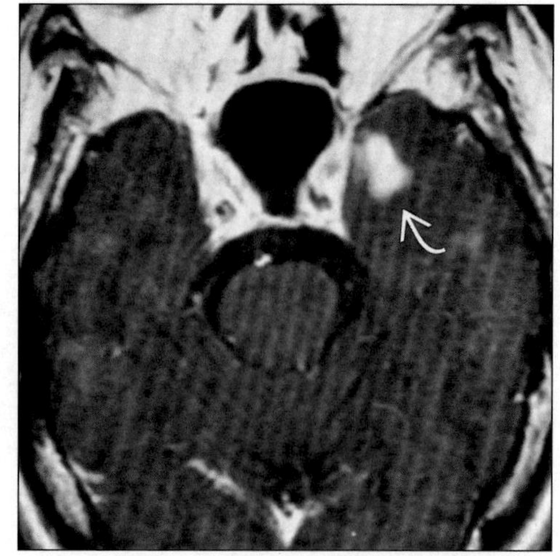

Axial T1WI MR post-contrast in the same patient as previous image, shows enhancement of the left temporal lobe lesion ➡. The nasopharyngeal radiation port had included the anterior temporal lobes.

TERMINOLOGY

Abbreviations and Synonyms

- Radiation-induced injury, radiation changes, X-ray therapy (XRT) changes

Definitions

- Includes radiation injury, leukoencephalopathy, diffuse necrotizing leukoencephalopathy, arteritis, radiation-induced tumors
- Radiation-induced injury may be divided into acute, early delayed injury, late delayed injury

IMAGING FINDINGS

General Features

- Best diagnostic clue
  - Radiation injury: Mild vasogenic edema to necrosis
  - Radiation necrosis: Irregular enhancing lesion(s)
  - Leukoencephalopathy: T2 WM hyperintensity
  - Necrotizing leukoencephalopathy: WM necrosis
  - Radiation arteritis: Vessel wall inflammation, obliterative endarteropathy, vascular malformations
- Location
  - Radiation injury occurs in radiation port
  - Periventricular WM especially susceptible
  - Subcortical U-fibers and corpus callosum spared

CT Findings

- NECT
  - Acute XRT: Confluent WM low density edema
  - Delayed XRT: Focal/multiple WM low densities
  - Leukoencephalopathy: Symmetric WM hypodensity
  - Necrotizing leukoencephalopathy: Extensive areas of WM necrosis; occasional Ca++
- CECT
  - Acute XRT: No enhancement
  - Delayed XRT: ± Patchy or ring-enhancement

MR Findings

- T1WI
  - Acute XRT: Periventricular WM hypointense edema
  - Early delayed XRT: Focal or multiple WM hypointensities
  - Late delayed XRT: Diffuse WM hypointensity or frank necrosis
  - Leukoencephalopathy: Diffuse, symmetric WM hypointensity; spares subcortical U-fibers

DDx: Radiation Vasculopathy, CNS

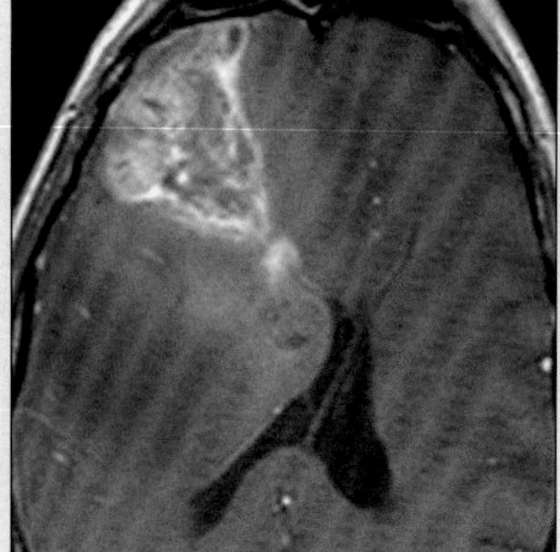

Glioblastoma Multiforme

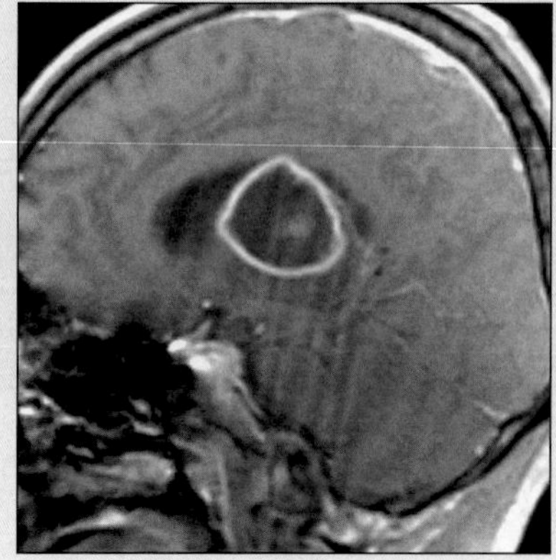

Abscess

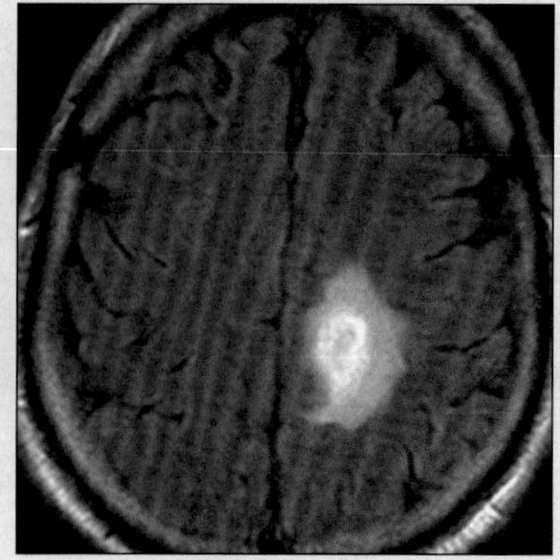

Multiple Sclerosis

RADIATION VASCULOPATHY, CNS

Key Facts

Terminology

- Includes radiation injury, leukoencephalopathy, diffuse necrotizing leukoencephalopathy, arteritis, radiation-induced tumors

Imaging Findings

- Radiation injury: Mild vasogenic edema to necrosis
- Radiation necrosis: Irregular enhancing lesion(s)
- Leukoencephalopathy: T2 WM hyperintensity
- Necrotizing leukoencephalopathy: WM necrosis
- Radiation arteritis: Vessel wall inflammation, obliterative endarteropathy, vascular malformations

Top Differential Diagnoses

- Residual/Recurrent Neoplasm
- Abscess
- Multiple Sclerosis
- Small Vessel Ischemic Disease

Pathology

- Acute: Mild and reversible, vasogenic edema
- Early delayed injury: Edema & demyelination
- Late delayed injury: More severe, irreversible, frank necrosis
- Radiation-induced tumors
- Radiation-induced cryptic vascular malformations

Clinical Issues

- Highly variable: Mild dementia to neurologic deficits

Diagnostic Checklist

- Distinguishing residual/recurrent neoplasm from XRT necrosis difficult using morphology alone
- MRS, MR PWI, PET or SPECT may help delineate recurrent tumor from radiation necrosis

---

- Necrotizing leukoencephalopathy: Extensive areas of WM necrosis
- Radiation-induced cryptic vascular malformations: Blood products of varying age, hypo-/hyperintense

- T2WI
  - Acute XRT: Periventricular WM hyperintense edema
  - Early delayed XRT: Focal or multiple hyperintense WM lesions with edema, demyelination
    - Spares subcortical U-fibers and corpus callosum
  - Late delayed XRT: Diffuse WM injury or frank necrosis
    - Hyperintense WM lesion(s), ± hypointense rim
    - Mass effect and edema
  - Leukoencephalopathy: Diffuse, symmetric involvement of central and periventricular WM, relative sparing of subcortical U-fibers
  - Necrotizing leukoencephalopathy: Extensive WM necrosis
  - Radiation-induced cryptic vascular malformations: Blood products of varying age, hypo-/hyperintense
- T2* GRE: Radiation-induced cryptic vascular malformations: Hypointense "blooming" related to short T2 blood products (SWI MR even more sensitive)
- T1 C+
  - Acute XRT: No enhancement
  - Early delayed XRT: ± Patchy enhancement
  - Late delayed XRT: May see nodular, linear, curvilinear, or "soap bubble" enhancement
    - May have multiple lesions remote from tumor site
    - Enhancement often resembles residual/recurrent tumor about resection cavity
- MRS
  - Radiation necrosis: Markedly reduced metabolites (NAA, Cho, Cr); ± elevated lactate/lipid peaks from cellular necrosis
    - Can be used to differentiate radiation effect from residual/recurrent neoplasm (neoplasm = ↑ Cho)
- Perfusion-weighted imaging (MR PWI)
  - Decreased cerebral blood volume (rCBV) in radiation necrosis from radiation arteritis and decreased neoplastic neoangiogenesis
    - Can be used to differentiate radiation effect from residual/recurrent neoplasm (neoplasm = ↑ rCBV)

Nuclear Medicine Findings

- FDG-PET: Radiation necrosis is hypometabolic
- Thallium 201 SPECT: Radiation necrosis is hypometabolic, decreased uptake
  - Can be used to differentiate radiation effect from residual/recurrent neoplasm (neoplasm = ↑ uptake)

Angiographic Findings

- Radiation-induced vasculopathy: Obliterative endarteropathy, progressive narrowing of supraclinoid ICA and proximal anterior circulation vessels may develop moyamoya pattern

Imaging Recommendations

- Best imaging tool: MR: T2/FLAIR, T1, T1 C+, GRE
- Protocol advice: PET, SPECT, MRS, MR PWI if question of XRT vs. recurrent neoplasm

DIFFERENTIAL DIAGNOSIS

Residual/Recurrent Neoplasm

- Enhancing mass with central necrosis, mass effect
- MRS shows increased Cho, decreased NAA, ± lactate
- MR PWI demonstrates elevated rCBV

Abscess

- Ring-enhancing mass, thinner margin along ventricle
- T2 hypointense rim, diffusion restriction characteristic
- MRS shows metabolites such as succinate, amino acids

Multiple Sclerosis

- Often incomplete, "horseshoe-shaped" enhancement
- Other lesions in typical perpendicular periventricular or subcallosal location, young patients
- Often lack significant mass effect, unless "tumefactive"

Small Vessel Ischemic Disease

- Typically old patients
- History of hypertension, diabetes or hyperlipidemia
- Associated lacunar infarcts, multifocal "microbleeds"

RADIATION VASCULOPATHY, CNS

Progressive Multifocal Leukoencephalopathy

- WM T2 hyperintensity, involves subcortical U-fibers
- May cross corpus callosum; nonenhancing typical
- Immunosuppressed patients

Foreign Body Reaction

- Granulomatous reaction to gelatin sponge, etc.
- Can mimic tumor recurrence, radiation necrosis

PATHOLOGY

General Features

- General path comments
  - Neurotoxic reaction to radiation therapy divided into acute, early delayed and late delayed injury
    - Acute: Mild and reversible, vasogenic edema
    - Early delayed injury: Edema & demyelination
    - Late delayed injury: More severe, irreversible, frank necrosis
  - XRT variables include: Total dose, field size, fraction size, number/frequency of doses, adjuvant therapy (intrathecal chemotherapy), survival duration, patient age
  - Most XRT injury is delayed (months/years)
  - Radiation-induced neoplasms: Meningiomas (70%), gliomas (20%), sarcomas (10%)
    - More aggressive tumors, highly refractory
  - Radiation-induced cryptic vascular malformations: Capillary telangiectasias, cavernous malformations
- Etiology
  - Radiation-induced neurotoxicity
    - Glial and WM damage (sensitivity of oligodendrocytes > > neurons)
    - Miscellaneous (effects on fibrinolytic system, immune effects)
  - Radiation-induced vascular injury
    - Permeability alterations, endothelial and basement membrane damage, accelerated atherosclerosis, telangiectasia formation
  - Radiation-induced tumors
    - Increased risk in patients with XRT ≤ 5 years old, those with genetic predisposition (NF1, retinoblastoma), BMT survivors
  - Radiation-induced cryptic vascular malformations
    - Altered venous endothelium, veno-occlusive disease
- Epidemiology
  - Overall incidence of radionecrosis 5-24%
    - External beam < 18%, radiosurgery 25-30%, brachytherapy 30-40%
  - Second neoplasms: 3-12%

Gross Pathologic & Surgical Features

- XRT: Spectrum from edema to cavitating WM necrosis
- Demyelination: Sharp interface with normal brain
- Radiation necrosis: Coagulative necrosis that favors WM, may extend to deep cortex

Microscopic Features

- Acute XRT injury: WM edema from capillary damage
- Early delayed injury: Vasogenic edema, demyelination
  - Demyelination: Macrophage infiltrates, loss of myelin, perivascular lymphocytic infiltrates, gliosis
- Late delayed injury: WM necrosis, demyelination, astrocytosis, vasculopathy
  - Radiation necrosis: Confluent coagulative necrosis, Ca++, telangiectasias, hyaline thickening and fibrinoid necrosis of vessels, thrombosis

CLINICAL ISSUES

Presentation

- Most common signs/symptoms: Highly variable: Mild dementia to neurologic deficits
- Radiation injury to the brain is divided into 3 groups
  - Acute injury: 1-6 weeks after or during treatment
  - Early delayed injury: 3 weeks to several months
  - Late delayed injury: Months to years after treatment

Natural History & Prognosis

- Younger patient at time of treatment: Worse prognosis
- Radiation necrosis is a dynamic pathophysiological process; often progressive, irreversible

Treatment

- Biopsy if cannot resolve tumor vs. radionecrosis
- Surgery if mass effect, edema
- Acute radiation injury may respond to steroids

DIAGNOSTIC CHECKLIST

Consider

- Distinguishing residual/recurrent neoplasm from XRT necrosis difficult using morphology alone

Image Interpretation Pearls

- MRS, MR PWI, PET or SPECT may help delineate recurrent tumor from radiation necrosis

SELECTED REFERENCES

1. Burn S et al: Incidence of cavernoma development in children after radiotherapy for brain tumors. J Neurosurg. 106(5 Suppl):379-83, 2007
2. Conill C et al: Incidence of radiation-induced leukoencephalopathy after whole brain radiotherapy in patients with brain metastases. Clin Transl Oncol. 9(9):590-5, 2007
3. Ullrich NJ et al: Moyamoya following cranial irradiation for primary brain tumors in children. Neurology. 68(12):932-8, 2007
4. Ruben JD et al: Cerebral radiation necrosis: incidence, outcomes, and risk factors with emphasis on radiation parameters and chemotherapy. Int J Radiat Oncol Biol Phys. 65(2):499-508, 2006
5. Chan YL et al: Dynamic susceptibility contrast-enhanced perfusion MR imaging in late radiation-induced injury of the brain. Acta Neurochir Suppl. 95:173-5, 2005
6. Weybright P et al: Differentiation between brain tumor recurrence and radiation injury using MR spectroscopy. AJR Am J Roentgenol. 185(6):1471-6, 2005
7. Tsuruda JS et al: Radiation effects on cerebral white matter: MR evaluation. AJR Am J Roentgenol. 149(1):165-71, 1987

IMAGE GALLERY

Typical

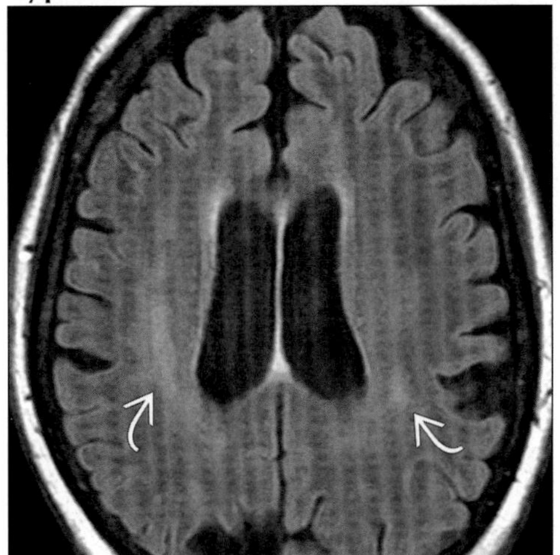

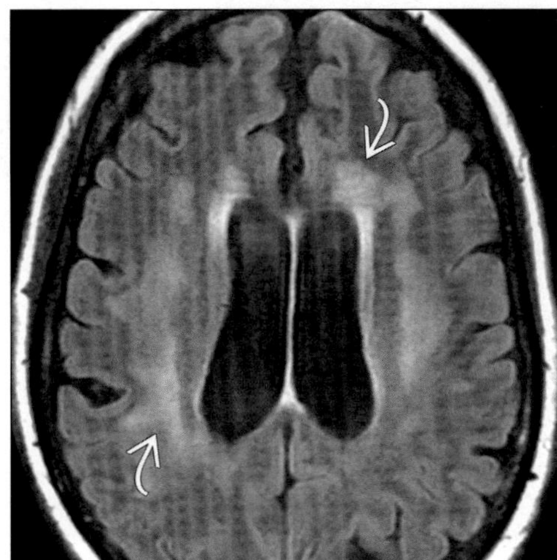

*(**Left**) Axial T2WI MR FLAIR shows mild diffuse deep white matter hyperintensity ➔ eight months following whole brain irradiation for metastatic breast carcinoma. (**Right**) Axial T2WI MR FLAIR in the same patient as previous image, thirteen months following radiation treatment, shows interval progression of the white matter disease ➔ from radiation induced leukoencephalopathy.*

Typical

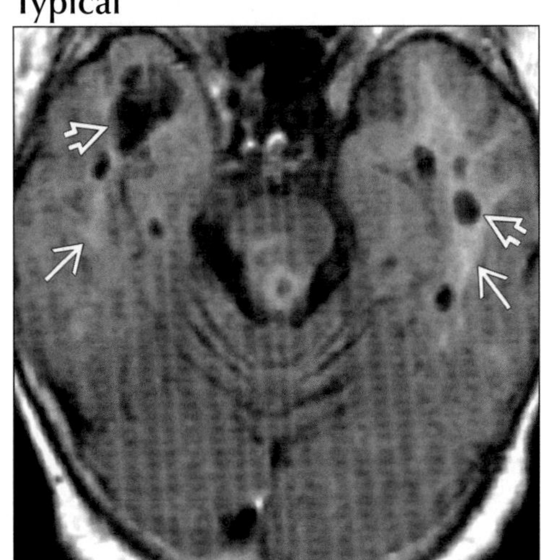

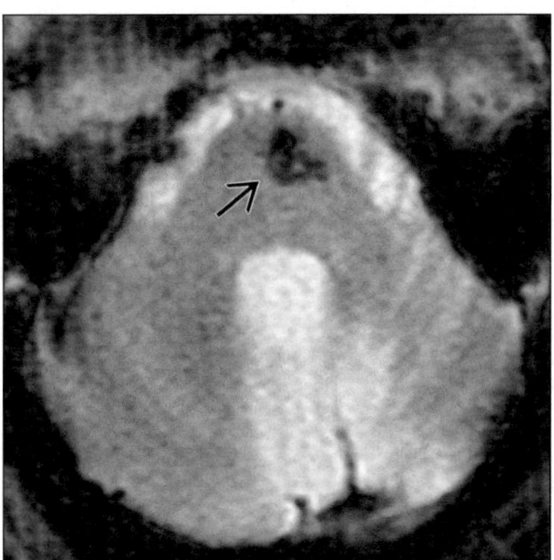

*(**Left**) Axial T2WI MR FLAIR shows hyperintense signal in the bitemporal white matter ➔ with associated hypointense signal from cystic encephalomalacia ➔ due to radiation vasculopathy. (**Right**) Axial T2WI MR GRE shows a focus of hypointense "blooming" in the pons ➔ from cavernous malformation secondary to radiation therapy following cerebellar medulloblastoma resection.*

Typical

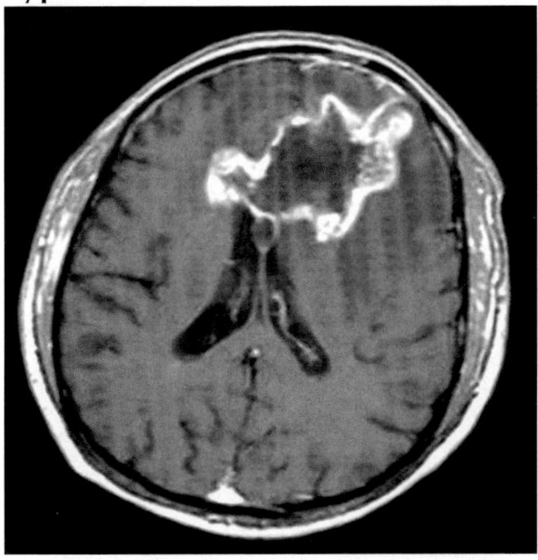

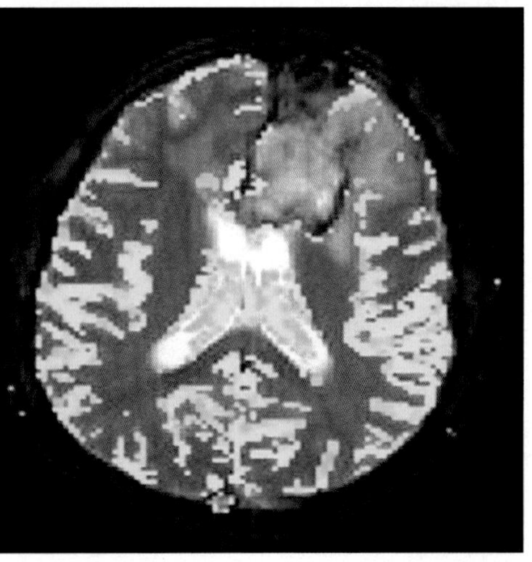

*(**Left**) Axial T1WI MR post-contrast shows bifrontal region of necrosis with nodular peripheral enhancement and surrounding vasogenic edema. Morphologic findings suspicious for recurrent neoplasm. (**Right**) Axial MR perfusion cerebral blood volume map in the same patient as previous image, depicts low rCBV in the frontal regions confirming radiation-induced necrotizing leukoencephalopathy (Courtesy A. Cianfoni, MD).*

SACCULAR ANEURYSM

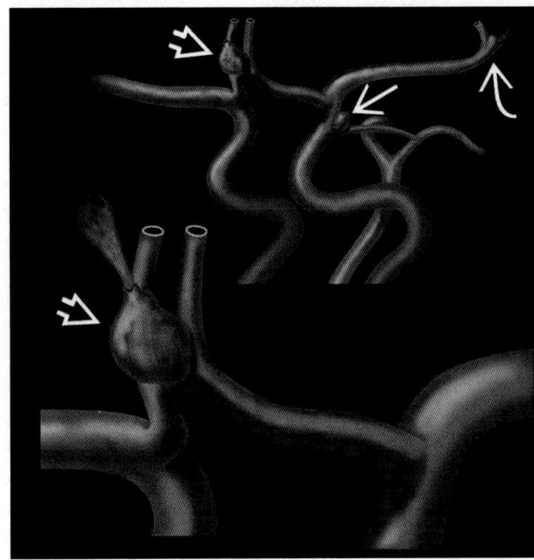

Anteroposterior graphic of the circle of Willis shows a large ACoA aneurysm ➲. The apex has ruptured, resulting in aSAH. Additional small IC-PCoA ➔ and MCA ➚ aneurysms are present.

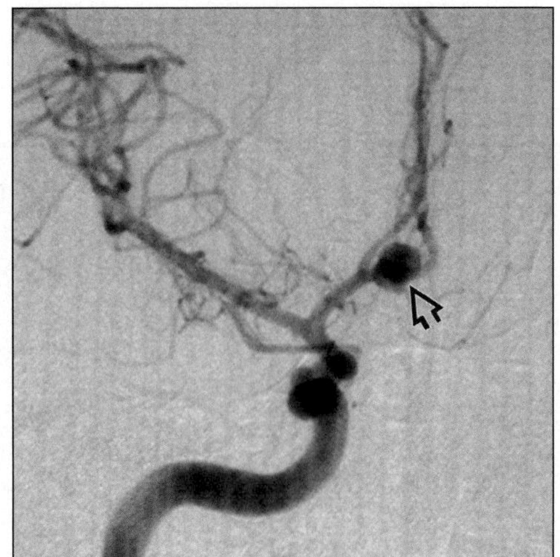

Anteroposterior DSA of a right internal carotid artery injection depicts a saccular aneurysm ➲ at the anterior communicating artery.

TERMINOLOGY

Abbreviations and Synonyms

- Intracranial saccular aneurysm (SA), true aneurysm, berry aneurysm

Definitions

- Arterial outpouching that lacks internal elastic lamina, muscular layers

IMAGING FINDINGS

General Features

- Best diagnostic clue: Round/lobulated outpouching from circle of Willis (COW), MCA bifurcation, or PICA origin
- Location
  - 90-95% arise from COW
    - 90% anterior circulation (IC-PCoA, ACoA most common sites; MCA less common)
    - 10% posterior (BA bifurcation, PICA most common sites)
    - 5% distal to COW (often traumatic, mycotic, oncotic)
  - Vessel bifurcation > lateral wall
- Size: Small (2-3 mm) to giant (> 2.5 cm)
- Morphology
  - Round, lobulated or bleb-like outpouching
  - Narrow or broad-based origin from parent vessel

CT Findings

- NECT
  - Ruptured SAs have acute high density aneurysmal subarachnoid hemorrhage (aSAH) in cisterns, sulci
    - Greatest concentration of aSAH can help identify location of aneurysm
  - Patent aneurysm
    - Well-delineated round/lobulated extra-axial mass
    - Slightly hyperdense to brain (may have mural Ca++)
  - Partially/completely thrombosed aneurysm
    - Moderately hyperdense (Ca++ common)
- CECT
  - Lumen of patent SA enhances strongly, uniformly
  - Completely thrombosed SA may have reactive rim enhancement

DDx: Saccular Aneurysm

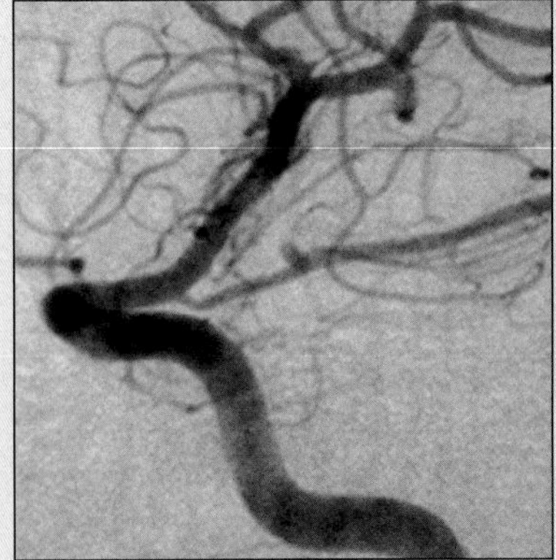

PCA Vessel Loop

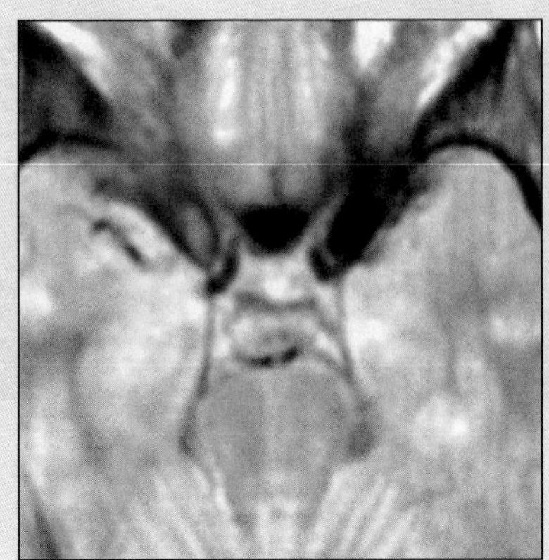

Aerated Clinoid

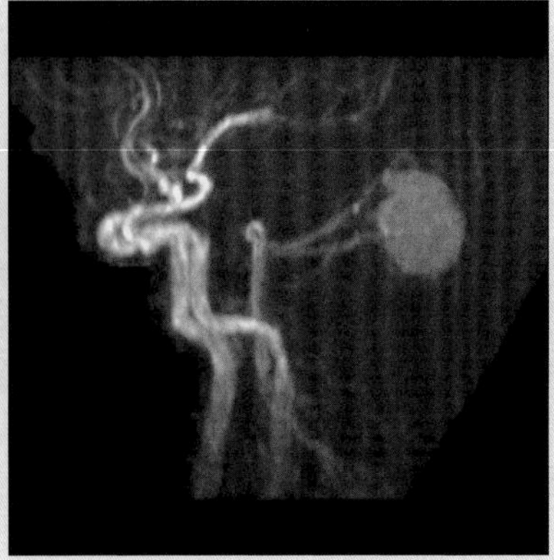

Lipoma

SACCULAR ANEURYSM

Key Facts

Terminology
- Arterial outpouching that lacks internal elastic lamina, muscular layers

Imaging Findings
- Best diagnostic clue: Round/lobulated outpouching from circle of Willis (COW), MCA bifurcation, or PICA origin
- Ruptured SAs have acute high density aneurysmal subarachnoid hemorrhage (aSAH) in cisterns, sulci
- Multi-slice CTA positive in 95% of patients with aSAH
- Typically hypointense on T2WI
- Flow in patent aneurysm produces phase artifact
- Best imaging tool: NECT for aSAH + multislice CTA

Top Differential Diagnoses
- Vessel Loop
- Vessel Origin Infundibulum
- Pseudoaneurysm
- "Flow Void" Mimic on MR
- Short T1 "Shine-Through" on MRA

Pathology
- SA development reflects complex combination of inherited susceptibility + acquired mechanically-mediated vessel wall stresses
- 10% prevalence in FIAs
- 1-2% incidental finding of unruptured SA at autopsy, angiography

Clinical Issues
- Low rupture risk if < 5 mm, high if > 2.5 cm
- ISAT: 22.6% relative, 6.9% absolute risk reduction (coiling vs. surgery) for ruptured aneurysms

- CTA
  - Positive in 95% of patients with aSAH
  - If screening for unruptured SA, negative CTA = very low probability of "clinically important" aneurysm

MR Findings
- T1WI
  - Patent aneurysm (signal varies)
    - 50% have "flow void" on T1WI
    - 50% iso/heterogeneous signal (slow/turbulent flow; saturation effects; phase dispersion)
  - Partially/completely thrombosed aneurysm
    - Signal depends on age(s) of clot
    - Common = mixed signal, laminated thrombus
- T2WI
  - Typically hypointense on T2WI
  - May be laminated with very hypointense rim
  - Flow in patent aneurysm produces phase artifact
- FLAIR: Acute aSAH = high signal in sulci, cisterns
- DWI: ± Foci of restricted diffusion secondary to vasospasm, ischemia
- T1 C+
  - Slow flow in patent lumen may enhance
  - Increases phase artifact in patent SAs
- MRA
  - 1.5T 3D TOF: > 90% for aneurysms 3 mm or greater
  - 3T 3D TOF C+ best (1024 x 1024 resolution)

Angiographic Findings
- Conventional
  - Role of DSA
    - Identify SA (round/lobulated, focal outpouching), define neck (narrow or broad-based)
    - Identify arteries that may arise from dome
    - Assess potential for collateral circulation
    - Rare = contrast extravasation with active aSAH
  - Multiple projections/injections: Complete 4-vessel evaluation
    - Detect multiple aneurysms
  - 3D DSA with shaded surface display optimal

Imaging Recommendations
- Best imaging tool: NECT for aSAH + multislice CTA
- Protocol advice
  - Thin slices, low pitch CTA; 3D TOF ± contrast-enhanced MRA
  - If CTA/MRA negative, DSA

DIFFERENTIAL DIAGNOSIS

Vessel Loop
- Use multiple projections

Vessel Origin Infundibulum
- < 3 mm, conical, small PCoA arises directly from apex

Pseudoaneurysm
- Often arises distal to COW
- May be indistinguishable from true SA

"Flow Void" Mimic on MR
- Aerated anterior clinoid or supraorbital cell
- No pulsation artifact in the phase encode direction

Short T1 "Shine-Through" on MRA
- Lipoma
- Pituitary gland (contrast-enhanced MRA)

PATHOLOGY

General Features
- General path comments
  - SA development reflects complex combination of inherited susceptibility + acquired mechanically-mediated vessel wall stresses
  - SA rupture risk also complex, multifactorial
- Genetics
  - Abnormal expression/polymorphism of some genes
    - Endoglin, MMP-9, apolipoprotein(a) genes
    - Overexpression of other genes encoding extracellular matrix components (such as collagen, α2(I) elastin)
    - Endothelial NO synthase (eNOS) gene
  - Familial intracranial aneurysms (FIAs)
    - No known heritable connective tissue disorder

SACCULAR ANEURYSM

- Occur in "clusters" (two first-order relatives)
- 10% prevalence in FIAs
- Younger patients, no female predominance
- Accounts for up to 20% of all aSAH

- Etiology
  - Aneurysm formation multifactorial
  - Flow-related "bioengineering fatigue" in vessel wall
  - Abnormal vascular hemodynamics
    - Arises at areas of high biomechanical stress
    - Abnormal slipstream vectors
    - Higher/disturbed flow, increased pulsatility
  - Larger aneurysms are likely to expand (LaPlace's law)
- Epidemiology
  - 1-2% incidental finding of unruptured SA at autopsy, angiography
  - 20% multiple
  - Annual risk of de novo aneurysm following previous clipping = 0.8%
- Associated abnormalities
  - Hereditary/connective tissue disorders
    - Fibromuscular dysplasia
    - Autosomal dominant polycystic kidney disease (10%)
    - Ehlers-Danlos type IV, NF1 (usually fusiform, not SA)
  - Anomalous/aberrant vessel
    - Intraoptic A1 ACA
    - Persistent trigeminal artery
    - ± Fenestrated vessel (usually basilar artery)
  - Flow-related (30-35% on feeding pedicle of AVM)
  - Trauma, infection, tumor, etc. (usually pseudoaneurysms)

Gross Pathologic & Surgical Features

- Round/lobulated sac, thin or thick wall, ± aSAH

Microscopic Features

- Disrupted/absent internal elastic lamina
- Muscle layer absent
- May have "bleb" of fragile adventitia

CLINICAL ISSUES

Presentation

- Most common signs/symptoms
  - aSAH 60-85%
    - Headache (often "thunderclap")
  - Cranial neuropathy 15-30%
    - Pupil-involving CN 3 palsy most common (PCoA aneurysm)
  - Other: "Migraine", TIA, seizure
- Clinical Profile: Middle-aged patient with "worst headache of my life"

Demographics

- Age
  - From 1.22/100,000 persons/yr (age 0-34) to 44.47/100,000 persons/yr (age 65-74)
  - Rare in children
    - 1-2% of all aneurysms
    - Different location (ICA bifurcation, M2 MCA)
    - Trauma most common cause
- Gender: Women > men (esp. multiple aneurysms)

Natural History & Prognosis

- Rupture risk
  - Size most important (but not only) factor
    - Low rupture risk if < 5 mm, high if > 2.5 cm
    - ENOS genotype may influence rupture size risk
  - Configuration vs. rupture risk increased if
    - Multilobed > round/ovoid shape
    - Apical "tit" or "bleb" present
    - Aspect ratio (length vs. neck) > 1.6
  - "Perianeurysmal environment" (contact with other structures)
  - Other (hypertension, female gender, smoking)
- Untreated "giant" aneurysm (> 2.5 cm)
  - 68% mortality rate at 2 y, 85% after 5 y
  - Most/all survivors have marked neurologic dysfunction

Treatment

- Endovascular (coiling, liquid embolics, stents)
  - ISAT: 22.6% relative, 6.9% absolute risk reduction (coiling vs. surgery) for ruptured aneurysms
- Clipping (high volume institutions and surgeons have significantly lower morbidity)

DIAGNOSTIC CHECKLIST

Consider

- aSAH vs. nonaneurysmal SAH or pseudoSAH

Image Interpretation Pearls

- "Angiogram-negative" aSAH may be caused by "blister-like" aneurysm
  - Look for mild asymmetric vessel wall bulge
- ACoA is most likely site of "initially occult aneurysm"

SELECTED REFERENCES

1. Ahn S et al: Fluid-induced wall shear stress in anthropomorphic brain aneurysm models: MR phase-contrast study at 3 T. J Magn Reson Imaging. 25(6):1120-30, 2007
2. El Khaldi M et al: Detection of cerebral aneurysms in nontraumatic subarachnoid haemorrhage: role of multislice CT angiography in 130 consecutive patients. Radiol Med (Torino). 112(1):123-37, 2007
3. Higashida RT et al: Treatment of unruptured intracranial aneurysms: a nationwide assessment of effectiveness. AJNR Am J Neuroradiol. 28(1):146-51, 2007
4. Lubicz B et al: Immediate intracranial aneurysm occlusion after embolization with detachable coils: a comparison between MR angiography and intra-arterial digital subtraction angiography. J Neuroradiol. 34(3):190-197, 2007
5. Wermer MJ et al: Risk of rupture of unruptured intracranial aneurysms in relation to patient and aneurysm characteristics: an updated meta-analysis. Stroke. 38(4):1404-10, 2007
6. Pannu H et al: The role of MMP-2 and MMP-9 polymorphisms in sporadic intracranial aneurysms. J Neurosurg. 105(3):418-23, 2006
7. Molyneux A et al: International Subarachnoid Aneurysm Trial (ISAT) of neurosurgical clipping versus endovascular coiling in 2143 patients with ruptured intracranial aneurysms: a randomised trial. Lancet. 360(9342):1267-74, 2002

SACCULAR ANEURYSM

IMAGE GALLERY

Typical

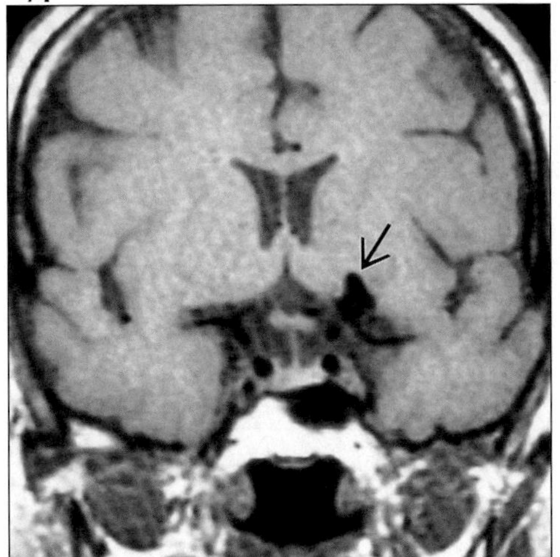

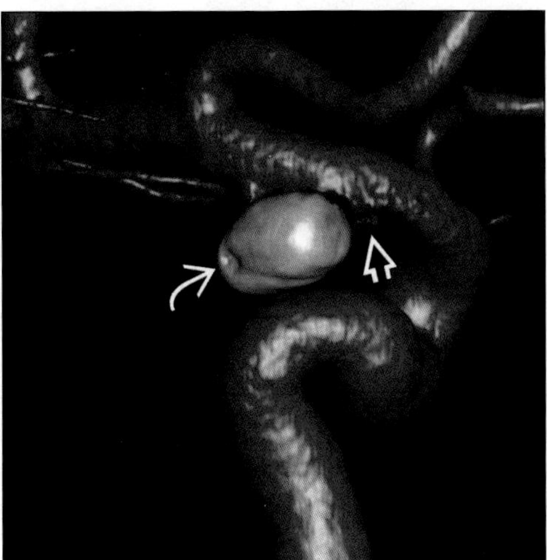

*(**Left**) Coronal T1WI MR demonstrates globular vascular flow void at the left internal carotid artery terminus ⇒ from an ICA bifurcation saccular aneurysm. (**Right**) Posteroanterior DSA rotational 3D acquisition, right ICA injection, shows a coiled 8 x 5 mm slightly wide-necked IC-PCoA aneurysm ➡. Note preserved posterior communicating artery ➡.*

Typical

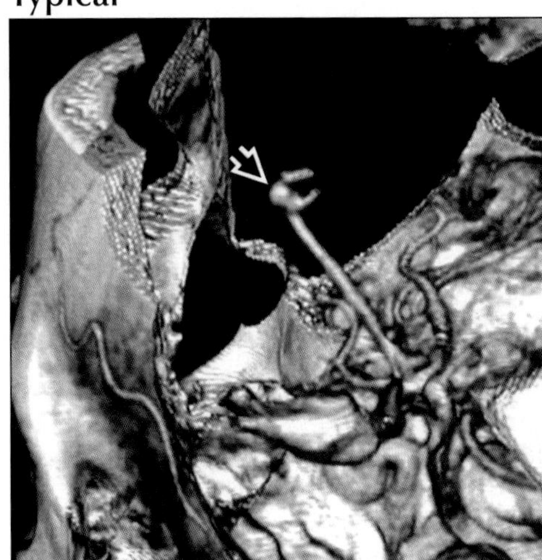

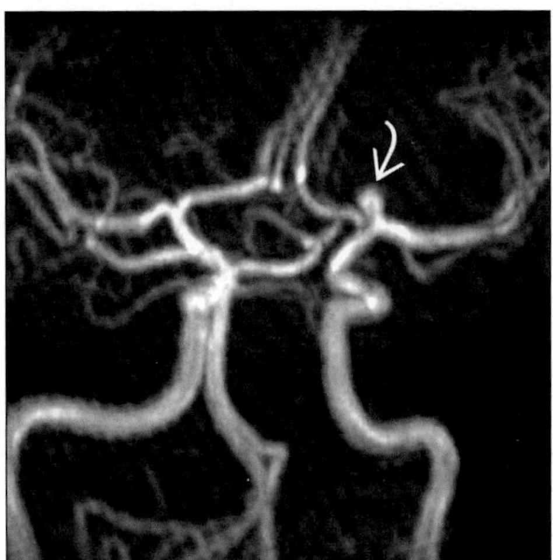

*(**Left**) Oblique CTA superolateral view shows an anterior cerebral artery A2 segment bifurcation aneurysm ➡. Aneurysms in this location can develop de novo or may be mycotic in origin. (**Right**) Coronal oblique conventional 3D time-of-flight MRA MIP image shows a left internal carotid artery terminus aneurysm ➡ (incidental finding).*

Variant

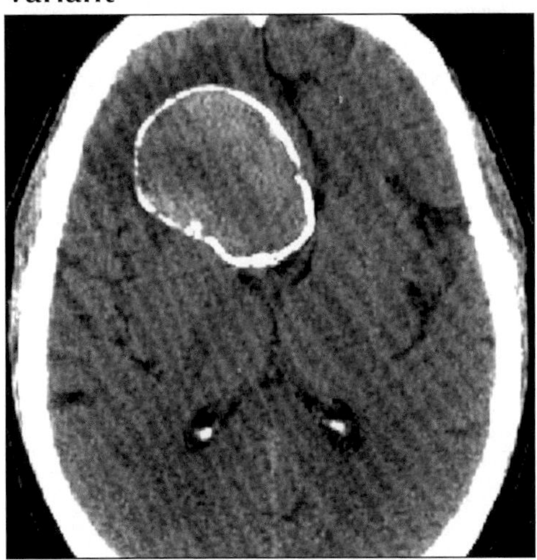

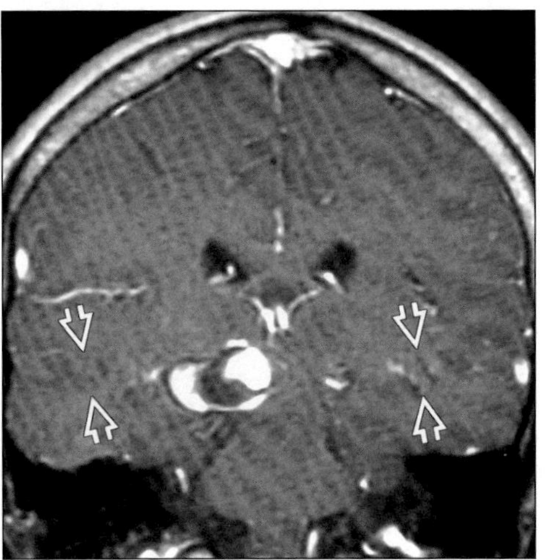

*(**Left**) Axial NECT shows a right frontal moderately hyperdense mass with peripheral calcification and adjacent parenchymal edema. This lesion was found to be a giant, mostly thrombosed, aneurysm. (**Right**) Coronal T1WI MR post-contrast shows a distal right posterior cerebral artery partially thrombosed aneurysm. Note pulsation artifact across the image in the phase encode direction ➡.*

FUSIFORM ANEURYSM

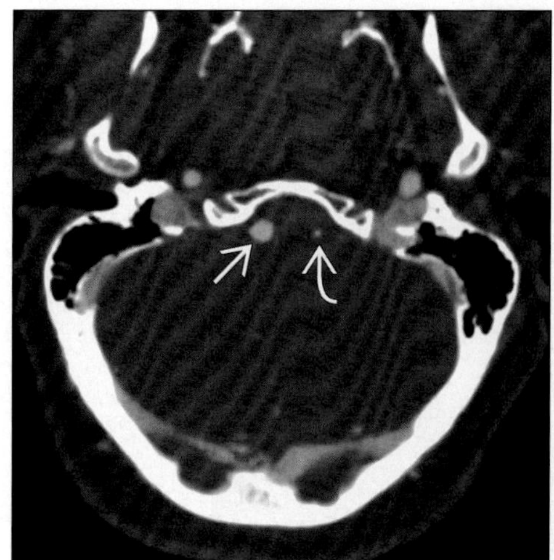

Axial CTA source image shows a FA of the right vertebral artery in a patient presenting with SAH ➡. Note size of the left vertebral artery ➡ for comparison.

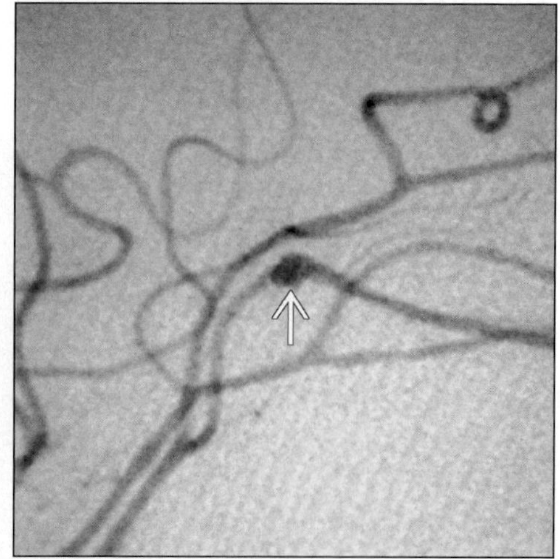

Magnified DSA in a different patient presenting with SAH and a history of head trauma shows a small pericallosal artery FA ➡.

TERMINOLOGY

Definitions

- Fusiform aneurysm (FA): Non-saccular dilatation of vessel with separate inflow and outflow pathways

IMAGING FINDINGS

General Features

- Best diagnostic clue
  - Fusiform or ovoid arterial dilatation on CTA/MRA/DSA
  - Slow/altered flow dynamics within lumen with swirling of contrast on DSA or inhomogeneous signal on MR/MRA ± intraluminal or intramural thrombus
- Location
  - Can occur anywhere there is vessel wall weakening in the head and neck
  - May be arterial or venous
- Size: Variable: Few mm to several cm

Radiographic Findings

- Radiography: May see Ca++ of aneurysm wall or intraluminal thrombus

CT Findings

- NECT
  - Vessel lumen ± intraluminal thrombus is hyperdense compared with brain parenchyma
  - Ca++ common
  - Subarachnoid hemorrhage (SAH) if FA is intradural (involves pial arteries or veins) and ruptures
- CECT: Lumen enhances strongly, intramural/intraluminal clot does not
- CTA: Multiplanar reconstructions ± shaded surface display (SSD) usually diagnostic of fusiform morphology

MR Findings

- Ectatic vessel ± more focal aneurysmal outpouching
- Mixed signal intensity on MR common, varies with
  - Flow velocity, direction, turbulence
    - Slow flow seen as high signal deep into imaged sections
  - Presence, age of mural hematoma

DDx: Fusiform Aneurysm

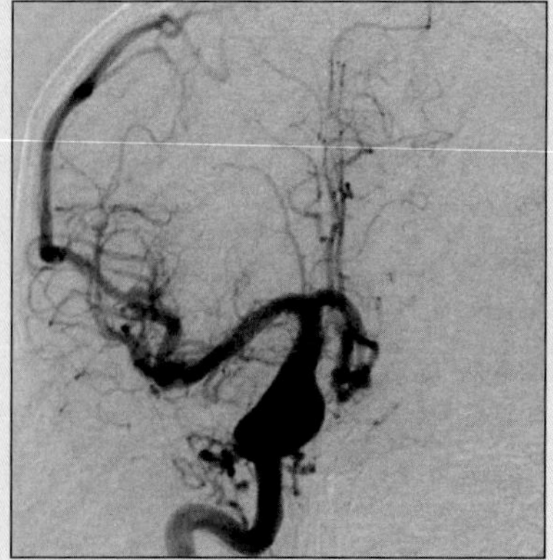

PHACES Syndrome

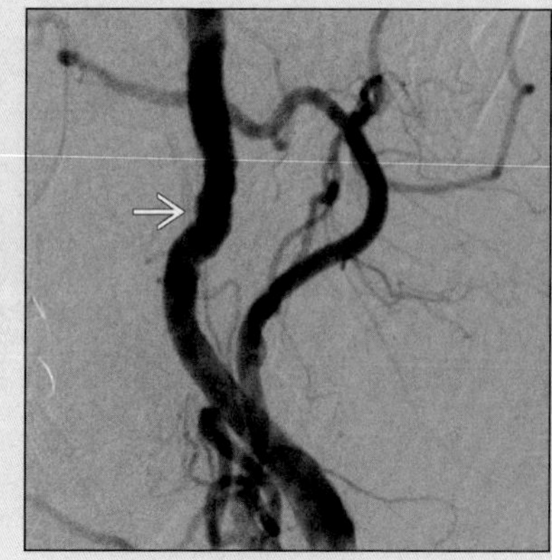

Fibromuscular Dysplasia

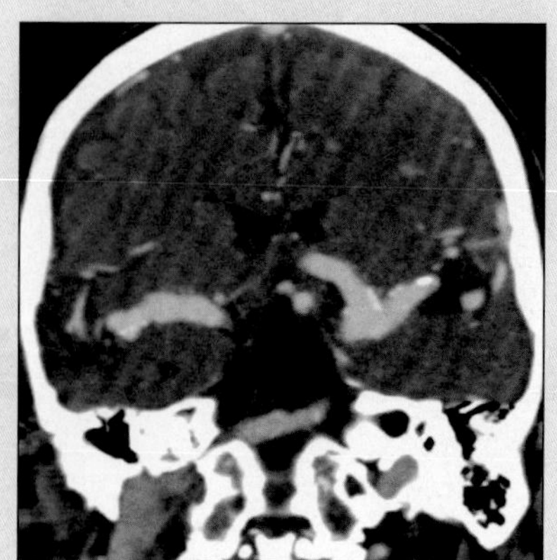

Dolichoectasia

FUSIFORM ANEURYSM

Key Facts

Terminology

- Fusiform aneurysm (FA): Non-saccular dilatation of vessel with separate inflow and outflow pathways

Imaging Findings

- Fusiform or ovoid arterial dilatation on CTA/MRA/DSA
- May be arterial or venous
- Radiography: May see Ca++ of aneurysm wall or intraluminal thrombus
- CECT: Lumen enhances strongly, intramural/intraluminal clot does not
- Multiplanar reconstructions ± shaded surface display (SSD) usually diagnostic of fusiform morphology
- DSA is gold standard for diagnosis

Pathology

- FA less common than saccular aneurysms
- Atherosclerosis usual cause of basilar FA in older adults
- Dissecting aneurysm
- Mycotic aneurysm
- Venous aneurysm/varix associated with AV shunts

Clinical Issues

- Often difficult proposition for surgery and endovascular techniques
- Mycotic aneurysm: Antibiotics may result in shrinkage and cure over time
- Venous aneurysm: Treatment of the underlying AV shunt results in ↓ venous flow and regression or thrombosis of FA

- Often hyperintense on T1WI, hypointense rim on T2WI
- Clot may be laminated (layers of organized thrombus at different stages of evolution)

- Residual lumen enhances strongly

Other Modality Findings

- MRA
  - Precontrast 3D-TOF may be inadequate because of
    - Flow saturation effects
    - Intravoxel phase dispersion
  - Giant FA usually requires dynamic contrast-enhanced sequences for improved delineation

Angiographic Findings

- Conventional
  - DSA is gold standard for diagnosis
  - Non-saccular or "sausage-shaped" dilatation of vessel lumen
  - Contained thrombus inferred by irregular contours of aneurysm lumen
  - May see associated stenosis if underlying etiology is dissection

DIFFERENTIAL DIAGNOSIS

Arterial Dolichoectasia

- Encompasses spectrum from mild fusiform ectasia → FA
- Typically associated with significant vessel tortuosity
- Vertebrobasilar 85%; carotid arteries 15%
- Usually older pt, underlying atherosclerotic vascular disease (ASVD)
- In younger patients, consider alternate underlying vasculopathy (e.g., Marfan, Ehlers-Danlos, fibromuscular dysplasia, autosomal dominant polycystic kidney disease)
- Ectasia may extends into branches of circle of Willis
- May rupture → SAH

Fibromuscular Dysplasia

- Classically alternating areas of arterial dilatation and stenoses → "beading"
- Affects renal > carotid > vertebral arteries
- Can predispose to fusiform aneurysms, particularly in the cavernous internal carotid artery (ICA)
  - May lead to arterial dissection → fusiform pseudoaneurysms (e.g., cervical ICA)

PHACES Syndrome

- Neurocutaneous association of anomalies
- Acronym for (P)osterior fossa malformation, (H)emangioma, (A)rterial anomalies, (C)ardiac defects, (E)ye abnormalities, (S)ternal clefts
- Arterial anomalies include intracranial arterial dilatations without arteriovenous shunting

PATHOLOGY

General Features

- General path comments
  - FA less common than saccular aneurysms
  - Can be acute (dissecting aneurysm) or chronic (ASVD, nonatherosclerotic vasculopathy)
  - May be bilateral (e.g., vertebral artery dissection) or multifocal (e.g., mycotic aneurysms)
  - May involve pial (cortical) veins if subjected to high pressure/flow as in AV shunts
  - Classification: Nonatherosclerotic fusiform and dissecting aneurysms
    - Type 1 = typical dissecting aneurysm
    - Type 2 = segmental ectasias
    - Type 3 = dolichoectatic dissecting aneurysms
    - Type 4 = atypically located saccular aneurysm (i.e., lateral wall, unrelated to branching zones)
- Genetics: Marfan syndrome: Mutation of fibrillin genes (FBN1)
- Etiology
  - Atherosclerosis usual cause of basilar FA in older adults
    - Lipid deposition is initial step

FUSIFORM ANEURYSM

- Internal elastic lamina (IEL): Muscle layers become disrupted
- Enhanced susceptibility to hemodynamic stress
- Dissecting aneurysm
  - Injury or tear to tunica intima permits entry of blood into vessel wall
  - Fusiform dilatation occurs when dissection not contained by tunica media
  - Vessel rupture or pseudoaneurysm when dissection extends through tunica adventitia
  - Intradural segment of vertebral arteries most commonly affected in head and neck, although can occur in any location
- Mycotic aneurysm
  - Uncommon complication of bacterial endocarditis, often associated with IV drug abuse
  - S. Aureus, Salmonella and Streptococcus common pathogens
  - May be multiple, bilateral, affect more than one organ system
  - Bacteria-laden thromboemboli lodge in small intracranial arteries and vessel wall destruction ensues
  - DDx based on location is traumatic intracranial aneurysm
  - SAH or intraparenchymal hematoma if aneurysm ruptures
- Venous aneurysm/varix associated with AV shunts
  - Dilatation of cortical (pial) veins commonly occur in the presence of AV shunts
  - Arteriovenous malformation (AVM), dural AV fistula (DAVF) subject these veins to arterial pressure → tortuosity, varicosities ± rupture (SAH)
- Miscellaneous
  - Immune deficiency (e.g., HIV)
  - Viral, other infectious agents (e.g., varicella)
  - Collagen vascular disorders (e.g., SLE)
  - Sickle cell anemia

Gross Pathologic & Surgical Features

- Focally dilated fusiform arterial ectasia(s)
- ± ASVD, arterial dissection

Microscopic Features

- Type 1 = widespread disruption of the IEL, no intimal thickening
- Type 2 = extended and/or fragmented IEL with intimal thickening
- Type 3 = IEL fragmentation, multiple dissections of thickened intima, organized thrombus
- Type 4 = absent IEL, muscular layer

CLINICAL ISSUES

Presentation

- Headache, SAH
- TIA, cranial neuropathy

Natural History & Prognosis

- Type 1: Rebleed common
- Type 2: Benign clinical course
- Type 3: Slow but progressive enlargement
- Type 4: Rerupture risk high

Treatment

- Often difficult proposition for surgery and endovascular techniques
- 80% of untreated giant aneurysms dead/disabled at 5 years
- Surgical
  - Bypass, vessel reconstruction (clips, wrapping), vessel sacrifice (Hunterian ligation)
- Endovascular
  - Vessel sacrifice (coils, liquid embolics)
  - Vessel reconstruction (covered stent, stent-supported coil embolization)
- Mycotic aneurysm: Antibiotics may result in shrinkage and cure over time
- Venous aneurysm: Treatment of the underlying AV shunt results in ↓ venous flow and regression or thrombosis of FA

DIAGNOSTIC CHECKLIST

Consider

- Atherosclerosis, arterial dissection (spontaneous or traumatic) and infection as underlying etiologies

Image Interpretation Pearls

- Differentiation from saccular/"berry" aneurysm on CTA/MRA is important for treatment planning; DSA may be required for clarification
- Characteristic location of FA is a clue to underlying etiology
  - Intradural (V4) segment of vertebral artery (dissecting aneurysm)
  - Distal intracranial arterial vasculature (mycotic or traumatic aneurysm)
  - Basilar artery (underlying ASVD dolichoectasia in older patients)

SELECTED REFERENCES

1. Ansari SA et al: Thrombosis of a fusiform intracranial aneurysm induced by overlapping neuroform stents: case report. Neurosurgery. 60(5):E950-1; discussion E950-1, 2007
2. Chen L et al: Management of complex, surgically intractable intracranial aneurysms: the option for intentional reconstruction of aneurysm neck followed by endovascular coiling. Cerebrovasc Dis. 23(5-6):381-7, 2007
3. Coert BA et al: Surgical and endovascular management of symptomatic posterior circulation fusiform aneurysms. J Neurosurg. 106(5):855-65, 2007
4. Ferroli P et al: Obliteration of a giant fusiform carotid terminus-M1 aneurysm after distal clip application and extracranial-intracranial bypass. Case report. J Neurosurg Sci. 51(2):71-76, 2007
5. Jager HR et al: Contrast-enhanced MR angiography of intracranial giant aneurysms. AJNR Am J Neuroradiol. 21(10):1900-7, 2000
6. Nakatomi H et al: Clinicopathological study of intracranial fusiform and dolichoectatic aneurysms : insight on the mechanism of growth. Stroke. 31(4):896-900, 2000
7. Mizutani T et al: Proposed classification of nonatherosclerotic cerebral fusiform and dissecting aneurysms. Neurosurgery. 45(2):253-9; discussion 259-60, 1999

FUSIFORM ANEURYSM

IMAGE GALLERY

Typical

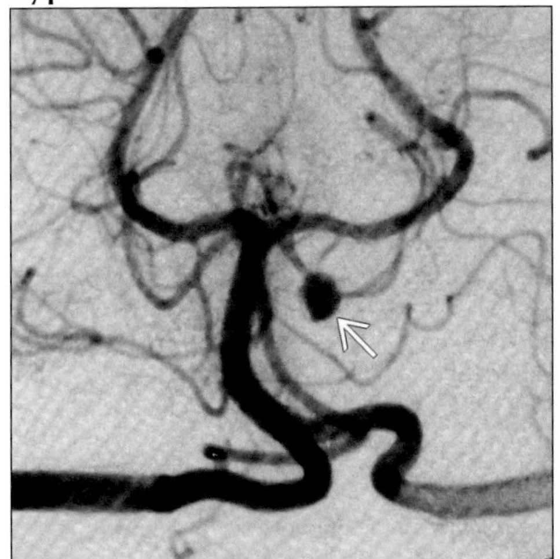

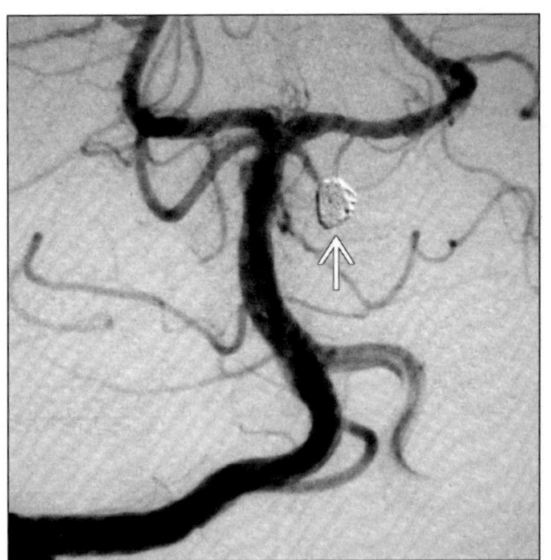

(Left) *Right vertebral artery DSA, Water's projection, in a patient with SAH shows a FA of the left superior cerebellar artery (SCA)* ➔. ***(Right)*** *Right vertebral artery DSA after embolization of the SCA FA using detachable coils and deliberate occlusion of the parent vessel* ➔. *The patient remained neurologically intact afterwards.*

Typical

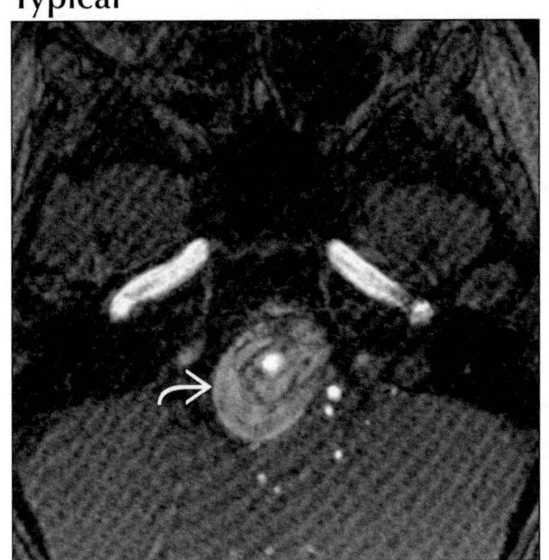

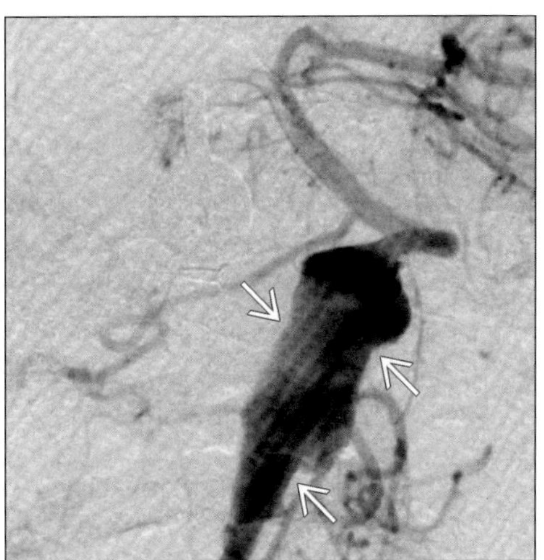

(Left) *Axial 3d-TOF MRA source image shows a large FA of the intracranial segment of the right vertebral artery* ➔. *The aneurysm contains considerable intraluminal ± intramural thrombus which appears as heterogeneous signal surrounding the residual vessel lumen.* ***(Right)*** *Oblique right vertebral artery DSA in the same patient shows irregular contours* ➔ *to the FA lumen due to contained thrombus.*

Typical

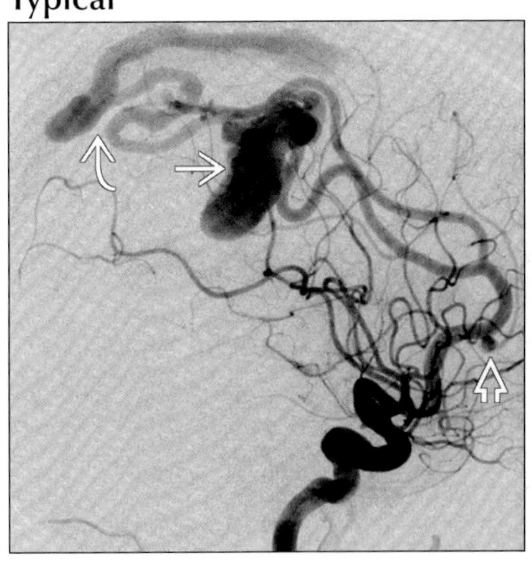

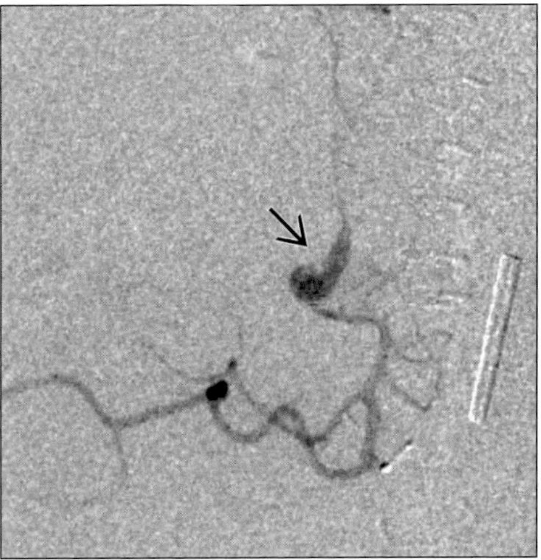

(Left) *Lateral left ICA DSA shows a pial AV fistula with associated large venous FA* ➔ *and associated tortuosity and dilatation of a cortical draining vein* ➔. *Note enlarged pericallosal artery supplying the fistula and associated flow related aneurysm* ➔. ***(Right)*** *Anteroposterior subselective right posterior temporal artery DSA shows a lobulated mycotic FA* ➔. *The aneurysm and parent vessel were subsequently occluded with Onyx™, a liquid embolic.*

POST-OP ANEURYSM

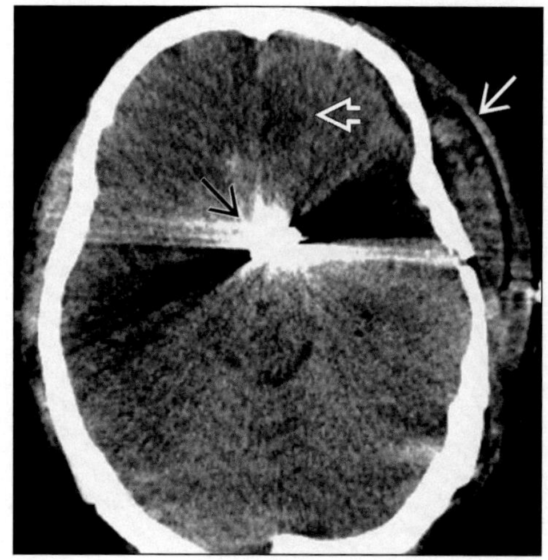

Axial NECT shows metallic star artifact S/P clipping of an ACoA aneurysm ➔. Note scalp soft tissue swelling ➔ and frontal lobe edema ➔.

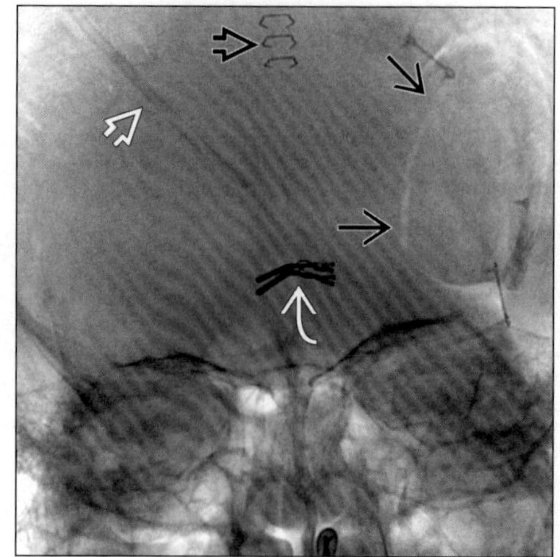

Frontal skull radiograph shows two aneurysm clips ➔, craniotomy defect ➔ and skin staples ➔ from recent craniotomy. A ventriculostomy is in situ ➔.

TERMINOLOGY

Definitions

- Clipped aneurysm: Metallic clip(s) placed via craniotomy across aneurysm neck to exclude aneurysm from circulation
- Coiled aneurysm: Platinum coils placed within aneurysm during endovascular surgery (embolization) to promote intra-aneurysmal thrombosis

IMAGING FINDINGS

General Features

- Best diagnostic clue
  - Clipped aneurysm: Metallic clip adjacent to vessel wall, craniotomy defect, edema (acute) or gliosis (chronic) along operative tract
  - Coiled aneurysm: Coil ball mass within aneurysm, no craniotomy defect
- Location
  - Berry aneurysms
    - Majority of berry aneurysms (> 85%) arise from circle of Willis + major branches
    - Common sites: ACoA (35%) > PCoA (30%) > MCA (20%) > carotid terminus > basilar apex
    - Other sites (5%): Pericallosal artery, PICA, SCA, AChA, AICA
- Size: Number + orientation of surgical clips or number and configuration of coils depends on aneurysm size, shape, geometry
- Morphology
  - Aneurysms: Smooth vs. lobulated, narrow vs. wide-necked, saccular (berry) vs. fusiform
  - Aneurysm clips: Straight, curved, right-angled, encircling
  - Embolization coils: Helical, straight, complex/3-dimensional

Radiographic Findings

- Radiography: Skull X-ray shows configuration of coil ball mass S/P embolization; may be useful for detection of coil compaction

CT Findings

- NECT
  - Used for routine post-op assessment after craniotomy
  - Metallic artifact arising from clip(s) or coils

DDx: Vascular Neurosurgical and Neurointerventional Procedures

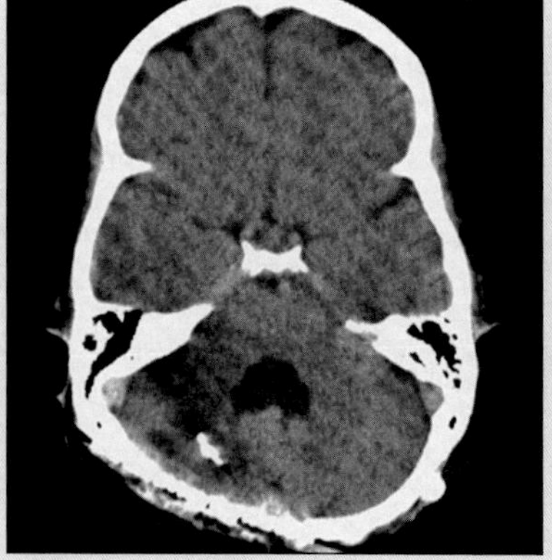

AVM Resection

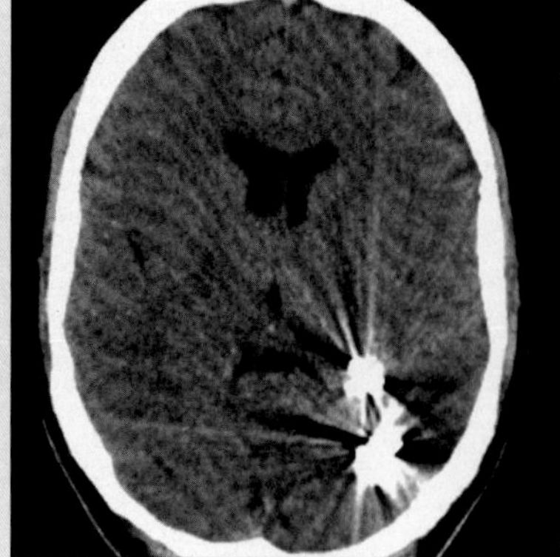

AVM Embolization

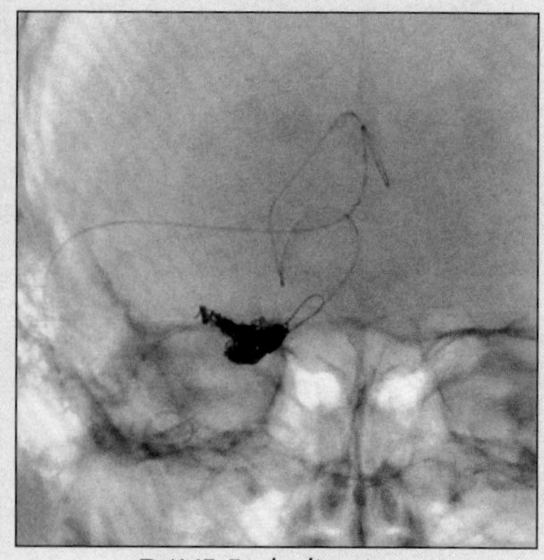

DAVF Embolization

POST-OP ANEURYSM

Key Facts

Terminology

- Clipped aneurysm: Metallic clip(s) placed via craniotomy across aneurysm neck to exclude aneurysm from circulation
- Coiled aneurysm: Platinum coils placed within aneurysm during endovascular surgery (embolization)

Imaging Findings

- Clipped aneurysm
  - Acute: Craniotomy/craniectomy defect, pneumocephalus, extra-axial blood beneath craniotomy flap, brain edema from surgical retraction, subgaleal fluid/hematoma, soft tissue swelling, proptosis, skin staples
  - Chronic: Gliosis along operative tract
- Coiled aneurysm: Coil ball mass within aneurysm, no craniotomy defect
- Potential danger with MR: If clip is ferromagnetic, it may torque in the magnetic field and can separate from the vessel result in SAH/death
- Trans-cranial Doppler
  - Useful for non-invasive monitoring of SAH-vasospasm

Clinical Issues

- SAH: Sudden onset, "worst headache of my life" (thunderclap headache)
- International subarachnoid aneurysm trial (ISAT): Endovascular coiling of ruptured aneurysms associated with greater chance of disability free survival compared with open neurosurgery
- Coil embolization of unruptured aneurysms associated with earlier return to baseline neurological function and employment compared with surgery

---

- Clipped aneurysm
  - Acute: Craniotomy defect, pneumocephalus, extra-axial blood, brain edema from surgical retraction, subgaleal fluid/hematoma
  - Chronic: Gliosis along operative tract
- Procedural complications: Intra-operative rupture → new SAH, edema/surgical retraction injury, infarction due to inadvertent branch vessel occlusion or emboli, extra-axial hematoma
- CTA: Metallic artifact from clips or coils hinders assessment of residual aneurysm and aneurysm recurrence

MR Findings

- MRA
  - Useful for follow-up of coiled aneurysms
  - Source images most helpful and not significantly degraded by susceptibility artifact from adjacent coils
  - Limited value after open surgical clipping due to susceptibility artifacts
- T1WI and T2WI: Metallic artifact arising from clip
  - Ferromagnetic clip → large artifact vs. nonferromagnetic → smaller artifact
- Potential danger with MR: If clip is ferromagnetic, it may torque in the magnetic field and can separate from the vessel result in SAH/death
- Must screen patients with possible ferromagnetic aneurysm clips before MR
  - History of type of aneurysm clip used may not be reliable
  - Important to verify with neurosurgeon directly the type of clip ± confirm with plain film if necessary
  - If clip is nonferromagnetic, MR can be performed safely but there will be local image distortion
- Most platinum embolization coils shown to be MR safe

Echocardiographic Findings

- Trans-cranial Doppler
  - Useful for non-invasive monitoring of SAH-vasospasm
  - Accuracy is operator dependent
  - Transtemporal "bone window" is absent in 10-15% of patients

Angiographic Findings

- Conventional
  - Gold-standard for detection of aneurysm remnant, regrowth, recurrence and de-novo aneurysms at other sites, SAH vasospasm
  - 3D DSA useful for determination of optimal projection for profiling of aneurysm neck/working views for coil embolization
  - Clipped aneurysm
    - Profiling of clip with blades overlapped provides best view of interface between the clip and parent vessel for detection of aneurysm remnant
    - Slow antegrade flow in adjacent vessel(s) ± retrograde flow in collateral vessels may indicate branch vessel occlusion or compromise (e.g., vasospasm, dissection, compression by clip)
  - Coiled aneurysm
    - Follow-up DSA or MRA essential as long-term durability of coiled aneurysms remains unproven
    - Coil compaction: Incidence 10-25% of treated aneurysms leading to aneurysm recurrence; appears as flattening/indentation of coil ball surface adjacent to parent vessel and/or change in configuration of coil ball mass compared with baseline
    - Coil prolapse into parent vessel may result in thrombus formation and distal embolization with branch occlusion(s)
    - "White line sign": Visible interface (thin white line) between parent vessel and coil ball mass indicative of neointimalization (healing) of aneurysm neck

Imaging Recommendations

- Best imaging tool
  - DSA for detection of aneurysm remnant/regrowth and SAH vasospasm
    - Initial follow-up post-clipping or coiling should be with DSA

POST-OP ANEURYSM

  - Subsequent follow-up of completely coiled aneurysms or those with stable remnant may be done with MRA
- NECT for routine post-op assessment S/P craniotomy
- CTA/MRA as first line investigation for work-up of berry aneurysms → determine if suitable for coil embolization vs. surgical clipping
- Protocol advice
  - DSA: Multiple projections preferably using biplane machine to profile aneurysm neck
    - 3D angiography with subtraction of mask + SSD can show aneurysm remnants, recurrences negating need for multiple projections

DIFFERENTIAL DIAGNOSIS

Arteriovenous Malformation (AVM)

- Congenital tangle of abnormal vessels (nidus) without intervening normal brain parenchyma
- AV shunt typically involving multiple feeding arteries and draining veins without intervening capillaries
- Flow-related and intranidal aneurysms ↑ risk of intracranial hemorrhage (ICH)

Dural Arteriovenous Fistula (DAVF)

- AV shunts associated with dural venous sinuses, meninges
- Typically numerous arterial feeders into a single venous pouch or dural sinus

PATHOLOGY

General Features

- General path comments
  - Aneurysm coils cause intra-aneurysmal blood flow stasis resulting in thrombosis
    - Neointimalization ("healing") at the aneurysm neck may be increased with the use of coils coated with a bioactive polymer (e.g., polyglycolic acid) that promotes an intense local inflammatory reaction
  - Regrowth of completely clipped aneurysms is 0.26% annually
  - Regrowth of incompletely clipped aneurysms is approx 1% annually
  - Coil compaction (aneurysm recurrence) occurs in 10-25% pts during follow-up
    - Incidence depends on aneurysm size, aneurysm site and morphology, density of initial coil packing
    - Possibly reduced with use of bioactive coils that induce an inflammatory/healing response at the aneurysm neck
  - De novo aneurysm formation after clipping/coiling of an aneurysm is 0.89% annually
- Aneurysm clip apposes intima and becomes functional wall of vessel

Microscopic Features

- Coiled aneurysm: Coil loops at neck covered by fibrin, fibrocellular matrix; fundus contains organized thrombus
- Bioactive coils: Polyglycolic acid coating on coils incite intense inflammatory response → leukocyte infiltration, collagen formation, smooth muscle cells, mature granulation tissue

CLINICAL ISSUES

Natural History & Prognosis

- Intraprocedural aneurysm rupture occurs in 2-4% during coil embolization although the majority of these will not have lasting clinical sequela
- 1% will have regrowth of the clipped aneurysm or develop new ones
- Aneurysmal SAH: Untreated aneurysms have high-risk of rebleeding (20% in first 2 weeks, 50% in first 6 months) if left untreated

Treatment

- International subarachnoid aneurysm trial (ISAT): Endovascular coiling of ruptured aneurysms associated with greater chance of disability free survival compared with open neurosurgery
- Coil embolization of unruptured aneurysms associated with earlier return to baseline neurological function and employment compared with surgery
- Multidisciplinary approach to aneurysm treatment comprising of interventional neuroradiologist and neurosurgeon optimizes management of aneurysm, sequela of SAH
  - Decide on coiling vs. clipping depending on aneurysm location, morphology, number and patient age, comorbidities

DIAGNOSTIC CHECKLIST

Consider

- 3D DSA for determination of optimal projection for assessment of aneurysm neck/working views for coil embolization
- MRA for long-term follow-up of stable aneurysms S/P coil embolization

Image Interpretation Pearls

- "White-line" sign is indicative of aneurysm neck healing (neointima formation) after coil embolization

SELECTED REFERENCES

1. Molyneux A et al: International Subarachnoid Aneurysm Trial (ISAT) of neurosurgical clipping versus endovascular coiling in 2143 patients with ruptured intracranial aneurysms: A randomized trial. J Stroke Cerebrovasc Dis. 11(6):304-314, 2002
2. Ng P et al: Endovascular treatment of intracranial aneurysms with Guglielmi detachable coils: analysis of midterm angiographic and clinical outcomes. Stroke. 33(1):210-7, 2002
3. Johnston SC et al: Treatment of unruptured cerebral aneurysms in California. Stroke. 32(3):597-605, 2001
4. Johnston SC et al: Endovascular and surgical treatment of unruptured cerebral aneurysms: comparison of risks. Ann Neurol. 48(1):11-9, 2000

POST-OP ANEURYSM

IMAGE GALLERY

Typical

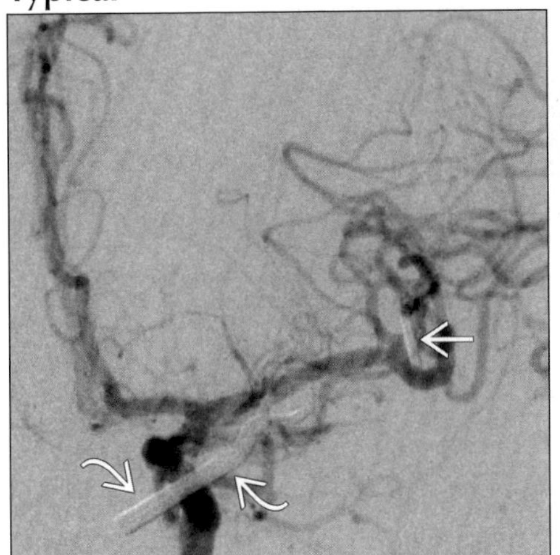

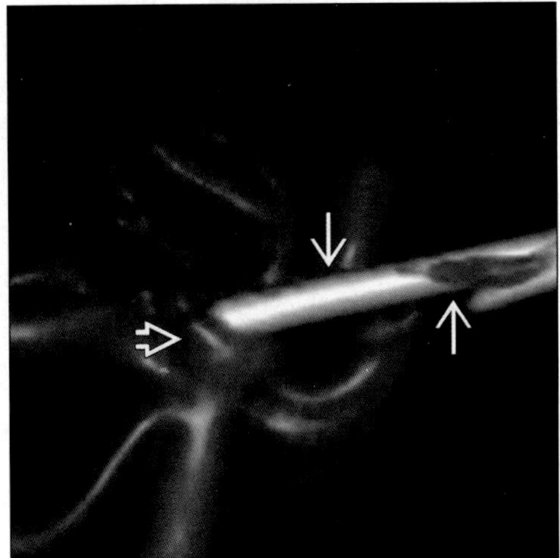

(Left) *Oblique left ICA DSA S/P clipping of an MCA aneurysm shows the outline of a metallic clip ➡ at the MCA bifurcation excluding the aneurysm from the circulation. An additional clip ➡ was placed to treat a basilar apex aneurysm.* ***(Right)*** *Left vertebral artery 3D DSA in the same patient as previous image, shows the a metallic clip ➡ at the basilar apex. A small aneurysm neck remnant is present below the clip ➡.*

Typical

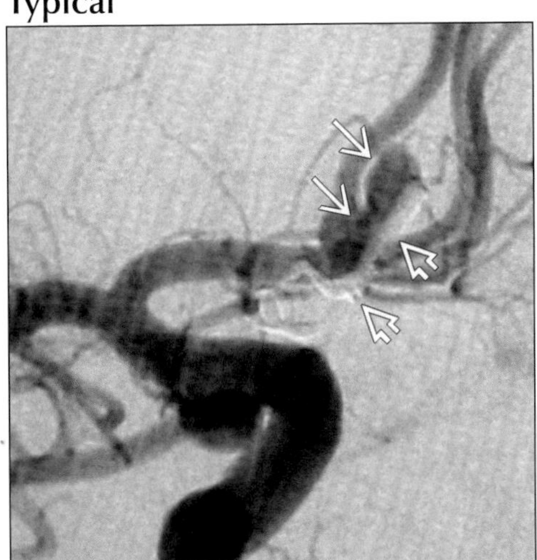

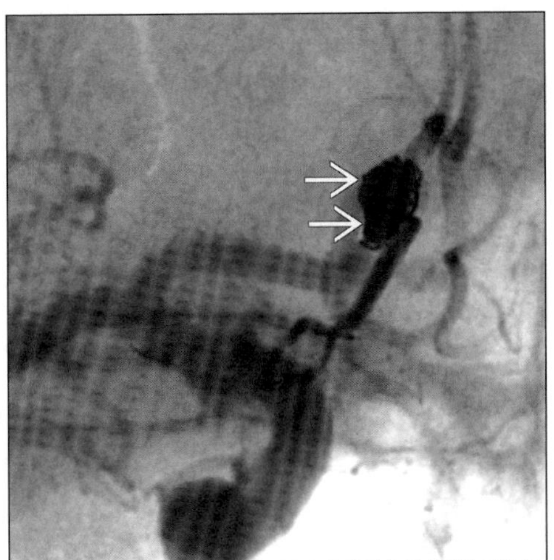

(Left) *Oblique right ICA DSA shows a lightbulb-shaped aneurysm remnant after partial clipping of an ACoA aneurysm ➡. An aneurysm clip is seen adjacent to the medial aspect of the aneurysm neck ➡.* ***(Right)*** *Unsubtracted image in the same projection shows occlusion of the aneurysm remnant after endovascular placement of 4 coils ➡. The patient was discharged home two days after treatment.*

Typical

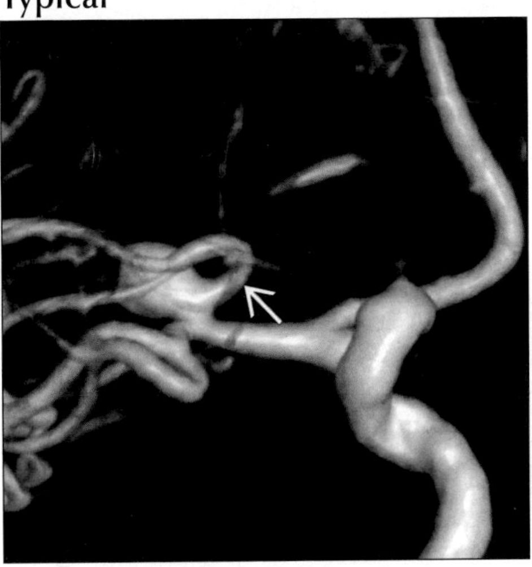

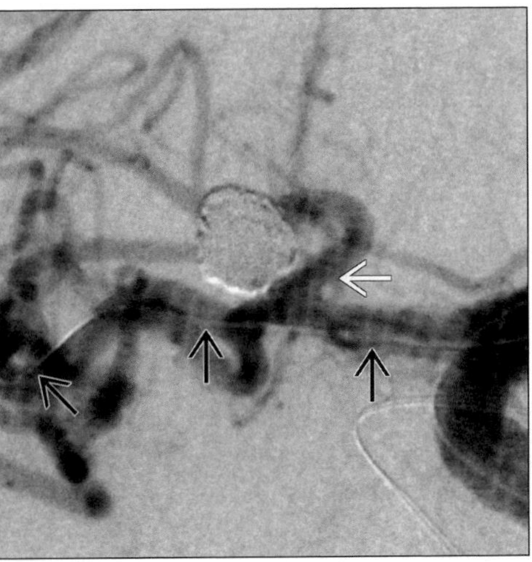

(Left) *3D DSA shows a right MCA bifurcation aneurysm with the superior MCA division incorporated into the aneurysm base ➡.* ***(Right)*** *Right ICA DSA after coil embolization shows complete aneurysm occlusion with preservation of the superior MCA division ➡. Note guidewire used for the balloon remodeling technique ➡. Bioactive coils were utilized as they have been shown to promote aneurysm neck healing in some patients.*

PRIMARY INTRACRANIAL HEMORRHAGE

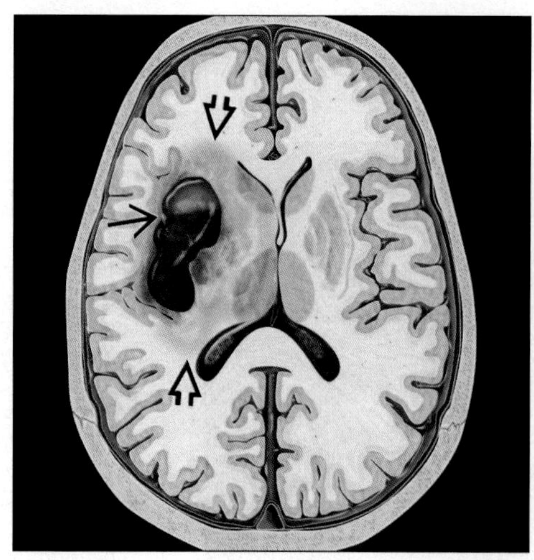

Axial graphic illustrates right external capsule/lentiform nucleus acute hematoma. Heme-fluid level →, peripheral edema ⇨ and mass effect on the right lateral ventricle are present.

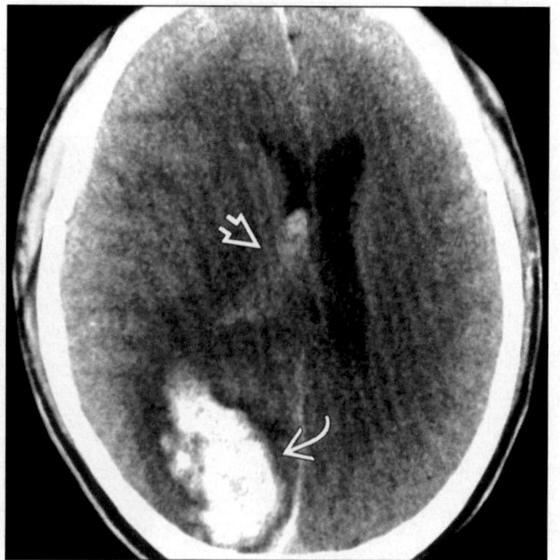

Axial NECT demonstrates a large right parietal hyperdense acute hematoma ➡ extending into the lateral ventricle ⇨. There is vasogenic edema and mass effect. Underlying AVM was found.

TERMINOLOGY

Abbreviations and Synonyms

- Primary intracranial hemorrhage (pICH), intracerebral hematoma (ICH), "stroke"

Definitions

- Acute intracranial hemorrhage of non-traumatic etiology
- Brain parenchymal blood collection secondary to local loss of vascular integrity

IMAGING FINDINGS

General Features

- Best diagnostic clue: Acute ICH without history of trauma
- Location
  - Varies: In general: Supra > infratentorial, solitary > multiple
  - Occurs from cortex to deep gray nuclei
    - Deep (ganglionic) hematoma common in hypertension (HTN)
    - Most spontaneous pontine hemorrhages also caused by HTN
    - Lobar/subcortical hematoma in cerebral amyloid angiopathy (CAA), cerebral vascular malformation (CVM), venous occlusion
- Size: Varies from sub-centimeter ("microbleeds") to multiple centimeters
- Morphology
  - Typically rounded or oval-shaped, fluid-fluid levels possible
  - Two distinct patterns seen with HTN hemorrhage
    - Acute focal hematoma
    - Multiple subacute/chronic "microbleeds"

CT Findings

- NECT
  - Acute (< 3 days): Round/elliptical hyperdense (50-70 HU) parenchymal mass
    - May have mixed isodensity if rapid bleeding, coagulopathy, low hematocrit
    - Peripheral low density (edema)
    - Ganglionic ICH may extend into lateral ventricle resulting in intraventricular hemorrhage (IVH)
  - Subacute (3 days-3 weeks): Isodense mass

DDx: Etiologies of Primary Intracranial Hemorrhage

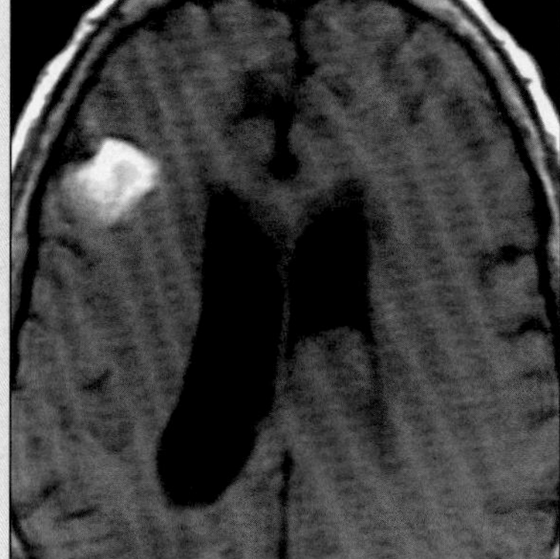

Cerebral Amyloid Angiopathy

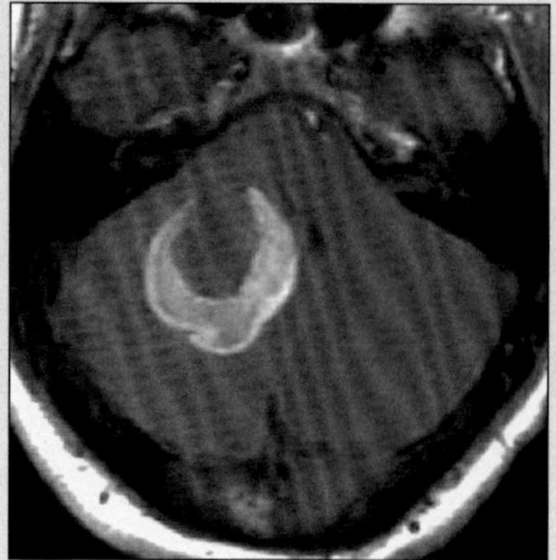

Cavernous Malformation

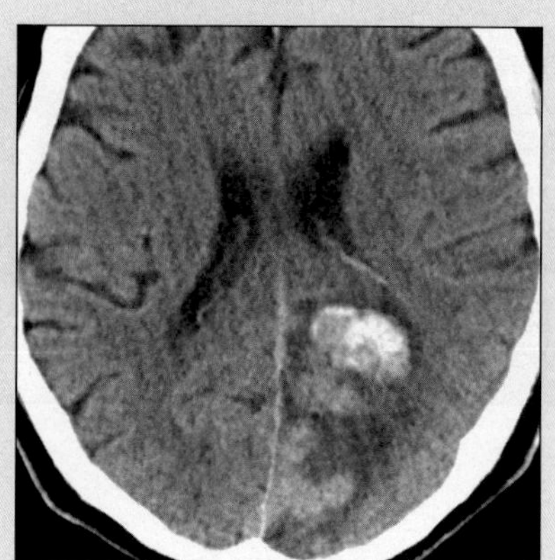

Left PCA Infarction

PRIMARY INTRACRANIAL HEMORRHAGE

Key Facts

Terminology
- Acute intracranial hemorrhage of non-traumatic etiology

Imaging Findings
- Acute (< 3 days): Round/elliptical hyperdense (50-70 HU) parenchymal mass
- If atypical hematoma or unclear history, do MR (GRE, T1 C+, MRA)
- DSA if suspicious for CVM

Top Differential Diagnoses
- Hypertensive Bleed
- Cerebral Amyloid Angiopathy (CAA)
- Vascular Malformation
- Neoplasm
- Ischemic Infarction
- Cortical Vein Thrombosis

Pathology
- May range from petechial "micro" hemorrhages to gross parenchymal hematomas
- Nontraumatic pICH causes 10% of acute "strokes"

Clinical Issues
- Large ICHs usually present with sensorimotor deficits, impaired consciousness
- Recovery poor; most survivors have significant deficits

Diagnostic Checklist
- Gross hemorrhage should prompt search for microbleeds with GRE or SWI (T2*) MR
- Microbleeds may signal a diffuse hemorrhage-prone vasculopathy (HTN, amyloid)

- Chronic (> 3 weeks): Hypodense mass, hyperdense calcifications possible (10%)
- CECT
  - Acute: Active bleeding → contrast pooling (rare)
  - Subacute: Peripheral "ring"-enhancement possible from vascularized capsule
- CTA: Usually normal; may be positive in setting of CVM

MR Findings
- T1WI
  - Hyperacute (< 24 hrs): Center: Oxy-hemoglobin (Hgb): Isointense; periphery: Deoxy-Hgb: Isointense
  - Acute (1-3 days): Deoxy-Hgb: Isointense
  - Early subacute (4-7 days): Intracellular met-Hgb: Hyperintense
  - Late subacute (1-3 weeks): Extracellular met-Hgb: Hyperintense
  - Chronic (> 3 weeks): Center: Extracellular met-Hgb: Hyperintense; periphery: Hemosiderin: Hypointense (proportion of hemosiderin increases over time)
- T2WI
  - Hyperacute: Center: Oxy-Hgb: Iso- to hyperintense; periphery: Deoxy-Hgb: Hypointense
  - Acute: Deoxy-Hgb: Hypointense
  - Early subacute: Intracellular met-Hgb: Hypointense
  - Late subacute: Extracellular met-Hgb: Hyperintense
  - Chronic: Center: Extracellular met-Hgb: Hyperintense; periphery: Hemosiderin: Hypointense (proportion of hemosiderin increases over time)
- T2* GRE: Multifocal hypointense lesions on T2* in setting of HTN and CAA (SWI MR even more sensitive)
- T1 C+
  - Subacute: Peripheral "ring"-enhancement possible
  - May see enhancement if hemorrhage secondary to neoplasm
- MRA
  - Usually normal, possible identification of CVM
  - Note: Intrinsic high T1 signal of met-Hgb may mask underlying lesion with TOF MRA; use PC MRA
- MRV: May show dural sinus thrombosis if hemorrhage from venous occlusion/venous infarct

Nuclear Medicine Findings
- PET: May demonstrate hypermetabolism if neoplastic etiology

Angiographic Findings
- Conventional: May demonstrate CVM (could be missed acutely if thrombosed), vasculitis, aneurysm, neoplasm

Imaging Recommendations
- Best imaging tool
  - NECT scan; if older patient with HTN and typical hematoma, stop
  - If no clear cause of hemorrhage or atypical appearance, consider MR
  - If MR shows co-existing multifocal "black dots," stop
  - If MR shows atypical hematoma, CTA or MRA
  - If CTA/MRA inconclusive, consider DSA
- Protocol advice
  - If atypical hematoma or unclear history, do MR (GRE, T1 C+, MRA)
  - MRV if suspicious for venous infarction
  - DSA if suspicious for CVM

DIFFERENTIAL DIAGNOSIS

Hypertensive Bleed
- More common in elderly, unusual in young patients unless drug abuse (e.g., cocaine)
- Usually ganglionic/external capsule, associated "microbleeds"

Cerebral Amyloid Angiopathy (CAA)
- Occurs in older patients
- May have evidence for previous hemorrhages
- Usually lobar
- Amyloid usually > 70 y, normotensive, demented

Vascular Malformation
- Arteriovenous malformation, cavernous malformation, capillary telangiectasia, developmental venous anomaly

PRIMARY INTRACRANIAL HEMORRHAGE

- Rate of ICH in patients with AVMs of the basal ganglia or thalamus (9.8% per year) much higher than rate in patients with AVMs in other locations
- The risk of incurring a neurological deficit with each hemorrhagic event is high

Neoplasm

- Often has disordered evolution of hemorrhage, foci of contrast-enhancement

Ischemic Infarction

- Hemorrhagic transformation of 15-45% of infarcts
- Delayed onset, 24-48 hours typical

Cortical Vein Thrombosis

- Adjacent dural sinus often (but not always!) thrombosed

Anticoagulation

- Check history
- "Growing" hematoma, fluid-fluid levels common

PATHOLOGY

General Features

- General path comments
  - May range from petechial "micro" hemorrhages to gross parenchymal hematomas
  - May be arterial or venous, cortical or deep, microscopic or gross
- Genetics
  - Matrix metalloproteinases (MMPs) are overexpressed in the presence of some neurological diseases in which blood-brain barrier disruption exists
  - Expression of MMP-9 is raised after acute spontaneous ICH
- Etiology
  - Older patients
    - HTN, CAA, infarction, neoplasm, coagulopathy
  - Younger patients
    - CVM, aneurysm, venous occlusion, vasculitis, drug use
- Epidemiology
  - Incidence: 15 per 100,000
  - Nontraumatic pICH causes 10% of acute "strokes"
  - 90% of patients with recurrent pICH are hypertensive
  - Neoplasm (2-14% of "spontaneous" ICH)

Gross Pathologic & Surgical Features

- Acute ganglionic/lobar hematoma
- May range from petechial hemorrhages to frank parenchymal hematomas

Microscopic Features

- Acute: Blood-filled cavity surrounded by inflammation
- Subacute: Organized clot with vascularized wall
- Chronic: Hemosiderin scar
- Co-existing microangiopathy common in CAA, HTN

Staging, Grading or Classification Criteria

- Clinical ICH score correlates with 30 day mortality
  - Admission GCS, age > 80 y, ICH volume, infratentorial location, presence of IVH

CLINICAL ISSUES

Presentation

- Most common signs/symptoms
  - Headache, vomiting, seizure
  - Large ICHs usually present with sensorimotor deficits, impaired consciousness

Demographics

- Age: May occur anytime from perinatal through adulthood
- Gender: No gender predisposition

Natural History & Prognosis

- Hematoma enlargement common in first 24-48 hrs
  - Risk factors = EtOH, low fibrinogen, coagulopathy, irregularly-shaped hematoma, disturbed consciousness
- Development of edema is known to contribute to poor outcome after ICH
- Mortality 30-55% in first month
- 30% of patients rebleed within 1 year
- Prognosis related to location, size of ICH
- Recovery poor; most survivors have significant deficits

Treatment

- Control of ICP/hydrocephalus, BP, seizures
- Surgical evacuation controversial

DIAGNOSTIC CHECKLIST

Consider

- Underlying etiology for hemorrhage (i.e., CVM, CAA, neoplasm, drug use, etc.)

Image Interpretation Pearls

- Gross hemorrhage should prompt search for microbleeds with GRE or SWI (T2*) MR
- Microbleeds may signal a diffuse hemorrhage-prone vasculopathy (HTN, amyloid)

SELECTED REFERENCES

1. Akter M et al: Detection of hemorrhagic hypointense foci in the brain on susceptibility-weighted imaging clinical and phantom studies. Acad Radiol. 14(9):1011-9, 2007
2. Ruiz-Sandoval JL et al: Grading scale for prediction of outcome in primary intracerebral hemorrhages. Stroke. 38(5):1641-4, 2007
3. Lee SH et al: Silent microbleeds are associated with volume of primary intracerebral hemorrhage. Neurology. 66(3):430-2, 2006
4. Auer RN et al: Primary intracerebral hemorrhage: pathophysiology. Can J Neurol Sci. 32 Suppl 2:S3-12, 2005
5. Abilleira S et al: Matrix metalloproteinase-9 concentration after spontaneous intracerebral hemorrhage. J Neurosurg. 99(1):65-70, 2003
6. Skidmore CT et al: Spontaneous intracerebral hemorrhage: epidemiology, pathophysiology, and medical management. Neurosurg Clin N Am. 13(3):281-8, v, 2002
7. Qureshi AI et al: Spontaneous intracerebral hemorrhage. N Engl J Med. 344(19):1450-60, 2001
8. Atlas SW et al: MR detection of hyperacute parenchymal hemorrhage of the brain. AJNR Am J Neuroradiol. 19(8):1471-7, 1998

IMAGE GALLERY

Typical

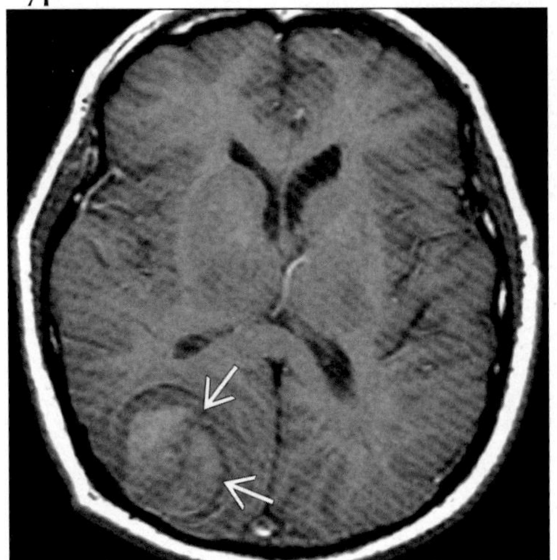

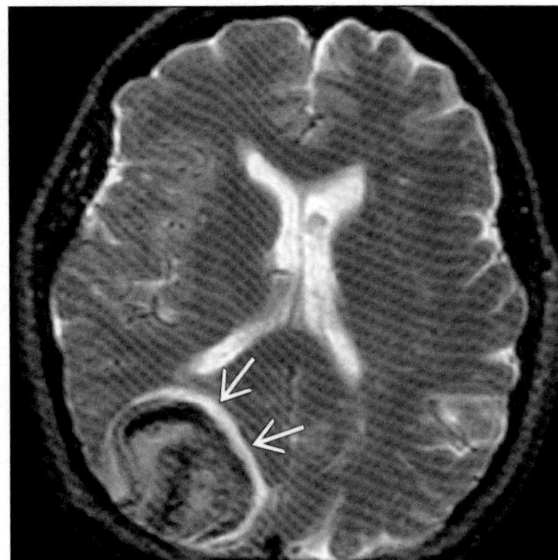

(Left) *Axial T1WI MR shows isointense mass ➡ in the right occipital and posterior temporal lobes from hyperacute primary intracranial hemorrhage.* ***(Right)*** *Axial T2WI MR in the same patient as previous image, shows mostly isointense signal centrally (oxyhemoglobin), hypointense signal peripherally (deoxyhemoglobin) and thin rim of adjacent hyperintense edema ➡.*

Typical

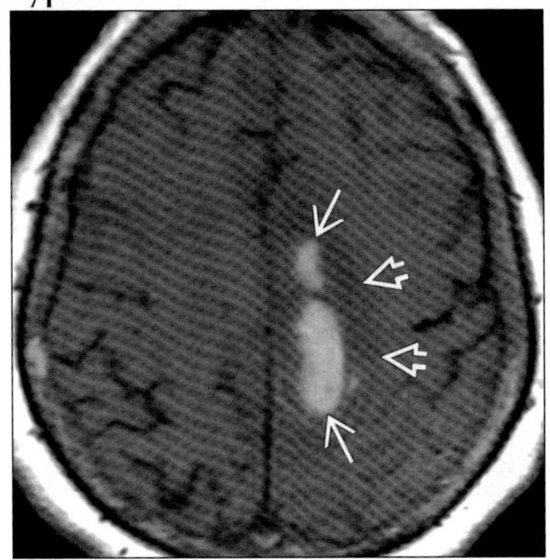

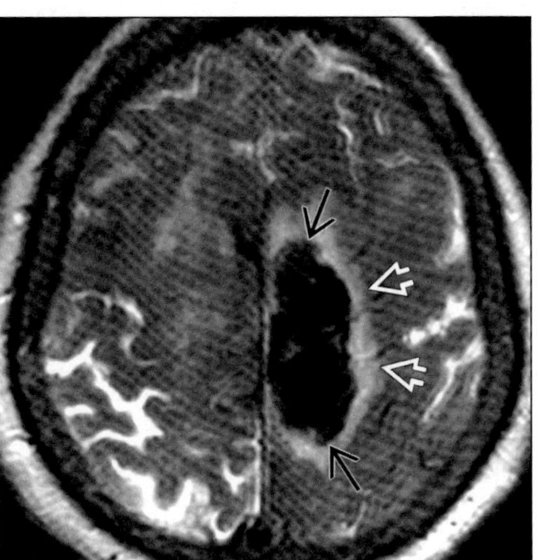

(Left) *Axial T1WI MR demonstrates hyperintense early subacute intracerebral hematoma ➡ with prominent peripheral hypointense edema ➡ in the medial left posterior frontal lobe.* ***(Right)*** *Axial T2WI MR in the same patient as previous image, depicts hypointense signal (intracellular methemoglobin) ➡ with associated surrounding hyperintense edema ➡. Edema is usually maximal at this time.*

Variant

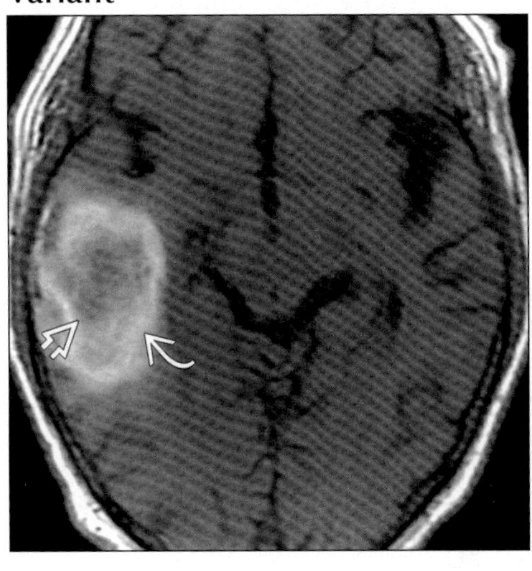

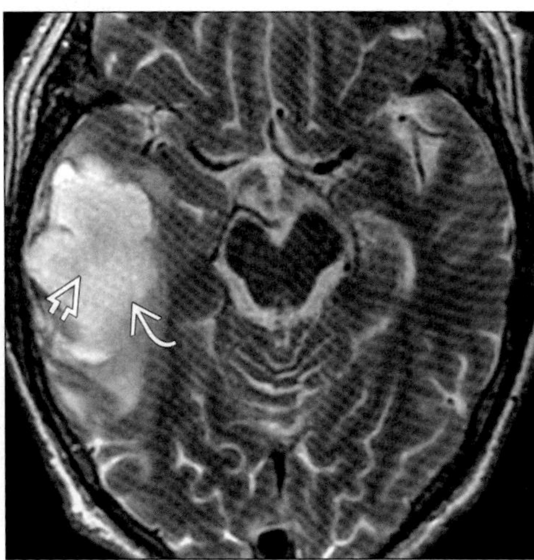

(Left) *Axial T1WI MR shows central isointense ➡ and peripheral hyperintense ➡ signal in the right temporal lobe from hyperacute hemorrhage superimposed on prior chronic intracranial hematoma.* ***(Right)*** *Axial T2WI MR shows isointense to hyperintense signal centrally (oxyhemoglobin) ➡, hyperintense signal peripherally (extracellular methemoglobin) ➡ and hyperintense surrounding edema.*

CEREBRAL AMYLOID ANGIOPATHY

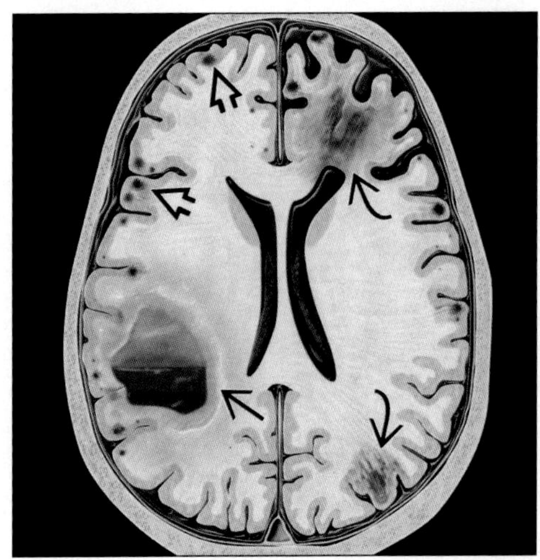

Axial graphic shows findings of cerebral amyloid angiopathy including acute hematoma with fluid level ➔, old lobar hemorrhages ➚ and multiple cortical/subcortical microbleeds ➲.

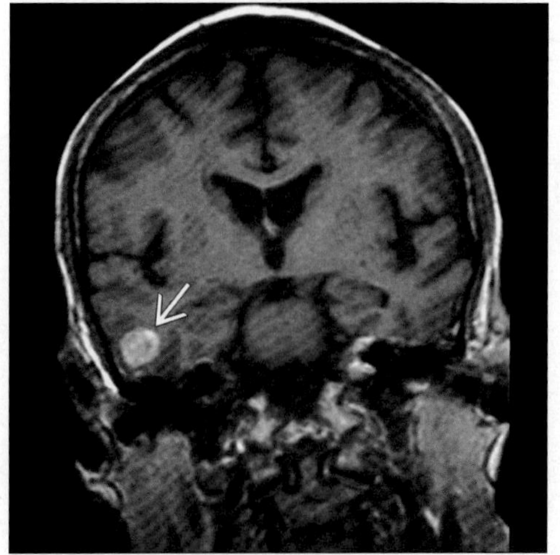

Coronal T1WI MR depicts hyperintense subacute lobar hematoma ➔, the typical location for hemorrhage from cerebral amyloid angiopathy in this non-hypertensive 75 year old man.

TERMINOLOGY

Abbreviations and Synonyms

- Cerebral amyloid angiopathy (CAA) = "congophilic angiopathy", also cerebral amyloidosis

Definitions

- Cerebral amyloid deposition occurs in 3 morphologic varieties
  - CAA (common)
  - Amyloidoma (rare)
  - Diffuse (encephalopathic) white matter (WM) involvement (rare)
- CAA is common cause of "spontaneous" lobar primary intracerebral hemorrhage (pICH) in elderly

IMAGING FINDINGS

General Features

- Best diagnostic clue
  - Normotensive demented patient with
    - Lobar hemorrhage(s) of different ages
    - Multifocal "black dots" (T2* GRE > T2 FSE), corresponding to chronic microbleeds (MB), particularly when subcortical
- Location
  - Subcortical WM (gray/white junction)
  - Parietal + occipital lobes most common at autopsy; also frontal + temporal on imaging
  - Less common in brainstem, deep gray nuclei, cerebellum, hippocampus
- Size
  - Acute lobar hemorrhage tends to be large
  - Punctate foci of hypointensity on T2*/susceptibility sequences (blooming) seen with chronic MB, but not specific for CAA
- Morphology: Acute hematomas are large, often irregular, with dependent blood sedimentation

CT Findings

- NECT
  - Patchy or confluent cortical/subcortical hematoma with irregular borders; surrounding edema (acute)
  - Hemorrhage may extend to subarachnoid space or into ventricles
  - Rare: Gyriform Ca++

DDx: Cerebral Amyloid Angiopathy

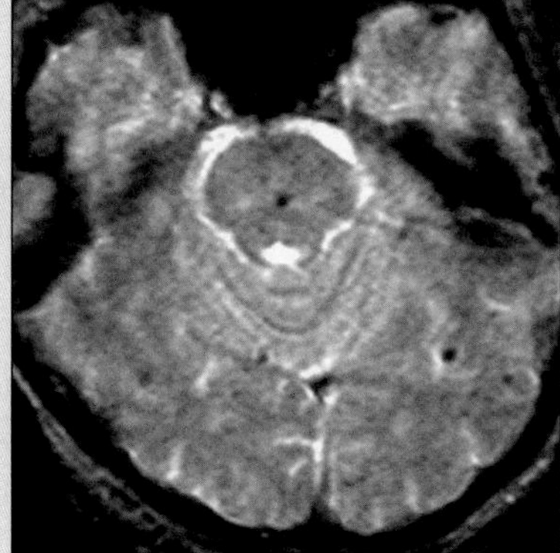

Hypertensive Microbleeds

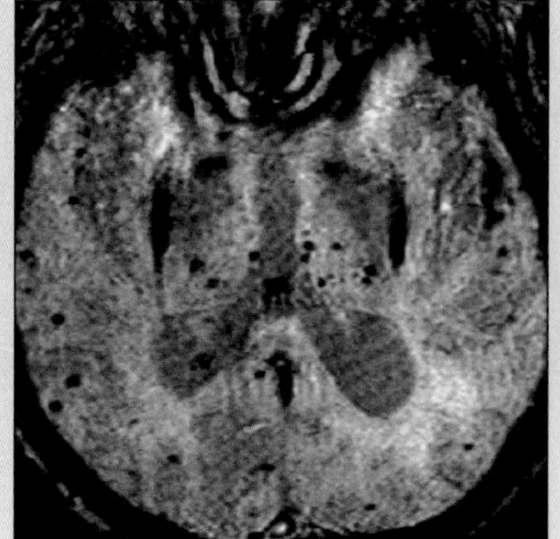

Cavernous Malformations

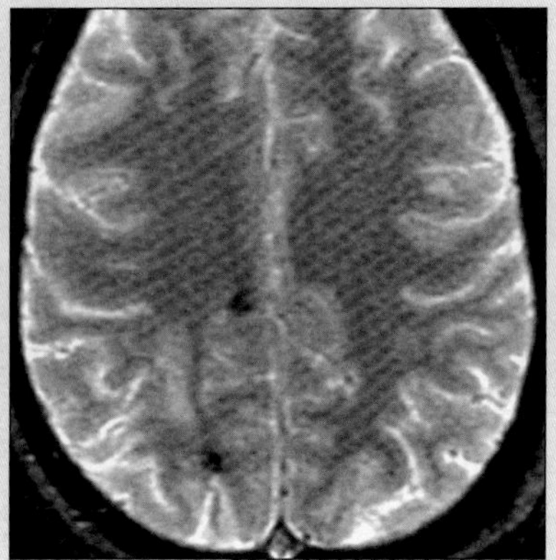

Diffuse Axonal Injury

CEREBRAL AMYLOID ANGIOPATHY

Key Facts

Terminology

- Cerebral amyloid angiopathy (CAA) = "congophilic angiopathy", also cerebral amyloidosis
- CAA is common cause of "spontaneous" lobar primary intracerebral hemorrhage (pICH) in elderly

Imaging Findings

- Lobar hemorrhage(s) of different ages
- Multifocal "black dots" (T2* GRE > T2 FSE), corresponding to chronic microbleeds (MB), particularly when subcortical
- Subcortical WM (gray/white junction)
- Less common in brainstem, deep gray nuclei, cerebellum, hippocampus
- Focal or patchy/confluent WM disease associated in nearly 70%
- Protocol advice: Include T2* weighted sequence in all patients > 60 y

Top Differential Diagnoses

- Hypertensive Microhemorrhages
- Ischemic Stroke with Microhemorrhage
- Multiple Vascular Malformations
- Other Causes of Multifocal "Black Dots"

Pathology

- APOE4 allele associated with CAA-related hemorrhage
- Amyloidosis = infrequent systemic disease caused by extracellular deposition of β-amyloid
- 1% of all strokes
- Causes up to 15-20% of pICH in patients > 60 y
- 27-32% of normal elderly (autopsy)
- 82-88% in patients with Alzheimer disease (AD)

  - Generalized atrophy common
- CECT: No enhancement, unless amyloidoma (rare)

MR Findings

- T1WI: Lobar hematoma (signal varies with age of clot)
- T2WI
  - Acute hematoma iso/hypointense
    - 1/3 also have old hemorrhages (lobar, petechial) seen as multifocal punctate "black dots"
  - Focal or patchy/confluent WM disease associated in nearly 70%
  - Rare form: Nonhemorrhagic diffuse encephalopathy: Confluent WM hyperintensities
  - MB: Small foci of dark T2 variably present; T2* much more sensitive
- T2* GRE
  - Multifocal "black dots" (T2* best type of sequence to detect chronic MB)
  - Susceptibility-weighted imaging (SWI): T2* sequence, even more sensitive to detect chronic MB than typical GRE
- T1 C+
  - CAA, lobar hemorrhages usually don't enhance
  - Amyloidoma (focal, nonhemorrhagic mass/masses)
    - Mass effect generally minimal/mild
    - May show moderate/striking enhancement, mimic neoplasm
    - Often extends medially to lateral ventricular wall with fine radial enhancing margins
    - Rare: Patchy, infiltrating

Angiographic Findings

- Conventional: Normal or avascular mass effect

Imaging Recommendations

- Best imaging tool
  - NECT = best initial screening study (for acute hemorrhage)
  - MR with T2* for non-acute evaluation (dementia)
- Protocol advice: Include T2* weighted sequence in all patients > 60 y

DIFFERENTIAL DIAGNOSIS

Hypertensive Microhemorrhages

- Deep structures (basal ganglia, thalami, cerebellum) > cortex, subcortical WM
- Often coexists with CAA
- Younger patients than CAA (< 65 y)

Ischemic Stroke with Microhemorrhage

- Multifocal hemosiderin deposits
  - Found in 10-15% of patients with ischemic strokes
- Hemorrhagic lacunar infarcts

Multiple Vascular Malformations

- Cavernous malformations
  - "Locules" of blood with fluid-fluid levels
  - Brain common, spinal cord rare
  - Type IV seen as multifocal "black dots"
    - Can occur following radiation therapy
- Capillary telangiectasias
  - Show faint, "brush-like" enhancement
  - Can occur anywhere but brainstem > lobar location

Other Causes of Multifocal "Black Dots"

- Traumatic diffuse axonal injury
  - History of trauma
  - Location in corpus callosum, subcortical/deep white matter, brainstem
- Hemorrhagic metastases
  - Location similar to CAA (gray-white junction)
  - Variable enhancement, edema
- CADASIL
  - Usually nonhemorrhagic
  - Young to middle-aged adults affected
  - Most common site = cortical-subcortical (up to 27% in thalami/brainstem)

PATHOLOGY

General Features

- Genetics
  - Sporadic

CEREBRAL AMYLOID ANGIOPATHY

    - APOE4 allele associated with CAA-related hemorrhage
    - Polymorphisms in presenilin-1 gene
  - Hereditary cerebral hemorrhage with amyloidosis
    - Autosomal dominant inheritance
    - Dutch type = mutated amyloid β precursor protein on chromosome 21, produces aberrant Abeta species and causes severe meningocortical vascular Abeta deposition
    - Other types include British, Flemish, etc.
- Etiology
  - Amyloidosis = infrequent systemic disease caused by extracellular deposition of β-amyloid
  - 10-20% localized form, including CNS
  - Can be idiopathic/primary
  - Can be reactive/secondary (e.g., dialysis-related amyloidosis)
- Epidemiology
  - 1% of all strokes
  - Causes up to 15-20% of pICH in patients > 60 y
  - Frequency of CAA in elderly
    - 27-32% of normal elderly (autopsy)
    - 82-88% in patients with Alzheimer disease (AD)
    - Common in Down syndrome
  - Other associations: Kuru, CJD, plasmacytoma

Gross Pathologic & Surgical Features

- Lobar hemorrhage(s)
- Multiple small cortical hemorrhages

Microscopic Features

- Interstitial, vascular/perivascular deposits of amorphous protein
  - Shows apple-green birefringence when stained with Congo red, viewed under polarized light
  - 3 components
    - Fibrillar protein component (varies, defines amyloidosis type)
    - Serum amyloid P
    - Charged glycosaminoglycans (ubiquitous)
- Microaneurysms
- Fibrinoid necrosis
- Hyaline thickening
- 15% have CAA-related perivascular inflammation

Staging, Grading or Classification Criteria

- WHO classification of amyloidoses
  - Primary systemic amyloidosis
  - Secondary amyloidosis
  - Hereditary systemic amyloidosis
  - Hemodialysis-related systemic amyloidosis
  - Medullary thyroid carcinoma
  - Type II diabetes

CLINICAL ISSUES

Presentation

- Most common signs/symptoms
  - Acute: Stroke-like clinical presentation with "spontaneous" lobar ICH
    - Incidence of CAA in such patients = 4-10%
  - Chronic: Dementia (CAA)
- Clinical Profile
  - CAA common in demented elderly patient
    - 2/3 normotensive; 1/3 HTN
    - 40% with subacute dementia/overt AD (overlap common)

Demographics

- Age
  - Usually older when sporadic (> 60 y)
  - Inflammatory CAA younger
- Gender: No gender predilection

Natural History & Prognosis

- Multiple, recurrent hemorrhages
- Progressive cognitive decline

Treatment

- Evacuate focal hematoma if patient < 75 y, no intraventricular hemorrhage, not parietal
- Consider immunosuppressive therapy in inflammatory CAA
- Adverse prognostic factors: Low Glasgow coma scale scores, APOE4 allele

DIAGNOSTIC CHECKLIST

Consider

- Susceptibility-weighted imaging (T2*) in all elderly

SELECTED REFERENCES

1. Haacke EM et al: Imaging cerebral amyloid angiopathy with susceptibility-weighted imaging. AJNR Am J Neuroradiol. 28(2):316-7, 2007
2. Herzig MC et al: BACE1 and mutated presenilin-1 differently modulate Abeta40 and Abeta42 levels and cerebral amyloidosis in APPDutch transgenic mice. Neurodegener Dis. 4(2-3):127-35, 2007
3. Lee SH et al: Cortico-subcortical distribution of microbleeds is different between hypertension and cerebral amyloid angiopathy. J Neurol Sci. 258(1-2):111-4, 2007
4. Maia LF et al: Clinical phenotypes of Cerebral Amyloid Angiopathy. J Neurol Sci. 257(1-2):23-30, 2007
5. Chao CP et al: Cerebral amyloid angiopathy: CT and MR imaging findings. Radiographics. 26(5):1517-31, 2006
6. Chen YW et al: Progression of white matter lesions and hemorrhages in cerebral amyloid angiopathy. Neurology. 67(1):83-7, 2006
7. Soffer D: Cerebral amyloid angiopathy--a disease or age-related condition. Isr Med Assoc J. 8(11):803-6, 2006
8. Wilcock DM et al: Quantification of cerebral amyloid angiopathy and parenchymal amyloid plaques with Congo red histochemical stain. Nat Protoc. 1(3):1591-5, 2006
9. Maat-Schieman M et al: Hereditary cerebral hemorrhage with amyloidosis-Dutch type. Neuropathology. 25(4):288-97, 2005
10. Miao J et al: Cerebral microvascular amyloid beta protein deposition induces vascular degeneration and neuroinflammation in transgenic mice expressing human vasculotropic mutant amyloid beta precursor protein. Am J Pathol. 167(2):505-15, 2005
11. Tanskanen M et al: Cerebral amyloid angiopathy in a 95+ cohort: complement activation and apolipoprotein E (ApoE) genotype. Neuropathol Appl Neurobiol. 31(6):589-99, 2005
12. Gandhi D et al: CT and MR imaging of intracerebral amyloidoma. AJNR Am J Neuroradiol. 24:519-22, 2003

CEREBRAL AMYLOID ANGIOPATHY

IMAGE GALLERY

Typical

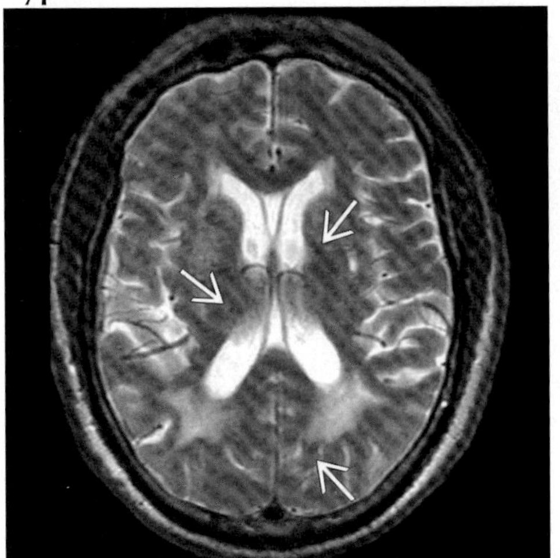

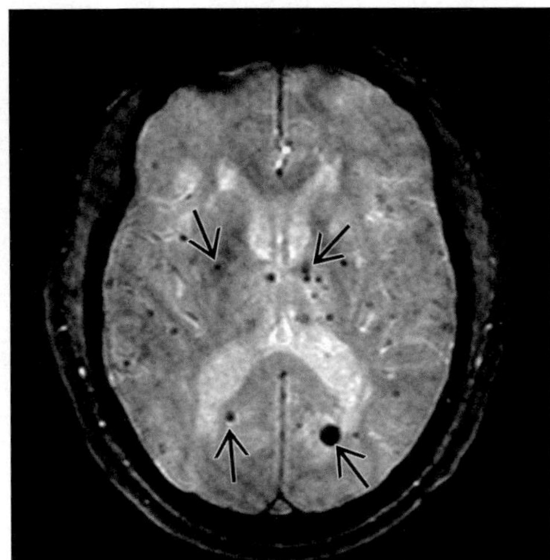

(Left) *Axial T2WI MR shows hyperintensity in the deep white matter but only a few foci of low signal intensity ➔, since fast spin echo images are insensitive to magnetic susceptibility effects.* ***(Right)*** *Axial T2* MR image in the same patient as previous image, more clearly depicts multiple hypointense foci from chronic microbleeds ➔ in this patient with cerebral amyloid angiopathy. (Courtesy M. Haacke, PhD).*

Typical

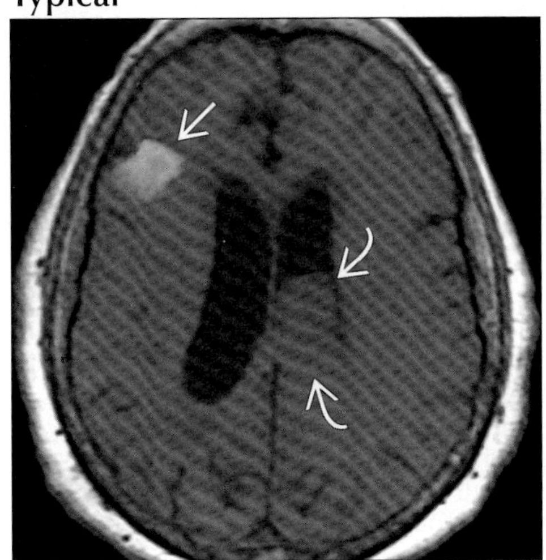

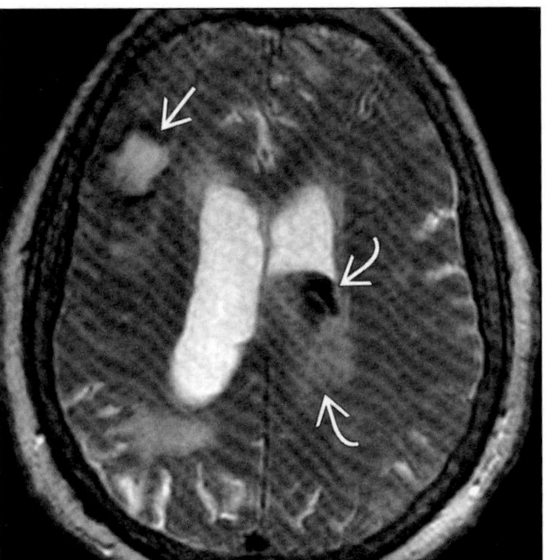

(Left) *Axial T1WI MR shows chronic lobar hemorrhage in the right frontal lobe ➔ from cerebral amyloid angiopathy as well as a focus of isointense signal superior to left lateral ventricle ➔.* ***(Right)*** *Axial T2WI MR in the same patient as previous image, shows the chronic hemorrhage ➔ but also depicts iso/hypointense signal ➔ in the left-sided lesion confirming additional focus of acute hemorrhage.*

Typical

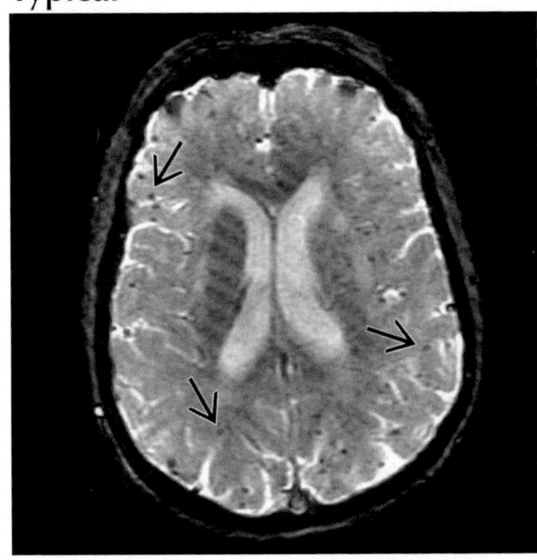

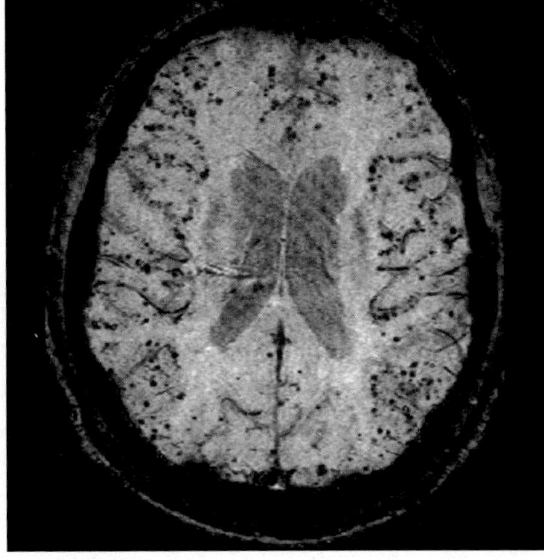

(Left) *Axial T2* MR GRE image shows multiple punctate primarily cortical/subcortical black dots ➔ from chronic microbleeds, the classic location and appearance of cerebral amyloid angiopathy.* ***(Right)*** *Axial T2* MR SWI in a different patient more easily depicts multiple black dots from chronic microbleeds due to extreme sensitivity to the susceptibility effects. (Courtesy M. Haacke, PhD).*

HYPERTENSIVE HEMORRHAGE

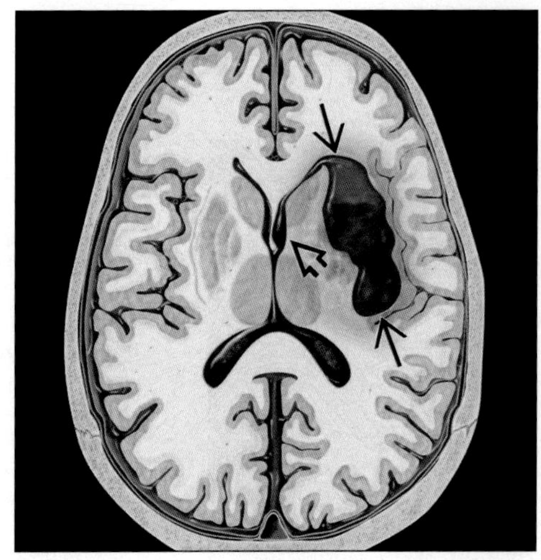

Axial graphic shows acute hypertensive hemorrhage ➔ centered in the left lentiform nucleus and subinsular region with extension into the left lateral ventricle ➪ and third ventricle.

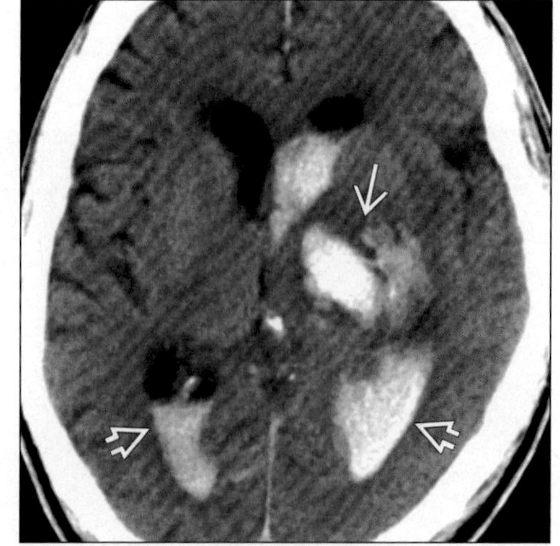

Axial NECT shows left lentiform/thalamic nucleus acute hypertensive hemorrhage ➔ with surrounding mild edema. There is intraventricular hemorrhage ➪ as well resulting in hydrocephalus.

TERMINOLOGY

Abbreviations and Synonyms

- Hypertensive intracranial hemorrhage (hICH)
- "Stroke" (common lay term for sudden onset of neurologic deficit)

Definitions

- Acute nontraumatic ICH secondary to systemic hypertension (HTN)

IMAGING FINDINGS

General Features

- Best diagnostic clue
  - Round/elliptical high density mass centered in basal ganglia/external capsule
  - Most characteristic sign = putamen/external capsule hematoma in patient with HTN
- Location
  - Striatocapsular (putamen/external capsule) 60-65%
  - Thalamus 15-25%
  - Pons, cerebellum 10%
  - Lobar 5-15%
  - Multifocal "microbleeds"
- Size: Varies from sub-centimeter ("microbleeds") to multiple centimeters
- Morphology
  - Typically rounded or oval-shaped
  - Two distinct patterns seen with hICH
    - Acute focal hematoma
    - Multiple subacute/chronic "microbleeds"

CT Findings

- NECT
  - Elliptical high density parenchymal mass
  - Most common = between putamen, insular cortex
  - Other sites = thalamus, brainstem, cerebellum
  - Acute ICH usually hyperdense
  - Mixed density if coagulopathy, active bleeding
  - Other: Intraventricular hemorrhage (IVH), hydrocephalus, herniation
- CECT
  - Usually no enhancement in acute hICH
    - Contrast extravasation = active hemorrhage
  - Hematoma may develop "rim"-enhancement in subacute stage

DDx: Hypertensive Hemorrhage

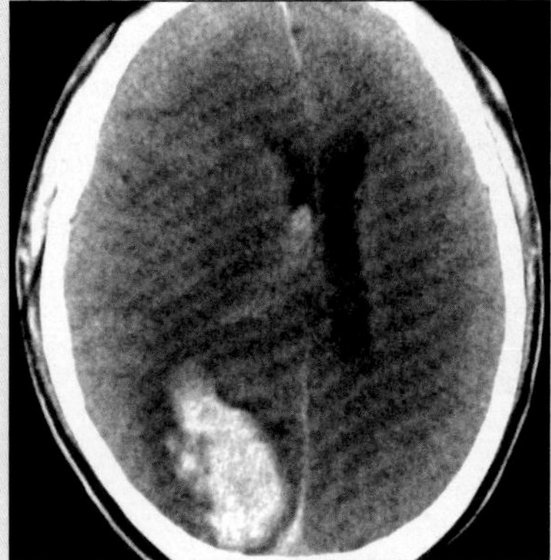

Arteriovenous Malformation

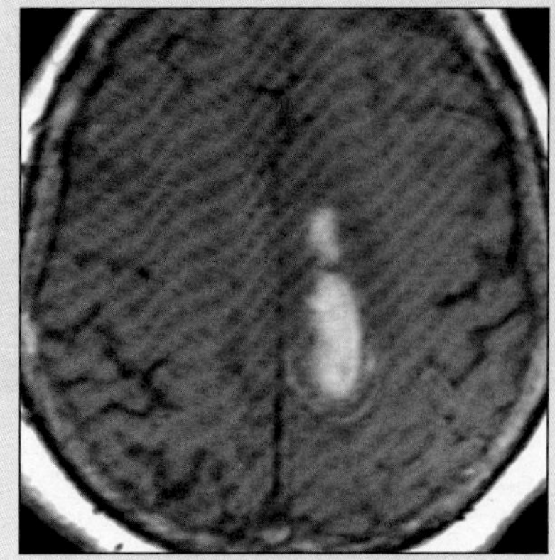

Cerebral Amyloid Angiopathy

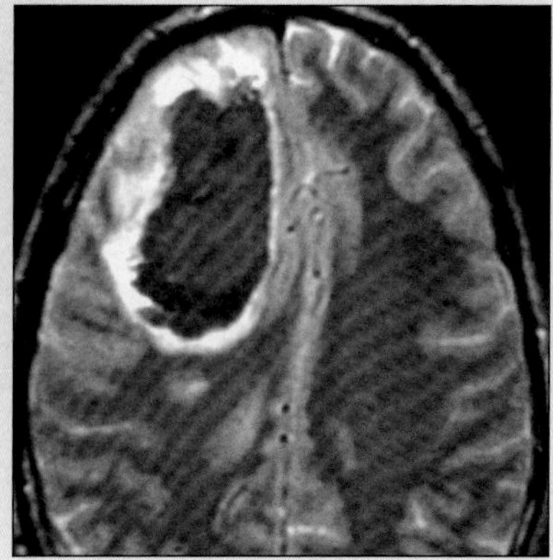

Moyamoya

HYPERTENSIVE HEMORRHAGE

Key Facts

Terminology
- Acute nontraumatic ICH secondary to systemic hypertension (HTN)

Imaging Findings
- Round/elliptical high density mass centered in basal ganglia/external capsule
- Striatocapsular (putamen/external capsule) 60-65%
- Thalamus 15-25%
- Pons, cerebellum 10%
- Lobar 5-15%
- Multifocal hypointense lesions ("black dots") on T2*
- Contrast extravasation = active hemorrhage

Top Differential Diagnoses
- Vascular Malformation, Aneurysm
- Amyloid Angiopathy
- Hemorrhagic Neoplasm

Pathology
- Striatocapsular hematoma is most common autopsy finding in patients with hICH
- 50% of primary nontraumatic ICHs caused by hypertensive hemorrhage
- HTN most common cause of spontaneous ICH between 45-70 years
- 5% of all cases of "stroke"; associated with highest mortality rate

Clinical Issues
- Large ICHs present with sensorimotor deficits, impaired consciousness
- 80% mortality in massive ICH with IVH
- Evacuation may improve outcome in some cases

MR Findings
- T1WI
  - Varies with age of clot
    - Hyperacute hematoma (< 24 hrs): Oxy-hemoglobin (Hgb) (isointense); note: Deoxy-Hgb (isointense) rim usually develops immediately from loss of oxygen to adjacent metabolically active brain parenchyma
    - Acute hematoma (1-3 days): Deoxy-Hgb (isointense)
    - Early subacute hematoma (4-7 days): Intracellular met-Hgb (hyperintense)
    - Late subacute hematoma (1-3 weeks): Extracellular met-Hgb (hyperintense)
    - Chronic hematoma (> 3 weeks): Extracellular met-Hgb (hyperintense) may persist indefinitely
    - Remote hematoma (months-years): Hemosiderin scar (hypointense) ± central CSF-filled cavity (hypointense) and peripheral gliosis (hypointense) more common final appearance
- T2WI
  - Varies with age of clot
    - Hyperacute hematoma (< 24 hrs): Oxy-Hgb (iso-/hyperintense); Deoxy-Hgb (hypointense) rim
    - Acute hematoma (1-3 days): Deoxy-Hgb (hypointense)
    - Early subacute hematoma (4-7 days): Intracellular met-Hgb (hypointense)
    - Late subacute hematoma (1-3 weeks): Extracellular met-Hgb (hyperintense)
    - Chronic hematoma (> 3 weeks): Extracellular met-Hgb (hyperintense) may persist indefinitely
    - Remote hematoma (months-years): Hemosiderin scar (hypointense) ± central CSF-filled cavity (hyperintense) and peripheral gliosis (hyperintense) more common final appearance
- T2* GRE
  - Multifocal hypointense lesions ("black dots") on T2*
  - Common with longstanding HTN
- DWI: Usually normal; may see restricted diffusion if hematoma results in acute ischemic infarction
- T1 C+
  - Typically no enhancement in acute hICH
    - Contrast extravasation = active hemorrhage
  - Hematoma may develop "rim"-enhancement in subacute stage
- MRA: Negative

Angiographic Findings
- Conventional
  - DSA almost always normal if HTN + deep ganglionic hemorrhage
  - May show avascular mass effect
  - Rare: "Bleeding globe" microaneurysm on lenticulostriate artery (LSA)

Imaging Recommendations
- Best imaging tool
  - If older patient with HTN and high suspicion for hICH, NECT
  - If hyperacute ischemic "stroke" suspected, MR
    - If MR shows classic hICH + co-existing multifocal "black dots," stop
  - If MR shows atypical hematoma, MRA or CTA
  - If MRA/CTA inconclusive, consider DSA
- Protocol advice: MR (include T2* GRE, DWI, ± MRA; T1 C+ optional)

DIFFERENTIAL DIAGNOSIS

Nonhypertensive Basal Ganglionic Hemorrhage
- Vascular malformation, aneurysm (younger patients)
- Hemorrhagic neoplasm (often mixed signal, enhancing)

Nonhypertensive Lobar Hemorrhage
- Amyloid angiopathy (elderly, demented, normotensive; rarely involves deep subcortical nuclei)
- Ruptured AVM or dAVFs (younger patients with enlarged vessels, early draining veins on angiography)
- Cortical vein thrombosis (co-existing dural sinus thrombosis often, but not always, present)
- Hemorrhagic neoplasm (primary or secondary)

HYPERTENSIVE HEMORRHAGE

- Other: Coagulopathy, trauma, hemorrhagic infarct, septic emboli, vasculitis, moyamoya, drug abuse

Multifocal "Black Dots" (Microbleeds)

- Cerebral amyloid angiopathy (CAA)
- Multiple cavernous/capillary malformations
- Hemorrhagic diffuse axonal injury
- Hemorrhagic metastases (rare)

PATHOLOGY

General Features

- General path comments
  - Striatocapsular hematoma is most common autopsy finding in patients with hICH
  - Diffuse "microbleeds" also common
- Etiology
  - Chronic HTN with atherosclerosis, fibrinoid necrosis, abrupt vessel wall rupture ± pseudoaneurysm formation
  - Charcot-Bouchard, "bleeding globe" microaneurysms (LSA, thalamoperforators, pontine perforators)
- Epidemiology
  - 50% of primary nontraumatic ICHs caused by hypertensive hemorrhage
  - HTN most common cause of spontaneous ICH between 45-70 years
  - 5% of all cases of "stroke"; associated with highest mortality rate
  - Of note: 10-15% of hypertensive patients with primary ICH have underlying aneurysm or AVM

Gross Pathologic & Surgical Features

- Large ganglionic hematoma ± IVH
- Subfalcine herniation, hydrocephalus common
- Co-existing small chronic hemorrhages, ischemic lesions common

Microscopic Features

- Fibrous balls (fibrosed miliary aneurysm)
- Severe arteriosclerosis with vessel hyalinization, smooth muscle layer hyperplasia, pseudoaneurysm formation (lacks media/internal elastic lamina)

CLINICAL ISSUES

Presentation

- Most common signs/symptoms
  - Large ICHs present with sensorimotor deficits, impaired consciousness
  - Seasonal, diurnal blood pressure variations cause higher incidence of ICH in colder months
- Clinical Profile: Most common in hypertensive, elderly African-American males

Demographics

- Age
  - Most common in older age group
  - May occur in younger age group (renovascular disease, pheochromocytoma, drugs, etc.)
- Gender: M > F
- Ethnicity: African-American > Caucasian

Natural History & Prognosis

- Bleeding can persist for up to 6 hr following ictus
- Neurologic deterioration common within 48 hr
  - Increasing hematoma
  - Edema
  - Development of hydrocephalus
  - Herniation syndromes
- Recurrent hICH in 5-10% of cases, usually different location
- Prognosis related to location, size of ICH
- 80% mortality in massive ICH with IVH
- Only one-third of patients with hICH survive first year
- One-third of survivors are severely disabled

Treatment

- Evacuation may improve outcome in some cases
- Control of ICP and hydrocephalus

DIAGNOSTIC CHECKLIST

Consider

- Does the patient have a history of poorly-controlled systemic HTN?
- Could there be an underlying coagulopathy, hemorrhagic neoplasm or vascular malformation?
- Check for history of substance abuse in young patients with unexplained hICH

Image Interpretation Pearls

- Underlying cause of lobar ICH is often difficult to determine
- Subarachnoid extension of lobar ICH on CT strongly indicates a non-hypertensive cause, more specifically it suggests hematoma caused by vascular abnormalities
- Definite diagnosis of CAA vs. HTN-related hemorrhage requires histopathological confirmation and should not be based solely on hemorrhage pattern

SELECTED REFERENCES

1. Ruiz-Sandoval JL et al: Hypertensive intracerebral hemorrhage in young people: previously unnoticed age-related clinical differences. Stroke. 37(12):2946-50, 2006
2. Fei Z et al: Secondary insults and outcomes in patients with hypertensive basal ganglia hemorrhage. Acta Neurochir Suppl. 95:265-7, 2005
3. Murthy JM et al: Decompressive craniectomy with clot evacuation in large hemispheric hypertensive intracerebral hemorrhage. Neurocrit Care. 2(3):258-62, 2005
4. Plesea IE et al: Study of cerebral vascular structures in hypertensive intracerebral haemorrhage. Rom J Morphol Embryol. 46(3):249-56, 2005
5. Ohtani R et al: Clinical and radiographic features of lobar cerebral hemorrhage: hypertensive versus non-hypertensive cases. Intern Med. 42(7):576-80, 2003
6. Dickinson CJ: Why are strokes related to hypertension? Classic studies and hypotheses revisited. J Hypertens. 19(9):1515-21, 2001
7. Yanagawa Y et al: Relationship between stroke and asymptomatic minute hemorrhages in hypertensive patients. Neurol Med Chir (Tokyo). 41(1):13-7; discussion 17-8, 2001

HYPERTENSIVE HEMORRHAGE

IMAGE GALLERY

Typical

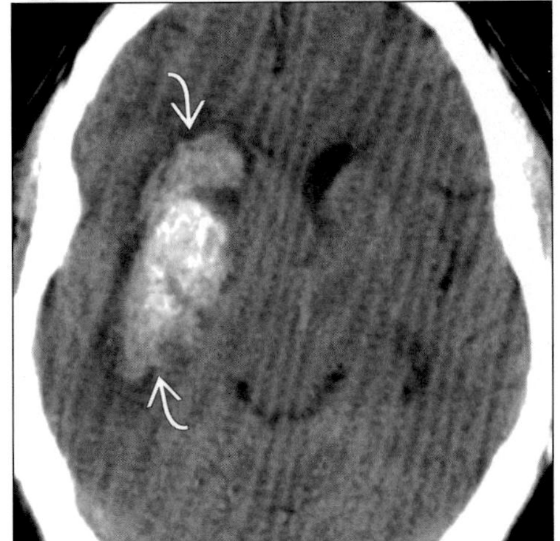

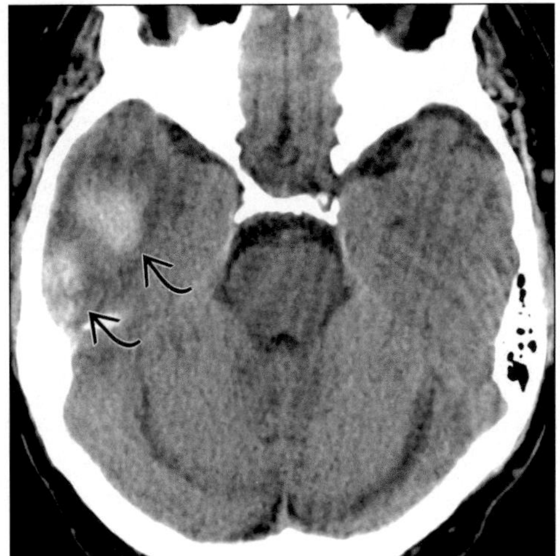

*(**Left**) Axial NECT shows subinsular acute hematoma ➢, location typical for hypertensive hemorrhage. There is resultant subfalcine herniation and compression of the right lateral ventricle. (**Right**) Axial NECT demonstrates temporal acute lobar hypertensive hemorrhage ➢. Only 5-15% of hICH are lobar but hypertension is so common that it should always be a diagnostic consideration.*

Typical

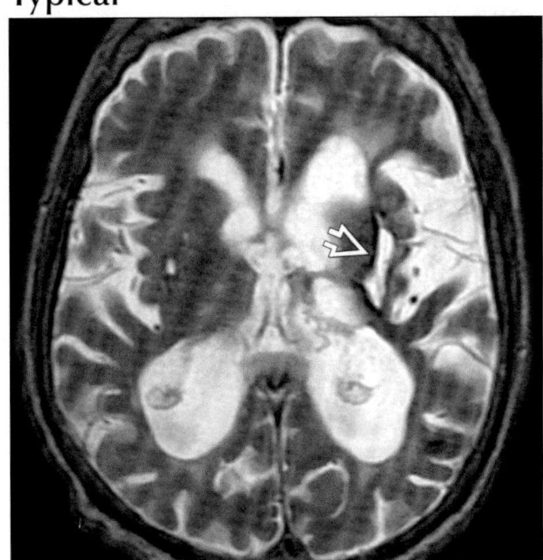

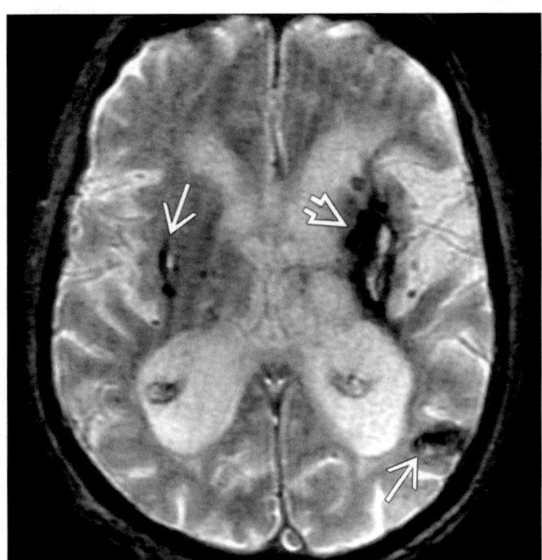

*(**Left**) Axial T2WI MR FSE shows left subinsular hypointense hemosiderin scar ➢ with central CSF-filled cavity from remote hypertensive hemorrhage. (**Right**) Axial T2WI MR GRE in the same patient as previous image, depicts hemosiderin scar ➢ but also more clearly demonstrates additional foci of chronic hICH ➔ due to "blooming" of short T2 blood products.*

Typical

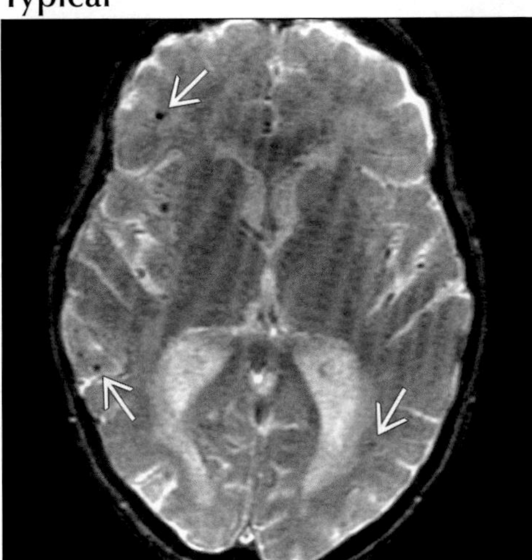

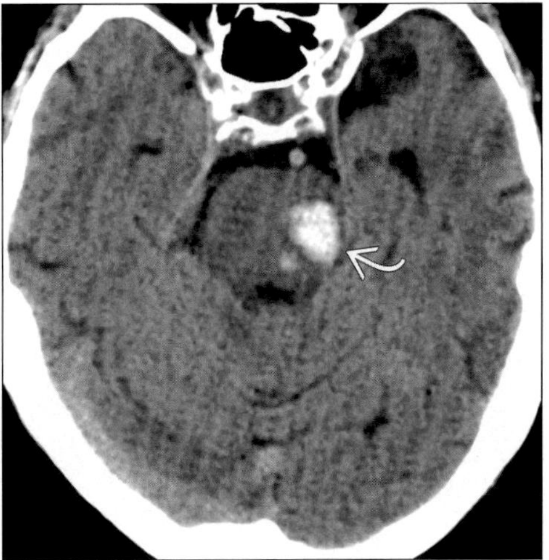

*(**Left**) Axial T2WI MR GRE demonstrates multiple punctate hypointense foci ➔ from chronic microbleeds, another imaging appearance of hypertensive hemorrhage. (**Right**) Axial NECT depicts acute hemorrhage ➢ with mild surrounding edema in the left pons, another common location for hypertensive hemorrhage due to rupture of the pontine perforating arteries.*

HYPERTENSIVE ENCEPHALOPATHY

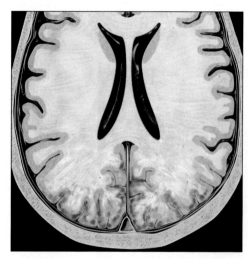

Axial graphic shows the classic posterior circulation cortical/subcortical vasogenic edema and petechial hemorrhages characteristic of hypertensive encephalopathy.

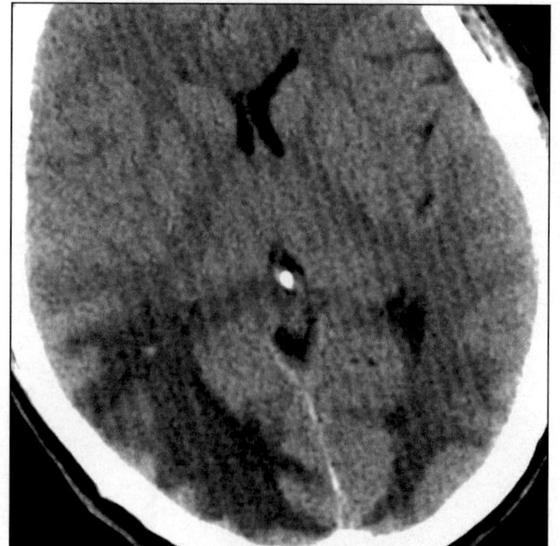

Axial NECT shows bilateral occipital and posterior temporal lobe hypodensity in the white matter and portions of the adjacent gray matter consistent with hypertensive encephalopathy.

TERMINOLOGY

Abbreviations and Synonyms

- Hypertensive encephalopathy (HE)
- HE is a subset of posterior reversible encephalopathy syndrome (PRES)/reversible posterior leukoencephalopathy syndrome (RPLS)

Definitions

- Cerebrovascular autoregulatory disorder characterized by headache, visual disturbances, altered mental function resulting from multiple etiologies, most of which are associated with acute hypertension (HTN)

IMAGING FINDINGS

General Features

- Best diagnostic clue: Patchy cortical/subcortical posterior circulation territory lesions in a patient with severe acute/subacute HTN
- Location
  - Most common: Cortex, subcortical white matter
    - Predilection for posterior circulation (parietal/occipital lobes, cerebellum)
    - At junctions of vascular watershed zones
    - Usually bilateral, often somewhat asymmetric
  - Less common: Basal ganglia
  - Rare: Predominate/exclusive brainstem involvement
- Size: Extent of abnormalities highly variable
- Morphology: Patchy > confluent

CT Findings

- NECT
  - Patchy bilateral nonconfluent hypodense foci
    - Posterior parietal, occipital lobes > basal ganglia, brainstem
  - Less common: Petechial cortical/subcortical or basal ganglionic hemorrhage
- CECT: With or without mild patchy/punctate enhancement
- CTA
  - Usually normal
  - Rare: Vasospasm with multifocal areas of arterial narrowing

MR Findings

- T1WI: Hypointense cortical/subcortical lesions

DDx: Hypertensive Encephalopathy

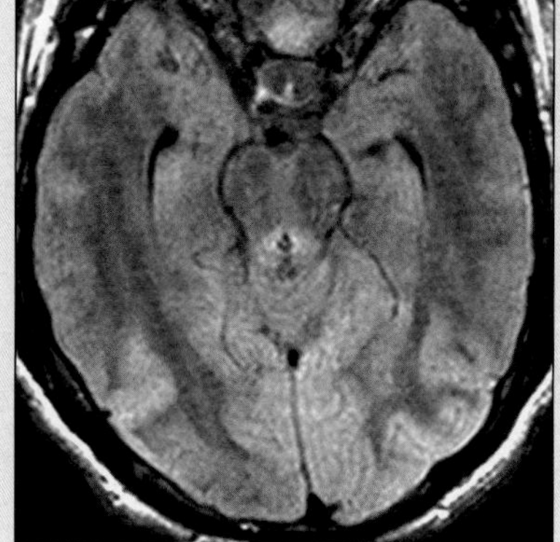

Bilateral PCA Infarcts

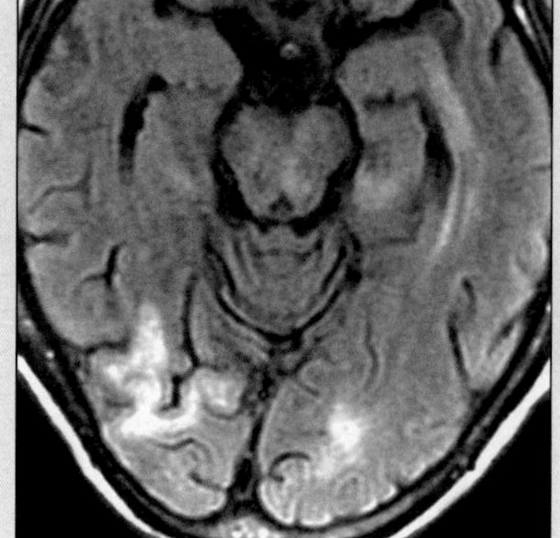

PML

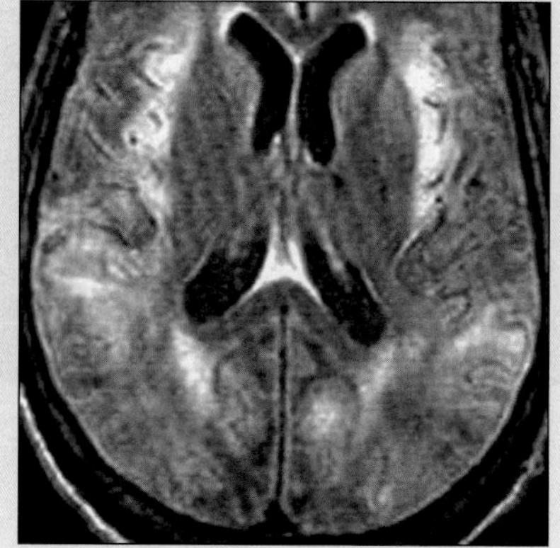

Hepatic Encephalopathy

HYPERTENSIVE ENCEPHALOPATHY

Key Facts

Imaging Findings

- Best diagnostic clue: Patchy cortical/subcortical posterior circulation territory lesions in a patient with severe acute/subacute HTN
- Parieto-occipital hyperintense cortical/subcortical lesions in 95%
- Usually normal (no restricted) diffusion
- T1 C+: Variable patchy enhancement
- Best imaging tool: MR with FLAIR, DWI, T1 C+

Top Differential Diagnoses

- Acute Cerebral Ischemia/Infarction
- Progressive Multifocal Leukoencephalopathy (PML)
- Metabolic Derangements
- Acute Demyelinating Disease
- Status Epilepticus
- Acute Cerebral Hyperemia Syndromes

Pathology

- Diverse causes, most clinical entities with HTN as common component
- Breakthrough of autoregulation causes blood-brain barrier disruption
- Result = vasogenic (not cytotoxic) edema
- Acute/subacute systemic HTN
- Preeclampsia, eclampsia
- Uremic encephalopathies
- Drug toxicity (many reported)

Clinical Issues

- HA, N/V, seizure, visual changes, altered MS
- Favorable outcome with prompt recognition, treatment of HTN
- Delayed diagnosis/therapy can result in chronic neurologic sequelae

- T2WI
  - Hyperintense cortical/subcortical lesions
  - Less common
    - Extensive brain stem hyperintensity
    - Generalized white matter edema
- PD/Intermediate: Multifocal hyperintensities
- FLAIR
  - Parieto-occipital hyperintense cortical/subcortical lesions in 95%
  - ± Symmetric lesions in basal ganglia
  - Does not discriminate between vasogenic, cytotoxic edema (both have increased signal intensity)
- T2* GRE: Blooms if short T2 hemorrhagic products present
- DWI
  - Usually normal (no restricted) diffusion
    - Less common: High signal on DWI with "pseudonormalized" ADC (may indicate irreversible infarction)
    - May progress to true restricted diffusion (infarction) if diagnosis is delayed
  - ADC map: Markedly elevated (increased diffusivity ± T2 "shine-through")
  - DTI (diffusion tensor imaging)
    - Shows foci of increased diffusion representing anisotropy loss
    - Vasogenic edema due to cerebrovascular autoregulatory dysfunction
- T1 C+: Variable patchy enhancement
- MRS
  - May show widespread metabolic abnormalities
    - Increased Cho, Cr; mildly decreased NAA
    - Usually returns to normal within 2 months
- Perfusion weighted imaging (PWI)
  - May show increased microvascular CBF

Nuclear Medicine Findings

- SPECT
  - Variable findings reported; some show hyper-, others hypoperfusion in affected areas

Imaging Recommendations

- Best imaging tool: MR with FLAIR, DWI, T1 C+
- Protocol advice: Repeat scan after BP normalized

DIFFERENTIAL DIAGNOSIS

Acute Cerebral Ischemia/Infarction

- Unlike HE, anterior circulation (MCA or ACA) more common than posterior circulation (PCA) distribution
- DWI usually shows restriction (high signal)

Progressive Multifocal Leukoencephalopathy (PML)

- Usually spares cortex, basal ganglia
- Immunocompromised patients

Metabolic Derangements

- History provides diagnostic clues
  - Dialysis disequilibrium syndrome, hepatic encephalopathy
- Locations somewhat different
  - Pons, basal ganglia, white matter in osmotic demyelination

Acute Demyelinating Disease

- Incomplete ring > patchy enhancement
- No predilection for posterior circulation

Status Epilepticus

- May cause transient gyral edema, enhancement
- Can mimic PRES, stroke, infiltrating neoplasm

Acute Cerebral Hyperemia Syndromes

- Rapid decompression of chronic SDH
  - Generally localized to cortex under the SDH
- Postcarotid endarterectomy, angioplasty or stenting
  - Hyperperfusion syndrome occurs in 5-9% of cases
  - Perfusion MR or CT scans show elevated CBF
  - Aggressive control of BP associated with clinical, radiological improvement

Gliomatosis Cerebri

- Entire lobe(s) involved rather than patchy cortical/subcortical lesions

HYPERTENSIVE ENCEPHALOPATHY

PATHOLOGY

General Features

- Etiology
  - Diverse causes, most clinical entities with HTN as common component
  - Acute HTN damages vascular endothelium
  - Breakthrough of autoregulation causes blood-brain barrier disruption
    - Primarily at arteriolar level
  - Result = vasogenic (not cytotoxic) edema
    - Arteriolar dilatation with cerebral hyperperfusion
    - Hydrostatic leakage (extravasation, transudation of fluid and macromolecules through arteriolar walls)
    - Interstitial fluid accumulates in cortex, subcortical white matter
    - Posterior circulation sparsely innervated by sympathetic nerves (predilection for parietal, occipital lobes); decreased ability to autoregulate arteriolar vasomotor tone
  - Infarction with cytotoxic edema ultimately possible
- Epidemiology
  - Pre-eclampsia in 5% of pregnancies
  - Eclampsia lower (< 1%)
- Associated abnormalities
  - Acute/subacute systemic HTN
  - Preeclampsia, eclampsia
    - Typically occurs after 20 weeks gestation
    - Rare: Headache, seizures up to several weeks postpartum
  - Uremic encephalopathies
    - Acute glomerulonephritis, hemolytic uremic syndrome, thrombotic thrombocytopenic purpura, lupus nephropathy, etc.
  - Drug toxicity (many reported)
    - Cyclosporin, FK-506 (tacrolimus), cisplatin, alpha-interferon, erythropoietin
  - Severe infection
    - 20-25% of patients with sepsis, shock
    - Blood pressure can be normal or elevated
  - Tumor lysis syndrome

Gross Pathologic & Surgical Features

- Common
  - Cortical/subcortical edema
  - ± Petechial hemorrhage in parietal, occipital lobes
- Less common: Lesions in basal ganglia, cerebellum, brainstem, anterior frontal lobes

Microscopic Features

- Usually no residual abnormalities after HTN corrected
- Autopsy in severe cases shows microvascular fibrinoid necrosis, ischemic microinfarcts, variable hemorrhage
- Chronic HTN associated with mural thickening, deposition of collagen, laminin, fibronectin in cerebral arterioles

CLINICAL ISSUES

Presentation

- Most common signs/symptoms
  - HA, N/V, seizure, visual changes, altered MS
  - Caution: Some patients, especially children, may be normotensive/minimally elevated BP!
- Clinical Profile
  - Young female with acute/subacute systemic HTN, headache, ± seizure
  - Child with kidney disease or transplant

Demographics

- Age: Any age but young > old
- Gender: M < F

Natural History & Prognosis

- Most cases resolve with adequate treatment
  - Reversibility not spontaneous but related to blood pressure normalization
  - Brainstem, deep white matter lesions less reversible than cortical/subcortical foci
  - Eclampsia more reversible than drug-related PRES
- May be life-threatening: Permanent infarction possible (even likely) if HE undiagnosed
- 4% of patients develop recurrent PRES

Treatment

- Favorable outcome with prompt recognition, treatment of HTN
- Delayed diagnosis/therapy can result in chronic neurologic sequelae

DIAGNOSTIC CHECKLIST

Consider

- Patchy bilateral low density foci in occipital lobes may be earliest manifestation of PRES

Image Interpretation Pearls

- Major ddx of PRES is cerebral ischemia; DWI is positive in the latter, usually negative in the former

SELECTED REFERENCES

1. Sweany JM et al: "Recurrent" posterior reversible encephalopathy syndrome: report of 3 cases--PRES can strike twice! J Comput Assist Tomogr. 31(1):148-56, 2007
2. Bartynski WS et al: Posterior reversible encephalopathy syndrome in infection, sepsis, and shock. AJNR Am J Neuroradiol. 27(10):2179-90, 2006
3. Ishikura K et al: Posterior reversible encephalopathy syndrome in children: its high prevalence and more extensive imaging findings. Am J Kidney Dis. 48(2):231-8, 2006
4. Narbone MC et al: PRES: posterior or potentially reversible encephalopathy syndrome? Neurol Sci. 27(3):187-9, 2006
5. Pande AR et al: Clinicoradiological factors influencing the reversibility of posterior reversible encephalopathy syndrome: a multicenter study. Radiat Med. 24(10):659-68, 2006
6. Striano P et al: Clinical spectrum and critical care management of Posterior Reversible Encephalopathy Syndrome (PRES). Med Sci Monit. 11(11):CR549-53, 2005
7. Kinoshita T et al: Diffusion-weighted MR imaging of posterior reversible leukoencephalopathy syndrome: a pictorial essay. Clin Imaging. 27(5): 307-15, 2003
8. Thambisetty M et al: Hypertensive brainstem encephalopathy: clinical and radiographic features. J Neurol Sci. 208(1-2): 93-9, 2003

IMAGE GALLERY

Typical

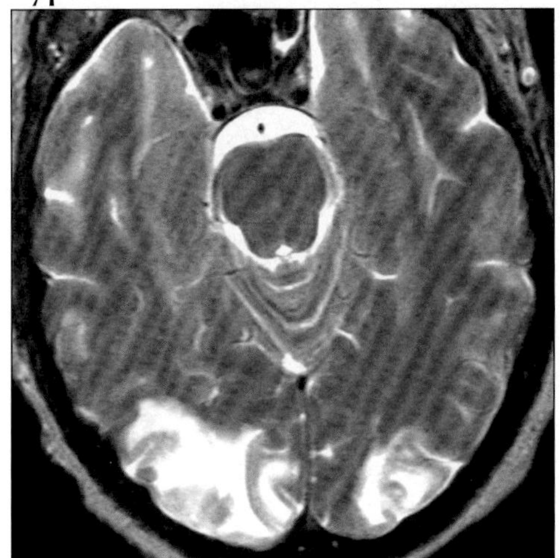

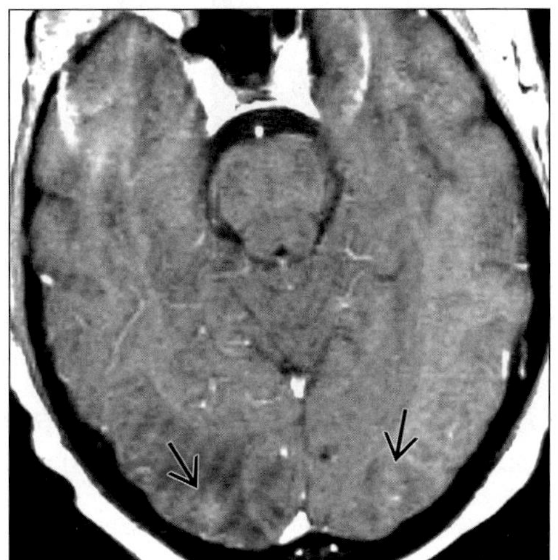

*(**Left**) Axial T2WI MR shows bilateral asymmetric high signal in the posterior white and gray matter in a 32 year old female on chemotherapy for acute myelogenous leukemia with new onset of seizure. (**Right**) Axial T1WI MR post-contrast in the same patient as previous image, demonstrates mild punctate/patchy enhancement of the lesions →. MR findings in conjunction with the patient's history are typical for PRES.*

Typical

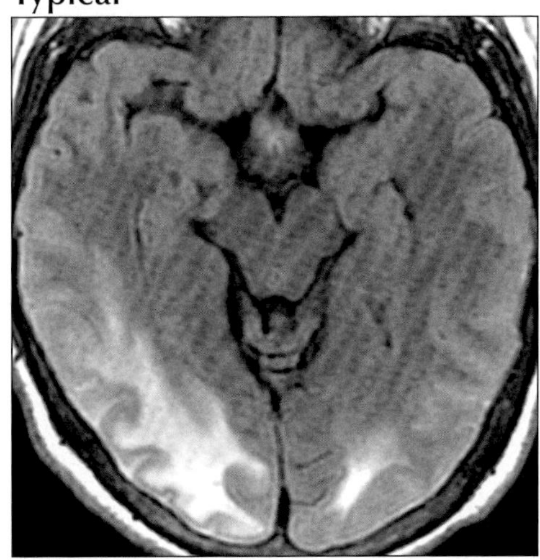

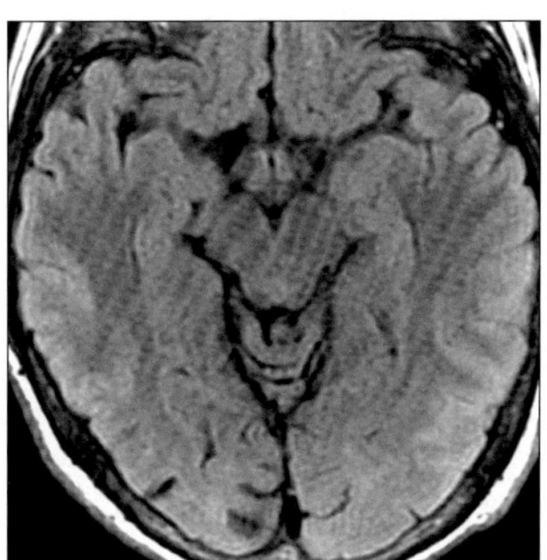

*(**Left**) Axial T2WI MR FLAIR shows high signal in the bilateral occipital and right posterior temporal lobes in a patient with HTN and vision loss who is on cyclosporine for renal transplant. (**Right**) Axial T2WI MR FLAIR in the same patient as previous image, shows near complete resolution of the lesions following blood pressure control and discontinuation of cyclosporin immunosuppression confirming prior HE.*

Variant

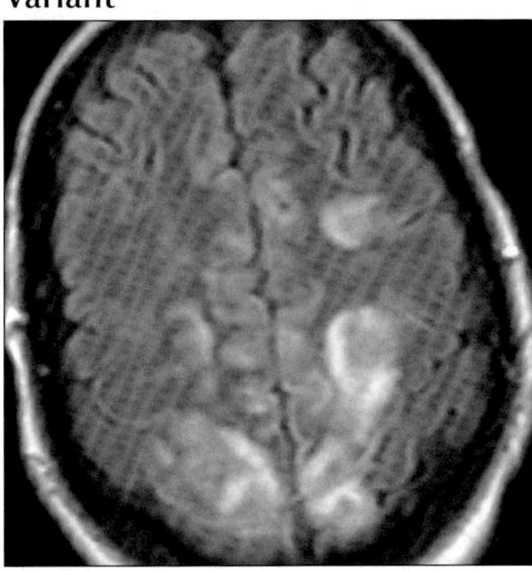

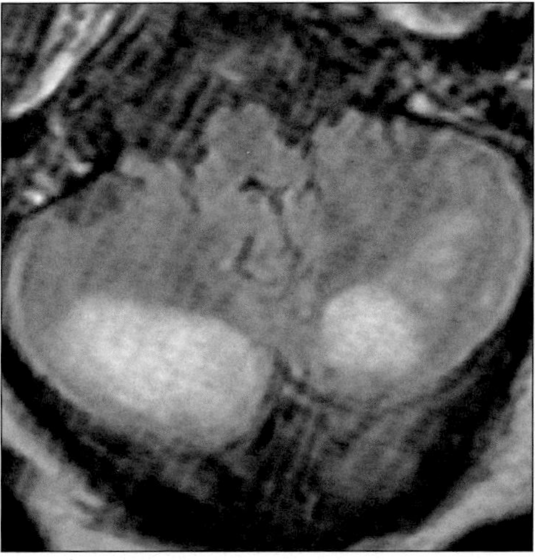

*(**Left**) Axial FLAIR MR depicts extensive cortical and subcortical high signal involving the posterior as well as anterior circulation territory in this patient with bone marrow transplant on FK-506. (**Right**) Axial FLAIR MR in the same patient as previous image, also demonstrates bilateral cerebellar lesions in this patient with extensive PRES. Findings resolved 6 months later following cessation of FK-506 treatment.*

SUPERFICIAL SIDEROSIS

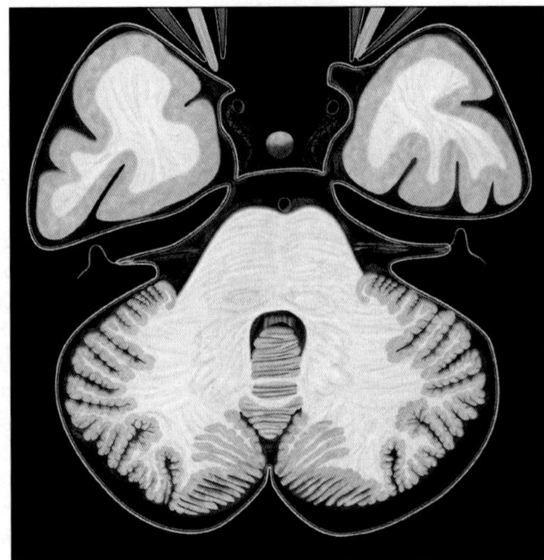

Axial graphic shows darker brown hemosiderin staining on all surfaces of the brain, meninges and cranial nerves. Notice 7th and 8th cranial nerves in the CPA-IAC are particularly affected.

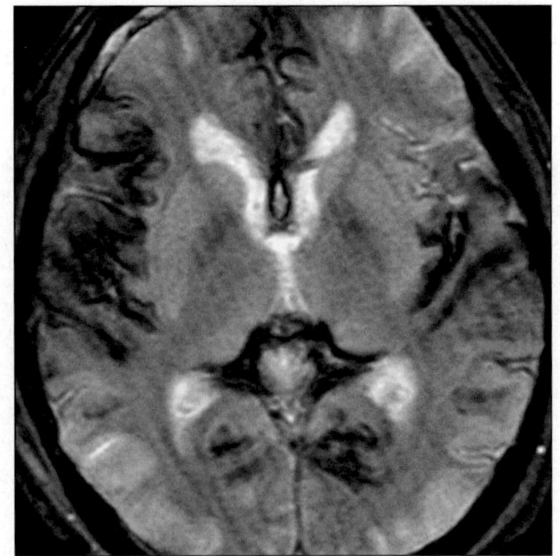

Axial GRE T2* MR image depicts a classic example of superficial siderosis with marked low signal along the surface of the brain due to hemosiderin deposition from multiple hemorrhages.

TERMINOLOGY

Abbreviations and Synonyms

- Central nervous system siderosis; siderosis; hemosiderosis

Definitions

- Recurrent subarachnoid hemorrhage (SAH) causes hemosiderin deposition on surface of brain, brainstem & cranial nerve leptomeninges

IMAGING FINDINGS

General Features

- Best diagnostic clue: Contours of brain & cranial nerves outlined by hypointense rim on T2 or T2* GRE MR images
- Location: Cerebral hemispheres, cerebellum, brainstem, cranial nerves & spinal cord may all be affected
- Size: Linear low signal along CNS surfaces varies in thickness but usually ≤ 2 mm
- Morphology: Curvilinear dark lines on CNS surfaces

CT Findings

- NECT
  - Cerebral and/or cerebellar atrophy
    - May be the only finding on CT
    - Especially marked in posterior fossa; cerebellar sulci often disproportionately large
  - Slightly hyperdense rim over brain surface
  - Relatively insensitive to presence of hemosiderin on CNS surfaces
- CECT: No enhancement typical

MR Findings

- T1WI: Hyperintense signal may be seen on CNS surfaces
- T2WI
  - High-resolution, thin section T2 MR images of CPA-IAC helpful
    - Cranial nerves 7 & 8 appear darker & thicker than normal
    - Adjacent cerebellar structures & brainstem show low signal surfaces
    - Less easily seen than on T2* GRE images
- FLAIR: Dark border on regional surfaces of brain, brainstem, cerebellum & cranial nerves

DDx: Superficial Siderosis

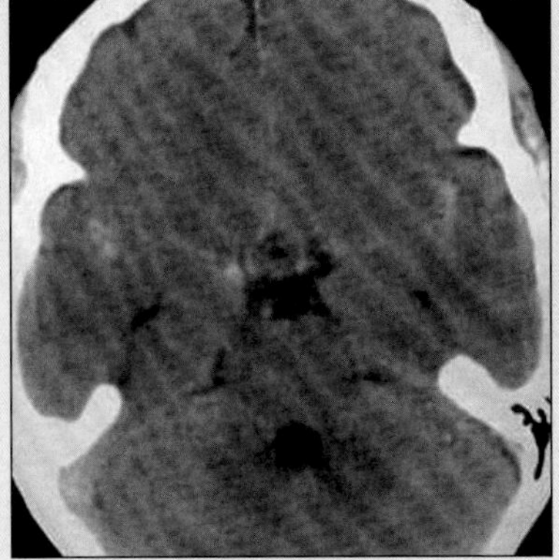

Acute Subarachnoid Hemorrhage

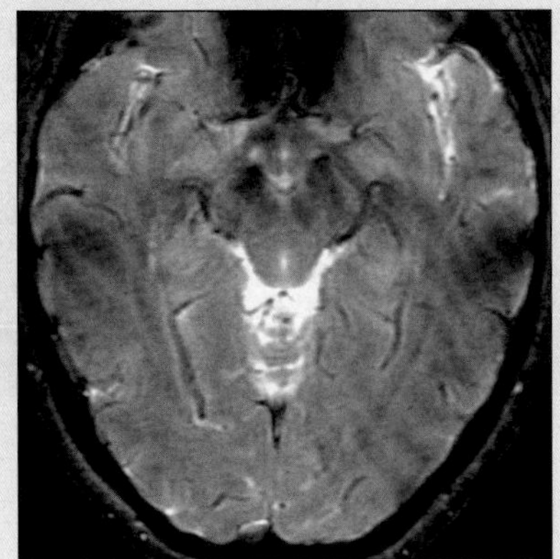

Normal Veins (3T)

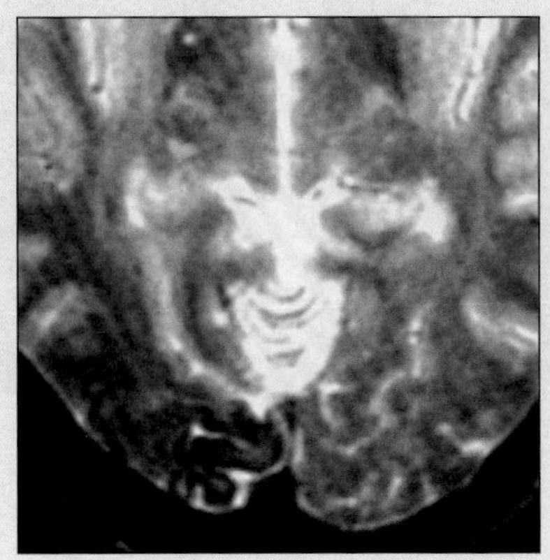

Sturge-Weber Syndrome

SUPERFICIAL SIDEROSIS

Key Facts

Terminology

- Recurrent subarachnoid hemorrhage (SAH) causes hemosiderin deposition on surface of brain, brainstem & cranial nerve leptomeninges

Imaging Findings

- Best diagnostic clue: Contours of brain & cranial nerves outlined by hypointense rim on T2 or T2* GRE MR images
- Location: Cerebral hemispheres, cerebellum, brainstem, cranial nerves & spinal cord may all be affected

Top Differential Diagnoses

- Acute Subarachnoid Hemorrhage (aSAH)
- MR Sequence Artifact
- Brain Surface Vessels
- Sturge-Weber Syndrome
- Neurocutaneous Melanosis
- Meningioangiomatosis (MA)

Pathology

- Hemosiderin is cytotoxic to neurons
- Causes of recurrent SAH found in ~ 50%
- CSF cavity lesion (surgical cavity) with fragile neovascularity most common
- Bleeding neoplasms (35%)
- Vascular abnormalities (18%)

Clinical Issues

- Classic presentation is adult patient with bilateral SNHL & ataxia
- Pre-symptomatic phase averages 15 years
- Treat source of bleeding

- T2* GRE
  - Most sensitive to hemosiderin deposition on CNS surfaces
  - "Blooming" dark signal; GRE makes it appear more conspicuous, thicker
- T1 C+: Surface of CNS does not enhance
- MR findings do not correlate with severity of disease

Imaging Recommendations

- Best imaging tool
  - Brain MR
    - Once diagnosis of superficial siderosis is made, search for cause of recurrent SAH must commence
    - Whole brain MR with contrast & MRA first
    - Total spine MR second if brain negative for underlying lesion
- Protocol advice
  - Brain MR
    - MR with FLAIR, ± T1 C+ initially
    - If suspect superficial siderosis, add T2* GRE sequences to confirm

DIFFERENTIAL DIAGNOSIS

Acute Subarachnoid Hemorrhage (aSAH)

- Can appear identical on CT
  - Patient history of sudden onset worst headache of life and acute neurological decline
- MR better to differentiate on imaging basis alone
  - Hyperintense signal in sulci on FLAIR with aSAH

MR Sequence Artifact

- Variably thick & prominent low signal on surface of brain
- Imaging clue: Artifact is not present on all sequences

Brain Surface Vessels

- Normal or abnormal surface veins
- Linear, focal area of low signal on surface of brain
- Appear even more pronounced with 3T

Sturge-Weber Syndrome

- Cortical calcification can appear low signal on MR
- Isolated parenchymal atrophy
- Cerebral (usually parieto-occipital) > > cerebellum
- Marked overlying leptomeningeal enhancement
- Ipsilateral choroid plexus enlargement

Neurocutaneous Melanosis

- Congenital syndrome
- Large or multiple congenital melanocytic nevi
- Benign or malignant pigment cell tumors of the leptomeninges may be low signal on surface of brain
- T1 high signal diffusely in pia-arachnoid
- T2 low signal diffusely in pia-arachnoid

Meningioangiomatosis (MA)

- Hamartomatous proliferation of meningeal cells into cerebral cortex via parenchymal perivascular spaces
- Leptomeninges are thick & infiltrated with fibrous tissue, may be calcified

PATHOLOGY

General Features

- General path comments
  - Hemosiderin staining of meninges
    - Hemosiderin is cytotoxic to underlying tissues
  - Xanthochromic CSF
- Etiology
  - Repeated SAH deposits hemosiderin on meningeal lining of CNS
    - Affects brainstem, cerebellum, cranial nerves, cerebrum & spinal cord
  - Hemosiderin is cytotoxic to neurons
    - "Free" iron with excess production of hydroxyl radicals is best current hypothesis explaining cytotoxicity
  - CN 8 is extensively lined with CNS myelin which is supported by hemosiderin-sensitive microglia
    - Increased exposure in CPA cistern
- Epidemiology
  - Rare chronic progressive disorder
  - 0.15% of patients undergoing MR imaging
- Associated abnormalities

SUPERFICIAL SIDEROSIS

- Causes of recurrent SAH pathologies include
  - Traumatic nerve root avulsion, bleeding CNS neoplasm, vascular malformations, aneurysms & arteriovenous fistulas

Gross Pathologic & Surgical Features

- Dark brown discoloration of leptomeninges, ependyma & subpial tissue
- Causes of recurrent SAH found in ~ 50%
  - Dural pathology (47%)
    - CSF cavity lesion (surgical cavity) with fragile neovascularity most common
    - Traumatic cervical nerve root avulsion
  - Bleeding neoplasms (35%)
    - Ependymoma, oligodendroglioma & astrocytoma
  - Vascular abnormalities (18%)
    - Arteriovenous malformation (AVM) or aneurysm
    - Multiple cavernous malformations near brain surface
    - Arteriovenous fistula; may occur in brain or spine
- Idiopathic (46%)

Microscopic Features

- Hemosiderin staining of meninges and subpial tissues to 3 mm depth
- Thickened leptomeninges
- Cerebellar folia: Loss of Purkinje cells and Bergmann gliosis

CLINICAL ISSUES

Presentation

- Most common signs/symptoms
  - Bilateral sensorineural hearing loss (SNHL) present in 95% of cases
  - Cerebellar ataxia common as are other cranial nerve palsies
- Clinical Profile
  - Classic presentation is adult patient with bilateral SNHL & ataxia
  - Seen less commonly as late complication of treated childhood cerebellar tumor
- Laboratory
  - CSF from lumbar puncture
    - High protein (100%), Xanthochromic (75%)
- Other symptoms
  - Ataxia (88%)
  - Bilateral hemiparesis
  - Hyperreflexia, bladder disturbance, anosmia, dementia & headache
    - Anosmia: Olfactory nerve particularly sensitive to hemosiderin deposition
  - Cognitive impairments affecting speech production, visual recall memory & executive functions
  - Pre-symptomatic phase averages 15 years

Demographics

- Age: Broad age range: 14-77 years
- Gender: M:F ratio = 3:1

Natural History & Prognosis

- Profound bilateral SNHL & ataxia within 15 years of onset
- Deafness almost certain if unrecognized
- 25% become bed-bound in years following 1st symptom
  - Result of cerebellar ataxia, myelopathic syndrome or both

Treatment

- Treat source of bleeding
- Surgically remove source of bleeding (surgical cavity, tumor, vascular lesion)
- Endovascular therapy for AVM, aneurysm or fistula
- Cochlear implantation for SNHL

DIAGNOSTIC CHECKLIST

Consider

- Remember that superficial siderosis is an effect, not a cause
- Look for source of recurrent SAH somewhere in brain or spine
- MR findings do not correlate with patient's symptom severity
  - MR diagnosis may be made in absence of symptoms

Image Interpretation Pearls

- CNS surfaces including cranial nerves appear "outlined in black" on T2 MR images with "blooming" on GRE

SELECTED REFERENCES

1. Kumar N: Superficial siderosis: associations and therapeutic implications. Arch Neurol. 64(4):491-6, 2007
2. Kim CS et al: Cochlear implantation in superficial siderosis. Acta Otolaryngol. 126(8):892-6, 2006
3. Ushio M et al: Superficial siderosis causing retrolabyrinthine involvement in both cochlear and vestibular branches of the eighth cranial nerve. Acta Otolaryngol. 126(9):997-1000, 2006
4. Miele VJ et al: Diagnostic pitfall of computed tomography in patients with superficial siderosis of the central nervous system. W V Med J. 101(4):172-5, 2005
5. van Harskamp NJ et al: Cognitive and social impairments in patients with superficial siderosis. Brain. 128(Pt 5):1082-92, 2005
6. Spengos K et al: Superficial siderosis of the brain as a late complication of subarachnoid haemorrhage. Cerebrovasc Dis. 17(1):87, 2004
7. Vibert D et al: Hearing loss and vertigo in superficial siderosis of the central nervous system. Am J Otolaryngol. 25(2):142-9, 2004
8. Anderson NE et al: Superficial siderosis of the central nervous system: a late complication of cerebellar tumors. Neurology. 52(1):163-9, 1999
9. Schievink WI et al: Surgical treatment of superficial siderosis associated with a spinal arteriovenous malformation. Case report. J Neurosurg. 89(6):1029-31, 1998
10. Maurizi CP: Superficial siderosis of the brain: roles for cerebrospinal fluid circulation, iron and the hydroxyl radical. Med Hypotheses. 47(4):261-4, 1996
11. Offenbacher H et al: Superficial siderosis of the central nervous system: MRI findings and clinical significance. Neuroradiology. 38 Suppl 1:S51-6, 1996
12. Tapscott SJ et al: Surgical management of superficial siderosis following cervical nerve root avulsion. Ann Neurol. 40(6):936-40, 1996

SUPERFICIAL SIDEROSIS

IMAGE GALLERY

Typical

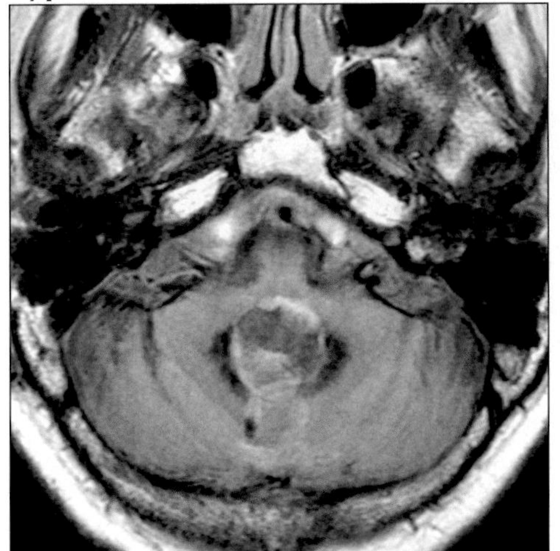

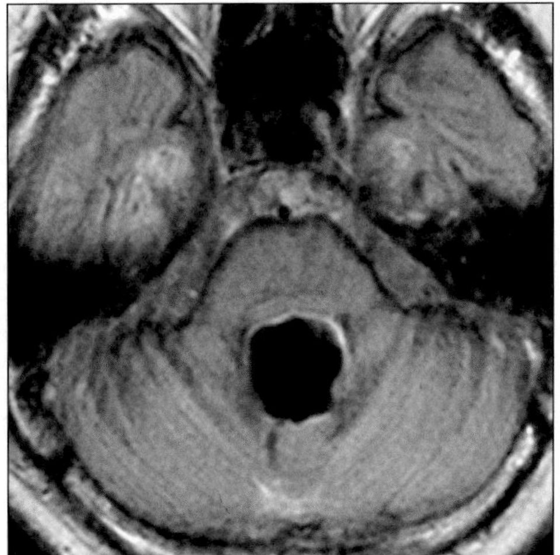

(Left) *Axial T2WI MR in a patient with prior midline cerebellar resection for juvenile pilocytic astrocytoma shows hypointense signal on the surface of the medulla, cerebellum and exiting nerves.* ***(Right)*** *Axial FLAIR MR image in the same case as previous image, more superior section, also demonstrates very low signal along the surface of the pons and within the cerebellar folia from superficial siderosis.*

Typical

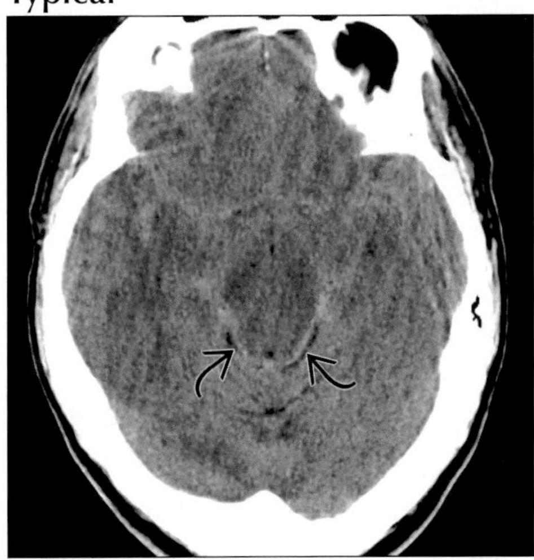

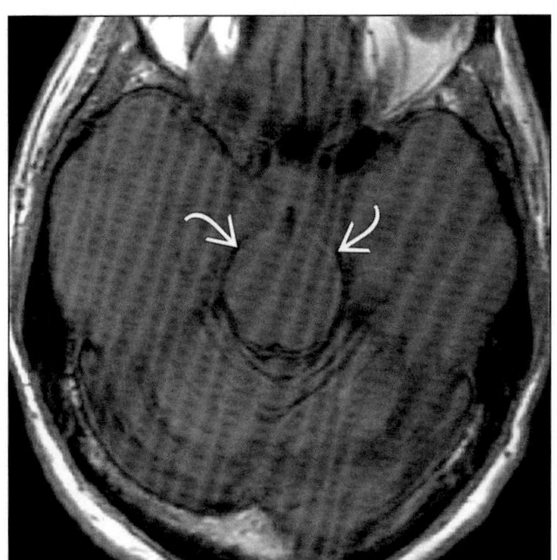

(Left) *Axial NECT shows high density in the sylvian and perimesencephalic cisterns suggesting acute subarachnoid hemorrhage. Note the high density is actually adherent to the midbrain ➚.* ***(Right)*** *Axial T1WI MR in the same case as previous image shows high signal intensity along the surface of the midbrain ➚ consistent with more chronic blood products due to superficial siderosis.*

Typical

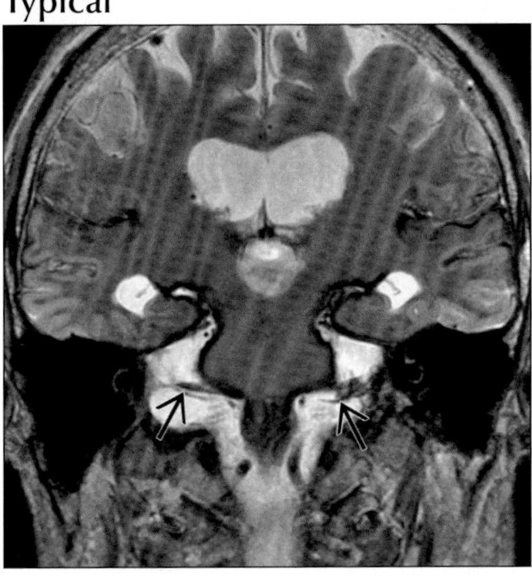

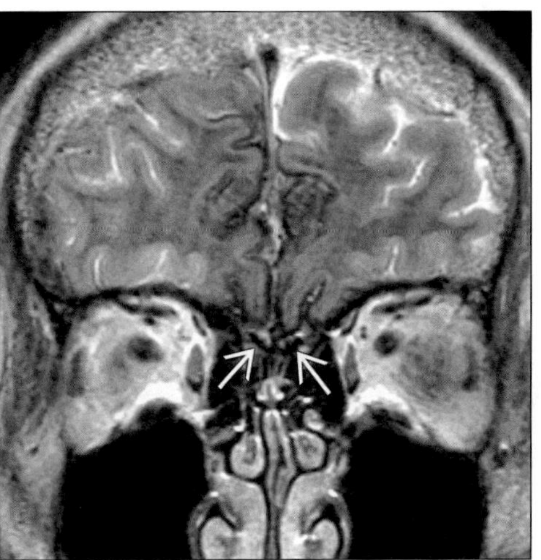

(Left) *Coronal T2WI MR in a patient with superficial siderosis shows hemosiderin staining on the 7th and 8th cranial nerve complexes ➔. The 8th cranial nerve is the most commonly affected.* ***(Right)*** *Coronal T2WI MR in the same case as previous image also demonstrates hemosiderin deposition on the bilateral 1st cranial nerves ➔. Olfactory nerves can be commonly involved as well resulting in anosmia.*

PERSISTENT TRIGEMINAL ARTERY

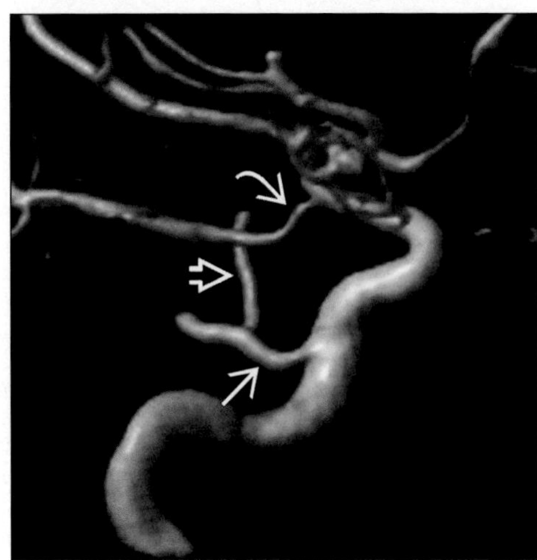

Lateral 3D ICA DSA shows an anomalous vessel arising from the pre-cavernous segment of the ICA ➔. Note fetal PCA ➔ and basilar artery ➔. Saltzman type II trigeminal artery.

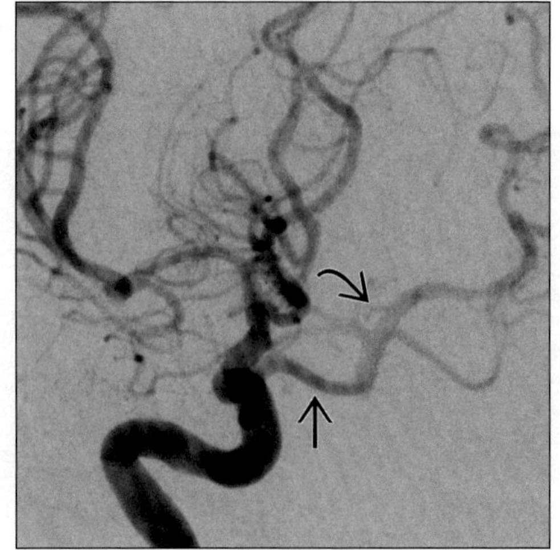

Oblique right ICA DSA in the same patient shows a trigeminal artery ➔ connecting the ICA to the basilar artery with opacification of the basilar caput and its branches ➔.

TERMINOLOGY

Definitions

- Persistent trigeminal artery (PTA): Persistent (fetal) carotid to vertebrobasilar (VB) anastomosis between pre-cavernous internal carotid artery (ICA) and basilar artery (BA)

IMAGING FINDINGS

General Features

- Best diagnostic clue
  - Anomalous vessel bridges anterior (ICA) and posterior (VB) circulations below level of posterior communicating artery (PCoA)
  - Sagittal MR shows "trident sign"
- Location: Pre-cavernous ICA to mid/distal-basilar artery or a cerebellar artery (AICA or SCA) in PTA variant
- Size: Variable; typically smaller in PTA variant
- Morphology: PTA may have irregular contour ± associated aneurysm

CT Findings

- NECT
  - PTA is not visualized
  - Subarachnoid hemorrhage (SAH) if associated aneurysm ruptures
- CECT: Large caliber vessel courses in pre-pontine cistern
- CTA: Delineates presence and course of vascular anomaly, associated abnormalities (e.g., saccular or fusiform aneurysm)

MR Findings

- Prominent flow void bridging anterior and posterior circulation
  - Sagittal T1WI: Looks like "Neptune's trident"
  - Axial T1, T2WI: Prominent but anomalous vessel passes posteriorly from ICA (either around or directly through dorsum sellae) to BA
- MRA readily depicts anatomical variant
- BA is often hypoplastic below the level of the anastomosis and enlarges to a more normal caliber above

DDx: Trigeminal Artery

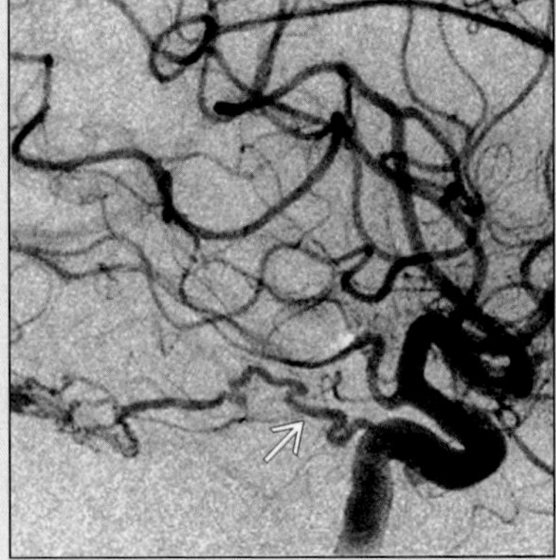

Tentorial Artery

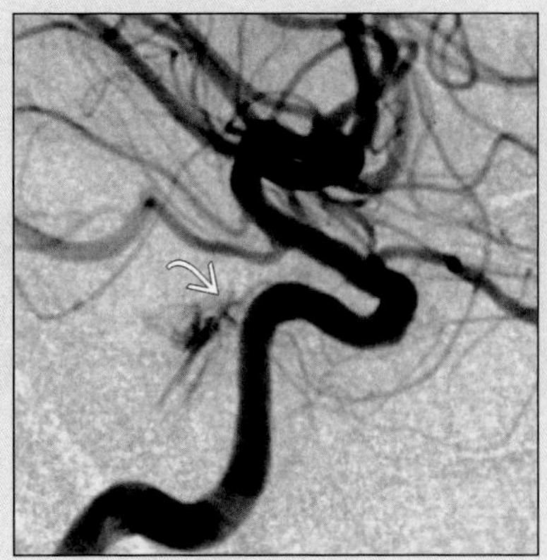

Indirect Carotid Cavernous Fistula

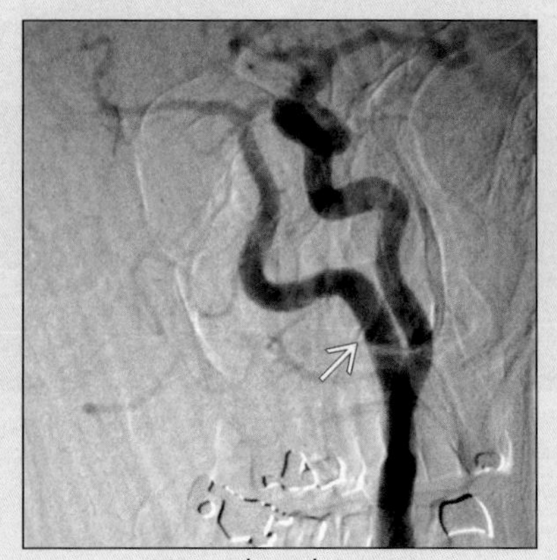

Hypoglossal Artery

PERSISTENT TRIGEMINAL ARTERY

Key Facts

Terminology

- Persistent trigeminal artery (PTA): Persistent (fetal) carotid to vertebrobasilar (VB) anastomosis between pre-cavernous internal carotid artery (ICA) and basilar artery (BA)

Imaging Findings

- Anomalous vessel bridges anterior (ICA) and posterior (VB) circulations below level of posterior communicating artery (PCoA)
- Sagittal MR shows "trident sign"
- Location: Pre-cavernous ICA to mid/distal-basilar artery or a cerebellar artery (AICA or SCA) in PTA variant
- Basilar artery caudal of primitive anastomosis may be hypoplastic
- MRA can define anatomy sufficiently for classification into medial, lateral, Saltzman types
- Look for associated aneurysm at PTA site

Pathology

- PTA: Most common CVBA
- Present in 0.2-0.6% of cerebral angiograms
- Vascular channel from pre-cavernous ICA courses posteriorly along trigeminal nerve or directly through dorsum sellae

Clinical Issues

- Most common presentation: Incidental finding at imaging (anomalous vessel noted on MR/CT/DSA)
- PTA aneurysms may be better treated with endovascular techniques due to location and difficult surgical access

Angiographic Findings

- Conventional
  - Anomalous vessel joining pre-cavernous ICA to mid/distal basilar artery vs. smaller caliber vessel from pre-cavernous ICA to AICA > SCA (trigeminal artery variant)
  - Basilar artery caudal of primitive anastomosis may be hypoplastic
  - Classification
    - Lateral type: Courses posterolaterally along the trigeminal nerve
    - Medial type: Courses posteromedially, may compress pituitary gland, penetrates dorsum sellae (a.k.a. "intrasellar" or "transhypophyseal" PTA); relevant for transsphenoidal surgery
    - Saltzman type 1: PCoA small or absent
    - Saltzman type 2: Fetal PCA from ipsilateral ICA

Imaging Recommendations

- Best imaging tool
  - MRA can define anatomy sufficiently for classification into medial, lateral, Saltzman types
  - Conventional angiography not indicated for further work-up of an incidentally discovered PTA on MR/MRA
- May be incidental finding on MR or CT
- Confirm with MRA or CTA
- Look for associated aneurysm at PTA site

DIFFERENTIAL DIAGNOSIS

Persistent Hypoglossal Artery

- Second most common carotid vertebrobasilar anastomoses (CVBA)
  - Found in 0.03-0.26% of angiograms
  - Connects cervical ICA (approximately C1-2 level) with BA
  - Courses through enlarged hypoglossal canal, not foramen magnum
  - Partly parallels CN12

Persistent Otic Artery (POA)

- Very rare; some authors dispute its existence
- Courses from petrous ICA through internal acoustic meatus to caudal BA
- Vertebral arteries may be absent or hypoplastic, therefore POA may be dominant or only supply to basilar artery

Proatlantal Intersegmental Artery (PIA)

- Most caudal of CVBAs
- Originates from cervical ICA (approximately C2-3 level) or (less commonly) from ECA
- Enters the intracranial compartment via the foramen magnum
- Vertebral arteries may be absent or hypoplastic, therefore PIA may be dominant or only supply to basilar artery
- Type I: Anomalous vessel arises from cervical segment of ICA
- Type II: Anomalous vessel arises from ECA

Hypertrophied Extradural ICA Branches

- Tentorial artery: May arise from cavernous ICA (meningohypophyseal trunk (MHT) ± inferolateral trunk (ILT); may be enlarged in vascular tumors (e.g., tentorial meningioma) or AV shunts (e.g., dural fistulas, AVMs)

Indirect Carotid Cavernous Fistula

- Lateral ICA DSA may show small fistulas as a vascular blush adjacent to the posterior aspect of the pre-cavernous ICA when supplied by MHT

PATHOLOGY

General Features

- General path comments
  - PTA: Most common CVBA
    - Present in 0.2-0.6% of cerebral angiograms
    - Trigeminal variant supplying only the ipsilateral AICA or SCA is less common

PERSISTENT TRIGEMINAL ARTERY

- Increased incidence of intracranial aneurysm at PTA site
- Embryology
  - Several transient segmental connections between primitive carotid & hindbrain circulations appear in early fetal development
  - Connections are named according to the cranial nerves they parallel (hypoglossal nerve, otic vesicle, trigeminal nerve)
  - Embryonic trigeminal artery supplies basilar artery before definitive PCoA and vertebral arteries develop
  - Embryonic trigeminal artery usually regresses as definitive circulation develops, approximately at 5-6 mm stage (29 days)
  - Failure to regress results in PTA
- Anatomy
  - PTA arises from pre-cavernous ICA near posterior genu
  - Vascular channel from pre-cavernous ICA courses posteriorly along trigeminal nerve or directly through dorsum sellae
  - Usually associated with small PCoA, vertebral arteries, proximally hypoplastic BA

- Associated abnormalities
  - 14-32% of patients with PTA have intracranial "berry" aneurysms involving PTA or at other sites
    - Incidence probably exaggerated due to selection bias (PTA found on angiography in patients having aneurysm work-up)
  - Likely some increase in risk of aneurysm formation at PTA site at vessel branch point (as with any berry aneurysm due to structural defects in vessel wall at bifurcations) but overall incidence around 3-5% is not increased from general population
  - Various case reports of association with intracranial arteriovenous malformations, facial hemangiomas, Klippel-Feil syndrome, Moya-Moya disease, Sturge-Weber syndrome, Dandy-Walker syndrome, cavum septum pellucidum, brain tumors, aortic arch anomalies but quite possibly coincidental

CLINICAL ISSUES

Presentation

- Most common signs/symptoms: Usually asymptomatic
- Other signs/symptoms
  - Trigeminal neuralgia (uncommon)
  - Isolated CN6 nerve palsy (rare)
- Most common presentation: Incidental finding at imaging (anomalous vessel noted on MR/CT/DSA)
- Medial type relevant if contemplating trans-sphenoidal surgery
- PTA has been reported to be a rare cause of brainstem and posterior circulation stroke resulting from carotid atherosclerotic disease
- PTA, like all CVBAs, are a contraindication to neuropsychological Wada testing via cervical ICA injection of sodium Amytal due to potential brainstem dysfunction (loss of consciousness, apnea)
  - Careful examination of preliminary DSA (AP and lateral views) during Wada test is required
  - If CVBA exists, injection of sodium Amytal via a microcatheter placed above the origin of the anomalous vessel may permit safe Wada testing by avoiding brainstem dysfunction

Treatment

- No treatment for PTA itself is required
- PTA aneurysms may be better treated with endovascular techniques due to location and difficult surgical access
- PTA may be used as a conduit to access the basilar artery from the ICA for endovascular treatment of posterior circulation aneurysms when the vertebral arteries and PCoAs are hypoplastic

DIAGNOSTIC CHECKLIST

Consider

- PTA and other CVBAs before ICA injection of Na Amytal for Wada test

Image Interpretation Pearls

- PTA is the most common and superiorly located of the 4 persistent fetal CVBAs
  - Anomalous vessel links pre-cavernous ICA to basilar artery

SELECTED REFERENCES

1. Agrawal D et al: Fusiform aneurysm of a persistent trigeminal artery. J Clin Neurosci. 12(4):500-3, 2005
2. Kalidindi RS et al: Persistent trigeminal artery presenting as intermittent isolated sixth nerve palsy. Clin Radiol. 60(4):515-9, 2005
3. Chan DT et al: Trispan-assisted coiling of a wide-necked Persistent Trigeminal Artery aneurysm. Acta Neurochir (Wien). 146(1):87-8; discussion 88, 2004
4. Pasco A et al: Persistent carotid-vertebrobasilar anastomoses: how and why differentiating them? J Neuroradiol. 31(5):391-6, 2004
5. Takase T et al: Surgically treated aneurysm of the trunk of the persistent primitive trigeminal artery--case report. Neurol Med Chir (Tokyo). 44(8):420-3, 2004
6. Ziyal IM et al: Trigeminal neuralgia associated with a primitive trigeminal artery variant: case report. Neurosurgery. 54(4):1033; author reply 1033, 2004
7. Patel AB et al: Angiographic documentation of a persistent otic artery. AJNR Am J Neuroradiol. 24(1):124-6, 2003
8. Ikushima I et al: Basilar artery aneurysm treated with coil embolization via persistent primitive trigeminal artery. Cardiovasc Intervent Radiol. 25(1):70-1, 2002
9. Mohammed MI et al: Stent-assisted coil placement in a wide-necked persistent trigeminal artery aneurysm with jailing of the trigeminal artery: a case report. AJNR Am J Neuroradiol. 23(3):437-41, 2002
10. Nishio A et al: Primitive trigeminal artery variant aneurysm treated with Guglielmi detachable coils--case report. Neurol Med Chir (Tokyo). 41(9):446-9, 2001
11. Cloft HJ et al: Prevalence of cerebral aneurysms in patients with persistent primitive trigeminal artery. J Neurosurg. 90(5):865-7, 1999
12. McKenzie JD et al: Trigeminal-cavernous fistula: Saltzman anatomy revisited. AJNR Am J Neuroradiol. 17(2):280-2, 1996
13. Silbergleit R et al: Persistent trigeminal artery detected with standard MRI. J Comput Assist Tomogr. 17(1):22-5, 1993

PERSISTENT TRIGEMINAL ARTERY

IMAGE GALLERY

Typical

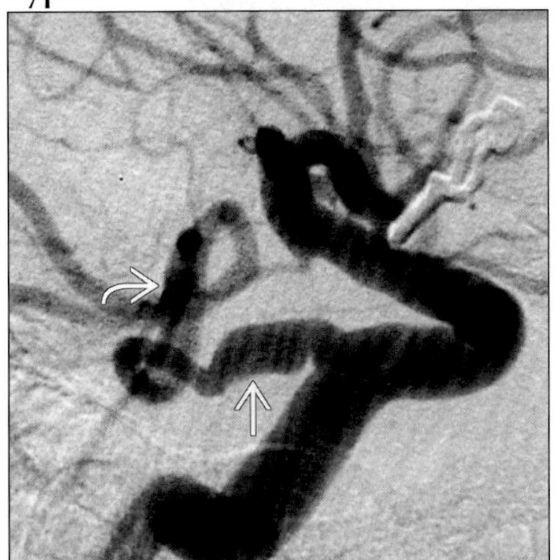

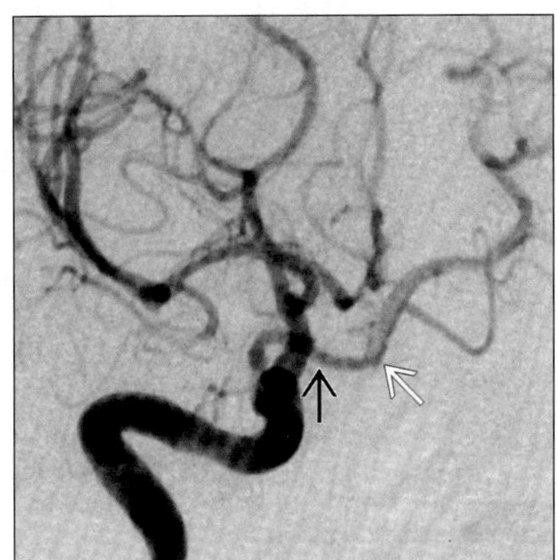

(Left) Lateral ICA DSA shows a large posteriorly directed branch arising from the pre-cavernous ICA opacifying the distal basilar artery ➡. Note dysplastic dilatation of a segment of the PTA ➡. *(Right)* Anteroposterior right ICA DSA shows a PTA ➡ arising from the ICA. The anomalous vessel courses posteromedially to join the distal basilar artery ➡.

Typical

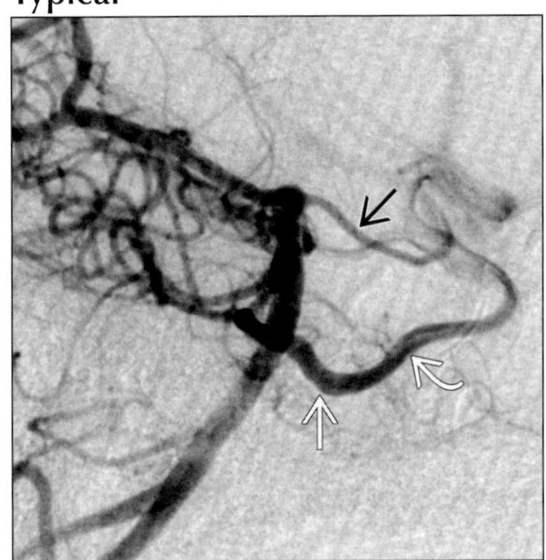

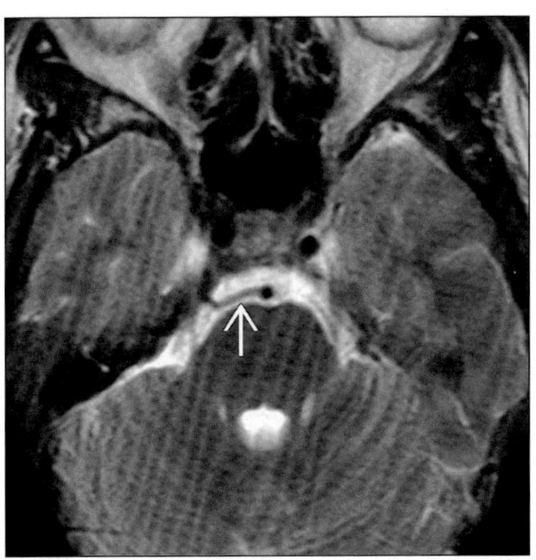

(Left) Lateral vertebral artery DSA shows a PTA as an anteriorly directed vessel ➡ opacifying the posterior genu of the carotid siphon ➡. Note PCoA located more superiorly ➡. *(Right)* Axial T2WI MR shows a prominent vessel running horizontally in the pre-pontine cistern into the basilar artery from the region of the petrous apex (trigeminal artery, lateral type) ➡. This vessel represents a lateral type PTA.

Typical

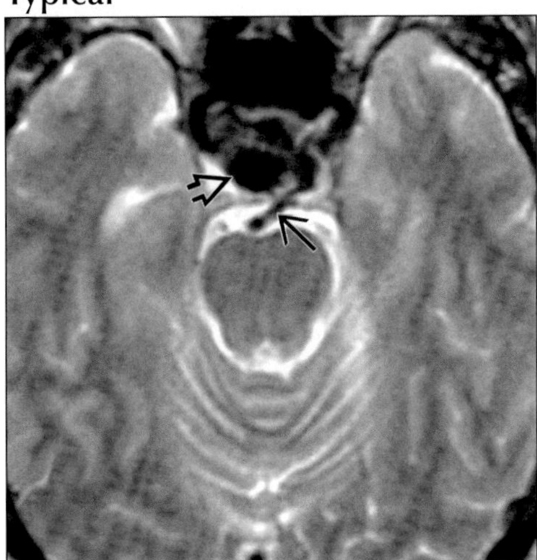

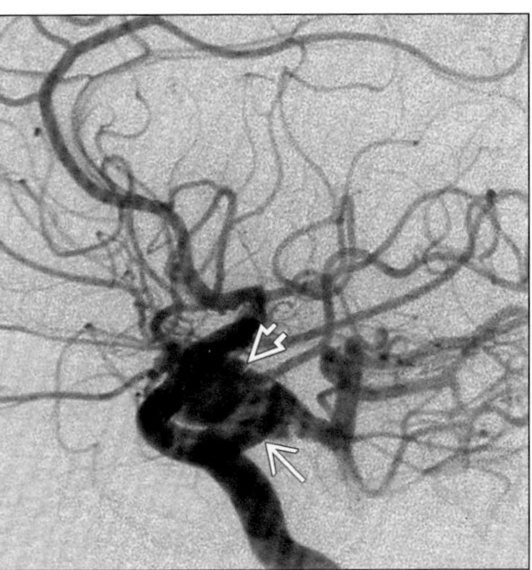

(Left) Axial T2WI MR shows a linear flow void ➡ that connects the left ICA with the basilar artery. A much larger area of signal loss is seen within the sella turcica ➡ representing an aneurysm associated with a PTA. *(Right)* Lateral angiography left ICA DSA in the same patient shows a PTA ➡ connecting the pre-cavernous ICA to the basilar artery. Note the large associated saccular aneurysm ➡ that is directed anteriorly into the pituitary fossa.

VENOUS SAMPLING: ENDOCRINE (NON-ADRENAL)

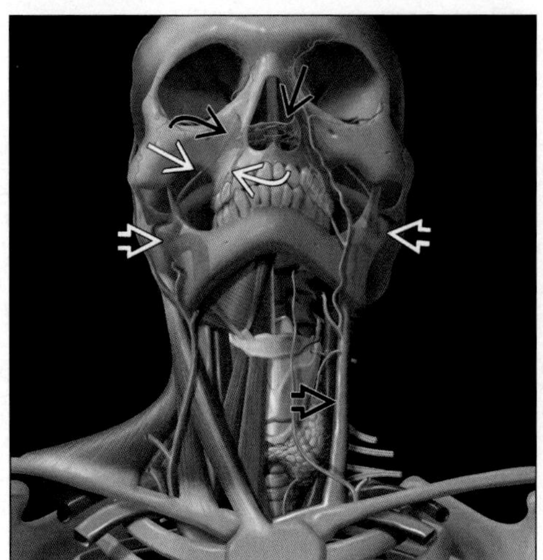

Graphic shows the pituitary venous plexus which drains into the cavernous sinuses. These drain via the superior and inferior petrosal sinuses into the sigmoid sinuses and the internal jugular veins.

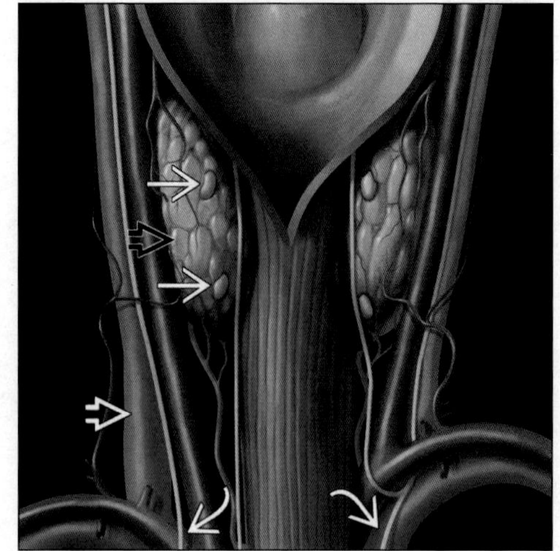

Graphic shows the normal location of the parathyroid glands on the posterior aspect of the thyroid gland. The thyroid and parathyroid glands drain into both internal jugular and brachiocephalic veins.

TERMINOLOGY

Abbreviations

- Bilateral inferior petrosal sinus sampling (BIPSS)
- Arterial stimulation and selective venous sampling (ASVS) for pancreatic endocrine tumors
- Selective venous sampling (SVS) for primary hyperparathyroidism

Definitions

- Bilateral inferior petrosal sinus sampling: Venous blood sampling from both inferior petrosal sinuses
  - Evaluates for ACTH secreting pituitary corticotrope adenoma as etiology for endogenous Cushing syndrome
  - Considered "gold standard" for confirming origin of ACTH secretion in Cushing syndrome
- Arterial stimulation and selective venous sampling
  - Used for pre-operative localization of pancreatic endocrine tumors
    - Evaluates for gastrinoma, insulinoma, VIPoma, glucagonoma, somatostatinoma, pancreatic polypeptide producing tumor (PPoma)
- Selective venous sampling for primary hyperparathyroidism
  - Used for pre-operative localization of functioning parathyroid adenoma that cannot be localized by noninvasive imaging
    - Used with negative or inconclusive noninvasive findings and prior noncurative neck surgery for primary hyperparathyroidism

PRE-PROCEDURE

Indications

- Cushing syndrome: Clinical complex resulting from prolonged, inappropriate exposure to glucocorticoids
  - Most frequently caused by administration of exogenous glucocorticoids or adrenocorticotrophic hormone (ACTH)
  - Endogenous causes include ACTH secreting pituitary tumor, adrenal neoplasm (benign or malignant) or ectopic ACTH secretion by tumor
    - Pituitary or ectopic sources generally have elevated serum ACTH levels
    - In endogenous Cushing syndrome, urinary cortisol excretion elevated; plasma levels fail to drop in response to dose of dexamethasone
  - 40-50% of pituitary Cushing disease cases will have no pituitary lesion on MR; also demonstrating a lesion does not imply functionality
    - 10% of population age 30-40 harbor incidental pituitary abnormality
    - BIPSS improves diagnostic accuracy in distinguishing pituitary vs. ectopic source of ACTH
- Pre-operative localization of pancreatic endocrine tumors
  - Insulinoma accounts for 50-60%
    - Symptoms: Hypoglycemia, palpitations, diplopia; elevated serum insulin and C-peptide levels
    - 75% solitary and benign; 10% malignant
  - Gastrinoma (20% incidence)
    - Causes Zollinger-Ellison syndrome: Severe peptic ulcer disease, gastric hypersecretion, elevated serum gastrin and non-B islet cell tumor
    - 60% of gastrinomas intrapancreatic and 40% extrapancreatic; often multiple
- Primary hyperparathyroidism
  - Estimated prevalence of 1:1,000
    - Corrected calcium > 2.65 mmol/L on 2 occasions
    - Inappropriately high or normal parathyroid hormone (PTH) level
    - Urine fractional calcium excretion ratio > 0.01
  - 85% of cases secondary to parathyroid adenoma

VENOUS SAMPLING: ENDOCRINE (NON-ADRENAL)

Key Facts

Terminology

- Inferior petrosal sinus sampling (BIPSS): Obtaining blood samples from both inferior petrosal sinuses
  - Evaluates for ACTH secreting pituitary adenoma as etiology for endogenous Cushing syndrome
- Arterial stimulation and selective venous sampling (ASVS)
  - Used for pancreatic endocrine tumor localization
- Selective venous sampling for primary hyperparathyroidism (SVS)
  - Used with negative or inconclusive noninvasive findings and prior noncurative neck surgery for primary hyperparathyroidism

Pre-procedure

- BIPSS improves diagnostic accuracy in distinguishing pituitary vs. ectopic source of ACTH

Procedure

- For BIPSS obtain venous samples simultaneously from both internal jugular veins for baseline followed by samples from both inferior petrosal sinuses
  - Basal ratio of central to peripheral ACTH ratio > 2 or stimulated interpetrosal sinus ratio of > 1.4 localizes pituitary microadenoma
- For ASVS, calcium secretogue causes rise in hepatic vein insulin or gastrin level (> 50% is positive)
  - Tumor site predicted by arterial injection locale
- For SVS for hyperparathyroidism obtain blood samples from neck and mediastinal veins at multiple levels
  - Positive sample is twice peripheral PTH measurement; reported by catheter position

---

    - 10% of parathyroid adenomas may be in ectopic location, with 5-10% of parathyroid glands in ectopic location
    - Ectopic locations: 10% anterior mediastinum, 3-5% posterior mediastinum, 1-3% within thyroid gland and 1% retroesophageal
  - Failure and complication rates of repeat parathyroid surgery are increased compared with initial operations because of scarring
  - Pre-operative localization studies used before repeat surgery for persistent hyperparathyroidism
    - Can reduce complexity of repeat surgical dissection and complication rate
    - Noninvasive localization procedures include ultrasonography, scintigraphy (technetium Tc-99m sestamibi), CT and MR
    - Invasive procedure of selective venous sampling (SVS) also used for localization
    - SVS frequently indispensable when noninvasive procedures have negative or inconclusive findings and has undergone prior neck surgery

Getting Started

- Medications
  - BIPSS: 100 micrograms of corticotrophin releasing hormone (CRH)
  - ASVS: 5 mL of calcium gluconate (0.025 mEq calcium/kg)
- Equipment List
  - Angiographic sheaths and catheters
  - Iodinated contrast medium
  - Blood sample collection vials

PROCEDURE

Patient Position/Location

- Best procedure approach
  - Introduction of two selective catheters from common femoral vein, via separate vascular sheaths
    - Both sheaths may be introduced from same femoral vein or from bilateral femoral approach

Procedure Steps

- Bilateral inferior petrosal sinus sampling
  - Obtain access from common femoral vein punctures, with introduction of two separate vascular sheaths
  - Introduce two separate selective catheters into the right and left internal jugular veins
    - Obtain venous samples simultaneously from both internal jugular veins for baseline followed by samples from both inferior petrosal sinuses
    - Inject 100 micrograms of stimulating agent, corticotrophin releasing hormone (CRH), intravenously
    - Obtain inferior petrosal sinus and peripheral blood samples 5 and 10 minutes after IV CRH stimulation
  - Label all tubes with attention to right vs. left
  - Submit samples for laboratory assays
- Arterial stimulation and selective venous sampling for pancreatic endocrine tumors
  - Obtain arterial and venous access from common femoral punctures, with introduction of two separate vascular sheaths
  - Introduce cobra catheter into right or middle hepatic vein
  - Introduce arterial catheter selectively into SMA, hepatic, gastroduodenal or splenic artery
    - Obtain two baseline hepatic venous blood samples
    - Perform selective angiography at each arterial site obtain hepatic venous samples every 30 seconds for three minutes; repeat in each arterial site
    - After each arteriogram inject 5 mL of calcium gluconate via arterial catheter; obtain hepatic vein samples every 30 seconds for three minutes
    - Allow 5 minutes between each calcium stimulation; repeat in each arterial site
- Selective venous sampling for 1° hyperparathyroidism
  - Obtain venous access from common femoral vein puncture, with introduction of vascular sheath
    - Introduce selective catheter for venous sampling
  - Obtain blood samples from neck and mediastinal veins at multiple levels

VENOUS SAMPLING: ENDOCRINE (NON-ADRENAL)

- Both internal jugular veins: Distal, mid and proximal
- Both subclavian veins: Distal and proximal
- Both brachiocephalic veins: distal and proximal
- Right and left inferior thyroidal veins
- Thymic vein
- SVC

Findings and Reporting

- Bilateral inferior petrosal sinus sampling
  - Basal ratio of central to peripheral ACTH ratio > 2 considered positive
  - Because ACTH secretion is episodic, CSH stimulation used to increase sensitivity; peak stimulated ratio > 3 strongly indicative of Cushing disease
  - Interpetrosal sinus ratio of > 1.4 indicative of ipsilateral localization of pituitary microadenoma
- Arterial stimulation and selective venous sampling for pancreatic endocrine tumors
  - Calcium secretogue will cause rise in insulin or gastrin level in hepatic vein (> 50% is positive)
  - Reported by which arterial injection site causes hormonal rise; predicts tumor site within pancreas
- Selective venous sampling for 1° hyperparathyroidism
  - Positive sample is twice peripheral PTH measurement; reported by catheter position
  - Peripheral serum measurement calculated as average of subclavian vein samples

Alternative Procedures/Therapies

- Radiologic
  - Alternatives to selective venous sampling in primary hyperparathyroidism
    - Parathyroid ultrasound can localize and distinguish enlarged glands but is operator dependent; less sensitive for ectopic locations
    - Tc-99m Sestamibi parathyroid scintigraphy uses radioisotope accumulation within thyroid and parathyroid tissue for localizing glands
    - Radioisotope clears more quickly from thyroid than parathyroid tissue enabling localization
    - Combined ultrasound and Tc-99m Sestamibi have greater sensitivity than as independent modalities
    - CECT and MR useful for ectopic gland detection
  - Alternatives to arterial stimulation and selective venous sampling for pancreatic endocrine tumors
    - CECT with imaging in arterial and venous phases
    - MR with fast spin echo, fat-saturation sequences and dynamic contrast-enhanced imaging more sensitive than CECT
    - Endoscopic ultrasound can precisely localize small lesions, but less sensitive in pancreatic tail; high false positive rate
    - Somatostatin-receptor scintigraphy (indium-111 pentotreotide); less sensitive for insulinoma
    - Transhepatic portal venous sampling has 0.7% mortality and 9.2% morbidity and thus abandoned in favor of ASVS
- Surgical
  - Alternatives to bilateral inferior petrosal sinus sampling in ACTH-dependent Cushing disease
    - ACTH-dependent Cushing disease and pituitary macroademona: Surgery without sampling
    - Normal scan or pituitary microadenoma: BIPSS prior to surgery

POST-PROCEDURE

Things To Do

- When obtaining venous samples, note time obtained and label all tubes with attention to right vs. left
- Collect samples in appropriate containers for laboratory analysis; conform to lab requirements for accurate sample analysis (e.g., refrigerated sample)

Things To Avoid

- False negative ASVS results in patients on diazoxide; stop medication prior to ASVS

PROBLEMS & COMPLICATIONS

Complications

- Most feared complication(s)
  - Complications common to all procedures include
    - Contrast reaction, contrast-induced nephropathy
    - Hematoma at puncture site, venous thrombosis
  - Complications of BIPSS include
    - Brainstem stroke, subarachnoid hemorrhage, cavernous sinus thrombosis, cranial nerve palsies
  - Complications of arterial stimulation and venous sampling for pancreatic endocrine tumors include
    - Hypoglycemia from systemic release of insulin during calcium stimulation, hypercalcemia from injection of calcium gluconate (both rare)

SELECTED REFERENCES

1. Ito F et al: The utility of intraoperative bilateral internal jugular venous sampling with rapid parathyroid hormone testing. Ann Surg. 245(6):959-63, 2007
2. Lad SP et al: The role of inferior petrosal sinus sampling in the diagnostic localization of Cushing's disease. Neurosurg Focus. 23(3):E2, 2007
3. Lau JH et al: The current role of venous sampling in the localization of endocrine disease. Cardiovasc Intervent Radiol. 30(4):555-70, 2007
4. Moriyama T et al: Diagnosis of a case of ectopic parathyroid adenoma on the early image of 99mTc-MIBI scintigram. Endocr J. 54(3):437-40, 2007
5. Tseng LM et al: The role of intra-arterial calcium stimulation test with hepatic venous sampling (IACS) in the management of occult insulinomas. Ann Surg Oncol. 14(7):2121-7, 2007
6. Eloy JA et al: Preoperative selective venous sampling for nonlocalizing parathyroid adenomas. Thyroid. 16(8):787-90, 2006
7. Ogilvie CM et al: Selective parathyroid venous sampling in patients with complicated hyperparathyroidism. Eur J Endocrinol. 155(6):813-21, 2006
8. Reidel MA et al: Localization of hyperfunctioning parathyroid glands by selective venous sampling in reoperation for primary or secondary hyperparathyroidism. Surgery. 140(6):907-13; discussion 913, 2006
9. Sung YM et al: Selective intra-arterial calcium stimulation with hepatic venous sampling for preoperative localization of insulinomas. Korean J Radiol. 4(2):101-8, 2003

IMAGE GALLERY

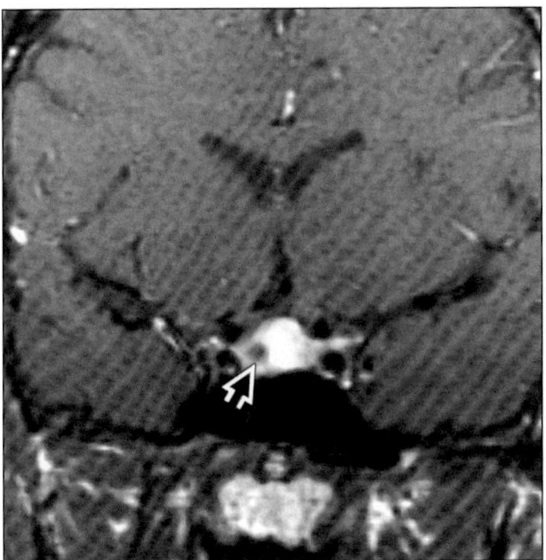

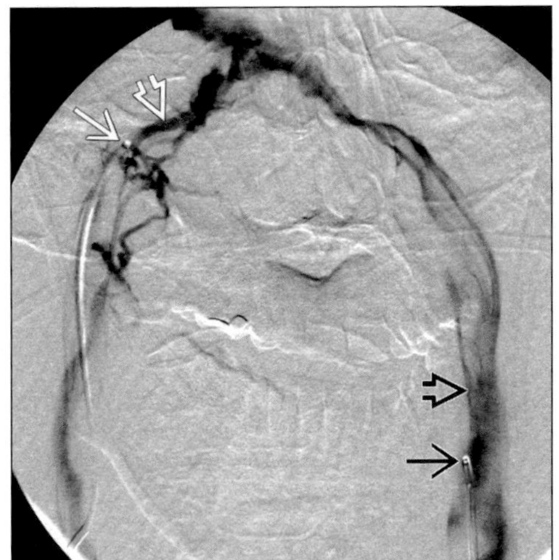

(Left) *Coronal T1WI MR with gadolinium shows a right-sided nonenhancing focus ➡ in the pituitary gland suspicious for a microadenoma in a patient with elevated serum ACTH levels.* ***(Right)*** *Venogram (same patient as previous image) during inferior petrosal sinus sampling shows a catheter ➡ in right inferior petrosal sinus ➡ & another catheter → in left internal jugular vein ⇨. Left catheter will be advanced into inferior petrosal sinus for simultaneous sinus sampling.*

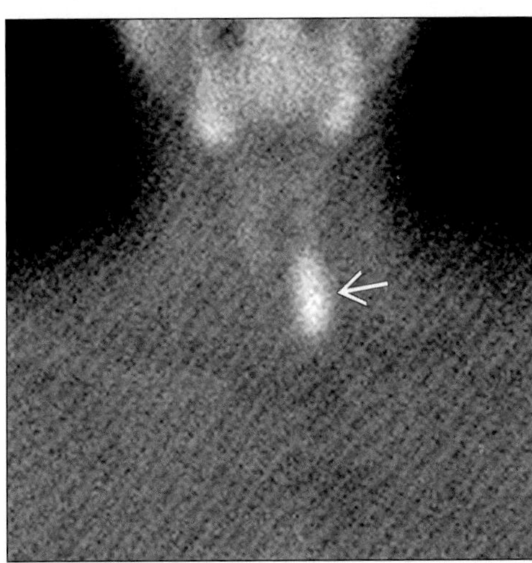

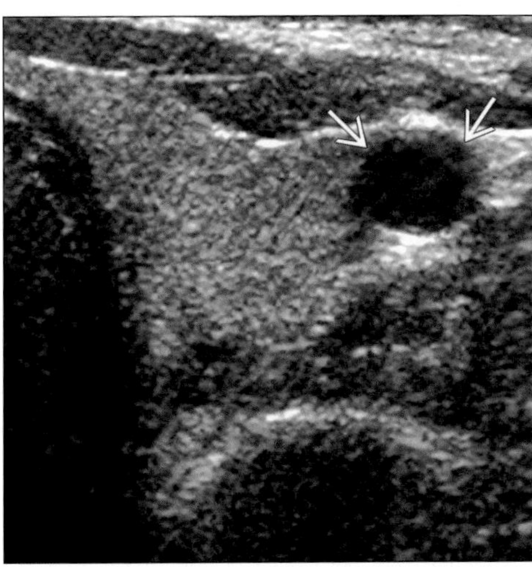

(Left) *Tc-99m sestamibi radionuclide scan obtained in a patient with primary hyperparathyroidism shows radioisotope accumulation ➡ over the lower left lobe of the thyroid gland, suspicious for a functioning parathyroid adenoma.* ***(Right)*** *Axial ultrasound examination shows a nodule ➡ in the lower left lobe of the thyroid gland, corresponding to the radioisotope accumulation on the radionuclide scan & confirming the suspected parathyroid adenoma.*

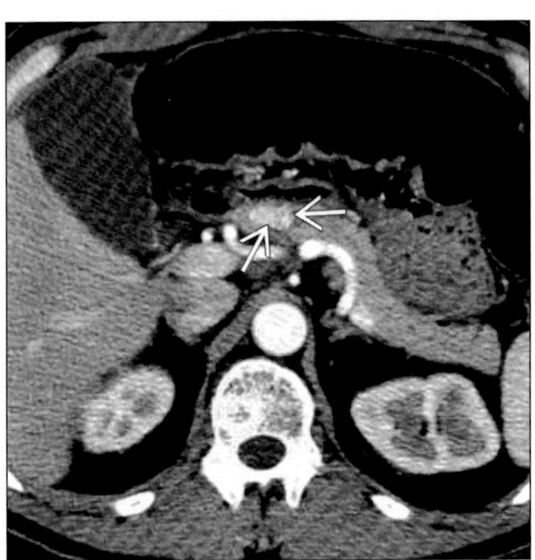

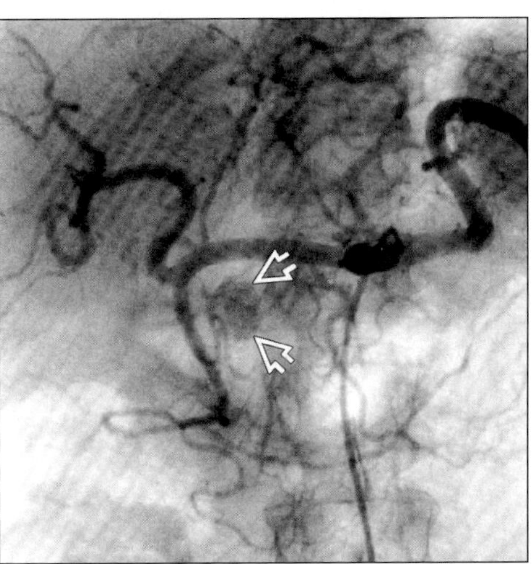

(Left) *Axial CECT shows an enhancing area ➡ in the pancreas in a patient with severe hypoglycemia, tachycardia and diplopia. Laboratory tests showed elevated serum insulin & C-peptide levels.* ***(Right)*** *Celiac arteriogram shows an enhancing mass ➡ corresponding to the CECT abnormality (previous image). Arterial stimulation & venous sampling were unnecessary, as the imaging findings & laboratory data were sufficient to diagnose an insulinoma.*

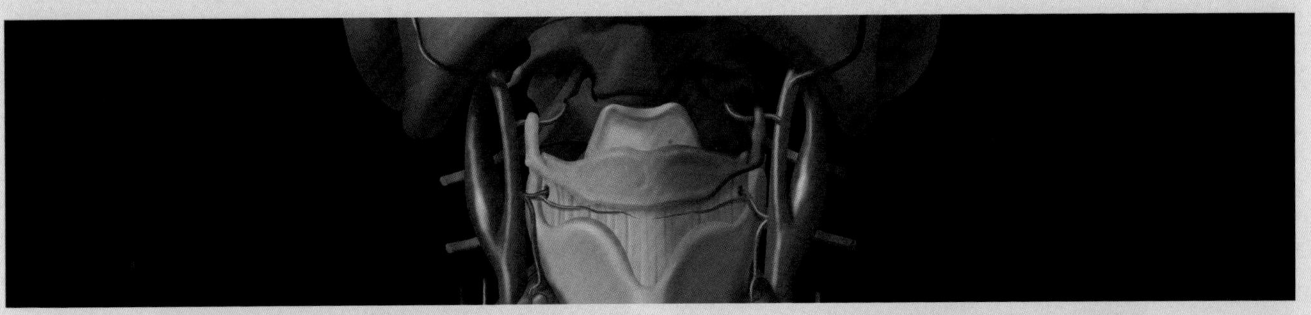

SECTION 2: Head & Neck

Introduction and Overview

Head & Neck

HEAD & NECK VASCULATURE

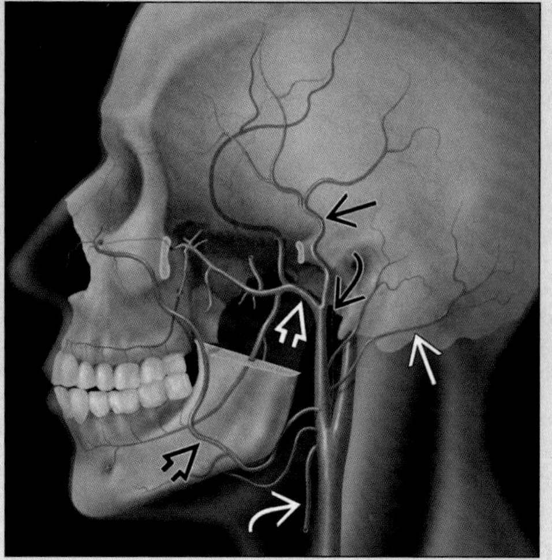
Lateral graphic of the carotid arterial system depicts branches of the ECA: SThA ➡, FA ➡, IMA ➡, OA ➡, APA ➡, STA ➡. LA below FA. PAA above OA. MMA 1st branch of IMA.

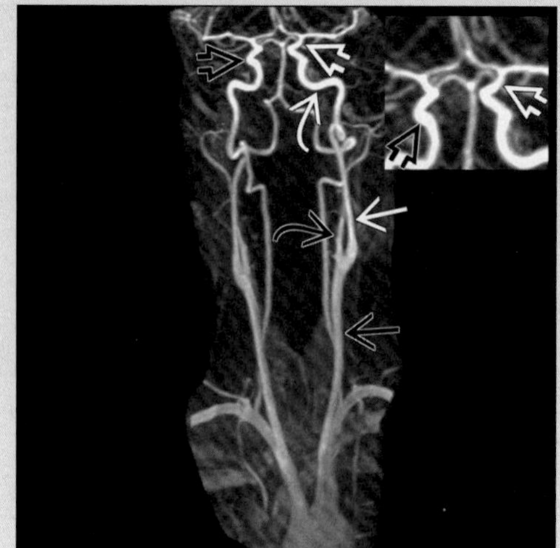
Anteroposterior 3D TOF MRA MIP image of the neck shows carotid arterial vasculature: CCA ➡, ECA ➡, cervical ICA ➡, petrous ICA ➡, cavernous ICA ➡, supraclinoid ICA ➡.

TERMINOLOGY

Abbreviations

- Aortic arch (AA); innominate artery (IA)
- Common/internal/external carotid, posterior cerebral arteries (CCA, ICA, ECA, PCA)
- Subclavian, vertebral, basilar, posterior inferior cerebellar arteries (SCA, VA, BA, PICA)
- Superior thyroid, ascending pharyngeal, lingual, facial, occipital, posterior auricular, superficial temporal, internal maxillary, middle meningeal arteries (SThA, APA, LA, FA, OA, PAA, STA, IMA, MMA)
- Caroticotympanic, vidian, superior hypophyseal, ophthalmic, posterior communicating, anterior choroidal arteries (CTA, ViA, SHA, OpA, PCoA, AChA)
- Meningohypophyseal, inferolateral trunks (MHT, ILT)
- Cavernous/sigmoid sinuses, pterygoid/vertebral venous plexuses (CS, SigS, PVP, VVP)
- Superficial temporal, superior/inferior orbital, facial, deep facial, maxillary, retromandibular, subclavian, brachiocephalic, internal/external jugular veins (STV, SOV, IOV, FV, DFV, MV, RV, SCV, BCV, IJV, EJV)

IMAGING ANATOMY

Anatomic Relationships

- Right CCA originates from IA (IA first branch of AA), left CCA from AA (second branch); course superiorly in carotid space of neck, anteromedial to IJV
- CCA divides into ICA, ECA; usually at C3-4
  - Variant: CCA bifurcation can be from T2 to C2
- ECA: Usually anteromedial to ICA; 8 branches
  - SThA: Arises from proximal anterior ECA (may arise from CCA); supplies superior thyroid, larynx
  - APA: Arises from proximal posterior ECA (or CCA bifurcation), courses between ECA/ICA in carotid sheath; supplies nasopharynx, oropharynx, middle ear, prevertebral muscles, CN 9-11
    - Anastomoses with MMA, CTA, ViA
  - LA: Second anterior ECA branch; supplies tongue, oral cavity, submandibular gland
  - FA: Originates above LA; supplies face, palate, lip
    - Anastomoses with OpA
  - OA: Second posterior ECA branch; supplies scalp, upper cervical musculature, posterior fossa meninges
    - Anastomoses with VA muscular branches
  - PAA: Originates above OA; supplies pinna, scalp, external auditory canal
  - STA: Smaller terminal ECA branch; supplies scalp
  - IMA: Larger terminal ECA branch, extends to pterygopalatine fossa; supplies cranial meninges (via MMA), deep face, nose
    - Anastomoses with ViA, ILT, OpA
- ICA: Usually posterolateral to ECA; 4 segments
  - Cervical segment: Courses superiorly within carotid space of neck; no named branches
    - Carotid bulb: Focal dilatation at ICA origin, has autonomic neural plexus (chemo-/baroreceptors)
  - Petrous segment: Within carotid canal of skull base; branches: CTA (supplies middle ear), ViA (supplies greater superficial petrosal nerve)
    - CTA, ViA anastomoses with IMA, APA
  - Cavernous segment: Portion of vessel within CS; branches: MHT (supplies pituitary, tentorium and clival dura), ILT (supplies CS dura, CN 3-6)
    - ILT anastomoses with IMA via foramen rotundum
  - Supraclinoid segment: Intracranial (subarachnoid) most distal part of vessel; branches: SHA (supplies optic nerve/chiasm, infundibulum, anterior pituitary), OpA (supplies ocular globe, orbit, rectus muscles, lacrimal gland), PCoA (joins with PCA), AChA (supplies posterior limb of internal capsule, temporal lobe choroid plexus)
    - OpA anastomoses with IMA, FA
  - Variant: Medial origin of ICA from CCA in 10-15%
  - Anomalies: Aberrant ICA: Petrous segment courses more posterolaterally, appears as hypotympanic mass; persistent stapedial artery: Arises from vertical petrous segment, enlarges tympanic segment of facial nerve canal, terminates as MMA (foramen spinosum absent); persistent carotid-vertebrobasilar anastomoses (trigeminal, otic, hypoglossal, proatlantal-intersegmental arteries)

HEAD & NECK VASCULATURE

Head & Neck Vascular Pathologic Entities

Vascular

- Carotid/vertebral stenosis, thrombosis
- Carotid/vertebral dissection, pseudoaneurysm
- Vertebrobasilar insufficiency, subclavian steal
- Carotid/vertebral fibromuscular dysplasia
- Arteriovenous fistula (carotid-cavernous fistula)
- Radiation vasculopathy
- Congenital vessel aplasia/hypoplasia, aberrant internal carotid artery, persistent stapedial artery
- Jugular vein thrombosis, thrombophlebitis
- Dehiscent jugular bulb, jugular bulb diverticulum
- Cervical spinal cord infarction, AVM, AV fistula

Neoplasm

- Juvenile nasopharyngeal angiofibroma
- Glomus jugulare/tympanicum paraganglioma
- Glomus vagale paraganglioma
- Carotid body paraganglioma
- Squamous cell carcinoma vascular invasion

- Right SCA originates from IA, left SCA from AA (third branch)
- VA: First branch of SCA, 4 segments
  - Extraosseous segment: SCA to C6 transverse foramen; cervical muscular/spinal artery branches
  - Foraminal segment: Ascends through C6-C3 foramina, turns superolaterally to course around C2, extends superiorly to C1 transverse foramen; anterior meningeal, muscular/spinal artery branches
  - Extraspinal segment: Exits top of C1, curves posteromedially around atlantooccipital joint, turns sharply anterosuperiorly to pierce dura at foramen magnum; posterior meningeal artery branch
    - Extraosseous to extraspinal segments have multiple anastomoses with ECA
  - Intradural (intracranial) segment: Courses supermedially behind clivus, unites with contralateral VA to form BA; anterior/posterior spinal artery, perforating medullary, PICA branches
  - Variants: Left dominant VA in 75%, right dominant 10-15%, co-dominant 10-15%; AA origin of left VA in 5% (usually hypoplastic VA)
  - Anomalies: Persistent carotid-vertebrobasilar anastomoses; VA/BA fenestration/duplication (increased prevalence of aneurysms)
- Extracranial veins
  - STV: Drains scalp and emissary/diploic veins
    - Emissary/diploic veins connect with meningeal veins, dural sinuses via transcranial channels
  - FV: Drains superficial orbit, face, jaw into IJV
  - SOV/IOV: Drains deep orbit structures to CS
  - DFV: Drains deep facial structures to PVP
  - PVP: Network of vascular channels in masticator space; connects DFV with CS, clival venous plexus; also drains superficially into MV
  - RV: Formed from union of STV, MV; lies within parotid space; drains into IJV, EJV
  - EJV: Drains RV, auricular/occipital veins from scalp/ear/face; size variable
  - IJV: Caudal continuation of SigS, courses inferiorly in carotid space of neck, joins SCV to form BCV
    - Jugular bulb: Dilatation at junction of SigS, IJV
  - VVP: Tributaries from clival/cervical epidural venous plexuses, cervical vertebral/muscular veins; interconnects with SigS; terminates in BCV
  - Variants: Extracranial venous drainage highly variable; Right/left IJV size asymmetry common

CLINICAL IMPLICATIONS

Clinical Importance

- Multiple anastomoses between ICA/ECA/VA possible collateral pathways but also potentially dangerous connections during endovascular embolization
- Horner syndrome from interruption of periarterial sympathetic plexus around ICA (e.g., dissection)
- Paraganglioma neoplasms derive from periarterial autonomic nerves/neural plexus
- Collateral enlargement of scalp/emissary veins, SOV/IOV with dural AV/carotid-cavernous fistula or dural sinus occlusion

IMAGE GALLERY

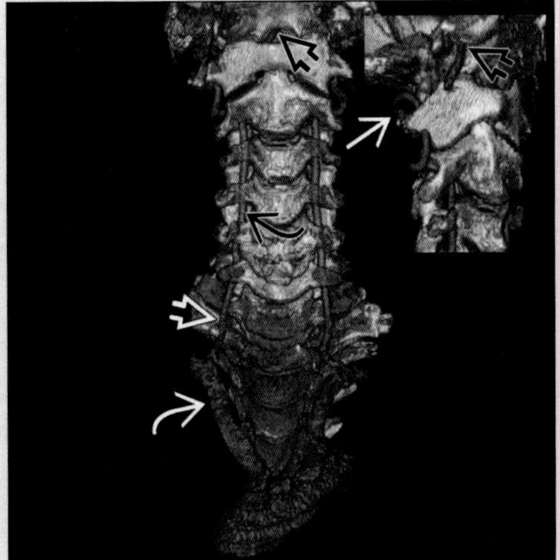

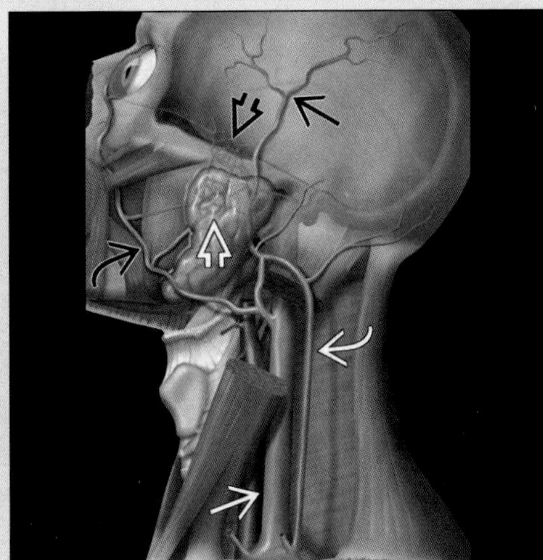

(Left) *Anteroposterior CTA 3D image of the neck (with AP oblique inset) shows VA vasculature: SCA, extraosseous VA, foraminal VA, extraspinal VA, intradural VA.* ***(Right)*** *Lateral graphic demonstrates the extracranial venous system: STV, FV, EJV, IJV, CS, PVP. SOV/IOV drain to CS. RV within parotid gland drains STV.*

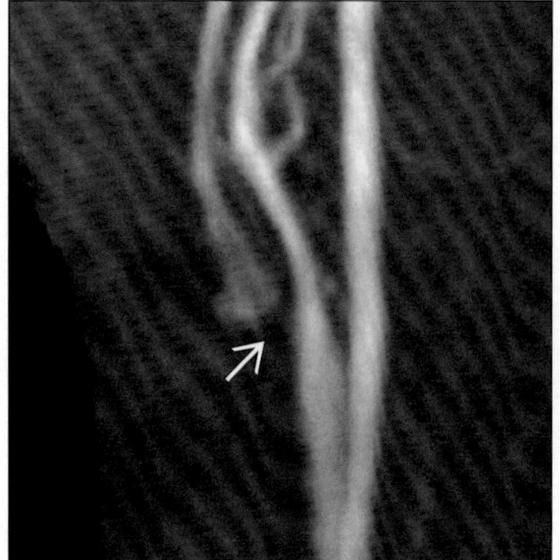

Sagittal Gd-enhanced MRA of the carotid bifurcation shows a "flow-gap" at the ICA origin ➡. MRA typically overestimates the degree of stenosis.

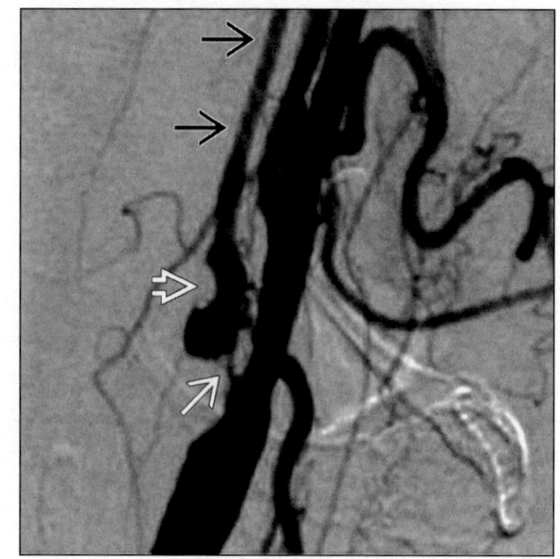

Lateral CCA DSA shows a high-grade stenosis of the ICA ➡ and indentation of vessel lumen by plaque ⮕. Note gracile cervical ICA ➔ due to proximal flow restriction.

TERMINOLOGY

Abbreviations and Synonyms

- Carotid atherosclerotic vascular disease (ASVD)

Definitions

- Narrowing of cervical segment of internal carotid artery (ICA) or common carotid artery (CCA)

IMAGING FINDINGS

General Features

- Best diagnostic clue: Carotid duplex US shows vessel narrowing with turbulent flow, increased peak systolic velocity, spectral broadening
- Location: Extracranial carotid ASVD most common at carotid bulb
- Size: Variable stenosis severity and length; usually < 3 cm
- Smooth or irregular narrowing ± ulceration ± intraluminal thrombus

CT Findings

- NECT
  - Calcified ASVD plaque at CCA bifurcation ± ICA
  - May see thromboembolic or hemodynamic cerebral infarction
    - Typically ipsilateral anterior circulation
    - Posterior cerebral artery (PCA) stroke possible via posterior communicating artery (PCoA) or fetal PCA
- CTA
  - Useful as screening tool
  - CTA allows estimation of stenosis severity
    - Multiplanar reformatted images in sagittal and coronal planes are helpful
    - Accuracy reduced if extensive lesional calcification is present
  - Dental amalgam artifacts may hinder visualization
  - May see intraluminal thrombus as filling defect within enhanced vessel
  - Unreliable visualization of plaque ulceration
  - Patchy/homogeneous low density in wall may be seen with large necrotic/lipid plaque

DDx: Non-ASVD Carotid Stenoses

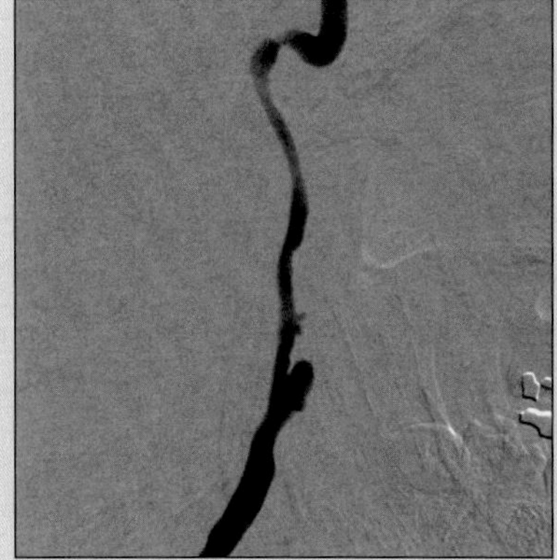

Carotid Dissection

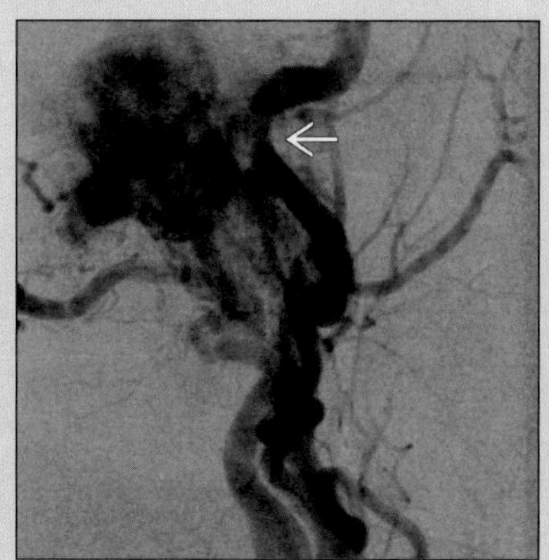

Tumor Compression

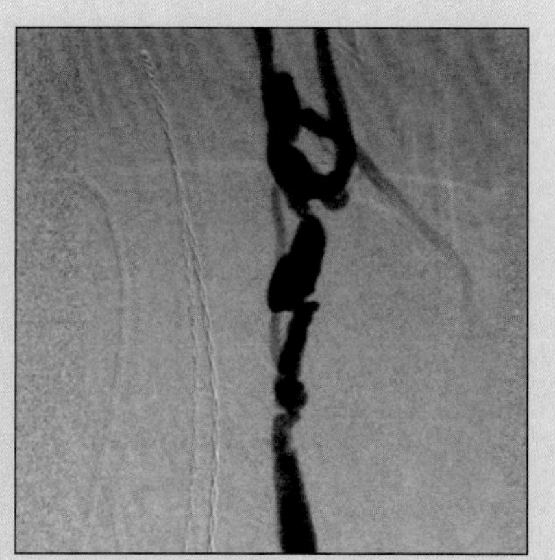

Fibromuscular Dysplasia

CAROTID STENOSIS, EXTRACRANIAL

Key Facts

Imaging Findings

- Best diagnostic clue: Carotid duplex US shows vessel narrowing with turbulent flow, increased peak systolic velocity, spectral broadening
- CTA allows estimation of stenosis severity
- Time of flight (TOF) MRA: Intravoxel dephasing causes signal loss with flow turbulence due to stenosis
- DSA = gold standard for evaluation of carotid stenosis severity
- "String sign" = very high-grade stenosis, slow antegrade "trickle" blood flow

Pathology

- Risk of stroke increases with stenosis severity, an indirect measure of plaque volume and potential for complicated plaque/embolization
- Irregular plaque surface: ↑ Stroke risk on medical treatment for all degrees of stenosis

Clinical Issues

- Stroke is the third most common cause of death in Western countries
- Transient ischemic attacks (TIA): Neurological deficit that spontaneously resolves in < 24 hrs
- Reversible ischemic neurological deficit (RIND): Neurological deficit > 24 hrs but < 3 wks
- Asymptomatic carotid bruit: 20% have > 60% ICA stenosis (3x normal population)
- Carotid artery stenting (CAS) becoming increasingly utilized and substantiated as a viable alternative to CEA
- CAS with distal protection device associated with risk of peri-procedural stroke ≤ CEA

MR Findings

- T1WI
  - Reduced caliber of ICA flow void ± intraluminal signal due to thrombus or slow flow
  - Fat-saturated sequence if dissection is suspected as alternate etiology
    - Intramural crescentic high signal represents methemoglobin in vessel wall (dissection)
- DWI: Most sensitive and specific for acute/subacute ischemic/infarction
- MRA
  - Provides multidirectional imaging (vs. conventional DSA)
  - Time of flight (TOF) MRA: Intravoxel dephasing causes signal loss with flow turbulence due to stenosis
    - Affects 2D > 3D TOF images
    - Accentuates stenosis severity
    - Gadolinium enhanced MRA superior to TOF sequences
  - "Flow gap" can occur in stenoses (> 95%) causing misdiagnosis of occlusion
- Brain T2WI, FLAIR, DWI may show "rosary-like" lesions in centrum semiovale ipsilateral to stenosis indicative of watershed ischemia/infarction

Ultrasonographic Findings

- Grayscale Ultrasound: Calcified plaque causes acoustic shadowing and may limit assessment of vessel lumen
- Pulsed Doppler
  - Duplex US: Flow velocity within stenosis proportional to stenosis severity
  - Flow turbulence within and beyond stenosis
  - Spectral broadening: Increased range of velocities seen in moderate to severe stenoses

Other Modality Findings

- CT/MR perfusion
  - Can provide assessment of collateral flow to the territory normally perfused by the stenotic carotid artery
  - Collateral circulation correlates with risk of hemodynamic ischemia/infarction
- Measurement of carotid stenosis severity
  - NASCET method widely accepted (> ECST)
  - NASCET: Denominator is normal post-stenotic ICA diameter
  - ECST: Denominator is estimated normal diameter of carotid bulb

Angiographic Findings

- Conventional
  - DSA = gold standard for evaluation of carotid stenosis severity
  - Use of "reverse-curve" catheters (e.g., Simmons) can avoid inadvertent crossing of carotid bifurcation stenosis with guidewire and dislodgement of plaque
  - Intraluminal thrombus seen as filling defect in contrast column
  - Can evaluate collateral flow to ischemic hemisphere from communicating arteries and leptomeningeal collaterals by studying contralateral ICA and dominant vertebral artery
  - "String sign" = very high-grade stenosis, slow antegrade "trickle" blood flow
    - Typically seen during after arterial phase of angiogram
    - May require prolonged DSA acquisitions for visualization
    - Preocclusive state with high risk of stroke
    - Important as carotid endarterectomy (CEA) or carotid artery stenting (CAS) may be an option if ICA still patent
  - More sensitive and specific than CTA and MRA for subtotal occlusion with "string sign"

Imaging Recommendations

- Ultrasound or CTA as screening tool
- CTA/MRA for comprehensive cerebrovascular evaluation
- DSA if US/CTA/MRA are equivocal or show "occlusion"

CAROTID STENOSIS, EXTRACRANIAL

DIFFERENTIAL DIAGNOSIS

Extrinsic Compressive Lesion (Rare)

- Carotid space neoplasm (e.g., carotid body paraganglioma, glomus jugulare tumor)

Dissection

- Typically spares carotid bulb and ICA origin
- Usually no Ca++ (dystrophic calcification is rare)
- Intimal flap with differential filling of true and false lumens on DSA
- Crescentic intramural high signal (methemoglobin) on T1WI MR

Fibromuscular Dysplasia

- Affects medium to large arteries
- M:F = 1:3
- Age peak: 25-50 yrs
- Classically see alternating segments of beading and stenoses involving extracranial ICA, ECA, vertebral & renal arteries

PATHOLOGY

General Features

- General path comments: Significant ICA narrowing identified in 20-30% of carotid territory strokes (vs. 5-10% of general population)
- Etiology
  - Risk of stroke increases with stenosis severity, an indirect measure of plaque volume and potential for complicated plaque/embolization
    - Larger plaques are complicated by hemorrhage, necrosis, disruption of fibrous cap and intima, causing embolization
  - Plaque composition and surface morphology also stroke risk factors
  - Irregular plaque surface: ↑ Stroke risk on medical treatment for all degrees of stenosis
  - Hypoperfusion may cause "watershed" infarcts, centrum semiovale lesions

Gross Pathologic & Surgical Features

- Fatty streak: Raised lesion due to fatty deposit in intima
- Fibrous (fibrolipid) plaque: Cholesterol + fibrous tissue with collagen cap
- Complicated plaque: Unstable, may rupture, thrombose, calcify, hemorrhage

Microscopic Features

- ASVD: Fatty streaks, lipid-laden macrophages & smooth muscle cells, fibrous cap, cholesterol deposits, foam cells, plaque rupture ± thrombus

CLINICAL ISSUES

Presentation

- Stroke is the third most common cause of death in Western countries
- Transient ischemic attacks (TIA): Neurological deficit that spontaneously resolves in < 24 hrs
  - 80% resolve in < 1 hr
  - Precede 30% of strokes
  - 50% of subsequent strokes occurs < 1 yr from TIA
- Reversible ischemic neurological deficit (RIND): Neurological deficit > 24 hrs but < 3 wks
- Amaurosis fugax (transient, monocular embolic blindness)
- Asymptomatic carotid bruit: 20% have > 60% ICA stenosis (3x normal population)

Natural History & Prognosis

- Progressive

Treatment

- Risk factor reduction (hypertension, smoking, diabetic control, hypercholesterolemia)
- Medical: Aspirin, statins
- NASCET (1991)
  - Symptomatic stenosis ≥ 70% associated with significant stroke risk, benefits from endarterectomy (CEA)
  - Symptomatic moderate stenosis (50-69%) also benefits from endarterectomy in selected cases
- ACAS (1995)
  - Asymptomatic patients benefit from endarterectomy with stenosis of 60%
- Carotid artery stenting (CAS) becoming increasingly utilized and substantiated as a viable alternative to CEA
- CAS with distal protection device associated with risk of peri-procedural stroke ≤ CEA
- SAPPHIRE (2004)
  - Compared CEA with CAS in "high-risk" patients (comorbidities, age > 80 yrs, recent surgery, etc.) with symptomatic and asymptomatic carotid stenoses
  - Lower complication rate with CAS, no difference in stroke incidence after 3 yrs (7.1% CAS vs. 6.7% CEA)

DIAGNOSTIC CHECKLIST

Consider

- Use of "reverse-curve" catheters for catheterization of CCA when carotid stenosis is suspected

Image Interpretation Pearls

- MRA often exaggerates degree of stenosis
- Look for intraluminal filling defect (CAS is contraindicated if intraluminal thrombus is present)

SELECTED REFERENCES

1. Halliday A et al: Prevention of disabling and fatal strokes by successful carotid endarterectomy in patients without recent neurological symptoms: randomised controlled trial. Lancet. 363(9420):1491-502, 2004
2. Yadav JS: Carotid stenting in high-risk patients: design and rationale of the SAPPHIRE trial. Cleve Clin J Med. 71 Suppl 1:S45-6, 2004
3. No authors listed: Carotid endarterectomy for patients with asymptomatic internal carotid artery stenosis. National Institute of Neurological Disorders and Stroke. J Neurol Sci. 129(1):76-7, 1995

CAROTID STENOSIS, EXTRACRANIAL

IMAGE GALLERY

Typical

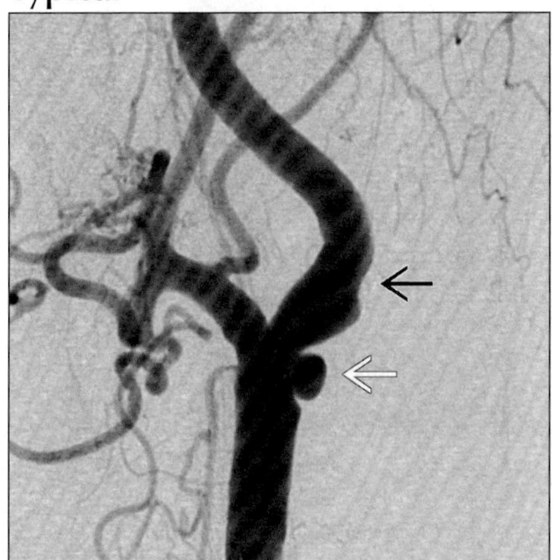

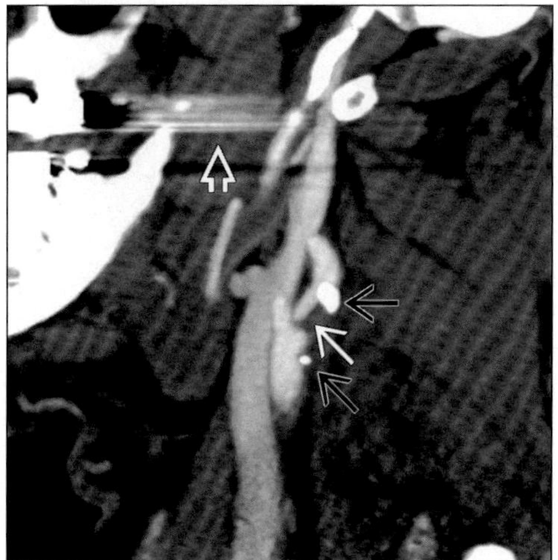

(Left) *Oblique CCA DSA shows an ulcerated ASVD plaque at the carotid bifurcation →. There is additional plaque distally → but no significant carotid stenosis.* ***(Right)*** *Sagittal CTA in a different patient shows a pinhole stenosis at the ICA origin →. Note adjacent calcification within ASVD plaque → and artifact from dental amalgam →.*

Typical

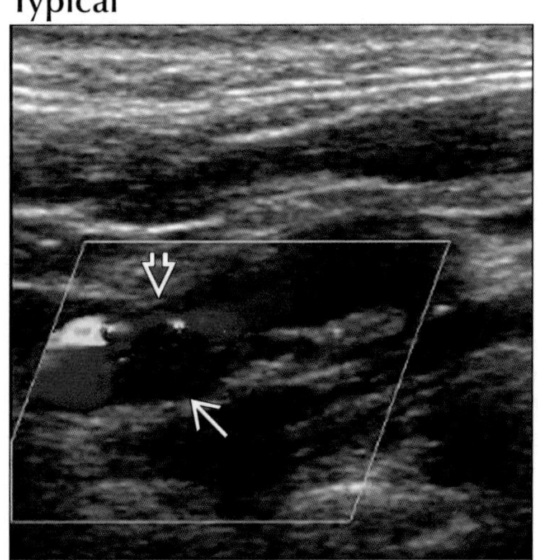

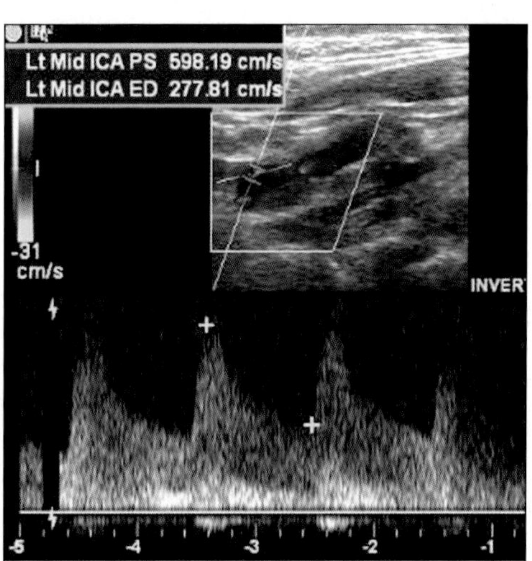

(Left) *Carotid duplex ultrasound of the proximal ICA shows moderate stenosis due to ASVD →. Within the stenotic segment there is flow turbulence as depicted by variations in color and intensity →.* ***(Right)*** *Carotid duplex spectral waveform in the same patient shows spectral broadening and a peak systolic velocity of 598 cm/s in keeping with a 70-99% stenosis.*

Typical

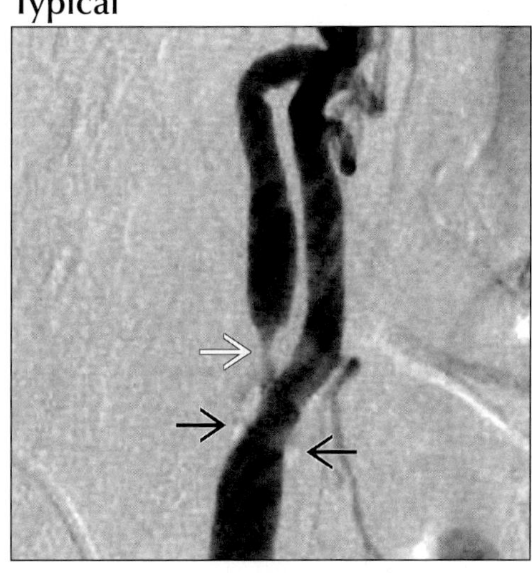

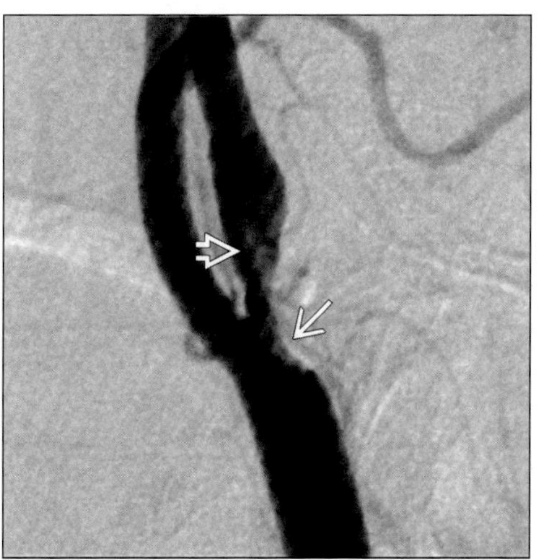

(Left) *Oblique CCA DSA shows a high-grade ASVD stenosis at the carotid bulb → with associated calcifications →.* ***(Right)*** *Oblique CCA DSA in a different patient shows calcified plaque at the carotid bifurcation extending into the ICA with associated stenosis →. An intraluminal filling defect → is seen. This represented thrombus for which the patient was anticoagulated. DSA 5 days later revealed resolution of the thrombus and CAS was undertaken at that time.*

CAROTID DISSECTION

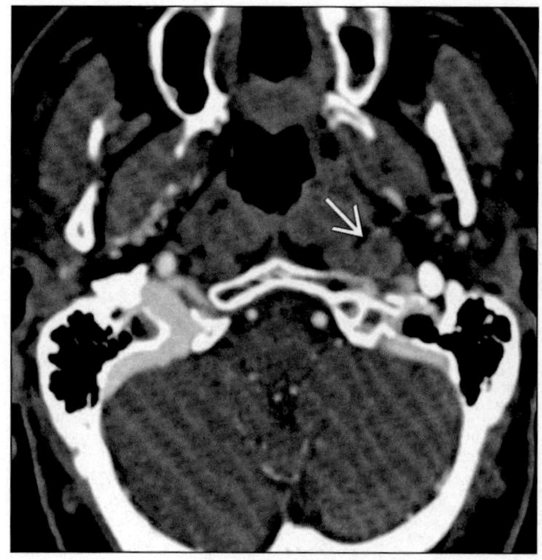

Axial CTA shows enlargement of the left ICA contour without enhancement of the vessel lumen ➡. Mild mural enhancement is seen.

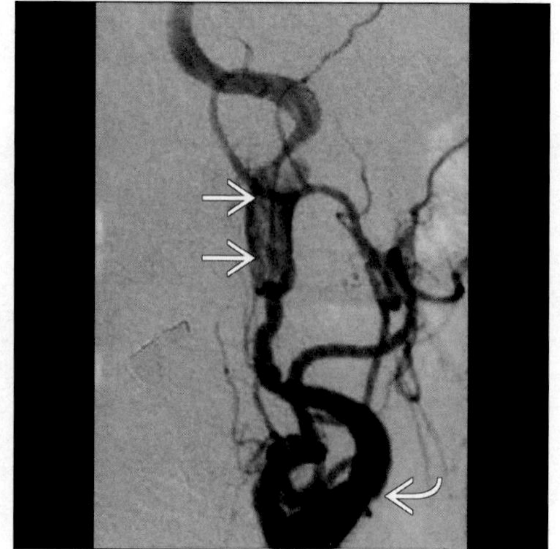

Oblique left carotid DSA shows cervical ICA dissection with stenosis of the true lumen by intramural thrombus ➡. The dissection extends to the carotid bulb ➦.

TERMINOLOGY

Definitions

- Delamination of wall of carotid artery from entry of blood (under arterial pressure) through a tear in intima

IMAGING FINDINGS

General Features

- Best diagnostic clue
  - Smooth, tapered ICA narrowing ± intimal flap ± adjacent vasospasm ± intramural thrombus ± pseudoaneurysm
  - Less commonly involves common carotid artery (CCA); may extend superiorly (from aortic arch dissection)
- Location: Cervical ICA near skull base = commonest

CT Findings

- NECT
  - May see associated pseudoaneurysm as iso- to slightly hyperdense carotid space mass
  - Look for fracture extending into carotid canal as clue to ICA injury
  - May see subarachnoid hemorrhage if supraclinoid ICA involved
  - End-organ injury = cerebral infarction
  - CT brain may be normal if no significant associated stenosis, collateral circulation adequate, no embolic ischemic sequela
- CTA
  - Narrowing of carotid artery (compression by intramural hematoma) ± intima flap separating true & false lumens ± pseudoaneurysm (contained extravasation beyond true arterial wall)
  - Non-enhancement of vessel if completely occluded ± distal reconstitution from cavernous ICA segment collaterals (from ECA) ± ophthalmic artery
  - No associated mural calcifications unlike atherosclerosis although rarely can see dystrophic calcification within mural thrombus

MR Findings

- T1WI
  - Subacute intramural thrombus (methemoglobin) is hyperintense

DDx: Carotid Vessel Irregularity

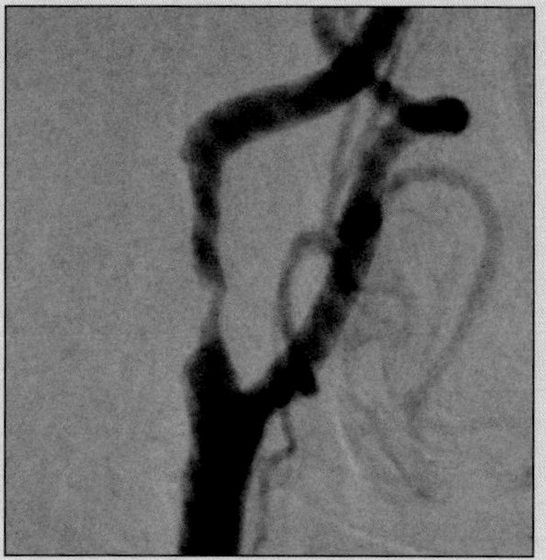

Atherosclerosis

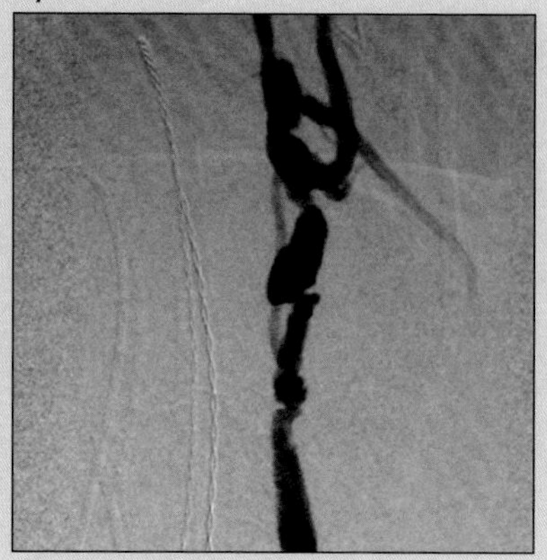

Fibromuscular Dysplasia

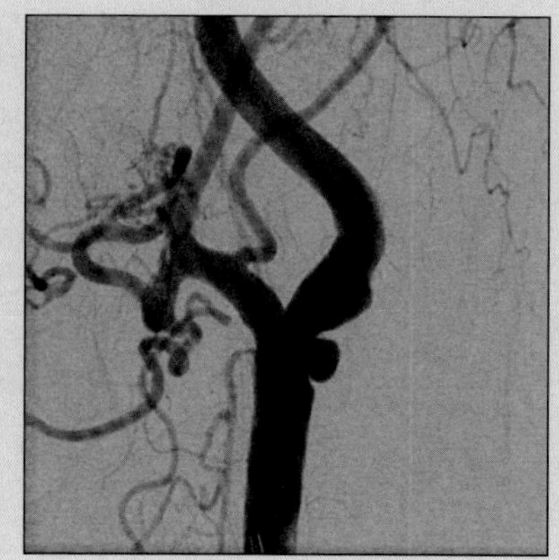

Ulcerated Plaque

CAROTID DISSECTION

Key Facts

Terminology
- Delamination of wall of carotid artery from entry of blood (under arterial pressure) through a tear in intima

Imaging Findings
- Look for fracture extending into carotid canal as clue to ICA injury
- Narrowing of carotid artery (compression by intramural hematoma) ± intima flap separating true & false lumens ± pseudoaneurysm (contained extravasation beyond true arterial wall)
- Non-enhancement of vessel if completely occluded ± distal reconstitution from cavernous ICA segment collaterals (from ECA) ± ophthalmic artery
- Crescentic intramural thrombus best seen on axial T1-weighted, fat-saturated images

Pathology
- CCA dissection usually due to extension of dissection from aortic arch
- ICA dissection: Most common site of head & neck arterial dissection
- Trauma: Most common cause
- Epidemiology: Annual incidence of ICA dissection = 3.5 per 100,000

Clinical Issues
- Consider in young/middle-aged patient with headache, TIA, stroke
- CCA dissection: Usually asymptomatic or presents with ipsilateral neck pain
- ICA dissection: Headache, neck/facial pain, Horner in 1/3

- Crescentic intramural thrombus best seen on axial T1-weighted, fat-saturated images
- DWI: Most sensitive and specific for detection of associated end-organ (cerebral) ischemia/infarction
- MRA
  - May see vessel stenosis, eccentrically narrowed lumen, occlusion or irregularity
  - Intramural methemoglobin may result in artifactual signal in TOF MRA; Gd-MRA superior

Ultrasonographic Findings
- Grayscale Ultrasound
  - Useful screening examination for carotid injury if CTA unavailable
  - May see smooth, tapered stenosis or occlusion
    - Increased flow velocities and turbulent flow if stenosis present
    - May see dissection flap; intervening septum may be thick or thin, movable or rigid, depending on wall components involved and chronicity

Angiographic Findings
- Conventional
  - Review CTA/MRA ± perform arch aortography prior to selective catheterization of dissected great vessel which could exacerbate stenosis, vasospasm or dislodge emboli
  - May see tapered stenosis or occlusion ± intimal flap ± pseudoaneurysm ± vasospasm
  - Look for associated intracranial thromboemboli + injury (dissection) of contralateral carotid artery + vertebral arteries
  - Endovascular stenting of hemodynamically significant stenosis can be performed ± coil embolization or covered-stent placement for carotid pseudoaneurysm

Imaging Recommendations
- Best imaging tool
  - MRA or CTA usually sufficient to make the diagnosis and for follow-up
  - DSA if MRA and CTA inconclusive or negative in the setting of high clinical suspicion, proven ischemic cerebral injury

DIFFERENTIAL DIAGNOSIS

Fibromuscular Dysplasia (FMD)
- "String of beads" appearance > long tubular narrowing
- FMD may predispose to dissection
- Often asymptomatic
- M:F = 1:1
- Renal > carotid > vertebral artery involvement

Carotid-Terminus Thromboembolus
- ICA thromboembolus beyond ophthalmic artery may result in complete occlusion or reduced flow in ICA
- Typically from primary cardiac source or via patent foramen ovale (PFO)
- CTA shows non-enhancement beyond proximal ICA
- DSA usually shows normal ICA beyond point of non-enhancement on CTA

Atherosclerosis
- Involves bulb
- Irregular > smooth tapered narrowing
- Calcifications often present
- ± Plaque ulceration
- ± Associated intraluminal thrombus

Vasospasm
- Vessel wall may be irritated by catheter tip or contrast injection during conventional angiography
- May result in vessel occlusion or stenosis around catheter tip
- Resolves with removal of irritant (catheter), time ± administration of vasodilators (e.g., nitroglycerin, verapamil)
- Failure to recognize catheter-induced vasospasm + continued injection into vessel wall may result in dissection

CAROTID DISSECTION

PATHOLOGY

General Features

- General path comments
  - Can occur between or within any layers, subintimal > subadventitial
  - CCA dissection usually due to extension of dissection from aortic arch
    - Occurs in 15% of aortic arch dissection, usually right side, not beyond bulb
  - ICA dissection: Most common site of head & neck arterial dissection
    - Upper cervical segment, near skull base most common
    - 15% multiple, simultaneous cervical arterial dissections (e.g., bilateral ICA, CCA or vertebral arteries involved)
- Etiology
  - Congenital or acquired defect in internal elastic lamina
  - Trauma: Most common cause
    - Penetrating or blunt, stretching/torsion (including chiropractic)
    - Minor neck torsion, trivial trauma in 25% (e.g., intense physical activity, coughing, sneezing)
    - Post endarterectomy (usually with patch graft)
  - Spontaneous
    - Underlying vasculopathy common (e.g., Marfan, Ehlers-Danlos)
    - Familial ICA dissection may occur
    - Hypertension in 1/3 of all patients
  - Iatrogenic
    - Angiography: Intimal injury with guidewire or catheter
    - Inadvertent puncture during placement of central venous catheters
- Epidemiology: Annual incidence of ICA dissection = 3.5 per 100,000

CLINICAL ISSUES

Presentation

- Most common signs/symptoms
  - Consider in young/middle-aged patient with headache, TIA, stroke
    - Dissection causes 10-25% of ischemic strokes in young adults
    - Stroke may occur from thromboembolic sequela or hemodynamic compromise from associated stenosis
- CCA dissection: Usually asymptomatic or presents with ipsilateral neck pain
  - Neurological deficit, stroke uncommon
- ICA dissection: Headache, neck/facial pain, Horner in 1/3
  - Onset within a few hours to 3-4 weeks
  - 70% of patients between 35-50 years old
  - M:F = 1:1
  - Uncommon: Cranial nerve palsy (CN 12 > 9, 10, 11)
  - Hemispheric ischemic symptoms may occur

Natural History & Prognosis

- May be asymptomatic, resolving spontaneously in 6-8 weeks
  - Even ICA occlusion frequently undergoes spontaneous flow restoration (lysis of thrombus, healing of intimal tear)
- No residual or mild neurologic deficit in 70%
- Disabling neurologic deficit in 25%
- Fatal in 5%

Treatment

- Anticoagulants (heparin, Coumadin)
- If hemodynamically significant stenosis/hypoperfusion symptoms then surgery (graft or bypass) or endovascular stenting is indicated
- Carotid pseudoaneurysms may be treated endovascularly using covered stents, coil embolization or vessel sacrifice

DIAGNOSTIC CHECKLIST

Consider

- Carotid dissection as a cause of stroke in young patients

Image Interpretation Pearls

- CTA or MRA usually sufficient for diagnosis and follow-up of treatment response
- Look for concurrent injury to other head and neck vessel in the context of trauma

SELECTED REFERENCES

1. Arnold M et al: Pain as the only symptom of cervical artery dissection. J Neurol Neurosurg Psychiatry. 77(9):1021-4, 2006
2. Binaghi S et al: Embolic stroke complicating cervical aneurysm. Cerebrovasc Dis. 22(2-3):196-8, 2006
3. Elijovich L et al: The emerging role of multidetector row CT angiography in the diagnosis of cervical arterial dissection: preliminary study. Neuroradiology. 48(9):606-12, 2006
4. Flis CM et al: Carotid and vertebral artery dissections: clinical aspects, imaging features and endovascular treatment. Eur Radiol. 2006
5. Matonti F et al: [Internal carotid artery dissection on arterial fibromuscular dysplasia causing a central retinal artery occlusion: a case report] J Fr Ophtalmol. 29(7):e15, 2006
6. Rizzo L et al: Dissection of cervicocephalic arteries: early diagnosis and follow-up with magnetic resonance imaging. Emerg Radiol. 12(6):254-65, 2006
7. Schonholz C et al: Stent-graft treatment of pseudoaneurysms and arteriovenous fistulae in the carotid artery. Vascular. 14(3):123-9, 2006
8. Wu HC et al: Spontaneous bilateral internal carotid artery dissection with acute stroke in young patients. Eur Neurol. 56(4):230-4, 2006
9. Lee WW et al: Bilateral internal carotid artery dissection due to trivial trauma. J Emerg Med. 19(1):35-41, 2000
10. Oelerich M et al: Craniocervical artery dissection: MR imaging and MR angiographic findings. Eur Radiol. 9(7):1385-91, 1999

IMAGE GALLERY

Typical

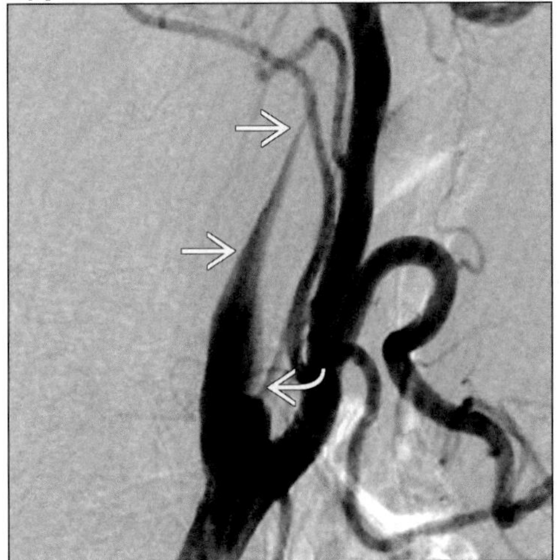

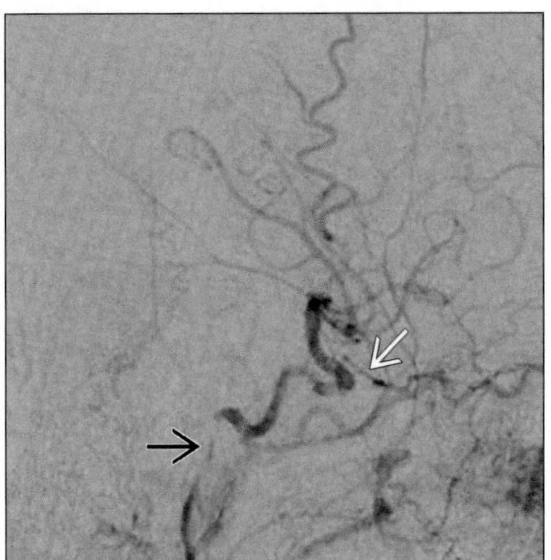

(Left) *Left carotid DSA shows irregularity of the carotid bulb* ➔ *and tapering of the cervical ICA due to dissection* ➔. ***(Right)*** *Lateral intracranial view of the same angiogram shows slow antegrade filling of the ICA with near-occlusion at the skull base due to dissection* →. *There is collateral flow to the supraclinoid ICA from the ECA via the ophthalmic artery* ➔.

Typical

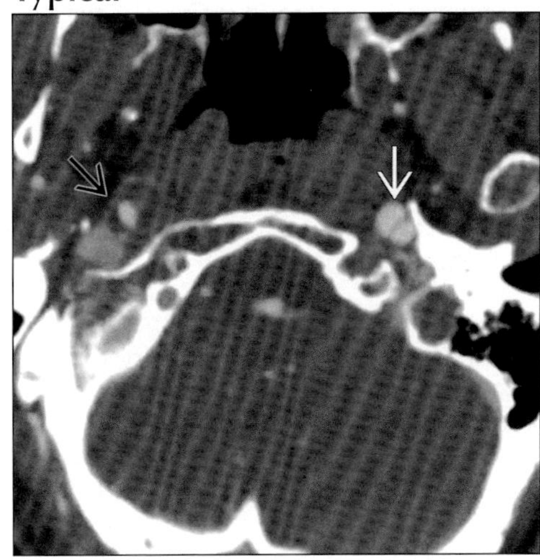

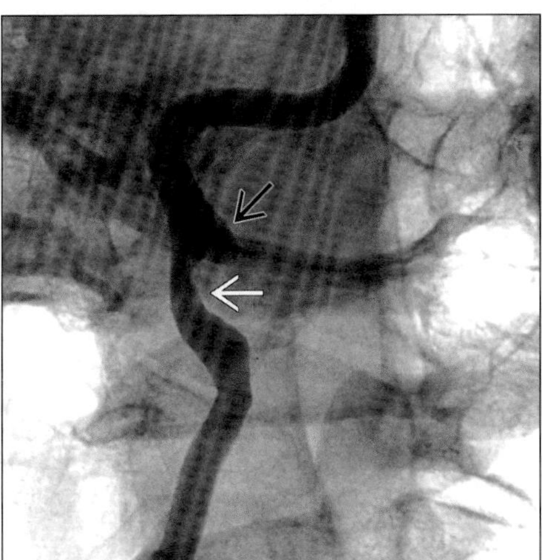

(Left) *Axial CTA shows bilateral internal carotid artery dissections. On the left a dissection flap* ➔ *is evident. On the right there is compression of the true lumen* → *by intramural thrombus.* ***(Right)*** *Oblique right ICA DSA in the same patient shows focal luminal irregularity of the cervical ICA with focal stenosis* ➔ *and adjacent pseudoaneurysm formation* →.

Typical

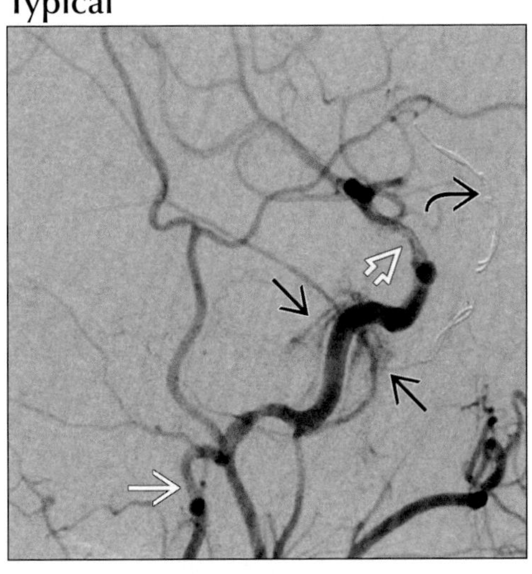

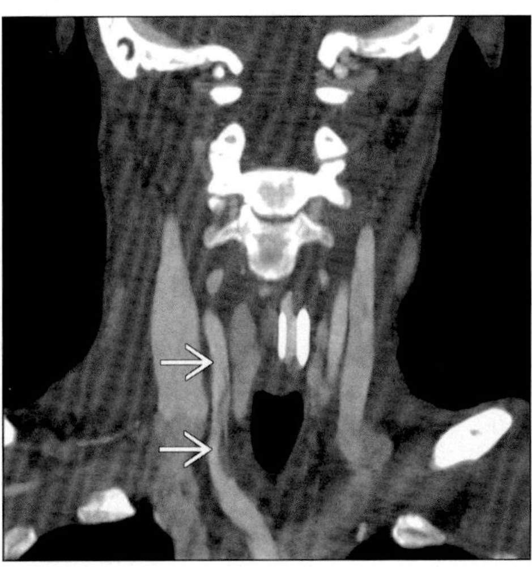

(Left) *Lateral CCA DSA in a patient with head trauma shows a gracile ICA* ➔ *as it enters the skull base due to dissection extending to the carotid bulb inferiorly. The supraclinoid ICA is also dissected and an intimal flap is visible* ➔. *Note carotid cavernous fistula* → *and embolization coils* → *in the middle meningeal artery used to treat a pseudoaneurysm.* ***(Right)*** *Coronal CTA in another patient shows dissection flap and intraluminal thrombus in the proximal CCA* ➔.

CAROTID PSEUDOANEURYSM, EXTRACRANIAL

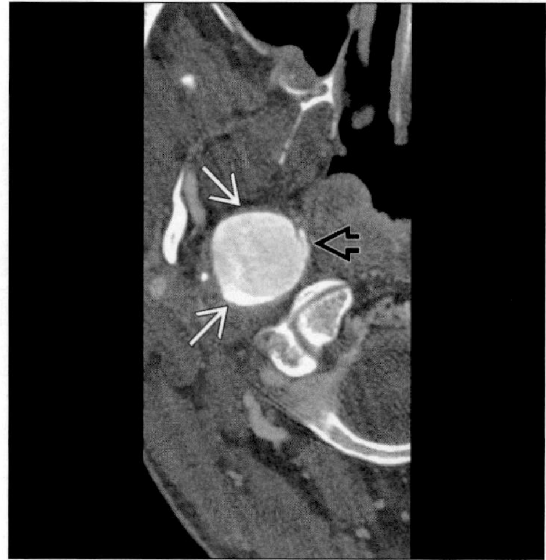

Axial CTA shows an enhancing carotid space mass consistent with a large saccular pseudoaneurysm of the cervical ICA ➡ with compression of the native ICA vessel lumen ⇨.

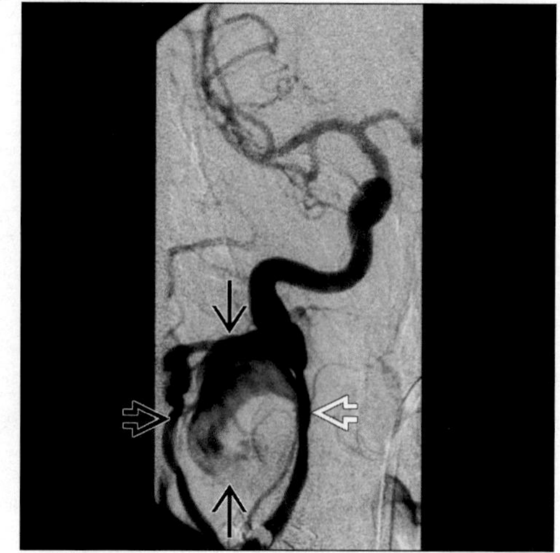

AP right CCA DSA shows a large pseudoaneurysm of the cervical ICA ➡. Note slow flow ± thrombus within the pseudoaneurysm with mass effect and displacement of the adjacent ICA ➡ and ECA ⇨.

TERMINOLOGY

Abbreviations and Synonyms

- "False" aneurysm

Definitions

- Paravascular cavitated clot in continuity with carotid artery
- Not contained by true vessel wall (tunica intima & media), hence "pseudo" or "false" aneurysm

IMAGING FINDINGS

General Features

- Best diagnostic clue: Contained contrast extravasation into a paravascular cavity lined by thrombus while in continuity with the carotid artery
- Location: Common carotid artery (CCA) and cervical segment of internal carotid artery (ICA) > petrous > cavernous > intradural ICA
- Morphology: May be fusiform dilatation vs. saccular outpouching
- Classic imaging appearance: Carotid space (CS) mass that communicates directly with carotid artery

CT Findings

- NECT
  - Round/ovoid/lobulated iso- to slightly hyperdense CS mass ± local bony expansion or remodeling if above skull base
  - May contain hyperdense thrombus
- CECT
  - Irregular widening of vessel contour
  - Outpouching of contrast from carotid artery
  - May compress carotid artery lumen
- CTA: Multiplanar reformats ± 3D reconstructions provide excellent visualization of pseudoaneurysm size + orientation of connection with carotid artery lumen ± contained thrombus

MR Findings

- T1WI: Inhomogeneous (usually isointense ± flow void, phase artifact)
- T2WI: Inhomogeneous (mixed hypo/hyperintense ± flow void)

DDx: Carotid Artery Pseudoaneurysm

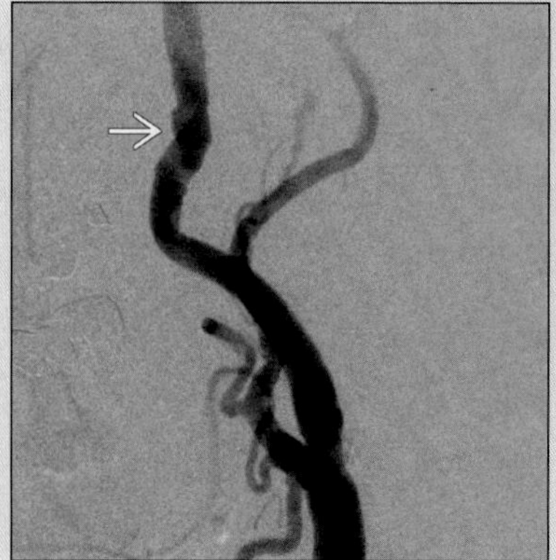

Fibromuscular Dysplasia

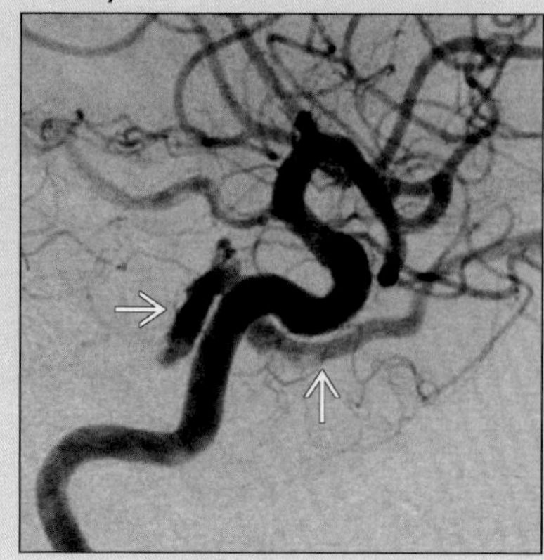

Carotid Cavernous Fistula

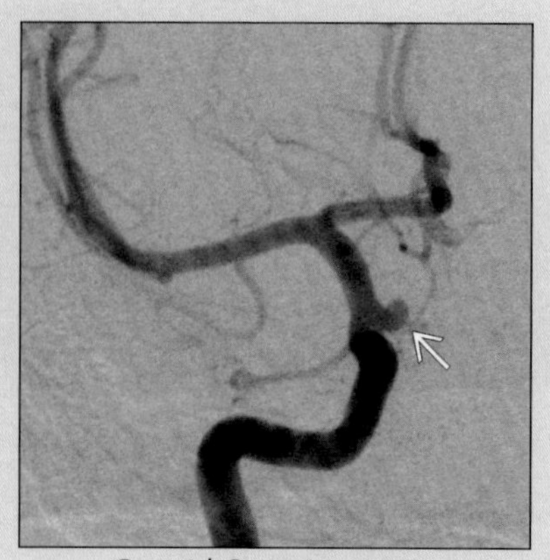

Carotid Cave Aneurysm

CAROTID PSEUDOANEURYSM, EXTRACRANIAL

Key Facts

Terminology
- "False" aneurysm
- Paravascular cavitated clot in continuity with carotid artery

Imaging Findings
- Best diagnostic clue: Contained contrast extravasation into a paravascular cavity lined by thrombus while in continuity with the carotid artery
- Classic imaging appearance: Carotid space (CS) mass that communicates directly with carotid artery
- DWI: Most sensitive for acute ischemia or infarction from thromboemboli or hypoperfusion
- DSA = gold standard for detection and characterization of carotid artery injury; useful for treatment planning: Surgical vs. endovascular vs. conservative/medical

Pathology
- "True" aneurysm contains layers of normal vessel wall; "false" or pseudoaneurysm does not
- > 80% of all cervical vascular injuries involve carotid arteries
- Usually occurs with trauma causing intimal dissection and subsequent vessel rupture contained by surrounding thrombus and soft tissues

Clinical Issues
- Can be occult, asymptomatic (2.5% of patients with blunt injury)
- 50-60% have palpable cervical mass (± pulsation)
- 40% neurologic symptoms
- Stent-supported coil embolization of pseudoaneurysm sac or placement of covered stent to exclude sac is usually curative

- FLAIR: Useful for detection of end-organ (brain) injury due to thromboemboli from pseudoaneurysm sac or hemodynamic compromise from compression of carotid artery lumen
- DWI: Most sensitive for acute ischemia or infarction from thromboemboli or hypoperfusion
- MRA
  - Visualization depends on flow dynamics within and adjacent to pseudoaneurysm
  - Flow turbulence may result in signal loss, reducing conspicuity
  - Gd-enhanced MRA superior to TOF

Ultrasonographic Findings
- Color Doppler
  - Duplex ultrasound useful as a screening tool
    - May see flow turbulence, pseudoaneurysm ± compression (stenosis) of carotid artery
- Power Doppler: Transcranial Doppler: May be utilized for real-time detection of thromboemboli arising from pseudoaneurysm sac

Angiographic Findings
- Conventional
  - DSA = gold standard for detection and characterization of carotid artery injury; useful for treatment planning: Surgical vs. endovascular vs. conservative/medical
  - Arch aortogram, arteriogram of carotid bifurcation should be considered prior to more distal selective catheterization of an injured carotid artery
  - Imaging of contralateral carotid ± vertebral artery(s) should be considered if concurrent injury is suspected in case of multi-trauma; necessary if carotid sacrifice being considered as a therapeutic option
  - Demonstration of sac morphology + size ± compression/stenosis of carotid artery lumen

Imaging Recommendations
- Best imaging tool: CTA useful as first line imaging tool for both extra + intracranial carotid injury
- Duplex sonography useful as a rapid screening examination in acute setting of suspected cervical vascular injury

DIFFERENTIAL DIAGNOSIS

Dissecting Aneurysm
- Intramural hematoma from rupture of vasa vasorum or intimal tear dilates and weakens vessel wall
- Is a true aneurysm as it is contained by tunica adventitia
- May see intimal flap between true and false lumens

Arteriovenous Fistula
- May occur as rare complication of carotid pseudoaneurysm rupture → AV shunt to neck veins or cavernous sinus
- More commonly associated with penetrating neck injury

Fibromuscular Dysplasia
- Irregular outpouchings from vessel lumen, usually along upper cervical ICA segment, bilateral in 60%
- Occurs in carotid circulation > vertebral arteries; renal artery involvement most common
- Often an asymptomatic finding
- M:F = 1:3
- Classic = "string of beads" with alternating segments of dilatation and strictures; less symmetric forms also occur

True Carotid Artery Aneurysm
- Contained by all layers of vessel wall as opposed to pseudoaneurysm
- CCA and cervical ICA locations extremely rare
- True cavernous ICA aneurysms associated with fibromuscular dysplasia, Ehlers-Danlos syndrome; rupture results in high-flow carotid cavernous fistula
- Supraclinoid ICA blister & berry aneurysms may rupture and cause subarachnoid hemorrhage

CAROTID PSEUDOANEURYSM, EXTRACRANIAL

PATHOLOGY

General Features

- General path comments
  - "True" aneurysm contains layers of normal vessel wall; "false" or pseudoaneurysm does not
  - > 80% of all cervical vascular injuries involve carotid arteries
  - Vessel wall disruption results in periluminal hemorrhage with contained extravasation
  - Paravascular clot forms, cavitates, communicates with parent vessel
- Etiology
  - Usually occurs with trauma causing intimal dissection and subsequent vessel rupture contained by surrounding thrombus and soft tissues
  - Rarely occurs as sequela of deep neck space infection with necrosis of vessel wall (mycotic pseudoaneurysm)
  - "Carotid Blowout syndrome"
    - Carotid pseudoaneurysm ± active bleeding into neck soft tissues or oral cavity
    - Related to aggressive primary and salvage surgery for head & neck cancer, irradiation
    - Requires emergent endovascular vessel occlusion or placement of covered stent
- Epidemiology: 1/3 of cervical ICA vascular injuries caused by penetrating trauma
- Associated abnormalities: Injury to other vessels possible due to traumatic etiology; should be sought on CTA/DSA

Gross Pathologic & Surgical Features

- Bluish-purple paravascular CS mass contained by fascia, organized hematoma ± adventitia

Microscopic Features

- Wall of pseudoaneurysm does not contain intima, internal elastic lamina, muscularis layers; adventitia may be present

CLINICAL ISSUES

Presentation

- Can be occult, asymptomatic (2.5% of patients with blunt injury)
- 50-60% have palpable cervical mass (± pulsation)
- 40% neurologic symptoms
  - Horner syndrome
  - CN IX-XI palsy
  - Jaw pain
  - Cerebral ischemia/infarction
- Cavernous ICA pseudoaneurysm rupture may cause
  - Massive epistaxis (rupture into sphenoid sinus); may be life-threatening
  - Direct carotid cavernous fistula (rupture into cavernous sinus) → ophthalmoplegia, proptosis, chemosis

Natural History & Prognosis

- Variable; may enlarge, resolve spontaneously, undergo thrombosis, rupture
- 45% combined stroke/mortality rate after ligation of parent vessel
- 23% stroke/mortality with observation only
- < 5% major morbidity/mortality if parent vessel repaired, reconstructed endovascularly

Treatment

- Goal: Occlusion of pseudoaneurysm with preservation of ICA if possible
- Alternative = therapeutic carotid sacrifice (occlusion) after ICA balloon test occlusion to ensure collaterals are adequate
- Stent-supported coil embolization of pseudoaneurysm sac or placement of covered stent to exclude sac is usually curative
- Placement of a non-covered stent may change hemodynamics within sac sufficiently to promote thrombosis without need for additional embolization with coils
- Endovascular embolization with Onyx® (a liquid embolic material) may also be curative

DIAGNOSTIC CHECKLIST

Consider

- History of trauma, surgery ± radiation therapy for head & neck cancer

Image Interpretation Pearls

- True cervical carotid aneurysms rare; look for associated trauma/dissection
- Multiplanar CTA reformats usually diagnostic; look for associated stenosis, contained thrombus
- Thromboembolic events best seen with MR (DWI for acute; FLAIR for chronic)

SELECTED REFERENCES

1. Asma A et al: Massive epistaxis secondary to pseudoaneurysm of internal carotid artery. Med J Malaysia. 61(1):84-7, 2006
2. Kaviani A et al: Infected carotid pseudoaneurysm and carotid-cutaneous fistula as a late complication of carotid artery stenting. J Vasc Surg. 43(2):379-82, 2006
3. Madan A et al: Traumatic carotic artery-cavernous sinus fistula treated with a covered stent. Report of two cases. J Neurosurg. 104(6): 969-73, 2006
4. Gorriz-Gomez E et al: [Internal carotid artery pseudoaneurysm and stenosis: treatment with stents and coils.] Neurocirugia (Astur). 16(6):528-32, 2005
5. Mordekar SR et al: Occult carotid pseudoaneurysm following streptococcal throat infection. J Paediatr Child Health. 41(12):682-4, 2005
6. Koyanagi M et al: Stent-supported coil embolization for carotid artery pseudoaneurysm as a complication of endovascular surgery--case report. Neurol Med Chir (Tokyo). 44(10):544-7, 2004
7. Alexander MJ et al: Treatment of an iatrogenic petrous carotid artery pseudoaneurysm with a Symbiot covered stent: technical case report. Neurosurgery. 50(3):658-62, 2002
8. Reisner A et al: Endovascular occlusion of a carotid pseudoaneurysm complicating deep neck space infection in a child. Case report. J Neurosurg. 91(3):510-4, 1999

IMAGE GALLERY

Typical

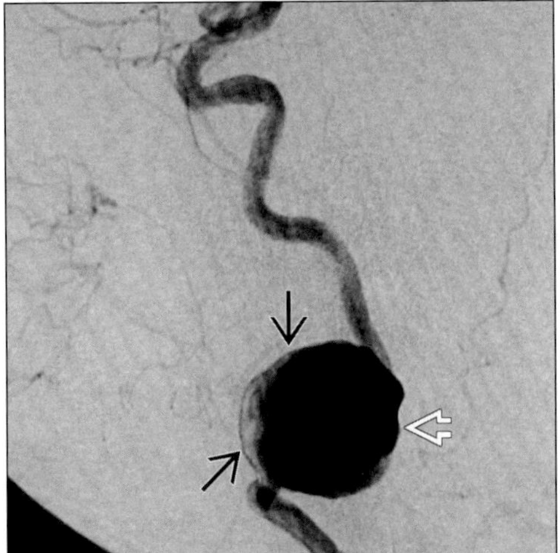

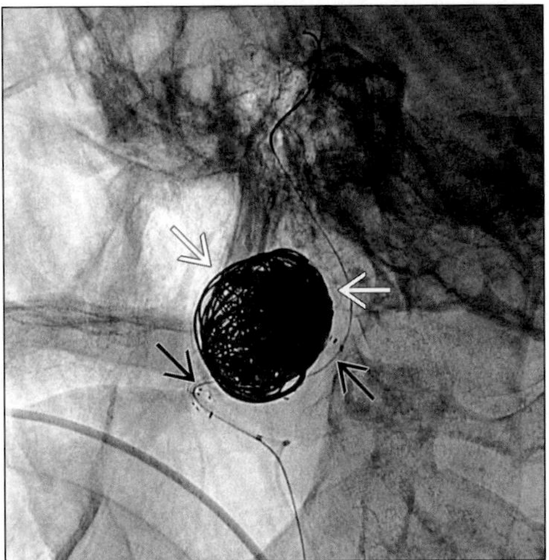

(Left) Lateral CCA DSA shows a fusiform pseudoaneurysm of the distal cervical ICA ⇒ in a patient with prior closed head injury. Irregularity of its wall ➡ is suggestive of contained thrombus. ***(Right)*** Unsubtracted image after stent-supported coil embolization shows coil packing ➡ within the pseudoaneurysm and a stent ⇒ within the ICA to maintain patency of the parent vessel.

Typical

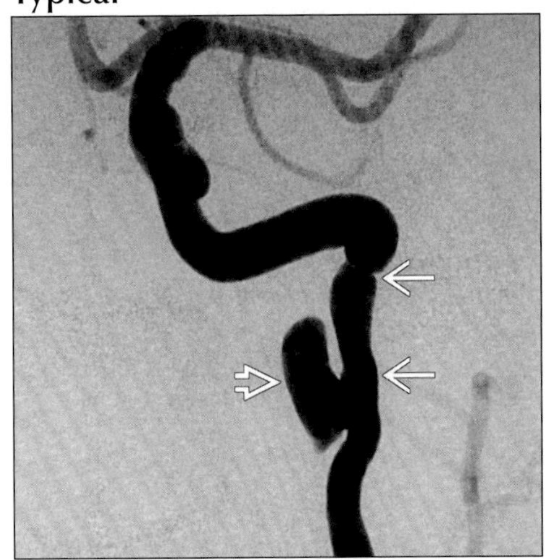

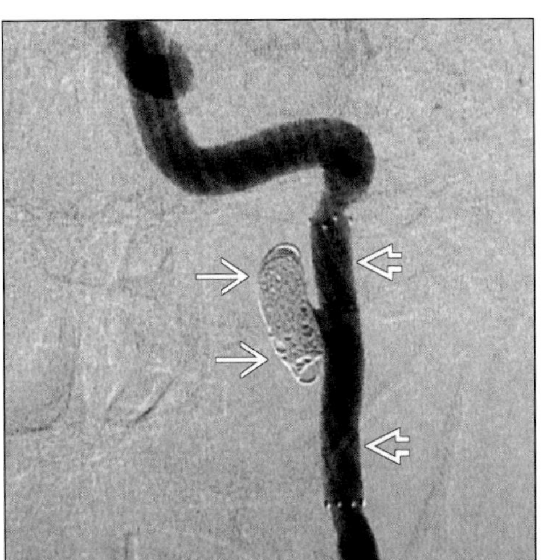

(Left) Left ICA DSA shows a boot-shaped saccular pseudoaneurysm ➡ with associated luminal irregularity of the adjacent parent vessel, probably the sequela of previous dissection ➡. ***(Right)*** Left ICA DSA after stent-supported coil embolization shows preservation of the parent vessel lumen by the stent ➡ and coil packing of the pseudoaneurysm lumen ➡.

Typical

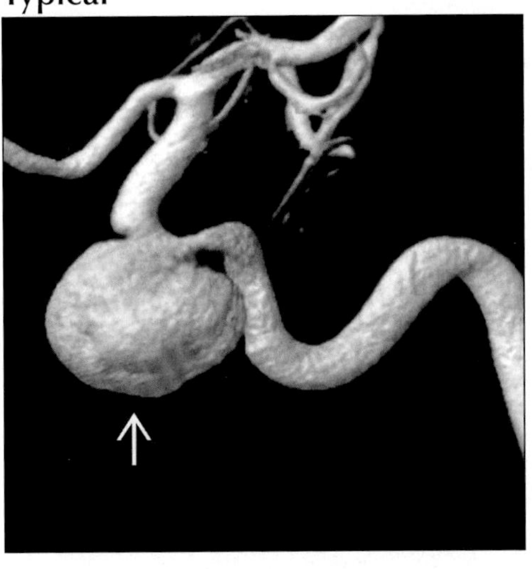

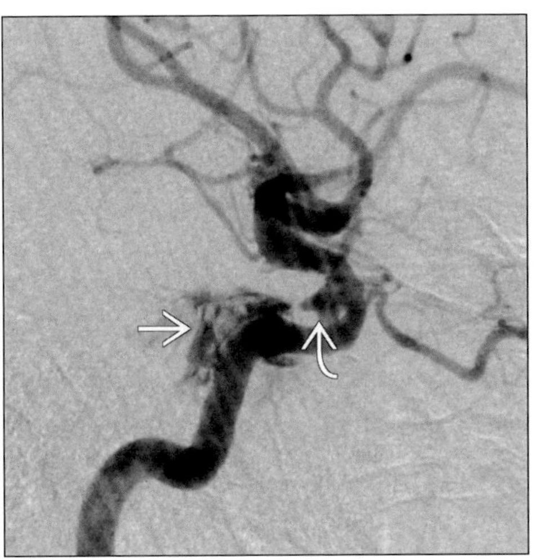

(Left) 3D DSA shows a large cavernous ICA pseudoaneurysm ➡ in a patient who underwent transsphenoidal pituitary surgery complicated by massive epistaxis. This was treated with a covered stent. ***(Right)*** Lateral ICA DSA in a different patient shows a direct carotid cavernous fistula ➡ and a lobulated paraclinoid ICA pseudoaneurysm ➡ which subsequently ruptured into the cavernous sinus (not shown).

ABERRANT INTERNAL CAROTID ARTERY

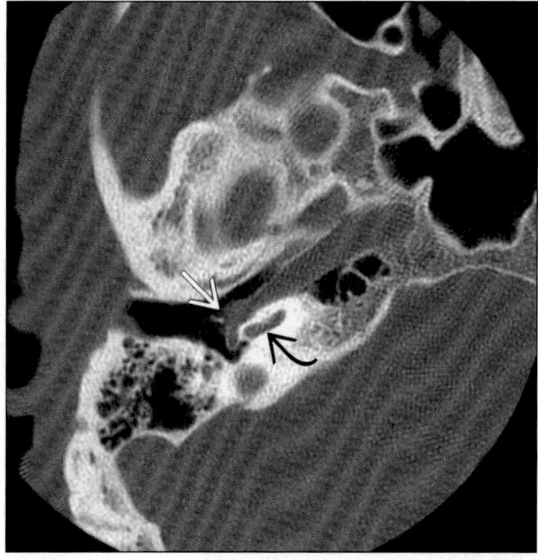

Axial NECT with bone windowing shows an aberrant internal carotid artery coursing through the middle ear cavity. The vessel is lateral to the cochlea ⇾. Note the absence of bone covering the vessel ➡.

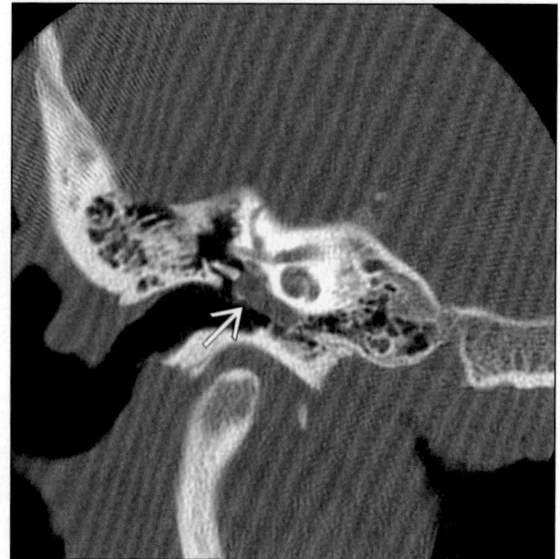

Coronal NECT with bone windowing shows an aberrant internal carotid artery coursing through the middle ear cavity ➡.

TERMINOLOGY

Abbreviations and Synonyms

- Aberrant internal carotid artery (AbICA)

Definitions

- Aberrant internal carotid artery: Congenital vascular anomaly resulting from regression of C1 segment of cervical ICA during embryogenesis

IMAGING FINDINGS

General Features

- Best diagnostic clue
  - AbICA enters posterior middle ear cavity from below, hugs cochlear promontory as it crosses middle ear, then joins posterior lateral margin of horizontal petrous ICA
  - Tubular nature of AbICA
- Location
  - Absent normal vertical segment of the petrous ICA
  - Reported right-sided preponderance
- Morphology: Tubular lesion crossing middle ear cavity from posterior to anterior

CT Findings

- NECT
  - CT appearance of AbICA is diagnostic
    - AbICA enters posterior middle ear through an enlarged inferior tympanic canaliculus
    - Courses anteriorly across cochlear promontory to join horizontal carotid canal through a dehiscence in carotid plate
    - Stenosis at the point where it rejoins horizontal carotid canal sometimes occurs & can lead to pulsatile tinnitus
  - Aberrant stapedial artery is often associated with AbICA
    - Absent foramen spinosum
    - Enlarged anterior tympanic segment of VII
  - Coronal CT shows a round soft-tissue density on cochlear promontory
    - Viewing multiple slices reveals tubular nature
    - On a single slice looks disturbingly like paraganglioma (hypotympanic mass)

DDx: Aberrant Internal Carotid Artery

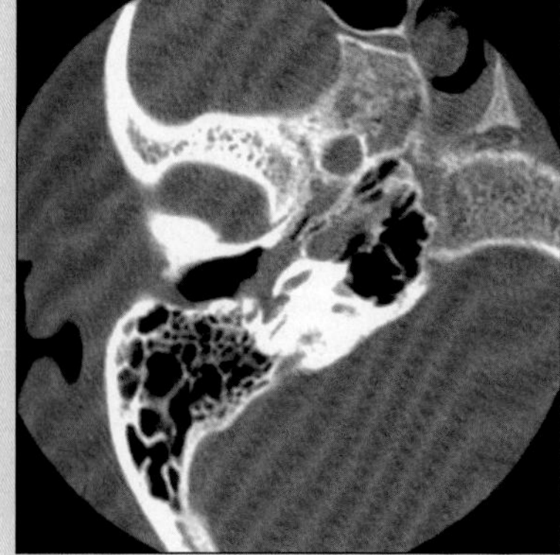

Glomus Tympanicum

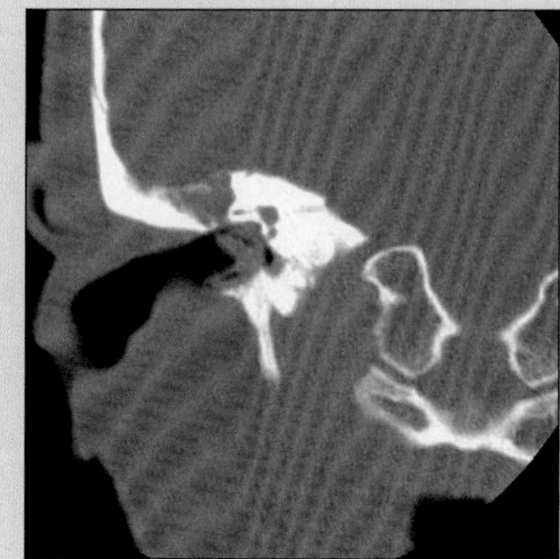

Cholesteatoma

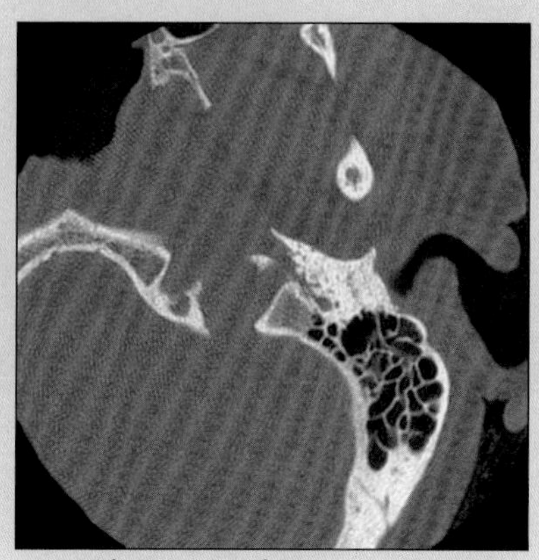

Glomus Jugulotympanicum

ABERRANT INTERNAL CAROTID ARTERY

Key Facts

Terminology

- Aberrant internal carotid artery: Congenital vascular anomaly resulting from regression of C1 segment of cervical ICA during embryogenesis

Imaging Findings

- AbICA enters posterior middle ear cavity from below, hugs cochlear promontory as it crosses middle ear, then joins posterior lateral margin of horizontal petrous ICA
- Morphology: Tubular lesion crossing middle ear cavity from posterior to anterior
- Aberrant stapedial artery is often associated with AbICA
- Coronal CT shows a round soft-tissue density on cochlear promontory
- MRA source & MIP images show aberrant course of artery
- Best imaging tool: Temporal bone CT makes this diagnosis

Top Differential Diagnoses

- Dehiscent Jugular Bulb
- Acquired Cholesteatoma, Middle Ear
- Paraganglioma
- Aneurysm, Petrous Internal Carotid Artery

Clinical Issues

- Most common signs/symptoms: Vascular retrotympanic mass in anterior inferior mesotympanum
- Inform clinician of this finding to prevent biopsy

    - Dehiscence of the bony plate that normally covers the tympanic portion of the ICA
- CECT: Same findings as NECT, vessel lumen enhances
- CTA: Aberrant course of artery can be seen, compare with contralateral side

MR Findings

- T2WI: Conventional MR does not reliably identify aberrant ICA but can be seen as an aberrant flow void
- MRA
  - MRA source & MIP images show aberrant course of artery
    - Side-to-side comparison shows AbICA enters skull base posterolateral to opposite normal side
    - Courses through middle ear across cochlear promontory
    - May get dephasing of spins from turbulence which can appear as a stenosis

Angiographic Findings

- Conventional
  - Line of Lapayowker: Vertical line dropped from lateral aspect of vestibular apparatus on AP skull film
    - Normal ICA lies medial
    - AbICA lies lateral
  - AbICA runs posterolateral to normal carotid canal + pinched appearance is characteristic
  - Angiography no longer necessary to confirm this imaging diagnosis
    - Primarily used for management of bleeding complications after injury to the AbICA

Imaging Recommendations

- Best imaging tool: Temporal bone CT makes this diagnosis
- Protocol advice: If MR done, MRA source and MIP images should be used

DIFFERENTIAL DIAGNOSIS

Dehiscent Jugular Bulb

- Focal absence of sigmoid plate
- Bud from superolateral jugular bulb enters middle ear cavity

Acquired Cholesteatoma, Middle Ear

- Soft tissue mass causing erosion of the scutum
- Lysis of middle ear ossicles
- No enhancement on post gadolinium images

Paraganglioma

- Glomus tympanicum
  - Focal enhancing mass on cochlear promontory
  - No tubular shape
- Glomus jugulotympanicum
  - Mass enters middle ear through medial floor
  - CT shows permeative bone changes between jugular foramen & middle ear mass

Aneurysm, Petrous Internal Carotid Artery

- Temporal CT shows focal smooth expansion of petrous carotid canal
- MRA/CTA is diagnostic of aneurysm

PATHOLOGY

General Features

- General path comments
  - Embryology-Anatomy
    - Regression or agenesis of cervical ICA during embryogenesis triggers a secondary anastomosis to occur between inferior tympanic branch of ascending pharyngeal artery and horizontal segment of petrous ICA
    - No normal vertical segment of petrous ICA is present
    - AbICA takes a posterolateral course as it runs through an enlarged inferior tympanic canaliculus accompanied by Jacobsen branch of CN9
    - Bony margin of posterolateral horizontal petrous ICA canal is dehiscent to allow AbICA to rejoin petrous ICA at this point
- Etiology
  - Alternate blood flow theory

        - C1 portion of the ICA involutes due to the persistence of the pharyngeal artery system
        - Blood flows via ascending pharyngeal artery to the enlarged inferior tympanic artery
        - Retrograde flow through the caroticotympanic vessels into the horizontal segment of the ICA
- Epidemiology: Very rare vascular anomaly
- Associated abnormalities
    - Persistent stapedial artery
        - Total reported incidence < 0.5%
        - Incidence of AbICA with persistent stapedial artery not known but multiple case reports exist

CLINICAL ISSUES

Presentation

- Most common signs/symptoms: Vascular retrotympanic mass in anterior inferior mesotympanum
- Other signs/symptoms
    - Objective pulsatile tinnitus (PT)
        - If stenosis is present at junction of AbICA and normal horizontal petrous ICA
        - If vessel abuts malleus handle
    - Subjective pulsatile tinnitus
    - Otalgia and fullness
    - Conductive hearing loss
    - Often asymptomatic
- Clinical Profile
    - Otoscopic appearance of this vascular-appearing retrotympanic lesion mimics glomus tympanicum & jugulotympanicum paraganglioma
    - Imaging appearances are pathognomonic: Must avoid biopsy!

Demographics

- Age: Congenital anomaly, present at birth
- Gender: Reported female preponderance

Natural History & Prognosis

- No long term sequelae reported with AbICA
- Often no symptoms and discovered incidentally during middle ear surgery
- Poor prognosis results only if misdiagnosis leads to biopsy
    - Severe bleeding and pseudoaneurysm formation
- If PT is loud, can be debilitating

Treatment

- Inform clinician of this finding to prevent biopsy
- A clinical-radiologic mistake in diagnosis with resultant surgical intervention can be disastrous
- Most patients have minor symptoms that do not require treatment however surgery can be performed to reduce tinnitus
    - Cover aberrant vessel with bone and fascia
    - Trim malleus handle that touches exposed carotid artery

DIAGNOSTIC CHECKLIST

Consider

- Look carefully for associated anomalies such as persistent stapedial artery

Image Interpretation Pearls

- Radiologist must hold onto correct imaging diagnosis against clinical impression of paraganglioma
- Temporal bone CT appearance is diagnostic

SELECTED REFERENCES

1. Endo K et al: Aberrant internal carotid artery as a cause of objective pulsatile tinnitus. Auris Nasus Larynx. 2006
2. Sauvaget E et al: Aberrant internal carotid artery in the temporal bone: imaging findings and management. Arch Otolaryngol Head Neck Surg. 132(1):86-91, 2006
3. Koesling S et al: Vascular anomalies, sutures and small canals of the temporal bone on axial CT. Eur J Radiol. 54(3):335-43, 2005
4. Moonis G et al: Otologic manifestations of petrous carotid aneurysms. AJNR Am J Neuroradiol. 26(6):1324-7, 2005
5. Lau CC et al: Combination of aberrant internal carotid artery and persistent stapedial artery. Otol Neurotol. 25(5):850-1, 2004
6. Kojima H et al: Aberrant carotid artery in the middle ear: multislice CT imaging aids in diagnosis. Am J Otolaryngol. 24(2):92-6, 2003
7. Roll JD et al: Bilateral aberrant internal carotid arteries with bilateral persistent stapedial arteries and bilateral duplicated internal carotid arteries. AJNR Am J Neuroradiol. 24(4):762-5, 2003
8. Jain R et al: Management of aberrant internal carotid artery injury: a real emergency. Otolaryngol Head Neck Surg. 127(5):470-3, 2002
9. Tien HC et al: Persistent stapedial artery. Otol Neurotol. 22(6):975-6, 2001
10. Botma M et al: Aberrant internal carotid artery in the middle-ear space. J Laryngol Otol. 114(10):784-7, 2000
11. Silbergleit R et al: The persistent stapedial artery. AJNR Am J Neuroradiol. 21(3):572-7, 2000
12. Koizuka I et al: Objective tinnitus caused by an aberrant internal carotid artery. Auris Nasus Larynx. 25(3):323-7, 1998
13. Waldvogel D et al: Pulsatile tinnitus--a review of 84 patients. J Neurol. 245(3):137-42, 1998
14. Davis WL et al: MR angiography of an aberrant internal carotid artery. AJNR Am J Neuroradiol. 12(6):1225, 1991
15. Lo WW et al: Aberrant carotid artery: radiologic diagnosis with emphasis on high-resolution computed tomography. Radiographics. 5(6):985-93, 1985

IMAGE GALLERY

Typical

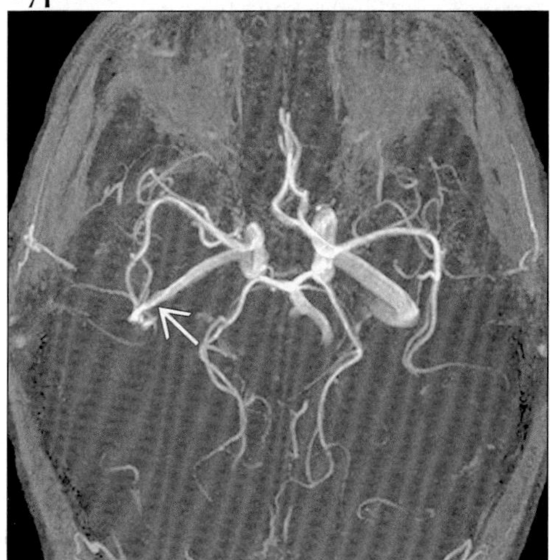

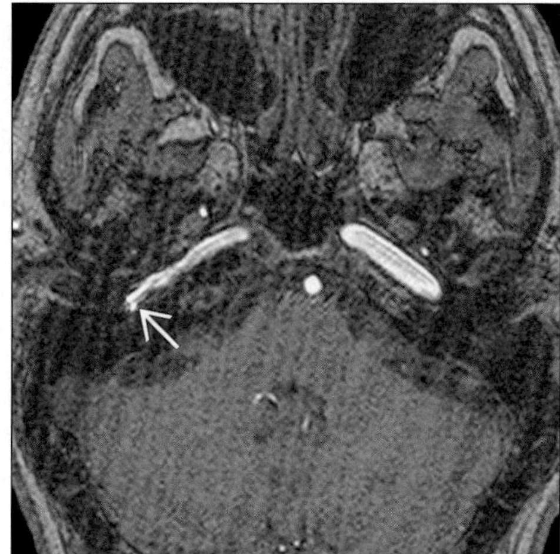

(Left) *Axial 3D TOF MRA collapsed view shows an aberrant right internal carotid artery ➔ coursing through the middle ear cavity.* ***(Right)*** *Axial 3D TOF MRA source image shows an aberrant right internal carotid artery coursing through the middle ear cavity ➔. Stenosis along its course in the middle ear is common and results in decreased flow ± turbulence. Thus there is reduced flow-related enhancement compared with the contralateral ICA.*

Typical

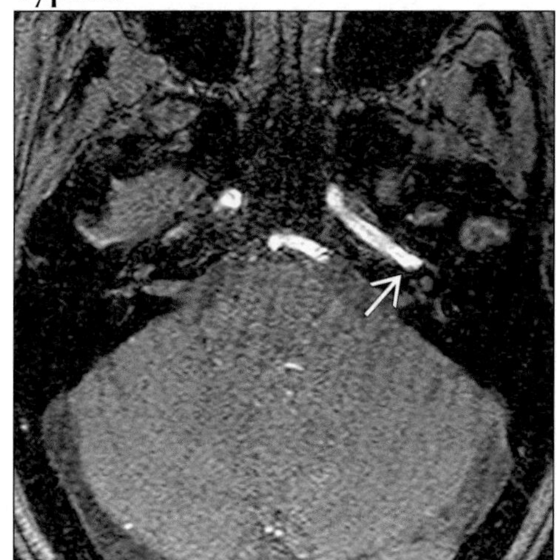

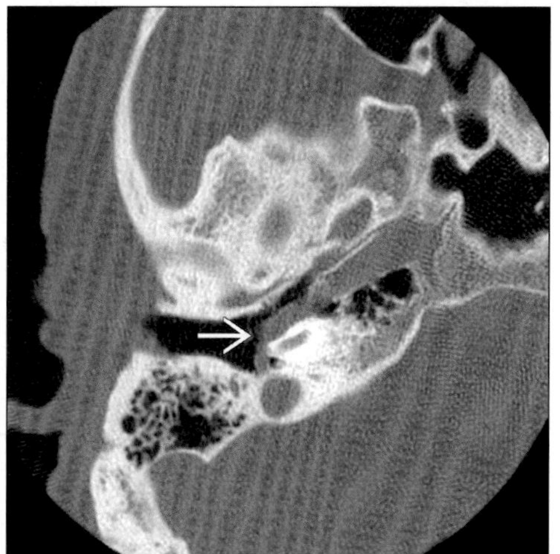

(Left) *Axial 3D TOF MRA shows an abnormal posterior course of the left internal carotid artery ➔.* ***(Right)*** *Axial NECT with bone windowing shows an aberrant internal carotid artery coursing through the middle ear cavity. Note the absence of bone covering the vessel ➔.*

Typical

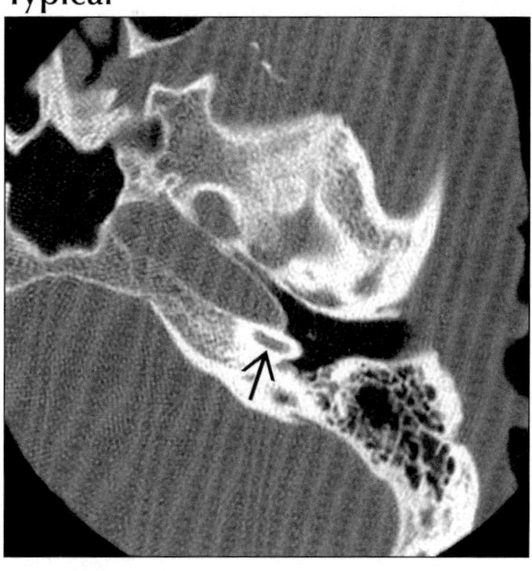

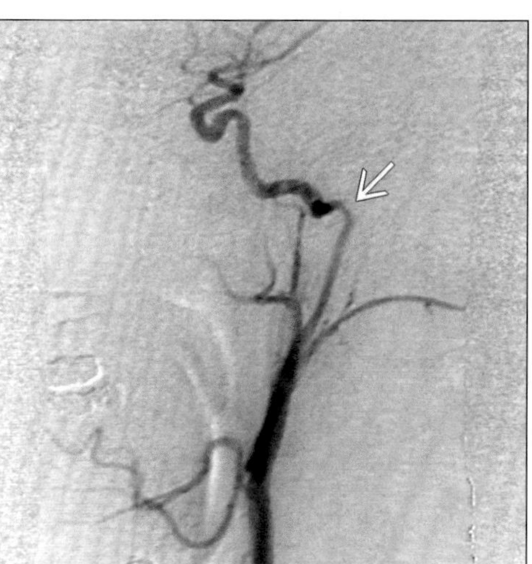

(Left) *Axial NECT shows an abnormally long petrous portion of the left internal carotid artery which extends posterior and laterally to cover a portion of the basal turn of the cochlea ➔.* ***(Right)*** *Lateral common carotid artery DSA shows a more posterior course of the ICA and an associated change in contour and caliber ➔ of the vessel as it enters the horizontal petrous carotid canal. Flow turbulence at this point can cause pulsatile tinnitus.*

VERTEBROBASILAR INSUFFICIENCY

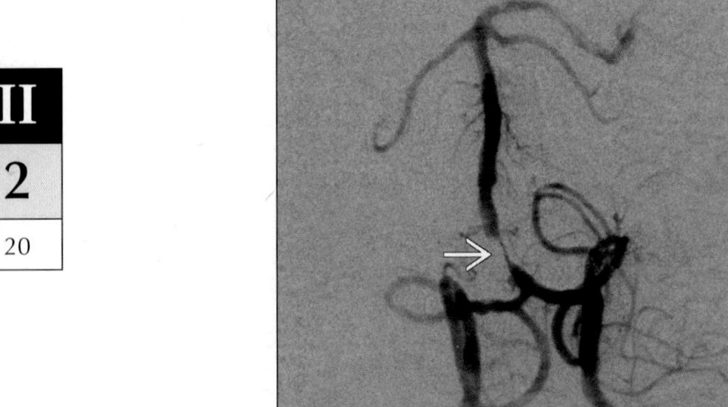

Left vertebral artery DSA shows a short-segment pin-point stenosis of the proximal basilar artery → in this patient presenting with episodic syncope.

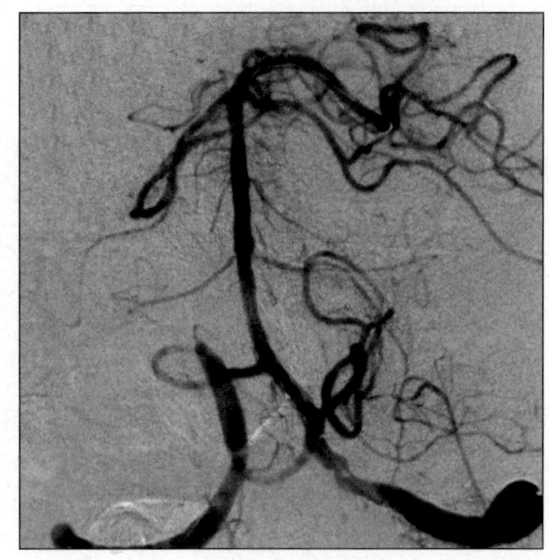

DSA following stent placement shows minimal residual stenosis. The patient's symptoms resolved.

TERMINOLOGY

Definitions

- Vertebrobasilar insufficiency (VBI): Posterior circulation ischemia of hemodynamic origin due to underlying vertebral artery (VA) or basilar artery stenosis

IMAGING FINDINGS

General Features

- Best diagnostic clue
  - Clinical history of postural symptoms (orthostatic hypotension exacerbates poor perfusion)
  - Posterior circulation (occipital lobe, cerebellar or brainstem) stroke on CT or MR
- Location: Stenosis at VA origin > intracranial vertebral artery > basilar artery > cervical segment of VA (rarely osteophytic compression)
- Size
  - Usually short-segment atherosclerotic stenosis (< 10 mm); longer segment if etiology is dissection
  - If VA stenosis: Contralateral VA is usually hypoplastic/absent/occluded for VBI to occur
- Morphology
  - Atherosclerotic vascular disease (ASVD): Smooth plaque, ulcerated plaque ± superimposed thrombus
  - Eccentric, tapered lumen in arterial dissection

CT Findings

- NECT
  - May see posterior circulation infarction (edema if acute vs. encephalomalacia if chronic)
  - Mural calcification of VA, basilar artery, or subclavian artery
- CECT: May see enhancement associated with acute/subacute infarction
- CTA
  - Multiplanar reformats of CTA provide excellent depiction of stenoses along the course of the vertebral and basilar arteries
  - Irregular or smooth short-segment stenosis of VA/basilar artery ± adjacent mural Ca++
  - Can visualize size of posterior communicating arteries (PCoA) as potential collateral pathway

DDx: Vertebrobasilar Lesions and Variants

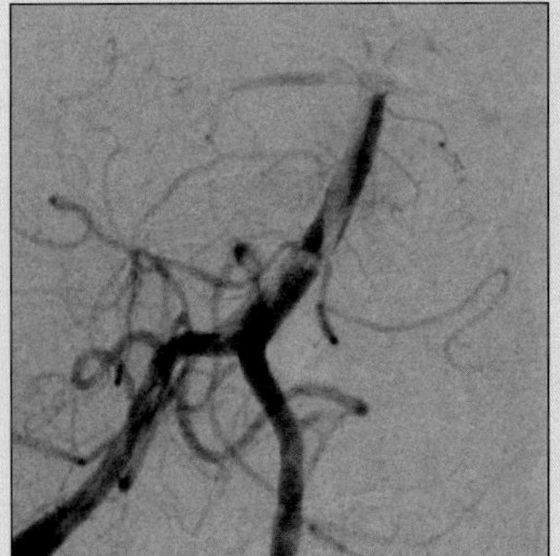

Basilar Artery Thromboembolism

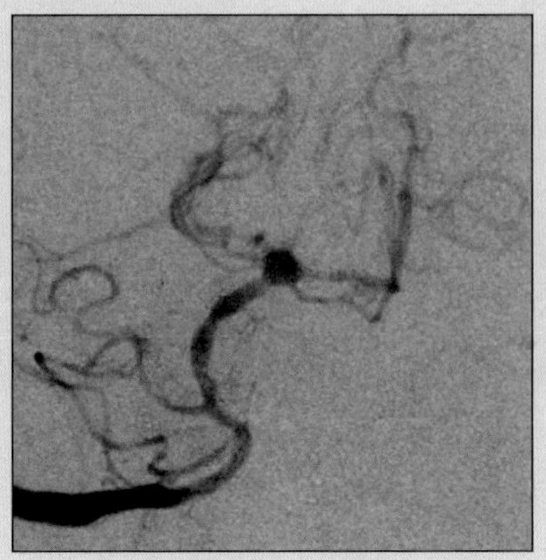

SAH Vasospasm

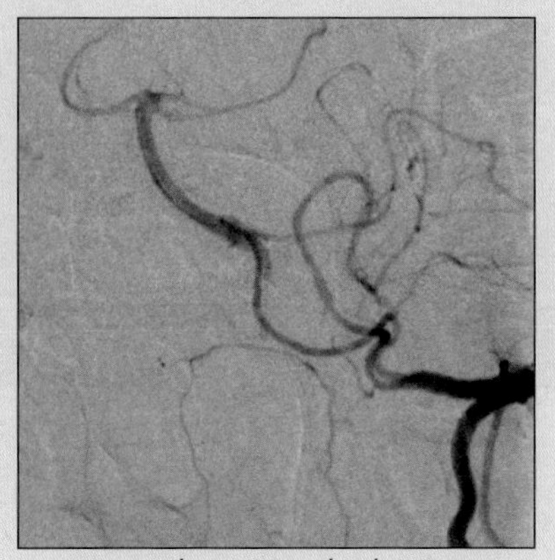

Hypoplastic Vertebral Artery

VERTEBROBASILAR INSUFFICIENCY

Key Facts

Terminology
- Posterior circulation ischemia of hemodynamic origin due to underlying vertebral or basilar artery stenosis
- Atherosclerotic etiology > dissection

Imaging Findings
- Posterior circulation (occipital lobe, cerebellar or brainstem) stroke on CT or MR
- Multiplanar reformats of CTA provide excellent depiction of stenoses along the course of the vertebral and basilar arteries
- MRA tends to accentuate stenosis: High grade stenosis may appear as signal void
- DSA: Typically irregular/smooth short segment stenosis ± adjacent Ca++ in ASVD
  - May see dissection flap or intramural hematoma compressing true lumen in cases of dissection

Top Differential Diagnoses
- Hypoplastic Vertebral Artery
- SAH Vasospasm
- Basilar Artery Thromboembolism

Pathology
- Atherosclerosis most common cause
- Less common: Takayasu, fibromuscular dysplasia, trauma, osteophyte compression, dissection, aneurysm, other arteritides

Clinical Issues
- Posterior circulation stroke or TIA
- Vertigo, ataxia, diplopia, syncope "drop attacks", dysphagia, alternating paresthesias, dysarthria
- Endovascular Rx: Angioplasty ± stenting of subclavian, vertebral and basilar arteries

  - Limited utility in follow-up of VA stent patency due to small size, high density of metallic stent obscuring visualization of lumen

MR Findings
- FLAIR: Sensitive for recent areas of ischemia/infarction
- T2* GRE
  - Useful for detection of hemorrhage associated with infarction
  - Petechial ± lobar hemorrhages may occur in subacute phase
- DWI: Most sensitive and highly specific for acute ischemia
- MRA
  - MRA tends to accentuate stenosis: High grade stenosis may appear as signal void
  - Not useful in follow-up of vessel patency S/P stent placement as metallic susceptibility from stent appears as a flow gap in the vessel
- T1WI and T2WI: Posterior circulation infarction
  - Acute: Mass effect in vascular territory
  - Subacute: No mass effect or volume loss; gyral enhancement with contrast
  - Chronic: Encephalomalacia, sulcal enlargement
- Perfusion imaging: ↓ rCBV and ↑ MTT in posterior circulation; rCBV may be normal or ↑ if collaterals adequate, ↓ if inadequate
- MRA
  - 3D TOF: Bilateral VA stenosis (> 70%), high grade stenosis in markedly dominant VA or basilar artery stenosis
  - Subclavian steal: Combination of TOF and Gd-enhanced MRA is diagnostic
    - TOF shows no flow on affected side due to saturation pulse while Gd-MRA shows enhancement of VA bilaterally

Ultrasonographic Findings
- Pulsed Doppler
  - Limited utility in assessment of VA stenosis as VA is obscured as it courses through the transverse foramina of C6-C1
  - Subclavian steal syndrome: Reversed flow direction within VA ipsilateral to subclavian artery stenosis

Angiographic Findings
- Conventional
  - Should image entire length of both vertebral arteries (look for bilateral stenoses, hypoplastic vertebral artery, dominance of affected vertebral artery)
  - DSA: Typically irregular/smooth short segment stenosis ± adjacent Ca++ in ASVD
    - May see dissection flap or intramural hematoma compressing true lumen in cases of dissection
  - Rarely postural VBI due to vertebral artery impingement by spinal osteophytes during neck rotation; stenosis may be visualized with DSA in various degrees of neck rotation
  - Subclavian steal
    - Retrograde flow into contralateral VA during injection of subclavian or vertebral artery contralateral to side of stenosis
    - Non-visualization of VA ± wash-in of unopacified blood from VA during injection of stenotic subclavian artery

Imaging Recommendations
- Best imaging tool
  - CTA or MRA as screening exam
  - DSA if CTA depicts a vertebrobasilar stenosis (for better delineation of lesion) or if CTA inconclusive
- Protocol advice
  - Gd-MRA better than TOF; do both to diagnose subclavian steal
  - DSA for definitive diagnosis, assessment of VA or basilar stent patency

DIFFERENTIAL DIAGNOSIS

Cardiac Insufficiency
- No postural symptoms; no evidence subclavian, vertebral or basilar stenosis on MRA
- CHF or arrhythmias

VERTEBROBASILAR INSUFFICIENCY

Postural Hypotension

- History of autonomic neuropathy, dehydration

Hypoplastic Vertebral Artery

- Left VA is dominant in 70%
- Non-dominant VA maybe markedly hypoplastic or end as the posterior inferior cerebellar artery
- Transverse foramina of C1-C6 will be correspondingly smaller than contralateral side

Benign Vertiginous State

- Ménière labyrinthitis, benign positional vertigo

SAH Vasospasm

- Smooth, tapered, long-segment narrowing of vertebral and basilar arteries typically 4-14 days post-SAH

Basilar Artery Thromboembolism

- Acute onset: Bilateral long-tract signs, ophthalmoplegia, reduced consciousness, dysarthria, "locked-in" syndrome
- Filling defect in BA on CTA or DSA
- Poor prognosis

PATHOLOGY

General Features

- General path comments
  - Vertebrobasilar insufficiency
    - If > 70% stenosis of both vertebral arteries and anterior circulation unable to compensate via circle of Willis
    - If > 70% subclavian stenosis proximal to origin of vertebral artery may have retrograde flow in ipsilateral VA (true "subclavian steal syndrome" only if VBI present clinically)
- Etiology
  - Atherosclerosis most common cause
  - Less common: Takayasu, fibromuscular dysplasia, trauma, osteophyte compression, dissection, aneurysm, other arteritides

Gross Pathologic & Surgical Features

- Stenosis of proximal subclavian artery, basilar artery, or both vertebral arteries and associated posterior circulation stroke

Microscopic Features

- Atherosclerosis: Fatty streaks, lipid-laden macrophages & smooth muscle cells, fibrous cap, cholesterol deposits, foam cells, plaque rupture ± thrombus

CLINICAL ISSUES

Presentation

- Most common signs/symptoms
  - Posterior circulation stroke or TIA
    - Hemi/quadrantanopsia (occipital lobe), sensory deficit (brainstem/thalamus), motor deficit (brainstem or cerebellum)
  - Vertigo, ataxia, diplopia, syncope "drop attacks", dysphagia, alternating paresthesias, dysarthria
  - If subclavian steal syndrome: Arm pain (ischemia) and VBI symptoms with arm exercise

Demographics

- Age
  - Usually elderly, 6th-8th decade
  - Consider dissection, underlying vasculopathy (e.g., fibromuscular dysplasia) if young patient

Natural History & Prognosis

- Risk of watershed infarction with reduction in mean arterial blood pressure
- Superimposed thrombosis in region of critical stenosis may complete occlusion of vessel

Treatment

- Indicated for symptomatic disease (vs. imaging diagnosis)
- Endovascular Rx: Angioplasty ± stenting of subclavian, vertebral and basilar arteries
  - Minimally invasive treatment
  - Risk of perforator occlusion during stenting of distal intracranial vertebral artery and basilar artery
  - Will need long-term antiplatelet therapy after stent placement
  - DSA follow-up required due to inability of MRA and CTA to visualize in-stent restenosis
  - Vertebral artery origin stenosis most problematic for recurrent stenosis after endovascular treatment; drug-eluting stents may reduce restenosis
- Surgery: Depends on level of disease
  - Proximal subclavian stenosis (subclavian steal): Reconstruction
  - V1 (ostial lesions): Vertebral artery reconstruction or bypass to ipsilateral carotid or subclavian arteries
  - V2 (within cervical foramina): Check for compressing osteophytes → excision
- Medical: Long-term anticoagulation ± antiplatelet therapy, permissive hypertension for atherosclerotic stenoses

DIAGNOSTIC CHECKLIST

Consider

- VBI in elderly patient with postural symptoms of posterior circulation ischemia ± stroke on imaging

Image Interpretation Pearls

- CTA or MRA sufficient to make diagnosis of significant vertebrobasilar or subclavian stenosis in most cases
- Further delineation ± intervention with catheter angiography

SELECTED REFERENCES

1. Berguer R et al: Surgical reconstruction of the extracranial vertebral artery: management. J Vasc Surg 31: 9-18, 2000
2. Caplan L: Posterior circulation ischemia: then, now, and tomorrow. Stroke. 31: 2011-23, 2000
3. Malek AM et al: Treatment of posterior circulation ischemia with extracranial percutaneous balloon angioplasty and stent placement. Stroke. 30: 2073-85, 1999

IMAGE GALLERY

Typical

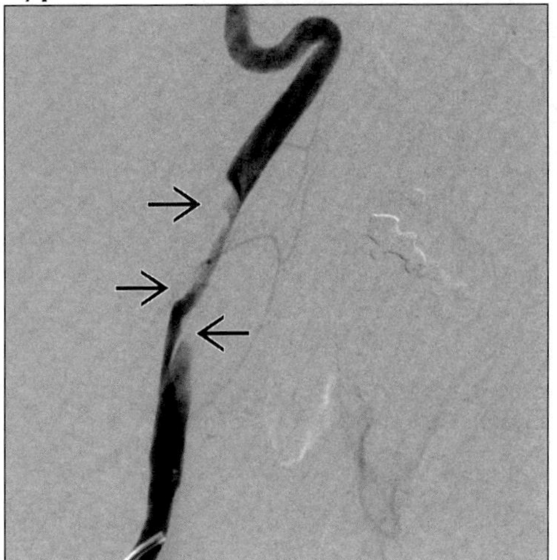

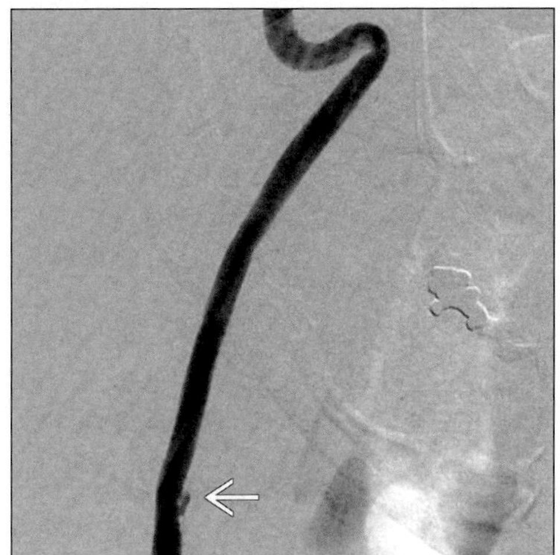

(Left) *Right vertebral artery DSA shows dissection of the cervical (V2) segment of the right vertebral artery. Note compression of the true lumen by intramural hematoma ⇒.* ***(Right)*** *Right vertebral artery DSA in the same patient as previous image, two months later, after treatment with Coumadin, shows impressive interval healing of the dissection with tiny residual pseudoaneurysm ➡.*

Typical

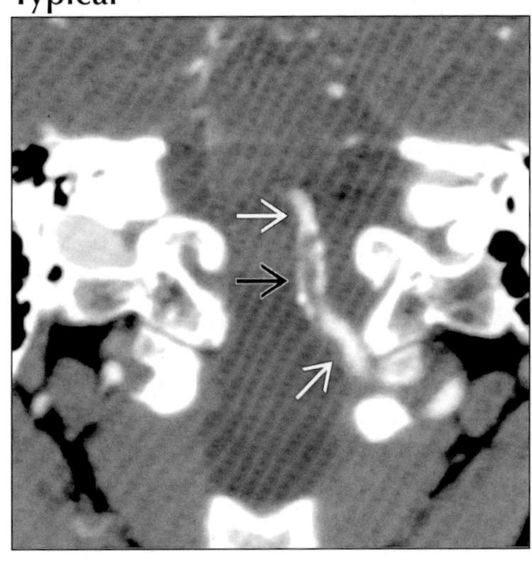

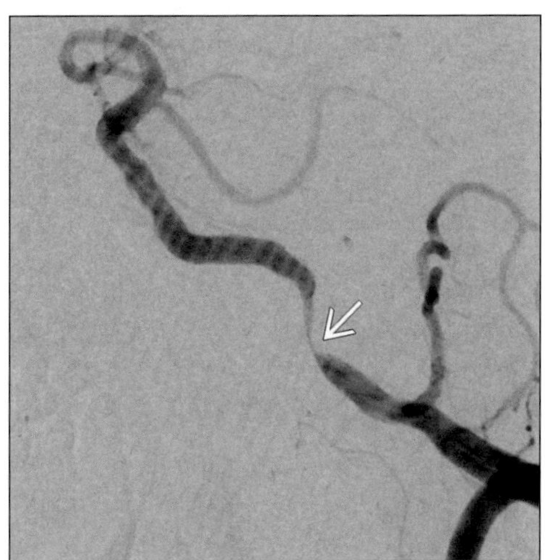

(Left) *Coronal CTA shows mural calcification along the left vertebral artery ⇒. Although no definite residual lumen is seen, enhancement and normal caliber of the adjacent vertebral artery ➡ suggests patency.* ***(Right)*** *Oblique right vertebral artery DSA in the same patient as previous image confirms patency with a pinpoint stenosis ➡. This was subsequently stented with resolution of symptoms.*

Typical

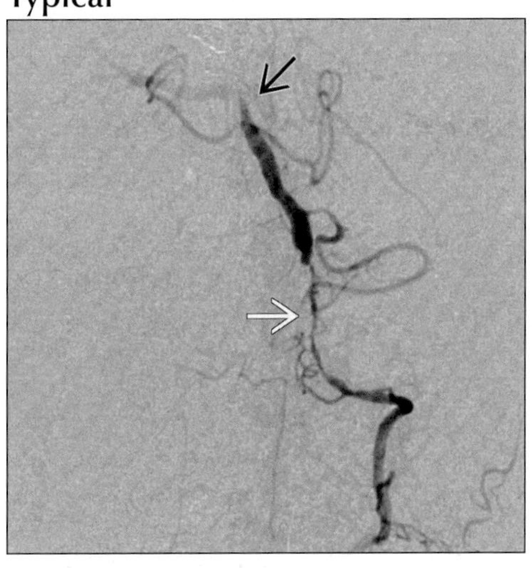

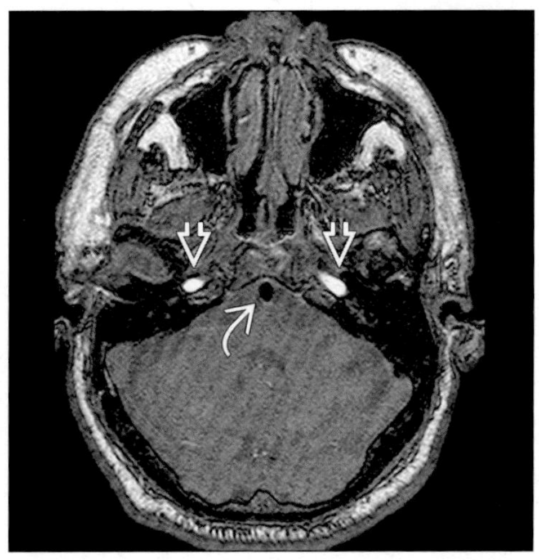

(Left) *Left VA DSA shows irregular stenosis of the V4 segment ➡. The right VA was occluded. Apparent tapering of the basilar tip ⇒ is due to slow antegrade flow and wash-in of unopacified blood from the PCoAs.* ***(Right)*** *Axial TOF MRA source image in a patient with basilar artery stent shows flow gap within the stent ➡ and flow-related enhancement of the carotid arteries ➡. MRA is not useful for determination of stent patency. DSA is required for follow-up.*

VERTEBRAL DISSECTION

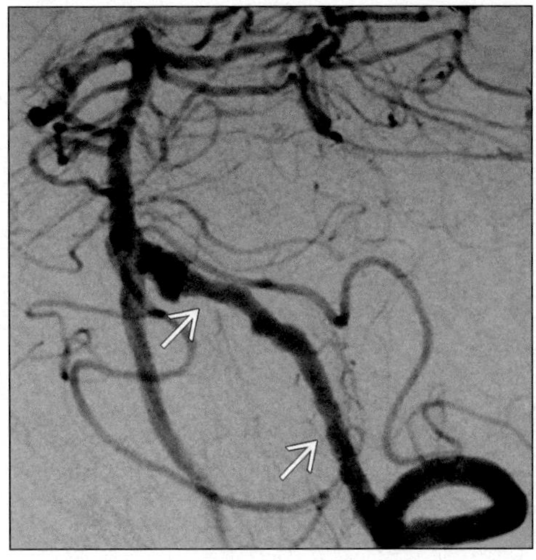

Left vertebral artery DSA shows a long segment of luminal irregularity along the V3-V4 segments ➡ consistent with dissection. The patient presented with subarachnoid hemorrhage.

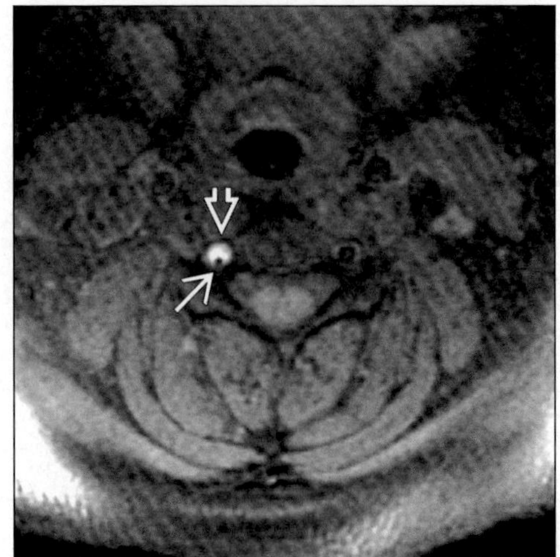

Axial T1WI FS MR in a patient with right vertebral artery dissection shows a small, eccentric flow-void ➡ representing the residual true lumen surrounded by a bright crescentic rim of methemoglobin ⇨.

TERMINOLOGY

Definitions

- Hemorrhage into damaged vessel wall with subsequent stenosis, pseudoaneurysm or rupture

IMAGING FINDINGS

General Features

- Best diagnostic clue
  - Eccentric vertebral artery stenosis associated with intramural hematoma ± intimal flap ± pseudoaneurysm on CTA
  - Intramural crescentic hyperintensity on fat-saturated T1WI MR surrounding a diminished flow void
- Location
  - Most common site is between C2 and skull base (V3/V4 segment)
    - May extend into origin of posterior inferior cerebellar artery (PICA)
  - May occur along cervical (V1-V2) segment from trauma ± fracture of C-spine transverse processes (vertebral artery traverses transverse foramina)

CT Findings

- NECT
  - Subarachnoid hemorrhage (SAH) ± focal clot adjacent to brainstem if there is extension of dissection through the tunica adventitia
  - Posterior circulation infarction due to thromboembolism ± hemodynamic compromise
  - Hyperdense subacute mural or intraluminal thrombus
- CTA: Irregular vessel lumen with associated stenosis or pseudoaneurysm

MR Findings

- T1WI: Fat-sat images most useful for diagnosis; high signal crescent or ring within vessel wall = methemoglobin (met-Hb)
- FLAIR: Sensitive for SAH if ruptured dissecting aneurysm or parenchymal injury from thromboembolic/hemodynamic infarction
- DWI: Specific for ischemic injury due to thromboemboli or hemodynamic insufficiency
- MRA
  - Variable appearances depending on degree of stenosis, morphology of pseudoaneurysm

DDx: Vertebral Artery Narrowing

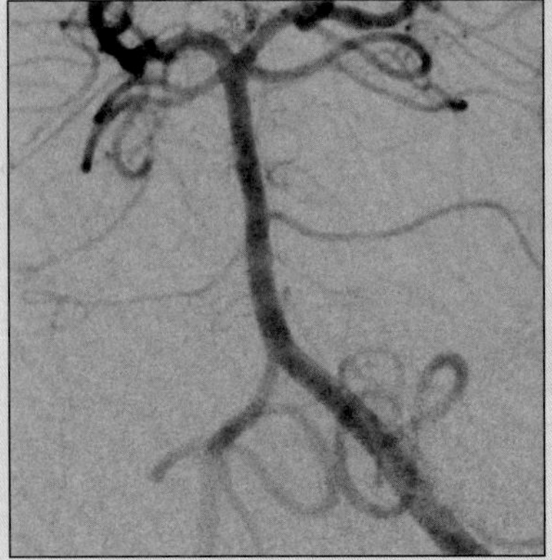

Hypoplastic Right Vertebral Artery

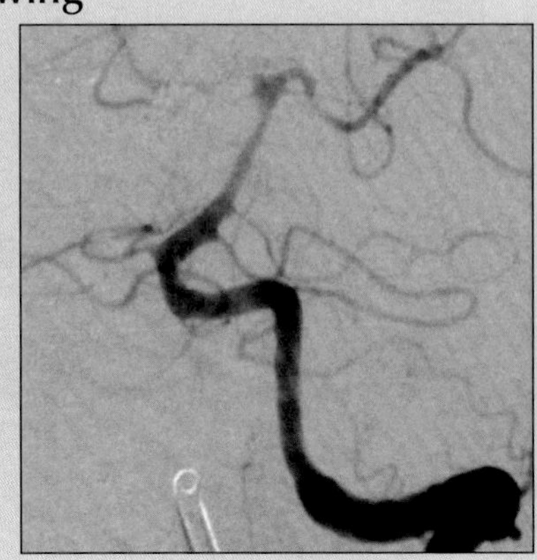

SAH Vasospasm

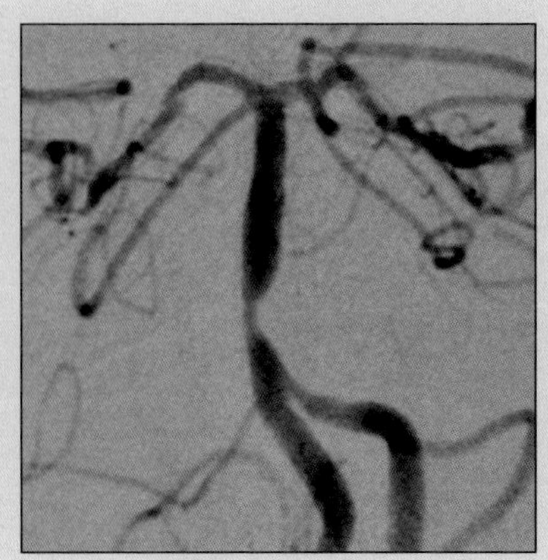

Atherosclerosis

VERTEBRAL DISSECTION

Key Facts

Terminology

- Hemorrhage into damaged vessel wall with subsequent stenosis, pseudoaneurysm or rupture

Imaging Findings

- Eccentric vertebral artery stenosis associated with intramural hematoma ± intimal flap ± pseudoaneurysm on CTA
- Intramural crescentic hyperintensity on fat-saturated T1WI MR surrounding a diminished flow void
- Most common site is between C2 and skull base (V3/V4 segment)
- May vary from mild stenosis → "string sign" → total occlusion

Top Differential Diagnoses

- Atherosclerotic Disease
- Fibromuscular Dysplasia (FMD)
- SAH Vasospasm

Pathology

- Fractures through transverse foramina associated with vertebral dissection
- Connective tissue diseases (CTDs) predispose to spontaneous dissection

Clinical Issues

- Most common signs/symptoms: Thromboembolic stroke
- SAH if intradural dissection and tear extends through tunica adventitia
- Hemodynamic stroke/ischemia if significant stenosis and poor collaterals (hypoplastic/absent contralateral vertebral artery, small PCoAs)

    - May see flow-related enhancement vs. signal loss if turbulent flow present
  - Thin, curvilinear, hypointense intimal flap
  - Normal or narrowed flow void (true lumen)
  - TOF images may give artifact from intramural met-Hb (high signal baseline, not flow-related enhancement)
  - PC images take longer to acquire + lower resolution but no baseline signal from met-Hb cf. TOF
  - Best resolution with Gd enhanced MRA; can also do subtracted Gd-MRA
    - Unable to differentiate direction of flow (e.g., subclavian steal) cf. TOF MRA
- Intramural hematoma
  - Hyperintense on fat-suppressed T1WI and T2WI
    - May be isointense initially
    - Intermediate signal intensity between flow-related enhancement and surrounding soft tissue
  - Crescentic, circumferential, or filling the entire lumen
  - May enhance after intravenous gadolinium

Angiographic Findings

- Conventional
  - Smooth or slightly irregular, tapered luminal narrowing
    - May vary from mild stenosis → "string sign" → total occlusion
  - Pseudoaneurysm (25-35%)
  - Intimal flap (10%) and double lumen
  - Branch vessel occlusion from thromboembolism or extension of dissection into vessel origin (e.g., PICA)
  - Relationship to PICA and anterior spinal artery (ASA) origins from vertebral artery important for stroke risk and therapeutic options
  - Imaging of contralateral vertebral artery is important to determine concurrent lesions + dominance of dissected vertebral artery, particularly if therapeutic vertebral artery sacrifice is contemplated
  - Size of posterior communicating arteries (PCoAs) may be important if dissection extends to vertebrobasilar junction (VBJ) or basilar artery if bilateral vertebral occlusion is contemplated as a therapeutic option

Imaging Recommendations

- Best imaging tool
  - CTA of neck with coronal + sagittal reconstructions usually diagnostic
  - MR including axial T1WI with fat-sat + TOF MRA will make the diagnosis in most cases; Gd MRA better
  - In equivocal cases or in cases where endovascular treatment is contemplated (SAH, hemodynamically significant stenosis) catheter angiography should be performed

DIFFERENTIAL DIAGNOSIS

Atherosclerotic Disease

- Often occurs at vertebral artery origin
- More focal, mural calcifications, other vessels involved
- No intramural hematoma

Fibromuscular Dysplasia (FMD)

- Can present with focal narrowing on conventional angiogram
- Vertebral artery involvement (7%) is less common than carotid arteries (85%)

Normal Dural Entry Zone

- Normal smooth constriction/change in caliber of vertebral artery as it enters the dura near the skull base → V4 segment
- Dural entry zone is usually at the foramen magnum but can be more caudal, hence extracranial vertebral artery dissection may result in SAH

SAH Vasospasm

- Peaks 4-14 days post-SAH

VERTEBRAL DISSECTION

PATHOLOGY

General Features

- General path comments
  - Embryology-anatomy
    - Vertebral artery divided into 4 segments: V1 = origin from subclavian artery to C6 transverse foramen; V2 = C6 to C2; V3 = C2 to dural entry between C1 and skull base; V4 = intradural segment to VBJ
    - Sites of greatest mobility are susceptible to injury (e.g., b/w dural entry and C2 transverse process; b/w origin from subclavian artery to C6 transverse process)
    - Fractures through transverse foramina associated with vertebral dissection
- Genetics
  - Connective tissue diseases (CTDs) predispose to spontaneous dissection
    - Ehlers-Danlos syndrome, Marfan syndrome, autosomal dominant polycystic kidney disease
  - Other arteriopathies
    - FMD
    - Cystic medial necrosis
- Etiology
  - Spontaneous
  - Hypertension: Primary or drug-induced, including over-the-counter, e.g., ephedrine
  - Major penetrating or blunt trauma
  - Trivial trauma (coughing, sneezing, roller-coaster ride, chiropractic = classic)
    - Prolonged or sudden neck hyperextension or rotation may be a precipitating factor
  - Iatrogenic from catheter angiography
    - Extreme care in patients with CTDs
    - Ehlers-Danlos type IV may have no peripheral stigmata → presents with vascular complication
  - Intimal tear or ruptured vasa vasorum → intramural hematoma → stenosis or pseudoaneurysm → thrombus formation → thromboembolic events ± hemodynamic compromise
- Epidemiology
  - Estimate of 1 to 1.5 per 100,000
  - Affects all ages, peak in the fifth decade of life

Microscopic Features

- Hematoma within tunica media of vessel wall
  - Compressing intima, distending ± rupture through adventitia

CLINICAL ISSUES

Presentation

- Most common signs/symptoms: Thromboembolic stroke
- Other signs/symptoms
  - SAH if intradural dissection and tear extends through tunica adventitia
  - Hemodynamic stroke/ischemia if significant stenosis and poor collaterals (hypoplastic/absent contralateral vertebral artery, small PCoAs)
- Dissection may affect other vessels if etiology is head/neck trauma or underlying collagen vascular disease
  - Should carefully examine entire course of both carotid and vertebral arteries in such patients
- Neurological symptoms may be delayed after initial injury
- Unilateral or bilateral occipital headache and posterior neck pain
- Unilateral arm pain or weakness
- Brainstem, cerebellar infarction
  - Lateral medullary syndrome of Wallenberg if PICA infarct
- Posterior cerebral artery territory infarction
  - Homonymous hemianopsia or Anton syndrome (cortical blindness) if bilateral

Demographics

- Age
  - Carotid and vertebral dissection responsible for 2% of all cerebrovascular accidents
    - Causes 10-25% of all infarcts in young and middle-aged patients

Natural History & Prognosis

- Spontaneously healing or recanalization in most cases
- Resolution or significant improvement of stenosis in 90% within the first 2 to 3 months

Treatment

- Anticoagulation, unless contraindications present
- If persistent ischemia
  - Endovascular stent or surgical bypass
- If recurrent emboli without pseudoaneurysm despite anticoagulation
  - Surgical ligation or endovascular occlusion if collateral blood flow sufficient
- If pseudoaneurysm source of emboli or associated mass effect
  - Consider covered stent, stent-supported coil embolization, vessel sacrifice

DIAGNOSTIC CHECKLIST

Consider

- Vertebral dissection in young patients with posterior circulation stroke

Image Interpretation Pearls

- Look for fractures that traverse transverse foramina of C1 to C6
- Multiplanar reformats of CTA diagnostic in most cases

SELECTED REFERENCES

1. Albuquerque FC et al: Endovascular management of intracranial vertebral artery dissecting aneurysms. Neurosurg Focus. 18(2):E3, 2005
2. Iihara K et al: Dissecting aneurysms of the vertebral artery: a management strategy. J Neurosurg. 97(2):259-67, 2002
3. Provenzale JM: Dissection of the internal carotid and vertebral arteries: imaging features. AJR Am J Roentgenol. 165(5):1099-104, 1995

IMAGE GALLERY

Typical

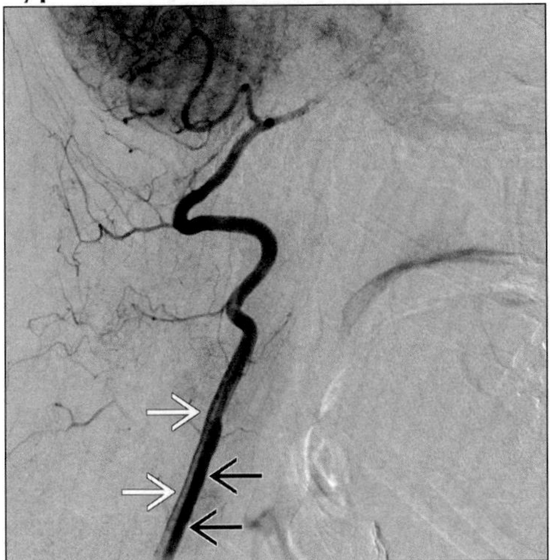

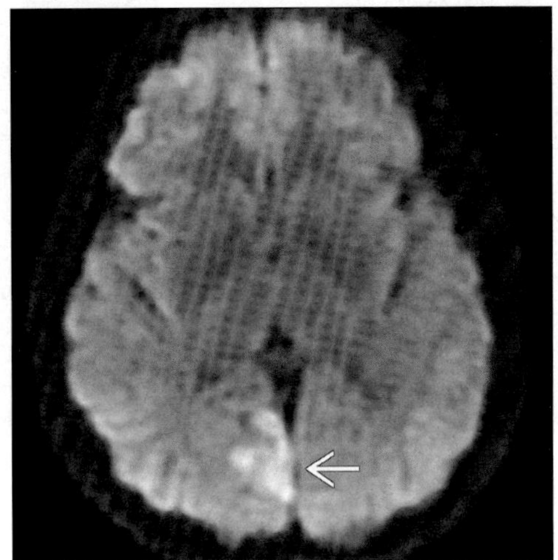

(Left) *Lateral right vertebral artery DSA shows dissection of the cervical (V2) segment with delayed washout of contrast from the false lumen, situated anteriorly ⇒ compared with the true lumen which is already partially filled with unopacified blood ➡ after contrast injection.* ***(Right)*** *Axial MR DWI in the same patient as previous image shows restricted diffusion in the right occipital lobe ➡ consistent with embolic infarction.*

Typical

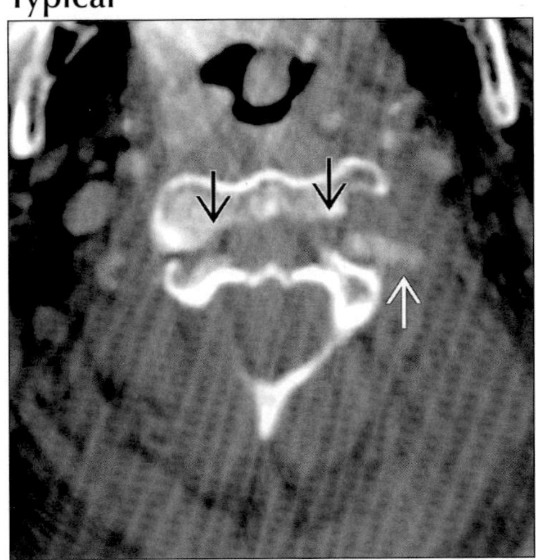

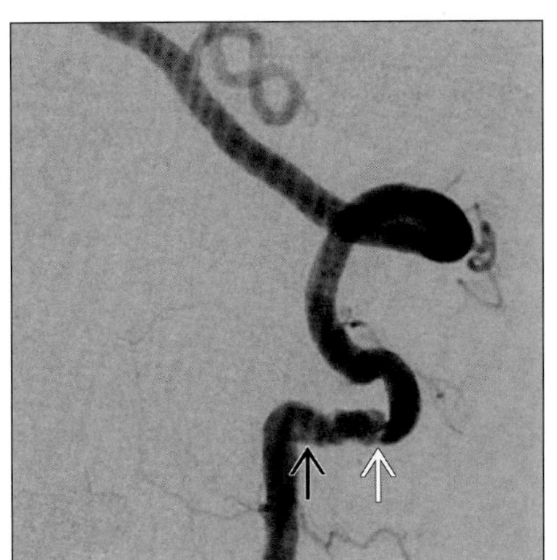

(Left) *Axial CTA shows a displaced fracture of C2 ⇒ extending into the foramen transversarium bilaterally. There is luminal irregularity of the left vertebral artery ➡ suggestive of traumatic dissection.* ***(Right)*** *Left vertebral artery DSA in the same patient as previous image confirms luminal irregularity within the left vertebral artery as it leaves the transverse foramen of C2. An intimal flap ➡ and mural thrombus ⇒ are seen.*

Typical

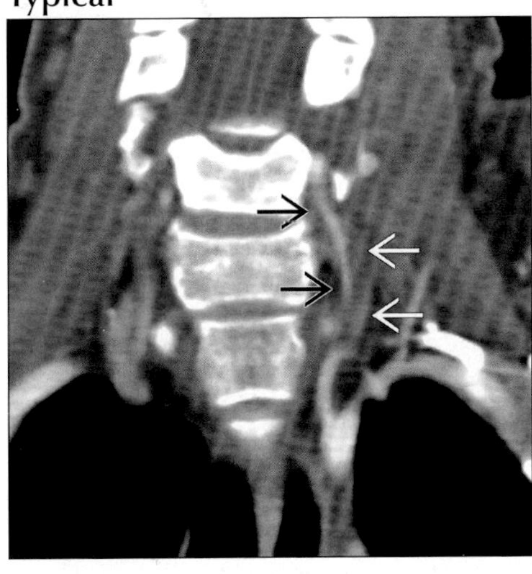

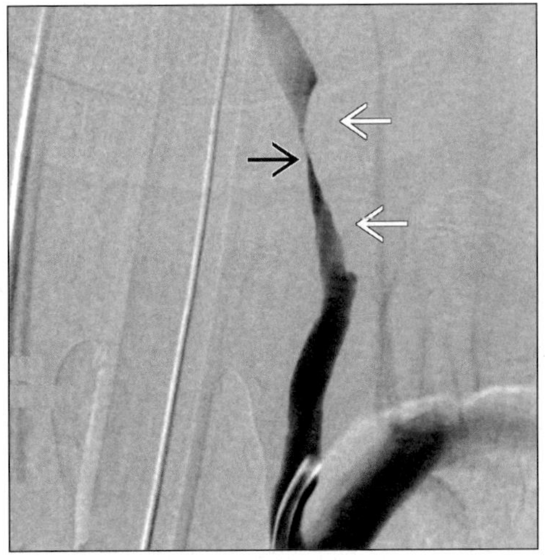

(Left) *Coronal CTA shows stenosis and luminal irregularity of the left vertebral artery at the C6-7 level ⇒. Note mural thrombus adjacent to the residual lumen ➡.* ***(Right)*** *Left vertebral artery DSA confirms arterial dissection with critical stenosis ⇒ of the true lumen from compression by intramural thrombus ➡. The patient presented with basilar artery embolic occlusion several days after neck manipulation.*

SUBCLAVIAN STEAL

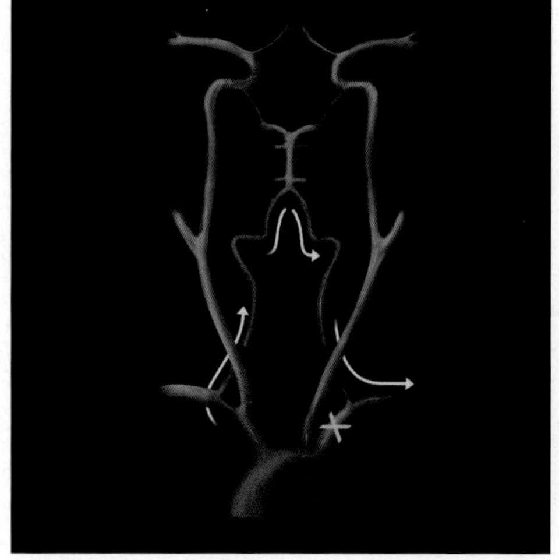

Anteroposterior graphic shows occlusion of left subclavian artery origin (X) with resultant "steal" of blood from left vertebral (via right vertebral) artery to supply the left extremity.

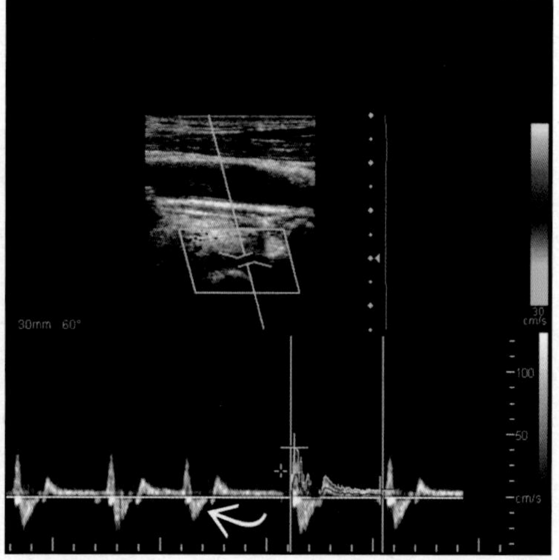

Color Doppler ultrasound of the left vertebral artery shows biphasic flow with late systolic reversal of flow ➔ indicative of moderate left subclavian steal.

TERMINOLOGY

Abbreviations and Synonyms

- Vertebral-to-subclavian steal

Definitions

- Collateral blood flow to the arm via the vertebral artery (VA) as a result of proximal subclavian artery (SCA) stenosis or occlusion

IMAGING FINDINGS

General Features

- Best diagnostic clue
  - Reversed or biphasic VA flow ipsilateral to stenosed or obstructed SCA; antegrade VA flow contralateral to stenosed or obstructed SCA
  - ↑ Volume/velocity of flow in contralateral VA
  - Exacerbated by increased arterial blood flow demand in the arm (i.e., arm exercise)
- Location: More common on the left but right-sided subclavian steal also possible

CT Findings

- NECT
  - May see calcification in vessel wall of stenotic or occluded proximal SCA
  - Large plaques may show low density foci (lipid)
- CECT
  - High-grade SCA stenosis or occlusion
    - Lesion must occur in the SCA proximal to the origin of the VA
- CTA
  - Permits 3D reconstruction of vasculature
    - Enables better estimation of degree of stenosis
    - Improves ability to differentiate severe stenosis from frank occlusion

MR Findings

- T1WI: May identify high signal lipid/hemorrhage in atherosclerotic plaque of stenosed SCA
- T2WI
  - Wall thickening and luminal narrowing in SCA
  - Absence of "flow-void" may occur if vessel severely stenotic or occluded
- MRA
  - Determine degree of SCA stenosis

DDx: Subclavian Steal

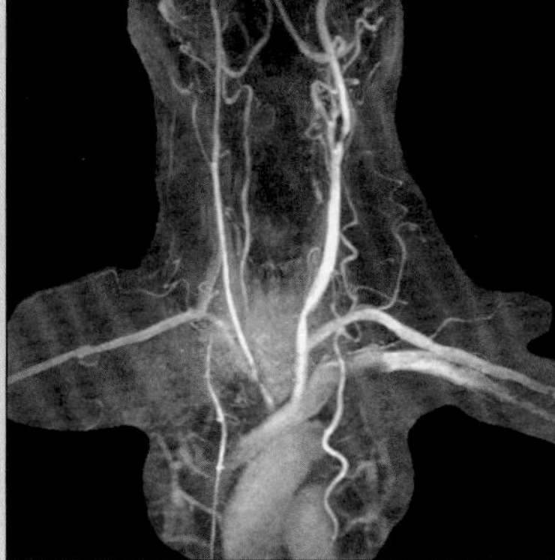

Right Common Carotid Artery Steal

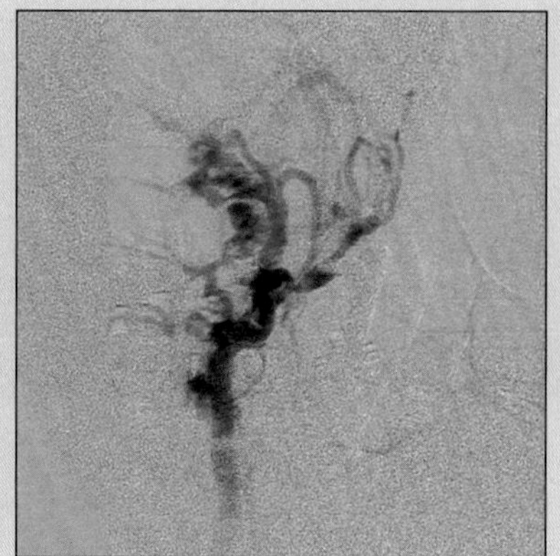

Right VA Arteriovenous Fistula

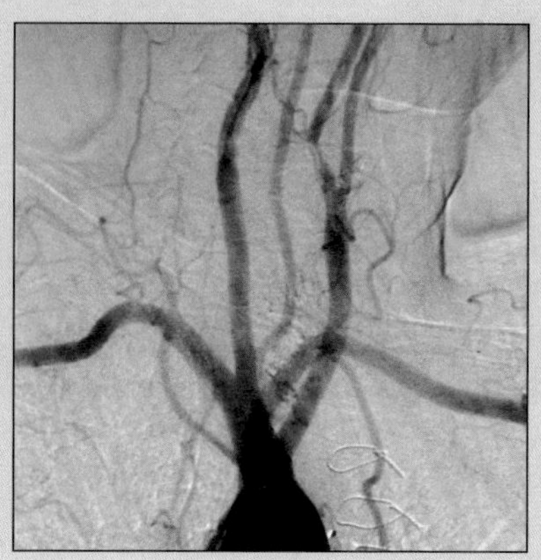

Occluded Right VA with Collaterals

SUBCLAVIAN STEAL

Key Facts

Terminology

- Collateral blood flow to the arm via the vertebral artery (VA) as a result of proximal subclavian artery (SCA) stenosis or occlusion

Imaging Findings

- 3D C+ MRA much better to delineate true presence and degree of stenosis
- Reversed flow in VA will be inapparent on noncontrast 2D time-of-flight MRA (due to superior saturation pulse used to remove inferiorly flowing venous signal); can mimic VA occlusion
- Phase contrast MRA can confirm vessel patency, reversal of VA flow, as well as regions of stenosis (anatomic and pathophysiologic abnormality!)
- Complete steal: Reversed flow in the affected VA on color and spectral Doppler
- If abnormal VA flow not detected at rest, then induce flow reversal with ipsilateral arm exercise or artificial arm hyperemia (following cuff compression)

Top Differential Diagnoses

- Right Common Carotid Artery Steal
- Vertebral Arteriovenous Fistula (AVF)
- Vertebral Artery Occlusion (or Very Severe Stenosis)

Pathology

- Atherosclerotic occlusive disease by far most common cause of SCA obstruction leading to subclavian steal

Clinical Issues

- Generally a harmless, asymptomatic phenomenon, but can be symptomatic in particular occurring with arm exercise
- Angioplasty/stenting of SCA

    - Intravascular signal may not be evident on noncontrast 2D time-of-flight MRA if high grade stenosis present; can mimic SCA occlusion
    - 3D C+ MRA much better to delineate true presence and degree of stenosis
  - Determine flow direction in VA
    - Reversed flow in VA will be inapparent on noncontrast 2D time-of-flight MRA (due to superior saturation pulse used to remove inferiorly flowing venous signal); can mimic VA occlusion
    - 3D C+ MRA demonstrates vessel patency but not flow direction ("time-resolved" 3D C+ MRA better to show retrograde VA flow)
    - Phase contrast MRA can confirm vessel patency, reversal of VA flow, as well as regions of stenosis (anatomic and pathophysiologic abnormality!)

Ultrasonographic Findings

- Duplex Doppler ultrasound
  - Complete steal: Reversed flow in the affected VA on color and spectral Doppler
  - Moderate steal: Alternating biphasic (to-and-fro) spectral Doppler flow in the affected VA at rest
    - Provocative dynamic tests with ipsilateral arm exercise or tourniquet-induced arm hyperemia may better demonstrate flow reversal
  - Mild steal: Systolic deceleration of VA flow
  - Increased blood flow in the contralateral VA (not precisely defined, but peak systolic velocity > 60 cm/sec suggests abnormality)
  - Damped Doppler waveforms (due to ischemia) in the affected SCA
  - Possible Doppler evidence of SCA stenosis (focal high velocity, turbulence)

Angiographic Findings

- DSA
  - Flow is reversed or to-and fro in the affected VA and antegrade in contralateral VA
  - High grade proximal SCA stenosis or occlusion ipsilateral to VA flow reversal

Imaging Recommendations

- Best imaging tool
  - Sonography alone able to diagnose subclavian steal
  - MRA, CTA or DSA for comprehensive pre-operative assessment
- Protocol advice
  - If abnormal VA flow not detected at rest, then induce flow reversal with ipsilateral arm exercise or artificial arm hyperemia (following cuff compression)
  - With MRA use phase-contrast technique to show flow direction/reversal in affected VA

DIFFERENTIAL DIAGNOSIS

Right Common Carotid Artery Steal

- Associated with high grade innominate artery stenosis or occlusion (right side only)
- Analogous to subclavian steal, but blood is "stolen" from the right common carotid artery (RCCA) as well as the right VA
- To-and-fro or reversed RCCA and right VA flow

Vertebral Arteriovenous Fistula (AVF)

- Abnormal direct communication between vertebral artery and vein
- High velocity turbulent flow with low resistance in the affected vessels
- Surrounding venous engorgement
- May demonstrate reversal of VA flow distal to the site of AVF

Vertebral Artery Occlusion (or Very Severe Stenosis)

- Flow not identified in VA
- Only venous flow noted (may be confused with slow reversal of flow in VA but will not demonstrate arterial waveform)
- Adjacent vessels usually from external carotid artery or proximal SCA may mimic VA patency and may even mimic reversal of VA flow

SUBCLAVIAN STEAL

- Cervical collateral vessels can also reconstitute VA distal to occlusion/stenosis resulting in distal VA dampened, high-resistance or alternating flow pattern

Vertebral Artery Hypoplasia

- Normal VA flow may not be detected in severe hypoplasia
- Usually right-sided but may occur on left side
- Hypoplastic left VA may arise directly from aortic arch
- Should demonstrate normal antegrade flow direction but may have high-resistance flow pattern due to increased flow friction in the small vessel and hypoplastic VA often only supplies ipsilateral PICA

PATHOLOGY

General Features

- General path comments
  - Anatomy
    - Subclavian steal occurs because of unique vertebrobasilar arterial system, with the two VAs combining at the foramen magnum to form the basilar artery
    - With proximal SCA occlusion or severe stenosis blood flow is conveniently "stolen" from the ipsilateral VA, supplying the arm with collateral blood flow
    - Thus, there is reversal of flow in the ipsilateral VA and hyperdynamic flow in the contralateral VA
    - Usually requires at least 70% SCA diameter stenosis
- Etiology
  - Atherosclerotic occlusive disease by far most common cause of SCA obstruction leading to subclavian steal
  - Rarely, steal-inducing SCA obstruction may result from vasculitis, dissection, trauma, or vessel compression from adjacent neoplastic mass

Staging, Grading or Classification Criteria

- Complete (persistent): Steal phenomenon is present at all times (implies SCA occlusion)
- Mild or moderate (intermittent): Steal phenomenon occurs only when arm exercise increases blood flow demand (implies SCA stenosis)

CLINICAL ISSUES

Presentation

- Most common signs/symptoms
  - Generally a harmless, asymptomatic phenomenon, but can be symptomatic in particular occurring with arm exercise
    - Arm claudication (pain with arm exercise)
    - If vertebrobasilar insufficiency/ischemia present may result in dizziness (most common), vertigo, imbalance, ataxia, drop attacks, diplopia, perioral numbness, tinnitus, alternating paresthesias, dysarthria, dysphagia, homonymous hemianopsia
- Other signs/symptoms
  - Very rarely causes vertebrobasilar infarct of brainstem, cerebellum or posterior cerebral hemispheres
    - Concomitant carotid/vertebral/cerebral vascular disease invariably present
- Diminished arm pulses and blood pressure ipsilateral to SCA obstruction (arm-to-arm blood pressure difference of 20-30 mm Hg)
- Predominately left side (85% of cases) but can occur on right

Demographics

- Age: Elderly (average age 60 years)
- Gender: M > F (slight male predominance)

Natural History & Prognosis

- Usually remains asymptomatic
- May become symptomatic with progression of atherosclerosis in the affected arm or the cerebral vasculature

Treatment

- Angioplasty/stenting of SCA
- Common carotid artery-to-SCA bypass, innominate artery-to-SCA bypass or axillary artery-to-axillary artery bypass
- Address atherosclerosis risk factors

DIAGNOSTIC CHECKLIST

Consider

- Subclavian steal likely if cerebral symptoms exacerbated with arm exercise
- SCA obstruction most likely due to atherosclerotic disease but vasculitis, dissection, trauma or adjacent neoplastic mass must be excluded

Image Interpretation Pearls

- Sonography easiest best test to confirm diagnosis
- If abnormal VA flow not detected at rest, then induce flow reversal with ipsilateral arm exercise or artificial arm hyperemia
- Reversed flow in VA will be inapparent on noncontrast 2D time-of-flight MRA: Use C+ MRA or better yet phase contrast MRA

SELECTED REFERENCES

1. Tan TY et al: Hemodynamic effects of subclavian steal phenomenon on contralateral vertebral artery. J Clin Ultrasound. 34(2):77-81, 2006
2. De Vries JP et al: Durability of percutaneous transluminal angioplasty for obstructive lesions of proximal subclavian artery: long-term results. J Vasc Surg. 41(1):19-23, 2005
3. Sheehy N et al: Contrast-enhanced MR angiography of subclavian steal syndrome: value of the 2D time-of-flight "localizer" sign. AJR Am J Roentgenol. 185(4):1069-73, 2005
4. Bitar R et al: MR angiography of subclavian steal syndrome: pitfalls and solutions. AJR Am J Roentgenol. 183(6):1840-1, 2004
5. Kliewer MA et al: Vertebral artery Doppler waveform changes indicating subclavian steal physiology. AJR Am J Roentgenol. 174(3):815-9, 2000
6. Pollard H et al: SUBCLAVIAN STEAL SYNDROME: A Review. Australas Chiropr Osteopathy. 7(1):20-8, 1998

SUBCLAVIAN STEAL

IMAGE GALLERY

Typical

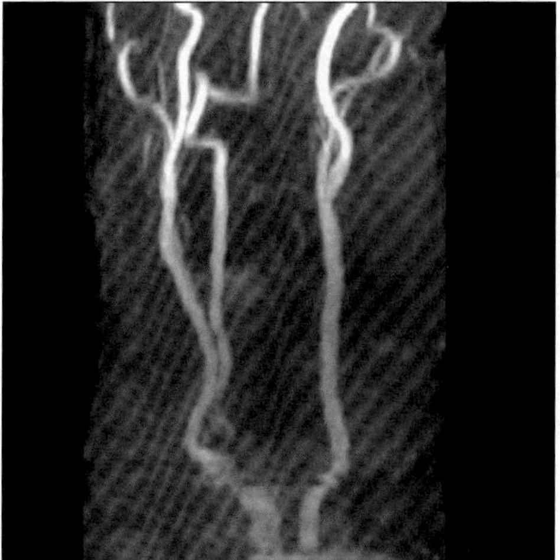

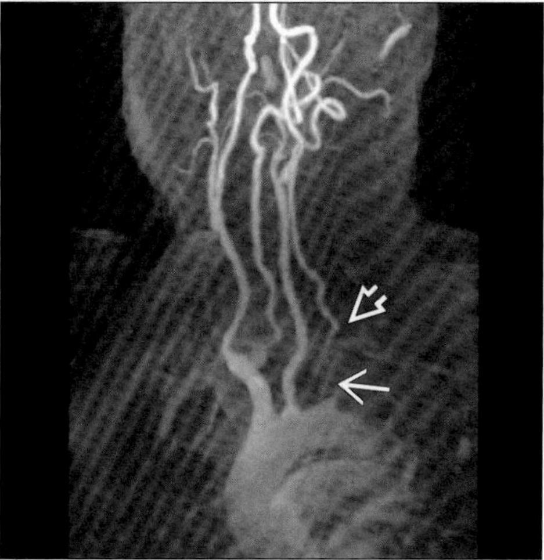

*(**Left**) Coronal oblique 2D TOF MRA MIP image shows lack of signal in left vertebral artery mimicking occlusion. This is actually due to superior saturation pulse nulling the signal of downward flow. (**Right**) Coronal oblique 3D TOF contrast-enhanced MRA MIP image in the same patient shows occlusion of proximal left SCA with reconstitution of SCA via reversal of flow in the left VA.*

Typical

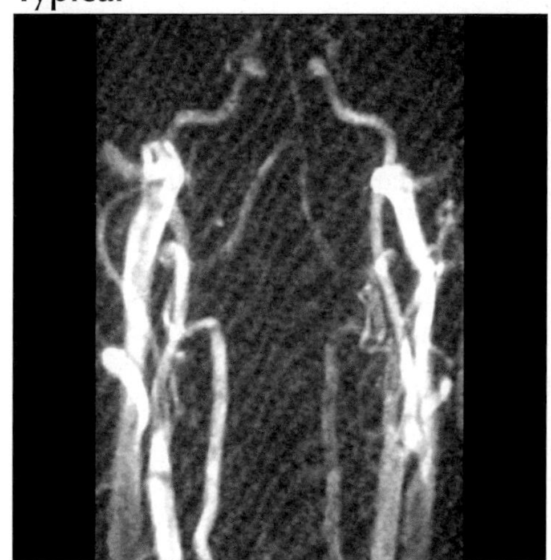

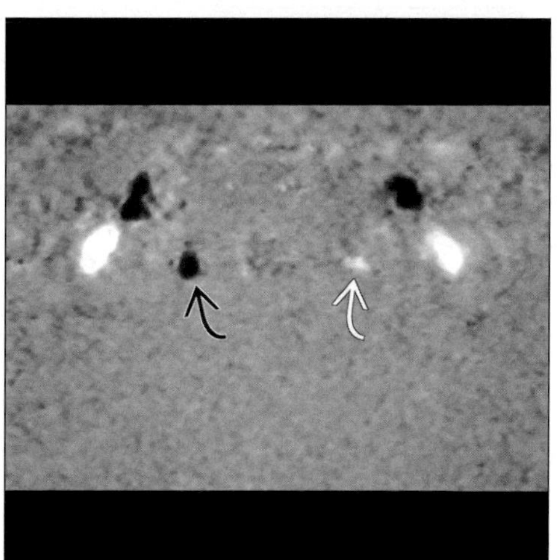

*(**Left**) Coronal PC MRA MIP image shows patency of the entire vertebrobasilar arterial system. 2D TOF MRA (not shown) demonstrated lack of flow in the left vertebral artery. Left subclavian steal. (**Right**) Axial 2D PC MRA image shows subclavian steal with upward flow (black) in carotid and right vertebral arteries and downward flow (white) in jugular veins and left vertebral artery.*

Typical

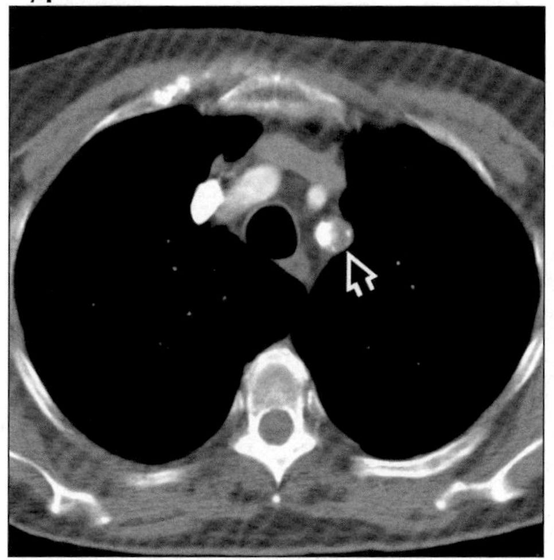

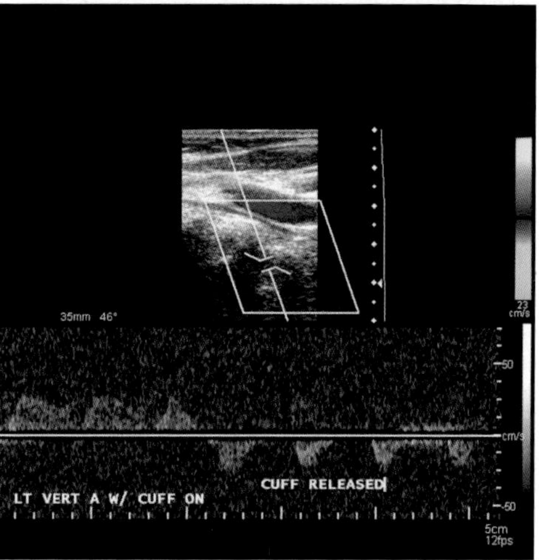

*(**Left**) Axial CECT shows stenosis of the proximal left subclavian artery with calcification (high density foci) and lipid (low density area) in the atheromatous plaque. (**Right**) Color Doppler ultrasound shows antegrade left vertebral artery flow with left arm cuff inflated and reversal of flow with cuff deflated, a provocative maneuver to evoke subclavian steal.*

CAROTID BODY PARAGANGLIOMA

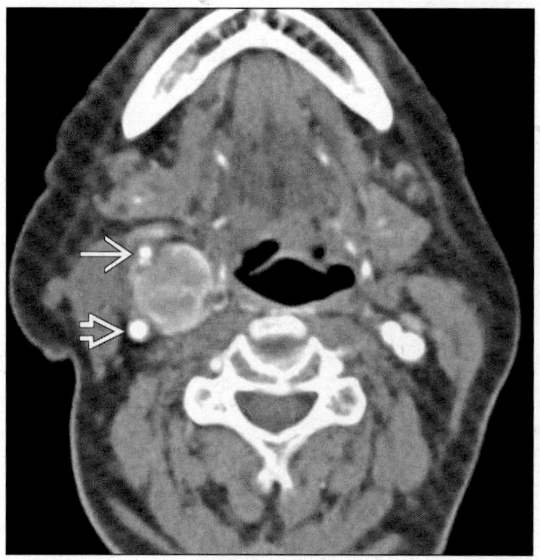

Axial CECT shows a heterogeneously enhancing mass splaying the ECA ➔ and ICA ➲. The patient presented with a painless neck lump and dysphagia.

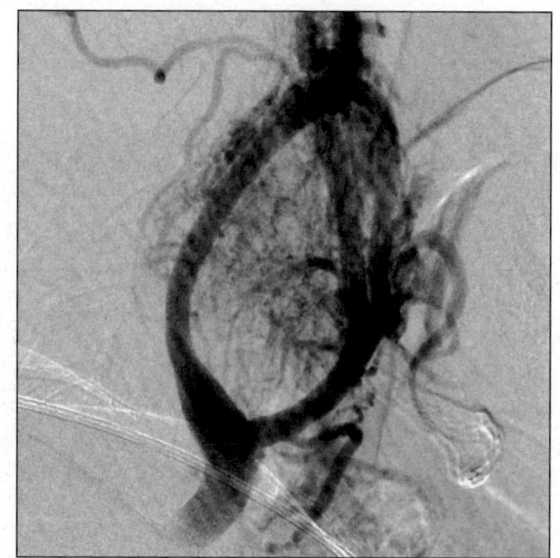

Lateral ICA DSA shows a large, hypervascular tumor splaying the carotid bifurcation.

TERMINOLOGY

Abbreviations and Synonyms

- Carotid body tumor, chemodectoma, non-chromaffin paraganglioma

Definitions

- Carotid body paraganglioma (CBP) is a benign vascular tumor derived from primitive neural crest tissue located in the glomus bodies at the common carotid artery (CCA) bifurcation

IMAGING FINDINGS

General Features

- Best diagnostic clue
  - External carotid artery (ECA) and internal carotid artery (ICA) are splayed
  - "Salt & pepper" appearance on both short and long T1 MR images
- Location: Carotid bifurcation, in the crotch between ICA and ECA
- Classic imaging appearance: Oropharyngeal carotid space mass splaying the ECA and ICA at the carotid bifurcation
  - ICA is characteristically displaced posterolaterally
  - Avid enhancement on CT, high velocity flow voids on T1 MR, highly vascular on color duplex US
- CT, MR and US appearances are diagnostic

CT Findings

- CECT: Avidly-enhancing mass in the crotch between the ECA and ICA at the carotid bifurcation

MR Findings

- T1WI
  - MR images may show "salt and pepper" in larger tumors (> 2 cm)
    - "Salt" is high-signal areas within the tumor parenchyma; secondary to subacute hemorrhage, tumor matrix, slow flow
    - "Pepper" is punctate or curvilinear, low-signal foci from high-velocity flow voids of feeding arteries
- T2WI: Larger tumors often have "salt and pepper" appearance as in T1WI
- T1 C+: Avidly-enhancing mass in the crotch between the ECA and ICA at the carotid bifurcation

DDx: Carotid Body Paraganglioma

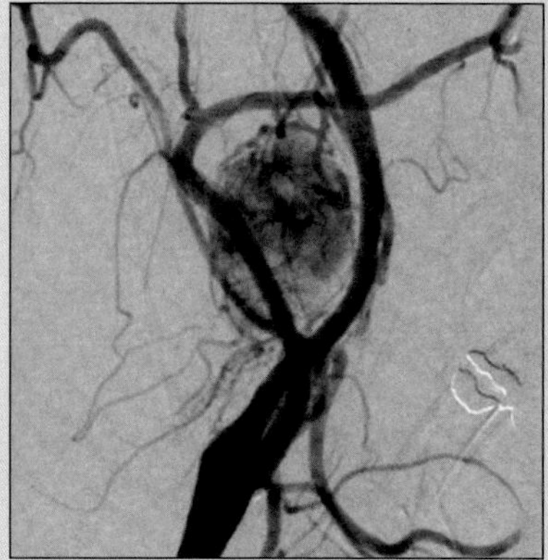

Glomus Vagale

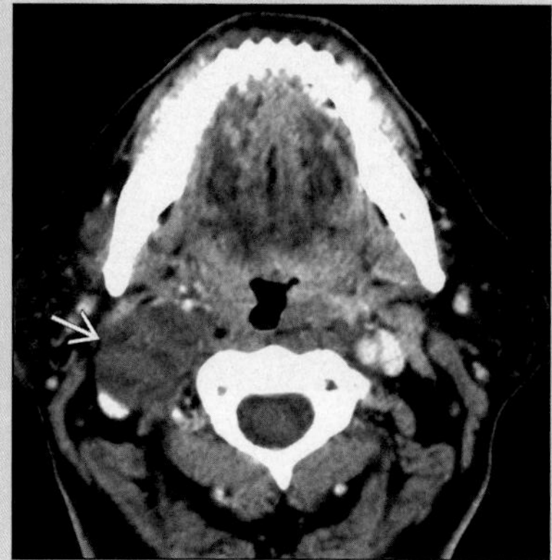

Neurofibroma

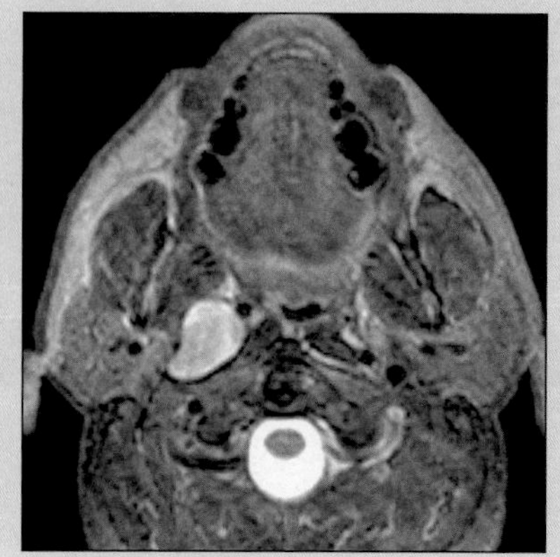

Schwannoma

CAROTID BODY PARAGANGLIOMA

Key Facts

Terminology

- Carotid body tumor, chemodectoma, non-chromaffin paraganglioma
- Carotid body paraganglioma (CBP) is a benign vascular tumor derived from primitive neural crest tissue located in the glomus bodies at the common carotid artery (CCA) bifurcation

Imaging Findings

- Classic imaging appearance: Oropharyngeal carotid space mass splaying the ECA and ICA at the carotid bifurcation
- Avid enhancement on CT, high velocity flow voids on T1 MR, highly vascular on color duplex US
- MR images may show "salt and pepper" in larger tumors (> 2 cm)
- DSA: Enlarged feeding vessels from ECA with prolonged, intense vascular blush ± early draining vein secondary to arteriovenous (AV) shunting

Clinical Issues

- Painless ± pulsatile neck mass
- Malignancy occurs in 6-12.5%: CBP is most frequently malignant head and neck paraganglioma
- Surgical excision is treatment of choice
- Pre-operative embolization with particulate emboli of major ECA feeders should be routine
- Resection complicated in 15-30% cases by CN10-12 injury; higher for tumors > 5 cm
- Radiotherapy is used for lesion control in poor surgical candidates

- MRA: Shows splayed ECA-ICA but not the capillary bed of CBP

Ultrasonographic Findings

- Color Doppler
  - Highly vascular tumor splaying the carotid bifurcation
  - Possible invasion or stenosis of branch vessels
  - Low resistance flow pattern in tumor vessels

Other Modality Findings

- In-111 Octreotide scan: May detect neuroendocrine tumors > 1.5 cm
  - Octreotide binds to somatostatin receptors in carcinoid, paraganglioma, medullary thyroid Ca, islet cell tumors, oat cell tumor, pheochromocytoma, pituitary adenoma
  - Useful for confirming/excluding CBP or other paraganglioma vs. neuroma, detection of recurrent disease, screening of patient with multiple endocrine neoplasia for additional tumors

Angiographic Findings

- Conventional
  - DSA: Enlarged feeding vessels from ECA with prolonged, intense vascular blush ± early draining vein secondary to arteriovenous (AV) shunting
  - Ascending pharyngeal artery branches are principal tumor feeder
  - May have contributions from facial, superior thyroid + occipital arteries
  - May see stenosis ± irregularity of ICA & ECA branches from tumor encasement
  - Pre-operative embolization is low risk and can significantly reduce intraoperative bleeding

Imaging Recommendations

- In familial patient group, screening MR beginning at 20 years old
- MR and angiography done before surgery
- Catheter angiography
  - Identifies ECA feeders suitable for embolization and those left for the surgeon to address
  - Evaluate collateral circulation of the brain, should intraoperative clamping or sacrifice of ICA be necessary; test balloon occlusion can be performed for further assessment
  - Search for multicentric tumors (glomus vagale, glomus jugulare & tympanicum): Perform bilateral carotid DSA
  - Pre-operative tumor embolization should be routine and is typically performed as single procedure with diagnostic DSA for minimization of intraoperative bleeding

DIFFERENTIAL DIAGNOSIS

Jugulodigastric (JD) Lymph Node Hyperplasia

- Enlarged, non-necrotic JD node pulsates against carotid bulb
- Clinically difficult to differentiate from CBP
- CT/MR shows enlarged lymph node without hypervascularity or flow-voids adjacent to a non-splayed carotid bifurcation

Vagal Schwannoma

- MR shows fusiform enhancing mass in carotid space
- MRA shows ICA bowed over anterior surface of mass
- DSA shows hypovascular tumor ± "puddling" of contrast without enlarged feeding arteries

Vagal Neurofibroma

- CECT shows low-density, well-circumscribed mass in carotid space (CS)
- MR imaging cannot differentiate from vagal schwannoma

Glomus Vagale Paraganglioma

- Mass centered approximately 2 cm below the skull base
- High-velocity flow voids
- "Salt and pepper" appearance on T1WI and T2WI
- ICA and ECA not splayed as with CBP but displaced, usually anteriorly

CAROTID BODY PARAGANGLIOMA

PATHOLOGY

General Features

- General path comments
  - Glomus tumors of head & neck are part of the extra-adrenal neuroendocrine system
  - At birth, small patches of paraganglionic cells derived from neural crest are widely dispersed throughout the body
    - In head & neck, such areas include the chemoreceptive areas (glomus tissue) at carotid bifurcation & temporal bone, orbit, pterygopalatine fossa, buccal mucosa, nasopharynx
    - Progressive involution occurs at these sites until puberty except for carotid bodies that detect changes in arterial concentrations of O^2, CO^2 and pH changes
  - Normal carotid bodies 3-5 mm: Function in autonomic control of respiratory and cardiovascular systems
- Genetics
  - Paragangliomas occur in a sporadic and a familial form
    - Familial paraganglioma is autosomal dominant
- Etiology: Arise from glomus bodies (paraganglia) in the carotid body
- Epidemiology
  - CBP is the most common location for paraganglioma
    - 40% of all paragangliomas are CBP
  - Increased incidence in people living at high altitudes
  - 5-10% of paragangliomas are multicentric in non-familial group
  - Familial incidence of multicentricity ~ 25%

Gross Pathologic & Surgical Features

- Dark tan-purple, usually well-circumscribed, lobulated, with thin fibrous capsule or pseudocapsule

Microscopic Features

- Type I (Chief) cells are APUD type cells with copious cytoplasm, and large round or oval nuclei: Release catecholamines with ↓ O^2, ↑ CO^2, ↓ pH
- Type II (sustentacular) cells are elongated cells that resemble Schwann cells: Function unclear
- Normal carotid body has cells arranged in clusters with core of chief cells surrounded by sustentacular cells embedded in a fibrovascular stroma
- In CBP: Clusters are larger (Zellballen formation), areas of spindle-shaped cells ("sarcomatoid foci"), highly vascular areas resembling angioma
- Electron microscopy shows neurosecretory granules

Staging, Grading or Classification Criteria

- Related to size and difficulty of resection (Shamblin, 1971)
  - Group I: Small, easily dissected from adjacent vessels
  - Group II: Medium size, intimately related to adjacent vessels but separable with careful subadventitial dissection
  - Group III: Large tumor, encases carotid, requiring partial or complete vessel resection or replacement

CLINICAL ISSUES

Presentation

- Most common signs/symptoms: Painless ± pulsatile neck mass
- Other signs/symptoms: Dysphagia, headaches, dizziness, pulsatile tinnitus, vagus nerve palsy, Horner syndrome
- 20% have vagal and/or hypoglossal neuropathy
- Catecholamine-secreting CBP is rare

Natural History & Prognosis

- Untreated may destroy recurrent laryngeal nerve or invade carotid vessels with risk of stenosis or carotid rupture
- Malignancy occurs in 6-12.5%: CBP is most frequently malignant head and neck paraganglioma

Treatment

- Surgical excision is treatment of choice
  - Pre-operative embolization with particulate emboli of major ECA feeders should be routine
  - Direct percutaneous tumor access and pre-operative embolization of liquid embolics has been reported
- Surgical cure without lasting post-operative cranial neuropathy is expected in CBP < 5 cm
- Resection complicated in 15-30% cases by CN10-12 injury; higher for tumors > 5 cm
- Radiotherapy is used for lesion control in poor surgical candidates

DIAGNOSTIC CHECKLIST

Consider

- Multicentric paragangliomas: Careful search on MR, CT ± bilateral carotid DSA

Image Interpretation Pearls

- Classic appearance: Highly vascular tumor splaying carotid bifurcation
- "Salt & pepper" appearance on MR due to flow voids in a background of tumor matrix ± hemorrhage

SELECTED REFERENCES

1. Sajid MS et al: A Multicenter Review of Carotid Body Tumour Management. Eur J Vasc Endovasc Surg. 2007
2. Dalainas I et al: Carotid body tumours. A 20-year single-institution experience. Chir Ital. 58(5):631-5, 2006
3. Kasper GC et al: A multidisciplinary approach to carotid paragangliomas. Vasc Endovascular Surg. 40(6):467-74, 2006
4. Muhm M et al: Diagnostic and therapeutic approaches to carotid body tumors. Review of 24 patients. Arch Surg. 132(3):279-84, 1997

CAROTID BODY PARAGANGLIOMA

IMAGE GALLERY

Typical

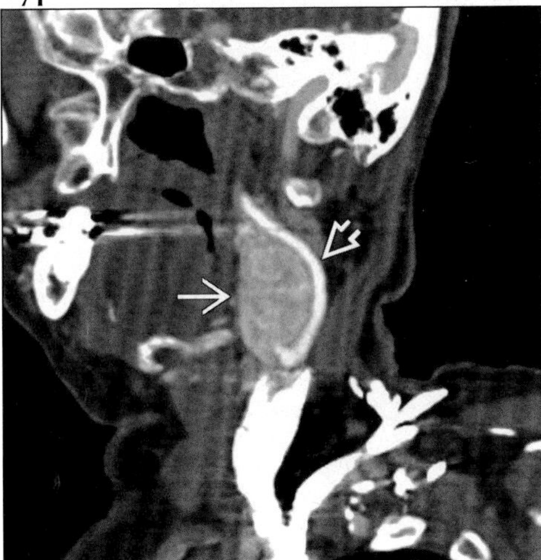

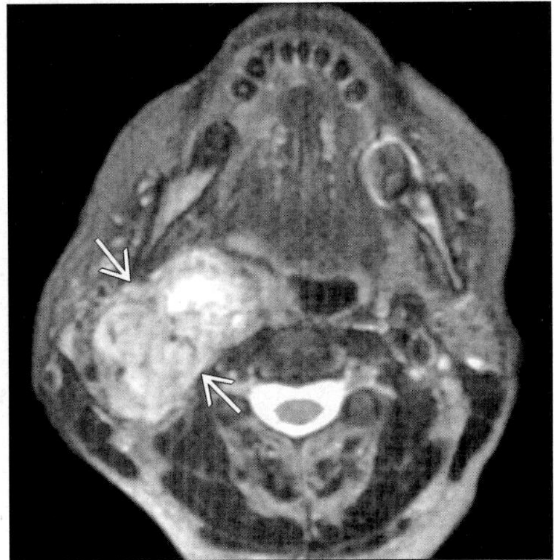

(Left) Sagittal CECT shows an enhancing mass at the crotch between the ECA and ICA origins ➔. The ICA ➔ is bowed posteriorly and separated from the ECA which is displaced anteriorly and out of plane in this image. **(Right)** Axial T2WI FS MR shows classic "salt and pepper" appearance of a CBP ➔. The tumor is lobulated and contains flow voids ("pepper") on a background of high signal tumor matrix ± blood products ("salt").

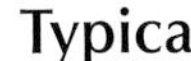

Typical

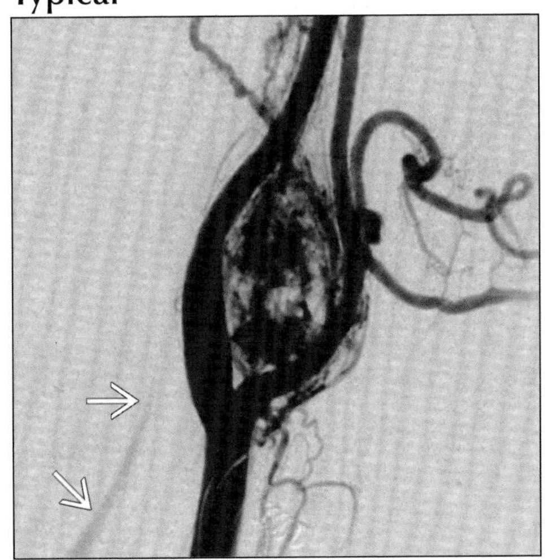

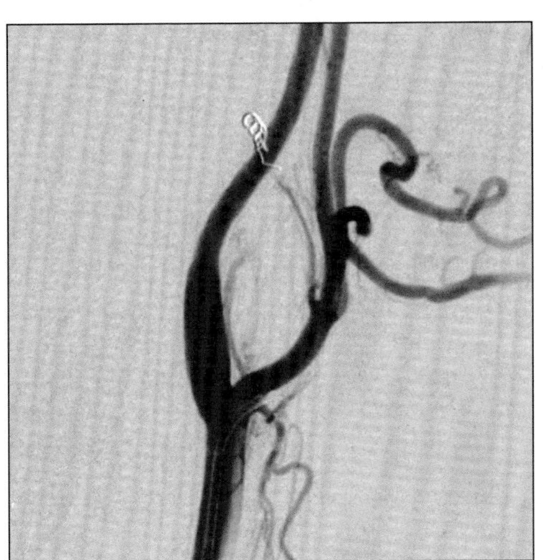

(Left) Lateral right common carotid artery (CCA) DSA shows a hypervascular tumor at the carotid bifurcation splaying the ICA and ECA. Note early filling of the internal jugular vein ➔ from AV shunting within the tumor. **(Right)** Right CCA DSA after pre-operative embolization utilizing polyvinyl alcohol (PVA) particles and fibered coils shows dramatic decrease in tumor vascularity.

Typical

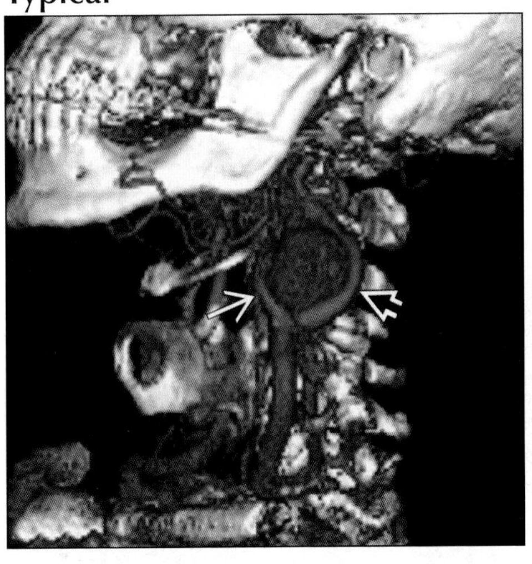

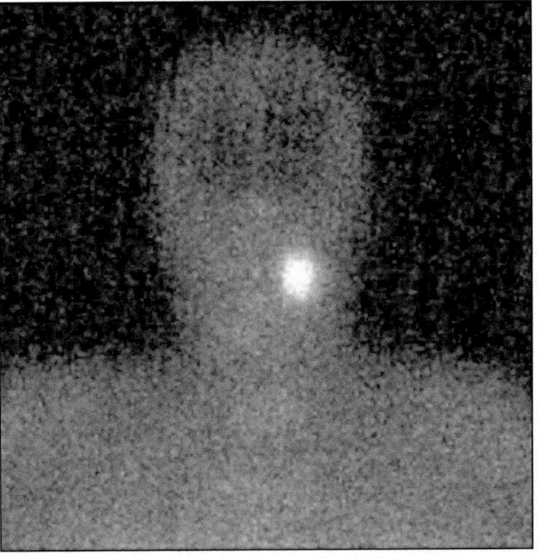

(Left) Lateral CTA 3D shaded surface display image shows an avidly enhancing tumor splaying the left carotid bifurcation. The ICA ➔ is displaced posteriorly and the ECA ➔ anteriorly. **(Right)** Anteroposterior 24 hr planar image from an In-111 labeled octreotide scan shows a focus of intense activity in the left side of the neck. Octreotide scans are useful for detection of multiple paragangliomas and differentiation from other neoplasms.

GLOMUS VAGALE PARAGANGLIOMA

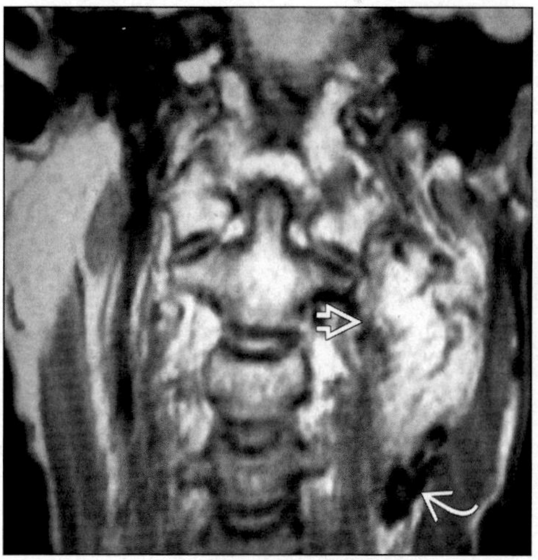

Coronal T1WI MR with intravenous gadolinium shows a large enhancing mass ➡ in the left carotid space with multiple low signal flow voids ➡.

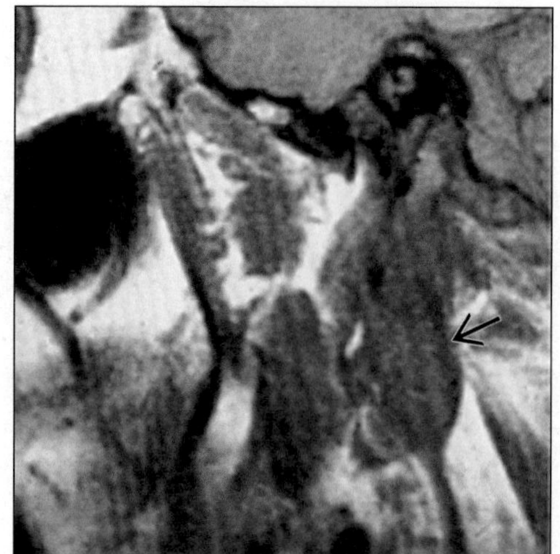

Sagittal T1WI MR shows a mass in the carotid space that is isointense to adjacent muscles ➡.

TERMINOLOGY

Abbreviations and Synonyms

- Vagal body tumors, glomus vagale, vagal paraganglioma, glomus intravagale tumor, chemodectoma

Definitions

- Benign vascular tumor derived from primitive neural crest that begins in the ganglia of the vagus nerve

IMAGING FINDINGS

General Features

- Best diagnostic clue: Carotid space mass displacing the parapharyngeal fat anteriorly, the ICA anteromedial; avid enhancement with CT, high-velocity flow voids on T1 MR
- Location
  - Carotid space mass displacing the parapharyngeal fat anteriorly and the internal carotid artery (ICA) anteromedial
  - Mass is typically centered 1-2 cm below jugular foramen
    - Usually near angle of mandible between the skull base and hyoid bone
  - Extends inferiorly along the carotid sheath
- Morphology: "Salt and pepper" appearance on MR

CT Findings

- CECT: Avidly-enhancing mass in carotid space

MR Findings

- T1WI: Low to intermediate signal intensity tumor with low signal foci from flow voids
- T2WI
  - "Salt and pepper" appearance
    - "Salt" = high signal from tumor stroma
    - "Pepper" = low signal foci from high velocity flow voids
- T1 C+
  - "Salt and pepper" appearance
    - "Salt" = enhancing tumor stroma
    - "Pepper" = low signal foci from high velocity flow voids

DDx: Glomus Vagale

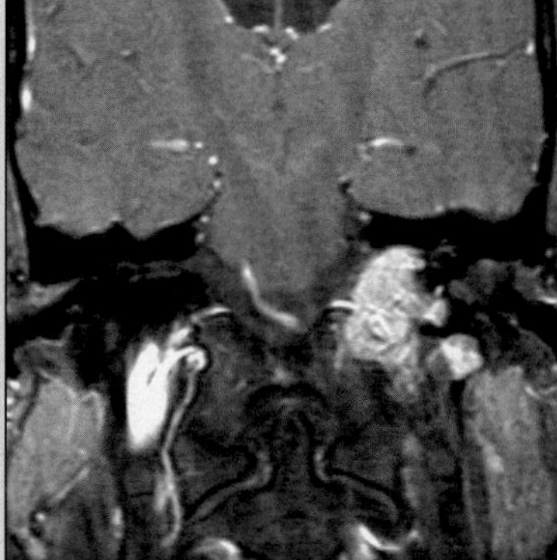

Glomus Jugulare

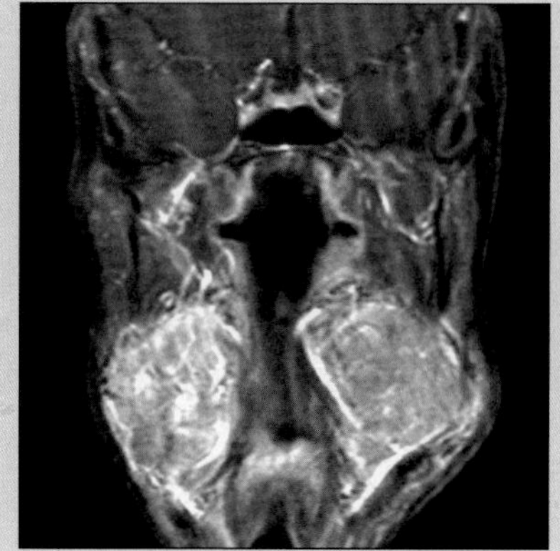

Carotid Body Tumors

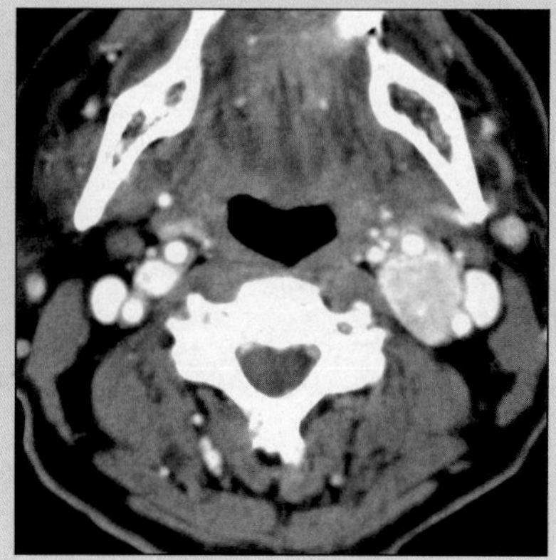

Carotid Body Tumors

GLOMUS VAGALE PARAGANGLIOMA

Key Facts

Terminology

- Vagal body tumors, glomus vagale, vagal paraganglioma, glomus intravagale tumor, chemodectoma
- Benign vascular tumor derived from primitive neural crest that begins in the ganglia of the vagus nerve

Imaging Findings

- Best diagnostic clue: Carotid space mass displacing the parapharyngeal fat anteriorly, the ICA anteromedial; avid enhancement with CT, high-velocity flow voids on T1 MR
- Mass is typically centered 1-2 cm below jugular foramen
- Morphology: "Salt and pepper" appearance on MR
- CECT: Avidly-enhancing mass in carotid space

Top Differential Diagnoses

- Vagal Schwannoma
- Meningioma of Carotid Space
- Glomus Jugulare Paraganglioma
- Carotid Body Paraganglioma

Pathology

- Arise from Nodose ganglion of the vagus nerve just below the level of the foramen magnum
- Rare; 2.5% of all paragangliomas

Clinical Issues

- Painless neck mass near the angle of the mandible
- Vocal cord paralysis
- Nearly 100% have unilateral vagus nerve paralysis from surgery

Other Modality Findings

- Indium-111 Octreotide sensitive for detecting paragangliomas
  - Useful for the detection of multiple tumors in familial cases and for detection of metastases
- MIBG can also be used but less sensitive than Octreotide

Angiographic Findings

- Conventional
  - Enlarged feeding vessels with prolonged, intense vascular blush ± early draining veins seen secondary to arteriovenous shunting
  - Ascending pharyngeal artery is typically the principal tumor feeder

Imaging Recommendations

- Best imaging tool: MR with contrast
- Protocol advice
  - MR and angiography done before surgery
  - In familial patient group, screening MR beginning at 20 years old
- Catheter angiography
  - Identify arterial feeders suitable for embolization and those that remain after embolization requiring surgical attention
  - Evaluate collateral arterial and venous circulation of the brain, should sacrifice of a major vessel become necessary
  - Search for multicentric tumors; requires bilateral carotid angiography
  - Pre-operative embolization for minimization of intraoperative bleeding

DIFFERENTIAL DIAGNOSIS

Vagal Schwannoma

- MR shows fusiform enhancing mass in carotid space
- MRA shows ICA bowed over anterior surface of mass
- Typically hypo- or avascular mass in angiography; displaces ± stretches adjacent vessels

Meningioma of Carotid Space

- Extends from jugular foramen above
- CT shows permeative sclerotic bony changes of the jugular foramen (JF) bony margins
- Dural thickening (tails) present along cephalad margin of JF
- Prolonged but mild tumor blush during angiography

Glomus Jugulare Paraganglioma

- Mass centered in JF with permeative bony margins (CT) and high velocity flow voids (T1 MR)

Carotid Body Paraganglioma

- Mass centered in crotch of ICA-ECA at the carotid bifurcation
- T1 MR images show high-velocity flow voids

PATHOLOGY

General Features

- Genetics
  - Paraganglioma occurs in a sporadic and a familial form
  - Familial paraganglioma (10-50% of paragangliomas)
    - Autosomal dominant with genomic imprinting
    - Frequently bilateral and multiple
    - Present at an earlier age
    - PGL 1 gene on 11q23 and PGL2 gene on 11q13 discovered
- Etiology
  - Arise from Nodose ganglion of the vagus nerve just below the level of the foramen magnum
  - Arise from glomus bodies = paraganglia
  - Glomus bodies are composed of chemoreceptor cells derived from the primitive neural crest
- Epidemiology
  - Rare; 2.5% of all paragangliomas
  - 5% multicentric in non-familial group
  - Familial incidence of multicentricity may reach 90%

Gross Pathologic & Surgical Features

- Lobulated, solid mass with fibrous pseudocapsule

- External surface is reddish-purple
- Cut surface shows multiple enlarged feeding arteries

Microscopic Features

- Biphasic pattern composed of chief cells and sustentacular cells surrounded by fibrovascular stroma
  - Chief cells arranged in characteristic compact cell nests or balls of cells (zellballen)
- Electron microscopy shows neuroendocrine granules

CLINICAL ISSUES

Presentation

- Most common signs/symptoms
  - Painless neck mass near the angle of the mandible
  - Vocal cord paralysis
    - Approximately 50% have vocal cord paralysis at presentation
- Other signs/symptoms
  - Horner syndrome
  - Dysphagia
  - Tongue hemiatrophy
  - Cough
  - Rarely hormonally active (3%)
    - Secrete catecholamines
    - Requires medical block prior to surgery
- Clinical Profile: Pulsatile lateral retropharyngeal mass

Demographics

- Age: 40-60 years
- Gender: Male:Female ratio = 1:3

Natural History & Prognosis

- Reported 16% malignancy rate is slightly higher than for other paragangliomas
- Nearly 100% have unilateral vagus nerve paralysis from surgery
- Deficits in CNs VII, IX-XII also possible following resection
- Vocal cord medialization and cricopharyngeal myotomy have been used to prevent aspiration when vagal nerve sacrifice required

Treatment

- Surgical excision is treatment of choice
- Radiotherapy is used for lesion control in poor surgical candidates
- Transcatheter embolization can decrease size of tumor and reduce intraoperative blood loss
  - Particulate emboli typically used
  - Direct percutaneous puncture of tumor and injection of n-BCA glue also reported
- If bilateral glomus vagale paraganglioma, surgery on one, radiotherapy on other to preserve unilateral vagus nerve function

DIAGNOSTIC CHECKLIST

Consider

- Familial form if multiple paragangliomas seen
- Look for sequela of cranial nerve injury on postoperative follow up scans

Image Interpretation Pearls

- "Salt and pepper" appearance on MR and avid enhancement very characteristic

SELECTED REFERENCES

1. Lowenheim H et al: Differentiating imaging findings in primary and secondary tumors of the jugular foramen. Neurosurg Rev. 29(1):1-11; discussion 12-13, 2006
2. Bradshaw JW et al: Management of vagal paraganglioma: is operative resection really the best option? Surgery. 137(2):225-8, 2005
3. Rajan GP et al: Intractable hemorrhage after incision of a vagal paraganglioma mimicking a peritonsillar abscess. Otolaryngol Head Neck Surg. 132(1):161-2, 2005
4. van den Berg R: Imaging and management of head and neck paragangliomas. Eur Radiol. 15(7):1310-8, 2005
5. Genc E et al: Radiology quiz case 2. Hypervascular vagal schwannoma mimicking paraganglioma. Arch Otolaryngol Head Neck Surg. 130(11):1341, 1343-4, 2004
6. Groblewski JC et al: Secreting vagal paraganglioma. Am J Otolaryngol. 25(4):295-300, 2004
7. Pellitteri PK et al: Paragangliomas of the head and neck. Oral Oncol. 40(6):563-75, 2004
8. van den Berg R et al: Head and neck paragangliomas: improved tumor detection using contrast-enhanced 3D time-of-flight MR angiography as compared with fat-suppressed MR imaging techniques. AJNR Am J Neuroradiol. 25(5):863-70, 2004
9. van den Berg R et al: The value of MR angiography techniques in the detection of head and neck paragangliomas. Eur J Radiol. 52(3):240-5, 2004
10. Carlsen CS et al: Malignant vagal paraganglioma: report of a case treated with embolization and surgery. Auris Nasus Larynx. 30(4):443-6, 2003
11. Jansen JC et al: Estimation of growth rate in patients with head and neck paragangliomas influences the treatment proposal. Cancer. 88(12):2811-6, 2000
12. Noujaim SE et al: Paraganglioma of the temporal bone: role of magnetic resonance imaging versus computed tomography. Top Magn Reson Imaging. 11(2):108-22, 2000
13. Weissman JL et al: Imaging of tinnitus: a review. Radiology. 216(2):342-9, 2000
14. Weissman JL: Case 21: glomus vagale tumor. Radiology. 215(1):237-42, 2000
15. Rao AB et al: From the archives of the AFIP. Paragangliomas of the head and neck: radiologic-pathologic correlation. Armed Forces Institute of Pathology. Radiographics. 19(6):1605-32, 1999
16. van den Berg R et al: Imaging of head and neck paragangliomas with three-dimensional time-of-flight MR angiography. AJR Am J Roentgenol. 172(6):1667-73, 1999
17. Netterville JL et al: Vagal paraganglioma: a review of 46 patients treated during a 20-year period. Arch Otolaryngol Head Neck Surg. 124(10):1133-40, 1998
18. Urquhart AC et al: Glomus vagale: paraganglioma of the vagus nerve. Laryngoscope. 104(4):440-5, 1994
19. van Gils AP et al: MR diagnosis of paraganglioma of the head and neck: value of contrast enhancement. AJR Am J Roentgenol. 162(1):147-53, 1994
20. Olsen WL et al: MR imaging of paragangliomas. AJR Am J Roentgenol. 148(1):201-4, 1987

GLOMUS VAGALE PARAGANGLIOMA

IMAGE GALLERY

Typical

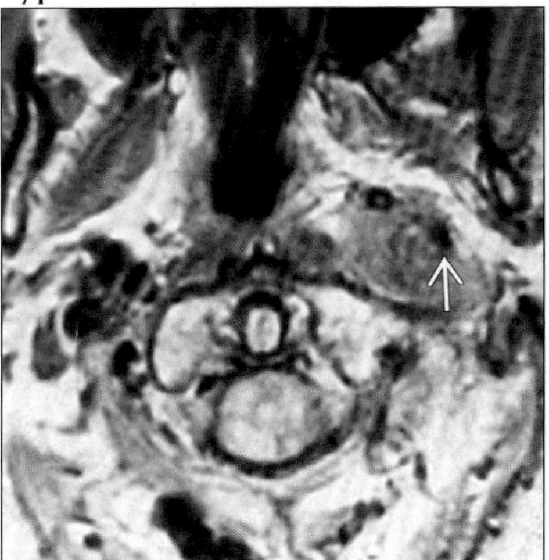

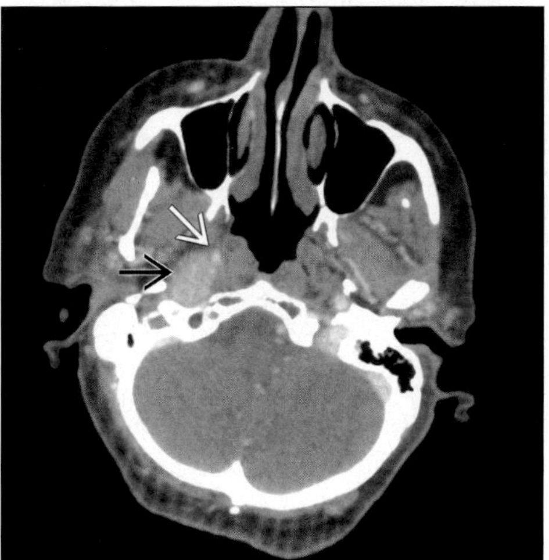

(Left) *Axial T2WI MR shows a mass in the left carotid space with large low signal intensity flow voids indicative of significant tumor vascularity ➡.* ***(Right)*** *Axial CECT shows a homogeneously-enhancing, soft tissue mass ➡ centered high in the neck at the skull base, displacing the right internal carotid artery anteromedially ➡.*

Typical

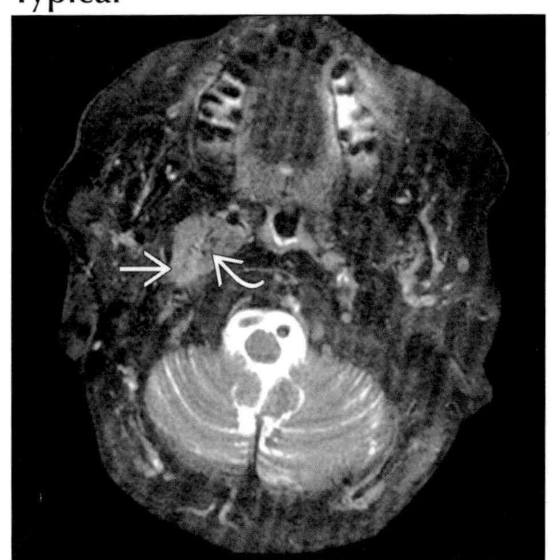

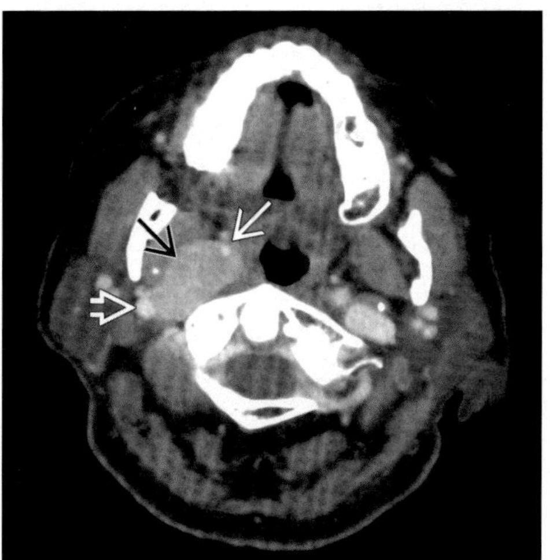

(Left) *Axial T2WI FS MR shows a soft tissue mass ➡ below the skull base with small focal signal voids ➡ indicating the presence of high-flow vessels.* ***(Right)*** *Axial CECT shows an enhancing soft tissue mass ➡ centered high in the neck at the skull base, displacing the right internal carotid artery anteromedially ➡ and the jugular vein laterally ➡.*

Typical

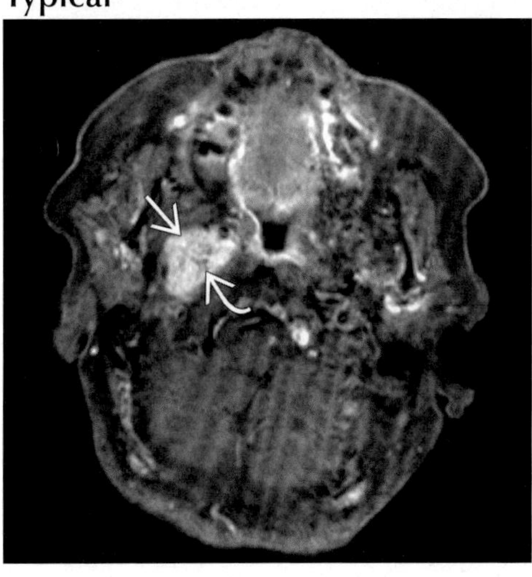

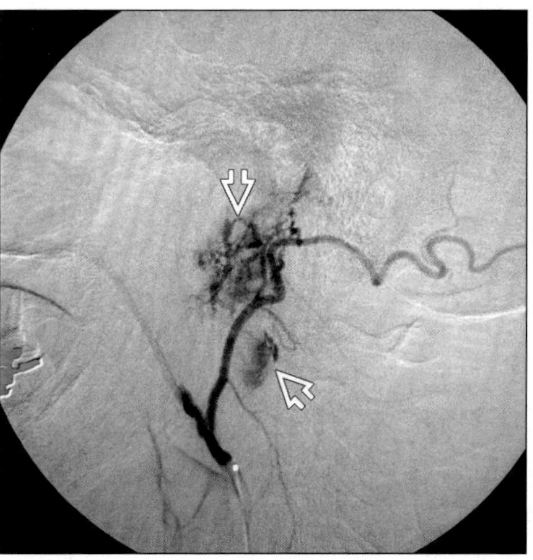

(Left) *Axial T1WI FS MR with intravenous gadolinium shows an enhancing mass in the right carotid ➡ space with small foci of low signal ➡ representing flow voids.* ***(Right)*** *Right external carotid artery DSA shows a hypervascular lesion with enlarged feeding vessels arising from the occipital artery and associated tumor blush ➡. Pre-operative embolization of these and other arterial feeders can significantly reduce intraoperative blood loss.*

GLOMUS JUGULOTYMPANICUM

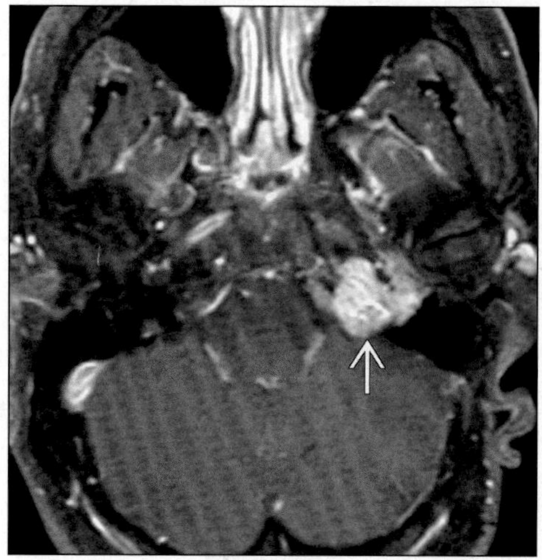

Axial gadolinium enhanced T1WI fat-saturated MR shows an enhancing mass centered on the left jugular foramen ➔.

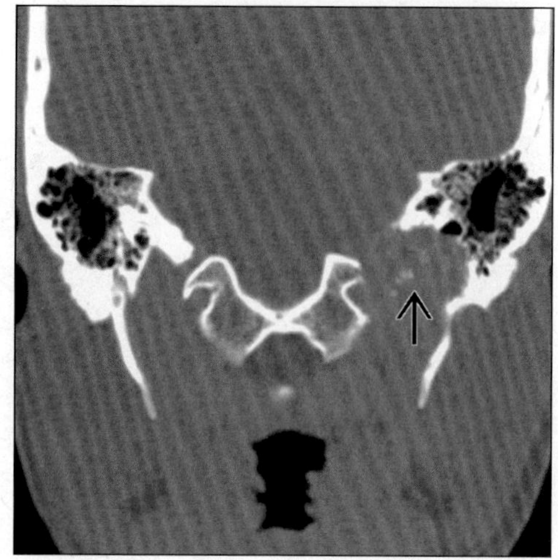

Coronal NECT shows a lytic and destructive lesion centered in the left jugular foramen ➔. There is extension into the middle ear and mastoid air cells.

TERMINOLOGY

Abbreviations and Synonyms

- Glomus jugulare & jugulotympanicum paraganglioma, chemodectoma

Definitions

- Glomus jugulotympanicum describes paraganglioma involving both jugular foramen (JF) & middle ear cavity

IMAGING FINDINGS

General Features

- Best diagnostic clue
  - CT: Permeative-destructive changes of bony margins of superolateral jugular foramen
  - MR: High-velocity flow voids, "salt and pepper" appearance
  - DSA: Early, intense tumor blush ± AV shunting
- Location
  - JF mass extends superolaterally into floor of middle ear cavity
  - Tumor spread vector is superolateral into middle ear cavity
- Morphology: "Salt and pepper" appearance on MR

CT Findings

- NECT
  - Permeative-destructive bone changes along superolateral margin of JF mark extent of tumor
    - Jugular spine and carotico-jugular crest erosion is common
    - Enlargement of JF
    - Vertical segment of petrous ICA posterior wall often dehiscent
    - Mastoid segment of facial nerve may be engulfed
- CECT: Enhancing mass within ± enlarging JF
- CTA: May see compression of internal jugular vein (IJV) or jugular bulb ± invasion ± thrombosis

MR Findings

- T1WI: Low to intermediate signal intensity tumor with low signal foci from flow voids
- T2WI
  - "Salt and pepper" appearance
    - "Salt": High signal of tumor stroma

DDx: Glomus Jugulare

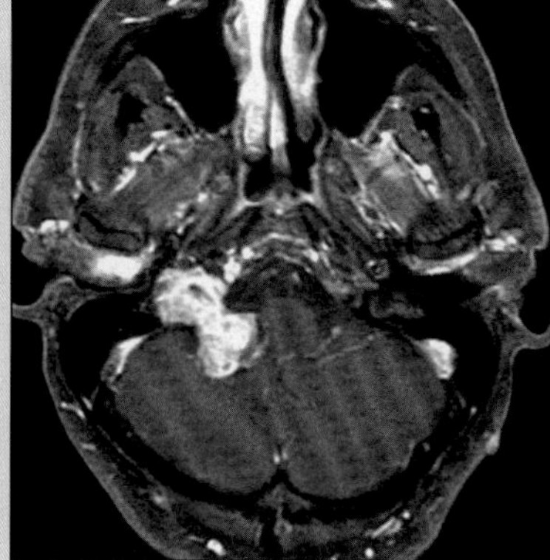

Schwannoma

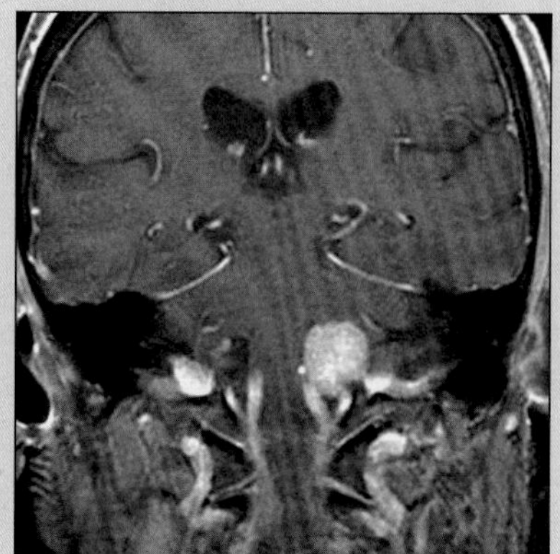

Meningioma

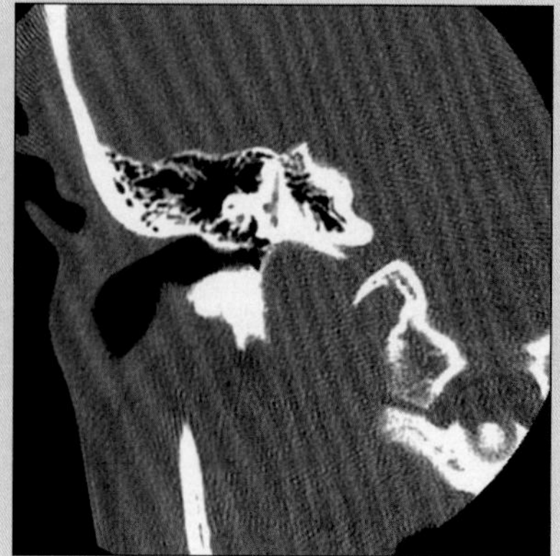

High Riding Jugular Bulb

GLOMUS JUGULOTYMPANICUM

Key Facts

Terminology

- Glomus jugulare & jugulotympanicum paraganglioma, chemodectoma

Imaging Findings

- CT: Permeative-destructive changes of bony margins of superolateral jugular foramen
- MR: High-velocity flow voids, "salt and pepper" appearance
- DSA: Early, intense tumor blush ± AV shunting
- CTA: May see compression of internal jugular vein (IJV) or jugular bulb ± invasion ± thrombosis
- Indium-111 Octreotide sensitive for detecting tumors > 1.5 cm

Top Differential Diagnoses

- High-Riding Jugular Bulb
- Dehiscent Jugular Bulb
- Meningioma of JF
- Schwannoma of JF

Pathology

- Arise from chemoreceptor tissue (paraganglia)
- Associated with parasympathetic fibers from CN 9 and CN 10

Clinical Issues

- Most common signs/symptoms: Pulsatile tinnitus
- Slow growing tumor can be watched in older patients
- Metastatic disease is rare (3%) to the lungs, liver, and bone
- Preoperative transcatheter embolization of arterial supply can significantly reduce intraoperative bleeding

---

    - "Pepper": Low-signal foci from high-velocity flow voids
- T1 C+
  - "Salt and pepper" appearance
    - "Salt": Enhancing tumor stroma
    - "Pepper": Low-signal foci from high velocity flow voids
  - Will show true extent of tumor in skull base & middle ear cavity
  - May show tumor extending intraluminally within internal jugular vein
  - Coronal images show tongue of tumor curving up from JF, through middle ear floor, terminating on cochlear promontory
  - Signal drop out can be seen after administration of high dose gadolinium

Other Modality Findings

- Indium-111 Octreotide sensitive for detecting tumors > 1.5 cm

Angiographic Findings

- Conventional
  - Enlarged feeding vessels with prolonged, intense, vascular blush with early draining veins seen secondary to AV shunting
  - Ascending pharyngeal artery = major feeding vessel

Imaging Recommendations

- Best imaging tool: MR reveals exact soft tissue extent of tumor
- Protocol advice
  - CT, MR and angiography all done before surgery
    - CT provides surgeon information about bony destruction, dehiscence, and landmarks not available from MR alone
- Conventional angiography
  - Evaluates collateral arterial & venous circulation of the brain
  - Searches for multicentric paragangliomas
  - Preoperative embolization useful for minimization of blood loss during surgery

DIFFERENTIAL DIAGNOSIS

High-Riding Jugular Bulb

- JF bony margins intact
- Increased signal within bulb does not persist in all MR sequences

Dehiscent Jugular Bulb

- Sigmoid plate is focally dehiscent
- Polypoid extension into middle ear is contiguous with jugular bulb

Meningioma of JF

- NECT: Permeative-sclerotic bony changes
- CE T1 MR: Enhancing mass with dural tails
- Vector of spread: Centrifugal spread along dural surfaces
- DSA: Early & prolonged tumor blush; AV shunting rare

Schwannoma of JF

- NECT: Smooth enlargement of JF
- T1 C+ MR: Fusiform enhancing mass ± intramural cysts
- Vector of spread: Spreads along course of CN 9-11
- Angio: Absence of tumor blush or enlarged feeding arteries on angiography; "puddling" on venous phase

PATHOLOGY

General Features

- Genetics: Autosomal dominant mode of inheritance has been suggested
- Etiology
  - Arise from chemoreceptor tissue (paraganglia)
    - Associated with parasympathetic fibers from CN 9 and CN 10
    - Embryologically derived from neural crest cells
- Epidemiology
  - Most common tumor found in jugular foramen (JF)
  - Synchronous or metachronous tumors approximately 10% of the time
  - When familial, multicentricity reaches 25%

- Associated abnormalities: Multiple Endocrine Neoplasia (MEN) syndromes

Gross Pathologic & Surgical Features

- Lobulated, solid mass with a fibrous pseudocapsule
- External surface is reddish-purple
- Cut surface shows multiple enlarged feeding arteries

Microscopic Features

- Biphasic cell pattern composed of chief cells & sustentacular cells surrounded by fibrovascular stroma
  - Chief cells arranged in characteristic compact cell nests or balls of cells (zellballen)
- Electron microscopy: Shows neurosecretory granules

Staging, Grading or Classification Criteria

- Fisch classification
  - A: Arise along tympanic plexus on promontory
  - B: Invasion of hypotympanum, cortical bone over jugular bulb intact
  - C1: Erosion of carotid foramen
  - C2: Destruction of carotid canal
  - C3: Invasion of carotid canal, foramen lacerum intact
  - C4: Invasion of foramen lacerum and cavernous sinus
  - De1/2: Intracranial extension, no infiltration of subarachnoid space; De1 or 2 according to displacement of dura
  - Di1/2/3: Intradural extension; Di 1-3 according to depth of invasion into posterior fossa

CLINICAL ISSUES

Presentation

- Most common signs/symptoms: Pulsatile tinnitus
- Other signs/symptoms
  - CN 9-11 palsies; CN 7 or 8 neuropathy less often
  - Conductive hearing loss
  - Vertigo

Demographics

- Age: 40-60 years
- Gender: M:F = 3:1

Natural History & Prognosis

- Slow growing tumor can be watched in older patients
- Metastatic disease is rare (3%) to the lungs, liver, and bone
- 60% of patients have postoperative cranial neuropathy

Treatment

- Surgery: Infratemporal fossa approach most commonly used
- Preoperative transcatheter embolization of arterial supply can significantly reduce intraoperative bleeding
- Conservative jugulopetrosectomy preserves normal anatomy of external and middle ear, used for small tumors
- Larger lesions may require surgery and radiation therapy
- Radiation therapy alone is palliative for older patients
  - Associated with lower morbidity of caudal cranial nerves

DIAGNOSTIC CHECKLIST

Consider

- Preoperative embolization for minimization of intraoperative blood loss

Image Interpretation Pearls

- Slow flow in the jugular bulb can be mistaken for a tumor on MR

SELECTED REFERENCES

1. Lowenheim H et al: Differentiating imaging findings in primary and secondary tumors of the jugular foramen. Neurosurg Rev. 29(1):1-11; discussion 12-13, 2006
2. Ramina R et al: Tumors of the jugular foramen: diagnosis and management. Neurosurgery. 57(1 Suppl):59-68; discussion 59-68, 2005
3. van den Berg R: Imaging and management of head and neck paragangliomas. Eur Radiol. 15(7):1310-8, 2005
4. Sanna M et al: Management of jugular paragangliomas: the Gruppo Otologico experience. Otol Neurotol. 25(5):797-804, 2004
5. van den Berg R et al: Head and neck paragangliomas: improved tumor detection using contrast-enhanced 3D time-of-flight MR angiography as compared with fat-suppressed MR imaging techniques. AJNR Am J Neuroradiol. 25(5):863-70, 2004
6. van den Berg R et al: The value of MR angiography techniques in the detection of head and neck paragangliomas. Eur J Radiol. 52(3):240-5, 2004
7. Pareschi R et al: Surgery of Glomus Jugulare Tumors. Skull Base. 13(3):149-157, 2003
8. Jansen JC et al: Estimation of growth rate in patients with head and neck paragangliomas influences the treatment proposal. Cancer. 88(12):2811-6, 2000
9. Noujaim SE et al: Paraganglioma of the temporal bone: role of magnetic resonance imaging versus computed tomography. Top Magn Reson Imaging. 11(2):108-22, 2000
10. Pipas JM et al: Treatment of progressive metastatic glomus jugulare tumor (paraganglioma) with gemcitabine. Neuro-oncol. 2(3):190-1, 2000
11. Weissman JL et al: Imaging of tinnitus: a review. Radiology. 216(2):342-9, 2000
12. Rao AB et al: Paragangliomas of the head and neck: Radiologic-pathologic correlation. RadioGraphics. 19:1605-32, 1999
13. van den Berg R et al: Imaging of head and neck paragangliomas with three-dimensional time-of-flight MR angiography. AJR Am J Roentgenol. 172(6):1667-73, 1999
14. van Gils AP et al: MR diagnosis of paraganglioma of the head and neck: value of contrast enhancement. AJR Am J Roentgenol. 162(1):147-53, 1994
15. Vogl TJ et al: Glomus tumors of the skull base: combined use of MR angiography and spin-echo imaging. Radiology. 192:103-10, 1994
16. Olsen WL et al: MR imaging of paragangliomas. AJR. 148:201-4, 1987

IMAGE GALLERY

Typical

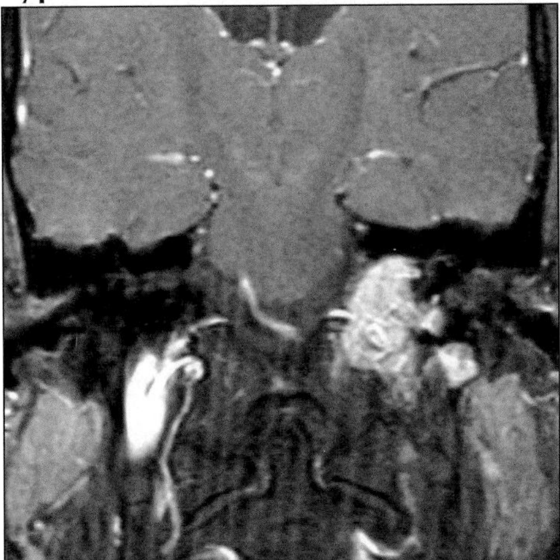

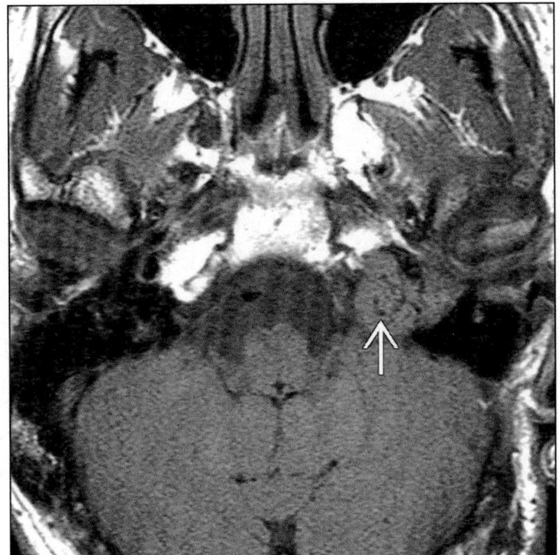

*(**Left**) Coronal T1WI FS MR with intravenous gadolinium shows an enhancing mass centered in the left jugular foramen which extends into the left middle ear cavity. (**Right**) Axial T1WI MR shows a mass with intermediate signal intensity centered in the left jugular foramen. Note the low signal intensity foci which represent flow voids ➡.*

Typical

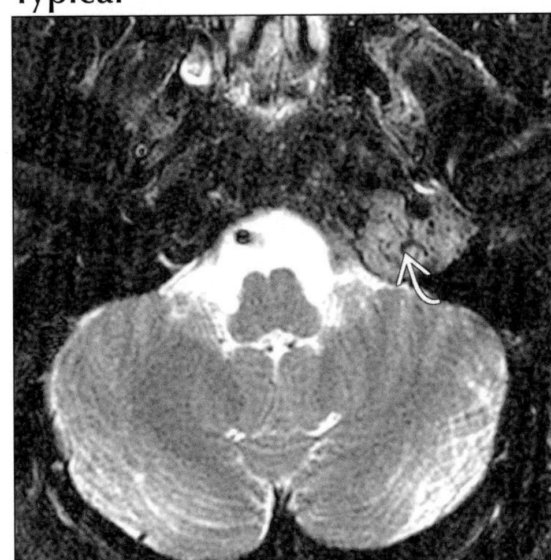

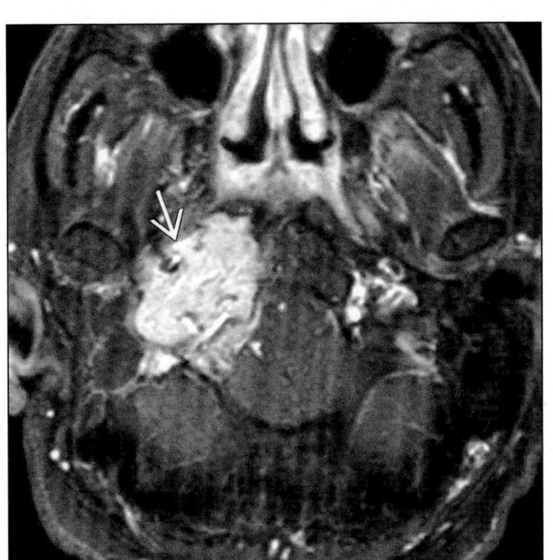

*(**Left**) Axial T2WI FS MR shows a mass with intermediate to high signal intensity centered in the left jugular foramen. Note the low signal intensity foci which represent flow voids ➡. (**Right**) Axial T1WI FS MR with intravenous gadolinium shows a large enhancing mass ➡ centered in the right jugular foramen.*

Typical

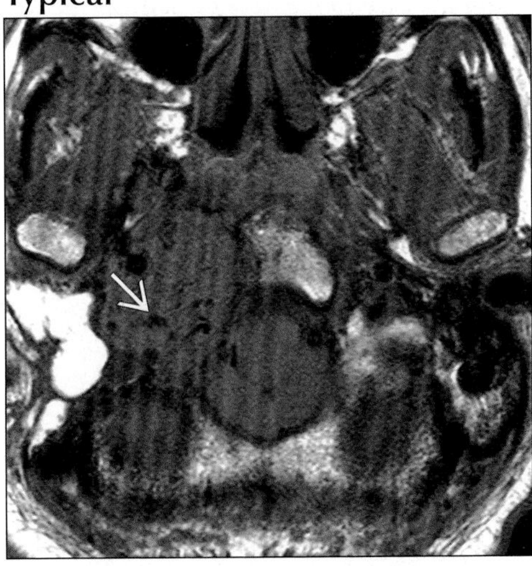

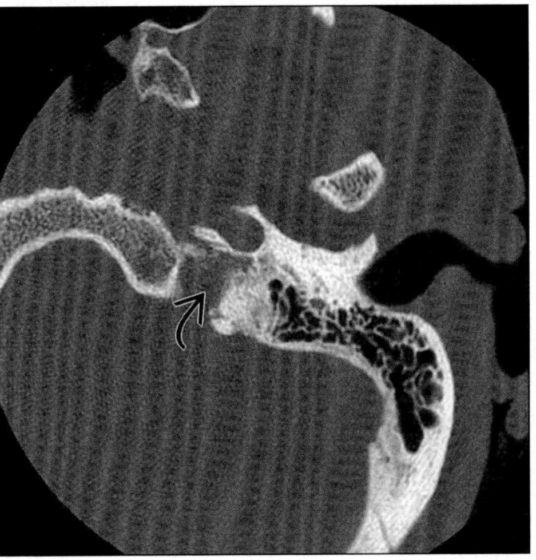

*(**Left**) Axial T1WI MR shows a large mass with intermediate signal intensity centered in the right jugular foramen. Note the multiple low signal intensity foci which represent flow voids ➡. (**Right**) Axial NECT with bone windowing shows erosive changes and widening of the left JF ➡. This feature is helpful in differentiating glomus tumors from schwannomas as the latter tends to remodel and expand the JF without erosive changes.*

GLOMUS TYMPANICUM

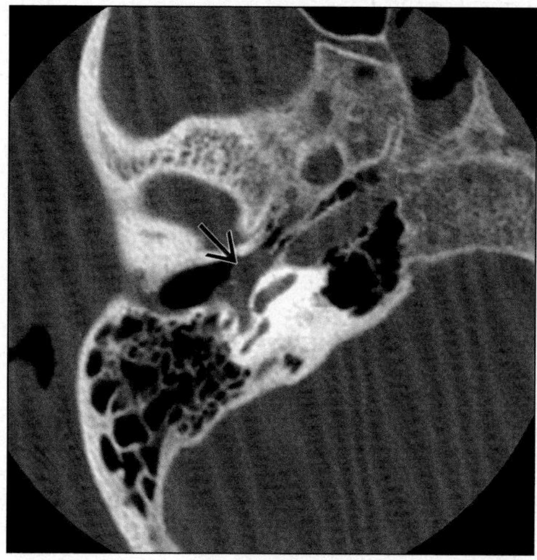

Axial NECT with bone windowing shows a soft tissue density mass ➔ centered at the cochlear promontory.

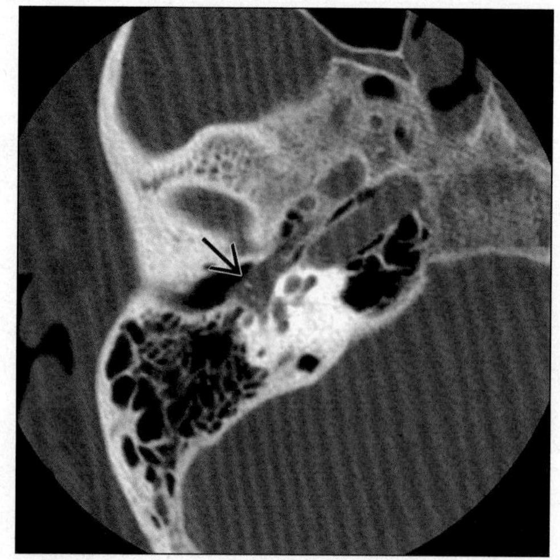

Axial NECT with bone windowing shows a soft tissue density mass ➔ in the middle ear cavity.

TERMINOLOGY

Abbreviations and Synonyms

- Glomus tympanicum paraganglioma (GTP), chemodectoma

Definitions

- Benign tumor that arises in glomus bodies situated on the cochlear promontory of medial wall of middle ear cavity

IMAGING FINDINGS

General Features

- Best diagnostic clue
  - Round mass with base on cochlear promontory
  - CT shows no bone erosion and T1 C+ MR shows intense enhancement
- Location
  - Vascular retrotympanic mass
  - Anteroinferior quadrant of tympanic membrane
  - Typically found lateral (but can also be anterior or inferior) to cochlear promontory (convexity of bone over basal turn of cochlea)
- Size: Usually small in size due to early presentation
- Morphology: Floor of middle ear cavity is intact; if eroded = glomus jugulotympanicum tumor

CT Findings

- NECT
  - Focal mass on cochlear promontory is characteristic
  - Small lesions: Fills lower middle ear, just reaches medial border of tympanic membrane (TM)
  - Large lesions: Fills middle ear cavity, creating attic block resulting in fluid collection in mastoid; margins of tumor not visible on CT
  - Bone erosion not usually present with GTP, even with larger lesions
  - Rare involvement of air cells along the inferior cochlear promontory may be mistaken for invasion
- CECT: Enhancing mass centered at the cochlear promontory

MR Findings

- T1WI: Intermediate signal mass centered at the cochlear promontory

DDx: Glomus Tympanicum

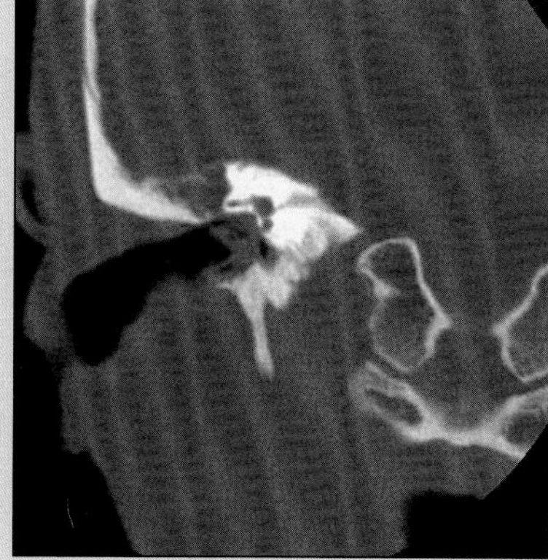

Cholesteatoma

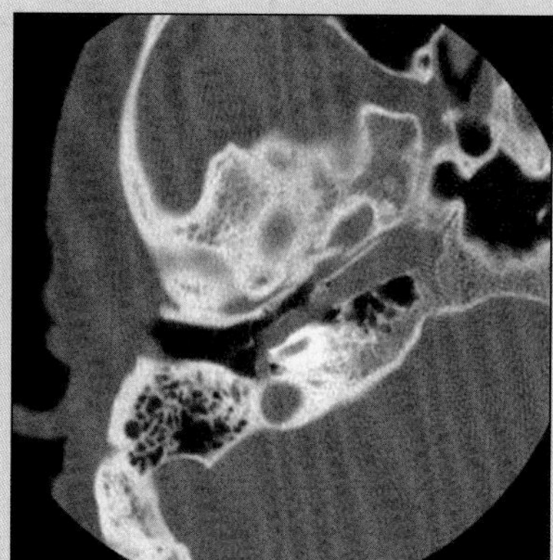

Aberrant ICA

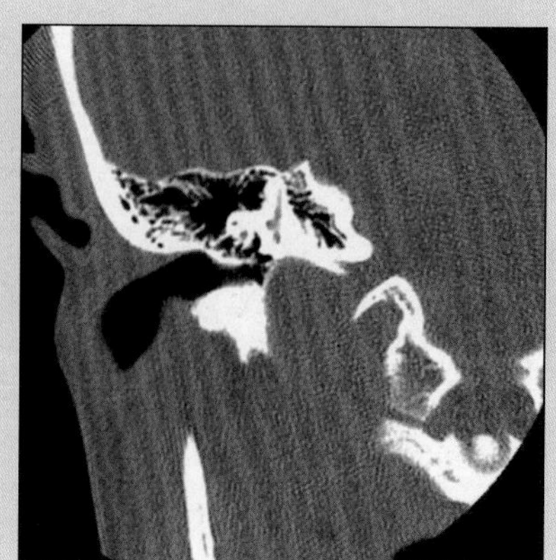

High-Riding Jugular Bulb

GLOMUS TYMPANICUM

Key Facts

Terminology

- Glomus tympanicum paraganglioma (GTP), chemodectoma
- Benign tumor that arises in glomus bodies situated on the cochlear promontory of medial wall of middle ear cavity

Imaging Findings

- Best diagnostic clue: Round mass with base on cochlear promontory; CT shows no bone erosion and T1 C+ MR shows intense enhancement
- Vascular retrotympanic mass
- Small lesions: Fills lower middle ear, just reaches medial border of tympanic membrane (TM)
- Focal enhancing mass on cochlear promontory
- Best imaging tool: Temporal bone CT without contrast best if GTP suspected clinically

Top Differential Diagnoses

- Aberrant Internal Carotid Artery
- Dehiscent Jugular Bulb
- Cholesteatoma of Middle Ear
- Glomus Jugulotympanicum Paraganglioma

Pathology

- Arise from chemoreceptor tissue (paraganglia) found along inferior tympanic nerve (Jacobson nerve) on cochlear promontory
- Embryologically derived from neural crest cells

Clinical Issues

- Most common signs/symptoms: Pulsatile tinnitus
- Age: 40-60 years of age at diagnosis
- Gender: M:F ratio = 1:3
- Malignant degeneration rare (< 5%)

- T2WI: High signal mass centered at the cochlear promontory
- T1 C+
  - Focal enhancing mass on cochlear promontory
  - Small GTP will be missed if slice thickness exceeds 3 mm
  - Very large GTP may leave middle ear via eustachian tube

Other Modality Findings

- Octreotide is an analogue of methyl-iodo-benzyl-guanidine (MIBG)
  - Taken up by chromaffin cells in paragangliomas
  - In-111 labeled octreotide scan maybe helpful in diagnosis of paragangliomas, extent of metastatic disease

Angiographic Findings

- Conventional
  - DSA not required for diagnosis
  - GTP supplied by enlarged ascending pharyngeal artery and its inferior tympanic branch, via inferior tympanic canaliculus
  - Large GTP or glomus jugulotympanicum tumors may be devascularized pre-operatively using transcatheter embolization to decrease intra-operative blood loss

Imaging Recommendations

- Best imaging tool: Temporal bone CT without contrast usually diagnostic
- Protocol advice
  - MR to define margins of large tumors
  - DSA ± pre-operative embolization of large tumors to minimize intra-operative bleeding

DIFFERENTIAL DIAGNOSIS

Aberrant Internal Carotid Artery

- Imaging: Tubular mass crosses middle ear cavity to rejoin horizontal petrous ICA; large inferior tympanic canaliculus
- Clinical: Vascular mass behind TM ± pulsatile tinnitus

Dehiscent Jugular Bulb

- Imaging: CT shows sigmoid plate is dehiscent; venous protrusion into middle ear cavity from superolateral jugular bulb
- Clinical: Asymptomatic incidental otoscopic observation

Cholesteatoma of Middle Ear

- Imaging: T1 C+ MR shows no enhancement, ↑ T2 signal, intermediate signal on T1
- Clinical: "White" mass behind intact TM (congenital) or disrupted TM (acquired)

Glomus Jugulotympanicum Paraganglioma

- Imaging: CT shows permeative change in bony floor of middle ear
- Clinical: Identical to GTP

PATHOLOGY

General Features

- Etiology
  - Arise from chemoreceptor tissue (paraganglia) found along inferior tympanic nerve (Jacobson nerve) on cochlear promontory
    - Embryologically derived from neural crest cells
  - Nonchromaffin (nonsecretory) in this location
- Epidemiology
  - GTP = most common primary neoplasm of middle ear
  - GTP not associated with multicentric paragangliomas

Gross Pathologic & Surgical Features

- Glistening, red polypoid mass centered near cochlear promontory
- Fibrous pseudocapsule

GLOMUS TYMPANICUM

Microscopic Features

- Biphasic cell pattern composed of chief cells and sustentacular cells surrounded by fibromuscular stroma
- Chief cells arranged in characteristic compact cell nests or balls of cells
  - Referred to as zellballen
- Electron microscopy: Shows neurosecretory granules

Staging, Grading or Classification Criteria

- Glasscock-Jackson Classification of GTP
  - Type I: Small mass limited to cochlear promontory
  - Type II: Mass completely fills the tympanic cavity
  - Type III: Mass fills the tympanic cavity and the mastoid air cells
  - Type IV: Mass fills the tympanic cavity, extending into the mastoid, the external auditory canal, or anterior to the carotid
- Fisch type A
  - No erosion of dome of jugular bulb
  - Important to distinguish from Fisch type B tumors such as glomus jugulare (erosion of dome of jugular bulb)
  - Different surgical approach for Fisch type B
  - Differentiate using CT of temporal bone

CLINICAL ISSUES

Presentation

- Most common signs/symptoms: Pulsatile tinnitus (90%)
- Other signs/symptoms
  - Conductive hearing loss (50%)
  - Facial nerve paralysis (5%)
  - Asymptomatic (5%)
- Clinical Profile
  - Vascular retrotympanic mass
  - GTP may be clinically indistinguishable from glomus jugulotympanicum paraganglioma or AbICA; imaging must differentiate these diagnoses and avoid biopsy of these vascular lesions

Demographics

- Age: 40-60 years of age at diagnosis
- Gender: M:F ratio = 1:3

Natural History & Prognosis

- Slow-growing, non-invasive tumor
- Spread along path of least resistance, can enter eustachian tube when large
- Average time from onset of symptoms to surgical treatment is 3 years
- Complete resection yields a permanent surgical cure
- Malignant degeneration rare (< 5%)

Treatment

- Tympanotomy for smaller lesions; mastoidectomy for larger lesions
- Consider pre-operative embolization of large GTP or jugulotympanicum paragangliomas
- Laser resection
- Radiation therapy can be employed as a conservative approach
- Octreotide directed radionuclide therapy may be useful in inoperable cases or for metastatic disease

DIAGNOSTIC CHECKLIST

Consider

- Temporal bone CT to confirm no erosion of jugular bulb (Fisch type B tumor)

Image Interpretation Pearls

- Enhancing mass centered near cochlear promontory without bone erosion
- Lesions can be very small at presentation

SELECTED REFERENCES

1. Boedeker CC et al: Paragangliomas of the head and neck: diagnosis and treatment. Fam Cancer. 4(1):55-9, 2005
2. Durvasula VS et al: Laser excision of glomus tympanicum tumours: long-term results. Eur Arch Otorhinolaryngol. 262(4):325-7, 2005
3. van den Berg R: Imaging and management of head and neck paragangliomas. Eur Radiol. 15(7):1310-8, 2005
4. van den Berg R et al: Head and neck paragangliomas: improved tumor detection using contrast-enhanced 3D time-of-flight MR angiography as compared with fat-suppressed MR imaging techniques. AJNR Am J Neuroradiol. 25(5):863-70, 2004
5. van den Berg R et al: The value of MR angiography techniques in the detection of head and neck paragangliomas. Eur J Radiol. 52(3):240-5, 2004
6. Lum C et al: Unusual eustachian tube mass: glomus tympanicum. AJNR Am J Neuroradiol. 22(3):508-9, 2001
7. Maroldi R et al: Computed tomography and magnetic resonance imaging of pathologic conditions of the middle ear. Eur J Radiol. 40(2):78-93, 2001
8. Jansen JC et al: Estimation of growth rate in patients with head and neck paragangliomas influences the treatment proposal. Cancer. 88(12):2811-6, 2000
9. Mafee MF et al: Glomus faciale, glomus jugulare, glomus tympanicum, glomus vagale, carotid body tumors, and simulating lesions. Role of MR imaging. Radiol Clin North Am. 38(5):1059-76, 2000
10. Noujaim SE et al: Paraganglioma of the temporal bone: role of magnetic resonance imaging versus computed tomography. Top Magn Reson Imaging. 11(2):108-22, 2000
11. Weissman JL et al: Imaging of tinnitus: a review. Radiology. 216(2):342-9, 2000
12. van den Berg R et al: Imaging of head and neck paragangliomas with three-dimensional time-of-flight MR angiography. AJR Am J Roentgenol. 172(6):1667-73, 1999
13. Weissman JL et al: Beyond the promontory: the multifocal origin of glomus tympanicum tumors. AJNR Am J Neuroradiol. 19(1):119-22, 1998
14. van Gils AP et al: MR diagnosis of paraganglioma of the head and neck: value of contrast enhancement. AJR Am J Roentgenol. 162(1):147-53, 1994
15. Larson TC 3rd et al: Glomus tympanicum chemodectomas: radiographic and clinical characteristics. Radiology. 163(3):801-6, 1987
16. Lo WW et al: High-resolution CT in the evaluation of glomus tumors of the temporal bone. Radiology. 150(3):737-42, 1984

IMAGE GALLERY

Typical

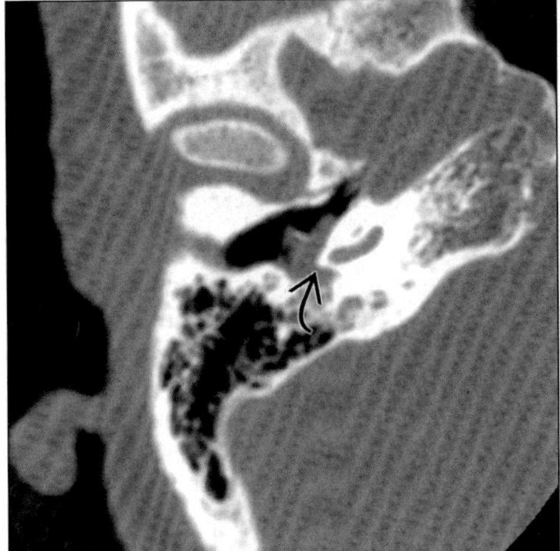

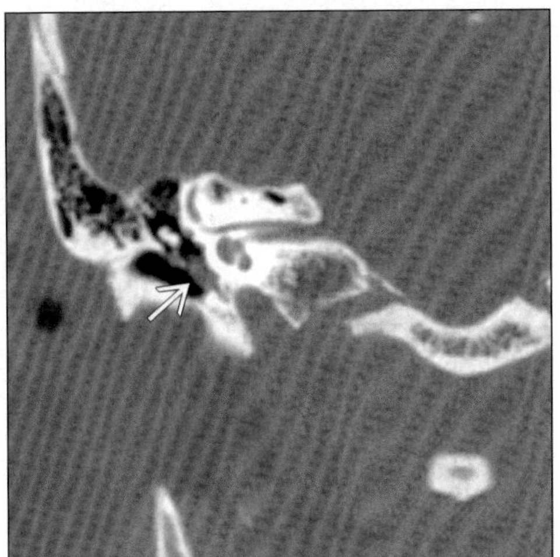

*(**Left**) Axial NECT with bone windowing shows a soft tissue density mass centered at the cochlear promontory ⇒. (**Right**) Coronal NECT with bone windowing shows a soft tissue density mass in the middle ear ➡.*

Typical

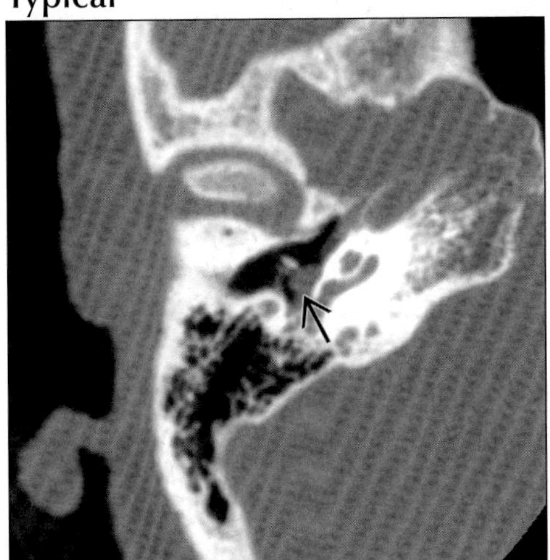

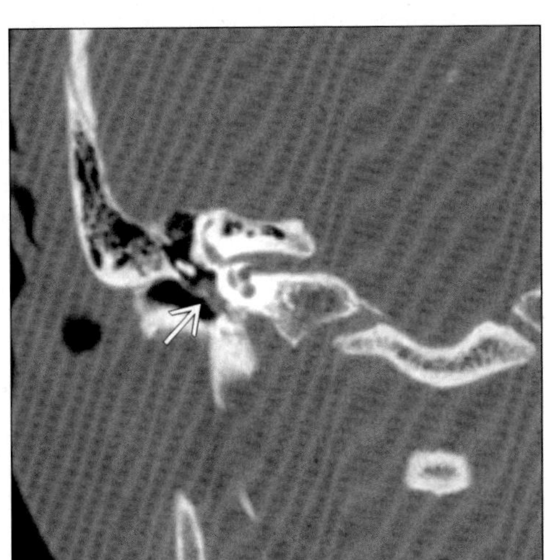

*(**Left**) Axial NECT with bone windowing shows a soft tissue density mass in the middle ear ⇒. (**Right**) Coronal NECT with bone windowing shows a soft tissue density mass in the middle ear ➡.*

Typical

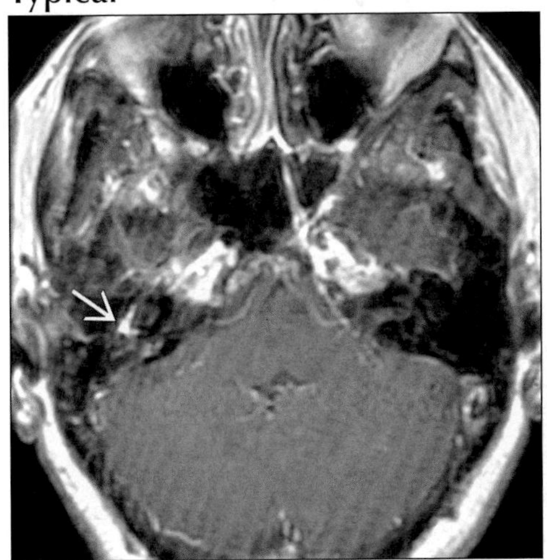

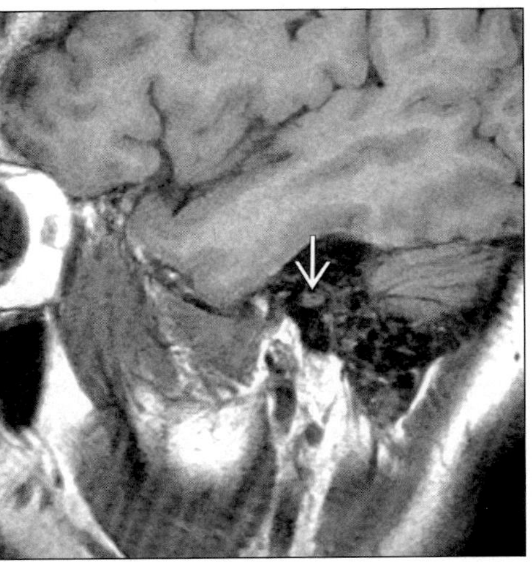

*(**Left**) Axial T1WI MR with intravenous gadolinium shows an enhancing mass in the right middle ear ➡. (**Right**) Sagittal FLAIR MR shows a soft tissue intensity mass in the middle ear ➡. The lesion localized to an enhancing mass on axial post gadolinium images. Small tumors such as these may be resected via a transmeatal or perimeatal approach. Alpha- & beta-blockers may prevent blood pressure lability & arrhythmias if given before surgery in hormonally active tumors.*

JUVENILE ANGIOFIBROMA

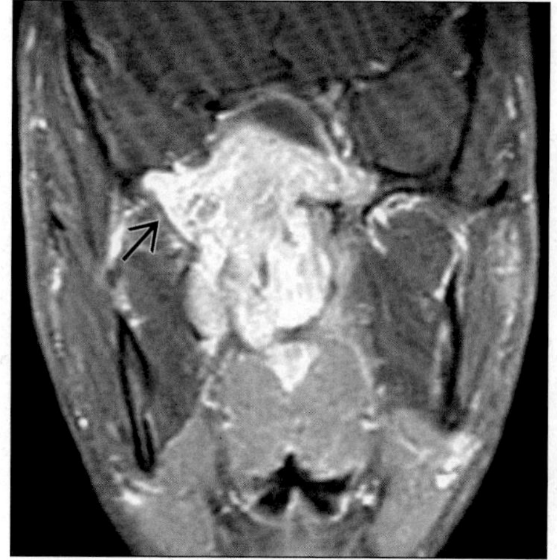

Coronal T1WI FS MR with intravenous gadolinium shows a large enhancing mass in the posterior nasal cavity and oropharynx, the sphenoid sinus, and the pterygopalatine fossa ➔.

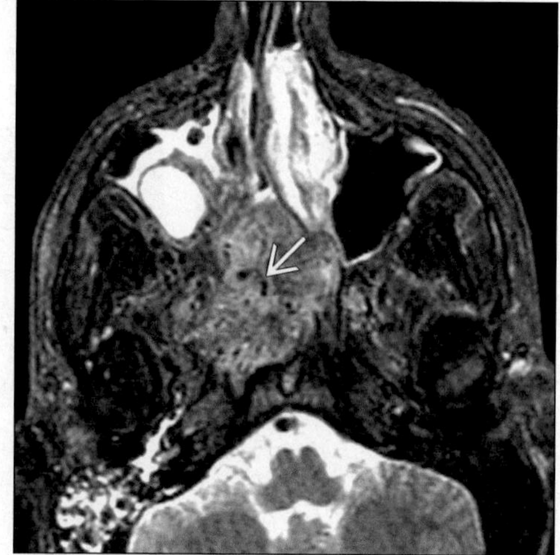

Axial T2WI FS MR shows a mass in the posterior nasal cavity extending into the sphenoid sinus, the right maxillary sinus and laterally into the right pterygopalatine fossa. Note flow voids ➔.

TERMINOLOGY

Abbreviations and Synonyms

- Juvenile nasopharyngeal angiofibroma (JNA); fibromatous or angiofibromatous hamartoma
  - JNA commonly used term but tumor begins in nose, (not in nasopharynx) and spreads secondarily into nasopharyngeal airway
  - Also called juvenile angiofibroma

Definitions

- Vascular, non-encapsulated, benign nasal cavity mass that is found almost exclusively in adolescent males

IMAGING FINDINGS

General Features

- Best diagnostic clue
  - Heterogeneous, intensely enhancing posterior nasal cavity, nasopharyngeal, maxillary and ethmoid sinus mass in a young male extending into pterygopalatine fossa, masticator space and orbit
  - Flow voids within mass on MR indicative of vascularity
- Location
  - Centered in posterior lateral wall of nasal cavity, at margin of sphenopalatine foramen
  - Penetrates the pterygopalatine fossa (PPF) early
  - Early involvement of upper medial pterygoid lamina
  - Intracranial spread in 10-20%
- Size: Usually large at diagnosis
- Morphology: Benign, vascular, locally aggressive nasal cavity mass

Radiographic Findings

- Radiography: Lateral plain film of face shows anterior displacement of posterior wall of maxillary antrum associated with nasal opacification

CT Findings

- NECT
  - Bone remodeling ± destruction by mass that is isodense to muscle
  - Ipsilateral nasal cavity and PPF enlarged
  - Posterior wall maxillary sinus bowed anteriorly

DDx: Juvenile Nasopharyngeal Angiofibroma

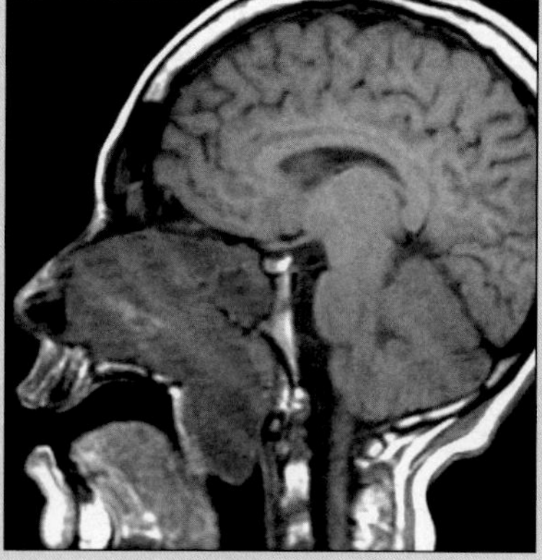

Antrochoanal Polyp

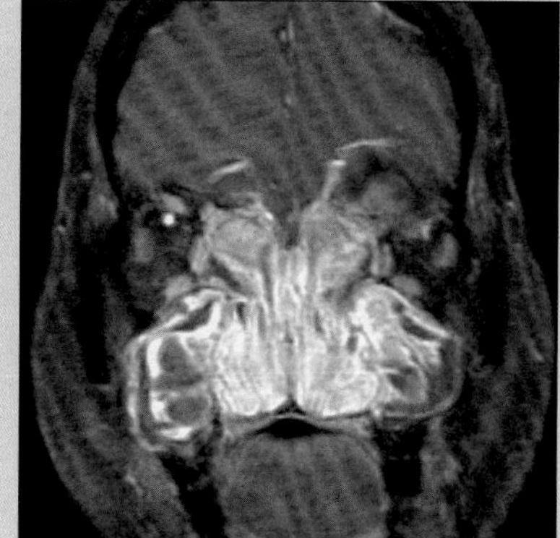

Polyposis

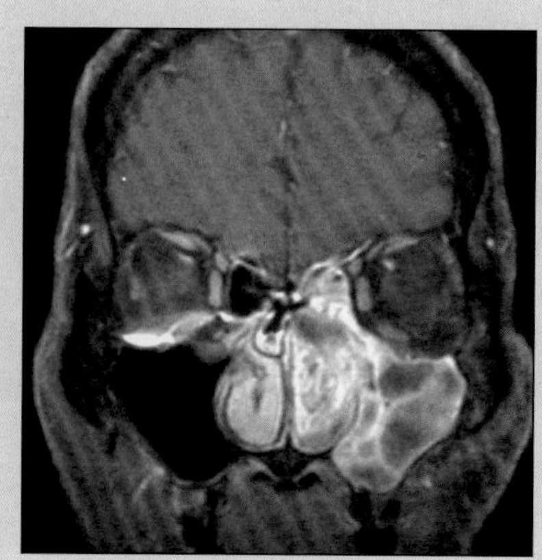

Inverting Papilloma

JUVENILE ANGIOFIBROMA

Key Facts

Terminology

- Juvenile nasopharyngeal angiofibroma (JNA); fibromatous or angiofibromatous hamartoma

Imaging Findings

- Heterogeneous, intensely enhancing posterior nasal cavity, nasopharyngeal, maxillary and ethmoid sinus mass in a young male extending into pterygopalatine fossa, masticator space and orbit
- Centered in posterior lateral wall of nasal cavity, at margin of sphenopalatine foramen
- Penetrates the pterygopalatine fossa (PPF) early
- Morphology: Benign, vascular, locally aggressive nasal cavity mass
- Bone remodeling ± destruction by mass that is isodense to muscle
- CECT: Markedly enhancing mass centered at sphenopalatine foramen
- T1WI: Heterogeneous signal with multiple flow voids within tumor

Top Differential Diagnoses

- Nasal Polyp
- Antrochoanal Polyp
- Inverting Papilloma
- Rhabdomyosarcoma

Clinical Issues

- Unilateral nasal obstruction
- Epistaxis
- Age: 10-25 years with peak at 15 years
- Gender: Almost exclusively males

  - If large, penetration of vidian canal ± foramen rotundum conveys tumor into pterygoid plate and medial middle cranial fossa respectively
- CECT: Markedly enhancing mass centered at sphenopalatine foramen

MR Findings

- T1WI: Heterogeneous signal with multiple flow voids within tumor
- T2WI
  - Heterogeneous signal with multiple flow voids within the tumor
  - Cystic changes sometimes seen, especially with larger tumors
- T1 C+
  - Intense enhancement
  - Coronal images necessary to show cavernous sinus, sphenoid sinus, or skull base/intracranial extension

Ultrasonographic Findings

- Color Doppler: Extensive vascularity can be seen

Angiographic Findings

- Conventional
  - Intense capillary blush is fed by enlarged feeding vessels from external carotid artery (ECA)
  - Internal maxillary artery (IMAX), ascending pharyngeal and accessory meningeal arteries from ECA are most common feeding vessels
    - Supply may be from contralateral ECA branches as well
  - Internal carotid artery (ICA) may supply tumor via mandibular artery (petrous segment) or meningohypophyseal trunk (cavernous segment) if skull base/cavernous sinus extension

Imaging Recommendations

- Best imaging tool
  - MR with contrast
  - CT shows bony destruction with more detail
- Protocol advice
  - Ideal workup to stage and characterize JNA includes
    - Maxillofacial MR with T1 C+ in axial and coronal planes
    - Bone algorithm non-contrast CT in axial and coronal planes
    - Catheter angiography of both ECA and ICA bilaterally to define blood supply prior to surgery
  - Embolization of ECA supply to tumor = low risk + minimizes intra-operative blood loss

DIFFERENTIAL DIAGNOSIS

Nasal Polyp

- Does not have aggressive bone destruction
- Enhances only peripherally

Antrochoanal Polyp

- Maxillary antrum is full; PPF not involved
- Lesion herniates into anterior nasal cavity, then nasopharynx
- Peripheral enhancement only

Inverting Papilloma

- Arises from maxillary sinus or lateral nasal wall
- Can show aggressive bone destruction and erode skull base
- Polypoid enhancement pattern without low signal flow voids

Rhabdomyosarcoma

- Homogeneous mass with bone destruction
- Not centered in posterolateral nasal cavity
- Does not usually penetrate the sphenopalatine foramen into PPF

PATHOLOGY

General Features

- General path comments
  - Angiomatous tissue in a fibrous stroma
  - Documented association with TGF-β, VEGF, and PCNA

JUVENILE ANGIOFIBROMA

- Genetics: Frequency of JNA increased in male FAP patients suggesting a possible association with alterations in the APC gene
- Etiology
  - Source of fibrovascular tissue of JNA is not known
  - Best current hypothesis: Primitive mesenchyme of sphenopalatine foramen is the source of JNA
- Epidemiology
  - Accounts for approximately 0.5% of all head and neck neoplasms
  - 5-20% extend to skull base, and may have skull base erosion

Gross Pathologic & Surgical Features

- Reddish-purple, compressible, mucosa-covered, nodular mass
- Cut surface has a "spongy appearance"

Microscopic Features

- Vascular and fibrous tissue
  - Myofibroblast is cell of origin
  - Fibrovascular stroma, with fine neovascularity
  - May be purely fibrous, with reduced vascularity
- Estrogen, testosterone or progesterone receptors may be present

Staging, Grading or Classification Criteria

- Several proposed classifications
- Fisch classification commonly used
  - Type I: Tumor limited to nasopharynx and nasal cavity, no bone destruction
  - Type II: Tumor invades pterygomaxillary fossa, maxillary, ethmoid, sphenoid sinuses with bone destruction
  - Type III: Tumor invades infratemporal fossa, orbit, parasellar region remaining lateral to cavernous sinus
  - Type IV: Tumor shows massive invasion of cavernous sinus, optic chiasm, or pituitary fossa

CLINICAL ISSUES

Presentation

- Most common signs/symptoms
  - Unilateral nasal obstruction
  - Epistaxis
- Other signs/symptoms
  - Pain or swelling in the cheek
  - Proptosis
  - Visual disturbances
- Clinical Profile
  - Adolescent male with average age at onset = 15 years
  - 10-25 years reported age range

Demographics

- Age: 10-25 years with peak at 15 years
- Gender: Almost exclusively males

Natural History & Prognosis

- May rarely spontaneously regress
- Local recurrence rate with surgery 6-24% usually seen within 2 years
- Local recurrence higher with large lesions, intracranial spread
- Rare reports of malignant change

Treatment

- Complete surgical resection using pre-operative embolization to decrease blood loss
- Radiation therapy
  - Adjuvant to surgery
  - Recommended for intracranial extension, incomplete resection or local recurrence
- Hormonal therapy
  - Not routine, as complete tumor regression does not occur
  - Feminization side-effects undesirable in adolescent male

DIAGNOSTIC CHECKLIST

Consider

- Pre-operative embolization to reduce blood loss during surgery

Image Interpretation Pearls

- Characteristic imaging findings obviate need for biopsy in most cases

SELECTED REFERENCES

1. McAfee WJ et al: Definitive radiotherapy for juvenile nasopharyngeal angiofibroma. Am J Clin Oncol. 29(2):168-70, 2006
2. Saylam G et al: Proliferation, angiogenesis and hormonal markers in juvenile nasopharyngeal angiofibroma. Int J Pediatr Otorhinolaryngol. 70(2):227-34, 2006
3. Kania RE et al: Early postoperative CT scanning for juvenile nasopharyngeal angiofibroma: detection of residual disease. AJNR Am J Neuroradiol. 26(1):82-8, 2005
4. Valanzano R et al: Genetic evidence that juvenile nasopharyngeal angiofibroma is an integral FAP tumour. Gut. 54(7):1046-7, 2005
5. Mann WJ et al: Juvenile angiofibromas: changing surgical concept over the last 20 years. Laryngoscope. 114(2):291-3, 2004
6. Vinaitheerthan M et al: Pathology teach and tell: nasopharyngeal angiofibroma. Pediatr Pathol Mol Med. 22(4):363-7, 2003
7. Yadav SP et al: Nasopharyngeal angiofibroma. J Otolaryngol. 31(6):346-50, 2002
8. Scholtz AW et al: Juvenile nasopharyngeal angiofibroma: management and therapy. Laryngoscope. 111(4 Pt 1):681-7, 2001
9. Chong VF et al: Radiology of the nasopharynx: pictorial essay. Australas Radiol. 44(1):5-13, 2000
10. Schick B et al: Radiological findings in angiofibroma. Acta Radiol. 41(6):585-93, 2000
11. Arslan H et al: Power Doppler findings in nasopharingeal angiofibroma. Clin Imaging. 22(2):86-8, 1998
12. Gullane PJ et al: Juvenile angiofibroma: A review of the literature and a case series report. Laryngoscope. 102:928-33, 1992
13. Harrison DF: The natural history, pathogenesis, and treatment of juvenile angiofibroma. Arch Otolaryngol Head Neck Surg. 113:936-42, 1987

IMAGE GALLERY

Typical

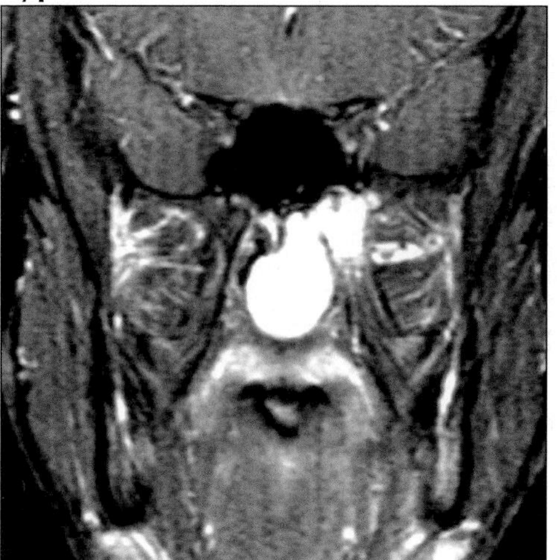

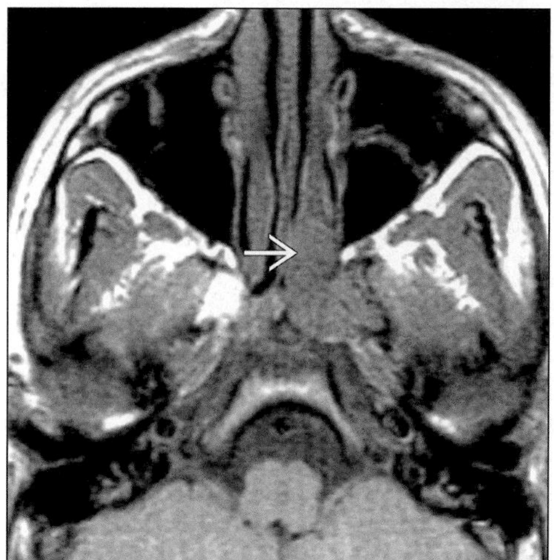

(Left) *Coronal T1WI FS MR with intravenous gadolinium shows an enhancing lobulated mass in the nasopharynx and left pterygopalatine fossa.* ***(Right)*** *Axial T1WI MR shows a mass arising from the posterior left nasal cavity ➔ which is isointense in signal with adjacent muscles. There is extension into the left pterygopalatine fossa.*

Typical

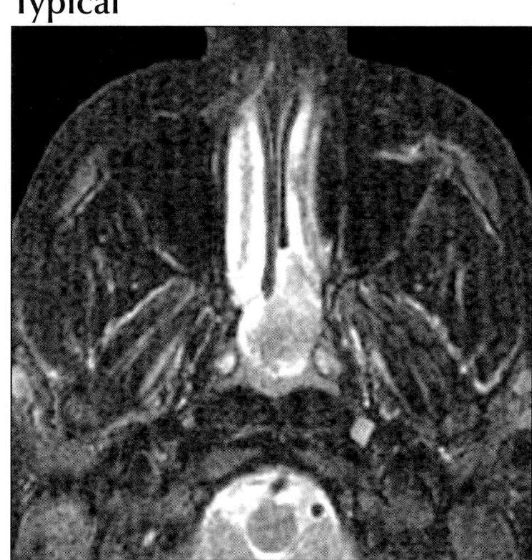

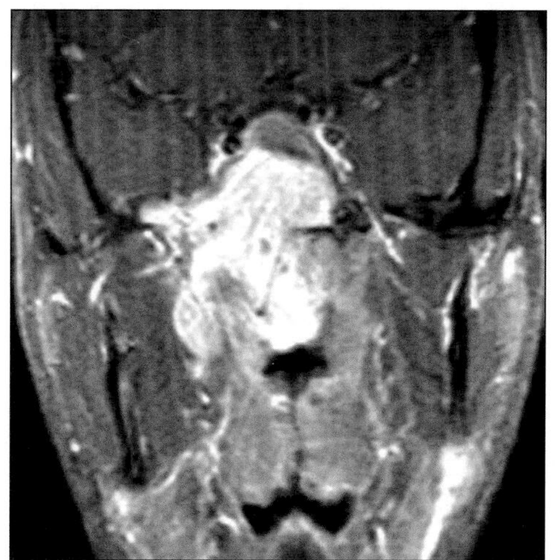

(Left) *Axial T2WI FS MR shows a heterogeneous mass arising from the posterior left nasal cavity which is extending into the nasopharynx.* ***(Right)*** *Coronal T1WI FS MR with intravenous gadolinium shows a large enhancing mass in the posterior nasal cavity and oropharynx, the sphenoid sinus, and the right pterygopalatine fossa.*

Typical

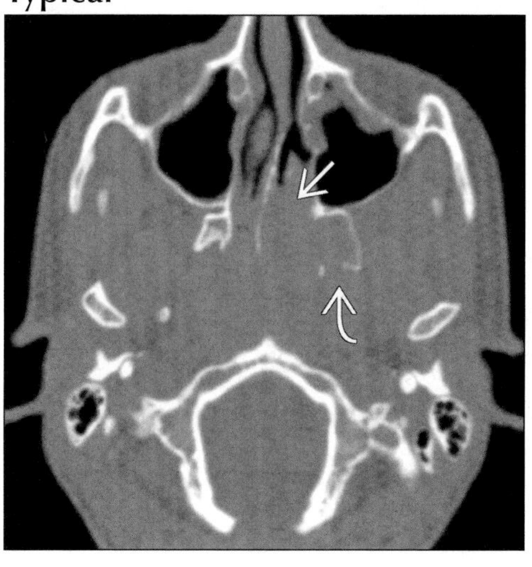

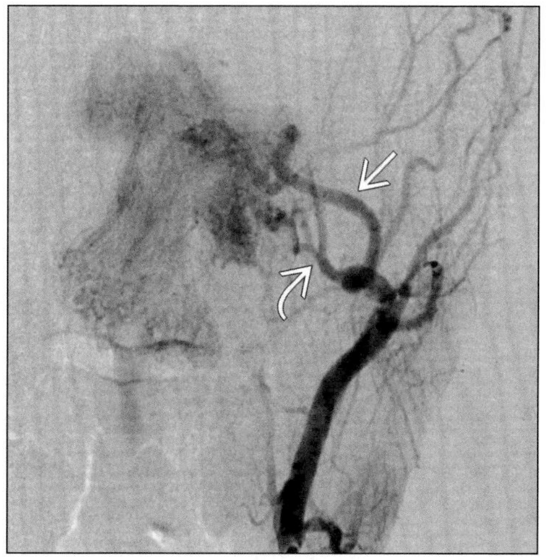

(Left) *Axial NECT shows a posterior nasal mass ➔ extending into the nasopharynx and crossing the midline. Note bone erosion and expansion of the left pterygoid plate ➔ and deviation of the bony nasal septum.* ***(Right)*** *Anteroposterior left ECA DSA in the same patient as previous image shows a hypervascular left nasal mass extending across the midline and supplied by branches of the IMAX ➔ and accessory meningeal artery ➔.*

FIBROMUSCULAR DYSPLASIA, CERVICAL

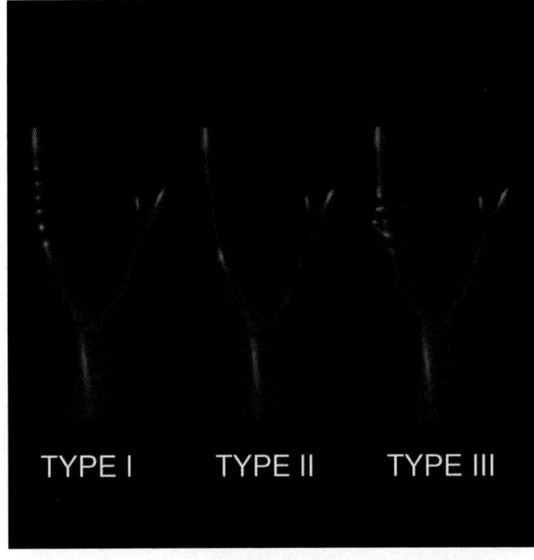

Graphic of the carotid bifurcation shows the principal subtypes of FMD. Type 1 appears as alternating areas of constriction and dilatation, type 2 as a tubular stenosis, and type 3 as focal corrugations ± diverticulum.

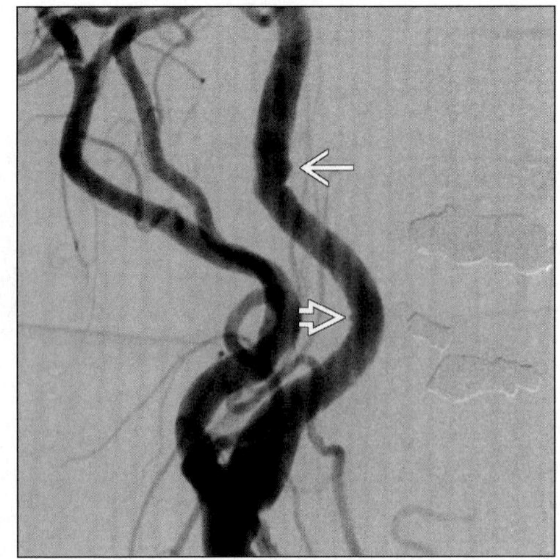

Oblique right CCA DSA shows short-segment luminal irregularity along the cervical ICA ➡ consistent with FMD. Note very subtle changes of FMD more inferiorly ⇨.

TERMINOLOGY

Definitions

- Fibromuscular dysplasia (FMD); fibromuscular hyperplasia (FMH); fibromuscular fibroplasia
- Arterial disease of unknown etiology affecting the medium & large arteries most commonly in young to middle-aged women
- Arteriopathy with dysplastic arterial wall characterized by overgrowth of smooth muscle & fibrous tissue

IMAGING FINDINGS

General Features

- Best diagnostic clue: Multifocal ± bilateral cervical carotid or vertebral artery irregularity on CTA/MRA/DSA; appears like a "string of beads"
- Location
  - Head & neck: Lesions most commonly at C1-C2 levels
    - Carotid artery involved in 30% (bilateral in 65%)
    - Vertebral artery involved in 10%
    - Intracranial involvement rare: Middle cerebral artery (MCA) commonest; anterior and posterior circulation can be affected
  - Peripheral vascular
    - Renal arteries most commonly affected (75%), 40% bilateral
    - Others: Hepatic, splenic, mesenteric, coronary
  - Affects > 1 vessel in 30% of patients
- Morphology
  - Classically alternating segments of stenosis and dilatation, "string of beads"
  - Others: Tubular stenosis, diverticular outpouching

CT Findings

- NECT
  - Not helpful in diagnosis
  - May see sequela of FMD (e.g., thromboembolic stroke, dissection) → cerebral infarction
  - Subarachnoid hemorrhage (SAH) from rupture of associated aneurysm or arterial dissection
- CTA
  - Morphological changes of FMD in carotid and vertebral artery circulations
    - Vessel beading/irregularities: "String of beads"

DDx: Fibromuscular Dysplasia, Cervical

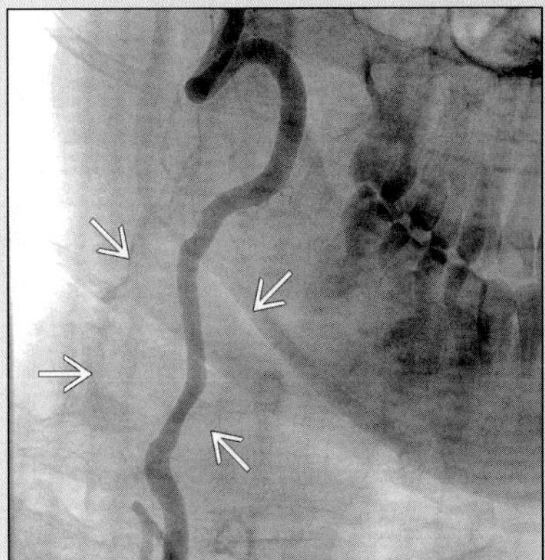

Tumor Encasement

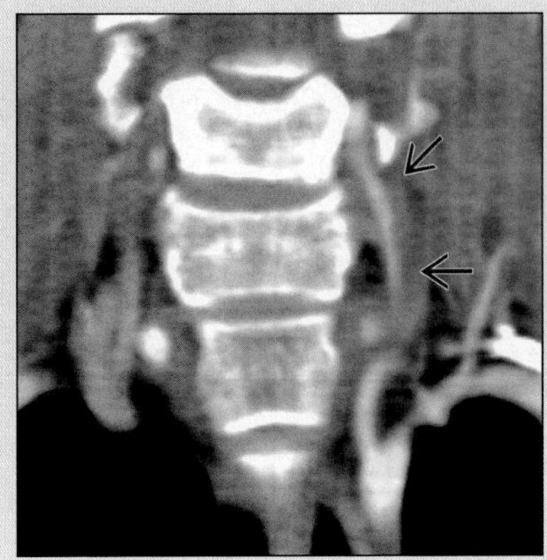

Vertebral Artery Dissection

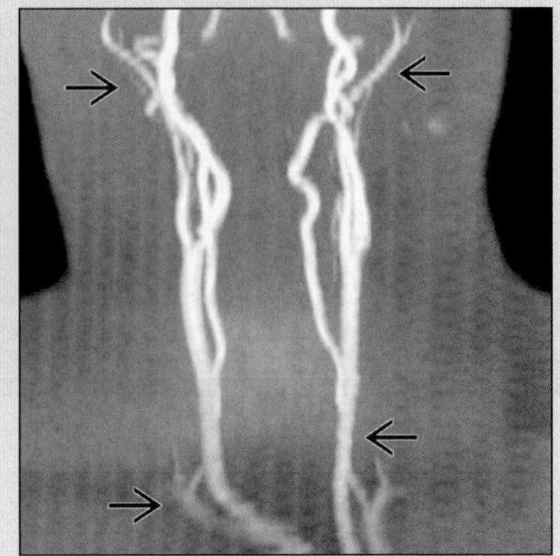

MRA Motion Artifact

FIBROMUSCULAR DYSPLASIA, CERVICAL

Key Facts

Terminology

- Arterial disease of unknown etiology affecting the medium & large arteries most commonly in young to middle-aged women

Imaging Findings

- Head & neck: Lesions most commonly at C1-C2 levels
  - Carotid artery involved in 30% (bilateral in 65%)
  - Vertebral artery involved in 10%
  - Intracranial involvement rare
- Peripheral vascular
  - Renal arteries most commonly affected (75%)
- Angiography shows 3 distinct appearances depending on FMD subtype
  - Type 1 (85%): Typical "string of beads"; medial fibroplasia
  - Type 2 (~ 10%): Long tubular stenosis; intimal fibroplasia
  - Type 3 (~ 5%): Asymmetric outpouching along one side of artery; periadventitial fibroplasia

Top Differential Diagnoses

- Atherosclerosis
- Arterial Dissection
- Standing Waves
- MRA Motion Artifact
- Tumor Encasement

Clinical Issues

- Hypertension (renal artery involvement → stenosis)
- Craniocervical FMD: Transient ischemic attack
- Antiplatelet ± anticoagulant therapy = conservative management for stroke prevention with cervical FMD

- Arterial stenosis without mural Ca++ (cf. ASVD)
- FMD associations: Dissection, pseudoaneurysm, intracranial aneurysms

MR Findings

- DWI: Detect end-organ injury (brain infarction) as sequela of FMD
- MRA
  - May see "string of beads" appearance of cervical vessels
  - Gd-MRA superior to TOF

Ultrasonographic Findings

- Grayscale Ultrasound
  - Distinguishing findings seen only in cases of excellent resolution
  - Visible ridges or thickening of carotid wall, with or without stenosis
  - Elevated velocity & disturbed flow in areas of stenosis
  - Abnormal supra-bifurcation ICA in young women suspicious for FMD

Angiographic Findings

- DSA: Gold standard for diagnosis
  - Angiography shows 3 distinct appearances depending on FMD subtype
    - Type 1 (85%): Typical "string of beads"; medial fibroplasia
    - Type 2 (~ 10%): Long tubular stenosis; intimal fibroplasia
    - Type 3 (~ 5%): Asymmetric outpouching along one side of artery; periadventitial or periarterial fibroplasia
  - FMD associations: May be seen on angio, CTA or MRA
    - Arterial dissection, pseudoaneurysm, berry aneurysms

Imaging Recommendations

- Best imaging tool
  - CTA or MRA for non-invasive assessment
  - DSA for definitive diagnosis ± endovascular intervention
- Protocol advice
  - 3D Gd-MRA superior to TOF for non-invasive assessment
  - If FMD found in any artery, consider study of cervical & intracranial arteries for FMD ± associated berry aneurysms

DIFFERENTIAL DIAGNOSIS

Atherosclerosis

- ASVD affects older vasculopaths
- Does not produce concentric ridges or "string of beads" appearance
- Usually focal, solitary stenosis at or above carotid bifurcation with mural Ca++

Arterial Dissection

- Post-traumatic or spontaneous
- Irregular stenosis ± outpouching from associated pseudoaneurysm

MRA Motion Artifact

- Patient movement, swallowing, coughing during TOF MRA acquisition
- Irregular or step-like outline to all vessels in region helps to differentiate from true pathology

Standing Waves

- Etiology uncertain
  - Oscillations from retrograde flow within an artery during cardiac cycle
  - Vasospasm during contrast injection at DSA
- May mimic type 1 FMD but regular periodicity and smoothness of vessel outpouchings helps to differentiate

Tumor Encasement

- Large head and neck tumors (e.g., carotid body tumor, glomus vagale, malignant nerve sheath tumor, sarcoma)
- Smooth, long-segment stenosis is typical

FIBROMUSCULAR DYSPLASIA, CERVICAL

- May mimic type 2 FMD

PATHOLOGY

General Features

- General path comments
  - Dysplastic disorder, not degenerative or inflammatory
  - May affect other medium-size arteries (peripheral, abdominal, cephalic)
  - Alternating zones of hyperplasia & weakening
    - Narrowing & dilatation = "sting-of-beads" appearance
  - Weakened areas may cause aneurysm formation or dissection
- Genetics
  - Not classically considered a genetic disorder
  - Possibly autosomal dominant with variable penetrance in males
  - Familial in 11% of cases
- Etiology
  - Unknown
  - Alpha-1 antitrypsin deficiency, hormonal effects on smooth muscle & mural ischemia in dysplastic vessels = current hypotheses
- Epidemiology
  - Renal artery > > carotid > vertebral > other arteries (lumbar, mesenteric, celiac, hepatic, iliac arteries)
  - In US, FMD incidence is 0.6% from angio data & 1.1% from autopsy
  - 4.4% asymptomatic incidence of FMD in adult renal transplant donors
- Associated abnormalities: Intracranial aneurysms present in 10% of patients with FMD
- Histopathology
  - Overgrowth of smooth muscle cells & fibrous tissue within arterial wall
  - Three principal histopathologic varieties; some authors describe 5 subtypes
    - Intimal fibroplasia: Intimal involvement
    - Medial fibroplasia: Medial layer involvement (85%), some authors subdivide into medial fibroplasia with aneurysm vs. without aneurysm
    - Perimedial fibroplasia: Involvement of adventitia adjacent to media, some authors subdivide into subadventitial and adventitial fibroplasias

Gross Pathologic & Surgical Features

- Vessels shows alternating aneurysmal outpouchings & stenoses in type 1 (commonest)
- Tubular stenosis in type 2
- Eccentric focal corrugations, vascular diverticulum in type 3

CLINICAL ISSUES

Presentation

- Most common signs/symptoms: Hypertension (renal artery involvement → stenosis)
- Craniocervical FMD: Transient ischemic attack
- Other presenting symptoms
  - Spontaneous ICA dissection in ~ 20%
  - Ischemic stroke
  - SAH (rupture of associated berry aneurysm or intracranial dissection)

Demographics

- Age
  - Onset of symptoms: 25-50 yrs
  - Any age (children, adolescents, elderly) may be affected
- Gender: M:F = 1:9 (medial subtype)

Natural History & Prognosis

- Slowly progressive disorder
- Long-term angioplasty results still pending

Treatment

- Antiplatelet ± anticoagulant therapy = conservative management for stroke prevention with cervical FMD
- Balloon angioplasty ± stenting is treatment of choice in patients with hemodynamically significant stenoses
  - Renal FMD typically responds well to balloon angioplasty without stenting
- Surgical bypass used infrequently

DIAGNOSTIC CHECKLIST

Consider

- FMD in younger patents with hypertension
- Non-invasive screening for intracranial aneurysms in patients with FMD

Image Interpretation Pearls

- "String of pearls" is classic appearance on CTA/MRA/DSA of most common subtype (type I)
- Standing waves are smooth, regular vessel wall irregularities cf. FMD (irregular, non-periodic)

SELECTED REFERENCES

1. Bhatt S et al: Hypertensive emergency in a young adult: diagnosis of FMD by renal angiography but not MRI/MRA. J Invasive Cardiol. 19(2):E31-3, 2007
2. Cohen JE et al: Petrous carotid artery pseudoaneurysm in bilateral carotid fibromuscular dysplasia: treatment by means of self-expanding covered stent. Surg Neurol. 68(2):216-20; discussion 220, 2007
3. de Bray JM et al: Fibromuscular dysplasia may herald symptomatic recurrence of cervical artery dissection. Cerebrovasc Dis. 23(5-6):448-52, 2007
4. Nerantzis CE et al: Post-mortem angiographic and histologic findings of coronary artery fibromuscular dysplasia. Int J Cardiol. 2007
5. Perdu J et al: Inheritance of arterial lesions in renal fibromuscular dysplasia. J Hum Hypertens. 21(5):393-400, 2007
6. Beregi JP et al: Fibromuscular dysplasia of the renal arteries: comparison of helical CT angiography and arteriography. AJR Am J Roentgenol. 172(1):27-34, 1999
7. Van Damme H et al: Fibromuscular dysplasia of the internal carotid artery. Personal experience with 13 cases and literature review. Acta Chir Belg. 99(4):163-8, 1999
8. Wong CY et al: Cerebral perfusion and vascular reserve in fibromuscular dysplasia of the internal carotid artery. J Stroke Cerebrovasc Dis. 7(5):364-6, 1998
9. Stewart MT et al: The natural history of carotid fibromuscular dysplasia. J Vasc Surg. 3(2):305-10, 1986

IMAGE GALLERY

Typical

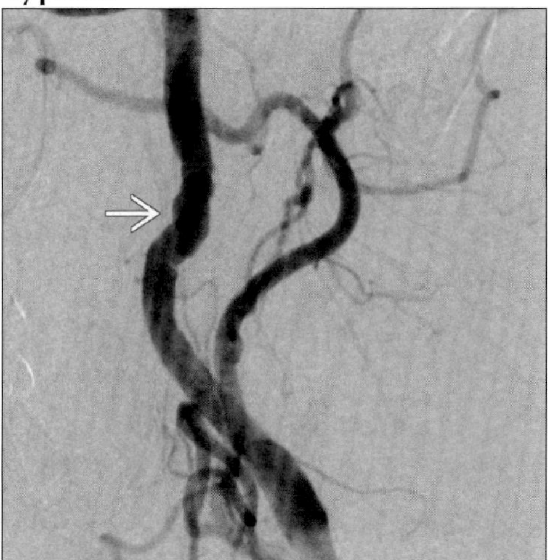
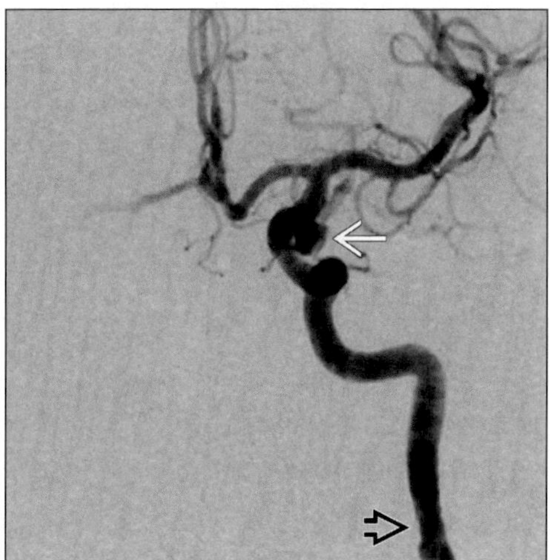

(Left) *Oblique left CCA DSA shows irregular outpouchings ➔ in the cervical ICA consistent with FMD.* ***(Right)*** *Anteroposterior left ICA DSA in the same patient as previous image, shows a 6 mm posterior communicating artery aneurysm ➔ which ruptured with resultant subarachnoid hemorrhage. Changes of FMD are again noted in the cervical ICA ⇨.*

Typical

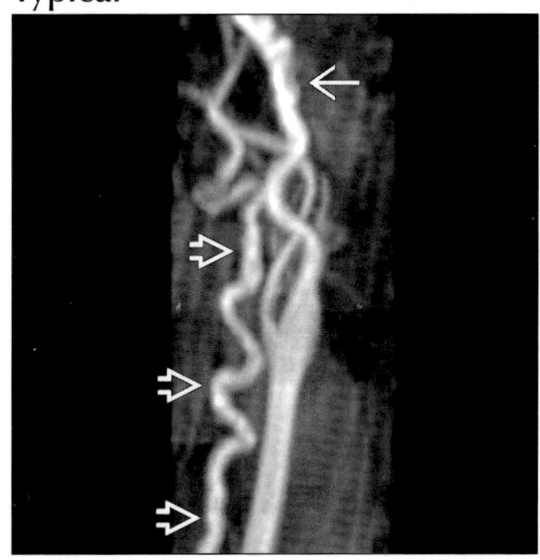
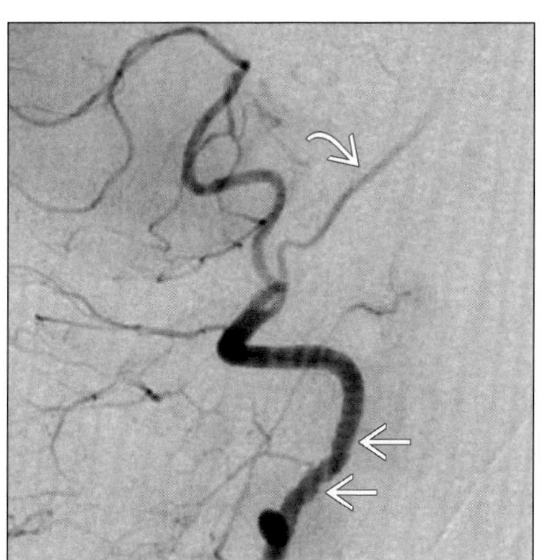

(Left) *TOF MRA shows extensive luminal irregularity of the cervical segments of the right vertebral ⇨ and internal carotid ➔ arteries in a patient with FMD. Note smooth outline of adjacent CCA and ECA making the changes in the ICA and vertebral artery unlikely to be artifactual.* ***(Right)*** *Lateral right vertebral artery DSA shows short segment luminal irregularity ➔ consistent with FMD. Note hypoplastic vertebral artery distal to the PICA ↷.*

Typical

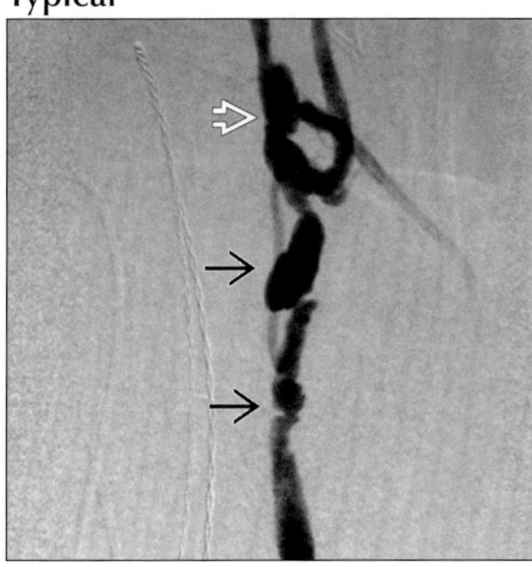
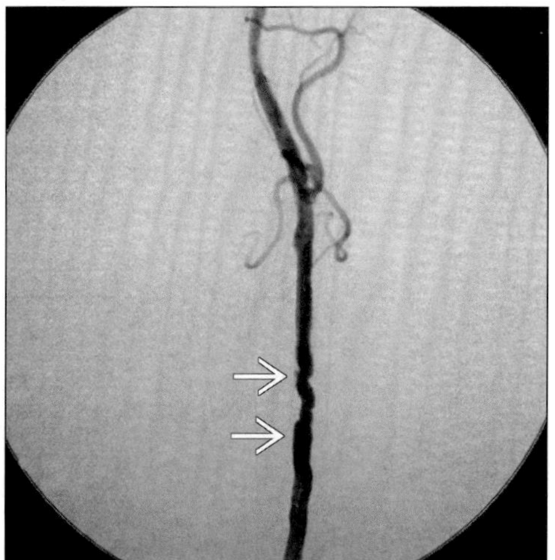

(Left) *Left CCA DSA shows bizarre irregularly spaced outpouchings and stenoses in the common ➔ and proximal internal ⇨ carotid arteries in a patient with TIAs.* ***(Right)*** *DSA immediately after deployment of overlapping self-expanding stents within the internal and common carotid arteries reveals minor residual luminal irregularity ➔ without significant residual stenosis.*

JUGULAR VEIN THROMBOSIS

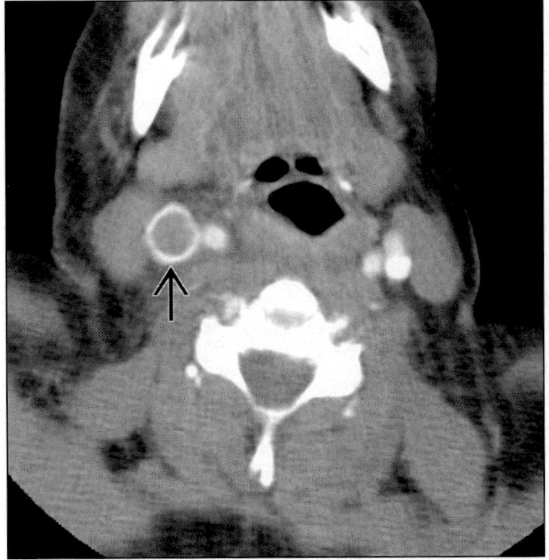

Axial CECT shows a large intraluminal filling defect with rim-enhancement of the right IJV wall ➡. Note inflammatory stranding in the adjacent fat planes.

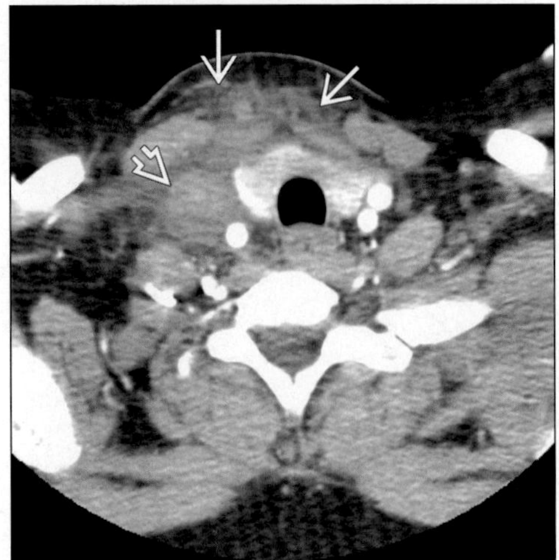

Axial CECT shows a distended right IJV without intraluminal contrast-enhancement ➡. Extensive adjacent soft tissue inflammatory changes ➡ are seen in the acute thrombophlebitic phase.

TERMINOLOGY

Definitions

- Jugular vein thrombophlebitis (JVT): Acute to subacute thrombosis of internal jugular vein (IJV) with associated adjacent tissue inflammation (myositis and fasciitis)
- Jugular vein thrombosis: Chronic IJV thrombosis (> 7 days) where clot persists within lumen but soft-tissue inflammation resolved

IMAGING FINDINGS

General Features

- Best diagnostic clue: Luminal clot present within IJV with soft-tissue inflammatory changes when acute-subacute (JVT)
- Findings depend on the stage of disease
- Acute-subacute thrombophlebitic phase (< 7 days): Imaging shows inflammation-induced loss of soft-tissue planes surrounding the enlarged, thrombus-filled IJV with vein wall rim-enhancement
- Chronic thrombotic phase (> 7 days): Imaging shows a well-marginated, tubular mass without adjacent inflammation
  - Multiple venous collaterals are seen bypassing the thrombosis
- Edema fluid may be present in retropharyngeal space (RPS) as a secondary sign of JVT

CT Findings

- NECT: Dense IJV
- CECT
  - Acute-subacute thrombophlebitic phase: CECT shows increased density in fat surrounding carotid space (CS)
    - IJV is enlarged and filled with low-density thrombus
    - Vasa vasorum of IJV wall enhances as a thin, hyperdense rim
  - Chronic thrombotic phase: Enhanced CT shows a tubular mass representing the thrombosed IV without increased density in adjacent fat

DDx: Jugular Vein Thrombosis

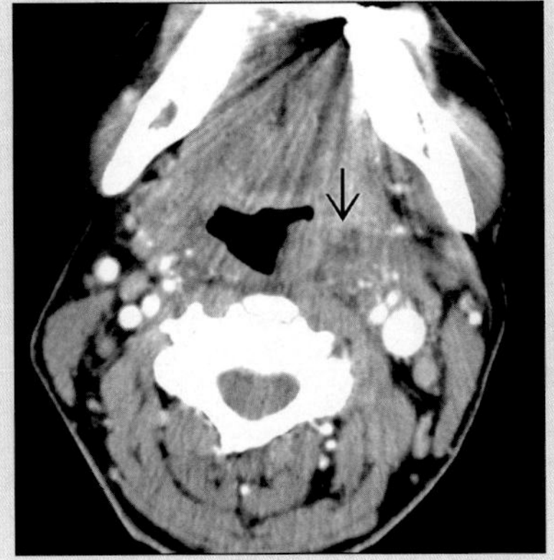

Abscess

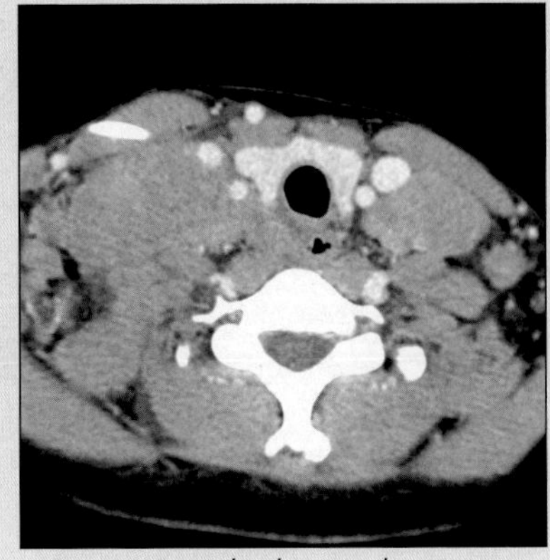

Lymphadenopathy

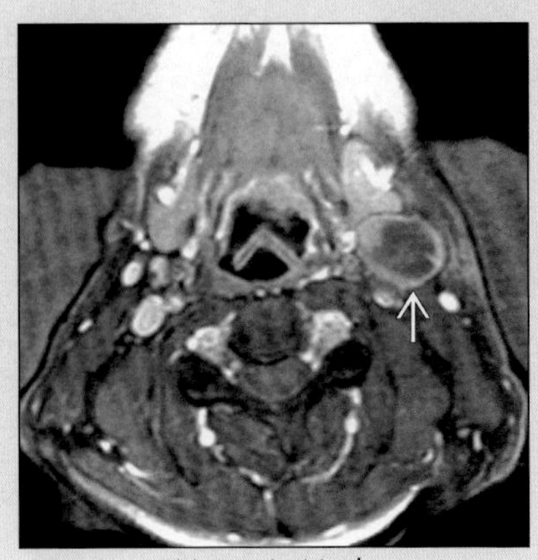

Necrotic Node

JUGULAR VEIN THROMBOSIS

Key Facts

Terminology

- Jugular vein thrombophlebitis (JVT): Acute to subacute thrombosis of internal jugular vein (IJV) with associated adjacent tissue inflammation (myositis and fasciitis)
- Jugular vein thrombosis: Chronic IJV thrombosis (> 7 days) where clot persists within lumen but soft-tissue inflammation resolved

Imaging Findings

- Best diagnostic clue: Luminal clot present within IJV with soft-tissue inflammatory changes when acute-subacute (JVT)
- Chronic thrombotic phase: Enhanced CT shows a tubular mass representing the thrombosed IV without increased density in adjacent fat
- T1WI: Subacute to chronic phase: Tubular mass in the posterolateral CS with high signal on T1 images secondary to T1 shortening from the paramagnetic effect of methemoglobin
- Absent signal in the region of thrombosis; may have artifactual signal from incorporation of high signal methemoglobin within thrombus on TOF MRV → underestimate extent of thrombosis
- Conventional: DSA: Partial or complete lack of filling of the IJV on venous phase; should compare with contralateral IJV

Clinical Issues

- JVT presents to radiologists in its acute phase as "rule out abscess"; in its chronic phase, as "evaluate tumor extent"

MR Findings

- T1WI: Subacute to chronic phase: Tubular mass in the posterolateral CS with high signal on T1 images secondary to T1 shortening from the paramagnetic effect of methemoglobin
- T2WI
  - Acute-subacute phase: May have a bizarre tumorous appearance, especially in coronal plane; adjacent fat appears infiltrated
  - High signal from methemoglobin can be seen
  - Loss of normal flow void
  - Edema in the retropharyngeal space
- T1 C+: Filling defect in the IJV
- MRV: Absent signal in the region of thrombosis; may have artifactual signal from incorporation of high signal methemoglobin within thrombus on TOF MRV → underestimate extent of thrombosis

Nuclear Medicine Findings

- PET: Variable but can demonstrate high accumulation of FDG

Ultrasonographic Findings

- Grayscale Ultrasound
  - Acute: Distended vein filled with hypoechoic thrombus
  - Subacute/chronic: Decreased vein size, increased thrombus echogenicity, variable recanalization
- Color Doppler
  - Flow is absent in the area of the thrombus, or the thrombus is surrounded by color of partially patent lumen
  - Collaterals are often visualized as prominent venous structures adjacent to the IJV
  - Spectral Doppler analysis may show loss of the normal biphasic venous waveform
    - Compare spectral waveform with contralateral side

Angiographic Findings

- Conventional: DSA: Partial or complete lack of filling of the IJV on venous phase; should compare with contralateral IJV

Imaging Recommendations

- Best imaging tool: Ultrasound or CTA/CTV in sick patients permits rapid diagnosis of JVT
- Protocol advice: MRV to evaluate for extension into dural venous sinuses especially in patients with mastoiditis as the primary etiology

DIFFERENTIAL DIAGNOSIS

Slow or Turbulent Flow in IJV

- High signal intensity on T1 MR images may be seen
- Look at all sequences, usually one will show flow
- If not, consider MRV or CTA/CTV to work this out

Reactive Adenopathy-Lymphadenitis

- Multiple focal masses along course of CS

Cervical Neck Abscess

- Focal walled-off fluid collection in any space of infrahyoid neck

SCCa Malignant Adenopathy

- Multiple focal, necrotic, and non-necrotic masses along the course of the cervical CS and posterior cervical space

Asymmetric/Heterogeneous Enhancement of the IJV

- Frequently seen pitfall during routine contrast-enhanced neck CT
- Can have normal asymmetry of IJVs (larger on side of dominant transverse-sigmoid sinus)
- May see bizarre enhancement pattern due to collateral flow in patients with subclavian vein or SVC stenosis/obstruction

JUGULAR VEIN THROMBOSIS

PATHOLOGY

General Features

- General path comments
  - In JVT there is lamination of thrombus, no hemosiderin deposition, and a delay in evolution of blood products (especially methemoglobin)
  - Lemierre syndrome
    - Septic thrombophlebitis of IJV associated with disseminated abscesses related to an acute oropharyngeal infection in a young patient
    - Fusobacterium necrophorum, an obligate anaerobic, pleomorphic, gram-negative rod is grown from blood or pus
  - Migratory IJV thrombophlebitis (Trousseau syndrome)
    - Associated with malignancy (pancreas, lung and ovary): Elevated factor VIII and accelerated generation of thromboplastin cause a hypercoagulable state
- Etiology
  - Pathogenesis: 3 mechanisms for thrombosis (Virchow triad)
    - Endothelial damage from an indwelling line or infection
    - Venous stasis from compression of the IJV in the neck (nodes) or mediastinum (SVC syndrome), dehydration
    - Hypercoagulability from Protein C and S deficiencies, Factor V Leiden or other etiology

CLINICAL ISSUES

Presentation

- Most common signs/symptoms: Swollen lateral infrahyoid neck
- Clinical diagnosis is unreliable
- JVT presents to radiologists in its acute phase as "rule out abscess"; in its chronic phase, as "evaluate tumor extent"
- Patient's history
  - Previous neck surgery, central venous catheterization, IJV access with drug abuse, hypercoagulable state or malignancy
  - May be spontaneous clinical event
  - Can be seen as a complication of ovarian hyperstimulation syndrome
- Acute thrombophlebitic phase: Tender, red mass with low grade fever; radiology requisition often reads "rule-out abscess"
- Chronic thrombotic phase: Hard, nontender mass; requisition reads "evaluate tumor extent"

Natural History & Prognosis

- IJV thrombophlebitis gives way to thrombosis over a 7-14 day period with decreased soft-tissue swelling

Treatment

- Aggressive antibiotics are given to treat any underlying infection; surgical or percutaneous drainage of focal abscess if seen on CT/MR
- Clinically significant thromboembolism to the lungs is relatively rare in IJV thrombosis; anticoagulant therapy is controversial and usually not used
- Prognosis is related to the underlying cause of the IJV thrombosis
- IJV thrombosis itself is self-limited, with venous collaterals forming to circumvent the occluded vein
- Percutaneous aspiration thrombectomy or mechanical embolectomy have been used successfully
- Superior vena cava filter can be considered in cases of bilateral IJV thrombosis

DIAGNOSTIC CHECKLIST

Consider

- History of previous neck surgery, central venous catheter placement, IV drug abuse, hypercoagulable state, malignancy

Image Interpretation Pearls

- Asymmetric/heterogeneous enhancement of the IJV on CECT
- Image artifact may arise from incorporation of signal from methemoglobin (subacute clot) on 2DTOF MRV → underestimate extent of thrombosis

SELECTED REFERENCES

1. Abbasi AA et al: An unusual swelling in the neck. Emerg Med J. 22(9):674-5, 2005
2. Chin EE et al: Sonographic evaluation of upper extremity deep venous thrombosis. J Ultrasound Med. 24(6):829-38; quiz 839-40, 2005
3. Wasay M et al: Neuroimaging of cerebral venous thrombosis. J Neuroimaging. 15(2):118-28, 2005
4. Berker B et al: Internal jugular vein thrombosis as a late complication of ovarian hyperstimulation syndrome in an ICSI patient. Arch Gynecol Obstet. 270(3):197-8, 2004
5. Bliss SJ et al: Clinical problem-solving. A pain in the neck. N Engl J Med. 350(10):1037-42, 2004
6. Kikuchi M et al: Case report: internal and external jugular vein thrombosis with marked accumulation of FDG. Br J Radiol. 77(922):888-90, 2004
7. Lin D et al: Internal jugular vein thrombosis and deep neck infection from intravenous drug use: management strategy. Laryngoscope. 114(1):56-60, 2004
8. Tajima H et al: Successful interventional treatment of acute internal jugular vein thrombosis. AJR Am J Roentgenol. 182(2):467-9, 2004
9. Wilkin TD et al: Internal jugular vein thrombosis associated with hemodialysis catheters. Radiology. 228(3):697-700, 2003
10. Chirinos JA et al: The evolution of Lemierre syndrome: report of 2 cases and review of the literature. Medicine (Baltimore). 81(6):458-65, 2002
11. Chiles C et al: Navigating the thoracic inlet. Radiographics. 19(5):1161-76, 1999
12. Sakai O et al: Asymmetrical or heterogeneous enhancement of the internal jugular veins in contrast-enhanced CT of the head and neck. Neuroradiology. 39(4):292-5, 1997
13. Poe LB et al: Acute internal jugular vein thrombosis associated with pseudoabscess of the retropharyngeal space. AJNR Am J Neuroradiol. 16(4 Suppl):892-6, 1995

JUGULAR VEIN THROMBOSIS

IMAGE GALLERY

Typical

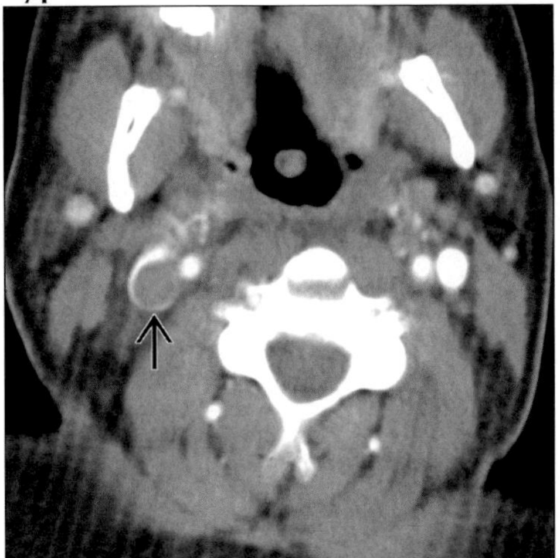

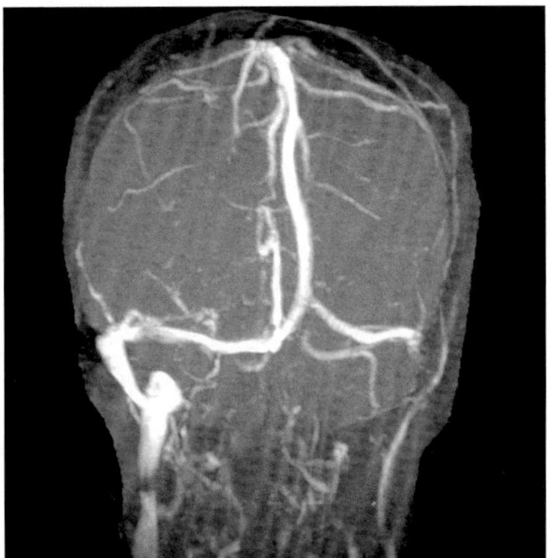

(Left) *Axial CECT shows a filling defect in the right internal jugular vein* ⇨. ***(Right)*** *2D TOF MR venogram in a different patient shows lack of flow related enhancement in the left sigmoid sinus and left internal jugular vein, consistent with thrombosis.*

Typical

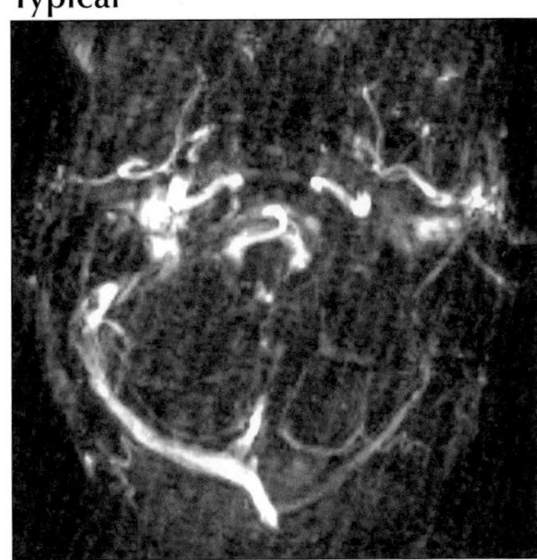

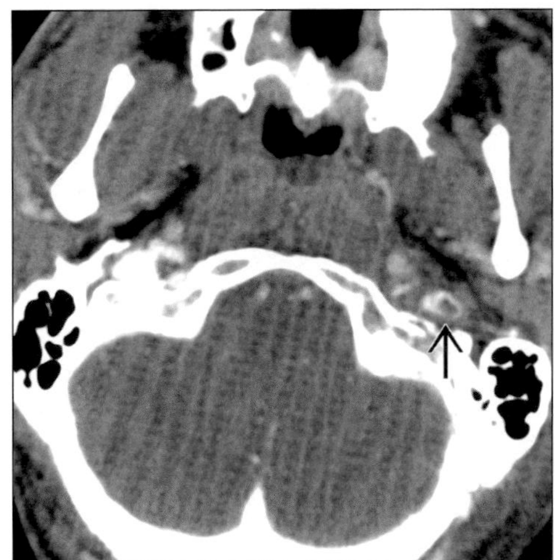

(Left) *Axial 2D TOF MR venogram shows lack of flow related enhancement in the left transverse sinus, sigmoid sinus, and left IJV, consistent with thrombosis.* ***(Right)*** *Axial CECT shows an intraluminal filling defect in the left IJV* ⇨*, consistent with contained thrombus.*

Typical

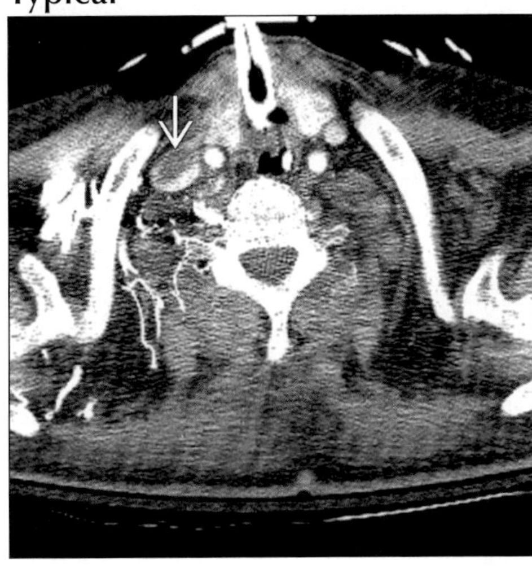

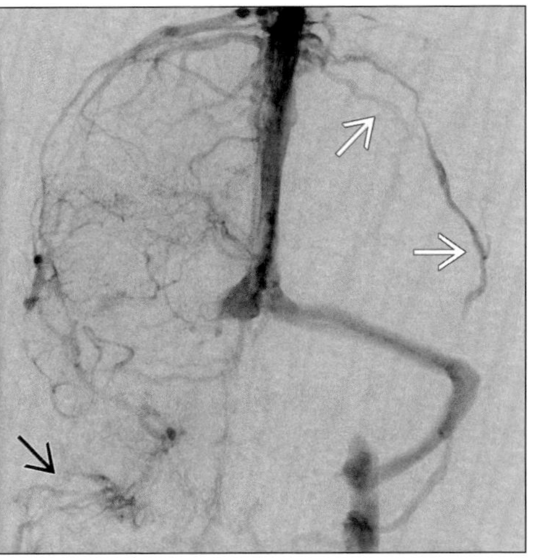

(Left) *Axial CECT shows a filling defect in the distal right IJV* ➡. ***(Right)*** *Anteroposterior right carotid DSA in a different patient shows non-filling of the right transverse-sigmoid sinus and IJV consistent with thrombosis. Note numerous collateral venous channels* ⇨*. There is also retrograde venous egress along cortical veins of the left cerebral hemisphere* ➡ *due to partial thrombosis of the superior sagittal sinus.*

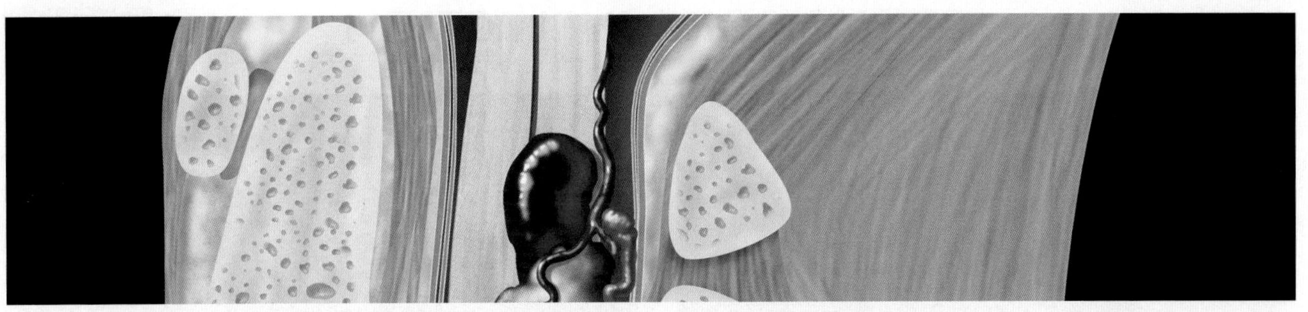

SECTION 3: Spine

SPINAL CORD INFARCTION

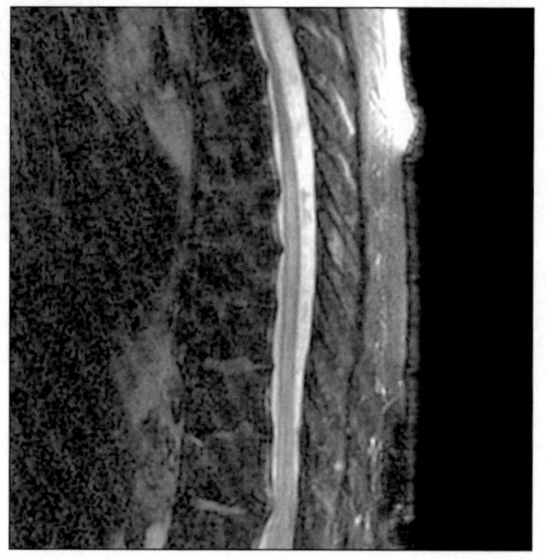

Sagittal T2WI FS MR shows central hyperintensity within the mid to lower thoracic spinal cord.

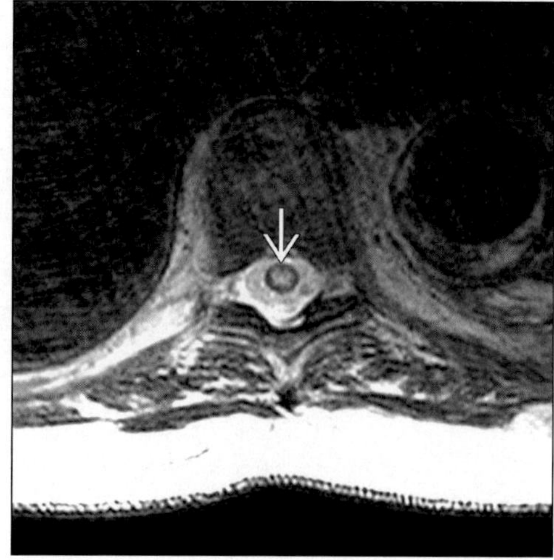

Axial T2WI MR shows central hyperintensity ➔ within the lower thoracic spinal cord.

TERMINOLOGY

Abbreviations and Synonyms

- Spinal cord infarction (SCI); cord ischemia; spinal stroke

Definitions

- Permanent tissue loss in spinal cord due to vessel occlusion, typically radicular branch of vertebral artery (cervical cord) or aorta (thoracic & lumbar cord)
- Venous ischemia common with spinal arteriovenous malformations (AVM) and may lead to infarction if prolonged venous hypertension, arterial steal

IMAGING FINDINGS

General Features

- Best diagnostic clue: Focal hyperintensity on T2WI in slightly expanded cord
- Location: Most frequent in thoracic cord because of arterial border zone between artery of cervical enlargement and artery of Adamkiewicz (arteria radicularis magna)
- Size: Variable, but usually > 1 vertebral body segment
- Morphology: Central hyperintensity on T2WI

Fluoroscopic Findings

- Myelography useful in diagnosis of spinal AVM if unable to perform MR
  - Serpiginous filling defects in thecal sac due to enlarged, tortuous draining veins

CT Findings

- NECT: Noncontributory
- CTA
  - Generally noncontributory
  - May see occlusion of intercostal arteries with aortic aneurysm + thrombosis
  - Visualization of anterior spinal artery (ASA) possible, but technically challenging

MR Findings

- T1WI
  - Slight cord expansion ± decreased signal
  - Early may have no significant T1 signal abnormality
  - Atrophy in late stage
  - Focal hemorrhagic conversion may occur with hyperintensity on T1WI & hypointensity on T2WI

DDx: Spinal Cord Infarction

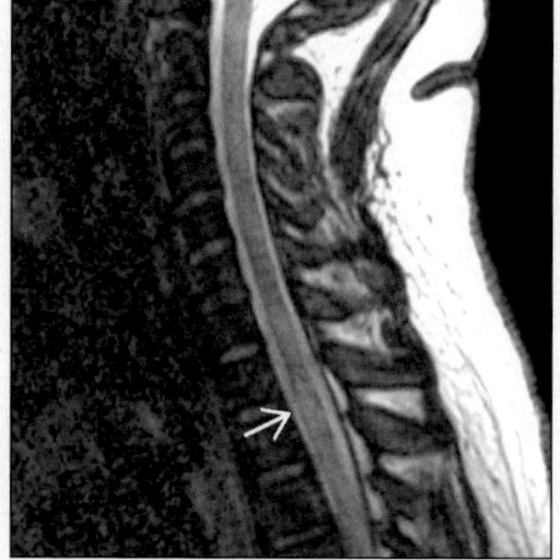

Multiple Sclerosis

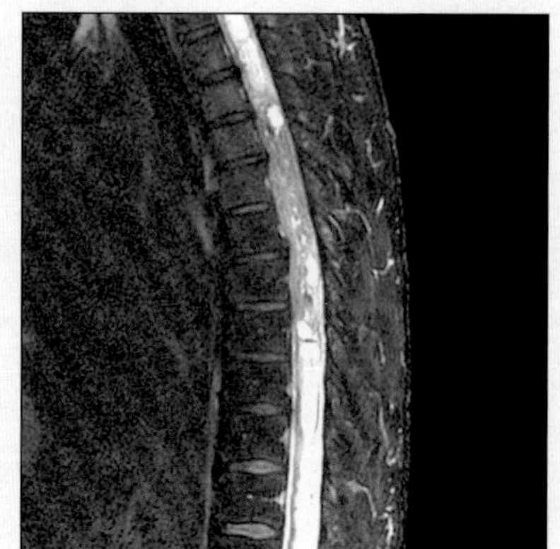

Ependymoma

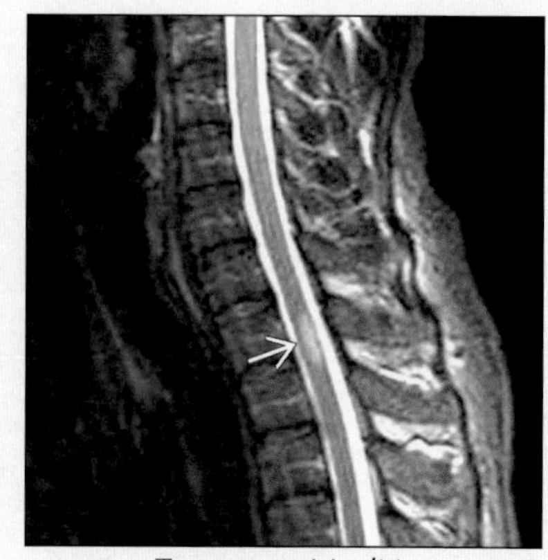

Transverse Myelitis

SPINAL CORD INFARCTION

Key Facts

Terminology

- Permanent tissue loss in spinal cord due to vessel occlusion, typically radicular branch of vertebral artery (cervical cord) or aorta (thoracic & lumbar cord)
- Venous ischemia common with spinal arteriovenous malformations (AVM) and may lead to infarction if prolonged venous hypertension, arterial steal

Imaging Findings

- Best diagnostic clue: Focal hyperintensity on T2WI in slightly expanded cord
- "Owl's eyes" appearance due to involvement of central gray matter
- Marrow T2 hyperintensity in anterior vertebral body or in deep medullary portion near endplate may be present due to vertebral body infarct
- Intradural serpiginous flow voids typically seen in spinal AVM (enlarged, tortuous perimedullary veins)
- DWI: Shows restricted diffusion (as in brain infarction)
- Best imaging tool: MR

Top Differential Diagnoses

- Multiple Sclerosis (MS)
- Spinal Cord Neoplasm
- Idiopathic Transverse Myelitis

Clinical Issues

- Sudden onset of neurologic deficits helps to make diagnosis of arterial spinal cord ischemia
- Progressive paraparesis is typical in venous cord ischemia due to underlying spinal AVM

- May see large vessel abnormalities such as aortic aneurysm or dissection
- T2WI
    - T2 hyperintensity in gray matter
        - "Owl's eyes" appearance due to involvement of central gray matter
        - With more extensive ischemia may see hyperintensity in gray matter and adjacent white matter, or entire cross-sectional area of cord
    - Marrow T2 hyperintensity in anterior vertebral body or in deep medullary portion near endplate may be present due to vertebral body infarct
    - Intradural serpiginous flow voids typically seen in spinal AVM (enlarged, tortuous perimedullary veins)
- STIR
    - Nonspecific increased signal in cord
    - Marrow hyperintensity may be present due to vertebral body infarct
- DWI: Shows restricted diffusion (as in brain infarction)
- T1 C+: May show patchy ill-defined enhancement in subacute phase
- MRA: Noncontributory since resolution of dynamic enhanced MRA not sufficient to define ASA

Angiographic Findings

- Conventional
    - Rarely indicated for suspected arterial ischemia
    - Variable findings, may see
        - Normal ASA
        - Absent ASA (occlusion at origin)
        - Occlusion along course of ASA due to thromboembolus
    - Gold standard for diagnosis/exclusion of spinal AVM if suspected venous ischemia by history or MR
        - AV shunts from ASA in type II, II, IV spinal AVMs
        - AV shunt from artery supplying dura of nerve root sleeve in type I spinal AVM (dural AV fistula)

Imaging Recommendations

- Best imaging tool: MR
- Protocol advice: T2WI sagittal and axial, 3 mm slice thickness; DWI of cord

DIFFERENTIAL DIAGNOSIS

Multiple Sclerosis (MS)

- Peripheral in location
- Less than two vertebral segments in length
- Less than half cross-sectional area of cord
- 90% incidence of associated intracranial lesions
- Relapsing & remitting clinical course

Spinal Cord Neoplasm

- Cord expansion invariably present
- Diffuse or nodular contrast-enhancement
- Extensive peri-tumoral edema
- Associated cystic changes
- Slower clinical onset

Idiopathic Transverse Myelitis

- Lesion centrally located
- 3-4 segments in length
- Occupying more than two-thirds of cord's cross-sectional area
- No associated intracranial lesions
- Onset not quite as sudden

PATHOLOGY

General Features

- General path comments
    - Embryology-anatomy
        - Seven to eight radicular arteries supply spinal cord in three territories
        - Cervicothoracic territory includes the cervical cord & first two or three thoracic segments, supplied by ASA from vertebral artery + branches of the costocervical trunk
        - Midthoracic territory includes fourth to eighth thoracic segments, supplied by radicular branch from aorta at T7 level
        - Thoracolumbar territory includes remainder of thoracic segments + lumbar cord, supplied by artery of Adamkiewicz

SPINAL CORD INFARCTION

- Artery of Adamkiewicz usually originates from T9-T12 intercostal artery (75%), usually on the left; may arise anywhere from T7 to L4
- Radicular arteries form one anterior & two posterior spinal arteries (PSA)
- ASA supplies gray matter + an adjacent mantle of white matter
- PSA supplies one-third to one-half of periphery of cord
- PSA infarction is rare

- Genetics
  - Rare: CADASIL (cerebral autosomal dominant arteriopathy with subcortical infarcts and leukoencephalopathy)
    - Mapped to chromosome 19q12
    - Subarachnoid vessel abnormalities including concentric thickening of media and adventitia
- Etiology
  - Idiopathic
  - Atherosclerosis
  - Thoracoabdominal aneurysm
  - Aortic surgery
  - Systemic hypotension
  - Infection
  - Embolic disease
  - Spinal arteriovenous malformation
  - Vasculitis
  - Dissection (vertebral artery or aorta)
  - Decompression sickness
  - Coagulopathy
  - Post anesthesia complication (epidural injection, celiac plexus block)
- Epidemiology: Rare, usually patients > 50
- Associated abnormalities: Atherosclerotic risk factors such as hypertension, diabetes, cigarette smoking

Gross Pathologic & Surgical Features

- Change with time
- Soft pale, swollen tissue with increasingly distinct margin with more normal tissue over time

Microscopic Features

- Acute: Ischemic neurons with cytotoxic + vasogenic edema, swelling of endothelial cells + astrocytes
- Subacute: Increasing numbers of phagocytic cells, activated microglia
- Chronic: Macrophages contain myelin breakdown products, progression of astrocytic reaction with protoplasmic extensions

CLINICAL ISSUES

Presentation

- Most common signs/symptoms
  - Anterior spinal syndrome presents with paralysis, loss of pain and temperature sensation, bladder & bowel dysfunction
  - Posterior spinal cord infarction characterized by loss of proprioception + vibration sense, paresis, sphincter dysfunction
  - Sudden onset of neurologic deficits helps to make diagnosis of arterial spinal cord ischemia
  - Progressive paraparesis is typical in venous cord ischemia due to underlying spinal AVM
  - Other signs/symptoms
    - Rarely spinal cord ischemia can manifest as Brown-Sequard syndrome (originally described with hemisection of cord)
- Clinical Profile
  - Arterial cord ischemia/infarction
    - Abrupt onset of weakness, loss of sensation
    - Rapid progression of neurologic deficits, reaching maximum impairment within hours
  - Venous cord ischemia/infarction
    - Insidious, progressive decline in mobility, sensation, bowel and bladder function over months

Demographics

- Age: > 50
- Gender: M = F

Natural History & Prognosis

- Acute arterial spinal cord ischemia syndrome has poor prognosis with likely permanent disabling sequelae
  - > 20% in-hospital mortality rate
- Venous ischemia secondary to AV shunt is progressive but reversible if treated before infarction ensues

Treatment

- Arterial ischemia/infarction
  - Antiplatelets (e.g., aspirin, clopidogrel)
  - Anticoagulation
  - Intravenous corticosteroids
  - Maintain systemic perfusion
  - Physical rehabilitation
- Venous ischemia/infarction
  - Definitive cure of spinal AVM
  - May require surgery, embolization or both

DIAGNOSTIC CHECKLIST

Consider

- Associated vertebral body infarction seen as T2 hyperintensity allowing specific diagnosis of otherwise nonspecific cord signal change

Image Interpretation Pearls

- Classic imaging appearance: T2 hyperintensity involving the anterior horn cells ("owl's eyes")
- Check for aortic aneurysm or dissection

SELECTED REFERENCES

1. Bornke C et al: Vertebral body infarction indicating midthoracic spinal stroke. Spinal Cord. 40(5): 244-7, 2002
2. Weidauer S et al: Spinal cord infarction: MR imaging and clinical features in 16 cases. Neuroradiology. 44(10): 851-7, 2002
3. Faig J et al: Vertebral body infarction as a confirmatory sign of spinal cord ischemic stroke: report of three cases and review of the literature. Stroke. 29(1): 239-43, 1998
4. Mascalchi M et al: Posterior spinal artery infarct. AJNR Am J Neuroradiol. 19(2): 361-3, 1998

IMAGE GALLERY

Typical

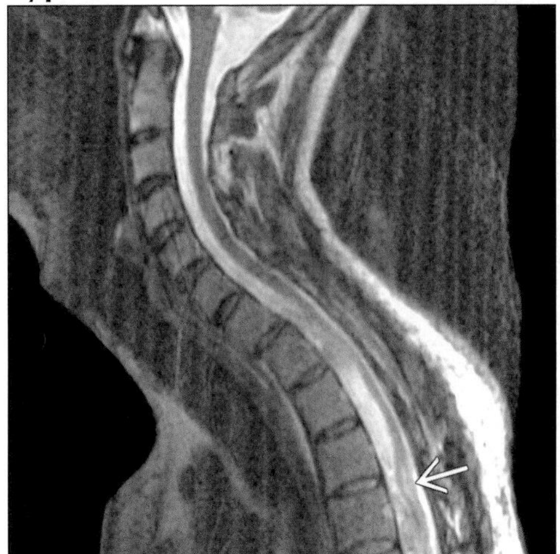

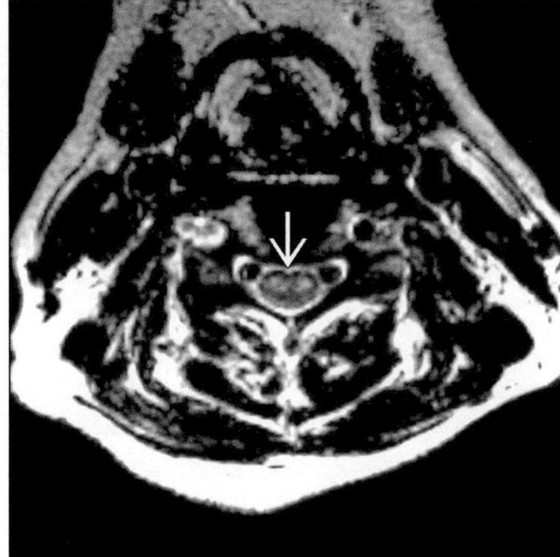

(Left) Sagittal T2WI MR shows atrophy of the lower cervical and upper thoracic spinal cord in addition to high T2 signal ➡ in the cord at the level of T4, consistent with late stage infarct. *(Right)* Axial T2WI MR shows central hyperintensity in the mid cervical spinal cord. The "owl's eyes" ➡ appearance of the anterior horn cells is typical early in the course of ischemia/infarction.

Typical

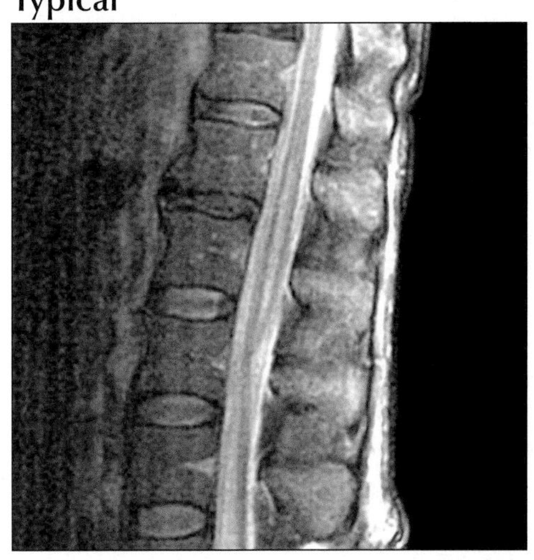

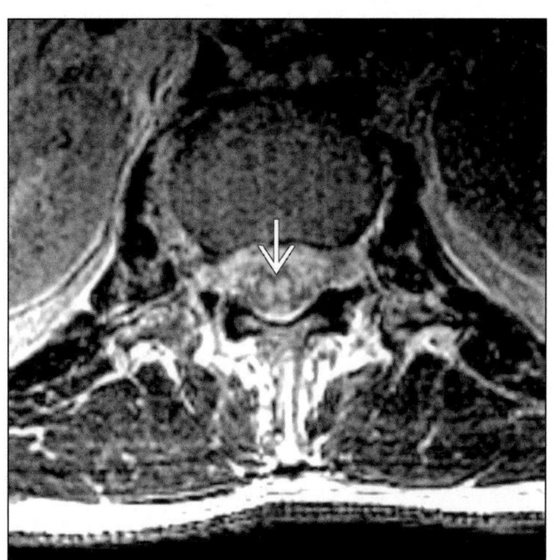

(Left) Sagittal T2WI MR shows central hyperintensity and some expansion of the lower thoracic spinal cord at the level of the conus medullaris. *(Right)* Axial T2WI MR shows central hyperintensity ➡ in the spinal cord at the level of the conus medullaris. The abnormality is confined to the central gray matter.

Typical

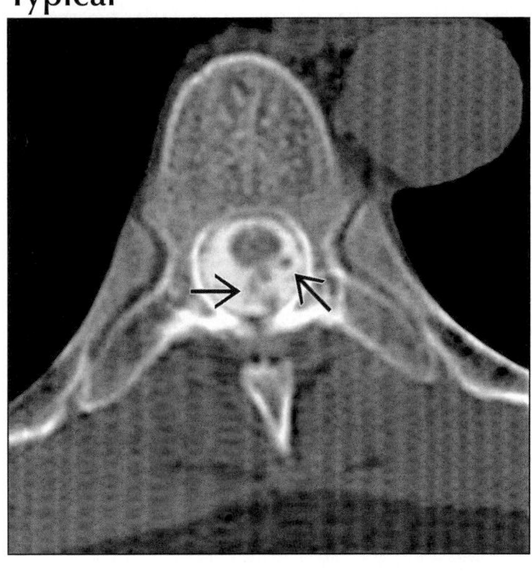

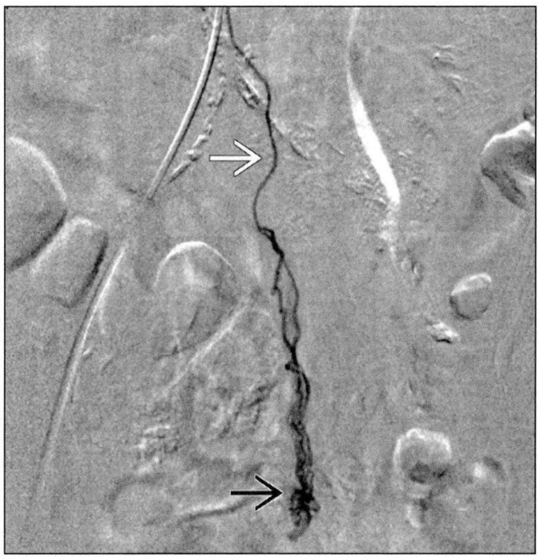

(Left) Axial thoracic CT myelogram in a patient presenting with progressive lower limb weakness and contraindications to MR shows serpentine and punctate filling defects ➡ within the subarachnoid space due to enlarged, tortuous perimedullary veins. *(Right)* Anteroposterior spinal DSA in the same patient shows an enlarged ASA ➡ supplying an AV fistula of the filum terminale ➡. Her symptoms rapidly improved after resection of the fistula.

ARTERIOVENOUS MALFORMATION, SPINE

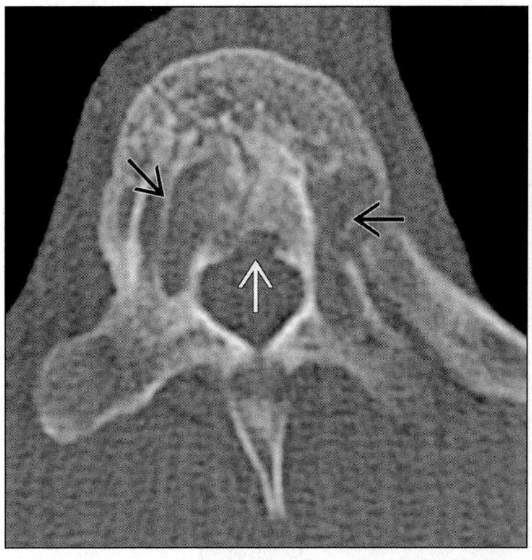

Axial NECT shows large cavities within the vertebral body ⇒ and enlargement of the foramen for the basivertebral vein ➡ in a patient with a metameric (type III) spinal AVM.

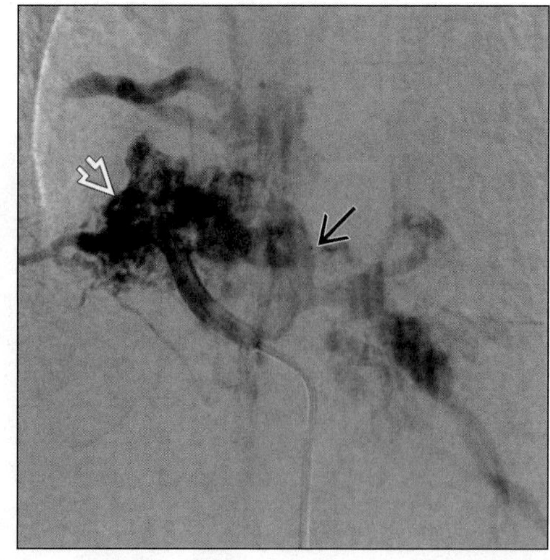

T9 intercostal artery DSA shows a large, predominantly extraspinal AVM nidus typical of metameric lesions ➡. Note large venous lakes ⇒ as depicted on CT.

TERMINOLOGY

Definitions

- Spinal arteriovenous malformation (AVM): Direct arteriovenous communications without intervening capillary bed
- Contemporary classification includes any AV shunt along the spinal axis (true AVM, dural AV fistula, perimedullary fistula)

IMAGING FINDINGS

General Features

- Best diagnostic clue
  - T2 weighted MR shows spinal cord swelling + intramedullary high signal due to venous hypertension, edema (non-specific)
  - Serpentine flow voids on MR due to dilated perimedullary venous plexus highly specific
  - Intramedullary, subdural + subarachnoid hemorrhage may occur with type II & III spinal AVMs; rare with type I & IV
- Location: Extradural, intradural, combined intra + extradural, ventral or dorsal to spinal cord depending on type I → IV
- Size: Variable sized shunts from single hole fistulas to diffuse AVM nidus

Radiographic Findings

- Radiography: Vertebral body erosion ± posterior body scalloping possible with type III AVMs

Fluoroscopic Findings

- Myelography: Serpentine filling defects within contrast column = dilated perimedullary veins within spinal subarachnoid space

CT Findings

- NECT: May see widened interpedicular distance, posterior vertebral scalloping with metameric AVMs, epidural fistulas with large venous varices
- CECT: May show enlarged cord with enhancing AVM nidus or non-specific patchy spinal cord enhancement
- CTA: May show dilated, tortuous perimedullary veins ± enlarged radiculomedullary artery (type I) or spinal artery (types II-IV)

DDx: Spinal Vascular Lesions

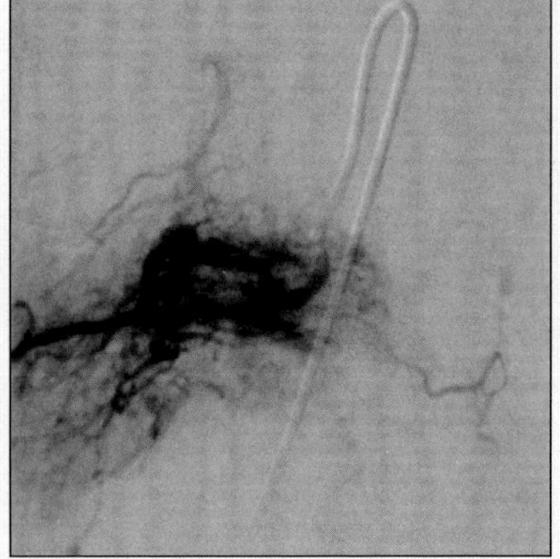

Vertebral Body Metastasis

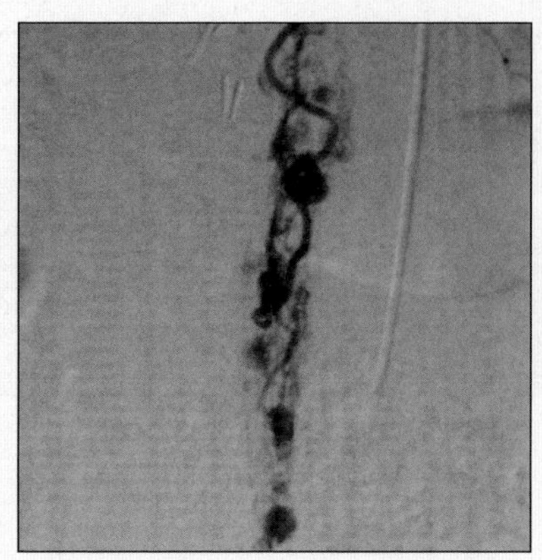

Spinal Cord Hemangioblastomas

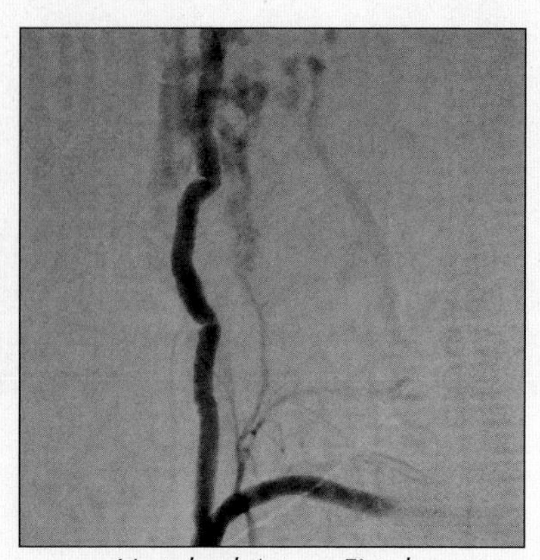

Vertebral Artery Fistula

ARTERIOVENOUS MALFORMATION, SPINE

Key Facts

Terminology
- Contemporary classification includes any AV shunt along the spinal axis (true AVM, dural AV fistula, perimedullary fistula)
- Spinal arteriovenous malformation (AVM): Direct arteriovenous communications without intervening capillary bed

Imaging Findings
- T2 weighted MR shows spinal cord swelling + intramedullary high signal due to venous hypertension, edema (non-specific)
- Serpiginous flow voids on MR due to dilated perimedullary venous plexus highly specific
- Myelography if MR contraindicated
- DSA required to confirm diagnosis, classify, define angioarchitecture

Top Differential Diagnoses
- Intramedullary Neoplasm
- Vertebral Body Metastasis
- Spinal Hemangioblastomas
- Vertebral Artery Fistula

Pathology
- AVMs account for < 10% of spinal masses
- Most common = type I (up to 80%)
- Second most common = type II > III (15-20%)
- Can be sporadic or syndromic

Clinical Issues
- Poor prognosis for juvenile (type III) AVM
- Depends on AVM type: Progressive paraparesis, pain, acute neurological deficit

MR Findings
- T1WI
  - Spinal cord swelling, low signal (edema) in types I&IV
  - Heterogeneous signal (blood products) in type II-III
  - Flow voids from enlarged arterial feeder(s) ± draining vein(s)
- T2WI
  - Intramedullary high signal (edema) ± cord swelling
  - Serpentine flow voids due to distension of tortuous perimedullary veins; often best appreciated on sagittal images
    - CSF flow artifact may look similar; axial images can help differentiate
  - Heterogeneous signal from blood products in type II-III
  - Spinal cord may be displaced or compressed by venous varices in extradural AVMs
- T2* GRE: May show blooming from blood products
- T1 C+
  - May see enhancement of distended perimedullary venous plexus (types I-IV) ± AVM nidus in types II & III
  - Non-specific patchy enhancement of spinal cord parenchyma may be seen

Angiographic Findings
- Conventional
  - DSA required to confirm diagnosis, classify, define angioarchitecture
  - Type I: Usually solitary arterial feeder (dorsal radiculomedullary artery) shunting into a dilated coronal venous plexus which in turn drains into epidural veins distant to fistula
  - Type II: Supplied by anterior spinal artery (ASA) ± posterolateral spinal artery (PLSA), nidus drains to coronal venous plexus (on cord surface) which in turn drains to epidural veins
    - Compact or diffuse nidus within spinal cord ± feeding artery/intranidal aneurysms
  - Type III: Large complex nidus (may have extramedullary or extraspinal component), multiple feeding vessels ± feeding artery/intranidal aneurysms
    - Additional soft tissue AVMs possible (metameric AVM)
  - Type IV: Direct single hole fistula between ASA and coronal venous plexus (no nidus)
    - Feeding artery aneurysms may be seen
  - Conus medullaris AVM: Multiple feeding arteries, multiple niduses, complex venous drainage
    - Usually extramedullary (pial-based) but may have intramedullary component
  - Epidural AV fistula: High-flow fistula(s) between epidural artery and distended epidural veins
  - Filum terminale AV fistula: ASA supplies fistula along filum, drains into perimedullary veins

Imaging Recommendations
- Best imaging tool
  - MR or spinal cord edema, serpentine flow voids (engorged perimedullary veins)
  - Myelography if MR contraindicated
  - DSA for definitive diagnosis, classification or exclusion of spinal AVM, treatment planning
- Protocol advice
  - DSA: One-frame per second filming rate sufficient during search for spinal AVM
    - May increase frame rate, obtain LAO/RAO/lateral projections once AV shunt is identified

DIFFERENTIAL DIAGNOSIS

Intramedullary Neoplasm
- Ependymoma: Heterogeneous (cysts, blood products)
- Astrocytoma: Multisegmental enhancing mass, no enlarged vessels

Vertebral Body Metastasis
- Hypervascular skeletal metastases from renal cell Ca, thyroid Ca, melanoma
- Pathological tumor blush ± AV shunting within spinal, paraspinal soft tissues

Spinal Hemangioblastomas

- Sporadic or associated with von-Hippel Lindau (often multiple lesions)
- Intramedullary tumor blush supplied by ASA, PLSA

Vertebral Artery Fistula

- Usually seen in penetrating injuries, iatrogenic during surgery
- Single-hole AV fistula between vertebral artery and adjacent veins ± reflux into epidural veins

PATHOLOGY

General Features

- General path comments
  - AVMs account for < 10% of spinal masses
    - Most common = type I (up to 80%)
    - Second most common = type II > III (15-20%)
  - Location
    - Type I: Thoracic
    - Type II (glomus): Cervical/upper thoracic (may occur anywhere)
    - Type III (juvenile): Cervical/upper thoracic (may occur anywhere)
    - Type IV: Conus medullaris (type A, B), thoracic (type C)
- Genetics
  - Can be sporadic or syndromic
  - Type II: Associated with cutaneous angiomas, Klippel-Trenaunay-Weber, Rendu-Osler-Weber syndromes
  - Type III: Associated with Cobb syndrome (metameric vascular malformation involving triad of spinal cord, skin, bone)
  - Type IV: Associated with Rendu-Osler-Weber syndrome

Microscopic Features

- Abnormal vessels with variable wall thickness, internal elastic lamina
- Reactive change in surrounding tissue: Gliosis, cytoid bodies, Rosenthal fibers; hemosiderin deposition ± Ca++

Staging, Grading or Classification Criteria

- Type I: Single (type A) or multiple (type B) radiculomedullary arteries supply the AVF in the subarachnoid space, along the dorsal nerve root sleeve
- Type II: Compact intramedullary nidus lacks normal capillary bed; no parenchyma within nidus; (nidus may have pial extension)
- Type III: Large, complex intramedullary lesion, normal neural parenchyma inside nidus (may involve extramedullary, extradural)
- Type IV: Direct fistula between ASA/PSA & draining vein, no nidus
  - IV-A: Small AVF with slow flow, mild venous enlargement
  - IV-B: Intermediate AVF, dilated feeding arteries; high flow rate
  - IV-C: Large AVF, dilated feeding arteries; dilated, tortuous veins
- Extradural (epidural) AV fistula: High-flow fistula(s) between epidural artery and vein
- Conus medullaris AVM: Usually mixed intra & extramedullary location with multiple glomus-type niduses supplied by spinal and radiculomedullary arteries
- Filum terminale AV fistula: ASA supplies fistula which drains into coronal venous plexus

CLINICAL ISSUES

Presentation

- Most common signs/symptoms
  - Depends on AVM type: Progressive paraparesis, pain, acute neurological deficit
    - Type I: M > F, 6th-7th decade, progressive myelopathy; hemorrhage very rare
    - Type II: M = F, 20-40 y, SAH most common symptom; pain, myelopathy
    - Type III: M = F, < 30 y, progressive neurologic decline (weakness), SAH
    - Type IV: M = F, 10-40 y, progressive conus/cauda equina syndrome, SAH

Natural History & Prognosis

- Good prognosis for type I (DAVF) if diagnosed early and treated before permanent venous ischemia/infarction of cord ensues
- Poor prognosis for juvenile (type III) AVM

Treatment

- Type I: Embolization or surgery are both effective
- Type II: Surgical resection, + pre-op embolization (aneurysms, nidus)
- Type III: Complete resection generally not possible; palliative therapy usually with embolization ± surgery to relieve cord compression
- Type IV: (A) surgical resection, (B) surgical resection or embolization, (C) embolization
- Epidural fistulas: Endovascular embolization

DIAGNOSTIC CHECKLIST

Consider

- Spinal AVM in middle-aged (type IV) and elderly (type I) patients with progressive paraparesis

Image Interpretation Pearls

- T2WI MR showing cord edema + intraspinal flow voids warrants DSA for definitive diagnosis/exclusion of spinal AVM

SELECTED REFERENCES

1. Caragine LP Jr et al: Vascular myelopathies-vascular malformations of the spinal cord: presentation and endovascular surgical management. Semin Neurol. 22(2):123-32, 2002
2. Spetzler RF et al: Modified classification of spinal cord vascular lesions. J Neurosurg. 96(2 Suppl):145-56, 2002

IMAGE GALLERY

Typical

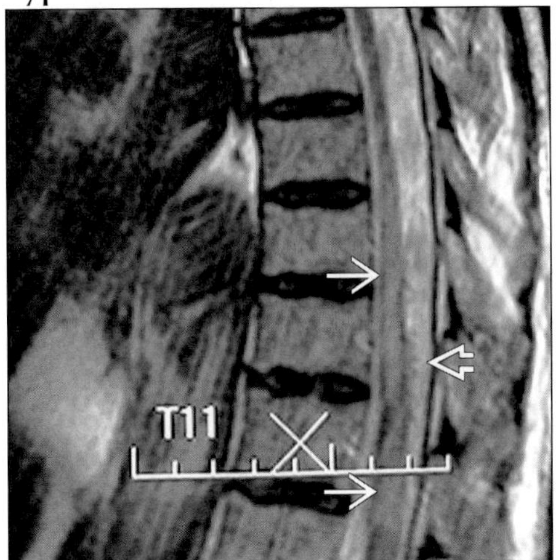

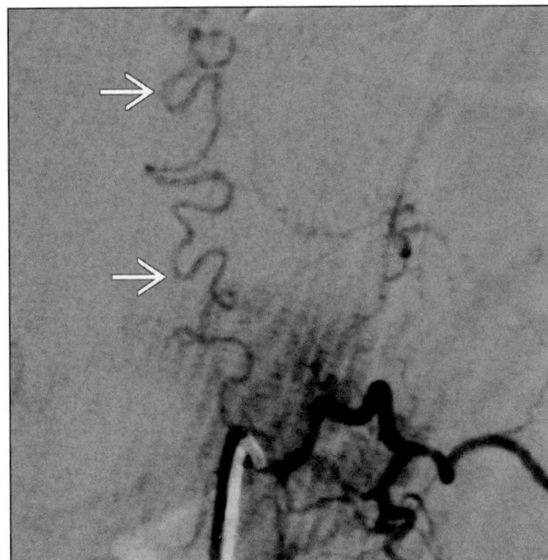

(Left) *Sagittal T2WI MR shows cord edema and expansion of the conus medullaris ➔. There are some flow voids ➔ along the dorsal aspect of the spinal cord suspicious for an underlying vascular malformation.* ***(Right)*** *Injection of the left T8 intercostal artery reveals prompt opacification of the perimedullary (coronal) venous plexus ➔ without an intervening nidus in keeping with a spinal DAVF (type I spinal AVM).*

Typical

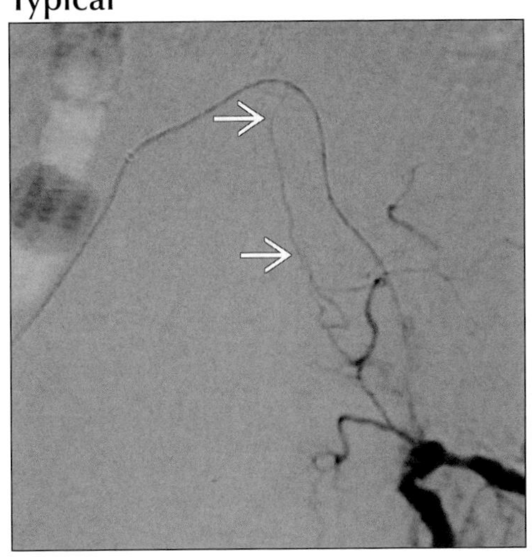

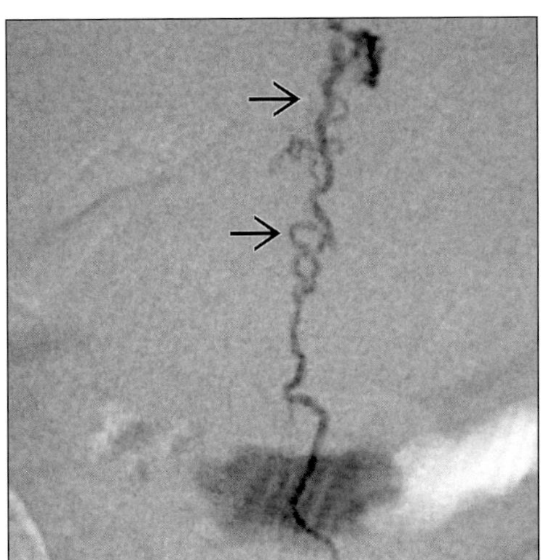

(Left) *Left internal iliac artery DSA reveals an anomalous vessel coursing superiorly ➔ in an elderly patient with progressive paraparesis and spinal cord edema on MR (not shown).* ***(Right)*** *Subselective injection of the lateral sacral artery in the same patient as previous image reveals opacification of a tortuous coronal venous plexus ➔ in keeping with a type I spinal AVM (DAVF).*

Typical

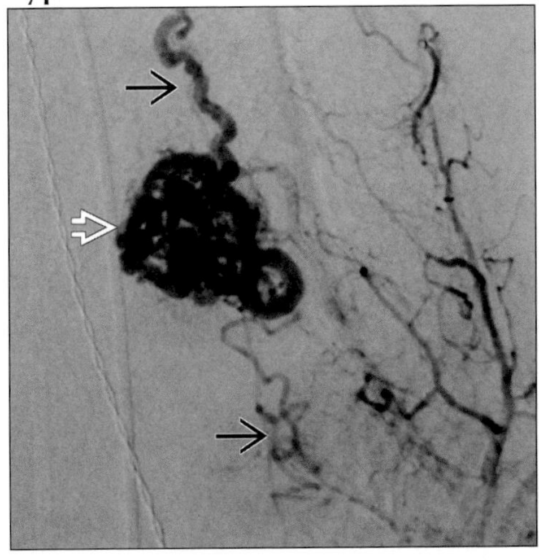

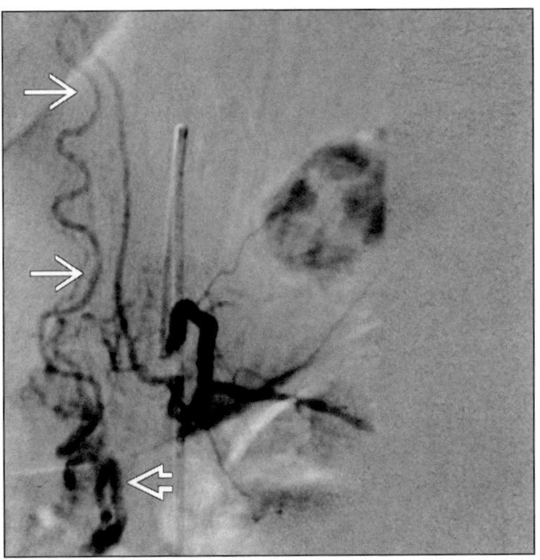

(Left) *Left costocervical artery DSA reveals a compact AVM nidus ➔ within the spinal cord (type II spinal AVM). Note venous drainage into the coronal venous plexus ➔.* ***(Right)*** *Selective injection of the left L1 lumbar artery in a different patient reveals an enlarged, tortuous anterior spinal artery ➔ supplying a perimedullary fistula (type IV spinal AVM) at the level of the conus medullaris. Note enlarged draining vein ➔.*

HEMANGIOBLASTOMA, SPINE

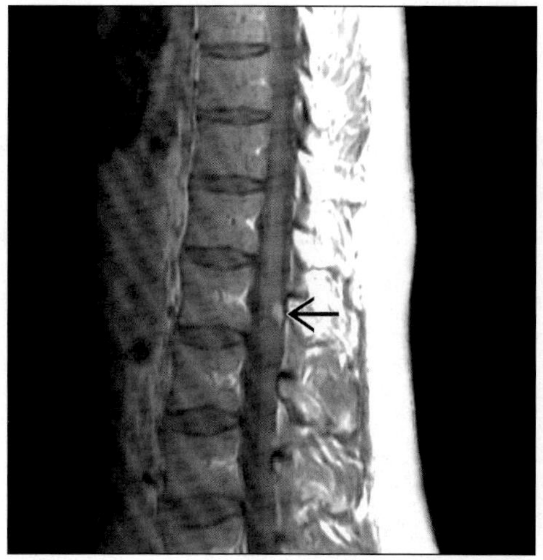

Sagittal T1WI MR with intravenous gadolinium shows an enhancing nodule in the dorsal aspect of the conus medullaris ⇒.

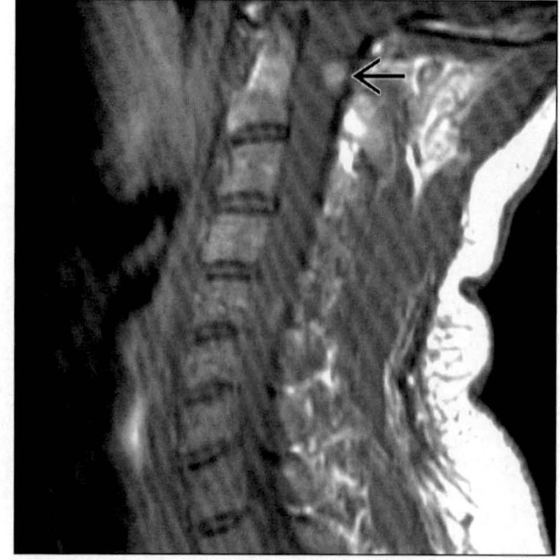

Sagittal T1WI MR with intravenous gadolinium shows an enhancing nodule at the cervicomedullary junction ⇒.

TERMINOLOGY

Abbreviations and Synonyms

- Capillary hemangioblastoma (HB); von Hippel-Lindau syndrome (VHL)

Definitions

- Low grade, capillary rich neoplasms of cerebellum and spinal cord that occur sporadically or in setting of von Hippel-Lindau syndrome

IMAGING FINDINGS

General Features

- Best diagnostic clue
  - Enhancing intramedullary mass ± adjacent cyst
  - Serpentine "flow voids" in larger lesions due to vascularity
  - May be associated with extensive adjacent spinal cord edema
- Location
  - Subpial
  - Posterior aspect of the spinal cord, often associated with intraspinal cyst
  - Rarely anterior aspect of cord
  - Thoracic cord most common followed by cervical cord
- Size
  - Few mm to several cm
  - Multiple tumors (often small) in VHL
- Morphology: Round, well-defined margins

CT Findings

- NECT: Intramedullary mass ± expanded/remodeled spinal canal
- CECT: May demonstrate enhancing nodule
- CTA: May show enlarged feeding vessels, enhancing mass

MR Findings

- T1WI
  - Depends on lesion size, presence of syrinx
  - Small
    - Isointense with cord (may be invisible unless hemorrhage has occurred)
    - Well-delineated syrinx (hypointense) may be present in > 50%

DDx: Spine Hemangioblastoma

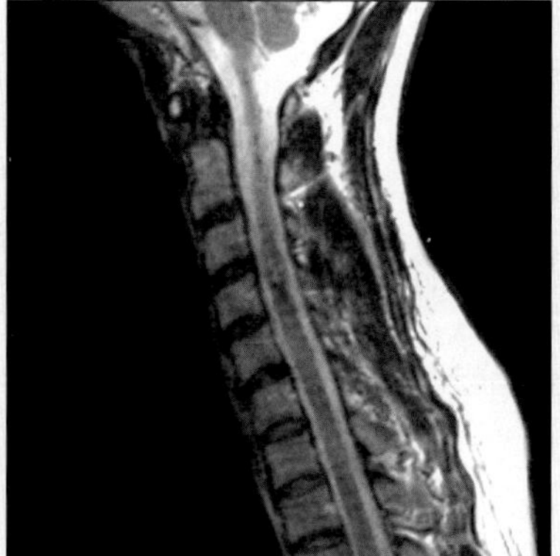

Cavernous Malformation

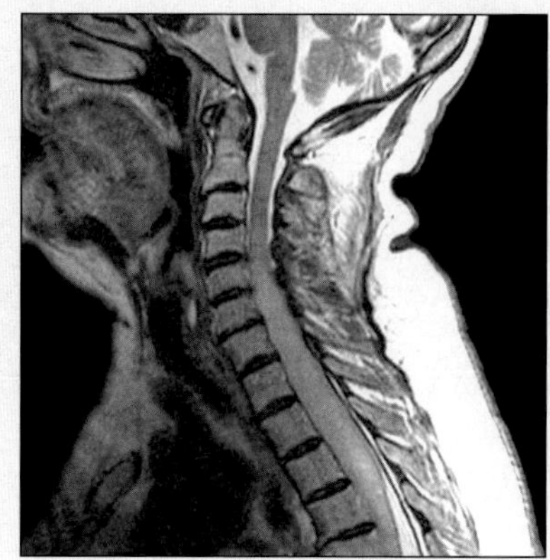

Astrocytoma

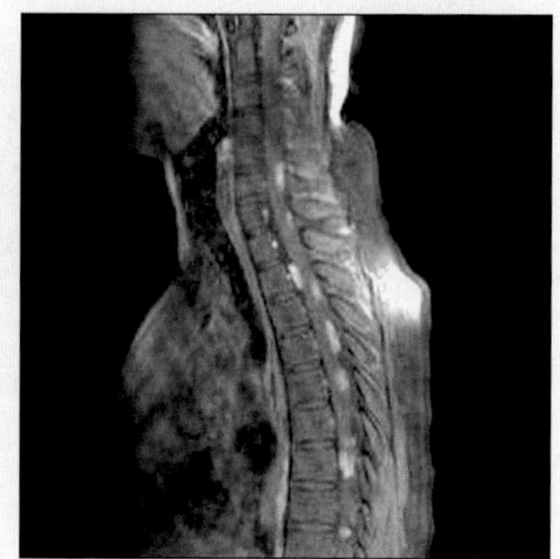

Hypervascular Metastases

Key Facts

Terminology

- Low grade, capillary rich neoplasms of cerebellum and spinal cord that occur sporadically or in setting of von Hippel-Lindau syndrome

Imaging Findings

- Enhancing intramedullary mass ± adjacent cyst
- Posterior aspect of the spinal cord, often associated with intraspinal cyst
- Heterogeneous areas of low signal (flow voids, hemorrhage common)
- May show extensive, long segment cord edema without syrinx
- Subpial nodule (often on surface of dorsal cord)
- Best imaging tool: Contrast-enhanced MR
- Scan brain, entire spine in patients with known/suspected VHL

Top Differential Diagnoses

- Arteriovenous Malformation (AVM)
- Cavernous Malformation
- Hypervascular Cord Neoplasms
- Intradural/Extramedullary Tumors

Pathology

- 1-5% of all spinal cord neoplasms
- 75% of spinal HBs are sporadic (25% VHL-associated)
- Often multiple (VHL usually has one large ± many small HBs)
- HBs are WHO grade I

Clinical Issues

- Clinical Profile: Young adult with family history of VHL
- Does not undergo malignant degeneration

  - Large
    - Mixed hypo/isointense
    - Lesions > 2.5 cm almost always show "flow voids" (enlarged feeding arteries and/or draining veins)
- T2WI
  - Small lesions usually uniformly hyperintense
  - ± Peritumoral edema
  - Cyst fluid may be hypo/hyperintense to CSF depending on concentration of contained proteins
  - Heterogeneous areas of low signal (flow voids, hemorrhage common)
  - May show extensive, long segment cord edema without syrinx
- T1 C+
  - Small
    - Subpial nodule (often on surface of dorsal cord)
    - Well-demarcated, intense, homogeneous enhancement
  - Large
    - Heterogeneous enhancement
    - If syrinx present, wall does not enhance

Other Modality Findings

- Intraoperative sonography may be useful in locating nodule

Angiographic Findings

- Conventional
  - Intense, prolonged vascular stain
  - ± Arteriovenous shunting
  - Enlarged spinal arteries (anterior > posterior) supply mass

Imaging Recommendations

- Best imaging tool: Contrast-enhanced MR
- Protocol advice
  - Scan brain, entire spine in patients with known/suspected VHL
  - DSA for large lesions ± pre-operative embolization to minimize blood loss

DIFFERENTIAL DIAGNOSIS

Arteriovenous Malformation (AVM)

- Cord often normal/small, gliotic
- Syrinx, focal nodule absent

Cavernous Malformation

- Mottled or speckled pattern of prior hemorrhage, hemosiderin rim
- Minimal enhancement

Hypervascular Cord Neoplasms

- Ependymoma (mass centrally located; no syrinx)
- Astrocytoma (usually not hypervascular; peritumoral edema common)
- Vascular metastasis (known primary, e.g., renal cell carcinoma)

Intradural/Extramedullary Tumors

- Meningioma/schwannoma rarely associated syrinx, flow voids uncommon
- Paraganglioma (filum > > cord but may be indistinguishable)

PATHOLOGY

General Features

- General path comments
  - VHL phenotypes
    - Type 1 = without pheochromocytoma
    - Type 2A = pheochromocytoma without renal cell carcinoma
    - Type 2B = pheochromocytoma with renal cell carcinoma
    - Type 2C = pheochromocytoma only
- Genetics
  - Familial HB (VHL)
    - Autosomal dominant
    - Chromosome 3p, other gene mutations common
    - VEGF highly expressed
    - Erythropoietin often upregulated

- Tumors arise after the loss or inactivation of wild type allele in a cell
- 20% of VHL families no deletion or mutation can be detected
  - Sporadic HB (unknown origin)
- Epidemiology
  - 1-5% of all spinal cord neoplasms
  - 75% of spinal HBs are sporadic (25% VHL-associated)
  - Often multiple (VHL usually has one large ± many small HBs)
- Associated abnormalities
  - VHL
    - Cerebellar HBs, retinal angiomas, pheochromocytoma, renal cell carcinoma, angiomatous or cystic lesions of the kidneys, pancreas, and epididymis

Gross Pathologic & Surgical Features

- Well-circumscribed vascular nodule
  - Dorsal surface of cord
  - Extramedullary spinal HBs occur but are rare
- Prominent arteries, veins
- ± Syrinx
- Extensive involvement of leptomeninges is rare: "Leptomeningeal hemangioblastomatosis"

Microscopic Features

- Large vacuolated stromal cells + rich capillary network

Staging, Grading or Classification Criteria

- HBs are WHO grade I

CLINICAL ISSUES

Presentation

- Most common signs/symptoms
  - Nonspecific clinical symptoms
  - Sensory/motor > pain
  - VHL patients usually have one dominant symptomatic lesion; may have other smaller, asymptomatic lesions
    - 95% symptom-producing spinal HBs associated with syringomyelia
  - Other signs/symptoms
    - May cause secondary polycythemia (erythropoietin upregulated)
- Clinical Profile: Young adult with family history of VHL

Demographics

- Age: Mean age at presentation = 30 years
- Gender: M = F

Natural History & Prognosis

- Grows slowly
- Does not undergo malignant degeneration

Treatment

- Microsurgical resection
- Pre-operative embolization of larger lesions with particulate emboli or liquid embolics can significantly reduce intraoperative bleeding

DIAGNOSTIC CHECKLIST

Consider

- Annual physical and ophthalmologic examinations should begin in infancy in patients with family history of VHL
  - Imaging of abdominal organs, CNS (brain and spine) to detect/exclude associated lesions in teenagers and adults

Image Interpretation Pearls

- Typical pattern of intensely enhancing small mass on dorsal pial surface of cord
- Large lesions have vessel flow voids

SELECTED REFERENCES

1. Kato M et al: Hemangioblastomatosis of the central nervous system without von Hippel-Lindau disease: a case report. J Neurooncol. 72(3):267-70, 2005
2. Lee DK et al: Spinal cord hemangioblastoma: surgical strategy and clinical outcome. J Neurooncol. 61(1):27-34, 2003
3. Pluta RM et al: Comparison of anterior and posterior surgical approaches in the treatment of ventral spinal hemangioblastomas in patients with von Hippel-Lindau disease. J Neurosurg. 98(1):117-24, 2003
4. Wanebo JE et al: The natural history of hemangioblastomas of the central nervous system in patients with von Hippel-Lindau disease. J Neurosurg. 98(1):82-94, 2003
5. Torreggiani WC et al: Von Hippel-Lindau disease: a radiological essay. Clin Radiol. 57(8):670-80, 2002
6. Chu BC et al: MR findings in spinal hemangioblastoma: correlation with symptoms and with angiographic and surgical findings. AJNR Am J Neuroradiol. 22(1):206-17, 2001
7. Conway JE et al: Hemangioblastomas of the central nervous system in von Hippel-Lindau syndrome and sporadic disease. Neurosurgery. 48(1):55-62; discussion 62-3, 2001
8. Hamazaki S et al: Metastasis of renal cell carcinoma to central nervous system hemangioblastoma in two patients with von Hippel-Lindau disease. Pathol Int. 51(12):948-53, 2001
9. Baker KB et al: MR imaging of spinal hemangioblastoma. AJR Am J Roentgenol. 174(2):377-82, 2000
10. Couch V et al: von Hippel-Lindau disease. Mayo Clin Proc. 75(3):265-72, 2000
11. Miller DJ et al: Hemangioblastomas and other uncommon intramedullary tumors. J Neurooncol. 47(3):253-70, 2000
12. Friedrich CA: Von Hippel-Lindau syndrome. A pleomorphic condition. Cancer. 86(11 Suppl):2478-82, 1999
13. Irie K et al: Spinal cord hemangioblastoma presenting with subarachnoid hemorrhage. Neurol Med Chir (Tokyo). 38(6):355-8, 1998
14. Bakshi R et al: Spinal leptomeningeal hemangioblastomatosis in von Hippel-Lindau disease: magnetic resonance and pathological findings. J Neuroimaging. 7(4):242-4, 1997
15. Eskridge JM et al: Preoperative endovascular embolization of craniospinal hemangioblastomas. AJNR Am J Neuroradiol. 17(3):525-31, 1996
16. Spetzger U et al: Hemangioblastomas of the spinal cord and the brainstem: diagnostic and therapeutic features. Neurosurg Rev. 19(3):147-51, 1996

IMAGE GALLERY

Typical

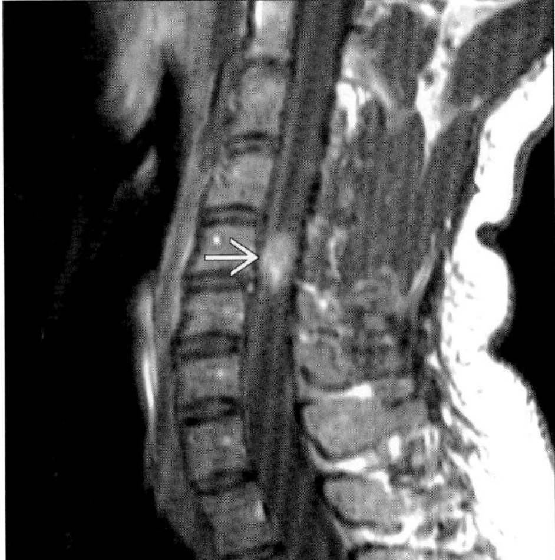

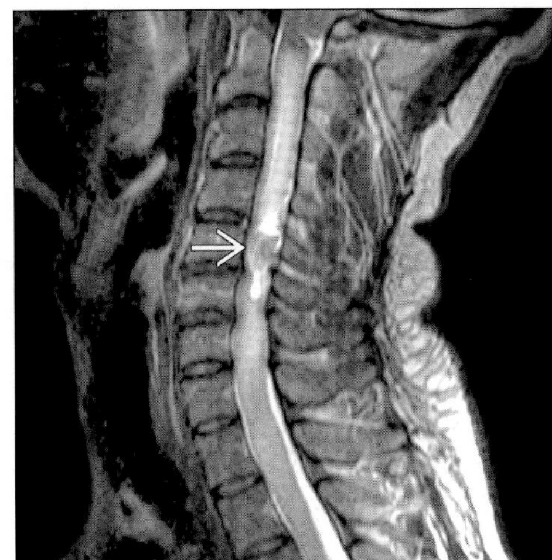

*(**Left**) Sagittal T1WI MR with intravenous gadolinium shows an enhancing mass ➔ in the mid cervical spinal cord. (**Right**) Sagittal T2WI MR in the same patient shows spinal cord enlargement due to a heterogeneous cystic lesion ➔ at C5 and associated extensive edema throughout the cervical spinal cord.*

Typical

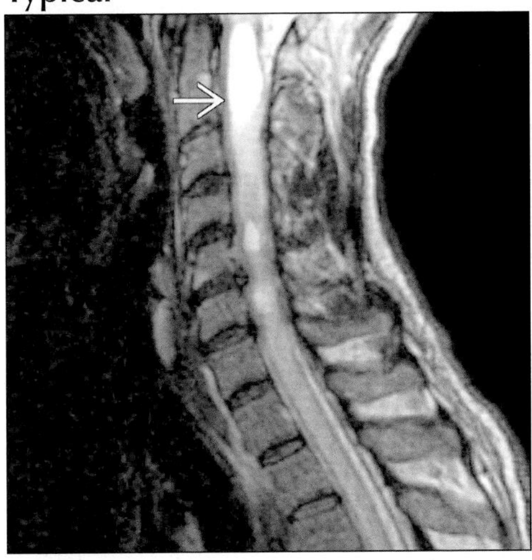

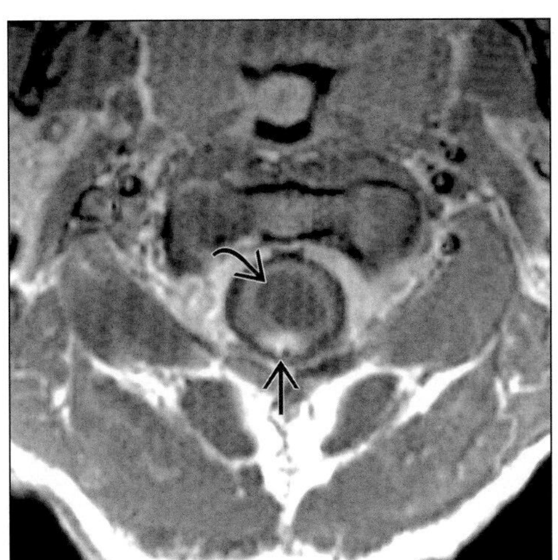

*(**Left**) Sagittal T2WI MR shows a large cystic mass ➔ in the upper cervical spinal cord associated with 2 smaller cystic areas in the mid cervical spinal cord and extensive cord edema. (**Right**) Axial T1WI MR with intravenous gadolinium shows cord expansion by a mass comprised of a dorsally situated, subpial enhancing nodule → and an adjacent intramedullary cyst ↷.*

Typical

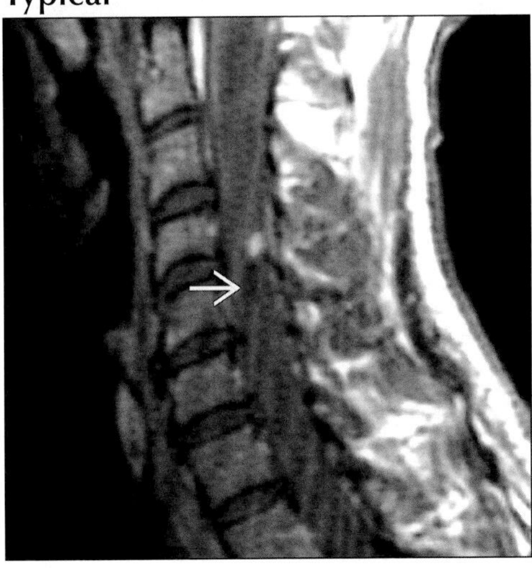

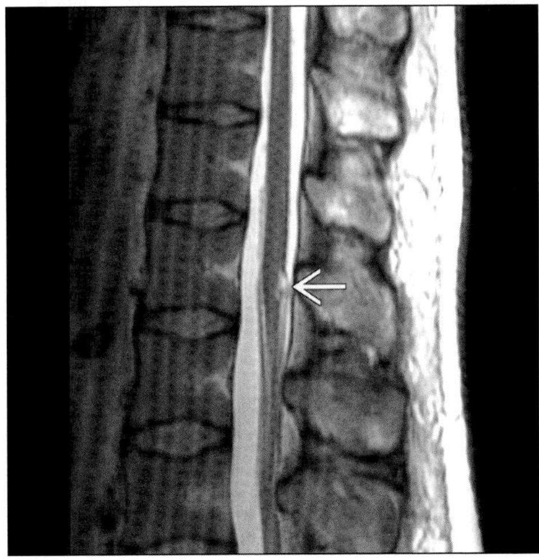

*(**Left**) Sagittal T1WI MR with intravenous gadolinium shows an enhancing nodule in the mid cervical spinal cord associated with a small low signal intensity cyst ➔. (**Right**) Sagittal T2WI MR shows a small hyperintense nodule ➔ on the dorsal subpial surface of the conus medullaris. In patients with known or suspected spinal HB on imaging, additional imaging of the brain, orbits and abdomen should be considered as 25% of patients with spinal HBs will have VHL.*

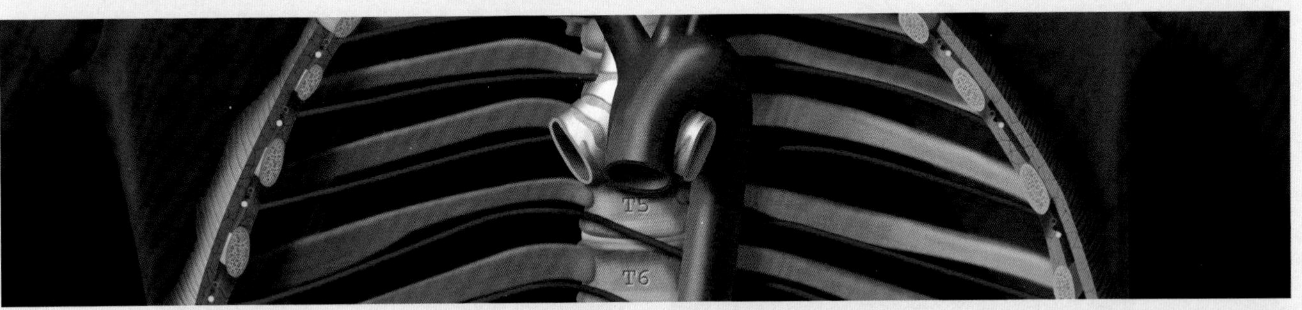

SECTION 4: Thorax

Introduction and Overview

Thorax

THORACIC AORTA AND GREAT VESSELS

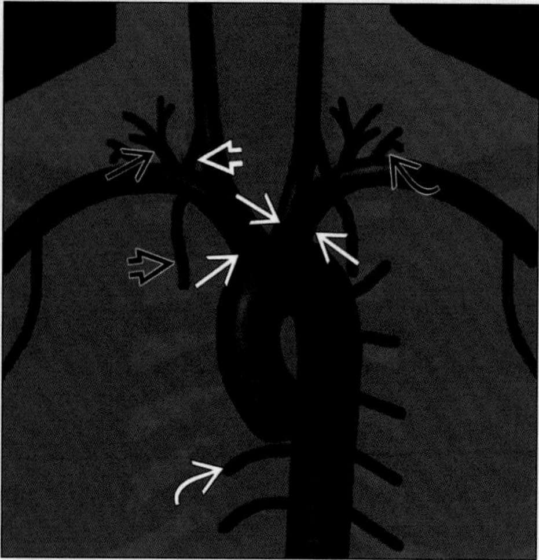

Graphic shows the great vessel origins ➡ from the aortic arch. The internal mammary ➡, thyrocervical ➡, costocervical ➡, and vertebral ➡ arteries are also noted. Descending aorta yields intercostal arteries ➡.

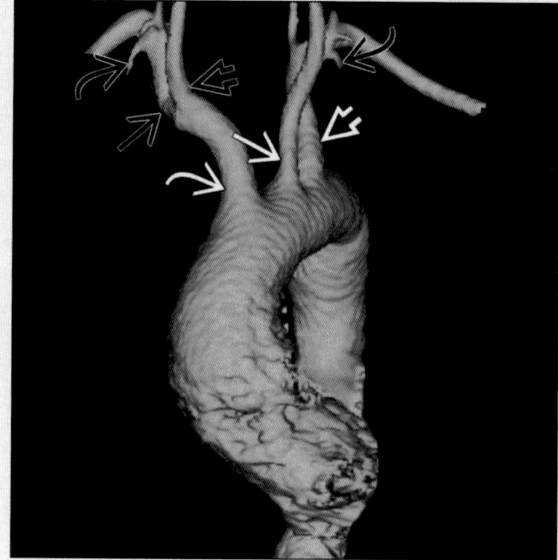

CTA shows normal origins of the innominate ➡, left CCA ➡, and left SCA ➡ from the aortic arch. The innominate artery divides into the right CCA ➡ and SCA ➡. The internal mammary arteries ➡ are visible.

TERMINOLOGY

Abbreviations

- Common carotid artery (CCA)
- Internal carotid artery (ICA)
- External carotid artery (ECA)
- Subclavian artery (SCA)
- Vertebral artery (VA)

IMAGING ANATOMY

General Anatomic Considerations

- Normal anatomy defined by left aortic arch
  - Innominate (brachiocephalic) artery arises as 1st of great vessels; divides into right CCA and SCA
    - Right SCA yields internal mammary,VA, thyrocervical, costocervical, long thoracic arteries; continues as axillary artery
    - Right CCA divides into ICA and ECA
  - Left CCA 2nd great vessel from arch
    - Divides into ICA and ECA
  - Left SCA 3rd great vessel from arch
    - Gives off internal mammary, VA, thyrocervical, costocervical, long thoracic arteries; continues as axillary artery
  - Rarely thyroid ima artery arises from aortic arch
    - Inconstant supply to thyroid isthmus
    - More commonly arises from innominate (3%) or right CCA (1%)
- Descending aorta gives off important small arteries
  - Bronchial arteries
  - Intercostal arteries
    - Supreme intercostals supply T1-T3; arise from costocervical trunk of SCAs
    - Paired intercostals from T4-T12
  - Thoracic spinal cord arterial supply comes from upper and lower descending aorta
    - Anterior spinal artery; supplied from intercostal and bronchial arteries at T4-5
    - Artery of Adamkiewicz arises from intercostal arteries at T6-T12 (75%)

Anatomic Relationships

- May have anatomic variations to aortic arch
  - Right aortic arch (< 0.1%); two types
    - Mirror image branching (65%); associated with cyanotic congenital heart disease (CHD) in 90%
    - Aberrant left SCA/other great vessel aberrant origin (35%); not associated with cyanotic CHD
    - Dilated origin of aberrant left SCA in 60%: Kommerell diverticulum; if also ligamentum arteriosum, vascular ring compresses trachea
  - Double (duplicated) aortic arch (< 0.1%)
    - Congenital anomaly resulting from persistence of left and right embryologic branchial arches
    - Accounts for > 40% thoracic vascular rings
    - Encircles and compresses trachea and esophagus
  - Cervical arch (< 0.1%)
    - Arises from 3rd rather than 4th branchial arch
    - High location in chest, near lung apex
    - May have anomalous great vessel origins
  - Coarctation (< 0.1%)
    - Congenital narrowing of aortic arch, usually distal to left subclavian
    - May be preductal (infantile), juxtaductal and postductal (adult)
- May have anatomic variants of great vessel origins
  - Left CCA may arise from innominate artery, rather than from aortic arch (bovine arch, incidence 20%)
  - Left VA may arise from aortic arch (5%)
    - Between left CCA and left SCA
  - Right SCA may arise separately from aortic arch, distal to left SCA (aberrant right SCA)
    - Aberrant right SCA often associated with Kommerell diverticulum

PATHOLOGIC ISSUES

General Pathologic Considerations

- Thoracic aortic aneurysms
  - Ascending aortic aneurysms
    - Atherosclerosis most common etiology in older patients; usually normal diameter aortic valve

Upper Extremity/Neck/Central Venous Anatomy

Jugular Veins
- Internal jugular veins drain head and neck; joined by external jugular veins draining face and scalp

Subclavian Veins
- Originate at axillary vein transition at 1st rib margin; typically valveless; joined by cephalic vein

Brachiocephalic Veins
- Formed by junction of subclavian and internal jugular veins; right short, vertical; left longer, crosses mediastinum anterior to great vessels
- Tributaries: Internal mammary, vertebral, pericardiophrenic, 1st intercostal, inferior thyroidal

Superior Vena Cava (SVC)
- Formed by right and left brachiocephalic veins
- 6-8 cm long, up to 2 cm diameter; azygos vein joins above pericardium; SVC enters right atrium

        - Post-stenotic dilatation from valvular stenosis
        - Marfan syndrome (dilated aortic valve, sinuses and ascending aorta)
        - Osteogenesis imperfecta, Ehlers-Danlos syndrome, rheumatoid arthritis, ankylosing spondylitis
        - Takayasu, giant cell arteritis
        - Syphilitic aortitis: Now uncommon, spares sinotubular junction, saccular aneurysm with extensive ascending calcification
        - Infection (acute or chronic; CABG/valve surgery)
    - Aortic arch
        - Atherosclerosis: Usually associated with ascending or descending aortic aneurysm
        - Arteritis (giant cell, Takayasu, Behçet disease) usually younger patients
        - Syphilis: 1/3 occur in aortic arch
    - Descending aorta
        - Atherosclerosis
        - Arteritis (giant cell, Takayasu, Behçet disease)
        - Trauma: Chronic pseudoaneurysm 2° to contained transection; deceleration, blunt, penetrating
        - Coarctation
        - Infection
        - Ductus diverticulum: Smooth bulge at site of obliterated ductus arteriosus; may become aneurysmal (> 3 cm)
        - Penetrating ulcer: Focal crater-like outpouching of lumen penetrates media; acute aortic syndrome
- Dissection
    - Aortic dissection classified by entry tear location, false lumen extent (Stanford/DeBakey classifications)
        - Surgical repair when ascending aorta involved; medical management or elective surgical or endovascular repair for descending involvement
    - Spontaneous dissection of CCA, ICA or VAs
- Atherosclerotic occlusive disease
    - Virtually non-existent in thoracic aorta; vasculitis most common cause of stenoses
    - Most common pathology in carotid/VA/SCA
    - SCA stenosis/occlusion may cause "subclavian steal"
- Fibromuscular dysplasia
    - ICA 2nd most involved artery
    - SCA, axillary and brachial arteries 5th
- Vasculitis
    - Takayasu arteritis may have long segment stenoses that involve proximal great vessels; rarely aneurysms, dissection
- Congenital
    - As delineated in anatomic variants section above

RELATED REFERENCES

1. Davies M et al: Developmental abnormalities of the great vessels of the thorax and their embryological basis. Br J Radiol. 76(907):491-502, 2003
2. Gil-Jaurena JM et al: Aortic coarctation, vascular ring, and right aortic arch with aberrant subclavian artery. Ann Thorac Surg. 73(5):1640-2, 2002

IMAGE GALLERY

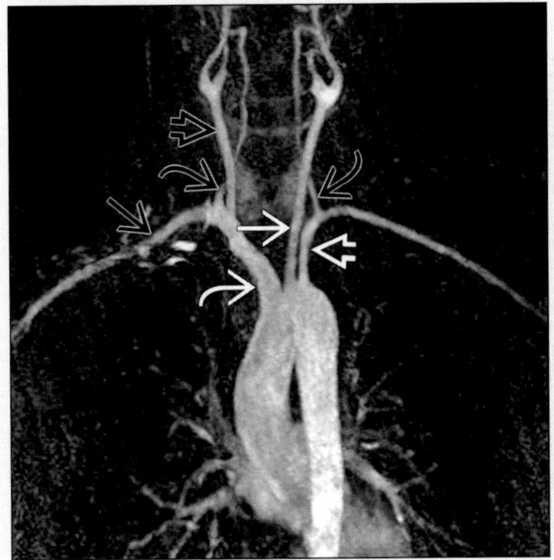

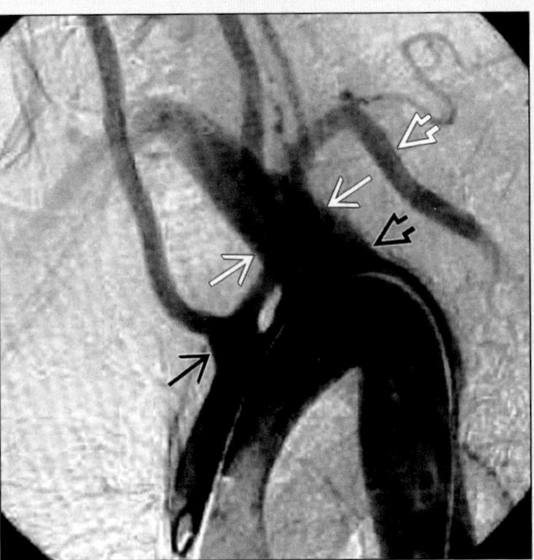

*(**Left**) Coronal TR MRA shows normal innominate ➔, left CCA ➔ and left SCA ➔ origins from the aortic arch. The innominate artery division into the right CCA ➔ and SCA ➔ and the origins of both vertebral arteries ➔ are well seen. (**Right**) DSA shows variant great vessel origins from the aortic arch. The left and right CCAs have a common origin ➔ (a variant of bovine arch, in which the left CCA arises from the innominate artery), and there is an aberrant right SCA origin ➔ distal to the left SCA ➔. The dilatation ➔ of the aberrant right SCA is a Kommerell diverticulum.*

THORACIC AORTIC ANEURYSM

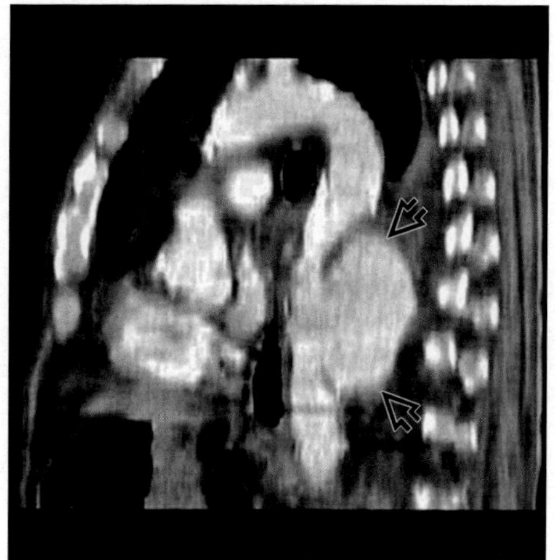

Sagittal CECT shows a large saccular aneurysm ⇨ in the descending aorta, extending posteriorly. Calcifications are present in the aorta, and this most likely represents an atherosclerotic aneurysm.

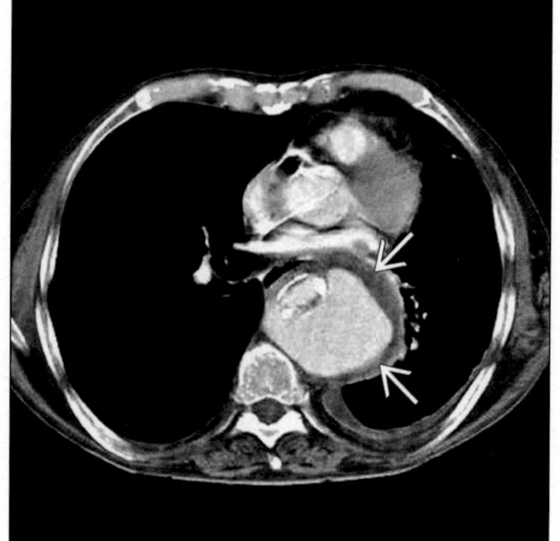

Axial CECT shows aneurysm extending from the aorta, with a thrombus ➡ in the periphery. Etiology is most likely atherosclerosis, but infection or aortic ulcer with contained rupture are also possible.

TERMINOLOGY

Abbreviations and Synonyms

- Thoracic aortic aneurysm (TAA)

Definitions

- Localized or diffuse dilation of aorta, diameter 50% > normal artery
- In thoracic aorta, diameter > 3.5 cm is dilated, diameter > 4.5 cm is aneurysmal

IMAGING FINDINGS

General Features

- Best diagnostic clue: Mediastinal mass with curvilinear rim calcification
- Location: 60% aortic root/ascending aorta; 10% aortic arch; 10% are thoracoabdominal; more than one region may be involved
- Size: > 6 cm at significant risk for rupture
- Morphology
  - Saccular (20%)
    - Eccentric focal dilatation of the aorta
  - Fusiform (80%)
    - Circumferential long segment spindle-shape dilatation of the aorta, eccentric thrombus

Radiographic Findings

- Radiography
  - Mass with curvilinear calcification
  - Left pleural effusion suggests rupture
  - Calcification of ascending aorta
  - Elevated hemidiaphragm suggests phrenic nerve compression
  - Ascending aorta aneurysm
    - Convex right paramediastinal anterior mass
    - Lateral films: Loss of the retrosternal air space
  - Aortic arch aneurysm
    - Enlarged or obscuration aortic arch
    - Mass in aortopulmonary window
    - Rightward tracheal deviation
  - Descending aorta aneurysm
    - Left paramediastinal or posterior mediastinal mass

CT Findings

- NECT

DDx: Thoracic Aortic Aneurysm

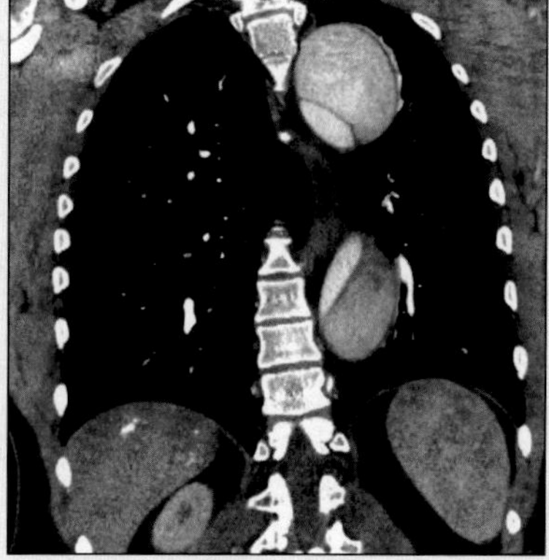

Aortic Dissection

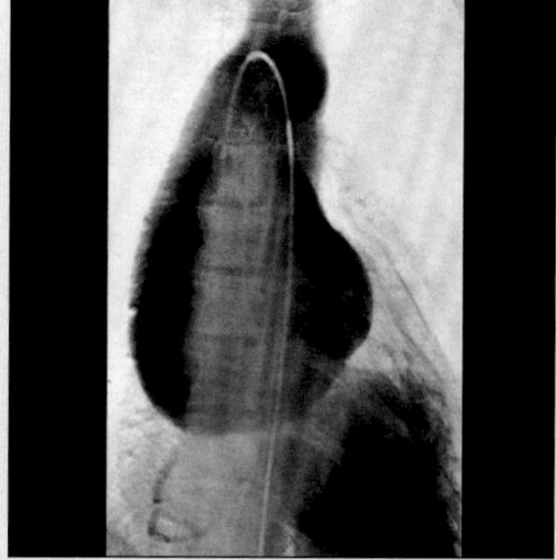

Marfan Syndrome

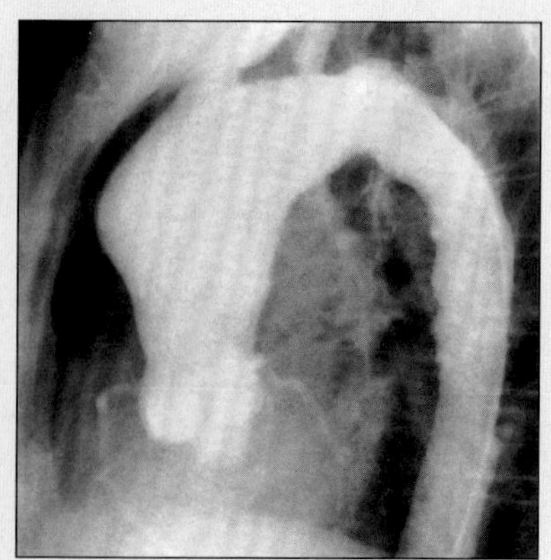

Syphilitic Aneurysm

THORACIC AORTIC ANEURYSM

Key Facts

Terminology
- Localized or diffuse dilation of aorta with a diameter at least 50% greater than the normal artery size
- 25% of patients with TAA also have an abdominal aortic aneurysm

Imaging Findings
- Size: > 6 cm significant risk for rupture
- Crescent sign: Peripheral high mural attenuation indicating early or impending rupture due to acute intramural hematoma

Top Differential Diagnoses
- Tortuosity (Aging) of the Aorta
- Post-Stenotic Dilatation from Aortic Valve Stenosis
- Patent Ductus Arteriosus
- Achalasia

Pathology
- True aneurysm: All layers of aortic wall involved
- Greatest hydraulic stress right lateral wall ascending aorta or descending aorta in proximity of ligamentum arteriosum
- Marfan: Ascending aortic aneurysm, involves the aortic root (annuloaortic ectasia), aortic valve insufficiency common when aortic root diameter exceed 5 cm
- Prevalence 3-4% in those older than 65 years
- Most cases are sporadic, may be genetic component, 19% of patients have family history of thoracic aortic aneurysm, present at a younger age

Diagnostic Checklist
- Any mediastinal mass should be considered as a vascular aneurysm until proven otherwise

    - Crescent sign: Peripheral high mural attenuation (acute intramural hematoma) indicates early or impending rupture
    - Calcification in aneurysm wall (75%)
    - Displacement of other mediastinal structures
    - Rupture - stranding around aorta, hematoma, or hemothorax
- CECT
    - Shows location, extent, relationship to major branch vessels and surrounding structures
    - Size, dissection, mural thrombus, intramural hematoma, free rupture, and contained rupture
- CTA: Delineates aortic lumen, defines extent of aneurysm, branch vessel involvement

MR Findings
- As on CECT
- Evaluate for aortic valvular regurgitation
- Sensitive for peri-aortic hematoma
- Useful for serial surveillance

Angiographic Findings
- DSA
    - Largely replaced by CT or MR
    - Primarily used prior to thoracic stent-grafting

Imaging Recommendations
- Best imaging tool
    - Multi-detector CT with volume rendering
        - Determines location, extent, and size of aneurysm, relationship to major branch vessels
        - Detects complications of dissection, mural thrombus, intramural hematoma, free rupture
- Protocol advice: Preliminary nonenhanced studies to evaluate for calcium in aortic wall, or valve leaflets

DIFFERENTIAL DIAGNOSIS

Tortuosity (Aging) of the Aorta
- No displacement intimal calcification, not dilated

Aortic Dissection
- May progress to aneurysmal dilation

Post-Stenotic Dilatation from Aortic Valve Stenosis/Bicuspid Valve
- Involves ascending aorta; aortic valve may be calcified

Patent Ductus Arteriosus
- Shunt vascularity or pulmonary artery hypertension
- Enlarged aortic arch and obliteration aorto-pulmonary window

Achalasia
- Air-fluid level upper mediastinum

PATHOLOGY

General Features
- General path comments
    - True aneurysm: All layers of aortic wall involved
    - False aneurysm: Disruption of intima and part of media with dilation of adventitia and/or media
    - Fusiform aneurysm: More diffuse aortic involvement
    - Saccular aneurysm: Discrete, localized region of aorta
- Genetics
    - Familial, 15% of first degree relatives
    - Inherited connective tissue disorders
- Etiology
    - Atherosclerosis (75%), trauma, infection, cystic medial necrosis, bicuspid aortic valve, hypertension, smoking
    - Trauma: 5% of transections present as late pseudoaneurysms
    - Infectious (mycotic)
        - Bacterial: Staphylococcus, Salmonella, Enterococcus, E. Coli, Aspergillus, etc.
    - Connective tissue disorder
        - Marfan: Ascending aortic aneurysm; involves aortic root, aortic valve
        - Ehlers-Danlos syndrome
    - Inflammatory aortitis/arteritis: Takayasu, giant cell
    - Ascending thoracic aneurysm
        - Family history of TAA without Marfan syndrome

  - Atherosclerosis (rare)
  - Infection - syphilis (rare), however with reemergence of syphilis, the late complications maybe seen more frequently
- Aortic arch thoracic aneurysm
  - Takayasu arteritis
  - Atherosclerosis
- Descending thoracic aortic aneurysm
  - Atherosclerosis, hypertension, smoking, hyperlipidemia, diabetes

- Epidemiology
  - Prevalence 3-4% in those older than 65 years
  - Most are sporadic; younger patients may be genetic

Gross Pathologic & Surgical Features

- Aging causes changes in collagen and elastin, leading to weakening of aortic wall and aneurysmal dilation
- Ascending aortic aneurysms
  - Cystic medial necrosis
- Aortic arch aneurysms
  - Involvement of innominate artery, left carotid, and left subclavian origins
- Descending thoracic aneurysms
  - May extend into abdomen
  - May compress or erode into surrounding structures: Trachea, bronchus, esophagus, vertebral body

Microscopic Features

- Elastic fiber fragmentation, loss of elastic fibers/smooth muscle cells, cystic medial necrosis, intraluminal thrombus, atherosclerotic plaque
- Common organisms in mycotic aneurysms: Staphylococcus aureus, Salmonella and Streptococcus

Staging, Grading or Classification Criteria

- Type (true or false), location, morphology, etiology
- Crawford classification for thoracoabdominal

CLINICAL ISSUES

Presentation

- Most common signs/symptoms
  - Asymptomatic and incidentally discovered
  - Most common complication is acute rupture
  - Most common presenting symptom: Pain
    - Acute: Impending rupture or dissection
    - Chronic: From compression of other structures
  - Ascending aorta ruptures into pericardium, resulting in acute tamponade
    - May erode into the sternum, compression of SVC, pulmonary arteries
  - Arch aneurysms: Hoarseness from stretching of recurrent laryngeal nerves
  - Descending thoracic aortic rupture may cause left hemothorax
- Other signs/symptoms
  - Peripheral embolization
    - Stroke or TIAs, bowel or extremity ischemia
  - Inflammatory or infectious aneurysms present with signs and symptoms of systemic disease
  - Aortic root dilatation gives symptoms of congestive heart failure from aortic insufficiency
  - 25% will also have an abdominal aortic aneurysm

Demographics

- Age
  - Increased prevalence in each decade of life
  - Mean patient age at diagnosis is 65 years
- Gender: Men affected 2-4 times more than women
- Ethnicity: TAA most common among whites

Natural History & Prognosis

- Symptomatic patients should undergo aneurysm resection regardless of size
- Growth rate ≥ 1 cm/y indicates surgical repair
- Rupture at 5 years: 0% if diameter < 4 cm, 16% if diameter 4-5.9 cm, 31% for aneurysms > 6 cm
- Patients at higher surgical risk: Elderly, end-stage renal disease, respiratory insufficiency, cirrhosis
- 5 year survival of untreated TAA 20%
- Survival < 20% if rupture occurs outside hospital

Treatment

- Risk reduction
  - Control hypertension
- Indications for surgery
  - Based on size, growth rate, or symptoms
  - Ascending aneurysms > 5.5 cm
  - Descending aneurysms > 6.5 cm
  - Surgery at smaller size if familial or Marfan
- Surgical repair
  - Mortality rates: Ascending aneurysms 5-10%, aortic arch 25%, descending aorta 5-15%
  - Complications
    - Stroke risk ascending aorta or arch repair
    - Spinal cord injury from descending aorta repair
- Thoracic stent-grafts
  - Descending aortic aneurysms
  - Can cross the left subclavian with stent grafts
  - GORE TAG is an FDA-approved stent graft for descending thoracic aneurysm repair
- Yearly serial CT or MR evaluation of aorta for recurrent aneurysms

DIAGNOSTIC CHECKLIST

Consider

- Infectious, inflammatory, cystic medial degeneration

Image Interpretation Pearls

- Any mediastinal mass should be considered as vascular aneurysm until proven otherwise

SELECTED REFERENCES

1. Milner R et al: Future of endograft surveillance. Semin Vasc Surg. 19(2):75-82, 2006
2. Bhalla S et al: CT of nontraumatic thoracic aortic emergencies. Semin Ultrasound CT MR. 26(5):281-304, 2005
3. Isselbacher EM: Thoracic and abdominal aortic aneurysms. Circulation. 111(6):816-28, 2005
4. Manghat NE et al: Multi-detector row computed tomography: imaging in acute aortic syndrome. Clin Radiol. 60(12):1256-67, 2005
5. Malouf JF et al: Mycotic aneurysms of the thoracic aorta: a diagnostic challenge. Am J Med. 115(6):489-96, 2003

THORACIC AORTIC ANEURYSM

IMAGE GALLERY

Variant

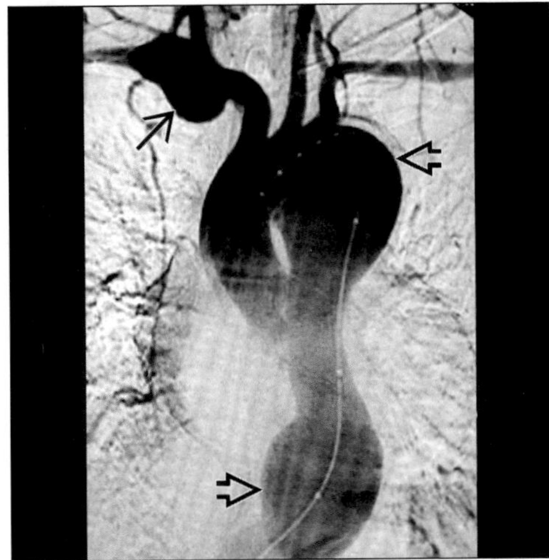

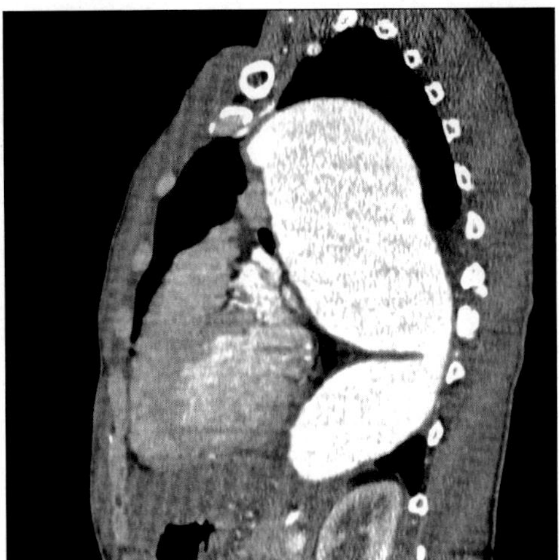

*(**Left**) DSA shows a very unusual aorta with multiple areas of dilatation in the descending aorta ⇨ and in the right subclavian artery →. The aorta and vessels do not show evidence of atherosclerotic disease. Marfan or Ehlers-Danlos could be considered. This patient had Takayasu aortitis. (Courtesy B. Katzen, MD). (**Right**) Sagittal CECT shows a very large descending aortic aneurysm. Again, no evidence of atherosclerotic disease. This patient had Marfan syndrome.*

Typical

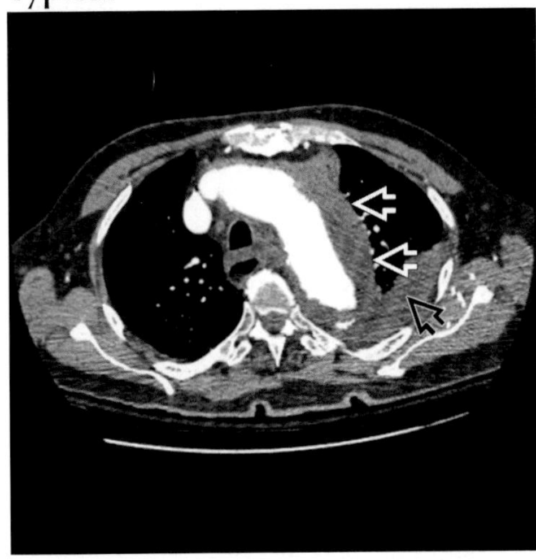

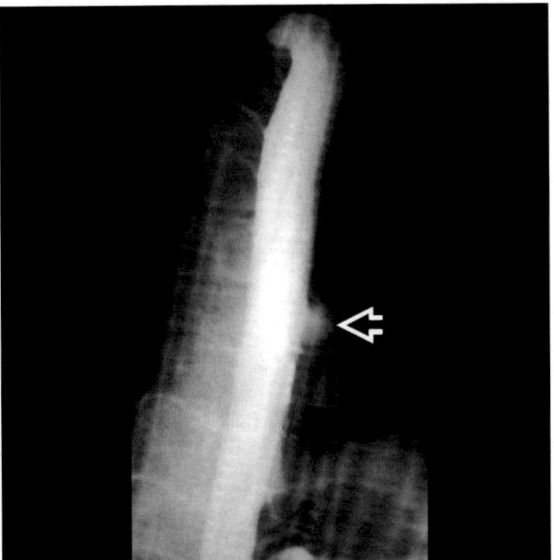

*(**Left**) Axial CECT shows an enlarged aortic arch with large amount of thrombus ➡. Represents a thoracic aortic aneurysm with a previous leak/bleed. Fluid seen in the pleural space ⇨. No high density material was identified in the fluid to suggest acute bleeding. (**Right**) Coronal catheter angiography shows a saccular outpouching in the distal thoracic aorta ➡. The rest of the aorta is smooth, no evidence of atherosclerotic disease. This is a mycotic aneurysm.*

Variant

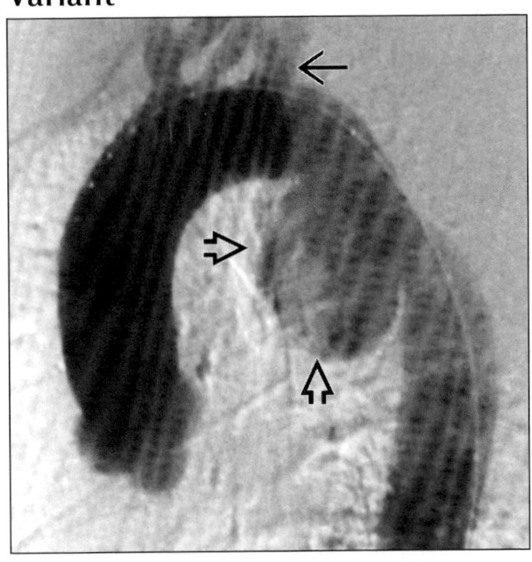

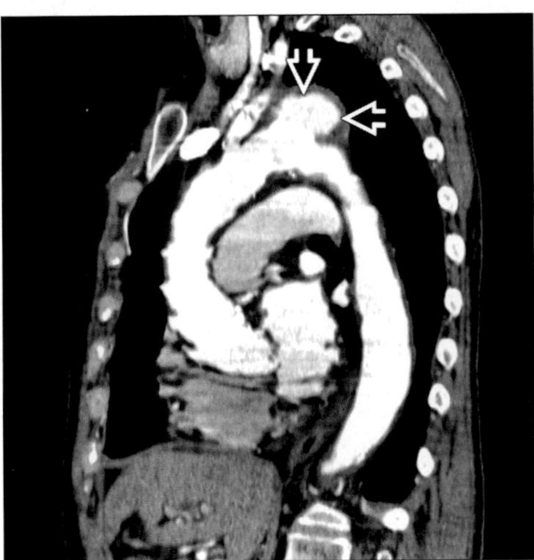

*(**Left**) DSA shows a saccular aneurysm ⇨ in the thoracic aorta just distal to the left subclavian artery →. This is a typical appearance of a late pseudoaneurysm of the aorta following trauma. Approximately 5% of aortic transections present as late pseudoaneurysms. (**Right**) Sagittal CECT shows an unusual appearance of a post-traumatic pseudoaneurysm ➡. Rather than extending below the aorta as in the prior image, the pseudoaneurysm extends above the aortic arch.*

MYCOTIC ANEURYSM

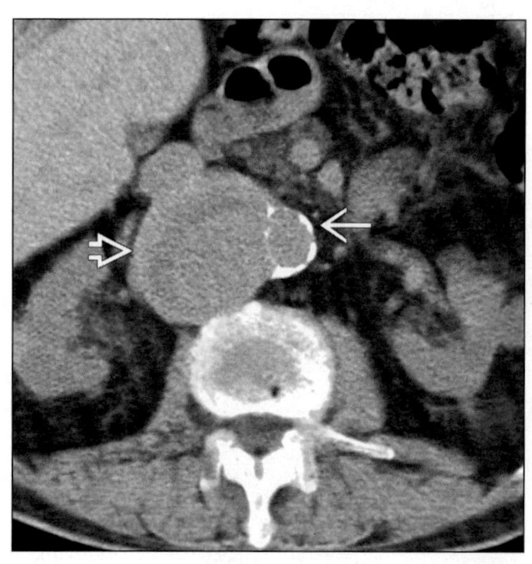

Axial NECT shows a saccular outpouching ➡ from the abdominal aorta ➡. This eccentric saccular appearance is typical of a mycotic aneurysm.

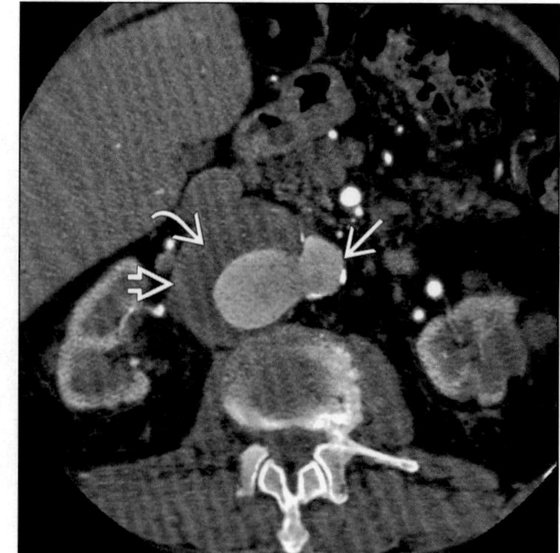

Axial CECT shows the saccular aneurysm ➡ with mural thrombus ➡, arising from the abdominal aorta ➡. Mycotic aneurysms typically involve a diseased segment of the arterial wall.

TERMINOLOGY

Abbreviations and Synonyms

- Infectious aneurysm (more appropriate term)

Definitions

- Aneurysm arising from infection of arterial wall, usually bacterial

IMAGING FINDINGS

General Features

- Best diagnostic clue: Rapidly growing saccular aneurysm arising eccentrically from aortic wall
- Location
    - Anywhere in aorta or other vessels
        - Tends to occur at major branchings of aorta
        - Thoracoabdominal aorta
        - Thoracic aorta
- Morphology
    - Usually saccular with focal involvement of the artery
    - Periaortic inflammation, abscess, mass
    - Periaortic gas
    - Adjacent vertebral body abnormalities due to spread of infection

Radiographic Findings

- Radiography: May identify increased size of aorta

CT Findings

- NECT
    - Bacterial aortitis is rarely calcified
    - Syphilitic aortitis shows curvilinear calcifications
    - Periaortic soft tissue stranding, edema and fluid are frequently present
    - Periaortic gas
    - Adjacent vertebral body abnormalities due to spread of infection
- CECT
    - One or more saccular aneurysms arising from aortic wall, usually focal involvement
    - Lobular contours of the aneurysm
    - Enhancement of periaortic soft tissue
    - Rim-enhancement in case of abscess

MR Findings

- T1WI

DDx: Mycotic Aneurysm

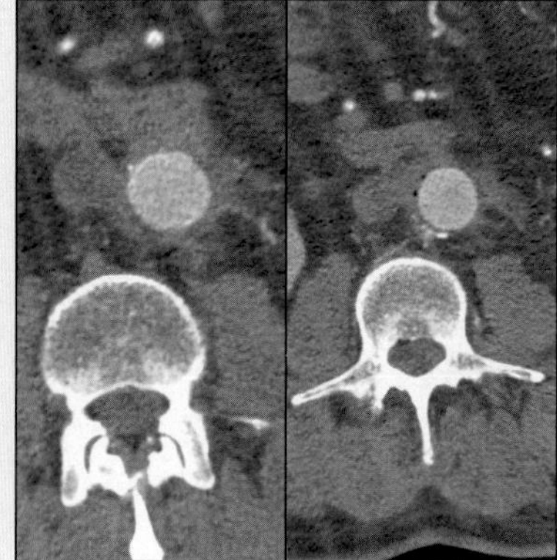

Aortoenteric Fistula

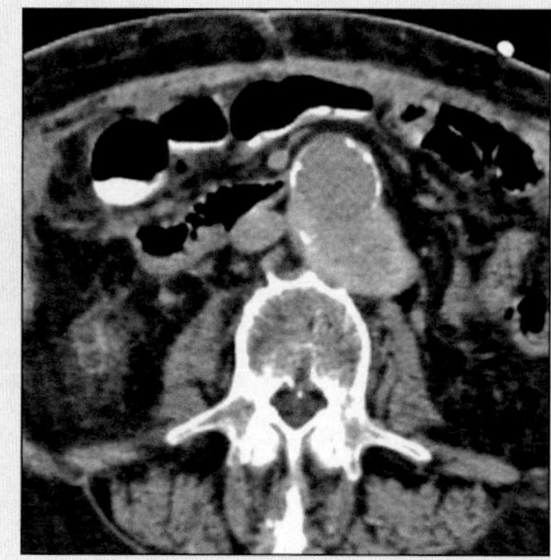

Contained Rupture AAA

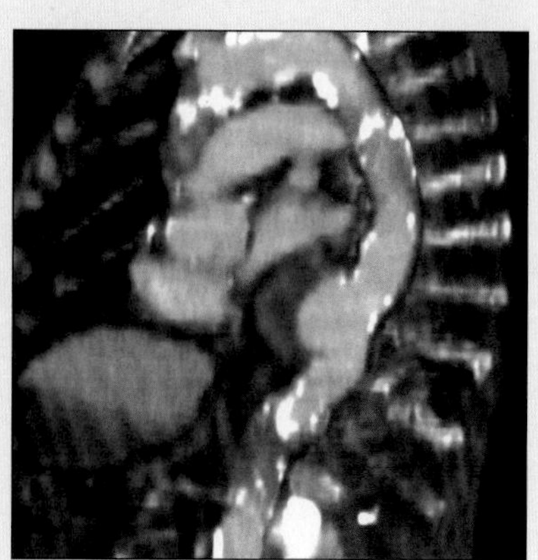

Atherosclerotic Aneurysm

MYCOTIC ANEURYSM

Key Facts

Terminology
- Infectious aneurysm (more appropriate term)
- Aneurysm arising from infection of arterial wall, usually bacterial

Imaging Findings
- Best diagnostic clue: Rapidly growing saccular aneurysm arising eccentrically from aortic wall
- Anywhere in aorta or other vessels
- Periaortic soft tissue stranding, edema and fluid are frequently present

Top Differential Diagnoses
- Atherosclerotic Aneurysm
- Inflammatory Aneurysm
- Contained Rupture
- Aortoenteric Fistula

Pathology
- Bacterial aortitis most commonly caused by Salmonella or Staph aureus
- Syphilitic aortitis involves the ascending aorta but spares the aortic sinus: Ascending aorta most common location
- Primary mycotic aneurysm arises from a distant, unknown, or remote source of infection
- Secondary mycotic aneurysm arises from specific source of infection

Clinical Issues
- In 25% of cases blood cultures are negative
- Acute rupture/hemorrhage seen in 75%
- Surgical resection/grafting following antibiotic therapy
- May need extra anatomic bypass grafting

- Periaortic low signal intensity in absence of gadolinium (Gd)
- Aortic and periaortic enhancement following Gd, especially evident on fat-suppressed images
- T2WI: Periaortic high signal intensity on fat-suppressed T2WI
- Contrast-enhanced MRA
  - One or more saccular aneurysms arising from aortic wall
  - Effacement of wall with possible leakage at rupture site
  - It is important to review MRA as well as delayed source images to identify areas of enhancement

Echocardiographic Findings
- Echocardiogram: Used to rule out endocarditis

Angiographic Findings
- Conventional: Focal, saccular aneurysm

Imaging Recommendations
- Best imaging tool: CT delineates aneurysms very well
- T1WI and T2WI MR followed by contrast-enhanced MRA

DIFFERENTIAL DIAGNOSIS

Atherosclerotic Aneurysm
- Slow growing
- More often fusiform
- Often calcified

Inflammatory Aneurysm
- Distal aorta and iliac involvement
- Fusiform aneurysm
- Retro-peritoneal fibrosis

Contained Rupture
- Focal disruption or gap in aortic wall
- High attenuation in wall or in periphery of aneurysm
- Lack of enhancement

Aortoenteric Fistula
- Most involve duodenum
- Periaortic soft tissue with periaortic gas
- Active contrast material extravasation or pseudoaneurysm
- Presenting as GI bleed

PATHOLOGY

General Features
- General path comments
  - Infection of major artery that weakens the wall
    - Septic embolus lodging on wall of artery, usually from endocarditis
    - Direct extension from an adjacent infected focus
    - Microorganisms directly infecting the arterial wall
  - Generally believed that mycotic aneurysm develops on already diseased aorta
- Etiology
  - Bacterial aortitis most commonly caused by Salmonella or Staph aureus
  - Syphilitic aortitis involves ascending aorta but spares aortic sinus: Ascending aorta most common location
  - Routes of infection
    - Most often caused by seeding of an existing lesion (atheroma or aneurysm) via vasa vasorum
    - Direct extension from infection in vessel wall, i.e., bacterial endocarditis
    - Invasion of aortic wall by extravascular contiguous infection
    - Lymphatic spread
- Epidemiology
  - 0.7-2.6% of all aortic aneurysms
  - Increased risk in
    - IV drug abusers
    - Patients with history of bacterial endocarditis
    - Immunocompromised patients
    - Patients with vascular prostheses (valves, grafts)

MYCOTIC ANEURYSM

Gross Pathologic & Surgical Features

- Bacterial aneurysm
  - Non-calcified, saccular aneurysm
  - Thinning of aortic wall with periaortic inflammatory changes
- Syphilitic aneurysm
  - Calcified lesion
  - "Tree bark" appearance when atheroma develops in infected areas

Microscopic Features

- Loss of intima and destruction of internal elastic lamina
- Media shows varying degrees of destruction
- Bacteria present on histology
- Common bacteria: Pseudomonas, Clostridia, Salmonella, Streptococcus, Aspergillus

Staging, Grading or Classification Criteria

- Classification system
  - Primary mycotic aneurysm arises from a distant, unknown, or remote source of infection
  - Secondary mycotic aneurysm arises from specific source of infection
    - Bacterial endocarditis (intravascular spread)
    - Tuberculosis (contiguous spread)

CLINICAL ISSUES

Presentation

- Most common signs/symptoms: Fever, signs of sepsis
- Symptoms vary greatly
- Nonspecific findings
- Low grade fever
- Localized pain
- Positive blood cultures
  - In 25% of cases blood cultures are negative

Natural History & Prognosis

- Nearly always fatal if untreated
- Acute rupture/hemorrhage seen in 75%
- Mortality rate estimated at 67%

Treatment

- Surgical resection/grafting following antibiotic therapy
- May need extra anatomic bypass grafting
- In some cases endovascular repair may be attempted

SELECTED REFERENCES

1. Guerrero ML et al: Endovascular repair of mycotic aneurysms of the aorta: an alternative to conventional bypass surgery in patients with acute sepsis. Scand J Infect Dis. 39(3):268-71, 2007
2. Iida H et al: Bacteremia causes mycotic aneurysm of the aortic arch in 110 days. Ann Thorac Surg. 83(5):1874-6, 2007
3. McPhee JT et al: The impact of gender on presentation, therapy, and mortality of abdominal aortic aneurysm in the United States, 2001-2004. J Vasc Surg. 45(5):891-9, 2007
4. Peterson BG et al: Five-year report of a multicenter controlled clinical trial of open versus endovascular treatment of abdominal aortic aneurysms. J Vasc Surg. 45(5):885-90, 2007
5. Taylor CF et al: Treatment options for primary infected aorta. Ann Vasc Surg. 21(2):225-7, 2007
6. Alpagut U et al: Endoluminal stenting of mycotic saccular aneurysm at the aortic arch. Tex Heart Inst J. 33(3):371-5, 2006
7. Froeschl M et al: Ruptured mycotic pseudoaneurysm of the thoracic aorta. Cardiovasc Pathol. 15(2):116-8, 2006
8. Kerzmann A et al: Infected abdominal aortic aneurysm treated by in situ replacement with cryopreserved arterial homograft. Acta Chir Belg. 106(4):447-9, 2006
9. Lee KH et al: Stent-graft treatment of infected aortic and arterial aneurysms. J Endovasc Ther. 13(3):338-45, 2006
10. Palanichamy N et al: Mycotic pseudo-aneurysm of the ascending thoracic aorta after cardiac transplantation. J Heart Lung Transplant. 25(6):730-3, 2006
11. Sirvanci M et al: Recurrent tuberculous pseudoaneurysm of the descending thoracic aorta--a case report. Angiology. 57(1):103-6, 2006
12. Ting AC et al: Endovascular stent graft repair for infected thoracic aortic pseudoaneurysms--a durable option? J Vasc Surg. 44(4):701-5, 2006
13. Villavicencio MA et al: Thoracic aorta false aneurysm: what surgical strategy should be recommended? Ann Thorac Surg. 82(1):81-9; discussion 89, 2006
14. Chan YC et al: The management of mycotic aortic aneurysms: is there a role for endoluminal treatment? Acta Chir Belg. 105(6):580-7, 2005
15. Gonzalez-Fajardo JA et al: Endovascular repair in the presence of aortic infection. Ann Vasc Surg. 19(1):94-8, 2005
16. Therasse E et al: Stent-graft placement for the treatment of thoracic aortic diseases. Radiographics. 25(1):157-73, 2005
17. Ting AC et al: Surgical treatment of infected aneurysms and pseudoaneurysms of the thoracic and abdominal aorta. Am J Surg. 189(2):150-4, 2005
18. Denguir R et al: [Mycotic aneurysm of the subrenal abdominal aorta: extra anatomical reconstruction in five patients] J Mal Vasc. 28(1):15-20, 2003
19. Malouf JF et al: Mycotic aneurysms of the thoracic aorta: a diagnostic challenge. Am J Med. 115(6):489-96, 2003
20. Čina ČS et al: Ruptured mycotic thoracoabdominal aortic aneurysms: a report of three cases and a systematic review. J Vasc Surg. 33(4):861-7, 2001
21. Locati P et al: Salmonella mycotic aneurysms: traditional and "alternative" surgical repair with arterial homograft. Minerva Cardioangiol. 47(1-2):31-7, 1999
22. Long R et al: Tuberculous mycotic aneurysm of the aorta: review of published medical and surgical experience. Chest. 115(2):522-31, 1999
23. Semba CP et al: Mycotic aneurysms of the thoracic aorta: repair with use of endovascular stent-grafts. J Vasc Interv Radiol. 9(1 Pt 1):33-40, 1998
24. Pasic M: Mycotic aneurysm of the aorta: evolving surgical concept. Ann Thorac Surg. 61(4):1053-4, 1996
25. Messa CA 3rd et al: Double clostridial mycotic aneurysms of the aorta. Cardiovasc Surg. 3(6):687-92, 1995
26. Schrander-vd Meer AM et al: Mycotic aneurysm of the suprarenal abdominal aorta. Neth J Med. 44(1):23-5, 1994
27. Fichelle JM et al: Infected infrarenal aortic aneurysms: when is in situ reconstruction safe? J Vasc Surg. 17(4):635-45, 1993

IMAGE GALLERY

Typical

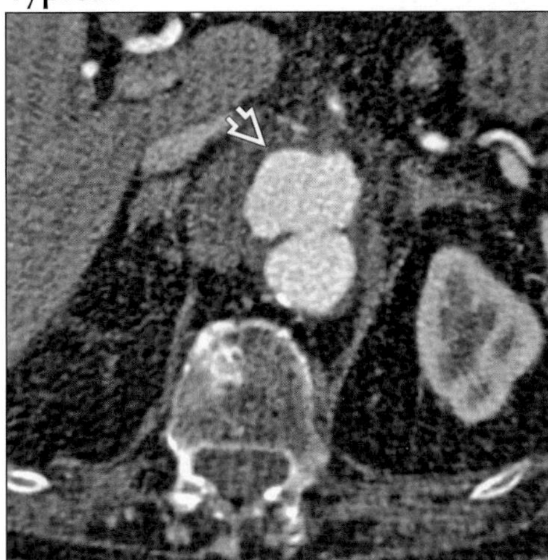

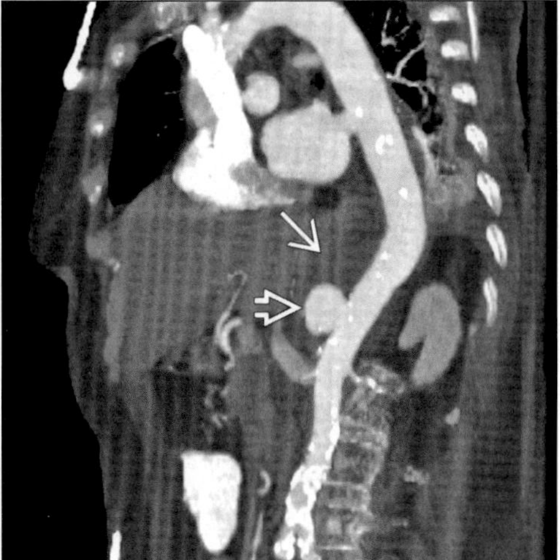

*(**Left**) Axial CECT shows a saccular aortic aneurysm → with mural thrombus. (**Right**) Oblique CTA shows a saccular aortic aneurysm → with peripheral mural thrombus →. Mycotic aneurysms are usually saccular and involve a focal arterial segment. Infection weakens the arterial wall and allows for the aneurysm formation.*

Typical

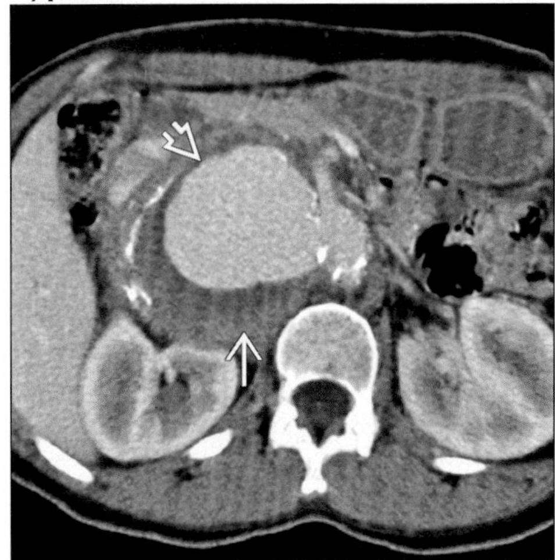

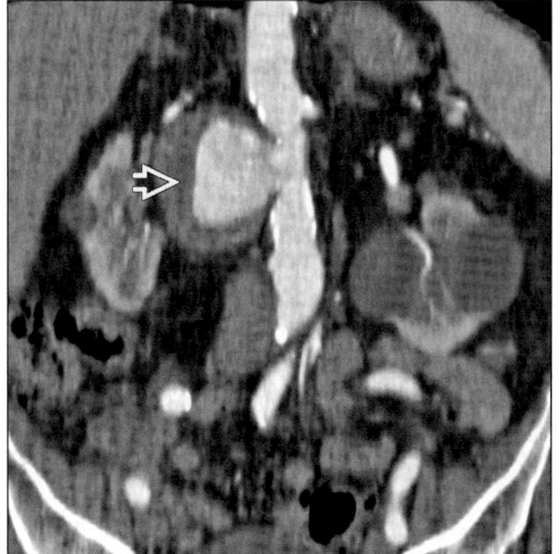

*(**Left**) Axial CECT shows a saccular aortic aneurysm → with mural thrombus and peri-aortic soft tissue →. (**Right**) Coronal CTA shows a saccular aortic aneurysm → arising from the lateral wall of the abdominal aorta. Mycotic aneurysms account for up to 2.6% of all aortic aneurysms. There is an increased risk for this type of aneurysm in IV drug abusers, immunocompromised patients, and in cases of bacterial endocarditis.*

Typical

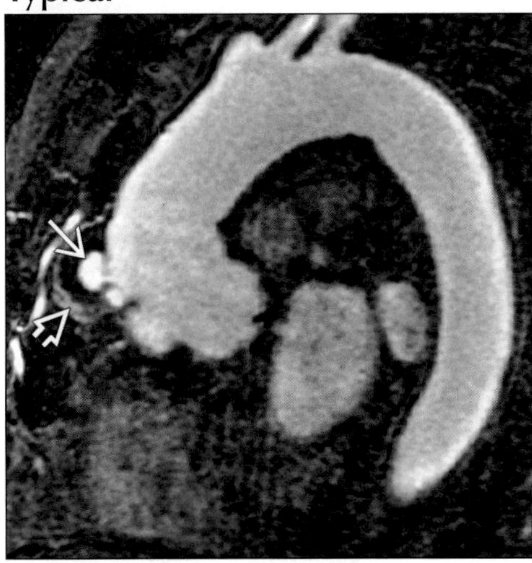

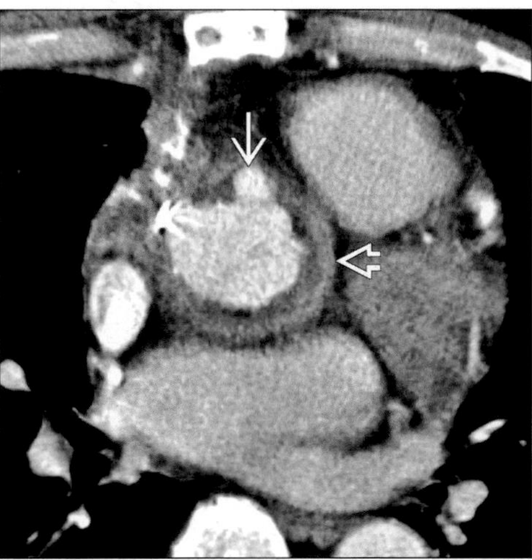

*(**Left**) Oblique MRA shows multiple, small, pseudoaneurysms →, following ascending aortic aneurysm repair. Also note enhancing soft tissue → surrounding the aneurysms. (**Right**) Axial CECT shows a pseudoaneurysm → and periaortic soft tissue → following surgical repair of an ascending aortic aneurysm.*

POST-TRAUMATIC PSEUDOANEURYSM

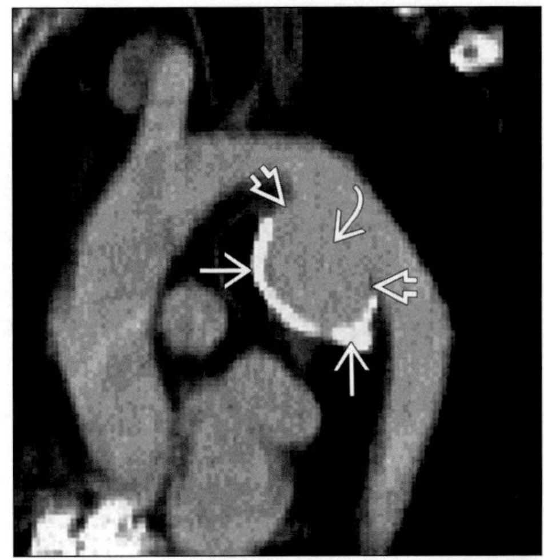

Sagittal CECT in a patient with a remote history of chest trauma shows a peripherally calcified ➡, eccentric, saccular outpouching ➡, with a large communicating channel ➡ located at the aortic isthmus.

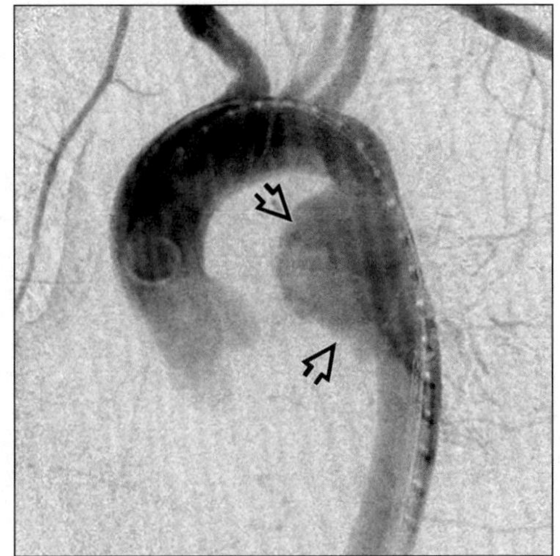

Sagittal DSA in the same patient shows contrast filling of the saccular outpouching ➡. The history combined with the CT and angiographic features are consistent with a post-traumatic thoracic aortic pseudoaneurysm.

TERMINOLOGY

Abbreviations and Synonyms

- Thoracic pseudoaneurysm
- Chronic post-traumatic aneurysm

Definitions

- Chronic pseudoaneurysm of thoracic aorta due to previous traumatic aortic injury
  - Typically located at isthmus with characteristic peripheral calcification

IMAGING FINDINGS

General Features

- Best diagnostic clue: Peripherally calcified vascular mass arising from aortic isthmus extending to aortopulmonic (AP) window
- Location
  - Immediately distal to left subclavian artery
    - Region of ligamentum arteriosum
    - Area of aorta susceptible to injury
  - Aortic isthmus: 1.5 cm long area between left subclavian artery origin and ligamentum arteriosum
  - May occur at diaphragmatic hiatus and aortic root
- Size: Variable: When small, often cryptic on conventional chest radiograph but with enlargement may manifest as aortopulmonic window mass
- Morphology
  - Usually saccular pseudoaneurysm
    - Commonly associated with mural calcification and/or thrombus

Radiographic Findings

- Radiography
  - May show soft tissue mass-like density along aortopulmonic window
  - Mediastinal widening
  - Curvilinear vascular calcification
  - Displacement of trachea to right
  - Rarely lung collapse

CT Findings

- NECT: Rim calcification is better identified
- CTA
  - Contrast-filled saccular aneurysm at isthmus

DDx: Post-Traumatic Pseudoaneurysm

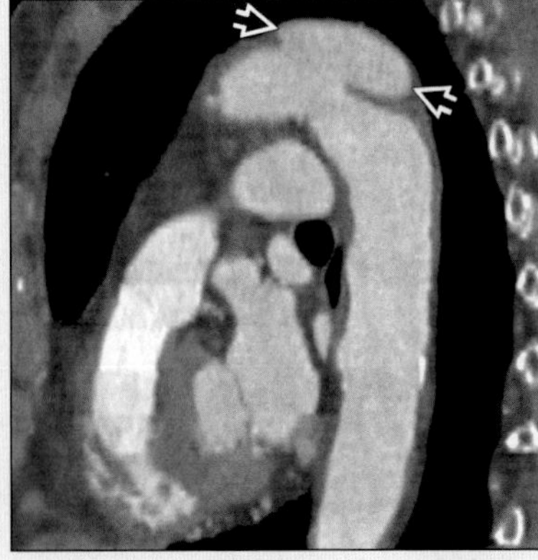

Atherosclerotic Pseudoaneurysm

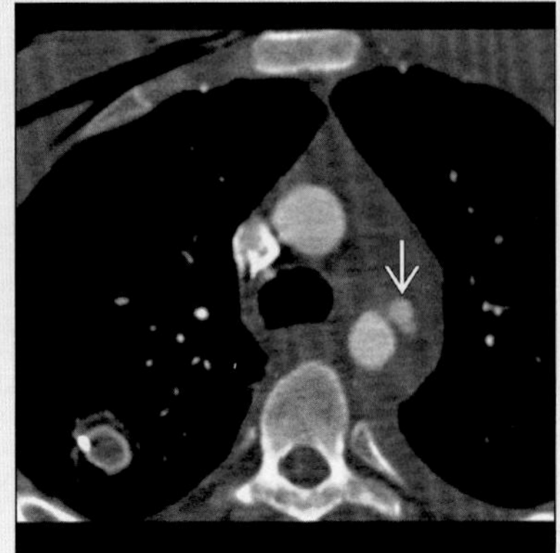

Traumatic Aortic Transection

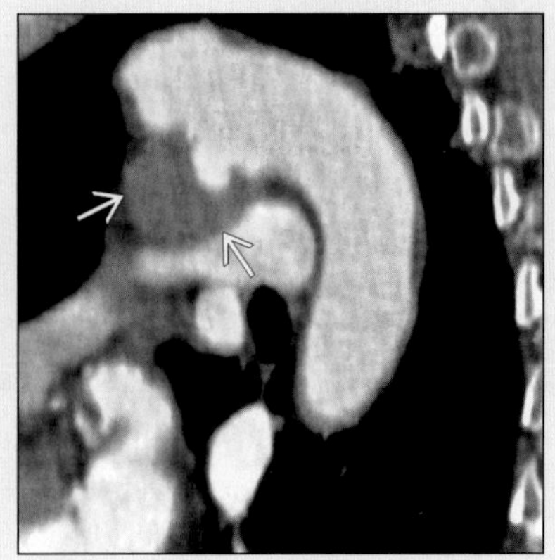

Ductus Diverticulum Aneurysm

POST-TRAUMATIC PSEUDOANEURYSM

Key Facts

Terminology
- Chronic pseudoaneurysm of thoracic aorta from prior trauma

Imaging Findings
- X-ray: Soft tissue mass along AP window
- CT: Contrast-filled saccular aneurysm at isthmus
  - Peripheral thrombus and calcification
  - No intimal flap
  - Remainder of aorta usually normal
- MR: Perfused saccular pseudoaneurysm; thrombus dark signal
  - Low signal peripheral thrombus on post T1WI GRE
  - Channel between aneurysm and aorta better seen
  - Presence of slow leak better seen on delayed passes
  - Perfused pseudoaneurysm lumen bright on SSFP and dark on Haste

Top Differential Diagnoses
- Atherosclerotic Aneurysm
- Mycotic/Septic Pseudoaneurysm
- Penetrating Ulcer with Pseudoaneurysm
- Traumatic Aortic Pseudoaneurysm

Pathology
- 2.5% of patients develop chronic post-traumatic pseudoaneurysm following initial trauma
- Saccular pseudoaneurysm contained by adventitia

Clinical Issues
- Signs/symptoms develop after 5 years in 40% of patients; after 20 yrs in 80%
- Usually asymptomatic
- May rupture especially if larger than 6 cm
- Treat with endovascular stent graft or open surgery

  - Low density thrombus and high density curvilinear calcification along pseudoaneurysmal wall
  - Arises anteromedial portion of isthmus and extends to AP window
  - No low density intimal flap
  - Extrinsic compression of left main bronchus
  - Reminder of the aorta is usually normal
- Cardiac Gated CTA: Helps to assess coronary arteries to plan for surgery

MR Findings
- T1 C+
  - Post T1WI GRE shows peripheral thrombus along pseudoaneurysmal wall as low signal
  - Channel between pseudoaneurysm and normal aorta better visualized
- MRA
  - Contrast-filled saccular outpouching from the isthmus, peripheral thrombus appears as dark signal
  - Communicating channel between pseudoaneurysm and aortic isthmus well seen
  - Slow leak well demonstrated on delayed passes (always obtain at least 2 passes of CEMRA)
  - TEMRA shows dynamic contrast filling and wash out of saccular pseudoaneurysm
- SSFP White Blood Cine: Bright signal (flowing blood) within saccular pseudoaneurysm, thrombus appears as low to intermediate signal
- Double IR FSE
  - Flowing blood within saccular pseudoaneurysm appears as dark signal
  - Thrombus or slow flowing blood appears as intermediate signal

Angiographic Findings
- "Gold standard"
- Confirms dynamic flow and communication between pseudoaneurysm and aorta
- Rapid clearing of contrast
- Thrombus not reliably evaluated
- Peripheral calcification better seen on non-subtracted images

Imaging Recommendations
- Best imaging tool
  - CTA or MR
  - MRI/MRA is better alternative technique
  - Catheter angiography remains "gold standard"
- Protocol advice
  - CT: 3 mm NECT followed by CECT/CTA
    - 1.5 mm thin section volumetric acquisition; at least 3 mm coronal and sagittal reconstructions
    - 80-100 mL contrast at 3 cc/sec
    - ECG gated scan can be performed to assess aortic root and coronary arteries
    - Always review sagittal or oblique sagittal reformatted images for pseudoaneurysm
  - MRI: Multiplanar SSFP, axial and sagittal pre- and post- T1 GRE, and coronal CE MRA
    - Axial, coronal, sagittal thin MIP (10 mm thickness with overlapping interval)
    - Time resolved MRA to show flow dynamics; needs < 5 cc of gadolinium
    - For CE MRA, use double dose to achieve good quality post contrast GRE images

DIFFERENTIAL DIAGNOSIS

Atherosclerotic Aneurysm
- Elderly
- No history of trauma
- Saccular or fusiform aneurysm, not restricted to isthmus
- Multiple calcifications of aorta
- Ulcerative plaques with small outpouchings of aorta

Mycotic/Septic Pseudoaneurysm
- Rapidly enlarging eccentric saccular pseudoaneurysm
  - Usually no peripheral calcification; disruption of mural calcification
  - Unusual locations
  - Rim-enhancement on CECT, C+ MR
- Peri/para-aortic soft tissue stranding
- Para-aortic gas pockets

POST-TRAUMATIC PSEUDOANEURYSM

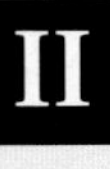

- Otherwise normal aorta
- Vertebral osteomyelitis (cause and effect)
- Look for source of infection; blood culture negative in 1/3 of patients

Penetrating Ulcer with Pseudoaneurysm

- Occurs anywhere in aorta
- Elderly, no history of trauma
- Severely atherosclerotic aorta; especially abdominal aorta
- Multiple ulcerations with small outpouchings
- Multiple focal calcified and non-calcified plaques
- Chronic mural hematoma appearing low density on CT

Acute Traumatic Aortic Pseudoaneurysm

- Acute
- Irregular contrast filling small pseudoaneurysm at isthmus
- Mediastinal and para-aortic hematoma
- No calcification
- High mortality

PATHOLOGY

General Features

- Etiology
  - Post-traumatic: Usually a history of trauma can be elicited from patient
    - Rapid deceleration injury
    - Aortic isthmus is "pinched" between anterior chest wall and thoracic spine
    - Transverse tear of aortic wall
    - Laceration involving anteromedial margin of aorta at ligament arteriosum may lead to pseudoaneurysm
    - Initial hematoma is contained within aortopulmonic window
- Epidemiology
  - 2.5% of patients develop chronic post-traumatic aortic pseudoaneurysm following aortic injury
    - May have symptom free period of months to years but usually symptoms eventually occur
- Associated abnormalities: Bony fractures

Gross Pathologic & Surgical Features

- Saccular pseudoaneurysm contained by adventitia or thrombus and fibrous tissue
  - Does not contain normal three vascular wall layers
- Mural calcifications

CLINICAL ISSUES

Presentation

- Most common signs/symptoms
  - Usually asymptomatic
    - Incidental finding on plain chest radiograph or CT
- Other signs/symptoms
  - Signs and symptoms develop after 5 years in 40% and after 20 yrs in 80% of patients
  - Symptoms due to pseudoaneurysm pressing on other structures, or other associated complications
    - Chest pain
    - Dyspnea from airway compression
    - Hoarseness from pressure on recurrent laryngeal nerve
    - Dysphagia from esophageal compression

Demographics

- Age: Adult
- Gender: M = F

Natural History & Prognosis

- May rupture especially if larger than 6 cm
- Risk of continual expansion
- Compression of left main bronchus and resultant lung collapse
- Other complications include aortic dissection, thromboemboli, bacterial endocarditis, and aorto-esophageal fistula
- 10 year survival rate < 70% without surgery, > 85% with surgery

Treatment

- Standard therapy is open surgical repair
- Endovascular stent graft may be appropriate in some patients and is increasingly first-line therapy
  - Requires satisfactory "landing zone" of healthy aortic tissue adjacent or distal to left subclavian artery origin

DIAGNOSTIC CHECKLIST

Consider

- Post-traumatic pseudoaneurysm in context of prior history of trauma and eccentric saccular outpouching at aortic isthmus

Image Interpretation Pearls

- Aneurysmal ductus diverticulum can resemble chronic post-traumatic pseudoaneurysm
  - Usually no calcification of ductus and no prior trauma

SELECTED REFERENCES

1. Salvolini L et al: Acute aortic syndromes: Role of multi-detector row CT. Eur J Radiol. 65(3):350-8, 2008
2. Garzon G et al: Endovascular stent-graft treatment of thoracic aortic disease. Radiographics. 25 Suppl 1:S229-44, 2005
3. Takahashi K et al: Multidetector CT of the thoracic aorta. Int J Cardiovasc Imaging. 21(1):141-53, 2005
4. Therasse E et al: Stent-graft placement for the treatment of thoracic aortic diseases. Radiographics. 25(1):157-73, 2005
5. Bortone AS et al: Endovascular treatment of thoracic aortic disease: four years of experience. Circulation. 110(11 Suppl 1):II262-7, 2004
6. Heystraten FM et al: Chronic posttraumatic aneurysm of the thoracic aorta: surgically correctable occult threat. AJR Am J Roentgenol. 146(2):303-8, 1986

POST-TRAUMATIC PSEUDOANEURYSM

IMAGE GALLERY

Typical

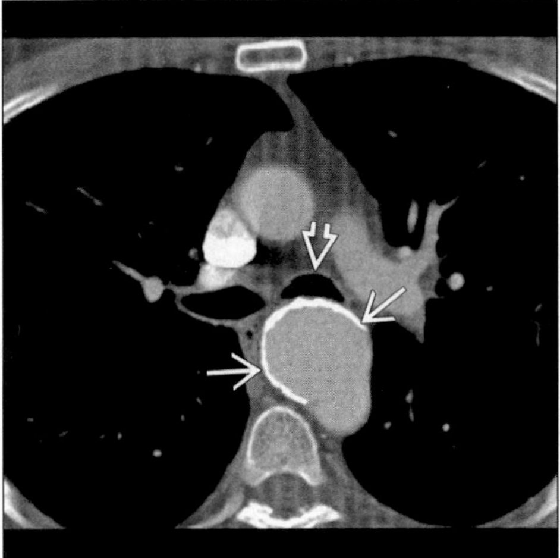

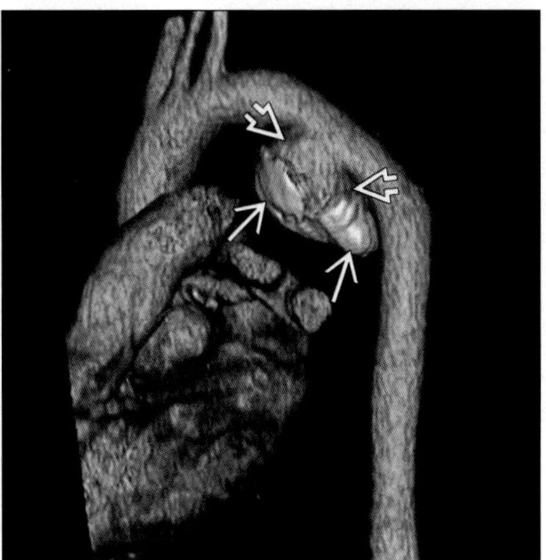

*(**Left**) Axial CECT shows a peripherally calcified enhancing saccular outpouching from the distal aortic arch with compression of the left main stem bronchus. Patients may develop clinical symptoms, such as dyspnea, from compression of adjacent structures by a pseudoaneurysm. (**Right**) Sagittal volume rendered CTA image (same patient) shows the post-traumatic pseudoaneurysm with eccentric peripheral calcification.*

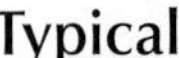

Typical

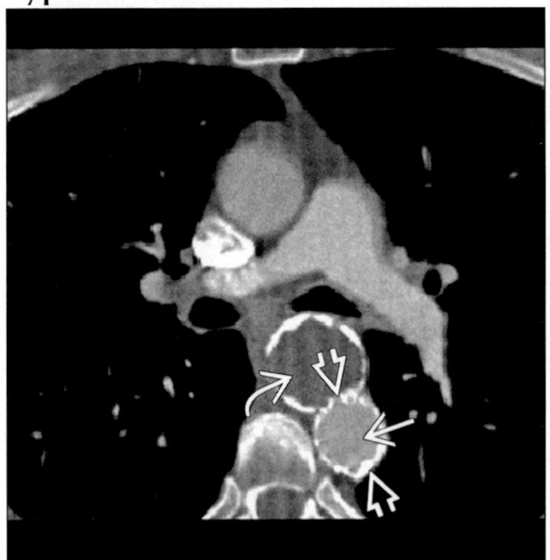

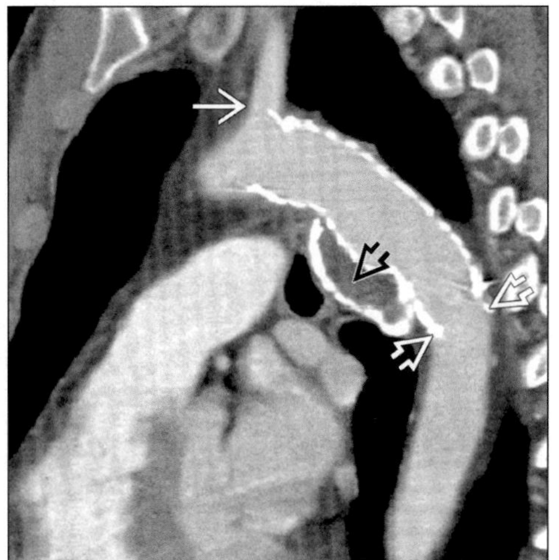

*(**Left**) Axial CECT of the same patient shows a thrombosed saccular pseudoaneurysm sac which has been excluded by an endovascular aortic stent graft that was used for treatment. The endovascular graft lumen is widely patent. (**Right**) Sagittal CECT in the same patient shows that the stent-graft extends from immediately distal to the left subclavian arterial origin to the descending aorta. The pseudoaneurysm is thrombosed and there is no endoleak.*

Typical

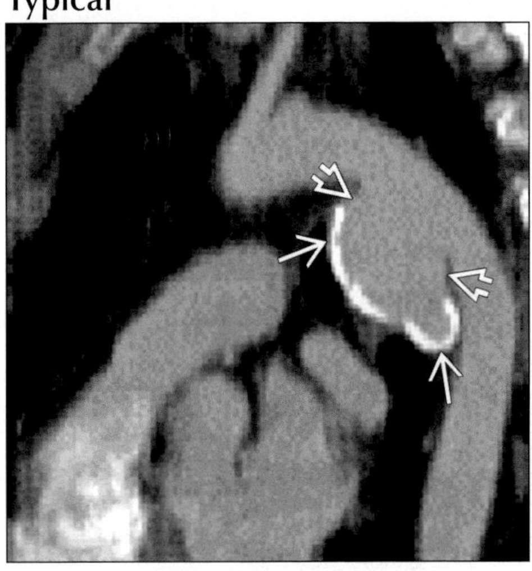

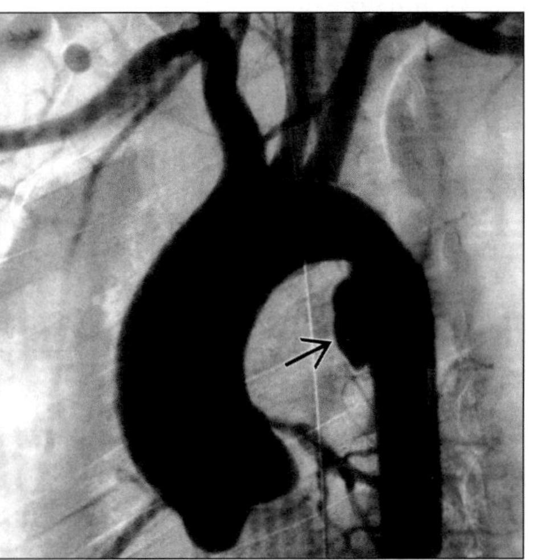

*(**Left**) Sagittal CECT in a patient with prior trauma shows a large saccular pseudoaneurysm along the aortic isthmus with peripheral rim calcification, consistent with a post-traumatic pseudoaneurysm. (**Right**) Left anterior oblique aortogram (same patient) shows contrast filling the aortic pseudoaneurysm. The location of the pseudoaneurysm allowed for successful endovascular treatment with an aortic stent-graft.*

AORTIC INTRAMURAL HEMATOMA

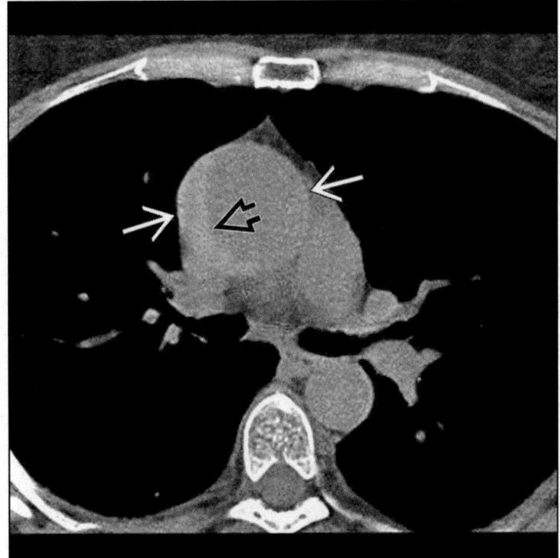

Axial NECT shows crescentic high density material ⊳ within the wall of an ascending aortic aneurysm ➡. The high density within the wall reflects hemorrhage from rupture of the vasa vasorum into the aortic media.

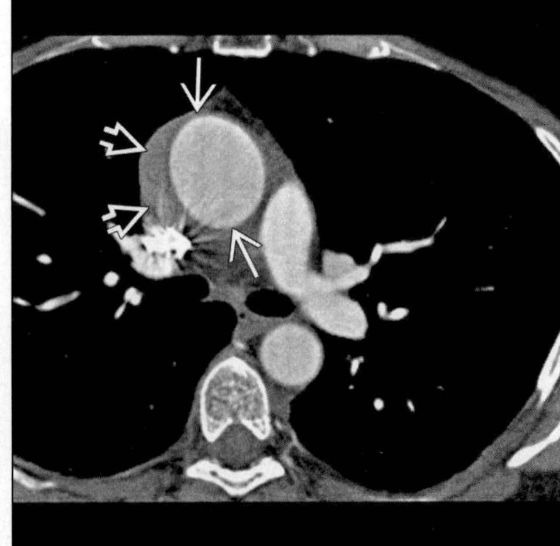

Axial CECT (same patient) shows crescentic low density aortic wall with smooth interface ⊳, elliptical-shaped aortic lumen ➡, ascending aortic aneurysm and no intimal flap, consistent with aortic intramural hematoma.

TERMINOLOGY

Abbreviations and Synonyms

- Intramural hematoma (IMH); atypical aortic dissection
  - Noncommunicating aortic dissection
- Variant of acute aortic syndrome (AAS)

Definitions

- Hemorrhage due to rupture of vasa vasorum within aortic media, resulting in noncommunicating dissection, with typical absence of intimal tear

IMAGING FINDINGS

General Features

- Best diagnostic clue
  - Crescentic or circular high density, mural thickening on NECT; appears hypodense after IV contrast with elliptical shape of perfused aortic lumen
  - No visible intimal flap
- Location: Ascending and descending thoracic aorta > abdominal aorta; commonly seen in descending aorta
- Size: Usually < 15 mm but > 4 mm mural thickness
- Morphology
  - Type A IMH always involves ascending aorta
  - Type B IMH involves only descending aorta
  - Mural hematoma may extend within media
    - May progress to aortic dissection
    - Saccular aortic aneurysm may form
  - Intimal displacement but no tear
  - Total diameter of aorta may be enlarged

Radiographic Findings

- Radiography
  - Chest film of limited value
    - New aneurysmal dilatation of aorta
    - Mediastinal widening
    - Displacement of intimal calcification
  - Pleural effusion commonly seen in true dissection or aortic rupture

CT Findings

- NECT
  - Acutely appears hyperdense, smooth crescentic area along aortic wall
  - Intimal calcifications may be displaced, best seen on narrow windows

DDx: Aortic Intramural Hematoma

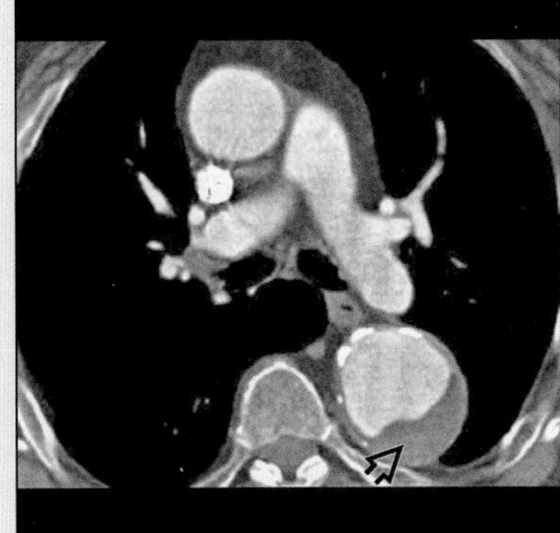

Atherosclerotic Mural Thrombus

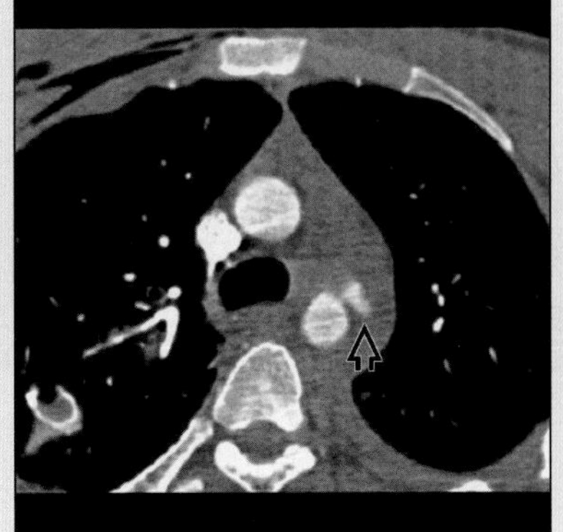

Acute Aortic Transection

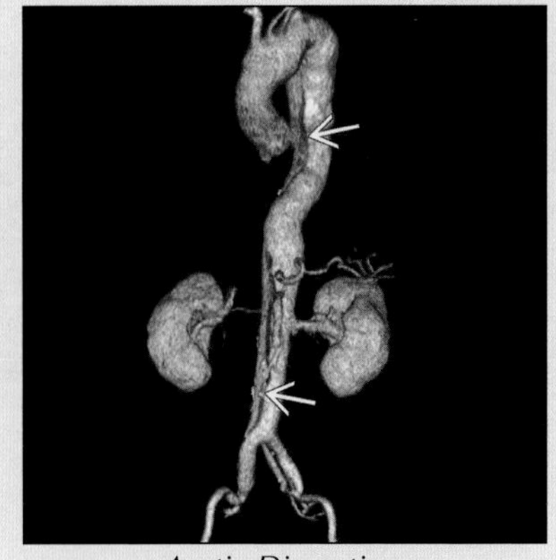

Aortic Dissection

AORTIC INTRAMURAL HEMATOMA

Key Facts

Terminology

- Rupture of vasa vasorum resulting in hematoma within aortic media

Imaging Findings

- CT is quick and primary modality of choice
- Crescentic hyperdense aortic wall on NECT
- Hypodense wall with elliptical aortic lumen on CECT
  - Smooth well-defined margin, no intimal flap
- High signal aortic wall thickening on pre-contrast T1WI
- IMH appears as low signal on post-contrast T1WI
- TE MRA shows only aortic lumen filling
- CE MRA shows lack of contrast in IMH

Top Differential Diagnoses

- Saccular Aortic Aneurysm with Mural Thrombus
- Dissection
- Traumatic Aortic Pseudoaneurysm
- Aortitis
- Penetrating Atherosclerotic Ulcer

Pathology

- Types A (ascending) and B (descending) aortic IMH
- Hemorrhage confined to media, with no intimal tear

Clinical Issues

- Typically hypertensive
- Acute chest pain: Severe, tearing, or migratory
- Treated similar to typical aortic dissection
  - Medical or surgical (open, EVAR) management
- May have complete resorption of hematoma (< 30%)
- CTA within 48 hrs of initial scan to check for progression to dissection

- Aneurysmal dilatation of aorta may or may not occur at level of IMH
- CTA
  - Circumferential or crescentic low density along aortic wall
  - Margin of this low density (hematoma) is well-defined and regular
  - Smooth inner margin of aorta
  - Displacement of intimal calcification
  - No intimal flap
  - No enhancement within aortic wall
  - Dilatation of aorta may occur secondary hematoma
  - Can be associated with penetrating ulcer

MR Findings

- T1WI
  - Pre-contrast T1WI GRE shows high signal crescentic aortic wall thickening
  - No low signal intimal flap
- T2WI: T2 haste shows intermediate to high signal aortic wall
- T1 C+
  - IMH appears as low signal on post-contrast T1 GRE (no perfusion)
  - Total wall-to-wall diameter of aorta better seen on this sequence than CE MRA
- MRA
  - TR MRA normally shows no false lumen and no perfusion of hematoma; only aortic lumen filling
  - CE MRA shows lack of contrast in IMH; seen as dark signal compared to high signal aortic lumen
  - Minimal compression of aortic lumen

Echocardiographic Findings

- Echocardiogram
  - TEE highly accurate
  - Smooth curvilinear luminal wall
  - No intimal flap, no flow communication
  - No rough irregular border (unlike penetrating ulcer)
  - Echo-free space within thickened aortic wall

Angiographic Findings

- Conventional
  - Intramural hematoma frequently missed
    - No intimal flap, no double lumen
    - Only seen if hematoma causes luminal compression

Imaging Recommendations

- Best imaging tool
  - MR is best technique, but time consuming and may be limited in critically ill patients
  - CT is quick and primary modality of choice
- Protocol advice
  - Non contrast CT with 3 mm slice thickness.
    - CTA with 1.5 mm slice collimation acquisition; 1.5 mm axial, 3 mm coronal and sagittal oblique reconstructions; ECG-gating is preferable
    - 80-100 mL contrast at flow rate of 3 cc/sec; bolus tracking with ROI in descending aorta
  - Essential MR sequences are precontrast T1WI GRE, SSFP (bright blood), contrast-enhanced MRA, post-contrast T1WI GRE
  - Time-resolved MRA to show flow dynamics
  - Cine SSFP axial and cine candy cane may be useful
  - Phase contrast GRE to asses flow and velocity

DIFFERENTIAL DIAGNOSIS

Saccular Aneurysm with Mural Thrombus

- Margins of mural thrombus inside aortic lumen
- Aneurysm involves all layers of aortic wall
- Usually calcified intimal plaque

Dissection

- Intimal tear or flap present
- True and false lumens have differential perfusion
- Direct flow communication between channels

Traumatic Aortic Pseudoaneurysm

- Acute presentation, often from deceleration injury
- Irregular margin, periaortic and mediastinal hematoma
- Pseudoaneurysm is contained by thin adventitia
- Typically located at areas of restricted aortic mobility

  - Isthmus, rarely at root, diaphragmatic hiatus
- Post-traumatic chronic pseudoaneurysm is associated with peripheral calcification

Aortitis

- Granulomatous inflammation of aortic wall
- Circumferential mural thickening and enhancement; latter appreciated on MR
- May have stenosis or occlusion of aortic lumen
- Small pseudoaneurysm, fat stranding and gas pockets in infective aortitis

Penetrating Atherosclerotic Ulcer

- Focal contrast-filled luminal outpouching
- Adjacent subintimal hematoma
- Calcified and inwardly displaced intima
- Ulcerative atheromatous plaque penetrates elastic lamina and extends into media

PATHOLOGY

General Features

- General path comments
  - Erroneous clinical diagnosis of dissection in 10-20%
  - Descending aorta involved in approximately 50-80%
- Etiology
  - Spontaneous rupture of vasa vasorum
  - Iatrogenic injury from catheter manipulations
  - Blunt chest trauma with aortic wall injury may lead to IMH
  - Atherosclerotic penetrating aortic ulcer
- Epidemiology
  - Common history of hypertension
  - More common in elderly
  - M = F
  - Older age at initial diagnosis has better long term prognosis
- Associated abnormalities: 30-40% associated with abdominal or thoracic aortic aneurysm

Gross Pathologic & Surgical Features

- Hemorrhage confined within media of aorta between intima and adventitia; no evidence of intimal tear
- Vasa vasorum penetrates outer 1/2 of aortic media and propagates along media layer of aorta

Staging, Grading or Classification Criteria

- Type A IMH, ascending aorta always involved
- Type B IMH, descending aorta alone involved

CLINICAL ISSUES

Presentation

- Most common signs/symptoms
  - Acute chest pain: Severe, tearing, or migratory
  - Intrascapular back pain
  - Similar to typical aortic dissection
- Other signs/symptoms: Diaphoresis, hypotension and tachycardia
- Clinical Profile: Typically hypertensive

Demographics

- Age: Mean age 66 years
- Gender: M = F

Natural History & Prognosis

- Intramural hematoma
  - May have complete resorption of hematoma (< 30%)
  - 25-45% may progress to aortic dissection
  - Wall configuration may change very rapidly
  - May progress to aneurysm
  - May progress to rupture

Treatment

- Current treatment similar to typical aortic dissection
  - Early surgery for type A
    - More likely to progress to dissection, contained rupture or aneurysm formation
  - Medical management for type B
    - Control hypertension
    - Careful, close follow-up
    - Endovascular or open surgery if there is aneurysmal dilatation or persistent chest pain
    - Endovascular stent grafts used in treatment of descending aorta involvement

DIAGNOSTIC CHECKLIST

Consider

- Factors predicting disease progression
  - Ascending aortic involvement, aortic diameter ≥ 50 mm, progressive thickening or increasing diameter of aortic wall, intimal ulceration, persistent pain

Image Interpretation Pearls

- No intimal flap or flow of contrast into wall with IMH
- Frequent follow-up imaging important in conservative therapy; CTA within 48 hrs of initial scan to check for progression to dissection
- Ulcerations > 2 cm wide, > 1 cm deep at higher risk; may require surgical or interventional repair

SELECTED REFERENCES

1. Nienaber CA et al: Aortic intramural haematoma: natural history and predictive factors for complications. Heart. 90(4):372-4, 2004
2. Song JK: Diagnosis of aortic intramural haematoma. Heart. 90(4):368-71, 2004
3. Castaner E et al: CT in nontraumatic acute thoracic aortic disease: typical and atypical features and complications. Radiographics. 23 Spec No:S93-110, 2003
4. Macura KJ et al: Pathogenesis in acute aortic syndromes: aortic dissection, intramural hematoma, and penetrating atherosclerotic aortic ulcer. AJR Am J Roentgenol. 181(2):309-16, 2003
5. Macura KJ et al: Role of computed tomography and magnetic resonance imaging in assessment of acute aortic syndromes. Semin Ultrasound CT MR. 24(4):232-54, 2003
6. Sawhney NS et al: Aortic intramural hematoma: an increasingly recognized and potentially fatal entity. Chest. 120(4):1340-6, 2001
7. Batra P et al: Pitfalls in the diagnosis of thoracic aortic dissection at CT angiography. Radiographics. 20(2):309-20, 2000
8. Coady MA et al: Pathologic variants of thoracic aortic dissections. Penetrating atherosclerotic ulcers and intramural hematomas. Cardiol Clin. 17(4):637-57, 1999

AORTIC INTRAMURAL HEMATOMA

IMAGE GALLERY

Typical

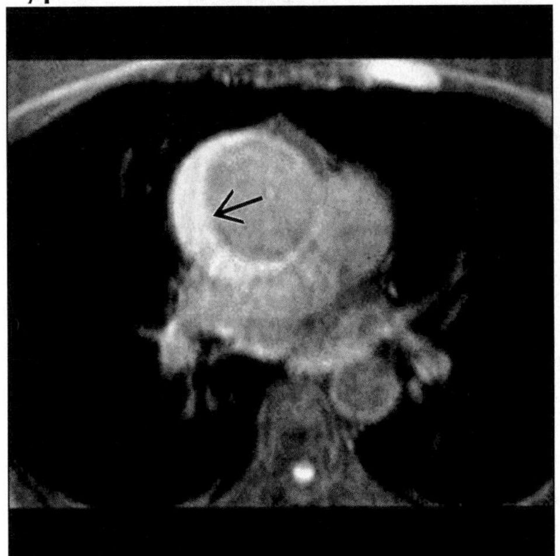

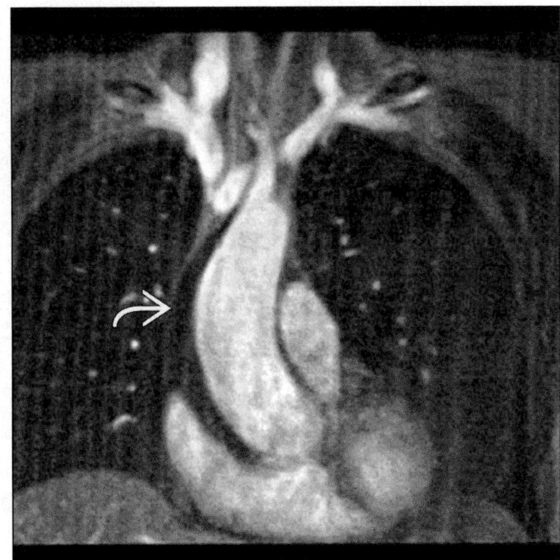

(Left) *Axial T1WI GRE shows a crescentic area of high signal → along the aortic wall consistent with an aortic intramural hematoma. Note the elliptical shape of the aortic lumen.* ***(Right)*** *Coronal CE MRA (same patient) shows a band of low signal along the ascending aortic wall adjacent to the contrast-enhanced lumen →. This confirms lack of flow within the aortic wall. When IMH involves the ascending aorta, there is a higher likelihood of progression to dissection & surgery may be necessary.*

Typical

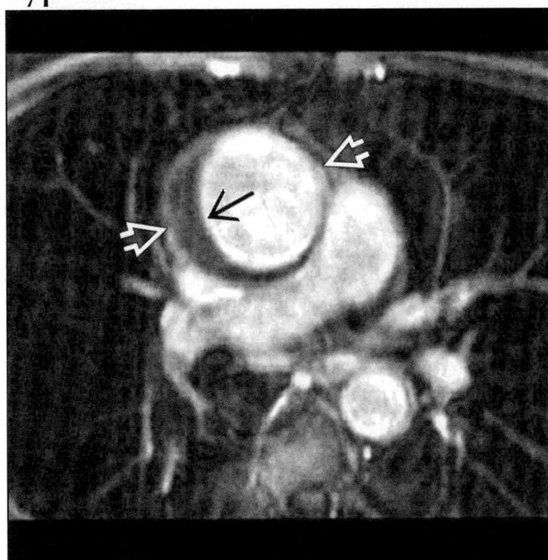

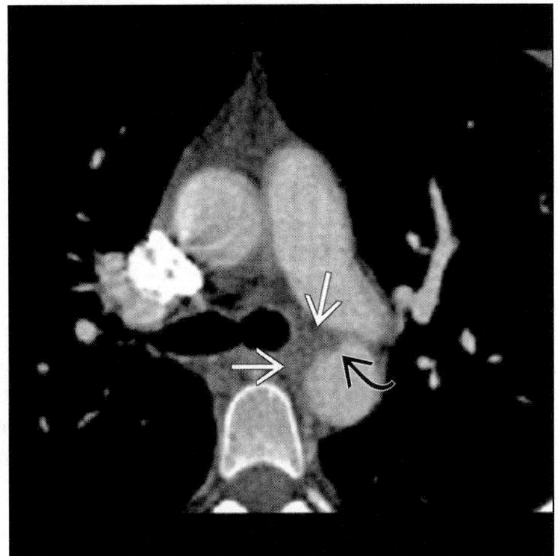

(Left) *Axial post-contrast T1WI GRE (same patient) shows corresponding low signal along the lateral wall of aorta → and resultant enlargement → of the ascending aorta.* ***(Right)*** *Axial CECT in a patient with acute trauma shows mural irregularity of the descending aortic wall → and crescentic low density →, consistent with an aortic intramural hematoma. 50-80% of cases of IMH involve the descending aorta and are often medically managed, but require close follow-up.*

Typical

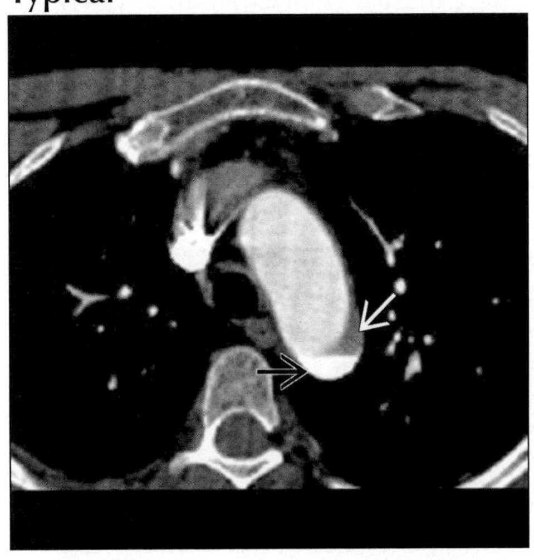

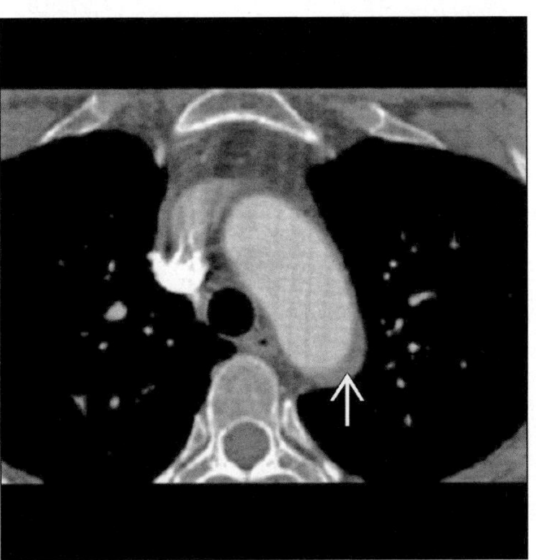

(Left) *Axial CECT shows dependent layering of contrast → with associated low density hematoma along the distal transverse arch following iatrogenic aortic injury → during a catheterization procedure.* ***(Right)*** *Axial CECT performed 48 hrs later (same patient as previous image) shows interval clearing of the contrast, but persistence of a small crescentic intramural hematoma →. Less than 30% of patients will have complete spontaneous resorption of an IMH.*

AORTIC ULCERATION

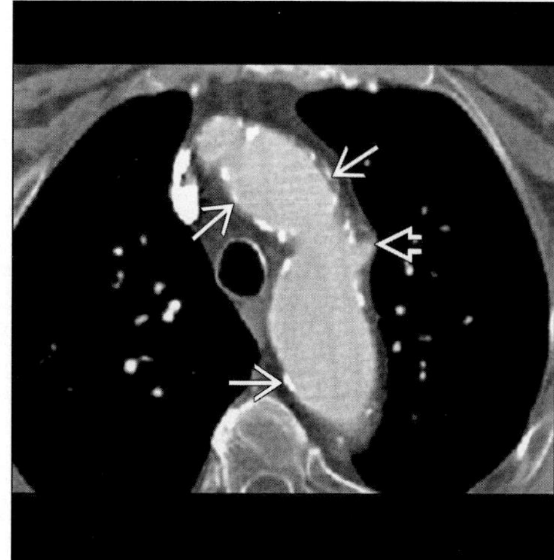

Axial CECT shows a diseased and ectatic transverse aorta with moderately heavy calcification ➡. There is a focal outpouching of contrast ➡ that projects from the lateral aortic wall and represents a penetrating ulcer.

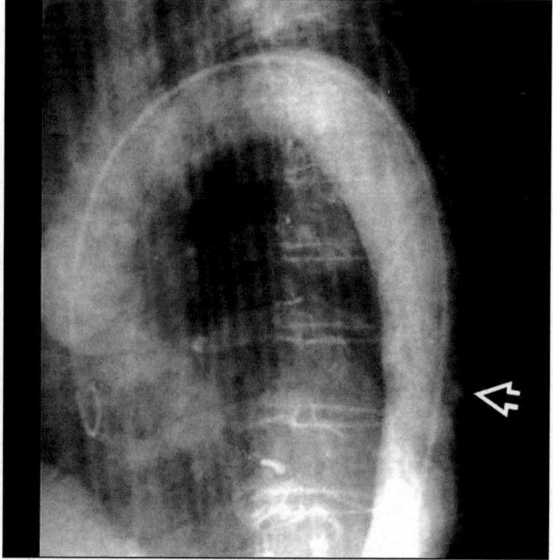

Oblique catheter angiography shows a small contrast outpouching ➡ on the wall of the descending thoracic aorta, representing an aortic ulceration. The aorta seems only mildly diseased on the aortogram.

TERMINOLOGY

Abbreviations and Synonyms

- Penetrating aortic ulcer, penetrating atherosclerotic ulcer

Definitions

- Mural ulceration that penetrates elastic lamina into media with associated aortic wall hematoma
- Distinct pathologic process from aneurysm or classic aortic dissection; one cause of acute aortic syndrome

IMAGING FINDINGS

General Features

- Best diagnostic clue
  - Focal involvement of aorta; crater-like outpouching of lumen, associated with subintimal hematoma and atherosclerotic disease
    - More common in descending thoracic aorta
- Location
  - Most common in descending aorta (94%)
  - Ascending aorta (11%)
  - Multiple ulcers in 10%
- Morphology: Focal outpouching of aortic wall; jagged edges, usually extensive aortic atheroma
- Intramural hematoma; often adjacent to ulceration, with short extension
- Severe atherosclerosis of surrounding aorta

CT Findings

- NECT: Extensive atherosclerosis, possible hyperdense intramural hematoma, displaced intimal calcifications, ulcer crater not demonstrated
- CECT: Focal defect within mural thrombus/plaque with acute margins
- CTA: Same as contrast enhanced CT
- Focal ulceration of aortic wall
- Contrast collection outside expected aortic lumen
- Thickening and enhancement of aortic wall
- Intramural hematoma
- Inward intimal displacement; intimal calcifications
  - Displacement of intimal calcification indicates sub-intimal hemorrhage
- Reconstructions may be helpful to delineate ulcer and any mural abnormalities

DDx: Aortic Ulceration

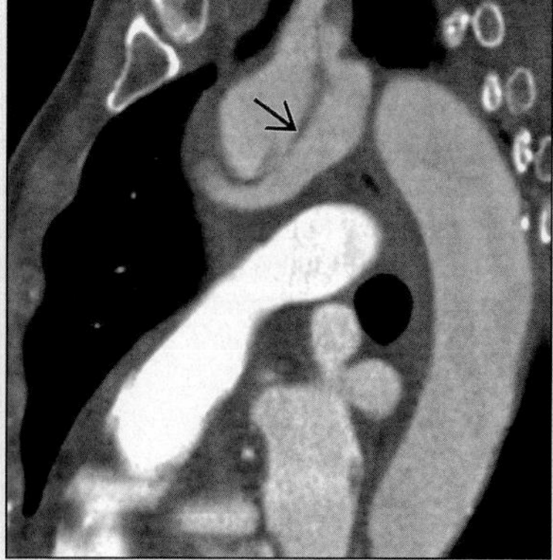

Aortic Dissection

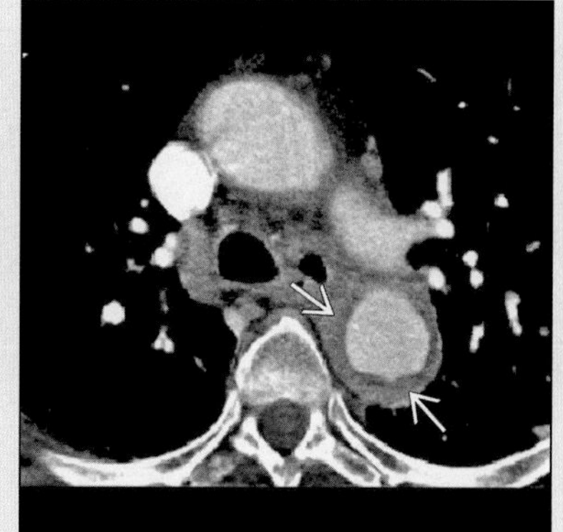

Mural Thrombus

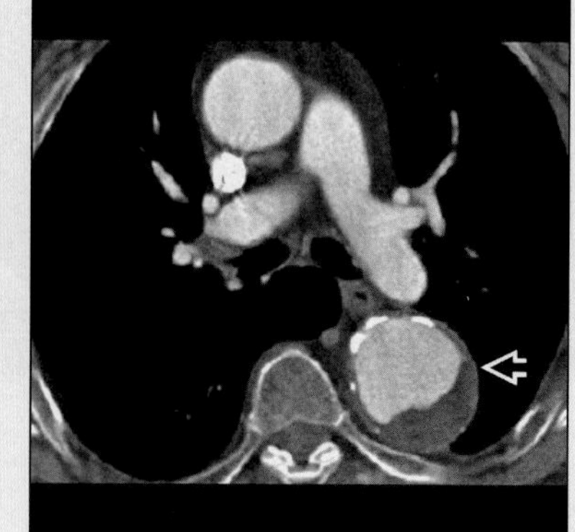

Aneurysm

AORTIC ULCERATION

Key Facts

Terminology

- Penetrating aortic ulcer, penetrating atherosclerotic ulcer
- Ulcerating atherosclerotic lesion penetrates elastic lamina; associated with hematoma formation within aortic media

Imaging Findings

- CECT/CTA best imaging tool
- Best diagnostic clue: Focal aortic involvement with crater-like luminal outpouching
  - Intramural hematoma often adjacent to ulceration
  - Usually evidence of severe adjacent atherosclerosis
  - Usually in descending thoracic aorta
- Imaging may reveal pleural/pericardial fluid, mediastinal hematoma, or pseudoaneurysm

Pathology

- Unknown true incidence; reported in 2-8% of symptomatic patients with suspected acute aortic syndrome

Clinical Issues

- Rate of aortic rupture as high as 40%
- Penetrating ulcer with initial diameter of ≥20 mm or depth of ≥10 mm has high risk of disease progression
- Penetrating ulcer in ascending, transverse and proximal descending aorta higher risk
- Treatment options include
  - Medical therapy (antihypertensive), close monitoring if pain resolves and no radiological evidence of progression
  - Surgical repair if ascending aorta involved
  - Endovascular therapy with aortic stent-graft

MR Findings

- T1 C+: In rare cases, chronic thrombus may enhance with contrast
- MRA
  - Similar findings to CECT/CTA
    - Wall may not be as well visualized as by CECT, depending upon sequence
- Superior to CT in differentiating acute intramural hematoma from atherosclerotic plaque and intraluminal thrombus
- Focal ulcerated contrast collection in aortic wall
- Intramural hematoma well seen
- Gadolinium enhancement improves recognition of ulcer

Echocardiographic Findings

- Transesophageal echocardiography
  - Focal outpouching in atherosclerotic wall; occurs in mid to distal portion of descending thoracic aorta

Ultrasonographic Findings

- Color Doppler: Focal outpouching of color, indicating flow beyond expected margin of lumen
- Intravascular ultrasound can be used to characterize plaque components

Angiographic Findings

- Conventional
  - Ulcerated lesion in descending thoracic aorta
  - Luminal irregularity from diffuse atherosclerotic plaque

Imaging Recommendations

- Best imaging tool: CTA, CECT
- Protocol advice
  - Obtain precontrast images
  - High flow rate (> 3 mL/sec for CT)
  - Compare to old studies if available
- Helical CECT recommended because of shorter examination time
- Gadolinium MR is modality of choice if iodinated contrast material contraindicated

DIFFERENTIAL DIAGNOSIS

Aortic Dissection

- Intimal flap extends across aorta; separates true and false lumens
  - False lumen may thrombose or compress true lumen
  - May have multiple fenestrations in intimal flap
- Length more extensive

Atheromatous Ulcer

- No extension beyond expected margin of aortic wall
- No hematoma present

Intramural Hematoma

- Concentrically located collection of blood within media of aortic wall
  - Hemorrhage involves vasa vasorum; localized noncommunicating intramural dissection
  - No intimal flap or ulcer crater

Mycotic Aneurysm

- More inflammatory appearance to ulcer
- Fever, elevated WBC, positive blood cultures

Pseudoaneurysm

- Usually occurs where aorta susceptible to trauma (e.g. ligamentum arteriosum, diaphragmatic hiatus, aortic root)
- Clinical history of trauma

PATHOLOGY

General Features

- General path comments
  - Location
    - Most commonly mid and distal descending thoracic aorta
    - Can occur at any point in aorta
    - Uncommon in abdominal aorta
  - Size
    - Diameter 5-25 mm
    - Depth 4-30 mm

AORTIC ULCERATION

- Etiology
  - Progression of atherosclerosis
    - Ulcer penetrates through elastic lamina and extends into media
    - Media exposed to pulsatile blood flow, causing intramural hematoma and variable degree of dissection
    - May extend into adventitia forming pseudoaneurysm, causing aortic dilatation or rupture
- Epidemiology
  - Unknown true incidence, reported in 2-8% of symptomatic patients with suspected acute aortic syndrome
  - Risk factors: Hypertension, advanced atherosclerosis, smoking history
  - Predominant age: Elderly
  - Predominant sex: Male > female
- Associated abnormalities
  - Advanced atherosclerosis
  - May have other co-existent aneurysms

Microscopic Features

- Extensive surrounding atherosclerosis
- Ulcer penetrating intima, rupturing internal elastic lamina and extending into media

Staging, Grading or Classification Criteria

- Classification based on Stanford classification of aortic dissection
  - Type A indicates involvement of ascending aorta
  - Type B indicates involvement of descending aorta
- Well-defined ulcer crater in aortic wall, subadventitial pseudoaneurysm extending beyond aortic wall, or transmural rupture with extra-aortic hematoma

CLINICAL ISSUES

Presentation

- Most common signs/symptoms: Similar to acute aortic dissection
- Maybe asymptomatic, patients commonly have hypertension, hyperlipidemia
- Symptoms in thoracic aorta
  - Sudden onset of severe chest/back pain
  - Embolization of atheroma (uncommon)
- Symptoms in abdominal aorta
  - Abdominal pain, back pain, flank pain

Demographics

- Age: Elderly
- Gender: M ≥ F

Natural History & Prognosis

- No change in 50-70% on follow-up
- May progress to dissection
- Rate of aortic rupture as high as 40%
  - Diameter of involved aortic segment maybe important risk factor for rupture
- Possibility of aortic dilation and aneurysm formation
  - Aneurysms develop in 50% of patients
  - Postulated most saccular aneurysms of aorta originate from penetrating ulcers
- Penetrating ulcer with initial diameter of ≥ 20 mm or depth of ≥ 10 mm has high risk of disease progression
- Penetrating ulcer in ascending aorta, arch, and proximal descending aorta more likely high risk
- Pain and/or increase in pleural effusion indicate disease progression

Treatment

- Medical therapy (antihypertensive agents) and close monitoring if pain resolves and no radiological evidence of progression
- Some type of intervention for larger and deeper ulcers, and continued symptoms
- Surgical intervention indications
  - Rapidly expanding aortic diameter
  - Hemodynamic instability
  - Persistent or recurring pain
  - Development of pseudoaneurysm, pericardial effusion, bloody pleural effusion or distal embolization
  - Surgical repair if ascending aorta involved
- Endovascular therapy
  - Aortic stent grafting
    - Reduces wall stress and provides stabilization of diseased aortic segment
    - Well suited for endovascular stent-graft since only very short aortic segment requires treatment

DIAGNOSTIC CHECKLIST

Consider

- Atheromatous ulcer, aortic intramural hematoma, aortic dissection, mycotic aneurysm, atherosclerotic aneurysm in differential diagnosis

Image Interpretation Pearls

- Ulcerated outpouching with associated subintimal hematoma, and atherosclerotic disease typical of penetrating aortic ulcer; usually in thoracic aorta

SELECTED REFERENCES

1. Batt M et al: Penetrating atherosclerotic ulcers of the infrarenal aorta: life-threatening lesions. Eur J Vasc Endovasc Surg. 29(1):35-42, 2005
2. Chiles C et al: Vascular diseases of the thorax: evaluation with multidetector CT. Radiol Clin North Am. 43(3):543-69, viii, 2005
3. Manghat NE et al: Multi-detector row computed tomography: imaging in acute aortic syndrome. Clin Radiol. 60(12):1256-67, 2005
4. Takahashi K et al: Multidetector CT of the thoracic aorta. Int J Cardiovasc Imaging. 21(1):141-53, 2005
5. Castaner E et al: CT in nontraumatic acute thoracic aortic disease: typical and atypical features and complications. Radiographics. 23 Spec No:S93-110, 2003
6. Eggebrecht H et al: Penetrating atherosclerotic ulcer of the aorta: treatment by endovascular stent-graft placement. Curr Opin Cardiol. 18(6):431-5, 2003
7. Macura KJ et al: Role of computed tomography and magnetic resonance imaging in assessment of acute aortic syndromes. Semin Ultrasound CT MR. 24(4):232-54, 2003

AORTIC ULCERATION

IMAGE GALLERY

Typical

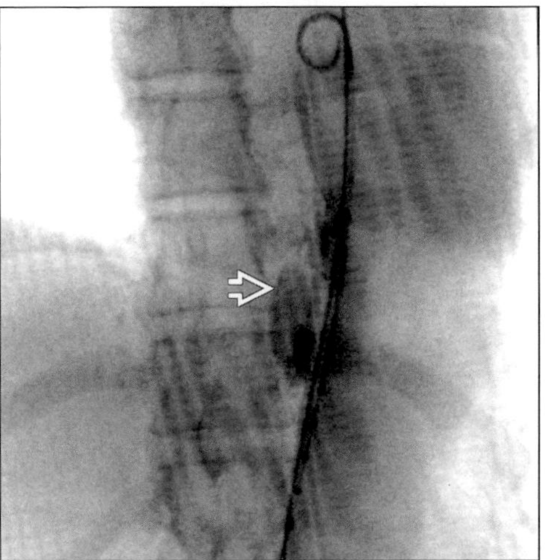

*(**Left**) Oblique CECT shows a large ulceration → in the transverse aortic arch. Additionally, the aorta has mild diffuse disease with scattered atherosclerotic calcifications →. (**Right**) DSA in a different patient shows a focal outpouching of contrast → in the descending thoracic aorta. This contrast collection persists after it has almost completely cleared from the remainder of the aorta. This abnormality could be treated with endovascular stent grafting.*

Typical

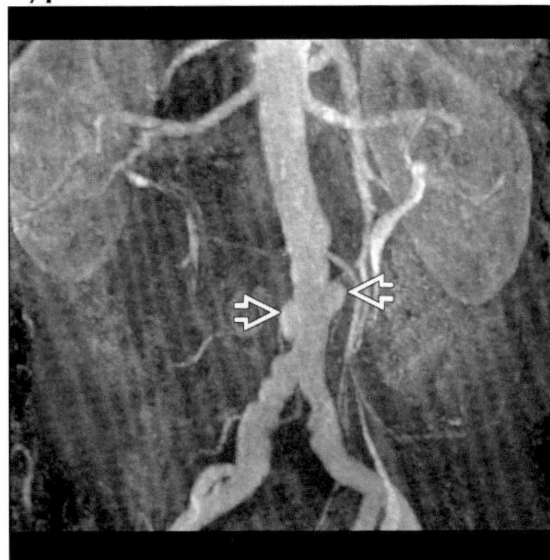

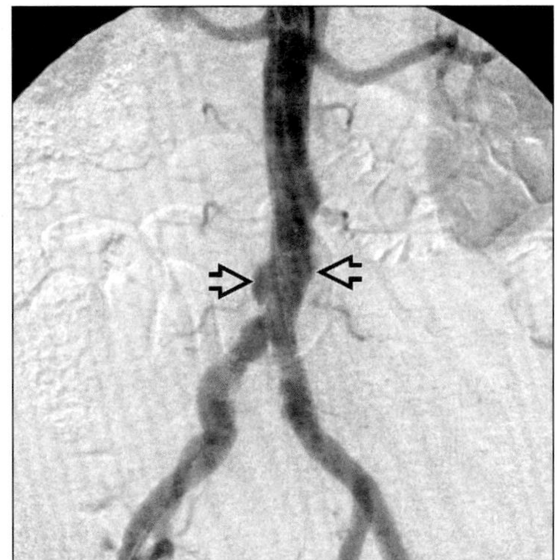

*(**Left**) Coronal MR cine shows two areas of focal outpouching → in the distal abdominal aorta. Although penetrating ulcers are uncommon in the abdominal aorta these areas are suspicious. There is also common iliac artery atherosclerotic disease. (**Right**) DSA corresponding to the previous MRA shows the outpouchings in the abdominal aorta →. There is mild common iliac artery atherosclerotic disease and more extensive disease involving the infrarenal aorta.*

Typical

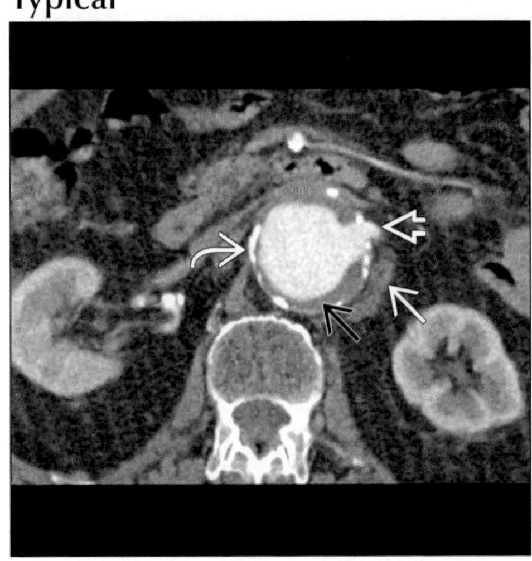

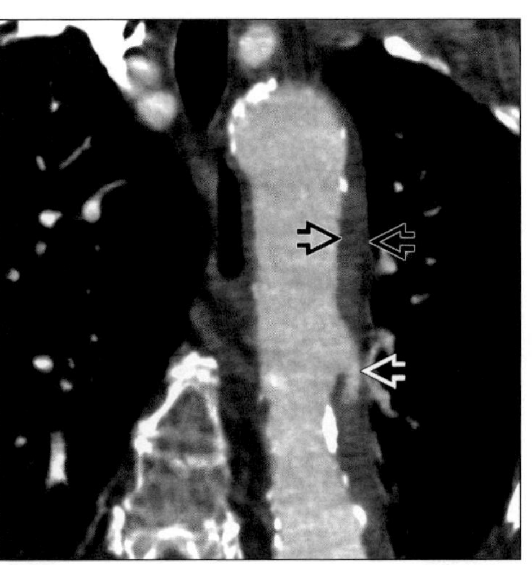

*(**Left**) Axial CECT shows contrast extending through a defect → in the mural thrombus → that lines the aortic lumen. There is calcification in the aortic wall → and an area of soft tissue density outside the aorta → which could represent bleeding. (**Right**) Coronal CECT shows atherosclerosis of the aorta with a collection of contrast → that projects outside of the expected aortic wall margins. There is also thickening of the aortic wall →. The descending aorta is typically involved.*

AORTIC DISSECTION

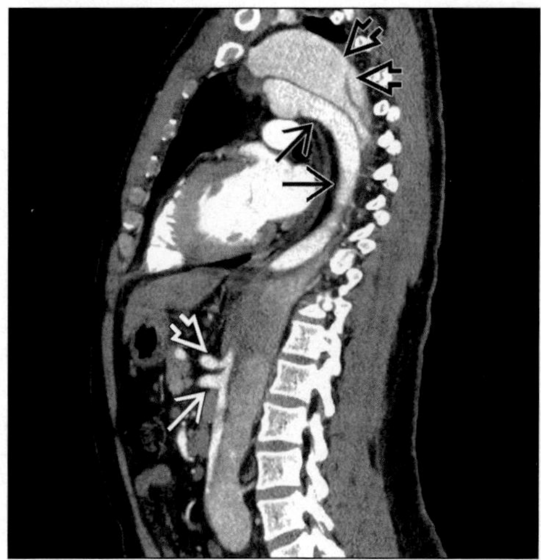

Sagittal CTA shows a dissection. True lumen ➔ is being compressed by the false lumen ➲. The celiac axis ➲ and superior mesenteric artery ➔ are being supplied by the true lumen.

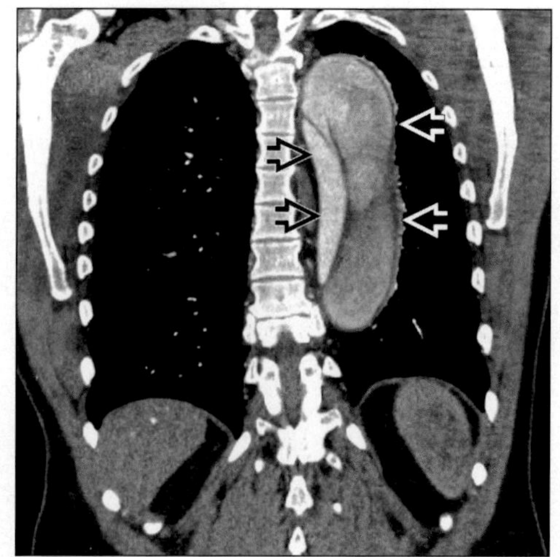

Coronal CTA shows marked compression of the true lumen ➲ by the false lumen ➲. There is partial thrombosis of the false lumen, although still with some enhancement.

TERMINOLOGY

Abbreviations and Synonyms

- Aortic dissection (AoD)

Definitions

- Blood enters media of aortic wall and splits it in a longitudinal fashion
- Stanford classification
  - Type A (60%): Involves at least ascending aorta, may or may not involve descending aorta; surgical treatment
  - Type B (40%): Limited to descending aorta; medical management
- DeBakey classification
  - Type I: Involves ascending aorta, aortic arch, and descending aorta
  - Type II: Ascending aorta
  - Type III: Descending aorta distal to the left subclavian artery

IMAGING FINDINGS

General Features

- Best diagnostic clue
  - "Double barrel" aorta with an interposed intimal flap
  - Aortic wall thickening with complete thrombosis of false lumen or intramural hematoma
  - Displacement of intimal calcification or compression or distortion of aortic lumen
- Location
  - Type A 90% within 10 cm of aortic valve
  - Type B is distal to left subclavian artery
- Additional imaging appearance
  - Imaging should evaluate great vessels, celiac, renal artery, SMA, iliac artery involvement

Radiographic Findings

- Radiography
  - Abnormal CXR (25% are normal) is nonspecific
  - Hemothorax occurs if rupture into pleural space
  - Widened mediastinum (> 8 cm)
  - Abnormal (blunted) aortic knob in 66%
  - Ring sign-displacement of aorta > 5 mm past the calcified aortic intima

DDx: Aortic Dissection

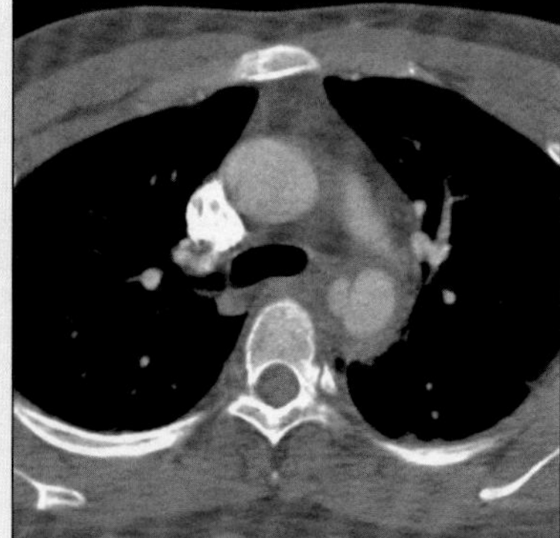

Traumatic Tear, Not Dissection

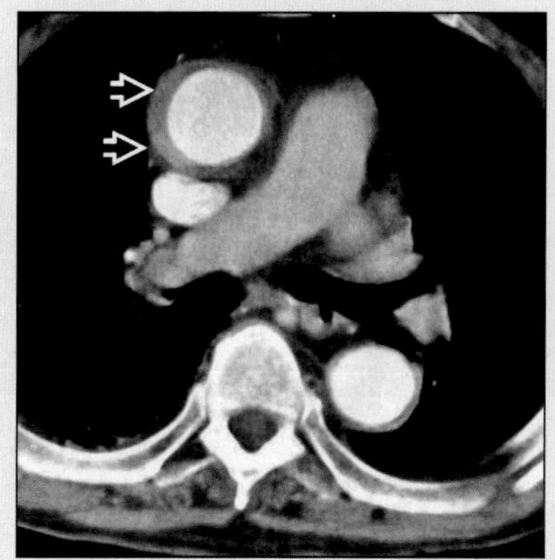

Intramural Hematoma

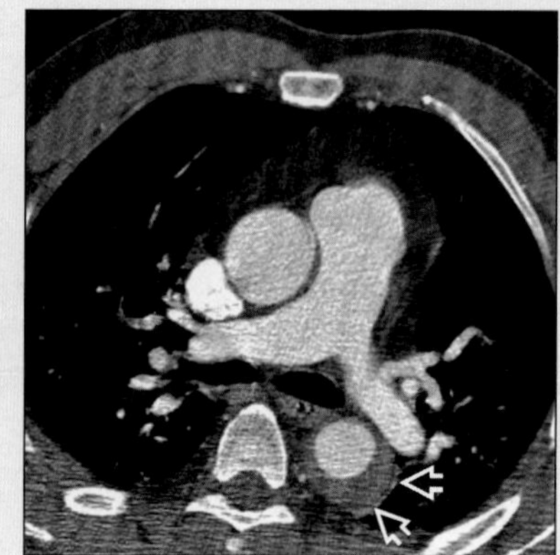

Hematoma vs. Dissection

AORTIC DISSECTION

Key Facts

Terminology

- Blood enters media of aortic wall and splits it in a longitudinal fashion
- Stanford classification
  - Type A (60%): Involves at least ascending aorta; surgical treatment
  - Type B (40%): Limited to descending aorta; medical management

Imaging Findings

- "Double barrel" aorta
- In addition to aorta, imaging should evaluate great vessels, celiac, renal artery, SMA, iliac artery involvement
- Important to exclude retrograde dissection into the aortic arch; presentation in 27% of type B dissections and associated with substantially higher mortality rates
- MR low signal intensity turbulent blood flow from the true lumen into the false lumen indicates the entry site

Clinical Issues

- Rupture of aorta
- Dissection into the pericardium with cardiac tamponade, occlusion of the coronary or supraaortic vessels, and severe aortic insufficiency with acute heart failure
- Type A: Requires surgery because of involvement of aortic root
- Type B: Control of hypertension is standard therapy

  - Left apical cap, tracheal deviation, depression of left main stem bronchus, esophageal deviation, loss of paratracheal stripe, pericardial effusion
  - Progressive aortic enlargement on serial images
    - Enlarged arch not specific for diagnosis; usually result of hypertension or atherosclerosis
    - Arch appears normal in 25% of cases
  - Apparent displacement of intimal calcification may be a projectional artifact

CT Findings

- NECT
  - Irregularity of aortic wall
  - Intramural or periaortic acute thrombus, cuff or crescent of high attenuation
  - Widening of aorta
  - Hyperattenuating mediastinal, pericardial, or pleural fluid collections
- CECT
  - Intimal flap between true and false lumens
  - Delayed flow in false lumen, and compression of true lumen by expanding false lumen
  - Identifies intraluminal thrombus, pericardial effusion
  - Infradiaphragmatic ischemic complications
  - Complete thrombosis and reduced flow in false lumen decreases risk of subsequent aortic dilatation
  - Atherosclerotic ulcer may progress to dissection
  - Important to exclude retrograde dissection into aortic arch; seen in 27% of type B dissections; this is associated with higher mortality rates (43%)

MR Findings

- T1WI
  - Shows site of intimal tear, type and extent of dissection, presence of aortic insufficiency
  - Signal intensity within false lumen is variable, depending on the blood flow, the presence, age, and composition of thrombus, and the pulse sequence
  - False lumen flow is slower, therefore the flap may be outlined by a signal void on one side and an increased intraluminal signal on the other
    - Slow flow in false lumen may resemble thrombus
  - Flap may be outlined by signal void on one side and increased intraluminal signal on other
  - Evaluation of abdominal artery involvement
  - Serial evaluation of progression of the initial dissection, or aneurysm formation
  - Identification of aortoannular ectasia
- T2* GRE
  - Intimal flap- low or medium signal intensity between two high-signal intensity blood-containing channels
  - Reentry site depicted by low-signal intensity turbulent flow between true and false lumens
  - False lumen with slow blood flow and/or thrombotic material; medium to low signal intensity

Echocardiographic Findings

- Echocardiogram
  - Transesophageal echocardiography (TEE)
    - Most important finding: Presence of an undulating intimal flap within aortic lumen
    - Identify entry site, presence of thrombus in false lumen, abnormal flow characteristics, involvement of coronary and arch vessels, pericardial effusion, and aortic valve regurgitation
    - False positives: Calcified aorta producing images resembling an intimal flap
- Color Doppler: Identifies flow in false lumen, site of intimal tear, and presence or absence of aortic insufficiency

Angiographic Findings

- Conventional
  - Evaluate extent of dissection, site of intimal tears, aortic valve regurgitation, coronary artery involvement, and filling of branch vessels
  - False lumen visualized in 87% intimal flap in 70%, and site of intimal tear in 56%
  - Indirect signs of AoD
    - Compression of true lumen by false lumen
    - Abnormalities of branch vessels
  - False negative angiogram due to
    - Thrombosis of false lumen

AORTIC DISSECTION

Imaging Recommendations

- CT scan highly accurate, slightly less accurate for ascending aorta dissection
- MR well-suited for follow-up
- TEE possible in most patients, including unstable
  - Highly dependent on operator's experience
  - Not used if esophageal varicosities or stenosis
  - Limited view of dissection

DIFFERENTIAL DIAGNOSIS

Thrombosed Aneurysm

- Calcification outside aortic shadow
- Large aorta and aortic lumen size

Aortic Wall Hematoma

- Hemorrhage within wall with no identifiable intimal flap or false lumen
- Caused by bleeding from vasa vasorum into media
- Imaging: Hyperdense aortic wall

Penetrating Aortic Ulcer

- Perforation of aortic wall in region of ulcerated atherosclerotic plaque
- Most common in descending aorta
- Clinical symptoms may mimic AoD
- May progress to dissection

Syndromes Associated with AoD

- Marfan syndrome, Ehlers-Danlos syndrome, Bicuspid aortic valve

PATHOLOGY

General Features

- General path comments
  - Dissections almost exclusively originate in thoracic aorta and secondarily involve abdominal aorta
  - Smooth muscle myosin heavy chain marker helpful in diagnosis
- Etiology
  - Medial degeneration is associated with many diseases that predispose to dissection
    - Atherosclerosis, hypertension (70%), structural collagen disorder (Marfan's, Ehlers-Danlos), congenital (aortic coarctation, bicuspid or unicuspid valve), pregnancy, collagen vascular disease (rare)
  - Syphilitic aortitis
  - Crack cocaine use may lead to AoD
  - Iatrogenic: Cardiac surgery, valve replacements, coronary artery bypass, or percutaneous catheter placement
- Epidemiology: If untreated, 33% die within 24h; 50% within 48h

Gross Pathologic & Surgical Features

- Tear in the intimal layer, leading to formation and propagation of subintimal hematoma
  - 5-10% are without intimal tear; dissection attributed to rupture of the aortic vasa vasorum
- Diseases that weaken aortic wall predispose to AoD

CLINICAL ISSUES

Presentation

- Most common signs/symptoms
  - Sudden onset of ripping or tearing chest pain
  - Anterior chest pain: Ascending AoD
  - Neck or jaw pain: Aortic arch dissection
  - Back tearing or ripping pain: Descending AoD
  - Myocardial infarction
  - 50% of AoD in women < 40 y related to pregnancy
- Sudden onset of aortic insufficiency
- Neurologic deficits: 20% of cases
- Ischemic extremity

Demographics

- Age: 75% in 40-70 years; peak at 50-65 years
- Gender: M:F, 3:1
- Ethnicity: African-Americans > Caucasians > Asians

Natural History & Prognosis

- Rupture of aorta
- Dissection into pericardium with cardiac tamponade, occlusion of coronary or supraaortic vessels, severe aortic insufficiency with acute heart failure
- 21% patients die before hospital admission
- < 10% of untreated patients with type A live 1 year
- Acute AoD: Diagnosed within 14 days
- Chronic AoD: Diagnosed after 14 days

Treatment

- Type A: Surgery due to involvement of aortic root
- Type B: Medical control of hypertension is standard
  - Surgery in complicated cases
    - Mesenteric, renal, extremity ischemia; rupture, aneurysmal enlargement of false lumen
- Percutaneous therapy for complicated non-surgical patients with type B dissections
  - Aortic stent graft
  - Fenestration of luminal flap
- Type A: Medically treated mortality 60%; surgically treated 30%
- Type B: Medically treated mortality 10%; surgically treated 30%

SELECTED REFERENCES

1. Liu Q et al: Three-dimensional contrast-enhanced MR angiography of aortic dissection: a pictorial essay. Radiographics. 27(5):1311-21, 2007
2. García A et al: MR angiographic evaluation of complications in surgically treated type A aortic dissection. Radiographics. 26(4):981-92, 2006
3. Bortone AS et al: Endovascular treatment of thoracic aortic disease: four years of experience. Circulation. 110(11 Suppl 1):II262-7, 2004
4. Batra P et al: Pitfalls in the diagnosis of thoracic aortic dissection at CT angiography. Radiographics. 20(2):309-20, 2000

IMAGE GALLERY

Typical

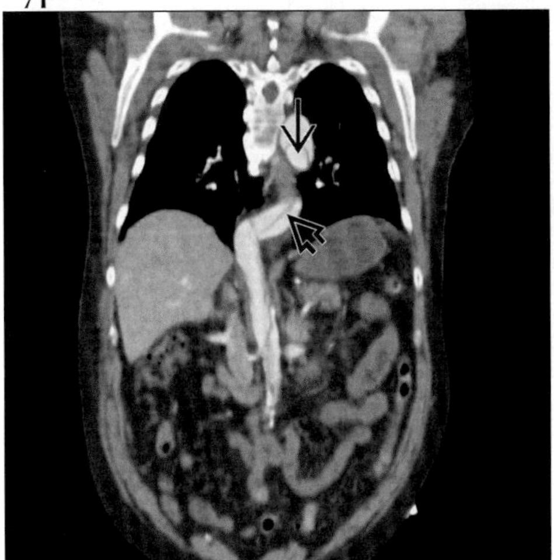

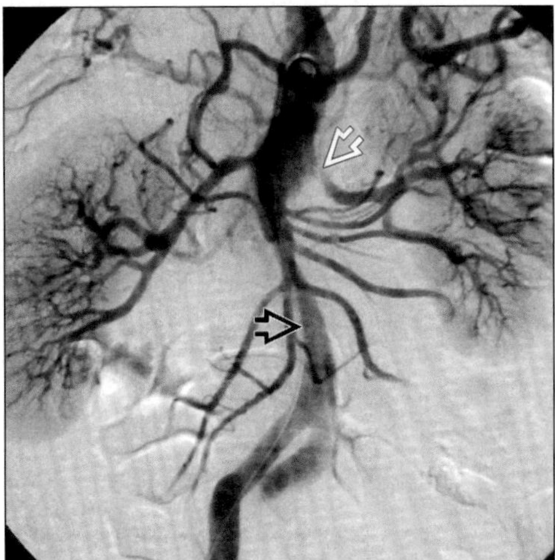

(Left) *Coronal CECT shows a dissection flap extending from the aortic arch ➙ into the descending aorta. The flap ➪ is spiraling down the aorta, with involvement of the aortic branches.* ***(Right)*** *DSA shows bizarre appearance of abdominal aorta. Marked smooth narrowing of the infrarenal aorta ➪ with change in caliber and contrast-enhancement. Narrowing of left renal artery ➪. May be related to involvement by dissection.*

Typical

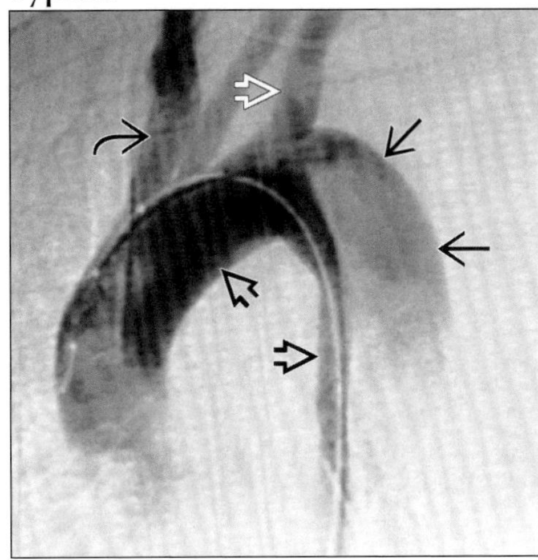

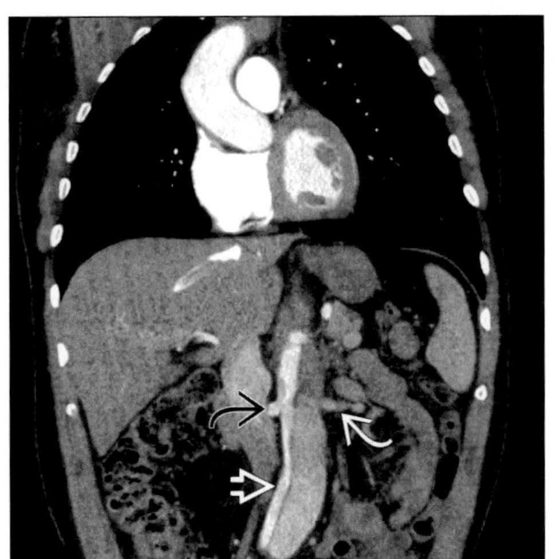

(Left) *Oblique catheter angiography shows both the true lumen ➪ and the false lumen ➙. There is a flap in the innominate artery ↷ and decreased flow in other great vessels ➪.* ***(Right)*** *Coronal CTA shows compression of true lumen in the abdominal aorta ➪. Right renal artery is supplied by the true lumen ↷. Left renal artery ↷ originates from the false lumen.*

Typical

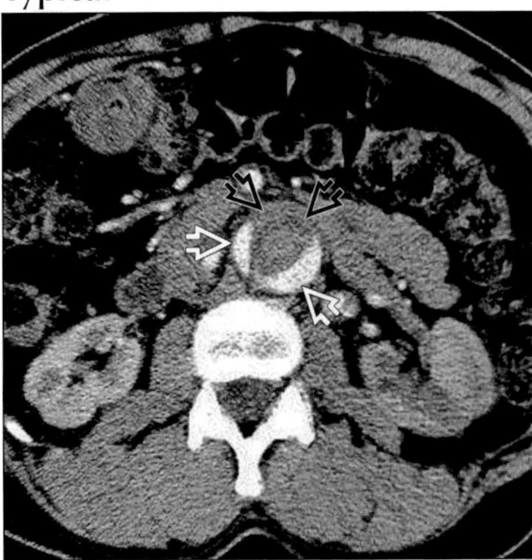

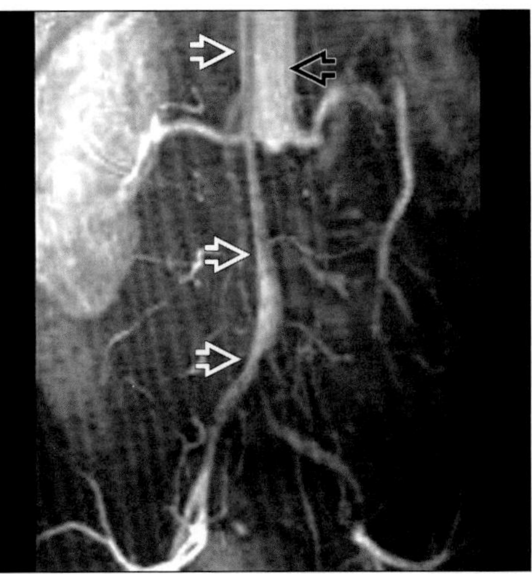

(Left) *Axial CECT shows a chronic dissection of the abdominal aorta. There are two regions of perfusion ➪ and the rest of the aorta is thrombosed ➪.* ***(Right)*** *Coronal MR cine shows the false lumen ➪ supplying the left renal artery. The small compressed true lumen ➪ supplies the right renal artery. The false lumen is thrombosed in the infrarenal area.*

TAKAYASU ARTERITIS

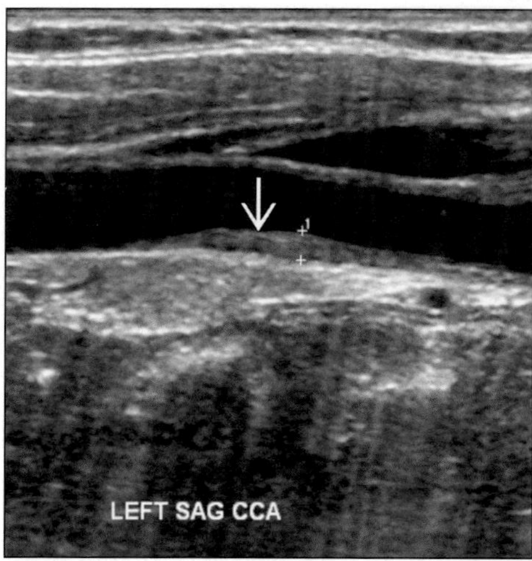

Sagittal grayscale ultrasound shows patchy thickening ➡ of the intima of the carotid artery.

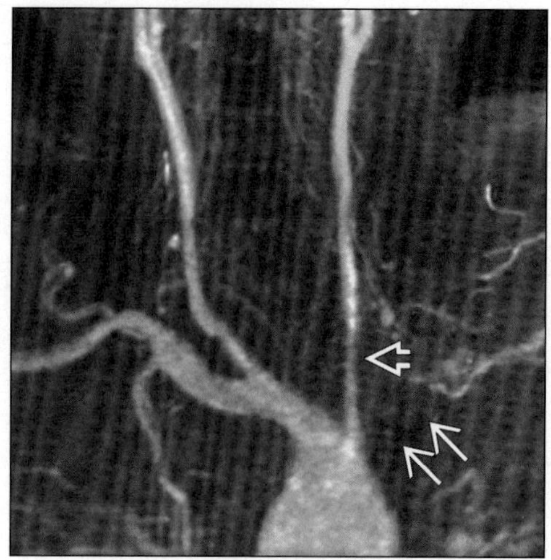

Coronal MRA of the great vessels shows occlusion of the proximal subclavian artery ➡ and irregular diffuse narrowing ➡ of the left common carotid artery.

TERMINOLOGY

Abbreviations and Synonyms

- Takayasu arteritis, pulseless disease, aortic arch syndrome, reverse coarctation, young female arteritis

Definitions

- Granulomatous inflammatory vasculitis affects walls of medium and large vessels, especially aorta and branches
  - Described in 1908 by a Japanese ophthalmologist
- Diagnosis may be problematic and delayed due to smoldering nature of disease

IMAGING FINDINGS

General Features

- Best diagnostic clue: Smooth narrowing of aorta and major vessels
- Location
  - Aorta and branches; left subclavian most common
  - Occasional pulmonary artery involvement
  - Distribution usually patchy, symmetric great vessel distribution common
- Morphology: Wall thickening of large and medium vessels

Radiographic Findings

- Radiography: Chest radiograph may show premature calcification of the aorta and rib notching due to formation of collateral vessels

CT Findings

- CECT
  - Great vessel changes
    - Stenosis or ostial arch vessel occlusion most common
    - Wall thickening, often concentric; wall may enhance
    - Aneurysm may be present
    - Calcification (dystrophic) of wall, different than arteriosclerotic plaque
  - Location: Aorta, brachiocephalic, subclavian, carotid, renal, and pulmonary arteries
  - Distribution patchy, symmetrical involvement of great vessels common

DDx: Asymmetric Vessel Wall Thickening

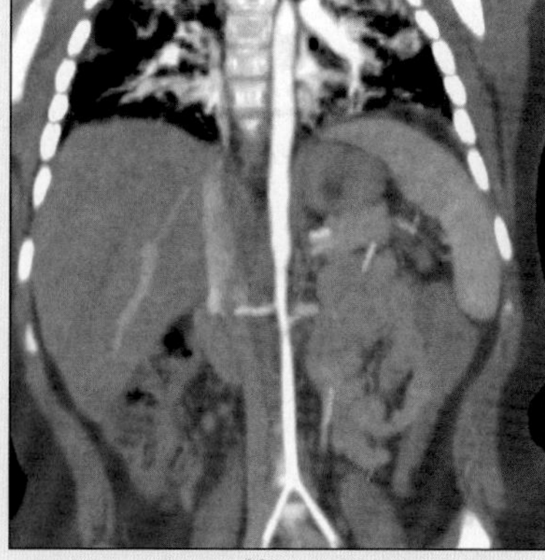

Neurofibromatosis

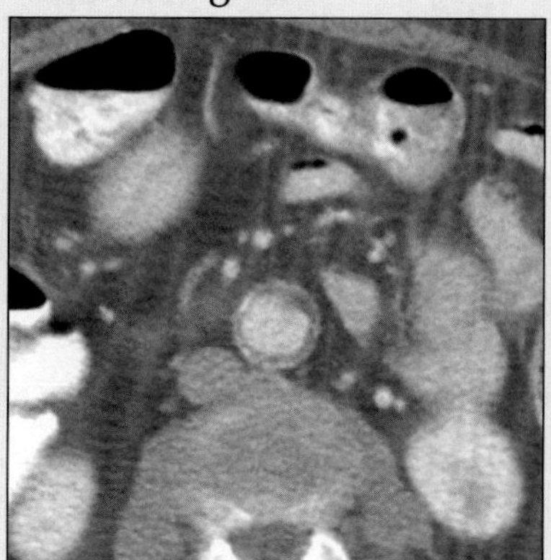

Atherosclerosis

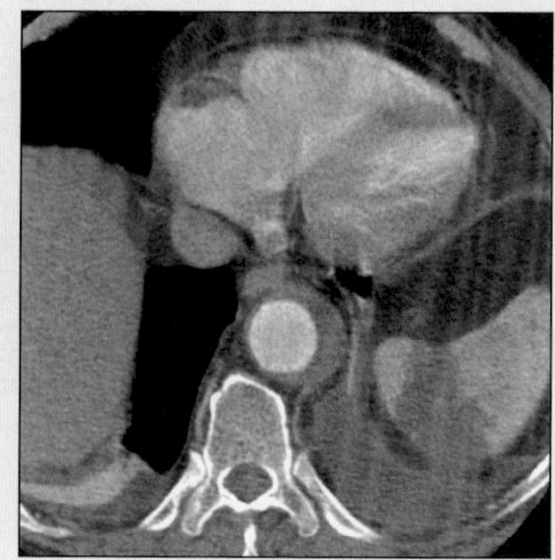

Intramural Hematoma

TAKAYASU ARTERITIS

Key Facts

Terminology
- Granulomatous inflammatory vasculitis affects walls of medium and large vessels, especially aorta and branches

Imaging Findings
- Best diagnostic clue: Smooth narrowing of aorta and major vessels
- Occasional pulmonary artery involvement
- Distribution usually patchy, symmetric great vessel distribution common

Top Differential Diagnoses
- Aortic Coarctation
- Other Vasculitis
- Aortic Aneurysm
- Fibromuscular Dysplasia
- Middle Aortic Syndrome

Pathology
- Most common in Asian countries
- Patchy thickening of large and medium size vessels

Clinical Issues
- Early phase inflammatory or prepulseless phase
- Late phase occlusive or pulseless
- Age < 30 in 90% of patients
- Gender: M:F = 1:8, but may be less female predominant in non-Asian countries
- Morbidity and mortality due to hypertension and stroke
- Corticosteroids are mainstay of therapy

- CTA: Multiplanar reconstruction useful for evaluation of wall thickness and stenosis

MR Findings
- T1WI
  - Great vessel changes similar to CT
    - Calcification less well-demonstrated than CT
  - Enhancement of wall on fat-suppressed post-contrast images suggests active disease
- MRA: Areas of focal stenosis or occlusion involving the aorta and great vessels

Nuclear Medicine Findings
- PET
  - May show increased activity in areas of active inflammation
  - Decreasing activity may be useful to monitor treatment response

Ultrasonographic Findings
- Grayscale Ultrasound
  - Shows thickening of carotid artery walls
  - May distinguish from atherosclerosis by paucity of plaque formation

Angiographic Findings
- Conventional
  - Focal areas of narrowing and occasionally dilatation
    - Aortic involvement in 75%; abdominal aorta in 53%
    - Left subclavian in 55%; right subclavian in 38%; left common carotid in 30%; right common carotid in 15%; renal artery in 38%; coronary artery in 15%
    - Pulmonary arteries may be involved (15-70% depending on series)
    - Mesenteric involvement occasionally, especially superior mesenteric artery
  - Stenotic areas focal, smooth
  - Aneurysms in 15%
  - Lesions often symmetric in great vessels
  - Distribution of lesions often patchy

Imaging Recommendations
- Best imaging tool
  - CT and MR have generally replaced angiography for diagnosis
    - Angiography used when percutaneous therapy is anticipated
- Protocol advice: Multiplanar and volumetric reconstructions may be valuable to assess wall thickness and occlusions

DIFFERENTIAL DIAGNOSIS

Aortic Coarctation
- Characteristic location in post-ductal variety is at ligamentum arteriosus
- Rib notching common

Other Vasculitis
- Giant cell or temporal arteritis typically affects large and medium size vessels in older patients

Aortic Aneurysm
- Occurs in men more than women, most > 40 years
- Mural calcification common; wall thickening eccentric and due to thrombus

Fibromuscular Dysplasia
- Artery commonly beaded; multiple arteries involved
- Spares aorta

Middle Aortic Syndrome
- Neurofibromatosis type 1: Dural ectasia, ribbon ribs
- William syndrome: Genetic disorder: Elfin facial features, neonatal hypercalcemia, supravalvular aortic stenosis, behavioral disorder
- Rubella more often affects middle and distal aorta

Kawasaki Disease
- Typically younger age with predominance in coronary arteries
- Mucocutaneous lymph node syndrome: Vasculitis of unknown etiology

TAKAYASU ARTERITIS

PATHOLOGY

General Features

- Genetics
  - May have hereditary component but not confirmed
    - Postulated link with various human leukocyte antigens (HLA) subtypes, HLA-B22
- Etiology: Unknown but may be CD4 T-cell mediated
- Epidemiology
  - Most common in Asian countries
    - 6 per 1,000 persons; 1 person per 1,000 in United States
  - Japanese: Higher incidence of aortic arch involvement
  - India: Higher incidence of thoracic and abdominal involvement
  - US: Higher incidence of great vessel involvement
- Associated abnormalities: Tuberculosis has been postulated as a cause in developing countries

Gross Pathologic & Surgical Features

- Patchy thickening of the large and medium size vessels
- Ridged, tree-bark appearance to intima

Microscopic Features

- Mononuclear infiltration of the adventitia early
- Cuffing of vasa vasorum
- Granulomatous changes in the tunica media
- Thickening and fibrosis of intima and media late

CLINICAL ISSUES

Presentation

- Most common signs/symptoms
  - Early phase inflammatory or prepulseless phase
    - Fever, tachycardia, fatigue (40%)
    - Pain of involved vessels (e.g., carotodynia)
    - Bruits; hypertension
    - Aortic insufficiency from dilated aortic root
  - Late phase occlusive or pulseless
    - Follows early phase by 5-20 years
    - Type 1: Involves arch vessels and is classic pulseless disease
    - Type 2: Involves aorta and arch vessels
    - Type 3: Involves aorta and may produce coarctation
    - Type 4: Involves aortic dilatation
    - Type 3 is most common (65% of patients)
    - Stroke; mesenteric ischemia; claudication; congestive heart failure
  - American College of Rheumatology (3 of 6 needed for diagnosis)
    - Age less than 40
    - Claudication of extremities
    - Decreased pulses of either brachial artery
    - Difference of at least 10 mm Hg in systolic blood pressure between arms
    - Bruit over one or both subclavian arteries or abdominal aorta
    - Radiographic narrowing or occlusion of aorta, great vessels, or large arteries in upper or lower extremities
- Other signs/symptoms
  - Often asymmetric pulses rather than truly pulseless
  - Retinopathy
  - Pulmonary hypertension in patients with pulmonary artery involvement

Demographics

- Age
  - Age < 30 in 90% of patients
  - Most common in 2nd and 3rd decade of life
- Gender: M:F = 1:8, but may be less female predominant in non-Asian countries

Natural History & Prognosis

- Morbidity and mortality are due to hypertension and stroke
  - Congestive heart failure primary cause of death
- 15 year survival 90-95%
- Minority have self-limited symptoms
  - 20% have monophasic episode and remit

Treatment

- Corticosteroids are mainstay of therapy
  - Cyclophosphamide and methotrexate are second-line
- Angioplasty or surgical bypass are options for narrowing or occlusion
  - Angioplasty should not be performed when the disease is active
  - Angioplasty usually performed when sedimentation rate is normal
- Stents have high failure rate

DIAGNOSTIC CHECKLIST

Consider

- Takayasu arteritis in a young woman with apparent atherosclerosis
- Takayasu arteritis in a young women with apparent coarctation at an unusual site

Image Interpretation Pearls

- Gadolinium-enhancement of the vessel wall may indicate the extent of disease activity
- PET scanning may be useful to determine disease activity

SELECTED REFERENCES

1. Kobayashi Y et al: Aortic wall inflammation due to Takayasu arteritis imaged with 18F-FDG PET coregistered with enhanced CT. J Nucl Med. 46(6):917-22, 2005
2. Teoh MK: Takayasu's arteritis with renovascular hypertension: results of surgical treatment. Cardiovasc Surg. 7(6):626-32, 1999
3. Tyagi S et al: Balloon angioplasty for renovascular hypertension in Takayasu's arteritis. Am Heart J. 125(5 Pt 1):1386-93, 1993
4. Pajari R et al: Treatment of Takayasu's arteritis: an analysis of 29 operated patients. Thorac Cardiovasc Surg. 34(3):176-81, 1986

IMAGE GALLERY

Typical

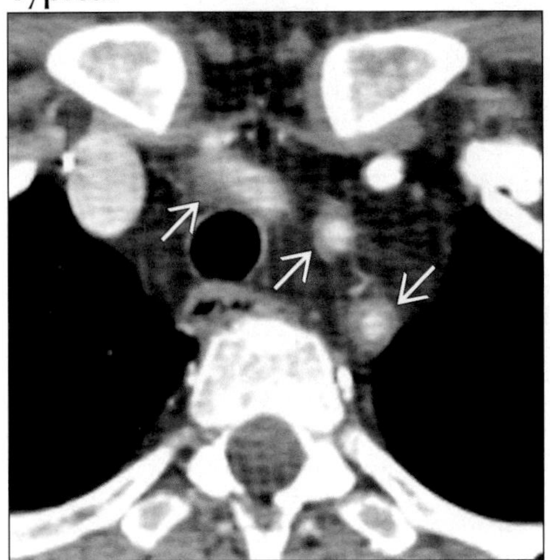

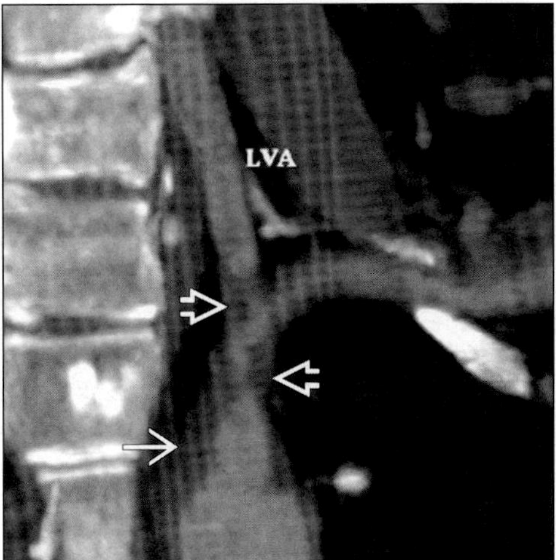

(Left) *Axial CECT shows diffuse circumferential thickening ➡ of the brachiocephalic, left common carotid and left subclavian arteries.* ***(Right)*** *Coronal CTA shows diffuse circumferential wall thickening ➡ affecting the aorta, left subclavian and vertebral arteries with focal stenoses ➡ at the origins of the left subclavian and vertebral arteries.*

Typical

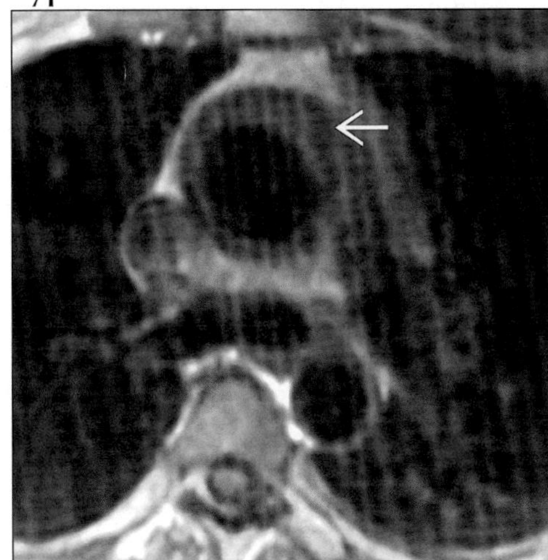

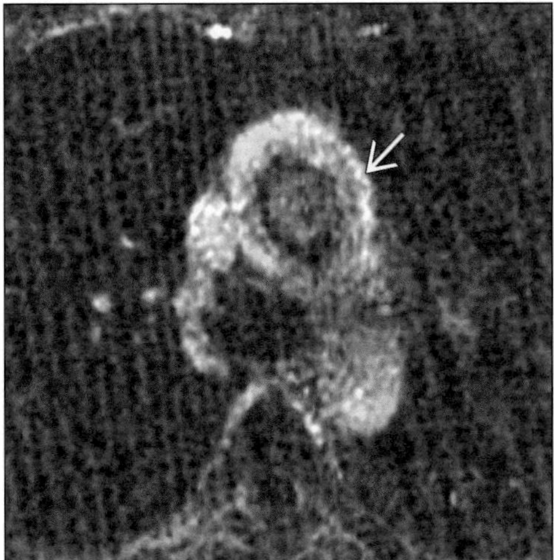

(Left) *Axial T1WI MR shows diffuse circumferential thickening ➡ of the wall of the ascending aorta.* ***(Right)*** *Axial T1WI FS MR following Gadolinium administration shows diffuse enhancement ➡ of the thickened wall of the ascending aorta. Wall enhancement such as this suggests active disease.*

Typical

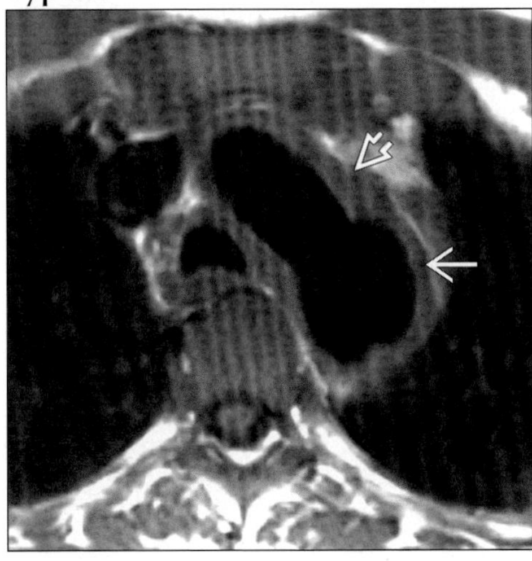

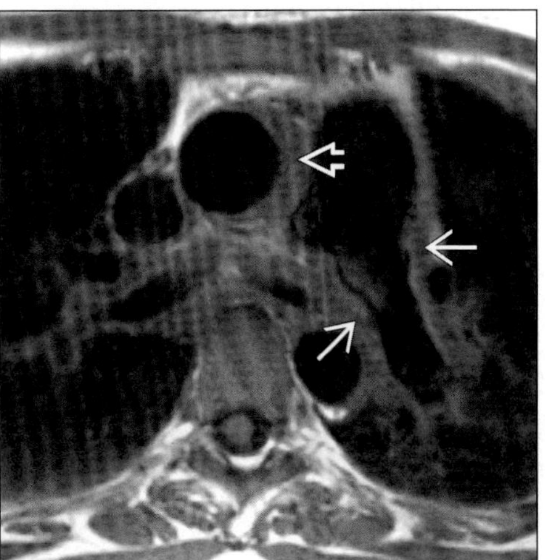

(Left) *Axial T1WI MR shows circumferential wall thickening ➡ of the arch of the aorta with focal aneurysm ➡ of the arch.* ***(Right)*** *Axial T1WI MR shows diffuse thickening of the ascending aorta ➡ and the pulmonary artery ➡. Patients with Takayasu arteritis who have pulmonary artery involvement may develop pulmonary arterial hypertension.*

GIANT CELL ARTERITIS

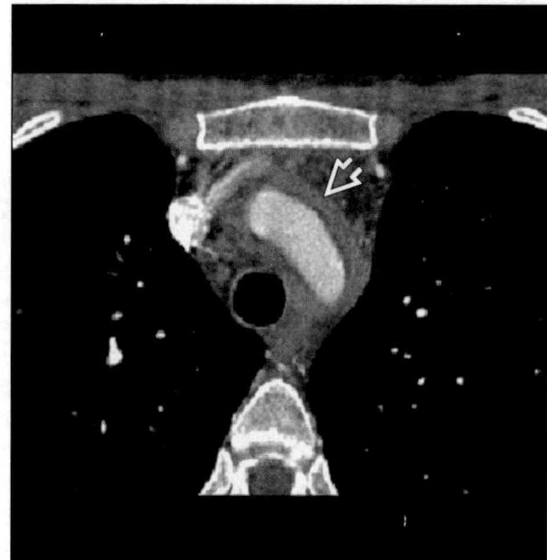

Axial CTA shows circumferential soft tissue thickening of aortic arch in a patient with giant cell arteritis (GCA). This represents an inflammatory reaction resulting in aortic mural thickening.

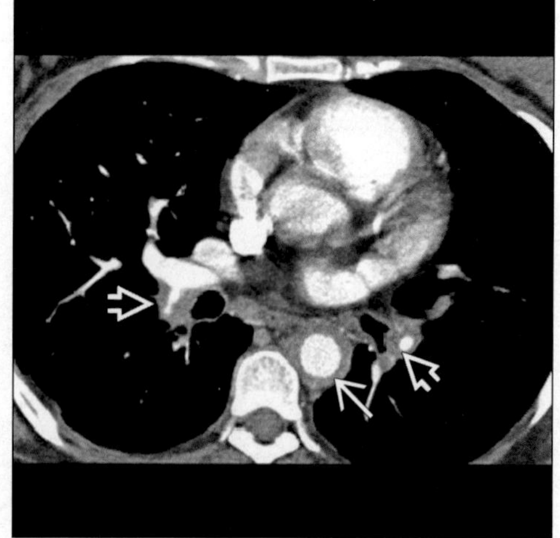

Axial CTA in a different patient shows irregular mural thickening of the descending thoracic aorta and the pulmonary arteries. Mural thickening represents a common sequela of inflammatory arteritis.

TERMINOLOGY

Abbreviations and Synonyms

- Giant cell arteritis (GCA)
- Temporal arteritis
- Cranial arteritis

Definitions

- Systemic granulomatous inflammatory vasculitis involving media of medium to large-sized arteries

IMAGING FINDINGS

General Features

- Best diagnostic clue
  - Smooth, bilateral tapering and stenosis/occlusion of subclavian and/or axillary arteries
  - Interspersed areas of mild luminal dilatation
  - Mural inflammation; vessel wall thickening and enhancement
- Location
  - Most commonly limited to extracranial carotid vessels (propensity for superficial temporal artery)
  - Rarely, thoracic/abdominal aorta, coronary, vertebral, subclavian, axillary, brachial, mesenteric, renal, iliac, or femoral arteries
- Morphology: Indistinguishable from Takayasu arteritis but latter more common in younger patients

CT Findings

- CTA
  - Often used in acute setting to exclude complications of large-vessel involvement
    - Aortic aneurysm, aortic dissection, intramural hematoma, acute luminal occlusion, coronary stenosis
  - Circumferential mural thickening
  - Limited utility in differentiation of mural thickening due to GCA involvement from that of atherosclerosis
  - May not demonstrate vessel wall enhancement

MR Findings

- T1WI: Spin-echo "black-blood" technique renders mural thickening conspicuous
- T2WI: Increased T2-signal intensity at site of vascular mural thickening indicates associated edema: Active vasculitis

DDx: Vasculitis

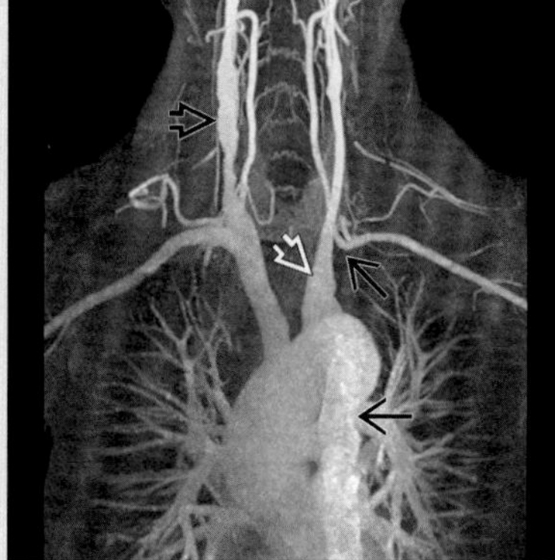

Takayasu Arteritis

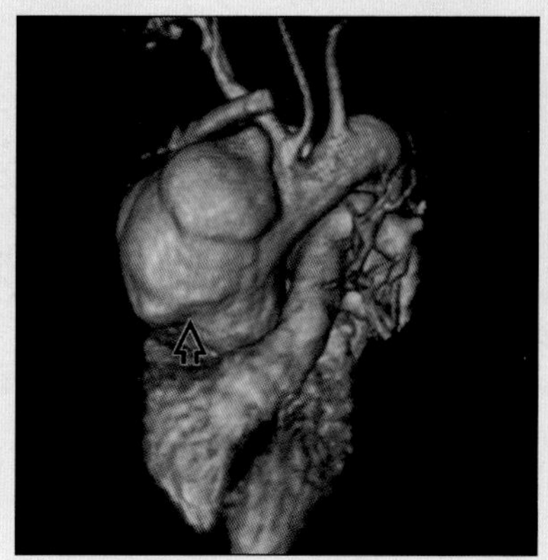

Syphilitic Aneurysm

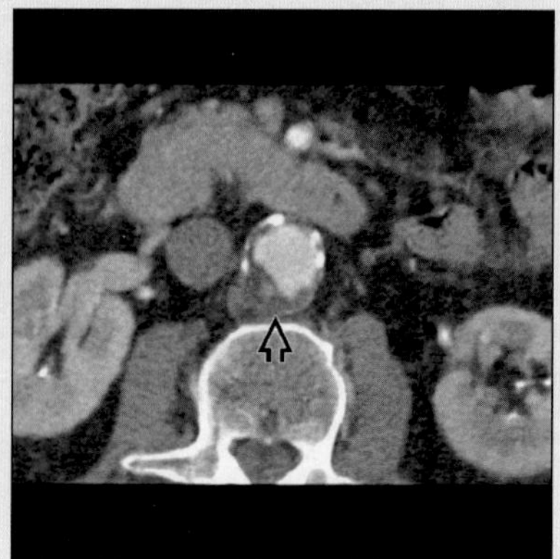

Mixed Atherosclerotic Plaque

GIANT CELL ARTERITIS

Key Facts

Terminology
- Systemic granulomatous inflammatory vasculitis involving media of medium to large-sized arteries

Imaging Findings
- Mural inflammation; vessel wall thickening and enhancement
- Indistinguishable from Takayasu arteritis but latter more common in younger patients
- Vital MR sequences are pre and post-contrast axial T1 GRE, TE-MRA, and high spatial resolution MRA
- Time resolved MRA may be helpful to show end organ perfusion defects
  - MR better than CT to differentiate active from chronic vasculitis
  - Irregular luminal configuration
- Varying degree of stenosis

Top Differential Diagnoses
- Takayasu Arteritis
- Atherosclerotic Disease
- Other Systemic Vasculidities (e.g., Polyarteritis Nodosa, Syphilitic Aortitis)

Pathology
- Rare before age 50, thereafter increasing frequency

Clinical Issues
- Fever, malaise, weight-loss
- Marked elevation in acute phase reactants (ESR, CRP)
- Male < Female
- Rapid response to corticosteroid treatment

Diagnostic Checklist
- Mural wall enhancement on T1 post-contrast MR

- STIR: May be more sensitive to mural edema than T2-weighted images
- T1 C+
  - High-resolution fat-saturated acquisitions
    - Wall thickening and mural enhancement (i.e., inflammation)
    - Degree of enhancement indicates inflammatory activity
  - Valuable modality in assessment of response of involved segments to medical treatment
- MRA
  - Evaluation of luminal patency for detection and follow-up of extent of segmental involvement
  - Irregular luminal configuration
  - Varying degree of stenosis
  - Segmental occlusion
  - Collaterals
  - Time-resolved MRA may be helpful to show end organ perfusion defects
    - Reverse flow in subclavian steal syndrome
- Respiratory suspension vital for optimal MR imaging

Nuclear Medicine Findings
- PET
  - Increasing evidence as to potential future role
  - Evaluation of initial disease extent and response to therapy (FDG-uptake parallels inflammatory activity)
  - Concomitant assessment of extravascular involvement
    - e.g., shoulder uptake due to perisynovitis in patients with polymyalgia rheumatica

Echocardiographic Findings
- Echocardiogram
  - Allows exclusion or evaluation of cardiac involvement
    - Aortic valve inflammation, resultant valvular insufficiency
    - Left ventricular dysfunction (myocarditis or secondary to coronary ischemia)
    - Aortic root evaluation for ectasia/aneurysmal dilatation

Ultrasonographic Findings
- Grayscale Ultrasound: Classic hypoechoic "halo-sign" surrounding superficial temporal artery, reflecting edema within inflamed vessel wall
- Color Doppler: May demonstrate luminal stenosis, though poor specificity for diagnosis of GCA

Angiographic Findings
- Conventional
  - Multiple smooth, segmental areas of luminal narrowing
  - Limited, if any role in diagnosis, reserved for endovascular intervention

Imaging Recommendations
- Best imaging tool
  - MR/MRA preferred due to availability/absence of ionizing radiation
  - CTA for exclusion of acute life- or limb-threatening complication (aortic dissection, coronary artery or subclavian occlusion)
  - MR better than CT to differentiate active from chronic vasculitis
- Protocol advice
  - Pre and post-contrast axial GRE images (for wall thickening and enhancement)
  - TE-MRA (flow direction and end organ perfusion) and high spatial resolution MRA (luminal configuration)
  - Respiratory suspension vital for optimal MR imaging of chest

DIFFERENTIAL DIAGNOSIS

Takayasu Arteritis
- Also involves both large and medium-sized arteries; histopathological features may be identical
- Tends to present at earlier age (< 30 years)
- Predominantly affects Asian population
- Aortic occlusion is highly specific

GIANT CELL ARTERITIS

Atherosclerotic Disease

- Similar age-group
- May be difficult to differentiate radiographically, though clinical symptoms often facilitate process

Other Systemic Vasculitides (e.g., Polyarteritis Nodosa, Syphilitic Aortitis)

- Occurs more in small and medium-sized arteries
- Biopsy and pattern of distribution often aid differentiation

Fibromuscular Dysplasia

- Most often affects renal arteries, but can involve carotid arteries also
- Results in stenoses; occasional spontaneous dissection

PATHOLOGY

General Features

- General path comments
  - Gold standard technique to establish diagnosis
  - "Skip lesions" may occur; segment of temporal artery required for confident diagnosis/exclusion
- Genetics: Associated with HLA-DR1-04 gene
- Etiology
  - Mycoplasma pneumoniae, Parvovirus B19, Chlamydia pneumoniae and Human Parainfluenza virus type 1 have been implicated
  - CD4+ T-Cells and macrophage response to antigenic stimulation
  - Initiation of inflammatory cascade results in vascular destruction, remodeling and deformity
- Epidemiology
  - Rare before age 50, thereafter increasing frequency
  - 2-6 times more frequent in women than men
  - Particularly common in Northern European descent
- Associated abnormalities: Frequently (approximately 40%) co-exists with Polymyalgia Rheumatica (PMR); suggested as different expression of same disorder

Microscopic Features

- Necrotizing panarteritis, featuring inflammatory infiltrate associated with marked disruption of internal elastic lamina
- Multinucleated giant cells

CLINICAL ISSUES

Presentation

- Most common signs/symptoms
  - Wide variability in symptoms at presentation
  - Constitutional
    - Fever, malaise, weight-loss
    - Symptoms of PMR (proximal muscle ache, stiffness, weakness, bursitis, tenosynovitis)
  - Vascular
    - Visual disturbance/blindness (optic nerve/retinal ischemia)
    - Jaw claudication, temporal tenderness, headache, ischemic neuropathy
    - Peripheral steno-occlusive signs/symptoms (claudication, rest pain, ulceration)
    - Complications: (17-fold risk thoracic aortic aneurysm; 2-fold risk abdominal aortic aneurysm, aortic dissection, myocardial infarction)
- Clinical Profile
  - Elevation in acute phase reactants (ESR, CRP)
  - Anemia, thrombocytosis
  - Clinically abnormal temporal artery

Demographics

- Age: Usually greater than 50 yrs
- Gender: Male < Female

Natural History & Prognosis

- Favorable prognosis if early treatment instigated
- Residual arterial stenosis persists despite resolution of inflammation
- Aortic ectasia/aneurysm requires intermittent follow-up (may continue to enlarge despite inflammatory suppression)

Treatment

- Rapid response to corticosteroid treatment
- Relapsing-remitting course not uncommon during steroid tapering
- Conflicting results have been obtained with methotrexate, when used as steroid-sparing measure
- Azathioprine therapy may be attempted in otherwise refractory cases

DIAGNOSTIC CHECKLIST

Consider

- GCA in patients presenting with low grade fever, weight loss, and transient neurological symptoms
  - Look for imaging evidence of associated mural inflammatory changes of medium and or large vessels

Image Interpretation Pearls

- Circumferential vessel wall thickening
- Mural wall enhancement on T1 post-contrast MR

SELECTED REFERENCES

1. Eberhardt RT et al: Giant cell arteritis: diagnosis, management, and cardiovascular implications. Cardiol Rev. 15(2):55-61, 2007
2. Levine SM et al: Giant cell arteritis. Curr Opin Rheumatol. 14(1):3-10, 2002
3. Salvarani C et al: Polymyalgia rheumatica and giant-cell arteritis. N Engl J Med. 347(4):261-71, 2002
4. Atalay MK et al: Magnetic resonance imaging of large vessel vasculitis. Curr Opin Rheumatol. 13(1):41-7, 2001
5. Evans JM et al: Increased incidence of aortic aneurysm and dissection in giant cell (temporal) arteritis. A population-based study. Ann Intern Med. 122(7):502-7, 1995
6. Hunder GG et al: The American College of Rheumatology 1990 criteria for the classification of giant cell arteritis. Arthritis Rheum. 33(8):1122-8, 1990

IMAGE GALLERY

Typical

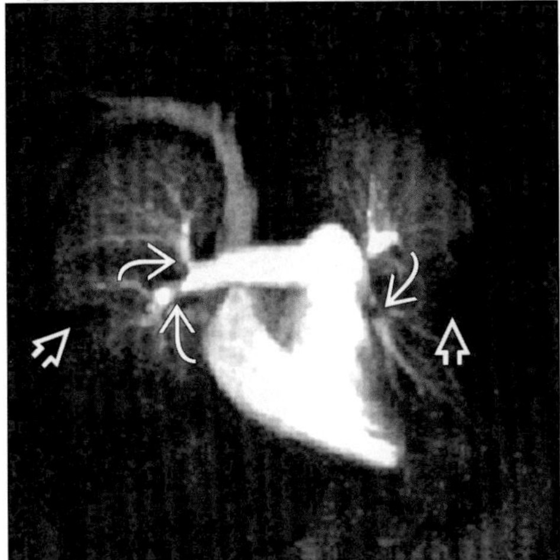

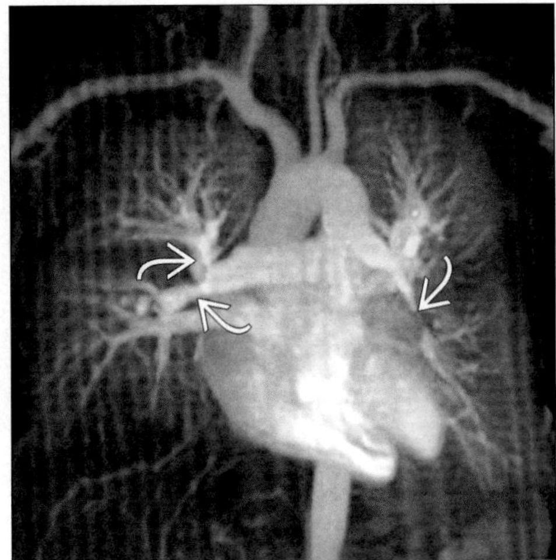

(Left) *Coronal TE-MRA frame shows irregularity and stenosis of the proximal pulmonary arteries in a patient with pulmonary vasculitis. Also note the presence of multiple segmental lung perfusion defects.* ***(Right)*** *Coronal CE-MRA MIP in the same patient as previous image confirms multiple stenoses of proximal pulmonary arteries without intraluminal thrombus. These are nonspecific features that are consistent with a pulmonary vasculitis including GCA.*

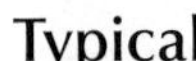

Typical

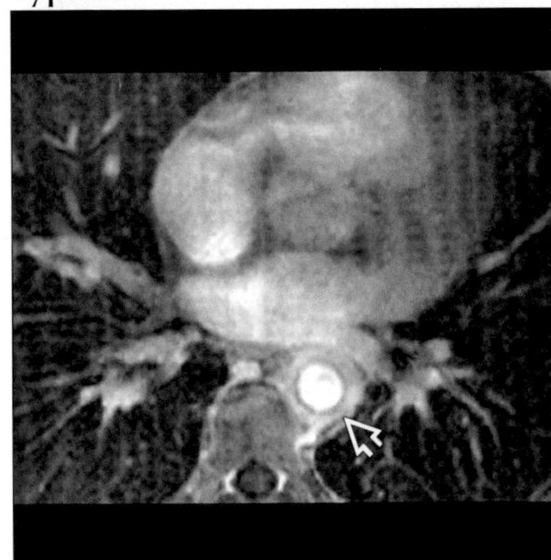

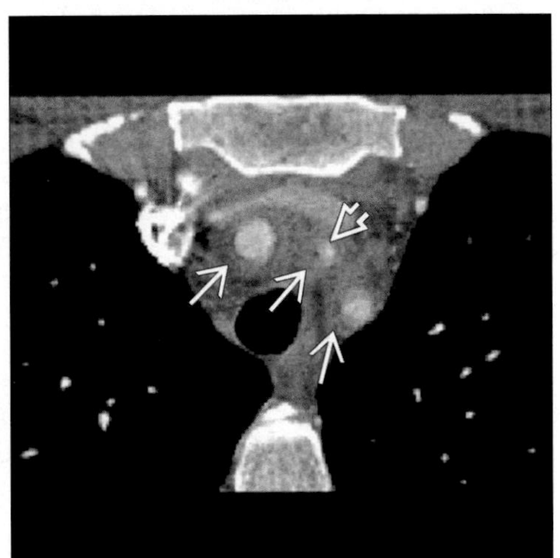

(Left) *Axial GRE MR following administration of gadolinium contrast-agent, in a different patient, shows marked circumferential mural thickening and enhancement of the descending thoracic aorta, consistent with an active arteritis.* ***(Right)*** *Axial CTA in a young patient shows mural thickening of the supra-aortic great vessels and stranding of the adjacent peri-vascular fat, due to a vasculitis. Note the stenosis of the left common carotid artery.*

Typical

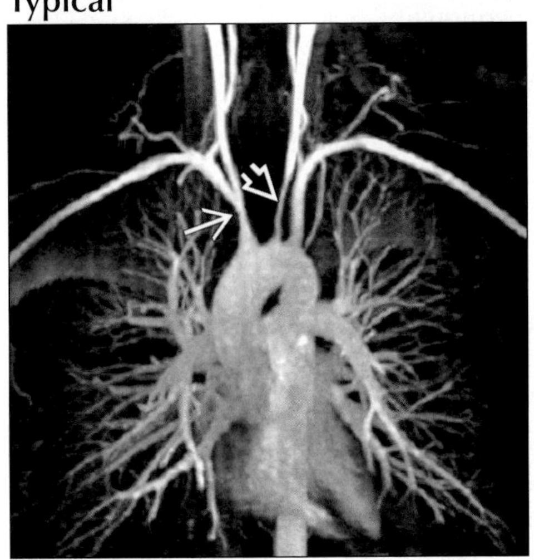

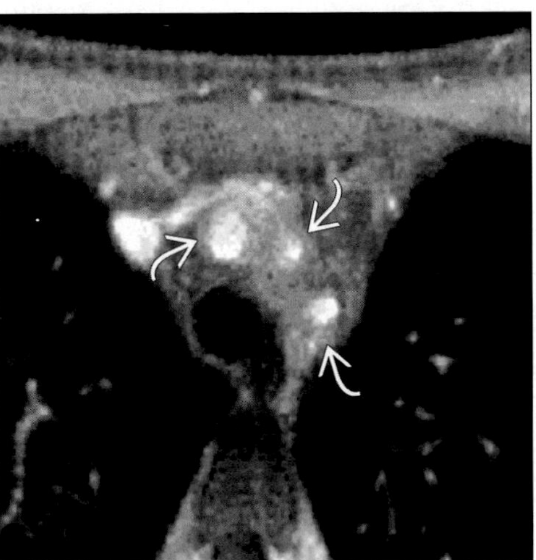

(Left) *Coronal CE-MRA (same patient as previous image) shows an irregular long-segment stenosis of the left common carotid artery and a moderate right subclavian artery stenosis, due to mural thickening. These findings are typical of GCA involving the great vessels.* ***(Right)*** *Axial GRE MR following gadolinium administration (same patient as previous image) confirms presence of mural thickening and enhancement of the supra-aortic arteries, consistent with active GCA.*

MARFAN SYNDROME

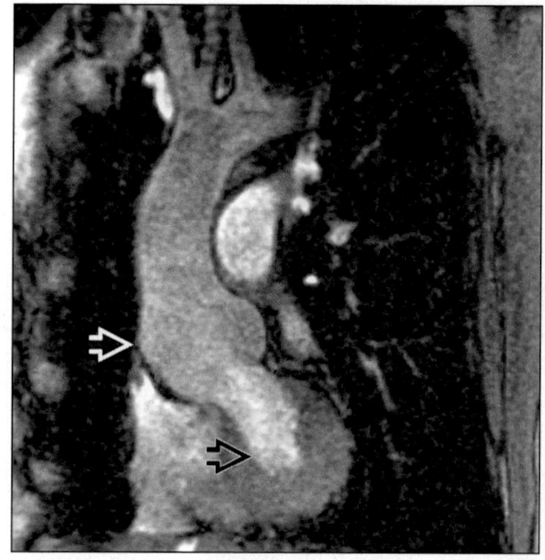

Coronal oblique MR demonstrates the appearance of annuloaortic ectasia with dilatation of the sinuses of Valsalva. Aortic regurgitation is also present.

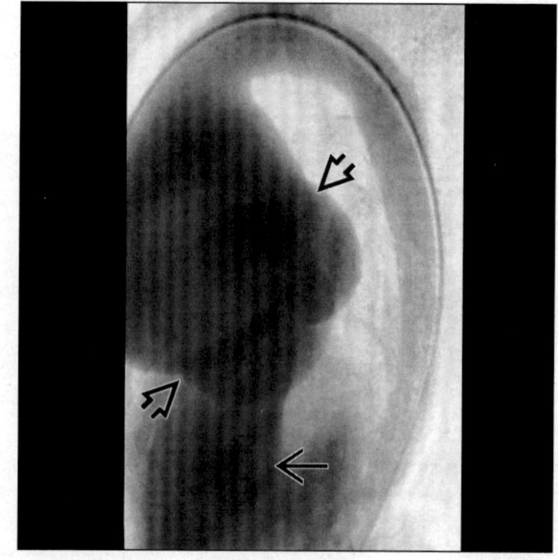

Catheter angiography shows massive dilatation of the sinuses of Valsalva. The aortic root is involved, but the rest of the aorta is normal in caliber. Aortic regurgitation is present.

TERMINOLOGY

Abbreviations and Synonyms

- Annuloaortic ectasia
- "Tulip bulb" aorta

Definitions

- Inherited autosomal dominant disorder of connective tissue characterized by skeletal, cardiovascular and ocular abnormalities

IMAGING FINDINGS

General Features

- Best diagnostic clue
  - Diagnosis of Marfan syndrome based on Ghent criteria which includes cardiovascular, ocular and pulmonary abnormalities
  - **Cardiovascular and valvular disease**: Seen in majority (> 90%) of patients and dominant cause of mortality
  - Major criteria
    - Annuloaortic ectasia: Prevalence 75%
    - Ascending aortic dissection
  - Minor criteria
    - Mitral valve prolapse (most prevalent valvular abnormality seen in 35-100% of patients)
    - Mitral annulus calcification (in patients < 40 years of age)
    - Main pulmonary artery dilatation (pulmonary valve normal)
    - Dilatation/dissection of descending thoracic or abdominal aorta
  - **Skeletal abnormalities** - major criteria
    - Pectus excavatum or carinatum severe enough to warrant surgery
    - Arm span to height ratio > 1.05
    - Scoliosis > 20° or spondylolisthesis (60%)
    - Limited elbow extension (< 170°)
    - Pes planus
    - Protrusio acetabuli
  - Minor criteria
    - Joint hypermobility
    - Pectus excavatum or carinatum of moderate severity
    - High-arched palate
  - Other: Arachnodactyly, long toes, thoracic lordosis

DDx: Marfan Syndrome

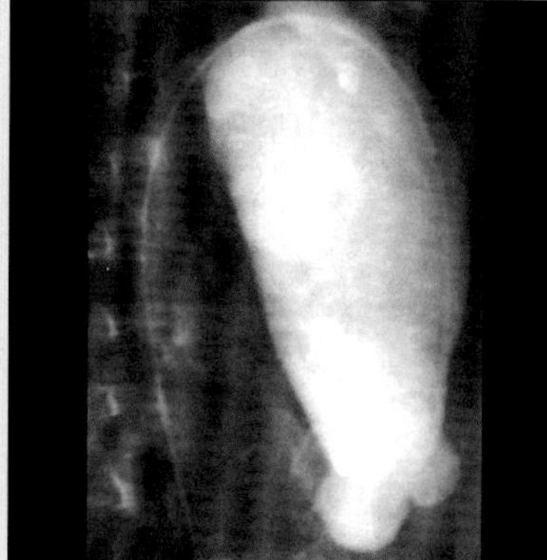

Syphilitic Aneurysm

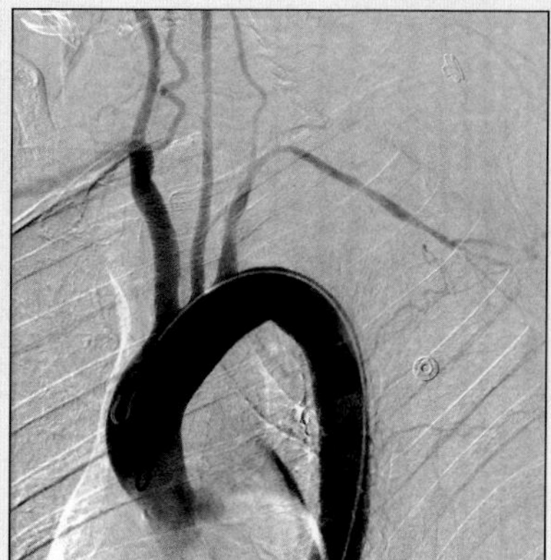

Giant Cell Aortitis

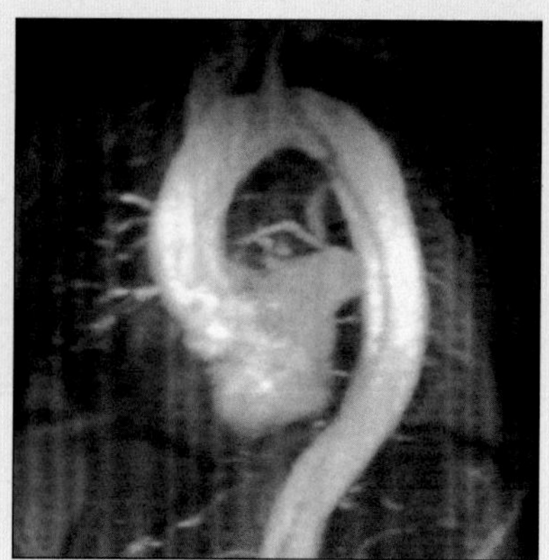

Dissection

MARFAN SYNDROME

Key Facts

Terminology
- Inherited autosomal dominant disorder of connective tissue characterized by skeletal, cardiovascular and ocular abnormalities
- Annuloaortic ectasia

Imaging Findings
- **Cardiovascular and valvular disease:** Seen in majority (> 90%) of patients and dominant cause of mortality
- Annuloaortic ectasia: Prevalence 75%
- Annuloaortic ectasia: Pear-shaped dilatation of the sinuses of Valsalva extending into the ascending aorta ("tulip-bulb")
- Mitral annulus calcification (in patients < 40 years of age)

Top Differential Diagnoses
- Neurofibromatosis Type 1
- Ankylosing Spondylitis
- Relapsing Polychondritis

Pathology
- Autosomal dominant inheritance with complete penetrance but variable expression
- Prevalence 1 in 3-5000 population

Diagnostic Checklist
- Aneurysmal dilatation precedes dissection and/or rupture
- Long term surveillance following aortic graft repair paramount; nearly 50% of late deaths due to anastomotic pseudoaneurysms

---

  - **Pulmonary disease**
  - Minor criteria
    - Apical blebs
    - Pneumothorax (recurrent and bilateral): Prevalence 5%
  - Other: Emphysema, recurrent lower respiratory tract infections, upper lobe fibrosis (rare)
  - **Ocular abnormalities**
  - Major criteria
    - Ectopia lentis (50%)
  - Other: Myopia, flattening of cornea, iris or ciliary muscle hypoplasia
  - Other diagnostic criteria include
    - Family history of first-degree relative who independently fulfills diagnostic criteria
    - Lumbosacral dural ectasia (major criterion)
    - Recurrent/incisional hernias (minor criteria)
- Location
  - Classically involving the root of the aorta and the ascending aorta
    - Involvement of the aortic root referred to as annuloaortic ectasia
- Morphology: "Tulip bulb" appearance - represents dilatation of the sinuses of Valsalva

Radiographic Findings
- Radiography
  - Chest radiograph
    - Long, elongated thorax with large-volume lungs
    - Dilatation ascending aorta
    - Cardiomegaly (due to aortic or mitral regurgitation, or spurious from pectus deformity)
    - Pectus deformity, either excavatum or carinatum
    - Apical blebs
    - Scoliosis and scalloping vertebral bodies

CT Findings
- CTA
  - More sensitive than chest radiography for
    - Annuloaortic ectasia: Dilatation of sinuses of Valsalva extending into ascending aorta
    - Dissecting aortic aneurysm
    - Subpleural blebs
    - Dural ectasia

MR Findings
- Similar to CT in sensitivity for major cardiovascular complications
- Better than CT for valve assessment
- Nonionizing radiation major advantage in following aortic root dilatation in young individuals

Echocardiographic Findings
- Standard surveillance for aortic root dilatation and assessment of aortic and mitral valve function

Imaging Recommendations
- Best imaging tool
  - Plain radiography for detection of skeletal anomalies
  - Serial chest radiography to demonstrate progressive aortic dilatation
  - 2D echocardiography for early diagnosis and monitoring of ascending aortic dilatation
  - Multi-detector row CT or magnetic resonance angiography for evaluation of aortic disease

DIFFERENTIAL DIAGNOSIS

Neurofibromatosis Type 1
- Inherited autosomal dominant neurocutaneous syndrome
- Also have dural ectasia and gibbus deformity (typically at thoracolumbar junction), lateral meningocele
- Essential hypertension, coarctation of the aorta
- Pulmonary valve stenosis
- Optic gliomas
- Ribbon ribs, rib notching

Ankylosing Spondylitis
- Seronegative arthritis possibly genetically related with predilection for the axial skeleton
- Syndesmophyte spinal fusion
- Aortitis may lead to aortic regurgitation
- Fibrocystic upper lobe disease (< 2%)

MARFAN SYNDROME

Relapsing Polychondritis
- Rare autoimmune inflammatory condition involving cartilage of the ear, tracheobronchial tree, eye, cardiovascular system and peripheral joints
- Tracheal involvement in 50%
- Also associated with aortic dissection and aortic or mitral regurgitation (25%)

Ehlers-Danlos Syndrome
- Genetic defect in collagen and connective tissue, much rarer than Marfan
- Affects skin, joints and blood vessels
- May also have aortic aneurysm, dissection and mitral valve prolapse

PATHOLOGY

General Features
- Genetics
  - Autosomal dominant inheritance with complete penetrance but variable expression
    - No family history in 25% of patients
  - Mutation in FBN1 gene, the extracellular matrix protein fibrillin-1 (encoding for large glycoprotein called fibrillin-1, a major component of microfibrils)
  - Animal studies demonstrate dysregulation of transforming growth factor-beta (TGF-β) activation & signaling, leading to apoptosis in developing lung
- Epidemiology
  - Prevalence 1 in 3-5000 population
    - Common genetic malformation

Gross Pathologic & Surgical Features
- Annuloaortic ectasia: Uniform dilatation all 3 sinuses of Valsalva extending into the ascending aorta obliterating the normal sinotubular ridge
  - Most aortic diseases do not cross the sinotubular ridge but involve either sinuses or ascending aorta
  - Also seen with Ehlers-Danlos and homocystinuria

Microscopic Features
- Cystic medial necrosis

CLINICAL ISSUES

Presentation
- Most common signs/symptoms
  - Cardiovascular disease
    - Acute onset chest pain (aortic dissection)
  - Pulmonary disease
    - Abrupt onset shortness of breath (spontaneous pneumothorax)
    - Dyspnea on exertion, substernal chest pain (severe pectus excavatum)
  - Ocular
    - Loss of vision (lens dislocation)

Demographics
- Gender
  - None
    - However, aortic root dilatation more common in men

Natural History & Prognosis
- Morbidity and mortality due to cardiovascular disease (aortic dissection)
  - Average age death untreated 35 years of age
- Prognosis improved with increased vigilance, plus current medical and surgical intervention
  - Average life expectancy up to 70 years
- Pregnant women at significant risk for aortic dissection
  - Surveillance echocardiography or MR every 6-10 weeks during pregnancy

Treatment
- Screening important for early detection of aortic vascular complications
- Β-adrenergic blocking drugs
  - Slows the rate of aortic dilatation
  - Lowers incidence of aortic regurgitation, dissection or need for surgery, congestive cardiac failure
  - Improves survival
- Exercise restriction
  - Avoidance of contact sports and isometric exercises
- Surgical intervention
  - Prophylactic aortic root surgery recommended when aortic diameter reaches 5 cm because of increased risk of rupture or dissection
  - With smaller aortic diameters, surgery still indicated if rapid growth (> 1 cm/year), a family history of dissection and moderate to severe aortic regurgitation
  - Surgical options include
    - Composite valve graft repair
    - Valve-sparing aortic root replacement
  - Genetic counseling: 50% offspring will have disease

DIAGNOSTIC CHECKLIST

Consider
- Diagnosis to be considered in patients with positive family history and combinations of cardiovascular, skeletal, ocular and possibly pulmonary disease

Image Interpretation Pearls
- Aneurysmal dilatation precedes dissection and/or rupture
- Long term surveillance following aortic graft repair paramount; nearly 50% of late deaths due to anastomotic pseudoaneurysms

SELECTED REFERENCES

1. Ammash NM et al: Marfan syndrome-diagnosis and management. Curr Probl Cardiol. 33(1):7-39, 2008
2. Ha HI et al: Imaging of Marfan syndrome: multisystemic manifestations. Radiographics. 27(4):989-1004, 2007
3. von Kodolitsch Y et al: Marfan syndrome: an update of genetics, medical and surgical management. Heart. 93(6):755-60, 2007

IMAGE GALLERY

Typical

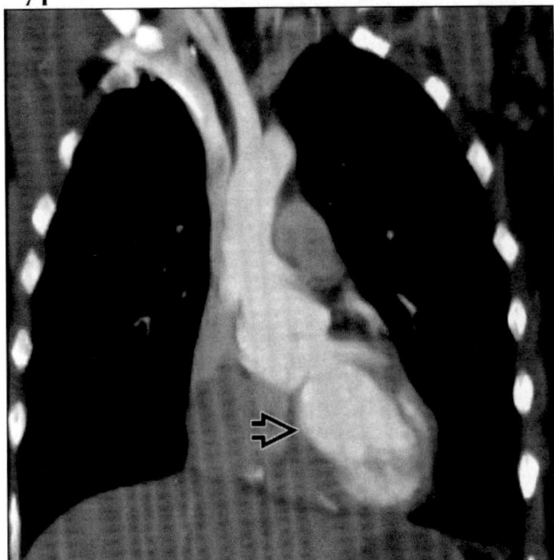

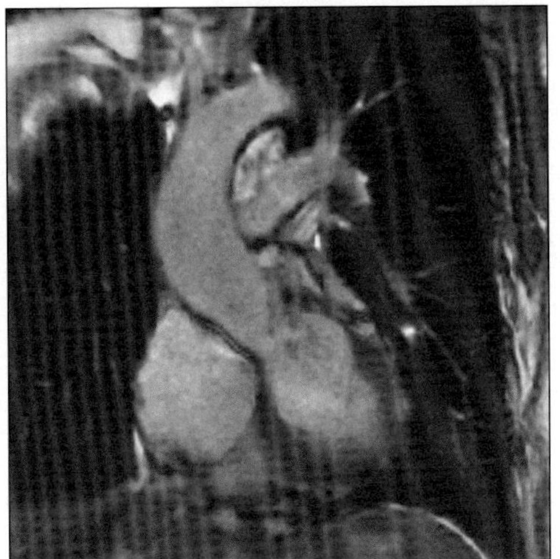

(Left) *Coronal CTA shows the dilated sinuses of Valsalva. When evaluating patients with Marfan syndrome, it is important to evaluate for potential complications, including aortic regurgitation,* ⇨ *ascending aortic dissection, and to compare with old studies since rapid growth is an indication for surgery.* ***(Right)*** *Coronal oblique MR cine shows similar findings of annuloaortic ectasia and aortic regurgitation. MR is an excellent way to follow young patients.*

Variant

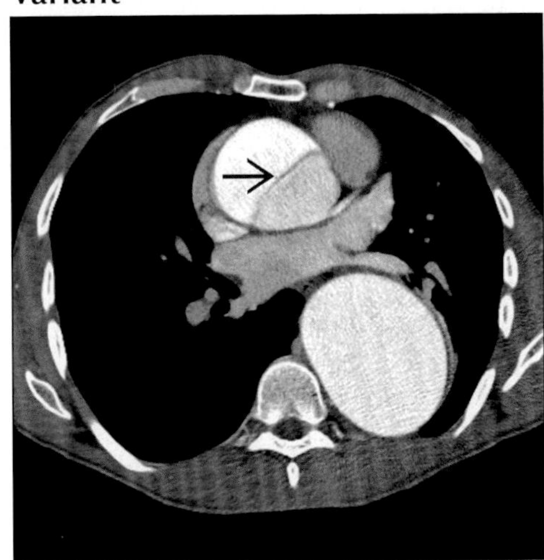

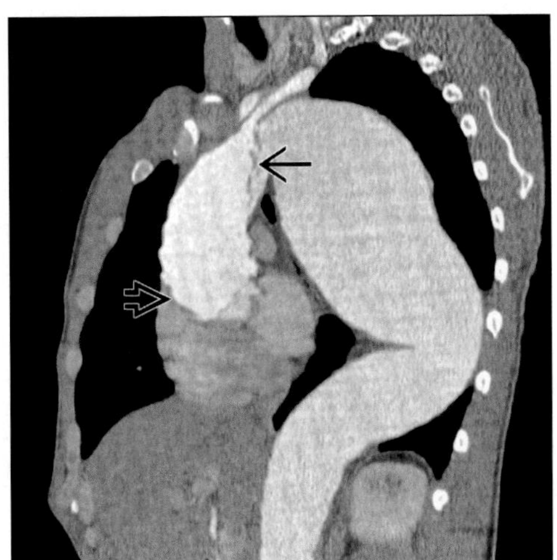

(Left) *Axial CECT shows markedly dilated ascending and descending aorta. There is a dissection flap in the ascending aorta* → *. No dissection flap is seen in the markedly aneurysmal descending aorta.* ***(Right)*** *Oblique CECT shows the dissection flap in the ascending aorta* → *. The dissection is extending up into the left subclavian. There is no flap demonstrated extending into the descending aorta. There is annuloaortic ectasia* ⇨ *present.*

Other

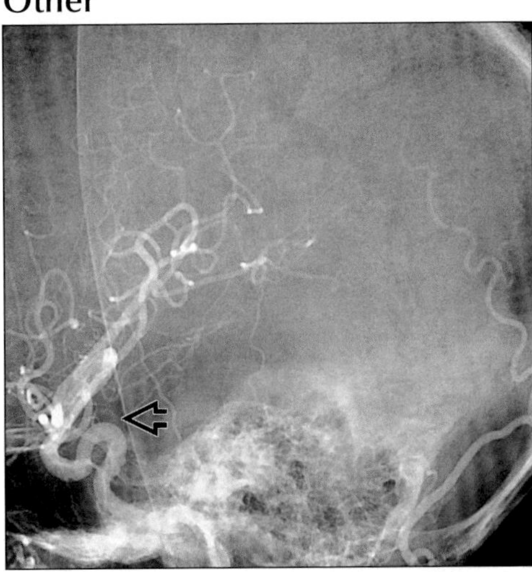

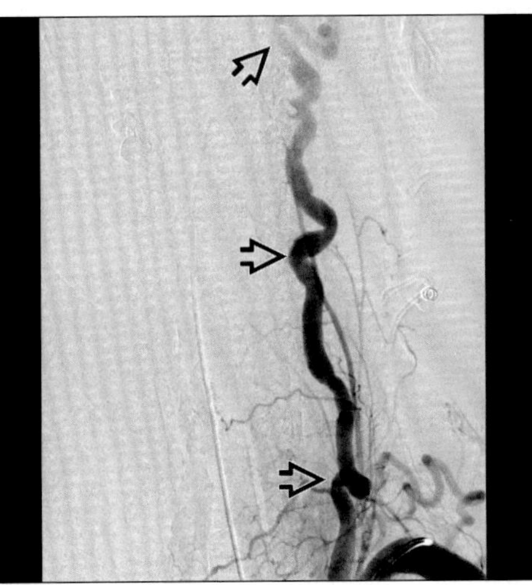

(Left) *DSA of the intracranial arteries shows the intracranial carotid artery as being markedly elongated, dilated and redundant in the supraclinoid segment* ⇨ *. Patients with Marfan may have aneurysms of the extracranial and intracranial carotid arteries. Redundancy in carotid arteries may be associated with dissection.* ***(Right)*** *DSA shows marked redundancy of the vertebral artery* ⇨ *. The redundancy is due to the structural abnormalities of the artery.*

PSEUDO-COARCTATION

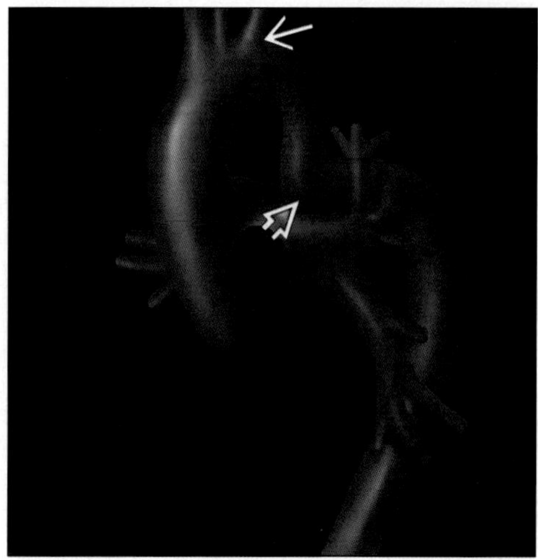

Coronal oblique graphic demonstrates an elongated, kinked, and buckled aortic arch ⇨, distal to the origin of the left subclavian artery ➡ at the level of the ductus arteriosus, consistent with aortic pseudo-coarctation.

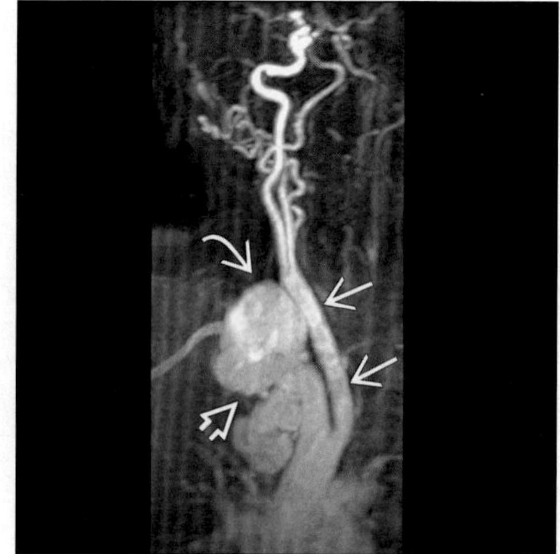

Coronal oblique thin MIP CEMRA shows aneurysmal dilatation and narrowing of the aortic arch ⇨, which extends to the supraclavicular space ➡. Also note the stretching ➡ of the supra-aortic arteries.

TERMINOLOGY

Abbreviations and Synonyms

- Redundant aortic arch
- Aortic kinking
- Aortic buckling
- Atypical coarctation
- Non-obstructive coarctation

Definitions

- Elongation of aortic arch with kinking of aorta distal to origin of left subclavian artery at level of ductus arteriosus

IMAGING FINDINGS

General Features

- Best diagnostic clue: Kinking and buckling of distal transverse arch with pressure gradient of less than 20 mmHg
- Location
  - Aortic isthmus at site of attachment of ligamentum arteriosum
  - Distal to origin of left subclavian artery
- Size
  - Normal caliber
  - Dilatation greater than 4 cm
  - Occasionally stenotic
- Morphology: Elongated and tortuous aortic arch without significant obstruction

Radiographic Findings

- Homogeneous left superior mediastinal soft tissue mass-like opacity
- Low-lying aortic knob
- Tubular and tortuous opacity with peripheral linear calcification
- On lateral radiograph, aortic arch is buckled forward at isthmus
- No rib notching
- No cardiomegaly

CT Findings

- NECT
  - Non-contrast CT may show elongated and tortuous aortic arch with possible multiple aneurysms and stenoses
  - Cervical aortic arch

DDx: Pseudo-Coarctation

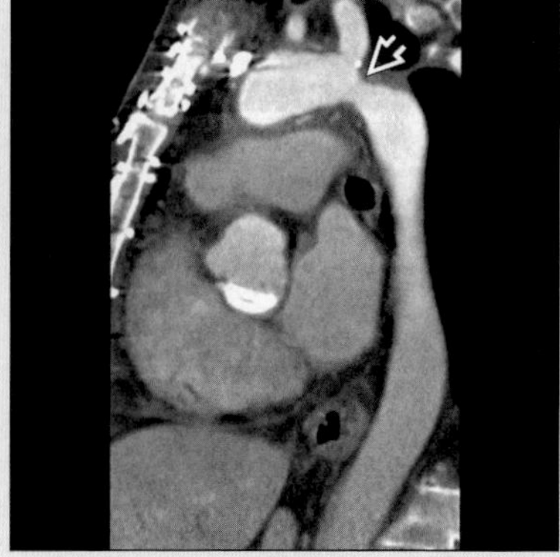

Recurrent Aortic Coarctation

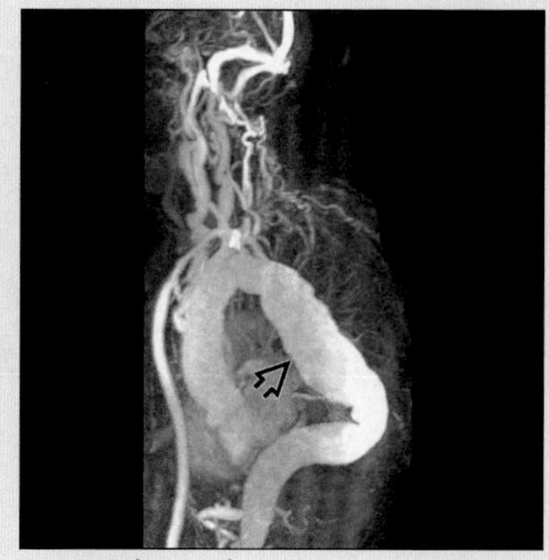

Atherosclerotic Aneurysm

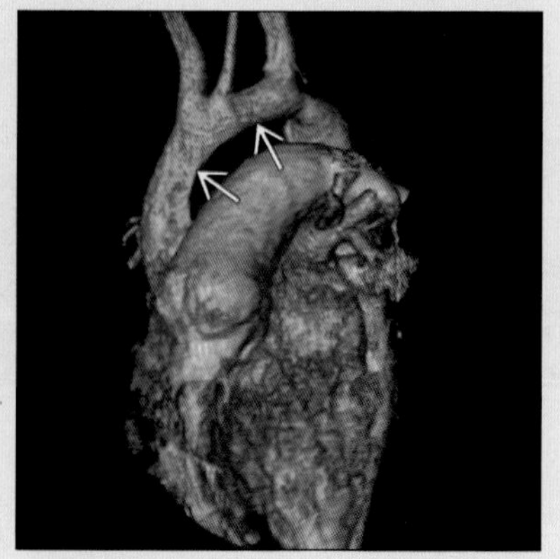

Hypoplastic Aortic Arch

PSEUDO-COARCTATION

Key Facts

Terminology

- Aortic buckling

Imaging Findings

- Contrast-enhanced 3D CTA and MRA show
  - Kinking and buckling of distal transverse arch; pressure gradient of less than 20 mmHg
  - Cervical aortic arch
  - Notch in distal transverse arch at attachment of short ligamentum arteriosum
  - Abnormal origins of supra-aortic arteries
  - No hemodynamically significant aortic narrowing and therefore no post-stenotic dilatation
- Homogeneous left superior mediastinal soft tissue mass-like opacity on plain films
  - No atherosclerotic calcification
  - Chimney-shaped high aortic arch extending into left supraclavicular region (children)
- Phase-contrast flow quantification MR may demonstrate no significant peak velocity; minimal or no pressure gradient across buckled segment
- "Figure 3 sign": Notch in descending aorta at attachment of short ligamentum arteriosum

Top Differential Diagnoses

- True Aortic Coarctation
- Aortic Aneurysm

Clinical Issues

- Usually asymptomatic and often recognized on routine chest X-ray
- No treatment required in asymptomatic patients

  - Anterior and medial displacement of distal aortic arch with a kink in posterior and lateral margins of aorta
  - Anterior displacement of the esophagus
- CTA
  - Elongated transverse aorta and kinking and buckling of aortic arch
  - Notch in distal transverse arch at attachment of short ligamentum arteriosum
  - No atherosclerotic calcification
  - Peripheral vascular calcification
  - No hemodynamically significant aortic narrowing and therefore no post-stenotic dilatation
  - No collateral vessels
  - No left ventricular enlargement
  - Chimney-shaped high aortic arch extending into left supraclavicular region (children)
  - May also demonstrate any associated aneurysm
  - Abnormal origins of the supra-aortic arteries
  - Dilatation of the brachiocephalic arteries

MR Findings

- MRA
  - Contrast-enhanced 3D MR angiography
    - Kinking and buckling of the elongated and tortuous transverse aorta
    - No collateral circulation or aortic narrowing of hemodynamic significance
    - No post-stenotic dilatation
    - No left ventricular enlargement
    - Associated aortic aneurysm
  - Time-resolved MRA
    - May show reverse flow in vertebral artery (steal phenomenon) in presence of subclavian artery stenosis
    - No collaterals
  - Phase-contrast flow quantification MR
    - Demonstrates absence of increased peak velocity (unlike true coarctation) and thus lack of pressure gradient across buckled segment
    - This technique is also useful for detection of flow reversal in "steal" syndrome

Angiographic Findings

- High position of aortic arch
- "Figure 3 sign": Notch in descending aorta at attachment of short ligamentum arteriosum

Imaging Recommendations

- Best imaging tool: Contrast-enhanced, three-dimensional (3D) CT and MR angiography
- Protocol advice
  - 3D CT angiography (CTA) preferably in sagittal orientation with MIP and MPR reconstructions
  - 3D high-resolution MR angiography (MRA) preferably in sagittal view with MIP and volume rendering algorithms
  - Time-resolved MR angiography for evaluation of flow patterns and collateral pathways
  - Phase-contrast flow quantification for measurement of peak velocities, flow direction, and pressure gradients
  - Axial images are useful for confident evaluation of a coexisting venous anomaly

DIFFERENTIAL DIAGNOSIS

True Aortic Coarctation

- Congenital narrowing of transverse arch distal to isthmus (post-ductal coarctation)
  - Diffuse hypoplasia of aortic arch distal to origin of innominate artery
- Post stenotic dilatation
- Reverse 3 sign and rib notching on CXR
- Collaterals on CTA and MRA in significant disease
- Raised peak velocity on phase contrast MR imaging resulting from increased pressure gradient
- Left ventricular enlargement
- Associated bicuspid aortic valve disease and other congenital cardiac abnormalities
- Normal supra-aortic arteries
- Commonly seen in younger patients

PSEUDO-COARCTATION

Aortic Aneurysm

- Usually seen in atherosclerotic aorta
  - Calcified intimal plaque usually present
- Saccular or fusiform dilatation
  - Mural thrombus often present within periphery of aneurysm
- Commonly seen in elderly patients

Mediastinal Mass

- Usually seen as vascular shadow on chest X-ray
- CT and MR angiography can differentiate a mass from pseudocoarctation

Hypoplastic Left Heart Syndrome

- Hypoplastic left heart syndrome (HLHS): Combination of cardiac malformations resulting from multiple developmental errors in early stages of cardiogenesis
  - Complex includes hypoplasia or atresia of aortic and mitral valves and hypoplasia of left ventricle and ascending aorta
  - If left untreated, invariably proves fatal
  - Great vessels have normal relationships
- Along with isolated coarctation and patent ductus arteriosus, HLHS is fourth most common cardiac malformation to manifest in 1st year of life

PATHOLOGY

General Features

- Etiology: Elongation of distal aortic arch caused by abnormal growth of preductal aorta
- Epidemiology: Very uncommon congenital anomaly
- Associated abnormalities
  - Bicuspid aortic valve, aneurysm of sinus of Valsalva
  - Patent ductus arteriosus (PDA), atrial septal defect (ASD), ventricular septal defect (VSD)
  - Aortic or subaortic stenosis may occur
  - Aortic coarctation may occur
  - Aortic aneurysms are usually associated with left-sided arches
  - Endocardial fibroelastosis
  - Subclavian steal syndrome also described as associated phenomenon as result of subclavian artery stenosis
  - May rarely have single ventricle

Microscopic Features

- Cystic medial necrosis is underlying cause rather than atherosclerosis in aortic aneurysms that are associated with pseudo-coarctation

CLINICAL ISSUES

Presentation

- Most common signs/symptoms
  - Usually asymptomatic and often recognized on routine chest X-ray films
    - May mimic mediastinal mass
- Other signs/symptoms
  - Patient may present with chest pain, exertional palpitation or dyspnea, fatigue, weakness, dysphasia, and syncope
  - Palpable supraclavicular pulsatile mass
  - Blood pressure discrepancy between both upper extremities
  - Hypertension
  - Ejection murmur

Demographics

- Age: 12-64 years
- Gender: No gender predominance

Natural History & Prognosis

- Pseudocoarctation usually asymptomatic and benign, but aneurysmal dilatations may develop
  - If aneurysms develop, must be monitored and treated

Treatment

- No treatment required in asymptomatic patients

DIAGNOSTIC CHECKLIST

Consider

- Pseudo-coarctation in young patient with left superior mediastinal soft tissue mass-like opacity and low-lying aortic knob on chest X-ray
  - On lateral radiograph, aortic arch is buckled forward at level of aortic isthmus

Image Interpretation Pearls

- Sagittal views for CTA and MRA are most useful for demonstrating pseudo-coarctation
  - 3D CTA with with MIP and MPR reconstructions
  - 3D MRA with MIP and volume rendering algorithms
- Lack of hemodynamically significant aortic narrowing and therefore no post-stenotic dilatation
  - Aids in differentiating from "true" aortic coarctation

SELECTED REFERENCES

1. Adaletli I et al: Pseudocoarctation. Can J Cardiol. 23(8):675-6, 2007
2. Matsui H et al: Anatomy of coarctation, hypoplastic and interrupted aortic arch: relevance to interventional/surgical treatment. Expert Rev Cardiovasc Ther. 5(5):871-80, 2007
3. Tanju S et al: Right cervical aortic arch and pseudocoarctation of the aorta associated with aneurysms and steal phenomena: US, CTA, and MRA findings. Cardiovasc Intervent Radiol. 30(1):146-9, 2007
4. Choi BW et al: Magnetic resonance angiography of pseudocoarctation. Heart. 90(10):1213, 2004
5. Sebastià C et al: Aortic stenosis: spectrum of diseases depicted at multisection CT. Radiographics. 23 Spec No:S79-91, 2003
6. Taneja K et al: Pseudocoarctation of the aorta: complementary findings on plain film radiography, CT, DSA, and MRA. Cardiovasc Intervent Radiol. 21(5):439-41, 1998
7. Lajos TZ et al: Pseudocoarctation of the aorta: a variant or an entity? Chest. 58(6):571-6, 1970

IMAGE GALLERY

Typical

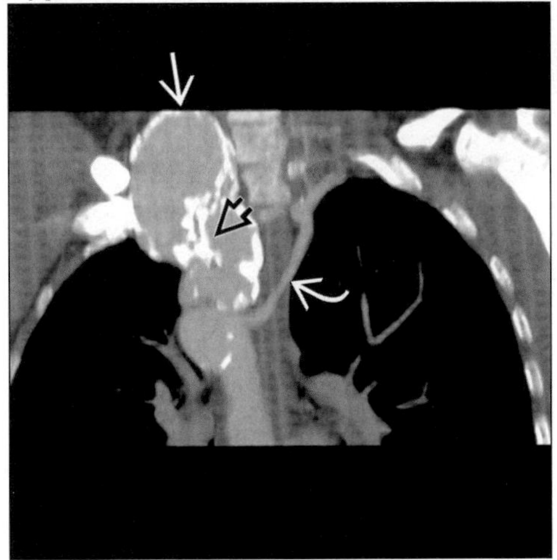

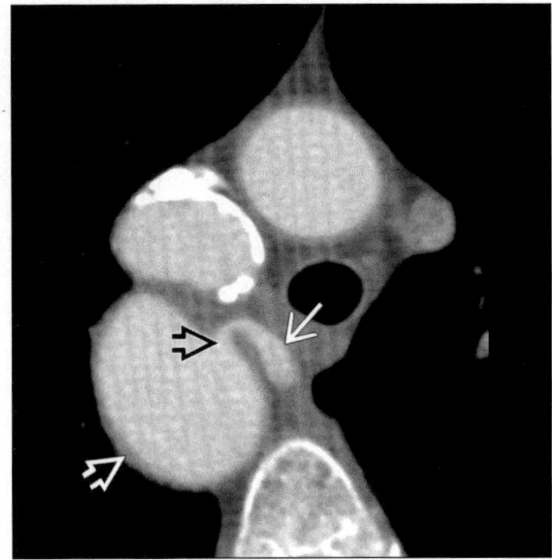

(Left) *Coronal CTA shows dilated and elongated right aortic arch → which is irregular and peripherally calcified. Note that there is extension of the aortic arch into the right lower neck → and also note the presence of an aberrant left subclavian artery →.* ***(Right)*** *Axial CTA (same patient as previous image) shows a dilated right aortic arch → and a high grade stenosis of the origin → of the aberrant left subclavian artery →. (Courtesy S. Tanju, MD).*

Typical

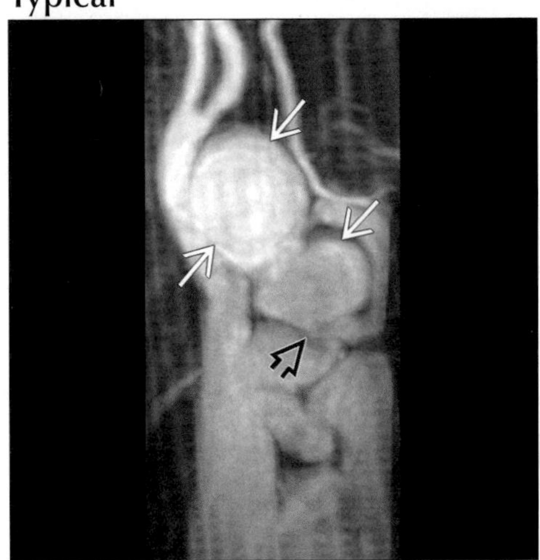

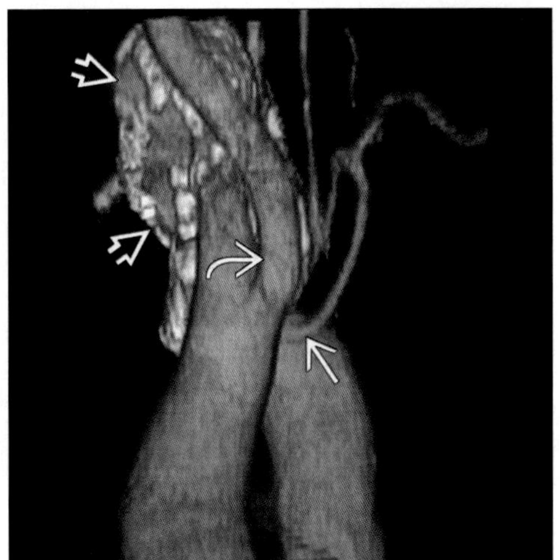

(Left) *Sagittal thin MIP CEMRA shows a very elongated and abnormal aortic arch with areas of dilatation → and narrowing →. Note the abnormal origin of left common carotid artery from the pseudo-coarctation.* ***(Right)*** *Sagittal CTA 3D volume rendered image of the same patient as previous image, shows an abnormally dilated and buckled aorta → and demonstrates the origins of the innominate → and the left subclavian arteries →. (Courtesy S. Tanju, MD).*

Typical

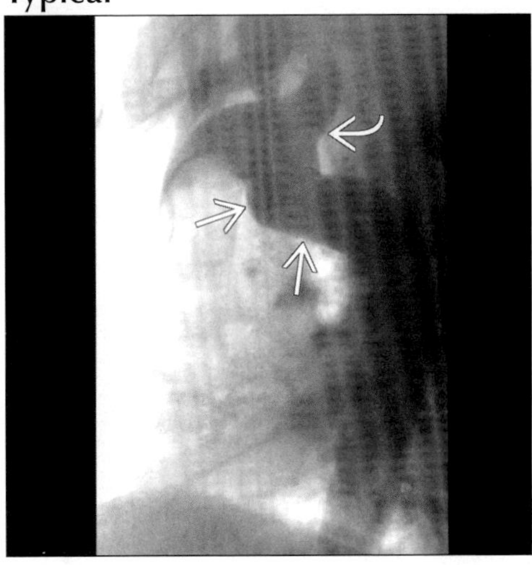

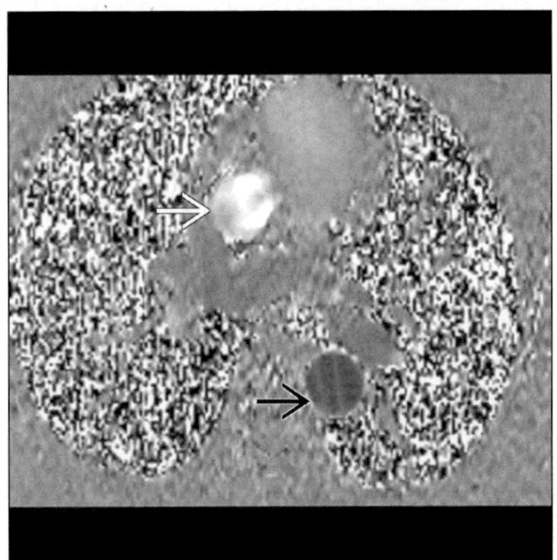

(Left) *Catheter angiography of pseudo-coarctation shows an elongated and kinked distal thoracic aortic arch → with an abnormally dilated origin of the left subclavian artery →.* ***(Right)*** *Axial PC MR obtained just distal the pseudo-coarctation shows an absence of increased flow velocity. Note: The bright signal in the ascending aorta indicates flow in the cephalad direction →, and the dark signal in the descending aorta indicates caudal flow →.*

TRAUMATIC AORTIC LACERATION

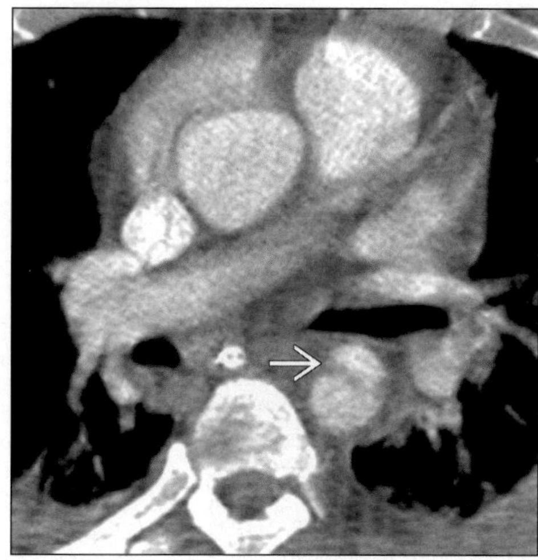

Axial CECT shows transection ➡ of the descending thoracic aorta following MVA. The linear lucency seen with traumatic laceration should not be mistaken for a dissection.

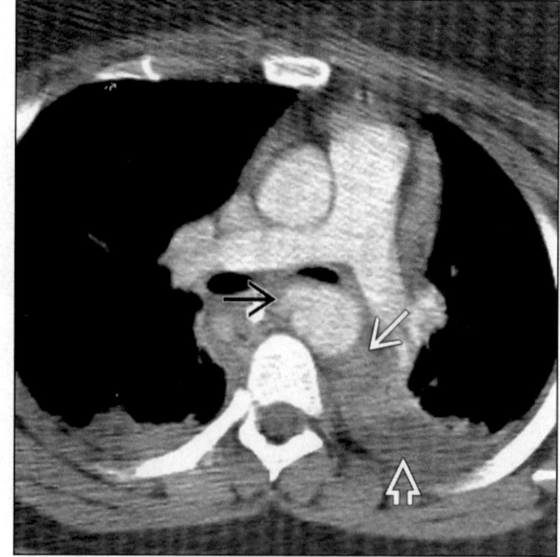

Axial CECT shows contour abnormality of the descending thoracic aorta with a pseudoaneurysm ➡. In addition, there is mediastinal hematoma ➡ and left pleural effusion ⇨.

TERMINOLOGY

Abbreviations and Synonyms

- Aortic pseudoaneurysm, aortic rupture, traumatic aortic aneurysm, aortic transection, traumatic aortic injury

Definitions

- Aortic laceration or rupture secondary to sudden horizontal (MVA) or vertical (fall from great height) deceleration injury of the thorax

IMAGING FINDINGS

General Features

- Best diagnostic clue
  - Mediastinal widening
  - Localized saccular outpouching of aorta
- Location
  - 88% aortic isthmus
  - 4.5% aortic arch with avulsion of brachiocephalic trunk
  - 2% descending thoracic aorta
  - 1% ascending aorta immediately above aortic valve
    - In autopsy series, there is a higher incidence of ascending aortic tears; this reflects the lethal nature of ascending aortic tears
  - Multiple tears may be present in a small number of patients

Radiographic Findings

- Radiography
  - Mediastinal widening > 8 cm (75%)
  - Indistinct aortic outline (75% at arch, 12% at descending)
  - Right paratracheal soft tissue density
  - Esophageal/nasogastric tube deviation to right (67%)
  - Tracheal displacement to right (61%)
  - Inferior displacement of left mainstem bronchus (53%)
  - Apical pleural cap (37%)
  - First or second rib fracture (17%)

CT Findings

- NECT
  - 55% sensitive, 65% specific
  - Obliteration of aortic-fat interface with increased attenuation suggesting mediastinal hemorrhage

DDx: Traumatic Aortic Injury

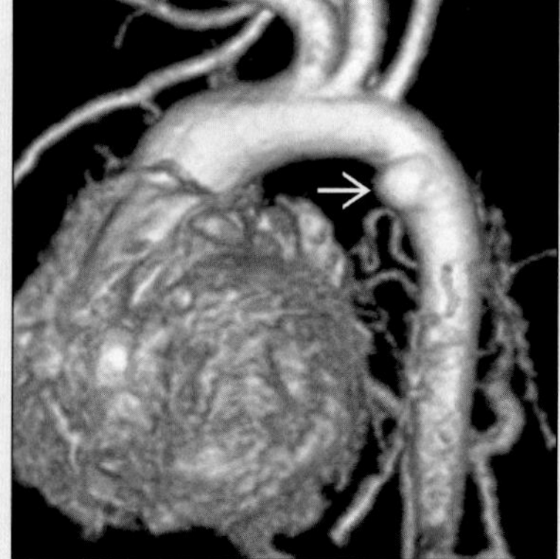

Ductus Diverticulum

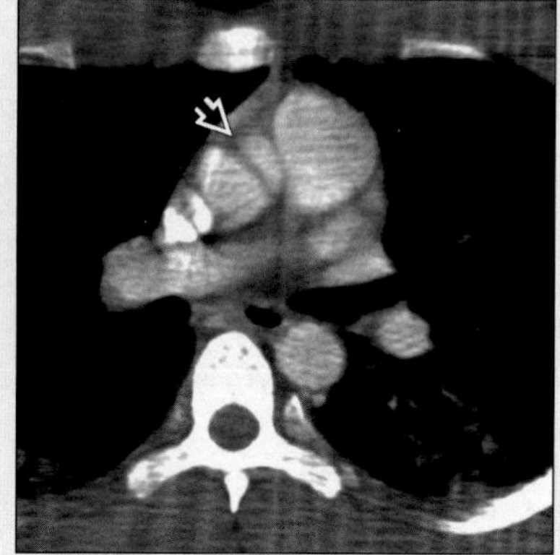

Aortic Pulsation Artifact

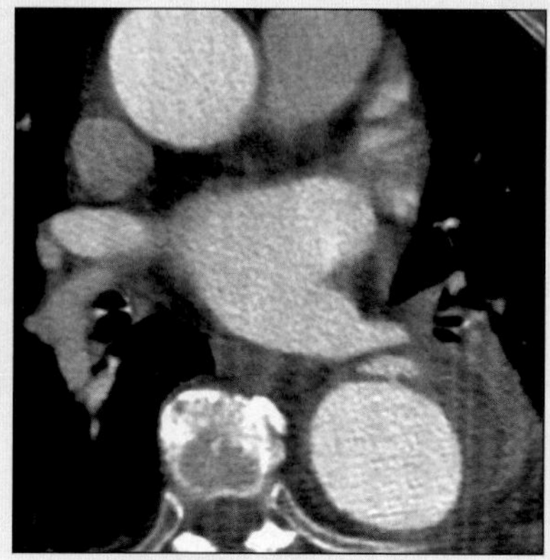

Penetrating Aortic Ulcer

TRAUMATIC AORTIC LACERATION

Key Facts

Terminology

- Aortic pseudoaneurysm, aortic rupture, traumatic aortic aneurysm, aortic transection, traumatic aortic injury

Imaging Findings

- Mediastinal widening
- Localized saccular outpouching of aorta
- 88% aortic isthmus
- 4.5% aortic arch with avulsion of brachiocephalic trunk
- 2% descending thoracic aorta
- 1% ascending aorta immediately above aortic valve
- Multiple tears may be present in a small number of patients
- Obliteration of aortic-fat interface with increased attenuation suggesting mediastinal hemorrhage
- Abrupt change of aortic contour
- Intimal flap
- Pseudoaneurysm

Top Differential Diagnoses

- Ductus Diverticulum
- Penetrating Atherosclerotic Ulcer

Diagnostic Checklist

- Critical not to mistake a linear lucency seen with traumatic laceration for a dissection
- Linear lucency seen on CT is localized, does not extend more than a few mm
- Treatment for dissection is control of blood pressure, treatment of a traumatic aortic laceration is surgical or endovascular repair

  - Hematoma displacing trachea and esophagus to the right
  - High attenuation in aorta wall: Intramural hematoma
  - Hemopericardium suggests ascending aortic or cardiac injury
- CECT
  - Negative CT has nearly 100% negative predictive value
  - Abrupt change of aortic contour
    - Descending aorta at level of left mainstem bronchus and left pulmonary artery
  - Intimal flap
  - Pseudoaneurysm
  - Intraluminal soft tissue densities or filling defects
  - Pseudocoarctation secondary to large pseudoaneurysm compressing lumen
  - Extravasation of contrast: Rare finding
  - May require multiplanar reformatting
    - Acquire using thin sections for CTA
    - Use rapid IV contrast bolus (2-5 cc/sec for 100-150 cc)

MR Findings

- MRA
  - Generally not used in acute setting
  - MR angiography may be used for equivocal cases if patient can undergo MR/MRA
  - Demonstrates delayed complications such as pseudoaneurysm, coarctation of aorta

Echocardiographic Findings

- Newer techniques in transesophageal echocardiogram (TEE) are accurate
  - Proximal ascending and descending aorta may be seen
  - May be performed at bedside

Angiographic Findings

- Conventional
  - Classically was gold standard but recent advances in CTA have led to limited role of angiography
  - Angiography reserved for equivocal cases, or in cases where endovascular repair is planned
  - Contour abnormality usually on undersurface of aorta, just distal to left subclavian
  - Intimal flap (5-10%)
  - Posttraumatic dissection is rare, maybe present in setting of atherosclerotic aorta
  - Rupture with extravasation of contrast material
  - Technique
    - At least two views optimal, prefer 45° lateral anterior oblique (LAO), AP and lateral view
    - Rate 20-30 cc/sec for total volume 40-60 cc
    - Consider brachial approach if there is any resistance encountered in passing wire or catheter in the region of the aortic isthmus

Imaging Recommendations

- Best imaging tool: Thin slice CT with image reformatting
- Initial study chest X-ray then consider CECT unless urgent surgery required due to unstable clinical status

DIFFERENTIAL DIAGNOSIS

Ductus Diverticulum

- Located at aortic isthmus in 10% of normal population
- Smooth contour with obtuse margin
- Broad-based outpouching
- Absence of any intimal flap or tear

Penetrating Atherosclerotic Ulcer

- Location usually not at inner aspect of aortic isthmus
- Look for associated calcified atherosclerotic plaque

PATHOLOGY

General Features

- General path comments
  - Shear stress at points of maximal fixation of aorta
  - Laceration most often transverse

 - Tear in one or more layers of the aorta
 - All layers of aortic wall involved in only 40%
- Etiology
 - Trauma
  - Rapid deceleration during motor vehicle accidents
  - Fall from great heights

Gross Pathologic & Surgical Features

- Intimal tear with mediastinal hematoma

CLINICAL ISSUES

Presentation

- Exsanguination before reaching hospital (85% of total)
- Chest pain
- Dyspnea
- Dysphagia
- Hypertension in upper extremities secondary to traumatic coarctation
- Systolic murmur in second left parasternal interface

Natural History & Prognosis

- 15-20% initial survival rate
- May develop chronic posttraumatic pseudoaneurysm
 - Defined as present > 3 months
 - Incidence: 2-5% patients surviving aortic transection > 24-48 hr
 - Most commonly at level of ligamentum arteriosum
- Incomplete rupture (15% of total)
 - Progression to complete rupture within 24 hours (50%)
 - False aneurysm formation (40-60%)
- With surgery 60-70% survival rate
- Without intervention
 - 80% death within 1 hour
 - 85% death within 24 hours
 - 98% death within 10 weeks

Treatment

- Surgical repair
 - Left thoracotomy with placement of interposition graft or primary anastomosis
- Endovascular stent grafting
 - Requires careful characterization of injury in order to plan approach

DIAGNOSTIC CHECKLIST

Image Interpretation Pearls

- Critical not to mistake a linear lucency seen with traumatic laceration for a dissection
- Linear lucency seen on CT is localized, does not extend more than a few mm
- Treatment for dissection is control of blood pressure, treatment of a traumatic aortic laceration is surgical or endovascular repair

SELECTED REFERENCES

1. Steenburg SD et al: Blunt traumatic injury of the ascending aorta: multidetector CT findings in two cases. Emerg Radiol. 13(4):217-21, 2007
2. Bruckner BA et al: Critical evaluation of chest computed tomography scans for blunt descending thoracic aortic injury. Ann Thorac Surg. 81(4):1339-46, 2006
3. Farber MA: Emergent stent-graft treatment for rupture. J Vasc Surg. 43 Suppl A:44A-47A, 2006
4. Field ML et al: Small vessel avulsion and acute aortic syndrome: A putative aetiology for initiation and propagation of blunt traumatic aortic injury at the isthmus. Med Hypotheses. 2006
5. Lin PH et al: Endovascular treatment of traumatic thoracic aortic injury--should this be the new standard of treatment? J Vasc Surg. 43 Suppl A:22A-29A, 2006
6. Malloy PC et al: Thoracic angiography and intervention in trauma. Radiol Clin North Am. 44(2):239-49, viii, 2006
7. Mirvis SE: Thoracic vascular injury. Radiol Clin North Am. 44(2):181-97, vii, 2006
8. Sayeed R et al: Magnetic resonance angiogram 3-D reconstruction in acute aortic transection. Emerg Med J. 23(2):e14, 2006
9. Manghat NE et al: Multi-detector row computed tomography: imaging in acute aortic syndrome. Clin Radiol. 60(12):1256-67, 2005
10. Amabile P et al: Surgical versus endovascular treatment of traumatic thoracic aortic rupture. J Vasc Surg. 40(5):873-9, 2004
11. O'Conor CE: Diagnosing traumatic rupture of the thoracic aorta in the emergency department. Emerg Med J. 21(4):414-9, 2004
12. Richens D et al: A finite element model of blunt traumatic aortic rupture. Eur J Cardiothorac Surg. 25(6):1039-47, 2004
13. Richens D et al: Rupture of the aorta following road traffic accidents in the United Kingdom 1992-1999. The results of the co-operative crash injury study. Eur J Cardiothorac Surg. 23(2):143-8, 2003
14. Parker MS et al: Making the transition: the role of helical CT in the evaluation of potentially acute thoracic aortic injuries. AJR Am J Roentgenol. 176(5):1267-72, 2001
15. Scaglione M et al: Role of contrast-enhanced helical CT in the evaluation of acute thoracic aortic injuries after blunt chest trauma. Eur Radiol. 11(12):2444-8, 2001
16. Trachiotis GD et al: Traumatic thoracic aortic rupture in the pediatric patient. Ann Thorac Surg. 62(3):724-31; discussion 731-2, 1996

IMAGE GALLERY

Typical

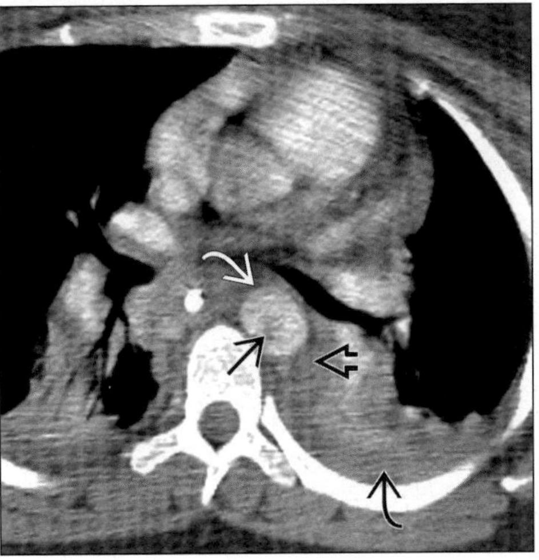

(Left) Axial CECT shows dissection flap in the descending aorta. In addition, peri-aortic hematoma and left pleural effusion are also seen. ***(Right)*** Axial CECT shows contour abnormality of the descending thoracic aorta with intraluminal filling defects, peri-aortic hematoma and a left pleural effusions.

Typical

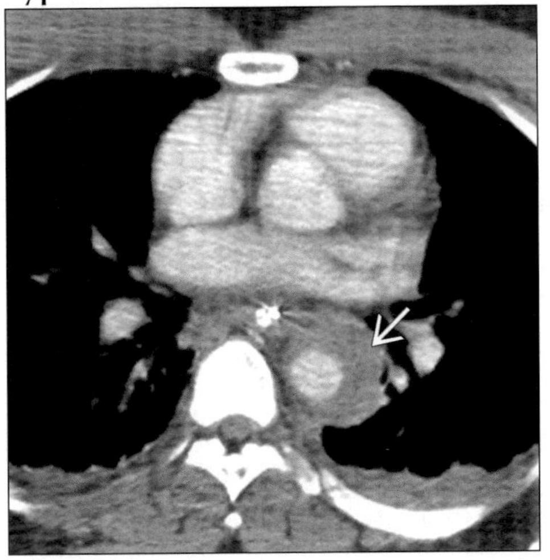

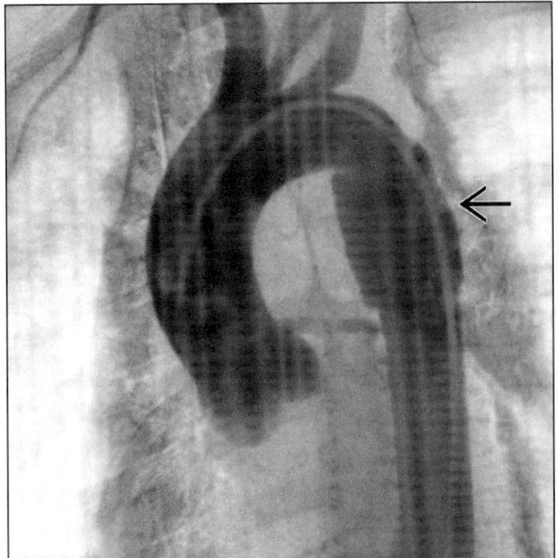

(Left) Axial CECT shows high attenuation in the wall of the descending thoracic aorta suggesting an intramural hematoma or thrombosed false lumen of an acute dissection. ***(Right)*** Left anterior oblique aortogram shows a pseudoaneurysm of the proximal descending thoracic aorta. 2-3% of patients will develop a chronic post-traumatic pseudoaneurysm aortic following an aortic laceration.

Typical

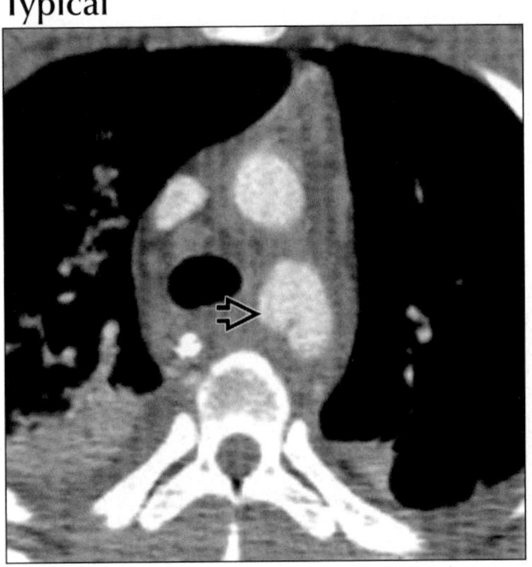

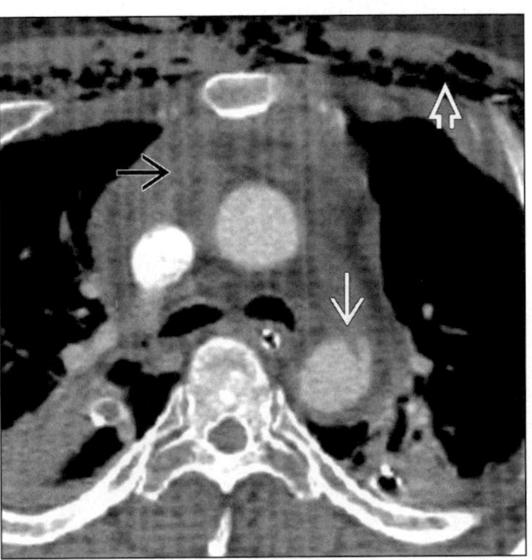

(Left) Axial CECT shows a pseudoaneurysm and contour deformity of the descending thoracic aorta. In addition, minimal periaortic hematoma is also seen. ***(Right)*** Axial CECT shows contour deformity of the descending thoracic aorta with a transection. Associated mediastinal hematoma and soft tissue emphysema are also seen in this patient who sustained a deceleration injury to the throat.

DUCTUS DIVERTICULUM

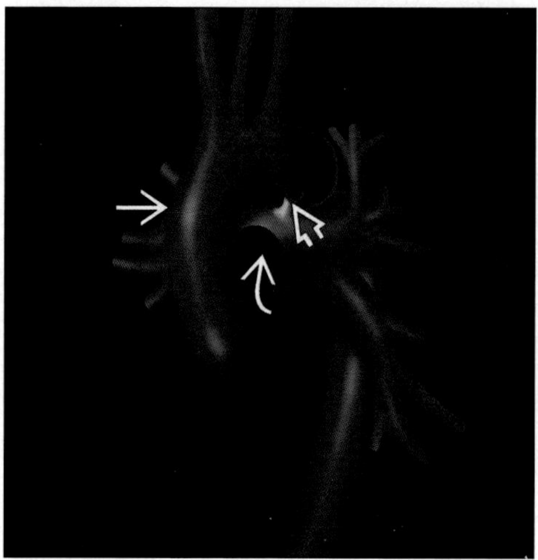

Graphic shows normal anatomy of the great vessels, and the location of the ductus diverticulum ➨, a remnant of the embryologic ductus arteriosus that connected the pulmonary arteries ➨ and the aorta ➨.

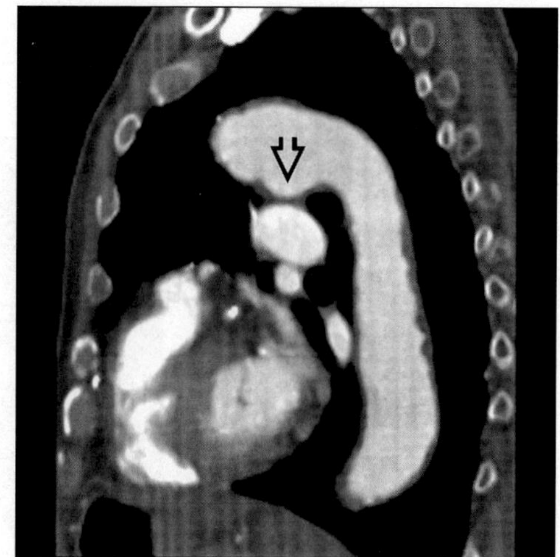

Sagittal CTA shows a smooth, well-defined outpouching ➨ along the aortic isthmus consistent with ductus diverticulum. The ductus diverticulum is located at the transition from transverse aorta to the descending aorta.

TERMINOLOGY

Abbreviations and Synonyms

- Ductus
- Ductus bulge
- Aortic diverticulum: Usually refers to diverticulum of Kommerell

Definitions

- Ductus diverticulum: Smooth focal bulge along anteromedial aspect of aortic isthmus at site of obliterated ductus arteriosus

IMAGING FINDINGS

General Features

- Best diagnostic clue
  - Well-defined smooth outpouching arising from distal transverse aortic arch at level of isthmus just after origin of left subclavian artery
  - Uninterrupted smooth margin: Best diagnostic clue
  - No sharp edges
  - Typically forms gentle obtuse angles with aortic wall
  - Otherwise normal mediastinum and aorta
  - Absence of intimal flap
  - Typically no contrast material retention on DSA
- Location: Along anteromedial aspect of transverse aortic arch at aortoductal junction (aortic isthmus)
- Size
  - Small bulge, can increase aortic diameter by average of 4.3 mm
  - Unusually enlarged ductus is called aneurysm
    - Aneurysmal dilatation of ductus diverticulum greater than 3 cm needs surgical intervention
- Morphology: Smooth bulging of aortic side of ductus arteriosus

Radiographic Findings

- Ductus is difficult to visualize on PA chest X-ray
  - Ductus aneurysm can sometimes be seen as aortopulmonary window soft tissue opacity or mass
- Lateral radiograph may show small bump-like vascular shadow at distal transverse aortic arch

CT Findings

- Typical appearance
  - No mediastinal or peri-aortic hematoma
  - No intimal flap

DDx: Ductus Diverticulum

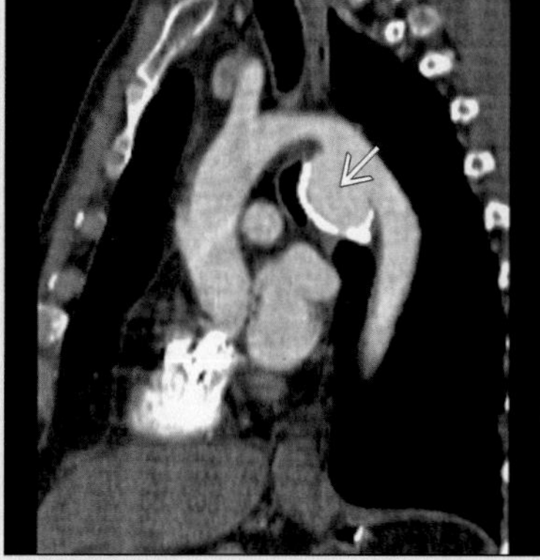

Post-Traumatic Pseudoaneurysm

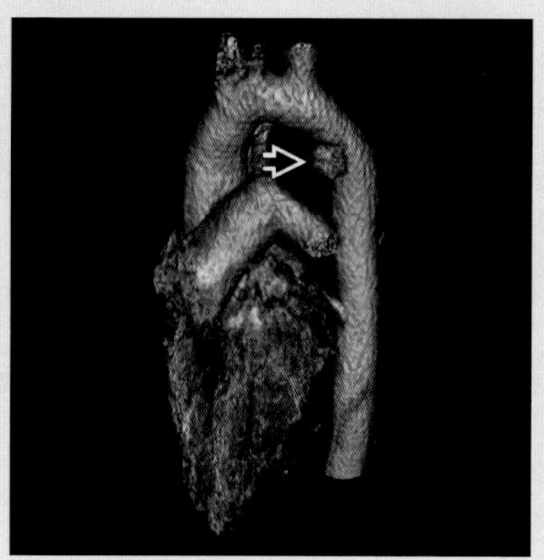

Aortic Transsection

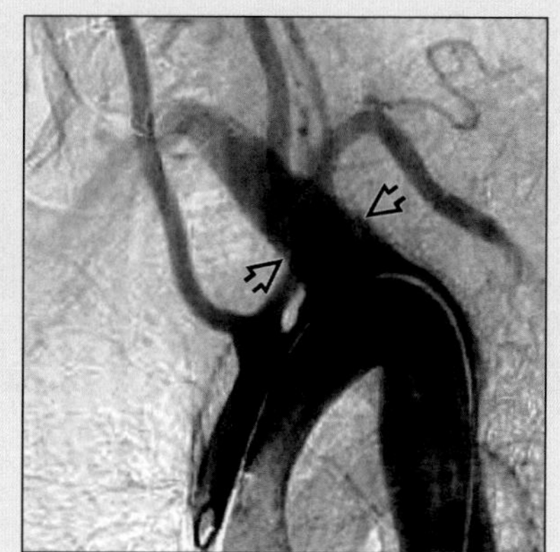

Diverticulum of Kommerell

DUCTUS DIVERTICULUM

Key Facts

Terminology

- Ductus diverticulum: Smooth focal bulge along anteromedial aspect of aortic isthmus at site of obliterated ductus arteriosus
  - Also termed ductus bulge, ductus

Imaging Findings

- Three dimensional (3D) CT or MR angiography
  - Smooth outpouching
  - Uninterrupted margin
  - Gently sloping symmetrical shoulders forming obtuse angles with inferior margin of aortic arch
- Atypical appearance
  - Acute angle at superior margin resulting in steep and asymmetrical sloping
  - Ductus may fold back against aorta and results in pseudo intimal flap

Top Differential Diagnoses

- Aortic (Traumatic) Pseudoaneurysm
- Ulcerated Atherosclerotic Plaque
- Diverticulum of Kommerell
- Atherosclerotic Aneurysm

Clinical Issues

- Diverticulum noted at infancy; usually shrinks over a period and stays as small residual bump at isthmus
- Treatment usually unnecessary unless aneurysmal
  - Usually no fatal sequelae
  - Rarely aneurysmal formation; especially in hypertensive and elderly patients with atherosclerotic aorta
  - Aneurysmal dilatation of ductus diverticulum needs intervention if size is greater than 3 cm

  - Wide-mouthed contrast-filled outpouching at anteromedial aspect of distal transverse aortic arch
  - Uninterrupted smooth margin/wall: Best diagnostic clue
  - Gently sloping symmetrical shoulders forming obtuse angles with inferior margin of aortic arch
  - Increase in aortic lumen not greater than 1 cm
- Atypical appearance
  - Acute angle at superior margin resulting in a steep and asymmetrical sloping
  - Ductus may fold back against the aorta and results in a pseudo intimal flap
- Best visualized on sagittal oblique reconstructed images; may be difficult to readily appreciate ductus diverticulum on axial images
- For exclusion of associated traumatic pseudoaneurysm in context of trauma and incidental ductus
  - Absence of mediastinal or periaortic hematoma and presence of uninterrupted smooth margin of diverticulum
  - Virtual angioscopy at workstation using a special post-processing software would help to identify intimal flap in setting of traumatic pseudoaneurysm
- Ductus diverticulum aneurysm is saccular dilatation along inferior margin of aortic arch
  - Superior margin of aneurysm extends to left subclavian artery
  - Axial CTA images may show a typical "3 star sign" at aortopulmonary window
    - Proximal arch, descending aorta and saccular aneurysm of diverticulum appear as a hook-shaped structure

MR Findings

- MRA
  - MRA and post-contrast GRE images are useful to exclude pseudoaneurysm from atypical ductus diverticulum
  - Findings are similar as described on CTA
    - No intimal flap
    - Smooth outpouching at anteromedial aspect of distal transverse aortic arch

Angiographic Findings

- Contrast-filled, well-defined smooth outpouching arising from inferior margin of aortic arch
- Contrast retention usually occurs in traumatic pseudoaneurysm but very rarely seen in atypical ductus diverticulum
- No intimal flap; pseudo intimal flap is seen with diverticulum fold over
- Aneurysm of ductus diverticulum is seen as saccular dilatation along inferior margin of distal transverse arch
  - Superior margin of aneurysm extends to left subclavian artery

Imaging Recommendations

- Best imaging tool: Three dimensional (3D) CT or MR angiography
- Protocol advice
  - Contrast-enhanced CT angiography with 1.5 mm collimation
  - Sagittal oblique thin MIP reconstruction images (3 mm slice thickness)
    - Essential to identify and assess relationship of ductus with pulmonary artery, aortic arch and subclavian artery
    - Also helps to see smooth shoulders of ductus diverticulum
  - Pre and post-contrast GRE and contrast-enhanced MRA (at least 2 passes)
    - Sagittal oblique thin MIP reconstruction images with 10 mm thickness; coronal thin MIP rotation

DIFFERENTIAL DIAGNOSIS

Aortic (Traumatic) Pseudoaneurysm

- Pseudoductus
- Traumatic pseudoaneurysm due to partial or complete aortic transection; hematoma is within media and is contained by adventitia of aortic wall
  - Presence of intimal flap

DUCTUS DIVERTICULUM

- Contrast-filled outpouching is irregular, and has varying size and shape
- Communication with aorta through narrow mouth; acute angles
- Intermediate to high density peri-aortic or mediastinal hematoma
- Pseudoaneurysm may compress aortic lumen
- Delayed clearance of contrast agent on catheter angiography

Ulcerated Atherosclerotic Plaque

- Elderly patients
- Contrast-filled irregular outpouching
- Commonly associated with mural thickening and calcification
- Solitary and multifocal lesions

Diverticulum of Kommerell

- Dilatation or aneurysm of aberrant subclavian artery origin at inferior margin of distal transverse arch
- May be associated with right-sided aortic arch and vascular ring

Atherosclerotic Aneurysm

- Elderly patients
- Saccular aneurysm usually involves anterolateral aspect of aorta
- Usually involves both sides of aortic wall

PATHOLOGY

General Features

- Genetics: No known genetic etiology is proposed; sporadic incidence
- Etiology
  - In developing fetus, ductus arteriosus is shunt connecting pulmonary artery to aortic arch
    - In utero allows most of blood from right ventricle to bypass fetus' fluid-filled lungs
    - Ductus arteriosus normally closes after birth
  - Ductus diverticulum is remnant of infundibular part of ductus arteriosus
    - Located at transition from transverse aorta to fixed descending aorta
- Epidemiology
  - 9-26% of all adults
  - 33% of infants
- Associated abnormalities
  - Aneurysm of ductus diverticulum
  - Persistent patent ductus arteriosus in infants

Microscopic Features

- Remnant of infundibular part of ductus arteriosus

CLINICAL ISSUES

Presentation

- Most common signs/symptoms
  - Asymptomatic
  - Nearly always noted as incidental finding on angiography such as CT, MR or DSA
- Other signs/symptoms: Aneurysmal dilatation may present with chest pain, embolic stroke, hemodynamic instability due to rupture

Demographics

- Age
  - All age groups
  - More common in children than adults
- Gender
  - Equally seen in males and females
  - No sex preponderance

Natural History & Prognosis

- Diverticulum noted at infancy, usually shrinks over period and stays as small residual bump at isthmus
- Usually no fatal sequelae
- Rare aneurysm formation; occurs in hypertensive and elderly patients with atherosclerotic aorta
  - Increased pressure load to aortic site of ductus diverticulum, eventually resulting in aneurysm
  - Rupture, thromboembolism, and infection of aneurysm may occur

Treatment

- None; leave it alone unless aneurysmal
- Aneurysmal dilatation of ductus diverticulum needs intervention if size is greater than 3 cm
  - Endovascular stent graft repair
  - Conventional open surgical repair

DIAGNOSTIC CHECKLIST

Image Interpretation Pearls

- Ductus diverticulum best visualized on sagittal oblique reconstructed images
  - May be difficult to readily appreciate ductus diverticulum on axial images
- Absence of periaortic hematoma and presence of uninterrupted smooth margin of diverticulum differentiates from traumatic pseudoaneurysm

SELECTED REFERENCES

1. Saito N et al: Successful endovascular repair of an aneurysm of the ductus diverticulum with a branched stent graft: case report and review of literature. J Vasc Surg. 40(6):1228-33, 2004
2. Sugimoto T et al: Aneurysm of the ductus diverticulum in adults: the diagnostic value of three-dimensional computed tomographic scanning. Jpn J Thorac Cardiovasc Surg. 51(10):524-7, 2003
3. Ferrera PC et al: Ductus diverticulum interpreted as traumatic aortic injury. Am J Emerg Med. 15(4):371-2, 1997
4. Fisher RG et al: "Lumps" and "bumps" that mimic acute aortic and brachiocephalic vessel injury. Radiographics. 17(4):825-34, 1997
5. Oxorn D et al: The ductus diverticulum: false-positive angiographic diagnosis of traumatic aortic disruption. J Cardiothorac Vasc Anesth. 11(1):86-8, 1997
6. Morse SS et al: Traumatic aortic rupture: false-positive aortographic diagnosis due to atypical ductus diverticulum. AJR Am J Roentgenol. 150(4):793-6, 1988
7. Goodman PC et al: Angiographic evaluation of the ductus diverticulum. Cardiovasc Intervent Radiol. 5(1):1-4, 1982

DUCTUS DIVERTICULUM

IMAGE GALLERY

Other

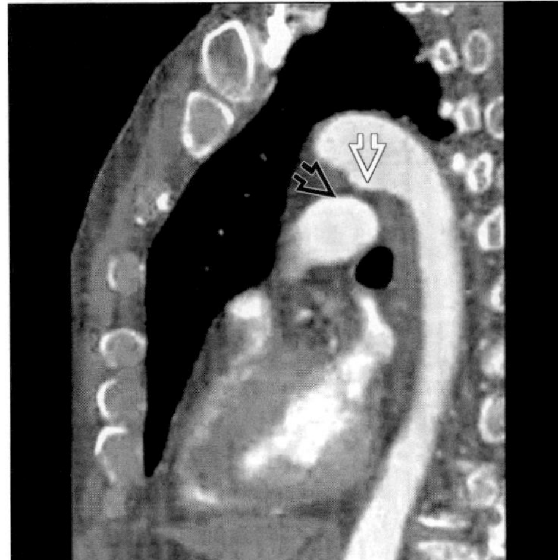

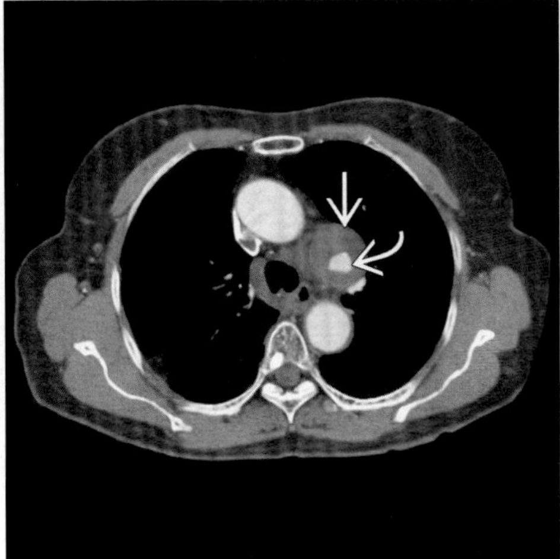

(Left) *Sagittal CTA shows a small bulge with gentle obtuse angles with the aortic wall which is typical for ductus diverticulum ⇨. The proximity of the ductus diverticulum to the main pulmonary artery ⇨ reflects that it is a remnant of the ductus arteriosus that connected the pulmonary artery to the aortic arch in utero.* ***(Right)*** *Axial CECT shows a thrombosed ductus diverticulum aneurysm →. The center of the thrombosed lumen is perfused ↪.*

Other

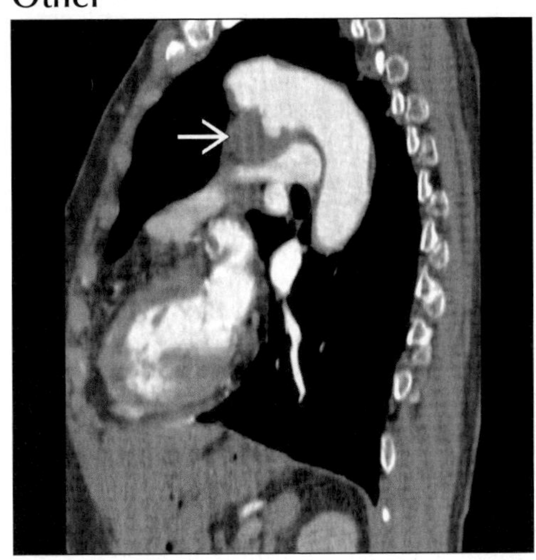

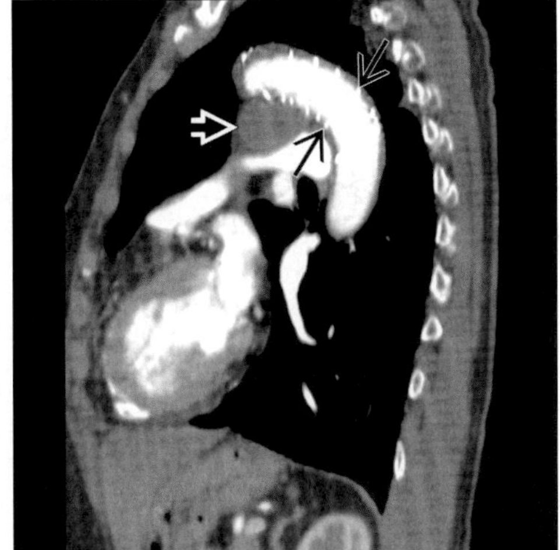

(Left) *Sagittal CTA (same as previous), shows the outpouching in the aortic isthmus which is consistent with a thrombosed ductus diverticulum aneurysm →. Although such aneurysms are rare, they can occur in elderly hypertensive patients with an atherosclerotic aorta.* ***(Right)*** *Sagittal CTA in the same patient as previous, following endovascular repair of the ductus diverticulum aneurysm shows a thoracic aortic stent graft → and exclusion of the ductus aneurysm ⇨.*

Variant

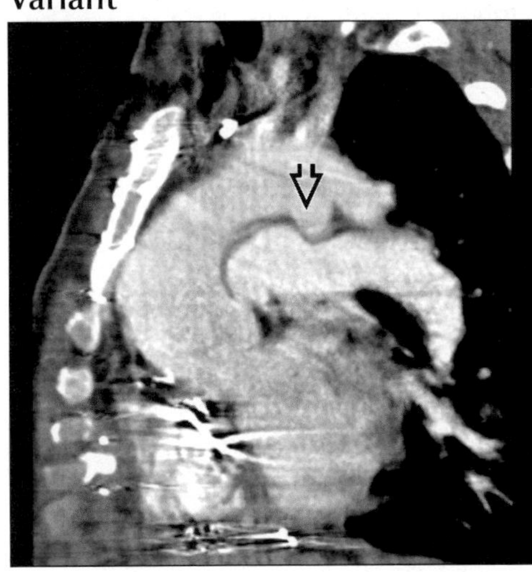

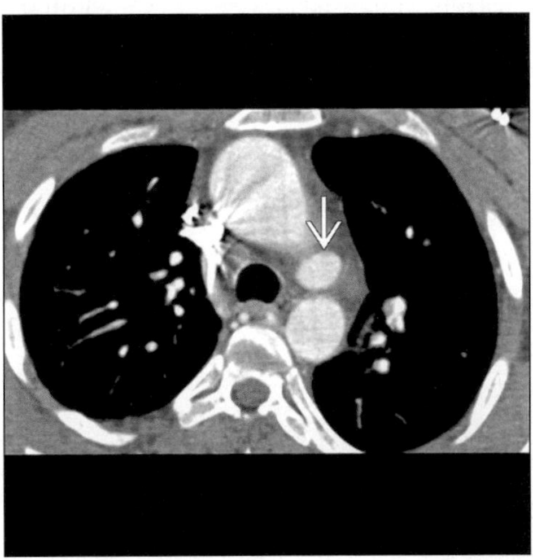

(Left) *Sagittal CTA demonstrates an atypical ductus diverticulum, which forms acute angles with the aortic wall. The smooth, uninterrupted margin with the aortic wall, however, is consistent with this benign diagnosis ⇨.* ***(Right)*** *Axial CECT (same patient as previous image) shows the atypical ductus diverticulum →. In a setting of trauma, the lack of periaortic or mediastinal hematoma and the absence of an intimal flap aid in differentiating this from aortic pseudoaneurysm.*

BRONCHIAL ARTERY PATHOLOGY

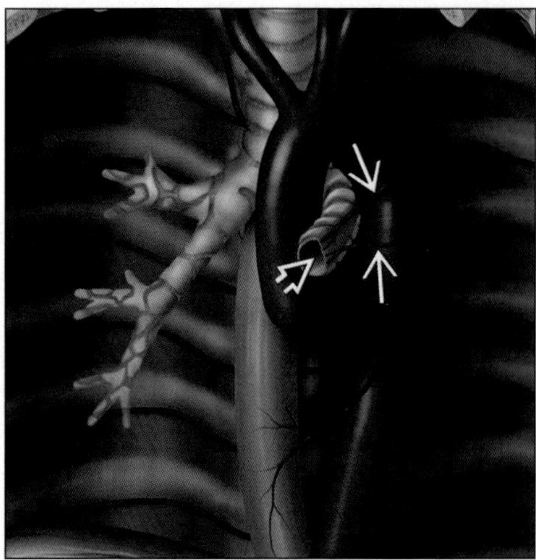

Graphic shows paired left bronchial arteries ➡ arising from the descending thoracic aorta supplying left mainstem bronchus ➡ and its divisions. The right bronchial arteries are not depicted in this graphic.

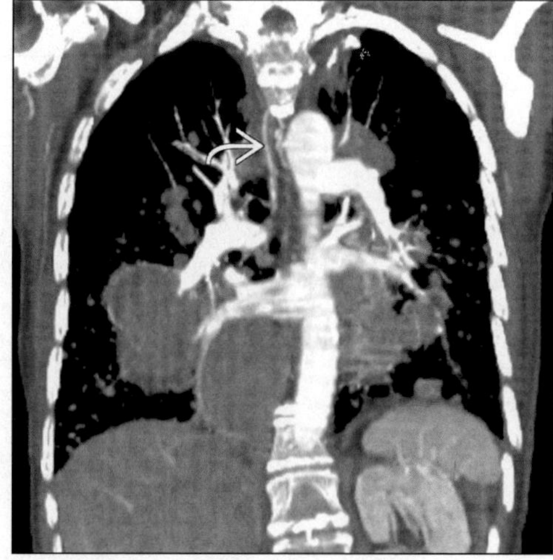

Coronal CTA shows a large bronchial artery on the right ➡ which courses upward, and then down along the bronchi. Patient with multiple lung masses from metastatic thyroid cancer.

TERMINOLOGY

Abbreviations and Synonyms

- Bronchial artery aneurysm (BAA)
- Bronchial artery embolization (BAE)

Definitions

- Arteries supplying bronchial structures
- Enlarged arteries commonly occurring with recurrent infections leading to potentially life-threatening hemoptysis
- Enlarged arteries which may occur in setting of lung cancer

IMAGING FINDINGS

General Features

- Best diagnostic clue
  - Abnormal lungs in patient with hemoptysis
    - Cystic fibrosis, tuberculosis, aspergillosis
  - Enlarged bronchial arteries seen on CT or angiography
- Location
  - Most common location is in thoracic aorta at level of carina
  - Originate directly from descending thoracic aorta, most commonly between T5-6 vertebrae
  - Right-sided bronchial artery frequently presents as an intercostobronchial trunk
  - Multiple branching patterns: Highly variable
    - Two on the left, one on the right (40%)
    - One on the left and one on right (21%)
    - Two on the left and two on the right (20%)
    - One on the left and two on the right (9.7%)
  - Supply trachea, airways, visceral pleura, esophagus and vasa vasorum of aorta, pulmonary artery and pulmonary vein
- Size
  - Normal bronchial arteries are very small, less than 1.5 mm
  - Bronchial artery larger than 2 mm is abnormal
- Morphology
  - Enhancing tubular structures within the mediastinum and around central airways
  - Retroesophageal area, retrotracheal area, retrobronchial area, aortopulmonary window

DDx: Causes of Hemoptysis

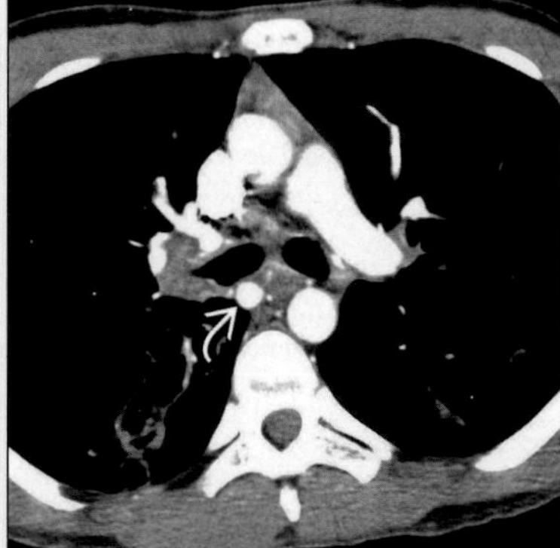

Aneurysm of Bronchial Artery

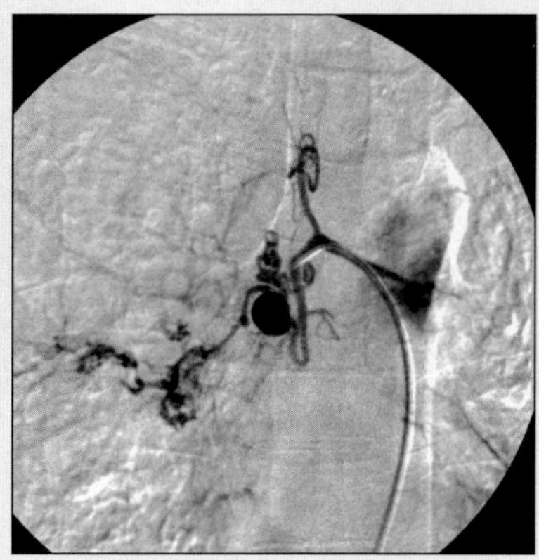

Angiogram: Bronchial Aneurysm

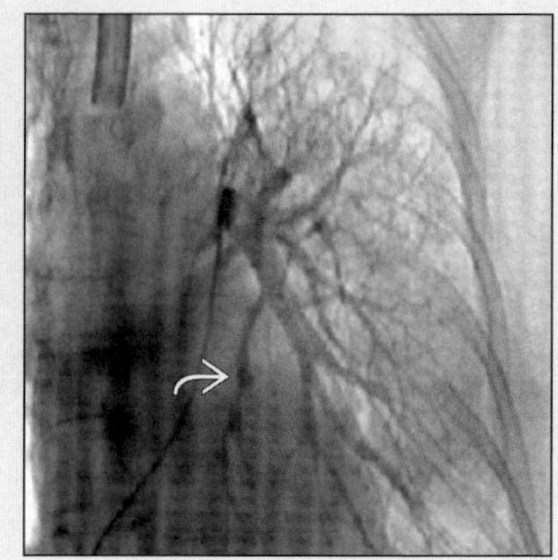

Pulmonary Artery Aneurysm

BRONCHIAL ARTERY PATHOLOGY

Key Facts

Imaging Findings
- Most common location is in thoracic aorta at level of the carina
- Multiple branching patterns: Highly variable
- Bronchial artery larger than 2 mm is abnormal
- MDCT excellent imaging tool
- Angiography required prior to therapy

Top Differential Diagnoses
- Causes of Massive Hemoptysis
  - Bronchial artery aneurysm or pseudoaneurysm
  - Pulmonary artery aneurysm (Rasmussen aneurysm)
  - Pulmonary arteriovenous malformations
  - Aortobronchial fistula
  - Ruptured aortic aneurysm

Pathology
- Bronchial arteries enlarge to provide circulation to diseased lung
- Pulmonary tuberculosis
- Aspergillosis
- Cystic fibrosis
- Bronchogenic cancer
- Chronic thromboembolic disease

Clinical Issues
- Other signs/symptoms
  - Bronchial artery embolization is an established procedure for management of massive hemoptysis
  - Most patients with massive hemoptysis are not surgical candidates because of their poor pulmonary reserve

Radiographic Findings
- Radiography
  - CXR: May demonstrate the side of bleeding
  - May demonstrate cause of bleeding
    - Tuberculosis, bronchogenic cancer, lung abscess, cystic fibrosis, aspergillosis, etc.

CT Findings
- CECT
  - MDCT excellent imaging tool
    - Diagnosis of underlying lung disease
    - Bronchiectasis, bronchogenic carcinoma, aspergilloma
    - May localize site of bleeding
    - Detect bronchial and nonbronchial systemic vessels
    - Pleural thickening and tortuous vascular structures in the extrapleural fat may be signs of nonbronchial systemic arterial supply
    - Nonbronchial arteries can be significant source of recurrent hemoptysis
  - Bronchial arteries usually arise from descending thoracic aorta, most commonly level T5-6
  - Right bronchial artery often a intercostobronchial trunk
    - Arises from right posteromedial aspect of the aorta
  - Left bronchial artery
    - Arises from anterior aspect of descending thoracic aorta
    - Short mediastinal length
    - 70% two left bronchial arteries
  - Anomalous bronchial arteries: Originate outside the T5-6 area are found in 8-21% of cases
    - Most arise from concavity of aortic arch
    - Also from lower thoracic aorta, subclavian arteries, thyrocervical trunk, internal mammary artery, pericardiophrenic artery or inferior phrenic artery
  - Evaluate for nonbronchial systemic arteries acting as collaterals
    - Abnormal, dilated, tortuous arteries in the lungs, but not going along the course of the bronchi
    - Commonly seen in association with pleural thickening
    - Particularly important in patients who have recurrent hemoptysis following bronchial artery embolization

Angiographic Findings
- DSA
  - Dilated, tortuous bronchial arteries
  - Hypervascularity in the lung
  - Bronchial artery to pulmonary artery or vein shunting
  - Unusual to see frank extravasation
  - Important to look for the anterior spinal artery (artery of Adamkiewicz) prior to treatment with embolization
    - Has a characteristic "hairpin" configuration
  - Evaluate for nonbronchial collaterals

Imaging Recommendations
- Best imaging tool
  - Preliminary evaluation with MDCT
  - Angiography required prior to therapy
    - Evaluate for bronchial and nonbronchial arterial supply
- Protocol advice
  - CECT
    - Overlapping axial thin-section images
    - Two-dimensional MIP reformatted images in coronal oblique and sagittal planes
    - Three-dimensional volumetric and shaded-surface-display useful prior to embolization therapy

DIFFERENTIAL DIAGNOSIS

Causes of Massive Hemoptysis
- Bronchial artery aneurysm or pseudoaneurysm
- Pulmonary artery aneurysm (Rasmussen aneurysm)
- Pulmonary arteriovenous malformations
- Aortobronchial fistula
- Ruptured aortic aneurysm

BRONCHIAL ARTERY PATHOLOGY

Nonbronchial Collaterals

- Internal mammary artery, thyrocervical trunk, subclavian artery, costocervical trunk, lateral thoracic artery, inferior phrenic, or abdominal aorta

PATHOLOGY

General Features

- Etiology
  - Lungs have dual arterial vascular system
    - Pulmonary arteries 99% of arterial blood supply to the lungs
    - Bronchial arteries responsible for supplying supporting structures of the airways
    - Anastomoses between bronchial and pulmonary arteries
  - Acute and chronic lung disease may lead to reduced pulmonary circulation because of hypoxic vasoconstriction
  - Bronchial arteries enlarge to provide circulation to diseased lung
  - Systemic arterial bleeding results in massive hemoptysis
  - Chronic inflammation also leads to increase in systemic arterial blood flow
- Epidemiology
  - Chronic inflammatory conditions
    - Pulmonary tuberculosis
    - Aspergillosis
  - Cystic fibrosis
    - Due to chronic infections
  - Bronchogenic cancer
  - Bronchial artery aneurysm
  - Conditions causing decreased arterial perfusion
    - Chronic thromboembolic disease
    - Vasculitis

Gross Pathologic & Surgical Features

- Enlarged, tortuous bronchial arteries

Microscopic Features

- Following embolization the histologic reaction to PVA may include fibrosis, mild chronic inflammation, localized foreign body reaction

CLINICAL ISSUES

Presentation

- Most common signs/symptoms
  - Massive hemoptysis
    - Defined as 240-600 mL/24 hours or greater than 100 mL/day persisting for 3 days or more

Natural History & Prognosis

- Mortality rate for massive hemoptysis managed conservatively is 50-100%

Treatment

- Bronchial artery embolization is an established procedure in the management of massive hemoptysis
  - Embolization usually with PVA particles (300-500 μm)
    - Avoid embolization material that will pass through bronchopulmonary anastomoses (usually < 300 μm)
  - Avoid liquid embolic agents because of high risk of tissue necrosis
  - Avoid coils because of proximal occlusion and preclude repeat embolization
  - Use microcatheter for good positioning and to be beyond any potential spinal arteries
- Aortogram may be useful for finding bronchial arteries of anomalous origin, or nonbronchial systemic arterial supply
- Complications of embolization
  - Chest pain, dysphagia
  - Spinal cord ischemia, rare 1.4-6.5%
  - Other rare complications: Bronchial necrosis, bronchoesophageal fistula, non-target embolization, transient cortical blindness
  - Transient cortical blindness maybe due to embolism of the occipital cortex via a bronchial artery-pulmonary vein shunt, or via collateral vessels between bronchial and vertebral arteries
- Bronchoscopy is usually used only for diagnosis and localization, not for treatment; use of bronchoscopy is being supplanted by MDCT
- Surgery is procedure of choice for some conditions: Aspergilloma, bronchial adenoma, vascular injury
  - Most patients with massive hemoptysis are not surgical candidates because of their poor pulmonary reserve

DIAGNOSTIC CHECKLIST

Image Interpretation Pearls

- Evaluate for number and position of bronchial arteries
- Look for nonbronchial systemic arterial supply

SELECTED REFERENCES

1. Khalil A et al: Role of MDCT in identification of the bleeding site and the vessels causing hemoptysis. AJR Am J Roentgenol. 188(2):W117-25, 2007
2. Andersen PE: Imaging and interventional radiological treatment of hemoptysis. Acta Radiol. 47(8):780-92, 2006
3. Bruzzi JF et al: Multi-detector row CT of hemoptysis. Radiographics. 26(1):3-22, 2006
4. Remy-Jardin M et al: Bronchial and nonbronchial systemic arteries at multi-detector row CT angiography: comparison with conventional angiography. Radiology. 2004
5. Tanaka K et al: Giant mediastinal bronchial artery aneurysm mimicking benign esophageal tumor: a case report and review of 26 cases from literature. J Vasc Surg. 38(5):1125-9, 2003
6. Yoon W et al: Bronchial and nonbronchial systemic artery embolization for life-threatening hemoptysis: a comprehensive review. Radiographics. 22(6):1395-409, 2002

BRONCHIAL ARTERY PATHOLOGY

IMAGE GALLERY

Typical

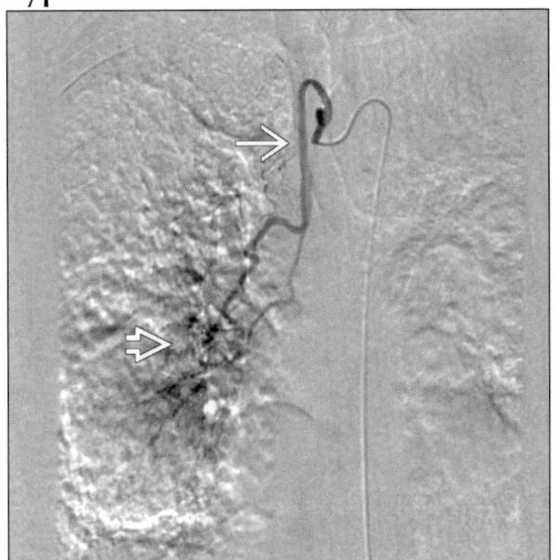

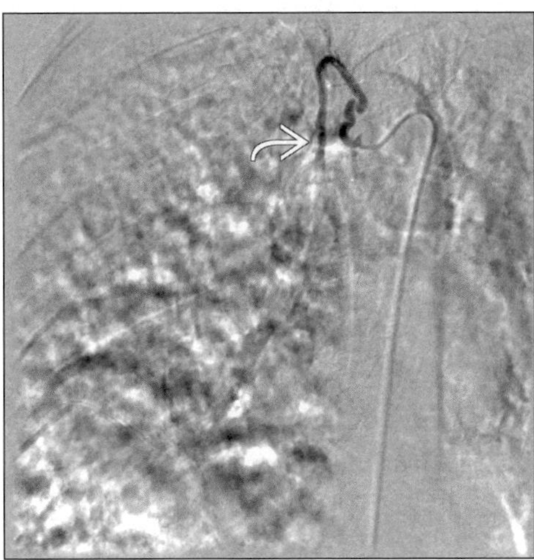

(Left) *DSA of a right bronchial artery in a patient with thyroid cancer and hemoptysis. Enlarged right bronchial artery ➡ with hypervascularity in the right lower lobe ➡.* ***(Right)*** *DSA following embolization with PVA particles. Proximal bronchial artery is occluded ➡. No vascularity identified in the right lower lobe. Bronchial artery embolization is an established procedure for managing massive hemoptysis.*

Other

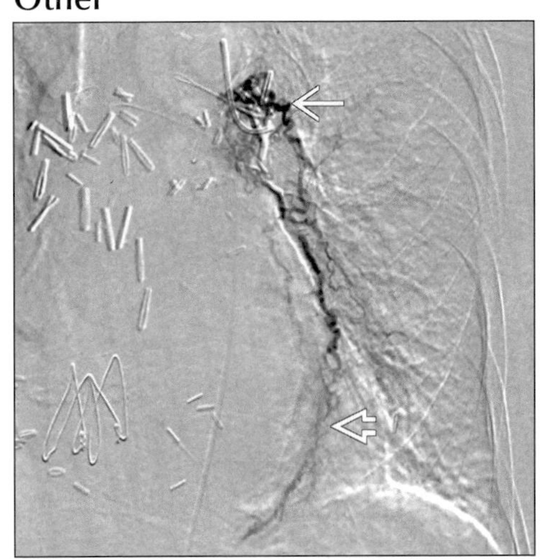

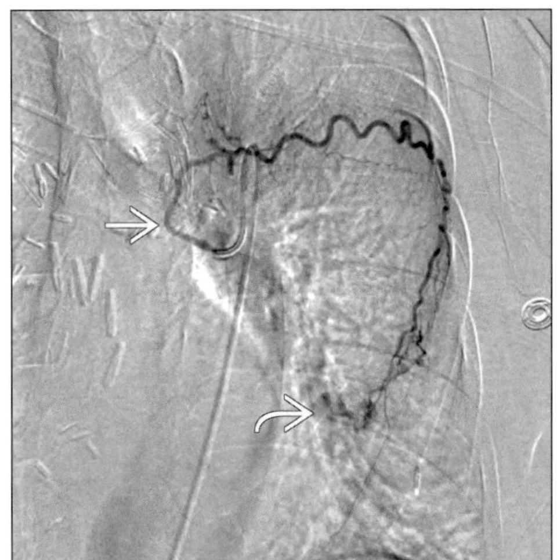

(Left) *DSA patient following lung transplant, now with left-sided hemoptysis. Unusual appearance of left bronchial artery ➡ with collaterals extending along the pericardium ➡.* ***(Right)*** *DSA with catheter in place in the left intercostal artery. Left intercostal artery ➡ supplying collaterals with hypervascularity in the left lung ➡. Non-bronchial collateral arteries can be a significant source of hemoptysis.*

Variant

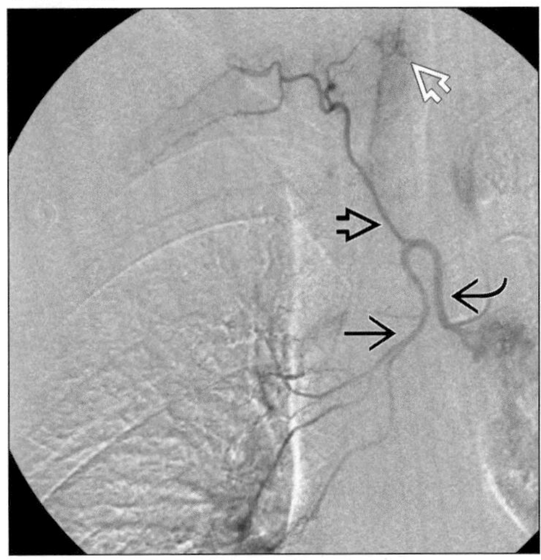

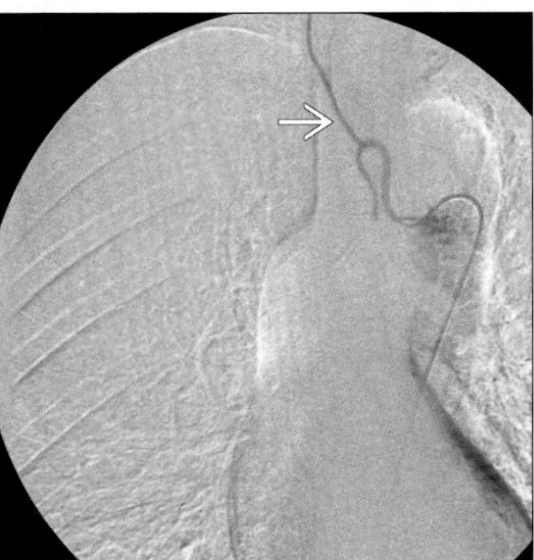

(Left) *DSA shows a common trunk ➡ supplying 2 right intercostals ➡ and a right bronchial artery ➡. Intercostal gives rise to a medially directed vessel probably supplying the trachea ➡.* ***(Right)*** *DSA post embolization with PVA via a microcatheter. The hypervascular bronchial vessels have been embolized. Flow to the intercostal artery ➡ remains.*

PULMONARY ARTERY ANEURYSM

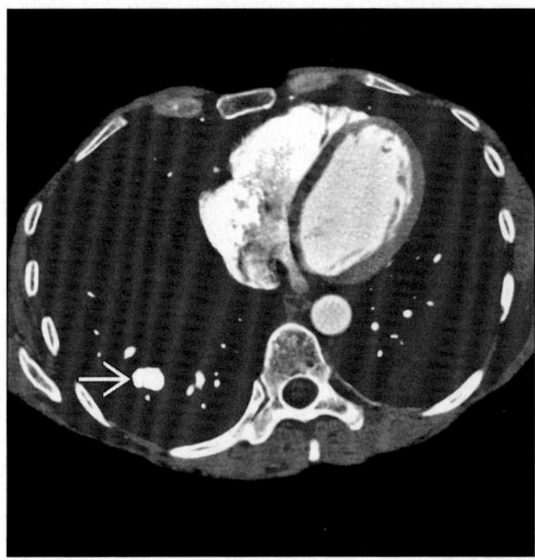

Axial CECT shows mass ➡ in the right lower lung which is strongly enhancing on the contrast CT, consistent with a vascular mass.

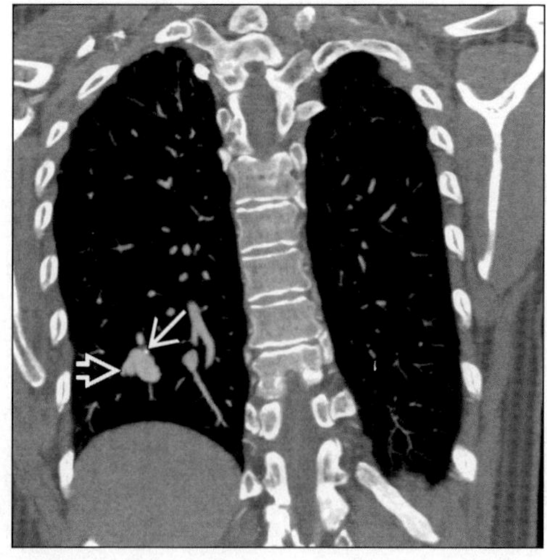

Coronal CECT shows a lobulated density in the lower right lung ➡ associated with a small fleck of calcification ➡. Density is enhanced, consistent with a vascular structure.

TERMINOLOGY

Abbreviations and Synonyms

- Pulmonary artery aneurysm (PAA); pulmonary artery (PA)

Definitions

- Focal enlargement of PA
- True aneurysm: All layers of the artery wall
- False aneurysm: Not all layers involved
- Dissecting aneurysm: Intimal disruption with extension into media of arterial wall

IMAGING FINDINGS

General Features

- Best diagnostic clue
  - Focal dilatation PA
  - Elliptical solitary pulmonary nodule adjacent to segmental PA
- Location
  - Main, hilar, lobar, segmental PAs
  - Peripheral PA less common

Radiographic Findings

- Radiography
  - Round perihilar opacity uni- or bilateral hilar enlargement
    - 1-3 cm in diameter
    - Maybe well-circumscribed or less well-defined
  - Areas of consolidation evolve into nodule or mass
    - Hemorrhage characterized by ill-defined margins or pulmonary consolidation surrounding nodule
  - Central PAA (main and lobar PAs)
    - Enlarged lobulated PAs
    - Asymmetric enlargement central PA
  - Peripheral PAA (segmental arteries to periphery)
    - Nonspecific solitary pulmonary nodule
    - Nodule adjacent to cavitary disease in mycotic aneurysms (Rasmussen)
- Swan-Ganz-induced false aneurysm
  - Most common right lower lobe (most frequent placement of Swan-Ganz catheter)
  - Sharply defined elliptical shape
  - Perihilar adjacent to segmental PA
  - Size usually < 3 cm
  - Rupture

DDx: Pulmonary Artery Aneurysm

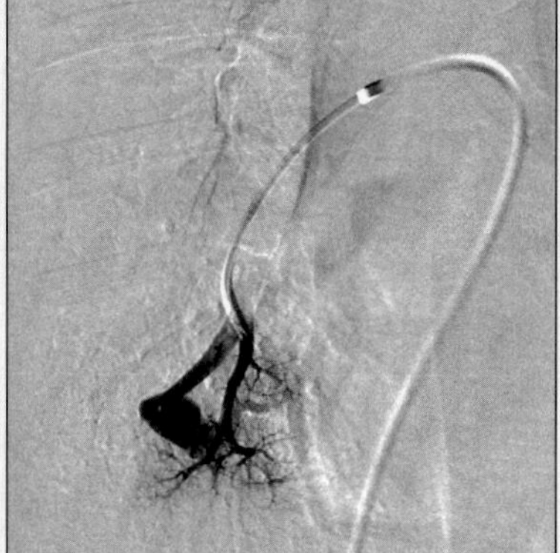

Looks Like Aneurysm

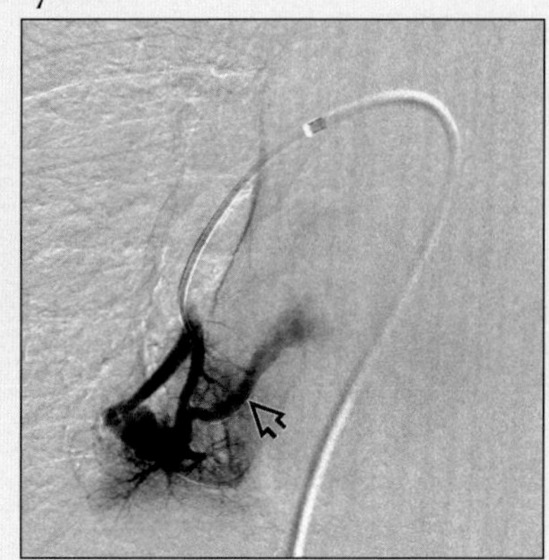

AVM - Early Draining Vein

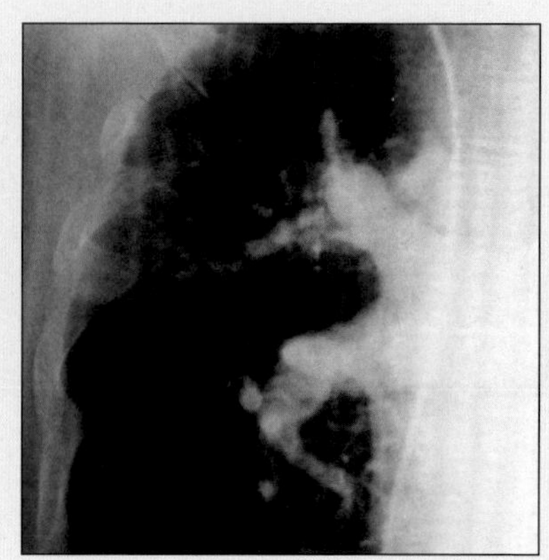

Chronic Pulmonary Emboli

PULMONARY ARTERY ANEURYSM

Key Facts

Imaging Findings
- Elliptical-shaped solitary pulmonary nodule (SPN) adjacent to segmental PA
- May be overlooked, mistaken as normal artery
- Aneurysm will enhance with intravenous contrast, identical to enhancement of adjacent PAs

Top Differential Diagnoses
- PA Stenosis
- PA Hypertension
- Carcinoid Tumors
- Chronic Pulmonary Emboli

Pathology
- Rasmussen aneurysm: Erosion of tuberculous cavity into artery producing a false aneurysm
- Direct rupture of vessel by inflated balloon or by catheter tip
- Mycotic aneurysms: TB, bacterial endocarditis, syphilis, septic emboli
- Systemic vasculitis

Clinical Issues
- Swan-Ganz aneurysm: Mortality rate 45-65%
- Peripheral and solitary aneurysms rupture in 60%
- Lesions enlarge rapidly and are susceptible to rupture

Diagnostic Checklist
- Pulmonary nodules adjacent to segmental arteries
- Carcinoid tumors may also intensely enhance

- Focal consolidation in area of Swan-Ganz catheter, size dependent on quantity of hemorrhage
- Hemothorax if rupture into pleural space

CT Findings
- NECT: Often misinterpreted as hilar adenopathy
- CECT
  - May be overlooked, mistaken as normal artery
  - Peripheral emboli may be detected
  - Aneurysm enhances identically adjacent PAs
  - Behçet disease
    - PA aneurysms (often multiple)
    - Thromboembolic disease
    - Intracardiac thromboses

MR Findings
- Multiplanar capability useful for small aneurysm
- White blood sequences better for characterization
- Black blood sequences less useful due to lack of signal from surrounding lung (poor conspicuity)

Angiographic Findings
- Depicts focal dilation of PA

Imaging Recommendations
- Best imaging tool: CTA with reformations to characterize pulmonary vascular lesions

DIFFERENTIAL DIAGNOSIS

PA Stenosis
- Enlarged main and left PA from jet effect across stenotic valve
- Left upper lobe arteries larger than mirror image arteries in the right upper lobe (due to increased flow)
- Calcified pulmonary valve (rare)

PA Hypertension
- Enlarged central PAs with pruning of distal arteries
- Generalized enlargement

Chronic Pulmonary Emboli
- Dilated proximal PAs
- Embolic material present distally
- Distal to embolus: Vessels appear thin
  - Oligemic regions distal to emboli

Carcinoid Tumors
- Location similar to Swan-Ganz induced false aneurysm
- May enhance, but not as intensely as false aneurysms
- May calcify (central nidus common)

Hereditary Hemorrhagic Telangiectasia
- AVM of pulmonary artery
- Simple form may appear as aneurysmal dilation of pulmonary artery

PATHOLOGY

General Features
- Genetics
  - Behçet disease
    - Associated with (HLA-B51)
  - Hugh-Stovin syndrome
    - Rare disorder
    - Large-vessel vasculitis
    - Multiple aneurysms of large and small PAs
    - Dural sinus and peripheral vein thrombosis
  - Behçet and Hugh-Stovin syndrome have similar pathology
    - Inflammation of vasa vasorum resulting in weakness of arterial wall
    - Fibrosis (thinning) of muscular and elastic arterial walls leading to aneurysms
  - Takayasu arteritis
    - Large-vessel vasculitis
  - Williams syndrome
    - Rare genetic disorder with large artery vasculitis
  - Marfan syndrome
    - Cystic medial necrosis
- Etiology
  - False aneurysms
    - Blunt or lacerating trauma
    - Swan-Ganz catheter false aneurysm

- Mycotic aneurysms: TB, bacterial endocarditis, syphilis, septic emboli, Aspergillus
  - Rasmussen aneurysm: Aneurysm of small to medium PA branches adjacent to tuberculous cavity
- Central PAA
  - True aneurysm
  - PA hypertension: Primary or secondary
  - Congenital anomalies: Left to right shunts, especially patent ductus arteriosus
  - Systemic vasculitis (Hughes-Stovin, Behçet)

- Epidemiology
  - Dissecting aneurysm
    - Pulmonary hypertension
    - Dissecting aneurysms occur with atherosclerosis of PA
    - Left-to-right shunt
    - Congenital defects of pulmonary valve
    - Primary and secondary pulmonary hypertension

Gross Pathologic & Surgical Features

- PA dissecting aneurysm
  - False lumen tends to rupture into the pericardium
  - Most located in main PA (80%); less common in intrapulmonary branches or peripheral vessels (20%)
  - Solitary or multiple
  - Aneurysms of main & lobar branches of PA are rare

Microscopic Features

- Mycotic aneurysms: Bacteria, infection
- Genetic aneurysms: Transmural/inflammation
- Necrotic-vasculitis
- Cystic medial necrosis
- Atherosclerosis

CLINICAL ISSUES

Presentation

- Most common signs/symptoms: Usually asymptomatic
- Other signs/symptoms: Cough, shortness of breath, dyspnea, hemoptysis (can be life threatening)
- Dissection PA
  - Pre-cordial pain
  - Rare and usually lethal complication of chronic pulmonary hypertension, rupture into pericardium tamponade and sudden death
- Behçet disease
  - Behçet triad: Oral ulcerations (99%), recurrent genital ulcers (60%), ocular lesions (70%)
  - Thrombophlebitis (15%), skin hypersensitivity (70%)

Demographics

- Age
  - Swan-Ganz false aneurysm
    - Older adult having hemodynamic monitoring
  - Behçet disease and Hugh-Stovin syndrome
    - Males (20-30 years)
- Gender
  - Swan-Ganz false aneurysm: M < F
  - Behçet disease and Hugh-Stovin syndrome: M > F, (2.3:1)
- Ethnicity: Behçet disease: Middle East, Eastern Mediterranean basin, and Japan

Natural History & Prognosis

- Swan-Ganz aneurysm: Mortality rate 45-65%
- Hughes-Stovin syndrome: Fever, hemoptysis, shortness of breath, dyspnea with exertion
- Underlying aneurysm causing massive hemoptysis (3-6%)
- Lesions enlarge rapidly and are susceptible to rupture
- Peripheral aneurysms rupture in 60% cases
- Cardiovascular symptoms may conceal pulmonary symptoms
- 50% of PAA related to congenital heart disease

Treatment

- Swan-Ganz or Rasmussen aneurysm
  - Interventional coil or balloon embolization
  - Surgical segmentectomy
- Main PA aneurysm: Surgical repair; high morbidity and mortality
  - Excision of the aneurysm and prosthetic patch replacement
- Corticosteroids and cytotoxic agents for vasculitis
- PA banding

DIAGNOSTIC CHECKLIST

Consider

- Determine underlying cause
  - Infection (mycotic aneurysms): Tuberculosis (Rasmussen aneurysm), syphilitic, bacterial, fungal
  - Structural heart disease
  - Structural vascular disease (Marfan syndrome, Behçet syndrome, vasculitis)
  - Pulmonary hypertension
  - Trauma (Swan Ganz catheter)
- Evaluate for left to right intracardiac shunt
- PAA if pulmonary nodules are adjacent to segmental artery

Image Interpretation Pearls

- Carcinoid tumors may also intensely enhance

SELECTED REFERENCES

1. Nguyen ET et al: Pulmonary artery aneurysms and pseudoaneurysms in adults: findings at CT and radiography. AJR Am J Roentgenol. 188(2):W126-34, 2007
2. Castañer E et al: Congenital and acquired pulmonary artery anomalies in the adult: radiologic overview. Radiographics. 26(2):349-71, 2006
3. Erkan D et al: Is Hughes-Stovin syndrome Behçet's disease? Clin Exp Rheumatol. 22(4 Suppl 34):S64-8, 2004

IMAGE GALLERY

Typical

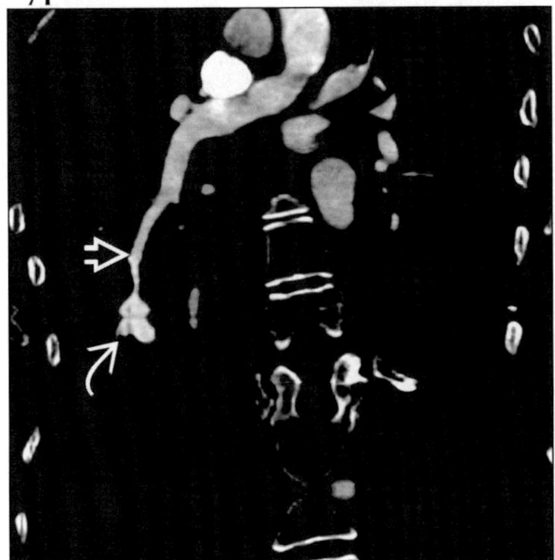

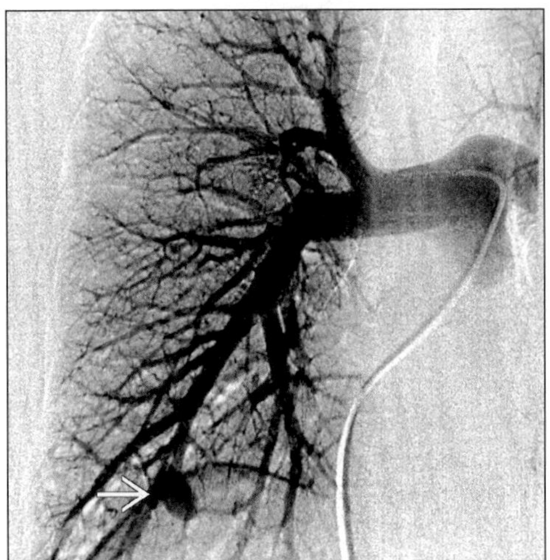

(Left) Coronal CECT that has been reformatted demonstrates the feeding artery ➩ into the aneurysm ➦. This is helpful for angiographic planning. *(Right)* DSA shows aneurysm ➡ arising from right lower lobe vessel. Note that there is no venous drainage to suggest a pulmonary arteriovenous malformation.

Typical

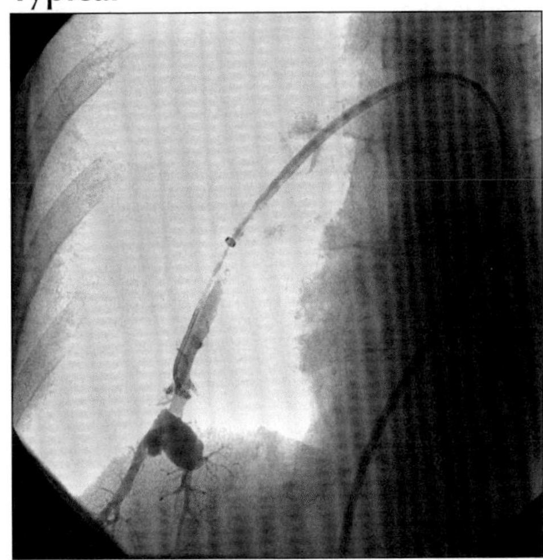

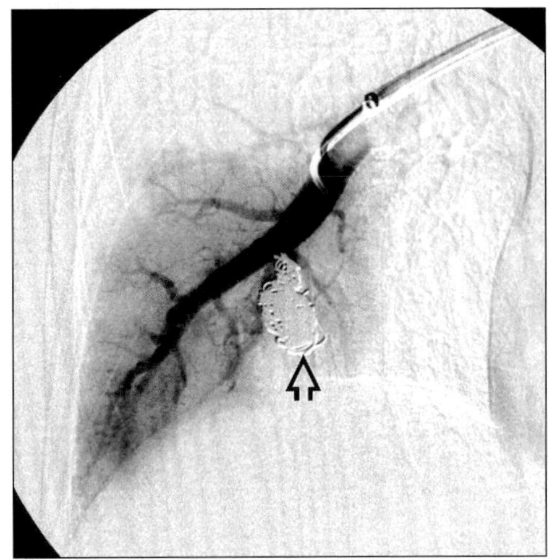

(Left) DSA performed with a subselective catheter position shows the aneurysm with no early venous filling. Very distal aneurysm which makes it a good candidate for embolization. *(Right)* DSA following coil embolization. Mass of coils ➩ that have been packed into the aneurysm to prevent recanalization. Good result with sparing of most of the lung parenchyma.

Typical

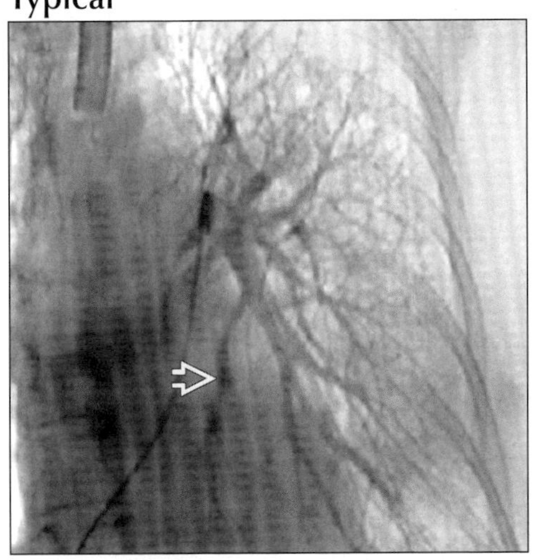

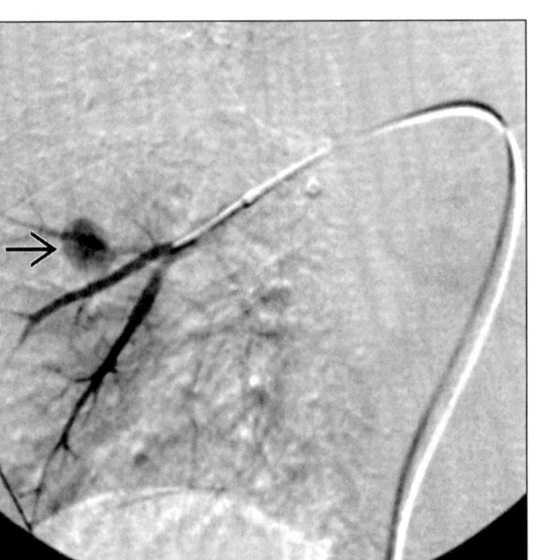

(Left) DSA shows small pulmonary artery aneurysm ➩. Patient had massive hemoptysis with no evidence of bronchial artery enlargement/bleeding. Pulmonary angiogram is an important consideration. *(Right)* DSA shows aneurysm ➡ which is present in a right pulmonary artery branch. The catheter has been placed subselectively in preparation for embolization.

ACUTE PULMONARY EMBOLISM

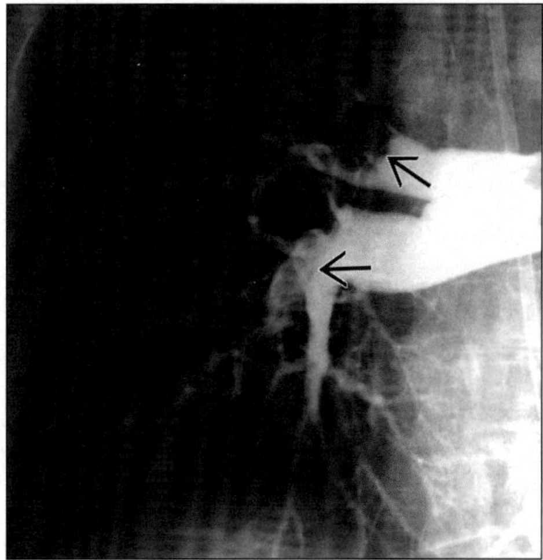

Catheter angiography shows intraluminal filling defects → in right pulmonary artery branches, consistent with PE. Angiography was the "gold standard" for diagnosis of pulmonary emboli, but has been replaced by CECT.

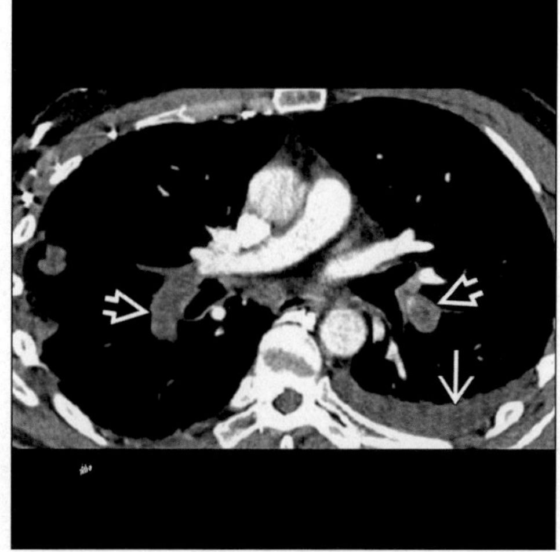

Axial CECT (same patient) shows filling defects in the segmental pulmonary arteries ➡, with distension of the vessel lumen consistent with acute pulmonary embolism. There is also a small left pleural effusion ➡.

TERMINOLOGY

Abbreviations and Synonyms

- Pulmonary embolus (PE), pulmonary thromboembolic disease, pulmonary thromboembolism
- Ventilation/perfusion (V/Q)
- Deep vein thrombosis (DVT)

Definitions

- Pulmonary arterial blockage with resultant segmental perfusion defect(s), most commonly caused by emboli arising from pelvic or lower extremity DVT

IMAGING FINDINGS

General Features

- Best diagnostic clue
  - Central low density filling defect within pulmonary arteries on CTA or angiography
  - Peripheral wedge-shaped consolidation
- Location
  - Commonly bilateral, may involve any portion of pulmonary vascular bed
    - Typically lodge at arterial bifurcations
- Size
  - May be of any size
    - Large emboli lodge proximally and may cause serious symptoms
    - Small emboli lodge where exceed vessel diameter; asymptomatic or may cause pulmonary infarct
- Morphology
  - Sharp interface with intravascular contrast material
  - Large emboli at pulmonary artery bifurcation termed saddle embolus

Radiographic Findings

- Radiography
  - Poor sensitivity and specificity; normal CXR in 10%
  - Vascular alteration
    - Enlargement of central pulmonary artery (knuckle sign) or right interlobar PA (Palla's sign)
    - Enlargement due to vascular distension by clot and increased proximal pulmonary pressure
    - Focal oligemia (Westermark sign) from vascular obstruction and decreased regional perfusion
    - Abrupt tapering or cut off of occluded artery
  - Atelectasis: 2° to decreased ventilation

DDx: Acute Pulmonary Embolism

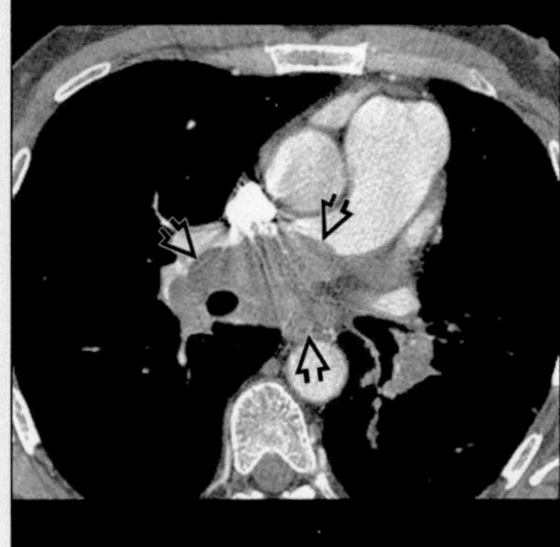

Pulmonary Artery Sarcoma

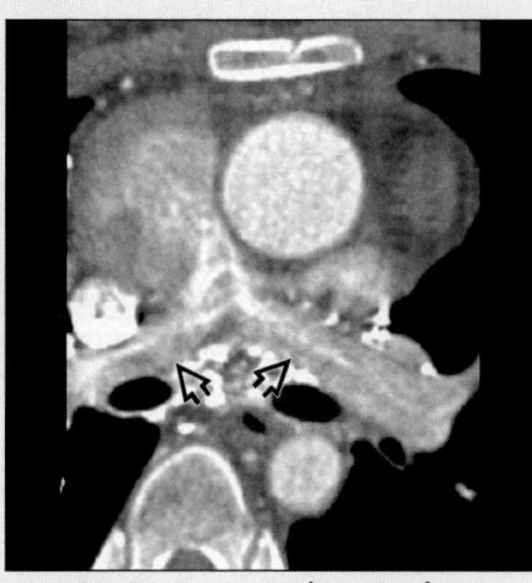

RA-PA Fontan, Flow Artifact

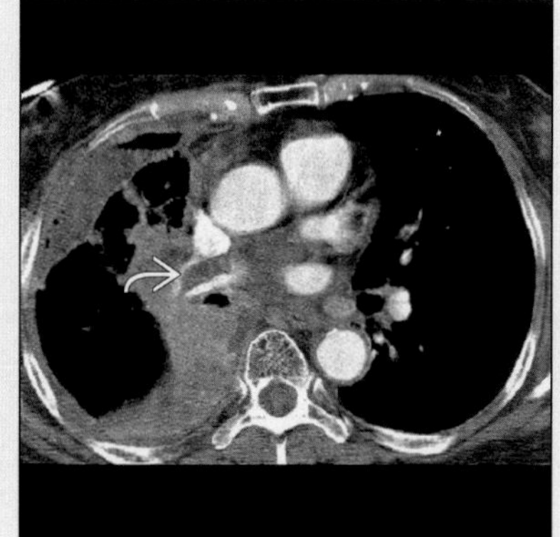

Tumor Thrombus

ACUTE PULMONARY EMBOLISM

Key Facts

Terminology
- Blockage of pulmonary artery, most commonly by emboli arising from pelvis or proximal LE

Imaging Findings
- Peripheral bubbly wedge-shaped consolidation
- Pleural effusion: Sometimes only radiographic finding
- Central hyperattenuating thrombus may be seen in hyperacute PE on NECT
- Complete or partial central low density filling defect within pulmonary arteries on CTA
- Large filling defect with occlusion of entire lumen and enlargement of involved artery; abrupt vessel cut off
- Partial filling defect surrounded by contrast material: "Railway track" sign and "polo mint" sign
- CE MRA and post T1WI GRE show pulmonary emboli as low signal intraluminal filling defects

Top Differential Diagnoses
- Tumor Thrombus
- Primary Pulmonary Artery Sarcoma
- Pulmonary Vasculitis

Pathology
- > 50% reduction in vascular bed leads to pulmonary hypertension and RHF

Clinical Issues
- Pleuritic chest pain, SOB, arterial hypoxia, raised D-dimer, tachycardia
- Anticoagulation mainstay of treatment
- Thrombolysis for patients with hemodynamic compromise

  - Pleural effusion: Approximately 1/2 of patients with PE, sometimes only radiographic finding
  - Pulmonary infarct: Ischemic necrosis with mixed hemorrhage and edema
    - < 10% embolic events result in infarction
    - Hampton's hump: Peripheral wedge-shaped pleural-based opacity with apex pointing toward hilum; usually in lower lung zones
    - Evolution: Can take months to resolve and leave linear scars (Fleischner lines) or pleural thickening
    - Infarcts "melt" (maintain shape, gradually shrink); pneumonia and edema "fade" away
    - Rarely cavitates unless 2° infection or sepsis

CT Findings
- CECT
  - Examination of choice, highly sensitive and specific, high interobserver agreement
  - Directly visualizes clot in pulmonary artery and helps to assess overall clot burden
    - Large filling defect with occlusion of entire lumen and enlargement of involved artery
    - Partial filling defect surrounded by contrast: "Railway track" sign (vessel viewed in long axis); "polo mint" sign (viewed in short axis)
    - Clot may be seen in right ventricle
    - Pulmonary artery enlargement (> 2.9 cm)
    - Right ventricle enlargement
    - Straightening or leftward bowing of interventricular septum, with D-shaped LV cavity
  - Negative CTPA outcomes good (< 1% embolic rate)
    - Negative CTPA rules out PE
  - Can combine with pelvic and thigh scan (2 minute delay from initial scan) for DVT evaluation
  - Pitfalls
    - Poor bolus, flow-related artifacts
    - Hilar lymph nodes
    - Respiratory motion artifacts
    - May miss subsegmental emboli

Nuclear Medicine Findings
- V/Q Scan findings
  - Abnormal perfusion and normal ventilation result in "mismatched" perfusion defect
  - High sensitivity but poor specificity
    - Normal perfusion scan excludes embolus
    - Matched defect can occur with pulmonary infarct
    - Other causes of V/Q mismatch include vasculitis, external compression of pulmonary artery, pulmonary hypertension, fibrosing mediastinitis
  - Interobserver agreement poor for low and indeterminate V/Q category (30%)

Echocardiographic Findings
- Echocardiogram: Assess right ventricular dysfunction

Ultrasonographic Findings
- Grayscale Ultrasound: Not useful for PE; excellent in evaluating for lower extremity DVT

Angiographic Findings
- Now primarily performed for thrombolysis; right heart and pulmonary artery pressures
- 25% false negative for small subsegmental emboli
- Poor interobserver agreement (30%) for subsegmental emboli

Imaging Recommendations
- Best imaging tool: CT angiography is study of choice
- Protocol advice
  - Bolus tracking with ROI at main pulmonary artery
  - 1.5 mm collimation following 80-100 mL IV contrast at rate of 3 cc/sec; 3 mm coronal/sagittal reformats
  - Essential MR sequences for PE evaluation are SSFP survey, contrast-enhanced MRA, post-contrast GRE
    - Add pre-contrast T1 GRE if suspicion of acute aortic syndrome

DIFFERENTIAL DIAGNOSIS

Tumor Thrombus
- Enhancing thrombus represents tumor thrombus; check for local tumor such as bronchogenic carcinoma
- Emboli may be large/central, or small/peripheral

Primary Pulmonary Artery Sarcoma

- Irregular, lobulated, and wall-adherent
- Enhancement of mass indicates vascularity
- Soft tissue density

Pulmonary Vasculitis

- Pulmonary arterial vasculitis can resemble PE
- Increased mural thickening and enhancement
- Usually spares central lumen
- Commonly involves other major vessels such as aorta

Laminar Flow Artifact

- Relatively low density linear filling defect; ill-defined margins, more common at vessel bifurcations
- Emboli are well-defined low density filling defects
- Commonly seen in patients with congenital heart disease having shunts/conduits (e.g., Fontan, Glenn)
  - Obtain arterial and delayed phase scans or utilize simultaneous foot and antecubital injections
  - MRI/MRA is an attractive alternative approach

PATHOLOGY

General Features

- General path comments: Pulmonary emboli arise from DVT, generally involving pelvis and lower extremities
- Genetics
  - Association with hypercoagulable states which may be stimulated by other stressors
  - Most common inherited predisposition is factor V Leiden
- Etiology
  - Usually thrombus from lower extremities
  - Non-thrombotic causes of pulmonary emboli
    - Fat embolism usually after trauma, long bone orthopedic procedures
    - Tumor embolus
    - Air embolus
    - Amniotic fluid embolus
    - Intravenous drug abuse with injection of foreign body material
- Epidemiology
  - Hospitalized patients have risk factors for PE
    - Immobilization
    - Surgery - particularly orthopedic and pelvic
    - Pregnancy, birth control pills
    - Malignancy
    - Obesity
    - Hypercoagulable state
    - Indwelling central venous catheters
    - Trauma
    - Incidental PE: 1-4% (4% in patients with cancer and/or undergoing chemotherapy)

Gross Pathologic & Surgical Features

- Hemodynamic effects: > 50% vascular bed reduction causes pulmonary hypertension, right heart failure

CLINICAL ISSUES

Presentation

- Most common signs/symptoms: Shortness of breath with tachypnea
- Other signs/symptoms: Cough, pleuritic chest pain, syncope, hypotension, tachycardia, cyanosis, hemoptysis, sudden death
- Clinical Profile
  - May have non-specific presentation
    - Arterial hypoxia, raised D-dimer, tachycardia, and a near normal chest X-ray favors PE

Demographics

- Age: All age groups; increased incidence in older patients

Natural History & Prognosis

- Good with appropriate therapy; maintain high index of suspicion as 20% mortality if untreated
- Outcomes for untreated subsegmental emboli unknown

Treatment

- Anticoagulation is mainstay of treatment
  - Hemorrhage complications in 2-15%
- Thrombolysis for severely symptomatic patients
  - May be delivered systemically via IV
  - Direct catheter delivery into clot
  - Contraindications: Intracranial disease (stroke, tumor, head trauma), ongoing GI bleeding
  - Relative contraindications: Recent surgery, trauma, obstetrical delivery, bleeding diathesis
- IVC filter if contraindications to drug therapy

DIAGNOSTIC CHECKLIST

Consider

- Chronic pulmonary emboli may have acute superimposed on chronic disease

Image Interpretation Pearls

- Thromboemboli are avascular; appear as near-occlusive intraluminal central filling defects in acute PE

SELECTED REFERENCES

1. Remy-Jardin M et al: Management of Suspected Acute Pulmonary Embolism in the Era of CT Angiography: A Statement from the Fleischner Society. Radiology. 245(2):315-329, 2007
2. Konstantinides S: Diagnosis and therapy of pulmonary embolism. Vasa. 35(3):135-46, 2006
3. Le Gal G et al: Contemporary approach to the diagnosis of non-massive pulmonary embolism. Curr Opin Pulm Med. 12(5):291-8, 2006
4. Schaefer-Prokop C et al: MDCT for the diagnosis of acute pulmonary embolism. Eur Radiol. 15 Suppl 4:D37-41, 2005
5. Wittram C et al: CT angiography of pulmonary embolism: diagnostic criteria and causes of misdiagnosis. Radiographics. 24(5):1219-38, 2004

IMAGE GALLERY

Typical

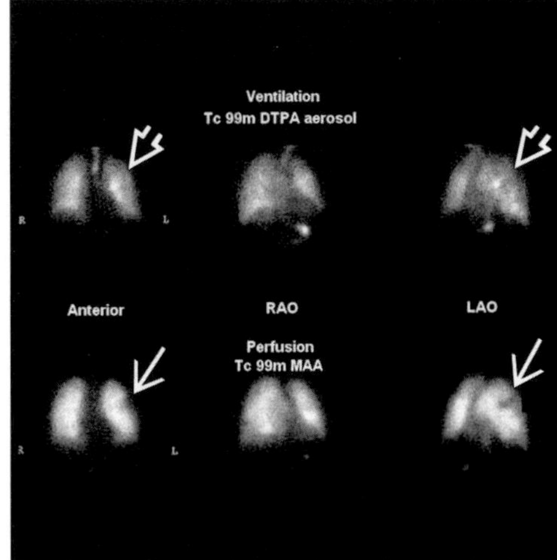

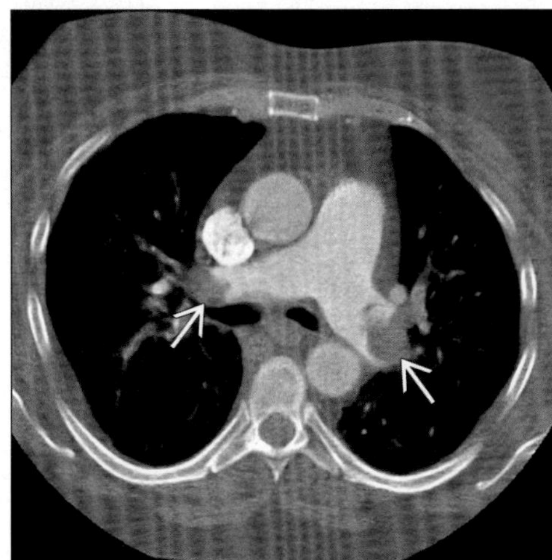

*(**Left**) Radionuclide V/Q lung scan shows a left upper lobe defect ➔ on the perfusion portion of the examination, and normal corresponding ventilation ➔. This ventilation/perfusion mismatch is considered "high probability" for pulmonary embolus. (**Right**) Axial CECT shows large bilateral emboli ➔ in the main pulmonary arteries. Contrast-enhanced CT has become the examination of choice in evaluating for pulmonary emboli as it is highly sensitive and specific.*

Typical

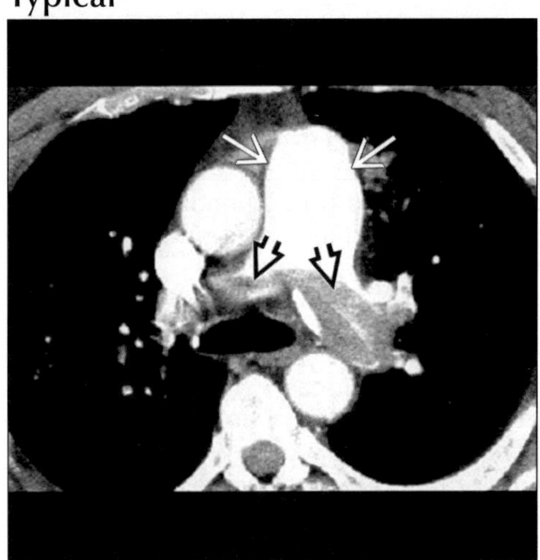

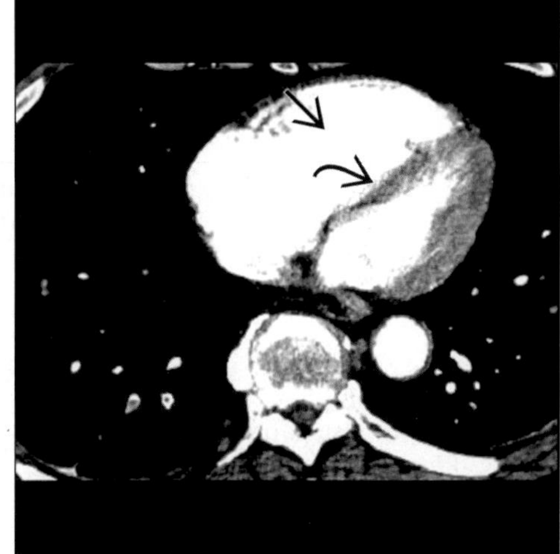

*(**Left**) Axial CTA shows a saddle embolus ➔ at the pulmonary artery bifurcation in a patient with acute PE. The main pulmonary artery is enlarged ➔ 2° to elevated pulmonary arterial pressure from outflow obstruction. (Courtesy K. Brown, MD). (**Right**) Axial CTA (same patient) shows right ventricular enlargement ➔ & leftward deviation of an abnormally straight interventricular septum ➔. These findings are consistent with right heart strain 2° to extensive pulmonary emboli.*

Typical

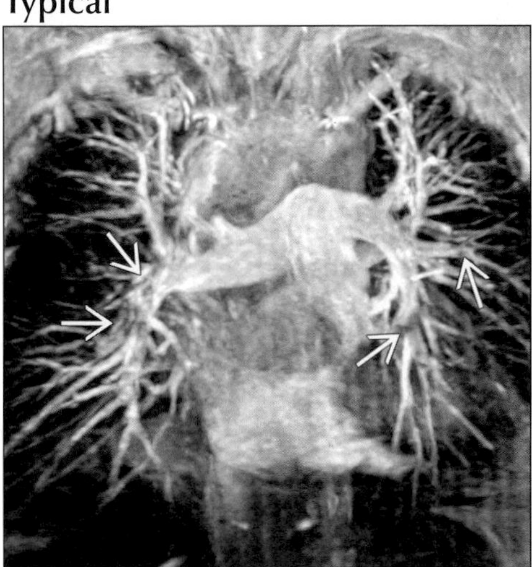

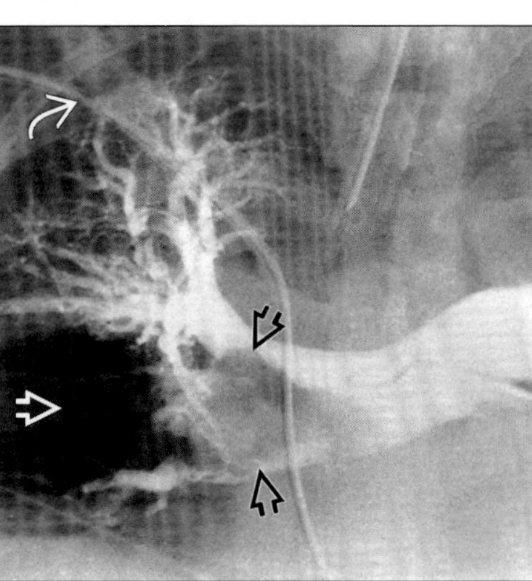

*(**Left**) MR cine shows defects ➔ in the pulmonary arteries, consistent with bilateral pulmonary emboli. Contrast-enhanced MRA and post-contrast GRE sequences are most useful in identifying pulmonary emboli. (**Right**) Catheter angiography from a subclavian venous approach ➔ shows a large filling defect in the right main and interlobar pulmonary arteries ➔ and lack of opacification ➔ of distal branch vessels consistent with a large PE. (Courtesy C. Aintree, MD).*

CHRONIC PULMONARY EMBOLISM

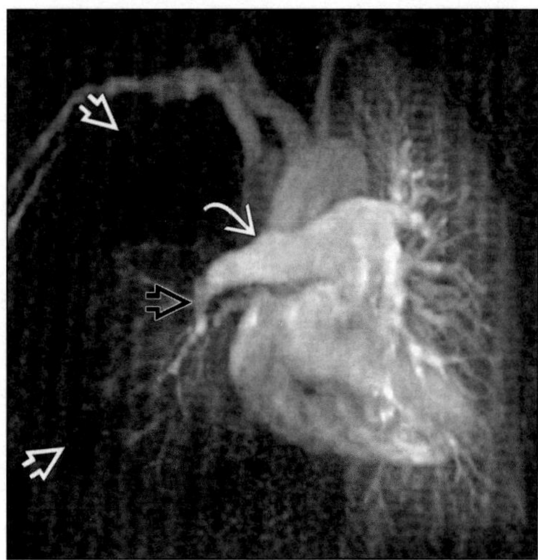

Coronal TR-MRA shows markedly decreased right lung perfusion due to small caliber right lower lobe pulmonary arteries, and right upper lobe pulmonary arterial occlusion in a patient with chronic PE.

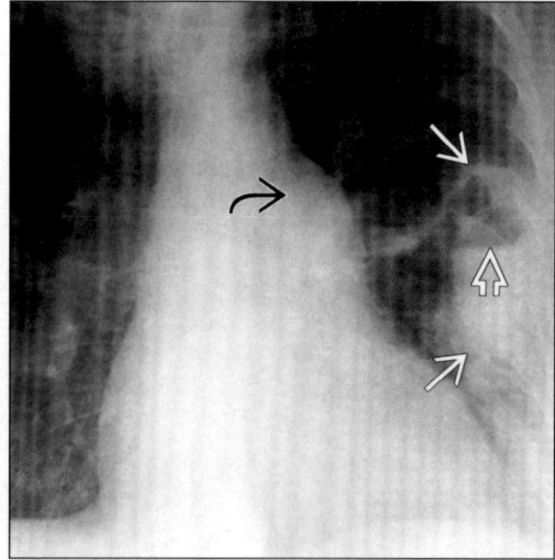

Radiograph shows a pulmonary infarct with cavitation in a patient with chronic PE. Pulmonary arterial enlargement and cardiomegaly reflect pulmonary hypertension. (Courtesy C. Aintree, MD).

TERMINOLOGY

Abbreviations and Synonyms

- Chronic pulmonary arterial thromboembolic disease
- Chronic thromboembolic pulmonary hypertension (CTEPH)
- Pulmonary arterial hypertension (PAH)
- Right ventricle enlargement (RVE)
- Pulmonary arteries (PA), pulmonary embolism (PE), Time-resolved MRA (TR-MRA)

Definitions

- Gradual formation of organized thromboemboli following acute pulmonary embolism with resultant pulmonary vascular obstruction/obliteration

IMAGING FINDINGS

General Features

- Best diagnostic clue: Eccentric, wall adherent, low density filling defect; dilated pulmonary artery(ies)
- Location: Pulmonary arteries, commonly bilateral
- Size: Usually smaller than in acute PE

Radiographic Findings

- Radiography
  - Normal CXR or abnormalities suggesting PAH
    - Pulmonary artery enlargement
    - Right heart enlargement
  - Subpleural opacities from prior pulmonary infarcts
  - Hypo- and hyperperfused lung regions
  - Rarely peripheral cavitary changes

CT Findings

- HRCT
  - Mosaic perfusion of pulmonary parenchyma
    - Heterogeneous attenuation of pulmonary parenchyma from variable perfusion
    - Decreased attenuation areas from decreased perfusion; small distal pulmonary arteries
  - Subpleural opacities from prior pulmonary infarcts
- CTA
  - CTA allows direct visualization of luminal thrombi, organized mural thrombi, occlusions, and webs
    - Emboli are eccentric in location
    - Smooth or nodular vascular wall thickening
    - Rarely eccentric wall-adherent PA calcifications

DDx: Chronic Pulmonary Thromboembolism

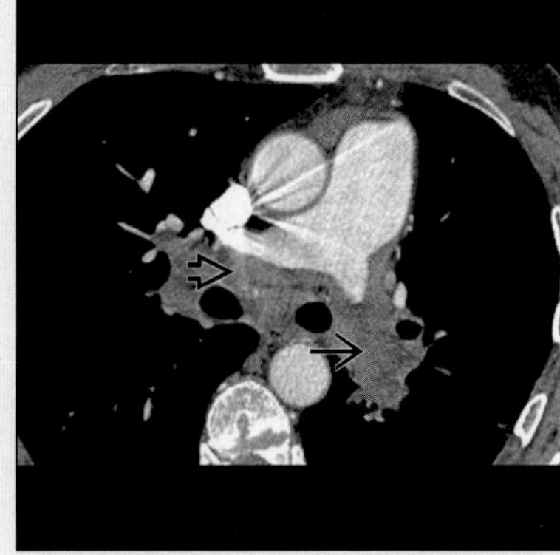

Pulmonary Artery Sarcoma

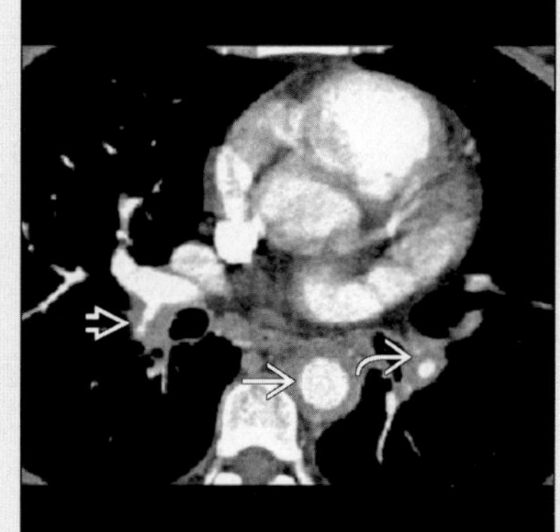

Vasculitis

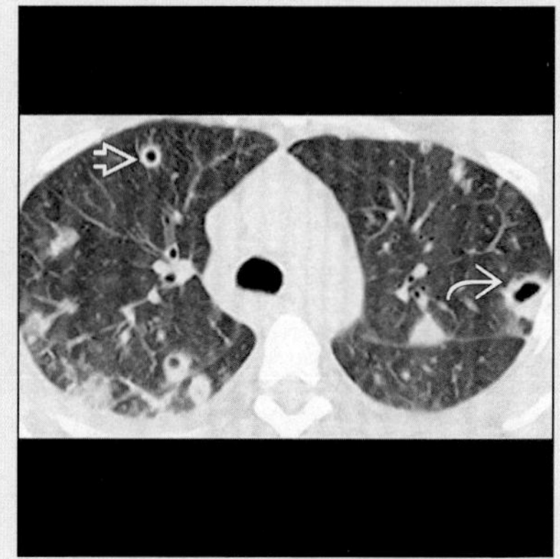

Septic Emboli

CHRONIC PULMONARY EMBOLISM

Key Facts

Terminology
- Chronic PE characterized by formation of organized thromboemboli following acute pulmonary embolism, with resultant pulmonary vascular obstruction/obliteration

Imaging Findings
- Best diagnostic clue: Eccentric, wall-adherent, low density thrombi with dilated main PA
- CTA & MRA show luminal thrombi, organized mural thrombi, occlusions, and webs
  - MRA cannot reliably detect subsegmental thrombi
- Right ventricular and pulmonary arterial enlargement
- Straight or left-bowing interventricular septum
- Abruptly narrowed or occluded vessels
- Mosaic perfusion of lung parenchyma on CT
- Eccentric, low-signal filling defect along arterial wall on MRI/MRA
- Decreased RV ejection fraction on cine SSFP
- Mismatched segmental or larger defects on V/Q

Top Differential Diagnoses
- Pulmonary Artery Sarcoma
- Large Vessel Arteritis (Takayasu Arteritis)
- Fibrosing Mediastinitis
- Septic Emboli
- Severe Intimal Hyperplasia in CHD

Clinical Issues
- Progressive exertional dyspnea
- Patients are anticoagulated for life
- Surgical option is pulmonary thromboendarterectomy

    - Webs seen as eccentric linear filling defects partially extending intraluminally
    - Abrupt narrowing or occlusion of vessels
    - "Pruning" of peripheral arteries
    - Peripheral neovascularity in long standing PAH
  - Enlarged pulmonary arteries related to PAH; aorta/PA ratio > 1 or main PA diameter > 29 mm
  - Evaluate cardiac chamber enlargement due to PAH
    - RV enlargement: RV/LV diameter > 1:1 at midventricular level
    - Straight or left-bowing interventricular septum
    - D-shaped LV cavity on short axis view
  - Size and distribution of bronchial arteries and non-bronchial systemic arteries
    - Visualization of increased bronchopulmonary collaterals distinguishes CTEPH from 1° PAH
    - Large bronchial blood supply can complicate surgery and predict poor surgical outcome
  - Exclude alternative causes of PAH
    - Congenital cardiovascular disease: Atrial septal defect, patent ductus arteriosus, anomalous pulmonary venous drainage
    - Pulmonary parenchymal disease: Emphysema, interstitial fibrosis
    - Other pulmonary vascular diseases: Veno-occlusive disease, capillary hemangiomatosis, vascular occlusions 2° to mediastinal fibrosis or PA sarcoma

MR Findings
- MRA
  - Correlates well with CTA to segmental level, cannot reliably detect smaller thrombi
  - Thrombi seen as eccentric, low-signal defects along arterial wall on SSFP, MRA and CE GRE sequences
  - Vessel occlusions, intraluminal webs and bands
  - TR-MRA useful for pulmonary perfusion pattern
- MR Cine
  - Allows qualitative and quantitative assessment of ventricular function
  - Phase-contrast imaging measures flow in systemic and pulmonary vessels; can assess surgery results:
    - Pre- and post pulmonary thromboendarterectomy

Nuclear Medicine Findings
- V/Q Scan
  - Normal V/Q scan rules out chronic PE
  - Multiple mismatched segmental or larger defects
  - Magnitude of perfusion defects often understate actual degree of obstruction
- PET: May aid in differentiating pulmonary arteritis (Takayasu) and chronic PE

Echocardiographic Findings
- Evidence of pulmonary arterial hypertension
- Right atrial and ventricular enlargement/dysfunction
- Tricuspid regurgitation
- Excludes cardiac causes of pulmonary arterial hypertension (e.g. patent foramen ovale, septal defect)

Angiographic Findings
- Vascular occlusions, webs, stenoses, mural thrombi
- Two orthogonal views essential for surgical planning
- Obtain right ventricular and PA hemodynamics

Imaging Recommendations
- Best imaging tool: CTA is most effective modality
- Protocol advice
  - Timing of contrast bolus should opacify pulmonary circulation more than systemic
    - Main PA as ROI for bolus tracking; 80-100 mL of contrast at 3 cc/sec; 1.5 mm collimation
    - ECG may be synchronized with CT scan to assess RV function; more radiation to patient
  - MRI/MRA sequences: Axial SSFP, cine SSFP of heart, coronal time resolved MRA (for perfusion), coronal CEMRA, axial and coronal post-contrast T1 GRE

DIFFERENTIAL DIAGNOSIS

Pulmonary Artery Sarcoma
- Sarcoma usually irregular, lobulated, wall-adherent
- Contrast-enhancement (best on MR) seen in sarcoma (vascular); not with thrombus (usually avascular)
- May involve pulmonary valve and extend retrograde into RV infundibulum; does not occur with chronic PE

CHRONIC PULMONARY EMBOLISM

Large Vessel Arteritis (Takayasu Arteritis)
- Mural thickening in pulmonary vasculitis can resemble eccentric thrombus
- Other vessels such as aorta involved in vasculitis
- CT and MR may identify circumferential inflammatory mural thickening
  - MR better than CT in assessing wall enhancement; differentiates active vs. chronic vasculitis
- FDG PET shows intense uptake in active disease

Fibrosing Mediastinitis
- CT shows mediastinal soft tissue obliterating fat planes
- Encases and compresses vascular structures
- Mediastinal calcification
- SVC stenosis

Septic Emboli
- Cavities are usually small, peripheral and multiple
- Usually no eccentric or central PA filling defects
- Patient clinically unwell, with fever
- Echo or cardiac MR indicated to rule out endocarditis

Laminar Flow Artifact
- Inappropriate timing of contrast bolus
  - Consider different injection protocols
- Linear central filling defects seen at vessel bifurcation

PATHOLOGY

General Features
- Etiology
  - Unresolved pulmonary emboli which organize, become adherent and incorporate into arterial wall
  - Secondary small-vessel arteriopathy in some patients
  - Proximal PA occlusion and arteriopathy contribute to elevated pulmonary vascular resistance
- Epidemiology: 5% incidence in patients with acute PE
- Associated abnormalities
  - Patients may have altered coagulation process
    - Factor VIII, high frequency of antiphospholipid antibodies, lupus anticoagulant may be risk factors
  - Splenectomy appears to increase the risk of chronic thromboembolic pulmonary hypertension

Gross Pathologic & Surgical Features
- Emboli transform into fibrous tissue; incorporation into pulmonary arterial intima and media
- Small vessel vasculopathy seen in remaining open vessels which are subjected to high flows

CLINICAL ISSUES

Presentation
- Most common signs/symptoms
  - Progressive exertional dyspnea
  - Exercise intolerance
- Other signs/symptoms: Exertional chest pain, presyncope, syncope, fatigue, palpitation, hemoptysis

Demographics
- Age: Commonly in elderly
- Gender: M = F

Natural History & Prognosis
- 2/3 of patients may have no history of acute PE
- Often misdiagnosed with asthma, CHF, COPD, physical deconditioning, or psychogenic dyspnea
- Extent of vascular obstruction a major determinant of development of PAH
- Low survival rate without intervention for PAH:
  - 5 year survival rate of 30% with mean pulmonary artery pressure ≥ 40 mm Hg
  - 5 year survival rate of 10% with main pulmonary artery pressure ≥ 50 mm Hg

Treatment
- Chronic PE is potentially correctable cause of PAH
- Patients should undergo IVC filter placement
  - Lifetime anticoagulation
- Medical therapy or angioplasty for non-surgical candidates
- Surgical thromboendarterectomy in some patients
  - Location/extent of proximal thromboembolic obstructions are critical determinants of operability
  - Occluding thrombi must involve main, lobar, or proximal segmental arteries

DIAGNOSTIC CHECKLIST

Consider
- Chronic PE in a patient with chronic shortness of breath, pulmonary arterial hypertension with eccentric or web-like thrombi or mosaic perfusion

Image Interpretation Pearls
- Eccentric web-like thrombi, differential lung perfusion, vessel calcifications, right heart strain favor chronic PE
- Intimal hyperplasia in congenital heart disease with central shunting may mimic chronic PE
  - Intravascular ultrasound helps to differentiate

SELECTED REFERENCES

1. Coulden R: State-of-the-art imaging techniques in chronic thromboembolic pulmonary hypertension. Proc Am Thorac Soc. 3(7):577-83, 2006
2. Hoeper MM et al: Chronic thromboembolic pulmonary hypertension. Circulation. 113(16):2011-20, 2006
3. Lang I et al: Risk factors for chronic thromboembolic pulmonary hypertension. Proc Am Thorac Soc. 3(7):568-70, 2006
4. Reddy GP et al: Imaging of chronic thromboembolic pulmonary hypertension. Semin Roentgenol. 40(1):41-7, 2005
5. Kreitner KF et al: Chronic thromboembolic pulmonary hypertension: pre- and postoperative assessment with breath-hold MR imaging techniques. Radiology. 232(2):535-43, 2004
6. Thistlethwaite PA et al: Pulmonary thromboendarterectomy surgery. Cardiol Clin. 22(3):467-78, vii, 2004
7. Jamieson SW et al: Pulmonary endarterectomy: experience and lessons learned in 1,500 cases. Ann Thorac Surg. 2003
8. Fedullo PF et al: Chronic thromboembolic pulmonary hypertension. N Engl J Med. 345(20):1465-72, 2001

IMAGE GALLERY

Typical

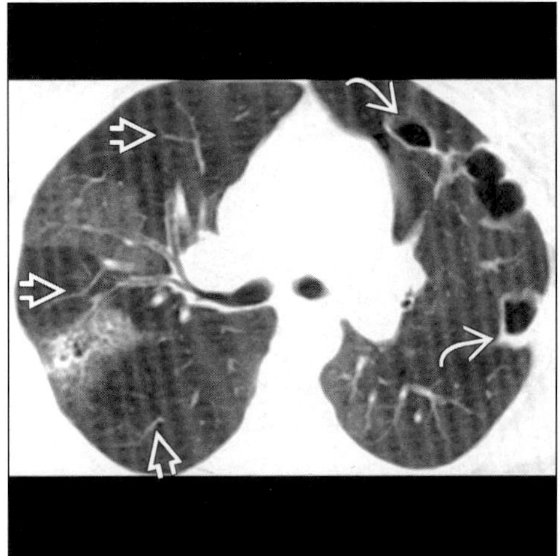

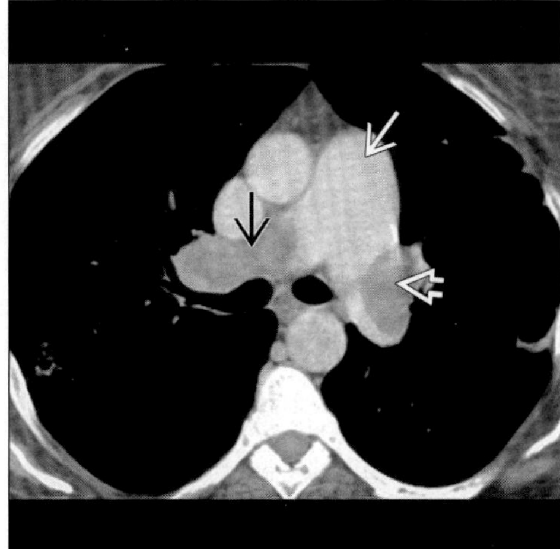

(Left) *Axial CECT shows a mosaic pattern of pulmonary perfusion due to oligemia (decreased vessel size) ➡ in areas involved by chronic emboli. Several cavities ➡ are due to resolving infarct.* ***(Right)*** *Axial CECT in the same patient as previous image, shows both eccentric ➡ and central ➡ occlusive emboli with an enlarged main pulmonary artery ➡, consistent with acute pulmonary emboli superimposed upon chronic pulmonary emboli. (Courtesy C. Aintree, MD).*

Typical

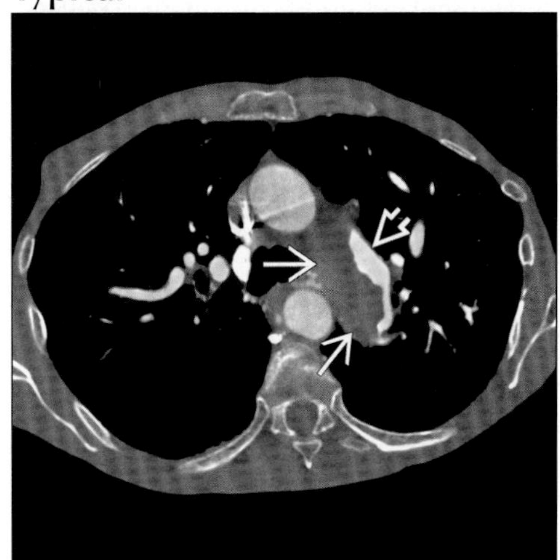

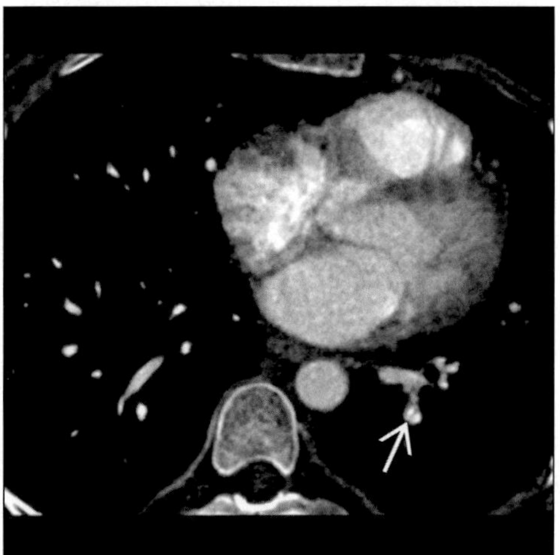

(Left) *Axial CECT in a patient with pulmonary arterial hypertension due to chronic PE shows a very large eccentric filling defect ➡ that is adherent to the wall of the left main pulmonary artery. Note that contrast ➡ courses adjacent to the thrombus, indicating that it is non-occlusive.* ***(Right)*** *Axial CECT shows an eccentric linear filling defect within a left lower lobe segmental pulmonary artery ➡ consistent with a web. This is typically seen in patients with chronic PE.*

Typical

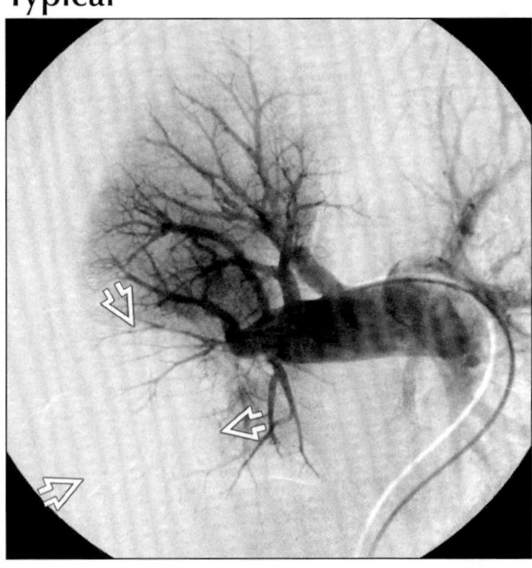

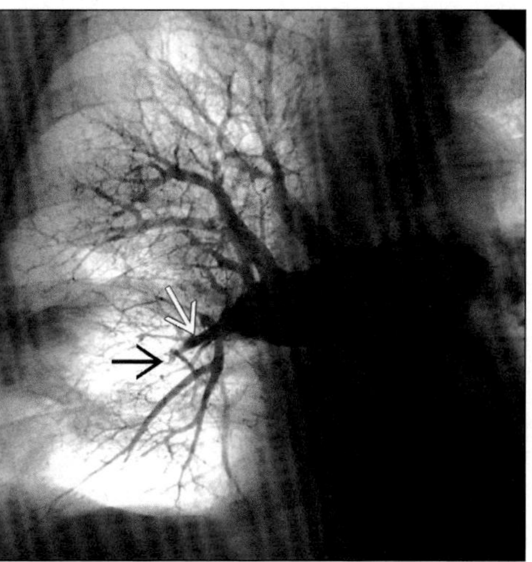

(Left) *Pulmonary arteriogram shows segmental non-perfusion of the right lower lobe ➡ due to chronic occlusion of the pulmonary arteries that would normally supply these portions of the lung.* ***(Right)*** *Pulmonary arteriogram (same patient as previous) obtained with a different obliquity shows tapering ➡ & occlusion ➡ of a right lower lobe pulmonary artery that has resulted in the segmental non-perfusion. These findings are typical of chronic pulmonary emboli.*

HEREDITARY HEMORRHAGIC TELANGIECTASIA

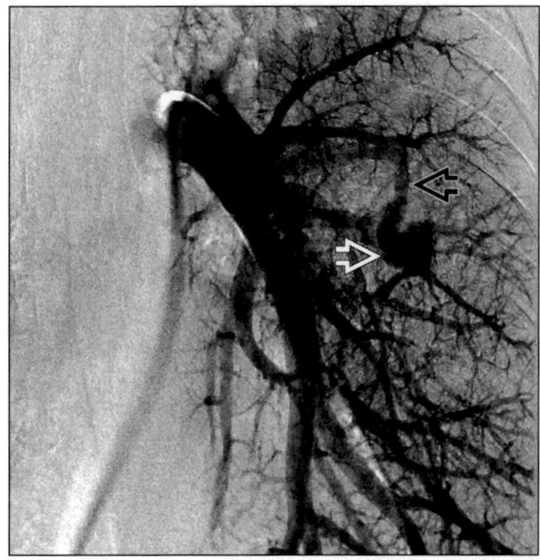

DSA shows a pulmonary AVM ➡. The arterial communication is not seen clearly on this non-selective view, but the draining vein ⇨ is seen easily. Typical appearance of a "simple" AVM.

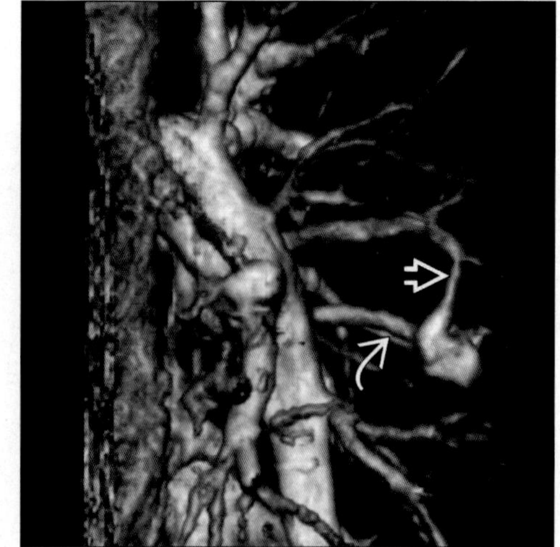

3D reconstruction shows the AVM in a similar view as the previous angiogram. The draining vein ➡ can be seen and the feeding artery is a little more visible ↗.

TERMINOLOGY

Abbreviations and Synonyms

- Hereditary hemorrhagic telangiectasia (HHT); Osler-Weber-Rendu

Definitions

- Autosomal dominant disorder with mucocutaneous & visceral telangiectasias/arteriovenous malformations (AVMs) in brain, lungs, GI tract, & liver
- AVMs and telangiectasias lack capillaries and consist of direct connections between arteries and veins

IMAGING FINDINGS

General Features

- Best diagnostic clue: Multiple pulmonary (pAVM) or cerebral (cAVM) arteriovenous malformations in patient with recurrent epistaxis

Radiographic Findings

- Radiography
  - Pulmonary AVM
    - Well-defined nodule, multiple, usually located at lung base
    - Tubular opacities contiguous with the pulmonary hilum, representing enlarged draining veins

CT Findings

- NECT
  - Lung: High-resolution multislice CT shows well-delineated vascular mass(es)
  - Brain
    - AVM = Isodense serpentine vessels
    - Abscess = Low density mass with iso-/hyperdense rim
- CECT
  - Dilated, tortuous hepatic artery with diffuse parenchymal telangiectasias
  - Prominent hepatic artery associated with dilated hepatic and/or portal veins
  - Splenomegaly
- CTA
  - Pulmonary AVM
    - Enlarged feeding/draining vessels
    - Simple AVMs fed by same segmental artery

DDx: Pulmonary Aneurysm

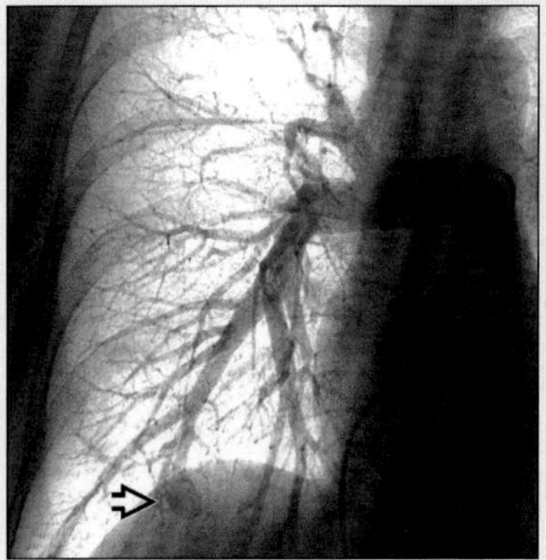

No Venous Drainage

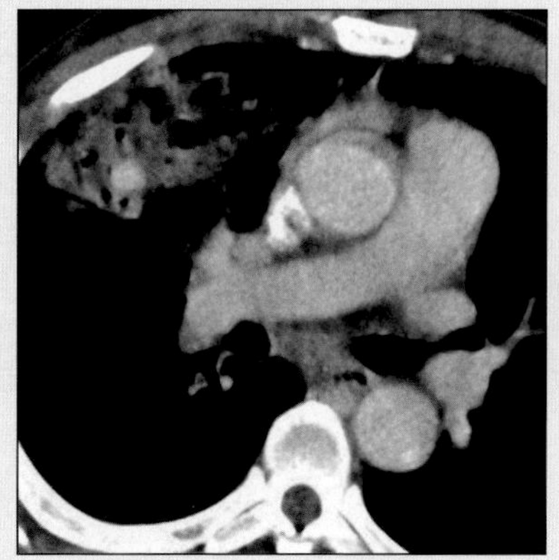

Hypervascularity in Pneumonia

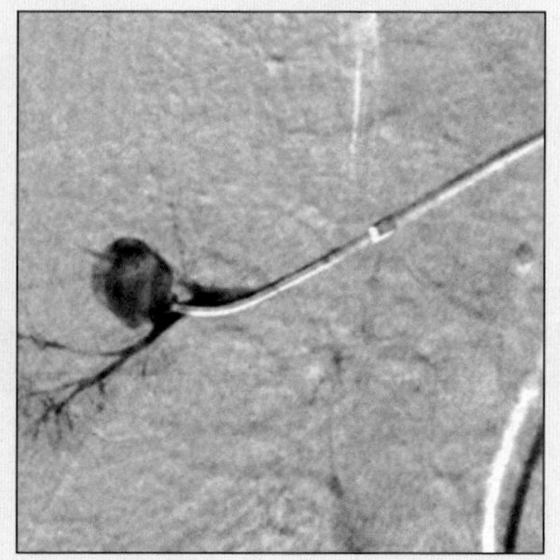

No Venous Drainage

HEREDITARY HEMORRHAGIC TELANGIECTASIA

Key Facts

Terminology

- Hereditary hemorrhagic telangiectasia (HHT); Osler-Weber-Rendu
- Autosomal dominant disorder with mucocutaneous & visceral telangiectasias/arteriovenous malformations (AVMs) in brain, lungs, GI tract, & liver

Imaging Findings

- Best diagnostic clue: Multiple pulmonary (pAVM) or cerebral (cAVM) arteriovenous malformations in patient with recurrent epistaxis
- 90% simple AVMs fed by branch(s) of the same segmental artery
- 10% complex AVMs supplied by 2 different segmental arteries
- Transthoracic echocardiography: Rapid appearance of microbubbles in left heart suggests intrapulmonary shunt
- Dilated, tortuous hepatic artery with diffuse parenchymal telangiectasias
- Patchy early sinusoidal filling and early opacified hepatic veins in hepatic arterial phase
- Poorly opacified hepatic parenchyma & dilated portal and hepatic veins in portal venous phase

Pathology

- HHT associated with two known mutations involved in the signaling of transforming growth factor (TGF-β)
- 70% of patients with pAVMs have HHT
- ≥ 50% of patients with multiple cAVMs have HHT

        - 10% complex AVMs supplied by 2 different segmental arteries
    - Hepatic AVM
        - Patchy early sinusoidal filling and early opacified hepatic veins in hepatic arterial phase
        - Poorly opacified hepatic parenchyma & dilated portal and hepatic veins in portal venous phase

MR Findings

- T1WI: "Flow voids" common, demonstrate intrahepatic vascular malformations
- T2* GRE: Demonstrates flow in cAVMs

Echocardiographic Findings

- Echocardiogram
    - Pulmonary AVM
        - "Bubble" test: Rapid appearance of microbubbles in left heart = intrapulmonary shunt

Ultrasonographic Findings

- Grayscale Ultrasound
    - Malformations depicted as dilated tubular structures with echogenic walls and prominent pulsations
    - Dilation of hepatic arteries (> 6 mm), celiac axis, portal veins, or hepatic veins
    - Elevated, turbulent celiac and hepatic arterial flows
- Color Doppler
    - High-velocity flow in hepatic artery and its branches
    - Hepatic artery to portal vein shunts
    - Hepatic artery to hepatic vein shunts

Angiographic Findings

- Conventional
    - Pulmonary AVMs
        - Single artery draining into an enlarged vein
        - Artery(ies) with drainage into multiple veins
    - Hepatic AVMs
        - Dilated, ectatic hepatic and celiac arteries
        - Diffuse telangiectases
        - Arteriovenous shunting or arterioportal shunting

Imaging Recommendations

- Multislice CT of lungs, liver
- MR, MRA of brain

DIFFERENTIAL DIAGNOSIS

Multiple Intracranial AVMs

- Rare; 50% not associated with HHT

Essential Telangiectasia

- Dilated blood vessel on skin or mucosal surface
- Absence of coexisting cutaneous or systemic disease
- Widespread anatomic distribution

Ataxia-Telangiectasia

- Autosomal recessive, complex, multisystem disorder
- Progressive neurologic impairment, cerebellar ataxia, variable immunodeficiency, ocular and cutaneous telangiectasia

Rothmund-Thomson Syndrome

- Autosomal recessive disorder
- Early photosensitivity and poikilodermatous skin changes, juvenile cataracts, skeletal dysplasias, and a predisposition to osteosarcoma and skin cancer

Louis-Bar Syndrome

- Genetic disease characterized by progressive cerebellar ataxia, oculocutaneous telangiectasia, and recurrent respiratory and sinus infections

PATHOLOGY

General Features

- General path comments: Abnormalities of vascular structure account for the manifestations of HHT
- Genetics
    - Autosomal dominant inheritance
    - Two known mutations involved in the signaling of transforming growth factor (TGF-β)
- Etiology: Abnormal intracellular signal transduction during angiogenesis
- Epidemiology
    - Rare; 1/15,000-20,000 births
    - 70% of patients with pAVMs have HHT
    - ≥ 50% of patients with multiple cAVMs have HHT

HEREDITARY HEMORRHAGIC TELANGIECTASIA

Gross Pathologic & Surgical Features

- Multiple telangiectasias of mucosa, dermis
- AVMs appear in only certain forms of HHT
  - Most pAVMs are actually AVFs (arteriovenous fistula): Direct connection between pulmonary artery and vein
  - Hepatic AV shunts less common presentation, often numerous

Microscopic Features

- Smallest telangiectasias = focal dilatations of post-capillary venules
- Larger lesions extend through entire dermis, often connect directly to dilated arterioles

Staging, Grading or Classification Criteria

- Most cAVMs in HHT are low-grade (Spetzler - Martin I or II)

CLINICAL ISSUES

Presentation

- Most common signs/symptoms
  - Recurrent epistaxis: Nasal mucosal telangiectasias
  - Gastrointestinal (GI) bleeding
    - Presents with iron deficiency anemia
    - Develops progressively with age (50-60 years)
    - Telangiectasia throughout GI tract; most common in stomach & duodenum
    - Massive gastrointestinal hemorrhage is rare
  - Hepatic involvement (30%)
    - Present with high output heart failure, portal hypertension, biliary disease
    - Large AVMs between hepatic artery and vein result in left to right shunt
    - Portal hypertension and hepatic encephalopathy due to shunts between hepatic artery and portal vein
  - Mucocutaneous telangiectasia (75%)
    - Face, lips, tongue, fingertips, buccal mucosa, conjunctival telangiectasia
    - Increasing in size and number with age
  - Pulmonary AVMs (30%)
    - Dyspnea, cyanosis, fatigue, polycythemia
    - Majority of patients with pAVM do not present with respiratory symptoms
    - PAVMs may hemorrhage
    - Neurological sequelae (cerebral emboli/abscess) due to paradoxical embolism
    - 36% are multiple and 50% bilateral
  - Cerebral AVMs (10-20%)
    - Headache, seizures, hemorrhage
    - Telangiectasias, cerebral AVMs, aneurysms, cavernous angiomas
    - Parenchymal or SAH with brain AVM
    - TIA, stroke, abscess as complications of pAVMs due to right-to-left shunt

Demographics

- Age: 71% develop some symptom by age 16 years; 90% by age 40 years: 97% manifest by age 60
- Gender: Equal frequency and severity in both sexes
- Ethnicity
  - United States: 1-2 cases per 100,000
  - Europe, Asia: 1 in 5-8,000
  - Dutch Antilles: 1:200; France: 1:2351

Natural History & Prognosis

- Epistaxis increases in frequency, severity
  - Recurrent epistaxis is observed in 50-80% of patients
  - 50% become more serious with age
  - Blood transfusions required in 10-30% of patients
- Strokes: Hemorrhagic or ischemic
  - Hemorrhagic due to cerebral AVMs
  - Ischemic strokes (2%), brain abscesses (1%) with pAVM
- Pulmonary dyspnea, fatigue
- GI bleeding occurring under age 50; many require multiple transfusions and endoscopies
- Hepatic AVM with heart failure have poor prognosis
- Fewer than 10% of patients die of complications

Treatment

- Mucocutaneous telangiectasias
  - Humidification, packing, transfusion, estrogen therapy, septal dermoplasty, laser, cautery, embolotherapy
- Pulmonary AVMs
  - Transcatheter embolotherapy, surgery rarely performed
- Cerebral AVMs
  - Neurovascular surgery, embolotherapy, stereotactic radiosurgery
- GI AVMs
  - Iron therapy; blood transfusion, laser therapy

DIAGNOSTIC CHECKLIST

Consider

- Spontaneously, recurrent nosebleeds/epistaxis
- Mucocutaneous telangiectasia
- Visceral lesions: GI telangiectasia, pulmonary AVM, hepatic AVM, cerebral AVM, spinal AVM
- Affected first degree relative (autosomal dominant inheritance)
- If AVM in pulmonary or cerebral circulation, think of HHT and evaluate other potential sites

Image Interpretation Pearls

- 3+ symptoms: Definite HHT
- 2+ symptoms: Suspected HHT

SELECTED REFERENCES

1. Garcia-Tsao G: Liver involvement in hereditary hemorrhagic telangiectasia (HHT). J Hepatol. 46(3):499-507, 2007
2. Ianora AA et al: Hereditary hemorrhagic telangiectasia: multi-detector row helical CT assessment of hepatic involvement. Radiology. 230(1):250-9, 2004
3. Hashimoto M et al: Angiography of hepatic vascular malformations associated with hereditary hemorrhagic telangiectasia. Cardiovasc Intervent Radiol. 26(2):177-80, 2003

IMAGE GALLERY

Other

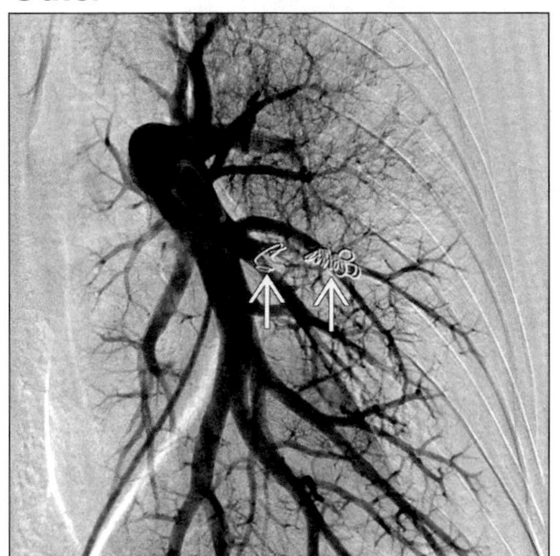

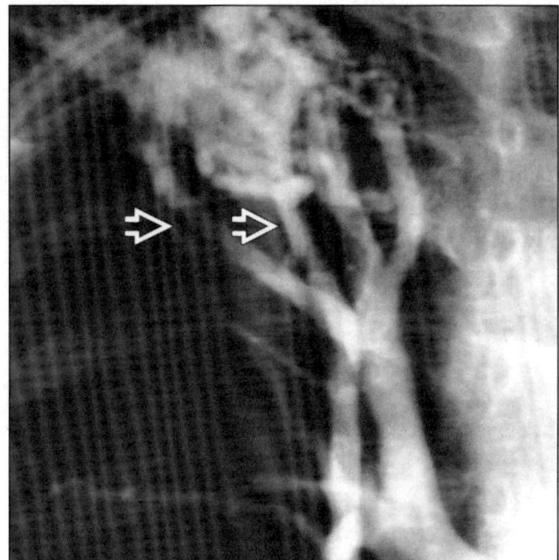

(Left) Continuing from the prior case, a DSA shows coils ➡ have been placed in the AVM. Coils are the most common embolization material to use in an AVM. Particulate embolization must be avoided. **(Right)** Catheter angiography shows a complex AVM ➡ with multiple feeding arteries and draining veins. These are less common than the simple AVMs (10%) and require embolization of all the feeding arteries.

Typical

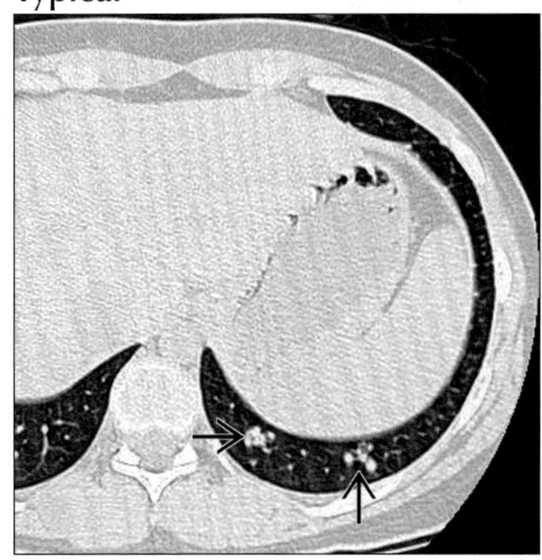

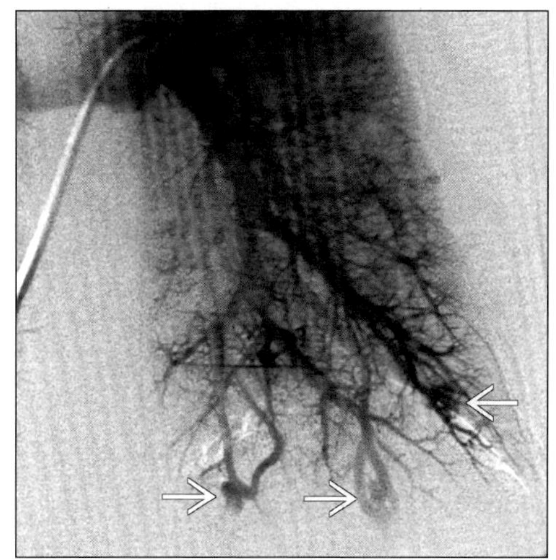

(Left) Axial CECT shows several lobular densities ➡ in the left lung base. These are small. The feeding artery and draining vein are not well seen. **(Right)** DSA shows the multiple small AVMs ➡ in the left lung base (seen on the previous CT image). These are simple AVMs, which are most common (90%). AVMs are frequently multiple.

Typical

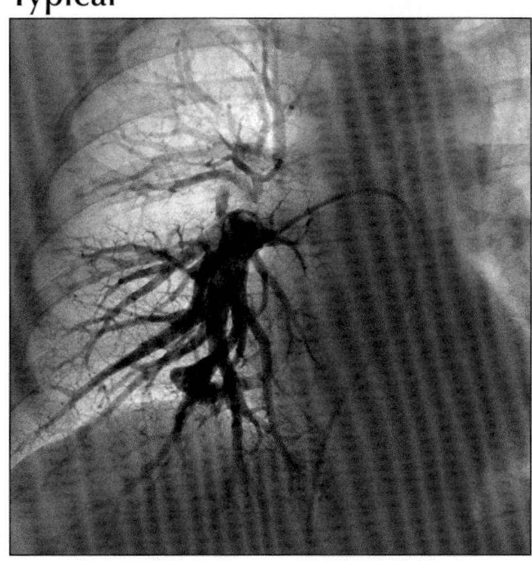

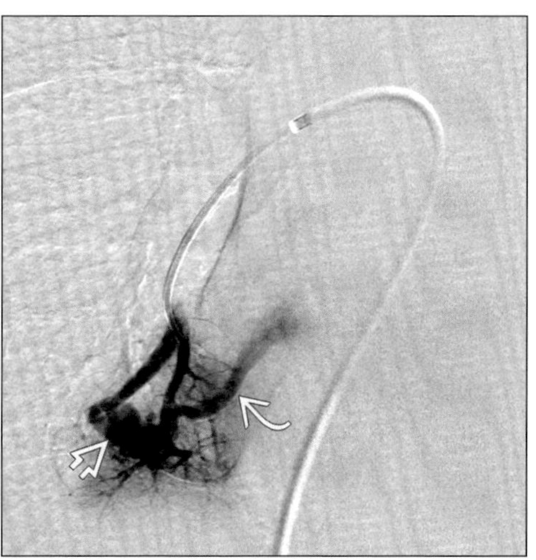

(Left) DSA of the pulmonary artery is done as the first part of the procedure to evaluate for the number and position of the AVMs. This will give a good overall view of the pulmonary arteries. **(Right)** DSA shows catheter now sub-selectively in the right lower lung with an aneurysmal filling area ➡ and with an early draining vein ➡. Findings: Simple AVM of the lung.

SEQUESTRATION

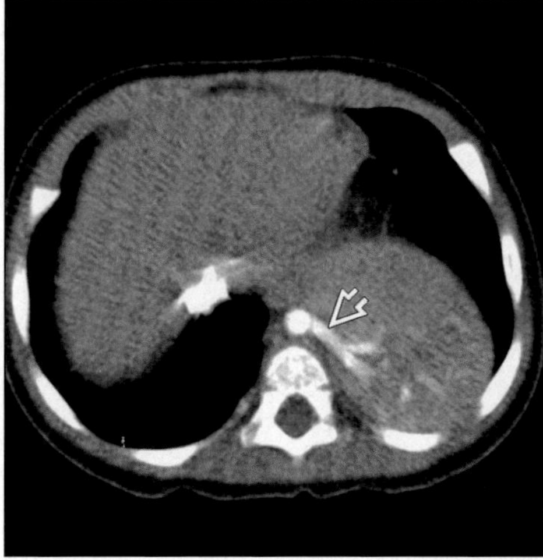

Axial CECT shows a large mass in the left chest with a very large artery ➡ originating from the aorta. The artery is supplying the mass, which is enhancing.

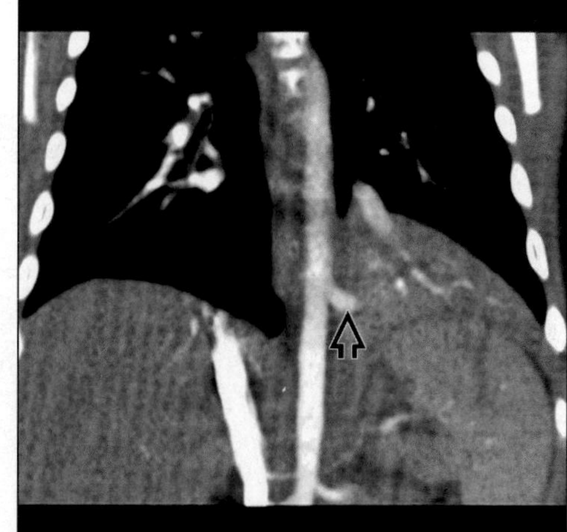

Coronal CECT shows the well-defined, triangular shaped, solid mass in the left chest. A large artery ➡ is originating from the aorta and extending into the mass. (Courtesy D. Frush, MD).

TERMINOLOGY

Abbreviations and Synonyms

- Bronchopulmonary sequestration
- Extralobar sequestration (ELS)
- Intralobar sequestration (ILS)

Definitions

- Pulmonary malformation with a portion of lung parenchyma separate from normal lobe
  - No normal communication with tracheobronchial tree
  - Blood supply from a systemic artery (aorta)
- Two major forms
  - ELS (25%)
    - Encased within own pleural membrane separate from normal lung
  - ILS (75%)
    - Shares visceral pleura of normal lung

IMAGING FINDINGS

General Features

- Best diagnostic clue
  - Persistent left-sided inferior paraspinal mass with history of recurrent pneumonia
  - CT or aortography demonstrates anomalous artery from aorta to sequestration
- Location
  - ELS
    - Posterior basal > medial basal segmental region
    - Left lower lobe (65%), right lower lobe (35%)
    - 10-15% intra-abdominal
    - 14% mediastinum
  - ILS
    - 98% lower lobes
    - 60% left side; bilateral rare
- Size: Variable: If cystic, often quite large

Radiographic Findings

- Uninfected sequestration: Well-circumscribed mass
- Infected sequestration: Ill-defined mass
- Pleural effusion (4%) and calcifications rare
- ELS

DDx: Sequestration

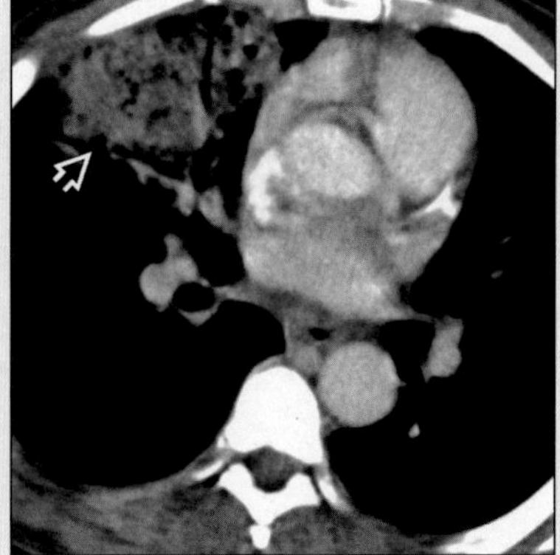

Pneumonia

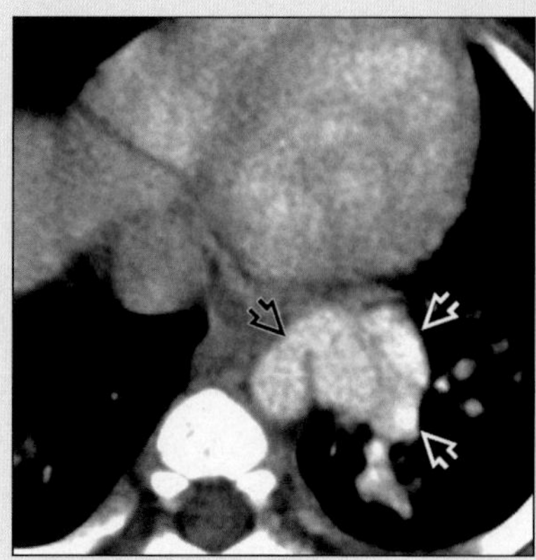

Isolated Systemic Supply (ISSNL)

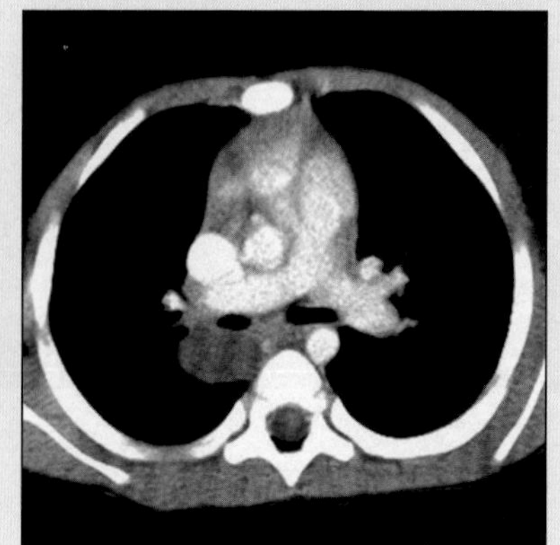

Bronchogenic Cyst

SEQUESTRATION

Key Facts

Terminology
- Bronchopulmonary sequestration
  - ELS (Extralobar sequestration)
  - ILS (Intralobar sequestration)
- ELS (25%)
  - Encased within own pleural membrane separate from normal lung
- ILS (75%)
  - Shares visceral pleura of normal lung

Imaging Findings
- Persistent left-sided inferior paraspinal mass with history of recurrent pneumonia
- Systemic artery identification from aorta is diagnostic
- Venous Drainage: 80% systemic venous system (IVC, Azygos, hemiazygos) creating left-to-right shunt
- Left lower lobe (65%), right lower lobe (35%)
- 14% mediastinum
- 10-15% intra-abdominal

Pathology
- ELS
  - Congenital systemic venous drainage
- ILS
  - Pulmonary venous drainage
  - Chronic infection with bronchial obstruction

Diagnostic Checklist
- Recurrent/persistent pneumonia in same region of lower lobe
- Multidetector CT angiography is the confirmatory diagnostic procedures

  - Sharply demarcated mass adjacent to left posterior medial hemidiaphragm
- ILS
  - Well-defined, triangular-shaped mass with long axis pointing medially, posterior in lung base
  - Hyperlucent (due to air-trapping)
  - Air containing single or multi-cystic mass
    - Air or air-fluid levels indicates pulmonary communication and/or infection
  - Chronic/recurrent bacterial pneumonia, mass left posterobasal lobe next to hemidiaphragm
  - Decrease in size with antibiotics, but no resolution
  - Focal bronchiectasis, subsegmental atelectasis, decreased lung volume, mediastinal shift, and prominence of the pulmonary hilum may be seen
- Limitations: Differentiating ELS from ILS is difficult; infradiaphragmatic ELS is difficult to detect

CT Findings
- Systemic artery identification from aorta is diagnostic
- Multiple small arteries may supply sequestration
- ELS
  - Lung bordering sequestration maybe hyperinflated
  - Well-circumscribed mass with homogeneous opacity that does **not** contain air-filled sacs
- ILS
  - Lesion with solid, fluid and/or cystic components
  - Heterogeneous enhancement
  - Hypervascularity or dilated vessels may be seen

MR Findings
- Excellent depiction of complex lesion
  - Cystic portions have variable signal manifestations
  - Hemorrhage
- May demonstrate abnormal systemic arterial supply

Angiographic Findings
- ELS
  - Arterial supply: Thoracic aorta or abdominal aorta 80%, brachiocephalic, subclavian, splenic, gastric, and intercostal arteries 15%, pulmonary artery 5%
  - Venous drainage: 80% systemic venous system (IVC, azygos, hemiazygos) creating left-to-right shunt
- ILS
  - Arterial supply: Thoracic aorta 75%, abdominal aorta, celiac axis or splenic artery 21%, intercostal artery 4%
    - No pulmonary or bronchial artery supply
  - Venous drainage: 95% pulmonary venous system creates left-to-left shunt

Imaging Recommendations
- Best imaging tool: Multidetector CT angiography
- Protocol advice: Multiplanar volume post processing to locate systemic artery supply

DIFFERENTIAL DIAGNOSIS

Chronic Pneumonia/Lipoid Pneumonia
- Chronic consolidative process in the lower lobe
  - No feeding artery will be present
- Fat density may be seen in lipoid pneumonia

Necrotizing Pneumonia/Abscess
- No feeding artery

Congential Cystic Adenomatoid Malformation (CCAM)
- Hamartomatous lesion often diagnosed in neonatal period or childhood
  - No systemic feeding artery
- Most have some cystic regions

Post Obstructive Pneumonia/Central Bronchial Neoplasm
- Ill-defined, consolidative or atelectatic area
- No dominant vessel arising from aorta
- Central obstructing lesion often seen

Scimitar Syndrome
- Abnormal connections of tracheobronchial airway, arterial supply, venous drainage, lung parenchyma

Bronchogenic Cyst
- Most common cystic lesion of mediastinum

- 75-85% mediastinum; 15-25% in lung; 36% with air
- Well-circumscribed, homogeneous, soft-tissue opacity, not vascular

Isolated Systemic Supply to the Normal Lung (ISSNL)

- Rare congenital malformation
- As with sequestration, ISSNL has a systemic arterial supply, but with ISSNL the lung is normal
- Often asymptomatic since the lung is normal, however hemoptysis or heart failure due to left to right shunt can occur

Additional Diagnosis

- Inferior paravertebral thoracic mass: Neurogenic tumor, lateral thoracic meningocele, extramedullary hematopoiesis, pleural tumor
- Cyst: Bronchiectasis, foregut cyst, pericardial cyst
- Infradiaphragmatic lesions: Neuroblastoma, teratoma, mesoblastic nephroma and foregut duplication

PATHOLOGY

General Features

- General path comments
  - Pulmonary parenchyma is separated from tracheobronchial tree
  - ELS
    - Systemic venous drainage
    - Most ELS is congenital in origin
    - Congenital anomalies 65%
  - ILS
    - Pulmonary venous drainage
    - Some may be congenital in origin (6-12%)
    - Majority secondary to bronchial obstruction from recurrent or chronic pneumonia
    - Chronic inflammation - hypertrophy of arteries with parasitization of systemic arteries

Gross Pathologic & Surgical Features

- ELS
  - Diseased tissue well-demarcated from surrounding lung parenchyma
    - Pleural thickening occurs with infection
  - Single lesion 0.5-15 cm (usually 3-6 cm)
  - Feeding artery possesses systemic structure
- ILS
  - Contiguous with normal lung, thick fibrinous visceral pleural lining with adhesions
  - Cystic spaces resemble ectatic bronchi
  - Pores of Kohn or a connection to normal small bronchi supply air within lesion
  - Parenchymal fibrosis and/or multiple cysts
  - Artery to sequestration is thin-walled

Microscopic Features

- ELS
  - Irregular bronchi/alveoli (2-5x > normal)
  - Bronchial structures absent, well-formed, or irregular
- ILS
  - Chronic inflammatory tissue and vascular sclerosis
  - Remnants of bronchioles surrounded by dense fibrous connective tissue infiltrated by lymphocytes

CLINICAL ISSUES

Presentation

- Most common signs/symptoms
  - ELS
    - 60% symptoms derived from associated anomalies
    - 15-20% are asymptomatic
    - Infection rare
    - Dyspnea, cyanosis, and feeding difficulties
    - Infants: Respiratory distress, feeding difficulties
    - Older children: Respiratory symptoms, congestive heart failure
  - ILS
    - 11% symptoms due to associated anomalies
    - Hemoptysis, which may be massive
    - Bruit found over sequestration
    - Recurrent respiratory infections caused by bacterial lower lobe pneumonia
    - Congestive heart failure

Demographics

- Age
  - ELS (25%)
    - M:F = 4:1
    - Age of onset: Infancy
    - 61% diagnosed by 6 months
  - ILS (75%)
    - Age of onset: Adulthood or older children
    - 50% diagnosed after adolescence
    - 85% symptomatic at time of diagnosis

Natural History & Prognosis

- Excellent prognosis following surgical excision

Treatment

- Surgical resection for symptomatic lesions
  - ELS: Sequestrectomy
  - ILS: Lobectomy rather than segmentectomy since sequestration crosses segmental planes
- Always search for multiple vessels vital prior to surgery
  - Pre-operative embolization of the aberrant artery

DIAGNOSTIC CHECKLIST

Consider

- Patients with recurrent/persistent pneumonia in same region of lower lobe may have sequestration

SELECTED REFERENCES

1. Agayev A et al: Extralobar pulmonary sequestration mimicking neuroblastoma. J Pediatr Surg. 42(9):1627-9, 2007
2. Deguchi E et al: Intralobar pulmonary sequestration diagnosed by MR angiography. Pediatr Surg Int. 21(7):576-7, 2005
3. Berrocal T et al: Congenital anomalies of the tracheobronchial tree, lung, and mediastinum: embryology, radiology, and pathology. Radiographics. 24(1):e17, 2004
4. Arenas J et al: Spiral CT diagnosis of isolated systemic supply to normal lung merging from the coeliac trunk. Clin Radiol. 2001

IMAGE GALLERY

Typical

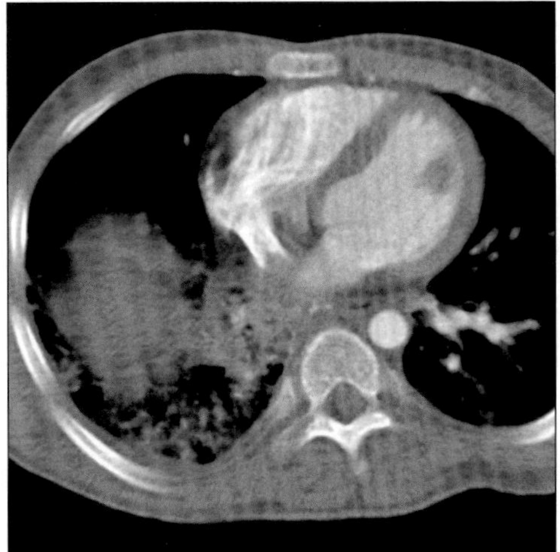

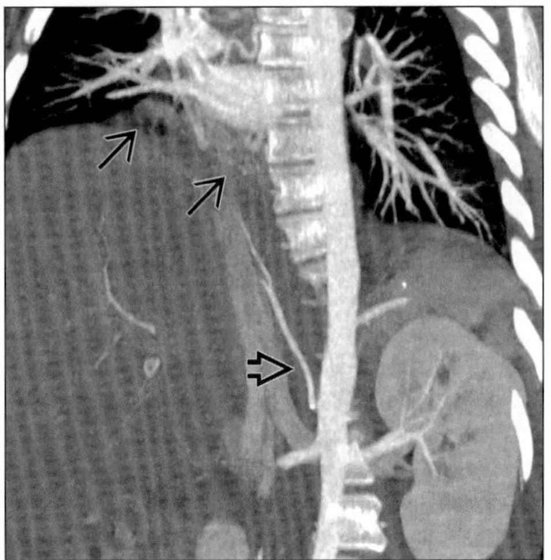

(Left) *Axial CECT shows area of consolidation in the base of the right lung with some cystic areas. Child with recurrent infections with improvement but without resolution. Now patient has hemoptysis.* ***(Right)*** *Coronal CTA shows an anomalous artery ⇨ arising above the level of the renal arteries and below the origin of the celiac and SMA. The vessel extends up to the diaphragm. The mass in the right lung base → appears to have small cysts within the mass.*

Typical

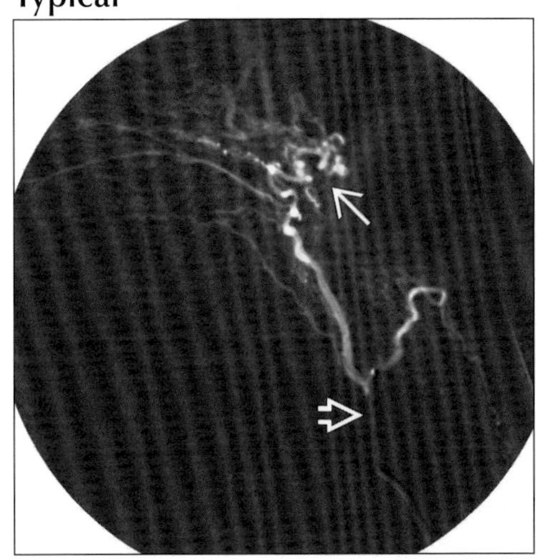

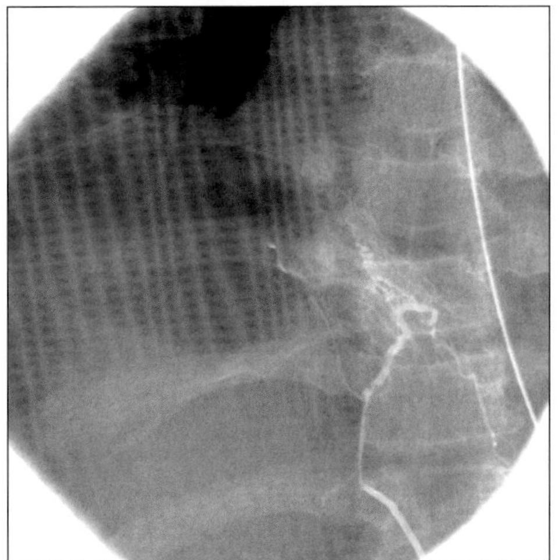

(Left) *DSA shows a microcatheter ➡ has been placed through the anomalous vessel and is now opacifying the multiple vascular branches ➡ that are supplying the right lung lesion. The patient has been having hemoptysis and the angiogram is in preparation for embolization.* ***(Right)*** *DSA shows the artery after embolization with polyvinyl alcohol (PVA) particles. The majority of the vessels that were supplying this mass are now occluded.*

Typical

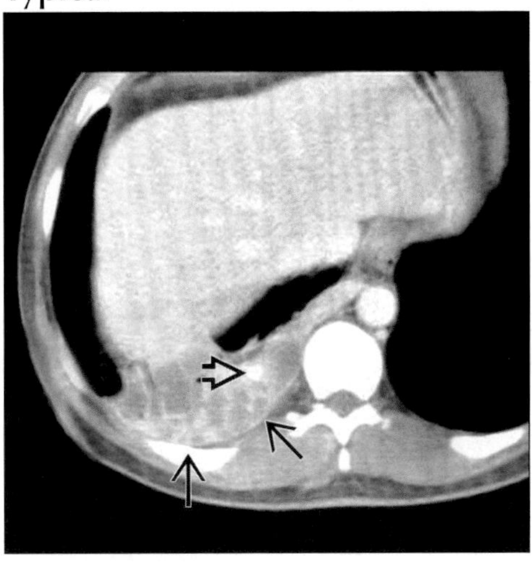

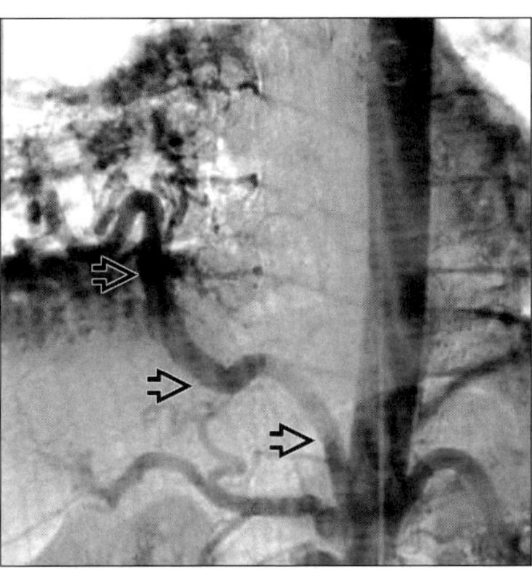

(Left) *Axial CECT shows a posterior, right lower lung mass →, triangular-shaped. The mass contains cystic components and is enhancing. There is a large artery ⇨ present.* ***(Right)*** *Catheter angiography shows a large artery ⇨ originating from the infradiaphragmatic aorta, just above the renal arteries. This artery corresponds to the vessel seen on the CT in the previous image. Treatment is surgical but preoperative embolization may decrease blood loss.*

SUPERIOR VENA CAVA SYNDROME

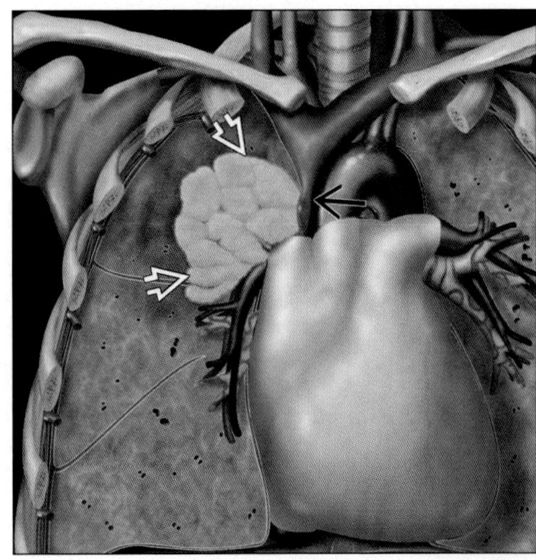

Graphic shows an anterior mediastinal mass ➡ causing extrinsic compression of the superior vena cava ➡. The resultant SVC narrowing may impair venous return from the head, neck and upper extremities.

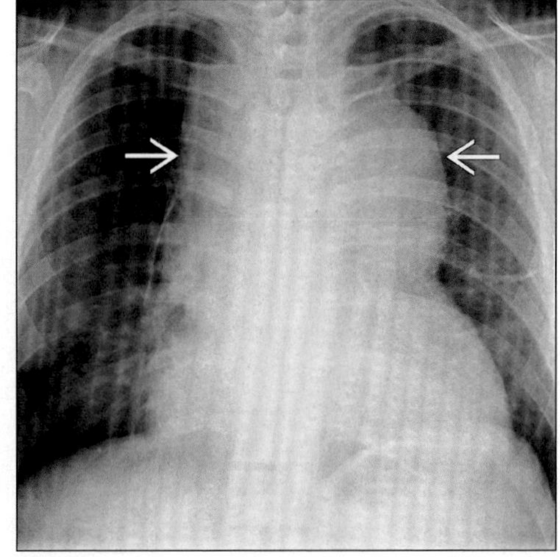

Posteroanterior radiograph of the chest demonstrates a widened mediastinum ➡, consistent with a mediastinal mass. Malignancy is the etiology of SVC syndrome in 80-90% of cases.

TERMINOLOGY

Abbreviations and Synonyms

- Superior vena cava syndrome (SVCS), superior vena cava obstruction (SVCO), superior vena cava stenosis

Definitions

- Obstruction or narrowing of superior vena cava (SVC) due to intraluminal, intramural or extrinsic disease
  - Impairs venous return from head, neck, upper extremities and trunk to right atrium
  - Can have benign or malignant etiology

IMAGING FINDINGS

General Features

- Best diagnostic clue
  - Non-visualization of superior vena cava with contrast administration
  - Multiple collateral vessels over upper chest
- Morphology
  - Narrowing or occlusion of superior vena cava
  - Impaired return of blood centrally

Radiographic Findings

- Radiography
  - Widened mediastinum secondary to mediastinal mass or dilated superior vena cava
  - Pleural effusion
  - Right hilar mass
  - Calcified lymphadenopathy
  - Prominent azygos arch
  - Normal chest X-ray in patient with SVCS is pathognomonic for chronic fibrous mediastinitis
    - In absence of a history of central venous catheters or prior surgery

CT Findings

- CECT
  - Absent or narrowed superior vena cava
  - Absent or decreased opacification of central venous structures distal to site of obstruction or narrowing
  - Extrinsic compression by adjacent masses
  - Intraluminal filling defects
  - Multiple collaterals, including central venous and subcutaneous collaterals
  - Prominent azygos arch and vein
  - Prominent superior intercostal vein

DDx: Impaired Trunk and Upper Extremity Venous Return

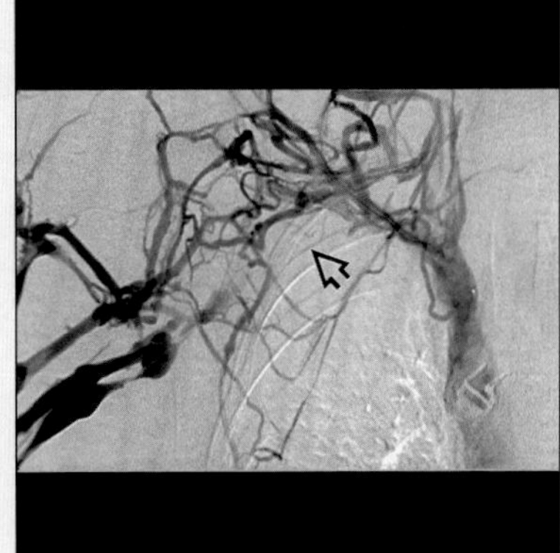

Occluded Subclavian Vein

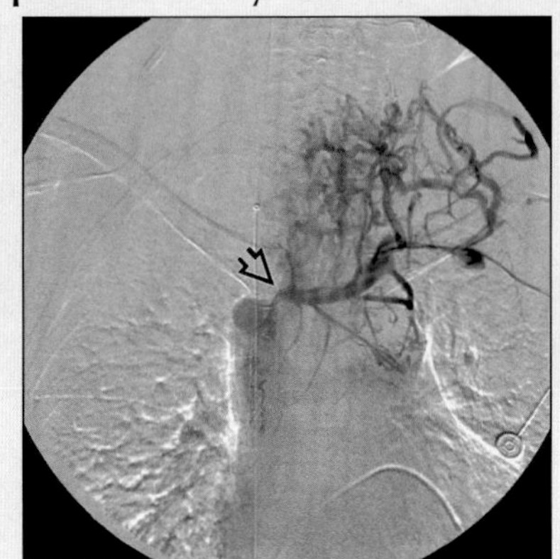

Innominate Vein Stenosis

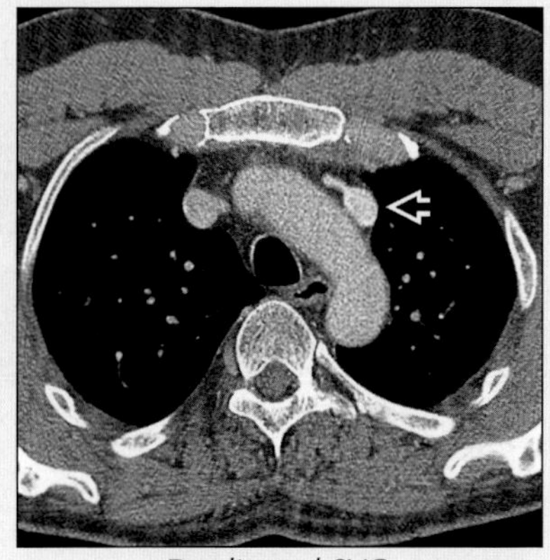

Duplicated SVC

SUPERIOR VENA CAVA SYNDROME

Key Facts

Terminology
- Superior vena cava syndrome (SVCS), superior vena cava obstruction (SVCO), superior vena cava stenosis
  - Obstruction or narrowing of the superior vena cava (SVC) due to intraluminal disease, intramural disease or extrinsic disease
  - Impaired venous return from head, neck, upper extremities and trunk to right atrium
  - Can have benign or malignant etiology

Imaging Findings
- Non-visualization of the superior vena cava with contrast administration

Pathology
- Intrathoracic malignancy including bronchogenic carcinoma
- Mediastinal tumors including lymphoma and metastases
- Infection including tuberculosis, histoplasmosis
- Benign etiologies include prior central venous catheters, presence of pacemakers, history of radiation or chemotherapy

Clinical Issues
- Enlarged and increased collateral vessels on chest wall with enlarged neck veins
- Edema of the face, neck, upper trunk and upper extremities
- Male preponderance for malignant etiologies, paralleling cancer incidences
- Equal distribution for benign etiologies
- Gradual and progressive narrowing or obstruction of superior vena cava

  - Inflow of contrast-enhanced blood into IVC

MR Findings
- MRV
  - Non-opacification of superior vena cava
  - Prominent azygos arch and vein
  - Multiple collateral vessels
- MR
  - Enhanced multiplanar MR can evaluate external causes of SVCS, and adjacent critical structures

Nuclear Medicine Findings
- Radionuclide venography can demonstrate obstruction and collaterals

Ultrasonographic Findings
- Grayscale Ultrasound
  - Entire superior vena cava cannot normally be directly evaluated with grayscale ultrasound
  - Dilatation of visualized portion of SVC
    - Lumen size unchanged with respirations or cardiac cycle
  - Increased intraluminal echogenicity suggests thrombus
  - Distended subclavian, brachiocephalic and jugular veins
- Pulsed Doppler
  - Altered spectral waveforms when evaluating the subclavian veins
  - Absent normal transmission of atrial waveform, respiratory phasicity, or response to provocative maneuvers
    - Monophasic antegrade flow
    - Low velocity flow
- Color Doppler: Sluggish or absent blood flow

Angiographic Findings
- DSA
  - Venography is performed superior or peripheral to obstruction or stenosis
  - Stasis or retrograde flow in subclavian or brachiocephalic veins if venography performed from upper extremity peripheral veins
    - May mimic subclavian or brachiocephalic vein occlusion
  - Mass effect and compression with luminal effacement is related to extrinsic masses
  - Long, smooth narrowing is related to indwelling devices such as central venous catheters and pacemakers
  - Filling defect is consistent with thrombus
  - Occlusion results in no flow of contrast through superior vena cava
  - Multiple collateral vessels are seen
  - Azygos arch and vein may be enlarged

Imaging Recommendations
- Best imaging tool
  - CT and MR may show etiology of narrowing, particularly in cases of malignancy
    - Permits evaluation of other critical structures, including airway, in cases of malignancy
  - Venography will accurately show site, degree of narrowing, and collateral blood flow to right atrium
    - Venography is done when cross-sectional imaging is non-diagnostic
    - Used in treatment planning for endovascular or surgical procedures
- Protocol advice
  - Contrast-enhancement identifies site of occlusion or narrowing, as well as collateral flow
  - Coronal or sagittal reconstructions can be helpful

DIFFERENTIAL DIAGNOSIS

Thoracic Outlet Syndrome
- Multiple collateral vessels seen over upper chest and neck
- Distinct area of narrowing at junction of clavicle and first rib
- Patent SVC demonstrated

Brachiocephalic Vein Occlusion or Stenosis
- Multiple collateral vessels seen over upper chest and neck

- Focal area of stenosis or occlusion in brachiocephalic vein
- Patent SVC demonstrated

Persistent Left Superior Vena Cava with Absent Right Superior Vena Cava

- Absence of SVC in expected location in mediastinum
- Absent collateral vessels
- Large venous structure in left anterior mediastinum which drains blood to right atrium via coronary sinus
- Inserted catheters or wires take aberrant course
- May also have duplicated SVC

Upper Extremity Deep Venous Thrombosis, Stenosis or Occlusion

- May clinically mimic SVCS with UE swelling
- Isolated, unilateral upper extremity edema
- Most often associated with previous/current PICC line
- Multiple collaterals present, but central veins and SVC are patent

PATHOLOGY

General Features

- Genetics: No genetic predisposition
- Etiology
  - Intrathoracic malignancy, including bronchogenic carcinoma
  - Mediastinal tumors including lymphoma and metastases
  - Atrial tumor or tumor extension
  - Infection including tuberculosis, histoplasmosis
  - Aortic aneurysm
  - Benign etiologies include prior central venous catheters, presence of pacemakers, history of radiation or chemotherapy
- Epidemiology
  - Malignancy is etiology in 80-90%
  - Benign causes are etiology in 10-20%
    - Mediastinal fibrosis is seen in 50% of benign cases of superior vena cava syndrome
    - With increasing use of central venous access devices, this etiology has increased in past twenty years

CLINICAL ISSUES

Presentation

- Most common signs/symptoms
  - Collateral vessels on chest wall; enlarged neck veins
  - Edema of face, neck, upper trunk and upper extremities
  - Headaches
  - Dyspnea, dysphagia, hoarseness
  - Coughing
- Other signs/symptoms
  - Syncope, seizures, visual changes
  - Coma in severe cases
- Clinical Profile
  - SVCS is a clinical diagnosis
    - Patients can be asymptomatic with well-compensated stenosis or occlusion

Demographics

- Age
  - 18 to 76 years, with a mean of 54 years
  - Malignant etiologies in older ages (40-60 years)
  - Benign etiologies in younger ages (30-40 years)
- Gender
  - Male preponderance for malignant etiologies, paralleling cancer incidences
  - Equal distribution for benign etiologies

Natural History & Prognosis

- Gradual, progressive narrowing or obstruction of SVC
  - Insidious onset of symptoms
- Rarely fatal: Most patients will die of their malignancy

Treatment

- External-beam radiation
- Chemotherapy depending on type of malignancy
- Anti-coagulation
- Endovascular therapy
  - Catheter-directed thrombolysis prior to endovascular stent placement
  - Percutaneous transluminal angioplasty; usually followed by large caliber intravascular stent
- Surgical therapy
  - Venous bypass
  - Venous transposition

DIAGNOSTIC CHECKLIST

Consider

- Non-invasive imaging prior to endovascular, surgical or radiation treatment

Image Interpretation Pearls

- Occluded superior vena cava
- Multiple collaterals in mediastinum and chest wall
- Enlarged azygous system
- Normal chest X-ray with SVCS indicates fibrosing mediastinitis
  - Unless patient has a history of central venous catheters or prior surgery

SELECTED REFERENCES

1. Eren S et al: The superior vena cava syndrome caused by malignant disease. Imaging with multi-detector row CT. Eur J Radiol. 59(1):93-103, 2006
2. Kalra M et al: Open surgical and endovascular treatment of superior vena cava syndrome caused by nonmalignant disease. J Vasc Surg. 38(2):215-23, 2003
3. Oderich GS et al: Stent placement for treatment of central and peripheral venous obstruction: a long-term multi-institutional experience. J Vasc Surg. 32(4):760-9, 2000
4. Kim HJ et al: CT diagnosis of superior vena cava syndrome: importance of collateral vessels. AJR Am J Roentgenol. 161(3):539-42, 1993
5. Parish JM et al: Etiologic considerations in superior vena cava syndrome. Mayo Clin Proc. 56(7):407-13, 1981
6. Webb WR et al: Catheter venography in the superior vena cava syndrome. AJR Am J Roentgenol. 129(1):146-8, 1977

SUPERIOR VENA CAVA SYNDROME

IMAGE GALLERY

Typical

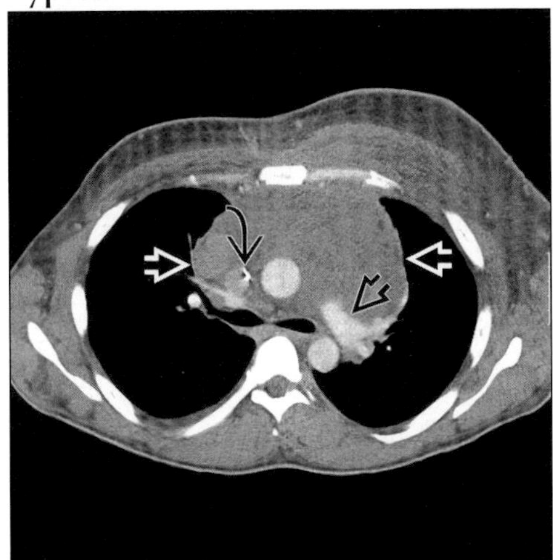

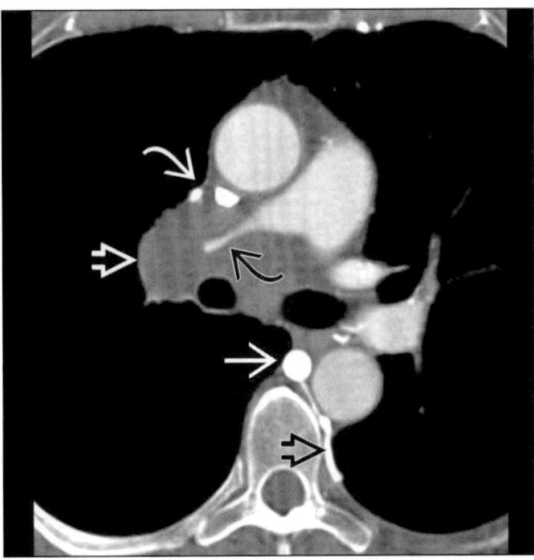

*(**Left**) Axial CECT shows a large anterior mediastinal mass encasing the vascular structures. A catheter is present in the narrowed superior vena cava. There is also mass effect involving the left pulmonary vein. (**Right**) Axial CECT shows a soft tissue mass narrowing the SVC and encasing the right pulmonary artery. The azygos vein is enlarged and there are prominent lumbar collateral veins present.*

Typical

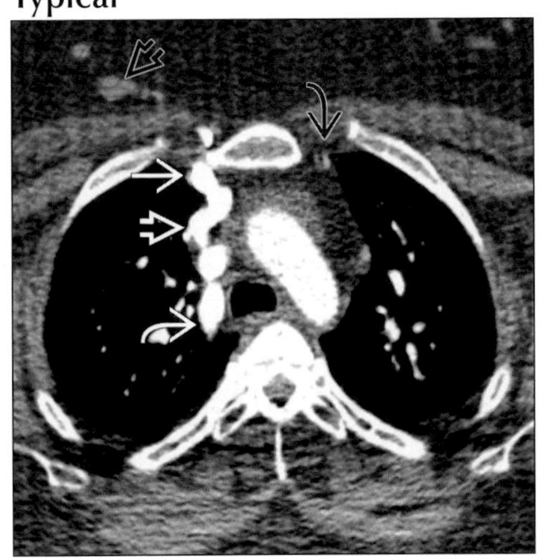

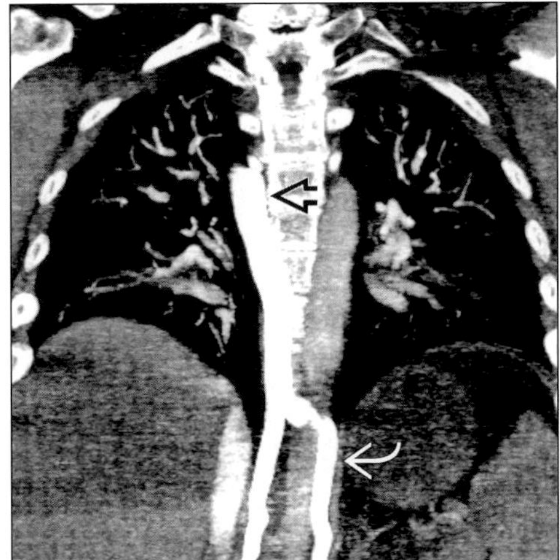

*(**Left**) Axial CECT shows a large collateral vessel between the azygos arch and the right internal mammary vein. There are also enlarged subcutaneous collateral veins. The left internal mammary vein is normal. (**Right**) Coronal CECT shows enlargement of the hemiazygos and azygos veins. These veins provide drainage of the head and neck, arms and trunk through chest and lumbar collaterals that communicate with the azygos system below the SVC obstruction.*

Typical

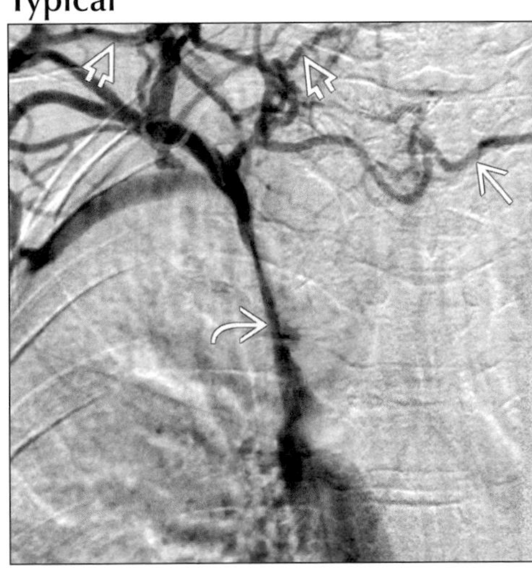

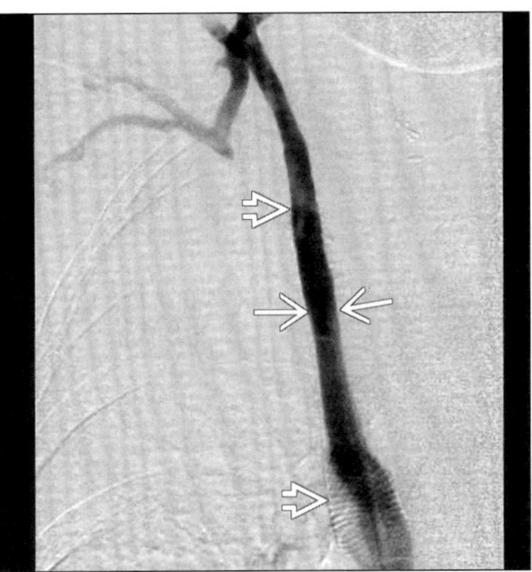

*(**Left**) Posteroanterior DSA via a catheter introduced into the SVC shows multiple collaterals over the neck and chest. The superior vena cava is markedly narrowed, as a result of tumor encasement. (**Right**) Posteroanterior DSA (same patient) after stent placement shows a normal caliber has been restored to the superior vena cava. Collateral vessels are much less prominent than on the initial venogram, indicating decompression of the previous venous obstruction.*

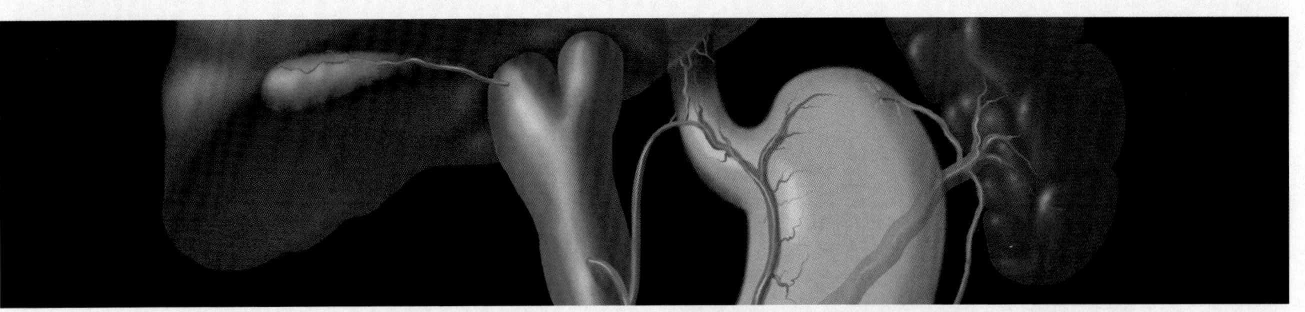

SECTION 5: Abdominal

ABDOMINAL AORTA AND VISCERAL VASCULATURE

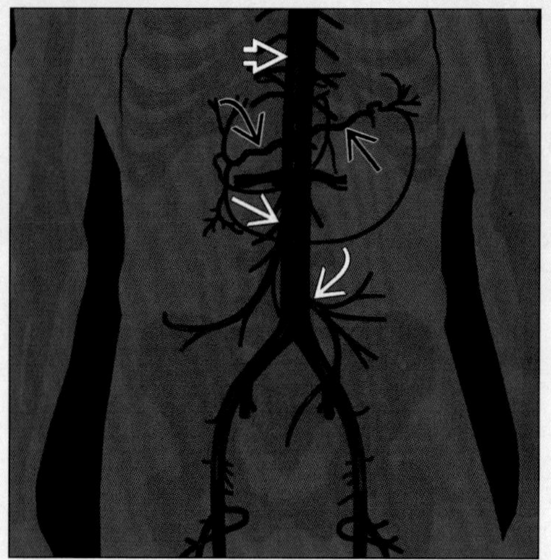

Graphic of the abdominal aorta shows the superior and inferior mesenteric arteries, which supply the small and large bowel. The splenic and common hepatic arteries also supply the gastrointestinal tract.

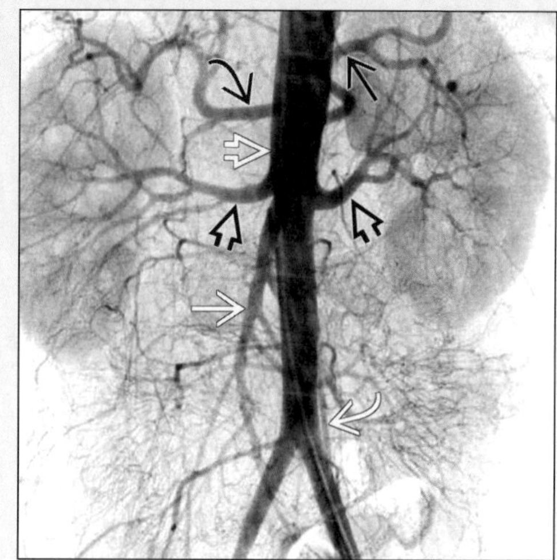

DSA shows the abdominal aorta and visceral arteries, including the SMA, IMA, common hepatic and splenic arteries. Both renal arteries are also well-demonstrated.

TERMINOLOGY

Abbreviations

- Superior mesenteric artery (SMA)
- Inferior mesenteric artery (IMA)
- Inferior vena cava (IVC)
- Gastroduodenal artery (GDA)
- Pancreaticoduodenal artery (PDA)

IMAGING ANATOMY

Arterial Anatomy

- Abdominal aorta
  - Extends from diaphragm to bifurcation into common iliac arteries
- Celiac artery (trunk)
  - Arises at T12-L1, courses under diaphragmatic crura
  - 1st branch is left gastric artery
    - Supplies gastric fundus/gastroesophageal junction
    - Anastomoses with right gastric artery
    - May arise directly from aorta (2%)
    - May give partial left hepatic arterial supply
  - Bifurcates into splenic and common hepatic arteries distal to left gastric artery origin (70%)
  - Dorsal pancreatic artery arises from celiac in 10%
    - Supplies body of pancreas
    - May also give blood supply to transverse colon
- Splenic artery
  - Posterior to pancreas; anterosuperior to splenic vein
  - Short gastric arteries arise near splenic hilum
  - Left gastroepiploic artery arises near splenic hilum
    - Anastomoses with right gastroepiploic artery
    - Supplies greater curvature of stomach
  - Contributes blood supply to pancreas
    - Yields dorsal pancreatic artery if not from celiac
    - Numerous small branches supply body and tail
    - Pancreatica magna from distal splenic artery
- Common hepatic artery
  - Contributes 1/3 hepatic blood supply, 2/3 oxygen; portal vein gives 2/3 blood supply, 1/3 of oxygen
  - Divides into proper hepatic, gastroduodenal arteries
- Proper hepatic artery
  - Divides into right, middle and left hepatic arteries
  - 45% variation in hepatic arterial supply
    - Right hepatic artery originates from SMA in 12%
    - Accessory right hepatic from SMA in 6%
    - Left hepatic from left gastric in 11%
    - Accessory left hepatic from left gastric in 11%
  - Hepatic arteries anterior to portal vein branches
  - Cystic artery (gallbladder) usually from right hepatic
- Gastroduodenal artery
  - Divides into superior pancreaticoduodenal and right gastroepiploic arteries
    - Pancreaticoduodenal arteries supply pancreatic head, part of body via transverse pancreatic artery
    - Superior and inferior PDA (from SMA) anastomose
    - Right and left gastroepiploic arteries anastomose
- Superior mesenteric artery (SMA)
  - Supplies duodenum, small bowel, colon
    - Colonic supply to cecum through splenic flexure
  - Arises below celiac artery; courses over left renal vein
    - Posterior to superior mesenteric vein in mesentery
  - 1st branch is inferior PDA or middle colic artery
  - Mid-portion of SMA supplies small bowel
    - 3rd-4th portions duodenum, jejunum, ileum
  - Right colic artery supplies ascending colon
  - Ileocolic artery is terminal branch of SMA
    - Supplies terminal ileum and cecum
  - Variant anatomy
    - Common celiacomesenteric trunk (1%)
    - Accessory or replaced right hepatic artery (20%)
    - Arc of Buehler (1%); persistent fetal celiac-SMA direct communication
    - Arc of Riolan: Collateral pathway connecting middle colic and left colic branch of IMA; runs centrally within mesentery
- Inferior mesenteric artery (IMA)
  - Arises from left side infrarenal aorta at L-3
    - 3-4 mm diameter; 2-3 cm above aortic bifurcation
  - 1st branch is left colic artery
    - Ascending branch of left colic artery supplies splenic flexure; middle colic artery anastomosis

Imaging of Visceral Arteries and Veins

Ultrasound
- Evaluation of portal, hepatic vein patency
- Less reliable in evaluating abdominal/pelvic vessels
  - May be limited by bowel gas, body habitus

CT
- CECT and CTA usually highly accurate in evaluating arterial and venous anatomy and pathology
- Assesses vascular calcifications
- 3-D, volume rendered and reformatted images

MR
- MRA excellent for evaluating origins and proximal portions of arteries
- MRV excellent for evaluating portal and hepatic veins; also evaluates hepatic parenchyma

Angiography
- "Gold standard" for evaluating arterial anatomy and pathology; only vascular lumen characterized
- May be combined with endovascular interventions

Venography
- Evaluation of venous anatomy and pathology usually requires selective catheterization
- Balloon-occlusion hepatic venography images small hepatic veins and portal vein; CO_2 may be used
- Indirect visualization achieved by arterioportography
  - Injection of SMA or celiac artery, with prolonged imaging sequences opacifies venous system
- Direct portal and mesenteric venography requires transhepatic or transjugular venous access; may be combined with intervention (e.g., embolization, TIPS)

    - Marginal artery of Drummond courses along mesenteric border of left colon
    - Descending branch of left colic artery supplies descending colon
  - Sigmoid artery branch of IMA
    - Supplies sigmoid colon
  - Superior hemorrhoidal artery
    - Terminal branch of IMA
    - Supplies superior rectum
- Phrenic arteries
- Intercostal and lumbar arteries
  - Paired arteries supply paraspinal, abdominal wall musculature; branches to vertebra, spinal canal
  - Provide collateral circulation in occlusive disease
- Renal/adrenal arteries
  - Described in separate section introduction
- Gonadal arteries
- Median sacral artery
  - Arises from posterior aorta proximal to bifurcation
- Common iliac arteries
- Internal iliac (hypogastric) arteries
  - Anterior division yields inferior gluteal, obturator, internal pudendal, vesicle, uterine arteries
    - Middle and inferior rectal arteries (terminal branches of anterior division) supply rectum
  - Posterior division yields superior gluteal, iliolumbar, lateral sacral arteries
- External iliac arteries

Portal Venous Anatomy
- Portal vein
  - Formed by confluence of superior mesenteric and splenic veins
  - Venous blood flows toward liver (hepatopetal flow)
    - 2/3 of hepatic blood supply, 1/3 of oxygen
    - Liver detoxifies gastrointestinal venous blood
  - Right and left portal veins perfuse each hepatic lobe
    - Hepatic segments perfused by portal branches
  - Normally 10-12 mm diameter and 8 cm length
- Splenic vein
  - Drains spleen and pancreas
  - Also partially drains stomach
    - Short gastric veins
- Left gastric (coronary) vein
  - Major drainage of stomach and lower esophagus
  - Enters portal vein in 2/3, splenic vein in 1/3
- Superior mesenteric vein (SMV)
  - Venous drainage that parallels SMA arterial anatomy
    - Drains duodenum, small bowel, right colon
- Inferior mesenteric vein
  - Venous drainage that parallels IMA arterial anatomy
  - Enters splenic vein in 2/3, enters SMV in 1/3
  - Drains left colon

Venous Anatomy of IVC and Branches
- Inferior vena cava (IVC)
  - Formed by confluence of common iliac veins
  - Located to right of midline, adjacent to aorta (97%)
    - Duplicated (1%); left sided (0.5%); absent (0.1%)
  - Retrohepatic segment courses in hepatic bare area; joined by hepatic veins below diaphragmatic hiatus
    - "Eustachian valve" at IVC/right atrial junction
- Hepatic veins
  - Drain hepatic lobes directly into IVC
  - Right, middle and left hepatic veins
    - Referred to as "upper group"
  - "Lower group" of hepatic veins drain caudate lobe and lower right hepatic lobe
- Renal/adrenal veins
  - Described in separate section introduction
- Right gonadal vein
  - Drains into anterior IVC below right renal vein
  - Left gonadal vein drains into left renal vein
- Lumbar veins (paired)
  - Drain vertebra and paraspinal musculature
  - Ascending lumbar veins anastomose with lumbars
    - Deep to psoas muscles, parallel to IVC
    - Arise from common iliac veins
    - Become azygos and hemiazygos veins in thorax
- Common iliac veins
  - Formed by internal & external iliac vein confluence
- Internal iliac veins
  - Tributaries include superior and inferior gluteal, obturator, vesical, uterine, vaginal, prostatic, middle and inferior rectal veins
- External iliac veins

ABDOMINAL AORTA AND VISCERAL VASCULATURE

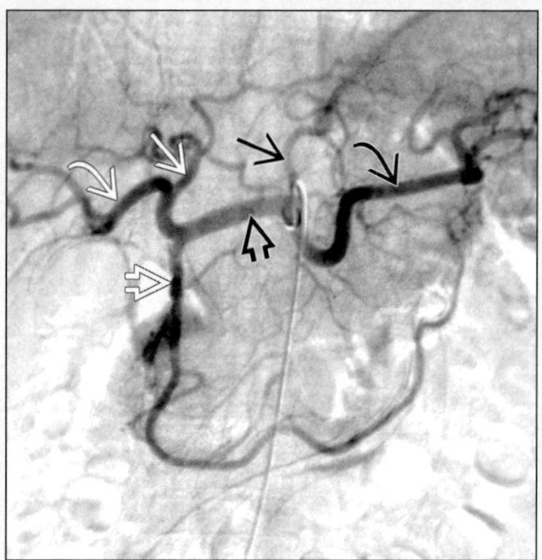

Celiac arteriogram shows the splenic ⇒, left gastric →, and common hepatic ⇒ arteries. The latter yields the GDA ⇒, continues as the proper hepatic artery, and divides into the right ⇒ and left ⇒ hepatic arteries.

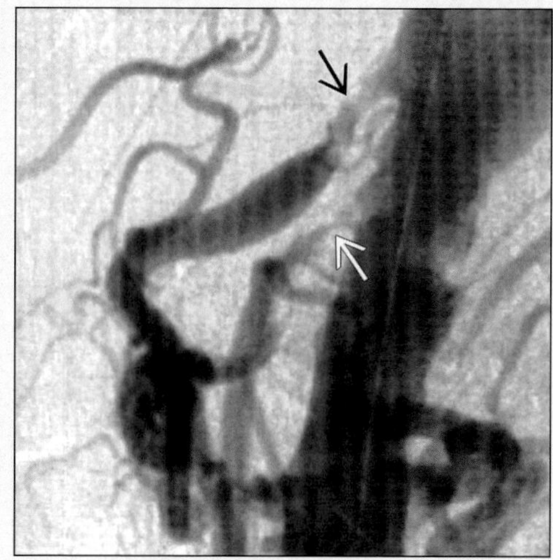

Lateral abdominal aortogram shows celiac → and SMA ⇒ stenoses in a patient with postprandial abdominal pain, typical of chronic mesenteric ischemia. The lateral view best demonstrates the origins of these vessels.

PATHOLOGIC ISSUES

Arterial Pathology

- Atherosclerotic occlusive disease
- Aneurysms
  - Abdominal aorta (AAA)
    - Suprarenal: Extends above renal arteries
    - Juxtarenal: Begins within 1 cm of renal arteries
    - Infrarenal: > 1 cm normal aorta below renals
    - Inflammatory AAA; uninfected but has enhancing circumferential inflammatory tissue (5% of AAA)
    - AAA treated with open or endovascular repair
  - Iliac
    - Dilatation > 1.5 cm normal arterial diameter
    - Common, internal iliac > external iliac arteries
    - Usually incidental finding; > 65% asymptomatic; however, rupture has 80% mortality
    - Open surgical or endovascular repair
  - Visceral
- Dissection
  - Isolated abdominal aortic or iliac dissection rare
    - Usually extension of thoracic dissection
    - Usually atherosclerotic etiology
    - Also 2° to Marfan, trauma, iatrogenic injury
  - Visceral artery dissection usually aortic extension
    - Spontaneous dissection associated with FMD, SAM
    - Iatrogenic and traumatic etiologies
- Fibromuscular dysplasia (FMD)
  - Visceral arteries 6th most frequent site
- Gastrointestinal hemorrhage
  - Much more common in upper than lower GI tract
    - Usually from gastritis, peptic ulcer disease
  - Inflammatory bowel disease (younger patients)
  - Diverticular disease (older patients)
- Neoplasms
- Mesenteric ischemia
  - Acute
    - 50% due to embolic SMA occlusion
    - Also from thrombosis of pre-existing stenosis
    - 10% from mesenteric venous thrombosis
    - Hypotension, low-flow states (nonocclusive mesenteric ischemia)
  - Chronic
    - Postprandial pain 2° to chronic arterial disease
    - Stenosis or occlusion of 2 mesenteric arteries
- Segmental arterial mediolysis (SAM)
  - Deficient media in arterial wall
  - Visceral artery dissections, aneurysms, stenoses
- Trauma
- Vasculitis
  - Polyarteritis nodosa involves visceral arteries
- Vascular malformations
  - May affect stomach, small bowel, colon
    - Angiodysplasia commonly affects right colon; dilated thin-walled submucosal malformation

Venous Pathology

- IVC obstruction
  - Usually involves infrarenal segment
  - Thrombosis most common etiology
  - May have extrinsic compression (e.g. tumor, adenopathy, retroperitoneal fibrosis)
- Iliac vein obstruction
  - May-Thürner syndrome
    - Artery compresses left common iliac vein
- Hepatic vein obstruction
  - Budd-Chiari syndrome
- Portal hypertension
  - Elevated portal venous pressure (> 10 mm Hg)
  - Cirrhosis most common etiology
    - Alcoholic liver disease, hepatitis
- Visceral venous thrombosis/occlusion
  - Portal, splenic, mesenteric vein thrombosis

RELATED REFERENCES

1. Grierson C et al: Multidetector CT appearances of splanchnic arterial pathology. Clin Radiol. 62(8):717-23, 2007
2. Wintersperger BJ et al: Multidetector-row CT angiography of the aorta and visceral arteries. Semin Ultrasound CT MR. 25(1):25-40, 2004

IMAGE GALLERY

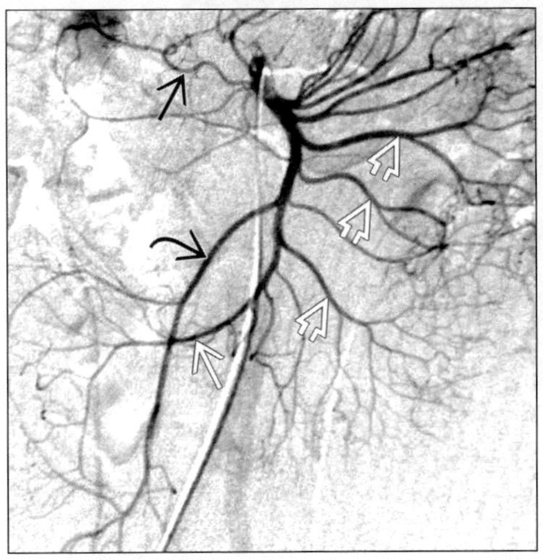

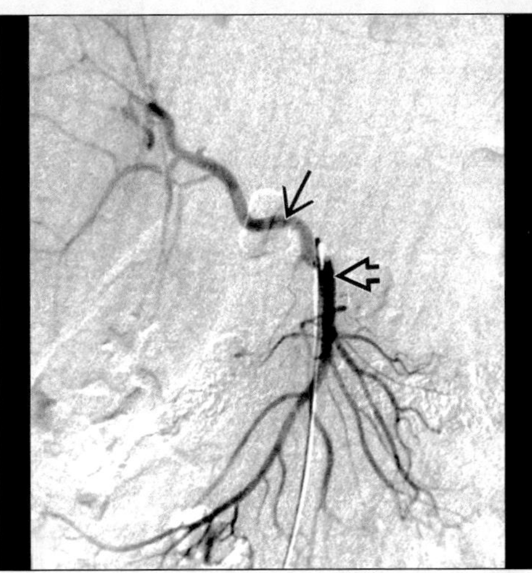

*(**Left**) SMA arteriogram shows the ileocolic ➡, right colic ➡ and middle colic ➡ arteries, which provide arterial supply to the terminal ileum, cecum, ascending and transverse colon. There are also multiple branches ➡ that supply the jejunal and ileal portions of the small bowel. (**Right**) SMA arteriogram in a different patient shows that the right hepatic artery ➡ arises from the proximal SMA ➡ rather than from the celiac trunk. This anatomic variant is seen in up to 20% of patients.*

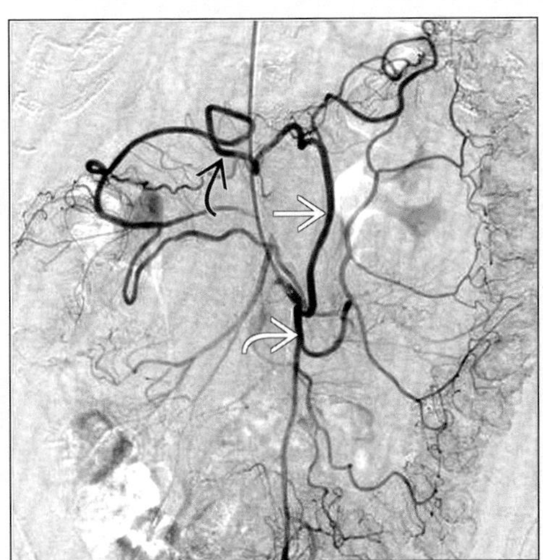

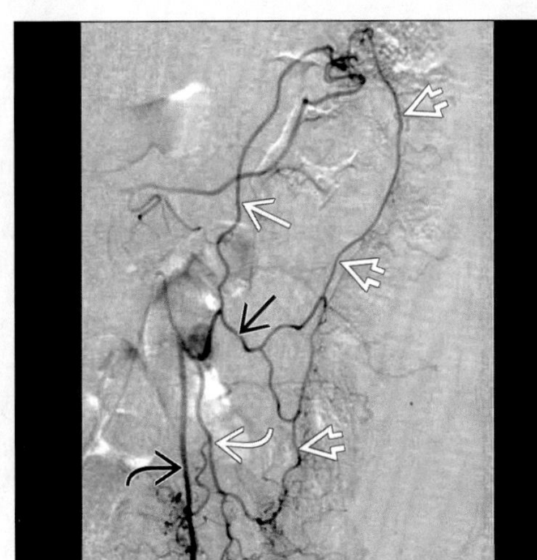

*(**Left**) DSA shows the Arc of Riolan ➡, a collateral between the IMA ➡ and the middle colic artery ➡. This arcade runs within the mesentery, rather than along the colonic border. (**Right**) IMA arteriogram shows the ascending ➡ and descending ➡ branches of the left colic artery, the sigmoid ➡ and the superior hemorrhoidal ➡ arteries. The marginal artery of Drummond ➡ courses along the mesenteric border of the colon and is an important collateral arcade.*

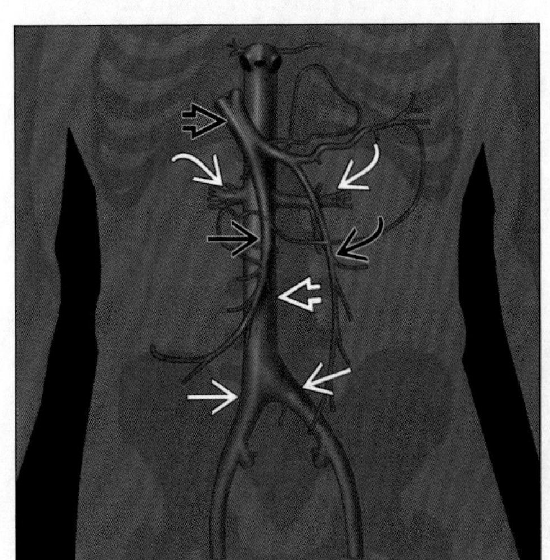

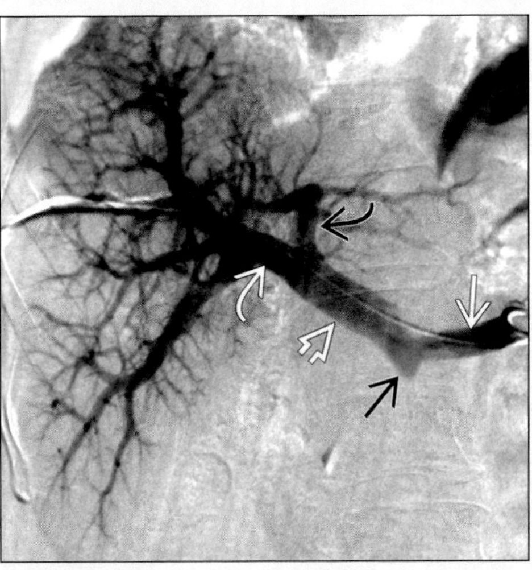

*(**Left**) Graphic shows the IVC ➡, formed by the iliac veins ➡. The renal veins ➡ drain into the IVC. The portal venous system drains the gastrointestinal tract. The superior ➡ and inferior ➡ mesenteric veins join with the splenic vein to form the portal vein ➡, which drains into the liver. (**Right**) Transhepatic portogram shows the splenic vein ➡, the main portal vein ➡ and the division into the right ➡ and left portal ➡ veins. There is trace reflux into the superior mesenteric vein ➡.*

ABDOMINAL AORTIC ANEURYSM

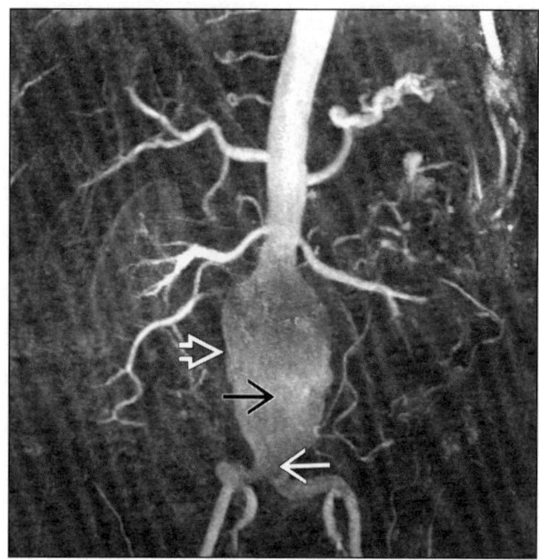

MR MIP shows an infrarenal AAA ➡ extending to the aortic bifurcation ➡. The decreased signal intensity ➡ in the aneurysm from turbulent flow. Aneurysm tortuosity is difficult to evaluate on the MIP.

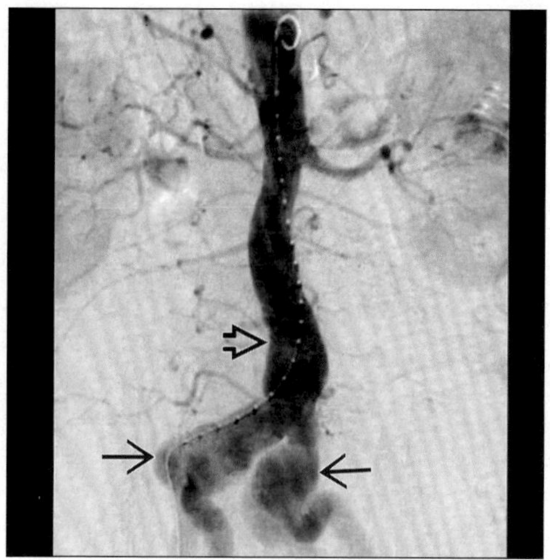

Catheter angiography shows an AAA ➡ and bilateral common iliac artery aneurysms ➡. Angiography may significantly underestimate the true diameter of an aneurysm, as only the lumen is displayed.

TERMINOLOGY

Definitions

- Abdominal aortic aneurysm (AAA)
  - Fusiform or saccular enlargement of aorta ≥ 1.5 times normal diameter (> 3 cm in abdominal aorta)
  - AAA described by relationship to renal arteries
    - Infrarenal: > 1 cm normal aorta below renals
    - Juxtarenal: Begins within 1 cm of renal arteries
    - Suprarenal: Extends above renal arteries
  - Inflammatory aneurysm: Uninfected AAA with enhancing circumferential inflammatory tissue
    - 5% of AAA; abdominal pain may mimic rupture
    - Adjacent structures involved (e.g., duodenum)
- Endovascular aneurysm repair (EVAR): Placement of intravascular endograft to bridge aortoiliac segments and depressurize AAA
- Endoleak: Persistent flow of blood outside endograft

IMAGING FINDINGS

General Features

- Best diagnostic clue: Focal or diffuse aortic dilatation
- Location
  - Most commonly involves infrarenal aorta
  - AAA can extend to involve iliac arteries (10-20%)
- Morphology
  - Fusiform (80%): Circumferential aortic dilatation
    - Degenerative etiology (e.g., atherosclerosis)
  - Saccular (20%): Focal, eccentric outpouching
    - May have infectious or post traumatic etiology
  - Measure at largest diameter, outer to outer wall
  - True aneurysm involves all three vessel wall layers: Intima, media, adventitia

Radiographic Findings

- Radiography
  - Widened aortic shadow
    - Curvilinear calcifications outlining aorta
    - > 55% have sufficient mural calcification to be seen on plain radiography
  - Additional cross-sectional imaging to evaluate aneurysms suspected on plain radiographs

CT Findings

- NECT
  - Increased attenuation area within mural thrombus may indicate acute hemorrhage

DDx: Enlarged Aorta

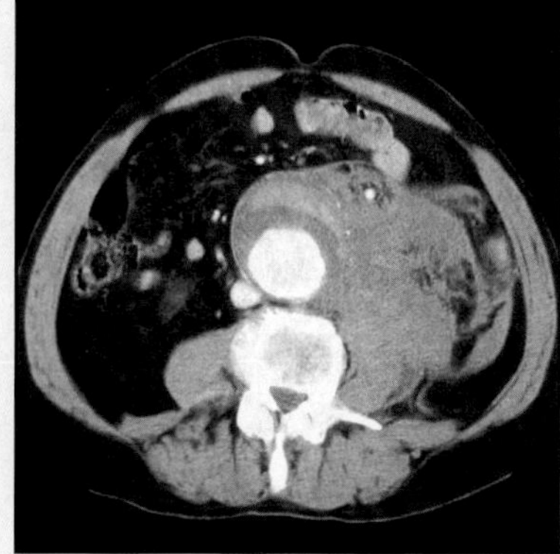

AAA Rupture

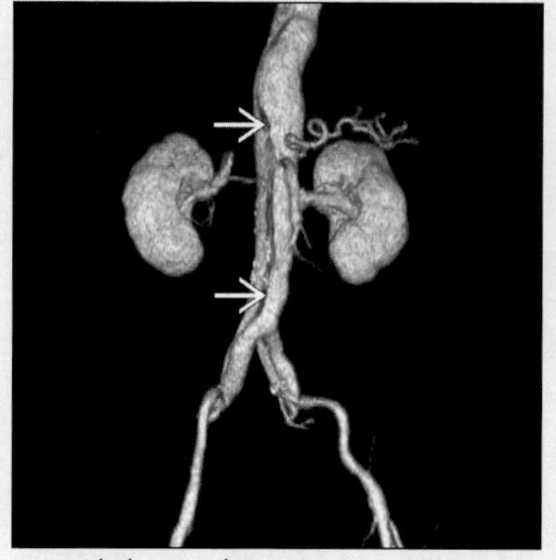

Abdominal Aortic Dissection

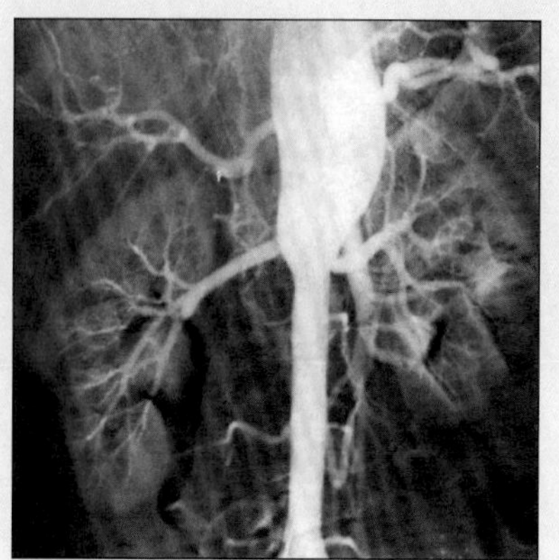

Takayasu Aortitis

ABDOMINAL AORTIC ANEURYSM

Key Facts

Terminology
- Abdominal aortic aneurysm (AAA)
  - Dilatation of aorta ≥ 1.5 times normal diameter
- AAA described by relationship to renal arteries

Imaging Findings
- Focal or diffuse aortic dilatation
- Most commonly involves infrarenal aorta
- Endoleak: Contrast outside graft but within aneurysm sac on delayed images
- CTA allows evaluation of aneurysm size and extent
  - Ideal for AAA repair planning, post-EVAR follow-up
  - Identifies endoleak; may categorize endoleak type
- US best method for following uncomplicated aneurysm; available, affordable and non-invasive
- Measure diameter perpendicular to long axis of aorta

Pathology
- Degenerative (atherosclerosis), traumatic, infectious or inflammatory etiologies for AAA
  - Atherosclerotic AAA most common

Clinical Issues
- Most AAAs asymptomatic and found incidentally
- Treatment
  - Close surveillance for aneurysms < 5 cm except under certain circumstances
  - EVAR for appropriate patient; needs suitable anatomy
  - Surgical open repair remains "gold standard"

Diagnostic Checklist
- Evaluate patient with popliteal aneurysm for AAA

  - Distinguishes periaortic hematoma from fibrosis
    - Periaortic fibrosis enhances on CECT
    - High attenuation, no enhancement to hematoma
  - Calcification within aortic walls
- CECT
  - Distinguishes residual lumen from mural thrombus
  - Leaking or ruptured aneurysm
    - Hematoma adjacent to or surrounding aneurysm; retroperitoneal hematoma; intraperitoneal blood
- CTA
  - Delineates branch vessel anatomy
    - Renal artery levels for pre-operative planning
    - Evaluate patency of inferior mesenteric artery
  - Define AAA neck, morphology, iliac involvement
- Surveillance after EVAR
  - Identifies graft fracture or component migration
  - Evaluates change in size of aneurysm sac
  - Identifies endoleak; may categorize endoleak type
  - NECT and CECT for pre and post-repair evaluation

MR Findings
- T1WI
  - Gadolinium enhanced MR useful in endoleak detection, characterization
  - High signal intensity lumen
  - Heterogeneous signal intensity mural thrombus
  - Calcium in aneurysm walls difficult to evaluate
  - Some limitations by artifacts from stents or coils
- MRA
  - Useful for anatomic evaluation pre-EVAR
    - TR MRA useful in characterizing post-EVAR endoleaks poorly seen on CECT

Ultrasonographic Findings
- Grayscale Ultrasound
  - Fusiform dilatation of aorta
  - Anechoic lumen; hyperechoic thrombus
- Color Doppler
  - Demonstrates residual lumen
  - Turbulent flow demonstrated within aneurysm sac
- Can monitor untreated aneurysm for growth
  - Limited by body habitus and overlying bowel gas

Angiographic Findings
- DSA
  - Opacifies only residual lumen; can underestimate true aneurysm size
    - May not demonstrate full extent of aneurysm due to intraluminal thrombus
  - Shows relationship of aneurysm to branch vessels (e.g., celiac, SMA, renal arteries)
    - Patency of IMA and lumbar arteries
    - Aneurysm extension into iliac arteries
  - Often performed for pre-EVAR embolization of internal iliac or inferior mesenteric artery
  - Less commonly used for pre-EVAR measurements

Imaging Recommendations
- Best imaging tool
  - CECT/CTA allows evaluation of aneurysm size, extent and residual lumen
    - Reformatted images evaluate branch vessels; aneurysm morphology
    - Ideal for EVAR planning and post-repair follow-up
- Protocol advice
  - CECT preferred to evaluate
    - Diameter and linear extent of aneurysm
    - Relationship of aneurysm to major aortic branches
    - Amount of intraluminal thrombus
    - Extravasation due to leak/rupture
    - Inflammatory changes in fat surrounding aorta
  - CECT for surgical or EVAR planning: 2.5 mm collimation with 1 mm overlap for reconstruction
    - Short axis diameter measurements of neck, AAA, iliac and femoral arteries
    - Centerline length measurements for selecting appropriate device
  - High index of suspicion for AAA rupture; unstable patient should undergo immediate repair
    - Stable patient should undergo CT then repair, if indicated
- MR C+ for iodine allergy, endoleak
- Ultrasound to detect, size and follow AAA
- Calcium best seen on lateral radiographs

ABDOMINAL AORTIC ANEURYSM

DIFFERENTIAL DIAGNOSIS

Aortic Dissection

- True and false lumens separated by intimal flap
- Aorta can be of normal diameter

Abdominal Aortic Trauma

- Normal or decreased aortic size and/or pseudoaneurysm
- Retroperitoneal hematoma or free peritoneal fluid

Aortitis (Vasculitis)

- Aortic wall thickening; may have narrowing or aneurysms, wall enhancement with contrast
- Atypical age and risks for atherosclerosis
- Etiologies include Takayasu, Behçet disease, radiation

PATHOLOGY

General Features

- Genetics: ~ 20% AAA incidence in 1st degree relatives
- Etiology
  - Degenerative, traumatic, infectious or inflammatory
  - Age-related deterioration of elastic media of aorta
    - Atherosclerosis causes medial fibrosis and atrophy
    - Weak media decreases wall strength; aorta dilates
  - Aortic wall infection causes mycotic aneurysm
    - Blood-borne microbes inoculate diseased atherosclerotic arterial wall
  - Traumatic aortic tear causes pseudoaneurysm
  - Dissection can lead to aneurysm formation
- Epidemiology: Incidence increased three-fold in last 3 decades
- Associated abnormalities
  - 50% of patients with popliteal aneurysm have AAA
  - 10-20% of AAA have iliac artery aneurysms

Gross Pathologic & Surgical Features

- Varied amounts of mural thrombus in aneurysms
  - Inner layer: Nonorganized thrombus
  - Outer layer: Loose cellular matrix

Microscopic Features

- Atherosclerotic degeneration: Thinned media, thickened intima
- Increased elastase, decreased medial and adventitial elastin

CLINICAL ISSUES

Presentation

- Most common signs/symptoms
  - Most asymptomatic and found incidentally
    - Widened aortic pulse or pulsatile abdominal mass
    - Found incidentally during unrelated imaging
  - First sign may be catastrophic rupture
    - Acute abdomen, back or flank pain
    - Rigid and/or distended abdomen
- Other signs/symptoms
  - Distal embolization and ischemia
  - Mass effect on adjacent structures
- Clinical Profile: Male, hypertensive, smoker, hypercholesterolemia, familial AAA history

Demographics

- Age: Older population (60-80 years)
- Gender: Male to female ratio 5:1
- Ethnicity: US prevalence: White male > black male; in females, equal prevalence

Natural History & Prognosis

- AAAs enlarge progressively at variable rate
- Elective AAA repair: Up to 5% mortality
  - Repair of ruptured aneurysm: Up to 80% mortality
- Mycotic and pseudoaneurysms: High rupture risk

Treatment

- Options, risks, complications: Rupture risk/year: 4-5 cm (1-3%), 5-7 cm (6-11%), > 7 cm (20%)
- Close surveillance for aneurysms < 5 cm, unless
  - Ruptured or symptomatic
  - Symptomatic and/or rapid growth (> 0.5 cm/6 mo)
    - Symptoms of back pain, thrombosis, occlusion
  - Atypical: Mycotic or saccular, or dissection present
- EVAR with stent-graft for appropriate patient
  - Poor surgical risk for open repair
  - All must have appropriate anatomy for EVAR repair
    - 60-80% AAAs qualify for EVAR
    - Adequate infrarenal "neck" for proximal graft fixation and seal
    - Circumferential thrombus, conical, dilated or excessively angled neck configuration problematic
    - Adequate distal fixation zone in iliac arteries
    - Need appropriate caliber access vessels (e.g., femoral and iliac arteries) for device introduction
    - Excessive access vessel tortuosity, calcification, occlusive disease problematic
  - May require adjunctive procedures (e.g., coil embolization, angioplasty, vascular conduit) pre-operatively or intraoperatively
  - 2° interventions post-EVAR may be necessary
    - Treatment of clinically significant endoleaks
    - Revascularization of limb thromboses
    - Conversion to open repair if endograft fails
- Surgical open AAA repair with graft placement
  - Remains "gold standard"
  - Durable procedure with good outcomes

DIAGNOSTIC CHECKLIST

Consider

- Evaluate patient with popliteal aneurysm for AAA

Image Interpretation Pearls

- Image AAA in multiple projections or > two planes
  - Measure perpendicular to aortic long axis

SELECTED REFERENCES

1. Blankensteijn JD et al: Two-year outcomes after conventional or endovascular repair of abdominal aortic aneurysms. N Engl J Med. 352(23):2398-405, 2005
2. LaRoy LL et al: Imaging of abdominal aortic aneurysms. AJR Am J Roentgenol. 152(4):785-92, 1989

IMAGE GALLERY

Typical

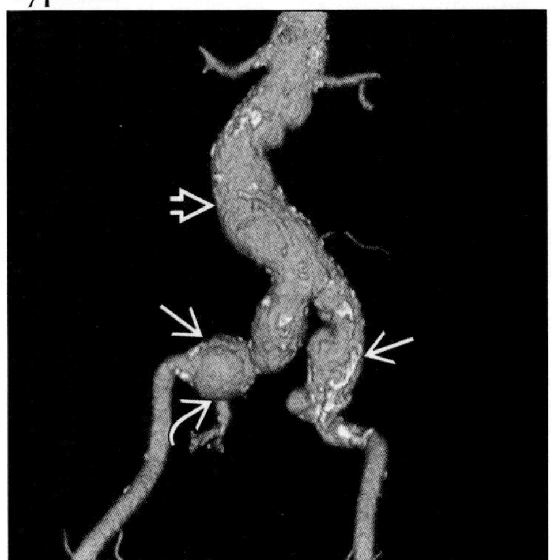

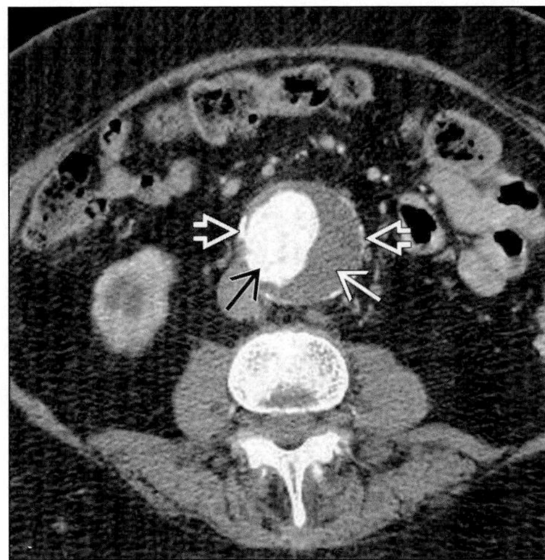

(Left) *3-D CTA shows abdominal aortic ➡ and bilateral common iliac artery ➡ aneurysms. There is appropriate anatomy for EVAR, but the common iliac artery aneurysms involve the iliac bifurcations ➡ and thus pre-operative internal iliac artery embolization is required.* ***(Right)*** *Axial CECT (same patient) shows the calcified wall ➡ of the AAA is significantly larger than the contrast-opacified lumen ➡ because of the extensive laminar thrombus ➡ within the aneurysm sac.*

Typical

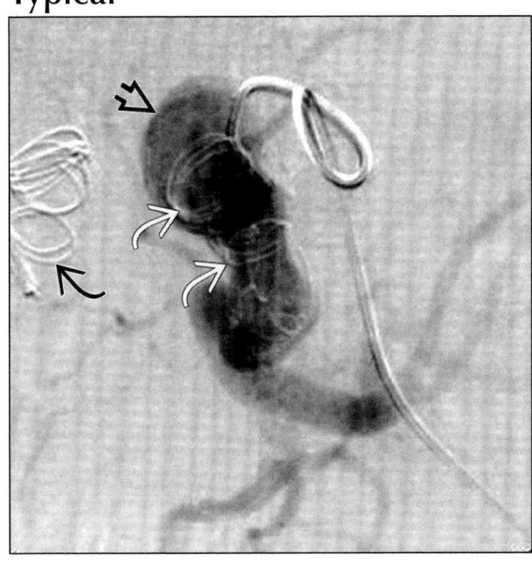

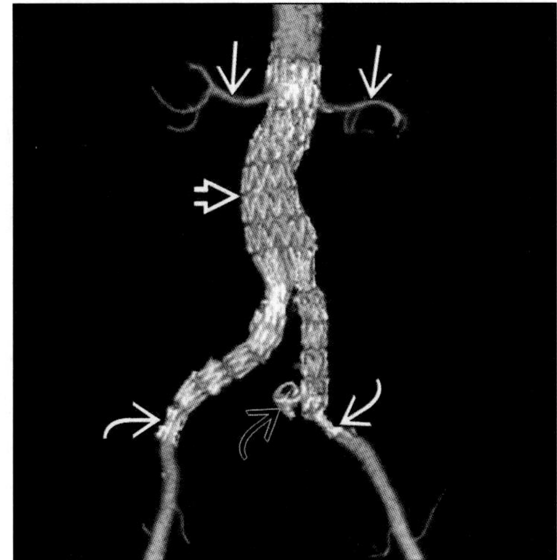

(Left) *Arteriogram shows coils ➡ in the left internal iliac artery ➡. Pre-operative embolization was necessary because the common iliac artery aneurysm involves the iliac bifurcation. Right internal iliac artery coils ➡ were also placed for this reason.* ***(Right)*** *3-D CTA after EVAR shows a stent graft ➡ extending from the renal ➡ to the external iliac ➡ arteries, excluding the AAA and bilateral common iliac artery aneurysms. Embolization coils are seen in the internal iliac artery ➡.*

Variant

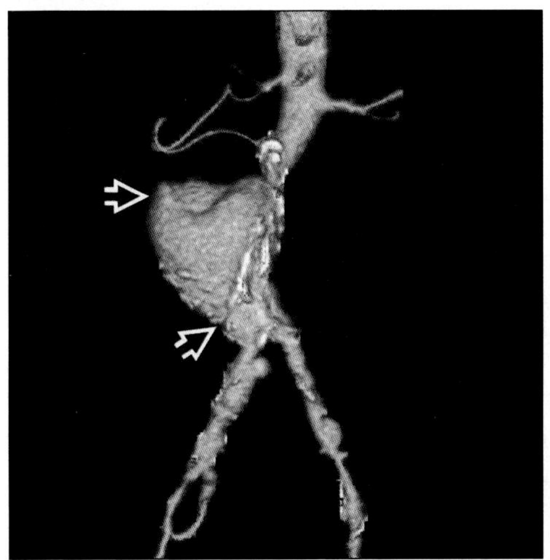

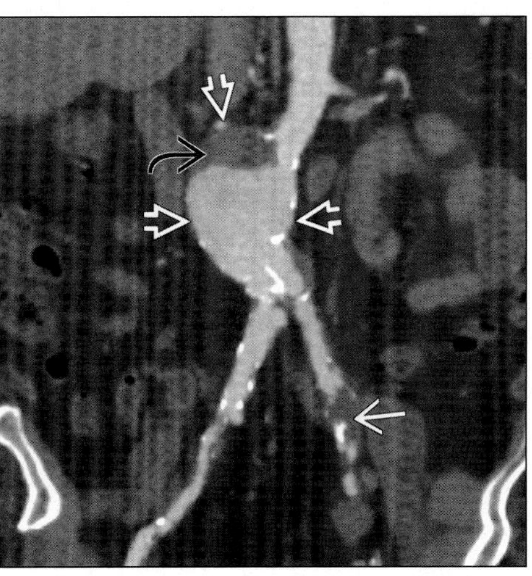

(Left) *3-D VR CTA shows an eccentric saccular AAA ➡. The unusual configuration suggests mycotic aneurysm. The diseased wall of an atherosclerotic aorta is susceptible to infection by blood-borne microbes.* ***(Right)*** *Coronal reformatted CTA (same patient) shows a thrombus ➡ superiorly in the aneurysm sac ➡. As a result, the volume rendered CTA underestimates the extent of the aneurysm. There is also thrombus ➡ in a severely diseased left common iliac artery.*

AAA WITH RUPTURE

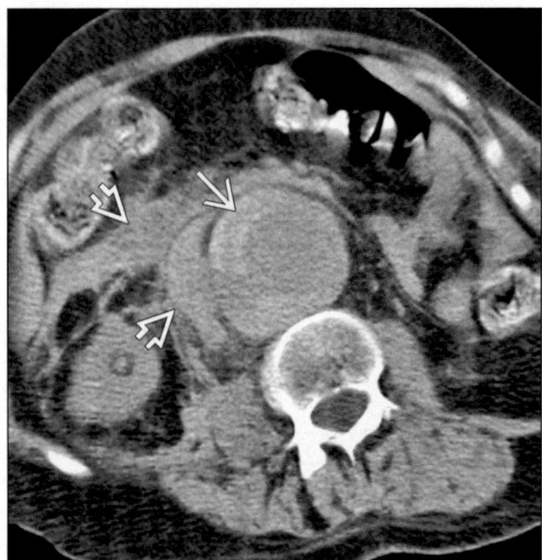

Axial NECT shows hyperattenuation ➔ in the wall of AAA associated with retroperitoneal hematoma ➲ consistent with rupture of the AAA.

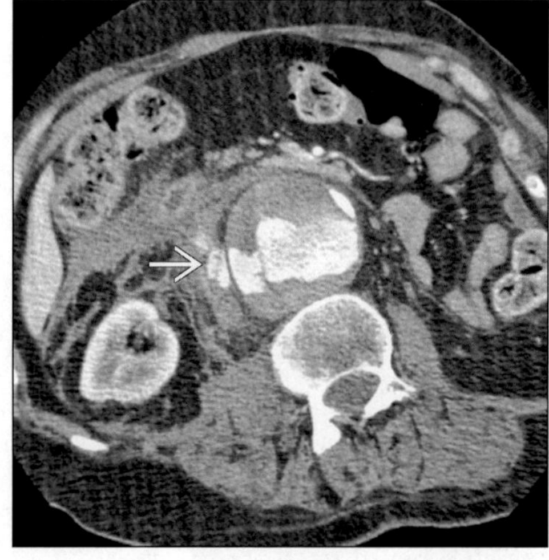

Axial CECT shows active extravasation ➔ of contrast material in the same patient as previous image.

TERMINOLOGY

Definitions

- Break in the wall of an abdominal aortic aneurysm (AAA)

IMAGING FINDINGS

General Features

- Best diagnostic clue
  - Acute: Crescentic collection of contrast in midst of extensive blood in mesentery and retroperitoneum
  - Chronic: Hematoma adjacent to aneurysm
- Morphology: In a chronic contained rupture (pseudoaneurysm) leak contained by retroperitoneal soft tissues
- Best imaging clue (CT)
  - Acute
    - Obscuration or anterior displacement of AAA by irregular high-density mass into one or both perirenal spaces, and less commonly pararenal spaces
  - Chronic
    - Noncontrast: Well-defined mass extending from aorta with attenuation value similar to or lower than that of native aorta
    - Post-contrast: Lumina of both aneurysm and pseudoaneurysm as well as their communication may be enhanced

CT Findings

- NECT
  - Acute
    - Large anteroposterior and transverse dimensions of aneurysm
    - Focal discontinuity in otherwise circumferential calcification
    - High attenuation crescents within mural thrombus
    - Retroperitoneal hematoma
    - Anterior displacement of kidney by hematoma
    - Enlargement or obscuration of psoas muscle
  - Chronic
    - Draping of posterior aspect of aorta over adjacent vertebral body
    - Erosion of adjacent vertebral body
- CECT

DDx: AAA with Rupture

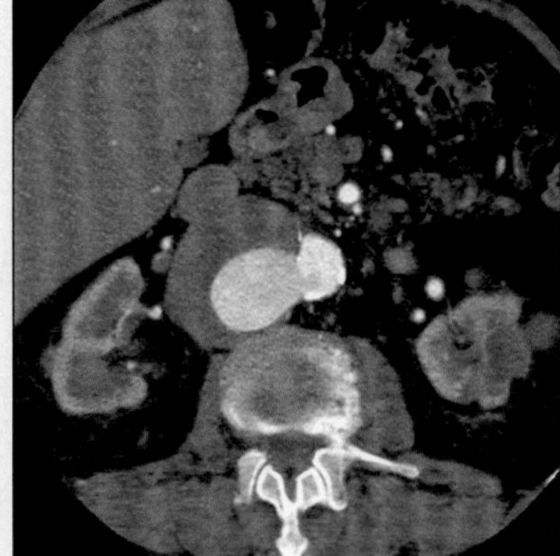

Mycotic Aneurysm

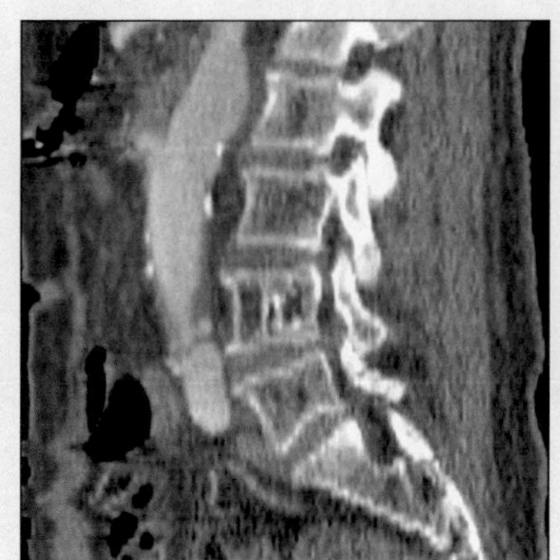

Aortoenteric Fistula

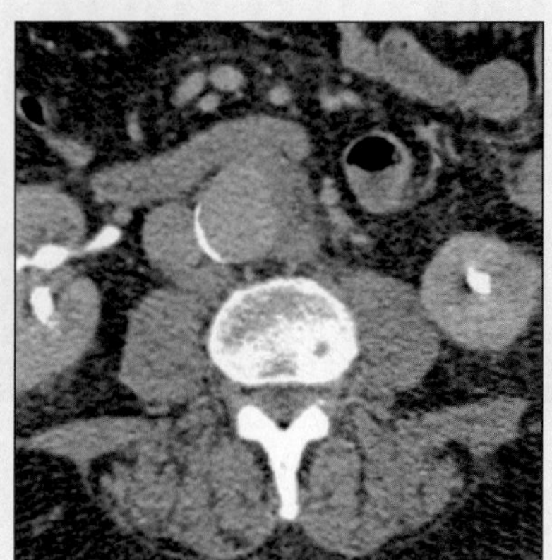

Inflammatory Aneurysm

AAA WITH RUPTURE

Key Facts

Terminology
- Break in the wall of an abdominal aortic aneurysm (AAA)

Imaging Findings
- Acute: Crescentic collection of contrast in midst of extensive blood in mesentery and retroperitoneum
- Chronic: Hematoma adjacent to aneurysm
- In chronic contained rupture (pseudoaneurysm) leak contained by retroperitoneal soft tissues

Top Differential Diagnoses
- Contained Rupture of Aorta
- Aortic Enteric Fistula
- Aortocaval Fistula
- Spontaneous Abdominal Hemorrhage Due to Anticoagulation
- Mycotic Aneurysm
- Inflammatory Aneurysm

Pathology
- Risk of rupture related to size of aneurysm

Clinical Issues
- Abrupt onset of severe central abdominal or back pain, occasionally localized to lower abdomen, groin, or testes
- Pulsatile, usually tender abdominal mass
- Operative mortality rates range from 50-75%
- Surgical repair must be performed as soon as diagnosis made

---

- Active extravasation of contrast material
- Focal pointing or pseudoaneurysm
- Findings predictive of impending rupture
  - Rapidly increasing aneurysm size
  - Relatively less thrombus in aneurysm
  - Relatively poorly calcified thrombus in aneurysm
  - Hyperattenuating crescents within mural thrombus

MR Findings
- MR has not been commonly used to evaluate patients suspected of having rupture of AAA
- Findings will be similar to CT findings, although calcifications will not be evident

Ultrasonographic Findings
- Grayscale Ultrasound
  - Findings of AAA, may demonstrate intraperitoneal fluid
  - Ultrasound not accurate for determining presence of rupture

Angiographic Findings
- Conventional: Active extravasation of contrast material

Imaging Recommendations
- Best imaging tool: CT
- Patients presenting with sudden onset of abdominal pain and pulsatile abdominal mass should be taken directly to surgery without any further diagnostic tests
- CT is imaging modality of choice for evaluation of suspected rupture

DIFFERENTIAL DIAGNOSIS

Contained Rupture of Aorta
- Rupture of aorta which is contained in retroperitoneum

Aortic Enteric Fistula
- Aortic aneurysm can rupture into GI tract causing massive GI bleeding
- Clinically may present with hypovolemia, abdominal pain, and pulsatile mass

Aortocaval Fistula
- Aortic aneurysm can rupture into inferior vena cava
- May present with cardiac decompensation, and a pulsatile mass in abdomen

Spontaneous Abdominal Hemorrhage Due to Anticoagulation
- Active contrast extravasation located within site of hematoma
- Iliopsoas or rectus sheath involvement common

Mycotic Aneurysm
- Usually at site of branching
- Focal saccular aneurysm with perianeurysmal soft tissue

Inflammatory Aneurysm
- Periaortic enhancing soft tissue

PATHOLOGY

General Features
- General path comments
  - Site of rupture
    - Posterolateral aorta with hemorrhage into retroperitoneum
    - Anterior or anterolateral aorta if rupture is intraperitoneal
- Etiology
  - Risk of rupture related to size of aneurysm
    - Size > 5 cm
    - Rapid increase in size: > 10 mm increase per year
  - Other risk factors for rupture
    - Hypertension, chronic obstructive pulmonary disease (COPD), bronchiectasis, smoking, family history of AAA
- Epidemiology
  - Approximate rates of rupture per year are
    - If less than 4 cm in diameter, 0%

- If 4-5 cm in diameter, 1-3%
- If 5-7 cm in diameter, 6-11%
- If greater than 7 cm in diameter, 20%

Gross Pathologic & Surgical Features

- Relatively less thrombus in aneurysm sac
- Relatively less calcified thrombus
- Chronic: Perianeurysmal organized hematoma

CLINICAL ISSUES

Presentation

- Abrupt onset of severe central abdominal or back pain, occasionally localized to lower abdomen, groin, or testes
- Pulsatile, usually tender abdominal mass
  - AAA may be palpable in 50%
  - May be absent due to hypotension
- Shock
  - Some patients with small, contained rupture may have stable blood pressure

Natural History & Prognosis

- Operative mortality rates range from 50-75%
- Death usually secondary to massive intra-operative hemorrhage and cardiac complications

Treatment

- Surgical repair must be performed as soon as diagnosis made
- Rapid and maintained replacement of blood loss with crystalloid and blood transfusion to correct hypotension
- Endovascular repair now being used in selected patients
  - Requires appropriate anatomy
  - Often involves aorto-uni-iliac endograft

SELECTED REFERENCES

1. Acosta S et al: Predictors for outcome after open and endovascular repair of ruptured abdominal aortic aneurysms. Eur J Vasc Endovasc Surg. 33(3):277-84, 2007
2. Bounoua F et al: Ruptured abdominal aortic aneurysm: does trauma center designation affect outcome? Ann Vasc Surg. 21(2):133-6, 2007
3. Champagne BJ et al: Incidence of colonic ischemia after repair of ruptured abdominal aortic aneurysm with endograft. J Am Coll Surg. 204(4):597-602, 2007
4. Dillon M et al: Endovascular treatment for ruptured abdominal aortic aneurysm. Cochrane Database Syst Rev. (1):CD005261, 2007
5. Hames H et al: The effect of patient transfer on outcomes after rupture of an abdominal aortic aneurysm. Can J Surg. 50(1):43-7, 2007
6. Holt PJ et al: Epidemiological study of the relationship between volume and outcome after abdominal aortic aneurysm surgery in the UK from 2000 to 2005. Br J Surg. 94(4):441-8, 2007
7. Holt PJ et al: Meta-analysis and systematic review of the relationship between volume and outcome in abdominal aortic aneurysm surgery. Br J Surg. 94(4):395-403, 2007
8. Klonaris C et al: Endovascular repair of late abdominal aortic aneurysm rupture owing to mixed-type endoleak following endovascular abdominal aortic aneurysm repair. Vascular. 15(3):167-71, 2007
9. Lederle FA et al: Systematic review: repair of unruptured abdominal aortic aneurysm. Ann Intern Med. 146(10):735-41, 2007
10. McPhee JT et al: The impact of gender on presentation, therapy, and mortality of abdominal aortic aneurysm in the United States, 2001-2004. J Vasc Surg. 45(5):891-9, 2007
11. McPhee JT et al: The impact of gender on presentation, therapy, and mortality of abdominal aortic aneurysm in the United States, 2001-2004. J Vasc Surg. 45(5):891-9, 2007
12. Mofidi R et al: Influence of sex on expansion rate of abdominal aortic aneurysms. Br J Surg. 94(3):310-4, 2007
13. Nguyen AT et al: Transperitoneal approach should be considered for suspected ruptured abdominal aortic aneurysms. Ann Vasc Surg. 21(2):129-32, 2007
14. Peterson BG et al: Five-year report of a multicenter controlled clinical trial of open versus endovascular treatment of abdominal aortic aneurysms. J Vasc Surg. 45(5):885-90, 2007
15. Rakita D et al: Spectrum of CT findings in rupture and impending rupture of abdominal aortic aneurysms. Radiographics. 27(2):497-507, 2007
16. Rakita D et al: Spectrum of CT findings in rupture and impending rupture of abdominal aortic aneurysms. Radiographics. 27(2):497-507, 2007
17. Schwartz SA et al: CT findings of rupture, impending rupture, and contained rupture of abdominal aortic aneurysms. AJR Am J Roentgenol. 188(1):W57-62, 2007
18. Tefera G et al: Effectiveness of intensive medical therapy in type B aortic dissection: A single-center experience. J Vasc Surg. 45(6):1114-9, 2007
19. Acosta S et al: Increasing incidence of ruptured abdominal aortic aneurysm: a population-based study. J Vasc Surg. 44(2):237-43, 2006
20. Acosta S et al: The Hardman index in patients operated on for ruptured abdominal aortic aneurysm: A systematic review. J Vasc Surg. 44(5):949-54, 2006
21. Berguer R et al: Refinements in mathematical models to predict aneurysm growth and rupture. Ann N Y Acad Sci. 1085:110-6, 2006
22. Dalainas I et al: Endovascular techniques for the treatment of ruptured abdominal aortic aneurysms: 7-year intention-to-treat results. World J Surg. 30(10):1809-14; discussion 1815-6, 2006
23. Salhab M et al: Impact of delay on survival in patients with ruptured abdominal aortic aneurysm. Vascular. 14(1):38-42, 2006
24. Vande Geest JP et al: Gender-related differences in the tensile strength of abdominal aortic aneurysm. Ann N Y Acad Sci. 1085:400-2, 2006
25. Visser JJ et al: Endovascular repair versus open surgery in patients with ruptured abdominal aortic aneurysms: clinical outcomes with 1-year follow-up. J Vasc Surg. 44(6):1148-55, 2006
26. Hartnell GG: Imaging of aortic aneurysms and dissection: CT and MRI. J Thorac Imaging. 16(1):35-46, 2001
27. Hallett JW Jr: Management of abdominal aortic aneurysms. Mayo Clin Proc. 75(4):395-9, 2000
28. Yeung BK et al: Surgical management of abdominal aortic aneurysm. Vasc Med. 5(3):187-93, 2000

AAA WITH RUPTURE

IMAGE GALLERY

Typical

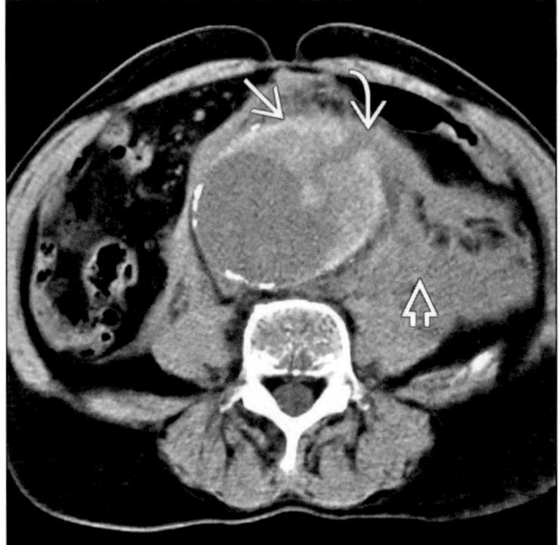

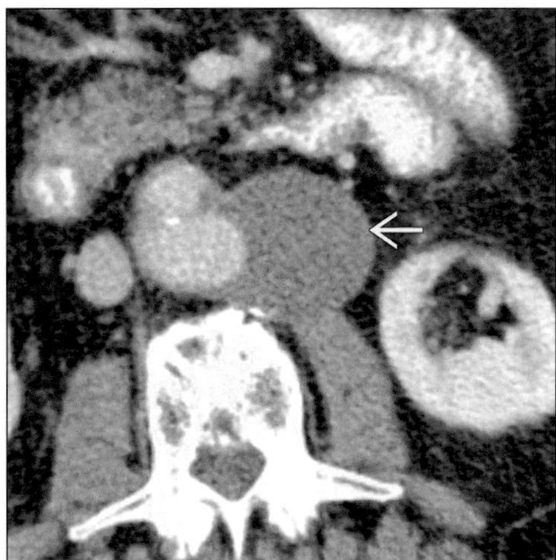

(Left) *Axial NECT shows intramural high attenuation in AAA with retroperitoneal hematoma consistent with ruptured AAA. The site of rupture is seen as discontinuity in the wall the AAA.* ***(Right)*** *Axial CECT shows AAA with contained chronic rupture. The eccentric enlargement with draping of the left psoas muscle suggests contained rupture.*

Typical

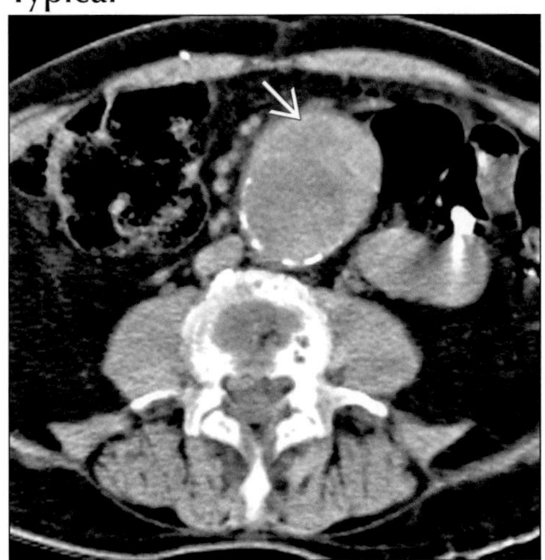

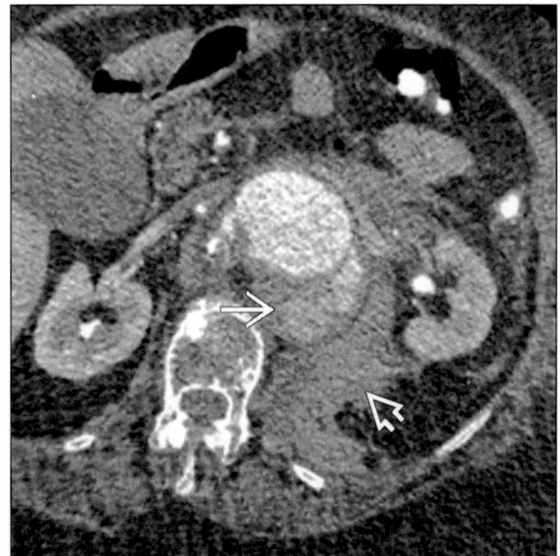

(Left) *Axial NECT shows intramural high attenuation with no retroperitoneal hematoma. This suggests either an impending rupture or an acute contained rupture.* ***(Right)*** *Axial CECT shows active contrast extravasation and retroperitoneal hematoma in a patient with AAA suggesting rupture of the AAA.*

Typical

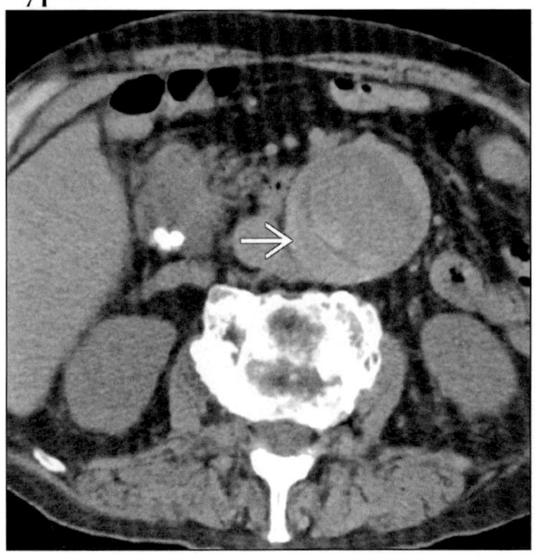

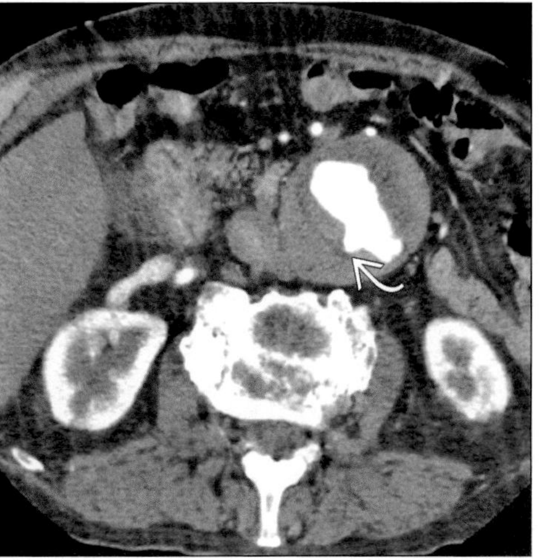

(Left) *Axial NECT shows intramural high attenuation in a patient with AAA suggesting an impending rupture or an acute contained rupture of AAA.* ***(Right)*** *Axial CECT in the same patient as previous image, shows focal pointing of the contrast-enhanced lumen of the AAA which is usually the site of rupture.*

ENDOLEAK POST AAA REPAIR

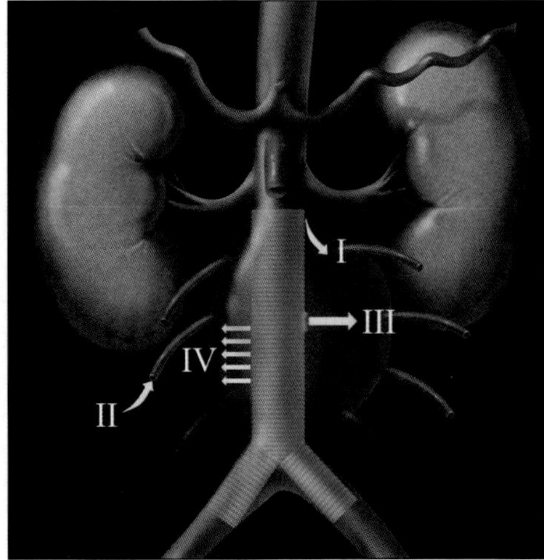

Graphic demonstration of various types of endoleaks.

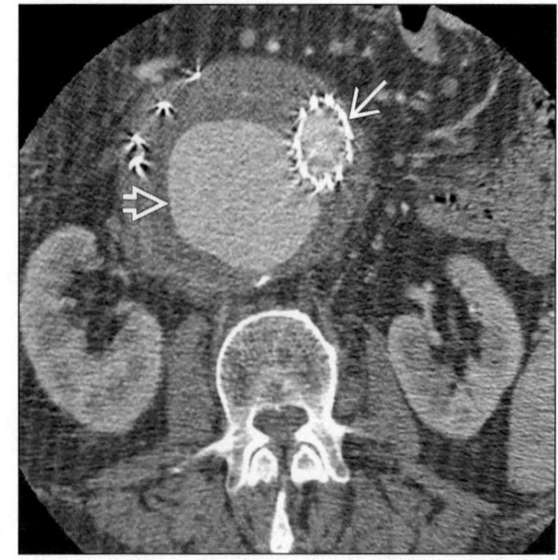

Axial CECT shows contrast material ⇨ in the aneurysm sac outside the endovascular stent ➔ consistent with an endoleak.

TERMINOLOGY

Definitions

- Persistent perfusion of aneurysmal sac after endovascular aneurysm repair (EVAR)
- Primary endoleak: Endoleak appearing during first 30 days after stent graft placement
- Secondary endoleak: Endoleak occurring after 30 days of stent graft implantation

IMAGING FINDINGS

General Features

- Best diagnostic clue
  - Leakage of contrast media outside endograft into aneurysm sac
    - Broad-based leakage near prosthesis often result of malposition of attachment of stent graft
    - Ventral leakage without direct communication to stent graft often supplied by inferior mesenteric artery (IMA)
    - Leakage at dorsolateral aneurysm sac often supplied by lumbar arteries
    - Large circumferential perigraft leakages often indicate dislocation of stent graft or prosthesis that is too short

CT Findings

- CT widely available, easily accessible, and well-tolerated by patients
- Reproducibility of CT measurements is excellent
- Delayed CT scan important to maximize sensitivity for detecting endoleaks, but increases radiation dose
- CT angiography shown to be superior to intraarterial DSA for detecting endoleaks
- CT protocol
  - Pre-contrast CT as comparison for detecting small changes in contrast associated with endoleak
  - CT angiography sequence during arterial phase of contrast-enhancement
  - Delayed CT angiography sequence performed 1-2 min following contrast administration to detect late endoleak
  - CT excellent for demonstrating relationship of stent graft material to branch vessels
  - Multiplanar reformations key for detecting separated modular components and type 1 endoleaks

DDx: Endoleak

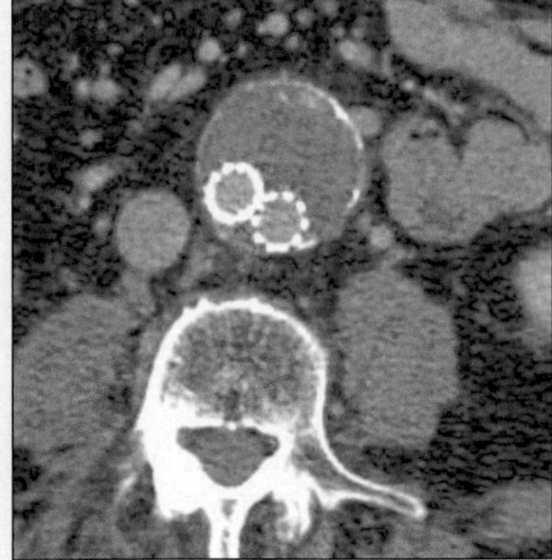

Calcified Mural Thrombus

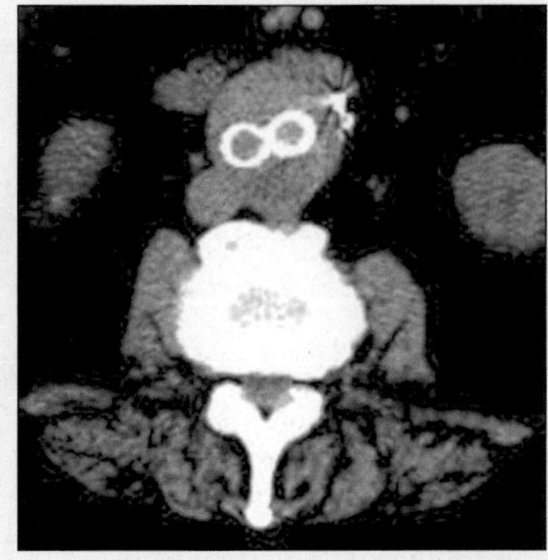

Hyperattenuating Thrombus

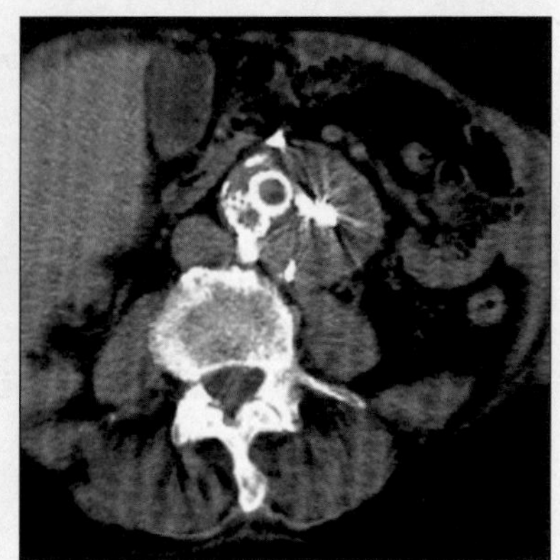

Coils/Glue Following Embolization

ENDOLEAK POST AAA REPAIR

Key Facts

Terminology
- Persistent perfusion of aneurysmal sac after endovascular aneurysm repair (EVAR)

Imaging Findings
- Leakage of contrast media outside endograft into aneurysm sac
- CT angiography is shown to be superior to intraarterial DSA for detecting endoleaks
- Delayed CT angiography sequence performed 1-2 min following contrast administration to detect late endoleak
- MR only in Nitinol based stent grafts
- MR greater sensitivity than CT for slow flow type II endoleaks
- Best surveillance method is CTA or MRA with aneurysm volume measurements

Top Differential Diagnoses
- Type I Endoleak (Graft-Related Endoleak)
- Type II Endoleak (Nongraft-Related Endoleak)
- Type III Endoleak (Device Failure)
- Type IV Endoleak (Graft Porosity)
- Type V Endotension

Pathology
- Epidemiology: Eurostar registry: Endoleaks occur in 2.4-45.5% of patients following endovascular repair of thoracic and abdominal aortic aneurysms

Clinical Issues
- Persistence of types I and III endoleak beyond 3-6 months increases the risk of aneurysm rupture
- Role of type II endoleaks relative to aortic rupture is controversial

MR Findings
- MR protocol
  - MR only in Nitinol based stent grafts
  - MR greater sensitivity than CT for slow flow type II endoleaks
  - Blood pool contrast agents useful for detecting small endoleaks
  - Pre- and post-contrast, fat-suppressed T1-weighted imaging to evaluate subtle contrast-enhancement
  - 3-D gradient recalled echo TR MRA sequence before, during, 2x following injection of gadolinium
  - Special attention required to minimize metal artifacts associated with the prosthesis, including short TE and large (45-90 degree) flip angle
  - Steady-state free procession (SSFP) imaging (white blood imaging) may differentiate endoleak from endotension

Angiographic Findings
- Conventional
  - Role of angiography primarily to characterize and treat endoleaks
  - Superior to CT for detection of outflow vessels in cases of type II endoleak
  - Aortography by placing a pigtail catheter initially above, and subsequently inside stent graft
  - Long acquisitions to detect slow flow endoleaks
  - Selective catheterization of IMA, lumbar, internal iliac arteries to detect type II endoleak

Imaging Recommendations
- Best surveillance method is CTA or MRA with aneurysm volume measurements
- CT provides mainstay for pre-operative evaluation and post-operative follow-up in aortic stent graft patients
- MRA useful in specific situations
  - Allergic reactions to iodine
  - Patients with life expectancy of more than 20 years due to radiation dose associated with serial follow-up studies
  - MRA more sensitive than CTA for endoleak (94% vs. 50%)
  - Nitinol grafts
  - MR not recommended in stainless steel grafts (Zenith-Cook)

DIFFERENTIAL DIAGNOSIS

Type I Endoleak (Graft-Related Endoleak)
- Inadequate seal at proximal or distal landing zones of graft
  - Type 1A: Proximal
  - Type 1B: Distal
  - Type 1C: Iliac occluder (aorto-uni-iliac EVAR)

Type II Endoleak (Nongraft-Related Endoleak)
- Persistent collateral blood pertusing aneurysm sac by flowing retrograde from
  - Lumbar arteries, inferior mesenteric arteries, other collateral vessels
    - Type 2A: Single vessel (simple)
    - Type 2B: Two or more vessels creating a circuit (complex)
- Complex architecture, often compared to arteriovenous malformation (sac being nidus fed by inflow and outflow vessels)

Type III Endoleak (Device Failure)
- Leakage of contrast through defect in graft fabric
- Leakage between segments of modular graft
- Mechanical failure of graft
  - Type 3A: Junctional separation of modular devices
  - Type 3B: Endograft fracture or holes

Type IV Endoleak (Graft Porosity)
- Minor blush of contrast through graft material
- Seen in early phase of commercial development of stent grafts, fabric leakage now rarely seen

Type V Endotension
- Continued aneurysm expansion in absence of confirmed endoleak

ENDOLEAK POST AAA REPAIR

PATHOLOGY

General Features

- General path comments: Endoleak results in "endotension", persistent elevated systemic pressures in aneurysm sac
- Etiology: Laplace law indicates that endotension (sac pressure) rather than flow causes expansion and rupture of aneurysm sac
- Epidemiology: Eurostar registry: Endoleaks occur in 2.4-45.5% of patients following endovascular repair of thoracic and abdominal aortic aneurysms

CLINICAL ISSUES

Presentation

- Usually asymptomatic
- Expanding aneurysm sac following endograft repair of aneurysm

Natural History & Prognosis

- High risk of endoleaks in
  - Complex anatomy of neck of aneurysm: Short, angulated, ulcerated, trapezoidal, and thrombus containing necks - increased risk of type 1 proximal endoleak
  - Tortuous, dilated and irregular iliac arteries - increased risk of type I distal endoleak
  - Patent IMA and branch vessels at time of stent graft placement - increased risk of type II endoleak
  - If patients on anticoagulation develop endoleak, endoleaks tend to persist in spite of treatment
- Persistence of types I and III endoleak beyond 3-6 months increases risk of aneurysm rupture
- Role of type II endoleaks relative to aortic rupture controversial

Treatment

- Type I endoleak
  - Extension of stent graft or cuff
  - Bare stent placement
  - Embolization
  - Surgery
- Type II endoleak
  - Embolization of inflow/outflow vessels or nidus; must thrombose central nidus; treat like AVM
    - Trans-arterial approach through SMA
    - Translumbar approach into sac
  - Embolic agents: Coils, cyanol-acrylate glue, thrombin, onyx
  - Open or laparoscopic surgical ligation of all inflow and outflow vessels
- Type III endoleak
  - Stent graft placement to cover separated modular components or hole in graft

DIAGNOSTIC CHECKLIST

Consider

- Enlarging sac after aortic endograft placement
- Delayed endoleaks possible with stent migration
- Treatment differs with type of endoleak

Image Interpretation Pearls

- Look for endoleak on delayed images
- Calcified thrombus or high density materials may mimic endoleak, non-contrast CT useful to exclude

SELECTED REFERENCES

1. Hiramoto JS et al: Long-term outcome and reintervention after endovascular abdominal aortic aneurysm repair using the Zenith stent graft. J Vasc Surg. 45(3):461-5; discussion 465-6, 2007
2. Hobo R et al: Influence of severe infrarenal aortic neck angulation on complications at the proximal neck following endovascular AAA repair: a EUROSTAR study. J Endovasc Ther. 14(1):1-11, 2007
3. Iyer VS et al: Reversible endotension associated with excessive warfarin anticoagulation. J Vasc Surg. 45(3):600-2, 2007
4. Leurs LJ et al: Long-term results of endovascular abdominal aortic aneurysm treatment with the first generation of commercially available stent grafts. Arch Surg. 142(1):33-41; discussion 42, 2007
5. Peterson BG et al: Five-year report of a multicenter controlled clinical trial of open versus endovascular treatment of abdominal aortic aneurysms. J Vasc Surg. 45(5):885-90, 2007
6. Springer F et al: Detecting endoleaks after endovascular AAA repair with a minimally invasive, implantable, telemetric pressure sensor: an in vitro study. Eur Radiol. 2007
7. Golzarian J et al: Endoleakage after endovascular treatment of abdominal aortic aneurysms: Diagnosis, significance and treatment. Eur Radiol. 16(12):2849-57, 2006
8. Choke E et al: Endoleak after endovascular aneurysm repair: current concepts. J Cardiovasc Surg (Torino). 45(4):349-66, 2004
9. Stavropoulos SW et al: Imaging modalities for the detection and management of endoleaks. Semin Vasc Surg. 17(2):154-60, 2004
10. Tonnessen BH et al: Late problems at the proximal aortic neck: migration and dilation. Semin Vasc Surg. 17(4):288-93, 2004
11. van Sambeek MR et al: Sac enlargement without endoleak: when and how to convert and technical considerations. Semin Vasc Surg. 17(4):284-7, 2004
12. Baum RA et al: Endoleaks after endovascular repair of abdominal aortic aneurysms. J Vasc Interv Radiol. 14(9 Pt 1):1111-7, 2003
13. Buth J et al: Endoleaks during follow-up after endovascular repair of abdominal aortic aneurysm. Are they all dangerous? J Cardiovasc Surg (Torino). 44(4):559-66, 2003
14. Thurnher S et al: Imaging of aortic stent-grafts and endoleaks. Radiol Clin North Am. 40(4):799-833, 2002
15. Baum RA et al: Diagnosis and management of type 2 endoleaks after endovascular aneurysm repair. Tech Vasc Interv Radiol. 4(4):222-6, 2001
16. Haulon S et al: Prospective evaluation of magnetic resonance imaging after endovascular treatment of infrarenal aortic aneurysms. Eur J Vasc Endovasc Surg. 22(1):62-9, 2001
17. Fillinger MF: Postoperative imaging after endovascular AAA repair. Semin Vasc Surg. 12(4):327-38, 1999
18. Gilling-Smith G et al: Endotension after endovascular aneurysm repair: definition, classification, and strategies for surveillance and intervention. J Endovasc Surg. 6(4):305-7, 1999

ENDOLEAK POST AAA REPAIR

IMAGE GALLERY

Typical

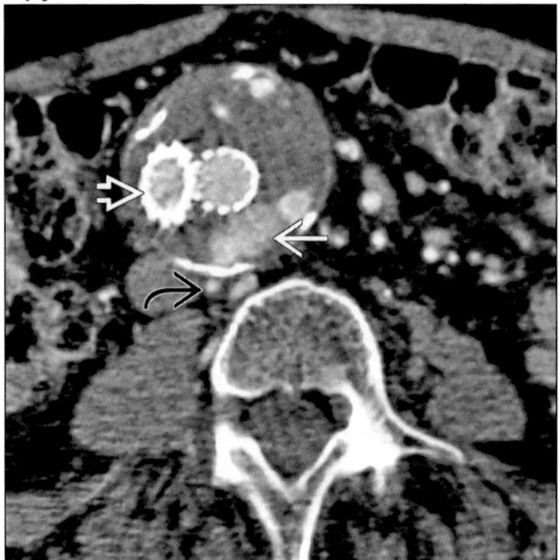

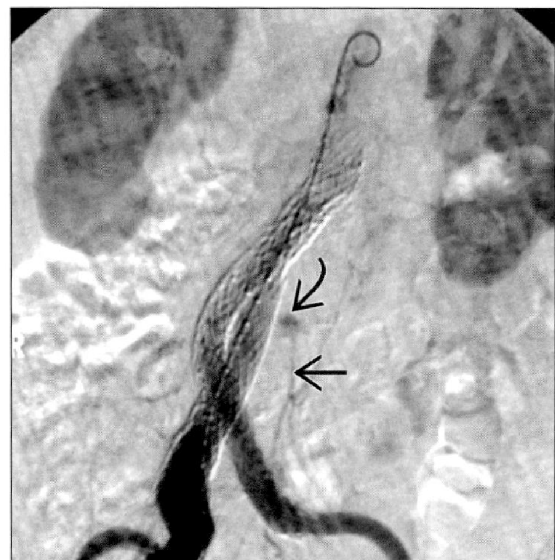

(Left) *Axial CECT shows type II endoleak following endovascular stent graft placement. The endoleak is contributed by the inferior mesenteric artery and the lumbar artery.* ***(Right)*** *Anteroposterior abdominal aortogram following endograft placement shows a type II endoleak contributed by retrograde flow in the inferior mesenteric artery.*

Typical

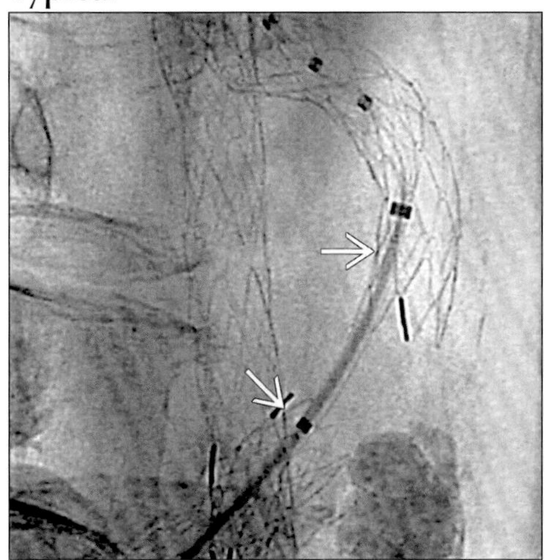

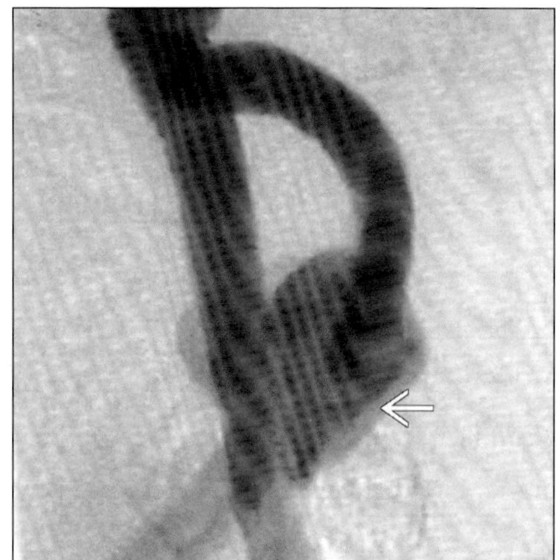

(Left) *Oblique radiograph shows separation of the stent graft components following endovascular repair of AAA.* ***(Right)*** *Oblique catheter angiography in the same patient as previous image, shows gross type III endoleak due to separation of the stent graft components. Treatment of this endoleak requires placement of a bridging stent-graft.*

Typical

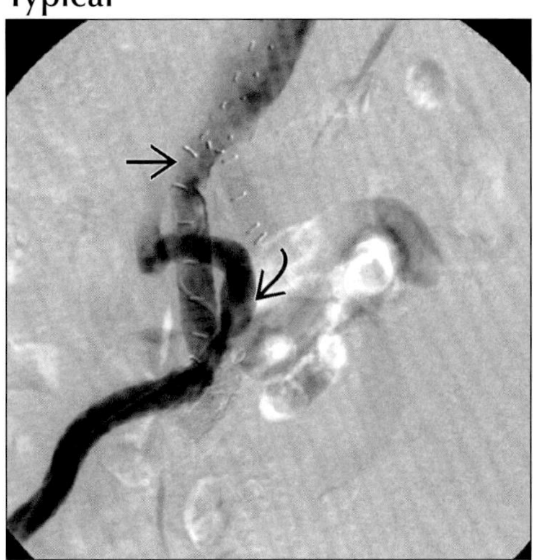

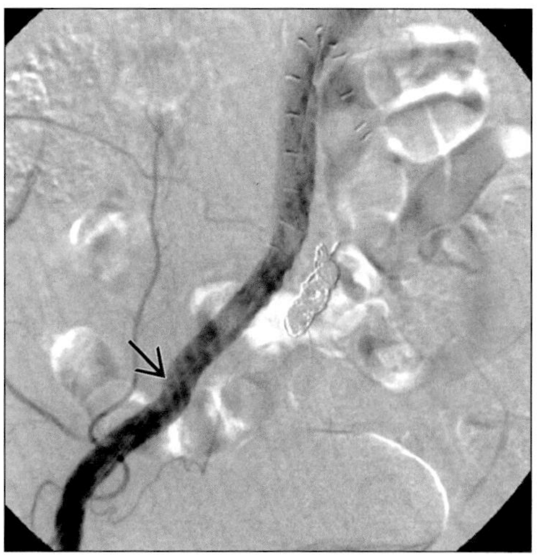

(Left) *Anteroposterior angiography demonstrates a type I endoleak at the distal attachment site of the stent graft.* ***(Right)*** *Anteroposterior angiography following repair of type I distal endoleak by extending the stent graft into the external iliac artery.*

AORTIC ENTERIC FISTULA

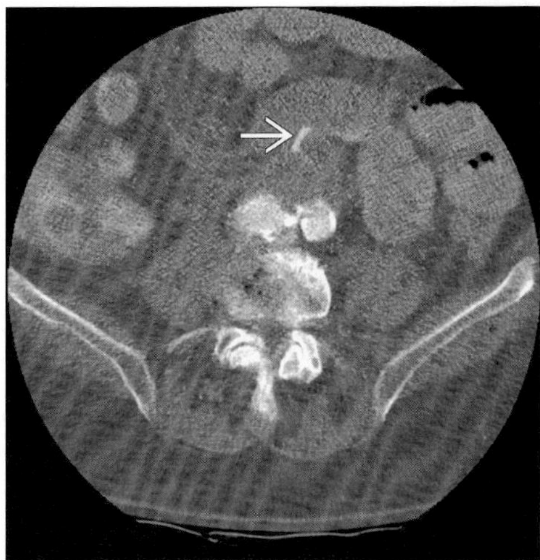

Axial CECT shows active extravasation ➔ of contrast material from the aneurysm sac into the bowel.

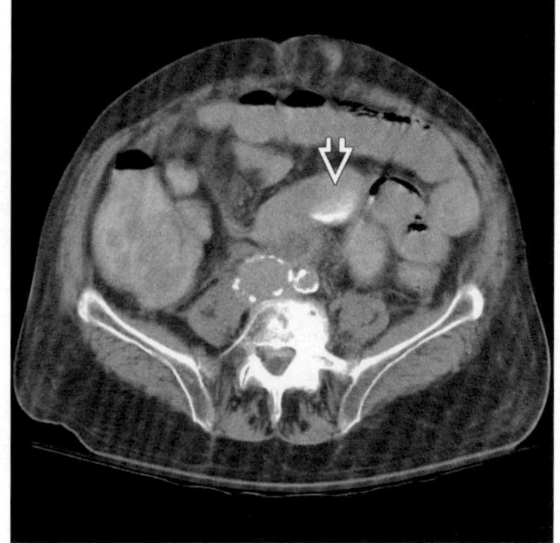

Axial CECT performed 3 minutes after the arterial phase shows increased amount of contrast material ➔ in the small bowel consistent with the diagnosis of aortoenteric fistula.

TERMINOLOGY

Abbreviations and Synonyms

- Aortic enteric fistula (AEF)

Definitions

- Abnormal communication between aorta & gastrointestinal (GI) tract
  - Primary aortoenteric fistula: Communication between native aorta or aortic aneurysm with GI tract
  - Secondary aortoenteric fistula: Communication between the aorta and GI tract following surgical or endovascular repair with prosthetic implants

IMAGING FINDINGS

General Features

- Best diagnostic clue: Inflammatory stranding and gas between abdominal aorta and third part of duodenum following aneurysm repair
- Location
  - Primary AEF: Duodenum (54%), esophagus (28%), small or large bowel (15%), stomach (2%)
  - Secondary AEF: Duodenum (73%), small bowel (19%), colon (6%), others (2%)
- Endoscopy Findings
  - Sensitivity 25-80%
  - Active bleeding
  - Ulcer
  - Fistulous tract
  - Visible graft material

Radiographic Findings

- Fluoroscopic-guided barium studies
  - Compression or displacement of third portion of duodenum by an extrinsic mass
  - Contrast extravasation: Wall of abdominal aorta outlined by extraluminal contrast medium tracking along graft into periaortic space (rare)

CT Findings

- Ectopic gas: Microbubble of gas adjacent to and/or in the aortic graft; may suggest perigraft infection
- Focal bowel wall thickening > 5 mm
- Perigraft soft tissue thickening > 5 mm (> 20 HU)
- Pseudoaneurysm formation

DDx: Air in the Sac

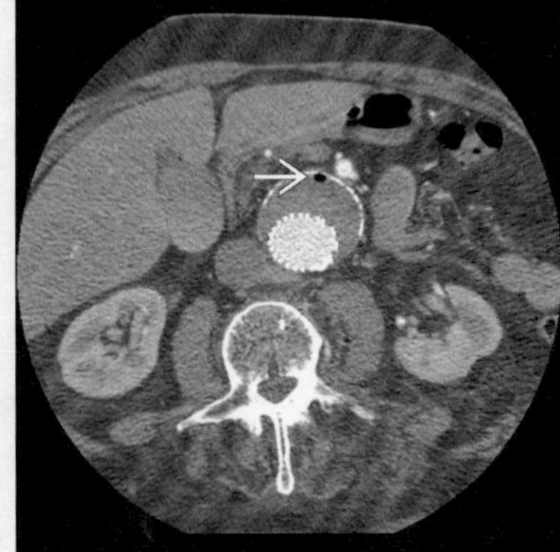

Post-Intervention

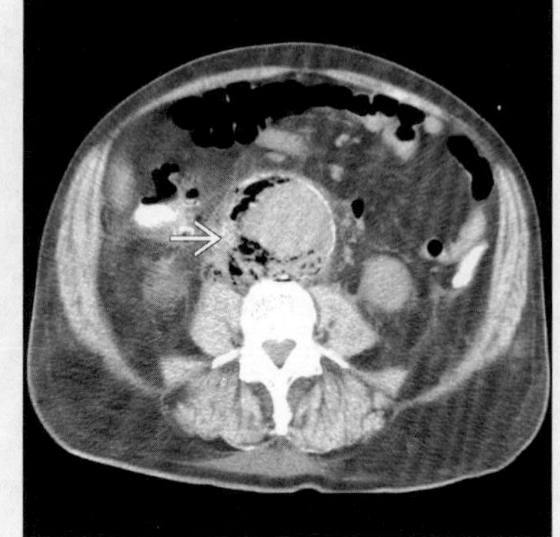

Infection with Clostridia

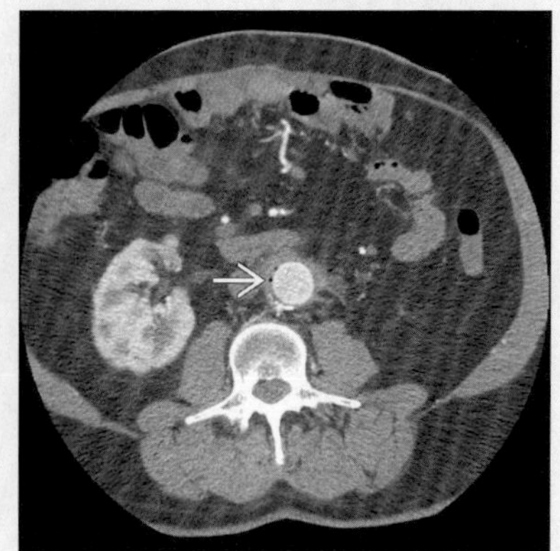

Aortoenteric Fistula

AORTIC ENTERIC FISTULA

Key Facts

Terminology

- Primary aortoenteric fistula: Communication between native aorta or aortic aneurysm with GI tract
- Secondary aortoenteric fistula: Communication between aorta and GI tract following surgical or endovascular repair with prosthetic implants

Imaging Findings

- Best diagnostic clue: Inflammatory stranding and gas between abdominal aorta and third part of duodenum following aneurysm repair
- Primary AEF: Duodenum (54%), esophagus (28%), small or large bowel (15%), stomach (2%)
- Secondary AEF: Duodenum (73%), small bowel (19%), colon (6%), others (2%)
- Best imaging tool: CT: 94% sensitive & 85% specific

Top Differential Diagnoses

- Periaortitis
- Post-Operation
- Post-Endovascular Stent
- Post-Intervention

Pathology

- Aortic reconstructive surgery (most common)
- Associated abnormalities: Perigraft infection

Clinical Issues

- "Herald" GI bleeding, followed by hours, days or weeks by catastrophic hemorrhage (most common)

Diagnostic Checklist

- Perigraft infection ↑ suspicion of fistula

- Disruption of aneurysmal wrap
- ↑ Soft tissue between graft and aneurysmal wrap
- Contrast in pseudoaneurysm (arterial phase)
- Increased attenuation of intestinal lumen contents (arterial phase); decreased attenuation (delayed phase)

Nuclear Medicine Findings

- Tagged RBC within abdominal aorta & enters bowel
- Indium labeled white cell scan shows increased uptake suggesting associated infection

Angiographic Findings

- Active extravasation of contrast material from aorta into intestine
- Pseudoaneurysm or nipple-like projection at site of fistula

Imaging Recommendations

- Best imaging tool: CT: 94% sensitive & 85% specific
- Protocol advice: Noncontrast CT, followed by CECT during arterial phase and delayed phase; no positive oral contrast material

DIFFERENTIAL DIAGNOSIS

Periaortitis

- Also known as inflammatory perianeurysmal fibrosis
- Soft tissue attenuation encasing aorta, inferior vena cava and other structures

Retroperitoneal Fibrosis

- Mantle of soft tissue enveloping aorta, IVC, ureters

Post-Operation

- "Normal" scarring with fluid between graft & aorta

Post-Endovascular Stent

- Endoleak: Blood flow outside stent, but within an aneurysm sac or adjacent vascular segment
- May have couple of gas bubbles between stent-graft and aortic wall soon after placement

Post-Intervention

- May have gas bubbles in sac following percutaneous puncture during endoleak embolization
- Other signs of intervention such as coils, access route inflammatory changes

PATHOLOGY

General Features

- Etiology
  - Primary
    - Abdominal aortic aneurysms
    - Infectious aortitis
    - Penetrating peptic ulcer
    - Tumor invasion
    - Radiation therapy
  - Secondary
    - Aortic reconstructive surgery (most common)
  - Pathogenesis
    - Third portion of duodenum is fixed & apposed to anterior wall of aortic aneurysm → pressure necrosis
    - Surgery → blood supply compromised
    - Pseudoaneurysm formation with erosion
    - Graft & suture line infection → anastomotic breakdown
    - Intraoperative injury to adjacent bowel
- Epidemiology
  - Incidence: 0.6-1.5% after aortic surgery
  - Onset after surgery: 3 years; 21 days up to 14 years
- Associated abnormalities: Perigraft infection

CLINICAL ISSUES

Presentation

- Most common signs/symptoms
  - "Herald" GI bleeding, followed by hours, days or weeks by catastrophic hemorrhage (most common)
  - Abdominal pain
  - Palpable and pulsatile mass

  - Intermittent rectal bleeding and recurrent anemia
  - Low-grade fever, fatigue, weight loss
  - Leukocytosis (infection of graft and perigraft area)
- Other signs/symptoms
  - Syncope, shock
  - Back pain
- Diagnosis
  - Esophagogastroduodenoscopy: Exclude obvious causes of bleeding
  - Helical CT: Definitive diagnosis

Demographics

- Age: > 55 years of age
- Gender: M:F = 4-5:1

Natural History & Prognosis

- Prognosis: Very poor, up to 85% mortality

Treatment

- Goals of treatment: To control hemorrhage, to control infection, and to maintain adequate distal perfusion
- Extra-anatomical bypass with resection of graft and closure of gastrointestinal perforation
- There have been case reports of treatment of AEF with covered stent graft and chronic antibiotic therapy

DIAGNOSTIC CHECKLIST

Consider

- Clinical and past surgical history; diagnosis requires emergent surgery

Image Interpretation Pearls

- Perigraft infection ↑ suspicion of fistula

SELECTED REFERENCES

1. Baril DT et al: Evolving strategies for the treatment of aortoenteric fistulas. J Vasc Surg. 44(2):250-7, 2006
2. Danneels MI et al: Endovascular repair for aorto-enteric fistula: a bridge too far or a bridge to surgery? Eur J Vasc Endovasc Surg. 32(1):27-33, 2006
3. Armstrong PA et al: Improved outcomes in the recent management of secondary aortoenteric fistula. J Vasc Surg. 42(4):660-6, 2005
4. Saers SJ et al: Primary aortoenteric fistula. Br J Surg. 92(2):143-52, 2005
5. Yoshimoto K et al: Secondary aortoenteric fistula. J Vasc Surg. 42(4):805, 2005
6. Cendan JC et al: Twenty-one cases of aortoenteric fistula: lessons for the general surgeon. Am Surg. 70(7):583-7; discussion 587, 2004
7. Ghansah JN et al: Complications of major aortic and lower extremity vascular surgery. Semin Cardiothorac Vasc Anesth. 8(4):335-61, 2004
8. Malinzak LE et al: Gastrointestinal complications following infrarenal endovascular aneurysm repair. Vasc Endovascular Surg. 38(2):137-42, 2004
9. Perks FJ et al: Multidetector computed tomography imaging of aortoenteric fistula. J Comput Assist Tomogr. 28(3):343-7, 2004
10. Bertges DJ et al: Aortoenteric fistula due to endoleak coil embolization after endovascular AAA repair. J Endovasc Ther. 10(1):130-5, 2003
11. Puvaneswary M et al: Detection of aortoenteric fistula with helical CT. Australas Radiol. 47(1):67-9, 2003
12. Chiesa R et al: Vascular prosthetic graft infection: epidemiology, bacteriology, pathogenesis and treatment. Acta Chir Belg. 102(4):238-47, 2002
13. Burks JA Jr et al: Endovascular repair of bleeding aortoenteric fistulas: a 5-year experience. J Vasc Surg. 34(6):1055-9, 2001
14. Busuttil SJ et al: Diagnosis and management of aortoenteric fistulas. Semin Vasc Surg. 14(4):302-11, 2001
15. Lenzo NP et al: Aortoenteric fistula on (99m)Tc erythrocyte scintigraphy. AJR Am J Roentgenol. 177(2):477-8, 2001
16. Tozzi FL et al: Primary aortoenteric fistula related to septic aortitis. Sao Paulo Med J. 119(4):150-3, 2001
17. Orton DF et al: Aortic prosthetic graft infections: radiologic manifestations and implications for management. Radiographics. 20(4):977-93, 2000
18. Pipinos II et al: Secondary aortoenteric fistula. Ann Vasc Surg. 14(6):688-96, 2000
19. Vogt PR et al: In situ repair of aortobronchial, aortoesophageal, and aortoenteric fistulae with cryopreserved aortic homografts. J Vasc Surg. 26(1):11-7, 1997
20. Kuestner LM et al: Secondary aortoenteric fistula: contemporary outcome with use of extraanatomic bypass and infected graft excision. J Vasc Surg. 21(2):184-95; discussion 195-6, 1995
21. Low RN et al: Aortoenteric fistula and perigraft infection: evaluation with CT. Radiology. 175(1):157-62, 1990
22. Wagner JR: Aortic graft-enteric fistula and paraprosthetic-enteric fistula: a review. Mt Sinai J Med. 56(2):150-6, 1989
23. Schutte HE: Angiographic signs of aortic graft-enteric fistulae. Clin Radiol. 38(5):503-8, 1987
24. O'Mara CS et al: Secondary aortoenteric fistula. A 20 year experience. Am J Surg. 142(2):203-9, 1981
25. Thompson WM et al: Aortoenteric and paraprosthetic-enteric fistulas: radiologic findings. AJR Am J Roentgenol. 127(2):235-42, 1976

AORTIC ENTERIC FISTULA

IMAGE GALLERY

Typical

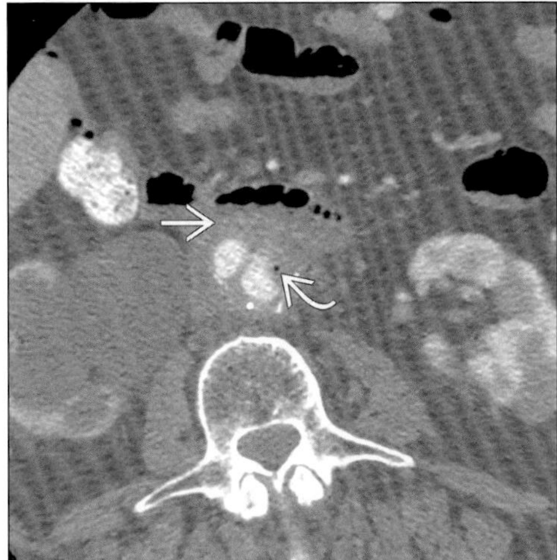

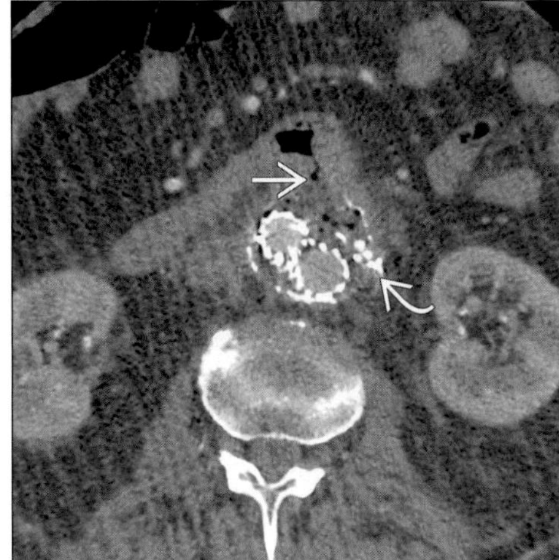

(Left) *Axial CECT in a patient with aorto-iliac-iliac graft and GI bleeding shows gas ➡ in the aneurysm sac and the duodenum in contact with the sac with loss of fat planes ➡ in between.* ***(Right)*** *Axial CECT shows a direct communication ➡ between the third part of duodenum and the aneurysm sac following an endoleak embolization with coils ➡. This represents an iatrogenic aortoenteric fistula.*

Typical

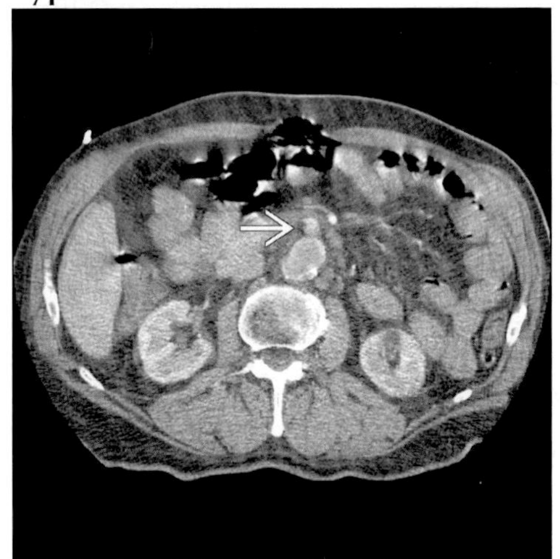

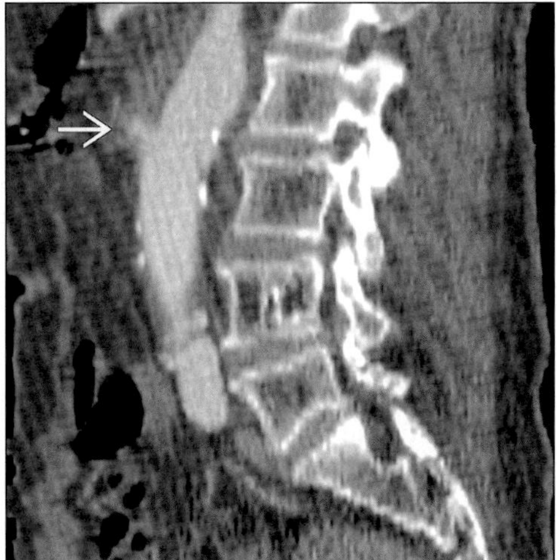

(Left) *Axial CECT shows small projection/nipple or pseudoaneurysm ➡ that protrudes into duodenum.* ***(Right)*** *Sagittal CECT in the same patient as previous image, shows a small pseudoaneurysm ➡ that projects into the duodenum. This "nipple-like" projection is typical of an aortoenteric fistula.*

Typical

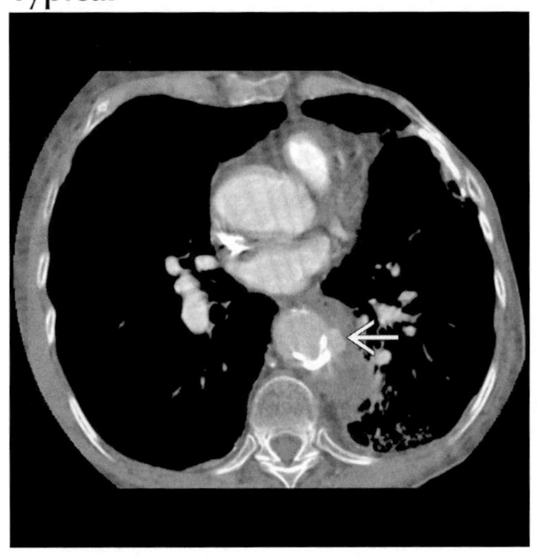

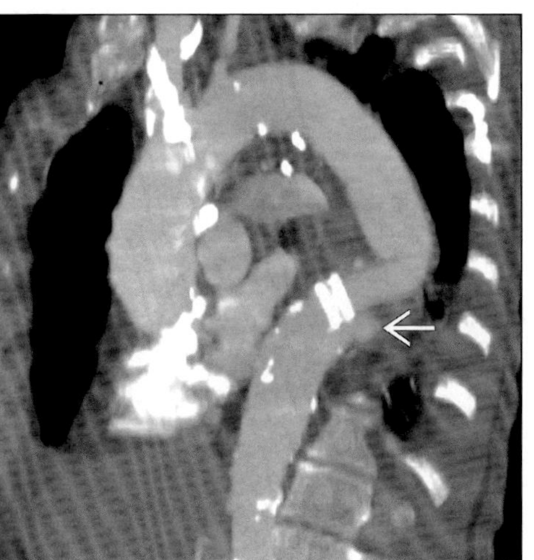

(Left) *Axial CECT shows a pseudoaneurysm ➡ at the site of the anastomosis of the thoracic graft in a patient with GI bleeding, suggesting an aorto-esophageal fistula.* ***(Right)*** *Oblique CTA in the same patient as previous image, shows the pseudoaneurysm ➡ at the site of the anastomosis of the thoracic graft.*

INFECTED AORTIC GRAFT

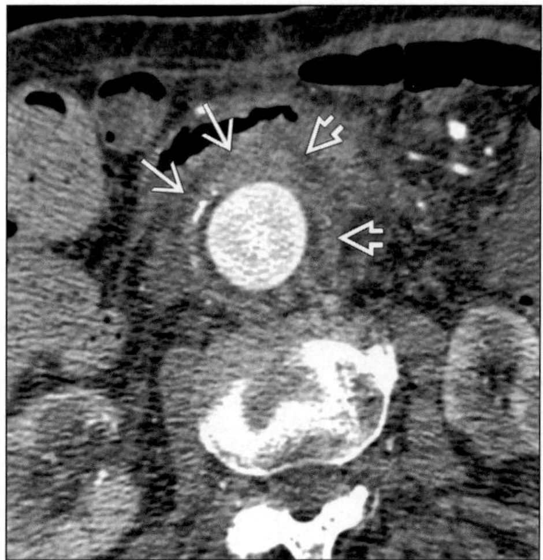

Axial CECT shows a perigraft enhancing soft tissue mass ➡ with associated loss of fat planes ➡ between the aorta and the duodenum. The latter finding is a much less specific one than the perigraft enhancement.

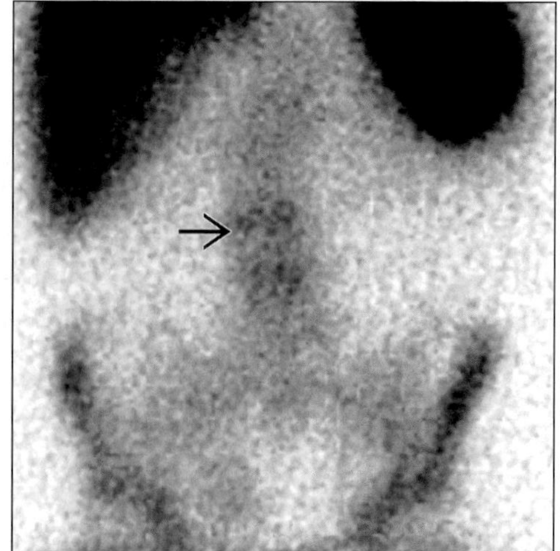

Indium-111 leukocyte scan shows increased uptake ➡ in the region of the aortic graft (same as prior patient). The patient history is important, as false positive scans occur during the early post-operative period.

TERMINOLOGY

Abbreviations and Synonyms

- Post-operative graft infection

Definitions

- Infection of prosthetic aortic graft

IMAGING FINDINGS

General Features

- Best diagnostic clue
  - Perigraft fluid, enhancing soft-tissue density, or ectopic gas increasing or persisting beyond four weeks after graft placement
    - Perigraft air more prevalent with aortoenteric fistula
- Location
  - Entire graft length may be involved or may be more focal and related to contiguous abscess
    - Most common site of aortoenteric fistula is third part of duodenum
    - Small bowel or colonic fistula can develop to iliac limbs of aortoiliac grafts

CT Findings

- NECT
  - Perigraft fluid collection
  - Perigraft soft tissue density
  - Stranding of retroperitoneal fat
  - Ectopic perigraft gas may represent aortoenteric fistula
  - Associated fluid collections in psoas
  - Lack of soft tissue plane between duodenum and aorta (less specific)
- CECT
  - Enhancement of perigraft soft tissue rind
  - Leakage of contrast into pseudoaneurysm, most pseudoaneurysms not infected
  - Leakage of contrast into bowel suggests aortoenteric fistula

MR Findings

- T1WI: Perigraft soft tissue mass, fluid collection low signal
- T2WI: Perigraft fluid collection high signal intensity
- Contrast-enhanced MR

DDx: Infected Aortic Graft

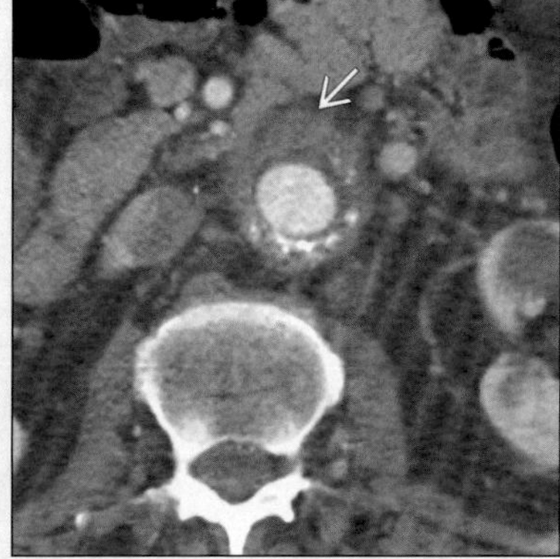

Inflammatory Aneurysm

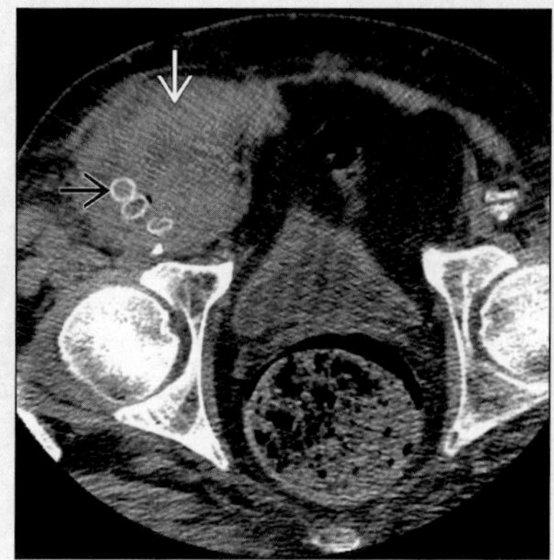

Post-Operative Hematoma

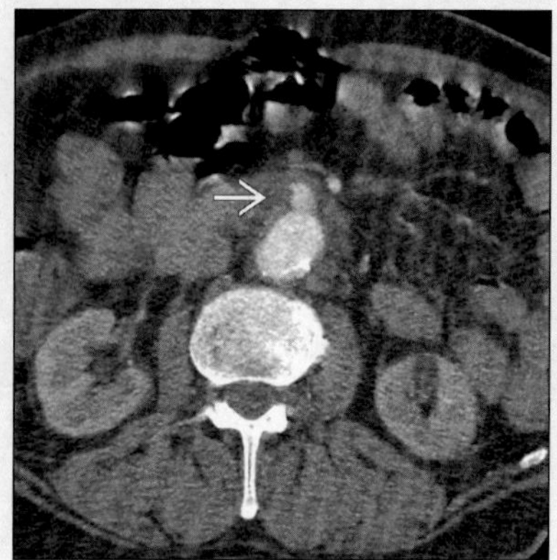

Aortoenteric Fistula

INFECTED AORTIC GRAFT

Key Facts

Terminology
- Post-operative graft infection
- Infection of prosthetic aortic graft

Imaging Findings
- Best diagnostic clue: Perigraft fluid, soft tissue density, or ectopic gas increasing or persisting beyond four weeks after graft placement
- Perigraft soft tissue density
- Ectopic perigraft gas may represent aortoenteric fistula
  - Perigraft air more prevalent with aortoenteric fistula
- Increased uptake with Indium-111 labeled leukocyte scan

Pathology
- Incidence is 1-6% of all post-operative aortic graft patients
  - Aortic enteric fistula is a subset of aortic graft infections
- Serious complication with mortality rates of 25-75%
  - Most common organism is staphylococcus epidermis
  - Graft infection 3x more common if aorta ruptured pre-operatively
- Hematoma after graft placement should resolve within 3 months

Clinical Issues
- Most effective current treatment is graft excision and placement of extra-anatomic bypass

  - Contrast-enhancement of perigraft inflammatory mass
  - Inflammatory changes in psoas, or fluid collection in psoas

Nuclear Medicine Findings
- Increased uptake with Indium-111 labeled leukocyte scan
- Gallium-67 scan less sensitive than Indium-111 leukocyte scan
- False positive scans occur during early post-op period

Ultrasonographic Findings
- Grayscale Ultrasound
  - Perigraft fluid collections and psoas fluid collections can be detected
    - Not helpful in diagnosing infection, as fluid collection nonspecific sign

Angiographic Findings
- Conventional
  - If aortoenteric fistula present, this is very rarely demonstrated
    - Pseudoaneurysm or "nipple" at site of aortoenteric fistula may be demonstrated
  - Useful for pre-operative road map of arteries for infected graft resection and extra-anatomic bypass graft surgery

Imaging Recommendations
- Best imaging tool: NECT and CECT should be used as first imaging tests
- In-111 labeled WBC scan important test if CT ambiguous
- MRA, CTA or angiography helpful to establish status of vessels distal to graft for secondary repair (e.g., axillary-femoral bypass procedure)

DIFFERENTIAL DIAGNOSIS

Anastomotic Pseudoaneurysm
- Incidence with AAA repair is 0.5-5.0%, when followed over 20-30 year period
- Etiologies include suture line disruption, graft or arterial wall failure, infection and technical error
  - Failure at suture line may be caused by excessive tension on anastomosis
  - Anastomotic pseudoaneurysms may result as secondary complication of graft infection
- Indications for repair include related complications (rupture, thrombosis or embolus), symptomatic pseudoaneurysms, large diameter pseudoaneurysm
- Femoral artery anastomotic pseudoaneurysms occur most frequently

Aortoenteric Fistula
- Primary aortoenteric fistula (AEF): Aortic communication with bowel lumen, occurring in absence of aortic surgery
  - Usually involves infrarenal AAA and duodenal sweep
  - Structures abut one another and with aneurysm expansion may allow erosive factors to form fistula
  - Usually secondary to aortic disease (70%)
    - Also association with GI disease, neoplasm, or inflammation (e.g., pancreatitis, radiation)
- Secondary AEF: Aortic communication with bowel lumen, occurring after aortic surgery
  - Much more common than primary AEF, although incidence less than 1%
  - Inciting event may be graft infection, pulsation from noncompliant graft, or duodenal process
  - Breakdown of graft repair with erosion of aortic contents into bowel
  - Duodenum is most common location of aortoenteric fistula
  - Classic clinical triad presentation of secondary AEF: GI bleeding, sepsis and abdominal pain
    - GI bleeding most common presentation, occurring in nearly 70%

Post-Operative Perigraft Hematoma
- Complete resolution of hematomas should occur within 3 months
- Ectopic gas in early post-operative period suspicious but not diagnostic; should be resorbed in 3-4 weeks

Inflammatory Abdominal Aortic Aneurysm

- Formerly believed to be distinct entity; currently considered an extreme in spectrum of AAA
  - Accounts for 5-15% of all AAAs; unknown etiology
- Thick fibrous anterior and lateral wall which may be up to 3 cm in maximum thickness
  - Usually very adherent to surrounding structures such as duodenum, IVC, left renal vein and occasionally ureters
  - Perianeurysmal enhancing soft tissue rind on CECT
    - Difficult to differentiate from infection

PATHOLOGY

General Features

- General path comments
  - Incidence is 1-6% of all post-operative aortic graft patients
  - Most infections believed to be result of contamination from abdominal incision
    - Most common organism is staphylococcus epidermis
    - Hematogenous seeding secondary to bacteremia may be a cause of late graft infection
  - Serious complication with mortality rates of 25-75%
    - Aortic enteric fistula is a subset of aortic graft infections
  - Graft infection 3x more common if aorta ruptured pre-operatively
  - Hematoma after graft placement should resolve within 3 months
- Etiology
  - Most common causative organism is staphylococcus epidermidis
    - Produces a slime that adheres to graft and thereby protects organism from both host natural defenses and antibiotics
    - Very difficult to eradicate
  - Many of organisms are fastidious and may require 14 days to culture

CLINICAL ISSUES

Presentation

- Signs and symptoms are not specific
  - Fever
  - Malaise
  - Back or abdominal pain
  - Gastrointestinal bleeding
  - Elevated sedimentation rate
  - Palpable mass
  - Draining sinus
- Patients may present days to years following surgery

Natural History & Prognosis

- High morbidity and mortality associated with operative repair of infected graft

Treatment

- Antibiotic therapy often not curative
  - Long-term suppressive antibiotic therapy mandatory if any chance for success
- Percutaneous aspiration of fluid around graft
  - Usually diagnostic to obtain fluid for microbiology examination, culture and sensitivity
  - Occasionally therapeutic
  - Installation of thrombolytics has been tried to attempt clearing staphylococcus epidermidis infection
- Graft excision and placement of extra-anatomic bypass is currently accepted standard treatment
  - Occasionally autogenous vein in situ, or very rarely rifampin-bonded prosthesis in situ used for constructing bypass

DIAGNOSTIC CHECKLIST

Image Interpretation Pearls

- Perigraft fluid with ectopic gas that is increasing or persisting beyond four weeks after graft placement highly suggestive of infected graft

SELECTED REFERENCES

1. Hsu RB et al: Surgical Pathology of Infected Aortic Aneurysm and Its Clinical Correlation. Ann Vasc Surg. 2007
2. Hulin SJ et al: Aortic endograft infection: open surgical management with endograft preservation. Eur J Vasc Endovasc Surg. 34(2):191-3, 2007
3. Mirzaie M et al: Surgical management of vascular graft infection in severely ill patients by partial resection of the infected prosthesis. Eur J Vasc Endovasc Surg. 33(5):610-3, 2007
4. Shahidi S et al: Detection of Abdominal Aortic Graft Infection: Comparison of Magnetic Resonance Imaging and Indium-Labeled White Blood Cell Scanning. Ann Vasc Surg. 21(5):586-592, 2007
5. Abouhamad P et al: Improved diagnosis of aortobifemoral vascular graft infection by In-111-labeled leukocyte SPECT. Clin Nucl Med. 31(6):338-9, 2006
6. O'Connor S et al: A systematic review and meta-analysis of treatments for aortic graft infection. J Vasc Surg. 44(1):38-45, 2006
7. Perera GB et al: Aortic graft infection: update on management and treatment options. Vasc Endovascular Surg. 40(1):1-10, 2006
8. Kitamura T et al: Management of infected grafts and aneurysms of the aorta. Ann Vasc Surg. 19(3):335-42, 2005
9. Wilson SE: New alternatives in management of the infected vascular prosthesis. Surg Infect (Larchmt). 2(2):171-5; discussion 175-7, 2001
10. Orton DF et al: Aortic prosthetic graft infections: radiologic manifestations and implications for management. Radiographics. 20(4):977-93, 2000
11. Calligaro KD et al: Graft preserving methods for managing aortofemoral prosthetic graft infection. Eur J Vasc Endovasc Surg. 14 Suppl A:38-42, 1997
12. Jausseran JM et al: Total prosthetic graft excision and extra-anatomic bypass. Eur J Vasc Endovasc Surg. 14 Suppl A:59-65, 1997
13. Pistolese GR et al: Conservative treatment of aortic graft infection. Eur J Vasc Endovasc Surg. 14 Suppl A:47-52, 1997
14. Low RN et al: Aortoenteric fistula and perigraft infection: evaluation with CT. Radiology. 175(1):157-62, 1990

IMAGE GALLERY

Typical

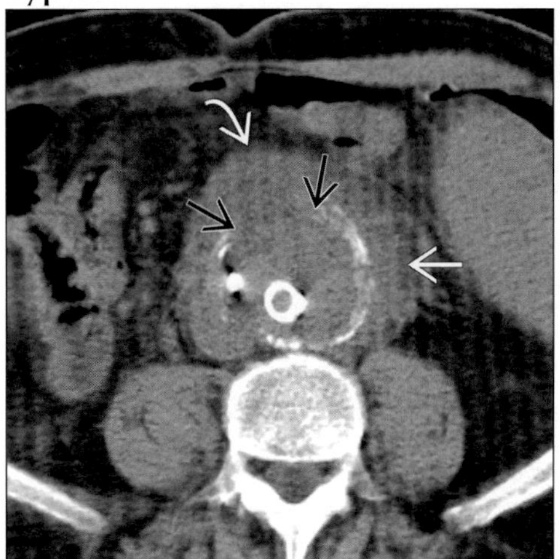

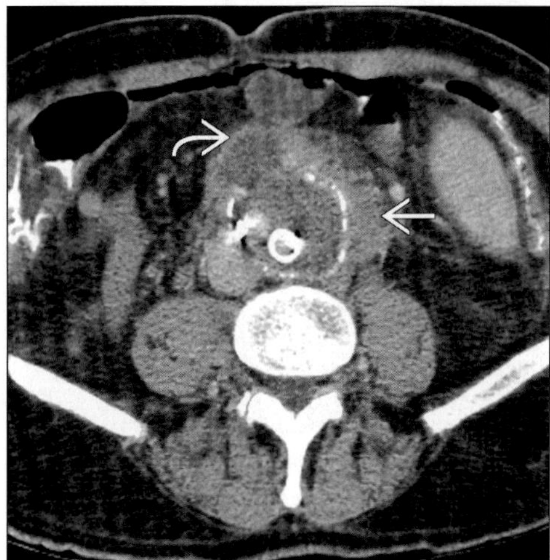

(Left) *Axial NECT in a patient with AAA who previously underwent aortic bypass surgery with plication of the residual aneurysm sac shows perianeurysmal soft tissue mass ➡ with focal outpouching ➡ anteriorly. Note the disruption ➡ in the anterior calcification of the plicated AAA.* ***(Right)*** *Axial CECT shows enhancement of the periaortic soft tissue mass ➡. The anterior focal bulging ➡ was an abscess on pathology. The residual AAA sac and the focal abscess are contiguous.*

Typical

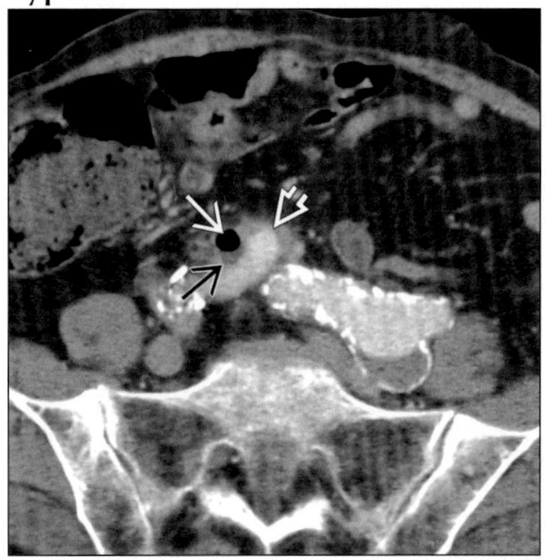

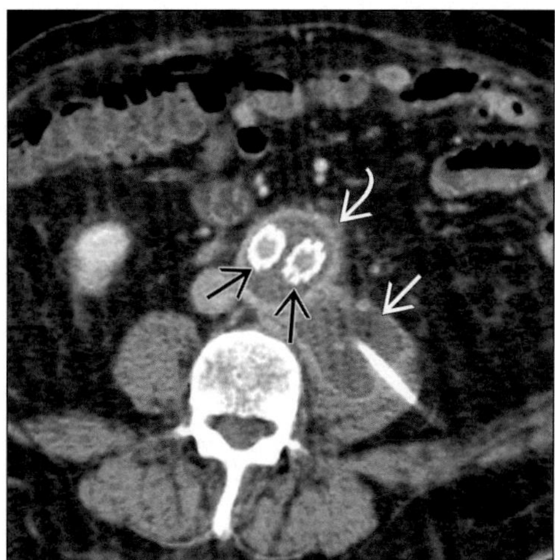

(Left) *Axial CECT shows air ➡ and fluid ➡ within the iliac limb ➡ of an aorto-bi-iliac bypass graft near the distal surgical anastomosis. This suggests an infected graft.* ***(Right)*** *Axial CECT in a patient who recently underwent endovascular AAA repair shows a left psoas abscess ➡ that abuts the enhancing perianeurysmal soft tissue mass ➡, consistent with infection. The endovascular graft limbs ➡ course through the infected residual AAA sac.*

Typical

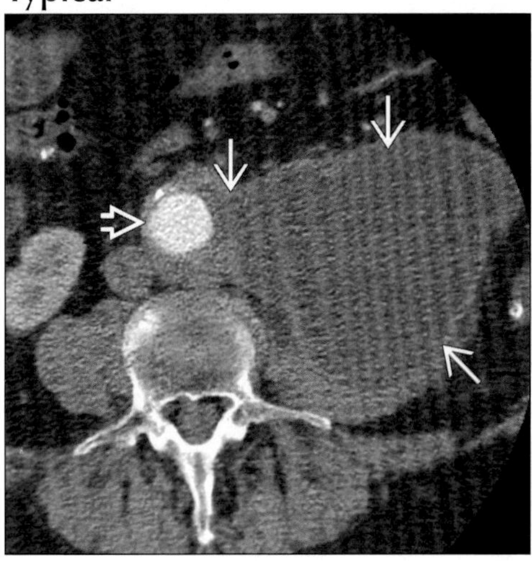

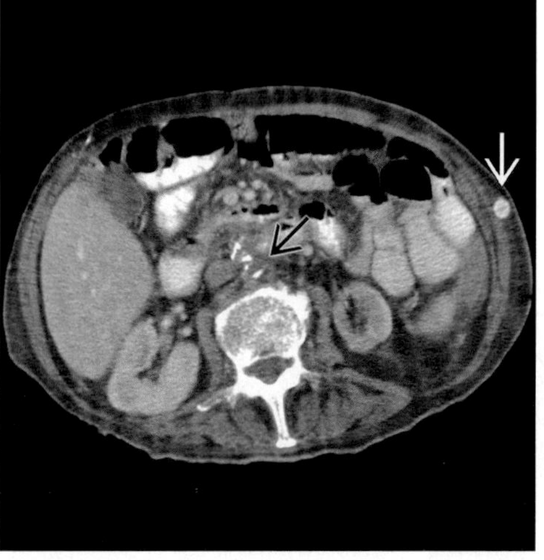

(Left) *Axial CECT shows a large left psoas fluid collection ➡ that is contiguous with an aortic graft ➡ suggesting a psoas abscess and aortic graft infection. Standard treatment consists of graft excision and extra-anatomic vascular bypass surgery.* ***(Right)*** *Axial CECT of the abdomen following resection of an infected aortic graft shows absence of the aorta ➡ and an extra-anatomic left axillary-femoral artery bypass graft ➡ in the subcutaneous soft tissues.*

ABDOMINAL AORTIC OCCLUSION

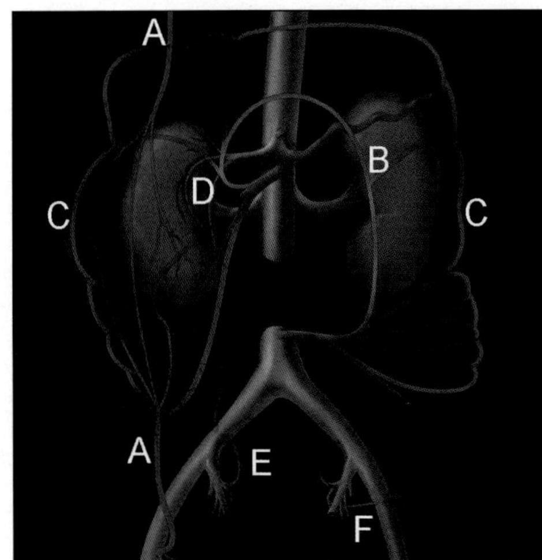

Graphic shows collaterals that may be seen in aortic occlusion. A) Superior to inferior epigastric, B) Arc of Riolan, C) Marginal artery of Drummond, D) Arc of Buhler, E) Iliolumbar, F) Gluteal.

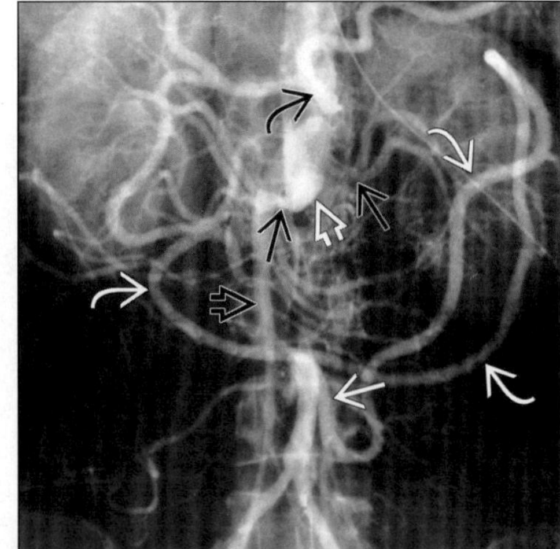

Catheter angiography shows aortic occlusion below the renal arteries. The superior mesenteric and celiac arteries reconstitute the distal aorta via large collaterals to the inferior mesenteric artery.

TERMINOLOGY

Abbreviations and Synonyms

- Aortic occlusion, aortoiliac occlusive disease, acute aortic occlusion, chronic aortic occlusion, Leriche syndrome

Definitions

- Acute or chronic total occlusion of abdominal aorta
- Leriche syndrome: Abdominal aortic or iliac artery occlusive disease causing absent femoral pulses, bilateral claudication and impotence

IMAGING FINDINGS

General Features

- Best diagnostic clue
  - Acute: Abdominal aortic occlusion with filling defect and few collaterals
  - Chronic: Abdominal aortic occlusion with extensive collaterals
- Location
  - Acute: Embolus in infrarenal aorta or bifurcation
  - Chronic: Distal aortic thrombosis propagating proximally to renal artery level

CT Findings

- NECT: Aortic wall calcification
- CECT
  - Acute and chronic
    - Normal contrast opacification of celiac axis, superior mesenteric (SMA) and renal arteries
  - Acute: Few collaterals, if relatively acute
    - Embolus: Partially occlusive intraluminal filling defect
    - Thrombo-emboli may be present in other vessels
    - Filling defect in infrarenal aorta, usually distally
  - Chronic
    - Thrombus: Totally occlusive intraluminal filling defect
    - Absent contrast opacification of infrarenal aorta; may extend into common iliac arteries
    - Multiple intra-abdominal collateral arteries reconstitute pelvic vessels
    - Distal aortic occlusion with proximal propagation of thrombus
- CTA

DDx: Abdominal Aortic Occlusion

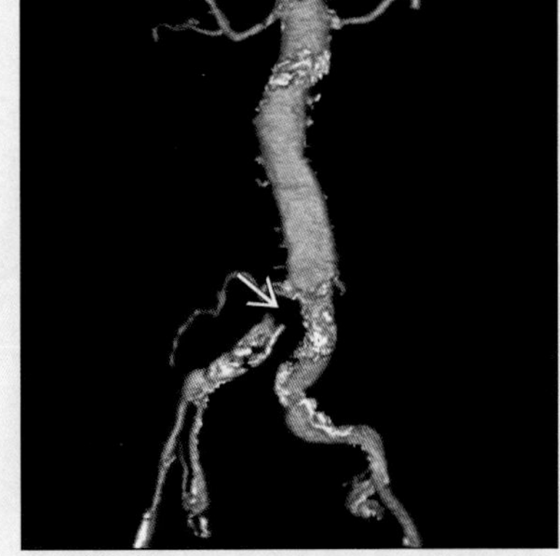

Common Iliac Artery Occlusion

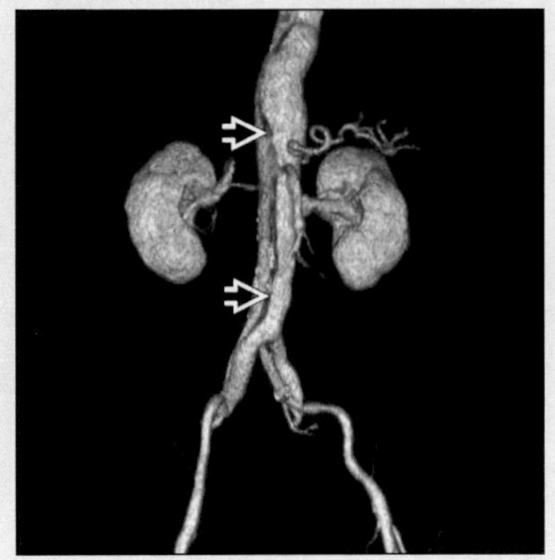

Aortic Dissection

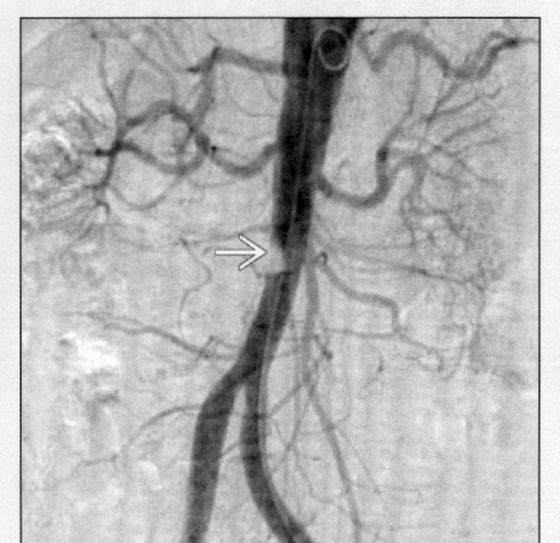

Aortic Stenosis

ABDOMINAL AORTIC OCCLUSION

Key Facts

Terminology

- Acute or chronic total occlusion of abdominal aorta
- Leriche syndrome: Abdominal aortic or iliac artery occlusive disease causing absent femoral pulses, bilateral claudication and impotence

Imaging Findings

- Acute: Abdominal aortic occlusion with filling defect and few collaterals
- Chronic: Abdominal aortic occlusion with extensive collaterals
- CTA with multiplanar reconstructions can determine extent of occlusion

Clinical Issues

- Development of collateral pathways around occlusion crucial
- Symptoms depend on acuteness of occlusion and presence of collaterals
    - Acute occlusion causes acute ischemia; chronic occlusion causes chronic ischemia
- Leriche syndrome triad: Absent femoral pulses, claudication, impotence
- Acute risk factors: Severe dehydration, hypercoagulable state, atrial myxoma
- Chronic risk factors: Atherosclerosis, hypertension, diabetes mellitus
- Surgical therapy is treatment of choice

Diagnostic Checklist

- Diagnosis may be delayed due to varied presentations
- Delayed diagnosis and delayed treatment yields poor outcome

---

- Absent segment of infrarenal aorta on MIPs or reconstructions
- Multiple collateral vessels connecting aortic side-branch arteries above and below occlusion

MR Findings

- T1 and T2WI: High signal intensity aortic thrombus with chronic thrombosis
    - Signal intensity may vary with age of thrombus
- Time-of-flight MRA technique inaccurate due to flow-related artifacts
- Contrast-enhanced MR angiography preferred for better accuracy
    - Acute occlusion
        - Abrupt termination of abdominal aorta
        - Filling defect/meniscus indicating embolus
    - Chronic occlusion
        - Infrarenal occlusion of aorta with collateral filling of distal vessels
        - Reconstitutes at iliac or common femoral arteries

Echocardiographic Findings

- Echocardiogram: Atrial myxoma or intracardiac mural thrombus can be seen in setting of embolic aortic occlusion

Ultrasonographic Findings

- Grayscale Ultrasound: Echogenic thrombus within occluded aorta
- Pulsed Doppler
    - Monophasic waveforms distal to occlusion
        - Reduced systolic velocities
- Color Doppler: Turbulent flow at occlusion; absent aortic flow below occlusion

Angiographic Findings

- DSA
    - Acute: Occlusion at bifurcation with or without extension into common iliac arteries
        - Fewer collaterals than with chronic occlusion
    - Chronic: Occlusion of aorta just below renal arteries
        - Multiple collateral vessels reconstitute lower extremity outflow
- Currently limited role in diagnosis with increased use of non-invasive modalities (CTA, MRA)
    - Requires access from upper extremity (radial, brachial or axillary puncture) or translumbar

Imaging Recommendations

- Best imaging tool
    - CTA with multiplanar reconstructions determines extent of occlusion
        - Use multidetector scanner, adequate contrast volume, rapid bolus injection and sophisticated post-processing
        - Reconstructions can delineate collateral flow
- Protocol advice: Gadolinium-enhanced 3D MRA; good signal to noise ratio, with decreased scanning time

DIFFERENTIAL DIAGNOSIS

Common Iliac Artery Occlusion or Stenosis

- Usually related to atherosclerotic vascular disease
    - Heavily calcified vessels
- May be unilateral or bilateral
- Multiple collaterals present

Aortic Dissection

- Usually an extension of thoracic dissection
- Characteristic intimal flap separating "true" and "false" lumens
    - Occlusion of true lumen by enlarging false lumen

Aortic Trauma

- Retroperitoneal and periaortic hematoma
- History of blunt force trauma to abdomen

Mid-Aortic (Coarctation) Syndrome

- Most lesions occur above or at level of renal arteries; proximal renal arteries involved in about 80% of cases
- Detected in 2nd or 3rd decade due to hypertension, claudication, or rarely mesenteric ischemia
- Etiologies include neurofibromatosis, radiation therapy, nonspecific aortitis and atherosclerosis

ABDOMINAL AORTIC OCCLUSION

Aortitis (Vasculitis)

- More frequent in younger patients
- Aortic involvement in Takayasu arteritis may extend from aortic root to include abdominal aorta and iliac arteries

PATHOLOGY

General Features

- General path comments: Most common cause of occlusion: Thrombosis superimposed on severe distal aortic atherosclerosis
- Etiology
  - Acute: 65% due to embolism; 35% due to thrombosis; other authors report reversed ratio
    - Embolism: Most likely cardiac origin; can be tumor embolus with known malignancy
    - Thrombosis: Acute thrombosis of atherosclerotic aorta or small AAA, hypercoagulable state, trauma
- Development of collateral pathways around occlusion crucial
  - Pancreaticoduodenal arcade (celiac to SMA)
  - Arc of Riolan (SMA to IMA)
  - Marginal artery of Drummond (SMA to IMA) along mesenteric side of colon
  - Iliolumbar (lumbar arteries to internal iliac branches)
  - Superior to inferior epigastric arteries
  - Gluteal collaterals

Gross Pathologic & Surgical Features

- Severe atherosclerosis of aorta, calcification

CLINICAL ISSUES

Presentation

- Most common signs/symptoms
  - Symptoms depend on acuteness of occlusion and amount of collateral blood flow
  - Leriche syndrome triad: Absent femoral pulses, claudication, impotence
  - Acute occlusion causes acute ischemia
    - Absent pulses and bilateral acute leg pain
    - Acute abdominal symptoms
  - Chronic occlusion causes chronic ischemia
    - Absent femoral or lower extremity pulses
    - Claudication
- Other signs/symptoms
  - Acute
    - Symptoms mimicking spinal cord compression
    - Acute onset hypertension
    - Cool skin
  - Chronic
    - Global lower extremity trophic changes in nails or skin
    - Claudication or rest pain; tissue loss
- Clinical Profile
  - Acute: Severe dehydration, hypercoagulable state, atrial myxoma
    - Cardiac dysfunction (associated with poor prognosis in aortic occlusion)
  - Chronic: Atherosclerosis, hypertension, diabetes mellitus, smoking history

Demographics

- Age: > 60 years of age
- Gender
  - Acute aortic occlusion: Females > males
    - Female gender a risk factor for embolism
  - Chronic aortic occlusion: Males > females
    - Male gender a risk for atherosclerosis

Natural History & Prognosis

- Acute aortic occlusion: > 50% mortality rate
- Chronic aortic occlusion: Lower morbidity and mortality rates than acute occlusion

Treatment

- Options, risks, complications: Cardiac complications, recurrent embolization, progression to thrombosis, renal failure, amputation
- Medical management: Alter risk factors; antiplatelet therapy or anticoagulation
  - Exercise regimen
- Endovascular therapy has limited role depending on chronicity, length of occlusion, distribution of disease
- Surgical therapy is "gold standard"
  - Aorto-bi-iliac bypass for occlusion reconstituting at iliac arteries
  - Aorto-bifemoral bypass for occlusion reconstituting at femoral arteries
  - Extra-anatomic bypass (e.g., axillo-bifemoral)
  - Endarterectomy (rarely performed)

DIAGNOSTIC CHECKLIST

Consider

- Diagnosis may be delayed due to varied presentations
- Delayed diagnosis and delayed treatment yields poor outcome
- Patients with chronic occlusion have high likelihood of arterial disease in other vessels

Image Interpretation Pearls

- Non-occlusive filling defect is embolus
- Occlusive filling defect is thrombus

SELECTED REFERENCES

1. Kao CL et al: Abdominal aortic occlusion: a rare complication of cardiac myxoma. Tex Heart Inst J. 28(4):324-5, 2001
2. Ruehm SG et al: Contrast-enhanced MR angiography in patients with aortic occlusion (Leriche syndrome). J Magn Reson Imaging. 11(4):401-10, 2000
3. Babu SC et al: Acute aortic occlusion--factors that influence outcome. J Vasc Surg. 21(4):567-72; discussion 573-5, 1995
4. Dossa CD et al: Acute aortic occlusion. A 40-year experience. Arch Surg. 129(6):603-7; discussion 607-8, 1994
5. Boender AC et al: An attempt to classify the collateral systems in total occlusions at different levels of the lumbar aorta and pelvic arteries: causes and consequences. Radiol Clin (Basel). 46(5):348-63, 1977

IMAGE GALLERY

Typical

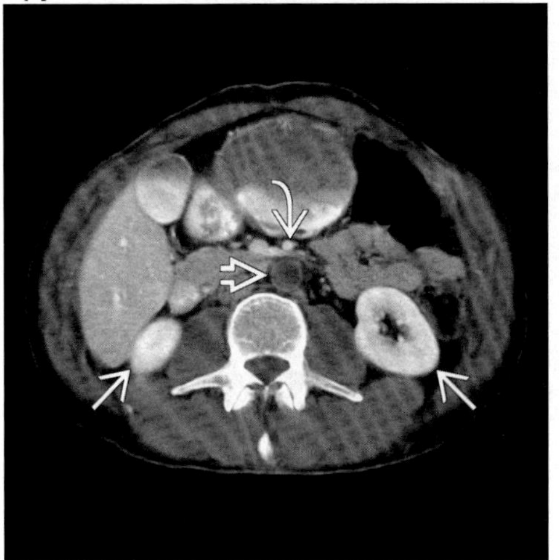

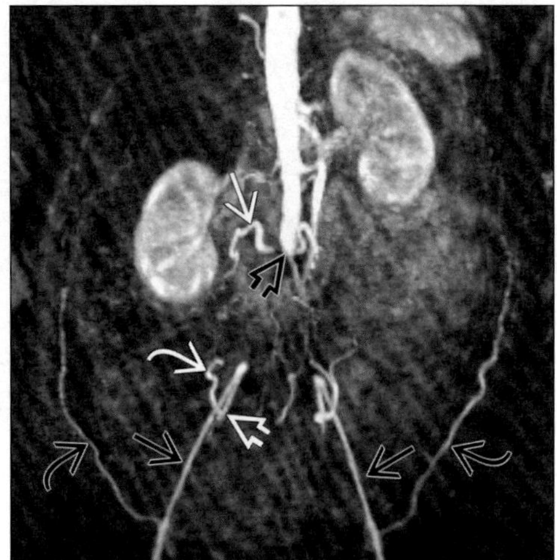

(Left) Axial CECT shows absence of contrast in the infrarenal aorta, consistent with occlusion. There is contrast opacification of the SMA and of the kidneys, indicating mesenteric and renal artery patency. *(Right)* MRA (same patient) shows distal aortic occlusion with reconstitution of the internal and external iliac arteries via lumbar to iliolumbar collaterals. Reconstitution is also through the deep circumflex iliac arteries.

Typical

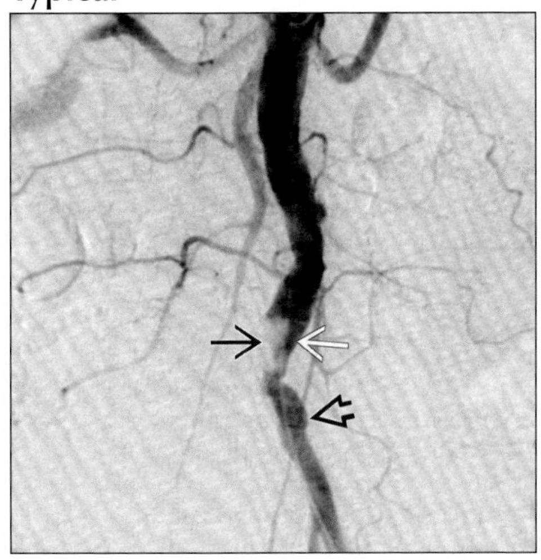

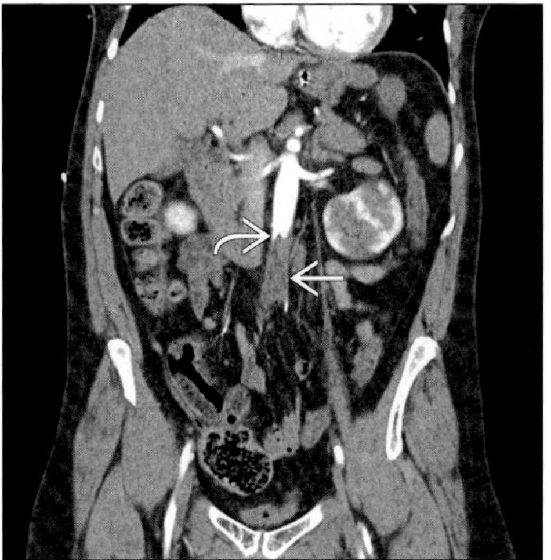

(Left) Catheter angiography shows a large filling defect in the distal abdominal aorta that occludes the right common iliac artery (non-opacified). The embolus does not occlude the entire aorta and allows left common iliac artery perfusion. There are poor collaterals. *(Right)* Coronal CTA (different patient) shows a meniscus sign and abrupt termination of the contrast column in the aorta, consistent with an acute embolus.

Typical

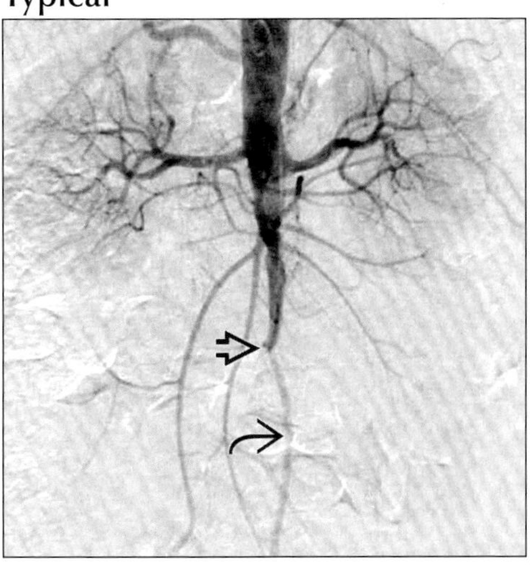

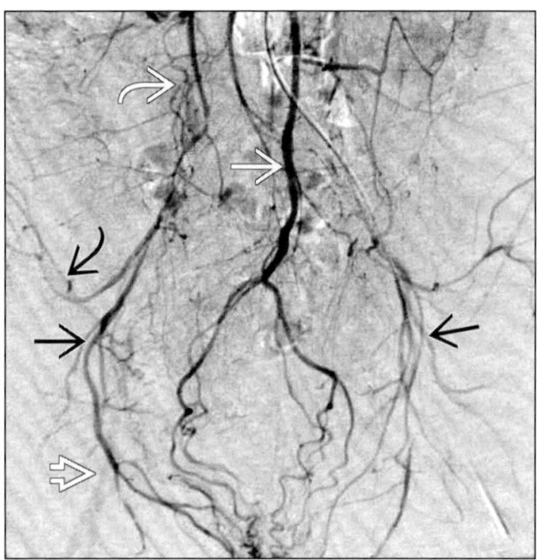

(Left) Catheter angiography of the abdominal aorta shows chronic occlusion of the distal infrarenal aorta, terminating in the inferior mesenteric artery. *(Right)* Catheter angiography of the pelvis (same patient) shows the IMA continues as the superior hemorrhoidal artery and communicates with multiple gluteal collaterals that reconstitute a faintly opacified right common femoral artery. There are also iliolumbar and deep circumflex femoral artery collaterals present.

ABDOMINAL AORTIC DISSECTION

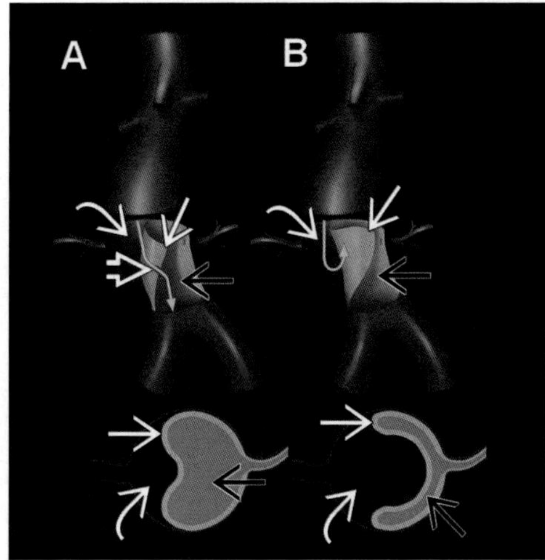

Graphic shows an abdominal aortic dissection with: (A) blood re-entering the true lumen via a fenestration in the intimal flap and (B) no blood re-entry, with the false lumen compressing the true lumen.

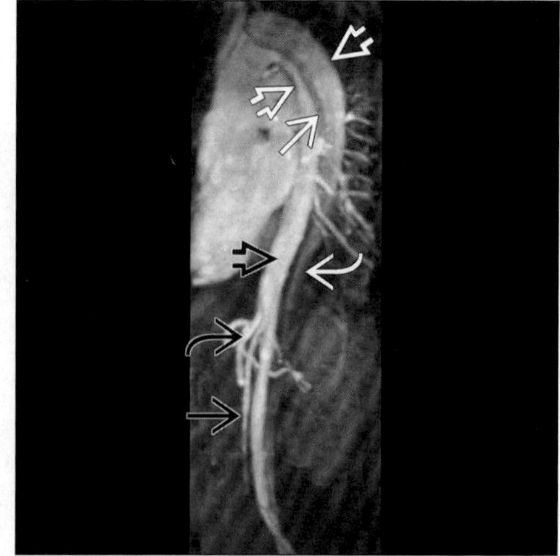

MRA shows a thoracic aortic dissection extending into the abdominal aorta. The celiac and SMA arise from the hyperintense true lumen separated by an intimal flap from the hypointense false lumen.

TERMINOLOGY

Abbreviations and Synonyms

- Isolated abdominal aortic dissection, abdominal aortic dissection, abdominal aortic aneurysm (AAA)

Definitions

- Separation of aortic intima from media by blood
  - Intimal flap divides into "true" and "false" lumens
    - True lumen circumferentially lined with intima
    - False lumen lies outside of intima
  - Re-entry: Return of blood from false into true lumen

IMAGING FINDINGS

General Features

- Best diagnostic clue: Intimal flap separating true and false lumens
- Location
  - Abdominal aorta below diaphragm
    - Most commonly involves infrarenal aorta
    - Rarely originates at SMA level
  - Dissections can terminate at IMA, above aortic bifurcation or extend into iliac arteries
- Morphology
  - Iliac and/or femoral artery extension in 50%
  - True and false lumens spiral around aortic axis
  - Distal re-entry site usually present
    - Smaller re-entry sites (fenestrations) exist; holes in intimal flap at separations from arterial orifices

CT Findings

- NECT
  - Hyperdense, crescentic intramural hematoma
  - Hyperdense periaortic/retroperitoneal hematoma
  - Calcification within aortic wall or lumen
    - Transmural calcification does not allow for separation of aortic wall layers
    - Calcification usually localizes to intima; calcification in outer wall and intimal flap indicates true lumen in acute dissection
- CECT
  - Low attenuation intimal flap
  - Enhancement pattern of true vs. false lumen
    - Larger diameter of false lumen from slow flow
    - False lumen may thrombose and not enhance

DDx: Complex Aortic Irregularity

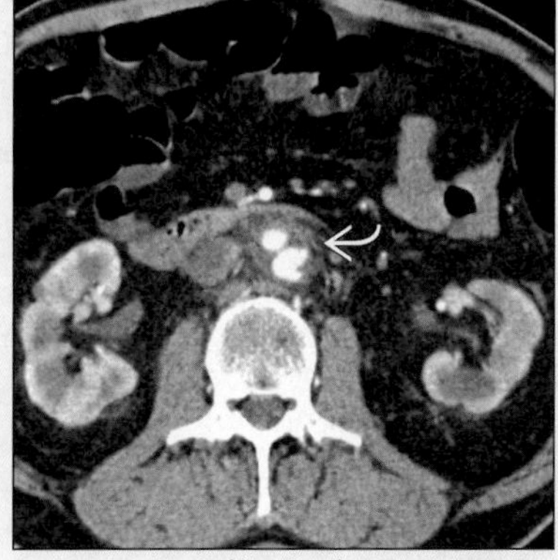

Aortitis with Pseudoaneurysm

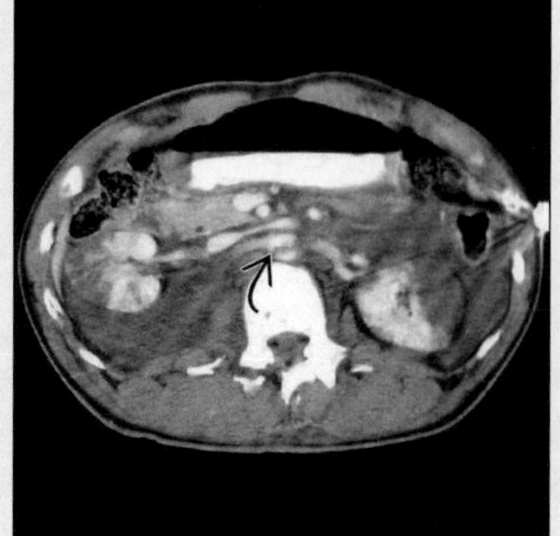

Abdominal Aortic Trauma

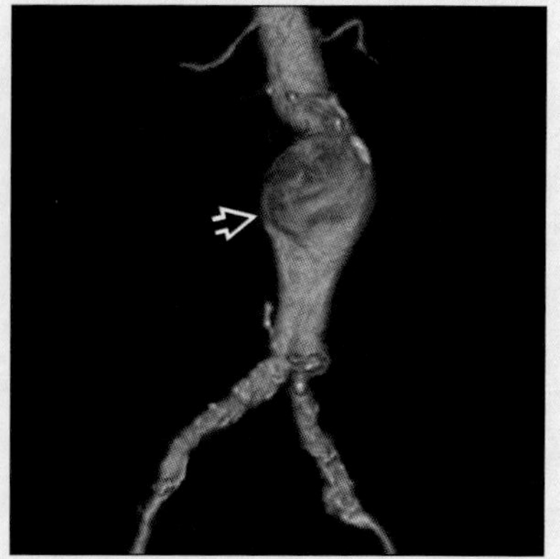

Abdominal Aortic Aneurysm

ABDOMINAL AORTIC DISSECTION

Key Facts

Terminology
- Isolated abdominal aortic dissection, abdominal aortic dissection, abdominal aortic aneurysm (AAA)
  - Aortic dissection originates below diaphragm
  - Separation of aortic intima from media by blood

Imaging Findings
- CECT with multiplanar reformations best imaging modality
- Most commonly involves infrarenal aorta
- Intimal flap separating true and false lumina
- Lumina will have different enhancement patterns
- Iliac and/or femoral artery extension occurs in 50%

Pathology
- Isolated abdominal aortic dissection post-traumatic (30%) or spontaneous (70%)

Clinical Issues
- Medical management: Descending aortic involvement only
- Surgical or endovascular management: Ascending and/or descending aortic involvement
  - Increased technical and clinical success rates for endovascular treatment; relatively decreased morbidity and mortality
  - Isolated abdominal aortic dissection with AAA treated due to rupture risk (28%)
- Chronic aortic dissection can lead to AAA formation

Diagnostic Checklist
- Identify proximal and distal extent of dissection
- Double-barreled aorta with differential enhancement in lumens suggests isolated abdominal aortic dissection

---

    - Delayed enhancement and washout of false lumen
    - Shows origins and involvement of branch vessels
  - Visceral involvement, ischemic changes
- CTA
  - "Double-barreled" aorta on axial imaging
  - Asymmetric aortic wall thickening
    - Seen adjacent to intimal flap

MR Findings
- T1WI: Thrombosed false lumen has increased signal intensity
- T1 C+: Delayed enhancement/washout in false lumen
- MRA: Maximum intensity projection (MIP) from gadolinium-enhanced 3-D MRA can demonstrate low signal intensity dissection flap and fenestration sites

Ultrasonographic Findings
- Grayscale Ultrasound
  - Echogenic intimal flap paralleling aortic walls
  - Differing echogenicities in aortic lumens, depending on presence of thrombus or flow rate
- Color Doppler
  - Discrepancy in flow between true and false lumens; decreased flow in false lumen
  - Absent flow in false lumen if thrombosed

Angiographic Findings
- Catheter "floats" in middle of aorta, settling against dissection flap instead of aortic wall
- Differential contrast filling of true and false lumens
  - Delayed filling and washout of false lumen
  - Differential filling of major branch vessels; depends on which lumen supplies them
- True lumen compression by filling of false lumen
- Important to identify true lumen
  - May require bilateral common femoral artery access
- Angiography can be performed from brachial approach
  - Avoids entering dissected segment
- Caution when injecting, if catheter is positioned within false lumen

Imaging Recommendations
- Best imaging tool
  - CECT with multiplanar reformations
    - Shows true and false lumens; extent of dissection
    - 95% sensitivity/specificity
- Protocol advice
  - Use contrast bolus timing in CECT to determine optimal scanning delay
    - Thin collimation to evaluate branch involvement
  - MR not recommended for acute isolated abdominal aortic dissection due to study duration
    - Good for monitoring chronic dissection
  - Trans-esophageal echocardiography has 80% sensitivity/specificity
- Catheter angiography was "gold standard"
  - Now infrequently used
  - Invasive, time consuming
  - Relatively limited ability to see multiple angles
- Dissection entry and exit points difficult to identify
  - Intravascular ultrasound can increase accuracy of entry and exit site detection
  - Surgery best defines extent of dissection

DIFFERENTIAL DIAGNOSIS

Aortitis
- Aorta can be stenotic, aneurysmal or occluded
- Diffuse aortic wall thickening

Aortic Trauma
- May be blunt, penetrating or iatrogenic
- Pseudoaneurysm or post-traumatic dissection
- Retroperitoneal hematoma

Abdominal Aortic Aneurysm
- No intimal flap
- Increased diameter of abdominal aorta
- May have laminar thrombus within aneurysm sac

ABDOMINAL AORTIC DISSECTION

PATHOLOGY

General Features

- Genetics
  - Inherited disorders associated with aortic dissection
    - Marfan syndrome
    - Ehlers-Danlos syndrome
    - Osteogenesis imperfecta
    - Polycystic renal disease
- Etiology
  - Defect in media allows blood to enter
    - Defect may be tear or atherosclerotic ulcer
    - Pressurized blood enters defect, dissects antegrade and/or retrograde
  - Extension from thoracic aortic dissection most common cause of abdominal aortic dissection
  - Isolated abdominal aortic dissection etiologies: Accidental (15%), iatrogenic (15%), trauma, or spontaneous (70%)
    - Reported rate of spontaneous occurrence < 2%

Gross Pathologic & Surgical Features

- Atherosclerosis found in region of dissection (> 75%)

Microscopic Features

- Medial degeneration

Staging, Grading or Classification Criteria

- DeBakey classification
  - DeBakey I: Both ascending and descending aorta
  - DeBakey II: Ascending aorta only
  - DeBakey III: Descending aorta only
- Stanford classification
  - Stanford A involves ascending aorta; may include descending aorta
  - Stanford B involves descending aorta only

CLINICAL ISSUES

Presentation

- Most common signs/symptoms
  - Acute abdominal, flank or back pain (70%)
  - Acute lower extremity ischemia (25%) without prior history of arterial insufficiency
  - Abdominal tenderness
  - Pulsatile abdominal mass
- Other signs/symptoms
  - May be asymptomatic
  - Abdominal bruit
  - Lower extremity neurological changes
  - Mesenteric ischemia or bowel infarction
- Clinical Profile
  - Hypertension in > 40% of patients with isolated abdominal aortic dissection
  - Poor survival when hypotensive upon presentation

Demographics

- Age: Middle age (50-70s)
- Gender: Male > female
- Ethnicity: Caucasian > other ethnicities

Natural History & Prognosis

- Chronic aortic dissection cause aneurysm from continuing expansion of false lumen (up to 30%)
- Due to rarity of condition, true natural history or treatment algorithm not yet determined

Treatment

- Options, risks, complications
  - Medical: Descending aortic involvement only (Stanford type B, DeBakey type III)
  - Surgical or endovascular: Ascending aortic involvement (Stanford type A, DeBakey types I-II)
  - Treatment indications
    - Aortic rupture or concurrent aneurysm
    - Lower extremity or visceral ischemia
    - Persistent pain (exclude other etiologies)
  - Abdominal aortic dissection in presence of AAA should be treated due to high risk of rupture (28%)
    - Aortic wall weakened by dissection
    - > 90% mortality risk with rupture
    - Rupture site coincides with junction of dissection and aneurysm (60%)
  - Surveillance post-treatment includes clinic visit, Doppler US and CT at 1, 3, 6 and 12 months
    - Lifetime annual surveillance recommended
- Medical management reported mortality rate of 75%, when dissection associated with trauma
  - For patients with uncomplicated dissection and absent trauma history
    - Antihypertensive medications and close follow-up
- Better technical and clinical success rates for endovascular therapy; decreased morbidity/mortality
  - Stent graft placement within true lumen
  - Balloon fenestration creates sites for re-entry
- Surgical management varies with presentation
  - Treats lower extremity ischemia
  - In patients with persistent abdominal pain, surgical exploration to rule out other sources of pain
  - Aortic rupture and dissection may require open repair in unstable patient
    - Aortoiliac or aortofemoral bypass if iliac extension

DIAGNOSTIC CHECKLIST

Consider

- False lumen may be thrombosed
- Identify proximal and distal extent of dissection
  - May affect treatment planning

Image Interpretation Pearls

- Double-barreled aorta with differential enhancement in lumens suggests isolated abdominal aortic dissection

SELECTED REFERENCES

1. Trimarchi S et al: Acute abdominal aortic dissection: insight from the International Registry of Acute Aortic Dissection (IRAD). J Vasc Surg. 46(5):913-919, 2007
2. Farber A et al: Isolated dissection of the abdominal aorta: clinical presentation and therapeutic options. J Vasc Surg. 36(2):205-10, 2002

IMAGE GALLERY

Typical

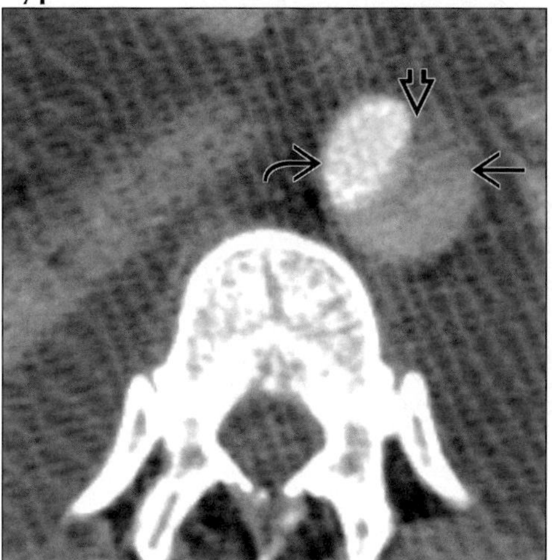

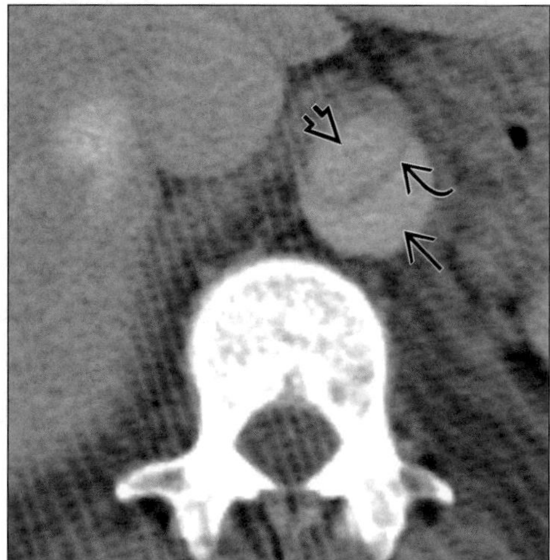

(Left) Axial CECT of an abdominal aortic dissection shows contrast opacification of the true lumen ⮫ and delayed opacification of the false lumen →. The intimal flap ⇨ is poorly seen due to a lack of contrast in the false lumen. (Right) Axial CECT with delayed imaging (same patient as previous image) clearly shows the intimal flap ⮫ with contrast in both the true ⇨ and false → lumens. The false lumen partially compresses the true lumen. There is delayed contrast washout in the false lumen.

Typical

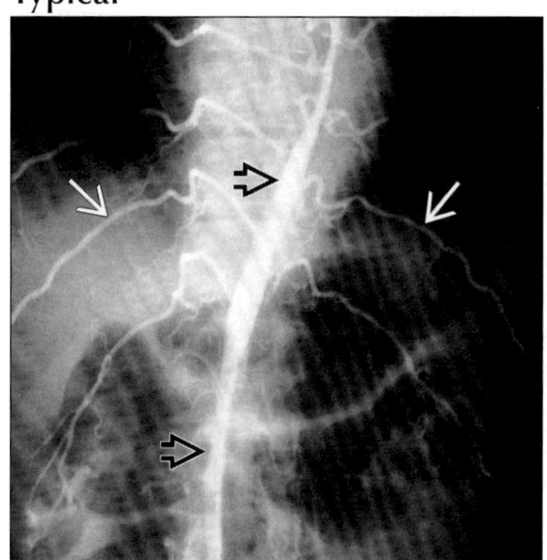

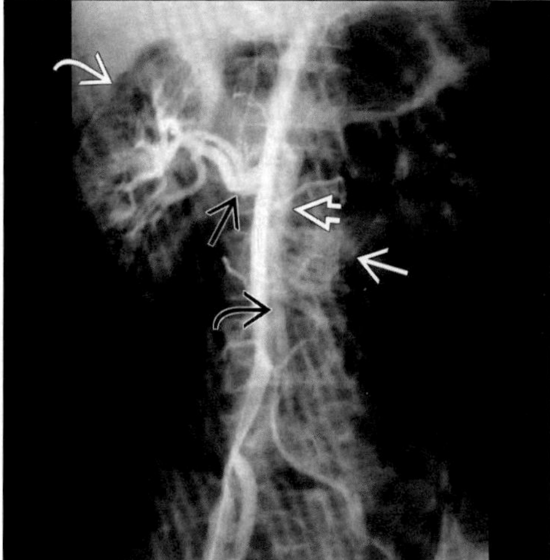

(Left) Catheter angiography of an aortic dissection shows an opacified, compressed, true lumen ⇨ in the initial phase of the contrast injection. Multiple intercostal arteries ➡ arise from this lumen, but no other aortic branches are seen. (Right) Later phase of the arteriogram (same patient) shows the less dense false lumen ⇨. The right renal artery →, SMA branches ➡ and a right nephrogram are now evident ⮫. The linear density ⮫ between the two lumens is the intimal flap.

Typical

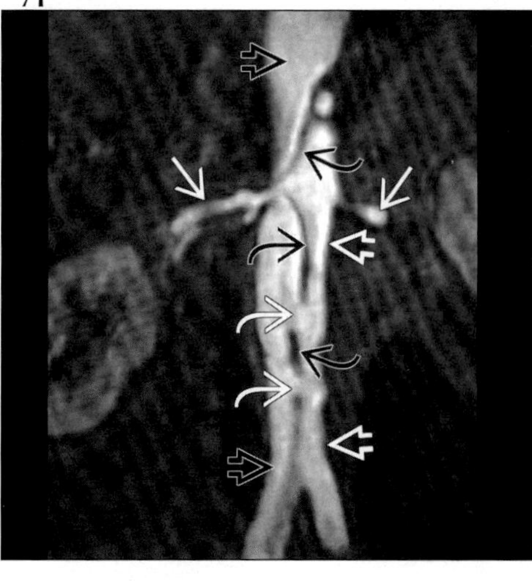

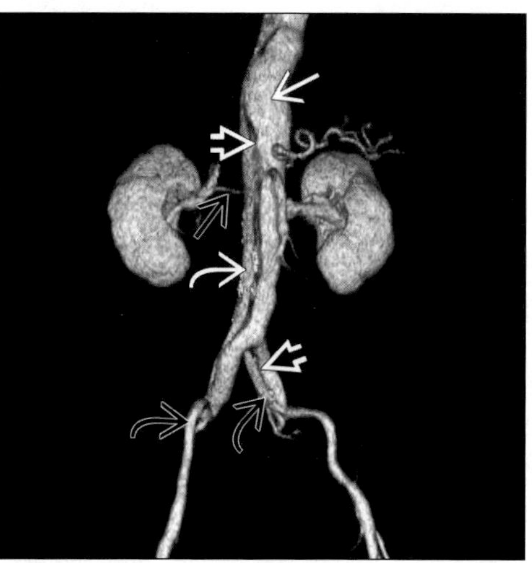

(Left) Coronal T2WI FSE MR shows an intimal flap ⮫ separating the true ⇨ and false ⇨ lumens, with fenestrations ⮫ that allow for re-entry points throughout the dissection. The renal arteries ➡ arise from the true lumen. (Right) 3-D CTA shows an intimal flap ⇨ separating the true ⮫ and false ➡ lumens of an aortic dissection. The right renal → and iliac arteries ⮫ arise from the true lumen, while the remaining branches originate from the false lumen.

ABDOMINAL AORTIC TRAUMA

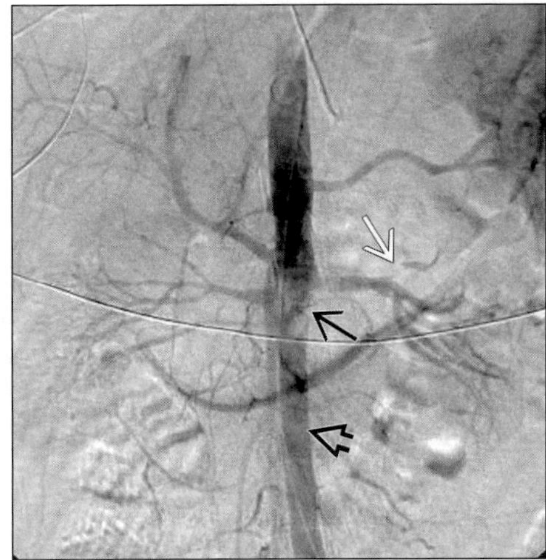

Posteroanterior DSA in a patient with severe trauma shows aortic irregularity ➔ near the renal arteries. The infrarenal aorta is less opacified ➔ than the segment above the injury. There is a left renal artery embolus ➔.

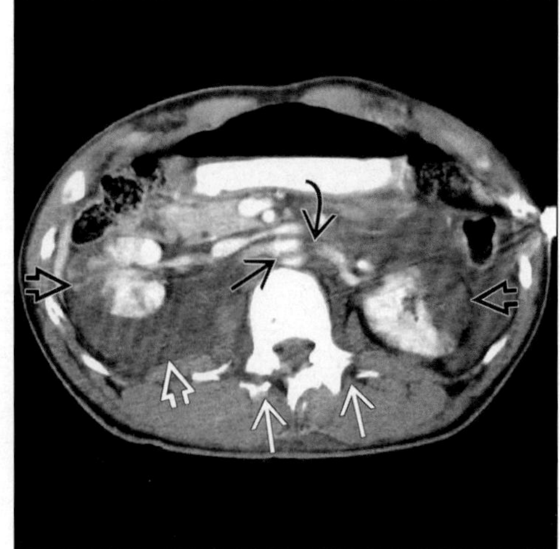

Axial CECT (same case as previous) shows an aortic transection ➔ involving the left renal artery ➔. Note: Bilateral renal infarcts ➔, right renal displacement by a retroperitoneal hematoma ➔, and spinal fractures ➔.

TERMINOLOGY

Abbreviations and Synonyms

- Abdominal aortic (Ao) rupture, transection, laceration; traumatic aortic dissection, seat belt syndrome

Definitions

- Trauma to abdominal aorta resulting in vascular injury
  - Commonly blunt force, can be penetrating

IMAGING FINDINGS

General Features

- Best diagnostic clue: Irregular appearance of abdominal aorta and retroperitoneal hematoma as well as appropriate clinical history
- Location
  - Abdominal aortic trauma accounts for 4.6% of aortic injuries
  - Infrarenal aorta most commonly involved
    - Most common site of injury: At or below origin of inferior mesenteric artery
    - Next most common: Renal artery level
  - Suprarenal aortic involvement relatively uncommon
    - Most common site of suprarenal involvement: Level of superior mesenteric artery

Radiographic Findings

- Radiography: Transverse fracture or dislocation of lumbar spine
- IVP
  - Abnormal nephrogram
    - Delayed or absent nephrogram ⇒ RA compromise
    - Wedge defects ⇒ emboli and infarct
    - Displaced kidney ⇒ retroperitoneal hematoma

CT Findings

- NECT
  - Abrupt caliber change of abdominal aorta
  - Periaortic hematoma
  - Retroperitoneal hematoma with or without kidney displacement
    - Fluid-fluid levels within hematoma show dependent high attenuation blood
  - High attenuation intramural hematoma
  - Peri-vascular stranding
  - Hemoperitoneum
  - Lumbar spine and other skeletal injury

DDx: Irregularity of Abdominal Aorta

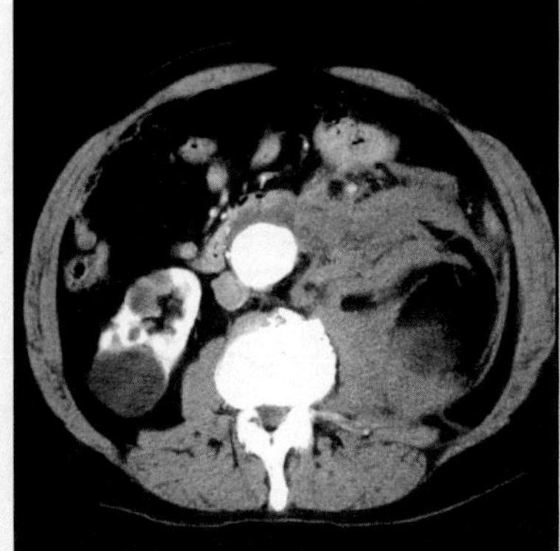

Ruptured Abdominal Ao Aneurysm

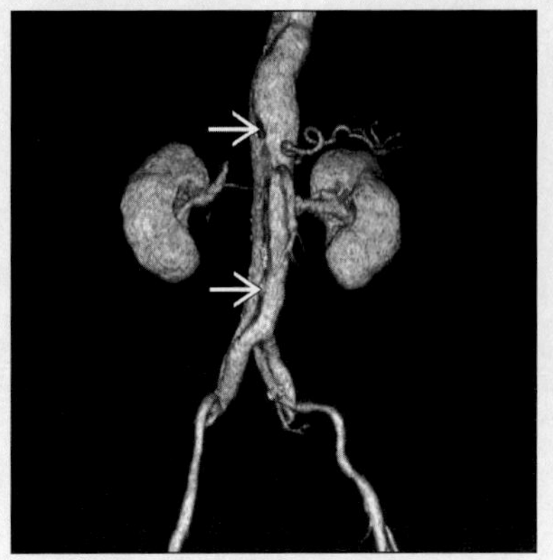

Aortic Dissection

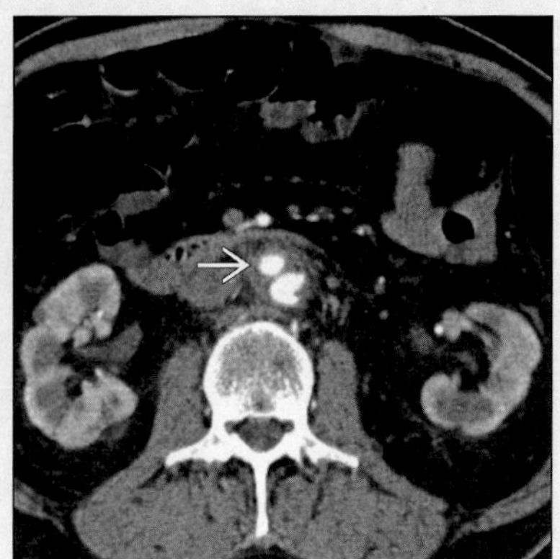

Aortitis with Pseudoaneurysm

ABDOMINAL AORTIC TRAUMA

Key Facts

Terminology
- Abdominal aortic (Ao) rupture, transection, laceration; traumatic aortic dissection, seat belt syndrome

Imaging Findings
- Best imaging clue: Irregular appearance of abdominal aorta and retroperitoneal hematoma as well as appropriate clinical history
- Most common site of injury: At or below origin of inferior mesenteric artery
- Abrupt caliber change of abdominal aorta
- Contrast-filled pseudoaneurysm
- Thrombosis

Pathology
- Direct crush injury of aorta against lumbar spine

Clinical Issues
- Acute blunt abdominal aortic trauma is frequently fatal
  - Significant morbidity for survivors of initial injury
- Absent/decreased peripheral pulses (94%), usually bilateral
- Solid organ and hollow viscus injury
- Bony injury, particularly transverse spinal fracture-dislocation
- Atherosclerotic aorta less distensible with weakened intima; more easily traumatized

Diagnostic Checklist
- Have high index of suspicion in patient with appropriate mechanism of injury
- Missed or delayed diagnosis (≤ 1/3 of cases) = higher mortality rate

- CECT
  - Low attenuation intimal flap in aortic lumen
  - Contrast-filled pseudoaneurysm
  - Thrombosis
  - Solid organ and hollow viscus injury
  - Intramural hematoma
  - Visceral vessel injury
  - Contrast extravasation
  - Aortic laceration
- CTA: Can have similar findings to CECT, but improved delineation of abnormality with higher density contrast

MR Findings
- T1WI
  - Acute retroperitoneal hematoma has same signal intensity as muscle
    - Large acute hematomas with fluid-fluid levels have hyperintense dependent segments relative to supernatant
  - Flow voids within aorta if not thrombosed
- T2WI
  - Acute retroperitoneal hematoma has hypointense signal
    - Hematomas with fluid-fluid levels have supernatant that is hyperintense relative to dependent portion
- T1 C+
  - Contrast within aortic lumen and pseudoaneurysm
  - Intimal flap
- MRA
  - Irregular aortic contour
  - Pseudoaneurysm
  - Intimal flap

Ultrasonographic Findings
- Grayscale Ultrasound
  - Echogenic thrombus within aorta
  - Echogenic intimal flap
  - Mixed echogenicity retroperitoneal hematoma surrounding aorta
- Color Doppler
  - Disorganized flow within aorta near intimal injury
  - Absent flow = thrombosis

Angiographic Findings
- DSA
  - Irregular aortic contour; caliber change
  - Dissection flap with true and false lumens
  - Thrombosis
  - Non-visualization of involved visceral branches
  - Distal embolization

Imaging Recommendations
- Best imaging tool: CECT with multiplanar reformations
- Protocol advice
  - NECT, CTA and delayed imaging, if feasible
  - Evaluation of hematoma, aortic injury and extravasation
  - Evaluation of other abdominal structures

DIFFERENTIAL DIAGNOSIS

Ruptured Abdominal Aortic Aneurysm
- Dilated infrarenal aorta(> 5 cm)
- Stranding of peri-aortic fat
- Retroperitoneal hematoma or fluid

Aortic Dissection
- Aortic size may be within normal limits
- Intimal flap with true and false lumens
- No retroperitoneal abnormality

Aortitis
- Normal to diminished caliber aorta
- Pseudoaneurysm formation
- Peri-aortic stranding

Abdominal Aortic Aneurysm
- Dilated infrarenal aorta (> 5 cm)
- Mural thrombus
- No retroperitoneal abnormality

Penetrating Aortic Ulcer
- Focal involvement of aorta

ABDOMINAL AORTIC TRAUMA

- Penetrates intima and involves media
  - Hematoma formation occurs within media
  - Intima is displaced centrally, and often calcified
- Can result in dissection, aneurysm or rupture

PATHOLOGY

General Features

- Etiology
  - Direct crush injury of aorta against lumbar spine
  - Automobile accidents
    - Seat belt or steering wheel injury
  - Blunt abdominal trauma of various etiologies
    - Fall from heights
    - Blow to abdomen
  - Penetrating trauma

Gross Pathologic & Surgical Features

- Intimal defects ± dissection
- Intraluminal thrombus ± thrombosis
- Pseudoaneurysm
- Aortic rupture
- Aortic contusion
  - Intramural hematoma
- Subintimal fibrosis
- Atheromatous emboli

CLINICAL ISSUES

Presentation

- Most common signs/symptoms
  - Acute blunt abdominal aortic trauma frequently fatal
    - Absent/decreased peripheral pulses (94%), usually bilateral
    - Acute abdomen (48%)
    - Lower extremity neurologic deficit (38%)
    - Abdominal wall contusion (38%)
    - Acute abdominal distension
    - Hypovolemic shock
  - Chronic or delayed diagnosis
    - Diminished pulses (52%)
    - Abdominal mass (43%)
    - Abdominal bruit (33%)
    - Claudication
- Other signs/symptoms
  - Acute
    - Abdominal wall defect (10%)
    - Abdominal mass (5%)
    - Abdominal bruit (5%)
    - Abdominal wall ecchymosis
  - Associated injuries
    - Solid organ and hollow viscus injury
    - Bony injury, particularly transverse spinal fracture-dislocation
    - Vascular injury with visceral ischemia ± infarct
    - Peripheral embolization
    - Paralysis and paresthesia

Demographics

- Age
  - Affects adults in third and fourth decades
  - Rarely involves pediatric population
  - Atherosclerotic aorta less distensible with weakened intima; more easily traumatized
- Gender: Male to female ratio ~ 2:1

Natural History & Prognosis

- High mortality with initial injury
  - ↑ Chance of death with diagnostic delay > 12 hours
  - ↑ Likelihood of death with increasing age
- Significant morbidity for survivors of initial injury
  - Related to initial arterial compromise or associated injuries
  - Neurologic deficits related to initial injury or surgical aortic cross clamp time
  - Sepsis
- Rarely, post-traumatic abdominal aortic pseudoaneurysm can occur years after initial trauma
  - Seen mostly with penetrating injuries
  - Rupture is main cause of mortality with diagnostic delay
- Aortic thrombosis

Treatment

- Endovascular repair with stent graft placement
- Surgical
  - Vascular bypass surgery
    - Temporary and extra-anatomic if bowel contamination present
  - Thrombectomy
  - Intimal repair
- Non-operative management
  - 75% mortality rate
  - Close observation for minor intimal injuries

DIAGNOSTIC CHECKLIST

Consider

- Have high index of suspicion in patient with appropriate mechanism of injury
  - Missed or delayed diagnosis (≤ 1/3 of cases) = higher mortality rate

Image Interpretation Pearls

- Retroperitoneal hematoma and lumbar fracture = significant aortic trauma may be present

SELECTED REFERENCES

1. Nucifora G et al: Blunt traumatic abdominal aortic rupture: CT imaging. Emerg Radiol. 2007
2. Borioni R et al: Posttraumatic infrarenal abdominal aortic pseudoaneurysm. Tex Heart Inst J. 26(4):312-4, 1999
3. Roth SM et al: Blunt injury of the abdominal aorta: a review. J Trauma. 42(4):748-55, 1997
4. Israel L et al: Abdominal aortic injury in blunt abdominal trauma. Emerg Radiol. 3(6):296-7, 1996
5. Lupetin AR et al: CT diagnosis of traumatic abdominal aortic rupture. J Comput Assist Tomogr. 14(2):313-4, 1990
6. Lock JS et al: Blunt trauma to the abdominal aorta. J Trauma. 27(6):674-7, 1987
7. Nizzero A et al: Blunt trauma to the abdominal aorta. CMAJ. 135(3):219-20, 1986
8. Lassonde J et al: Blunt injury of the abdominal aorta. Ann Surg. 194(6):745-8, 1981

IMAGE GALLERY

Typical

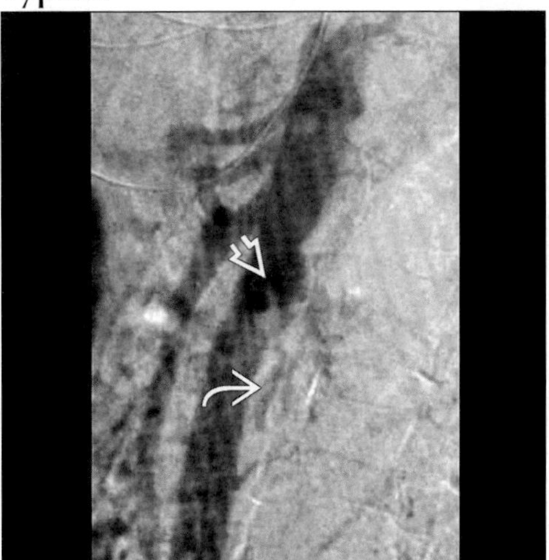

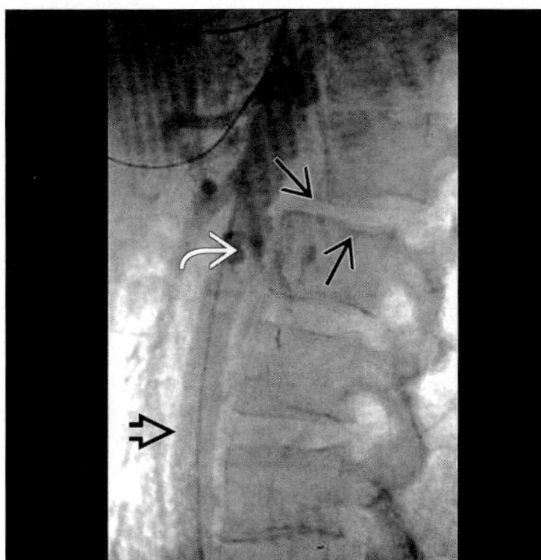

*(**Left**) Lateral DSA in a patient who suffered a seatbelt injury during a high impact automobile accident shows aortic irregularity ➡ at the level of the renal arteries. The right renal artery ➡ is displaced anteriorly as a result of a very large retroperitoneal hematoma. (**Right**) Lateral DSA (same case as previous) shows a spinal fracture-dislocation ➡ with aortic narrowing ➡ at L2 level. Note decreased contrast ➡ within infrarenal aorta below injury.*

Typical

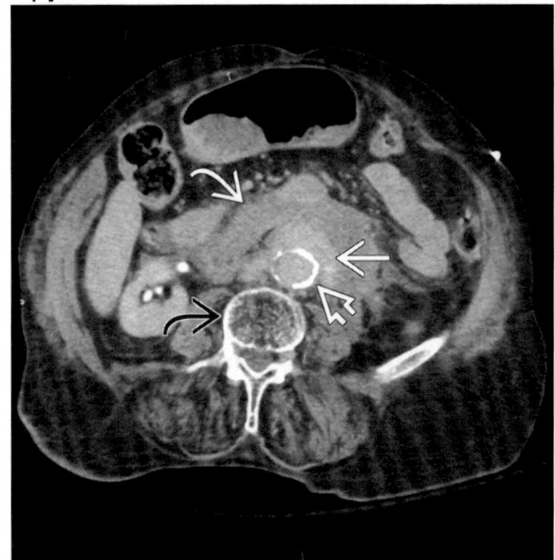

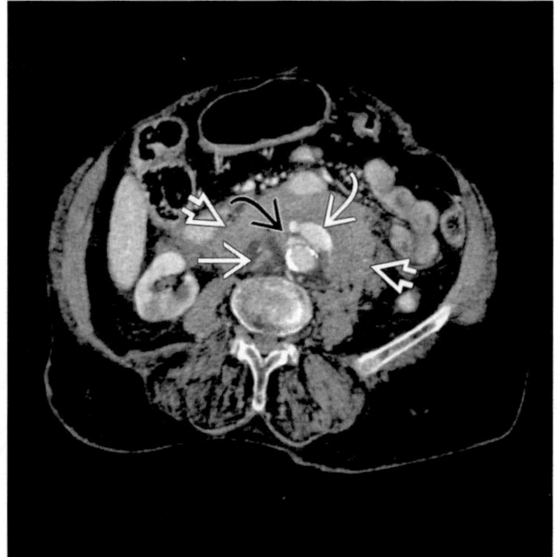

*(**Left**) Axial NECT shows a highly calcified, nonaneurysmal abdominal aorta ➡ surrounded by mixed attenuation hemorrhage ➡. Higher attenuation hemorrhage ➡ is more acute. Adjacent lumbar vertebra ➡ is intact. (**Right**) Axial CECT in the same case as previous, shows a retroperitoneal hematoma ➡ surrounding the aorta. The aorta is calcified with dissection flap ➡ and a pseudoaneurysm ➡. The IVC ➡ also has an irregular appearance.*

Typical

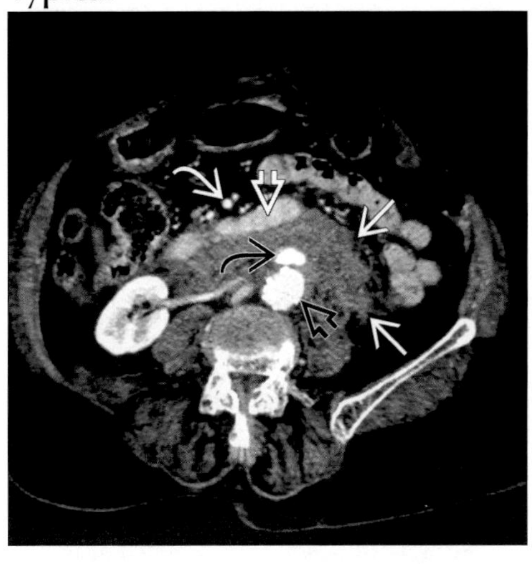

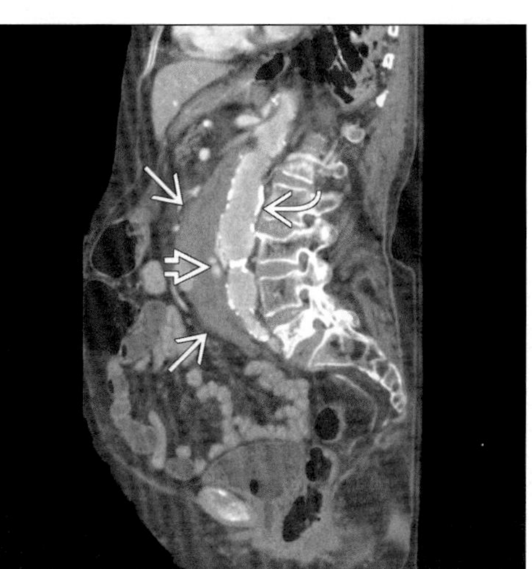

*(**Left**) Axial CTA shows contrast in the abdominal aorta ➡. Anterior to the aorta there is a contrast-filled pseudoaneurysm ➡. A retroperitoneal hematoma ➡ displaces the bowel ➡ anteriorly. SMA branches ➡ remain perfused. (**Right**) Sagittal CECT (same case as previous) shows narrowing ➡ of the distal aorta and a pseudoaneurysm ➡ anterior to the aorta. Note the retroperitoneal hematoma ➡ and the calcified aortic wall ➡. The lumbar alignment is intact.*

SUPERIOR MESENTERIC ARTERY EMBOLUS

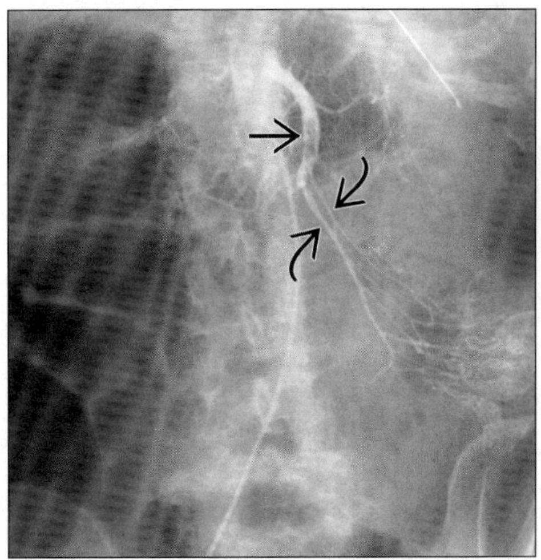

Abdominal aortogram shows a large embolus ➔ within the proximal SMA, occluding almost all distal branches. Only two small jejunal branches ➚ remain perfused. This patient expired from massive bowel infarction.

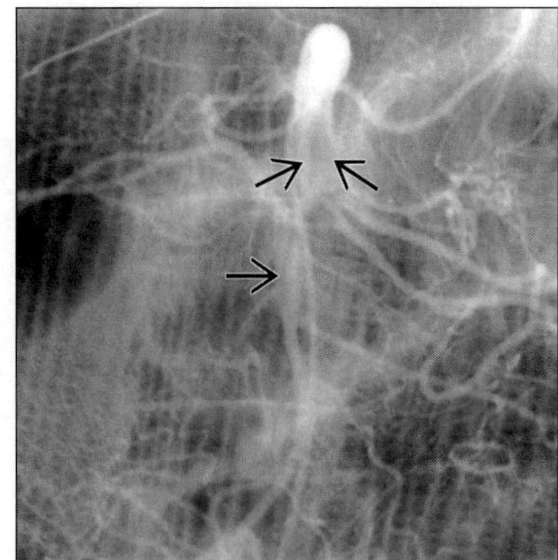

Selective superior mesenteric arteriogram shows a large filling defect ➔ within the main trunk of the SMA. The jejunal and distal SMA branches are contrast filled, indicating that this embolus is only partially occlusive.

TERMINOLOGY

Abbreviations and Synonyms

- Superior mesenteric artery (SMA) embolus
- Acute mesenteric ischemia (AMI)
- Intestinal angina

Definitions

- SMA embolus results in acute mesenteric ischemia from obstruction of arterial supply to bowel

IMAGING FINDINGS

Radiographic Findings

- Ileus may be early finding and later may show evidence of bowel wall edema ("thumbprinting") or pneumatosis

CT Findings

- CECT
  - CTA may show filling defect in SMA and poor filling of arterial branches distally
  - Focal lack of bowel wall enhancement, bowel dilatation and bowel wall thickening
  - Mesenteric inflammatory changes, pneumatosis intestinalis, free intraperitoneal air or free fluid

Angiographic Findings

- Intraluminal filling defect corresponding to embolus
- Poorly filling or non-opacified SMA arterial branches distally
- Lack of bowel enhancement in nonperfused vascular territories
- May help in surgical planning by identifying appropriate sites for vascular bypass grafts

Imaging Recommendations

- Best imaging tool
  - Noninvasive imaging modalities: CECT with CTA and occasionally gadolinium-enhanced 3-D MR
  - Angiography remains valuable imaging modality in suspected acute mesenteric ischemia
    - Definitive in confirming embolic occlusion and in demonstrating which arteries remain patent
    - Use is controversial and must be individualized, as delay in treatment may outweigh benefits

DDx: Mesenteric Ischemia

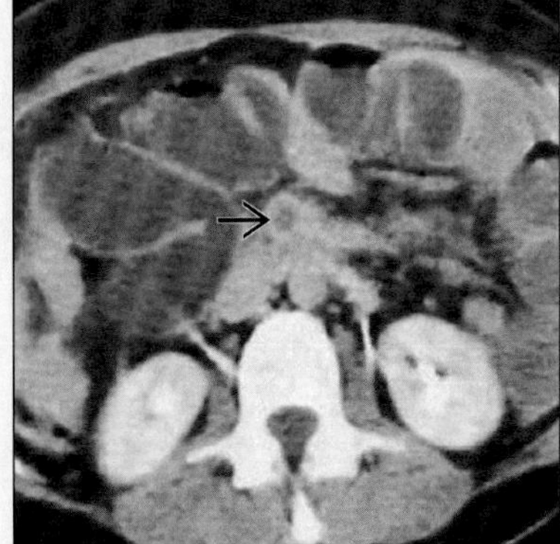

Mesenteric Venous Thrombosis

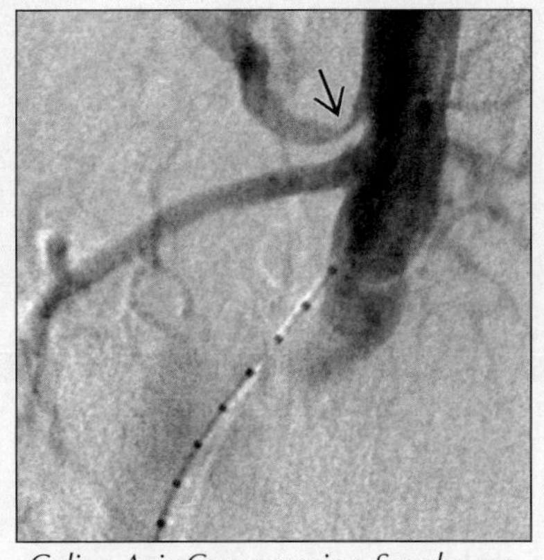

Celiac Axis Compression Syndrome

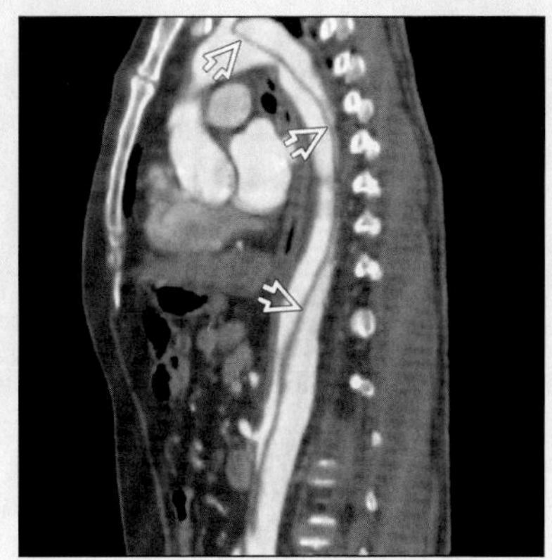

Aortic Dissection

SUPERIOR MESENTERIC ARTERY EMBOLUS

Key Facts

Imaging Findings

- Angiography remains valuable imaging modality in suspected acute mesenteric ischemia
- Definitive in confirming embolic occlusion and demonstrating which arteries remain patent
- Use is controversial and must be individualized, as delay in treatment may outweigh benefits

Top Differential Diagnoses

- Acute Mesenteric Ischemia from other causes
- Chronic Mesenteric Ischemia
- Celiac Axis Compression Syndrome
    - Controversial entity with often poorly manifested symptoms; in only 1/3 of patients abdominal pain clearly postprandial
- Other Causes of Severe Abdominal Pain

Clinical Issues

- Severe abdominal pain with sudden dramatic onset
- Accompanying onset of diarrhea (often bloody)
- Associated simultaneous peripheral vascular embolus in approximately 20% of patients
- Clinical Profile: Older patient with history of cardiac disease who presents with sudden dramatic onset of severe abdominal pain accompanied by diarrhea
- Mortality rate of acute intestinal ischemia from all causes exceeds 80%, with time to diagnosis and treatment as primary survival determinant
- In most patients, surgical embolectomy or bypass, with resection of nonviable bowel usually necessary
- Extent of intestinal infarction is a predictor of adverse outcome, but neither age nor gender is a determinant for extent of infarction

DIFFERENTIAL DIAGNOSIS

Acute Mesenteric Ischemia from Other Causes

- Non-occlusive mesenteric ischemia
    - Responsible for approximately 20-30% of cases of acute mesenteric ischemia, with high mortality rate
    - Usual setting of systemic illness with circulatory insufficiency, end-organ shock, and splanchnic vasoconstriction from systemic hypotension
    - May persist after correcting cause of hypotension, as normal autoregulatory mechanisms fail to allow reperfusion before intestinal necrosis occurs
    - Intestinal mucosal permeability increases in direct proportion to duration and severity of vasoconstriction
    - Angiography shows diffuse arterial vasospasm, impaired filling of distal arterial branches and delayed mesenteric vein filling
    - In absence of intestinal infarction, best treated with stabilization of cardiovascular status
    - Further treatment with selective intra-arterial SMA papaverine bolus (45-60 mg) followed by continuous transcatheter infusion therapy
    - Following infusion therapy, exploratory laparotomy and resection of infarcted bowel as necessary
- Superior mesenteric artery thrombosis
    - Usually occurs in patients with underlying atherosclerotic lesion
    - History of intestinal angina in 50% of patients
    - Angiography may demonstrate
        - SMA typically occluded near origin, without a meniscus or intraluminal filling defect
        - Collaterals sometimes reconstituting distal SMA beyond the acute occlusion
    - If peritoneal signs present, treat surgically with thromboendarterectomy or bypass
    - In absence of peritoneal signs may consider thrombolysis followed by angioplasty or intravascular stent
- Mesenteric venous thrombosis
    - Accounts for 5-10% of acute mesenteric ischemia
    - Associated with portal hypertension, trauma, hypercoagulability, abdominal inflammatory disease, oral contraceptives and prior surgery
    - If inadequate venous collaterals, will develop intestinal mucosal edema and resultant arterial hypoperfusion
    - Angiographic findings of arterial flow resistance, prolonged arterial phase, lack of mesenteric vein opacification, and mesenteric or portal thrombus
    - Treat by stabilizing cardiovascular status, volume replacement, resection of nonviable bowel, and pre-operative and post-operative anticoagulation
- Aortic dissection
    - Acute mesenteric ischemia seen in 5% of patients with aortic dissection
    - High-operative mortality (90%)
    - Dissection flap extends to occlude mesenteric arteries, resulting in poorly perfused bowel
    - May attempt endovascular treatments (angioplasty, stents) to re-establish perfusion

Chronic Mesenteric Ischemia

- Less common than acute mesenteric ischemia because of rich mesenteric collateral circulation
- Significant stenosis or occlusion of at least two mesenteric arteries usually necessary
- Failure to achieve normal postprandial arterial intestinal flow is basic mechanism of chronic intestinal ischemia
- Postprandial pain is defining symptom with onset 30 to 45 minutes following meal; may be associated with nausea, vomiting, diarrhea or malabsorption
- Angiography is definitive imaging modality, but CECT with CTA and gadolinium-enhanced MRA also employed
- Duplex ultrasonography may identify high grade stenotic lesions by demonstrating elevated fasting SMA and/or celiac arterial peak systolic velocities
- Treatment consists of either surgical revascularization (endarterectomy or mesenteric bypass) or endovascular treatment (angioplasty and stent)

Celiac Axis Compression Syndrome

- Compression of celiac artery by median arcuate ligament of diaphragm, pronounced during expiration
- Controversial entity with often poorly manifested symptoms; in only 1/3 of patients abdominal pain clearly postprandial
- Some argue compression merely a marker of excessive celiac ganglion splanchnic nerve entrapment
- Pain relief from surgical decompression may actually result from destruction of splanchnic nerves
- Many patients have history of psychiatric disorder, substance abuse or prior abdominal surgery

Other Causes of Severe Abdominal Pain

- Arteritis, inflammatory bowel disease, neoplasm, pancreatitis, peptic ulcer disease etc.

PATHOLOGY

General Features

- Etiology
  - Most emboli originate from a cardiac source
    - Other sources of emboli are aneurysms, proximal aortic atherosclerotic or thrombotic disease and iatrogenic emboli from intravascular procedures
    - Emboli from noncardiac sources tend to be smaller and thus lodge more distally affecting bowel more locally
- Epidemiology: SMA embolus is most common cause of acute mesenteric ischemia (40-50% of cases)

CLINICAL ISSUES

Presentation

- Most common signs/symptoms
  - Severe abdominal pain with sudden dramatic onset
  - Accompanying onset of diarrhea (often bloody)
  - Frequent history of cardiac arrhythmia
- Other signs/symptoms
  - Associated simultaneous peripheral vascular embolus in approximately 20% of patients
  - Prior history of another embolic event in 30-40% of patients
- Clinical Profile: Older patient with history of cardiac disease who presents with sudden dramatic onset of severe abdominal pain accompanied by diarrhea

Demographics

- Age: Often affects elderly patients with ischemic heart disease and atrial fibrillation

Natural History & Prognosis

- Mortality rate of acute intestinal ischemia from all causes exceeds 80%, with time to diagnosis and treatment as primary survival determinant
- Slightly more favorable prognosis with SMA embolus vs. SMA thrombosis, as emboli often lodge distally in SMA, allowing partial perfusion of proximal intestine
  - Large emboli may initially lodge in proximal SMA, then progress distally and stop beyond first jejunal branches, sparing proximal jejunum from ischemia
  - Proximal occlusion and obstruction of potential collateral pathways causes profound ischemia
- Bowel ischemia can rapidly progress to infarction
- High clinical suspicion, early diagnosis and aggressive intervention are keys to favorable outcome

Treatment

- Options, risks, complications
  - In most patients, surgical embolectomy or bypass, with resection of nonviable bowel usually necessary
    - Proximal occlusions likely to be more accessible to vascular reconstructions than distal occlusions
    - After revascularization, bowel is assessed for viability and infarcted bowel resected
    - Bowel of uncertain viability is left and later reassessed with second-look surgery, so as to preserve as much bowel as possible
    - High frequency of cardiac thrombi after embolic occlusion of SMA emphasizes importance of prophylaxis with optimal anticoagulation
  - May consider catheter-based intervention when clinical status and imaging suggest viable bowel; thrombolysis and suction embolectomy utilized
- Extent of intestinal infarction is a predictor of adverse outcome, but neither age nor gender is a determinant for extent of infarction
- Early diagnosis and treatment are most important factors associated with morbidity and mortality

DIAGNOSTIC CHECKLIST

Consider

- SMA embolus in patient with history of cardiac disease who presents with sudden onset of profound abdominal pain accompanied by bloody diarrhea
- Very selective and judicious use of angiography given high mortality rate if delay in diagnosis and treatment
- Urgent surgical exploration if high clinical suspicion for SMA embolus

SELECTED REFERENCES

1. Acosta S et al: Clinical implications for the management of acute thromboembolic occlusion of the superior mesenteric artery: autopsy findings in 213 patients. Ann Surg. 241(3):516-22, 2005
2. Yasuhara H: Acute mesenteric ischemia: the challenge of gastroenterology. Surg Today. 35(3):185-95, 2005
3. Bingol H et al: Surgical therapy for acute superior mesenteric artery embolism. Am J Surg. 188(1):68-70, 2004
4. Wakabayashi H et al: Emergent treatment of acute embolic superior mesenteric ischemia with combination of thrombolysis and angioplasty: report of two cases. Cardiovasc Intervent Radiol. 27(4):389-93, 2004
5. Sato O et al: Emergency CT scan for the diagnosis of superior mesenteric artery embolism. Report of 2 cases. Int Angiol. 22(4):438-40, 2003
6. Barakate MS et al: Management of acute superior mesenteric artery occlusion. ANZ J Surg. 72(1):25-9, 2002
7. Greenwald DA et al: Ischemic bowel disease in the elderly. Gastroenterol Clin North Am. 30(2):445-73, 2001
8. Alaeddini J et al: Thoraco-abdominal aortic thrombosis and superior mesenteric artery embolism. Tex Heart Inst J. 27(3):318-9, 2000

SUPERIOR MESENTERIC ARTERY EMBOLUS

IMAGE GALLERY

Variant

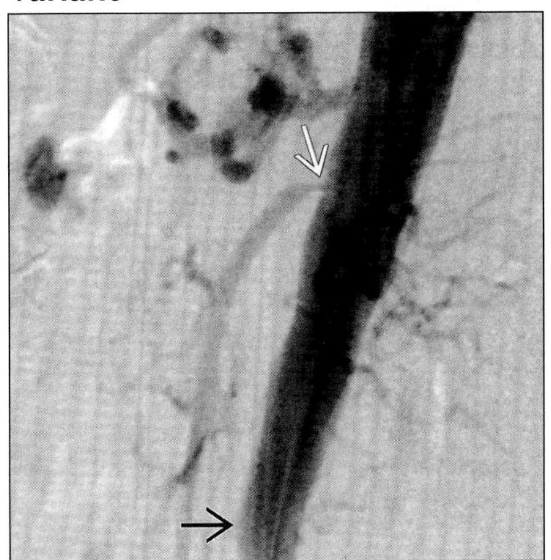

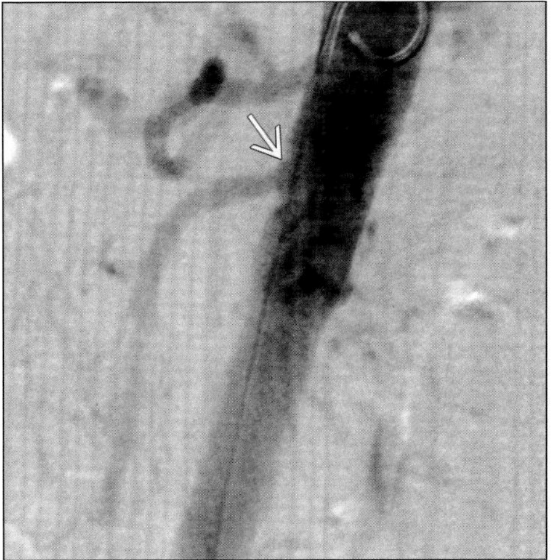

(Left) *Lateral abdominal aortogram shows a high grade stenosis at the origin of the superior mesenteric artery* → *and occlusion of the inferior mesenteric artery* →*. This patient had classic symptoms of chronic mesenteric ischemia.* ***(Right)*** *Lateral abdominal aortogram in the same patient as previous image, shows that the previously demonstrated SMA origin stenosis has been treated and corrected* → *with intravascular stent placement.*

Variant

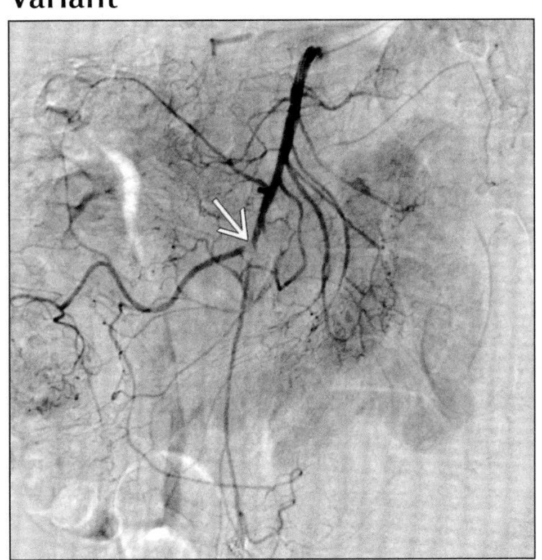

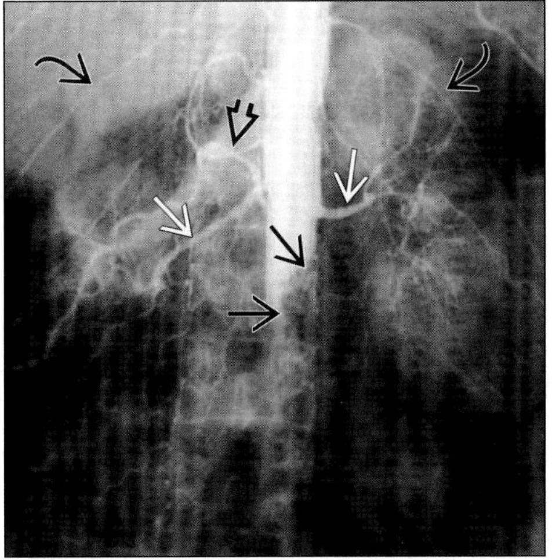

(Left) *SMA arteriogram (same patient as previous image) shows small distal embolus* →*. This was an iatrogenic complication of stent placement, but because embolus was only partially occlusive, patient was asymptomatic.* ***(Right)*** *Aortogram in another patient shows massive occlusive embolus* → *in infrarenal aorta. Renal* →*, intercostal* → *& lumbar* → *arteries are patent but visceral vessels are occluded by emboli. Patient expired from massive bowel infarction.*

Typical

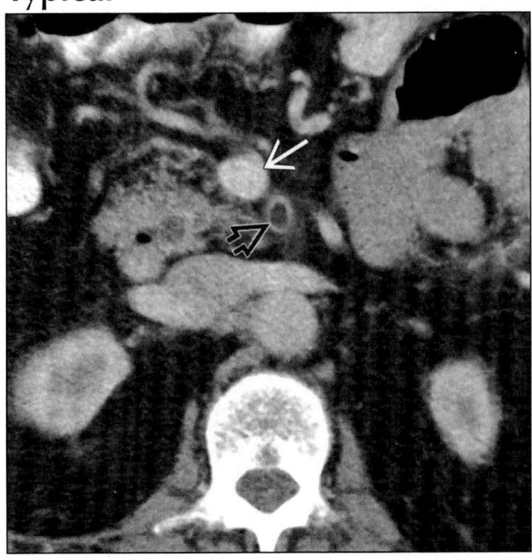

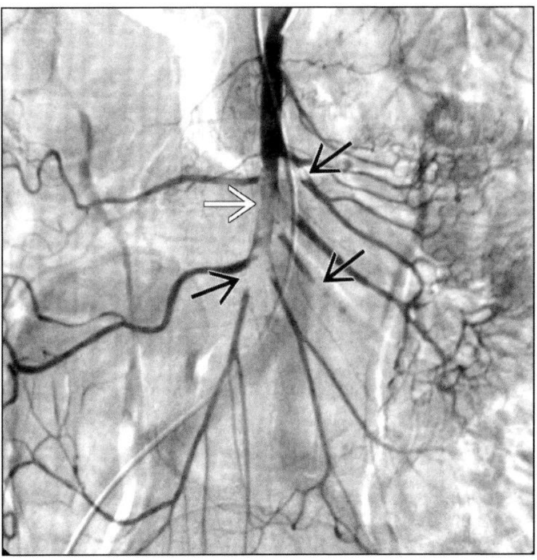

(Left) *Axial CECT shows an embolus* → *in the main trunk of the SMA. The superior mesenteric vein* → *is adjacent. This patient with known atrial fibrillation presented with acute severe abdominal pain.* ***(Right)*** *Superior mesenteric arteriogram in the same patient as previous image shows the large embolus* → *within the main trunk of the SMA. As the embolus traveled distally, portions extended into branch vessels* → *with resultant multifocal areas of arterial occlusion.*

NONOCCLUSIVE MESENTERIC ISCHEMIA

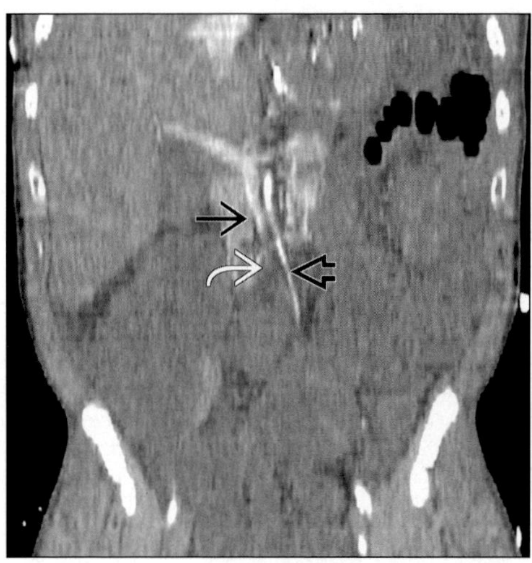

Coronal CECT shows some flow through the proximal SMA ➪, but this appears to become more attenuated, and no branch vessels are seen. SMV ➔ filling close to portal vein, but not distally ➦.

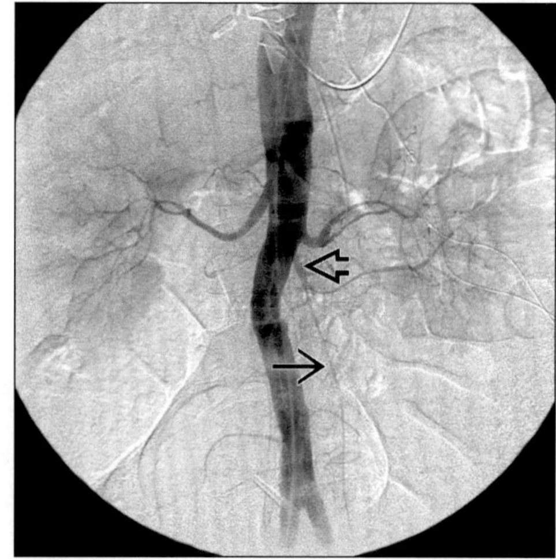

DSA shows relatively normal aorta with narrowing of all the vessels, consistent with shock. The SMA is seen proximally ➪, but extremely small vessels are seen distally ➔.

TERMINOLOGY

Abbreviations and Synonyms

- Nonocclusive mesenteric ischemia (NOMI), shock bowel

Definitions

- Intestinal gangrene with patent arterial tree
- Mesenteric ischemia without occlusion of mesenteric arteries

IMAGING FINDINGS

General Features

- Best diagnostic clue: Narrowing of mesenteric arteries

Imaging Recommendations

- Best imaging tool
  - Mesenteric angiography
    - Due to microvascular constriction, angiography most reliably demonstrates early NOMI diagnosis
    - Hypotensive or hypovolemic patients show mesenteric vasoconstriction
    - Origins of mesenteric vessels usually patent; narrowing of proximal vessels; poor visualization of distal vessels
    - Delayed filling of peripheral branches of mesenteric vessels
    - Delayed opacification of mesenteric veins
    - In severe NOMI, vasoconstriction present in superior and inferior mesenteric arteries, celiac trunk; possibly, renal arteries
    - Reflux of contrast into abdominal aorta when injection done into mesenteric arteries due to resistance to forward flow
    - Spread out segmental arteries due to distension of bowel loops
    - "Pruned" appearance of mesenteric tree
    - Narrowing of at least two branches of superior mesenteric artery (SMA)
    - "String of sausages sign": Alternating dilation and constriction of major arteries
    - Reversibility of angiographic findings with administration of papaverine
  - Abdominal film

DDx: Nonocclusive Mesenteric Ischemia

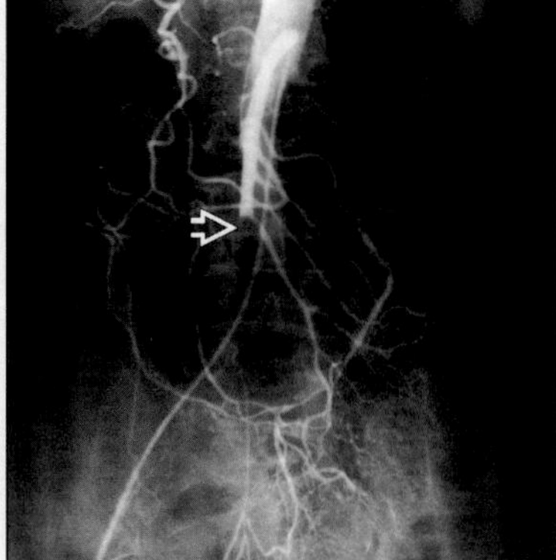

SMA Embolus, Abrupt Cutoff

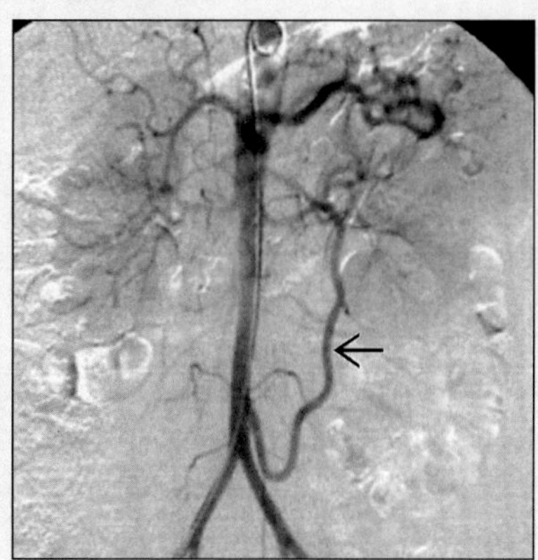

Chronic SMA Occlusion Collateral

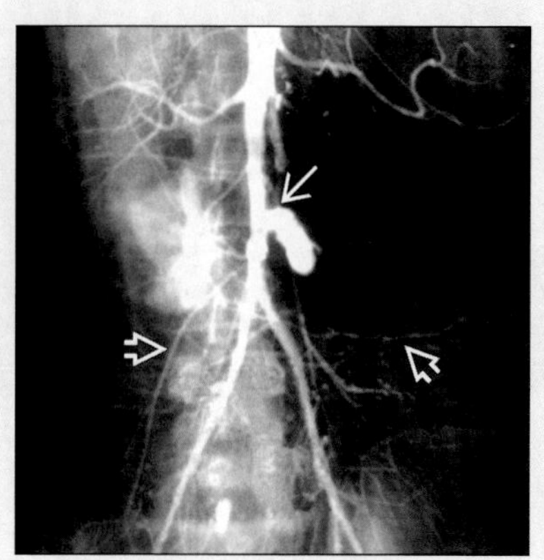

Shock: Aortoenteric Fistula

NONOCCLUSIVE MESENTERIC ISCHEMIA

Key Facts

Terminology

- Intestinal gangrene with patent arterial tree
- Nonocclusive mesenteric ischemia (NOMI); shockbowel

Imaging Findings

- Mesenteric angiography
  - Origins of mesenteric vessels patent; narrowing of proximal vessels; poor visualization of distal vessels
  - Delayed opacification of mesenteric veins
  - Delayed filling of peripheral branches of mesenteric vessels
- Computed tomography
  - SMA enhancement may be markedly diminished
  - Absence of bowel wall enhancement, thickening of bowel wall

Pathology

- Blood shunted to central circulation to maintain perfusion of brain and heart
- Mesenteric vasoconstriction
- Most have underlying cardiovascular disease
- Most have had hypotension or sepsis event
- High mortality rate (40-100%)

Clinical Issues

- Gradual onset of cramping, periumbilical abdominal pain out of proportion to minimal physical findings
- Mesenteric angiography and direct infusion of papaverine via superior mesenteric artery to treat mesenteric vasoconstriction and reverse bowel ischemia

---

- "Thumb-printing" of bowel wall, intramural air, portal venous air, free intraperitoneal air; usually present at late stage, possible bowel infarction
- Intramural gas bubbles in portal vein
- Ultrasonography
  - Lack of flow in proximal mesenteric arteries
- Computed tomography
  - See proximal mesenteric arteries but poor visualization of smaller branches
  - Superior mesenteric artery enhancement may be markedly diminished
  - Superior mesenteric vein enhancement will also be markedly diminished
  - Demonstrates findings of mesenteric ischemia
  - Absence of bowel wall enhancement, thickening of bowel wall
  - Intramural hemorrhage
  - Focal or diffuse intraperitoneal fluid collections
  - Intestinal pneumatosis
  - Portal venous gas collections
  - Inhomogeneous contrast-enhancement of mucosa with venous thrombosis
  - Exclude other causes of mesenteric ischemia

DIFFERENTIAL DIAGNOSIS

Mesenteric Arterial Occlusion

- Thrombosis
  - Occlusion of mesenteric vessels
  - Atherosclerotic changes
- Embolism
  - Filling defect in mesenteric vessels

Splanchnic Venous Thrombosis

- Thrombosis of superior mesenteric vein

Causes of Low Flow State and Decreased Cardiac Output

- Septic shock
- Hypovolemic shock
- Hemorrhagic shock
- Anaphylaxis

PATHOLOGY

General Features

- Etiology
  - Mesenteric vasoconstriction
    - Shunts blood into central circulation to maintain perfusion of brain and heart during systemic hypotension
    - If NOMI fails to resolve, may result in bowel infarction
  - Intestinal hypoxia
  - Ischemia-reperfusion injury
    - Hypoxia followed by generation of oxygen free radical metabolites during reperfusion
  - Increased intestinal metabolic demand
  - Infection
    - Seen in young males who ingest large amounts of pork: "Pig-belly"
    - Spontaneously reversible; can lead to necrosis and death (rare)
    - Clostridium welchii present in most cases
  - Pancreatitis
    - Superior mesenteric artery in close proximity to celiac plexus to the pancreas; inflamed pancreas stimulates vasoconstriction
  - 9-20% of deaths in dialysis-dependent patients due to NOMI
    - Triggering factor of NOMI in hemodialysis patients is a hypotensive episode
- Epidemiology
  - Most have underlying cardiovascular disease
  - Most have had hypotension or sepsis event
  - High mortality rate (40-100%)
  - Causes for vasoconstriction including digitalis, ergots, vasopressin or other pressors, amphetamine, cocaine
  - NOMI accounts for 20-60% of patients with intestinal ischemia

Gross Pathologic & Surgical Features

- Splanchnic vasoconstriction leading to decreased mesenteric blood flow

NONOCCLUSIVE MESENTERIC ISCHEMIA

- Ischemic necrosis
  - Reperfusion injury may lead to ischemic damage
  - Superoxide and hydrogen peroxide generated during metabolism of ATP lead to lipid peroxidation and damage to biological membranes

CLINICAL ISSUES

Presentation

- Most common signs/symptoms
  - Patient hypotension, decreased cardiac output, shock, preceding development of abdominal pain
  - Gradual onset of cramping, periumbilical abdominal pain out of proportion to minimal physical findings; progresses to dull ache
  - Transition of pain to severe pain as mucosal ischemia moves toward transmural infarction resulting in perforation and peritonitis
  - Nausea, diarrhea
  - Decreased bowel sounds
  - Hypotension
  - Gastrointestinal bleeding
  - Leukocytosis
  - Fever, metabolic acidosis, hypovolemic shock present later
  - If related to enteral feedings, abdominal distension and feeding intolerance
- Other signs/symptoms
  - Lactic acidosis results from anaerobic glycolysis occurring during hypoxia
  - Increased beta-galactosidase-activity seen as early as 90 minutes following onset of NOMI

Demographics

- Age: > 60 years

Natural History & Prognosis

- Progressive ischemia of intestine causing infarction, sepsis; if untreated, septic shock
- Mortality rate high, even if diagnosed early

Treatment

- Correct predisposing causes (congestive heart failure, cardiac arrhythmias, hypotension, hypovolemia)
  - Systemic vasodilators for congestive heart failure: Hydralazine, prazosin, nitroglycerin, nitroprusside
- Hemodialysis patients
  - Ultrafiltration, may be an may be an inciting factor in patients on hemodialysis
  - More frequent dialysis sessions, but decreased length of dialysis sessions will lessen hemodynamic changes and volume shifts
- Early NOMI
  - Improving perfusion should be primary therapy since intestinal mucous membrane not yet necrotic
  - Mesenteric angiography and direct infusion of papaverine via superior mesenteric artery to treat mesenteric vasoconstriction and reverse bowel ischemia
  - Parenteral antibiotics
  - Nasogastric compression
  - Fluid resuscitation
- Late NOMI
  - Infarction or peritonitis
    - Laparotomy or bowel resection
    - Laparotomy used for unresolved symptoms following papaverine treatment

DIAGNOSTIC CHECKLIST

Consider

- Chronic mesenteric ischemia
- Mesenteric artery thrombosis
- Mesenteric venous thrombosis

Image Interpretation Pearls

- Diffusely narrowed mesenteric artery and branches
- Poor enhancement of bowel
- Poor enhancement of mesenteric veins

SELECTED REFERENCES

1. Archodovassilis F et al: Nonocclusive mesenteric ischemia: a lethal complication in peritoneal dialysis patients. Perit Dial Int. 27(2):136-41, 2007
2. Bozlar U et al: Nonocclusive mesenteric ischemia: findings at multidetector CT angiography. J Vasc Interv Radiol. 18(10):1331-3, 2007
3. Horton KM et al: Multidetector CT angiography in the diagnosis of mesenteric ischemia. Radiol Clin North Am. 45(2):275-88, 2007
4. Shih MC et al: CTA and MRA in mesenteric ischemia: part 1, Role in diagnosis and differential diagnosis. AJR Am J Roentgenol. 188(2):452-61, 2007
5. Wildermuth S et al: Multislice CT in the pre- and postinterventional evaluation of mesenteric perfusion. Eur Radiol. 15(6):1203-10, 2005
6. Lee R et al: CT in acute mesenteric ischaemia. Clin Radiol. 58(4):279-87, 2003
7. Trompeter M et al: Non-occlusive mesenteric ischemia: etiology, diagnosis, and interventional therapy. Eur Radiol. 12(5):1179-87, 2002
8. Rha SE et al: CT and MR imaging findings of bowel ischemia from various primary causes. Radiographics. 20(1):29-42, 2000

IMAGE GALLERY

Typical

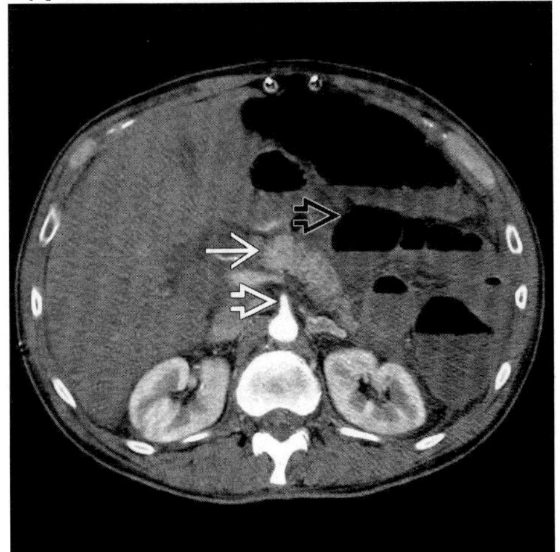

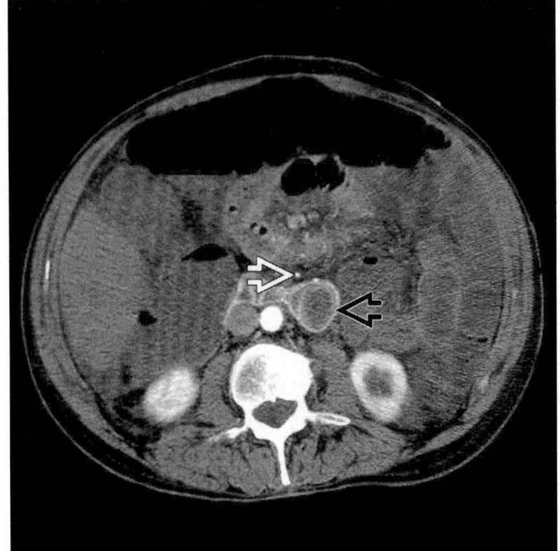

(Left) *Axial CECT shows patent origin of SMA ➡ with opacification of the duodenum ➡. More distal bowel is dilated, with air-fluid levels ➡, and appears to have relatively minimal opacification with contrast. Patient had severe coronary disease and was recently post-operative from cardiac surgery with the development of abdominal pain.* ***(Right)*** *Axial CECT shows a more caudal image in the same patient. SMA is very small ➡. Enhancement of the proximal bowel ➡.*

Typical

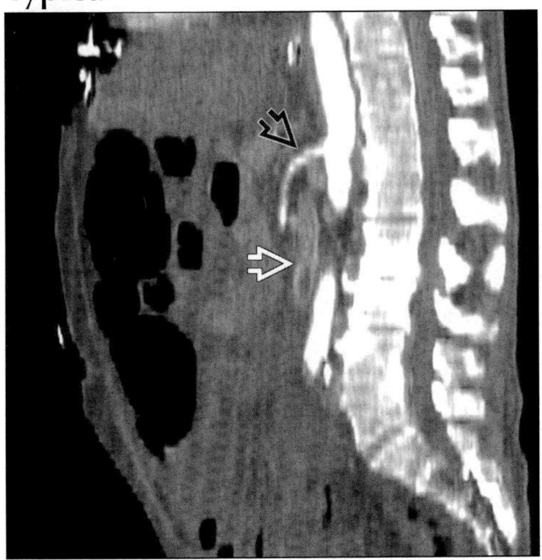

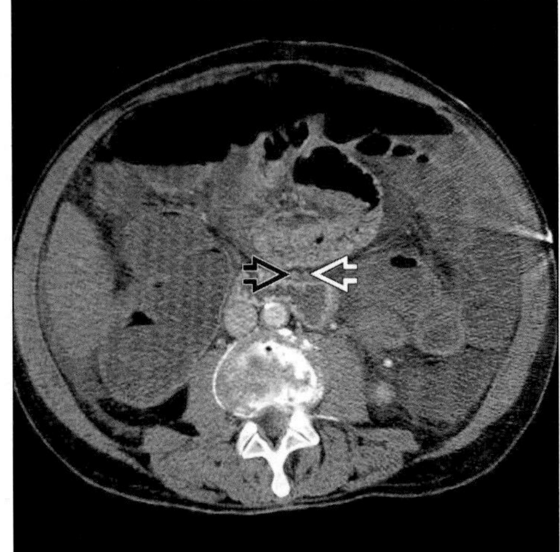

(Left) *Sagittal CECT shows patent proximal SMA without evidence of filling defect ➡. However, the SMA begins to taper. Inferior pancreatic-duodenal vessels are present which opacify proximal bowel ➡. There is minimal opacification of the distal bowel, although this is relatively early in the injection.* ***(Right)*** *Axial CECT shows, in later images, the distal bowel with minimal enhancement compared to the proximal bowel. SMA ➡ and SMV ➡ without contrast-enhancement.*

Typical

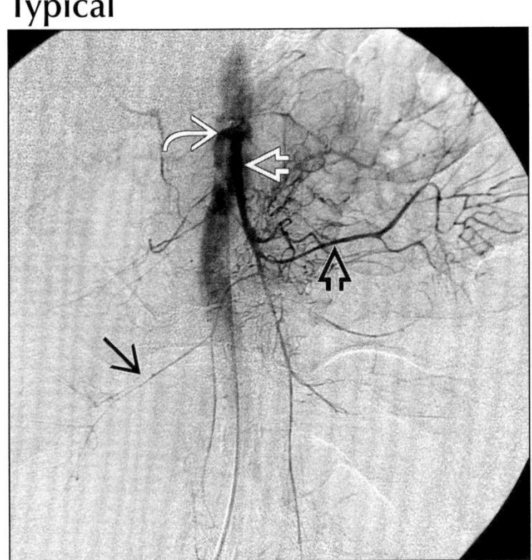

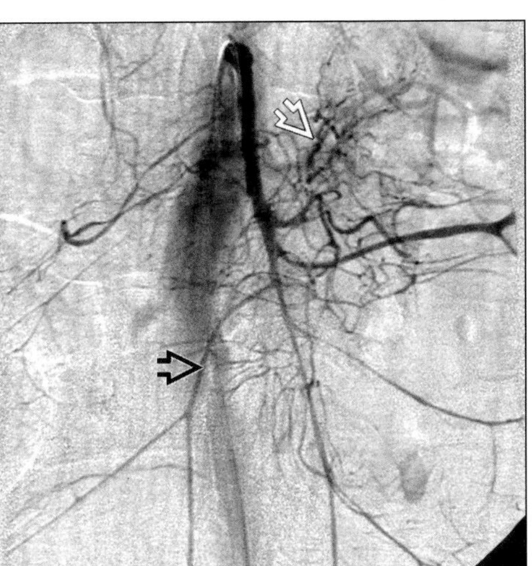

(Left) *DSA shows patent proximal SMA ➡ with moderate perfusion of proximal bowel ➡ but distal bowel arteries with very little flow ➡. Large amount of reflux into the aorta ➡ on this selective SMA injection.* ***(Right)*** *DSA shows some improvement in the distal vasculature ➡ following papaverine infusion. There still remains significant reflux into the aorta on this selective injection. Continued better perfusion of proximal vessels ➡ is still evident.*

CHRONIC MESENTERIC ISCHEMIA

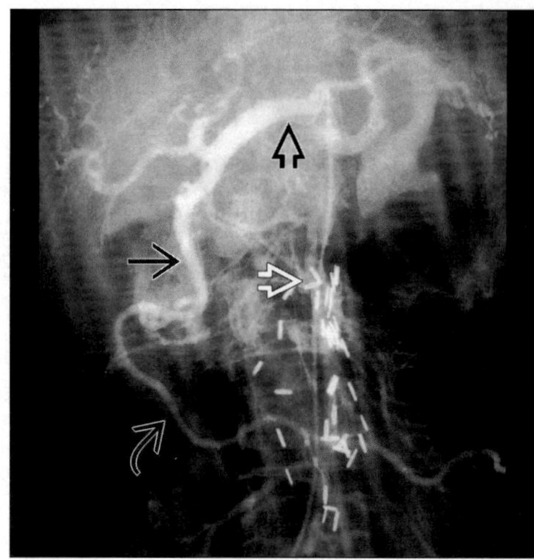

Catheter angiography shows multiple surgical clips. There is a very large celiac axis ⇨ with a very large gastroduodenal artery → and a large collateral ↗ which reconstitutes the SMA ➡.

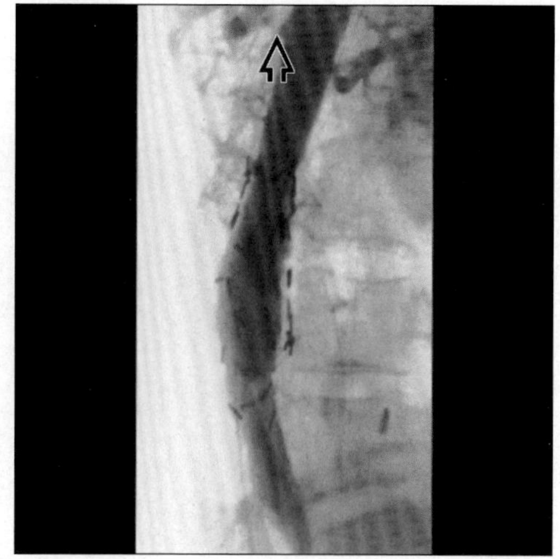

DSA shows the lateral aortogram. The superior mesenteric artery is not present, the inferior mesenteric artery is not present. The celiac is at the very top of the image and is patent ⇨.

TERMINOLOGY

Abbreviations and Synonyms

- Abdominal angina
- Intestinal angina
- Chronic mesenteric ischemia (CMI)

Definitions

- Insufficient blood flow to the gut to satisfy metabolic demands of post-prandial bowel activity
- Reduction in blood flow due to hypoperfusion, occlusion, or vasospasm of the mesenteric vasculature
- CMI results from insufficient blood flow to the intestinal wall
  - Leading to decreased levels of oxygen and nutrients required for cellular metabolism
- 2 of 3 visceral arteries must be occluded: Superior mesenteric artery (SMA), inferior mesenteric artery (IMA), celiac artery (CA)

IMAGING FINDINGS

General Features

- Best diagnostic clue
  - Stenosis or occlusion of at least two of the three mesenteric arteries associated with classic symptoms of abdominal pain with meals, weight-loss, and food avoidance
  - Identification of mesenteric artery occlusive disease alone does not indicate mesenteric ischemia
  - Visualization of luminal thrombus
  - Presence of extensive arterial collaterals

CT Findings

- CECT
  - Useful for demonstrating mesenteric artery stenosis
  - Heavy calcification of the mesenteric arteries origins
  - Visualization of arterial collaterals
  - Decreased contrast-enhancement of SMV

MR Findings

- T1WI: Useful for excluding other causes of abdominal pain

DDx: Chronic Mesenteric Ischemia

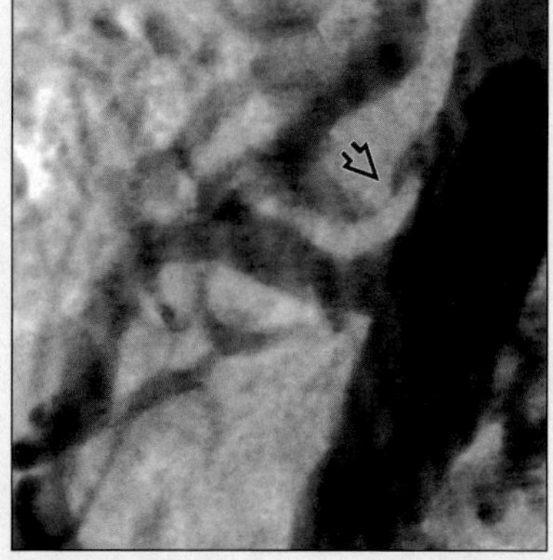

CA Compression Syndrome

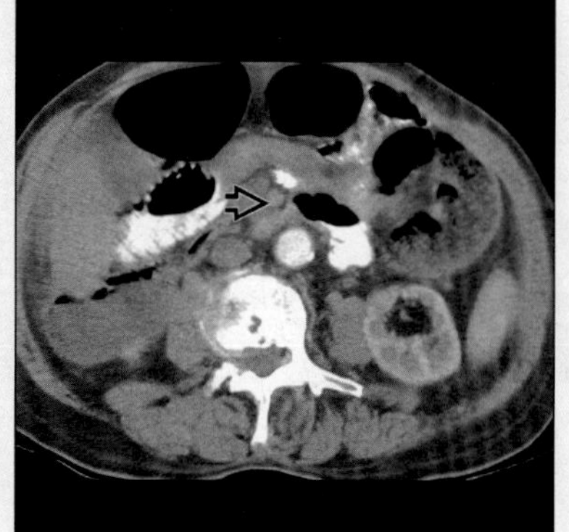

Embolus into SMA

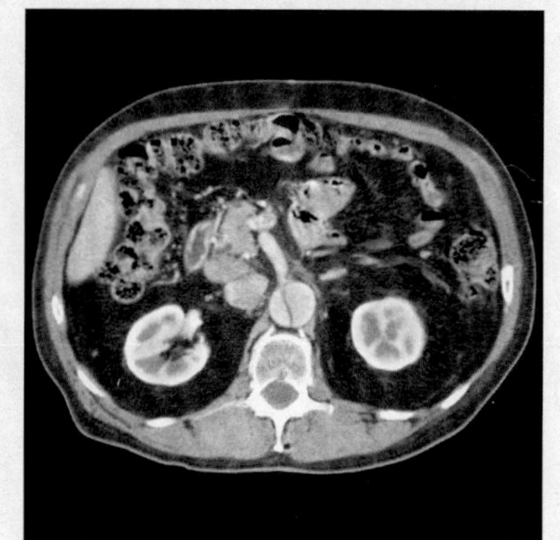

Dissection, into Visceral Arteries

CHRONIC MESENTERIC ISCHEMIA

Key Facts

Terminology
- Abdominal angina
- Intestinal angina
- Insufficient blood flow to the gut to satisfy needs after meals

Imaging Findings
- Stenosis or occlusion of at least two of the three mesenteric arteries associated with classic symptoms of abdominal pain, weight-loss, and avoidance of food
- Identification of mesenteric artery occlusive disease alone does not indicate mesenteric ischemia
- Presence of extensive arterial collaterals
- Heavy calcification of the mesenteric arteries origins
- Decreased contrast-enhancement of SMV
- Contrast-enhanced MRA: Method of choice for characterizing mesenteric artery stenotic disease

Clinical Issues
- Presentation
  - Chronic post-prandial abdominal pain
  - 75% have signs of peripheral vascular disease (e.g., decreased pulses, extremity ischemia)
  - Cardiac: Coronary artery disease (43%) myocardial infarction, atrial fibrillation
  - Cerebral: Carotid bruits, TIAs, CVA
- 90% have initial spontaneous symptomatic relief; recurrence rates < 10%
- Surgical or endovascular treatment options include endarterectomy, bypass, stenting

- Contrast-enhanced MRA: Method of choice for characterizing mesenteric artery stenotic disease
  - Aortic atherosclerosis, involving ostia of mesenteric arteries
  - Stenosis or occlusion of at least two of three mesenteric arteries
  - Evidence of collateral circulation
    - Pancreaticoduodenal arcade [celiac to superior mesenteric artery (SMA)]
    - Arc of Riolan [SMA to inferior mesenteric artery (IMA)]
    - Marginal artery of Drummond (SMA to IMA)

Ultrasonographic Findings
- Grayscale Ultrasound
  - Stenoses at origins of superior mesenteric and celiac arteries
  - Hemodynamically significant stenosis in celiac axis (CA) is suggested if peak systolic velocity (PSV) > 200 cm/s and end-diastolic velocity > 55 cm/s
    - For the SMA, PSV > 275-300 cm/s and end-diastolic velocity > 45 cm/s

Angiographic Findings
- Conventional
  - Occlusion of 2 of 3 visceral branches of aorta
  - Atherosclerotic calcified plaques at or near the origins of proximal splanchnic arteries
  - Remains gold standard, with increased risk of catheter-induced complications in these patients with extensive aortic atherosclerosis

DIFFERENTIAL DIAGNOSIS

Celiac Artery Compression Syndrome
- Extrinsic compression of celiac artery by median arcuate ligament
- Controversial diagnosis as cause of abdominal pain
- Classic imaging appearance
  - Impression along superior aspect of celiac artery with normal inferior aspect
  - Worse on expiration compared to inspiration

Mesenteric Thrombosis
- Chronic venous thrombosis of SMV may present as chronic mesenteric ischemia
- Venous thrombosis accounts for 5-15% of CMI
- Requires use of arterial and venous phase imaging when evaluating patients

Mesenteric Ischemia due to Other Causes
- Aortic dissection with occlusion or stenosis of mesenteric artery origins
- Vasculitis
- Vasoactive drugs causing vasoconstriction
- Fibromuscular dysplasia
- Aortic coarctation syndromes

PATHOLOGY

General Features
- General path comments
  - Atherosclerosis in proximal visceral arteries
  - Atherosclerosis of mesenteric branches is relatively frequent, but chronic mesenteric ischemia is relatively uncommon
  - Development of arterial collateral circulation
  - Usually a minimum of two visceral arteries are occluded or severely stenosed
  - 85% of cases involve the celiac axis and SMA vessels
  - Ischemic changes of intestines
  - 50% of all acute intestinal ischemic events due to embolic disease of SMA
  - 10% of CMI from the development of thrombosis in mesenteric arteries
  - Concomitant splanchnic stenosis in celiac trunk
- Genetics
  - Hereditary cause of atherosclerosis
  - Hereditary hypercoagulation disorders cause primary thrombosis of mesenteric artery or SMV
  - Inflammatory or malignant conditions may cause secondary thrombosis of the mesenteric vessels

        - Trauma, pancreatitis, inflammatory bowel disease, postoperative states, paraneoplastic disorders, cirrhosis and portal hypertension
- Etiology
    - 5% intestinal ischemic events are due to CMI
    - Atherosclerosis giving rise to stenotic or occlusive disease of mesenteric arteries
    - Smoking in 75% of CMI patients
    - Hypertension in 37% of CMI patients
    - Hyperlipidemia, hypercholesterolemia
    - Diabetes mellitus 10% of CMI patients
    - Inflammatory arterial disease (Takayasu)
    - Atherosclerosis, hyperlipidemia
    - Mid-aortic syndrome
        - Chronic renal failure in 20% of CMI patients
        - Peripheral vascular disease in 55% of CMI patients
        - Previous vascular surgery in 52% of CMI patients
    - Fibromuscular dysplasia
    - Cocaine abuse, rarely
- Epidemiology
    - M:F, 1:3
    - Average age of presentation is 65 years
    - Atherosclerosis in 95%
    - Acute thrombosis leads to increased mortality
    - Risk of developing symptoms from asymptomatic CMI is 86%; 40% mortality rate

Gross Pathologic & Surgical Features

- Atherosclerosis involving aorta, ostia, and proximal mesenteric arteries
- Dense calcification of aortic wall
- Blood flow varies from 25% (fasting) to 35% (postprandial phase)
    - Ischemic symptoms occur when blood flow demands increase following a meal
- Collateral vascularization occurs among the three main arteries

Microscopic Features

- Mesenteric vessels show diffuse atherosclerosis
    - Atrophy of villi tips leads to loss of absorptive surface in small bowel

CLINICAL ISSUES

Presentation

- Most common signs/symptoms
    - Triad of post-prandial upper abdominal pain (98%), weight loss (78%), and an epigastric bruit (60%)
    - Malnutrition, sitophobia (fear of eating)
    - Intensity of pain related to size of meal
- Other signs/symptoms
    - Nausea, vomiting 33%
    - Diarrhea 36%
    - Constipation 18%
- Chronic postprandial abdominal pain (epigastric or periumbilical) (94%)
    - Intestinal ischemia due to increased secretory, digestive, and motility activities following eating
- Other signs of vascular disease
    - Cardiac: Coronary artery disease (43%), myocardial infarction, atrial fibrillation
    - Cerebral: Carotid bruits, TIAs
    - Peripheral-decreased pulses, extremity ischemia

Treatment

- Low-fat diet
- Surgery is preferred and most durable form of therapy
    - Endarterectomy of the celiac or SMA
    - Aorto-mesenteric bypass
    - Retrograde bypass from the external iliac artery
    - Mesenteric reimplantation (distal aorta or iliac arteries)
    - 90% associated with initial symptomatic relief; recurrence rates < 10%
    - Surgical mortality rate: 4-10%
- Percutaneous therapy
    - Possible if artery not completely occluded, short stenosis, and not due to external compression
    - Stenting of visceral vessels may be helpful
    - Technical success rate variable (30-90%)
    - Recurrence rates with angioplasty: 10-67%
    - Catheter-induced complications occur up to 30%
    - Acceptable alternative for high risk surgical patients

DIAGNOSTIC CHECKLIST

Image Interpretation Pearls

- Untreated or undiagnosed CMI may develop into acute ischemia with bowel infarction, which is a surgical emergency

SELECTED REFERENCES

1. Sreenarasimhaiah J: Chronic mesenteric ischemia. Best Pract Res Clin Gastroenterol. 19(2):283-95, 2005
2. Cognet F et al: Chronic mesenteric ischemia: imaging and percutaneous treatment. Radiographics. 22(4):863-79; discussion 879-80, 2002
3. Rha SE et al: CT and MR imaging findings of bowel ischemia from various primary causes. Radiographics. 20(1):29-42, 2000

IMAGE GALLERY

Typical

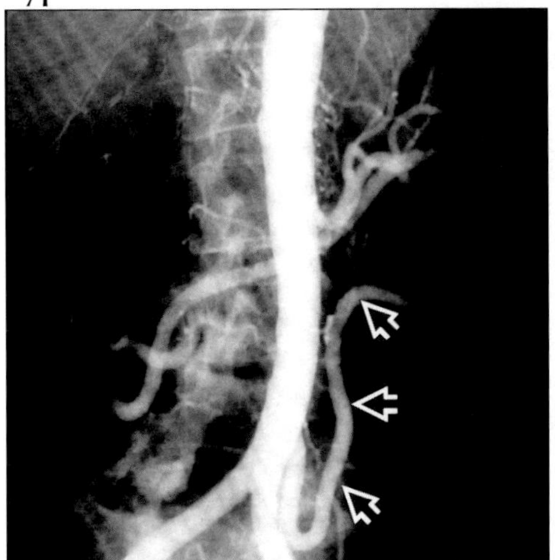

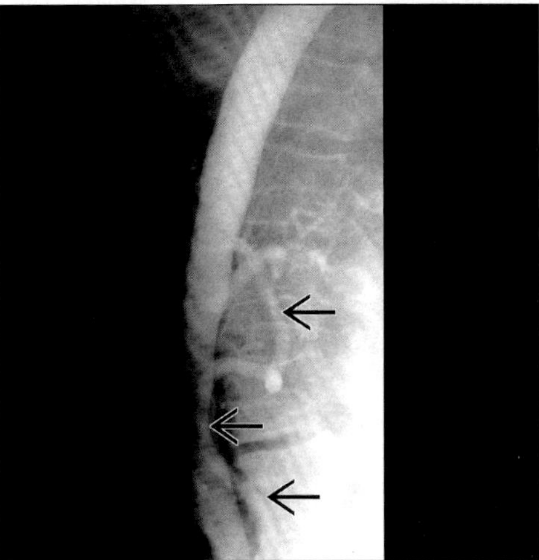

(Left) *Catheter angiography shows large IMA collateral, no SMA demonstrated, no celiac axis. All of the bowel, spleen and liver is being supplied by this single artery.* ***(Right)*** *Catheter angiography shows the lateral view. The anterior surface of the aorta is without any evidence of the SMA or celiac arteries. There is a very large collateral which is seen extending up from the low abdomen and which represents the large IMA seen on the AP angiogram.*

Typical

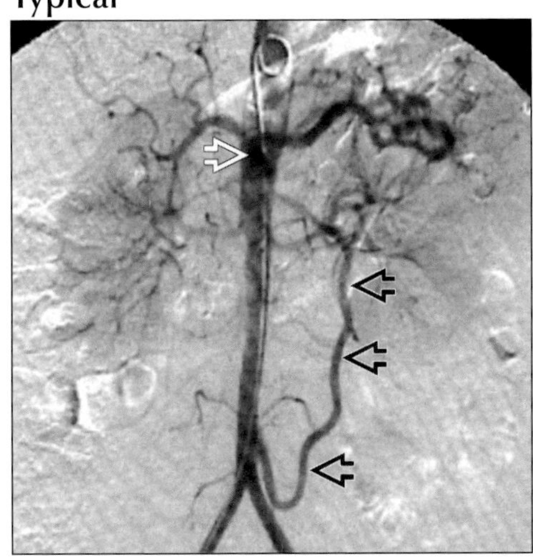

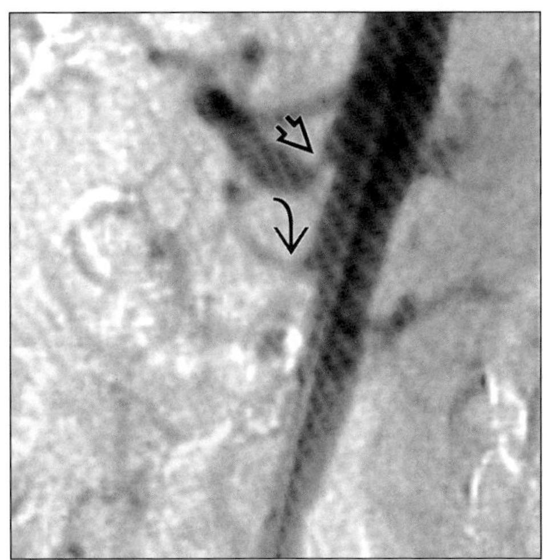

(Left) *DSA shows same patient. Large IMA with large collateral to the SMA. Celiac axis is also seen, but narrowing is not identified. This demonstrates importance of lateral image.* ***(Right)*** *DSA shows narrowing of the celiac axis, very diminutive SMA, and no IMA identified. The narrowing of the superior and inferior aspect of the celiac excludes compression by the median arcuate ligament as the cause.*

Typical

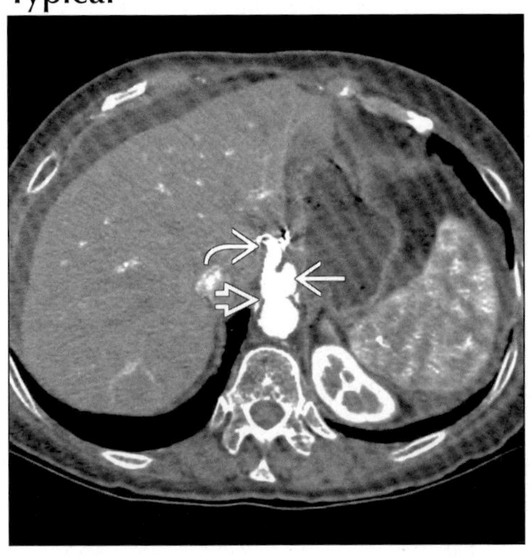

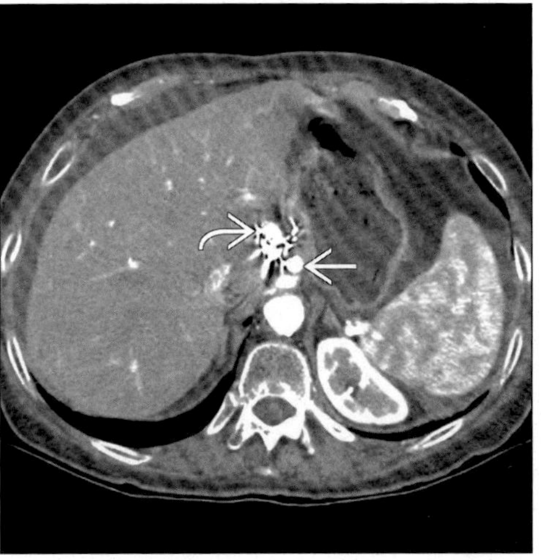

(Left) *Axial CECT shows a graft that has been used to correct mesenteric ischemia. The graft is placed as an end of graft to side of aorta at a level just at the diaphragmatic hiatus. The graft extends anteriorly and has two limbs - one to the celiac and the other to the SMA.* ***(Right)*** *Axial CECT is at a slightly lower level, the two limbs of the graft can be more clearly seen. The anterior limb extends to the celiac axis and the other connects to the SMA.*

CELIAC ARTERY COMPRESSION SYNDROME

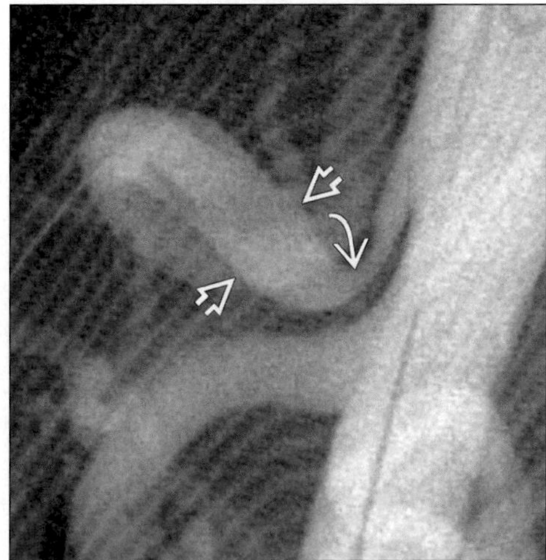

Catheter angiography on expiration shows a focal significant stenosis of the celiac axis ➢ with upward hooking of a dilated post-stenotic segment ➢, in a patient with post-prandial abdominal pain.

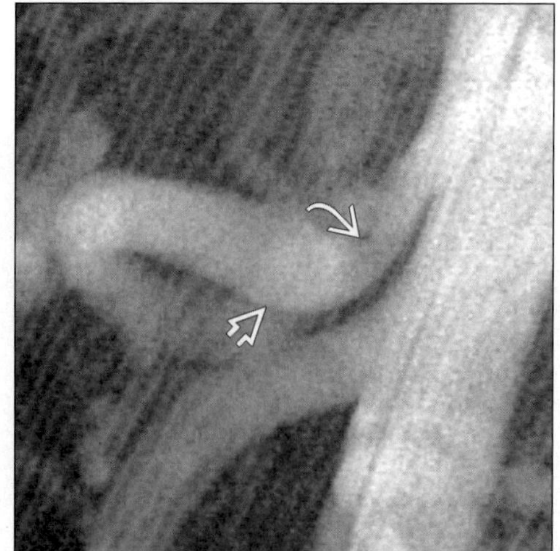

Catheter angiography on inspiration in the same patient shows persistent but mildly decreased stenosis ➢, post-stenotic dilation, and hooking of celiac artery ➢, consistent with celiac artery compression syndrome.

TERMINOLOGY

Abbreviations and Synonyms

- Median arcuate ligament syndrome (MALS), median arcuate ligament (MAL), celiac artery (CA)
  - Celiac artery compression syndrome (CACS)

Definitions

- Extrinsic celiac axis compression by median arcuate ligament of diaphragm causing luminal stenosis, post-stenotic dilatation, collaterals, abdominal pain
  - Median arcuate ligament forms anterior margin of aortic hiatus; muscular/fibrous tissue band connecting right and left crus of diaphragm

IMAGING FINDINGS

General Features

- Best diagnostic clue
  - Narrowing and hooking of celiac axis during end-inspiration
  - Fibrous band crossing proximal celiac axis
  - During expiration, cephalad motion of ligament, aorta and celiac artery results in compression of superior aspect of celiac axis: Normal variant
    - Presence of narrowing of celiac artery during end-inspiration abnormal
- Location
  - Median arcuate ligament found at T12-L1; bridges right and left crus of diaphragm, anterior to aorta and above celiac artery origin
  - In celiac artery compression syndrome, ligament lies slightly lower than T2/L1 level and crosses over anterior aspect of proximal celiac artery
- Size: Focal stenosis/kinking

CT Findings

- CTA
  - Focal narrowing of celiac artery, usually 5 mm from origin from aorta
    - Characteristic upward hooking of celiac artery
    - Dilatation of celiac axis distal to focal stenosis
  - Prominent, tortuous and dilated collateral vessels from SMA to celiac artery branches
    - Usually prominent pancreaticoduodenal arcade

DDx: Celiac Artery Compression Syndrome

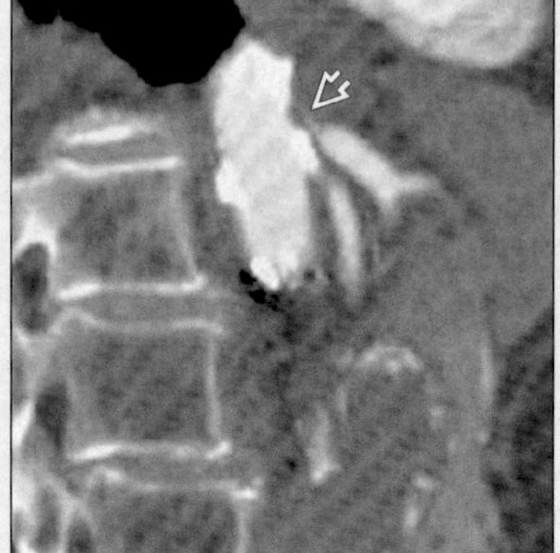

Atherosclerotic Stenosis

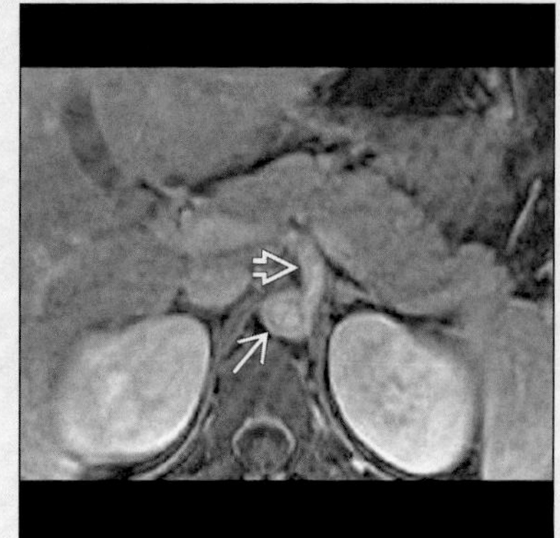

Vasculitis (Mural Thickening)

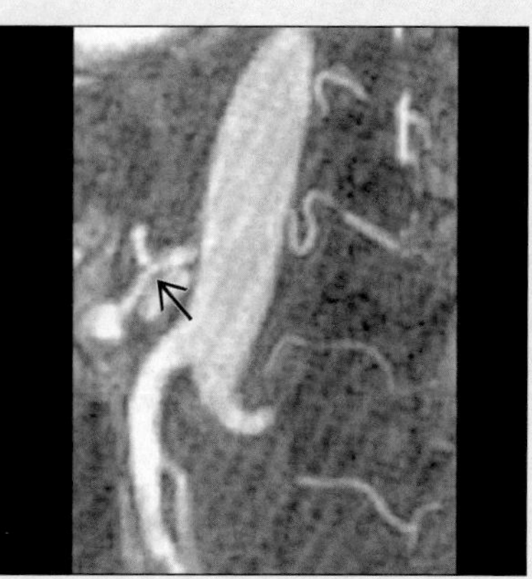

Dissection

CELIAC ARTERY COMPRESSION SYNDROME

Key Facts

Terminology
- Celiac artery compression by median arcuate ligament with abdominal pain
- Median arcuate ligament is muscular band joining right and left diaphragmatic crura

Imaging Findings
- Celiac compression best seen in sagittal projection
- Acquire data during end-inspiration
- Narrowing of celiac axis during end-inspiration
- Upward hooking of celiac artery
- Post-stenotic dilatation
- Usually prominent pancreaticoduodenal arcade
- Supra-celiac ligament course best seen on MR and CT
  - Shows both median arcuate ligament and celiac artery stenosis

Top Differential Diagnoses
- Atherosclerosis
- Vasculitis
- Dissection

Clinical Issues
- Symptomatic celiac artery compression = syndrome
  - More common in thin women
  - Post-prandial epigastric pain, varying abdominal bruit
- Surgery is treatment of choice

Diagnostic Checklist
- Compression of celiac axis in expiration is normal variant
  - 1-2% show severe and persistent stenosis on inspiration with symptoms

---

  - Ligament seen as intermediate density constricting superior aspect celiac axis
  - Best seen on sagittal reconstructed images, difficult to appreciate on coronal and axial images

MR Findings
- MRA
  - Pre-contrast T1 and T2 images may show medial arcuate ligament as low to intermediate signal
  - TR-MRA can show collateral flow and prominent pancreaticoduodenal arcade
  - CE-MRA shows similar findings as CTA
    - Ligament difficult to see on MRA images
  - Upward hooking accentuated on end-expiration images
  - Post-contrast T1 GRE images show no mural thickening or enhancement of celiac artery, may show low signal MAL crossing over artery

Ultrasonographic Findings
- Grayscale Ultrasound
  - Focal luminal narrowing accentuated on expiratory phase
    - Ligament connecting right and left crus of diaphragm can be seen compressing celiac axis
- Pulsed Doppler: Varying degree of raised velocity distal to stenosis; worse during expiration

Angiographic Findings
- Conventional
  - Considered "gold standard"
    - Angiography should be obtained in both inspiration and expiration in lateral projection
    - Focal constriction of celiac axis accentuated on expiration
    - Upward orientation of post-stenotic dilatation in inspiration
    - Collaterals feeding celiac branches via SMA better evaluated
    - Medial arcuate ligament not seen

Imaging Recommendations
- Best imaging tool
  - CTA
    - Shows both medial arcuate ligament and characteristic appearance of celiac artery stenosis
  - MRA better alternative technique to assess artery in both expiration and inspiration, especially in younger patient (avoids radiation exposure)
  - Previously catheter angiography was considered prime diagnostic tool, but limited in showing ligament course
  - Best seen on sagittal images/projection
- Protocol advice
  - Always acquire data during end-inspiration for suspected MALS
  - CTA: Thin section 1.5 mm collimation volumetric data acquisition at end-inspiration
    - Bolus tracking, with ROI in descending aorta, 80-100 mL contrast at 3 cc/sec
    - Sagittal reconstructions: Best plane to see ligament crossing over celiac artery
    - At least 3 mm slice thickness with overlap interval
  - MRA: First pass during end-inspiration and second pass during end-expiration
    - Axial and sagittal post-contrast T1 GRE to assess arterial wall, and median arcuate ligament
  - Selective catheter angiography with separate injections during end-expiration and end-inspiration

DIFFERENTIAL DIAGNOSIS

Atherosclerosis Stenosis
- Elderly
- Calcified and non-calcified mural plaque
- Aortic calcification and ulceration

Vasculitis
- Middle age
- Circumferential mural thickening
- Mural enhancement
- Usually associated with aortitis

CELIAC ARTERY COMPRESSION SYNDROME

Celiac Artery Dissection
- Usually associated with aortic dissection
- Differential perfusion of true and false lumen
- Intimal flap

Extrinsic Compression
- Soft tissue mass
- Lymphoma
- Pancreatic tumor may encase celiac axis

PATHOLOGY

General Features
- General path comments: Compression of celiac artery causes intimal fibrosis, luminal stenosis and impaired splanchnic blood flow
- Etiology
  - Exact etiology unknown: Two main theories for etiology of symptoms; thought partly related to embryologic migration of celiac origin
    - Mesenteric ischemia from celiac compression arises from either foregut ischemia or post-prandial steal from SMA to celiac collaterals
    - Neurogenic = compression of celiac ganglion and plexus leading to splanchnic vasoconstriction from direct irritation of sympathetic pain fibers
- Epidemiology
  - Normal variant in 13-50% of patients
    - Only 1-2% show severe and persistent stenosis on inspiration and develop symptoms
- Associated abnormalities
  - Patients often thin
  - Patients with celiac artery compression who undergo orthotopic liver transplantation have increased incidence of hepatic artery thrombosis

CLINICAL ISSUES

Presentation
- Most common signs/symptoms
  - Symptoms often vague and patients may complain of abdominal fullness or abdominal bruit
  - Varying abdominal bruit on respiration
  - Epigastric pain, particularly post-prandial and with expiration, weight loss and emesis

Demographics
- Age: Younger patients, 20-40 years
- Gender: F:M = 3:1
- Ethnicity: More common in thin women

Natural History & Prognosis
- No spontaneous recovery
- Signs and symptoms may gradually progress
- Prognosis good following surgical resection
- Celiac artery compression with symptoms defined as syndrome

Treatment
- Ligament excision/division by open or laparoscopic surgery, ganglion blockage or bypass surgery
- In severe ligamentous constriction of celiac artery, vessel reconstruction may be required
- Angioplasty with stent placement may not cure condition; recurrence possible

DIAGNOSTIC CHECKLIST

Consider
- True celiac artery compression syndrome if
  - Symptomatic patient
  - Focal stenosis and hooked post-stenotic dilatation of celiac artery with associated prominent pancreaticoduodenal arcade

Image Interpretation Pearls
- Mild narrowing of celiac axis in end-expiratory phase only is normal variant
- If suspected ischemic bowel, images should be obtained in end-inspiratory phase

SELECTED REFERENCES

1. Duncan AA: Median arcuate ligament syndrome. Curr Treat Options Cardiovasc Med. 10(2):112-6, 2008
2. Jarry J et al: [Laparoscopic management of median arcuate ligament syndrome.] J Mal Vasc. [Epub ahead of print] French, 2008
3. Delis KT et al: Median arcuate ligament syndrome: open celiac artery reconstruction and ligament division after endovascular failure. J Vasc Surg. 46(4):799-802, 2007
4. Gloviczki P et al: Treatment of celiac artery compression syndrome: does it really exist? Perspect Vasc Surg Endovasc Ther. 19(3):259-63, 2007
5. Ilica AT et al: Median arcuate ligament syndrome: multidetector computed tomography findings. J Comput Assist Tomogr. 31(5):728-31, 2007
6. Karahan OI et al: Celiac artery compression syndrome: diagnosis with multislice CT. Diagn Interv Radiol. 13(2):90-3, 2007
7. Horton KM et al: Median arcuate ligament syndrome: evaluation with CT angiography. Radiographics. 25(5):1177-82, 2005
8. Lee VS et al: Celiac artery compression by the median arcuate ligament: a pitfall of end-expiratory MR imaging. Radiology. 228(2):437-42, 2003
9. Bech FR: Celiac artery compression syndromes. Surg Clin North Am. 77(2):409-24, 1997
10. Cornell SH: Severe stenosis of the celiac artery. Analysis of patients with and without symptoms. Radiology. 99(2):311-6, 1971
11. Dunbar JD et al: Compression of the celiac trunk and abdominal angina. Am J Roentgenol Radium Ther Nucl Med. 95(3):731-44, 1965

CELIAC ARTERY COMPRESSION SYNDROME

IMAGE GALLERY

Typical

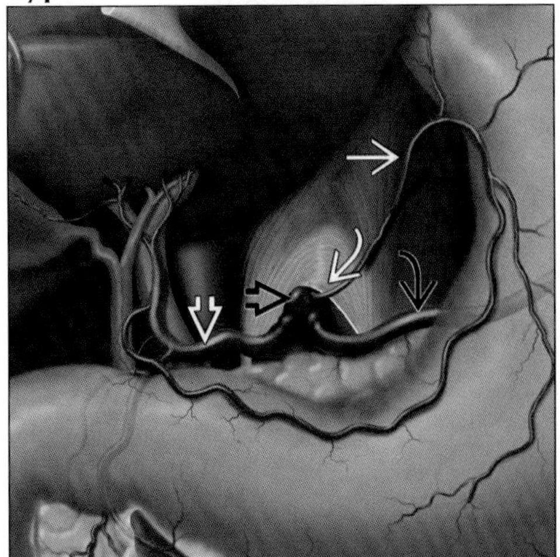

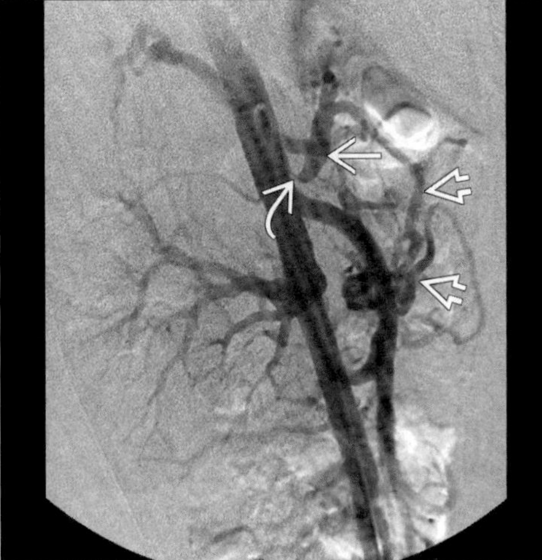

(Left) *Graphic shows the median arcuate ligament connecting the crura of the diaphragm and crossing over the proximal celiac axis. The common hepatic left gastric and splenic arteries are also seen.* ***(Right)*** *DSA obtained in the lateral projection on inspiration in a patient with celiac artery compression syndrome shows cephalad celiac artery deviation, a proximal stenosis, post-stenotic dilation, and a prominent pancreaticoduodenal arcade.*

Typical

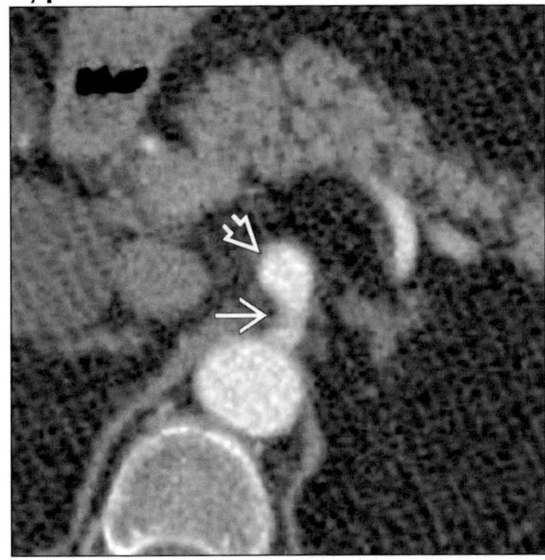

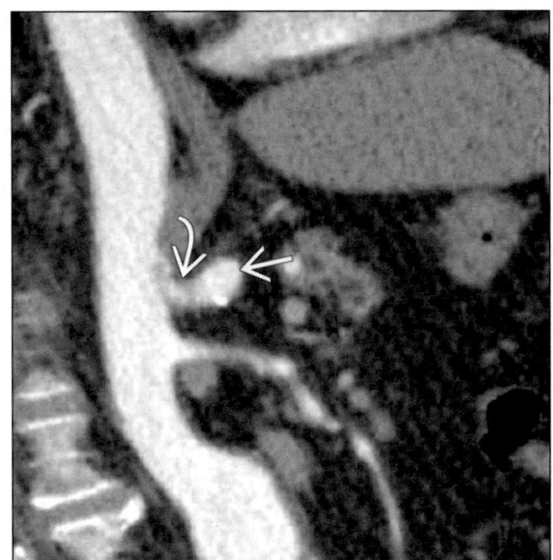

(Left) *Axial CECT shows mild focal stenosis at the origin of the celiac artery due to compression by the median arcuate ligament. Note the post-stenotic dilatation of the celiac artery. The median arcuate ligament typically is not well-appreciated on axial images.* ***(Right)*** *Sagittal CECT (same patient) better demonstrates the hooking of the dilated post-stenotic segment of the celiac artery & median arcuate ligament compression. These were incidental findings.*

Typical

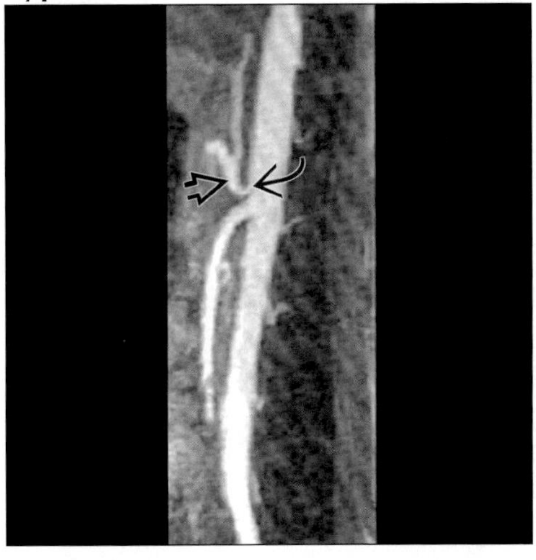

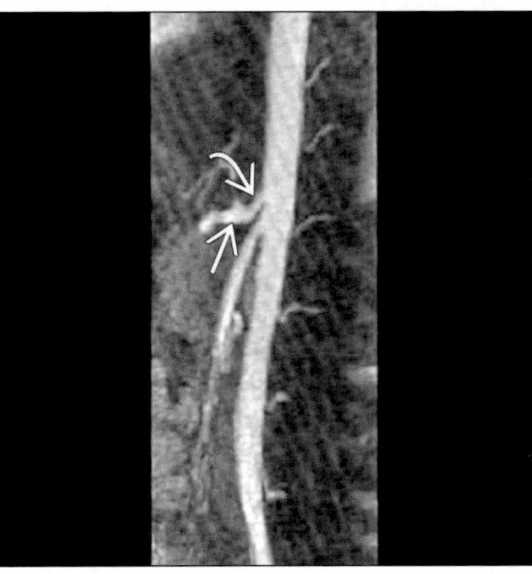

(Left) *Sagittal thin MIP CE MRA obtained during expiration shows the narrowing of the celiac artery origin with characteristic hooking of the post-stenotic segment in a young female patient with epigastric pain.* ***(Right)*** *Sagittal CE MRA of the same patient obtained during inspiration shows a persistent but mild stenosis and hooking of the celiac artery with post-stenotic dilatation. These findings are consistent with true celiac artery compression syndrome.*

UPPER GI BLEEDING

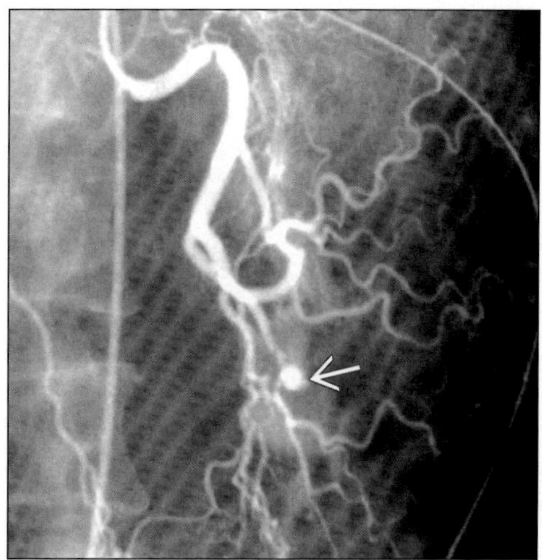

Selective left gastric arteriogram shows a round focus of contrast ➔ corresponding to a bleeding ulcer along the lesser curvature of the stomach. Additionally, there is diffuse vascular hyperemia, consistent with gastritis.

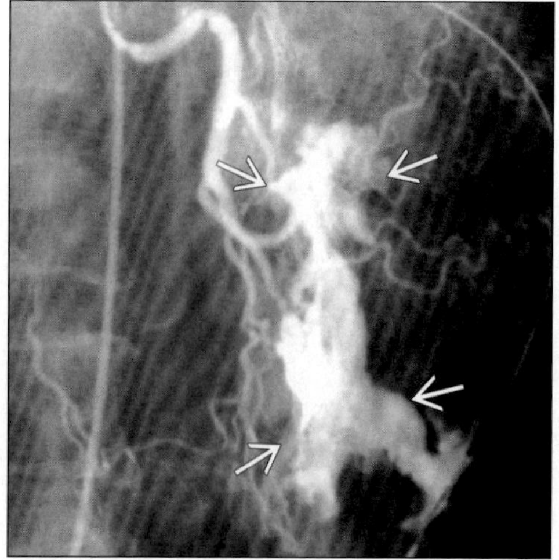

Later phase of left gastric arteriogram in same patient as previous image, shows massive contrast extravasation ➔ at site of bleeding ulcer. Subsequent transcatheter embolization stabilized this hypotensive patient.

TERMINOLOGY

Definitions

- Acute or chronic hemorrhage from gastrointestinal tract proximal to ligament of Treitz

IMAGING FINDINGS

Radiographic Findings

- Very limited value of barium studies
  - Large quantities of blood in lumen make interpretation difficult
  - Abnormalities detected may not be etiology of current bleeding episode
  - Presence of barium precludes subsequent angiography and interferes with endoscopy

CT Findings

- Active bleeding appears as linear, pooled or swirled focal collection of extravasated intraluminal or extraluminal contrast on CECT

Nuclear Medicine Findings

- Tc-99m Sulfur Colloid
  - Extravasation of isotope at active bleeding site
  - Bleeding rate of 0.05-0.1 mL/min detected
    - Better sensitivity than Tc-99m labeled RBC scan
    - Usually only valid for lower GI bleeding because activity in liver and spleen obscures upper GI tract
  - Intravascular half-life of 2.5 minutes
    - By 15 min isotope cleared from vascular system, producing significant contrast between bleeding site and surroundings
- Tc-99m Labeled Red Cell Scintigraphy
  - Bleeding rate of 0.1-0.2 mL/min detected
  - 5-10 mL of extravasated blood required for detection
  - Sensitivity (85-95%) and specificity (70-85%) for all sources of GI bleeding (upper and lower)
    - 50% sensitivity in upper GI bleeding
  - Continuous dynamic imaging (large FOV camera)
    - 15 min dynamic "flow" image sequence followed by 1 minute interval scans for 1 hour
    - Repeat until bleeding identified or study stopped
  - Labeled RBCs outside of normal areas of blood pool constitutes a positive study

DDx: Upper GI Bleeding

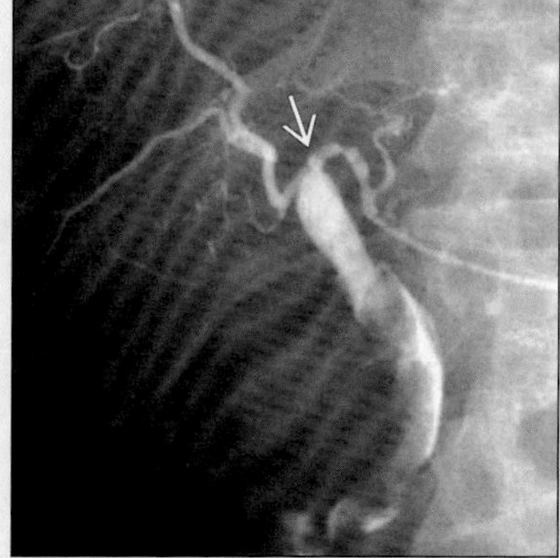

Hemobilia

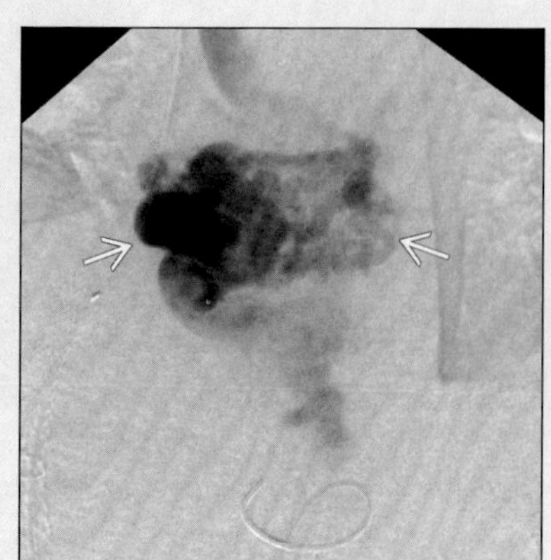

Esophageal Varices

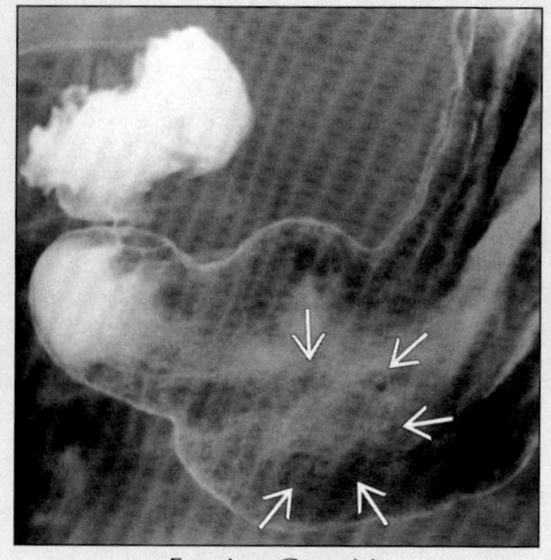

Erosive Gastritis

UPPER GI BLEEDING

Key Facts

Terminology
- Acute or chronic hemorrhage from gastrointestinal tract proximal to ligament of Treitz

Top Differential Diagnoses
- Peptic Ulcer Disease
- Erosive Gastritis
- Gastroesophageal Varices

Pathology
- Upper GI bleed accounts for 76% of GI hemorrhage
  - Usually present with hematemesis, melena

Clinical Issues
- 80% of patients requiring hospitalization for GI bleeding respond to conservative management with sedation, bedrest and blood volume replacement
- Angiographic diagnosis and treatment
  - For evaluation and treatment of upper GI bleeding that is refractory to medical and endoscopic management, for inconclusive endoscopy and for transcatheter intervention
- Angiographic treatment options include transcatheter embolization and vasopressin infusion
- Embolization provides rapid and definitive control
- Transcatheter vasopressin infusion may be used if embolization is not possible or bleeding is diffuse
- Surgical treatment for bleeding refractory to endoscopic or angiographic control

Diagnostic Checklist
- Scintigraphy for hemodynamically stable cases
- Angiography for hemodynamically unstable cases

  - Advantages of RBC scan
    - Active bleeding unnecessary at time of injection
    - Higher detection rate for intermittent bleeding
    - Ability to monitor over prolonged period
  - Disadvantages of RBC scan
    - Origin of bleed unclear on delayed scans as tagged cells may travel in antegrade or retrograde fashion
    - Vascular organs may interfere with detection
    - Loss of tag can produce false ±
    - Less sensitive than Tc-99m sulfur colloid (SC) scan

Angiographic Findings
- Conventional
  - Diagnostic accuracy: 70-95%
  - Bleeding rate of > 0.5 mL/min required for detection
  - Active bleeding appears as localized contrast extravasation during arterial phase
  - Major limitations in identifying bleeding source
    - Intermittent nature of GI hemorrhage, with negative study if temporary cessation of bleeding
    - Inability to demonstrate venous or variceal bleeding from selective arterial injection

DIFFERENTIAL DIAGNOSIS

Peptic Ulcer Disease
- Barium collection with radiating folds within surrounding mound of edema
- Giant ulcers, usually located in duodenal bulb, have increased risk of hemorrhage
- Wall thickening, luminal narrowing or deformity

Erosive Gastritis
- Predilection for gastric antrum
- Scalloped or nodular antral folds
- Multiple punctate or slit-like collections of barium

Gastroesophageal Varices
- Tortuous, serpiginous filling defects on barium studies
- Scalloped esophageal mural masses on NECT
- Tortuous peri-esophageal, peri-gastric and splenic hilar vascular channels on CECT

Mallory-Weiss Tear
- Bleeding secondary to longitudinal mucosal lacerations at gastroesophageal (GE) junction
- Occurs from rapid and transient transmural pressure gradient across GE junction, as caused by vomiting
- Bleeding stops spontaneously in 80-90%

Iatrogenic
- Biopsies, gastrostomies, bariatric surgery

Hemobilia
- Bleeding from biliary tree, often iatrogenic in etiology
- May be treated with transcatheter embolization

Aortoenteric Fistula
- Communication between aorta and bowel (usually duodenum) resulting from disease at either site
- Classified as primary (rare and usually caused by an untreated abdominal aortic aneurysm) or secondary (complication of abdominal aortic surgery)
- Endoscopy is most helpful method for diagnosis
- Requires surgical treatment, with high mortality if not performed promptly

Arteriovenous Malformation
- Rare cause of upper GI bleeding, but can occur in stomach, duodenum or pancreas
- Erosion of overlying mucosa results in bleeding from friable vessels

Dieulafoy Lesion
- Single large tortuous submucosal arteriole with abnormal branching or a caliber of 1-5 mm (> 10 times normal diameter of mucosal capillaries)
- Bleeds into upper GI tract through minute mucosal defect caused from the submucosal surface by the pulsatile arteriole protruding into the mucosa
- 95% occur in upper stomach, commonly in lesser curvature, but can occur anywhere

Pseudoaneurysm
- Caused by inflammatory processes such as pancreatitis
- Transcatheter embolization for treatment

UPPER GI BLEEDING

PATHOLOGY

General Features

- Epidemiology: > 400,000 annual US hospitalizations
- Upper GI bleed accounts for 76% of GI hemorrhage
  - Usually present with hematemesis, melena
  - Most common cause: Peptic ulcers (> 50% cases) followed by gastritis
  - Other causes include portal hypertension (varices), Mallory-Weiss tear, marginal ulcer, iatrogenic injury, neoplasm, pseudoaneurysm, hemobilia, aortoenteric fistula, AVM and Dieulafoy lesion
- Risk factors for upper GI bleeding
  - Alcohol, tobacco, anticoagulants, aspirin, non-steroidal anti-inflammatory agents

Staging, Grading or Classification Criteria

- Classification based on onset & presentation
  - Acute: Hematemesis, hematochezia, melena
  - Chronic: Iron deficiency anemia

CLINICAL ISSUES

Presentation

- Most common signs/symptoms
  - Upper GI bleeding
    - Hematemesis: Bloody vomitus with red or "coffee grounds" appearance
    - Melena: Black, tarry stools requiring 100-200 mL of blood in upper GI tract for occurrence
    - Hematochezia: Red blood per rectum (usually lower GI source) may result from severe upper GI hemorrhage
  - Symptoms and signs of blood loss include dizziness, tachycardia, hypotension and shock
- Laboratory data
  - Occult blood in stool, iron deficiency anemia
  - ↓ CBC count, hematocrit, serum electrolytes
  - Abnormal coagulation parameters

Demographics

- Age: More common in older age group

Natural History & Prognosis

- 80% of patients requiring hospitalization for GI bleeding respond to conservative management with sedation, bedrest and blood volume replacement
- Good prognosis with early detection, resuscitation & treatment; poor with delay
- Mortality rate in upper GI bleeding from gastroesophageal varices is 30-50%
- Massive GI bleeding may result in shock and death

Treatment

- Medical
  - Conservative management with bedrest, sedation, fluid and blood replacement
  - Correction of any underlying coagulopathy
  - Peptic ulcer disease and gastritis now less frequently encountered because of aggressive preventive therapy with histamine H2-receptor antagonists
  - Endoscopy should be initial diagnostic procedure
    - Source identified in > 95%
    - Bleeding source treated with electrocautery, injection sclerotherapy, mechanical clips or sutures, topical agents or banding
- Angiographic diagnosis and treatment
  - For evaluation and treatment of upper GI bleeding that is refractory to medical and endoscopic management, for inconclusive endoscopy and for transcatheter intervention
  - Selective injection of artery supplying most likely bleeding source, based on clinical data and other prior diagnostic studies (endoscopy, nuclear scan)
    - Celiac arteriogram for most upper GI sources
    - SMA arteriogram to evaluate small bowel and collateral supply to stomach and duodenum
  - Angiographic treatment options include transcatheter embolization and vasopressin infusion
  - Embolization provides rapid and definitive control
    - Decreases arterial pressure and flow to bleeding source, allowing hemostasis to occur without creating symptomatic ischemia
    - Embolic agents typically used are large particles, Gelfoam pledgets or microcoils
    - Rich gastric arterial collaterals allows for embolization with relative impunity
    - Can empirically embolize left gastric artery in endoscopically proven fundal lesions
    - Therapeutic failure may occur when treating a site that has a dual arterial supply
  - Transcatheter vasopressin infusion may be used if embolization is not possible or bleeding is diffuse
    - Causes contraction of smooth muscles of GI tract and vascular bed
    - Selective infusion of 0.2-0.4 U/min generally sufficient to stop arterial or mucosal bleeding
    - Treatment may require infusions up to 48 hours
- Surgical treatment for bleeding refractory to endoscopic or angiographic control
- Transjugular intrahepatic portosystemic shunt (TIPS)
  - Treatment of portal hypertension; gastroesophageal varices

DIAGNOSTIC CHECKLIST

Consider

- Scintigraphy for hemodynamically stable cases
- Angiography for hemodynamically unstable cases
  - Can evaluate and treat bleeding that is refractory to medical and endoscopic management

SELECTED REFERENCES

1. Wang HH et al: Interventional therapy for acute hemorrhage in gastrointestinal tract. World J Gastroenterol. 12(1):134-6, 2006
2. Hastings GS: Angiographic localization and transcatheter treatment of gastrointestinal bleeding. Radiographics. 20(4):1160-8, 2000
3. Maurer AH et al: Effects of in vitro versus in vivo red cell labeling on image quality in gastrointestinal bleeding studies. J Nucl Med Technol. 26(2):87-90, 1998
4. Whitaker SC et al: The role of angiography in the investigation of acute or chronic gastrointestinal haemorrhage. Clin Radiol. 47(6):382-8, 1993

IMAGE GALLERY

Typical

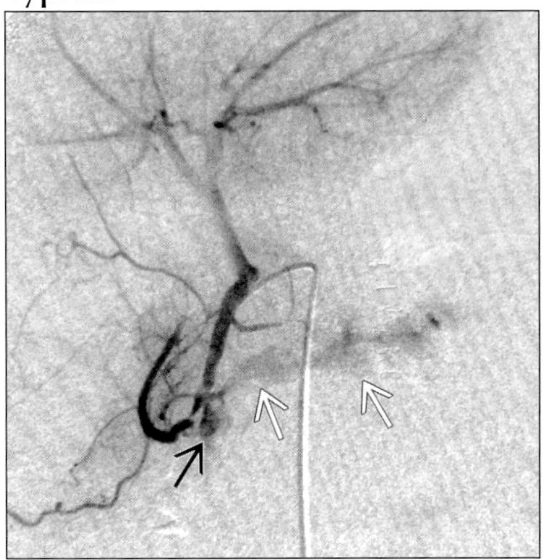

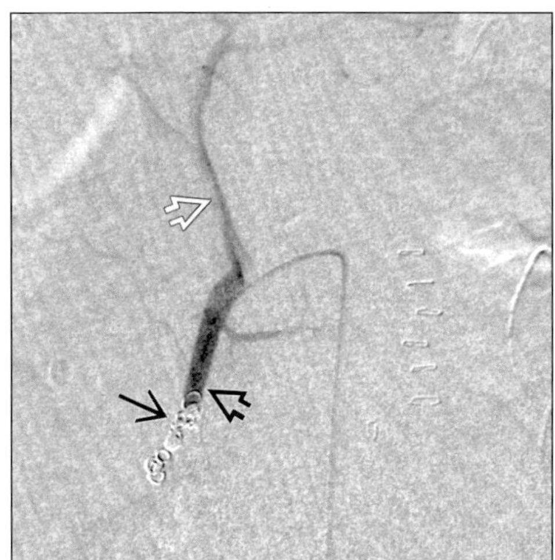

(Left) Selective gastroduodenal arteriogram in a patient with severe pancreatitis and massive upper GI bleeding demonstrates contrast extravasation ➡ and a pseudoaneurysm ➡ as the source of hemorrhage. *(Right)* Selective arteriogram after embolization shows coils ➡ in the distal gastroduodenal artery ➡ that were deployed proximal to the pseudoaneurysm for control of hemorrhage. The proper hepatic artery ➡ is seen coursing cephalad.

Typical

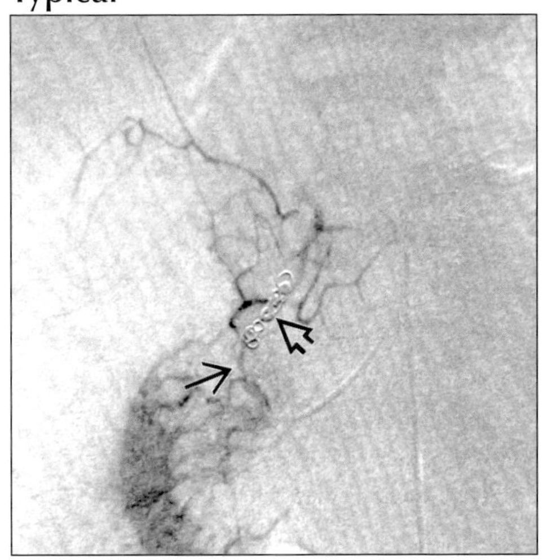

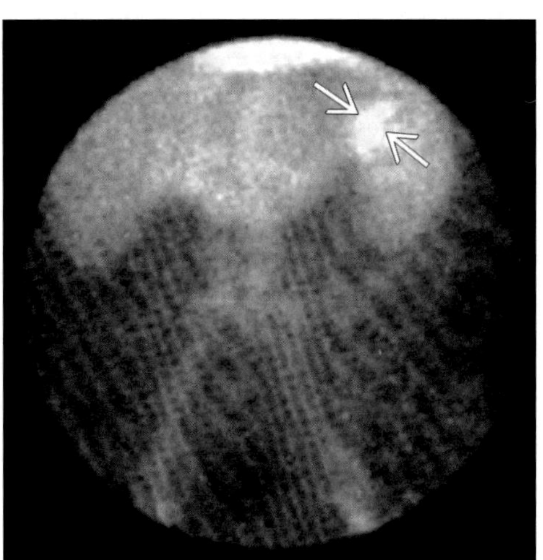

(Left) Selective inferior pancreaticoduodenal artery ➡ angiogram following the embolization ➡ confirms control of bleeding from the pseudoaneurysm, despite the dual blood supply from the pancreaticoduodenal arcade. *(Right)* Tc-99m labeled RBC nuclear scan in a different patient with hematemesis shows radioisotope accumulation ➡ in the gastric region of the left upper quadrant. Because the stomach was blood-filled, no bleeding source was identified at endoscopy.

Typical

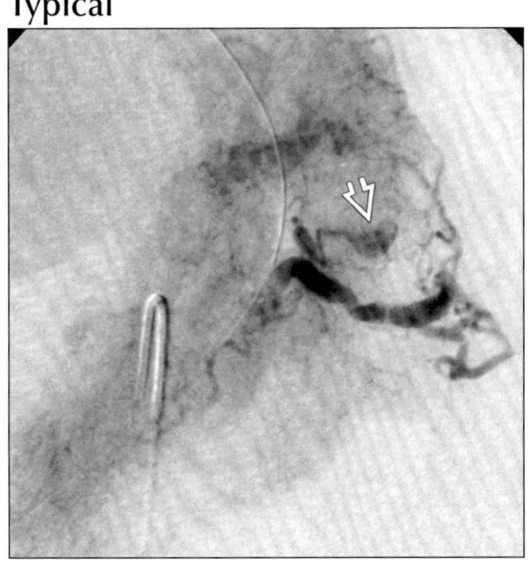

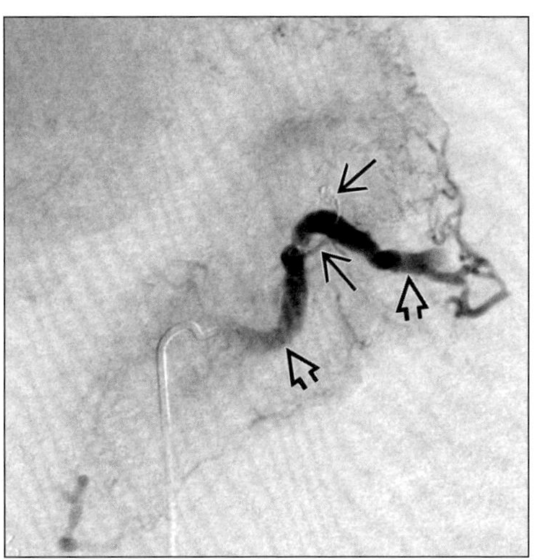

(Left) Arteriogram following nuclear scan (previous image) shows contrast extravasation ➡ in the stomach at the site of upper GI bleeding. With significant intragastric blood accumulation, extravasated contrast may layer between clots or within gastric rugal folds and assume a "pseudovein" appearance. *(Right)* Arteriogram after coil embolization ➡ shows there is no longer active bleeding. Source of bleeding was from a short gastric artery, arising from the splenic artery ➡.

LOWER GI BLEEDING

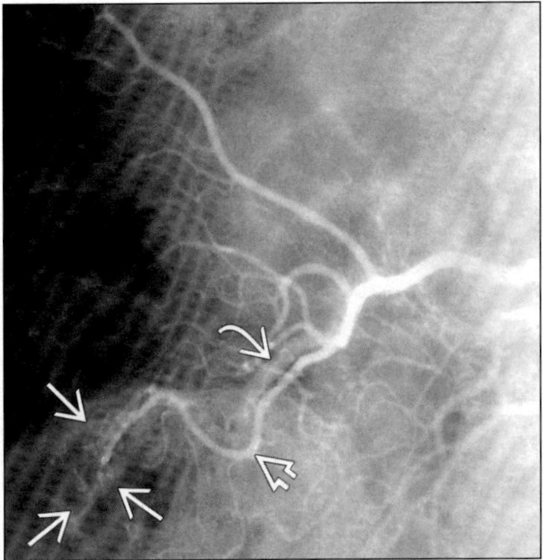

Selective ileocolic arteriogram shows angiodysplasia in the cecum ➡ as the cause of chronic anemia and bleeding in an elderly patient. There is a prominent feeding artery ➡ and an early draining vein ➡.

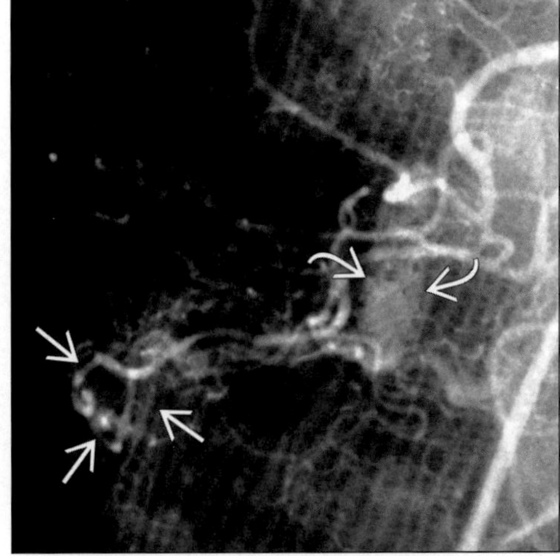

A more magnified view from the arteriogram shows that the angiodysplasia is an AVM, characterized by a tangle of small arteries ➡ and a prominent early draining vein ➡. These are seen to better advantage in this view.

TERMINOLOGY

Definitions

- Acute or chronic bleeding from gastrointestinal tract distal to ligament of Treitz

IMAGING FINDINGS

Radiographic Findings

- Very limited value of barium studies
  - Large quantities of blood in lumen make interpretation difficult
  - Abnormalities detected may not be etiology of current bleeding episode
  - Presence of barium precludes subsequent angiography and interferes with endoscopy

CT Findings

- Active bleeding appears as linear, pooled or swirled focal collection of extravasated intraluminal or extraluminal contrast on CECT

Nuclear Medicine Findings

- Tc-99m Sulfur Colloid
  - Extravasation of isotope at active bleeding site
  - Bleeding rate of 0.05-0.1 mL/min detected
    - More sensitive than Tc-99m labeled RBC scan
    - Usually valid only for localizing lower GI bleeding
  - Intravascular half-life: 2.5 minutes
    - By 15 min isotope cleared from vascular system, producing significant contrast between bleeding site and surroundings
- Tc-99m Labeled Red Cell Scintigraphy
  - Bleeding rate of 0.1-0.2 mL/min detected
  - 5-10 mL of extravasated blood required for detection
  - Sensitivity (85-95%) and specificity (70-85%) for all sources of GI bleeding (upper and lower)
  - Continuous dynamic imaging (large FOV camera)
    - 15 min dynamic "flow" image sequence followed by 1 minute interval scans for 1 hour
    - Repeat until bleeding identified or study stopped
  - Labeled RBCs outside of normal areas of blood pool constitutes a positive study
  - Advantages of RBC scan
    - Active bleeding unnecessary at time of injection

DDx: Lower GI Bleeding

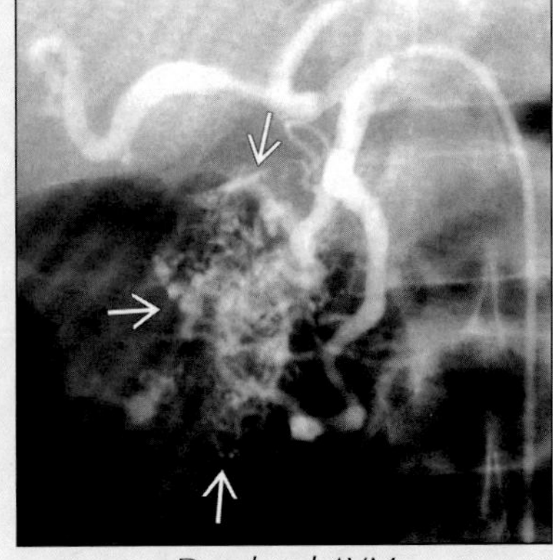

Duodenal AVM

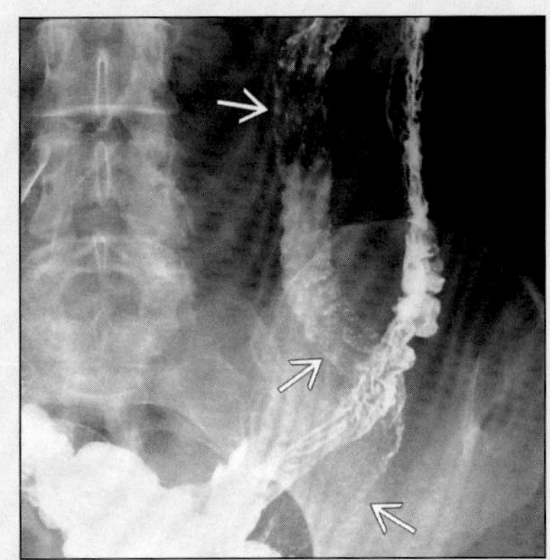

Inflammatory Bowel Disease

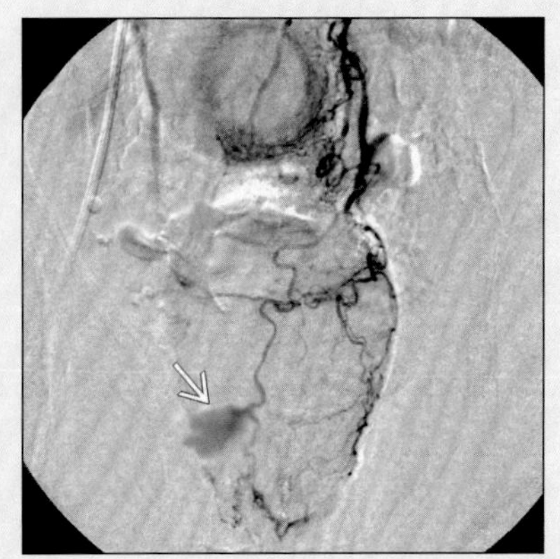

Iatrogenic (Rectal Biopsy)

LOWER GI BLEEDING

Key Facts

Terminology
- Acute or chronic bleeding from gastrointestinal tract distal to ligament of Treitz

Imaging Findings
- Nuclear scintigraphy is usually the procedure of choice following inconclusive or negative endoscopy
- Angiography may be used in hemodynamically unstable patients with active bleeding

Top Differential Diagnoses
- Diverticulosis
- Colonic Angiodysplasia

Clinical Issues
- Angiographic diagnosis and treatment
  - For evaluation and treatment of lower GI bleeding that is refractory to medical and endoscopic management, for inconclusive endoscopy and for transcatheter intervention
  - Can evaluate small bowel between duodenum and ileocecal valve, an endoscopically difficult area to assess and an uncommon site of hemorrhage
- Angiographic treatment options include transcatheter embolization and vasopressin infusion
- Surgical treatment for bleeding refractory to endoscopic or angiographic control
- Hard to localize lesions and may also miss lesions

Diagnostic Checklist
- Scintigraphy for hemodynamically stable cases
- Angiography for hemodynamically unstable cases

    - Higher detection rate for intermittent bleeding
    - Ability to monitor over prolonged period
  - Disadvantages of RBC scan
    - Origin of bleed unclear on delayed scans as tagged cells may travel in antegrade or retrograde fashion
    - Vascular organs may interfere with detection
    - Loss of tag can produce false ±
    - Less sensitive than Tc-99m sulfur colloid (SC) scan

Angiographic Findings
- Conventional
  - Usually preceded by Tc-99m-labeled RBC scan
  - Diagnostic accuracy: 70-95%
  - Bleeding rate of > 0.5 mL/min for detection
  - Active bleeding appears as localized contrast extravasation during arterial phase
  - Major limitations in identifying bleeding source
    - Intermittent nature of GI hemorrhage, with negative study if temporary cessation of bleeding
    - Inability to demonstrate venous or variceal bleeding from selective arterial injection

Imaging Recommendations
- Nuclear scintigraphy is usually the procedure of choice following inconclusive or negative endoscopy
  - Active gastrointestinal hemorrhage must be present in a hemodynamically stable patient
  - Enhances the efficacy of angiography
  - May delineate obscure sources and intermittent bleeding
- Angiography may be used in hemodynamically unstable patients with active bleeding

DIFFERENTIAL DIAGNOSIS

Diverticulosis
- 75% of diverticula occur in left colon but 70% of diverticular bleeding occurs in right colon
- Diverticula are small sac-like outpouchings of mucosa and submucosa along antimesenteric surface of colon
  - Diverticular bleeding occurs when there is erosion into a blood vessel at base of a diverticulum
- Bleeding in 10-30% of patients with diverticulosis
  - 80% resolve spontaneously
  - Persistent severe bleeding requiring intervention occurs in 5%
  - Selective transcatheter embolization or selective vasopressin infusion controls bleeding in 80-90%
  - Emergency colectomy carries high morbidity and mortality, as this is a disease of the elderly

Colonic Angiodysplasia
- Tend to be small lesions of vascular ectasia that occur in the cecum, ascending or proximal transverse colon
- Symptoms of intermittent low-grade bleeding, but occasionally have episodes of massive rectal bleeding
- Visible on colonoscopy and selective arteriography
  - Angiographically a cluster or tangle of small arteries is seen in arterial phase, with early filling and delayed emptying of dilated veins
- Decision to surgically resect ascending and proximal transverse colon in these patients made on basis of colonoscopy and occasionally angiography

Bleeding from an Upper GI Source
- Peptic ulcer disease
- Gastritis
- Gastroesophageal varices
- Less common entities such as portal hypertension (varices), Mallory-Weiss tear, marginal ulcer, iatrogenic injury, neoplasm, pseudoaneurysm, hemobilia, aortoenteric fistula, AVM and Dieulafoy lesion
- Massive upper GI bleeding can result in hematochezia

Bleeding from a Small Bowel Source
- 3-5% of all GI tract bleeding
- Undiagnosed iron deficiency anemia or episodic melena with normal endoscopy and colonoscopy
- Most common etiologies are neoplasm, AVM and mesenteric varices

Neoplasms
- Tumor invasion or mucosal erosion results in bleeding

Inflammatory Bowel Disease
- Rectal bleeding may be first manifestation of colitis

LOWER GI BLEEDING

- Bleeding may also occur with ischemic colitis

Iatrogenic

- Bleeding following endoscopic biopsy, polypectomy
- Bleeding from a surgical site

PATHOLOGY

General Features

- Etiology
  - Diverticulosis (43%), angiodysplasia (20%)
  - Idiopathic (12%), neoplasia (9%)
  - Colitis (radiation, ischemic, ulcerative) 9%
- Epidemiology
  - Annual incidence of 20.5/100,000
  - Accounts for < 1% of all hospital admissions in US
- Lower GI bleed accounts for 24% of GI hemorrhage

Staging, Grading or Classification Criteria

- Classification based on onset & presentation
  - Acute: Hematochezia, melena
  - Chronic: Iron deficiency anemia

CLINICAL ISSUES

Presentation

- Most common signs/symptoms
  - May present acutely with hematochezia (bright red blood per rectum) or melena (black, tarry stools that typically are seen with chronic blood loss)
  - May also present with occult blood loss, detected by chemical testing of stool
    - Unexplained iron deficiency anemia and intermittent episodic melena are signs of chronic bleeding
  - Symptoms and signs of blood loss include dizziness, tachycardia, hypotension and shock
- Lab data
  - Fresh blood or occult blood in stool
  - Iron deficiency anemia
  - ↓ CBC count, hematocrit, serum electrolytes
  - Abnormal coagulation profile (aPTT, PT, platelet count, bleeding time)

Demographics

- Age: More common in older age group
- Gender: M > F

Natural History & Prognosis

- Prognosis
  - Good prognosis with early detection, resuscitation & treatment; poor with delay
  - Acute massive GI bleeding can result in shock and death
  - Mortality rate in lower GI bleeding ranges from 0-21%

Treatment

- Medical
  - Conservative management with bedrest, sedation, fluid and blood replacement
  - Correction of any underlying coagulopathy
  - Endoscopy should be initial diagnostic procedure
    - Source identified in > 95%
    - Bleeding source treated with electrocautery, injection sclerotherapy, mechanical clips or sutures, topical agents or banding
  - Capsule endoscopy: Pitfalls
    - May fail in bowel with strictures or prior surgery
    - Lengthy study requiring 8 hrs of prior preparation and 8 hrs to compile and interpret data
    - Hard to localize lesions and may also miss lesions
- Angiographic diagnosis and treatment
  - For evaluation and treatment of lower GI bleeding that is refractory to medical and endoscopic management, for inconclusive endoscopy and for transcatheter intervention
  - Can evaluate small bowel between duodenum and ileocecal valve, an endoscopically difficult area to assess and an uncommon site of hemorrhage
  - Selective injection of artery supplying most likely bleeding source, based on clinical data and other prior diagnostic studies (endoscopy, nuclear scan)
    - Celiac arteriogram for most upper GI sources
    - SMA arteriogram to evaluate small bowel and collateral supply to stomach and duodenum
    - IMA arteriogram
  - Angiographic treatment options include transcatheter embolization and vasopressin infusion
  - Embolization provides rapid and definitive control
    - Decreases arterial pressure and flow to bleeding source, allowing hemostasis to occur without creating symptomatic ischemia
    - Embolic agents typically used are large particles, Gelfoam pledgets or microcoils
  - Transcatheter vasopressin infusion may be used if embolization not possible or bleeding is diffuse
    - Causes contraction of smooth muscles of GI tract and vascular bed
    - Selective infusion of 0.2 0.4 U/min generally sufficient to stop arterial or mucosal bleeding
    - Treatment may require infusions up to 48 hours
- Surgical treatment for bleeding refractory to endoscopic or angiographic control

DIAGNOSTIC CHECKLIST

Consider

- Scintigraphy for hemodynamically stable cases
- Angiography for hemodynamically unstable cases

SELECTED REFERENCES

1. Tew K et al: MDCT of acute lower gastrointestinal bleeding. AJR Am J Roentgenol. 182(2):427-30, 2004
2. Hastings GS: Angiographic localization and transcatheter treatment of gastrointestinal bleeding. Radiographics. 20(4):1160-8, 2000
3. Maurer AH et al: Effects of in vitro versus in vivo red cell labeling on image quality in gastrointestinal bleeding studies. J Nucl Med Technol. 26(2):87-90, 1998
4. Bunker SR: Cine scintigraphy of gastrointestinal bleeding. Radiology. 187(3):877-8, 1993
5. Whitaker SC et al: The role of angiography in the investigation of acute or chronic gastrointestinal haemorrhage. Clin Radiol. 47(6):382-8, 1993

IMAGE GALLERY

Typical

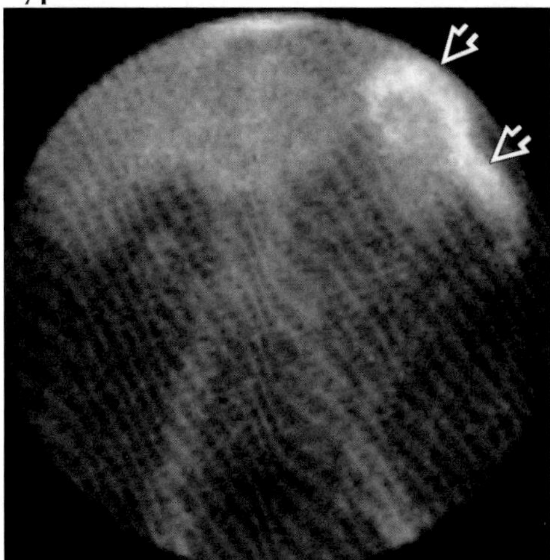

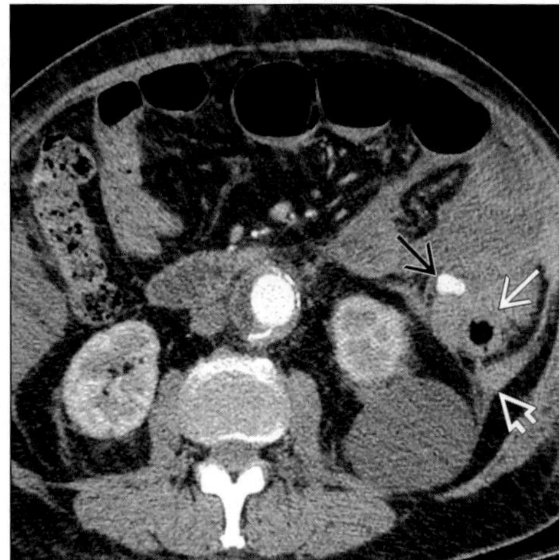

*(**Left**) Tc-99m labeled RBC scan shows radioisotope accumulation ➡ in the left upper abdomen, at a site of active bleeding in the splenic flexure or descending colon. Tagged RBCs may travel antegrade or retrograde in the bowel lumen. (**Right**) Axial CECT shows a focal contrast collection → in the left mid-abdomen adjacent to the descending colon ➡ in a patient who presented with hypotension and hematochezia. There is blood in the left paracolic gutter ➡.*

Typical

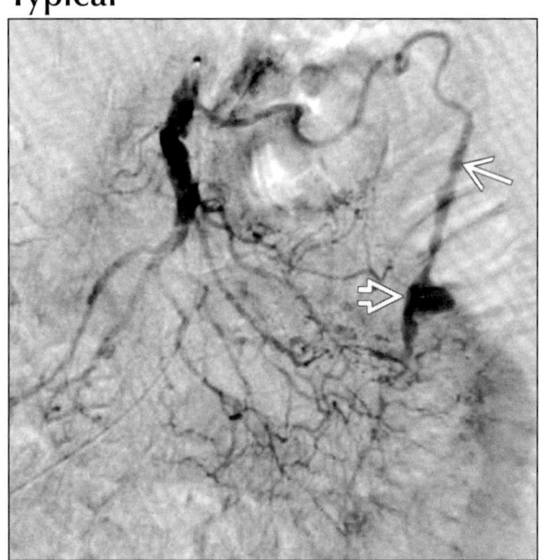

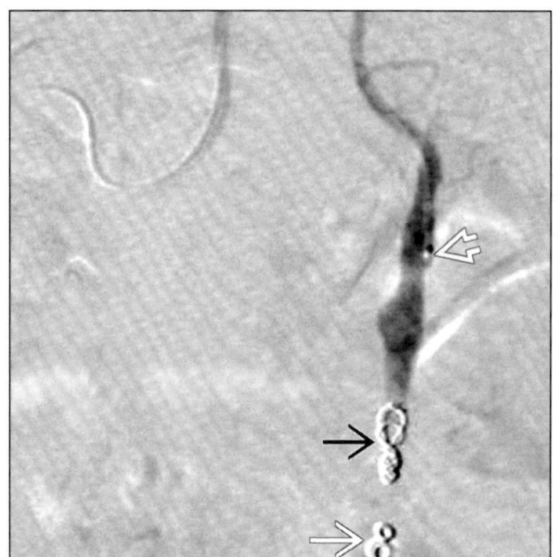

*(**Left**) Superior mesenteric arteriogram shows an ovoid contrast collection ➡ arising from the left colic artery ➡, corresponding to the collection on the CECT. This represents contrast that has collected within a bleeding diverticulum. (**Right**) Left colic arteriogram via a microcatheter ➡ introduced from the SMA shows embolization coils proximal → and distal ➡ to the bleeding diverticulum. Contrast no longer fills the diverticulum and symptoms resolved.*

Typical

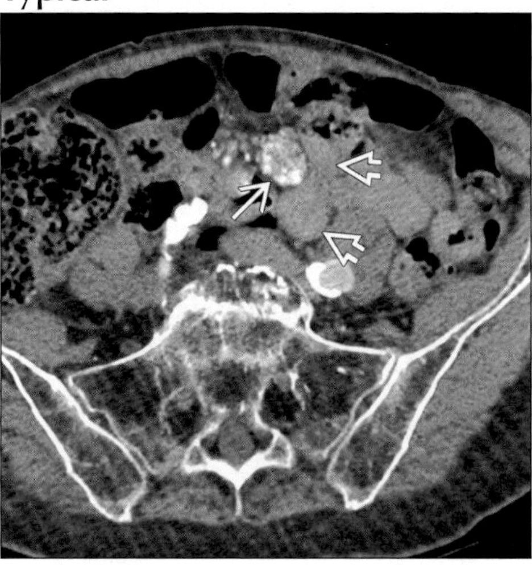

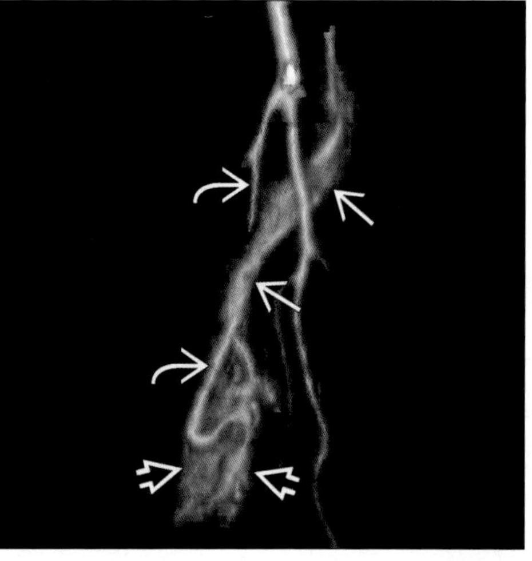

*(**Left**) Axial CECT in another patient shows a vascular mass ➡ adjacent to a pelvic small bowel loop ➡. There was a history of chronic iron deficiency anemia and intermittent melena. Upper endoscopy and colonoscopy were negative. (**Right**) Volume rendered 3-D CTA shows that the CECT abnormality is a small bowel AVM ➡. Note the feeding artery ➡ and the draining vein ➡. Erosion of the overlying bowel mucosa results in chronic bleeding from friable vessels.*

HEPATIC ARTERY TRAUMA

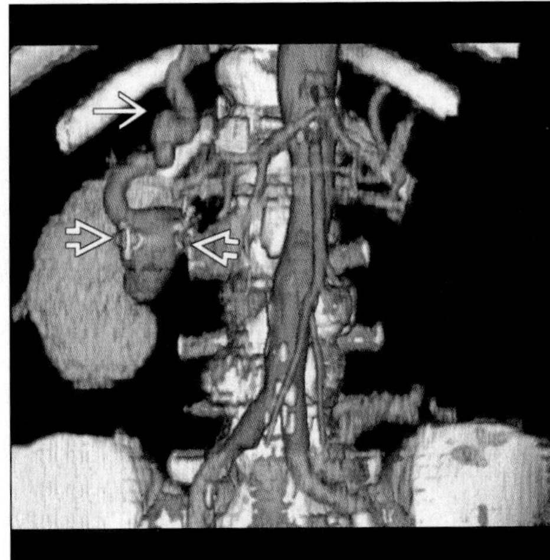

CTA volume rendered reconstruction shows a saccular post-traumatic pseudoaneurysm ⇨ of the right hepatic artery. There is tortuous venous drainage ➡. (Courtesy A. Lemos, MD).

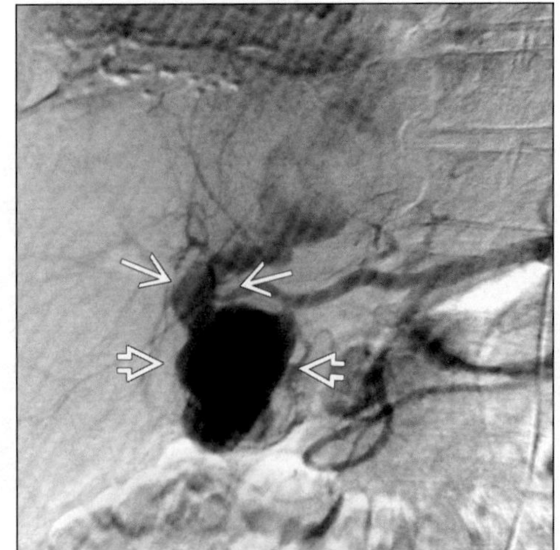

DSA same patient (45 year old man victim of blunt trauma) with a pseudoaneurysm of the right hepatic artery ⇨ and formation of an arteriovenous fistula. Venous drainage ➡.

TERMINOLOGY

Abbreviations and Synonyms

- Hepatic artery (HA) laceration, hepatic artery transection, hepatic artery injury

Definitions

- Injury to abdominal visceral vessel at the porta hepatis
  - Injuries to abdominal vessels are uncommon but devastating entities

IMAGING FINDINGS

General Features

- Best diagnostic clue: CT scan reveals active hemorrhage
- Location
  - Porta hepatis
  - Intrahepatic

CT Findings

- NECT: Hemoperitoneum surrounding porta hepatis, celiac axis, pancreas, lesser sac and gallbladder fossa
- CECT
  - Extravasation of contrast material in area of celiac axis or portal triad
  - Active hemorrhage can manifest as extravasation of contrast inside liver parenchyma (parenchymal hematoma) or freely into peritoneal space as "jet"
  - Trauma CT protocol: Abdominal scanning performed 70 seconds after start of intravenous contrast administration
    - Follow-up CT examination after 6-8 hours to catch abdominal arterial injuries missed in previous scan
  - CT angiography: Sensitivity is between 91% and 97% and specificity between 95% and 99%

Angiographic Findings

- If dissection is proven, precise anatomical delineation and assessment of collateral vessels is done with angiography
- Also helpful for planning of further treatment

Imaging Recommendations

- Best imaging tool: CECT scan has sensitivity 70% compared to US (sensitivity 40%)
- Protocol advice

DDx: Injuries Associated with Hepatic Artery Trauma

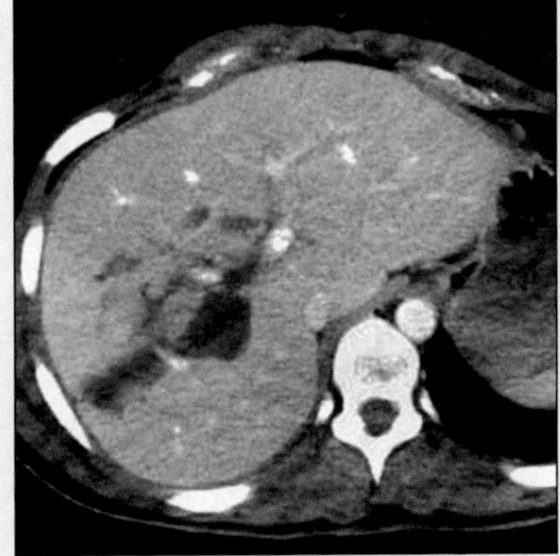

Biloma Following Trauma

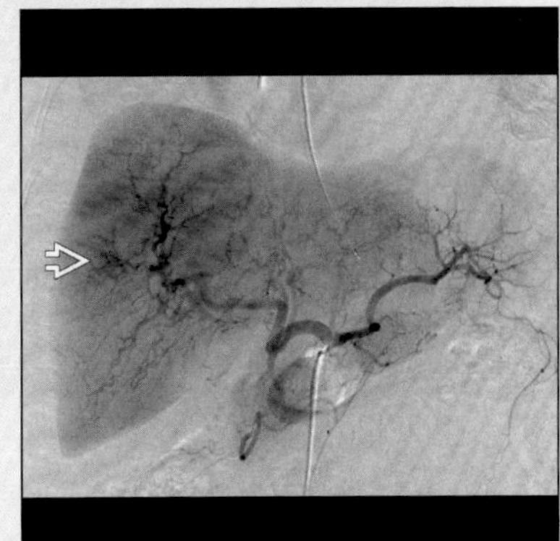

Parenchymal Extravasation

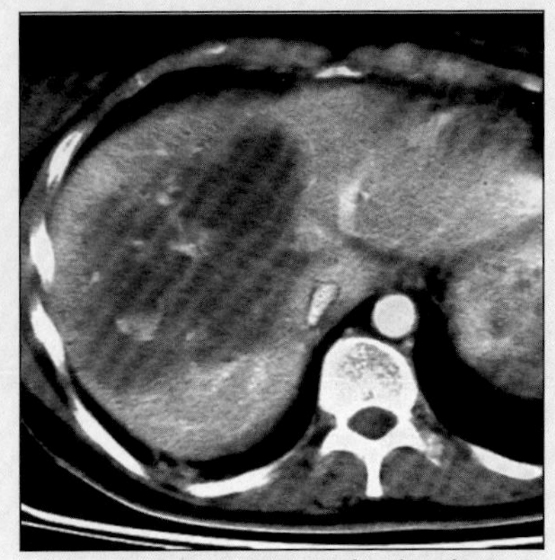

Large Hematoma with Bleeding

HEPATIC ARTERY TRAUMA

Key Facts

Terminology

- Injuries to abdominal vessels are uncommon but devastating entities

Imaging Findings

- CECT scan has sensitivity of 70% compared to US (sensitivity of 40%)
- Active hemorrhage following blunt liver trauma identified at early phase CECT
  - Focal high attenuation area representing contrast material collection secondary to arterial bleeding
- Re-imaging may be helpful in immediate post-injury period to better evaluate findings such as fever, anemia, or laboratory abnormalities
- Trauma CT protocol: Abdominal scanning performed 70 seconds after start of intravenous contrast administration
- Follow up CT examination after 6-8 hours to catch any abdominal arterial injuries missed in previous scan
- CT angiography: 91% up to 97% and specificity between 95% and 99%

Pathology

- HA is least commonly injured structure, accounting for only 1-2% of all vascular injuries
- HA is least injured structure (23%) during blunt trauma of the porta hepatis
  - Superior mesenteric artery is most frequently injured
- When blunt hepatic injuries occur, most commonly result in pseudoaneurysm formation; less often occlusion, partial, or complete transection occurs

  - Active hemorrhage following blunt liver trauma is identified at early phase CECT
    - Focal high attenuation area representing contrast material collection secondary to arterial bleeding
  - Re-imaging may be helpful in immediate post-injury period to better evaluate findings such as fever, anemia or laboratory abnormalities
  - Active arterial extravasation can be differentiated from clotted blood by measuring CT attenuation
    - Active arterial extravasation attenuation range: 91-274 HU (mean 155 HU)
    - Clotted blood attenuation range: 28-82 HU (mean 54 HU)

DIFFERENTIAL DIAGNOSIS

Parenchymal (Subcapsular, Intraparenchymal) Hematoma

- Subcapsular hematoma
  - Lenticular configuration, often involving right lobe
  - Creates indentation or flattening of underlying liver margin where perihepatic hemorrhage does not
  - NECT: Liver is hyperattenuating compared to hematoma
  - CECT: Hematoma is low attenuating collections compared with hyperattenuating liver parenchyma
- Intraparenchymal hematoma: If acute, presents as irregular high attenuation area (clotted blood) at CECT surrounded by low attenuating unclotted blood or bile
  - Over time, when attenuation is reduced, hematoma forms well-defined serous fluid collection

Parenchymal Laceration

- Linear streaking area involving parenchymal areas contiguous to intraparenchymal portal branches and suprahepatic veins
- Parallel to hepatic veins or posterior segmental right branch of portal vein
- Acute lacerations have sharp or jagged margins
  - If multiple and parallel, due to compression forces (bear claw lacerations)

Other Vascular Injuries (Portal Venous System)

- Injuries to major hepatic veins and retrohepatic IVC are uncommon after blunt trauma
- CT shows lacerations extending into major hepatic veins and IVC or retrohepatic hemorrhage extending near diaphragm or lesser sac

Biloma

- Small in volume but may increase in size if supplied by a large biliary duct; it can form inside or outside the liver parenchyma
- Bilomas < 3 cm do not require therapeutic intervention
- Bilomas > 3 cm are cured with US/CT-guided drainages

Gallbladder Injury

- Occurs in 2-8% of patients with blunt liver trauma
- CT findings: Ill-defined or irregular wall contour, wall thickening, intraluminal blood, pericholecystic fluid, collapsed gallbladder, contrast-enhancement of gallbladder wall or mucosa, mass effect on duodenum, free intraperitoneal fluid

PATHOLOGY

General Features

- Etiology
  - Penetrating (gunshot) trauma (90-95%)
  - Blunt trauma (5-10%): Possible mechanisms of injury in restrained passengers
    - Sudden increase of intra-abdominal pressure with diaphragm elevation
    - Compression of celiac artery by median arcuate ligament (MAL)
    - Deceleration injury of celiac artery against MAL
  - Surgery: True incidence of vascular injuries during cholecystectomy is unknown
    - Autopsy study shows incidence of right hepatic artery injury after open cholecystectomy is 7%

- Biopsy: Iatrogenic, vascular, and bile duct injuries have increased in number due to
  - Laparoscopic operations
  - Endoscopic procedures
  - Percutaneous interventions such as drainages, biopsies, TIPS
- Epidemiology
  - HA is least commonly injured structure, accounting for only 1-2% of all vascular injuries
    - HA is least injured structure (23%) during blunt trauma of the porta hepatis; superior mesenteric artery (SMA) is most frequently injured
    - HA injuries are equally distributed between the right, left, proper and common hepatic artery
- Associated abnormalities: Hemobilia

Gross Pathologic & Surgical Features

- When blunt hepatic injuries occur they most commonly result in pseudoaneurysm formation
  - Less often in either occlusion, partial, or complete transection

Microscopic Features

- Since arterial injury generally initiated at interface with circulating blood, the layer most frequently involved is inner layer (intima)
  - Adventitial layer can play major role as well (fibroblasts play a critical role in the adventitial response to injury)
  - Fibroblasts convert into myofibroblasts and lead to perivascular fibrosis

CLINICAL ISSUES

Presentation

- Most common signs/symptoms
  - Transections (partial or complete) result in significant blood loss and patients are invariably hemodynamically unstable
  - Pseudoaneurysms may not manifest for several days to months after injury
    - Pseudoaneurysms present with abdominal pain, jaundice (if biliary ducts are obstructed), and melena, because of hemobilia
- Other signs/symptoms: Right upper quadrant pain, hypotension, hemorrhagic shock, biliary peritonitis with diffuse pain, absence of intestinal paresis

Natural History & Prognosis

- Fewer than 10% of patients with major liver trauma have life-threatening bleeding
- Regardless of whether penetrating or blunt trauma, exsanguination is the most common cause of death
- Mortality rates up to 50% with isolated triad injuries and 80% with combined injuries (Western Trauma Association)

Treatment

- Conservative treatment possible for limited dissections and when serial examinations have demonstrated no evidence of rupture or expansion
- Management of HA injuries includes surgical ligation, primary repair (reconstruction with a patch or graft interposition) and hepatic embolization
  - HA ligation: Performed in those patients who exhibit hemodynamic instability and are in operating room
    - Liver tolerates HA ligation well
    - Incidence of subsequent hepatic necrosis is relatively low
    - Collateral flow from translobar, subcapsular collaterals, phrenicoabdominal and intercostal arteries will reconstitute arterial flow as early as 24 hours after injury
  - Injuries to other structures, especially portal vein, must be evaluated in conjunction with HA injury, as ligation of both structures will result in liver necrosis
  - Evaluation for evidence of hepatic ischemia after ligation should be considered
    - When portal vein inflow has been compromised
    - When patient suffered from prolonged period of shock
- Endovascular treatment should be considered, particularly if patient does not require other abdominal surgery
- Hemorrhage from other intra-abdominal vessels such as aorta, renal arteries or veins or inferior vena cava may complicate vascular control
- Embolization of HA injuries within liver parenchyma well-established
- Extraparenchymal HA injuries with higher rate of bleeding and lack of tamponade effect may preclude embolization

DIAGNOSTIC CHECKLIST

Consider

- Injuries to hepatic vessels can be devastating and need to be diagnosed and rapidly treated, especially in hemodynamically unstable patients

Image Interpretation Pearls

- Active hemorrhage following blunt liver trauma is identified at early phase CECT

SELECTED REFERENCES

1. Michel JB et al: Topological determinants and consequences of adventitial responses to arterial wall injury. Arterioscler Thromb Vasc Biol. 27(6):1259-68, 2007
2. Moreno RD et al: Late presentation of a hepatic pseudoaneurysm with hemobilia after angioembolization for blunt hepatic trauma. J Trauma. 62(4):1048-50, 2007
3. Miglietta MA et al: Hepatic artery transection after blunt trauma: case presentation and review of the literature. J Pediatr Surg. 41(9):1604-6, 2006
4. Ripley RT et al: Hepatic artery avulsion secondary to blunt abdominal trauma. J Trauma. 61(4):1022, 2006
5. Yoon W et al: CT in blunt liver trauma. Radiographics. 25(1):87-104, 2005
6. Romano L et al: Hepatic trauma: CT findings and considerations based on our experience in emergency diagnostic imaging. Eur J Radiol. 50(1):59-66, 2004

IMAGE GALLERY

Typical

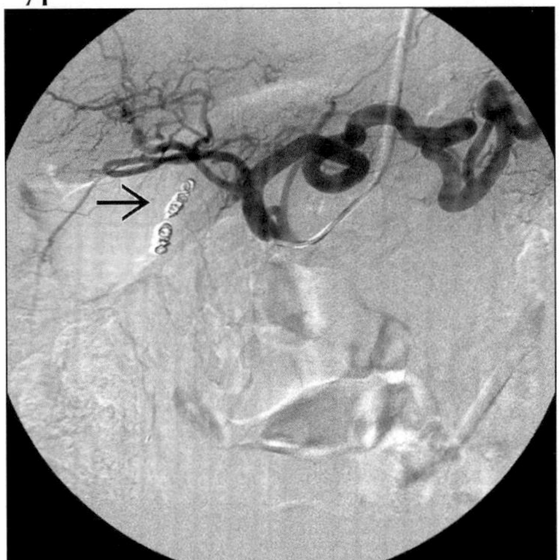

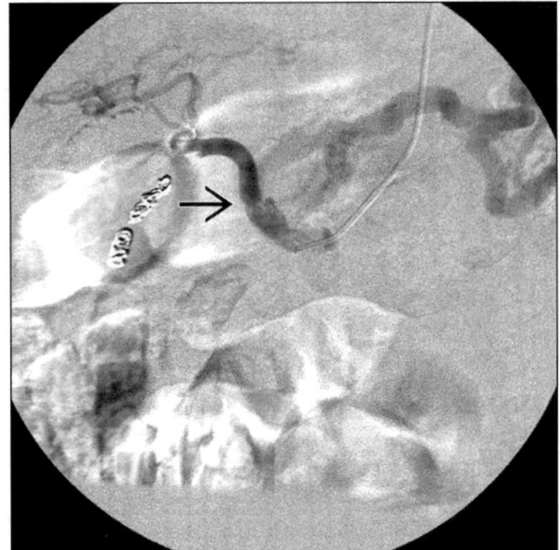

*(**Left**) DSA shows catheterization of the celiac trunk to visualize prior embolization of gastroduodenal artery (GDA) ➔ in patient with liver metastasis. (Courtesy S.C. Rose, MD). (**Right**) Late arterial phase DSA (same patient as previous image), shows complication of procedure. Non occlusive intimal flap of the celiac trunk due to catheterization ➔.*

Typical

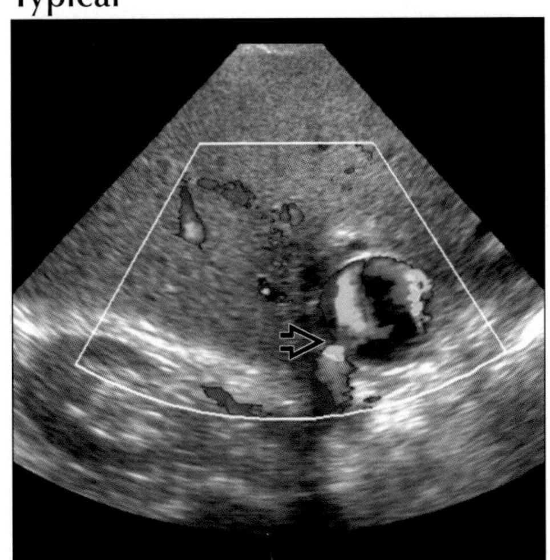

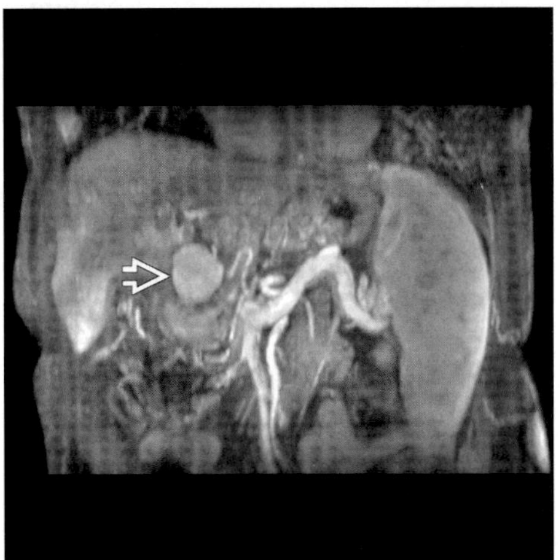

*(**Left**) Color Doppler ultrasound shows a pseudoaneurysm ⇨ in a patient following a liver biopsy. Notice "the ying-yang" appearance of a pseudoaneurysm caused by the to-and-fro flow in the pseudoaneurysm. (**Right**) MR MPR coronal display demonstrates the hepatic artery pseudoaneurysm ⇨ arising just on the outer edges of the liver. MPR is very helpful for evaluating the position of the pseudoaneurysm.*

Other

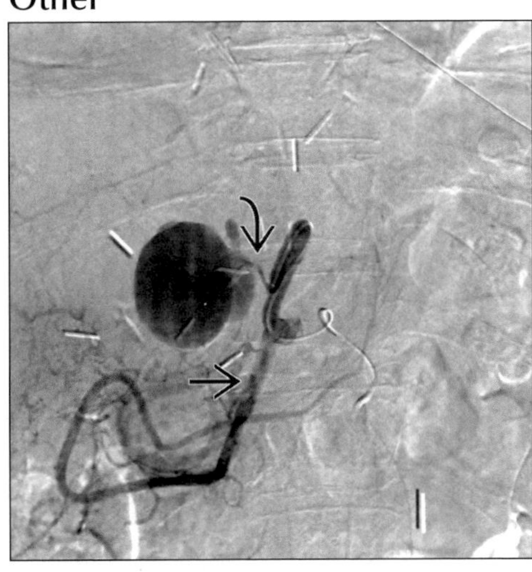

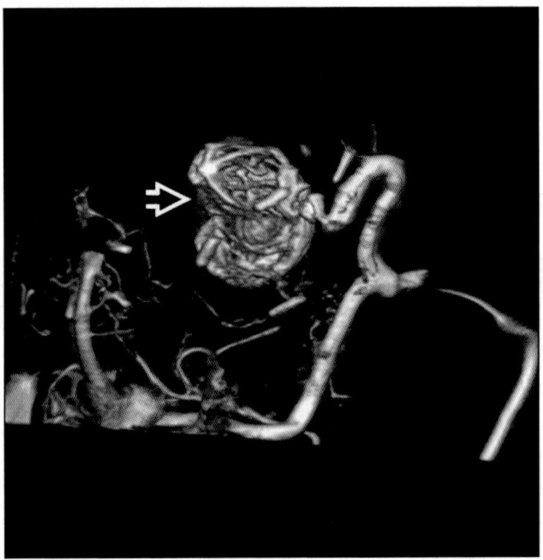

*(**Left**) DSA shows the very narrow neck of the pseudoaneurysm ➔ which is arising from the very beginning of the proper hepatic artery just following the take off of the gastroduodenal artery ➔. (**Right**) 3D reconstruction of the pseudoaneurysm following coil embolization ⇨. Such reconstructions can be useful in evaluating the structure of the coils within the pseudoaneurysm.*

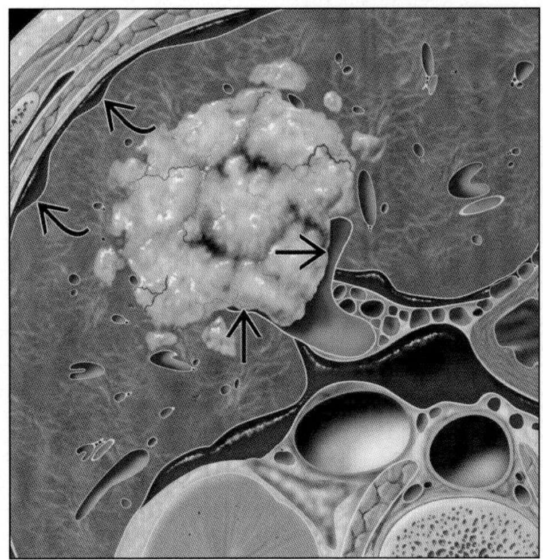

Graphic shows tumor in the hepatic parenchyma extending into the portal vein ➔. Nodularity of the liver ➔ representing cirrhotic changes is demonstrated.

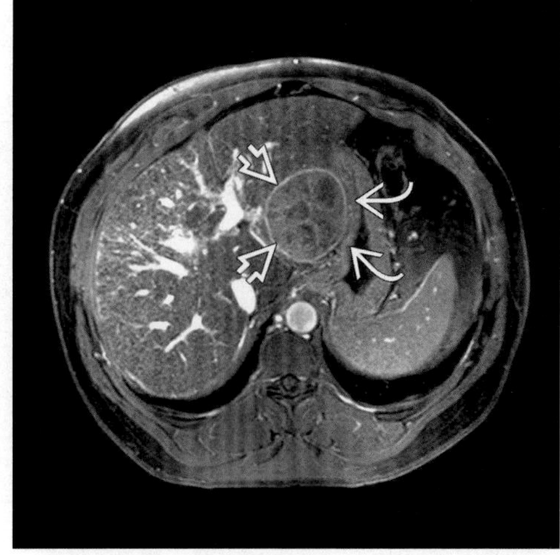

Axial MR FSE demonstrates a large, relatively well-encapsulated lesion ➔. It is compressing the stomach wall ➔ but on this and other series appears to be separate from the stomach.

TERMINOLOGY

Abbreviations and Synonyms

- Hepatocellular carcinoma (HCC)
- Hepatic (liver) lesion, hepatic (liver) nodule, focal liver lesion (FLL)

Definitions

- Hypervascular mass
- Most frequent primary malignant tumor of the liver

IMAGING FINDINGS

General Features

- Best diagnostic clue
  - Early enhancement in arterial phase and washout during portal and delayed phases of contrast-enhanced dynamic imaging including CT and MR
  - Multidetector spiral CT and fast MR techniques permit rapid imaging of the entire abdomen in a single breath hold
  - Ability to perform rapid scanning is particularly important in evaluation of hepatic neoplasms
    - Imaging can be conducted during arterial, portal venous and equilibrium phases of contrast-enhancement

CT Findings

- CECT
  - Transient hepatic attenuation difference (THAD)
    - Attenuation difference of liver appearing during bolus-enhanced dynamic CT
    - Caused by dual flow (arterial and portal flow)
    - Associated with hepatic tumors
    - Generally characteristic of malignant tumors
    - However, benign focal lesions may be accompanied by THADs
  - HCC is most common primary hepatic tumor associated with THAD
    - Because associated with arterio-portal shunts in 63% of cases

Ultrasonographic Findings

- Color Doppler
  - Color and power Doppler have limited ability in depicting intralesional vascularity

DDx: Hepatic Neoplasm

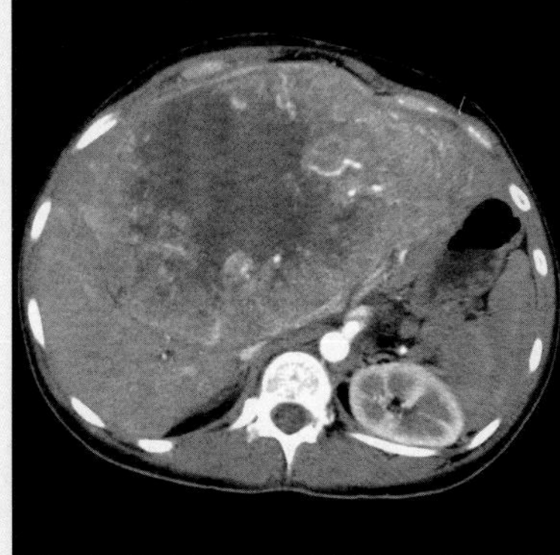

Neuroendocrine Tumor

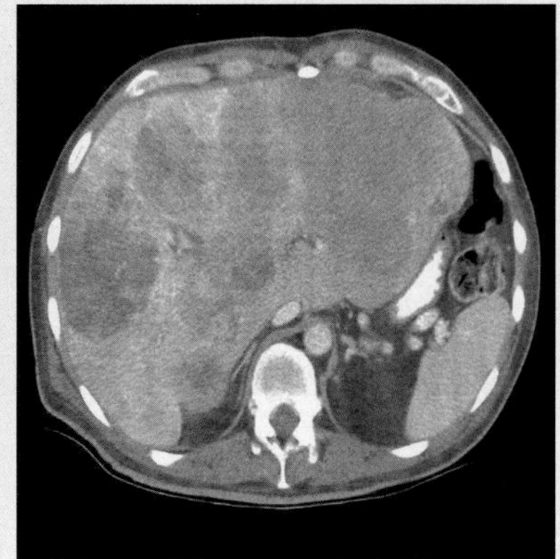

Carcinoid Tumor Metastases

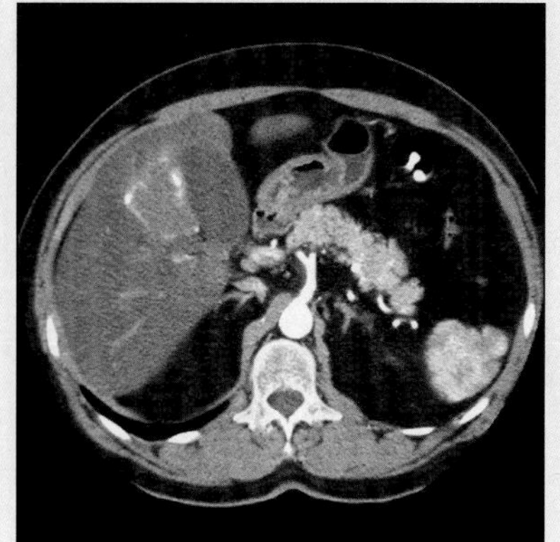

Cavernous Hemangioma

HEPATIC NEOPLASM

Key Facts

Terminology
- Hepatocellular carcinoma (HCC)

Imaging Findings
- Early enhancement in arterial phase and washout during portal and delayed phases of contrast-enhanced dynamic imaging including CT and MR
- Protocol advice: Non-invasive diagnostic criteria: Lesion > 2 cm on two imaging tests (dynamic US, MR, CT scanning) showing hypervascularity or
- α-fetoprotein > 400 ng/mL and one imaging test showing hypervascularity

Pathology
- Chronic HCV infection most common cause of liver cancer (HCC)
- Liver cancer 6th most common newly diagnosed cancer, 3rd most common cause of cancer mortality worldwide

Clinical Issues
- Most common signs/symptoms: Right upper quadrant (RUQ) pain, early satiety and weight loss, vascular bruit in the RUQ if hypervascular tumor
- If lesion is resectable, then surgery offers best option for cure
  - Liver transplantation is an option for lesions meeting criteria
- Transarterial chemoembolization (TACE) and radioembolization are commonly used in patients who are not surgical candidates

    - Insensitive to slow flow and deeply located blood vessels
    - Associated with significant artifacts
  - Contrast-enhanced US (CEUS) overcomes limitations of conventional color Doppler sonography
    - Has been shown to improve assessment of vascularity in FLL

Imaging Recommendations
- Best imaging tool: CECT, MR imaging with gadolinium-based agents
- Protocol advice
  - Hepatic lesions < 2 cm require biopsy confirmation if typical pattern for HCC is not identified in two imaging tests
  - Noninvasive diagnostic criteria
    - Lesion > 2 cm on two imaging tests (dynamic US, MR, CT scanning) showing hypervascularity or
    - α-fetoprotein > 400 ng/mL and one imaging test showing hypervascularity

DIFFERENTIAL DIAGNOSIS

Liver Metastatic Disease
- Most frequent hepatic malignancy (18x more common that primary HCC)
- Variable in size and appearance depending on tissue of origin
- Hypervascular metastases: Carcinoid tumors, pancreatic islet cell tumors, melanoma, choriocarcinoma, pheochromocytoma, thyroid carcinoma, and renal cell carcinoma
- Hypovascular metastases include colon, breast, lung carcinoma, and pancreatic adenocarcinoma

Hemangioma
- Most common benign hepatic neoplasm with incidence of 1-20% in autopsy series
- Often asymptomatic if small; large hemangiomas may cause abdominal discomfort
- NECT: Low attenuation lesions compared with adjacent parenchyma
- CECT: Peripheral, discontinuous, globular enhancement that progresses toward central aspect of lesion with time
- MR: Relative to liver - low signal intensity on T1WI; high signal intensity on T2WI

Focal Nodular Hyperplasia (FNH)
- Second most common benign liver lesion (8% of all benign lesions)
- Well-circumscribed lesion that contains a central scar and abnormally arranged hepatocytes, Kupffer cells, and abnormal bile ductules
- Growth promoted by use of oral contraceptives
- CECT: Hypervascular lesions with rapid washout; central scar is detected more frequently in large lesion than in small lesions
- Signal intensity of FNH is similar to or indistinguishable from adjacent liver on T1WI and T2WI; enhancement pattern identical to CT

Cholangiocarcinoma
- Rare malignancy with wide variation in incidence rates throughout the world
- 10% of patients with cholangiocarcinoma have risk factors such as
  - Infestation with liver flukes, primary sclerosing cholangitis, choledochal cysts, hepatolithiasis, or cirrhosis
- When located adjacent to hilar portion of liver it frequently shows THAD of lobar distribution hepatic arterial phase images
  - THAD is an important indirect sign of vascular invasion

Dysplastic Nodules (DN)
- DNs are nodules in cirrhotic liver that are macroscopically distinct from surrounding cirrhotic nodules (because larger than cirrhotic nodules)
  - High grade DNs are precursors of HCC
- DNs have mainly portal vein blood supply compared with surrounding parenchyma

- MR perfusion seems to be best noninvasive imaging method to differentiate liver nodules (like regenerative nodules from DNs)

PATHOLOGY

General Features

- Etiology
  - Chronic hepatitis C virus (HCV) infection is most common cause of liver cancer (HCC)
  - Factors independently associated with HCC development are: α Feto-protein (AFP) > 20 ng/mL, γ glutamyl transferase (GGT) > 58 U/I and male gender
  - Recent studies have proved that previous exposure to HBV in patients with chronic HCV and cirrhosis increases risk of HCC
- Epidemiology
  - Liver cancer is sixth most common newly diagnosed cancer and third most common cause of cancer mortality in world
  - In US incidence of HCC among white, black and Hispanic population increased by > 90% between 1976 and 2000
  - Racial group with highest risk of liver cancer and with fastest growth rate in US is API (Asian/Pacific Islanders)
  - Because of lag time between onset of infection and development of cirrhosis, incidence of HCV-related HCC will continue to increase over next 20 years
- Associated abnormalities: Easy bruising and bleeding

Gross Pathologic & Surgical Features

- Classic macroscopic classification (Eggel) mainly used on autopsy cases (used since 1901): HCC classified as nodular, massive and diffuse
  - Nodular tumors are smaller, more distinct with sharper margins to liver
  - Massive lesions are either composed of confluent smaller tumors or consist of one large lesion that often occupies entire liver
  - Diffuse lesions are multiple infiltrating lesions

Microscopic Features

- HCC has been classified according to predominant histologic pattern
  - Trabecular (43% of cases), pseudoacinar (13%), compact small cell (10%), undifferentiated (10%)
- HCC consists of polymorphous hepatocyte-like cells with loss of normal parenchymal architecture of liver

CLINICAL ISSUES

Presentation

- Most common signs/symptoms: Right upper quadrant (RUQ) pain, early satiety and weight loss, vascular bruit in the RUQ if hypervascular tumor
- Other signs/symptoms
  - Uncommon presentations
    - Spontaneous rupture of tumor into peritoneal cavity, obstructive jaundice, bony pain from metastasis
  - Paraneoplastic syndromes associated with HCC
    - Erythrocytosis (erythropoietin) hypoglycemia (insulin-like growth factor) hypercalcemia (parathyroid-related protein)

Demographics

- Age
  - Male adults in sixth decade of life
  - Fibrolamellar type of HCC typically occurs in young patients; rare variant.
  - HCC in young adults is more likely to be extensive and the prognosis for these patients is poor
- Gender: Male > Female
- Ethnicity
  - Prevalence of HCV in United States is highest among the African American (AA) population (3.2%) in comparison to non AA
  - Incidence of HCC is 2-3x higher in AA than in Caucasians as is rate of age-standardized mortality due to HCC

Natural History & Prognosis

- > 90% of patients with HCC have underlying cirrhosis of the liver
  - Functional impairment of underlying liver has a significant impact on prognosis and on types of treatments indicated due to functional reserve of the liver

Treatment

- If lesion is resectable, then surgery offers best option for cure
  - Liver transplantation is an option for lesions meeting criteria
- Transarterial chemoembolization (TACE) and/or embolization with radioactive particles commonly used in non-surgical candidates

DIAGNOSTIC CHECKLIST

Consider

- Incidence of hepatitis C related HCC will continue to increase and careful attention should be paid to all liver lesions

SELECTED REFERENCES

1. Colagrande S et al: Transient hepatic intensity differences: part 1, Those associated with focal lesions. AJR Am J Roentgenol. 188(1):154-9, 2007
2. Jepsen P et al: Incidence rates of hepatocellular carcinoma in the U.S. and Denmark: Recent trends. Int J Cancer. 2007
3. Kemmer N et al: Ethnic Differences in Hepatocellular Carcinoma: Implications for Liver Transplantation. Dig Dis Sci. 2007
4. Kim YK et al: Three-phase dynamic CT of pelioid hepatocellular carcinoma. AJR Am J Roentgenol. 189(3):W160-2, 2007
5. Kulik LM: Advancements in hepatocellular carcinoma. Curr Opin Gastroenterol. 23(3):268-74, 2007
6. Sultana S et al: Hypervascular hepatocellular carcinomas: bolus tracking with a 40-detector CT scanner to time arterial phase imaging. Radiology. 243(1):140-7, 2007

IMAGE GALLERY

Other

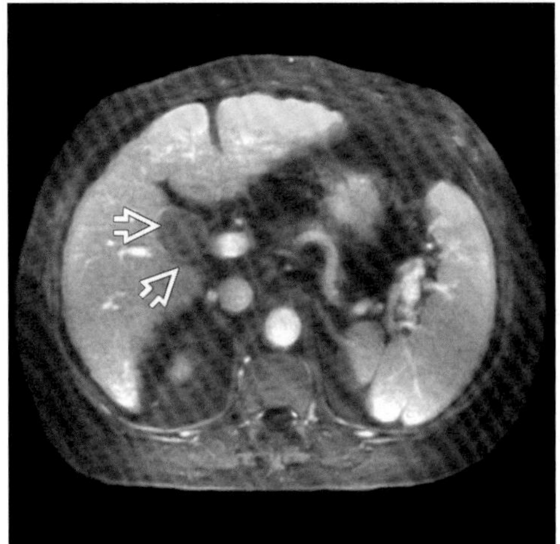

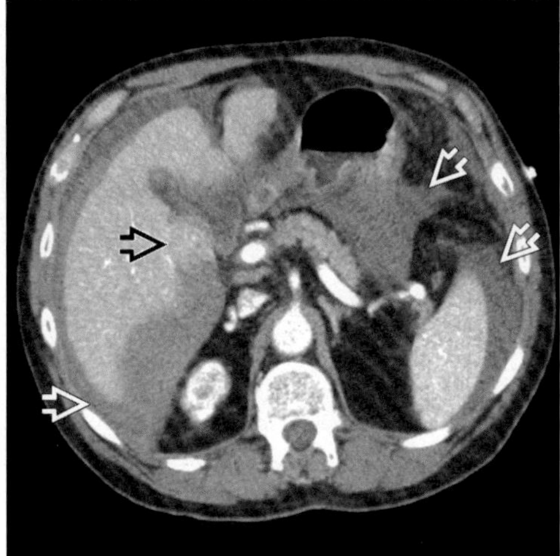

(Left) *Axial T1WI MR with contrast shows focal lesion in the liver ➡ of a patient with markedly elevated AFP. The lesion has heterogeneous enhancement. The liver is small, with some nodularity suggesting cirrhosis.* ***(Right)*** *CECT shows same patient as previous image, a few days later. The hypervascular mass is again visible ➡ and now there is fluid in the abdomen ➡. This patient has had a large hematocrit drop. There has been spontaneous bleeding of hepatoma.*

Typical

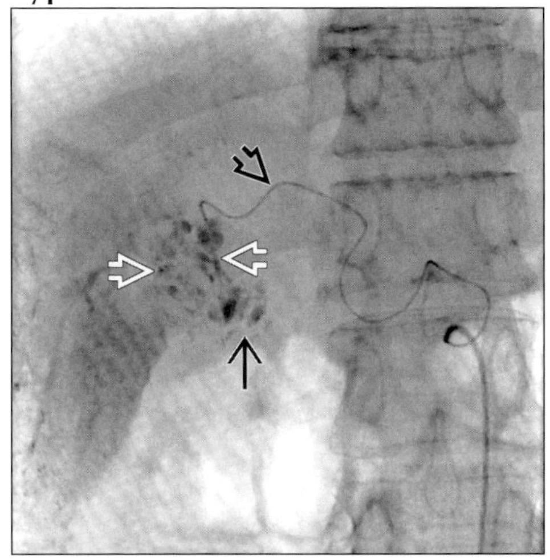

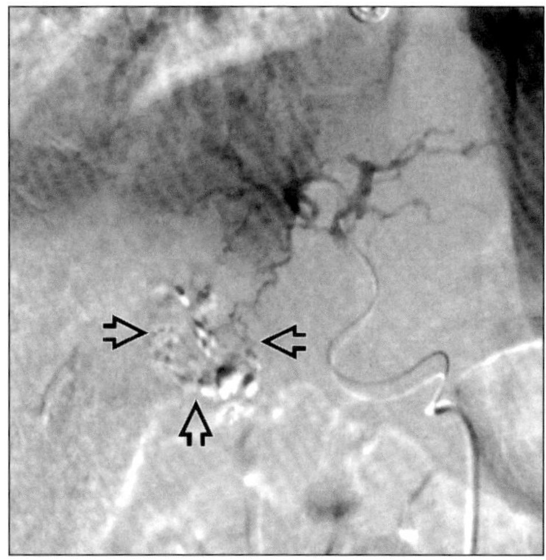

(Left) *DSA shows a microcatheter ➡ in the vessel supplying the hepatoma. Contrast is both within ➡ & outside → the tumor consistent with extravasation & explaining the increased fluid in the abdomen.* ***(Right)*** *DSA shows reinjection of the hepatic artery following chemoembolization. The Ethiodol oil is seen as a subtraction artifact ➡. No further extravasation is seen. The patient's hematocrit stabilized & no further transfusions were required.*

Typical

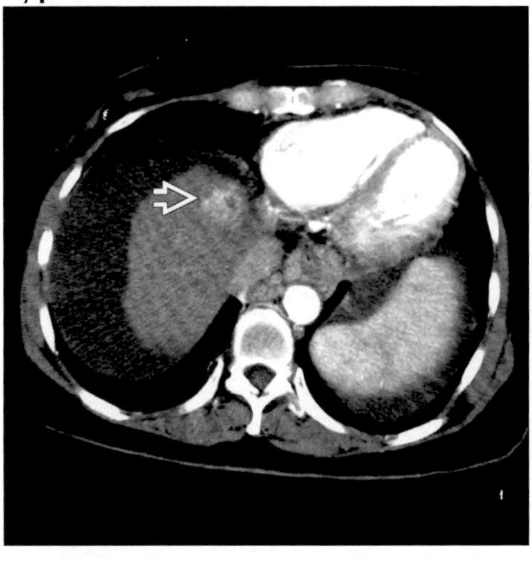

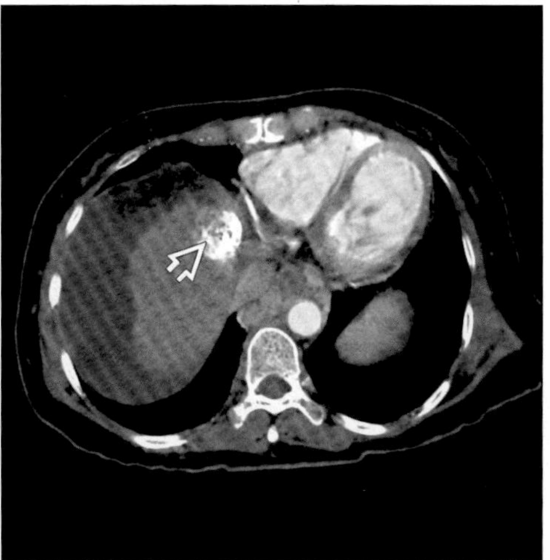

(Left) *Axial CECT shows an enhancing mass ➡ in the dome of the liver. The patient had an elevated AFP level. A history of hepatitis C is the most common cause of liver cancer.* ***(Right)*** *Axial CECT shows the same lesion following chemoembolization (TACE). The high density ➡ is due to the accumulation of Ethiodol within the lesion. The Ethiodol is taken up by the cancer cells. Followup after TACE frequently needs to be performed with MR because of the artifact of the Ethiodol.*

SPLENIC TRAUMA

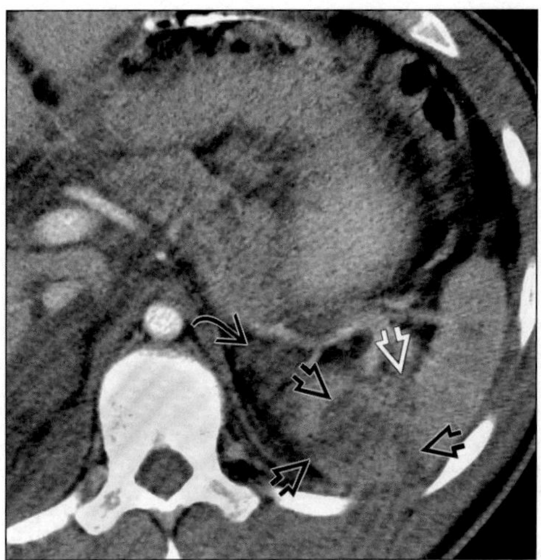

Axial CECT shows grade III splenic hematoma ⇨, with laceration extending to splenic hilum ➡. Intraperitoneal perisplenic hematoma is present ↪.

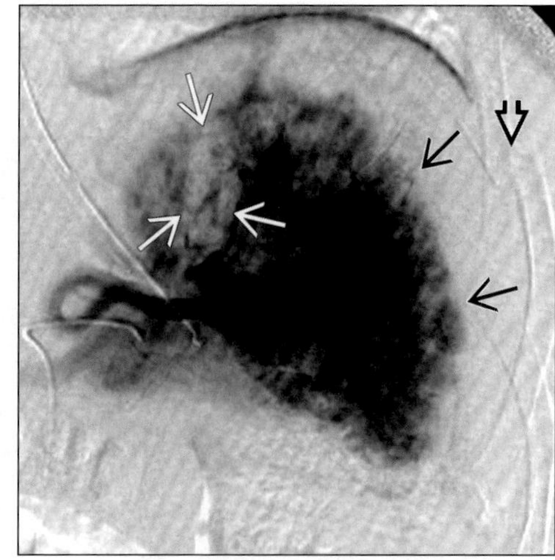

Late phase splenic arteriogram in different patient shows avascular area ➡ corresponding to grade III hematoma, rib fracture ⇨ and medial displacement of spleen → from subcapsular hematoma.

TERMINOLOGY

Abbreviations and Synonyms

- Splenic hematoma
- Splenic laceration
- Splenic fracture

Definitions

- Parenchymal injury to spleen, with or without capsular disruption, usually resulting from blunt trauma to left upper quadrant of abdomen

IMAGING FINDINGS

General Features

- Best diagnostic clue: Low attenuation splenic laceration with high density active hemorrhage; heterogeneous contrast-enhancement on dual phase CECT
- Morphology
  - Subcapsular hematoma: Flattened contour of splenic parenchyma, with hemorrhage contained by splenic capsule
  - Laceration: Linear or irregular edges
  - Fracture: Laceration extending from outer cortex to hilum

CT Findings

- NECT: High attenuation (> 30 HU) hemoperitoneum or perisplenic thrombus (> 45 HU)
- CECT
  - Dual-phase CECT with images obtained 60-70 seconds and 5 minutes after IV contrast administration
    - Active arterial extravasation: High attenuation focus surrounded by lower attenuation hematoma
    - Delayed phase helps differentiate contained vascular injury from active hemorrhage with extravasation
  - Subcapsular hematoma: Compresses lateral margin of parenchyma
  - Parenchymal laceration: Irregular linear area of non-enhancement due to hematoma
  - Splenic fracture: Deep laceration extending from outer capsule through splenic hilum

DDx: Splenic Trauma

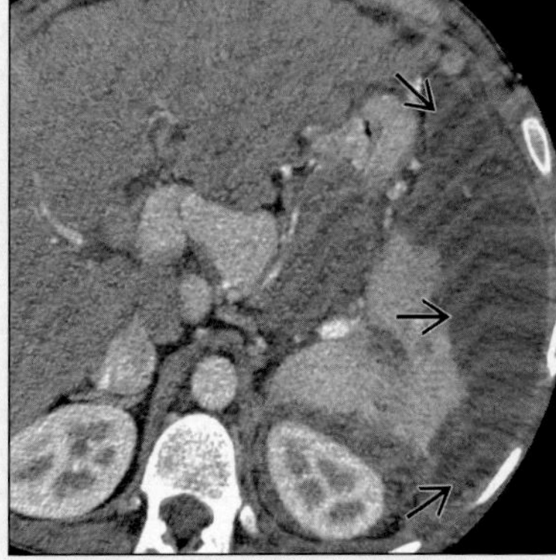

Splenic Infarct

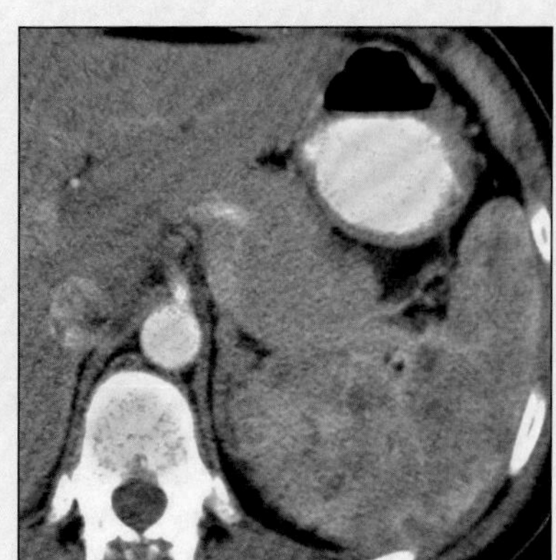

Splenic Lymphoma

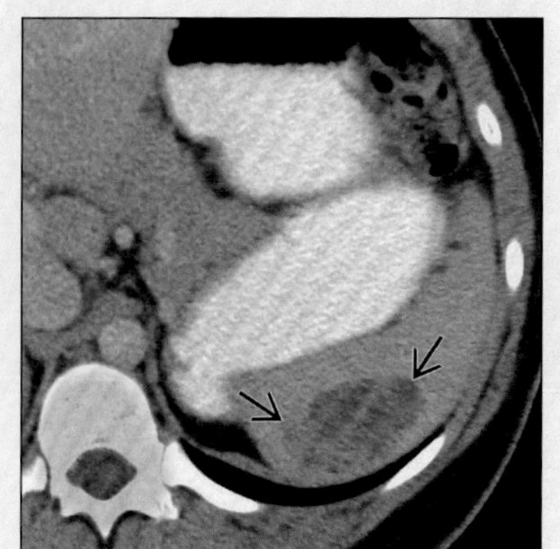

Splenic Abscess

SPLENIC TRAUMA

Key Facts

Terminology
- Parenchymal injury to spleen, with or without capsular disruption, usually resulting from blunt trauma to left upper quadrant of abdomen

Imaging Findings
- Best diagnostic clue: Low attenuation splenic laceration with high density active hemorrhage; heterogeneous contrast-enhancement on dual phase CECT
- Best imaging tool: CECT
- 100-150 mL IV contrast at 4 mL/sec with 5 mm collimation
- Dual-phase CECT with images obtained 60-70 seconds and 5 minutes after IV contrast administration
- 50% of CT findings not demonstrated by angiography, suggesting CT more predictive of outcome

Pathology
- Epidemiology: Most common abdominal organ injury requiring surgery

Clinical Issues
- Prone to develop delayed hemorrhage
- Excellent prognosis with early diagnosis & intervention (surgery or embolization)
- Non-operative management is standard of care in hemodynamically stable patients and has minimal long-term complications
- Transcatheter embolization if active arterial extravasation on CT

  - Extremely sensitive for contrast extravasation but much less sensitive for pseudoaneurysm and A-V fistula than angiography

MR Findings
- T2WI
  - Acute splenic hematoma hyperintense with prolonged T2
  - Blood products evolve over time into methemoglobin, deoxyhemoglobin with concomitant signal intensity changes
- Not typically used in initial assessment of abdominal trauma but distinguishes acute from chronic hematoma, as well as other DDx

Ultrasonographic Findings
- Grayscale Ultrasound: FAST (Focused Assessment with Sonography in Trauma) used for rapid detection of free abdominal fluid but poor sensitivity and specificity for splenic trauma

Angiographic Findings
- Avascular parenchymal laceration
- Flattened lateral parenchymal contour 2° to subcapsular hematoma
- Rounded contrast collections (pseudoaneurysms), A-V fistulas
- Amorphous parenchymal extravasation
- 50% of CT findings not demonstrated by angiography, suggesting CT more predictive of outcome

Imaging Recommendations
- Best imaging tool: CECT
- Protocol advice
  - 100-150 mL IV contrast at 4 mL/sec with 5 mm collimation
  - Dual phase images at 60-70 seconds and 5 minutes after IV contrast administration

DIFFERENTIAL DIAGNOSIS

Splenic Abscess
- Clinical signs of infection
- Rounded, irregular, non-enhancing low attenuation lesion on CECT

Splenic Cyst
- Well-defined, rounded, hypoechoic lesion on US
- No enhancement on CECT, low T1 and high T2 signal

Splenic Infarct
- Associated with splenomegaly, systemic embolization
- Wedge-shaped area of non-enhancing low attenuation on CECT

Splenic Neoplasm
- Lymphoma
  - Splenomegaly
  - Single or multiple hypodense lesions on CECT
- Metastasis (rare)
  - Other sites of metastatic involvement
  - Evidence of primary neoplasm
- Vascular neoplasms
  - Hemangioma, hamartoma, angioma, lymphangioma, angiosarcoma (rare)

PATHOLOGY

General Features
- Etiology: Spleen contains approximately 1 unit of blood, is supplied by splenic artery and a rich collateral network and thus susceptible to parenchymal injury and hemorrhage from blunt LUQ trauma
- Epidemiology: Most common abdominal organ injury requiring surgery
- Associated abnormalities: Injuries to left hemithorax, tail of pancreas, left hepatic lobe and/or mesentery

Gross Pathologic & Surgical Features
- Varies according to extent of injury

Microscopic Features
- Necrotic injured tissue with surrounding hematoma

SPLENIC TRAUMA

Staging, Grading or Classification Criteria

- Grading may be misleading; minor injuries may go on to devastating delayed hemorrhage
- Splenic hematoma grade
  - Grade I: Subcapsular hematoma < 10% of surface area
    - Intact capsule without active bleeding or expanding hematoma
  - Grade II: Subcapsular hematoma 10-50% of surface area; parenchymal hematoma < 5 cm in diameter
    - Intact capsule without active bleeding or expanding hematoma
  - Grade III: Subcapsular hematoma > 50% surface area, subcapsular rupture, or rupture of capsule; parenchymal hemorrhage > 5 cm diameter
    - Capsule may or may not be intact; active bleeding, expanding hematoma
  - Grade IV: Parenchymal rupture
    - Capsular disruption and active bleeding with hemoperitoneum
- Splenic laceration grade
  - Grade I: < 1 cm depth
    - No active bleeding or vessel involvement
  - Grade II: 1-3 cm depth
    - Active bleeding but no vessel involvement
  - Grade III: > 3 cm depth
    - Active bleeding and trabecular vessel involvement
  - Grade IV: Major devascularization (> 25% parenchyma)
    - Active bleeding with segmental or hilar vessel involvement
  - Grade V: Shattered spleen with complete devascularization
    - Active bleeding with hilar vessel involvement

CLINICAL ISSUES

Presentation

- Most common signs/symptoms: Blunt abdominal trauma; LUQ pain; hypotension

Demographics

- Age
  - Pediatric spleen has thicker and more elastic capsule and is thus more tolerant of blunt trauma
    - Fairly responsive to conservative management regardless of severity of injury
  - Adult spleen progressively less elastic and more vulnerable to significant injury, particularly after 50
    - Greater transfusion risk and compromised shock response with increasing age, thus conservative management success rates vary

Natural History & Prognosis

- Innocuous injury may lead to life-threatening delayed hemorrhage, especially with anticoagulation
- Prone to develop delayed hemorrhage
- Excellent prognosis with early diagnosis & intervention (surgery or embolization)

Treatment

- Options, risks, complications
  - Non-operative management is standard of care in hemodynamically stable patients and has minimal long-term complications
  - Transcatheter embolization if active arterial extravasation on CT
    - Selective diagnostic splenic arteriogram
    - Proximal coil embolization stabilizes splenic hemorrhage through transient reduction in parenchymal perfusion pressure, yet allows for collateral perfusion
    - Avoid coil reflux into celiac trunk or distal embolization by oversizing first coil, allowing for a stable initial embolization
    - More distal or superselective embolization may be indicated with massive extracapsular extravasation or extravasation from major interpolar branch
    - High success rate (87-100%) even in grade IV and V spleens
    - Distal coil embolization or particulate (e.g., Gelfoam slurry) embolization increases risk of significant parenchymal infarction
  - Splenorrhaphy preferred when surgery required; splenectomy only if necessary
    - Splenic preservation if possible, given late risks associated with splenectomy, particularly in pediatric population as spleen has immunologic role in clearing blood borne encapsulated bacteria
- Close monitoring for delayed rupture regardless of intervention
  - With higher grade splenic injury, repeat CT used to assess adequacy of treatment, predict late failure or determine need for re-intervention
  - Patients with low grade splenic injury and stable hematocrit may not require repeat CT

DIAGNOSTIC CHECKLIST

Image Interpretation Pearls

- When high attenuation intraperitoneal fluid seen on NECT in clinical setting of blunt trauma to left upper quadrant, obtain dual phase CECT to evaluate for splenic injury

SELECTED REFERENCES

1. Anderson SW et al: Blunt splenic trauma: delayed-phase CT for differentiation of active hemorrhage from contained vascular injury in patients. Radiology. 243(1):88-95, 2007
2. Haan JM et al: Follow-up abdominal CT is not necessary in low-grade splenic injury. Am Surg. 73(1):13-8, 2007
3. Impellizzeri P et al: [Conservative treatment of pediatric spleen trauma. Twenty years of experience] Pediatr Med Chir. 29(1):38-43, 2007
4. Kristoffersen KW et al: Long-term outcome of nonoperative pediatric splenic injury management. J Pediatr Surg. 42(6):1038-41; discussion 1041-2, 2007
5. Schroeppel TJ et al: Diagnosis and management of blunt abdominal solid organ injury. Curr Opin Crit Care. 13(4):399-404, 2007
6. Rajani RR et al: Improved outcome of adult blunt splenic injury: a cohort analysis. Surgery. 140(4):625-31; discussion 631-2, 2006
7. Elsayes KM et al: MR imaging of the spleen: spectrum of abnormalities. Radiographics. 25(4):967-82, 2005

SPLENIC TRAUMA

IMAGE GALLERY

Typical

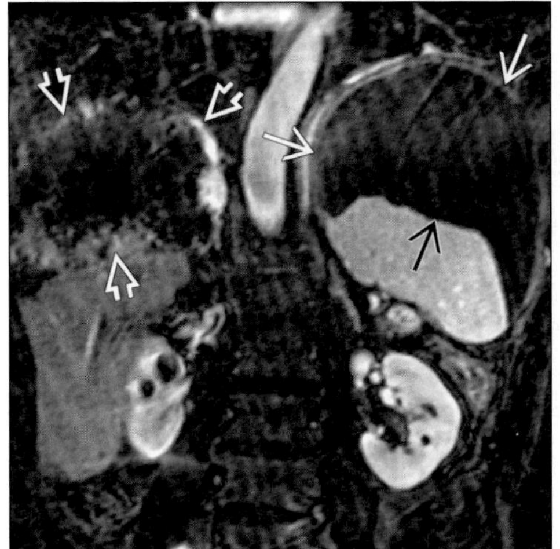

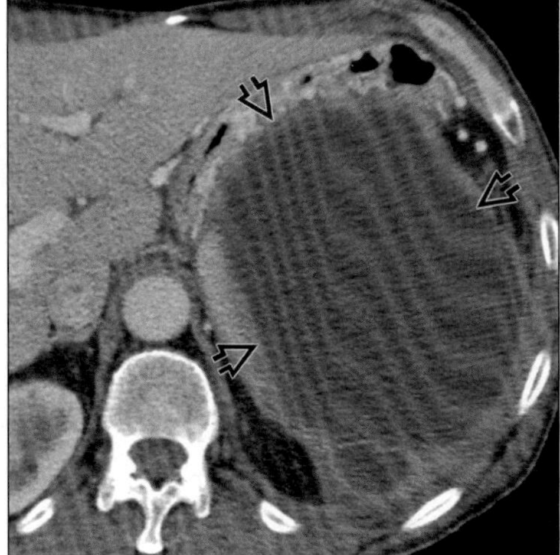

(Left) *Coronal T1WI MR shows both a large chronic subcapsular hematoma* → *compressing the lateral splenic margin* → *and a hepatic injury* →. *MR is not typically used in initial evaluation of suspected splenic trauma.* ***(Right)*** *Axial CECT in same patient as previous image, shows the large subcapsular splenic hematoma* →. *This chronic hematoma resembles a large cyst, but the subcapsular location and mass effect are atypical for splenic cyst.*

Typical

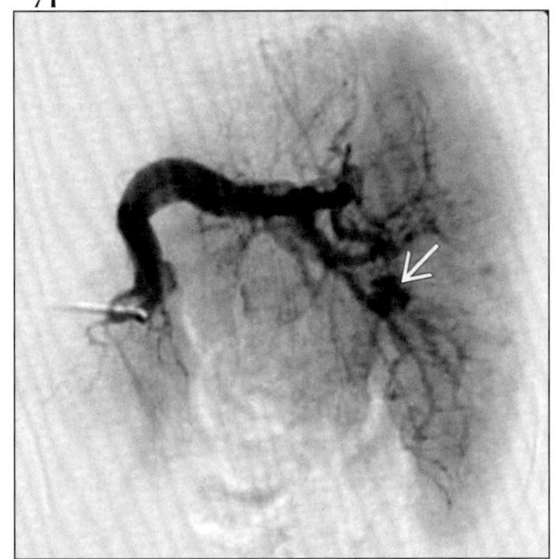

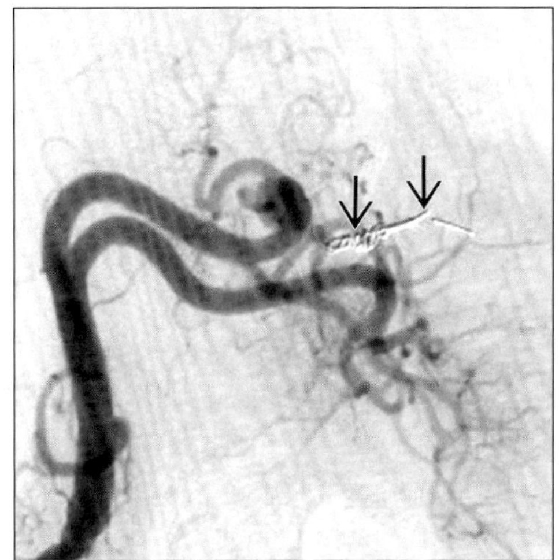

(Left) *Selective splenic arteriogram shows focal contrast extravasation* → *originating from an interpolar arterial branch in a patient with a grade IV splenic laceration.* ***(Right)*** *Splenic arteriogram following transcatheter embolization shows coils* → *within the injured interpolar branch of the splenic artery. Note that there is no longer any contrast extravasation and there is good splenic arterial perfusion.*

Typical

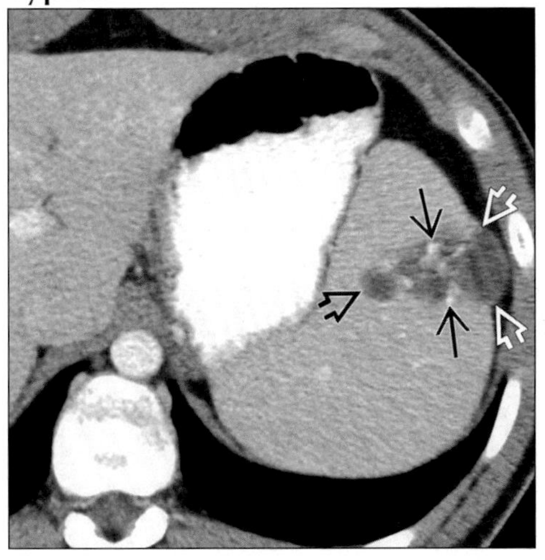

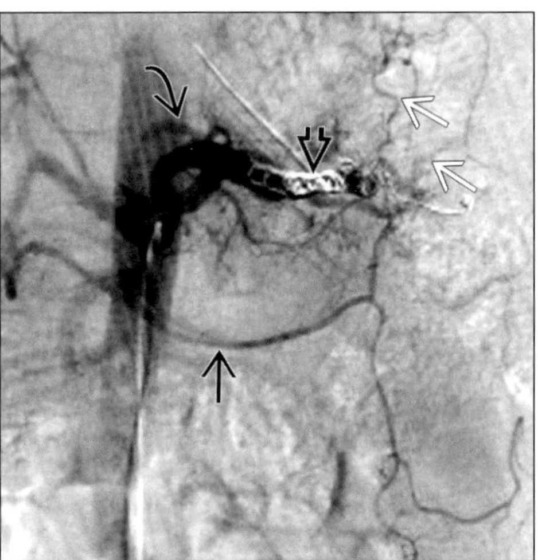

(Left) *Axial CECT shows grade II splenic subcapsular hematoma* → *with active extravasation* → *at the margins of the grade III splenic laceration* →. ***(Right)*** *Celiac arteriogram shows embolization coils* → *within the main trunk of splenic artery. Collaterals perfuse the spleen through the short gastric arteries* → *that arise from the gastroepiploic* → *and left gastric* ↷ *arteries.*

SPLENIC ARTERY ANEURYSM

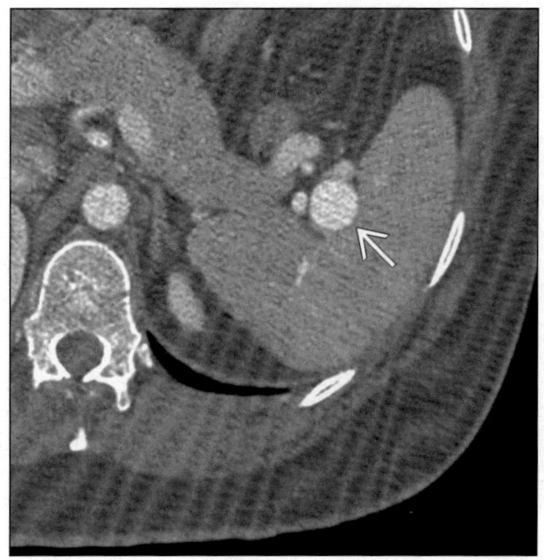

Axial CTA shows a hyperattenuating rounded structure in splenic neck ➡. The mass is enhancing at the same rate as the other arteries, which is consistent with splenic artery aneurysm.

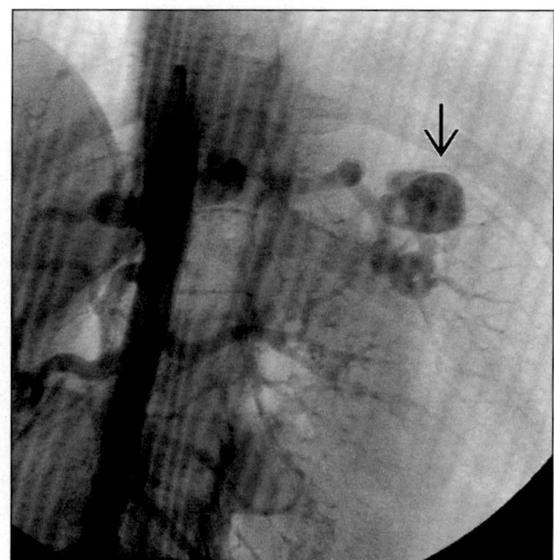

Left anterior oblique catheter angiography shows the same aneurysms ➡ prior to coil embolization. Treatment is indicated in splenic artery aneurysms larger than 2 cm.

TERMINOLOGY

Abbreviations and Synonyms

- Splenic artery aneurysm (SAA)

Definitions

- Focal circumscribed dilation involving all three layers of the splenic arterial lumen (intima, media, and adventitia)
  - Splenic artery pseudoaneurysm involves the intima and media only

IMAGING FINDINGS

General Features

- Best diagnostic clue: 80% contain peripheral rim of calcification
- Location
  - Most (75%) are located in the distal third of the splenic artery, 20% in middle third (usually near the body and tail regions of pancreas)
  - Frequently at an arterial bifurcation point
  - Giant SAAs typically located in middle third of splenic artery
- Size: Mean diameter 2.2 cm, rarely greater than 3 cm, but a few case of giant SAAs have been documented at greater than 10 cm
- Morphology: Most are solitary (80%) and saccular

Radiographic Findings

- Radiography: Round lesion with peripheral calcification in LUQ, in region of splenic artery

CT Findings

- NECT: Low-density mass in region of the splenic artery with or without peripheral calcification
- CECT
  - Early and marked enhancement of the aneurysm
  - Nonenhancing mural thrombus
  - Extravasation due to leakage or rupture
  - Thrombosed aneurysm can appear as a mass

MR Findings

- Nonenhanced
  - Mass lesion
  - Low signal intensity peripheral rim

DDx: Splenic Artery Aneurysm

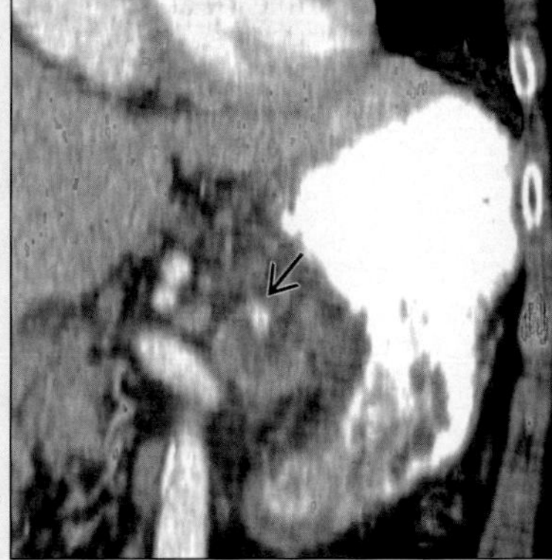

Pseudoaneurysm

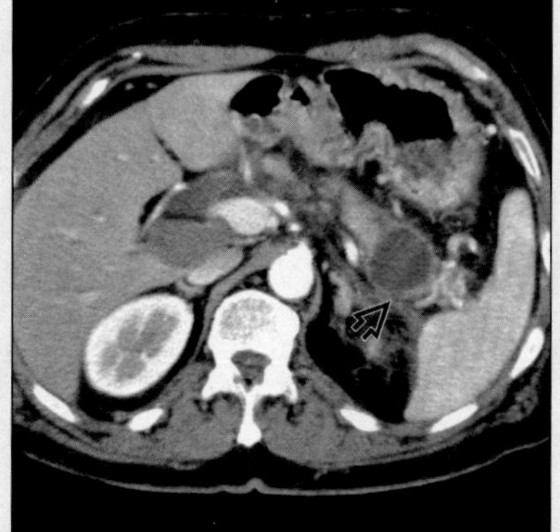

Pancreatic Pseudocyst

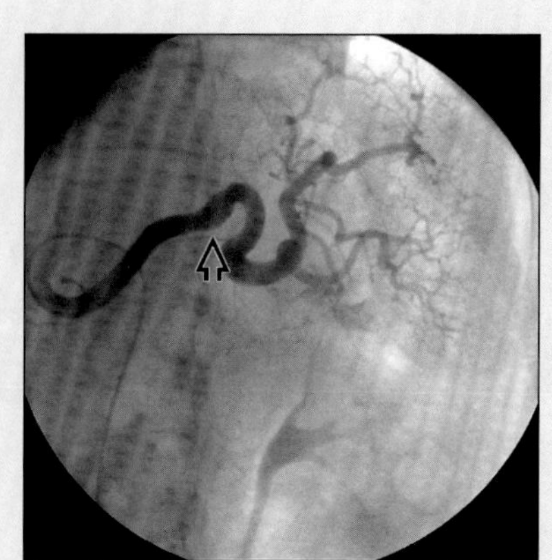

Very Subtle Aneurysm

SPLENIC ARTERY ANEURYSM

Key Facts

Imaging Findings

- Most (75%) are located in the distal third of the splenic artery, 20% in middle third (usually near the body and tail regions of pancreas)
- Most are solitary (80%) and saccular
- Early and marked enhancement of the aneurysm
- No color Doppler signal if aneurysm filled with large clot and sluggish vascular flow through aneurysm, or when aneurysm wall heavily calcified

Top Differential Diagnoses

- Pseudoaneurysm
- Pancreatic Pseudocyst

Pathology

- Most common visceral artery aneurysms, accounting for 60-71%
- Third most common intra-abdominal aneurysm (after aortic and iliac aneurysms)

Clinical Issues

- Frequency of rupture is increased with liver transplantation, portal hypertension, and pregnancy
- Rupture carries mortality risk between 20% and 36%
- Embolization is the primary approach to treatment

Diagnostic Checklist

- Important to differentiate SAA from other neoplasms, or pseudocysts prior to intervention

---

 - Signal intensity at the center depends on flow alteration, mural thrombus, etc.
- Enhanced
  - Early enhancement

Ultrasonographic Findings

- Grayscale Ultrasound
  - Anechoic mass with or without peripheral echogenic rim (calcification)
  - With or without mural thrombus
  - Donut-like appearance with US: Thick outer wall with an anechoic central region
  - Ultrasound is operator dependent, and may be limited due to spatial resolution, obesity, shadowing from bowel gas, and arteriosclerosis
- Color Doppler
  - Weak, turbulent, pulsatile flow
    - No color Doppler signal if aneurysm filled with large clot and sluggish vascular flow through aneurysm, or when aneurysm wall heavily calcified

Angiographic Findings

- Saccular dilatation (mostly) at the convexity of the arteries (road map for endovascular treatment)

Imaging Recommendations

- Best imaging tool
  - Celiac artery angiography considered gold standard for diagnosis, however, spiral CT with multislice reconstructions reported to be more sensitive
    - Angiography usually performed prior to intervention
- Protocol advice: Spiral CT with multiplanar reconstruction

DIFFERENTIAL DIAGNOSIS

Pseudoaneurysm

- Pancreatitis and peptic ulcer disease are known causes of pseudoaneurysms
- Coexisting pseudocyst present in 41% of cases
- Almost always present with symptoms (unlike SAA)
  - Symptoms usually due to underlying etiology, e.g., pancreatitis

Pancreatic Pseudocyst

- No central enhancement with CECT
  - May be diffuse generalized enhancement or rim enhancement
- Other pancreatic cystic lesions including benign and malignant neoplasms
  - Islet cell tumors can be markedly enhancing in the arterial or pancreatic phase of CT (use 3D rendering to help distinguish from an aneurysm

Gastric Neoplasia

- Appears as a mass with possible diffuse enhancement

PATHOLOGY

General Features

- Etiology
  - Hormonal and hemodynamic alterations specific to pregnancy likely contribute to intimal hyperplasia and fragmentation
    - May in turn lead to aneurysm formation
  - SAAs are more common in patients with large diameter splenic arteries
    - Suggests relationship with increased flow and SAA formation
  - Inflammatory reactions from the adjacent pancreas can also cause SAAs
- Epidemiology
  - Most common visceral artery aneurysm, accounting for 60-71%
  - Third most common intra-abdominal aneurysm (after aortic and iliac aneurysms)
  - Prevalence uncertain, but ranges from 0.16-10.4% in general population
    - Prevalence as high as 7-20% in patients with portal hypertension
- Associated abnormalities
  - Pregnancy

SPLENIC ARTERY ANEURYSM

- Portal hypertension with splenomegaly, cirrhosis, liver transplantation
- Atherosclerosis, hypertension
- Connective tissue disorders
  - F-1-antitrypsin deficiency
  - Ehlers-Danlos syndrome
  - Polyarteritis nodosa
  - Fibromuscular dysplasia
  - Arterial fibrodysplasia
  - Congenital anomalies
  - Any primary or secondary vasculitides
- Infections: Mycotic aneurysms, pancreatitis
- Trauma

Gross Pathologic & Surgical Features

- 80-90% of SAAs show atherosclerosis

CLINICAL ISSUES

Presentation

- Most common signs/symptoms
  - Most are asymptomatic (90%) and diagnosed incidentally
    - SAAs have slow growth rates
  - If symptomatic, can present with
    - Left upper quadrant, epigastric, or back pain
    - Pulsatile mass
    - Rupture of SAA will present with sudden onset of LUQ pain and possible hemodynamic instability
    - Rupture occurs in 2-10% of SAAs and is three times more common in men
    - Frequency of rupture increased with liver transplantation, portal hypertension, and pregnancy
    - Double rupture can occur when initial rupture into lesser sac tamponaded, followed by hemodynamic instability when bleeding occurs into peritoneal cavity
    - Occasionally, GI bleeding occurs due to SAA communication with gastro-intestinal tract or with pancreatic ductal system

Demographics

- Age: Mean age at presentation is 61 years
- Gender: M:F = 1:4 (particularly prevalent among multiparous women)

Natural History & Prognosis

- Most are stable, however, rupture has been reported to occur in 2-10% of cases of SAA
- Rupture carries a mortality risk between 20% and 36%

Treatment

- Indications for treatment include
  - Symptomatic SAAs
  - Documented enlargement
  - Pregnancy or anticipation of pregnancy
  - Portal hypertension
  - Planned liver transplantation
  - Diameter greater than 2 cm
- Treatment options are individualized and include
  - Open or laparoscopic surgery for aneurysmectomy and ligation (with or without splenectomy)
  - Endovascular therapy including stent graft exclusion, embolization, or thrombin injection
    - Embolization is the primary approach to treatment
    - Stent grafts usually used for proximal aneurysms
    - Thrombin is reserved for difficult situations and usually administered percutaneously

DIAGNOSTIC CHECKLIST

Consider

- Important to differentiate SAA from other neoplasms, or pseudocysts prior to intervention

SELECTED REFERENCES

1. Agrawal GA et al: Splenic artery aneurysms and pseudoaneurysms: clinical distinctions and CT appearances. AJR Am J Roentgenol. 188(4):992-9, 2007
2. Casadei R et al: Thrombosed splenic artery aneurysm simulating a pancreatic body mass: can two entities be distinguished preoperatively thus avoiding diagnostic and therapeutic mistakes? JOP. 8(2):235-9, 2007
3. Varadarajulu S et al: Diagnosis of an aneurysm masquerading as a pancreatic-cyst lesion at EUS. Gastrointest Endosc. 65(4):721-5, 2007
4. De Schepper AM et al: Vascular pathology of the spleen, part I. Abdom Imaging. 30(1):96-104, 2005
5. Madoff DC et al: Splenic arterial interventions: anatomy, indications, technical considerations, and potential complications. Radiographics. 25 Suppl 1:S191-211, 2005
6. Pescarus R et al: Giant splenic artery aneurysms: case report and review of the literature. J Vasc Surg. 42(2):344-7, 2005
7. Pilleul F et al: Diagnosis of splanchnic artery aneurysms and pseudoaneurysms, with special reference to contrast enhanced 3D magnetic resonance angiography: a review. Acta Radiol. 45(7):702-8, 2004
8. Tessier DJ et al: Clinical features and management of splenic artery pseudoaneurysm: case series and cumulative review of literature. J Vasc Surg. 38(5):969-74, 2003
9. Abbas MA et al: Splenic artery aneurysms: two decades experience at Mayo clinic. Ann Vasc Surg. 16(4):442-9, 2002

SPLENIC ARTERY ANEURYSM

IMAGE GALLERY

Typical

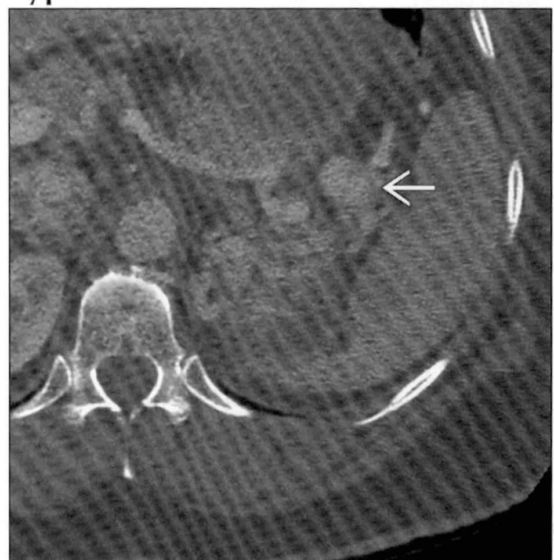

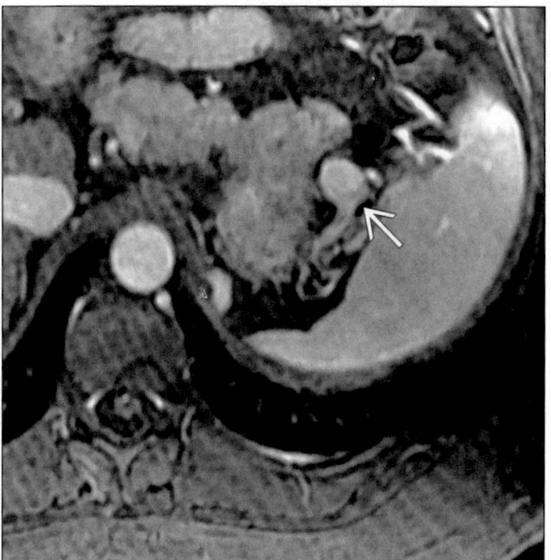

*(**Left**) Axial CECT shows a high density rounded mass ➡ which is enhancing at the same rate as with the other arterial structures. Mass is much larger than other vessels in same area. It is removed from other structures such as pancreas, or splenic parenchyma. The appearance is consistent with a 2.2 cm aneurysm in the distal splenic artery. (**Right**) Axial T1WI FS MR shows an aneurysm ➡ in the distal splenic artery which is demonstrating marked enhancement.*

Typical

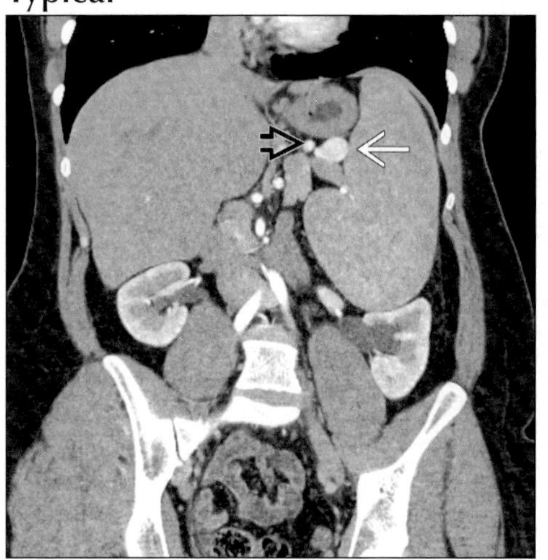

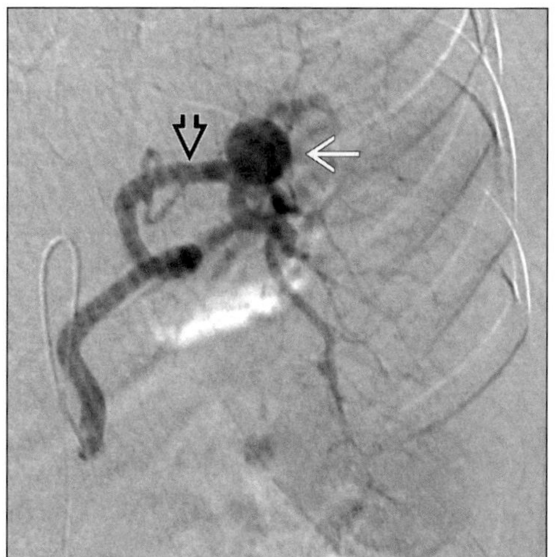

*(**Left**) Coronal CECT nicely demonstrates a strongly enhancing mass in the region of the splenic hilum. It is separated from the stomach above, and from the splenic parenchyma. It is also considerably larger than the adjacent artery ⇨. This represents a splenic artery aneurysm ➡ in the splenic hilum. (**Right**) DSA shows a splenic artery aneurysm ➡. Note the difference in size compared to the splenic artery ⇨. Tortuosity can mimic this appearance, so oblique imaging is important*

Typical

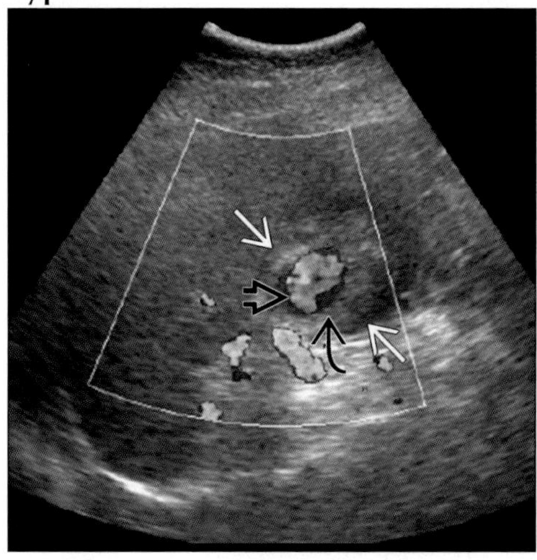

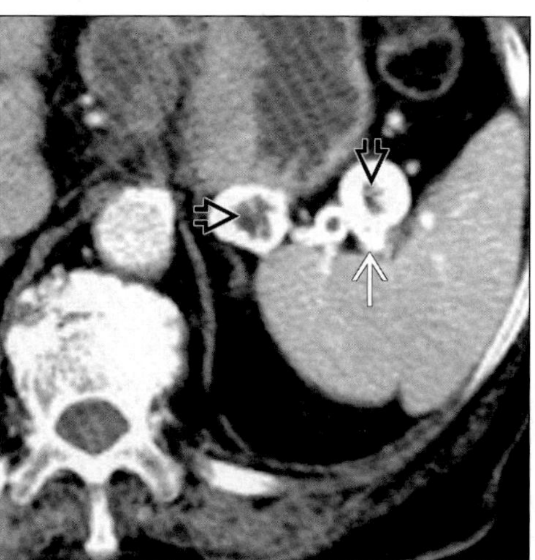

*(**Left**) Sagittal color Doppler ultrasound shows a partially thrombosed splenic artery aneurysm with thickened outer walls ➡. The lumen contains an area of high flow ⇨ but also contains region which is anechoic ↷. (**Right**) Axial CECT shows rim of peripheral dense calcification in splenic artery aneurysm ➡. There is thrombus in the proximal dilated artery and in the more circular aneurysm ⇨.*

PORTAL HYPERTENSION

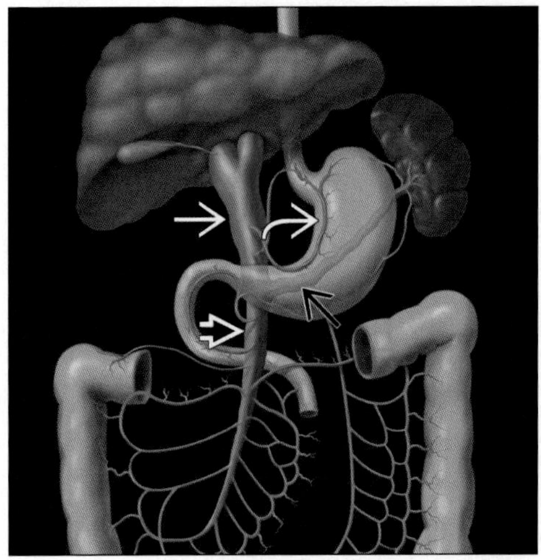

Graphic shows the tributaries of the SMV emptying into the SMV ➡ which then joins the splenic vein ➡ to form the portal vein ➡. A normal coronary vein (left gastric vein) is also seen ➡.

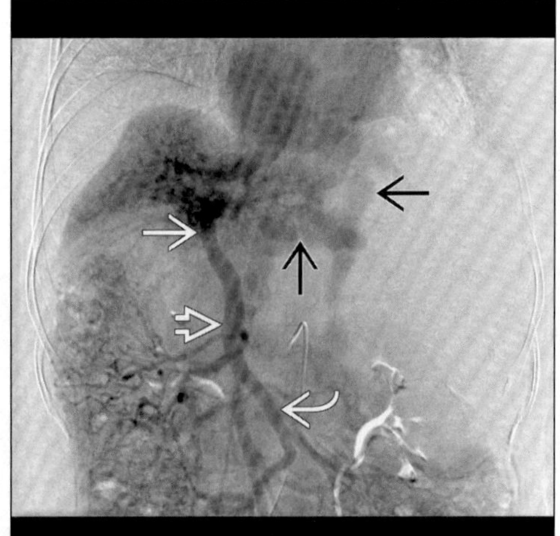

DSA shows the venous phase of an SMA injection. Filling of the venous tributaries of the SMV ➡, the SMV ➡, and the portal vein ➡. Gastric varices ➡, in patient with portal hypertension.

TERMINOLOGY

Abbreviations and Synonyms

- Portal vein (PV)
- Portal hypertension (PH)

Definitions

- Elevated pressure (> 10 mm Hg) in the portal venous system
- Increased resistance to blood into the liver
  - Prehepatic
    - PV thrombosis (PVT)
    - Portal compression or occlusion by biliary and pancreatic neoplasms and metastases
  - Intrahepatic: Acute, chronic liver diseases
    - Presinusoidal resistance: Schistosomiasis
    - Sinusoidal: Liver fibrosis, usually cirrhosis (increased resistance at level of sinusoids due to perisinusoidal deposition of collagen)
    - Hepatoportal fibrosis
    - Nodular regenerative hyperplasia
  - Posthepatic
    - Thrombosis of posthepatic hepatic veins (Budd Chiari), posthepatic portion of IVC; congestive heart failure, constrictive pericarditis
  - Increased portal flow
    - Arteriovenous fistula
    - Hepatoma with arterioportal shunt
    - Massive splenomegaly
- Wedged pressure measurement
  - Pre-sinusoidal: Normal wedged pressure
  - Sinusoidal: Increased wedged pressure, normal free hepatic venous pressure
  - Post-sinusoidal: Increased wedged pressure, increased free hepatic venous pressure

IMAGING FINDINGS

General Features

- Best diagnostic clue
  - Reversal of flow in PV
  - Dilatation of the PV, splenic and mesenteric veins
  - Porto-systemic collaterals
  - Splenomegaly
- Morphology: Irregular and lobulated hepatic contour

DDx: Variants of Portal Hypertension

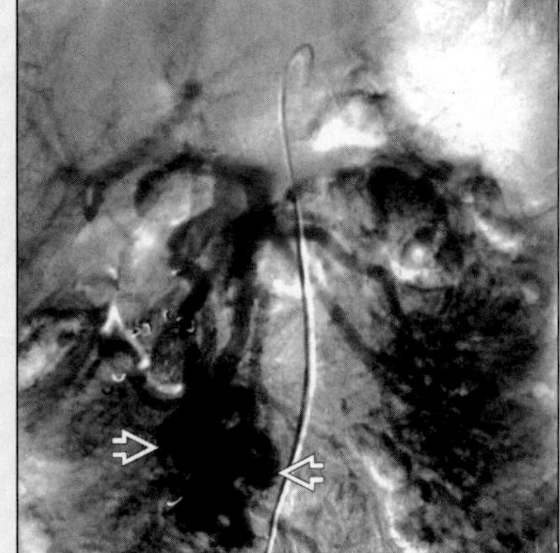

Mesenteric Varices

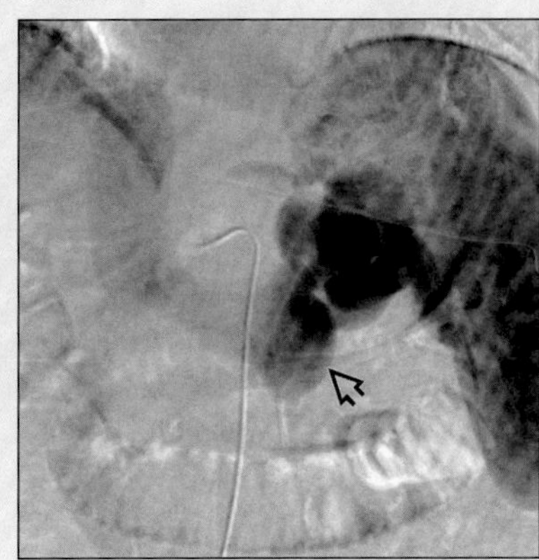

Spontaneous Spleno-Renal Shunt

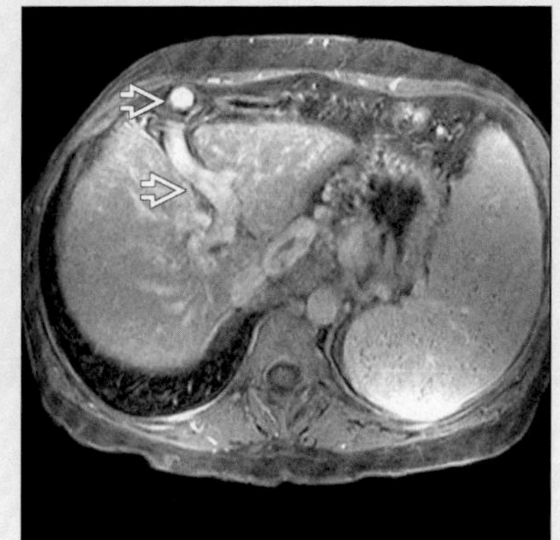

Large Recanalized Umbilical Vein

PORTAL HYPERTENSION

Key Facts

Terminology
- Elevated pressure (> 10 mm Hg) in the portal venous system
- Increased resistance to blood into the liver
  - Prehepatic
  - Intrahepatic: Presinusoidal, sinusoidal
  - Posthepatic

Imaging Findings
- Dilatation of the PV, splenic and mesenteric veins
- Porto-systemic collaterals
- Splenomegaly
- Reversal of flow in PV
- CT/MR if US technically impaired, and pre-transplantation
- Ultrasound for primary diagnosis of PH/PV occlusion

Pathology
- Most commonly caused by hepatic cirrhosis

Clinical Issues
- PH often an important incidental finding on imaging studies
- 90% with cirrhosis develop varices, and 30% of these varices bleed
- First episode of variceal hemorrhage has mortality rate of 30-50%
- Endoscopic sclerotherapy for gastroesophageal hemorrhage
- Transjugular intrahepatic portocaval shunt (TIPS) is an excellent treatment in patients who fail endoscopic control of varices, and can also be used in patients with intractable ascites

CT Findings
- CT/MR Findings
  - Dilated PV (> 17 mm with deep inspiration)
  - Portosystemic collaterals
    - Gastroesophageal (coronary vein/left gastric, right gastric/splenogastric)/perisplenic/retrogastric
    - Spontaneous splenorenal shunt entering and enlarging the left renal vein may simulate a mass in renal hilum
    - Recanalized umbilical vein: Travels caudally toward anterior abdominal wail; may terminate in a subcutaneous "caput medusae" appearance
    - Mesenteric/retroperitoneal varices
  - Hepatic cirrhosis
    - Surface nodularity, small right lobe, enlarged left/caudate lobes
  - Splenomegaly
  - Ascites
  - Decrease in overall liver volume
  - Increase in size and prominence of intrahepatic fissures
  - Caudate: Right lobe ratio (C:RL)
    - Accuracy for cirrhosis close to biopsy
    - Normal liver with C:RL of 0.47
    - Cirrhotic liver with C:RL of 1.00
  - Dilatation of the IVC

MR Findings
- MRA
  - As in CT
  - Intense MR signal (spin-echo imaging technique) in extrahepatic PV: Indicates abnormal flow state
  - Dilated hepatic artery from increased compensatory arterial flow
  - Enlarged azygos vein (4-6 mm in diameter) indicates collateral circulation (gastro-esophageal)
  - Dilation of superior mesenteric vein
  - Stenosis of the intrahepatic segment of the IVC
  - Portal and draining hepatic veins narrowed
  - Extrahepatic PH: Absence of PV trunk, collateral vessels around thrombosed PV

Ultrasonographic Findings
- Grayscale Ultrasound
  - As in CT
  - Flow reversal in PV (definitive finding)
  - PV > 13 mm in quiet respiration, supine subject
  - < 20% increase in splenic vein/SMV diameter from quiet respiration to deep inspiration (normally increase 50-100%)
  - Recanalized umbilical vein a central anechoic focus within the falciform ligament
  - Changes in normal triphasic hepatic venous waveform with patterns of turbulent, diminished, reversed PV blood flow

Other Modality Findings
- Liver-Spleen Scan
  - Colloidal shift from the liver to the spleen or bone marrow

Angiographic Findings
- Conventional
  - Wedge hepatic vein (portal sinusoid) pressure 10 mm Hg > IVC
  - Corrected sinusoidal pressure = wedged hepatic venous pressure minus free hepatic venous pressure (> 5 mm Hg)

Imaging Recommendations
- Ultrasound for primary diagnosis of PH/PV occlusion
- CT/MR if US technically impaired, and pre-transplantation
- Angiography/interventional for therapy

DIFFERENTIAL DIAGNOSIS

Splenic Vein Occlusion
- Mimics portal hypertension findings
  - Large spleno-renal, spleno-gastric, gastroesophageal collateral veins
  - Splenomegaly
  - Gastroesophageal hemorrhage

Right Heart Failure
- Distended hepatic veins, PVs, IVC
- Hepatomegaly
- Ascites

Hepatoma
- Increased arterial flow leads to arterioportal shunting
- Portal vein invasion and thrombosis by tumor

Budd-Chiari Syndrome
- Absence of hepatic veins, comma-shaped intrahepatic collateral vessels, constriction of the intrahepatic IVC

Schistosomiasis
- Most common cause of PH worldwide
- Granulomatous reaction to deposition of parasite eggs in portal venules
- PH results from fibrosis due to inflammatory response

PATHOLOGY

General Features
- General path comments
  - Anatomy
    - Sinusoidal system
  - Increased resistance to blood flow
    - Caused by intraparenchymal fibrosis and architectural distortion
    - Develops variceal bleeding when portocaval gradient increases above 12 mm Hg
- Etiology
  - Most commonly caused by hepatic cirrhosis
  - Development of extensive portal-systemic venous collateral channels
    - Gastroesophageal, hemorrhoidal, periumbilical, retroperitoneal, umbilical vein, splenorenal
    - Varices at high risk for bleeding
  - Progressive hepatic fibrosis
    - Severity of chronic liver disease related to collagen deposits leading to liver fibrosis
- Epidemiology: Chronic active hepatitis and schistosomiasis are major cause of PH morbidity and mortality

CLINICAL ISSUES

Presentation
- Most common signs/symptoms
  - Enlarged spleen
  - Abdominal swelling when there is ascites
  - Bleeding from gastroesophageal varices
  - Anorectal varices, rectal hemorrhoids
  - Caput medusae (tortuous collaterals around the umbilicus)
  - Portal hypertension gastropathy (PHG)
    - Dilatation of capillaries and venules of gastric mucosa
    - Prevalence: 70% in advanced cirrhosis
  - Variceal bleeding
    - Hematemesis or melena (gastroesophageal varices, portal gastropathy), rectal varices
- Encephalopathy
- Peripheral clinical evidence of chronic liver disease (firm liver, enlarged spleen, spider angiomas, clubbing of fingers, palmar erythema)
- Hepatic hydrothorax
- PH often an important incidental finding on imaging studies
  - Risk of hemorrhage at surgery
  - Risk of spontaneous variceal hemorrhage

Demographics
- Age: 40-60 years
- Gender
  - Alcohol-related cirrhosis (M:F, 2:1)
  - Primary biliary cirrhosis: Females > 90%
- Ethnicity
  - North America: Alcohol, Hepatitis C
  - Africa, Middle East, Far East: Cirrhosis PH are virus-related
  - Noncirrhotic idiopathic PH more common in India and Japan

Natural History & Prognosis
- Progressive when due to cirrhosis
- 50% of patients with cirrhotic ascites will die in two years if they do not receive a liver transplant
- 90% with cirrhosis develop varices, and 30% of these varices bleed
  - First episode of variceal hemorrhage has mortality rate of 30-50%
  - Incidence of esophageal varices increases 5% per year
- Risk for varices bleeding associated with variceal size
  - Small varices: Bleeding increases 5% per year
  - Medium, large varices: Bleeding increases 15% per year

Treatment
- Diuretics
- Beta-blockers reduce portal and collateral blood flow, cardiac output; splanchnic vasoconstriction
- Endoscopic sclerotherapy for GI hemorrhage
- Transjugular intrahepatic portocaval shunt (TIPS)
- Surgical portosystemic (portocaval, mesocaval) shunt, distal splenorenal shunt (DSRS)

DIAGNOSTIC CHECKLIST

Consider
- Tumor when a cirrhotic patient with no history of GI bleeding starts bleeding

SELECTED REFERENCES

1. Baik SK et al: Recent variceal bleeding: Doppler US hepatic vein waveform in assessment of severity of portal hypertension and vasoactive drug response. Radiology. 240(2):574-80, 2006
2. Halpern EJ: Science to practice: Noninvasive assessment of portal hypertension--can US aid in the prediction of portal pressure and monitoring of therapy? Radiology. 240(2):309-10, 2006
3. Abraldes JG et al: The management of portal hypertension. Clin Liver Dis. 9(4):685-713, vii, 2005

IMAGE GALLERY

Typical

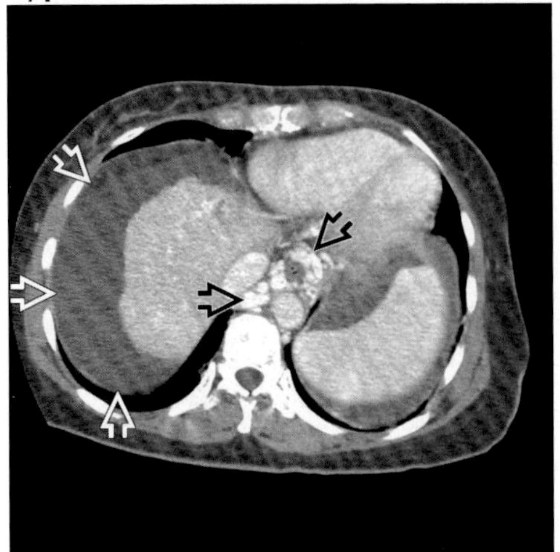

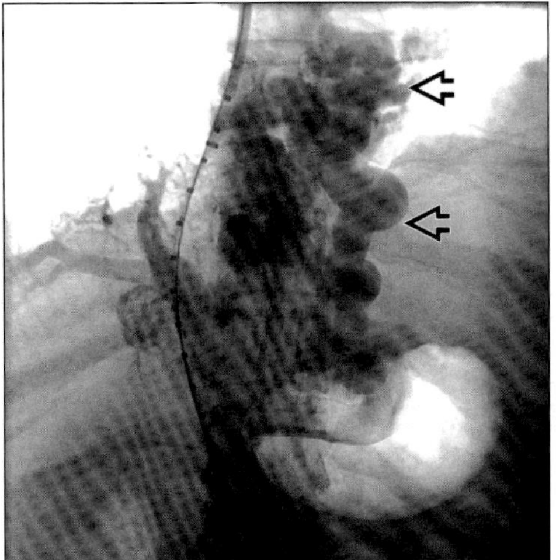

(Left) *CECT shows large esophageal varices ⇨ & a large amount of ascites ➡. Liver is small and somewhat nodular in appearance consistent with cirrhosis in this patient with hepatitis B.* ***(Right)*** *DSA shows massive esophageal varices ⇨. Patient with recurrent esophageal bleeding who had undergone multiple banding procedures. Now undergoing TIPS procedure which was successful in decompressing varices & lowering portal pressure gradient.*

Typical

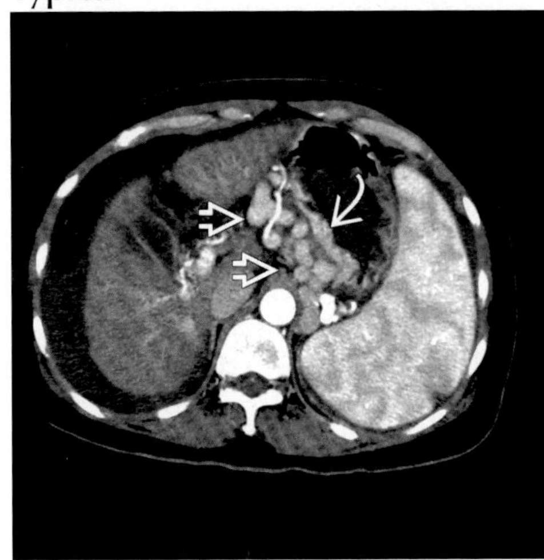

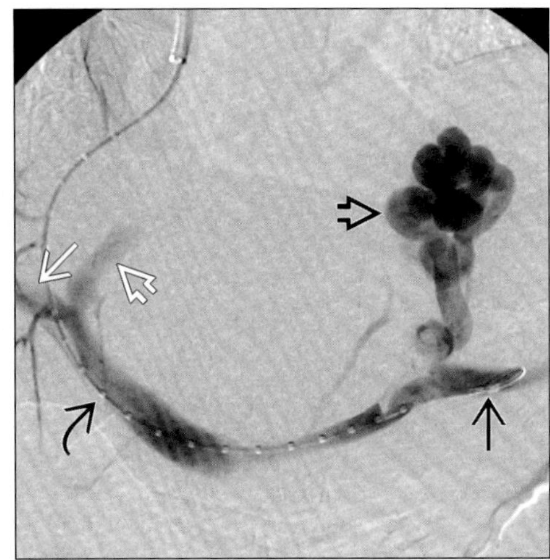

(Left) *Axial CECT shows large gastrohepatic varices ➡ involving the posterior wall of the stomach ➡. Spleen is very enlarged. Small liver which is slightly nodular.* ***(Right)*** *DSA from TIPS study. Catheter → is in the splenic vein and shows filling of large gastric varices ⇨. The TIPS stent has not yet been placed. Filling of the portal vein ⇨ and the right ➡ and left ➡ portal veins. Varices that do not decompress after TIPS will be embolized.*

Typical

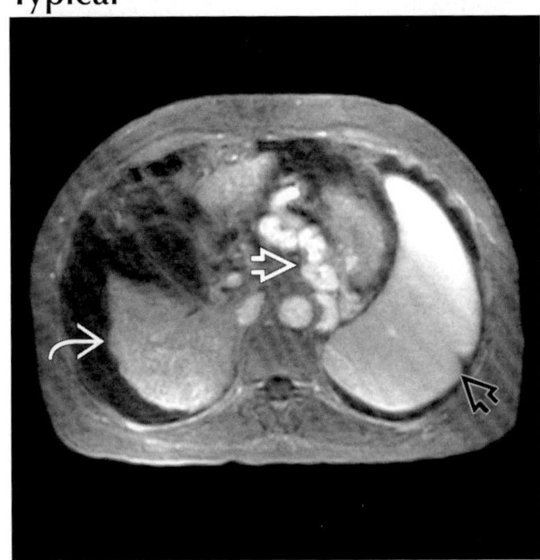

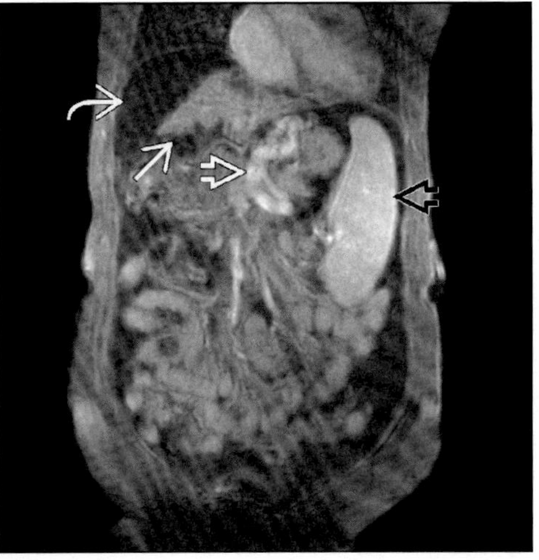

(Left) *Axial contrast-enhanced MR demonstrates the large gastrohepatic varices ➡. The nodularity of the liver is demonstrated ➡ indicative of cirrhosis. The spleen is very enlarged ⇨ consistent with portal hypertension.* ***(Right)*** *Coronal MR demonstrates the gastric varices ➡. It also shows the small liver ➡, large amount of ascites ➡, and large spleen ⇨, all evidence of cirrhosis and portal hypertension in this patient with Hepatitis C.*

PORTAL VEIN OCCLUSION

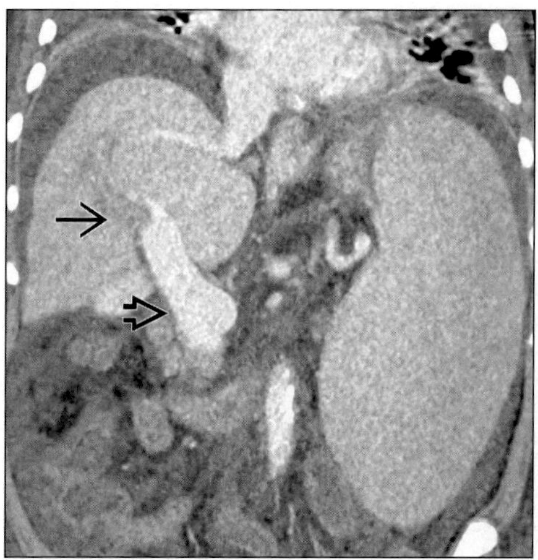

Coronal CECT shows a large portal vein with thrombus in the intrahepatic portal vein, and extending out to the right. Patient with portal hypertension - ascites, large spleen, small liver.

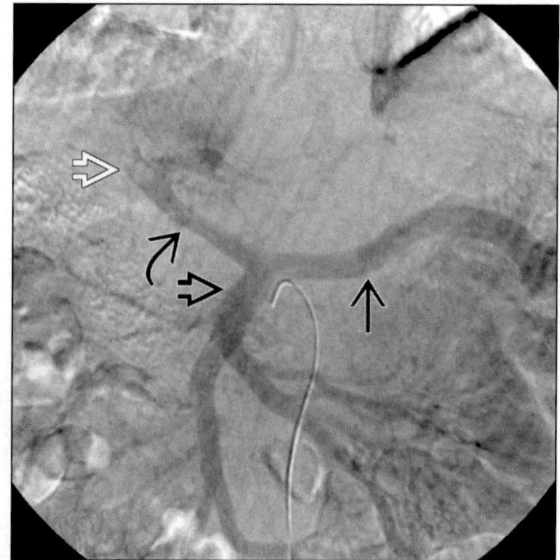

DSA shows venous phase of a SMA arteriogram. There is filling of the SMV, retrograde flow into the splenic vein, diminished flow in portal vein, and thrombus in right portal vein.

TERMINOLOGY

Abbreviations and Synonyms

- Portal vein (PV) occlusion (PVO)
- Portal hypertension (PH)

Definitions

- PV occlusion by thrombosis or tumor invasion

IMAGING FINDINGS

General Features

- Best diagnostic clue
  - Absence of blood flow or flow void in the PV
  - Non-visualization of the PV (chronic occlusion)
  - Cavernous transformation of the PV (collateralization in the porta hepatitis)

Radiographic Findings

- Radiography
  - Plain films
    - Calcification in PV - parallel radiodense lines along expected course of PV
    - PV clot has calcification throughout
    - Calcification implies PVO

CT Findings

- NECT: Lobar hypodensity
- CECT: Thrombus demonstrated as a nonenhanced intraluminal-filling defect
- Acute PV thrombosis (PVT)
  - Non-occlusive: Thrombus partially filling PV
  - Occlusive: Thrombus filling dilated PV
    - Congested mesenteric veins distal to thrombus
    - Bowel wall edema, ileus, ascites, splenomegaly
- Chronic PV thrombosis
  - Non-visualization of PV
  - Cavernous transformation of PV: Collaterals along the usual course of PV, hepatoduodenal ligament
  - Peripheral enhancement of PV
  - Well-developed portosystemic collaterals
  - Increased hepatic artery size and flow
  - Possible splenomegaly
- PV tumor invasion
  - Variable degree of contrast-enhancement of intraluminal tumor
  - Primary tumor usually visible in vicinity

DDx: Cavernous Transformation

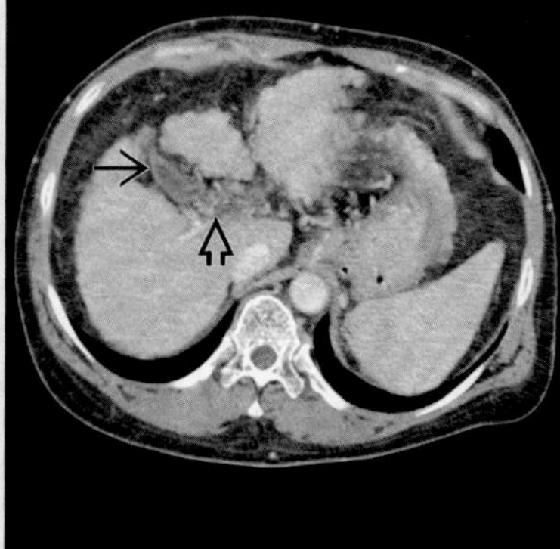

Portal Vein Thrombus - Collaterals

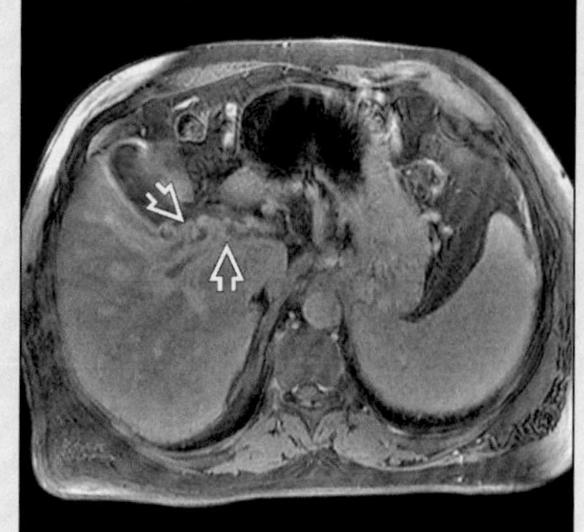

Portal Vein Collaterals

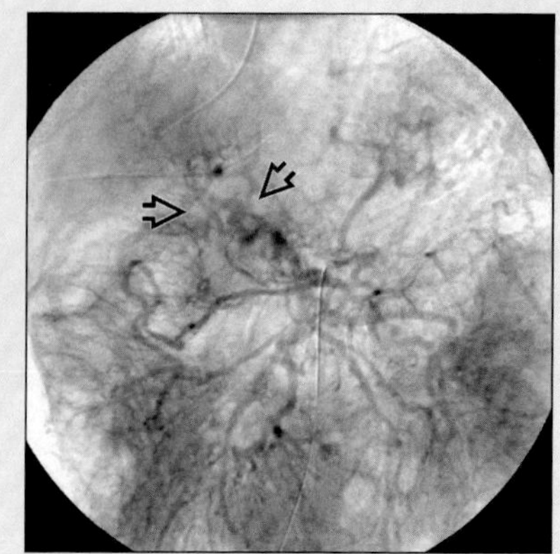

SMV Collaterals

PORTAL VEIN OCCLUSION

Key Facts

Terminology
- Occlusion of the PV due to thrombosis or tumor invasion

Imaging Findings
- Absence of blood flow or flow void in the PV
- Cavernous transformation of the PV (collateralization in the porta hepatitis)
- Thrombus demonstrated as a nonenhanced intraluminal-filling defect
- PVO shown as a nonopacification of central portion of vein, enhancement of periphery, transient inhomogeneous enhancement of periportal parenchyma

Pathology
- Commonly associated with hepatic cirrhosis and pancreatitis
- PV occlusion = extensive portosystemic collateral network
- Thrombosis
- Tumor thrombus

Clinical Issues
- Presentation varies from acute symptoms to unrecognized clinically
- Blockage of the portal vein gives rise to PH
- Patients with cirrhosis and varices have a 20-30% 2 year bleeding risk with a mortality rate of 30-70%

- Arterioportal shunting opacification of the involved portal branch occurs prematurely in arterial phase
- When small, the periportal collaterals may not be recognized and the porta hepatis will appear "empty"
- CTA may show unusual enhancement
  - Some segments of liver supplied by hepatic artery, some by PV

MR Findings
- T1WI
  - Acute clot (< 5 week) appears hyperintense
  - Acute PVO: Absent flow in PV lumen
  - Chronic thrombosis (cavernous transformation) periportal collaterals with flow voids
  - Valuable sign of portal vein patency is a uniform, signal-free ring surrounding an inner bright zone
- T2WI: Tumor thrombi; more hyperintense on T2-weighted images and enhance with gadolinium
- MRA
  - Presence of large venous collaterals in the hepatoduodenal ligament
  - Flow enhancement absent in all imaging planes
  - High sensitivity for detection of submucosal, serosal, paraesophageal collaterals
- Contrast-enhanced MRA more accurate than TOF and phase contrast

Ultrasonographic Findings
- Grayscale Ultrasound
  - Triad of findings in PVO
    - Nonvisualization of extrahepatic portal vein
    - Bright echogenic band representing either thrombus or periportal fibrosis in region of PV
    - Periportal collaterals appearing as multiple vascular channels in porta hepatis
  - Ancillary findings: Splenomegaly, varices, spontaneous splenorenal shunts, gallbladder varices
    - Doppler of collateral channels detect hepatopetal flow patterns characteristic of PV
  - Tumor in PV may appear identical to thrombosis
    - Arterial flow in the thrombus suggests tumor
    - Enlargement of portal vein, lymphadenopathy or adjacent mass
  - String sign (thickening of the PV with narrowing of its lumen) due to portal phlebitis
  - Duplex Doppler
    - No Doppler signal in the portal vein
    - Enlarged hepatic arteries
  - 10-33% cases have fresh thrombosis and vein appears anechoic
  - Cavernous transformation of portal vein
    - Multiple collateral channels formed: Periportal (vasa vasorum) or within thrombus (due to recanalization)
- Color Doppler: Tumor thrombosis shows numerous small lucencies within the echogenic clot; tumor vessels usually visible in intraluminal tumor

Angiographic Findings
- Conventional
  - Celiac arteriography shows dilation of hepatic artery and branches
  - Arterial portography shows portosystemic and portal-portal collaterals
  - Portal-portal collateral pathways
    - Splenic vein to short gastric veins to coronary vein to remaining patent segment of portal vein
    - Splenic vein to gastroepiploic vein to portal vein
    - Splenic vein to omental vein (arc of Barkow) to PV
    - Pancreaticoduodenal veins and cystic veins to hilar PV
  - Splenoportography allows best visualization of cavernous transformation
  - Pressure measurements
    - Hepatic wedge pressure is normal and hepatic venography is normal
    - Measurement with direct portography

Imaging Recommendations
- US initially: Highly accurate and cost effective
- Contrast CT for comprehensive evaluation/search
- MR as alternative for CT

PORTAL VEIN OCCLUSION

DIFFERENTIAL DIAGNOSIS

Sluggish PV Flow Due to Cirrhosis

- Mimic occlusion on Duplex US and non-contrast MRA
- No cavernous transformation

Splenic Vein Occlusion

- Massive splenic-systemic collateral network mimics PV occlusion
- Patent PV, absence of splenic vein

PATHOLOGY

General Features

- General path comments
  - PV occlusion uncommon
  - Anatomy
    - PV occlusion = portosystemic collateral network
    - Increased hepatic artery size and flow due to decreased PV flow
- Genetics: Prothrombin gene G20210A, antithrombin III, anticoagulation factors (proteins C, S) defects
- Etiology
  - Thrombosis
    - Stasis from cirrhosis
    - Acute pancreatitis, hypercoagulable states, myeloproliferative disorders
    - Pyelophlebitis: Seeding of PV by infected material (acute appendicitis, intraperitoneal abscess, etc.)
  - Tumor thrombus
    - Hepatocellular carcinoma most common 30%
    - Pancreatic carcinoma, liver metastases, leiomyosarcoma of PV
- Epidemiology
  - Extrahepatic PVO: 5-10% of all cases of PH
  - PH in developing countries, 40% attributed to PVO

Gross Pathologic & Surgical Features

- Cavernous transformation of PV occurs with chronic PVO

CLINICAL ISSUES

Presentation

- Most common signs/symptoms
  - Blockage of portal vein gives rise to PH
    - Esophageal varices, bleeding varices, splenomegaly
  - Acute PVO
    - Sudden onset RUQ pain, nausea, fever
    - Progressive ascites, intestinal ischemia resulting from propagation of thrombus
    - Intestinal edema secondary to acute PH
  - Chronic PVO
    - PH complications
    - 90% of cases present with variceal bleeding, splenomegaly in 75-100% of patients
    - Intra-abdominal malignancies: Bleeding is less common; more common are sudden ascites, anorexia, RUQ or epigastric pain, and weight loss
- Other signs/symptoms
  - Schistosomiasis
  - Mesenteric venous thrombosis extends into the PV and results in intestinal angina
- Common incidental finding in advanced cirrhosis

Demographics

- Age: PVO predominantly affects young children, but it can occur in persons of any age
- Gender: Slight male predominance in patients whose obstruction is secondary to cirrhosis
- Ethnicity
  - U.S. rare (0.05-0.5%)
  - No racial differences have been reported
  - Incidence of PVO in cirrhotics is 5-18% (U.S.)

Natural History & Prognosis

- Non-occlusive PV thrombosis may lyse = no residua or minor PV scarring
- PV tumor invasion is fatal
- Patients without cirrhosis, the 2-year bleeding risk from esophageal varices is 0.25% with a mortality rate of 5%
- Patients with cirrhosis and varices have a 20-30% 2-year bleeding risk with a mortality rate of 30-70%
- 10-year survival rate is 38-60% in adults, > 70% in children

Treatment

- Reduce pressure in PV, preventing bleeding of esophageal varices
- Anticoagulation for acute thrombosis
- Acute bleeding
  - Octreotide infusion: Bleeding control in 85%
  - Propranolol
  - Variceal banding or sclerotherapy
  - Recanalization of acute PVO via transhepatic route: Thrombolytic followed by anticoagulation therapy
- Shunt between PV & IVC reduces pressure in PV
  - Distal splenorenal shunt, portocaval shunt
  - Operative mortality with cirrhosis: (18%), without cirrhosis: (2%)
  - Post-operative complications rate (30%)
  - TIPS indicated for complications due to PVO, if possible
- Liver transplantation

DIAGNOSTIC CHECKLIST

Image Interpretation Pearls

- Look for collaterals along the usual course of the portal vein, portal vein may not be visualized
- Thrombus in the portal vein with enhancement - need to differentiate PV thrombosis from tumor thrombus

SELECTED REFERENCES

1. Hidajat N et al: Portal vein thrombosis: etiology, diagnostic strategy, therapy and management. Vasa. 34(2):81-92, 2005
2. Wang JT et al: Portal vein thrombosis. Hepatobiliary Pancreat Dis Int. 4(4):515-8, 2005
3. Ishigami K et al: Portal vein occlusion with aberrant left gastric vein functioning as a hepatopetal collateral pathway. J Vasc Interv Radiol. 15(5):501-4, 2004

IMAGE GALLERY

Typical

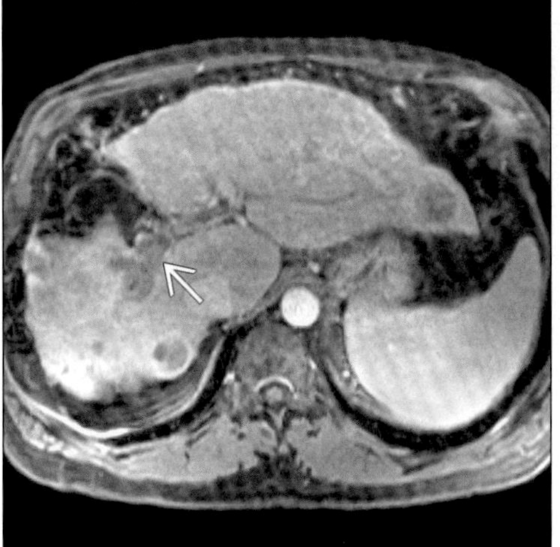

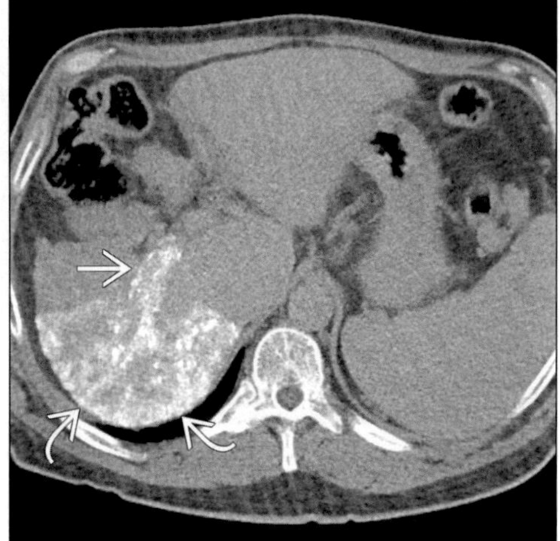

*(**Left**) Axial T1WI MR shows thrombus in the right PV ➔. The liver is small and nodular consistent with cirrhosis. The right lobe has some increased enhancement, and there is some heterogeneous enhancement of thrombus. Findings are suggestive of tumor thrombus. (**Right**) Axial NECT shows area of high density ➔ which represents Ethiodol from TACE procedure. Thrombus in portal vein ➔ has taken up Ethiodol confirming that this represents tumor thrombus.*

Typical

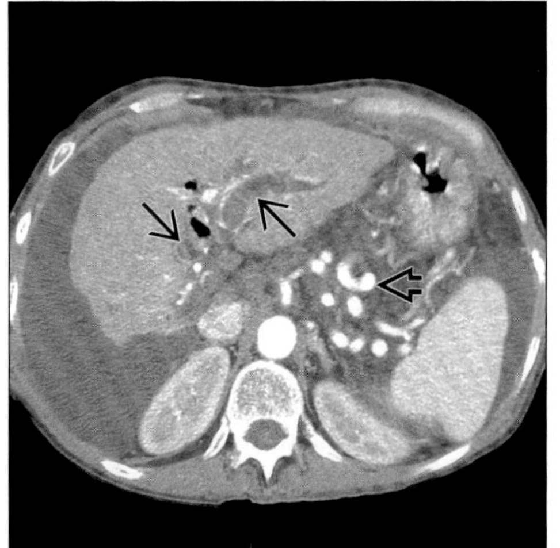

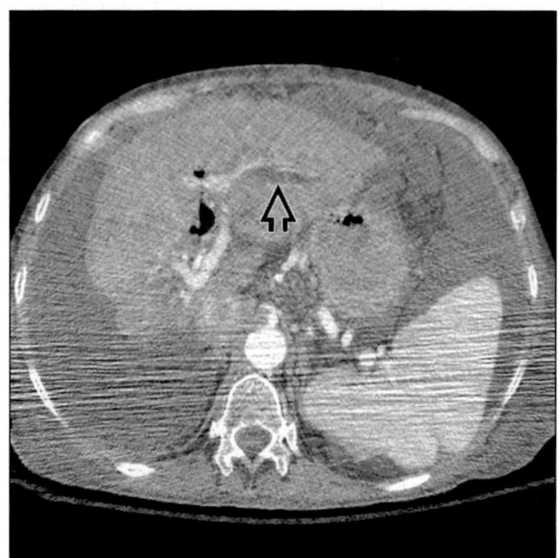

*(**Left**) Axial CECT shows thrombus in the branches of the portal vein ➔. There is a small liver, massive ascites, and gastrohepatic varices ➔ in patient with hepatitis C. (**Right**) Axial CECT 3 weeks following previous scan demonstrates some resolution of the portal vein thrombus ➔. The patient's severe liver disease had precluded any aggressive treatment and partial resolution occurred with conservative therapy.*

Typical

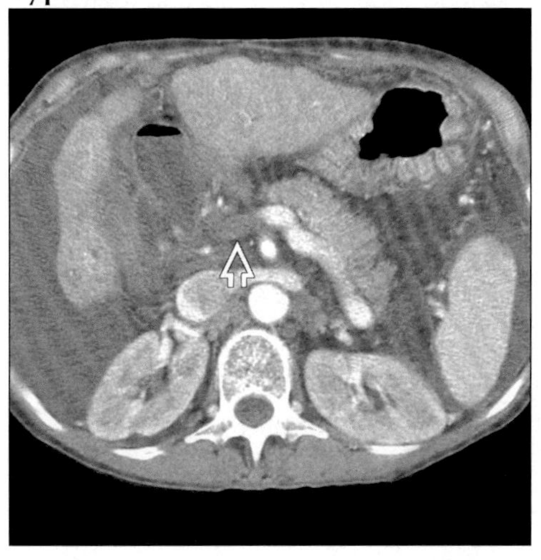

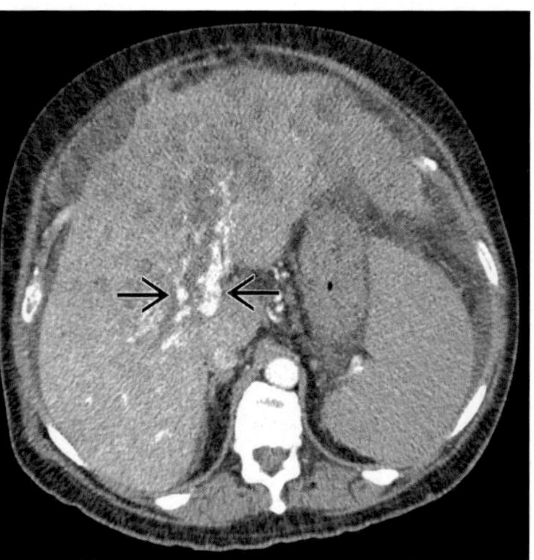

*(**Left**) Axial CECT shows thrombus ➔ in the splenic vein and extending to the SMV/splenic vein confluence. From this level the thrombus extended up into the intrahepatic PV. (**Right**) Axial CECT shows an enlarged PV filled with thrombus. In addition there is enhancement of the edges of the thrombus ➔. This enhancement is in the arterial phase of the CT indicating arterioportal shunting. There is also a mass diffusely involving the liver. This represents HCC.*

TIPS FOLLOW-UP

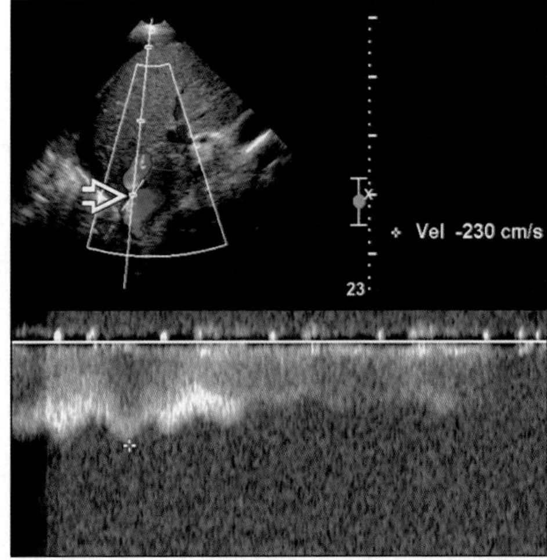

Sagittal color Doppler ultrasound shows very high velocity of 230 cm/s at the hepatic vein of the TIPS just at the point where it enters the hepatic vein ➡. This is a common failure point.

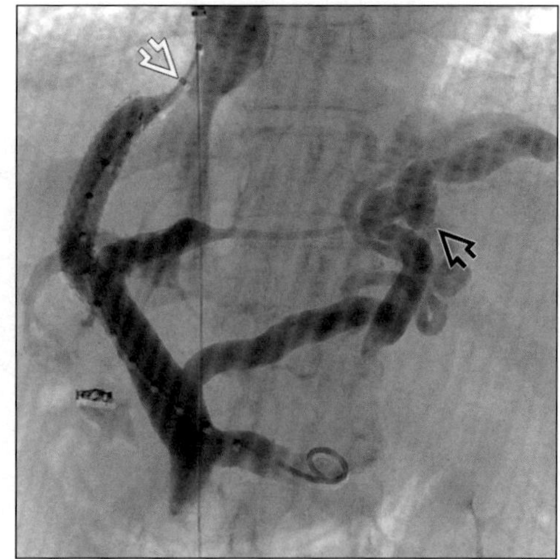

DSA shows a study of a TIPS with a very tight stenosis of the hepatic vein end of the stent ➡. Because of the tight stenosis there is marked filling of the left gastric (coronary) vein ⇨.

TERMINOLOGY

Abbreviations and Synonyms

- Transjugular intrahepatic portosystemic shunt (TIPS)
- Portal vein (PV)
- Hepatic vein (HV)

Definitions

- Percutaneous access via jugular vein, with shunt created by placement of stent between PV and HV
- TIPS placed to reduce portal pressure in patients with complications related to portal hypertension
  - Variceal bleeding
  - Portal gastropathy
  - Ascites
  - Budd-Chiari syndrome
- Goal of TIPS is to divert portal blood flow into hepatic vein, reducing pressure in portal circulation
- Bare metal stents originally used to create shunt between PV and HV
- Stent-grafts being used commonly now to create TIPS

IMAGING FINDINGS

General Features

- Best diagnostic clue: Intrahepatic metallic stent or stent graft connecting the hepatic venous system with the portal venous system
- Location: Stent usually extends from right PV to the right HV
- TIPS failure
  - Stent malposition or kink
  - Focal stenosis
    - Midportion of the stent; due to biliary duct fistula
    - Intimal hyperplasia within or at ends of stents
    - Most often at HV end of stent
  - Diffuse stenosis from neointimal hyperplasia
- Susceptibility artifact from stent limits MR follow-up

CT Findings

- Post-TIPS CT Findings
  - IV contrast-enhancement, timing for portal phase essential (triple-phase liver technique)
  - Functional stent
    - Ends of stent squarely centered HV, PV
    - Smooth curve, no kinks

DDx: TIPS Follow-Up

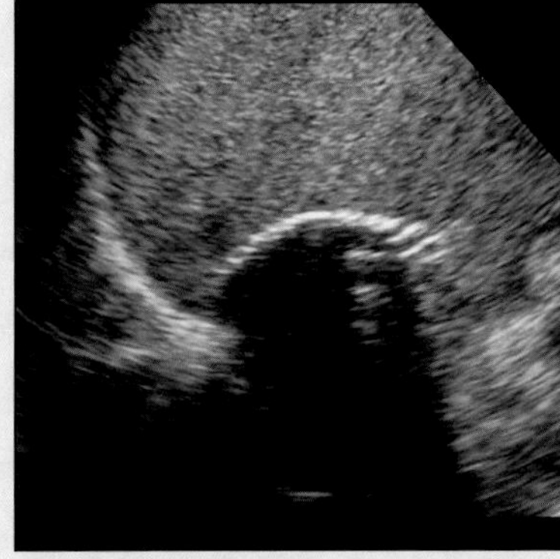

Newly Placed Viatorr Stent Graft

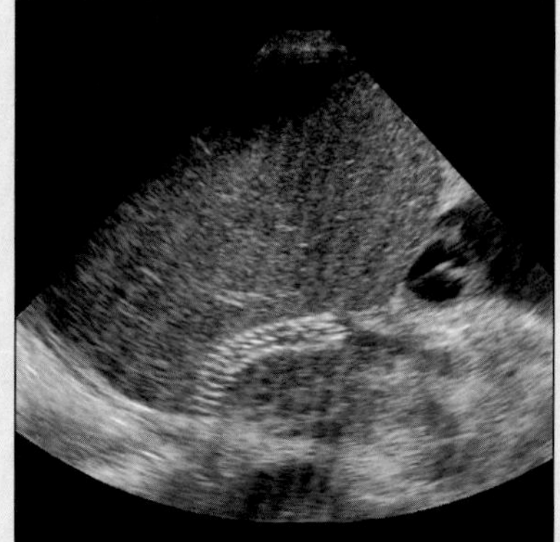

Viatorr Several Weeks Later

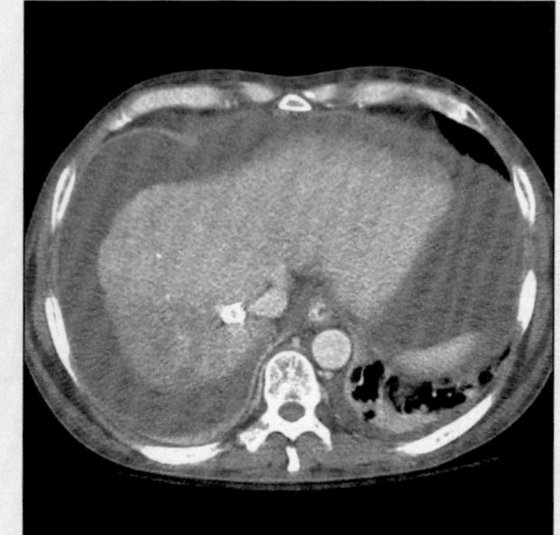

CT: Large Amount of Ascites

TIPS FOLLOW-UP

Key Facts

Terminology

- TIPS is placed to reduce portal pressure in patients with complications related to portal hypertension
- Percutaneous access via jugular vein, with shunt created by placement of stent between PV and HV

Imaging Findings

- Stent usually extends from right HV to right PV, near confluence with main PV
- TIPS failure: Findings on ultrasound
  - Diffuse stenosis from neointimal hyperplasia
  - Stent malposition or kink
  - Focal stenosis
  - Midportion of the stent; due to biliary duct fistula
  - Intimal hyperplasia within or at ends of stents
  - Most often at HV end of stent
  - Localized stenosis with high velocity/turbulence
- Diffuse narrowing, with or without high velocity
- Generalized low velocity
- Decreased PV velocity from baseline (< 30 cm/sec)
- Stent velocity (peak): Similar at portal and hepatic ends; usually 90-120 cm/sec; minimal normal: 50-60 cm/sec
- Hepatofugal flow in PV, may be biphasic
- Absence of flow in shunt
- Assess direction of PV flow and velocities through the shunt and within HV

Clinical Issues

- Treatment for poorly functioning TIPS
- Stent or stent-graft placement
- Additional TIPS shunt
- Continued alcohol abuse

    - Prompt contrast opacification of stent
    - Contrast extends to stent walls (no filling defect)
    - Uniform vein/stent caliber (no focal narrowing)
    - Hepatopetal flow in main PV and splenic vein
  - Nonfunctional stent
    - Poor centering or kinking of stent
    - Absence of stent flow
    - Delayed stent opacification
    - Stenosis: Fusiform or focal, within stent or HV
    - Hepatofugal flow in portal vein

Ultrasonographic Findings

- Grayscale Ultrasound
  - TIPS stenosis
    - Flow reversal
    - Jet lesion
    - Decreased flow in the TIPS or portal vein
- Color Doppler
  - Assess direction of PV flow and velocities through the shunt and within HV
    - Absent flow in malfunctioning stent
    - Low peak shunt velocity (< 50 to 90 cm/s)
    - High peak shunt velocity (190 cm/s)
    - Low mean PV velocity (< 30 cm/s)
    - Antegrade flow in the intrahepatic PVs
    - Change in shunt velocity (> 50 cm/s)
- Pre-TIPS US Evaluation
  - Confirm patency of
    - Internal jugular vein
    - HV, PV patency
  - Confirm right and left portal branches unite within liver (risk of hemorrhage with extrahepatic union)
  - Document
    - Flow direction in right, left and main PVs, and splenic vein
    - Peak flow velocity in main PV
- Post-TIPS Ultrasound Findings
  - Stent grafts cannot be visualized for at least 1 week post-placement due to air bubbles in graft
  - Satisfactory
    - Stent velocity (peak): Similar at portal and hepatic ends; usually 90-120 cm/sec; minimal normal: 50-60 cm/sec
    - PV velocity (peak): Usual range 35-45 cm/sec; minimum 30 cm/sec
    - Hepatopetal PV, splenic vein flow (left PV may remain reversed)
    - Turbulence and pulsatility common
  - Unsatisfactory
    - Localized stenosis with high velocity/turbulence
    - > 100 cm/sec increase in velocity from one point to another in stent
    - Diffuse narrowing, with or without high velocity
    - Generalized low velocity
    - Decreased PV velocity from baseline (< 30 cm/sec)
    - Hepatofugal flow in PV, may be biphasic
    - Absence of flow in shunt

Angiographic Findings

- Stent placed as follows
  - Cannulation of right internal jugular vein
  - Catheterization of HV
  - Penetration of liver by needle into right PV, wire then catheter placed into PV forming intrahepatic tract
  - Intrahepatic tract balloon dilatated
  - Placement of balloon-expandable covered stent in intrahepatic tract; noncovered end of stent extending into PV
- TIPS venography
- Direct portal and right atrial pressure measurements

Imaging Recommendations

- US for primary pre/post TIPS assessment
- CT when US technically compromised
- DSA for confirmation and treatment

DIFFERENTIAL DIAGNOSIS

Surgical Porto-Systemic Shunt

- Extrahepatic location

Spontaneous Porto-Hepatic Shunt

- No stent

TIPS FOLLOW-UP

PATHOLOGY

General Features

- Epidemiology
  - Primary patency after TIPS placement after 1 yr (66%); 2 yr (42%)
    - Primary-assisted patencies at 1 yr (83%); 2 yr (79%)
    - Secondary patency at 1 yr (96%); 2 yr (90%)
  - Survival rates in patients with Child grades of A, B, and C, respectively, were 75%, 68%, and 49% at 1 yr; 75%, 55%, and 43% at 2 yr
  - Complete resolution of ascites (63%), marked decrease in diuretic (83%)
  - Risk for encephalopathy is 9-25% after TIPS
    - Rates of encephalopathy associated with medical therapy (17-44%); surgical therapy (24-49%)

CLINICAL ISSUES

Presentation

- TIPS patients should enter routine US surveillance
  - Baseline scan within 24 hr of placement; look for complications
  - 6 month follow-up
  - If patient's US findings are unsatisfactory, then refer for TIPS venographic study and treatment
- Early complications
  - Thrombosis of the TIPS may occur within 24 hours of TIPS creation (10-15%)
  - Early shunt thrombosis is believed to be caused by leakage of bile into the shunt, hypercoagulable syndromes, or inadequate coverage of the TIPS tract with stents
  - Acute hepatic failure
  - Portal vein thrombosis
  - Arteriovenous fistula in liver
  - Hepatic artery injury, bile duct injury, capsular hematoma, hemoperitoneum
  - Portal venous puncture in an extrahepatic location can result in hemoperitoneum
  - Deterioration of hemodynamic status because of acute increases in cardiac output & increased central venous & pulmonary pressures; right-sided heart failure
  - Loss of PV decompression due to shunt stenosis or occlusion
- Late complications
  - Stenosis of stent
  - Occlusion of stent
  - Thrombosis or intimal hyperplasia
    - 17% loss of shunt patency at 5-year follow-up
  - Hepatic encephalopathy (25%)
  - Hepatoma

Natural History & Prognosis

- Progressive hepatic diseases
- 2, 3 and 5 year survival rates are 51%, 49%, and 42%
- High stenosis/occlusion rate with bare metal stents
  - 66% one-year patency without intervention
  - 96% one-year patency with intervention
- Decreased stenosis/occlusion with stent grafts
- Reduction or loss of portal liver perfusion
- Overall flow to liver is an important factor in determining survival after TIPS
- Best indicator of TIPS dysfunction is recurrence of original problem for which TIPS was placed
- Rebleeding
  - Variceal rebleeding rate seen with TIPS is 19%
  - Shunt stenosis and occlusion commonly develops within 6 months after TIPS creation
  - Causes of shunt stenosis and occlusion
    - Acute shunt thrombosis
    - Development of pseudointimal hyperplasia in parenchymal tract of shunt
    - Narrowing of outflow hepatic vein
- Predictors of poor patient survival
  - Advanced liver disease
    - Child-Pugh score, elevated transaminases, hyperbilirubinemia, decreased albumin, ascites, preexisting encephalopathy
  - Elevated serum creatinine
  - Age
- Predictors of shunt failure
  - Fistula with biliary tract
  - High platelet count
  - Continued alcohol abuse
- Successful TIPS placement
  - Results in portosystemic gradient of < 12 mm Hg & immediate control of variceal-related bleeding
  - Repeated interventions required to maintain function in majority of TIPS patients

Treatment

- Treatment for poorly functioning TIPS
  - Angioplasty
  - Stent or stent-graft placement
  - Additional TIPS shunt
  - Thrombolysis followed by new stent/stent-graft for occluded shunt
  - Surgical portosystemic shunt
  - Liver transplantation

DIAGNOSTIC CHECKLIST

Consider

- TIPS malfunction when patient has recurrent ascites, or bleeding

SELECTED REFERENCES

1. Bureau C et al: Patency of stents covered with polytetrafluoroethylene in patients treated by transjugular intrahepatic portosystemic shunts: long-term results of a randomized multicentre study. Liver Int. 27(6):742-7, 2007
2. Carr CE et al: Role of ultrasound surveillance of transjugular intrahepatic portosystemic shunts in the covered stent era. J Vasc Interv Radiol. 17(8):1297-305, 2006
3. Barrio J et al: Comparison of transjugular intrahepatic portosystemic shunt dysfunction in PTFE-covered stent-grafts versus bare stents. Eur J Radiol. 55(1):120-4, 2005

IMAGE GALLERY

Typical

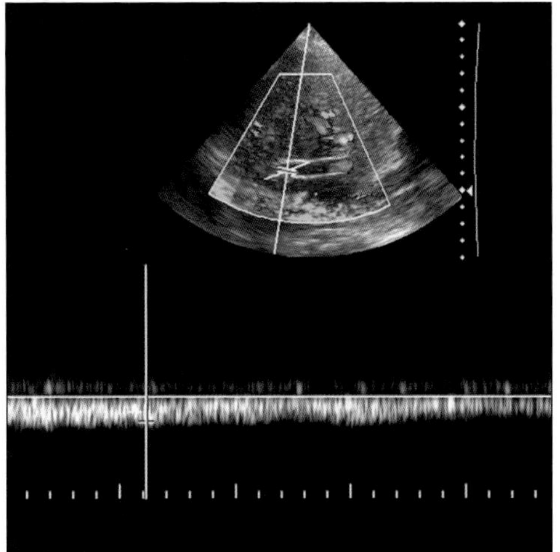

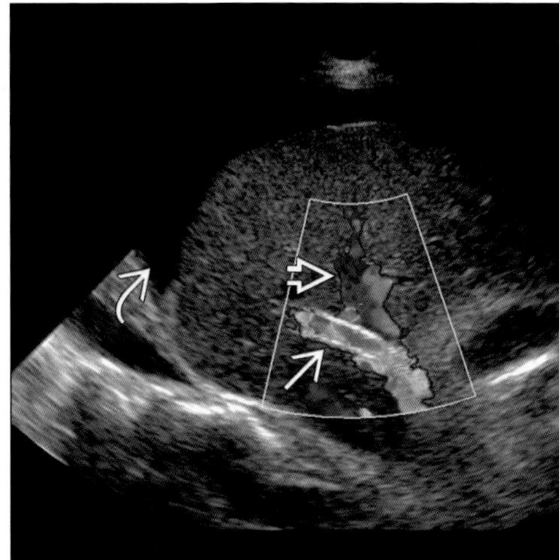

(Left) *Sagittal color Doppler ultrasound shows low velocities at the distal end of the TIPS. This is the most common area for the TIPS to fail. Velocities should not be below 30 cm/s.* ***(Right)*** *Sagittal color Doppler ultrasound shows the TIPS in place ➡ and the right portal vein ➡. Portal vein flow should be hepatofugal (towards the TIPS). In a failing TIPS, as in this case, the flow in the RPV is hepatopetal (towards the liver). Note the ascites ➡.*

Typical

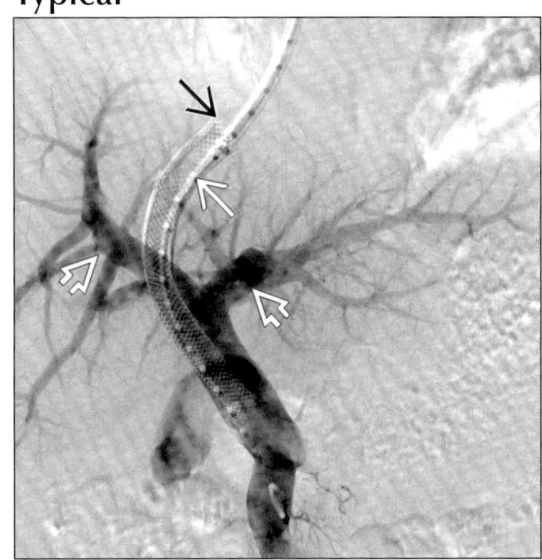

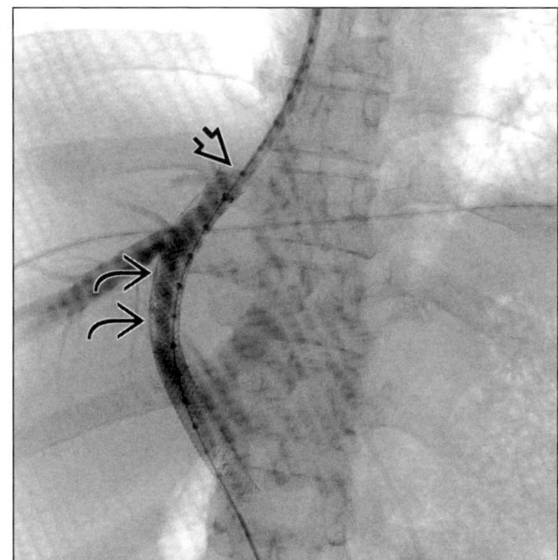

(Left) *DSA shows malfunctioning TIPS. Flow in the portal vein branches ➡ is hepatopetal, away from the TIPS shunt. There is no flow in TIPS shunt ➡, because the stent is short, not to the distal hepatic vein ➡.* ***(Right)*** *With a selective injection into the TIPS above the portal veins, the stenosis of the hepatic vein at the distal end of the TIPS can be seen ➡. This is a typical malfunction of the TIPS. A small amount of intimal hyperplasia is also seen ➡.*

Typical

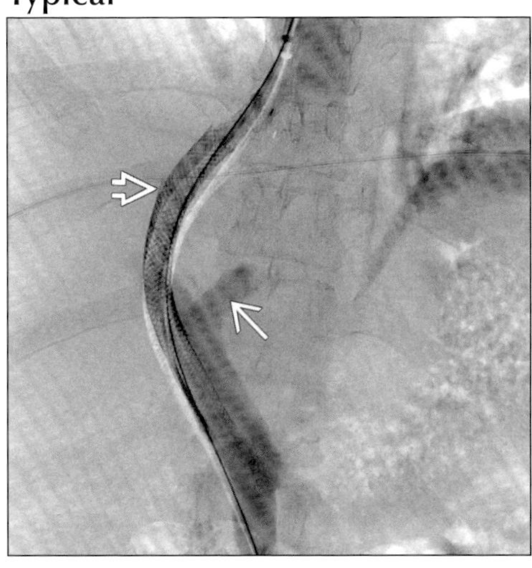

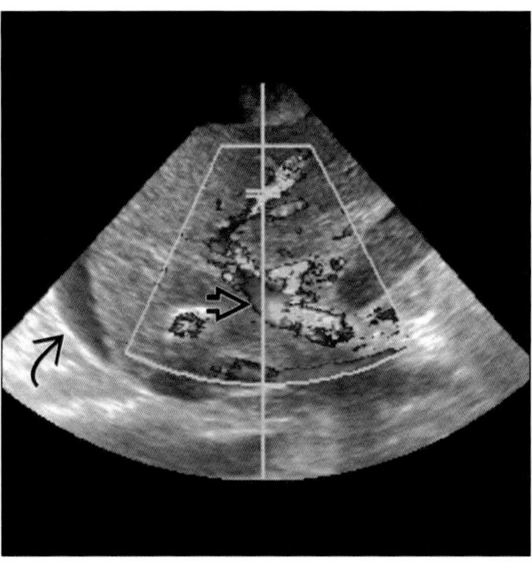

(Left) *DSA shows the appearance of the TIPS following angioplasty and restenting of the distal portion of the TIPS. Now the blood flow is through the TIPS ➡ and there is only very minimal flow into the left portal vein ➡. This is an appropriate result following treatment.* ***(Right)*** *Color Doppler ultrasound now shows the left portal vein ➡ with hepatofugal flow. The flow is now towards the TIPS which is appropriate. Still a small amount of ascites ➡.*

BUDD-CHIARI SYNDROME

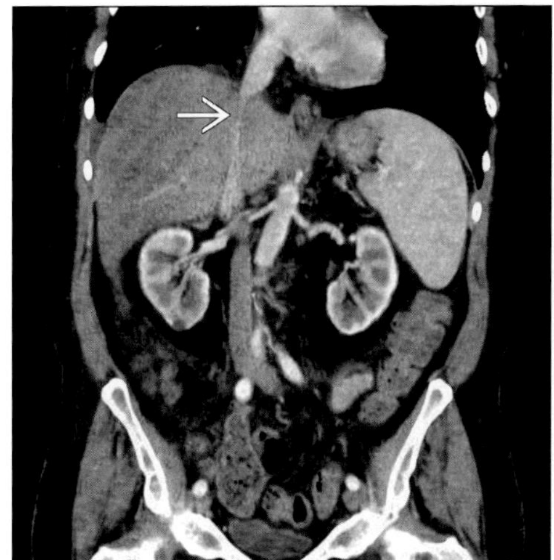

Coronal CECT shows marked narrowing of the IVC ➔ as it passes through the liver. This represents a type I classification, with narrowing of the IVC as a cause for the Budd-Chiari syndrome.

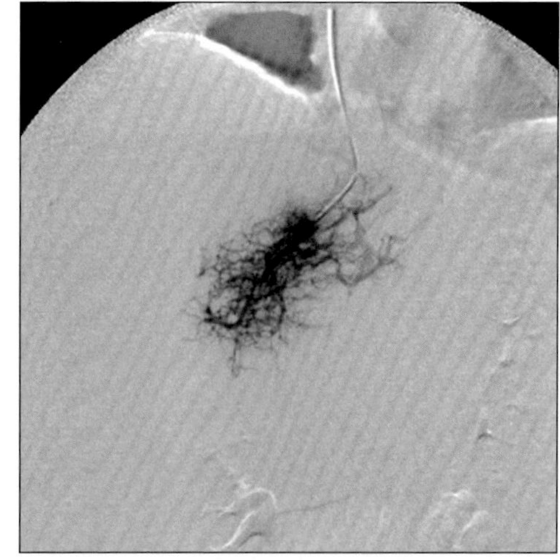

DSA shows the classic appearance of the venoocclusive type of Budd-Chiari syndrome. This represents the type III classification, with occlusion of the small hepatic veins.

TERMINOLOGY

Abbreviations and Synonyms

- Budd-Chiari syndrome (BCS)

Definitions

- Venous outflow obstruction to large hepatic veins
- Obstruction of suprahepatic segment of IVC
- Venoocclusive disease

IMAGING FINDINGS

General Features

- Best diagnostic clue: "Bicolored" hepatic veins on color Doppler sonography
- Location: Hepatic veins, centrilobar veins, or IVC
- Key concepts
  - Caudate lobe often spared due to separate venous drainage

CT Findings

- NECT
  - Acute phase
    - Diffusely hypodense enlarged liver
    - Enlarged caudate lobe
    - Ascites
    - Hyperdense IVC & hepatic veins (thrombus)
    - Mild splenomegaly
  - Chronic phase
    - As in acute phase
    - Atrophy of peripheral liver segments
    - Portosystemic and intrahepatic collateral vessels
- CECT
  - Changes as with NECT
  - Acute phase
    - Classic "flip-flop" pattern: Early enhancement of caudate lobe & central portion around IVC, with decreased liver enhancement peripherally; later decreased enhancement centrally with increased enhancement peripherally
    - Low density thrombi seen in hepatic veins, IVC, portal vein, splenic vein, superior mesenteric vein
  - Chronic phase
    - Total obliteration of IVC & hepatic veins
    - Hypoperfused liver parenchyma
    - Large intrahepatic collateral vessels
    - Chronic thrombosis calcification

DDx: Types of Budd Chiari Syndrome

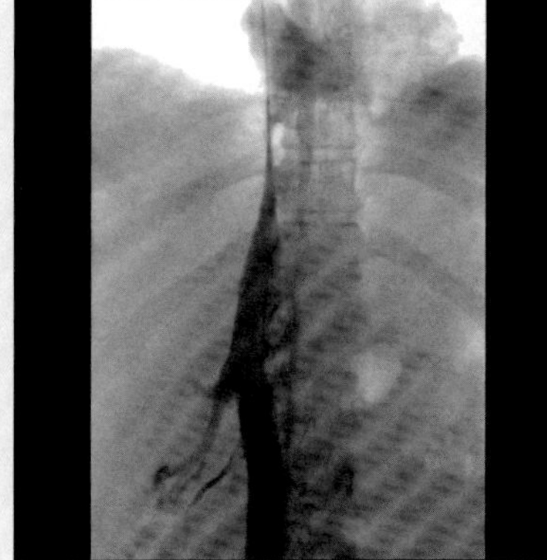

Type I Occlusion of IVC

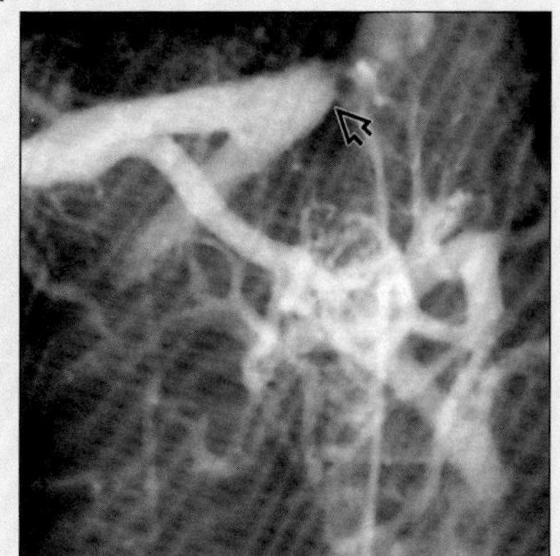

Type II Major Hepatic Vein

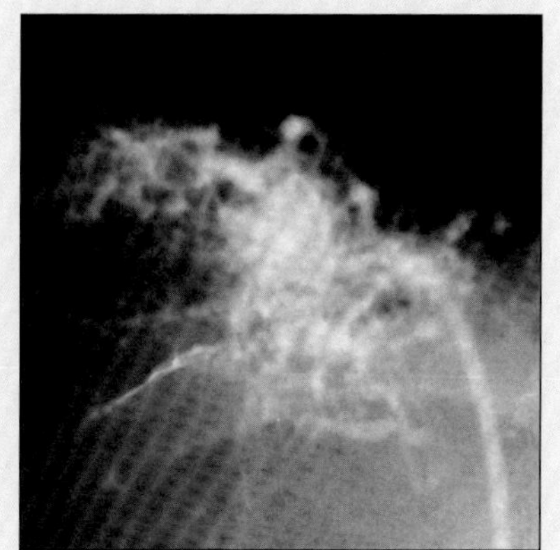

Type III Venoocclusive

BUDD-CHIARI SYNDROME

Key Facts

Terminology
- Hepatic venous outflow obstruction
- Venous outflow obstruction to large hepatic veins

Imaging Findings
- Best diagnostic clue: "Bicolored" hepatic veins on color Doppler sonography
  - Intrahepatic collateral pathways
- Ascites
- Enlarged caudate lobe
- Stenosis or occlusion of hepatic veins, centrilobar veins, and/or IVC
- Non-visualization of IVC & hepatic veins
- Venoocclusive "spider web" pattern of hepatic venous collaterals on venography

Top Differential Diagnoses
- Hepatic Cirrhosis

Pathology
- Primary: Membranous obstruction hepatic vein
- Secondary: Hypercoagulable, venoocclusive, etc.
- Type I: Occlusion of IVC ± hepatic veins
- Type II: Occlusion of major hepatic veins ± IVC
- Type III: Occlusion of small centrilobar veins

Clinical Issues
- Medical management
  - Steroids, nutritional therapy, anticoagulants
- Liver decompression
  - Surgical, angioplasty, stenting, TIPS

    - Hyperintense regenerative nodules
  - Membranous IVC or hepatic venous obstruction
    - Narrowing or occlusion of IVC above web
    - Enlarged retroperitoneal collaterals
  - Partial BCS (obstruction of a single vein)
    - Affected liver is hypodense, simulates a mass lesion

MR Findings
- T1WI: Findings as in CT
- T2WI
  - Heterogeneously increased signal intensity in periphery compatible with congestion and edema
  - Absence of flow signal in hepatic veins and IVC
  - Islands of preserved signal intensity correlates with less compromised drainage adjacent to periportal triads
- T2* GRE: Fails to show flow in hepatic veins or IVC
- T1 C+: As in CECT
- MRA: Depicts thrombus & level of venous obstruction

Ultrasonographic Findings
- Grayscale Ultrasound
  - Findings as seen with CT
  - Hepatic veins
    - Stenosis, proximal dilation, thick wall echoes, thrombosis, tortuosity, extrahepatic anastomosis
    - Stagnant, reversed or turbulent flow
    - Intrahepatic or subcapsular collaterals
  - Portal vein flow may be hepatopetal or hepatofugal
  - IVC changes
    - Reduced bidirectional or no flow in IVC
    - Thrombus or tumor within IVC
    - Compression by caudate lobe
    - Echogenic membrane or fibrous cord in the IVC
    - Narrowing or loss of IVC at the intrahepatic level
- Color Doppler
  - Hepatic veins & IVC
    - "Bicolored" hepatic veins-intrahepatic collateral pathways

Angiographic Findings
- Inferior venacavography
  - Constriction of the intrahepatic IVC
  - IVC obstruction by a web, thrombus, tumor
  - Thrombus in hepatic veins or IVC
  - Hepatic venogram
    - Proximal hepatic vein stenosis
    - Hepatic vein occlusion may be caused by tumor (usually associated with hepatocellular carcinoma)
    - Venoocclusive "spider web" pattern of hepatic venous collaterals
- Arterial portography
  - Sluggish hepatopetal flow
  - Thrombi in major splanchnic veins

Imaging Recommendations
- Best imaging tool: Color Doppler sonography, MR/MRV, or angiography for pressures or treatment

DIFFERENTIAL DIAGNOSIS

Hepatic Cirrhosis
- Hypertrophy: Caudate & lateral segment of left lobe
- Atrophy: Right lobe & medial segment of left lobe
- Varices, ascites, splenomegaly
- Patent hepatic veins & IVC
- Regenerative nodules
  - Usually small in size compared to BCS

Hepatocellular Carcinoma
- Contrast-enhancing on arterial phase

Primary Vascular Abnormality
- Primary IVC thrombosis, heart failure, constrictive pericarditis

PATHOLOGY

General Features
- Genetics
  - Thrombogenic condition, hypercoagulability
  - Factor V Leiden
    - Most common cause of hereditary thrombophilia

BUDD-CHIARI SYNDROME

- Second most common cause of thrombotic occlusion of hepatic and caval vessels
- Etiology
  - Primary
    - Membranous obstruction of hepatic vein
  - Secondary
    - Intrinsic obstruction (tumor or parasitic mass)
    - Extrinsic compression (tumor, abscess, cyst)
    - Hypercoagulable states
    - Venoocclusive disease: Bone marrow transplantation, antineoplastic drugs, toxins, consumption of herbal teas containing senecio
  - Tumors
    - Hepatocellular, renal cell, Wilms tumor, adrenal carcinoma, leiomyosarcoma of IVC
    - Right atrial myxoma
  - Hematological disorders
    - Polycythemia rubra vera, paroxysmal nocturnal hemoglobinuria, myeloproliferative disorders
  - Inherited thrombotic diathesis
    - Protein C, S, Antithrombin III, factor V Leiden
  - Chronic infections
    - Hydatid cysts, amebic abscess, aspergillosis, tuberculosis, syphilis
  - Chronic inflammatory diseases
    - SLE, sarcoidosis, inflammatory bowel disease
- Epidemiology
  - Primary (congenital-membranous type)
    - Common in Japan, India, Israel & South Africa
  - Secondary (thrombotic)
    - Most common in Western countries
    - Usually due to hypercoagulable state

Gross Pathologic & Surgical Features

- Acute phase
  - Liver enlarged, congested
  - Occlusion of hepatic veins and/or IVC
- Chronic phase
  - Liver: Nodular
  - Hypertrophy of caudate lobe (80%)
    - Organized thrombi in main hepatic veins

Microscopic Features

- Centrilobular congestion, dilated sinusoids
- Fibrosis, necrosis & cell atrophy
- Hepatic venoocclusive disease

Staging, Grading or Classification Criteria

- Classified into three types based on location
  - Type I: Occlusion of IVC ± hepatic veins
  - Type II: Occlusion of major hepatic veins ± IVC
  - Type III: Occlusion of small centrilobar veins
    - "Venoocclusive disease"

CLINICAL ISSUES

Presentation

- Most common signs/symptoms
  - No symptoms
    - Obstruction of only one hepatic vein
    - Slow obstruction of 2-3 hepatic veins with collaterals formation
  - Acute phase
    - Rapid obstruction ≥ 2 major veins or thrombus superimposed on long-standing partial obstruction
    - Triad: RUQ pain, ascites, hepatomegaly
    - Tender liver, hypotension, abdominal pain, fever, nausea, vomiting
  - Chronic phase (> 6 months)
    - More common than acute presentation
    - RUQ pain, hepatomegaly, splenomegaly
    - Jaundice, ascites, varices, bleeding
    - Encephalopathy, coagulopathy, malnutrition
    - Hepatorenal syndrome

Demographics

- Age: Any age group
- Gender: M < F

Natural History & Prognosis

- Complications
  - Acute: Liver failure, emboli from IVC thrombus
  - Chronic: Cirrhosis, variceal bleeding, portal hypertension
- Prognosis based on degree of obstruction
  - Acute early phase: Good with treatment
  - Chronic phase: Poor (with or without treatment)
  - Untreated, death of hepatic failure ~ 3 years

Treatment

- Goal: Relieve venous obstruction; preserve hepatic function by eliminating congestion
- Medical management
  - Steroids, nutritional therapy, anticoagulants
- Liver decompression
  - Angioplasty, stenting, TIPS
- Surgical decompression
  - Cavo-, meso-, splenoatrial; mesojugular shunts
  - Direct surgical correction of stenosis/occlusion
- Long term anti-coagulation post-transplant
- 10 year survival rates BCS below 55%

DIAGNOSTIC CHECKLIST

Consider

- Rule out cirrhosis

Image Interpretation Pearls

- Absent, reversed or flat flow in hepatic veins & reversed flow in IVC on color Doppler sonography
- Characteristic large benign regenerative nodules

SELECTED REFERENCES

1. Kamath PS: Budd-Chiari syndrome: Radiologic findings. Liver Transpl. 12(11 Suppl 2):S21-2, 2006
2. Bogin V et al: Budd-Chiari syndrome: in evolution. Eur J Gastroenterol Hepatol. 17(1):33-5, 2005
3. Brancatelli G et al: Benign regenerative nodules in Budd-Chiari syndrome and other vascular disorders of the liver: radiologic-pathologic and clinical correlation. Radiographics. 22(4):847-62, 2002

IMAGE GALLERY

Typical

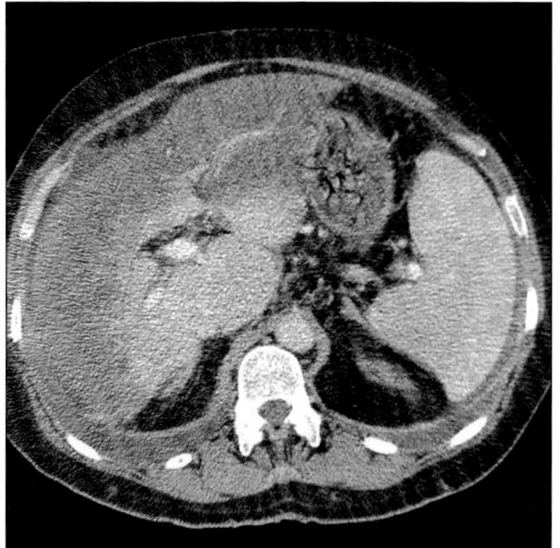

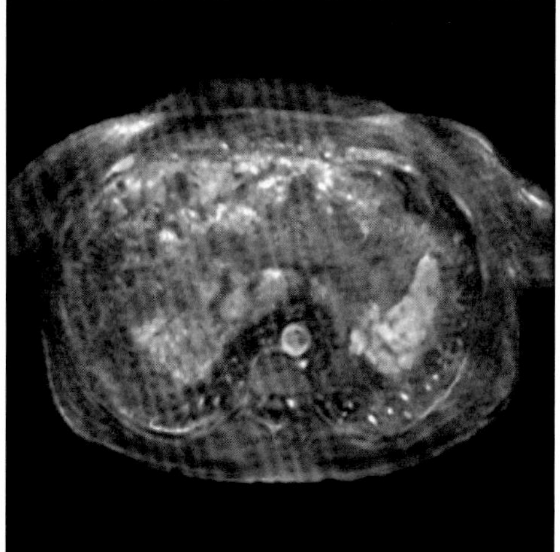

(Left) Axial CECT shows pattern of early enhancement of the caudate lobe and central portion of the liver, with decreased liver enhancement peripherally. *(Right)* Axial GRE MR shows heterogeneously increased signal intensity in the periphery, compatible with congestion and edema. Preserved signal intensity in areas of liver adjacent to periportal triads.

Other

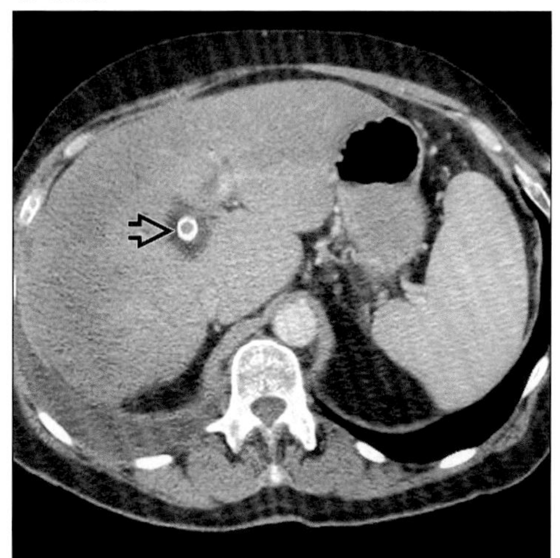

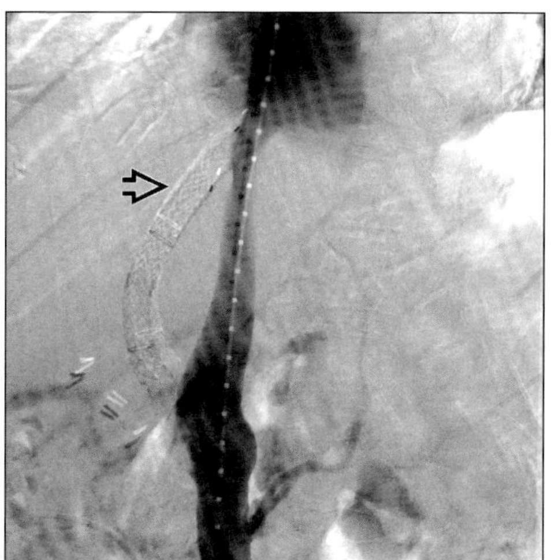

(Left) Axial CECT shows TIPS shunt ⇨ which was placed 2 weeks ago. Ascites has resolved, cava not visible on previous image, is now slightly visible. Still decreased peripheral enhancement. *(Right)* DSA shows TIPS shunt ⇨ in place. There is increased diameter of IVC with decreasing size of caudate lobe, decreasing constriction of the intrahepatic IVC.

Other

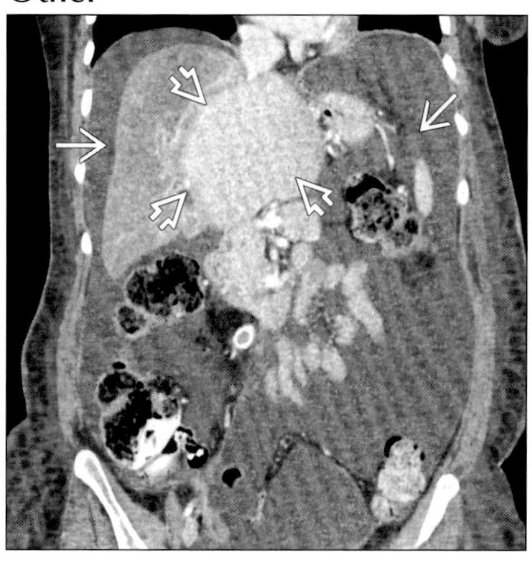

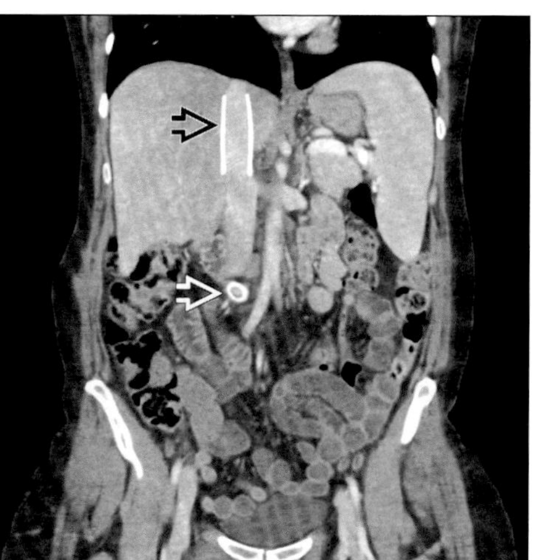

(Left) Coronal CECT shows multiple findings of Budd-Chiari syndrome: Ascites ➡, markedly enlarged caudate lobe ➡, decreased liver enhancement in the periphery with central enhancement. *(Right)* Coronal CECT shows IVC stent ⇨ in the intrahepatic IVC. This is the treatment for type I Budd-Chiari. Ascites has resolved. Liver more normal in appearance. Previous meso-atrial shunt ➡.

IVC ANOMALIES

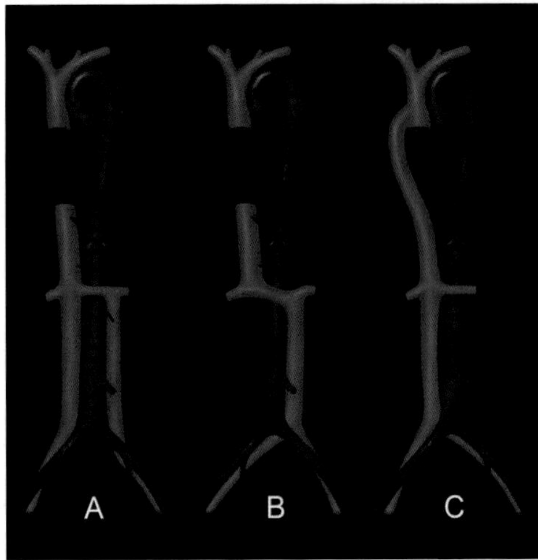

Graphic shows three types of IVC anomalies, with venous structures rendered blue. Figure A shows duplication of the IVC, figure B shows a left-sided IVC and figure C shows azygos continuation of the IVC.

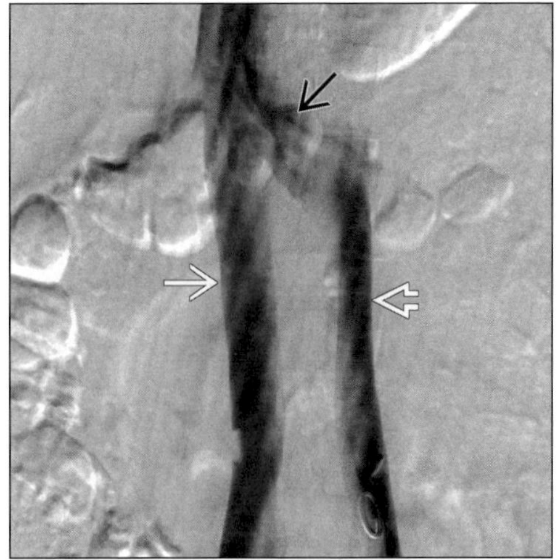

Conventional catheter venography through bilateral femoral vein catheterization shows duplicated vena cava. The left IVC ➡ joins the right IVC ➡ through the left renal vein →.

TERMINOLOGY

Definitions

- Congenital anomalies of inferior vena cava (IVC)

IMAGING FINDINGS

General Features

- Best diagnostic clue: Malposition or duplication of IVC inferior to renal veins
- Types of IVC anomalies
  - Duplication of IVC (double IVC)
  - Left IVC
  - Azygos continuation of IVC
  - Circumaortic left renal vein
  - Retroaortic left renal vein
  - Duplication of IVC with retroaortic right renal vein and hemiazygos continuation of IVC
  - Duplication of IVC with retroaortic left renal vein and azygos continuation of IVC
  - Circumcaval, retrocaval or transcaval ureter
  - Absence of infrarenal or entire IVC

CT Findings

- Duplication of IVC
  - Left and right IVC inferior to renal veins
  - Usually left IVC ends at left renal vein, which crosses anterior to aorta in normal fashion to join right IVC
  - Left and right IVC may have significant size asymmetry
- Left IVC
  - Left IVC ends at left renal vein, which crosses anterior to aorta in normal fashion, uniting with right renal vein to form normal right suprarenal IVC
  - ↑ Enhancement of right renal vein relative to left renal vein (dilution from unenhanced venous return from lower extremities)
- Azygos continuation of the IVC (absence of hepatic segment of IVC with azygos continuation)
  - IVC passes posterior to diaphragmatic crus to enter thorax as azygos vein
  - Azygos vein joins superior vena cava at normal location in right peribronchial location
  - Hepatic veins drain directly into right atrium and intrahepatic IVC is absent

DDx: IVC Anomalies

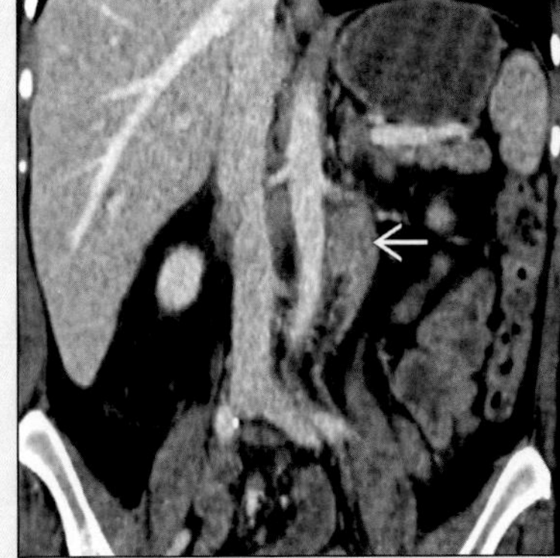

Retroperitoneal Lymph Nodes

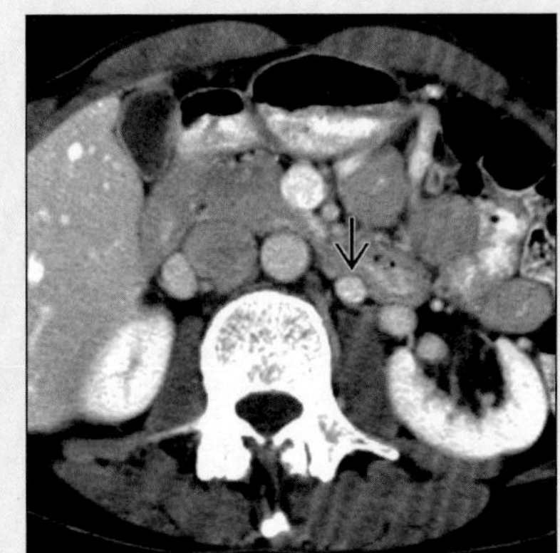

Dilated Gonadal Vein

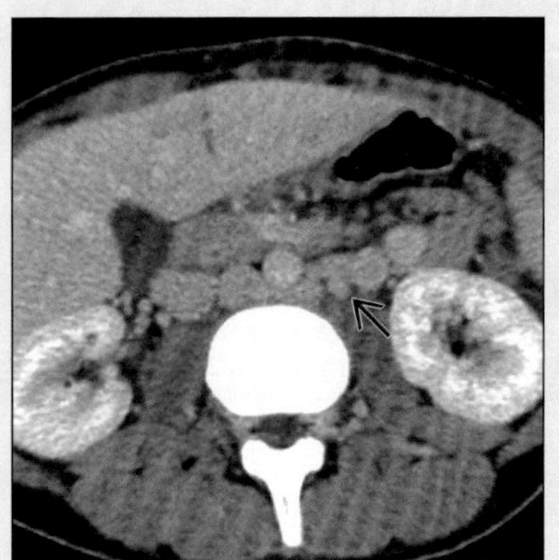

Retroperitoneal Collaterals

IVC ANOMALIES

Key Facts

Terminology
- Congenital anomalies of inferior vena cava (IVC)

Imaging Findings
- Best diagnostic clue: Malposition or duplication of IVC inferior to renal vein
- Usually, left IVC ends at left renal vein, which crosses anterior to aorta in normal fashion to join right IVC
- Left and right IVC may have significant asymmetry in size
- Best imaging tool: CT; consider multiplanar reformations

Top Differential Diagnoses
- Retroperitoneal Lymphadenopathy
- Varices/Collaterals
- Gonadal Vein

Pathology
- Duplication of IVC: 0.2-3% of general population

Clinical Issues
- Asymptomatic and usually incidentally diagnosed by imaging

Diagnostic Checklist
- Duplication of IVC should be suspected in recurrent pulmonary embolism following IVC filter placement
- Pre-operative imaging and recognition of IVC anomalies important in planning abdominal surgery and abdominal organ transplantation
- Important to recognize IVC anomalies in certain interventional procedures (e.g., IVC filters, varicocele sclerotherapy, venous renal or adrenal sampling)

  - Enlarged azygos vein is similar in attenuation to superior vena cava
  - Gonadal veins drain to ipsilateral renal veins
- Duplication of IVC with retroaortic right renal vein and hemiazygos continuation of IVC
  - Left and right IVC inferior to renal vein
  - Right IVC ends at right renal vein, which crosses posterior to aorta to join left IVC
  - Suprarenal IVC passes posterior to diaphragmatic crus to enter thorax as hemiazygos vein
  - In thorax, collateral pathways for hemiazygos vein include
    - Crosses posterior to aorta at T8-9 to join azygos vein
    - Continues superiorly to join coronary vein of heart via persistent left superior vena cava
    - Accessory hemiazygos continuation to left brachiocephalic vein
- Duplication of IVC with retroaortic left renal vein and azygos continuation of IVC
  - Mixture of findings previously mentioned
- Circumaortic left renal vein (common variant)
  - 2 left renal veins
    - Superior renal vein joined by left adrenal vein and crosses aorta anteriorly
    - Inferior renal vein (1-2 cm below superior renal vein) joined by left gonadal vein and crosses aorta posteriorly
- Retroaortic left renal vein
  - 1 left renal vein which crosses aorta posteriorly
- Circumcaval ureter
  - Proximal ureter courses posterior IVC, emerges to right of aorta and lies anterior to right iliac vessels
- Absence of infrarenal or entire IVC
  - External and internal iliac veins join to form enlarged ascending lumbar veins
  - Venous return from lower extremities to azygos and hemiazygos vein via anterior paravertebral collateral veins
  - ± Suprarenal IVC formed by left and right renal veins
  - May be acquired abnormality following thrombosis of IVC

MR Findings
- Flow voids or flow-related enhancement may distinguish aberrant vessels from masses
- Other findings similar to CT

Ultrasonographic Findings
- Hepatic veins drain directly into right atrium when intrahepatic IVC is absent
- Duplicated IVC may be detected as two IVCs adjacent to aorta on either side

Angiographic Findings
- Venography is most accurate method for diagnosis and demonstrates course of major abdominal venous drainage

Imaging Recommendations
- Best imaging tool
  - CECT; consider multiplanar reformations
  - Venous phase imaging is key for diagnosis

DIFFERENTIAL DIAGNOSIS

Retroperitoneal Lymphadenopathy
- Metastases, lymphoma, granulomatous disease
- Left-sided para-aortic adenopathy may mimic duplication of IVC or left IVC
  - Differentiate by renal vein drainage or contrast-enhancement of IVC
- Retrocrural adenopathy may mimic enlarged azygos vein in retrocrural space
  - Differentiate by tubular structure of azygos vein extending from diaphragm to azygos arch
  - Retrocrural adenopathy lacks enhancement
- Retroperitoneal adenopathy may mimic circumaortic left renal vein

Varices/Collaterals
- Seen in cirrhosis, IVC obstruction

Gonadal Vein

- May appear as para-aortic soft tissue "mass" or mimic left-sided IVC
- Follow inferiorly: Does not "join" left iliac vein

PATHOLOGY

General Features

- General path comments
  - Embryology
    - 6-8th gestational weeks: Infrahepatic IVC develops from appearance and regression of three paired embryonic veins; postcardinal, subcardinal and supracardinal veins
    - Normal IVC comprised of hepatic, suprarenal, renal and infrarenal segments
    - Hepatic segment develops from vitelline vein
    - Suprarenal segment develops from right subcardinal vein through subcardinal-hepatic anastomosis
    - Renal segment develops from right supra-subcardinal and post-subcardinal anastomoses
    - Infrarenal segment develops from right supracardinal vein
    - In thorax, supracardinal veins form azygos and hemiazygos veins
    - In abdomen, subcardinal and supracardinal veins progressively replace postcardinal veins
    - In pelvis, postcardinal veins form common iliac veins
- Genetics: Congenital with first degree relatives as risk factor
- Etiology
  - Duplication of IVC
    - Persistence of both supracardinal veins
  - Left-sided IVC
    - Regression of right supracardinal vein with persistence of left supracardinal vein
  - Azygos continuation of the IVC
    - Failure to form right subcardinal-hepatic anastomosis with resulting atrophy of right subcardinal vein
  - Circumaortic left renal vein
    - Persistence of dorsal limb of embryonic left renal vein and of dorsal arch of renal collar (intersupracardinal anastomosis)
  - Retroaortic left renal vein
    - Persistence of dorsal arch of renal collar and regression of ventral arch (intersubcardinal anastomosis)
  - Duplication of IVC with retroaortic right renal vein and hemiazygos continuation of IVC
    - Persistence of left lumbar and thoracic supracardinal vein and left suprasubcardinal anastomosis
    - Failure to form right subcardinal-hepatic anastomosis
  - IVC duplication and azygos continuation with retroaortic left renal vein
    - Persistent left supracardinal vein and dorsal limb of renal collar
    - Regression of ventral arch and failure forming subcardinal-hepatic anastomosis
- Epidemiology
  - Prevalence
    - Duplication of IVC: 0.2-3% of general population
    - Left IVC: 0.2-0.5%
    - Azygos continuation of the IVC: 0.6%
    - Circumaortic left renal vein: 8.7%
    - Retroaortic left renal vein: 2.1%

CLINICAL ISSUES

Presentation

- Most common signs/symptoms
  - Asymptomatic
  - Circumcaval ureter: Partial right ureteral obstruction or recurrent urinary tract infections
  - Absence of infrarenal or entire IVC: Venous insufficiency of lower extremities or idiopathic deep venous thrombosis
- Diagnosis
  - Usually incidentally diagnosed by imaging

Treatment

- Usually no treatment
- Circumcaval ureter: Surgical relocation of ureter anterior to IVC

DIAGNOSTIC CHECKLIST

Consider

- Duplication of IVC should be suspected in recurrent pulmonary embolism following IVC filter placement

Image Interpretation Pearls

- Pre-operative imaging may be important in planning abdominal surgery, liver or kidney transplantation
- Important to recognize IVC anomalies in certain interventional procedures (e.g., IVC filters, varicocele sclerotherapy, venous renal or adrenal sampling)

SELECTED REFERENCES

1. Basile A et al: Embryologic and acquired anomalies of the inferior vena cava with recurrent deep vein thrombosis. Abdom Imaging. 28(3):400-3, 2003
2. Yilmaz E et al: Interruption of the inferior vena cava with azygos/hemiazygos continuation accompanied by distinct renal vein anomalies: MRA and CT assessment. Abdom Imaging. 28(3):392-4, 2003
3. Brochert A et al: Unusual duplication anomaly of the inferior vena cava with normal drainage of the right IVC and hemiazygous continuation of the left IVC. J Vasc Interv Radiol. 12(12):1453-5, 2001
4. Bass JE et al: Spectrum of congenital anomalies of the inferior vena cava: cross-sectional imaging findings. Radiographics. 20(3):639-52, 2000
5. Mayo J et al: Anomalies of the inferior vena cava. AJR Am J Roentgenol. 140(2):339-45, 1983

IVC ANOMALIES

IMAGE GALLERY

Typical

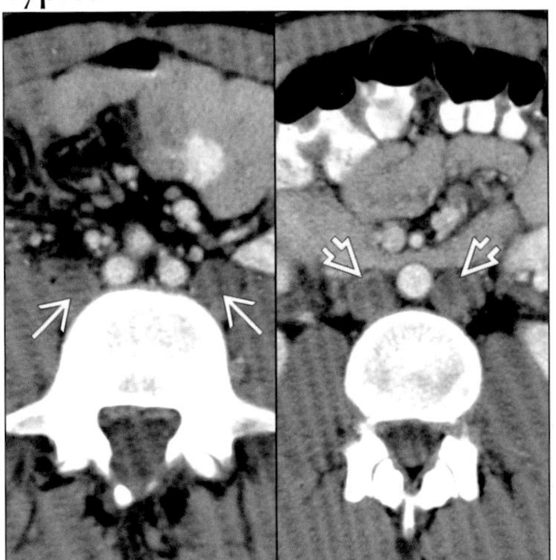

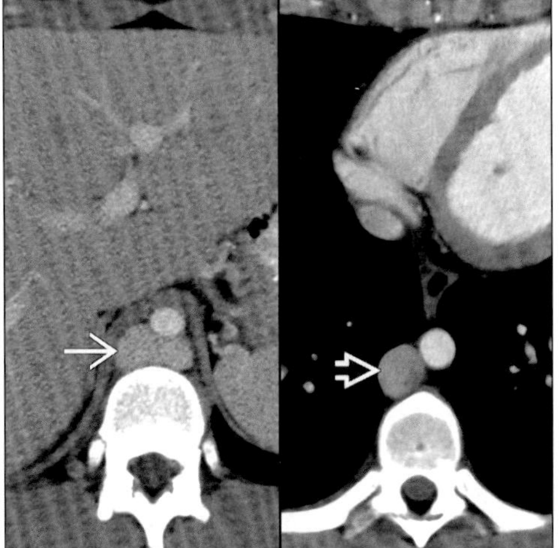

(Left) *Axial CECT shows the iliac veins (seen in left image) continuing cephalad as a duplicated IVC (seen in the right image). The venous structures are not yet opacified on this CECT, as these images were obtained in the arterial phase.* ***(Right)*** *Axial CECT in same patient as previous, obtained at a more cephalad level, shows that the duplicated IVC join together, course under the diaphragmatic crura & continue as the azygos vein. This is the "double IVC with azygos continuation".*

Typical

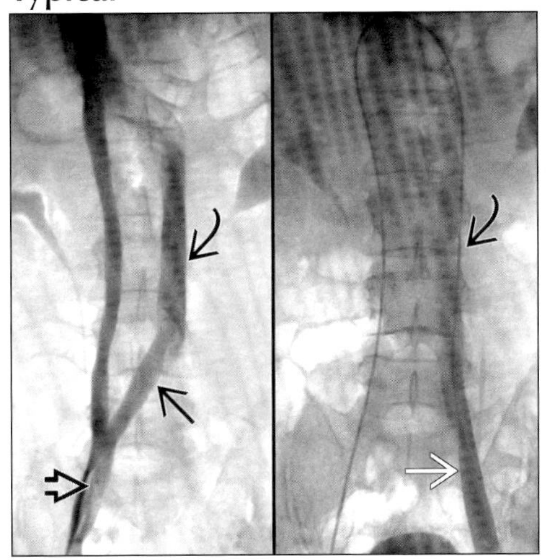

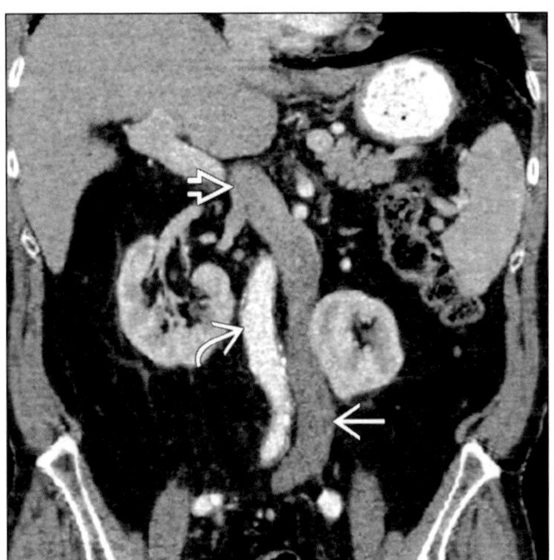

(Left) *Variant of duplicated IVC on venography. This variant, termed an "H-shaped IVC", results from a tributary from the right iliac vein joining the left IVC. The continuation of the left iliac vein into the left IVC is also shown in the left-sided image.* ***(Right)*** *Coronal CTA shows a left IVC that crosses the aorta anteriorly as the left renal vein and continues as the right suprarenal IVC. This is the usual venous drainage in this anatomic variant.*

Typical

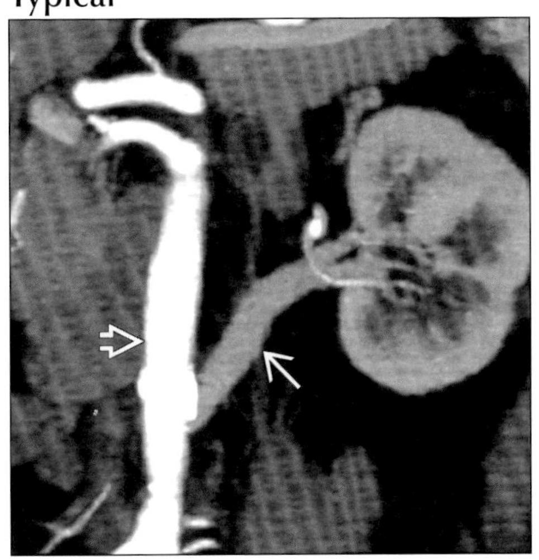

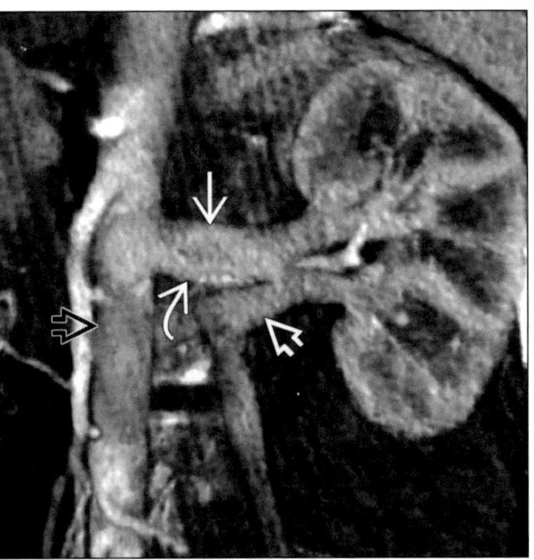

(Left) *CTA shows retroaortic left renal vein that courses inferiorly and crosses the aorta posteriorly to join the IVC. As with other IVC anomalies, this is usually asymptomatic and is incidentally discovered.* ***(Right)*** *CTA shows circum-aortic left renal vein. The superior left renal vein crosses the aorta anteriorly and joins the IVC. The inferior left renal vein crosses the aorta posteriorly. The left renal artery is seen coursing between the two left renal veins.*

IVC OCCLUSION

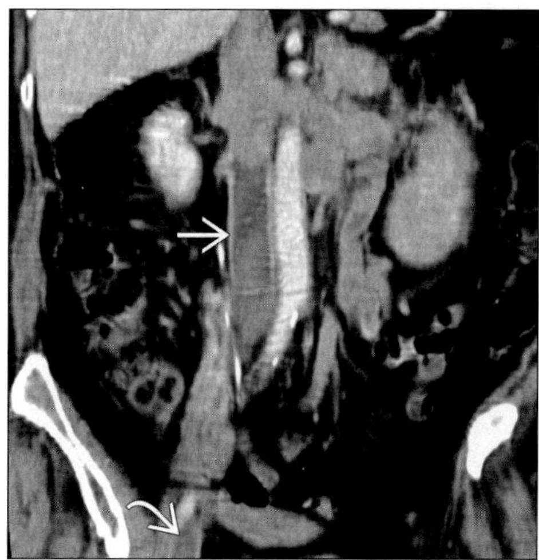

Coronal CTA shows acute thrombotic occlusion ➡ of the infrarenal IVC. Note the thrombus ➡ in the right external iliac vein. The thrombosed portion of the IVC is slightly distended, which is typical in acute thrombosis.

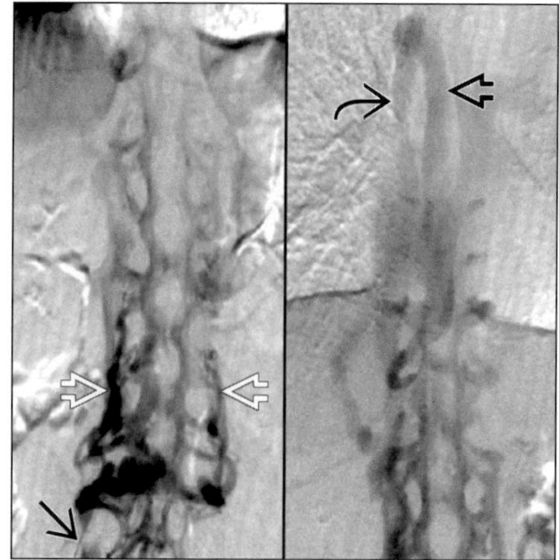

Conventional venogram through a catheter ➡ placed in the right iliac vein. The IVC is occluded and the venous drainage is through retroperitoneal collaterals ➡ which drain into the SVC ➡ via azygos vein ➡.

TERMINOLOGY

Abbreviations and Synonyms

- Inferior vena cava (IVC) occlusion
- IVC obstruction

Definitions

- Obstruction or occlusion of inferior vena cava from acute or chronic thrombosis or extrinsic compression

IMAGING FINDINGS

General Features

- Best diagnostic clue
  - Intraluminal filling defect (thrombus) within IVC in acute occlusion
  - Small IVC with multiple retroperitoneal collaterals in chronic occlusion
- Location
  - Infrarenal IVC more often involved in occlusive processes than suprarenal IVC
  - Thrombus generally propagates cephalad into IVC from iliac veins
    - In situ thrombus in IVC is secondary to foreign body (filter) or extrinsic compression (IVC clip or mass)
- Size
  - Diameter of IVC varies with respiration and blood volume
    - Mean diameter of normal infrarenal IVC is 20 mm (range 13-30 mm)
    - Mega cava refers to diameters > 30 mm
  - Most current filters approved for IVC diameter of 28-30 mm except for Bird's Nest Filter which is approved for IVC diameter up to 40 mm
- Ultrasonography
  - Acute thrombus
    - Presence of thrombus in the IVC
    - Distension of IVC
    - Echogenicity varies with age: Fresh thrombus is anechoic or hypoechoic; subacute to chronic thrombus is hyperechoic
    - Tongue-like projection at tip of thrombus suggests free floating clot
    - Absence of color flow if complete thrombus
    - Peripheral rim of flow if incomplete thrombus

DDx: IVC Occlusion

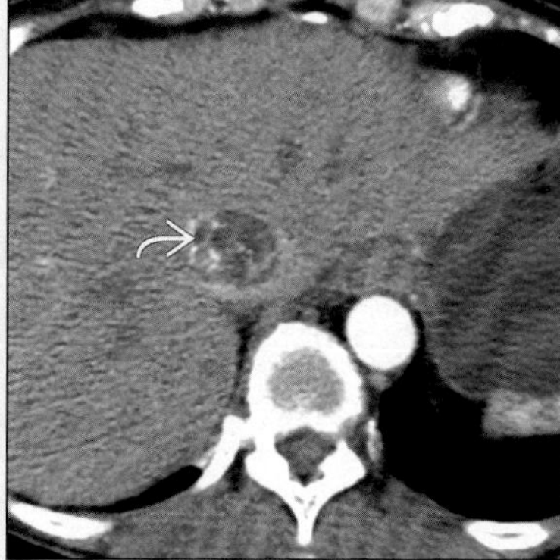

Primary Tumor (Sarcoma) of IVC

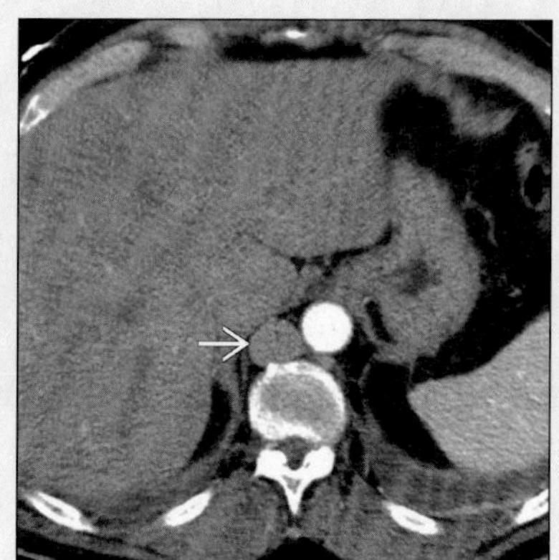

Azygos Continuation of IVC

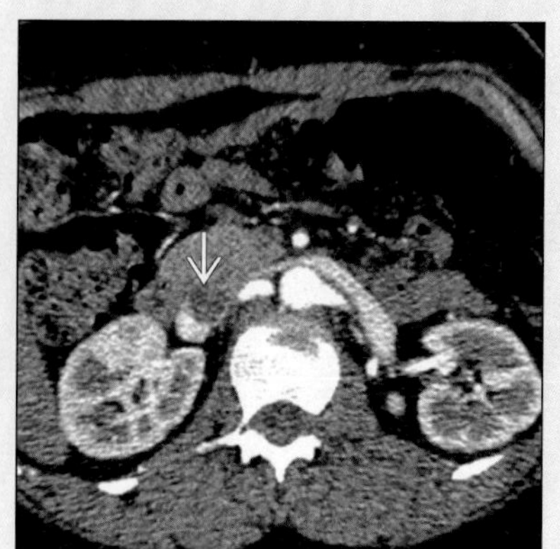

Inflow of Non-Opacified Blood

IVC OCCLUSION

Key Facts

Terminology

- Obstruction or occlusion of inferior vena cava from acute or chronic thrombosis or extrinsic compression

Imaging Findings

- Intraluminal filling defect (thrombus) within IVC in acute occlusion on US, CECT and angiography
  - Ultrasonic echogenicity of thrombus varies with age: Fresh thrombus is anechoic or hypoechoic; subacute to chronic thrombus is hyperechoic
- Small IVC with multiple retroperitoneal collaterals in chronic occlusion
  - Infrarenal IVC more often involved in occlusive processes than suprarenal IVC

Top Differential Diagnoses

- Primary Tumor of IVC
- Tumor Extension into IVC
- Inflow of Unopacified Blood
- Congenital Anomalies of IVC

Clinical Issues

- Treatment for thrombotic IVC occlusion includes
  - Anticoagulation therapy with heparin or Coumadin
  - IVC filter placement
  - Catheter directed thrombolysis and stenting

Diagnostic Checklist

- Acute thrombus on ultrasound can be anechoic and can be missed on grayscale ultrasound
- Delayed CT 90-120 sec after contrast administration useful to accurately diagnose, and assess the extent of thrombus in IVC

- Distal to occluding thrombus, Doppler may show absence of respiratory flow variations in IVC
  - Chronic occlusion
    - Difficult to evaluate with ultrasound
    - Absent or small caliber IVC
    - Multiple vessels in normal location of IVC may represent partially recanalized thrombus
    - Multiple retroperitoneal collaterals
- CT
  - Acute thrombus
    - Distended IVC with complete or partial thrombus
    - Fresh thrombus hyperdense on non-contrast CT
    - Thrombus surrounded by contrast material on CECT indicates partial IVC thrombosis
    - Associated extrinsic compression from mass may be seen
    - Enhancement of wall with distension of IVC suggest intrinsic obstruction with thrombus
    - Enhancement of thrombus suggests tumor thrombus
    - Thrombus in filter best assessed with CT
    - Best examination to assess extent of thrombus
  - Chronic occlusion
    - Small or absent IVC
    - Commonly affects infrarenal IVC
    - Multiple retroperitoneal collaterals
- MR
  - Findings similar to CT
  - Chronic occlusion better appreciated on contrast enhanced MRV
- Intravascular ultrasound
  - Useful to accurately assess extent of thrombus
- Angiography
  - Acute thrombus
    - Filling defect on venacavography
    - Extent, size and involvement of tributaries can be assessed
    - Inflow from renal veins should be differentiated from thrombus
    - Catheter injection should be performed at the site of suspected thrombus/stenosis
  - Chronic thrombus
    - Small caliber IVC with multiple retroperitoneal collaterals
    - Stenosis of IVC

Imaging Recommendations

- Best imaging tool: Contrast-enhanced CT
- Protocol advice: Delayed CT imaging at 90-120 sec after contrast administration useful to accurately diagnose extent of thrombosis

DIFFERENTIAL DIAGNOSIS

Primary Tumor of IVC

- Sarcoma or leiomyomatosis
- Enhancement of the thrombus

Tumor Extension into IVC

- From renal cell carcinoma, hepatocellular carcinoma, uterine sarcoma or retroperitoneal sarcomas
- Continuity of mass with primary tumor
- Enhancement of the thrombus

Inflow of Unopacified Blood

- Inflow from renal veins may mimic thrombus on CT or angiography
- Angiography: Filling defect from renal vein inflow changes with each image frame and is not consistent
- CECT: Central filling defect in IVC due to rapid inflow of contrast-enhanced blood from renal veins and unopacified blood from lower extremities
  - Delayed imaging helpful for differentiation

Congenital Anomalies of IVC

- Congenital absence of IVC with azygos continuation
- Left IVC

PATHOLOGY

General Features

- Etiology
  - Intrinsic
    - Thrombus extending from lower extremities

- Hypercoagulable states
- Primary tumor of IVC: Leiomyomatosis, sarcoma
- Secondary tumor extension from renal cell carcinoma, hepatoma, retroperitoneal sarcoma, adrenal carcinoma
- Congenital membrane of IVC
  - Extrinsic
    - Enlarged lymph nodes from neoplasm or infection
    - Retroperitoneal mass (e.g., neoplasm, hematoma)
    - Aortic aneurysm
    - Retroperitoneal fibrosis
    - Pregnancy
    - Hepatomegaly
    - Surgical ligation or plication of IVC
- Associated abnormalities
  - May Thurner syndrome
  - Congenital anomalies of the IVC

CLINICAL ISSUES

Presentation

- Most common signs/symptoms
  - Acute occlusion
    - Pain and swelling of both lower extremities
    - Hypotension
  - Subacute or chronic occlusion
    - Asymptomatic if sufficient venous collaterals
    - Multiple collaterals may be present in anterior abdominal wall
    - Swelling of lower extremities
    - Venous stasis dermatitis or ulcers in legs

Treatment

- Anticoagulation therapy with heparin or Coumadin
- IVC filter placement
  - Filter placed in infrarenal IVC above thrombus
    - Suprarenal IVC filter if thrombosis extends to renal vein level or involves renal or gonadal veins
  - Acute thrombosis of IVC may result from filter catching a massive embolus
- Catheter directed thrombolysis with t-PA
  - May be supplemented with intravascular stent placement following successful thrombolysis
  - Ascending lumbar veins have been stented in cases of chronic total IVC occlusion
- Mechanical thrombectomy
- Surgery
  - IVC ligation
  - IVC plication or IVC clip placement
- Treatment of extrinsic compression as cause of IVC obstruction or occlusion
  - Surgical resection of tumor or mass
  - Radiotherapy or chemotherapy of adenopathy or tumor
  - Stent placement in IVC

DIAGNOSTIC CHECKLIST

Consider

- Catheter directed thrombolysis with t-PA, followed by intravascular stents in severely symptomatic patient

Image Interpretation Pearls

- Acute thrombus on ultrasound can be anechoic and can be missed on grayscale ultrasound
- Delayed CT useful to assess and correctly diagnose thrombus in IVC and its extent
- Abdominal wall collaterals can be due to SVC or IVC obstruction or portal venous hypertension

SELECTED REFERENCES

1. Delis KT et al: Successful iliac vein and inferior vena cava stenting ameliorates venous claudication and improves venous outflow, calf muscle pump function, and clinical status in post-thrombotic syndrome. Ann Surg. 245(1):130-9, 2007
2. Koc Z et al: Interruption or congenital stenosis of the inferior vena cava: prevalence, imaging, and clinical findings. Eur J Radiol. 62(2):257-66, 2007
3. Protack CD et al: Long-term outcomes of catheter directed thrombolysis for lower extremity deep venous thrombosis without prophylactic inferior vena cava filter placement. J Vasc Surg. 45(5):992-7; discussion 997, 2007
4. Ushijima T et al: Successful surgical treatment of chronic inferior vena caval thrombosis following blunt trauma. Gen Thorac Cardiovasc Surg. 55(6):255-8, 2007
5. Healey CT et al: Endovascular stenting of ascending lumbar veins for refractory inferior vena cava occlusion. J Vasc Surg. 44(4):879-81, 2006
6. Healey CT et al: Endovascular stenting of ascending lumbar veins for refractory inferior vena cava occlusion. J Vasc Surg. 44(4):879-81, 2006
7. Raju S et al: Obstructive lesions of the inferior vena cava: clinical features and endovenous treatment. J Vasc Surg. 44(4):820-7, 2006
8. te Riele WW et al: Endovascular recanalization of chronic long-segment occlusions of the inferior vena cava: midterm results. J Endovasc Ther. 13(2):249-53, 2006
9. te Riele WW et al: Endovascular recanalization of chronic long-segment occlusions of the inferior vena cava: midterm results. J Endovasc Ther. 13(2):249-53, 2006
10. Yamada N et al: Pulse-spray pharmacomechanical thrombolysis for proximal deep vein thrombosis. Eur J Vasc Endovasc Surg. 31(2):204-11, 2006
11. Hilliard NJ et al: Leiomyosarcoma of the inferior vena cava: three case reports and review of the literature. Ann Diagn Pathol. 9(5):259-66, 2005
12. Robbins MR et al: Endovascular stenting to treat chronic long-segment inferior vena cava occlusion. J Vasc Surg. 41(1):136-40, 2005
13. Jost CJ et al: Surgical reconstruction of iliofemoral veins and the inferior vena cava for nonmalignant occlusive disease. J Vasc Surg. 33(2):320-7; discussion 327-8, 2001
14. Okuda K: Membranous obstruction of the inferior vena cava (obliterative hepatocavopathy, Okuda). J Gastroenterol Hepatol. 16(11):1179-83, 2001
15. Patel T et al: Successful stenting of a complex inferior vena cava stenosis using a modified sharp recanulization technique. Catheter Cardiovasc Interv. 52(4):492-5, 2001
16. Kazmers A et al: Duplex examination of the inferior vena cava. Am Surg. 66(10):986-9, 2000
17. Razavi MK et al: Chronically occluded inferior venae cavae: endovascular treatment. Radiology. 214(1):133-8, 2000
18. Victor S et al: Dorsal cavoatrial bypass graft for coarctation of inferior vena cava-trial of aortic occlusion technique. Trop Gastroenterol. 12(3):148-52, 1991
19. Hadar H et al: CT findings in chronic post-thrombotic obstruction of the inferior vena cava. J Comput Tomogr. 6(1):11-6, 1982

IVC OCCLUSION

IMAGE GALLERY

Typical

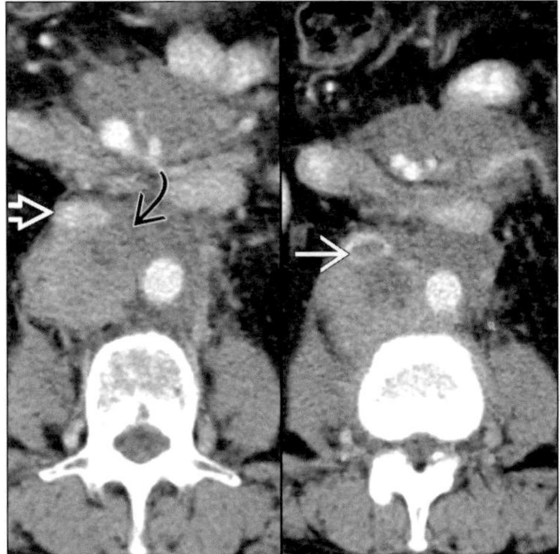

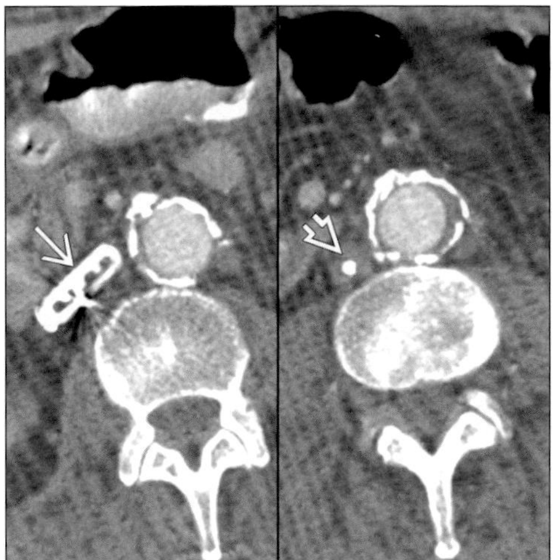

(Left) *Axial CECT shows a retroperitoneal mass → extrinsically compressing the IVC → (left image), resulting in thrombus → within the IVC more inferiorly (right image). The thrombus is surrounded by contrast medium, indicating partial IVC thrombosis.* ***(Right)*** *Axial CECT shows a Dewees IVC plication clip → (left image), which resulted in chronic occlusion of the IVC. Note calcium within the IVC → which occurred as a result of the chronic thrombotic occlusion (right image).*

Typical

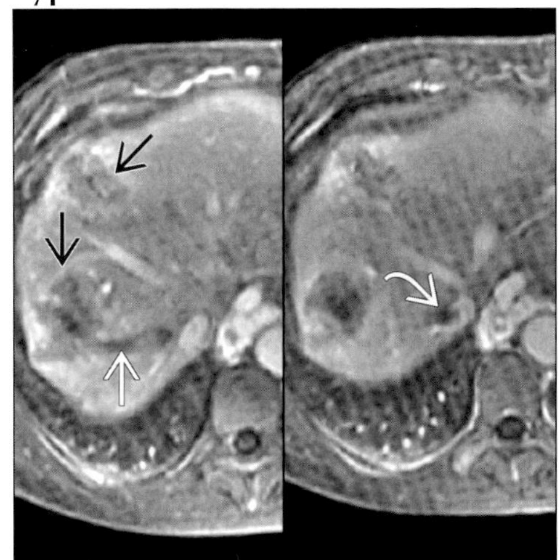

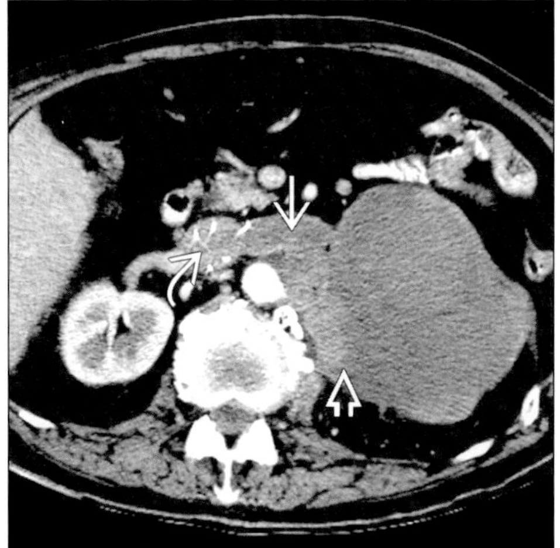

(Left) *Axial gadolinium enhanced MR shows multiple intrahepatic tumors →, with tumor thrombus extending through the hepatic veins → (left image) into the IVC → (right image).* ***(Right)*** *Axial CECT shows renal cell carcinoma → extending into the IVC → through the left renal vein →. The tumor thrombus shows slight enhancement on the contrast study. Also note that there is a filter within the IVC →.*

Typical

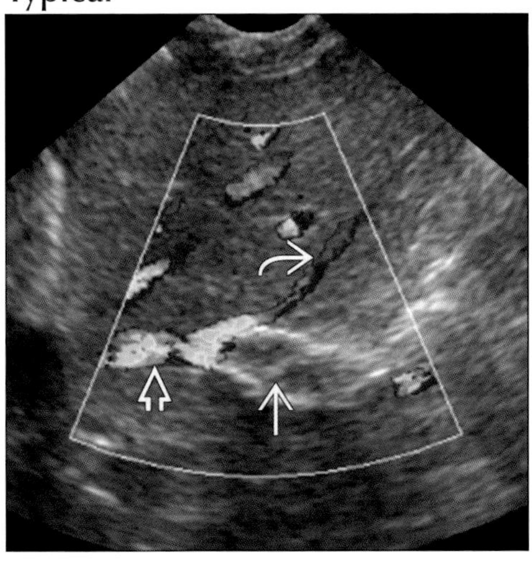

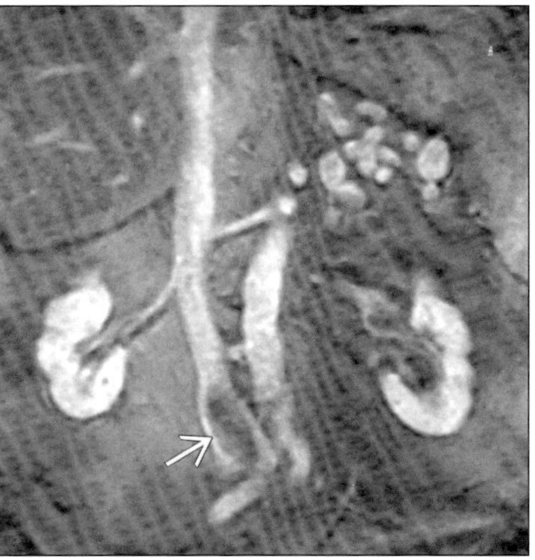

(Left) *Sagittal color Doppler ultrasound shows thrombus → within the IVC. Thrombus echogenicity varies with age, appearing anechoic or hypoechoic when acute, and hyperechoic when chronic. Note patent upper IVC → and inflow → from the hepatic vein.* ***(Right)*** *Coronal MRA shows thrombus → in the infrarenal segment of the IVC. Above the thrombus the IVC is patent. The infrarenal segment of the IVC is more frequently involved in occlusive processes than the suprarenal segment.*

VARICOCELE

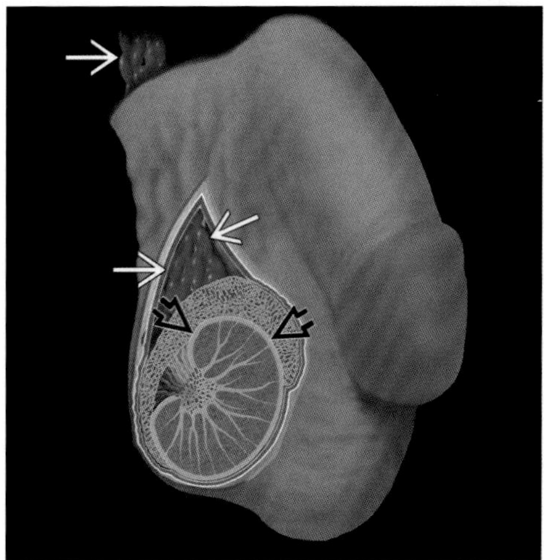

Oblique graphic shows serpiginous dilated veins ➔ coursing posterior to the superior pole of the testis ⇨. Varicoceles result from flow reversal in the testicular vein, with dilatation of the pampiniform plexus.

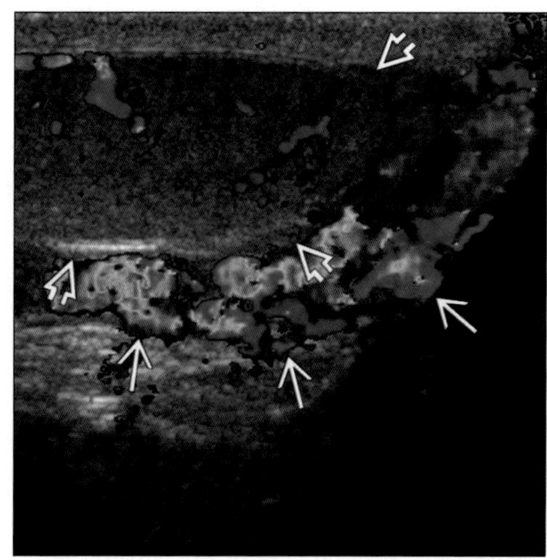

Sagittal color Doppler ultrasound shows dilated veins ➔ posterior to the testis ⇨, typical of a varicocele. The images were obtained during a Valsalva maneuver, resulting in venous distension from flow reversal.

TERMINOLOGY

Abbreviations and Synonyms

- Testicular vein, gonadal vein, internal spermatic vein all same entity

Definitions

- Varicocele is the abnormal dilatation of veins of the pampiniform plexus as a result of retrograde flow in testicular vein

IMAGING FINDINGS

General Features

- Best diagnostic clue
  - Dilated serpiginous veins posterior to superior pole of testis on color Doppler US
  - Distension during Valsalva maneuver as a result of retrograde flow
- Location
  - Testicular venous drainage has multiple routes
    - Pampiniform plexus (spermatic venous plexus), formed by multiple venous sinuses coalesces to form internal spermatic vein
    - Internal spermatic vein (major drainage route) drains into renal vein on left and directly into infrarenal IVC on right
    - Three additional drainage routes: External pudendal vein, ductus deferens (vasal) vein, and cremasteric (external spermatic) vein
    - Collateral vessels around internal spermatic vein may anastomose to systemic circulation at multiple sites and may aberrantly perfuse varicoceles
    - Collaterals may cause recurrences in patients treated with embolization or surgical ligation
- Size: Veins in pampiniform plexus normally ≤ 2 mm; diagnosis of varicocele if multiple veins > 2-3 mm in diameter and size increases with Valsalva maneuver
- Morphology: Tortuous vascular channels representing dilated veins

Ultrasonographic Findings

- Grayscale Ultrasound

DDx: Scrotal/Testicular Mass

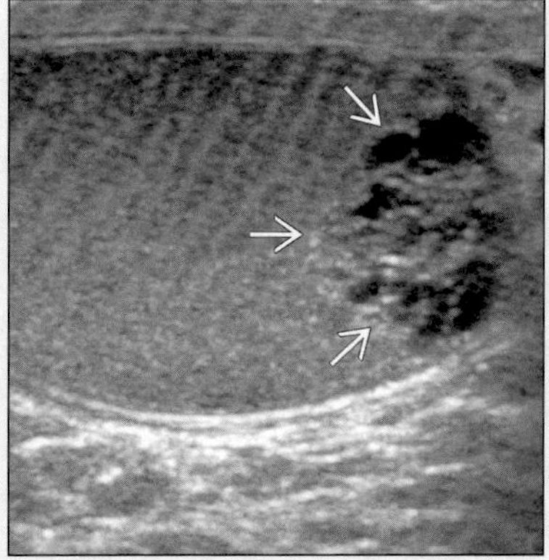

Rete Testis

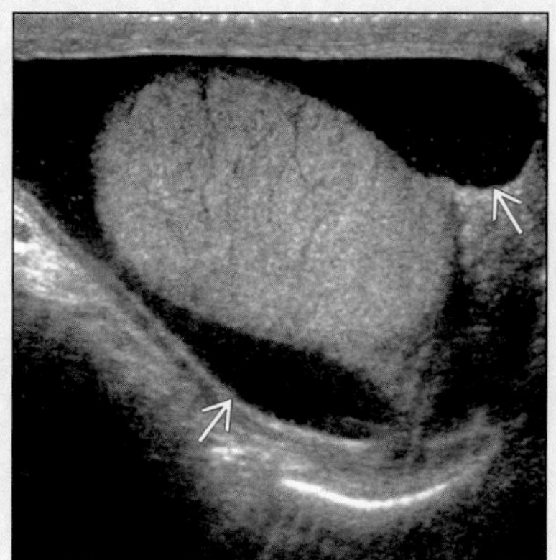

Hydrocele

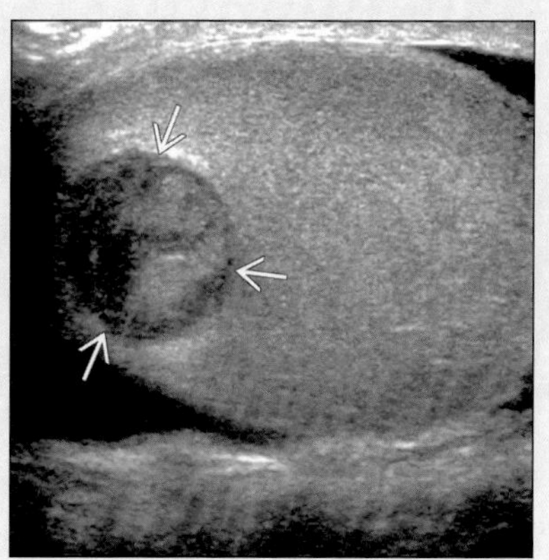

Testicular Neoplasm

VARICOCELE

Key Facts

Terminology

- Varicocele is the abnormal dilatation of veins of the pampiniform plexus as a result of retrograde flow in testicular vein

Imaging Findings

- Distension during Valsalva maneuver as a result of retrograde flow
- Protocol advice: Resting and Valsalva color Doppler images of pampiniform plexus using dedicated, small parts transducer (5-10 MHz) to demonstrate a dilated plexus and venous reflux into the varicosities
- Catheter venography with contrast injection into left renal vein and into the testicular vein demonstrates retrograde flow into dilated venous channels

Pathology

- Most frequent cause of male infertility
- Majority (90%) of varicoceles are left-sided; bilateral in 10-15% of patients

Clinical Issues

- Vague scrotal discomfort, pressure or pain, particularly when standing
- Surgical correction was mainstay of treatment prior to transcatheter embolization, with ligation of the internal spermatic vein at one of three levels
- Transcatheter embolization of testicular vein if symptomatic or causing low sperm count

Diagnostic Checklist

- Valsalva maneuver during color Doppler imaging essential for diagnosis of small varicoceles

---

  - Tubular serpiginous vessels posterior to testis on grayscale ultrasound
  - Dilated pampiniform plexus with veins larger than 2-3 mm in diameter
- Color Doppler: Prominent color flow within vessels during Valsalva maneuver as a result of retrograde flow

Angiographic Findings

- Catheter venography with contrast injection into left renal vein and into the testicular vein demonstrates retrograde flow into dilated venous channels
- Considered "gold standard" for demonstrating reflux in the testicular vein
- Catheter tip position and variable injection rates may or may not represent physiologic conditions in testicular vein or left renal vein

Imaging Recommendations

- Best imaging tool
  - US with color Doppler
    - Can detect 93% of venographically evident, subclinical varicoceles when compared to physical examination
- Protocol advice: Resting and Valsalva color Doppler images of pampiniform plexus with 5-10 MHz small parts transducer showing dilated plexus and venous reflux

DIFFERENTIAL DIAGNOSIS

Tubular Ectasia/Rete Testis

- Normal variant of dilated seminiferous tubules in mediastinum of testis
- No flow on color Doppler
- May be associated with spermatocele

Tumor

- Focal intra-testicular mass on grayscale images
- Abnormal pattern of vasculature on color Doppler

Epididymitis/Orchitis

- Enlarged hypoechoic epididymis with increased flow on color Doppler
- Associated clinical signs and symptoms of infection
- Most often due to retrograde extension of organisms from vas deferens and rarely result of hematogenous spread

Hydrocele

- Anechoic, nonvascular scrotal fluid collection
- Communicating hydrocele: Patent processus vaginalis permits peritoneal fluid to flow into scrotum
- Noncommunicating hydrocele: Patent processus vaginalis present, but no communication with peritoneal cavity
- Cord hydrocele: Defective closure of tunica vaginalis, with distal end of processus vaginalis closing correctly, but patent mid portion
- Adult onset hydroceles are usually secondary and may result from trauma, orchitis, epididymitis; may also be associated with tumor or torsion
- Usually painless and asymptomatic unless large

Testicular Torsion

- Absent or decreased flow to testis on color Doppler
- Hypoechoic testis in late stage
- Testicular infarction if unrecognized and not treated

PATHOLOGY

General Features

- Etiology
  - Primary: Incompetent venous valves in testicular vein
  - Secondary: Extrinsic venous compression or obstruction of veins draining pampiniform plexus, with resultant elevation of venous pressures
- Epidemiology
  - Most frequent cause of male infertility
  - Incidence of varicocele in healthy males is 8-23%
  - Majority (90%) of varicoceles are left-sided; bilateral in 10-15% of patients
  - Subclinical varicocele in 40-75% of infertile men
- Associated abnormalities
  - Low sperm count

- Varicocele causes elevated scrotal and testicular temperature, with adverse effect on spermatogenesis
- Reflux of adrenal and renal toxic metabolites may also be a cause of testicular dysfunction

Gross Pathologic & Surgical Features

- Dilated veins within pampiniform plexus

Staging, Grading or Classification Criteria

- Pathophysiology of varicoceles either primary or secondary
  - Primary
    - Idiopathic (incompetent valves): 98% from this cause occur on left
    - Most common cause of correctable male infertility
  - Secondary
    - Compression of veins draining pampiniform plexus from pelvic or abdominal pathology such as tumor or adenopathy
    - Obstruction or compression of left renal vein by extrinsic process such as "nutcracker phenomenon" or retroaortic left renal vein
- Varicoceles diagnosed by palpation and then graded
  - Subclinical varicoceles cannot be palpated, but patient is infertile with abnormal semen analysis: Diagnosed by duplex and color Doppler ultrasound
  - Grade 1 (small) palpable with Valsalva maneuver
  - Grade 2 (moderate) palpable without Valsalva
  - Grade 3 (large) visible without palpation

CLINICAL ISSUES

Presentation

- Most common signs/symptoms
  - Vague scrotal discomfort, pressure or pain, particularly when standing
  - Infertility
- Other signs/symptoms: Testicular atrophy, scrotal enlargement

Demographics

- Age: > 15 yrs
- Gender: Exclusively male

Treatment

- No effective medical treatment for this entity
- Surgical correction was mainstay of treatment prior to transcatheter embolization, with ligation of the internal spermatic vein at one of three levels
  - High retroperitoneal (Palomo or modified Palomo procedure)
  - Low retroperitoneal (Ivanissevich procedure)
  - Subinguinal (Marmar procedure)
    - With these procedures, surgical recurrence rate of 10-20% following ligation, usually resulting from collateral flow around ligature, a missed collateral or additional internal spermatic vein or a loose ligature
- Transcatheter embolization of testicular vein if symptomatic or causing low sperm count
  - Outpatient procedure with conscious sedation
  - Selective left renal venogram to assess for reflux into testicular vein, followed by selective left and right gonadal venography
    - Catheter advanced to level of inguinal canal and multiple embolization coils placed along course of internal spermatic vein
    - Attempt to block all collaterals that could result in recurrence
    - Multiple embolic agents used for treatment; with sclerosants avoid reflux into scrotum as may lead to swelling, phlebitis and testicular damage
  - Technical success rate of transcatheter embolization exceeds 90%, with a 10% recurrence rate
    - Sperm counts improve in 70-80% of patients
    - Minor complications of nontarget embolization, contrast reactions, pain, phlebitis, and puncture site related problems
- Variable successful pregnancy rates (0-70%) after varicocele surgery or embolization; mixed results for improved fertility, perhaps less effective than thought

DIAGNOSTIC CHECKLIST

Consider

- Imaging to exclude retroperitoneal pathology for an isolated right varicocele or sudden onset of varicocele
- Tumor invasion of left renal vein in elderly male
- Nutcracker syndrome
- Retroaortic left renal vein

Image Interpretation Pearls

- Valsalva maneuver during color Doppler imaging essential for diagnosis of small varicoceles

SELECTED REFERENCES

1. Al-Buheissi SZ et al: Predictors of success in surgical ligation of painful varicocele. Urol Int. 79(1):33-6, 2007
2. Beutner S et al: Treatment of varicocele with reference to age: a retrospective comparison of three minimally invasive procedures. Surg Endosc. 21(1):61-5, 2007
3. Shindel AW et al: Does the number and size of veins ligated at left-sided microsurgical subinguinal varicocelectomy affect semen analysis outcomes? Urology. 69(6):1176-80, 2007
4. Chen C: Varicocele in male factor infertility: role of laparoscopic varicocelectomy. Int Surg. 91(5 Suppl):S90-4, 2006
5. Gazzera C et al: Radiological treatment of male varicocele: technical, clinical, seminal and dosimetric aspects. Radiol Med (Torino). 111(3):449-58, 2006
6. Beddy P et al: Testicular varicoceles. Clin Radiol. 60(12):1248-55, 2005
7. Evers JL et al: Assessment of efficacy of varicocele repair for male subfertility: a systematic review. Lancet. 361(9372):1849-52, 2003
8. Naughton CK et al: Pathophysiology of varicoceles in male infertility. Hum Repro Update. 7(5): 473-81, 2001
9. Munden MM et al: Scrotal pathology in pediatrics with sonographic imaging. Curr Probl Diagn Radiol. 29(6): 185-205, 2000

IMAGE GALLERY

Typical

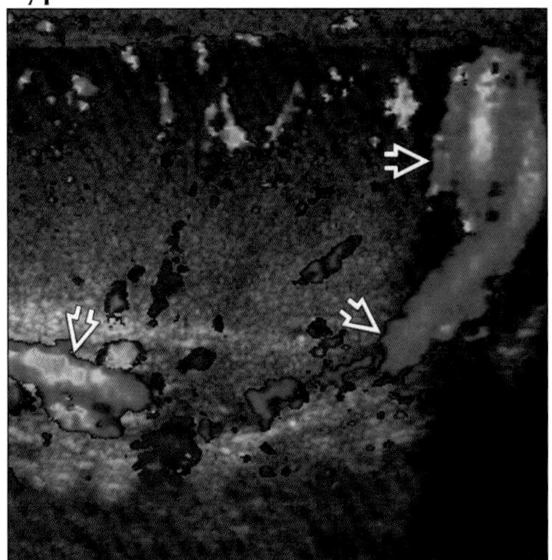

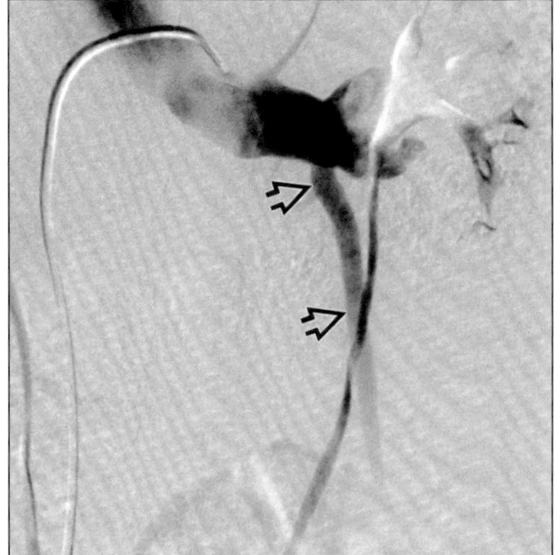

(Left) *Color Doppler ultrasound shows a large left-sided varicocele ➡. This 27 year old male had chronic left testicular pain that was exacerbated when standing. His symptoms had progressively worsened, prompting him to seek medical attention.* **(Right)** *Selective left renal venogram shows reflux into a dilated left testicular vein ➡, indicating that there is venous valvular incompetence.*

Typical

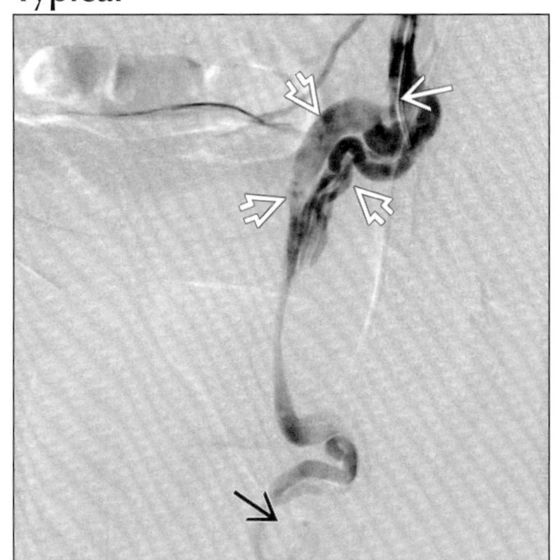

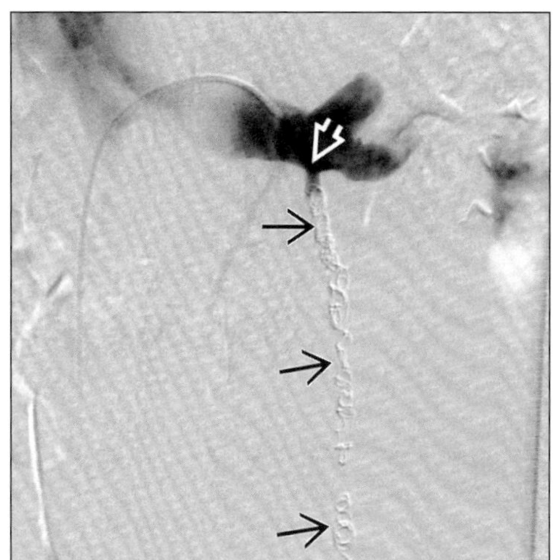

(Left) *Left testicular venogram shows an angiography catheter ➡ within the distal portion of the vein at the level of the inguinal canal. Multiple dilated veins ➡ extend into the scrotum adjacent to the location of the testis ➡.* **(Right)** *Selective left renal venogram following left testicular vein transcatheter embolization shows multiple embolization coils ➡ within the vein. Only the origin of the vein fills with contrast ➡ because there is no longer any reflux.*

Typical

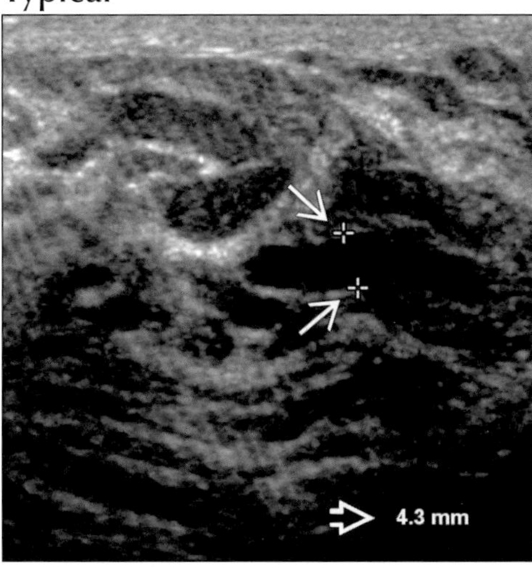

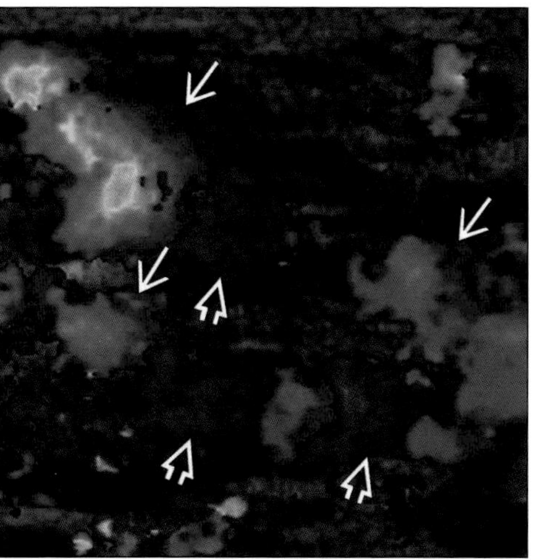

(Left) *Sagittal grayscale US of pampiniform plexus of patient with chronic testicular pain shows characteristic dilated veins of varicocele. Cursor measurement ➡ shows venous diameter of 4.3 mm ➡, exceeding normal value of veins in this plexus.* **(Right)** *Color Doppler US of pampiniform plexus (same patient as previous) obtained during Valsalva maneuver, shows mixed antegrade ➡ & retrograde ➡ flow within venous plexus characteristic of varicocele.*

PELVIC CONGESTION SYNDROME

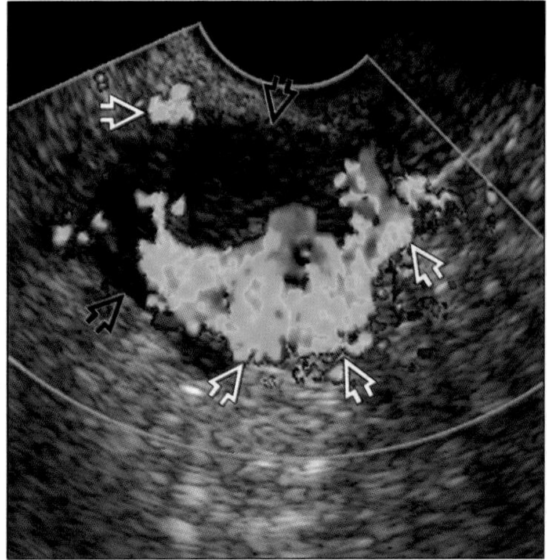

Color Doppler ultrasound shows dilated veins ➡ surrounding the ovary ➡ of a patient with a history of pelvic pain and dyspareunia. Further evaluation with venography confirmed pelvic and ovarian vein varices.

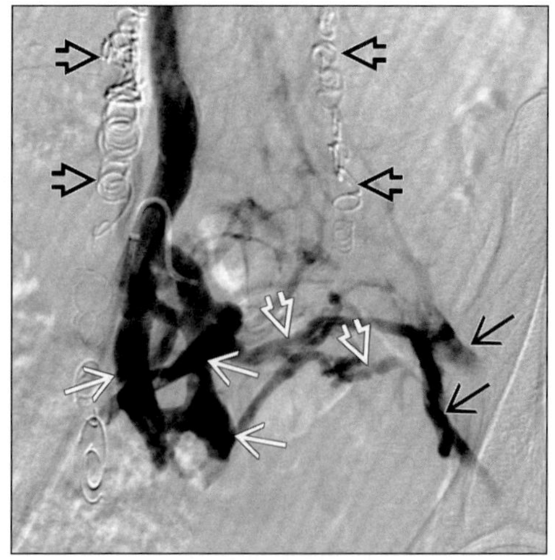

Right internal iliac venogram prior to sclerotherapy shows dilated pelvic veins ➡ and contralateral venous filling ➡ via transpelvic venous collaterals ➡. There has been prior bilateral ovarian vein embolization ➡.

TERMINOLOGY

Abbreviations and Synonyms

- Pelvic congestion syndrome (PCS)
- Pelvic venous incompetence (PVI)

Definitions

- Chronic syndrome characterized by dull pelvic pain, pressure, and heaviness
  - Results from retrograde flow through incompetent valves in ovarian veins, producing dilated, tortuous, and congested pelvic and periuterine veins

IMAGING FINDINGS

General Features

- Location
  - Normal pelvic venous drainage via common iliac, external iliac, internal iliac and ovarian veins
  - Internal iliac veins have visceral and parietal branches
    - Visceral branches: Vesical, vaginal and uterine plexi, rectal, labial and clitoral branches
    - Parietal branches: Iliolumbar, superior and inferior gluteal, and obturator veins, sacral venous plexus
  - Left ovarian vein drains into left renal vein and right ovarian vein drains into IVC below right renal vein
    - Left side may communicate with inferior mesenteric vein (implications for embolotherapy)
    - Often multiple ovarian venous trunks bilaterally
- Size
  - Traditional view that ovarian venous incompetence requires ovarian vein diameter > 10 mm
    - However, diameter does not seem to correlate with pelvic venous incompetence
    - Frequent communication between ovarian and internal iliac varices and thus ovarian vein trunks may not be dilated

MR Findings

- T1WI
  - Pelvic varices have no signal intensity on T1WI because of flow-void artifact
  - 3-D T1 gradient-echo sequences following IV gadolinium most effective sequence for pelvic varices

DDx: Chronic Pelvic Pain

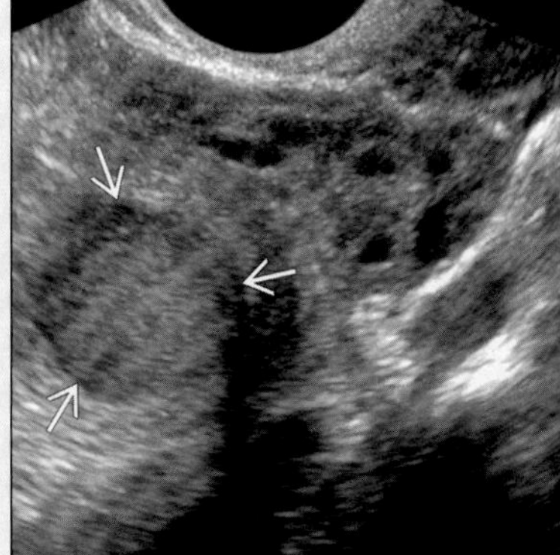

Ovarian Endometrioma

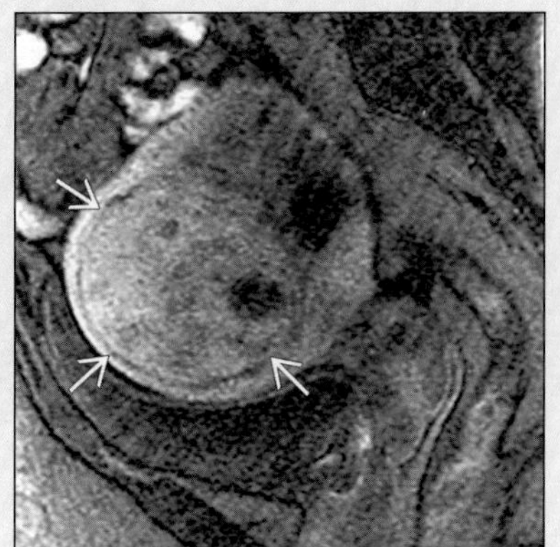

Uterine Fibroids

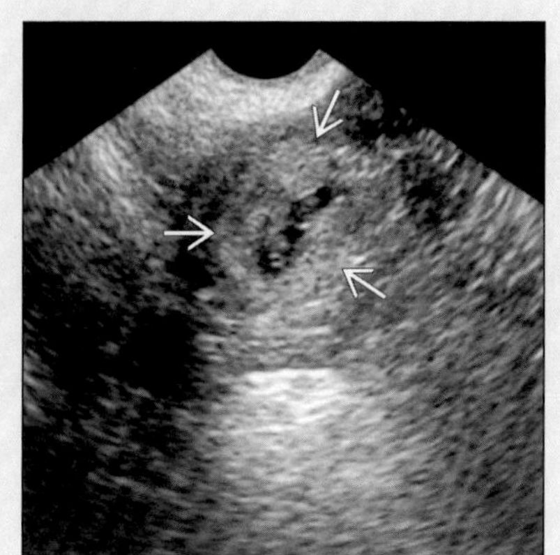

Ectopic Pregnancy

PELVIC CONGESTION SYNDROME

Key Facts

Terminology

- Chronic syndrome characterized by dull pelvic pain, pressure, and heaviness
  - Results from retrograde flow through incompetent valves in ovarian veins producing dilated, tortuous, and congested pelvic and periuterine veins

Imaging Findings

- Venous phase CECT, MRV or ultrasonography all used as screening imaging modalities
- If high clinical suspicion of ovarian and pelvic varices and equivocal imaging studies, consider venography
  - Direct visualization of tortuous dilated ovarian and pelvic veins by venography is definitive imaging modality for diagnosis

Pathology

- Primary problem is reflux in dilated, incompetent ovarian veins, with resultant chronic dilatation of pelvic veins producing pelvic pressure and heaviness
- Epidemiology: Prevalence related to ovarian varices occurring in 10% of female population; 60% of these may develop pelvic congestion syndrome

Clinical Issues

- Treatment includes
  - Laparoscopic transperitoneal ovarian vein ligation
  - Hysterectomy and oophorectomy
  - Transcatheter ovarian vein embolization
- Reported rates of symptomatic relief are approximately 75%, with about 60% of patients experiencing complete resolution of symptoms

  - High signal intensity blood flow in pelvic varices on GRE images
- T2WI: Pelvic varices usually have low signal intensity, but may also have hyperintensity or mixed signal because of relatively slow flow

Ultrasonographic Findings

- Grayscale Ultrasound: Initial modality used for evaluating patients with pelvic pain
- Color Doppler
  - Pelvic varices can be identified by using transvaginal US with color Doppler and Doppler spectral analysis
    - Multiple dilated tubular structures around uterus and ovary with venous Doppler signal
    - Tortuous pelvic veins with diameter greater than 4 mm with slow blood flow (about 3 cm/sec)
    - Transpelvic collateral venous communication between bilateral pelvic varicose veins

Angiographic Findings

- Direct visualization of tortuous dilated ovarian and pelvic veins by venography is definitive imaging modality for diagnosis
- Selective catheterization of contrast injection into ovarian veins demonstrating
  - Reflux of contrast from left renal vein into ovarian vein, often with venous dilatation
  - Uterine venous engorgement
  - Congestion of ovarian venous plexus
  - Filling of ipsilateral and contralateral pelvic veins
  - Vulvovaginal or thigh varicosities

Imaging Recommendations

- Best imaging tool
  - Ovarian and pelvic varices often poorly demonstrated by imaging modalities in which patient is supine
    - Reduced hydrostatic pressure in supine position results in venous decompression
  - Venous phase CECT, MRV or ultrasonography all used as screening imaging modalities
  - If high clinical suspicion of ovarian and pelvic varices and equivocal imaging studies, consider venography

DIFFERENTIAL DIAGNOSIS

Pelvic Mass

- Uterine: Leiomyoma, adenocarcinoma, leiomyosarcoma
- Adnexal: Ectopic pregnancy, ovarian neoplasm, tubo-ovarian abscess
- Bladder: Neoplasm, neurogenic bladder
- Bowel: Inflammatory disease, neoplasm

Endometriosis

- Occurs during reproductive years; present in 7-10% of general female population
- Endometrial tissue implanted on surface of organs outside of uterine musculature that responds to hormonal stimuli
- Most frequent sites: Ovary, uterine ligament, pouch of Douglas, pelvic peritoneum and fallopian tubes
- Symptoms in 50-80% of patients include infertility, dysmenorrhea, dyspareunia and abnormal menses
- Transvaginal US for initial evaluation: Helpful in assessment of endometriotic cysts but limited for peritoneal implants
- MR imaging more effective for identifying endometrial implants
  - Classic features are cystic mass with high signal intensity on T1WI and loss of signal intensity on T2WI, due to high protein and iron concentration from recurrent hemorrhage in endometrioma

Adenomyosis

- Migration of glands from basal layer of endometrium into myometrium, with these glands surrounded by smooth muscle hyperplasia
- High-resolution transvaginal US and MR imaging can help accurately establish diagnosis, since appearance closely correlates with histopathologic characteristics

PELVIC CONGESTION SYNDROME

PATHOLOGY

General Features

- General path comments
  - Primary problem is reflux in dilated, incompetent ovarian veins, with resultant chronic dilatation of pelvic veins producing pelvic pressure and heaviness
  - Higher left-sided incidence of pelvic congestion syndrome due to 15% absence of ovarian venous valves on left, compared to 6% on right
- Etiology
  - Pathogenesis most likely multifactorial
    - May result from obstructing anatomic anomalies such as retroaortic left renal vein, nutcracker syndrome or common iliac vein compression
    - Secondary congestion seen in various disorders, including portal hypertension, valvular incompetence or acquired IVC syndrome
    - Risk factors may include heredity, hormonal influence, pelvic surgery, retroverted uterus, history of varicose veins and multiple pregnancies
    - Ovarian dysfunction proponents claim induced or natural low estrogen states lead to smaller varicose vein diameters, suggesting estrogen is a venous dilator that exacerbates venous congestion
    - High incidence of anxiety and depression
- Epidemiology: Prevalence related to ovarian varices occurring in 10% of female population; 60% of these may develop pelvic congestion syndrome
- Associated abnormalities: Cystic ovaries in over 50%

CLINICAL ISSUES

Presentation

- Most common signs/symptoms
  - Deep prolonged dull ache often associated with movement, posture, and activities that increase abdominal pressure
  - Chronic unilateral, bilateral or asymmetric pain with no obvious source
  - Associated with dyspareunia (71%), dysmenorrhea (66%), and postcoital ache (65%)
  - Suggestive physical findings include varicose veins (vulva, buttocks, and legs) and ovarian point tenderness upon palpation
- Other signs/symptoms: Rectal discomfort and increased urinary frequency
- Clinical Profile
  - Reproductive-aged female with pelvic pain described as "heaviness or fullness"
    - Worsens when upright and improves when supine; may worsen with intercourse or menses

Natural History & Prognosis

- One hallmark of pelvic congestion syndrome is its disappearance after menopause
  - Syndrome may occur as a result of gonadal dysfunction, combined with factors of venous dilatation and congestion

Treatment

- Medical treatment of underlying disorder, such as hormonal imbalance, may be possible with medroxyprogesterone or goserelin (GnRH analog)
  - Estrogen is a venous dilator, and low estrogen states or antagonizing estrogen with progesterone may result in improvement
- Surgical treatment includes
  - Laparoscopic transperitoneal ovarian vein ligation
    - Complete pain remission and absence of pelvic varicosities for 12 months in one study
  - Hysterectomy and oophorectomy
    - Longer hospitalization and post-op recovery time; fertility issues in reproductive-aged patients
- Transcatheter ovarian vein embolization
  - Indications for embolization in patient include
    - Chronic pain and otherwise negative work-up
    - Dyspareunia and otherwise negative work-up
    - Severe labial and perineal varicosities
  - Selective bilateral ovarian vein catheterization
    - Sclerosant injected into pelvic ovarian vein plexus followed by coil embolization of main ovarian veins
  - Selective bilateral internal iliac vein catheterization
    - Sclerotherapy using occlusion balloon catheter to achieve stasis; coils used infrequently
  - Technical success rates of 96-99%, with few immediate or long-term complications
  - Few immediate or long-term complications
    - Most common complaint is transient pelvic pain, likely related to pelvic venous thrombosis
    - Most complications usually do not require hospital admission for treatment
  - Reported rates of symptomatic relief are approximately 75%, with about 60% of patients experiencing complete resolution of symptoms

DIAGNOSTIC CHECKLIST

Consider

- Pelvic imaging in patient with thigh or vulvar varices and competent greater saphenous vein

SELECTED REFERENCES

1. Kwon SH et al: Transcatheter Ovarian Vein Embolization Using Coils for the Treatment of Pelvic Congestion Syndrome. Cardiovasc Intervent Radiol. 2007
2. Ahmed K et al: Current trends in the diagnosis and management of renal nutcracker syndrome: a review. Eur J Vasc Endovasc Surg. 31(4):410-6, 2006
3. Kim HS et al: Embolotherapy for pelvic congestion syndrome: long-term results. J Vasc Interv Radiol. 17(2 Pt 1):289-97, 2006
4. Nicholson T et al: Pelvic congestion syndrome, who should we treat and how? Tech Vasc Interv Radiol. 9(1):19-23, 2006
5. Rudloff U et al: Mesoaortic compression of the left renal vein (nutcracker syndrome): case reports and review of the literature. Ann Vasc Surg. 20(1):120-9, 2006
6. Kuligowska E et al: Pelvic pain: overlooked and underdiagnosed gynecologic conditions. Radiographics. 25(1):3-20, 2005

PELVIC CONGESTION SYNDROME

IMAGE GALLERY

Typical

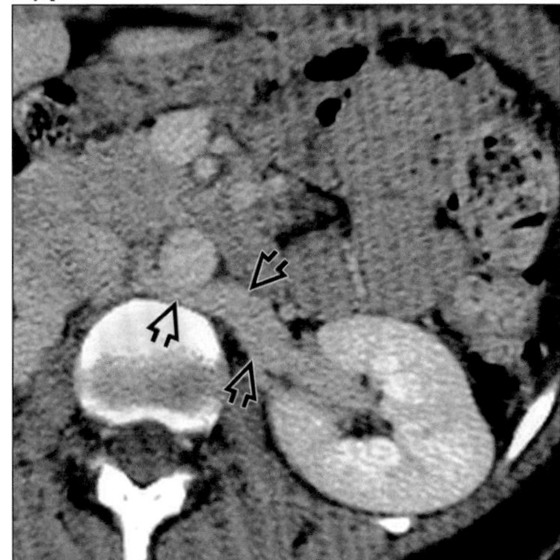

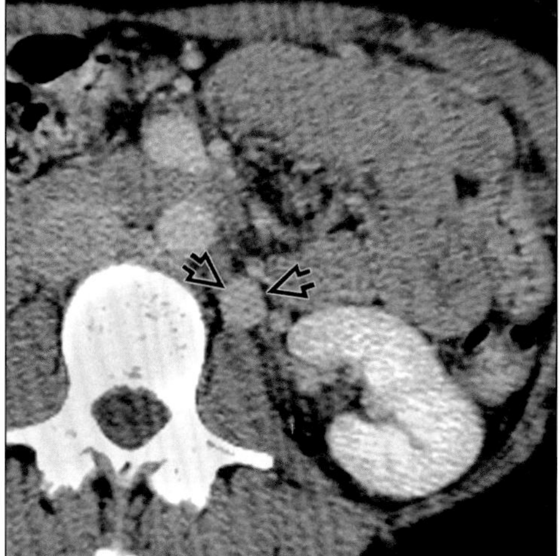

(Left) *Axial venous phase of CECT shows dilated retroaortic left renal vein ⇨ in a young patient with history of chronic left-sided pelvic discomfort. Aortic compression of left renal vein may result in elevated venous hydrostatic pressure & ovarian vein reflux.* ***(Right)*** *Axial venous phase of CECT (same patient as previous) shows dilated left ovarian vein ⇨. Ovarian vein reflux may result in pelvic venous engorgement & symptoms that characterize pelvic congestion syndrome.*

Typical

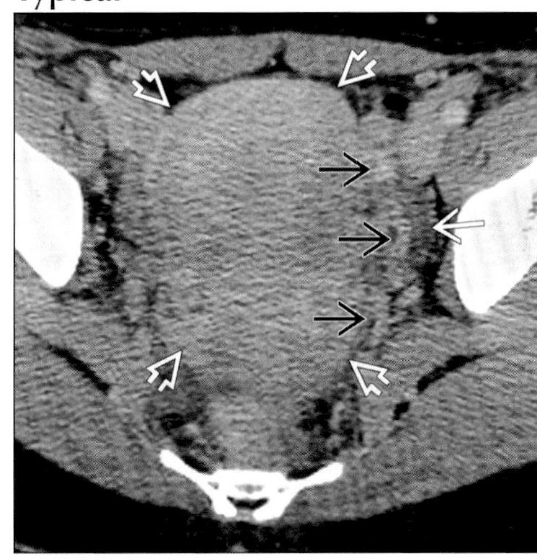

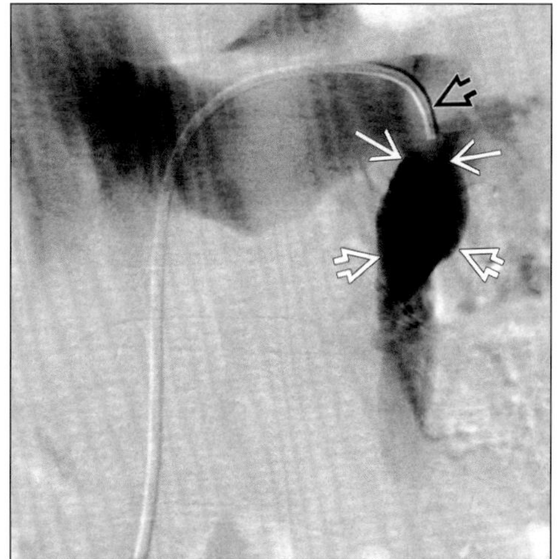

(Left) *Axial venous phase of CECT (same patient as previous image) shows dilated veins → adjacent to the uterus ➡ & left ovary ➡. There are no abnormal veins on the right, correlating with the patient's unilateral symptoms.* ***(Right)*** *Left renal venogram (same patient as previous image) obtained with catheter tip ⇨ adjacent to the left ovarian vein origin ➡ shows reflux of contrast into the dilated ovarian vein ➡. This reflux is indicative of left ovarian venous valvular incompetency.*

Typical

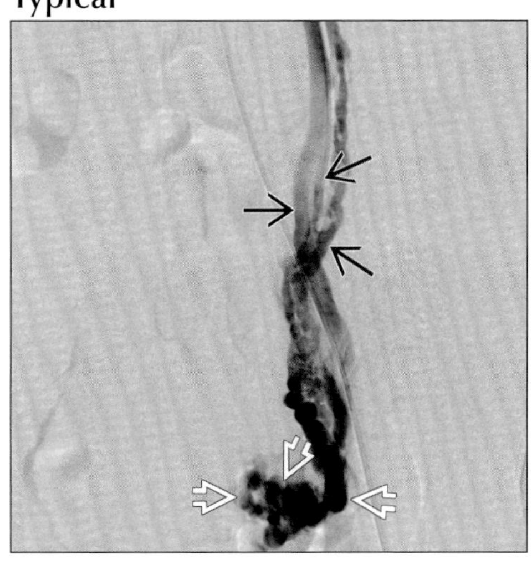

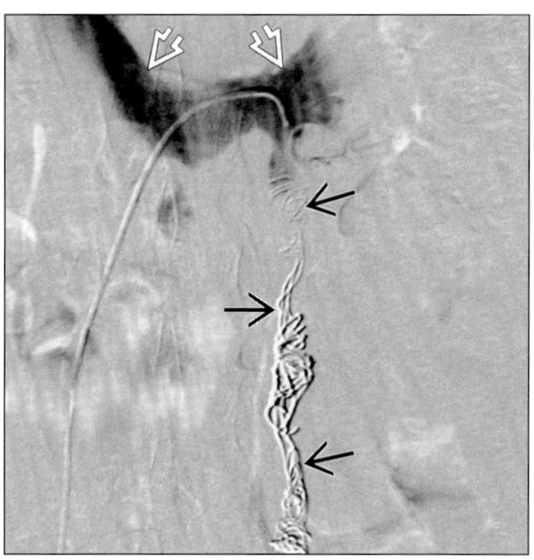

(Left) *Left ovarian venogram shows multiple dilated veins ➡ within the pelvis, supplied from numerous venous channels → arising from an incompetent ovarian vein. The ovarian pelvic venous plexus was treated with a sclerosant.* ***(Right)*** *Left renal venogram ➡ following transcatheter embolization shows multiple embolization coils → in the left ovarian vein. There is no longer any contrast reflux into the vein after embolization. The patient had complete resolution of her symptoms.*

OVARIAN VEIN THROMBOSIS

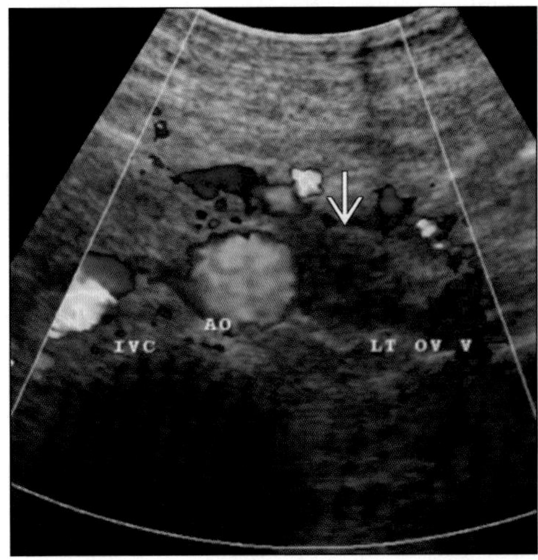

Color Doppler ultrasound in transverse orientation shows a filling defect in the left ovarian vein ➔. The ovarian vein is just lateral to the aorta.

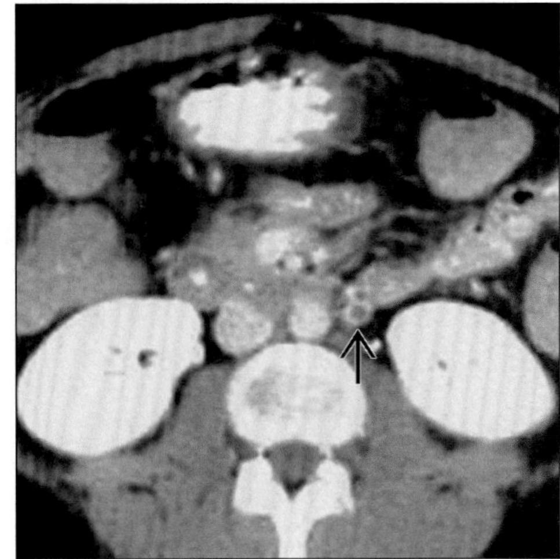

Axial CECT in the same case confirms thrombosis in the left ovarian vein ➔.

TERMINOLOGY

Abbreviations and Synonyms

- Ovarian vein thrombosis (OVT); post partum ovarian vein thrombosis (POVT); right ovarian vein (ROV)
- Septic pelvic thrombophlebitis (SPT): Inflammation of pelvic veins with infected thrombosis
  - Theory of continuum existing between OVT and SPT; SPT initially involving smaller pelvic vessels not detectable by currently available imaging techniques

Definitions

- Rare, serious post-partum condition associated with thrombosis of one or both ovarian veins

IMAGING FINDINGS

General Features

- Best diagnostic clue
  - Fever not responding to adequate broad spectrum antibiotics, "enigmatic fever"
  - Lower abdominal pain
  - Abdominal tenderness
- Location: Right ovarian vein or left ovarian vein

CT Findings

- CECT
  - Ovarian vein appears as a rounded or oval hypodense mass surrounded by hyperdense ring
  - Sausage-shaped structure in paracolic gutter disappearing at level of renal veins
  - Dilated ovarian vein may be larger than inferior vena cava (IVC)
  - Accurate evaluation of extension of thrombus into IVC or iliac veins
  - Sensitivity: 77.8%, specificity: 62.5% in evaluating OVT

MR Findings

- T1WI: Low signal intensity tubular mass
- T2WI: Moderate signal intensity tubular mass
- Axial images are well-suited to exploit in flow effects because of cranio-caudal direction of flow in ovarian veins
  - Placing spacial saturation band superior to the slice being acquired virtually eliminates all arterial signals
- Limitations: Not used for severely ill patients
- Sensitivity and specificity in evaluating OVT: 100%

DDx: Right Lower Quadrant Pain in Post-Partum Women

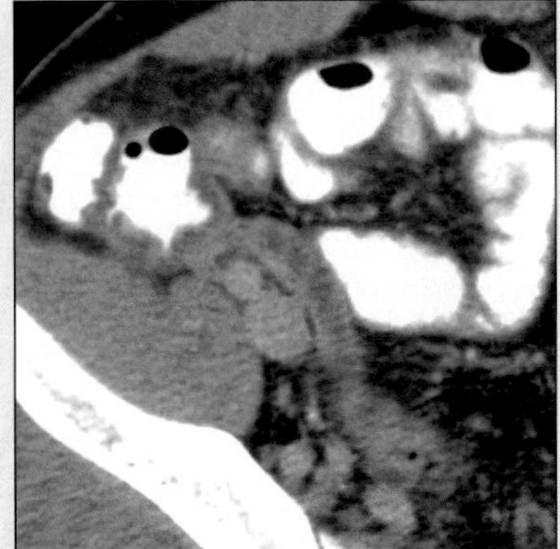

Appendicitis

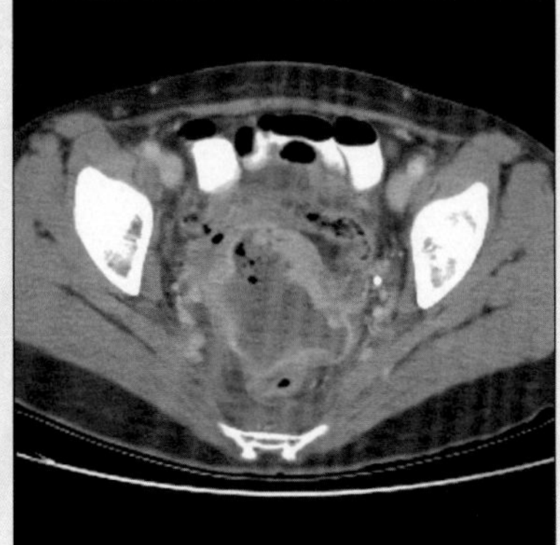

Pelvic Abscess

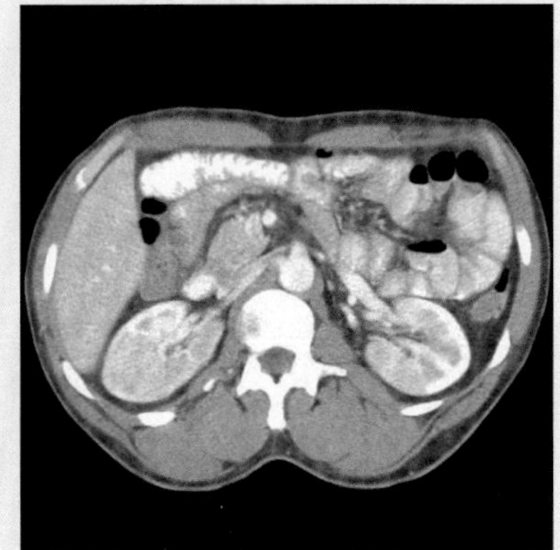

Pyelonephritis

OVARIAN VEIN THROMBOSIS

Key Facts

Terminology
- Rare, serious post-partum condition associated with thrombosis of one or both ovarian veins

Imaging Findings
- CECT: Rounded or oval hypodense mass surrounded by hyperdense ring in right ovarian vein
- CECT: Sensitivity: 77.8%, specificity: 62.5% in evaluating OVT
- T1WI: Low signal intensity tubular mass
- T2WI: Moderate signal intensity tubular mass
- Sensitivity and specificity in evaluating OVT: 100%

Top Differential Diagnoses
- Acute Appendicitis
- Adnexal Torsion
- Adnexal Abscess
- Pyelonephritis
- Endometritis

Pathology
- Involves right ovarian vein in 90% of cases
- Complicates 0.05-0.18% of deliveries

Clinical Issues
- Early diagnosis of ovarian vein thrombosis is essential to prevent life-threatening sequelae
- Women (4-7 days from delivery) presenting with pyrexia not responding to antibiotic therapy

Diagnostic Checklist
- CECT: Tubular mass between right adnexa and renal hilum with low density lumen and sharply defined walls

Ultrasonographic Findings
- Color Doppler
  - Anechoic, hypoechoic mass between adnexa and IVC, absence of blood flow within mass
  - Limitations: Obesity, gaseous intestinal distension, operator dependent
  - Sensitivity: 55.6%, specificity: 41.2% in evaluating OVT

Imaging Recommendations
- Best imaging tool: CECT - readily available
- Protocol advice: Avoid noncontrast CT to minimize radiation exposure

DIFFERENTIAL DIAGNOSIS

Acute Appendicitis in Pregnancy
- Symptoms: Lower abdominal pain (sometimes the pain is located in other quadrants because gravid uterus displaces appendix), nonspecific leukocytosis
- Diagnosis: US with graded compression technique is the modality of choice (limitation: Not feasible during third trimester)
- Appendiceal perforation is much more common in pregnant women than in general population (up to 55%)

Adnexal Torsion
- 2.7% of all gynecological emergencies usually affecting child bearing age women
- Symptoms: Sudden, continuous nonspecific pain in lower abdomen, nausea and vomiting
- Diagnosis
  - Ultrasound (first imaging tool): Nonspecific US findings
  - In almost all cases a pelvic mass is demonstrated with US, CT and MR
  - CECT and MR additional findings: Fallopian tube thickening, ascites, uterine deviation towards twisted side
- Treatment: Urgent surgical intervention is indicated
  - Despite "necrotic" appearance of twisted ischemic ovary, detorsion is the only procedure which should be performed at surgery
    - Oophorectomy should be avoided because ovarian function is preserved in 88-100% of cases

Adnexal Abscess
- Symptoms: Pain (88%), fever (35%), adnexal mass (35%), diarrhea (24%), nausea and vomiting (18%), irregular menses (12%), difficult voiding (6%)
- Diagnosis
  - US and CT: Useful tools to identify the mass but do not establish definitive diagnosis
  - MR and radionuclide scanning using indium-111: More accurate diagnostic tools
- Treatment: Hospitalization, intravenous antibiotics, surgery in complicated cases

Pyelonephritis
- Pregnant women are at increased risk of UTI for anatomical and hormonal changes
  - Pyelonephritis is the most common severe bacterial infection that can lead to maternal and perinatal complications
- Diagnosis
  - Urine culture: Gold standard
  - US: Good screening tool, sensitive for identification of dilated collecting system; may miss abscesses or perinephric diseases
  - CT: Gives excellent anatomic details, can identify stones and can evaluate ureters and perinephric disease
    - Findings: Focal area of decreased attenuation and decreased function
- Treatment: Hospitalization, parenteral antibiotics treatment and supportive care

Endometritis
- Infection of endometrium or decidua with extension into myometrium and parametrial tissues
- PID is a common predecessor of endometritis in nonobstetric population

- Transvaginal ultrasound (TVUS) findings of endometritis are non specific, possible thickened irregular appearing endometrium with fluid, debris and gas apparent
  - Appearance of gas is highly suggestive of anaerobic endometritis

PATHOLOGY

General Features

- General path comments
  - OVT involves right ovarian vein in 90% of cases
    - Anatomy: ROV crosses in front of right ureter at L4 level
    - Post-partum setting: Retrograde flow in left ovarian vein (LOV), antegrade flow into ROV increases bacterial inoculum especially in presence of endometritis
- Etiology
  - Virchow triad: Vessel wall injury, stasis, hypercoagulation
    - Vessel wall injury: Direct surgical trauma, local infection or inflammation
    - Stasis: ROV longer than LOV with less competent valves
    - During pregnancy uterine dextrorotation with compression of ROV; diameter of ROV increases to 3 times; blood flow declines immediately after delivery
    - Hypercoagulation during pregnancy: Elevated coagulation factor levels (I, II, VII, VIII, IX, X), increased platelets adhesion, decreased fibrinolysis with return to normal levels 2 to 6 weeks post-partum
- Epidemiology
  - OVT complicates 0.05-0.18% of deliveries
  - Symptoms develop within 4 weeks of delivery, most frequently within the first 4 days
- Associated abnormalities: OVT can present as complication of streptococcal group B infection of the vagina or endometrium

Gross Pathologic & Surgical Features

- Right lateral flank incision used to exposed the dilated ovarian vein with semi-formed and gelatinous content (thrombus)

CLINICAL ISSUES

Presentation

- Most common signs/symptoms
  - Mild to moderate fever: First 48-96 hours after delivery (80%); tachycardia
  - "Cord-like" tender lower abdominal mass (55%)
  - Lower abdominal quadrant pain (right lower quadrant 55%, left lower quadrant 3.6%)
  - Nausea and vomiting
- Other signs/symptoms: Ureteral obstruction and leakage and involvement of IVC or renal vein
- Clinical Profile: Women (4-7 days from delivery) presenting with pyrexia not responding to antibiotic therapy

Demographics

- Age: Child bearing women (post-partum complication)
- Gender: Women after delivery at any gestational age

Natural History & Prognosis

- Early diagnosis of ovarian vein thrombosis is essential to prevent life-threatening sequelae
- Mortality from OVT is less than 5% and is usually associated with cases of pulmonary embolism or metastatic abscesses

Treatment

- Options, risks, complications
  - Broad spectrum antibiotics
    - Intravenous agents: Clindamycin, gentamicin, imipenem, ampicillin, sulbactam
  - Anticoagulation
    - Heparin
    - Low molecular weight heparins (LMWHs) have replaced traditional heparin therapy for both prophylaxis and treatment of thromboembolism
  - Antibiotics and heparin are continued until the patient is afebrile for 24-48 hours
  - Pulmonary embolism in 13-33% of reported cases
    - Use of IVC filter when anticoagulation therapy is contraindicated
    - An IVC filter would have to be placed in a suprarenal IVC position

DIAGNOSTIC CHECKLIST

Consider

- Rare but serious disease that requires an awareness by physicians, combined with a careful history and physical examination
- Disease with potential for significant morbidity and mortality if treatment is not promptly instituted

Image Interpretation Pearls

- CECT: Tubular mass between right adnexa and renal hilum with low density lumen and sharply defined walls

SELECTED REFERENCES

1. Carr S et al: Surgical treatment of ovarian vein thrombosis. Vasc Endovascular Surg. 40(6):505-8, 2006
2. Humes DJ et al: Acute appendicitis. BMJ. 333(7567):530-4, 2006
3. Kominiarek MA et al: Postpartum ovarian vein thrombosis: an update. Obstet Gynecol Surv. 61(5):337-42, 2006
4. Pedrosa I et al: MR imaging evaluation of acute appendicitis in pregnancy. Radiology. 238(3):891-9, 2006
5. Takach TJ et al: Ovarian vein and caval thrombosis. Tex Heart Inst J. 32(4):579-82, 2005
6. Dessole S et al: Postpartum ovarian vein thrombosis: an unpredictable event: two case reports and review of the literature. Arch Gynecol Obstet. 267(4):242-6, 2003
7. Kubik-Huch RA et al: Role of duplex color Doppler ultrasound, computed tomography, and MR angiography in the diagnosis of septic puerperal ovarian vein thrombosis. Abdom Imaging. 24(1):85-91, 1999

IMAGE GALLERY

Typical

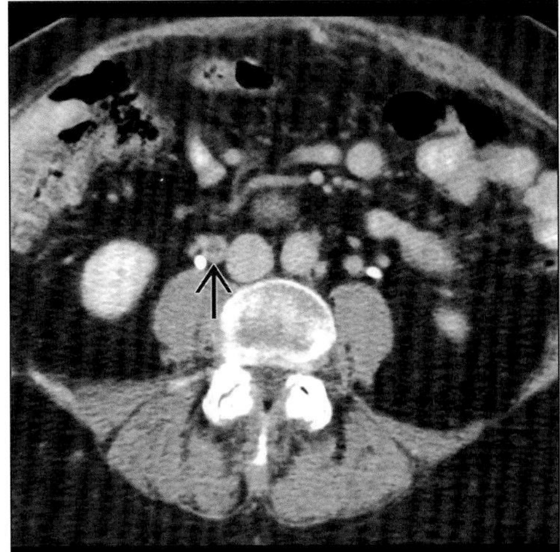

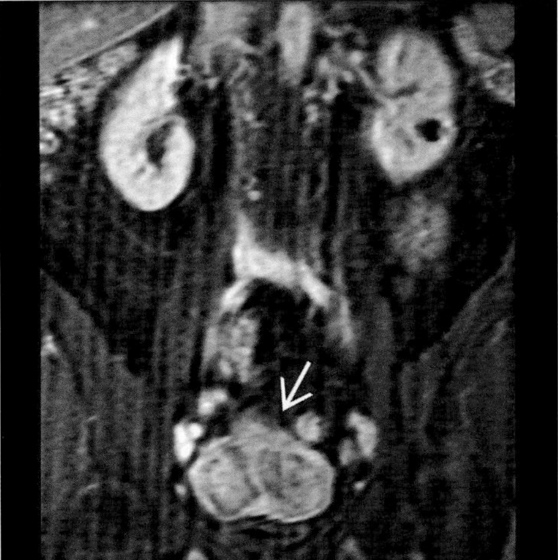

*(**Left**) Axial CECT shows a dilated right ovarian vein containing low density thrombus in a patient with ovarian carcinoma. (**Right**) Coronal CECT reconstruction on the same case shows the ovarian cancer. The ovarian vein thrombosis is not well seen on the coronal images.*

Typical

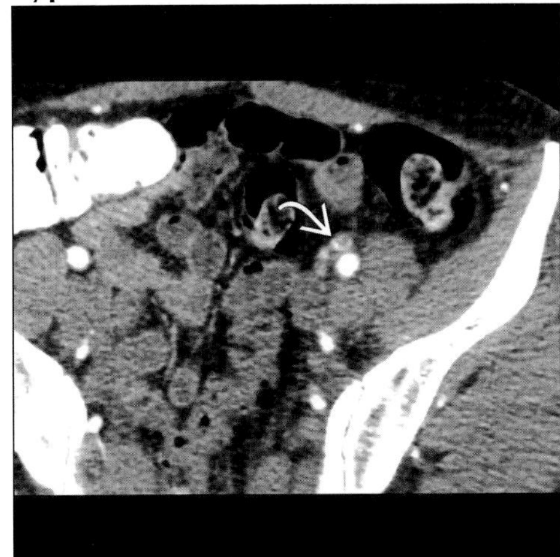

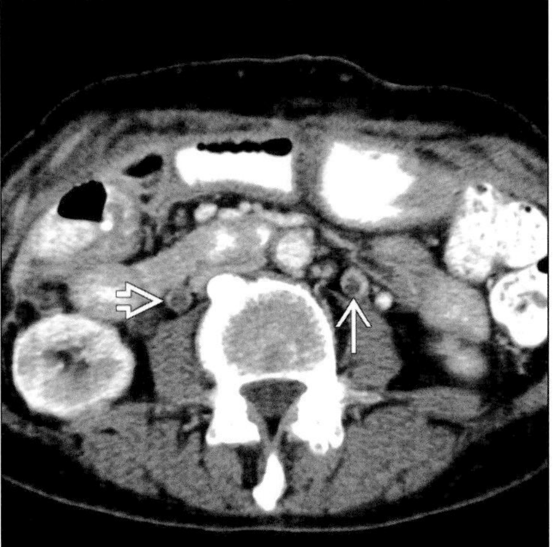

*(**Left**) Axial CECT shows thrombosis of the left ovarian vein in the pelvis. It has an enhancing periphery and low density interior consistent with thrombus. (**Right**) Axial CECT shows bilateral ovarian vein thrombosis. The right ovarian vein is almost completely thrombosed. The left ovarian vein has a small amount of enhancement in periphery.*

Typical

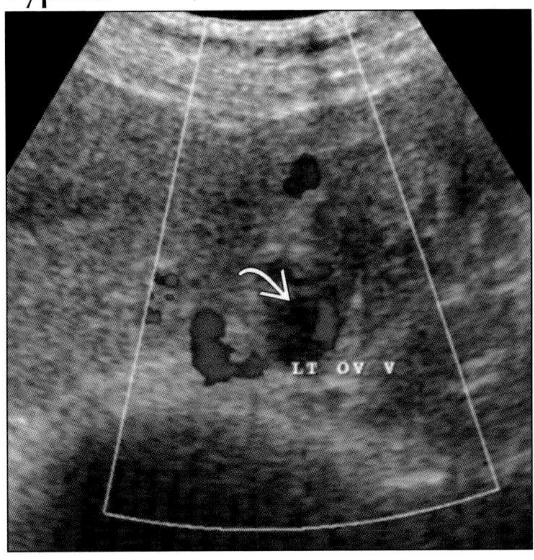

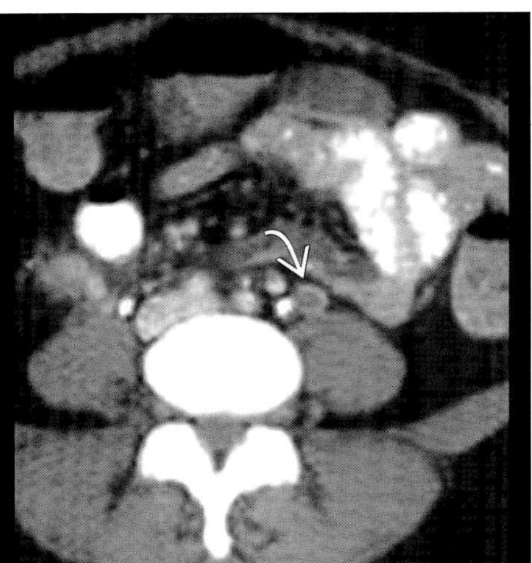

*(**Left**) Color Doppler ultrasound performed in the lower abdomen demonstrates thrombosis of the left ovarian vein. Bowel gas and adipose tissue often makes the diagnosis of ovarian vein thrombosis with ultrasound difficult. CT may be required to make a definitive diagnosis. (**Right**) Axial CECT shows CT from the same case confirms left ovarian vein thrombus. (Courtesy M. O'Boyle, MD).*

MAY THURNER SYNDROME

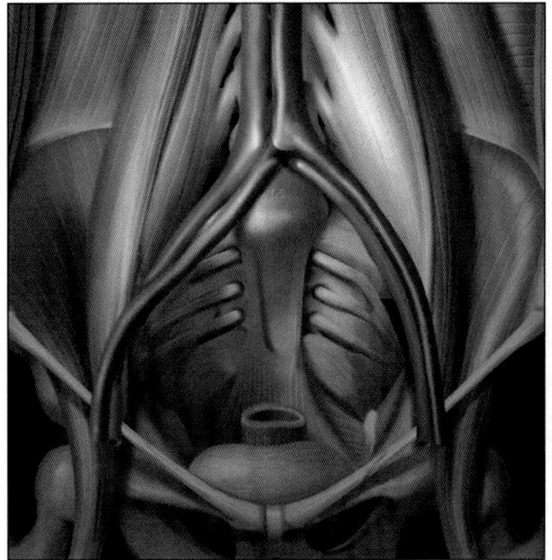

Graphic shows the crossing of the right common iliac artery over the left common iliac vein. This same appearance is beautifully demonstrated on the following MR image.

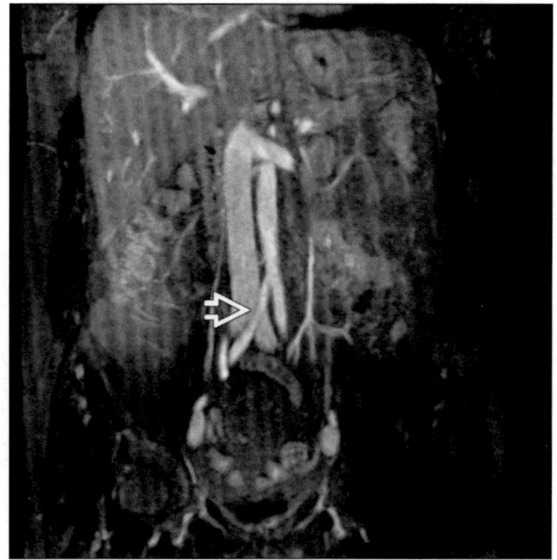

Coronal shows course of the right common iliac artery ➡ crossing over and compressing the left common iliac vein. Classic image of May-Thurner syndrome.

TERMINOLOGY

Abbreviations and Synonyms

- May-Thurner syndrome, iliac vein compression syndrome (IVCS), Cockett syndrome, iliocaval vein syndrome

Definitions

- Compression of left common iliac vein (CIV) by right common iliac artery (CIA)

IMAGING FINDINGS

General Features

- Best diagnostic clue: Young women with persistent left lower leg edema
- Location: Left common iliac vein

CT Findings

- CECT
  - Extrinsic compression of left CIV by right CIA
  - Diameter of left CIV at origin smaller than normal
  - Presence of collaterals crossing midline to join contralateral veins
  - Tortuosity of aortoiliac arteries
  - Calcified foci in iliac arteries and/or aorta
  - Mild to moderate degenerative changes in lumbar vertebrae

MR Findings

- MRV
  - Easily depicts the area of compression or obstruction and documents the presence of collaterals
  - Disadvantages
    - Vascular region above bifurcations have disturbed non laminar flow and can present a confusing picture mimicking intraluminal filling defects

Ultrasonographic Findings

- Color Doppler
  - Standard test to diagnose deep vein thrombosis (DVT)
  - Difficult visualization of iliac vessels
  - 20% of iliac vein ultrasound studies are non diagnostic in best vascular laboratories

DDx: May-Thurner

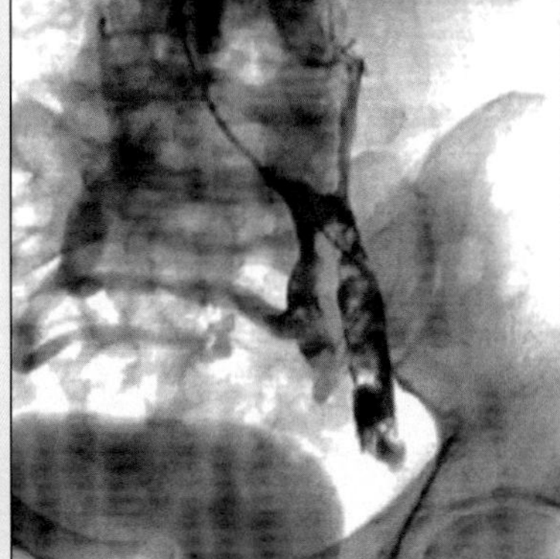

Thrombosis of Vein

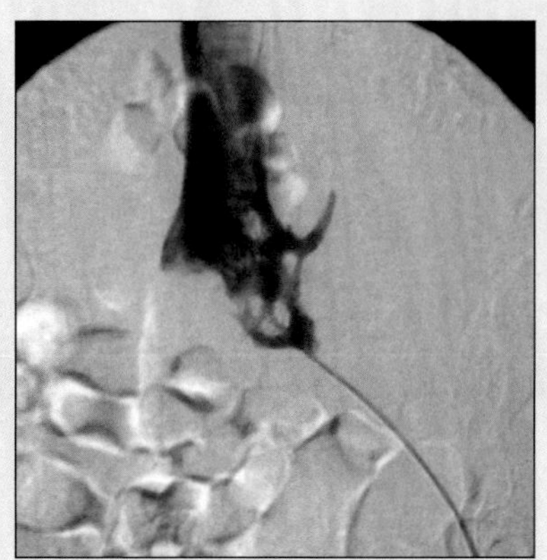

Synechiae within Iliac Vein

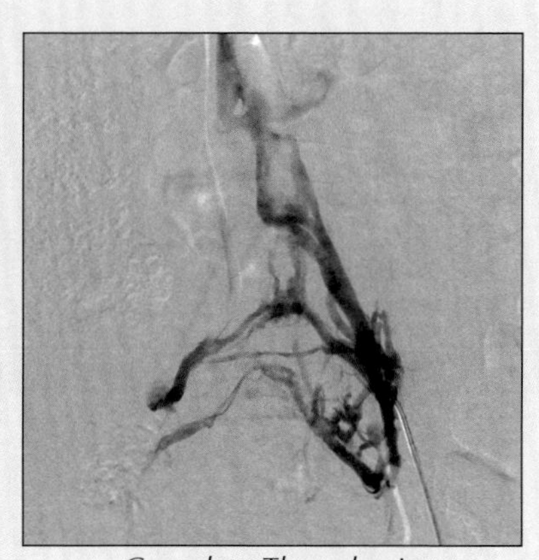

Complete Thrombosis

MAY THURNER SYNDROME

Key Facts

Terminology

- Compression of left common iliac vein (CIV) by right common iliac artery (CIA)

Imaging Findings

- Best diagnostic clue: Young women with persistent left lower leg edema
- Extrinsic compression of left CIV by right CIA
- Best imaging tool: Femoral venography

Top Differential Diagnoses

- Trauma
- Surgery
- Pelvic Tumors

Pathology

- General path comments: Physical entrapment of left CIV between right CIA and fifth lumbar vertebra
- DVT occurs 3-8 times more frequently in left side

Clinical Issues

- Treatment goals
  - With chronic symptoms: Resolve significantly improve or prevent chronic pain, aching or edema, venous claudication or ulceration
  - Improve quality of life
- With acute iliofemoral DVT: Prevention of PE, restoration of unobstructed venous return, preservation of valve function, prevention of recurrence

Other Modality Findings

- Intravascular ultrasound (IVUS)
  - 12.5 MHz or 20 MHz transducer introduced through a sheath into the lumen of veins
  - IVUS can determine the vessel size and internal wall morphology, may demonstrate intraluminal "spur" and assist with treatment planning (stent placement)
- Air plethysmography (APG)
  - To investigate and determine cause and severity of venous complaints and to find evidence of proximal obstruction
  - May also be non diagnostic because of collateralization or insufficient narrowing to change the flow dynamics
- IVCS can be encountered as incidental finding during electrophysiologic studies

Angiographic Findings

- Venography (femoral, popliteal or pedal access)
  - Used as diagnostic and therapeutic tool
  - Direct pressure measurement across iliofemoral stenosis during venography
    - Significant stenosis: Difference greater than 2 mm Hg at rest or 3 mm Hg with exercise
    - Non diagnostic pressure gradient does not exclude the diagnosis of IVCS
  - Standard amount of dye injected into foot is not sufficient to evaluate iliac veins in pelvis

Imaging Recommendations

- Best imaging tool: Femoral venography
- Protocol advice
  - Use venography to diagnose IVCS first and plan the treatment last (thrombolysis and stenting)
  - IVCS is often a diagnosis by exclusion of other possible causes
    - Presenting symptoms (swelling, DVT and possible PE) whether acute or chronic may be due to several causes (see differential diagnosis)

DIFFERENTIAL DIAGNOSIS

Immobilization

- Risk of developing lower extremities DVT during conventional lower limb immobilization: 4.5-71.4% depending on
  - Indication for immobilization
  - Method of diagnosing DVT
- Very important to prevent DVT during lower limb immobilization

Trauma

- Polytraumatized patients have an increased risk of developing DVT and PE
- Current methodological imperfections make it impossible to correctly assess incidence of DVT and PE in multiple trauma population
  - Studies with rigorous methodology using precise stratification of the trauma injuries are required to determine real risk for DVT/PE in trauma patients and to assess impact of early systematic prophylaxis

Surgery

- Cancer-related surgery increases risk of DVT complications because of frequent venous trauma
- Post surgery risk of developing DVT ranges from 15-40% (in most surgery patients) to as high as 60% in orthopedic surgery patients

Radiation, Chemotherapy and Hormonal Therapy

- Patients with malignancies have an increased risk of thromboembolism
  - DVT and PE may present as a complication after diagnosis of cancer
- Risk factors include radiotherapy, chemotherapy and hormonal therapy

Catheterization

- Presence of peripheral catheters increases the risk of developing DVT (rate ranging: 2-40%)

Pelvic Tumors

- Patients with active cancer have a 4x increased risk of developing venous thromboembolism (VTE) compared with individuals without cancer
  - Risk increases to 6.5x with chemotherapy

PATHOLOGY

General Features

- General path comments: Physical entrapment of left CIV between right CIA and fifth lumbar vertebra
- Epidemiology
  - 2-5% of women undergoing evaluation for lower extremities venous disorder
  - DVT occurs 3-8 times more frequently on left side
- Associated abnormalities: DVT

Gross Pathologic & Surgical Features

- Compression of left iliac veins against lumbar vertebrae can cause chronic irritation of the vascular endothelium
  - Leads to endothelial proliferation and hyperplasia

Microscopic Features

- Collagen and elastin deposition result in the formation of "spurs"
  - Spurs: Replacement of normal intima and media of the vein by well-organized connective tissue covered with endothelium
  - Spurs create mechanical obstruction to flow and increase risk of left-sided iliofemoral thrombosis

Staging, Grading or Classification Criteria

- Three stages
  - Asymptomatic compression at the left iliocaval confluence without intrinsic changes or development of venous collateral vessels on venography
  - Development of intraluminal filling defects (spurs)
  - Iliofemoral thrombosis

CLINICAL ISSUES

Presentation

- Most common signs/symptoms
  - Unilateral swelling, pain and aching of left leg
  - Venous stasis and ulcers
- Other signs/symptoms: Phlegmasia cerulea dolens

Demographics

- Age: 2nd-4th decade
- Gender: M < F

Natural History & Prognosis

- Progressive disease with long term disabling complications
- Diagnosis of compression before insurgence of thrombosis and insufficiency is essential for a good prognosis

Treatment

- Options, risks, complications
  - Treatment goals
    - With chronic symptoms: Important to resolve, significantly improve, or prevent chronic pain, aching, edema, venous claudication or ulceration
    - Improve quality of life
  - With acute iliofemoral DVT: Prevention of PE, restoration of unobstructed venous return, preservation of valve function, prevention of recurrence
  - Treatment options
    - Standard: Anticoagulation, compression
    - Higher level of care: Catheter directed thrombolysis followed by endovascular intervention, (balloon angioplasty, stenting)
    - Surgery: Thrombectomy, direct surgical reconstruction or bypass (Palma crossover), vein patch angioplasty (long term success as patency of left CIV documented between 40-88%)
  - Complications
    - Pulmonary embolism
    - Retroperitoneal hemorrhage

DIAGNOSTIC CHECKLIST

Consider

- May-Thurner syndrome in young to middle age women with swelling of left lower extremity

Image Interpretation Pearls

- Venography: Stenosis of left CIV and presence of venous collaterals crossing the midline

SELECTED REFERENCES

1. Billakanty S et al: May-Thurner syndrome: A vascular abnormality encountered during electrophysiologic study. Pacing Clin Electrophysiol. 29(11):1310-1, 2006
2. Raffini L et al: May-Thurner syndrome (iliac vein compression) and thrombosis in adolescents. Pediatr Blood Cancer. 47(6):834-8, 2006
3. Oguzkurt L et al: Computed tomography findings in 10 cases of iliac vein compression (May-Thurner) syndrome. Eur J Radiol. 55(3):421-5, 2005
4. Shebel ND et al: Diagnosis and management of iliac vein compression syndrome. J Vasc Nurs. 23(1):10-7; quiz 18-9, 2005
5. Forauer AR et al: Intravascular ultrasound in the diagnosis and treatment of iliac vein compression (May-Thurner) syndrome. J Vasc Interv Radiol. 13(5):523-7, 2002
6. Wolpert LM et al: Magnetic resonance venography in the diagnosis and management of May-Thurner syndrome. Vasc Endovascular Surg. 36(1):51-7, 2002

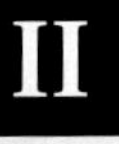

IMAGE GALLERY

Typical

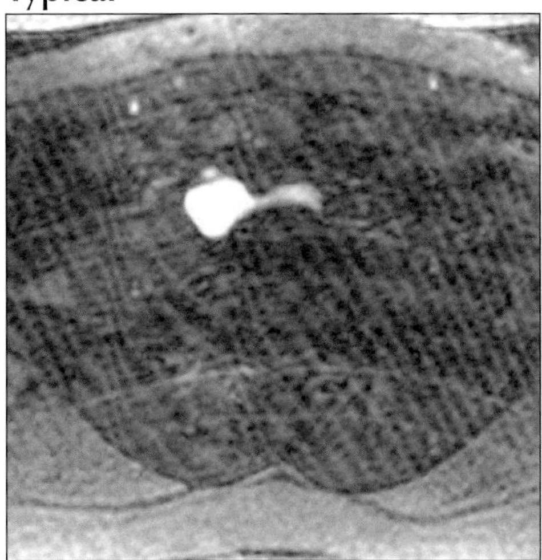

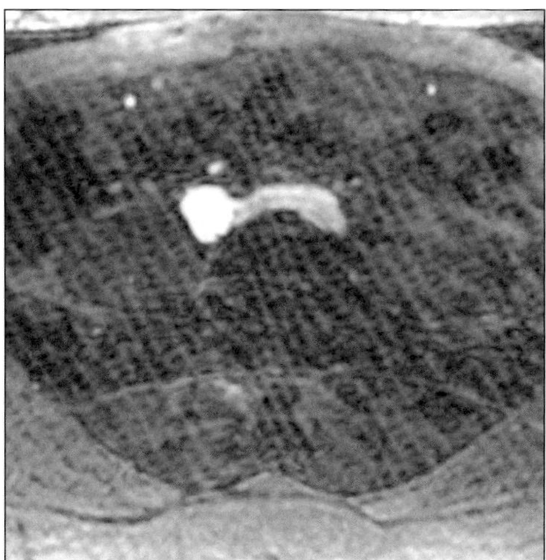

(Left) *Axial ECG-gated 2D TOF with MIP shows narrowing of the left CIV at the IVC origin. (Courtesy C. Sirlin, MD).* ***(Right)*** *Axial (same patient as previous image), caudal cut shows narrowing of the left CIV at the confluence with right CIV. (Courtesy C. Sirlin, MD).*

Typical

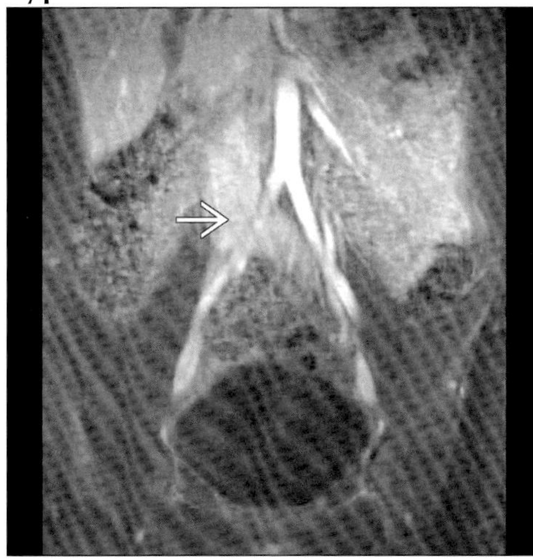

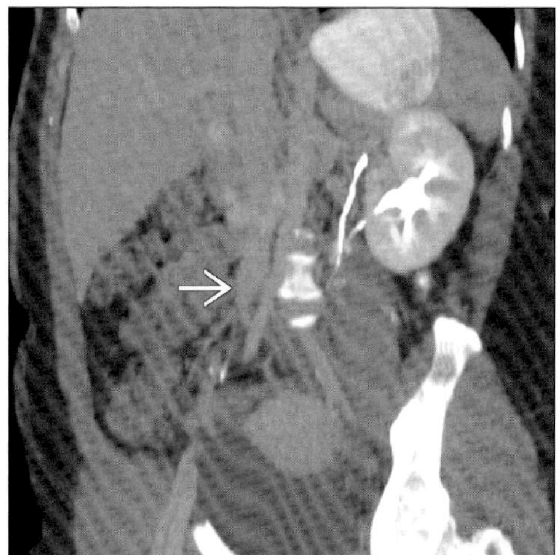

(Left) *Coronal MRA shows mild narrowing ➔ of the left CIV from extrinsic compression by right CIA in a 26 year-old female with bilateral LE pain made worse with exercise. (Courtesy C. Sirlin, MD).* ***(Right)*** *Coronal oblique CECT shows site of compression ➔ of left CIV (by right CIA) against lumbar vertebrae (L4-L5). (Courtesy C. Sirlin, MD).*

Typical

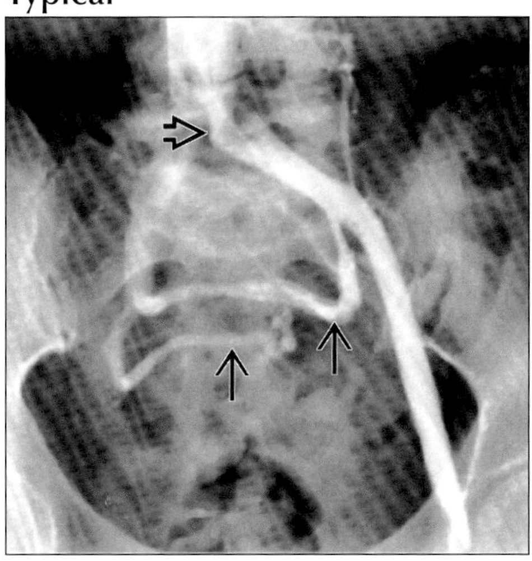

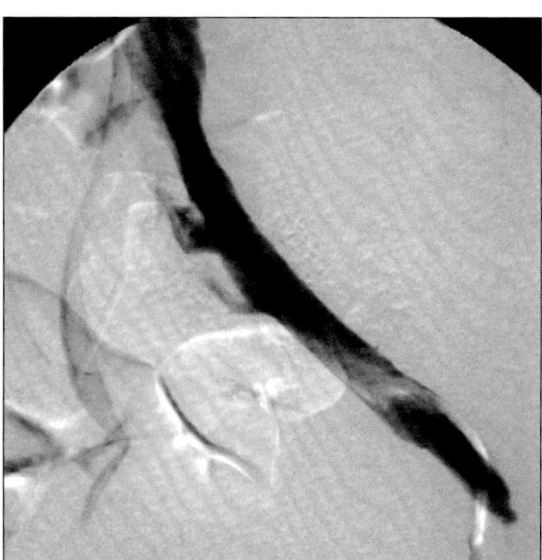

(Left) *DSA shows narrowing of the left common iliac vein ➪ This represents compression by the crossing right common iliac artery. Cross pelvic collaterals ➔ indicate a significant obstruction.* ***(Right)*** *DSA shows improvement in the narrowing of the left common iliac vein by placement of a self-expanding stent. The cross pelvic collaterals have resolved.*

NUTCRACKER SYNDROME

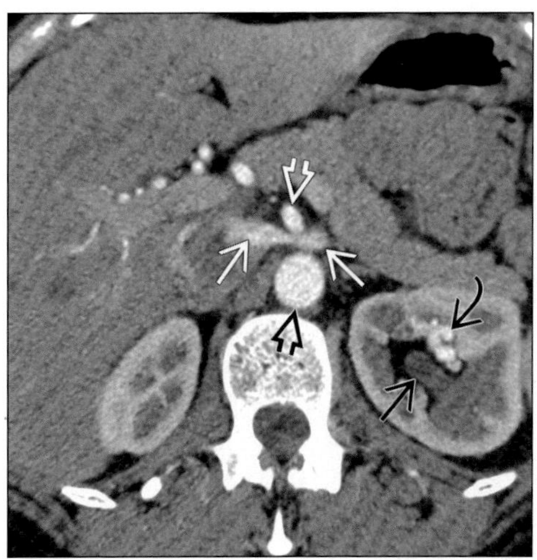

Axial CECT shows compression of the left renal vein ➡ between the abdominal aorta ⇨ and the SMA ➡ that is typical of nutcracker syndrome. Note the renal hilar varices ↗ adjacent to the renal collecting system ➡.

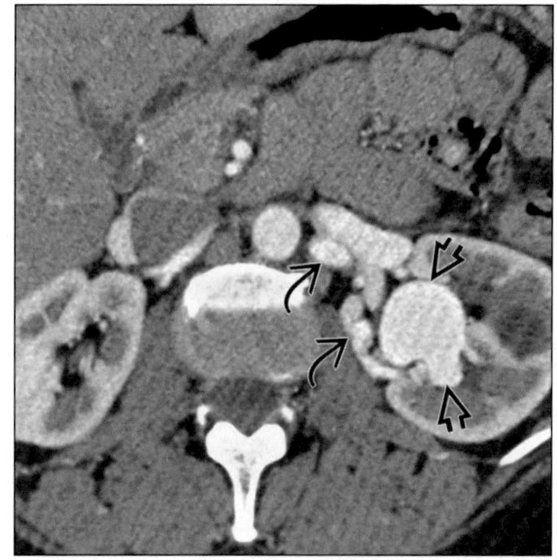

Axial CECT (same patient as previous image) shows more extensive renal varices ↗ inferiorly, adjacent to the renal collecting system ⇨. These may rupture into the collecting system with resultant hematuria.

TERMINOLOGY

Definitions

- Compression of left renal vein as it passes between aorta and superior mesenteric artery (SMA), with resultant left renal venous hypertension and accompanying hematuria

IMAGING FINDINGS

General Features

- Best diagnostic clue
  - Flank, pelvic or abdominal pain with accompanying hematuria, proteinuria; and intrarenal, perirenal varices or a left varicocele
  - Urine cytology, ureteroscopy, ultrasound and renal biopsy used in assessing etiology of unilateral hematuria
- Location: Left renal vein courses between anterior aspect of abdominal aorta and dorsal aspect of the SMA

CT Findings

- CECT
  - 50% or greater compression of left renal vein between abdominal aorta and SMA
  - Extensive left intrarenal and perirenal varicosities or venous collaterals may be present
  - CT venography findings are similar to those of left renal venography

MR Findings

- MRV: Similar findings as on DSA or CT venography

Ultrasonographic Findings

- Color Doppler
  - High sensitivity of renal Doppler US as initial non-invasive test
  - Peak velocity measurements within renal vein and IVC to assess for gradient

Angiographic Findings

- DSA

DDx: Enlarged Left Renal Vein

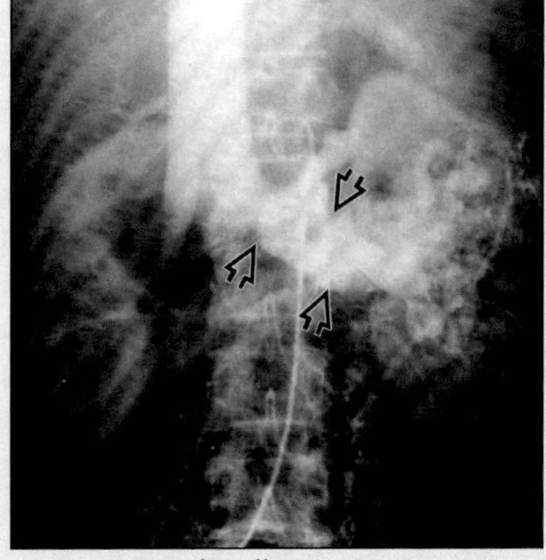

Renal Cell Carcinoma

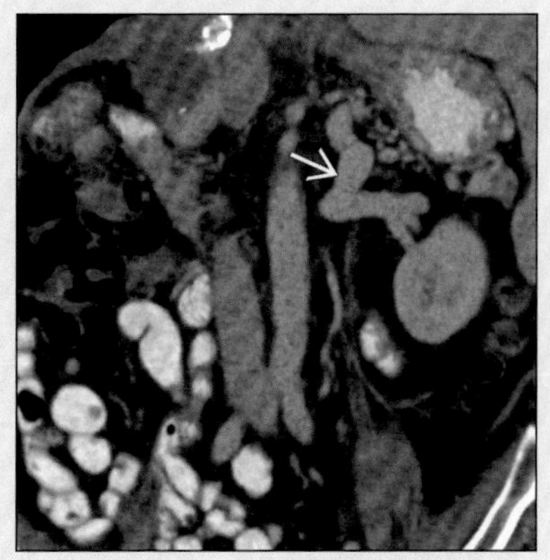

Spontaneous Splenorenal Shunt

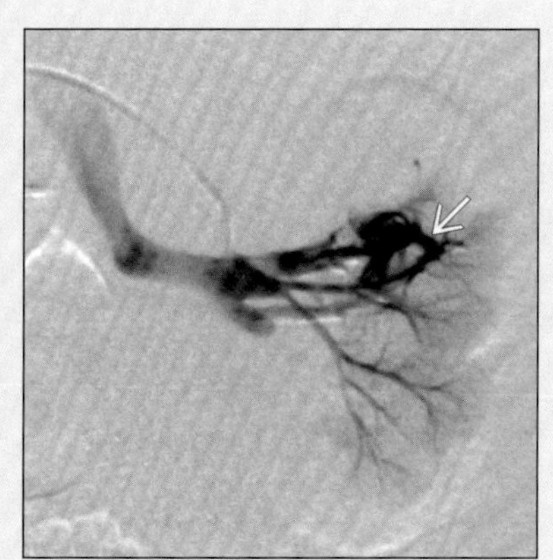

Arteriovenous Fistula

Key Facts

Terminology

- Compression of left renal vein as it passes between aorta and superior mesenteric artery (SMA), with resultant left renal venous hypertension and accompanying hematuria

Imaging Findings

- Left renal venography with measurement of pressure gradient between inferior vena cava and left renal vein used to confirm nutcracker syndrome in selected cases
- Pressure gradient > 2 mm Hg suggestive of renal venous hypertension due to outflow obstruction
- High sensitivity of renal Doppler US as initial non-invasive test

Pathology

- An important cause of non-glomerular hematuria to be considered in the pediatric age group

Clinical Issues

- Most common signs/symptoms: Left flank and abdominal pain, with or without unilateral hematuria
- Patients with mild, tolerable symptoms may be treated conservatively as left renal vein hypertension may eventually resolve with development of collateral veins
- Persistent, recurrent or massive hematuria is an indication for treatment
- Open surgical and transcatheter endovascular treatments designed to lower intrarenal venous pressure by removing renal vein outflow obstruction

- Left renal venography with measurement of pressure gradient between inferior vena cava and left renal vein used to confirm nutcracker syndrome in selected cases
- Pressure gradient > 2 mm Hg suggestive of renal venous hypertension due to outflow obstruction
- Enlarged tortuous renal hilar varices draining into retroperitoneal collaterals may be present

Imaging Recommendations

- Best imaging tool
  - Color Doppler sonography with peak velocity measurements within renal vein and IVC should be initially obtained as screening examination
  - Left renal venous hypertension confirmed with selective catheter pressure measurements within left renal vein and IVC

DIFFERENTIAL DIAGNOSIS

Congenital Venous Malformation

- May be extensive, with numerous points of communication with retroperitoneal veins

Renal Vein Thrombosis

- Acute thrombosis results in renal dysfunction, back pain and hematuria
- Frequently associated with a systemic disease
  - Hypercoagulable state
  - Dehydration
  - Neoplasm
- May be associated with intrinsic renal disease
  - Nephrotic syndrome
  - Glomerulonephritis
  - Tumor

Arteriovenous Fistula

- Rapid flow hemodynamics and high venous pressures within enlarged renal vein

Vascular Renal Tumor

- Arteriovenous shunting within tumor such as renal cell carcinoma may result in renal vein varices

Spontaneous Splenorenal Shunt

- Relatively rare condition occurring in and complicating hepatic cirrhosis
- Elevated pressure within splenic vein spontaneously decompresses into left renal vein
- Results in pressurized and dilated left renal vein, with accompanying renal vein and retroperitoneal varices

Obstructing Renal or Ureteral Calculus

- Obstructive uropathy from calculus causing unilateral flank, pelvic or abdominal pain and hematuria mimics symptoms of nutcracker syndrome

Retroaortic Left Renal Vein

- Compression by aorta may result in left renal venous hypertension

PATHOLOGY

General Features

- General path comments
  - An important cause of non-glomerular hematuria to be considered in the pediatric age group
  - Severe left renal vein compression and resultant left renal venous hypertension can result in congestion of the left gonadal vein
- Etiology
  - Left renal venous hypertension results from compression of left renal vein by aorta and SMA where it passes between these arteries
  - Venous hypertension leads to development of collaterals with intrarenal and perirenal varicosities
  - Microscopic or gross hematuria can result from rupture of collateral veins into collecting system
  - May be exacerbated in upright position
- Associated abnormalities
  - Left flank or abdominal pain
  - Hematuria
  - Mild to moderate proteinuria
  - Pediatric chronic fatigue syndrome
  - Female pelvic varicosities

- Male varicoceles

Gross Pathologic & Surgical Features

- Fibrosis may be present between aorta and SMA, where left renal vein courses

Microscopic Features

- Renal biopsy shows spectrum from normal to mild or moderate mesangial proliferative nephritis

CLINICAL ISSUES

Presentation

- Most common signs/symptoms: Left flank and abdominal pain, with or without unilateral hematuria
- Other signs/symptoms
  - If left ovarian vein congestion and pelvic varicosities occur, can produce symptoms similar to pelvic congestion syndrome
  - If varicocele occurs in male can produce testicular pain, infertility
- Clinical Profile
  - Two age distributions, with somewhat different presentations
    - Thin young woman with recent substantial weight loss who has new onset of vague flank pain and hematuria
    - Pediatric patient with microscopic hematuria and associated mild to moderate proteinuria that may be orthostatic, or with sudden onset of dark urine

Demographics

- Age: Pediatric and young adult
- Gender: Males and females equally affected

Natural History & Prognosis

- Childhood nutcracker syndrome may be a transient phenomenon resolving spontaneously with time by physical development
- As venous collateral vessels develop, left renal venous hypertension may resolve
- Extensive venous collateral development may result in female pelvic congestion syndrome or male varicocele

Treatment

- Options, risks, complications
  - Patients with mild, tolerable symptoms may be treated conservatively as left renal vein hypertension may eventually resolve with development of collateral veins
  - Persistent, recurrent or massive hematuria is an indication for treatment
  - Open surgical and transcatheter endovascular treatments designed to lower intrarenal venous pressure by removing renal vein outflow obstruction
    - Surgical treatments in severe cases have included nephrectomy, left renal vein reanastomosis to IVC and autotransplantation of the left kidney
    - Reported endovascular treatments have included angioplasty and intravascular stent placement
    - Currently no consensus on indication for and success of endovascular treatment

DIAGNOSTIC CHECKLIST

Consider

- Nutcracker syndrome in pediatric patient with hematuria and proteinuria
- Nutcracker syndrome in differential diagnosis of young female who presents with vague flank, pelvic or abdominal pain and hematuria
- Nutcracker syndrome as a possible etiology or a contributing factor to symptoms of pelvic congestion syndrome in female patients or left-sided varicocele in male patients

Image Interpretation Pearls

- Compression of left renal vein between aorta and SMA on US, CECT or MRV is non-diagnostic for nutcracker syndrome in absence of intrarenal or perirenal varices unless pressure gradient demonstrated by Doppler measurements or direct venous manometry

SELECTED REFERENCES

1. Fitoz S et al: Nutcracker syndrome in children: the role of upright position examination and superior mesenteric artery angle measurement in the diagnosis. J Ultrasound Med. 26(5):573-80, 2007
2. Scholbach T: From the nutcracker-phenomenon of the left renal vein to the midline congestion syndrome as a cause of migraine, headache, back and abdominal pain and functional disorders of pelvic organs. Med Hypotheses. 68(6):1318-27, 2007
3. Shin JI et al: Doppler ultrasonographic indices in diagnosing nutcracker syndrome in children. Pediatr Nephrol. 22(3):409-13, 2007
4. Shin JI et al: Effect of renal Doppler ultrasound on the detection of nutcracker syndrome in children with hematuria. Eur J Pediatr. 166(5):399-404, 2007
5. Zhang H et al: The left renal entrapment syndrome: diagnosis and treatment. Ann Vasc Surg. 21(2):198-203, 2007
6. Ahmed K et al: Current trends in the diagnosis and management of renal nutcracker syndrome: a review. Eur J Vasc Endovasc Surg. 31(4):410-6, 2006
7. Culafic D et al: Spontaneous splenorenal shunt in a patient with liver cirrhosis and hypertrophic caudal lobe. J Gastrointestin Liver Dis. 15(3):289-92, 2006
8. Rudloff U et al: Mesoaortic compression of the left renal vein (nutcracker syndrome): case reports and review of the literature. Ann Vasc Surg. 20(1):120-9, 2006
9. Chang CT et al: Nutcracker syndrome and left unilateral haematuria. Nephrol Dial Transplant. 20(2):460-1, 2005
10. Cuellar i Calabria H et al: Nutcracker or left renal vein compression phenomenon: multidetector computed tomography findings and clinical significance. Eur Radiol. 15(8):1745-51, 2005
11. Hartung O et al: Endovascular stenting in the treatment of pelvic vein congestion caused by nutcracker syndrome: lessons learned from the first five cases. J Vasc Surg. 42(2):275-80, 2005
12. Kim SJ et al: Long-term follow-up after endovascular stent placement for treatment of nutcracker syndrome. J Vasc Interv Radiol. 16(3):428-31, 2005
13. Yu G et al: The nutcracker syndrome. J Urol. 169(6):2293-4, 2003

IMAGE GALLERY

Typical

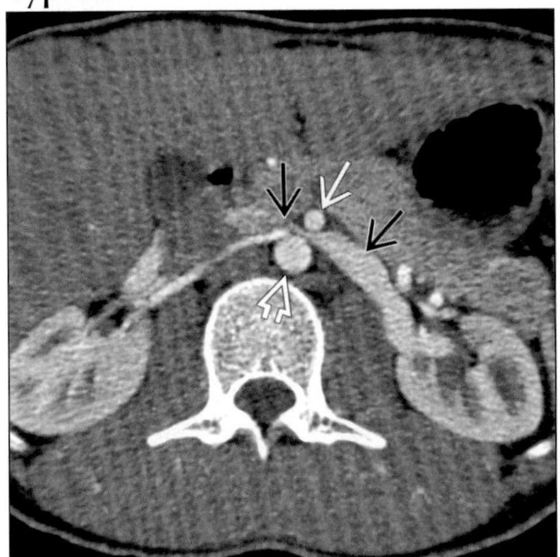

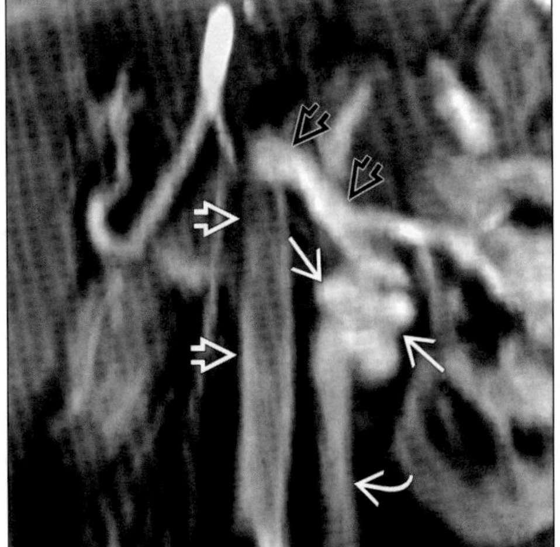

(Left) *Axial CECT shows left renal vein ⇒ compressed between the abdominal aorta ➡ and the superior mesenteric artery ➡. Note that the degree of compression exceeds 50%.* ***(Right)*** *Coronal reformatted 3-D CTA in the same patient as previous image, shows the dilated left renal vein ⇒ coursing anterior to the abdominal aorta ➡. Note the extensive perihilar renal varices ➡ and the dilated gonadal vein ➡.*

Typical

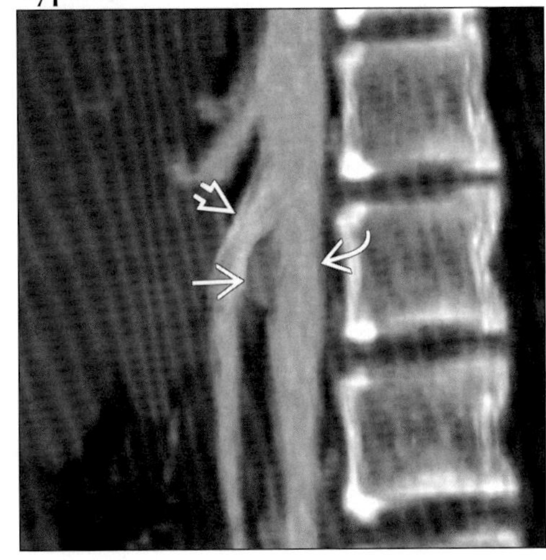

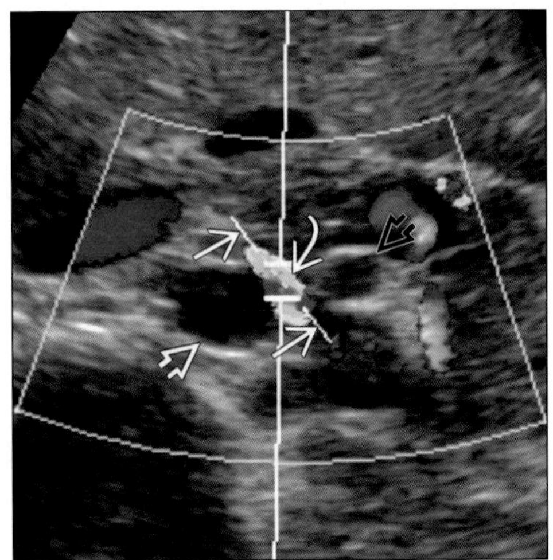

(Left) *Sagittal reformatted 3-D CTA in the same patient as previous image, shows the left renal vein ➡ compressed within the fork formed by the abdominal aorta ➡ and the superior mesenteric artery ➡.* ***(Right)*** *Color Doppler ultrasound shows cursor ➡ positioned within the left renal vein ➡ where it is compressed between the abdominal aorta ➡ and the SMA ⇒. Velocity measurements confirmed a gradient produced by the compression.*

Typical

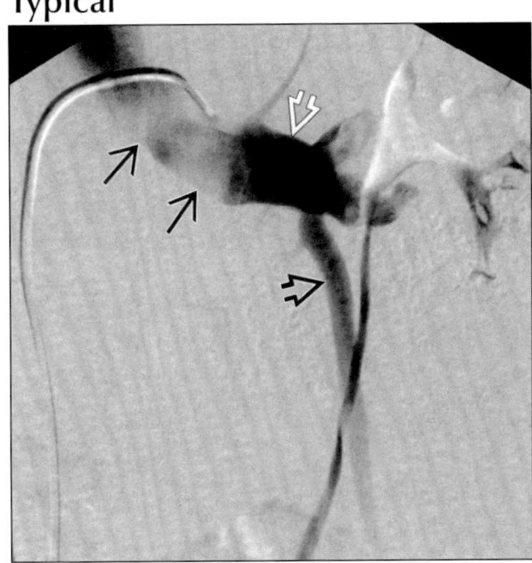

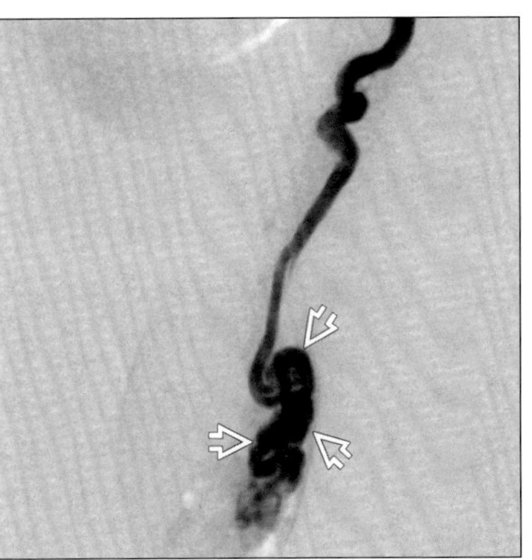

(Left) *Left renal venogram shows dilated renal vein ➡ and contrast reflux into the left gonadal vein ⇒. The contrast is less dense in the middle 1/3 of the renal vein ⇒ where it is compressed between the aorta and the SMA.* ***(Right)*** *Left gonadal venogram in the same patient as previous image, shows a varicocele ➡ that has resulted from the venous hypertension produced by compression of the left renal vein between the aorta and the SMA.*

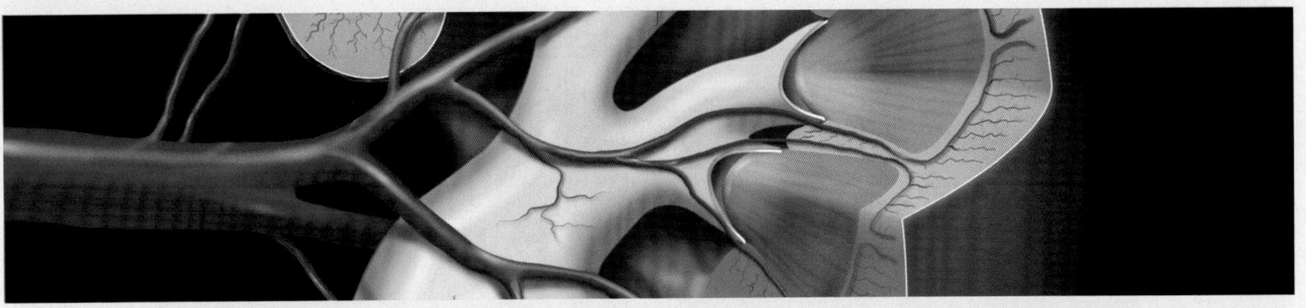

SECTION 6: Renal

Introduction and Overview

Renal

RENAL VASCULATURE

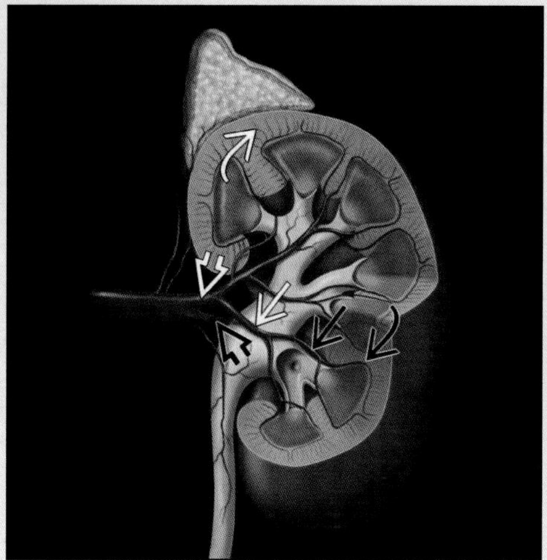

Graphic shows anterior and posterior divisions of the renal artery, dividing into segmental branches and then into interlobar arteries. These yield arcuate arteries that terminate as interlobular arteries.

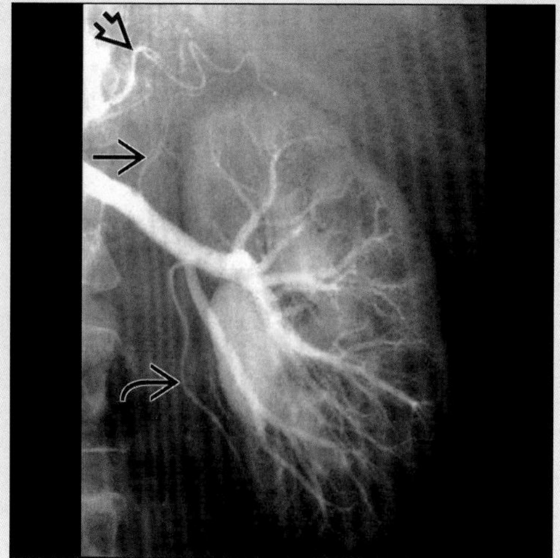

Catheter angiography shows the normal renal arterial branching pattern, as depicted in the graphic. Additionally, the inferior adrenal, ureteral, and renal capsular arteries are well-demonstrated.

TERMINOLOGY

Abbreviations

- Renal artery (RA)
- Renal vein (RV)
- Arteriovenous malformation (AVM)
- Arteriovenous fistula (AVF)
- Fibromuscular dysplasia (FMD)
- Segmental arterial mediolysis (SAM)
- Superior mesenteric artery (SMA)
- Inferior vena cava (IVC)

IMAGING ANATOMY

Anatomic Relationships

- Each kidney typically supplied by main renal artery
  - Originate from abdominal aorta below SMA
    - Right RA arises anterolaterally from aorta; courses posterior to IVC and right RV
    - Left RA origin more lateral; posterior to left RV
  - Each RA usually 4-6 cm long, 5-6 mm diameter
  - RA bifurcates at renal hilus into anterior and posterior divisions
    - Anterior division supplies upper and lower poles, anterior mid-kidney
    - Posterior division supplies posterior renal parenchyma; some additional upper and lower pole supply
  - Anterior and posterior divisions yield segmental (apical, upper, middle, lower, posterior) arteries
    - Segmental arteries yield interlobar arteries
    - Interlobar arteries divide into arcuate arteries at corticomedullary junction
    - Arcuate arteries terminate as interlobular arteries that supply glomeruli
- Kidneys may have one or more accessory renal arteries
  - Variability to amount of perfused renal parenchyma
- Superior adrenal arteries arise from phrenic arteries; middle adrenal arteries directly from aorta
- Inferior adrenal, renal capsular and ureteral arteries arise from proximal main RAs
- Left renal vein crosses anterior to aorta to join IVC; short right renal vein drains directly into IVC
  - Left adrenal and gonadal veins drain into main renal vein; on right drain directly into IVC

ANATOMY-BASED IMAGING ISSUES

Imaging Approaches

- Ultrasound images renal parenchyma, collecting system, vascular structures
  - Color flow duplex assesses renal arteries
  - Doppler evaluation of arterial waveforms, velocities, resistive indices
- Nuclear medicine evaluates renal function
  - Assesses glomerular filtration of isotope bound agent
- CECT/CTA highly sensitive in detecting vascular pathology, masses
  - Depicts normal/abnormal vascular anatomy
  - Characterizes vascularity, components of renal mass
- MRI provides detailed vascular anatomic information
  - MRA characterizes vascular pathology, renal masses
- Conventional angiography confirms suspected vascular pathology
  - May be combined with catheter-based interventions

PATHOLOGIC ISSUES

General Pathologic Considerations

- Renal arteries are end arteries; poor collateral pathways
  - In presence of stenosis may form capsular, ureteral, adrenal and retroperitoneal collaterals
    - Sufficient to perfuse kidney but inadequate for normal renal function

Pathology Involving Renal Vasculature

- Renal artery occlusive disease
  - Atherosclerosis
    - Most common cause of stenosis/occlusion (90%)
    - Older patients; more commonly male
  - Dissection

RENAL VASCULATURE

Imaging of Renal Vasculature

Ultrasound
- Color-flow duplex imaging of renal arteries; Doppler analysis used in screening for renal artery stenosis
- Excellent for imaging renal parenchyma; characterizing masses as solid vs. cystic

CECT/CTA
- High sensitivity and specificity for identifying and characterizing renal vascular pathology, masses

MRI/MRA
- Delineates parenchymal and vascular pathology
- Gadolinium enhancement expands sensitivity

Angiography
- Usually follows positive non-invasive imaging study
- Provides imaging for endovascular interventions

Nuclear Medicine
- Functional information; infers presence of stenosis

        - Spontaneous, associated with thoracoabdominal aortic dissection
        - Iatrogenic; catheter-associated procedures
    - Fibromuscular dysplasia (FMD)
        - Younger patients; more commonly female
        - Medial fibroplasia in 80% of patients
    - Neurofibromatosis
        - May cause abdominal aortic coarctation; associated visceral and renal artery stenoses
    - Segmental medial arteriolysis (SAM)
        - Nonatherosclerotic, noninflammatory arterial entity; medial necrosis and mediolysis
        - Resultant arterial dissections, aneurysms; similar appearance to FMD; poor response to angioplasty
    - Vasculitis
        - Polyarteritis nodosa most common vasculitis affecting peripheral visceral and renal arteries
        - Takayasu arteritis may affect renal and visceral artery origins
- Renal arteriovenous malformation and fistulas
    - Congenital AVM rare; AVF usually acquired
    - Iatrogenic or trauma causes > 70% AVF
- Renal artery aneurysm
    - Rare lesions; most often degenerative (atherosclerosis) or associated with FMD
    - Other associations: Vasculitis, trauma, iatrogenic, neoplasms, mycotic, Ehlers-Danlos syndrome
- Renal neoplasm
    - Benign
        - Angiomyolipoma
        - Oncocytoma
        - Adenoma
    - Malignant
        - Renal cell carcinoma
        - Transitional cell carcinoma
        - Wilm tumor
        - Lymphoma
        - Metastasis
    - Renal vein thrombosis
        - Benign
        - Associated with renal neoplasm
- Nutcracker syndrome
    - Compression of left RV between aorta and SMA
- Trauma
    - Iatrogenic
    - Blunt
    - Penetrating

RELATED REFERENCES

1. Ardalan MR et al: Do mechanical fluid laws dictate the branching pattern of the renal artery? Transplant Proc. 40(1):111-3, 2008
2. Herborn CU et al: MR angiography of the renal arteries: intraindividual comparison of double-dose contrast enhancement at 1.5 T with standard dose at 3 T. AJR Am J Roentgenol. 190(1):173-7, 2008
3. Lockhart ME et al: Renal vascular imaging: ultrasound and other modalities. Ultrasound Q. 23(4):279-92, 2007
4. Sabharwal R et al: Multidetector spiral CT renal angiography in the diagnosis of renal artery fibromuscular dysplasia. Eur J Radiol. 61(3):520-7, 2007

IMAGE GALLERY

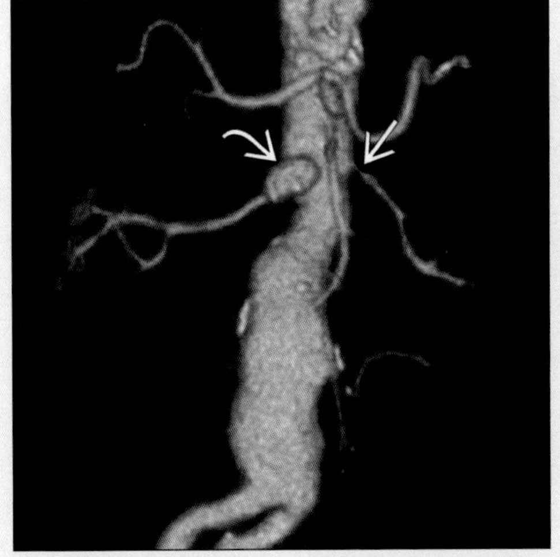

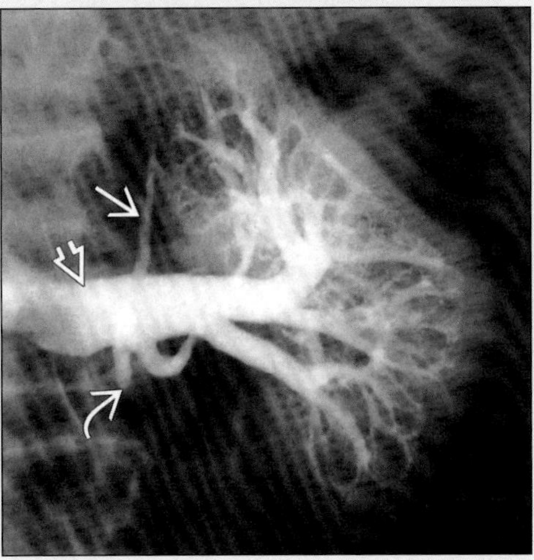

(Left) *VR 3-D CTA shows a severe left renal artery origin stenosis ➔ and an aneurysm ➔ of the right renal artery origin. High quality reformatted CECT and CTA images provide excellent anatomic detail of the renal arteries and may be used in planning surgical or endovascular therapy.* ***(Right)*** *Normal left renal venogram shows the left adrenal vein ➔ draining into the main left renal vein ➔. Each adrenal gland normally has a single vein, in contrast to the multiple arteries that are typically present. There is trace reflux into a normal appearing left gonadal vein ➔.*

RENAL ARTERY ATHEROSCLEROSIS

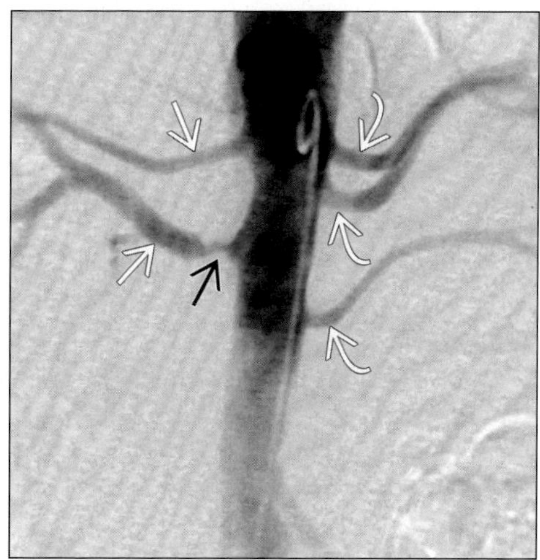

DSA abdominal aortogram shows a high grade right renal artery stenosis involving the arterial ostium. The right kidney is supplied by two renal arteries and the left kidney by three renal arteries.

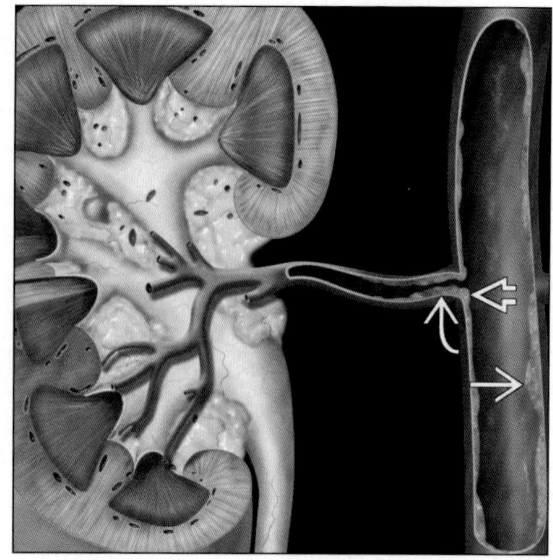

Graphic shows atherosclerotic plaque in the aorta and right renal artery. The aortic plaque causes ostial narrowing. The plaque extends from the aorta into the renal artery lumen, causing proximal stenosis.

TERMINOLOGY

Abbreviations and Synonyms

- Renal artery atherosclerosis, atherosclerotic renal artery stenosis, renal artery stenosis (RAS)

Definitions

- Narrowing of renal artery lumen
- Occlusion of renal arterial lumen

IMAGING FINDINGS

General Features

- Best diagnostic clue
  - Focal or segmental luminal narrowing of renal artery
  - Smaller ipsilateral kidney
- Location
  - Renal artery ostium or within proximal 2 cm
    - Renal artery branch involvement not common
  - Can be bilateral in up to 75% of patients
- Size: Discrepancy in renal size of > 2 cm

Radiographic Findings

- Radiography
  - Asymmetric renal shadows; smaller kidney has renal artery stenosis
  - Aortic or renal artery calcification
- IVP
  - Kidney: Normal (mild RAS); atrophic (high-grade stenosis or occlusion)
  - Delayed/absent nephrogram
  - Delayed contrast excretion and clearing from collecting system
    - Increased density of contrast
  - Ureteral notching from collateral arteries

CT Findings

- NECT
  - Unilateral or bilateral renal atrophy
  - Aortic and renal artery wall calcification
    - Calcified hard plaque; low density soft plaque
- CECT
  - Delayed nephrogram and contrast excretion
  - Hyperdense or persistent nephrogram
  - Cortical and parenchymal thinning
- CTA

DDx: Renal Artery Narrowing

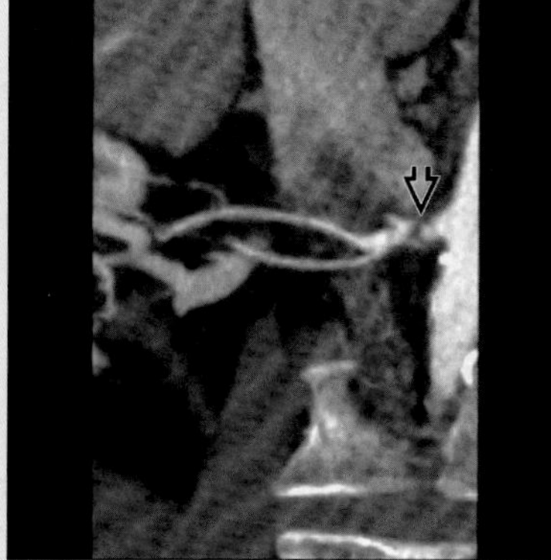

Dissection with Thrombus

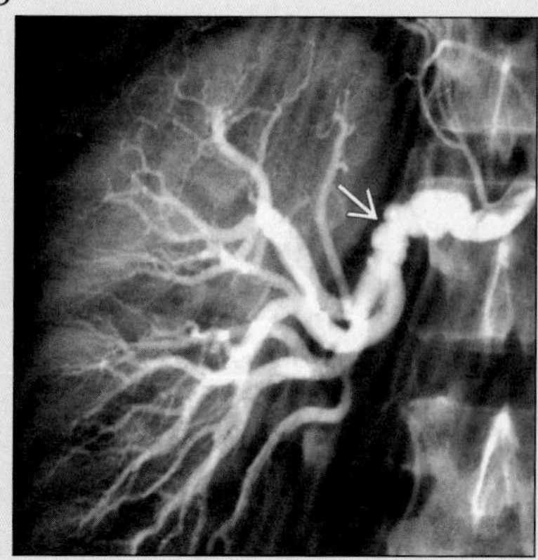

Fibromuscular Dysplasia

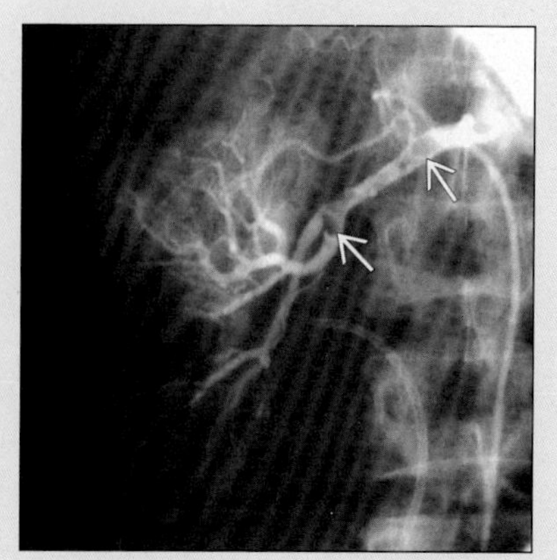

Renal Artery Thromboemboli

RENAL ARTERY ATHEROSCLEROSIS

Key Facts

Terminology

- Atherosclerotic renal artery stenosis

Imaging Findings

- Focal or segmental renal artery narrowing at ostium or within 2 cm
- > 2 cm discrepancy in renal size
- Delayed contrast excretion and clearing from collecting system
- Cortical and parenchymal thinning
- Absent cortico-medullary differentiation
- CTA with MIP, volume-rendering, and reformatted images demonstrate origins of all renal arteries
- US: Elevated peak systolic velocity: 100-200 cm/sec ⇒ < 50% stenosis; > 200 cm/sec ⇒ 50-99% stenosis
- Angiography "gold standard" for renovascular hypertension diagnosis; invasive, reserved for endovascular treatment
- > 50% renal artery stenosis corresponds to ~ 20 mmHg gradient between renal artery and aorta

Clinical Issues

- Intervention may be indicated when one or more 1° renal functions affected
- Hypertension
  - Correction of stenosis can result in resolution, improvement or no change

Diagnostic Checklist

- Consider renal artery stenosis in patient with asymmetric renal size
- Rule out other causes of renal artery stenosis

  - Renal artery narrowing within 2 cm of ostium
  - Truncal renal artery stenosis beyond proximal 2 cm
  - Locations and origins of all renal arteries

MR Findings

- T1WI
  - Small kidney, with variable signal intensity
  - Absent cortico-medullary differentiation
  - Cortical thinning with 2° parenchymal thinning
- T2WI: Small kidney, with variable signal intensity
- T1 C+: Decreased and delayed nephrogram

Nuclear Medicine Findings

- ACE inhibitor renography
  - Delayed radiotracer uptake and excretion in affected kidney; time to peak > 30 minutes
  - Ratio of 20 min/peak cortical activity > 0.3

Ultrasonographic Findings

- Grayscale Ultrasound
  - Smaller kidney with chronic, significant stenosis
  - Increased echogenicity of parenchyma
- Pulsed Doppler
  - Increased peak systolic velocity: 100-200 cm/sec ⇒ < 50% stenosis; > 200 cm/sec ⇒ 50-99% stenosis
  - Renal-to-aortic ratio of peak systolic velocity > 3.5
  - Post-stenotic turbulence and spectral broadening with or without flow reversal
  - Absent flow denotes occlusion
  - Early systolic acceleration: < 20-30 cm/sec (best predictor)
  - Pulsus tardus-parvus: Low velocity renal artery waveform with delayed acceleration
  - Resistive index: < 5% on affected side compared to normal side
- Color Doppler
  - Color aliasing at stenosis (systolic turbulence)
  - Soft tissue "thrill" or vibration

Angiographic Findings

- DSA
  - "Gold standard" for diagnosis, intervention
    - Focal, segmental, eccentric or concentric stenoses
    - Ostial lesion: Proximal 2 cm of renal artery
    - Post-stenotic dilatation; collateral vessels
    - > 50% renal artery stenosis corresponds to ~ 20 mmHg gradient between renal artery and aorta
    - Option for transcatheter intervention
  - CO_2 angiography in patients with renal failure
- Renal vein sampling can be performed at same time
  - Infrequently used technique

Imaging Recommendations

- Best imaging tool
  - Angiography "gold standard"; used for endovascular treatment
  - CTA with MIP, volume-rendering, reformatting
    - Limited in patient with renal insufficiency
- Protocol advice
  - Imaging after appropriate history and physical, high index of suspicion
  - MR: Multiplanar, 3-D C+, dark blood, 2-D TOF, phase contrast sequences
    - Include adrenal glands to exclude adrenal pathology as etiology for hypertension
  - Color Doppler US (3.5-MHz curvilinear probe); requires accurate Doppler angle of ≤ 60°
  - CECT/MR: Confirm findings on multiple images

DIFFERENTIAL DIAGNOSIS

Arterial Dissection

- Aortic dissection extending into renal artery, post-traumatic or iatrogenic renal artery dissection
- False or occluded lumen and intimal flap

Vasculitis

- Polyarteritis nodosa; Takayasu arteritis

Thromboembolism

- Filling defects in main renal artery or branches
- Acute onset of symptoms

Fibromuscular Dysplasia

- Classic "string-of-beads" appearance to renal artery
- Typically young female, acute onset of hypertension

RENAL ARTERY ATHEROSCLEROSIS

PATHOLOGY

General Features

- Etiology: Atherosclerosis (60-90%)
- Epidemiology
  - Renovascular hypertension: 2° to renal artery occlusive disease
    - Accounts for 1-4% of patients with hypertension
    - Most common cause of 2° hypertension
  - Atherosclerotic disease
    - Most common cause of RAS (65-70%)
    - Uncommon cause of hypertension (5%)

Gross Pathologic & Surgical Features

- Eccentric plaque in ostium or proximal renal artery
- Mild renal artery stenosis: Normal-sized kidney
- Moderate-severe renal artery stenosis: Atrophic kidney
- Post-stenotic dilatation of main renal artery; collaterals

Microscopic Features

- Complex fibrous plaque with calcification, hemorrhage, cholesterol, and thrombus

Staging, Grading or Classification Criteria

- ≥ 50% narrowing of renal artery diameter thought to be hemodynamically significant

CLINICAL ISSUES

Presentation

- Most common signs/symptoms
  - Hypertension
    - New onset or malignant
    - Requires > 3 medications to control hypertension
    - Acute worsening of previously controlled hypertension
  - Progressive or acute renal impairment
  - Mild stenoses may be asymptomatic
- Other signs/symptoms
  - Stenotic renal artery with embolization causes acute occlusion
    - Acute flank or abdominal pain
    - Acute renal insufficiency or failure
    - Fever, nausea, and vomiting
- Clinical Profile
  - Patients with peripheral vascular disease (PVD) and/or coronary artery disease (CAD)
  - Risk factors: Hypertension, hyperlipidemia, smoking, diabetes mellitus
- Lab data
  - Positive captopril test
    - Exaggerated increased plasma renin activity

Demographics

- Age: > 50 years
- Gender: M > F

Natural History & Prognosis

- Stenosis progression in untreated patients (40-50%)
  - Progression to thrombosis or occlusion
- Complications
  - Severe hypertension: Chronic untreated hypertension results in nephrosclerosis
  - Renal insufficiency or renal failure 2° to ischemic nephropathy

Treatment

- Options, risks, complications
  - Intervention may be indicated when one or more 1° renal functions affected
    - Refractory blood pressure control; worsening or malignant hypertension
    - Volume control may cause recurrent congestive heart failure, flash pulmonary edema
    - Decreased glomerular filtration may cause progressive renal insufficiency or failure
  - Treatment of stenosis can result in resolution, improvement or no change in hypertension
    - If no change, diagnose hypertension as "essential"
    - Mixed response with renal insufficiency/failure
    - Intervention has somewhat controversial role; 1/3 of patients improve, but 1/3 unchanged and 1/3 worsened; atheroemboli to renal bed may occur
- Medical management
  - Angiotensin-converting enzyme (ACE) inhibitors, diuretic therapy, β-blockers
- Endovascular management
  - Percutaneous transluminal angioplasty treatment of choice when intervention indicated
    - Minimally invasive; 80% success rate in non-ostial lesions, 30% in ostial lesions
  - Primary stent placement with ostial lesions
    - Stents also used if suboptimal PTA result or complications
- Surgical management
  - Anatomic or extra-anatomic bypass: Extra-anatomic more common because of decreased morbidity
  - Endarterectomy: Technically challenging, high risk
  - Surgical revascularization: 80-90% success rate
  - Nephrectomy: Typically reserved for kidneys with < 10% renal function

DIAGNOSTIC CHECKLIST

Consider

- Rule out other causes of renal artery stenosis
- Renal artery stenosis with asymmetric renal size

Image Interpretation Pearls

- Renal artery narrowing at ostium or within 2 cm of ostium typical of atherosclerotic stenosis

SELECTED REFERENCES

1. Gray BH: Intervention for renal artery stenosis: endovascular and surgical roles. J Hypertens Suppl. 23(3):S23-9, 2005
2. Gross CM et al: Determination of renal arterial stenosis severity: comparison of pressure gradient and vessel diameter. Radiology. 220(3):751-6, 2001
3. Prince MR et al: Hemodynamically significant atherosclerotic renal artery stenosis: MR angiographic features. Radiology. 205(1):128-36, 1997

IMAGE GALLERY

Typical

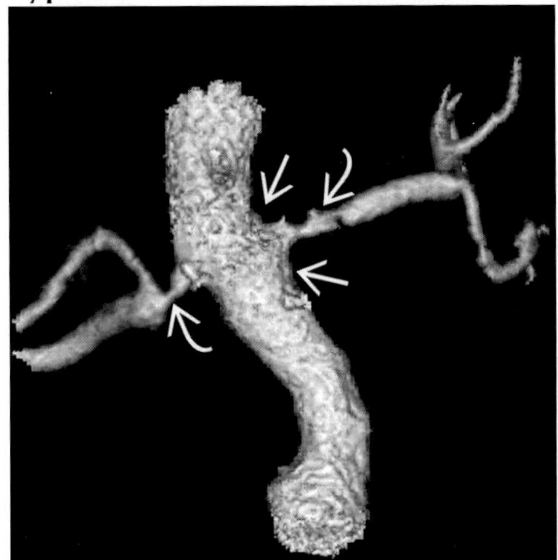

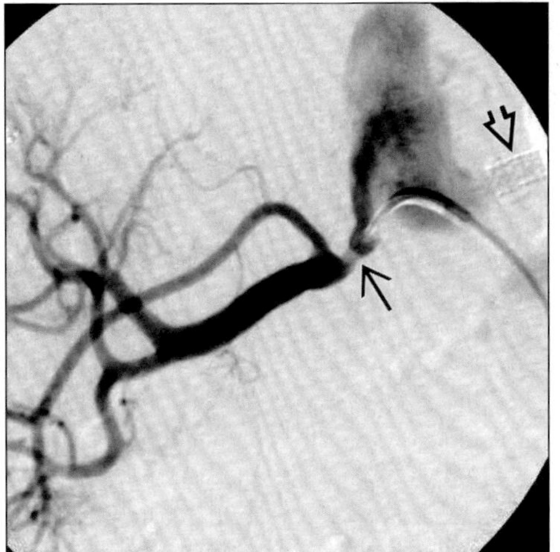

(Left) *3-D CTA shows stenoses of the ostia and proximal portions of both renal arteries, typical of atherosclerotic disease. Note the scalloped margins of the aortic wall adjacent to the renal arterial origin, consistent with aortic plaque encroaching on the ostium.* ***(Right)*** *Selective right renal arteriogram shows a high grade right renal artery stenosis, corresponding to the CTA findings. The left renal artery had been stented two weeks before this study.*

Typical

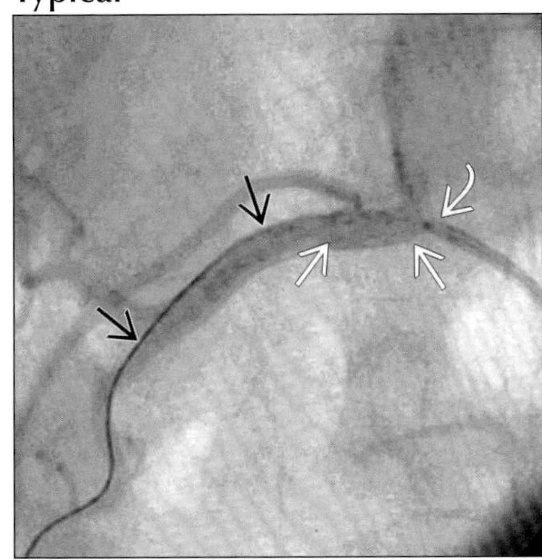

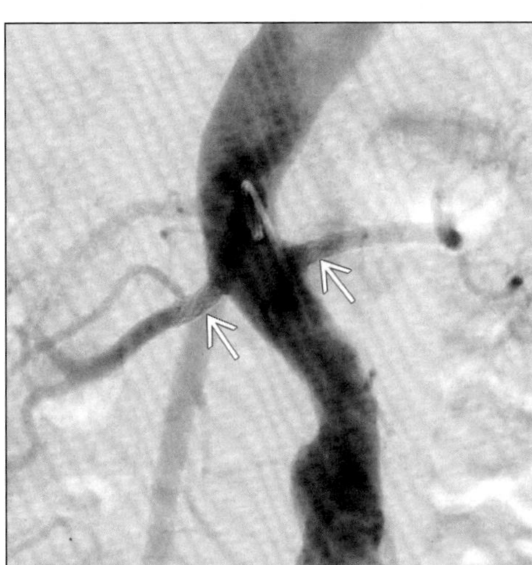

(Left) *Right renal arteriogram shows a guiding catheter at the right renal artery origin. A balloon mounted stent has been introduced over the guidewire and placed across the stenosis. When intervention is indicated, primary stenting is the treatment of choice for renal ostial lesions, as they respond poorly to primary angioplasty.* ***(Right)*** *Abdominal aortogram following bilateral renal artery stents shows patent main renal arteries.*

Typical

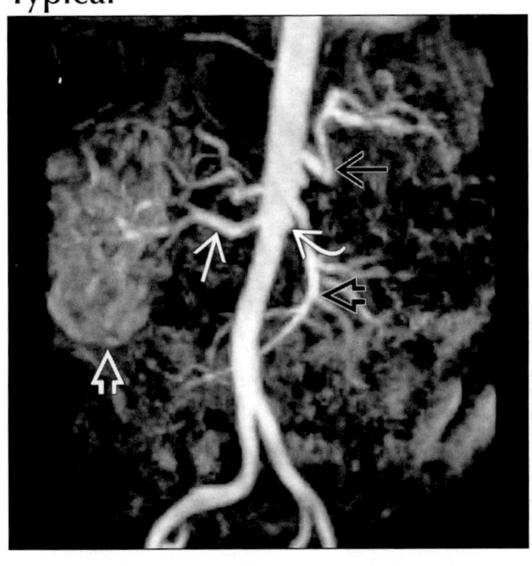

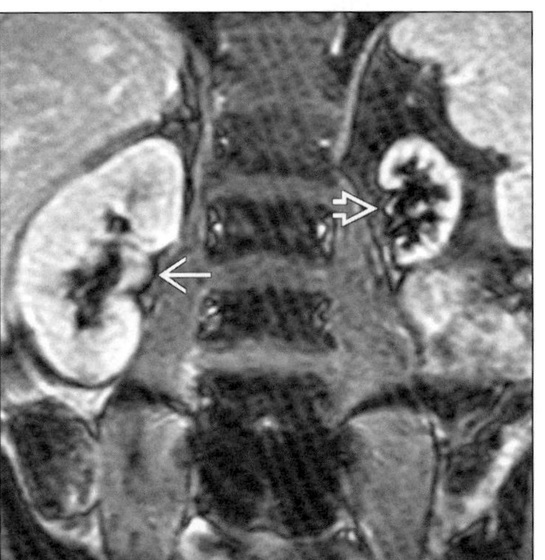

(Left) *Coronal oblique MIP MRA shows complete occlusion of the left renal artery at the origin. The left kidney is not seen, while the right renal artery and the right kidney are visible. The celiac and superior mesenteric arteries are patent.* ***(Right)*** *Coronal T1WI FS MR in the same patient shows marked asymmetry of the kidneys. The left kidney is severely atrophic, consistent with chronic ischemia from renal artery occlusion. The right kidney is normal in appearance.*

FIBROMUSCULAR DYSPLASIA, RENAL

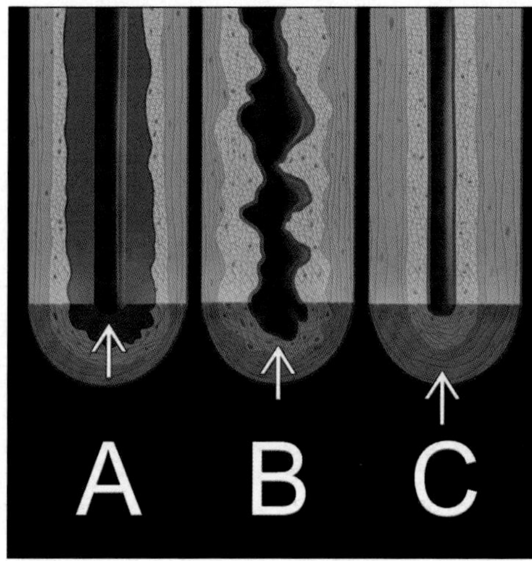

Graphic shows the three main subtypes of fibromuscular dysplasia or FMD: A) Intimal B) Medial C) Perimedial. The ➔ indicates the layer involved in the disease process.

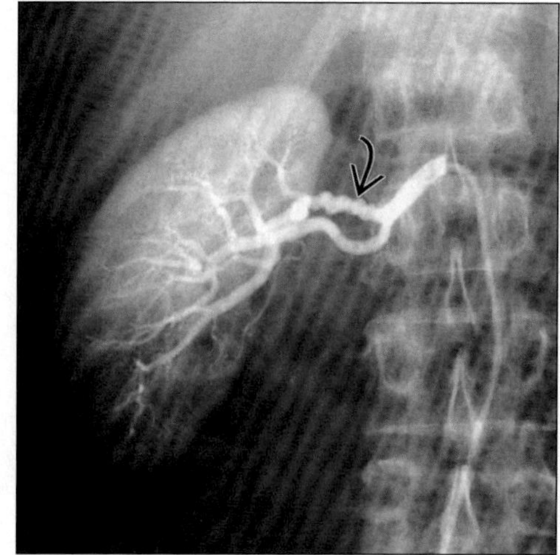

Posteroanterior conventional angiography shows classic beaded appearance ⇗ of right renal artery FMD. The affected area of involvement is the mid-to-distal segment of the renal artery, which is typical of FMD.

TERMINOLOGY

Abbreviations and Synonyms

- Fibromuscular dysplasia (FMD); fibromuscular hyperplasia; fibromuscular fibroplasia; arterial fibrodysplasia; medial hyperplasia

Definitions

- Idiopathic non-inflammatory, non-atherosclerotic disorder of small to medium-sized arteries
  - Characterized by dysplastic segmental overgrowth of smooth muscle and fibrous tissue

IMAGING FINDINGS

General Features

- Best diagnostic clue
  - Multifocal renal artery (RA) stenoses and aneurysms
    - "String-of-beads" angiographic appearance
    - Serial circular ridges encroach on arterial lumen
    - Diameter of aneurysmal portion > native vessel
- Location
  - Principally affects mid to distal main RA in 79%
    - Can occasionally affect renal artery branches
  - Bilateral in 50-65%; unilaterally more on right
  - Can affect carotid, visceral, extremity arteries
  - Rarely involves coronaries, pulmonary artery, aorta
- Morphology
  - Sequential areas of narrowing and dilatation resulting in "string-of-beads" appearance (62%)
  - Smooth, long-segment stenoses (14%)
  - Focal (< 1 cm) stenoses (7%)
  - Multiple morphologies (17%)

Radiographic Findings

- IVP
  - KUB and nephrogram shows small or asymmetric kidneys suggesting renal artery stenosis
  - Irregular renal contour suggests atrophy or infarct
  - Unilateral delayed nephrogram with delayed contrast excretion and washout

CT Findings

- CECT
  - Discrepant renal sizes
  - Evidence of prior renal infarct or global ischemia
- CTA
  - Multifocal stenoses, ringed ridges, "string of beads"

DDx: Beaded Appearance of Renal Artery

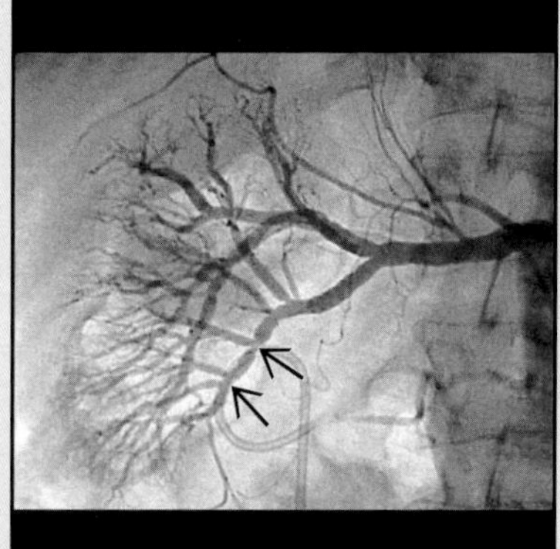

Irregularity of Vasculitis

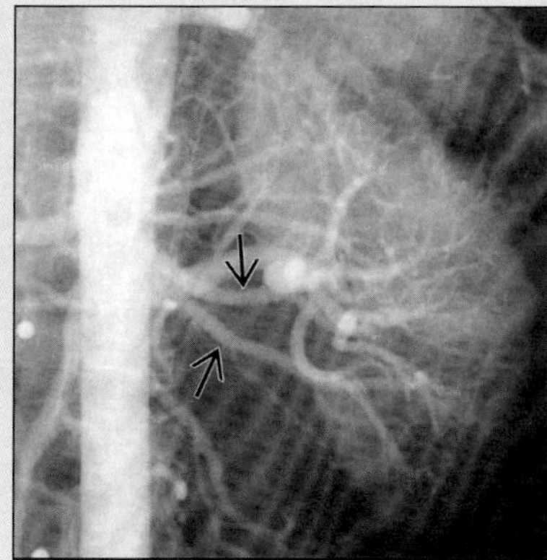

Standing Waves

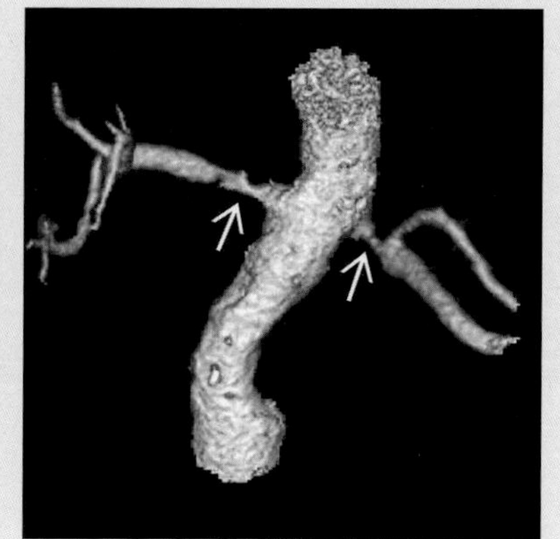

Atherosclerotic Stenosis

FIBROMUSCULAR DYSPLASIA, RENAL

Key Facts

Terminology
- FMD, fibromuscular hyperplasia, fibromuscular fibroplasia, arterial fibrodysplasia, medial hyperplasia
- Dysplastic arterial wall disorder characterized by overgrowth of smooth muscle and fibrous tissue

Imaging Findings
- "String-of-beads" angiographic appearance
- Principally affects mid to distal main RA in 79%
- CT angiography with reformations is the best non-invasive imaging tool for FMD
- DSA remains the "gold standard" for diagnosis of FMD
- DSA performed with intent to treat abnormality

Pathology
- Classification of FMD based on which arterial wall layer is predominantly involved

Clinical Issues
- Female predominance (1:3-5) in all types of FMD except intimal fibroplasia
- Most commonly presents in young to middle age adults
- Renovascular HTN
- Majority of patients with FMD are asymptomatic
- Indolent, slowly progressive disorder
- Balloon angioplasty is treatment of choice
- Long-term angioplasty and surgical results are excellent

Diagnostic Checklist
- "String-of-beads" appearance of renal artery in young female with new onset hypertension suggests FMD
- FMD should be considered in child or young adult with acute or refractory HTN

    - Involves mid to distal main RA or hilar branches
  - Accessory renal arteries may also be affected by FMD

MR Findings
- T1WI
  - Atrophic kidney if significant chronic ischemia
  - Cortico-medullary thinning
- T1 C+: Delayed nephrogram and excretory phases
- MRA: Similar findings demonstrated by CTA with beaded appearance or stenosis
- MIP images evaluate arteries in multiple obliquities

Nuclear Medicine Findings
- Tc-99m MAG-3 or Tc-99m DTPA Captopril renography
  - Positive scan seen in patients with renovascular hypertension (HTN) and hemodynamically significant RAS (< 60-70% luminal narrowing)
    - Delayed or decreased perfusion of affected kidney
    - Delayed excretion of affected kidney
    - Prolonged washout of affected kidney
  - Difficulty diagnosing bilateral disease due to symmetric findings

Ultrasonographic Findings
- Grayscale Ultrasound
  - Distinguishing findings only seen with excellent resolution (e.g., in children)
  - Visible ridges, thickening of artery wall, +/- stenosis
  - Small or asymmetric renal size suggests RA stenosis
- Color Doppler
  - Elevated velocity, disturbed flow in areas of stenosis
  - Spectral broadening
  - Flow reversal or absent diastolic flow
- Intravascular ultrasound (IVUS)
  - Endoluminal filling defects
    - Membranous webs, folds, eccentric ridges

Angiographic Findings
- DSA
  - Beaded appearance of renal artery
    - May also have long and short segment stenoses
  - Curvilinear lucencies within vessel are intra-luminal webs; contribute to functional stenosis
  - Post-stenotic dilatation or aneurysms
  - Dissection or occasionally occlusion
  - Nephrogram and excretory findings as on IVP

Imaging Recommendations
- Best imaging tool
  - CT angiography with reformations is best non-invasive imaging tool
    - 92% specificity and 64% sensitivity
  - DSA remains "gold standard" for diagnosis
    - Performed with intent to treat
- MRA, CTA for noninvasive assessment; less accurate than DSA
- 3D contrast-enhanced MRA required for accurate RA diagnosis
- CTA is evolving; multidetector technology with reconstruction algorithms will improve accuracy
- Visualization of hilar RA branches essential
- US not 1° diagnostic method except in small children

DIFFERENTIAL DIAGNOSIS

Atherosclerosis
- Does not produce "string-of-beads" appearance
- Usually focal orificial renal artery stenosis
  - Up to 30% bilateral lesions
- Multifocal, distal or hilar branch stenosis uncommon
- Involves other vessels (e.g., aorta, carotid, coronary)

Arteritis or Vasculitis
- Other vessels involved
- Does not produce "string-of-beads" appearance
- Long segment narrowing mimics intimal FMD

Genetic Syndromes (Ehlers-Danlos, Williams)
- Renal and visceral arterial stenosis resembles FMD
- Diagnosis relies on physical findings associated with specific syndrome

Neurofibromatosis
- Neurofibromas in renal artery adventitia

- Aneurysms
- Involves renal artery origin; may be bilateral

Segmental Arterial Mediolysis

- Fundamentally a variant of fibromuscular dysplasia
  - Arterial wall thickening, dissection and multiple aneurysms of small abdominal arteries
  - Involves mesenteric and renal arteries
- Angiographic appearance may be indistinguishable from FMD; may have "string-of-beads"
- Responds poorly to angioplasty

Standing Waves

- String-of-beads appearance, but symmetrically spaced; more regular appearance of "beads"
- Transient finding

PATHOLOGY

General Features

- General path comments
  - Dysplastic, not degenerative or inflammatory
  - Characterized by overgrowth of smooth muscle cells and fibrous tissue within arterial wall
  - RA predominance, carotid & iliac arteries distant 2nd & 3rd in frequency
  - Alternating zones of hyperplasia and weakness; narrowing and dilatation appear as "string-of-beads"
  - Weakened areas may cause aneurysms or dissection
- Genetics
  - Not classic genetic disorder
    - 11% of cases familial; female predominance (90%)
- Etiology
  - Idiopathic
  - Studies suggest effects of environmental factors (smoking, hormones, renal mobility) and genetics

Microscopic Features

- Three main subtypes of FMD
  - Intimal FMD demonstrates erratically arranged mesenchymal cells, loose matrices of subendothelial connective tissue, fragmented internal elastic lamina
    - Manifests as focal, tubular narrowing
  - Medial FMD demonstrates homogeneous elastic tissue with areas of stenosis and outpouching; internal elastic lamina remains intact
    - Manifests as classic "string of beads"
  - Perimedial FMD demonstrates prolific tissue deposition at medial-adventitial junction
    - Manifests as tubular narrowing
- Combined subtypes can exist in same arterial segment

CLINICAL ISSUES

Presentation

- Most common signs/symptoms
  - Renovascular hypertension
  - Bruit over kidneys with auscultation
  - Majority of patients with FMD are asymptomatic
    - 0.4% prevalence of symptomatic renal FMD
    - 4.4% prevalence of asymptomatic renal FMD
- Other signs/symptoms
  - Symptoms mainly due to arterial stenosis/occlusion
    - Elevated plasma renin levels
    - Persistent flank or abdominal pain
    - Rarely acute dissection occurs causing renal infarct (acute flank pain, hematuria and escalating HTN)
    - Can have ischemia in other affected arterial beds
  - Complications include: Occlusion, post-stenotic aneurysm formation, dissection, distal embolization

Demographics

- Age
  - Presents at any age; most common in young/middle age adults: Age overlaps with atherosclerosis
  - Can be seen in pediatric population
- Gender: Female predominance in all types of FMD except intimal fibroplasia, which has equal or slightly higher male predominance

Natural History & Prognosis

- Indolent, slowly progressive disorder
  - Stenoses may worsen; occlusion rare
  - Microvasculature remains normal
    - Less renal failure/atrophy than atherosclerosis
- Excellent long-term angioplasty and surgical results

Treatment

- Balloon angioplasty is treatment of choice
  - > 95% cure/improvement of renovascular HTN
- Primary stenting of FMD not currently advocated
  - Stents used for angioplasty failure or complication
- Surgical bypass used infrequently; reserved for complex, distal involvement
- Medical management for long standing HTN and residual HTN post revascularization

DIAGNOSTIC CHECKLIST

Consider

- FMD in young adult with acute or refractory HTN

Image Interpretation Pearls

- "String-of-beads" appearance of renal artery in young female with new onset hypertension suggests FMD
- Cortical/medullary thinning reflect ischemic change

SELECTED REFERENCES

1. Plouin PF et al: Fibromuscular dysplasia. Orphanet J Rare Dis. 2:28, 2007
2. Moore WS: Vascular surgery: a comprehensive review, ed 6. Philadelphia, WB Saunders. 142-3, 295, 306-7, 2002
3. Beregi JP et al: Fibromuscular dysplasia of the renal arteries: Comparison of helical CT angiography and arteriography. AJR. 72:27-34, 1999
4. Papachristopoulos G et al: Breath-hold 3D MR angiography of the renal vasculature using a contrast-enhanced multiecho gradient-echo technique. Invest Radiol. 34: 731-8, 1999
5. Kincaid OW et al: Fibromuscular dysplasia of the renal arteries. Arteriographic features, classification, and observations on natural history of the disease. Am J Roentgenol Radium Ther Nucl Med. 104(2):271-82, 1968

FIBROMUSCULAR DYSPLASIA, RENAL

IMAGE GALLERY

Typical

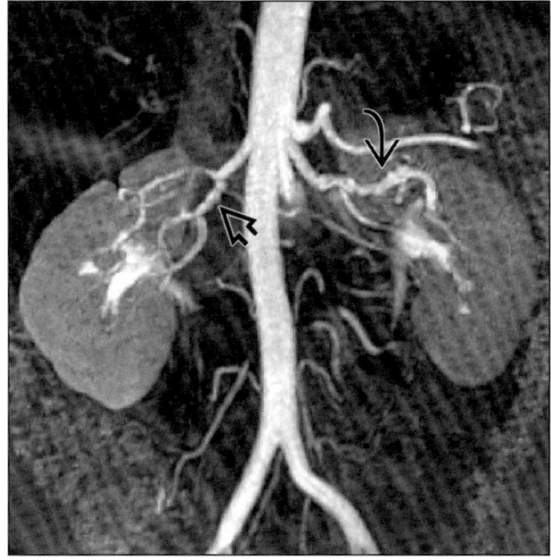

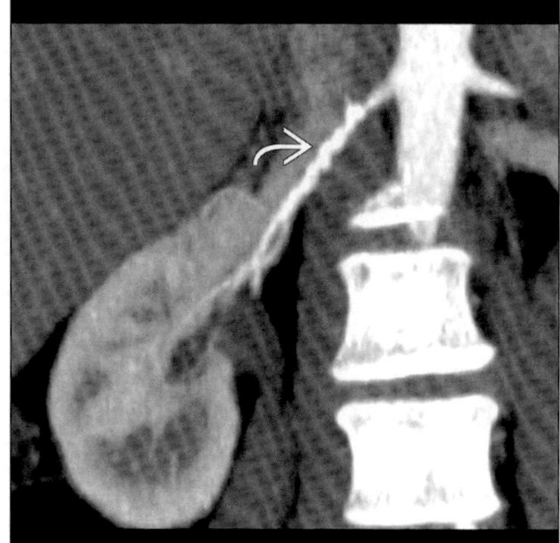

(Left) *Coronal MIP image show beaded appearance of the lower branch of the right renal artery and the upper branch of the left renal artery, a pattern that fits the classic description of FMD.* ***(Right)*** *Coronal oblique CTA shows irregular, beaded appearance of the right renal artery consistent with FMD. CTA and MRA are used for screening, but are currently less sensitive and specific than DSA, which remains the "gold standard".*

Other

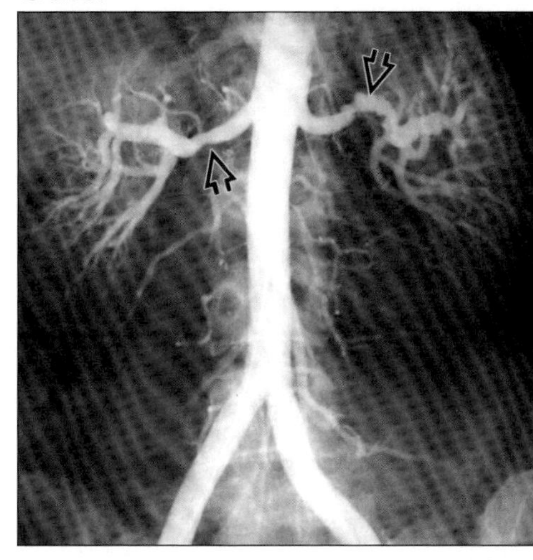

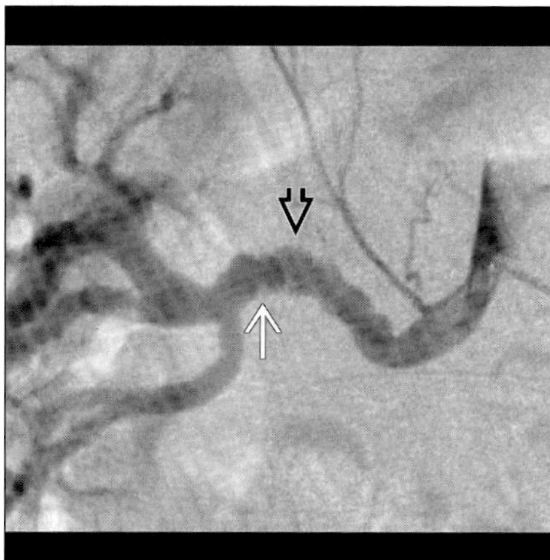

(Left) *Abdominal aortogram shows bilateral involvement of the renal arteries with FMD. Note that the right renal lesion is more focal, whereas the left lesion has the classic "string of beads" appearance. The remaining vessels are unremarkable. Renal size and contour are symmetric.* ***(Right)*** *Posteroanterior DSA of the right renal artery shows beaded appearance of FMD. Areas of attenuated contrast can represent intraluminal webs.*

Typical

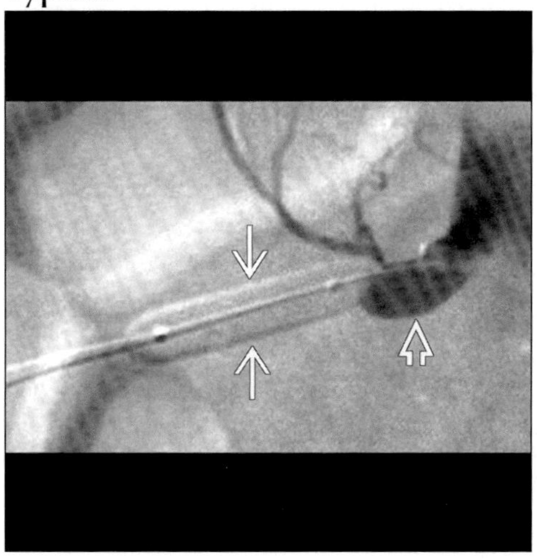

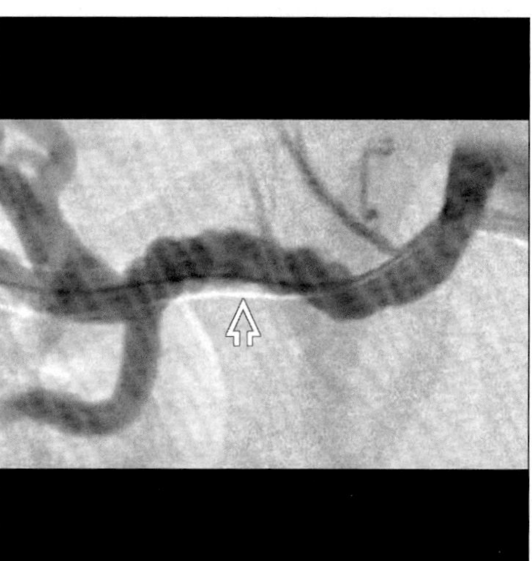

(Left) *Posteroanterior DSA shows inflated angioplasty balloon. Angioplasty is the primary treatment for FMD. Contrast is noted in the right renal artery, proximal to the angioplasty balloon.* ***(Right)*** *Posteroanterior DSA of the right renal artery (same patient as previous image) shows persistent but decreased irregularity after percutaneous transluminal angioplasty. FMD typically responds well to angioplasty; intravascular stents are not routinely used.*

SEGMENTAL ARTERIAL MEDIOLYSIS

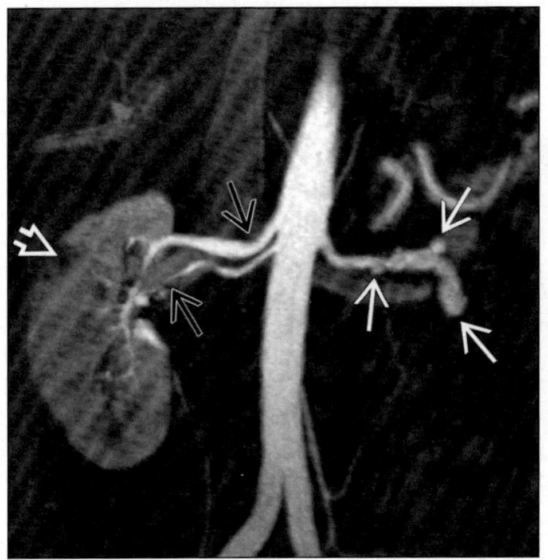

Coronal MRA shows aneurysms ➡ in the left renal artery and caliber changes ⇨ in the two right renal arteries. There is also a right renal infarct ⮕. The appearance is typical of segmental arterial mediolysis.

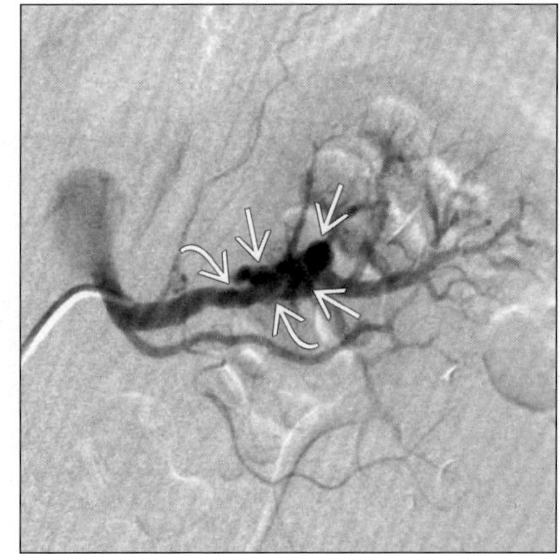

Renal arteriogram (same patient), shows the aneurysms ➡, dissections ⮕ and luminal irregularity that are characteristic of SAM. These lesions respond poorly to angioplasty due to a weakened, deficient arterial wall.

TERMINOLOGY

Abbreviations and Synonyms

- Segmental arterial mediolysis (SAM)
- Segmental mediolytic arteriopathy

Definitions

- Segmental arterial mediolysis: Rare nonatherosclerotic and noninflammatory arterial disease
  - Fundamentally a variant of fibromuscular dysplasia (FMD)
  - Described as distinct pathologic entity by Slavin et al in 1976

IMAGING FINDINGS

General Features

- Best diagnostic clue
  - Arterial wall thickening, dissection, and multiple saccular aneurysms of small abdominal arteries
  - Involvement of multiple arterial beds
- Location
  - Small to medium-sized abdominal arteries
    - Most frequently involves mesenteric, then renal arteries

CT Findings

- CTA will have similar findings to angiography
  - NECT or CECT will also demonstrate any associated pathology such as retroperitoneal hemorrhage

MR Findings

- MRA will have similar findings to angiography

Angiographic Findings

- Characteristic findings include dissections and multiple saccular aneurysms or microaneurysms
  - Arteries may become elongated and kinked
  - Angiographic appearance may be indistinguishable from that of vasculitis or FMD
    - Occasionally has "string of beads" appearance that is seen in FMD
    - Involvement of multiple arteries in different vascular beds characteristic of SAM
  - Arteriovenous fistula occurs rarely

Imaging Recommendations

- Best imaging tool

DDx: Renal Artery Stenosis

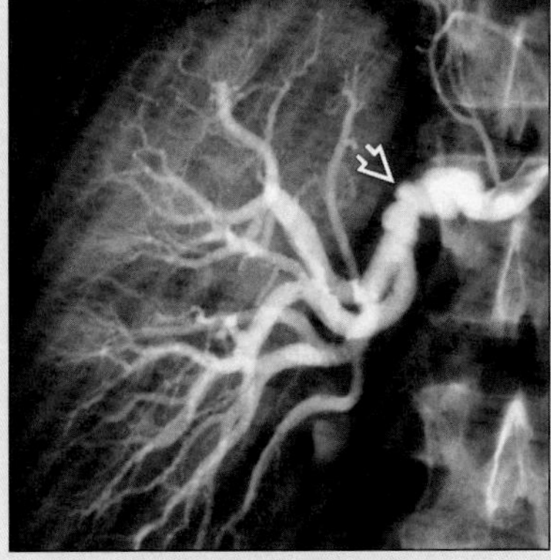

Fibromuscular Dysplasia

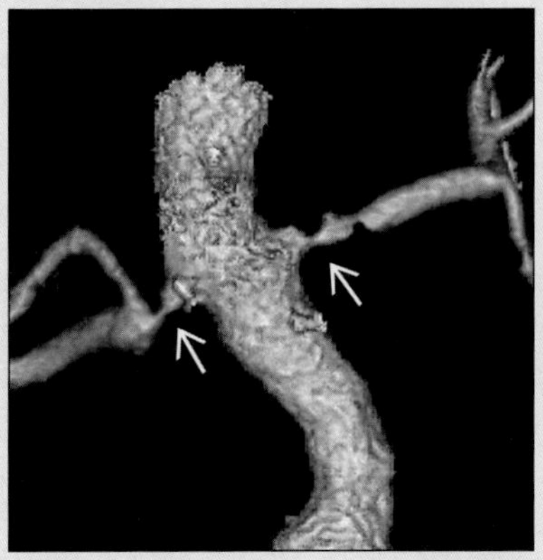

Atherosclerotic Renal Artery Stenosis

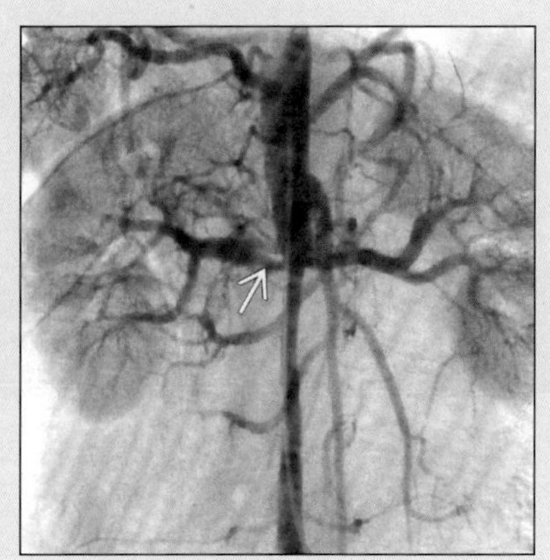

Takayasu Arteritis (Vasculitis)

SEGMENTAL ARTERIAL MEDIOLYSIS

Key Facts

Terminology

- Segmental arterial mediolysis (SAM)
  - Rare, noninflammatory arterial disease
  - Fundamentally a variant of fibromuscular dysplasia

Imaging Findings

- Arterial wall thickening, dissection, and multiple saccular aneurysms of small abdominal arteries
  - Most frequently involves mesenteric, then renal arteries
- Angiographic appearance may be indistinguishable from that of vasculitis or FMD
  - May have characteristic "string of beads" as well as dissections and microaneurysms
  - Involvement of multiple arteries in different vascular beds characteristic of SAM

Pathology

- Correct diagnosis can be made only after histopathologic evaluation of the arterial lesions

Clinical Issues

- 5th decade or older for SAM; 3rd-4th decade for FMD
- Thrombosis, arterial wall hemorrhage, and dissection are complications of segmental arterial mediolysis
- Nonocclusive ischemic bowel disease or retroperitoneal bleeding from rupture of splanchnic artery aneurysm most frequent severe complications
- Intervention deferred unless severe end-organ ischemia
  - Weakened, deficient arterial wall responds poorly to angioplasty; may rupture or cause more dissections

---

- CTA or MRA for initial evaluation
  - Catheter angiography for further evaluation and confirmation

DIFFERENTIAL DIAGNOSIS

Fibromuscular Dysplasia

- Younger patients in 3rd to 5th decade
  - Females affected more than males
- Nonatherosclerotic, noninflammatory arterial disease caused by overgrowth of fibrous tissue and smooth muscle cells within arterial wall
  - Histological classification of three main subtypes: Intimal, medial and perimedial
    - Medial fibroplasia is pathology in 80%
  - Alternating zones of hyperplasia and weakening produce characteristic "string of beads" appearance
    - Aneurysms or dissections may occur in weakened areas of arterial wall
    - Bilateral renal artery disease in > 50%
- Affects predominantly renal, carotid and iliac arteries
  - Carotid and iliac arteries affected, but less frequently
  - Also rarely affects other medium-sized arteries, including mesenteric vessels
- Renovascular hypertension is most common manifestation of renal artery FMD
- Complications of cervicocranial FMD are dissection or stroke
  - Can be associated with intracerebral aneurysms with risk of subarachnoid or intracerebral hemorrhage
- Responds well to angioplasty

Atherosclerotic Disease

- Most common cause of renal artery stenosis
  - Typically affects vessel origin or proximal portion of the renal artery
    - In majority of patients, atherosclerotic stenosis involves initial 1 cm of renal artery
    - Usually caused by aortic plaque encroaching upon vessel origin and termed "ostial stenosis"
    - Intrarenal branch involvement with severe atherosclerosis or longstanding hypertension
  - < 10% of lesions confined to renal artery proper
  - Renal artery disease is etiology in only 5% of patients with hypertension
- Patient usually in 6th decade or older
  - Males affected more than females
- May also affect origins of celiac, SMA and IMA with resultant stenoses or occlusions

Arterial Trauma

- Iatrogenic trauma to renal or visceral vessels
  - Can occur during surgery or diagnostic and therapeutic angiographic procedures
    - Intimal flap, dissection, pseudoaneurysm, thrombosis, distal embolization
    - More serious hemorrhage, AV fistulas and rupture may occur
  - Common cause of renal arterial trauma are renal biopsy, nephrostomy or nephrolithotomy
- Non-iatrogenic injuries can occur with blunt or penetrating trauma
- Deceleration injuries may result in intimal tear and subsequent stenosis, aneurysm or thrombosis

Inflammatory Pseudoaneurysm

- Renal or mesenteric artery pseudoaneurysms are rare and complex complications of inflammatory disease
  - Can be associated with compression or erosion into adjacent structures and may result in life-threatening hemorrhage
  - Noninflammatory pseudoaneurysms may also occur following abdominal surgery or trauma
- Traditional management is open surgical ligation, aneurysm resection with interposition grafts, or resection/partial resection of involved end organ
  - Endovascular repair has been reported as alternate treatment

Renal Artery Aneurysm

- Rare lesions with incidence of approximately 0.1%
  - 20% bilateral and 30% multiple
- Aneurysms in atherosclerosis, FMD and SAM typically involve extraparenchymal renal artery branches

- Extraparenchymal aneurysms predominate, comprising approximately 85%
  - Of the extraparenchymal type, 70% saccular, 20% fusiform, and 10% dissecting
- Symptomatic patients may have hematuria, hypertension and flank pain
  - Incidence of hypertension may be as high as 90%
- Treatment of symptomatic or ruptured aneurysms may be surgical or endovascular

Vasculitis

- Polyarteritis nodosa may have renal artery aneurysms that are typically intraparenchymal and peripheral
  - Commonly are microaneurysms
  - Clinical findings in polyarteritis nodosa and SAM are similar
    - Multiple aneurysms and abdominal pain from rupture of lesions
- Takayasu arteritis, a non-specific giant-cell vasculitis, affects aorta and main branches
  - Renal involvement manifested by renovascular hypertension followed by ischemic nephropathy
    - Angiographically has long smooth stenoses
  - Typically is younger female patient
  - Immunosuppressive treatment can improve prognosis and delay complications

PATHOLOGY

General Features

- Etiology
  - Condition may be result of inappropriate vasoconstrictive response to shock or severe hypoxemia in splanchnic vascular bed
    - Hypothesis is supported by morphologic and clinical findings in SAM
    - Arterial changes from vasospasm have histologic similarities to segmental arterial mediolysis
- Epidemiology: Majority of abdominal visceral artery aneurysms may be secondary to SAM as definite clinical and pathological entity

Gross Pathologic & Surgical Features

- No predilection for vascular branch points
  - Lesions often have concomitant deposition of loose fibrous tissue, resulting in focal arterial weakening, aneurysm, dissecting hemorrhage, and rupture
  - Segmental lysis of abdominal splanchnic arteries resulting in aneurysms, and acute bleeding in a skip pattern

Microscopic Features

- Correct diagnosis can be made only after histopathologic evaluation of arterial lesions
  - Focal vacuolization of media and internal elastic lamina of only portions of arterial circumference
  - Inflammation, eosinophilic infiltrates, and immunoglobulin complexes not consistently found
  - Medial necrosis and transmural mediolysis result in gaps in arterial wall
    - Allows development of dissecting hematomas and aneurysms

CLINICAL ISSUES

Presentation

- Most common signs/symptoms: Hypertension, abdominal pain, spontaneous retroperitoneal or intraperitoneal hemorrhage

Demographics

- Age: 5th decade or older

Natural History & Prognosis

- Thrombosis, arterial wall hemorrhage, and dissection are complications of segmental arterial mediolysis
- Nonocclusive ischemic bowel disease or retroperitoneal bleeding from rupture of splanchnic artery aneurysm most frequent severe complications
  - Lytic degeneration of arterial media results in intra-abdominal bleeding
  - Clinical presentation may be catastrophic as a result of vascular occlusion or rupture

Treatment

- Intervention deferred unless end-organ ischemia
  - Weakened, deficient arterial wall responds poorly to angioplasty; may rupture or cause more dissections
- Medical control of hypertension, if present

DIAGNOSTIC CHECKLIST

Consider

- Diagnosis of segmental arterial mediolysis if arterial dissections, stenoses and/or aneurysms are seen involving multiple arteries in different vascular beds

SELECTED REFERENCES

1. Slavin RE et al: Segmental arterial mediolysis with accompanying venous angiopathy: a clinical pathologic review, report of 3 new cases, and comments on the role of endothelin-1 in its pathogenesis. Int J Surg Pathol. 15(2):121-34, 2007
2. Michael M et al: Segmental arterial mediolysis: CTA findings at presentation and follow-up. AJR Am J Roentgenol. 187(6):1463-9, 2006
3. Obara H et al: Reconstructive surgery for segmental arterial mediolysis involving both the internal carotid artery and visceral arteries. J Vasc Surg. 43(3):623-6, 2006
4. Phillips CK et al: Spontaneous retroperitoneal hemorrhage caused by segmental arterial mediolysis. Rev Urol. 8(1):36-40, 2006
5. Hirakawa E et al: Asymptomatic dissecting aneurysm of the coeliac artery: a variant of segmental arterial mediolysis. Histopathology. 47(5):544-6, 2005
6. Frauenfelder T et al: Nontraumatic emergent abdominal vascular conditions: advantages of multi-detector row CT and three-dimensional imaging. Radiographics. 24(2):481-96, 2004
7. Soulen MC et al: Segmental arterial mediolysis: angioplasty of bilateral renal artery stenoses with 2-year imaging follow-up. J Vasc Interv Radiol. 15(7):763-7, 2004
8. Ryan JM et al: Coil embolization of segmental arterial mediolysis of the hepatic artery. J Vasc Interv Radiol. 11(7):865-8, 2000
9. Lee SI et al: Splanchnic segmental arterial mediolysis. AJR Am J Roentgenol. 170(1):122, 1998

SEGMENTAL ARTERIAL MEDIOLYSIS

IMAGE GALLERY

Typical

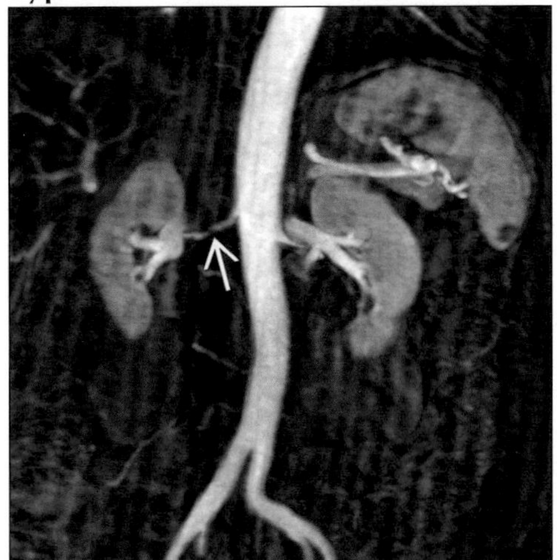

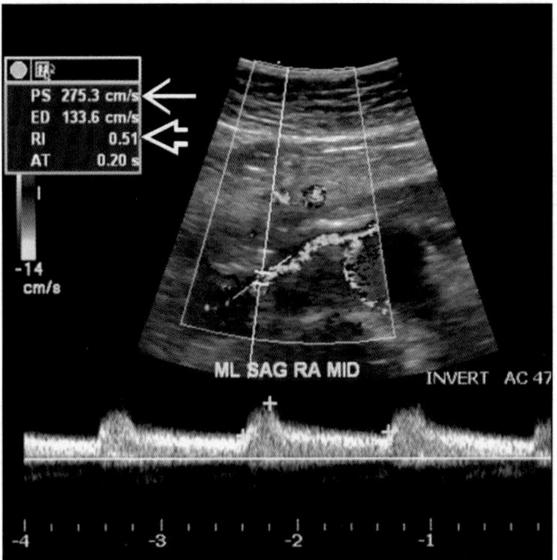

(Left) *Coronal MRA in severely hypertensive young patient shows right renal artery stenosis →, suspicious for fibromuscular dysplasia. Additional imaging was obtained.* ***(Right)*** *Color Doppler ultrasound of renal artery (same patient as previous image) shows elevated peak systolic velocity (PS) of 275.3 cm/sec →. Value > 180 cm/sec suggests renal artery stenosis > 60%. Low resistive index (RI) of 0.51 → predicts a positive outcome with revascularization.*

Typical

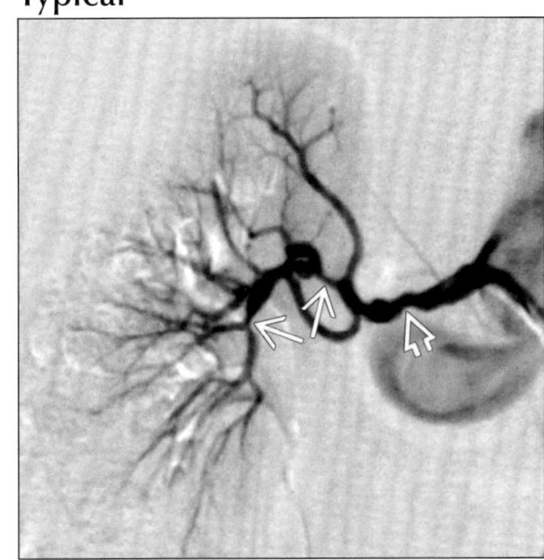

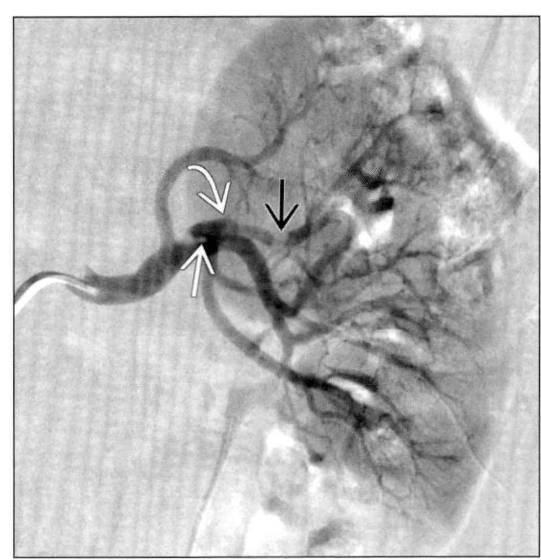

(Left) *Right renal arteriogram (same patient as previous image) confirms stenosis seen on MRA →, & demonstrates additional stenoses → of intrarenal arterial branches.* ***(Right)*** *Left renal arteriogram (same patient as previous image) shows focal renal artery dissection → with associated aneurysm → & intrarenal artery branch stenosis →. FMD & SAM may appear almost identical by angiography, but the above findings are more typical of the latter.*

Typical

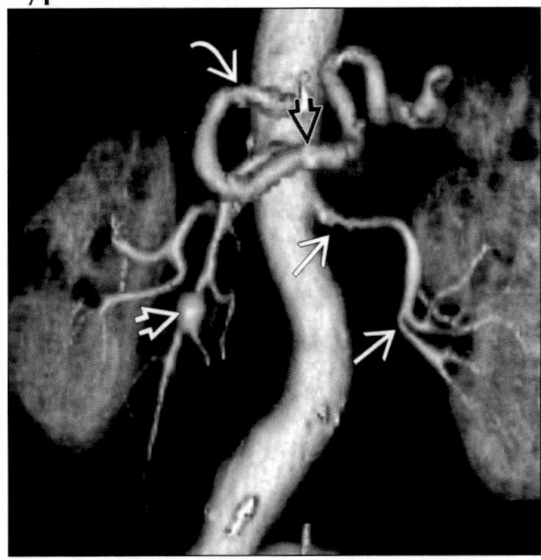

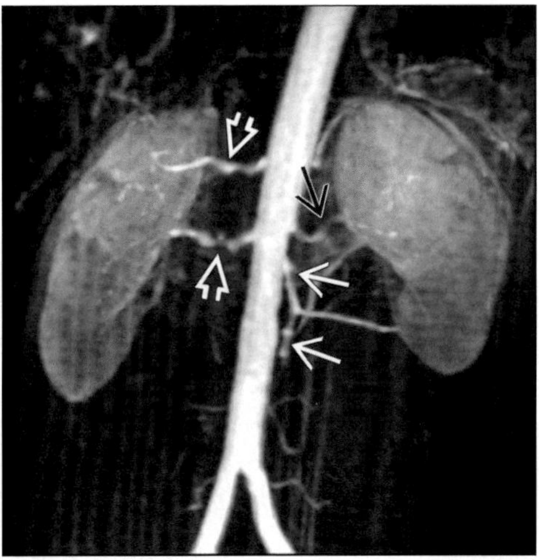

(Left) *Coronal CTA shows an aneurysm of the distal SMA → and luminal irregularities in the left renal artery →. There is also disease of the celiac → and the splenic → arteries. Involvement of multiple arterial beds is typical of segmental arterial mediolysis.* ***(Right)*** *MRA (different patient) again shows the involvement of multiple arteries with SAM. There are stenoses and aneurysms of the SMA → and of the right renal arteries →. There may also be a left renal artery stenosis →.*

POLYARTERITIS NODOSA

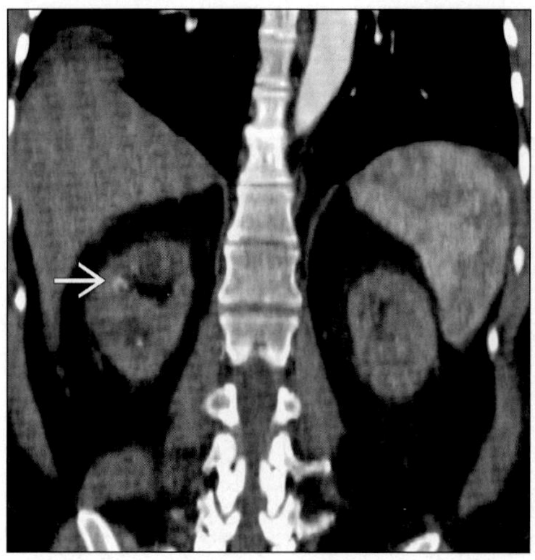

Coronal CECT shows small high density regions in the kidneys bilaterally although more distinct in the right kidney ➡. In some cases hemorrhage may be present, or evidence of inflammation.

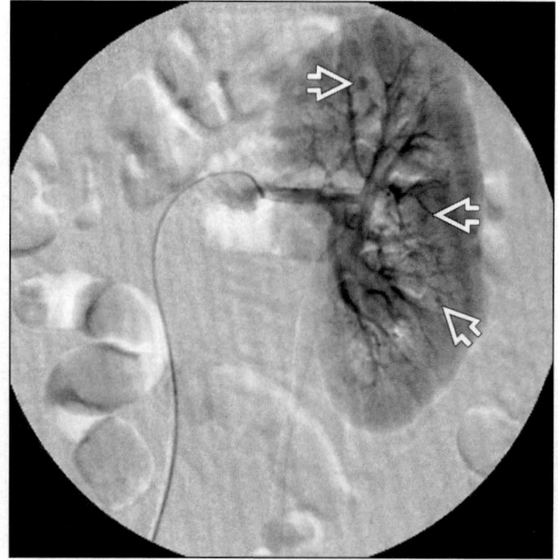

DSA shows multiple small aneurysm scattered throughout the kidney ⇨. The arteries also appear slightly irregular.

TERMINOLOGY

Abbreviations and Synonyms

- Polyarteritis nodosa (PAN); Kussmaul-Maier disease

Definitions

- Systemic vasculitis causing necrotizing inflammation of small and medium-sized vessels, resulting in microaneurysms, occlusions, and strictures

IMAGING FINDINGS

General Features

- Best diagnostic clue
  - Multiple 1-5 mm peripheral aneurysms
  - Occlusions
  - Irregular stenoses
- Location
  - Kidneys (70-80%)
  - GI tract, peripheral nerves, skin (50%)
  - Skeletal muscles and mesentry (30%)
  - CNS (10%)
  - Heart, testicles, lung, and spleen rarely involved

CT Findings

- NECT
  - Multiple, often less than 1 cm, renal and hepatic aneurysms appear as low attenuation structures
  - Wedge-shaped infarcts may be seen in kidney
- CECT
  - Often see thickening of the wall of medium-sized arteries
  - Multiple small renal infarcts consistent with fibrinoid necrosis and vascular thrombosis
  - May see perirenal and retroperitoneal hemorrhage from aneurysm rupture
  - Infarcted bowel may appear thickened, perforated, or obstructed from stricture
  - Liver aneurysm formation may result in interstitial hepatitis and cirrhosis
- CTA
  - Multiple aneurysms of varying sizes
  - Smooth segmental narrowing of vessels; stenosis and occlusions of larger vessels
  - Thickening of wall of medium-sized arteries
  - May provide noninvasive, rapid diagnosis

DDx: Polyarteritis Nodosa

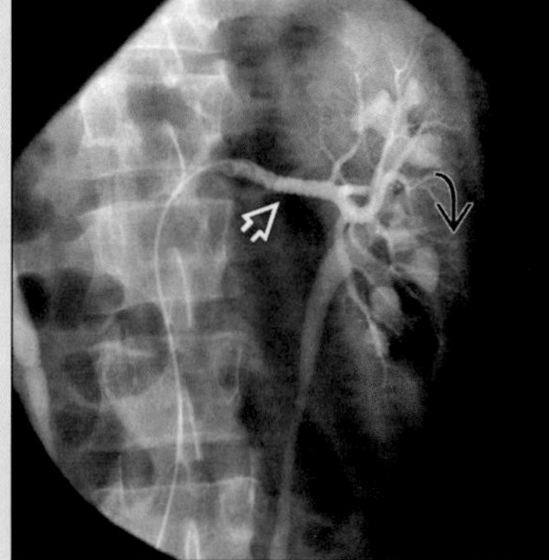

FMD Main Artery and PAN Distal

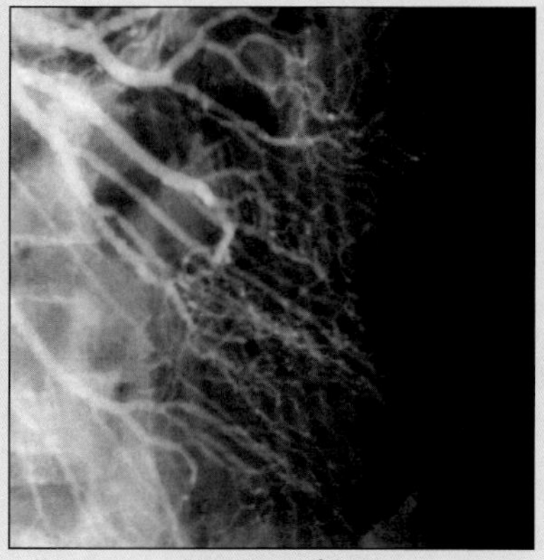

SLE Vasculitis

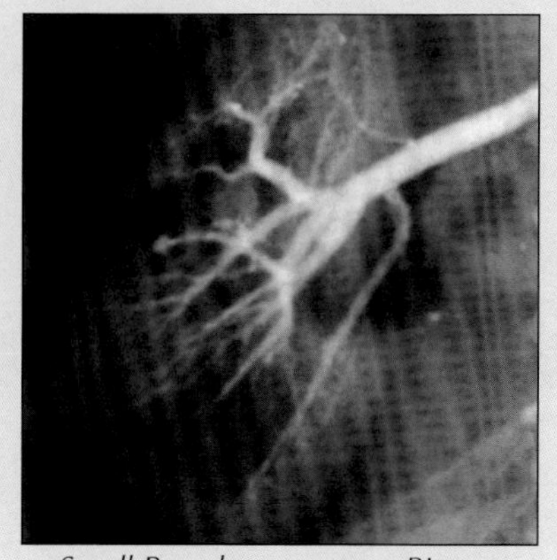

Small Pseudoaneurysm - Biopsy

POLYARTERITIS NODOSA

Key Facts

Terminology

- Systemic vasculitis causing necrotizing inflammation of small and medium-sized vessels, resulting in microaneurysms, occlusions, and strictures

Imaging Findings

- Multiple aneurysms of varying sizes
- Smooth segmental narrowing of vessels; stenosis and occlusions of larger vessels

Pathology

- Diagnosis made by performing tissue biopsy in association with angiography
- Aneurysms typically seen at vessel branch points
- Necrotizing arteritis with pleomorphic cellular infiltrate in vessel walls

Clinical Issues

- Subacute presentation with vague symptoms: fever, weight loss, malaise, headache, myalgia
- Spectrum of disease from single organ involvement to polyvisceral failure
- Glucocorticoids as first line treatment, remission in 50% of patients
- Addition of cyclophosphamide if necessary; remission or cure in 90%

Diagnostic Checklist

- Rapid diagnosis necessary due to progression to life threatening complications
  - CNS hemorrhage, GI hemorrhage or perforation, acute appendicitis, liver infarct, acute renal failure, renal/perirenal hematomas, and cardiac failure

MR Findings

- MRA
  - Multiple aneurysms of varying sizes
  - Demonstrates organ involvement, with regions of ischemia/infarction
  - Less invasive than angiography; no contrast, no radiation
  - Useful to suggest diagnosis, monitor disease progression and response to therapy
  - New technology overcomes traditional limitations of flow artifacts, long acquisition times, and misregistration due to multiple breath-holds

Ultrasonographic Findings

- Color Doppler
  - Operator dependent
  - Microaneurysms appear as small hyperechoic structures
    - Spectral analysis may demonstrate vascular lesions with arterial flows
    - Occasionally aneurysms are too small to detect with color flow

Angiographic Findings

- Conventional
  - Multiple microaneurysms, ectasia, stenoses, intra-arterial thrombosis, and occlusions
    - Aneurysms may be small, difficult to detect, or isolated to one organ
    - Aneurysms may resolve in disease remission
  - Findings predominately in visceral arteries
  - Extremities and small branches of aorta rarely involved
  - Helps confirm clinical impression when biopsy is lacking or results are inconclusive

Imaging Recommendations

- Best imaging tool
  - Angiography considered traditional gold standard
  - CT and MR are less invasive and provide evidence of end-organ damage

DIFFERENTIAL DIAGNOSIS

Microscopic Polyangiitis (MPA)

- Systemic vasculitis with clinical features similar to PAN
- Histologically similar to PAN except for involvement of smaller vessels
- Results in glomerulonephritis, not seen in PAN
- Imaging often does not reveal microaneurysms

Systemic Lupus Erythematosus (SLE)

- Small vessel inflammation associated with antigen-antibody complexes
- Angiographic appearance similar to PAN with multiple microaneurysms
- Vessels show tapered or abrupt occlusions with few collateral vessels.
- CT demonstrates dilated bowel, bowel wall thickening, ascites, LAD, and hydronephrosis

Wegener Granulomatosis

- Granulomatous vasculitis of upper and lower respiratory tract with glomerulonephritis
- Multiple microaneurysms on imaging
- Often ANCA positive

Churg-Strauss Syndrome

- Granulomatous vasculitis of multiple organ systems
- Multiple microaneurysms on imaging
- Often ANCA positive

Drug Abuse

- May manifest as multiple microaneurysms in various organs
- Often severe renal, GI, cardiac, and neurologic involvement

Fibromuscular Dysplasia (FMD)

- Angiography may demonstrate multiple aneurysms
- "String-of-beads" appearance
- Acute phase reactants often elevated in PAN and normal in FMD

POLYARTERITIS NODOSA

PATHOLOGY

General Features

- General path comments: Diagnosis made by tissue biopsy in association with angiography
- Etiology
  - Unknown; possibly associated with immune-complex deposition
  - Often associated with Hepatitis B
  - Occasional reports with HIV, CMV, HTLV-1, AND HCV
- Epidemiology
  - Annual incidence: 2-9 cases per million
  - Up to 77 per million in areas of hyperendemic hepatitis B

Gross Pathologic & Surgical Features

- Aneurysms typically seen at vessel branch points
- Complete occlusion may occur secondary to endothelial proliferation and thrombosis

Microscopic Features

- Necrotizing arteritis with pleomorphic cellular infiltrate in vessel walls
- Destruction of external and internal elastic lamina with fibrinoid necrosis of media

CLINICAL ISSUES

Presentation

- Most common signs/symptoms
  - Subacute presentation with vague symptoms: Fever, weight loss, malaise, headache, myalgia
  - Spectrum of disease from single organ involvement to polyvisceral failure
    - Renal: Hypertension, renal insufficiency, vascular nephropathy (HTN, oliguric renal failure), hemorrhage
    - GI: Ischemia, abdominal pain, weight loss, infarction, bowel perforation, hemorrhage, pancreatitis, appendicitis, and cholecystitis
    - Peripheral neuropathy: Mononeuritis multiplex, often asymmetric neuropathy with sciatic involvement
    - Cardiac: Coronary arteritis, congestive heart failure
    - Skin: Palpable purpura, infarctions, and ulcerations
    - Ophthalmologic: Retinal vasculitis, retinal detachment, cotton-wool spots
  - Brain, eyes, pancreas, lungs, testicles, ureters, breasts, and ovaries rarely involved
- Clinical Profile
  - Clinical symptoms related to ischemia
  - Arthralgia and peripheral neuropathies often symptomatic early
  - No association with ANCA
  - ESR and CRP may correlate with disease activity

Demographics

- Age: Most common in 5th-7th decade
- Gender: 2:1 male to female

Natural History & Prognosis

- Fulminant disease, 5-year survival < 15%
- Relapse in 40% of patients; median survival 33 months
- 50% of patients with abdominal involvement develop acute surgical abdomen with mortality of 12.5%
- Five factor score (FFS) estimates prognosis
  - Scores renal, GI, cardiac, and CNS involvement
  - Low score correlates with better 5-year survival

Treatment

- Glucocorticoids as first line treatment; remission in 50% of patients
- Addition of cyclophosphamide; remission or cure in 90%
- HBV associated PAN requires the addition of antivirals
- Plasma exchange/plasmapheresis may have added benefit in refractory cases
- Large aneurysms may be treated by catheter embolization to avoid risk of rupture
- Surgery may be needed to treat GI complications

DIAGNOSTIC CHECKLIST

Consider

- Rapid diagnosis necessary due to progression to life threatening complications
  - CNS hemorrhage, GI hemorrhage or perforation, acute appendicitis, liver infarct, acute renal failure, renal/perirenal hematomas, and cardiac failure

Image Interpretation Pearls

- Multiple aneurysms seen in 50-60% of cases, often at artery bifurcations
- CTA and MRA provide less invasive alternative to angiography

SELECTED REFERENCES

1. Lin J et al: Whole-body three-dimensional contrast-enhanced magnetic resonance (MR) angiography with parallel imaging techniques on a multichannel MR system for the detection of various systemic arterial diseases. Heart Vessels. 21(6):395-8, 2006
2. Ozcakar ZB et al: Polyarteritis nodosa: successful diagnostic imaging utilizing pulsed and color Doppler ultrasonography and computed tomography angiography. Eur J Pediatr. 165(2):120-3, 2006
3. Kato T et al: A case of polyarteritis nodosa with lesions of the superior mesenteric artery illustrating the diagnostic usefulness of three-dimensional computed tomographic angiography. Clin Rheumatol. 24(6):628-31, 2005
4. Stone JH: Polyarteritis nodosa. JAMA. 288(13):1632-9, 2002
5. Stanson AW et al: Polyarteritis nodosa: spectrum of angiographic findings. Radiographics. 21(1):151-9, 2001
6. Ha HK et al: Radiologic features of vasculitis involving the gastrointestinal tract. Radiographics. 20(3):779-94, 2000
7. Jee KN et al: Radiologic findings of abdominal polyarteritis nodosa. AJR Am J Roentgenol. 174(6):1675-9, 2000

IMAGE GALLERY

Typical

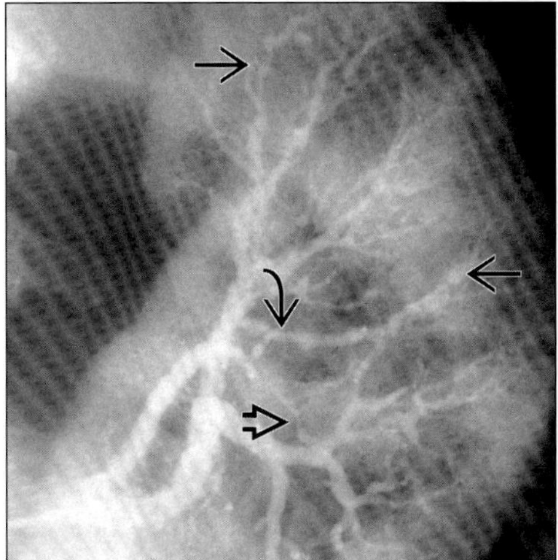

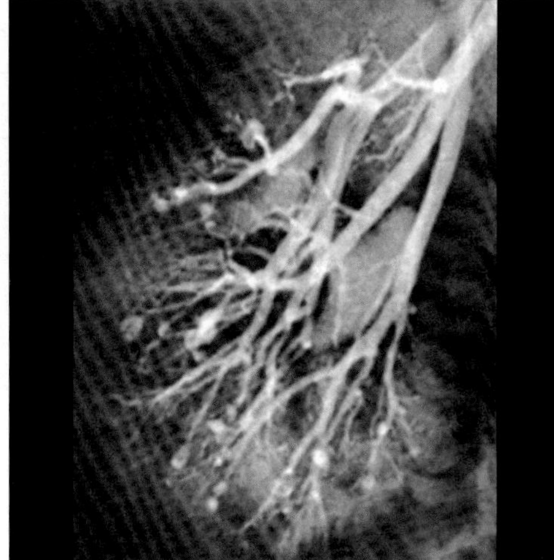

*(**Left**) Catheter angiography shows very severe involvement of renal vessels with multiple microaneurysms →, beading appearance of vessels ↷, and stenoses ⇨. All characteristic signs of PAN. (**Right**) Catheter angiography shows florid case of polyarteritis nodosa. Multiple aneurysms throughout the kidney, multiple subsegmental branches. Larger vessels are not involved in this process.*

Typical

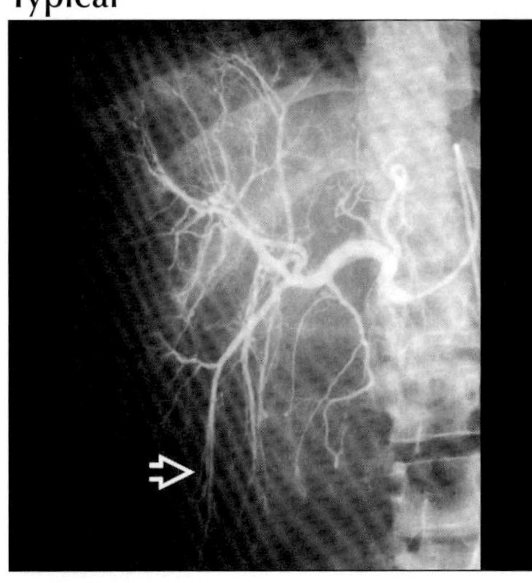

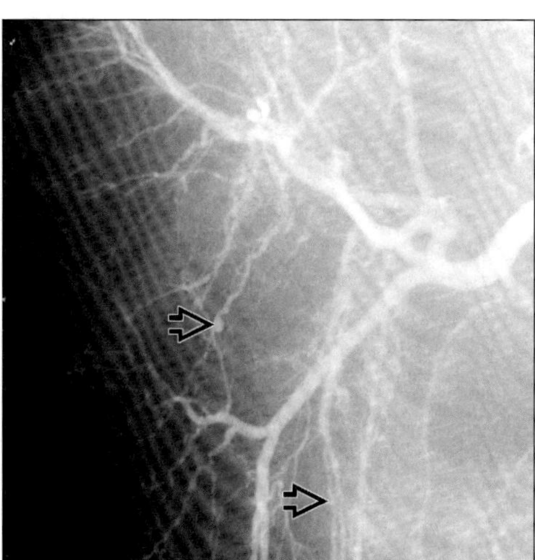

*(**Left**) Catheter angiography shows minimally abnormal appearance of some branches of hepatic artery ⇨. However it would be difficult to see abnormality without magnification views or a subselective evaluation. (**Right**) DSA magnification shows hepatic artery involvement. Arteries have a very irregular, beaded appearance. Several small aneurysms ⇨ represent necrotic process involving arterial wall. These findings would be very difficult to see on CT or MR.*

Typical

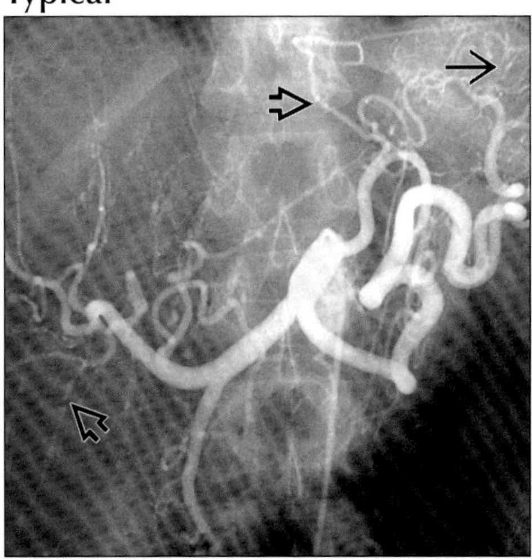

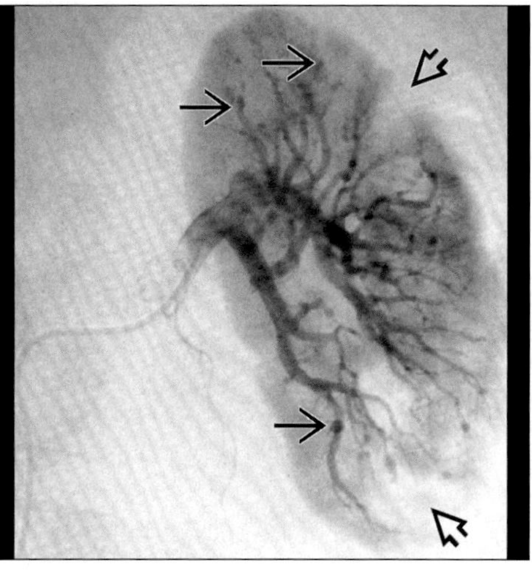

*(**Left**) Catheter angiography shows more subtle liver involvement. Multiple segmental branches have a beaded appearance with multiple small aneurysms ⇨. Splenic vessels may also be involved →. (**Right**) DSA shows the characteristic multiple microaneurysms →. There are also areas within the kidney parenchyma with decreased perfusion consistent with infarcts ⇨. Infarcts may represent necrosis or thrombosis. Hemorrhage may occur if the aneurysms rupture.*

RENAL ARTERY ANEURYSM

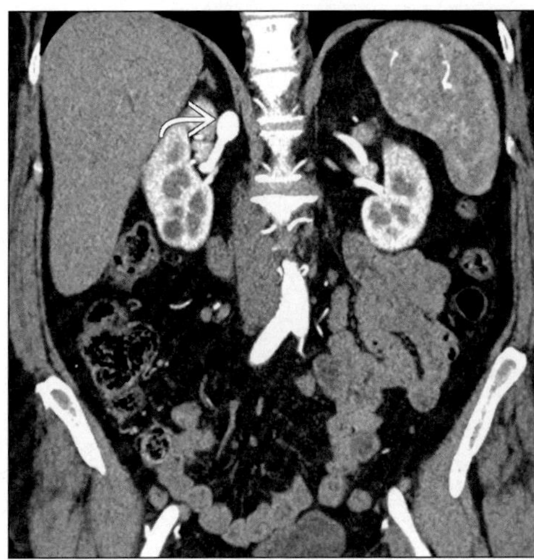

Coronal CTA shows rounded enlargement of the right renal artery consistent with a saccular renal artery aneurysm.

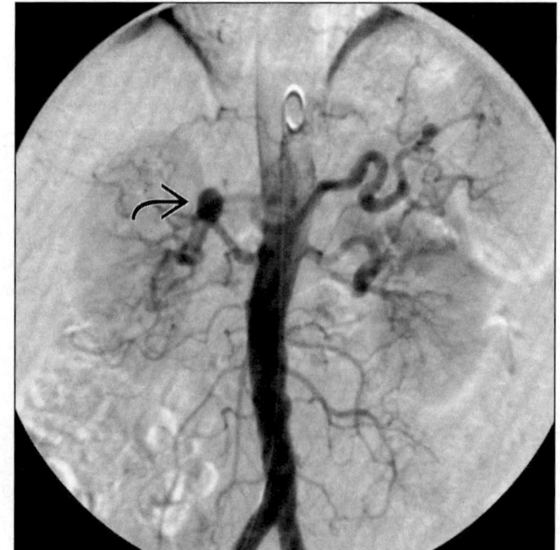

DSA shows an aortogram demonstrating a focal, saccular aneurysm of the right renal artery. It is difficult to determine the exact relationship of the aneurysm to the renal artery.

TERMINOLOGY

Abbreviations and Synonyms

- Renal artery aneurysm (RAA)

Definitions

- Dilation of the renal artery with a diameter at least twice that of a normal segment

IMAGING FINDINGS

General Features

- Best diagnostic clue: Studies demonstrating a mass-like lesion that is vascular in origin
- Location
  - May be extraparenchymal (most common), intraparenchymal, and bilateral
  - Commonly located at bifurcation of the main renal artery
- Size
  - Variable
  - 2 cm or larger is considered high risk of rupture
- Morphology
  - 80% saccular
  - 20% fusiform
  - False aneurysm associated with blunt trauma

CT Findings

- NECT: May show mass-like lesion with soft tissue attenuation and rim calcification in region of renal artery
- CECT
  - Helps determine if mass is vascular in origin
  - Varying contrast-enhancement may be due to thrombus within aneurysm
- CTA
  - Images acquired during arterial phase of enhancement
  - High quality images acquired utilizing thin collimation and overlapping reconstruction
  - Clear demonstration of 3D anatomy often useful for preintervention planning

MR Findings

- MRA
  - Advantages of MRA
    - Lack of ionizing radiation
    - Absence of potential renal toxic contrast agent

DDx: Renal Artery Aneurysm

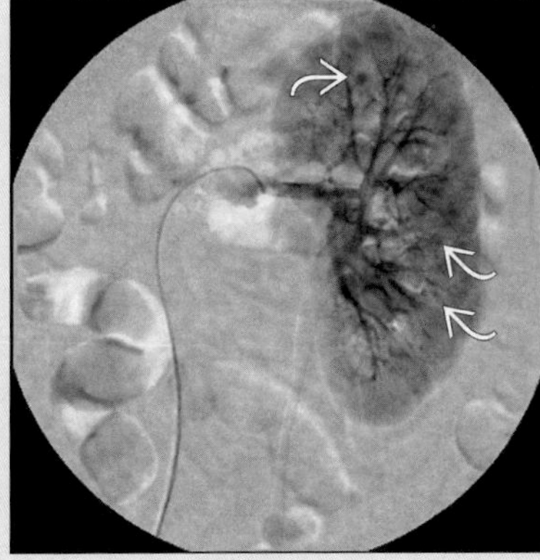

Polyarteritis Nodosa (PAN)

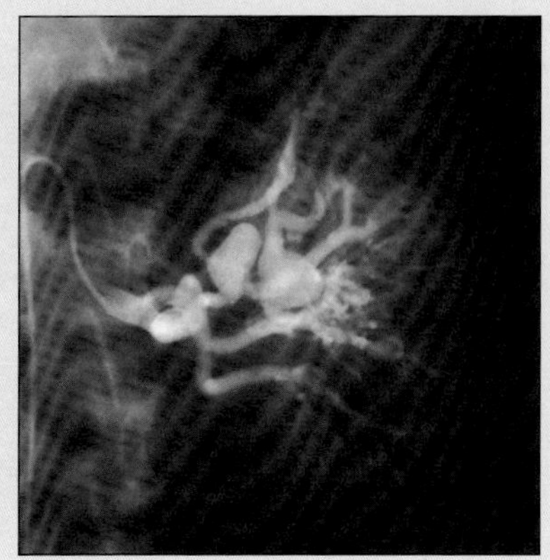

Aneurysms in Neurofibromatosis

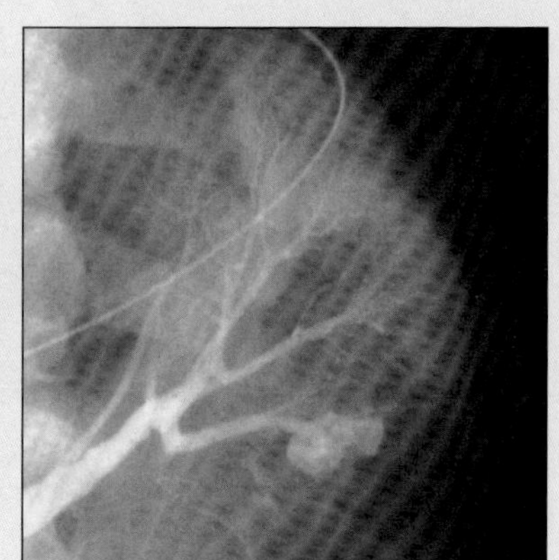

Traumatic Pseudoaneurysm

RENAL ARTERY ANEURYSM

Key Facts

Terminology

- Dilation of the renal artery with a diameter at least twice that of normal

Imaging Findings

- Studies demonstrating a mass-like lesion that is vascular in origin
- Commonly located at bifurcation of main renal artery
- Best imaging tool: MRA or CTA depending on radiologist preference and patient tolerance of radiation dose and contrast agents
- Images acquired during arterial phase of enhancement can generate high-quality 3D images
- Clear demonstration of 3D anatomy often useful for preintervention planning

Pathology

- True aneurysms often caused by atherosclerosis, fibromuscular dysplasia, and collagen disorders
- Epidemiology: 0.3%-0.7% of autopsies and up to 1% of renal arteriographic procedures

Clinical Issues

- Majority asymptomatic
- Associated with hypertension in up to 73% of cases
- Diameter greater than 1.5 cm requires repair
- Pregnant females present high risk of rupture and mortality
- Surgical repair with low morbidity and mortality
- Endovascular treatment (coils and/or stent grafts) are reserved for aneurysms with narrow necks that are not at vessel branch points
- Aneurysm repair cures hypertension in 20-50%

        - Avoidance of radiation dose
    - Produces 3D images with similar quality to CTA
    - Potential modality for following small aneurysms

Ultrasonographic Findings

- Color Doppler
    - Outpouching along artery containing color flow
    - Slow velocities and a turbulent pattern often observed
    - Provides a rapid, noninvasive alternative to CTA and MRA
    - Results operator dependent
- Power Doppler: Helps visualize entire vascular tree from main RA to arcuate arteries and interlobular arteries
- 3D
    - Excellent alternative to conventional invasive angiography
    - Avoids contrast agents, ionizing radiation, arterial catheterization, and cost/time of MRA

Angiographic Findings

- Traditional gold standard
- Clearly outlines renal vasculature and provides detailed relationships to surrounding structures
- Invasive procedure requiring contrast and ionizing radiation
- Important for assessing endovascular therapies

Imaging Recommendations

- Best imaging tool: MRA or CTA depending on radiologist preference and patient tolerance of radiation dose and contrast agents

DIFFERENTIAL DIAGNOSIS

Polyarteritis Nodosa (PAN)

- Necrotizing inflammation of small and medium-sized arteries
- Often associated with multiple renal aneurysms

Fibromuscular Dysplasia (FMD)

- Angiopathy of unknown etiology that often affects renal arteries
- Dilated renal artery segments with a "string of beads" appearance on angiography

Type I Neurofibromatosis

- Associated with arterial ectasia, aneurysms, stenosis, and arteriovenous malformations
- Arterial pathology most common in renal artery; presents with hypertension

Ehler-Danlos Syndrome

- Disorder of collagen metabolism
- Aneurysms in association with skin hyperextensibility, joint hypermobility, and poor wound healing

Atherosclerosis

- Often fusiform aneurysm of main renal artery
- Found in association with other atherosclerotic lesions

Trauma

- Commonly seen with gun shots, stab wounds, and iatrogenic catheter manipulations
- Often an extraparenchymal pseudoaneurysm

Renal Angiomyolipoma

- Benign neoplasm composed of fat, vascular, and smooth muscle elements
- Abnormal tumor vessels predisposed to aneurysms

Dilated Renal Vein

- May be mistaken for aneurysm on US
- Can be differentiated by its appearance on contrast-enhanced CT during excretory phase

PATHOLOGY

General Features

- Etiology
    - True aneurysms often caused by atherosclerosis, fibromuscular dysplasia, and collagen disorders

- Pseudoaneurysm often results from trauma, inflammation, infection, or vasculitis
- Epidemiology: 0.3-0.7% of autopsies and up to 1% of renal arteriographic procedures

Microscopic Features

- Atherosclerotic changes often observed in vessel wall
- Fusiform aneurysms often with fibroplasia-type changes in media associated with FMD

CLINICAL ISSUES

Presentation

- Most common signs/symptoms
  - Majority asymptomatic
  - Incidental finding during investigation with CT, MR, or angiography for abdominal pathology
- Other signs/symptoms: May present with flank pain, hematuria, collecting system obstruction, renal infarction, shock (from rupture), hypertension, embolization of peripheral vascular bed, or arterial thrombosis
- Clinical Profile
  - Associated with hypertension in up to 73% of cases
  - HTN may be secondary to coexisting renal artery stenosis, microembolization, compression of renal artery, or turbulent flow

Demographics

- Age: Average 40-60 years old
- Gender
  - Approximately equal in men and women
  - Hormones released in pregnancy may alter vessel matrix and predispose to RAA formation

Natural History & Prognosis

- Asymptomatic, small (less than 1.5 cm) RAA may be followed closely
- Indications for intervention
  - Symptoms indicating rapid expansion
  - Association with significant renal artery stenosis and hypertension
  - Pregnant females (high risk of rupture and mortality)
  - Diameter greater than 1.5 cm
  - Enlarging aneurysm
  - Renal ischemia or embolization
  - Acute dissection

Treatment

- Options, risks, complications
  - 1.0-1.5 cm RAAs without hypertension may be followed by spiral CT or MR imaging every 1-2 years
  - Most aneurysms 1.5-2.0 cm regardless of BP status should be treated surgically
    - Goals of therapy are to exclude the aneurysm from arterial circulation and pressure
    - Emergency surgery required for rupture
    - Mortality of rupture in pregnancy: Up to 56% in mother and 78% in fetus
  - Surgical options
    - Aneurysmectomy with primary vessel wall closure
    - Aneurysmectomy with bypass
    - Extracorporeal reconstruction with autotransplantation
    - Nephrectomy
  - Surgical repair with low morbidity and mortality
    - Perioperative complications include: Post-operative hemorrhage requiring re-operation, DVT, pneumonia requiring intubation, heart block, and post-operative pancreatitis
    - Primary patency greater than 90% at 48 months
  - Endovascular treatment (coils and/or stent grafts) are reserved for aneurysms with narrow necks that are not at vessel branch points
    - Arterial bypass or covered stent may be required if collateral flow does not exist
    - Risks include: Graft occlusion and renal dysfunction from warm ischemia time
- Most patients have a significant reduction in blood pressure
  - Cure rate of hypertension: 20-50%
  - Majority of patients no longer require medication

DIAGNOSTIC CHECKLIST

Consider

- Controversy exists on size to repair (in absence of other definitive indication for repair): Reports vary from 1.5-3.0 cm

Image Interpretation Pearls

- Multidetector CT
  - Dramatically faster scan acquisition
  - Low dose of contrast medium
  - Improved spatial resolution
- MR advantages
  - Avoidance of contrast material
  - Avoidance of radiation

SELECTED REFERENCES

1. Nosher JL et al: Visceral and renal artery aneurysms: a pictorial essay on endovascular therapy. Radiographics. 26(6):1687-704; quiz 1687, 2006
2. Browne RF et al: Renal artery aneurysms: diagnosis and surveillance with 3D contrast-enhanced magnetic resonance angiography. Eur Radiol. 14(10):1807-12, 2004
3. English WP et al: Surgical management of renal artery aneurysms. J Vasc Surg. 40(1):53-60, 2004
4. Rha SE et al: The renal sinus: pathologic spectrum and multimodality imaging approach. Radiographics. 24 Suppl 1:S117-31, 2004
5. Sheth S et al: Multi-detector row CT of the kidneys and urinary tract: techniques and applications in the diagnosis of benign diseases. Radiographics. 24(2):e20, 2004
6. Willmann JK et al: Aortoiliac and renal arteries: prospective intraindividual comparison of contrast-enhanced three-dimensional MR angiography and multi-detector row CT angiography. Radiology. 226(3):798-811, 2003
7. Henke PK et al: Renal artery aneurysms: a 35-year clinical experience with 252 aneurysms in 168 patients. Ann Surg. 234(4):454-62; discussion 462-3, 2001
8. Zubarev AV: Ultrasound of renal vessels. Eur Radiol. 11(10):1902-15, 2001

RENAL ARTERY ANEURYSM

IMAGE GALLERY

Typical

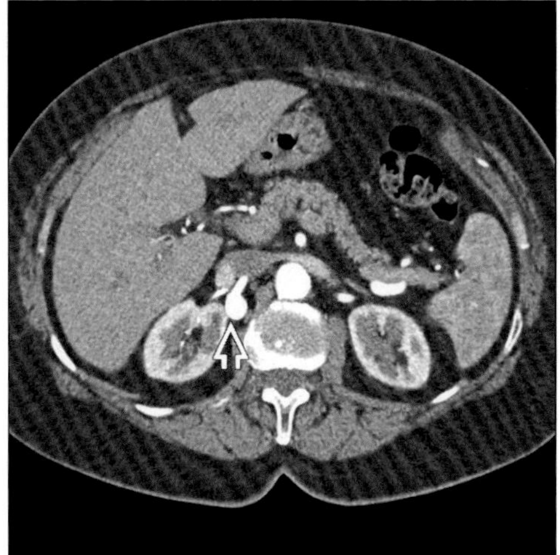

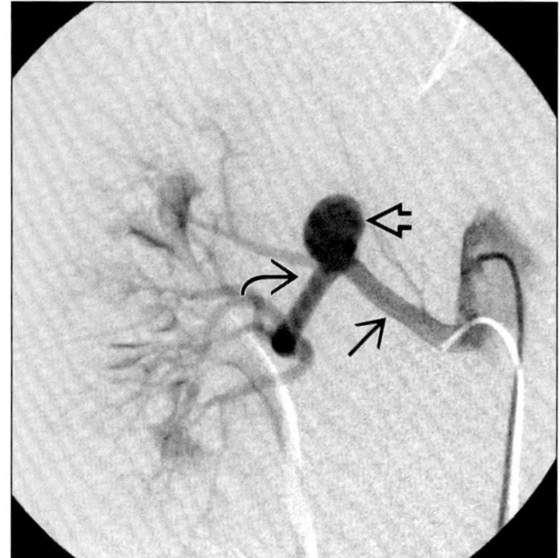

(Left) *Axial CTA shows a focal saccular aneurysm. It is difficult to determine on this scan what portion of the renal artery is giving rise to the aneurysm.* ***(Right)*** *DSA shows a saccular aneurysm which extends off the main right renal artery in a region of a bifurcation. Treatment would be difficult because of concern for occluding artery.*

Variant

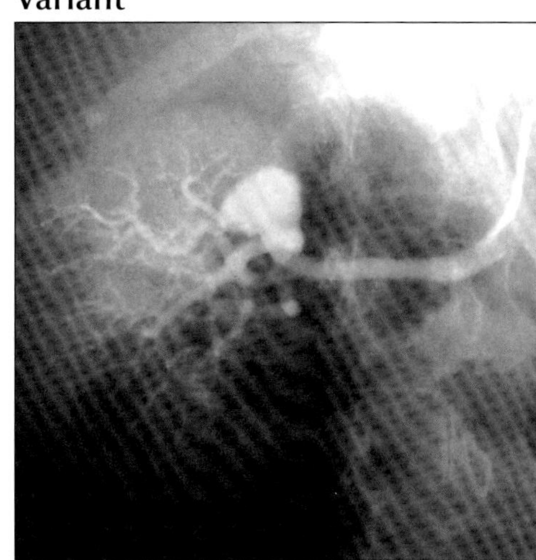

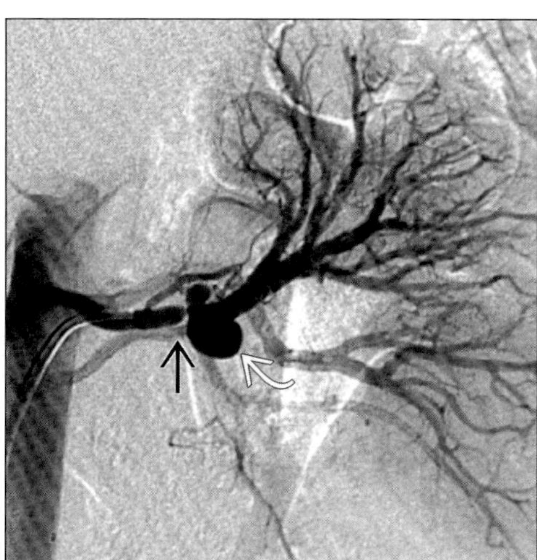

(Left) *Catheter angiography shows an aneurysm arising from a branch vessel. The patient presented without any other evidence of underlying vascular disease and with a history of remote trauma, probably pseudoaneurysm.* ***(Right)*** *DSA shows stenosis in the renal artery and an aneurysm more distally. The patient has fibromuscular dysplasia with an aneurysm.*

Variant

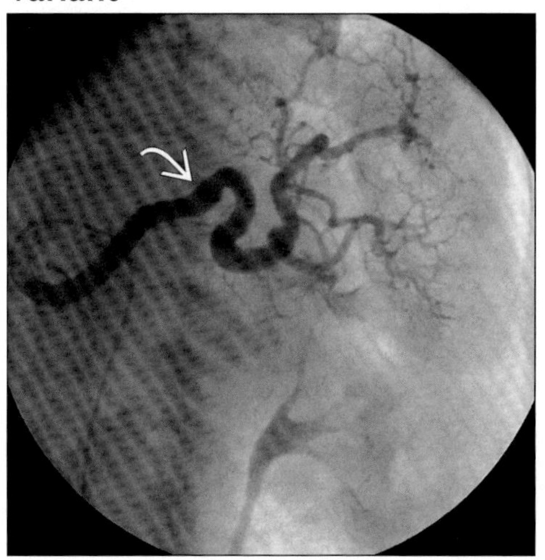

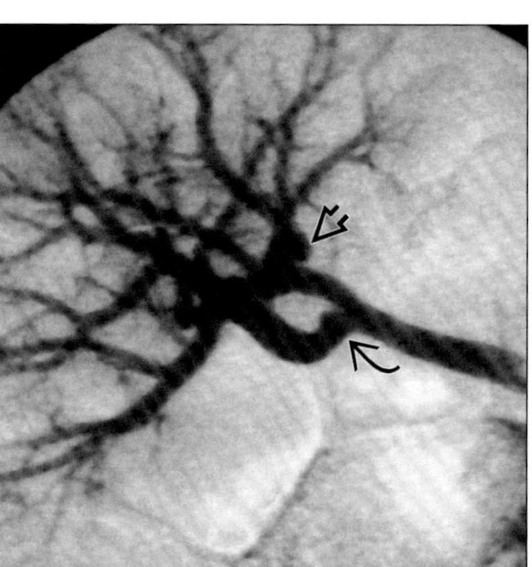

(Left) *DSA shows subtle aneurysmal disease in a patient with atherosclerotic disease. An area of focal enlargement is present. An angiogram may underestimate the degree of dilatation.* ***(Right)*** *DSA shows a patient with multiple aneurysms in the renal arteries. This patient also had fibromuscular dysplasia, with a more typical beaded appearance in the other renal artery.*

RENAL TRAUMA

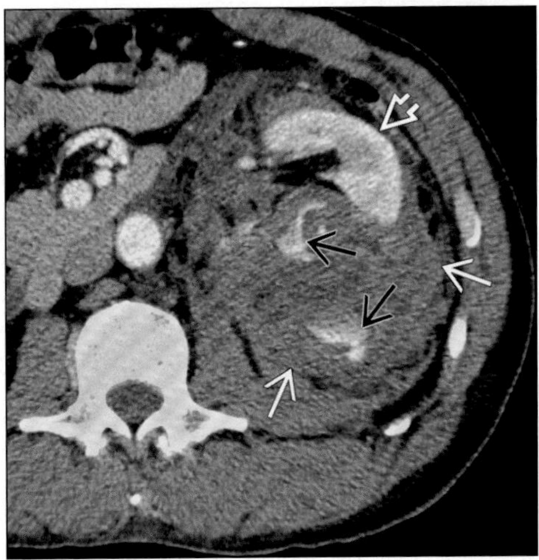

CECT shows a retroperitoneal hematoma ➡ displacing the left kidney ➡ anteriorly. Contrast extravasation ➡ within the hematoma indicates active bleeding. Renal perfusion is intact despite the severe injury.

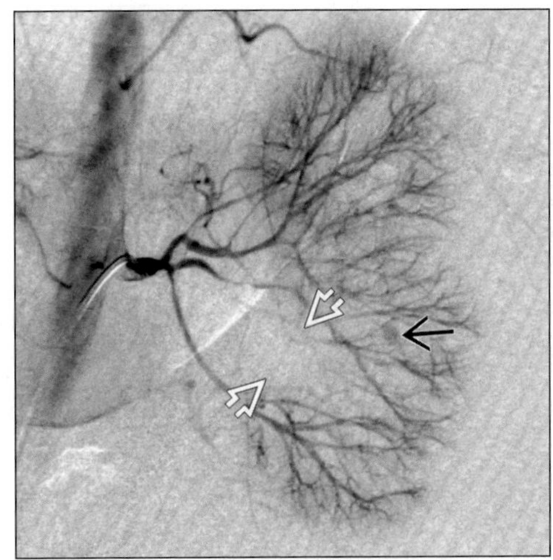

Left renal arteriogram (same patient as previous image) shows an avascular area ➡ corresponding to the deep renal laceration in this class IV injury. Small collection of contrast ➡ is seen at site of active bleeding.

TERMINOLOGY

Abbreviations and Synonyms

- Renal contusion
- Renal hematoma or subcapsular hematoma
- Renal laceration
- Renal fracture

Definitions

- Parenchymal injury to the kidney, the renal vascular pedicle, or both, as a result of blunt trauma, penetrating injury or iatrogenic trauma

IMAGING FINDINGS

General Features

- Best diagnostic clue: Defect within the renal parenchyma, with intrarenal or perirenal hemorrhage

Radiographic Findings

- IVP
  - With minor injury (class I and II) is usually normal
  - With more severe injury (class III-V) may have delayed or absent contrast excretion or extravasation

CT Findings

- CECT
  - Findings vary according to severity of injury
    - Class I-II may have intrarenal, subcapsular or perinephric hematoma; small hypodense areas
    - Class III may have irregular linear hypodense area with associated hematoma, larger areas of hemorrhage
    - Class IV may have multiple lacerations, segmental wedge-shaped areas of decreased enhancement secondary to infarction, vascular injury with extravasation or partial nonperfusion of kidney
    - Class V may have segmental or global nonperfusion of kidney with infarction, diffuse contrast extravasation, circumferential urinoma if collecting system has been avulsed

MR Findings

- T2WI
  - Acute hematoma hyperintense with prolonged T2

DDx: Renal Trauma

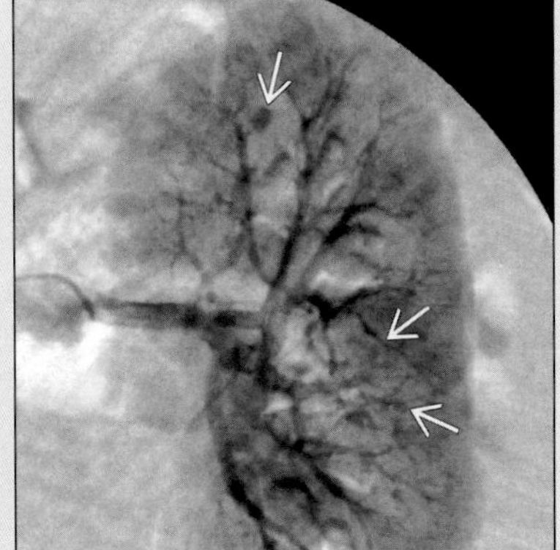

Polyarteritis Nodosa

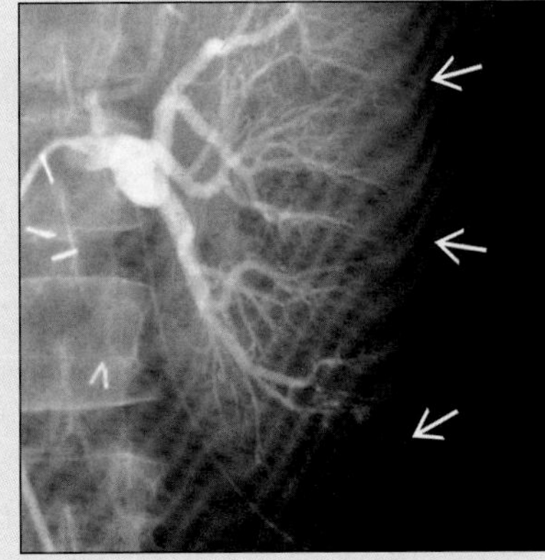

Renal Cell CA with Hematoma

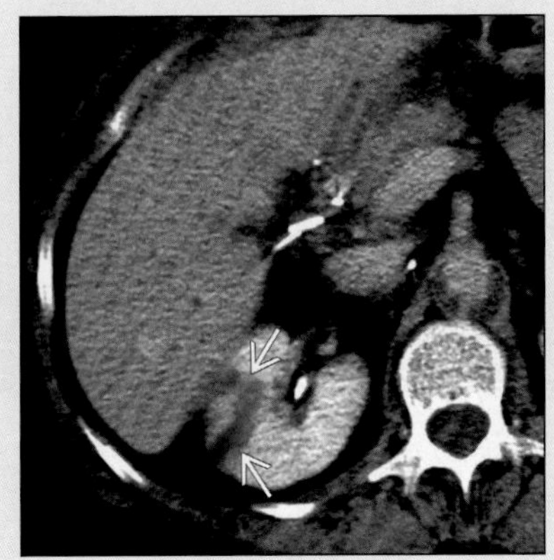

Renal Infarct

RENAL TRAUMA

Key Facts

Terminology

- Parenchymal injury to the kidney, the renal vascular pedicle, or both, as a result of blunt trauma, penetrating injury or iatrogenic trauma

Imaging Findings

- Best imaging tool is CECT; obtain delayed images if laceration identified
- Angiography used if persistent retroperitoneal hemorrhage amenable to transcatheter embolization is suspected
  - Selective renal arteriography for evaluation and potential treatment of renal vascular injury

Pathology

- Gunshot and stab wounds likely to require intervention
- Common causes of penetrating renal trauma include percutaneous renal biopsy, percutaneous nephrostomy, and percutaneous nephrolithotomy

Clinical Issues

- Almost 90% of renal pedicle injuries occur in children and young adults
- Class I and II injuries treated conservatively since most renal contusions and minor lacerations heal spontaneously
- Transcatheter embolization of renal artery branch injuries has high success rate
- Low complication rate for transcatheter embolization
- Successful surgical repair of renal pedicle injury requires revascularization within 4-6 hours of injury

- Over time, blood products evolve into methemoglobin, deoxyhemoglobin with concomitant signal intensity changes
- Infrequently used in assessment of abdominal trauma but may distinguish acute from chronic changes

Ultrasonographic Findings

- Grayscale Ultrasound: FAST (Focused Assessment with Sonography in Trauma) used for rapid detection of free intra-abdominal fluid

Angiographic Findings

- Indications for angiography
  - Active arterial extravasation identified on CECT
  - Patients with persistent or recurrent hematuria
  - Persistent retroperitoneal hemorrhage amenable to transcatheter embolization is suspected
  - When diagnosis of a correctable vascular lesion is uncertain
- Aortography essential to delineate basic renal vascular anatomy and detect any associated vascular injuries
- Selective renal arteriography for evaluation and potential treatment of renal vascular injury
  - Avascular parenchymal laceration
  - Flattened parenchymal contour secondary to subcapsular hematoma
  - Amorphous parenchymal extravasation
  - A-V fistulas, pseudoaneurysms
  - Intimal injury, arterial occlusion

Imaging Recommendations

- Best imaging tool: CECT
- Protocol advice: Obtain delayed images when laceration identified on CECT, so as to evaluate for vascular or urinary extravasation

DIFFERENTIAL DIAGNOSIS

Renal Abscess

- Clinical signs of infection
- Irregular, non-enhancing low attenuation area on CECT

Renal Infarct

- Wedge-shaped area of non-enhancing low attenuation on CECT

Renal Neoplasm

- Vascular neoplasms
  - Renal cell carcinoma
  - Renal adenoma
  - Oncocytoma
  - Angiomyolipoma
- Lymphoma

Vasculitis

- Polyarteritis nodosa, SLE, segmental arterial mediolysis

PATHOLOGY

General Features

- Etiology
  - Blunt renal trauma
    - More common than penetrating trauma
    - Kidney is one of most frequently injured organs in blunt abdominal trauma
    - Requires surgery or intervention in < 10%
    - Extreme force required given kidney's protected position
    - Associated injuries common and seen in approximately 20% of blunt trauma patients
  - Penetrating injuries
    - Gunshot and stab wounds likely to require intervention
    - 70% cause major injury
    - Frequently associated with injury to other organs
  - Iatrogenic trauma
    - Common causes of penetrating renal trauma include percutaneous renal biopsy, percutaneous nephrostomy, and percutaneous nephrolithotomy
    - These interventions cause some degree of hemorrhage in high percentage of patients
    - Majority of injuries managed conservatively

- More serious hemorrhage, A-V fistulas and renal rupture seen in small percentage of patients
  - Direct trauma to renal artery
    - Can occur with blunt or penetrating trauma
    - Can occur during diagnostic and therapeutic angiographic procedures
    - Intimal flap, laceration, thrombosis, distal embolization
    - Can occur with deceleration injuries with resultant intimal tear and subsequent delayed thrombosis
- Associated abnormalities: Serious or severe renal trauma often results in injuries to other organs such as liver, spleen, pancreas and bowel

Gross Pathologic & Surgical Features

- Renal contusion, laceration, hematoma, infarction, vascular or ureteropelvic injury

Staging, Grading or Classification Criteria

- Organ injury classification system of American Association for Surgery of Trauma
- Class I
  - Minor parenchymal contusions
  - Stable small subcapsular hematoma without parenchymal injury
- Class II
  - Cortical laceration < 1.0 cm deep without extension into collecting system
  - Stable perirenal hematoma
- Class III
  - Cortical laceration > 1.0 cm deep without extension into collecting system
- Class IV
  - Parenchymal lacerations involving cortex, medulla and collecting system
  - Contained vascular injuries to main renal artery or vein, e.g. dissection flaps or small pseudoaneurysms
- Class V
  - Completely shattered kidney
  - Avulsion of renal hilum with vascular pedicle injury devascularizing kidney

CLINICAL ISSUES

Presentation

- Most common signs/symptoms
  - Flank pain, ecchymosis
  - Persistent or recurrent hematuria, anuria, uremia
  - Decreasing hematocrit, shock

Demographics

- Age
  - Children more susceptible to renal trauma, even without pre-existing pathology
    - Pediatric kidney is relatively large, more mobile and thus more vulnerable
    - Adult kidney protected by ribs and heavy musculature of flank and back
  - Almost 90% of renal pedicle injuries occur in children and young adults

Treatment

- Options, risks, complications
  - Class I and II injuries treated conservatively since most renal contusions and minor lacerations heal spontaneously
  - Many major injuries also managed conservatively
    - Monitor for hypotension, dropping hematocrit, sepsis or other signs requiring intervention
  - Transcatheter embolization of renal artery branch injuries has high success rate
    - Assess whether vessel can be sacrificed
    - Occlusion of branch vessel will result in infarct in that vascular territory, therefore embolization should be as selective as possible
    - Gelatin sponge (Gelfoam) or coils most often used as embolic agents
    - Alternative surgical treatment would typically result in either equal or greater tissue loss
  - Low complication rate for embolization
    - Nontarget embolization causes greatest concern; small infarcts usually asymptomatic
    - Rare occurrence of transient hypertension
    - Roughly 10% develop self-limited postembolization syndrome (transient pain, leukocytosis and fever)
  - Class V injuries may require emergent surgical revascularization
    - Renal function severely affected after 3 hours of total ischemia and 6 hours of partial ischemia
    - Successful repair of renal pedicle injury requires revascularization within 4-6 hours of injury
    - Results following revascularization generally poor
  - Early complications after renal trauma include sepsis, urinoma, abscess, A-V fistula, pseudoaneurysm
  - Late complications include hypertension, calculus, hydronephrosis, chronic pyelonephritis, renal failure, atrophy

DIAGNOSTIC CHECKLIST

Consider

- Arteriography if evidence of contrast extravasation on CECT, or if there is persistent retroperitoneal hemorrhage that may require embolization
- Associated injuries are common in blunt abdominal trauma

SELECTED REFERENCES

1. Brandes SB: Management of high grade renal trauma: 20-year experience at a pediatric level-I trauma center. Int Braz J Urol. 33(3):437-8, 2007
2. Delgado Oliva FJ et al: [Conservative approach in major renal trauma] Actas Urol Esp. 31(2):132-9; discussion 140, 2007
3. Henderson CG et al: Management of high grade renal trauma: 20-year experience at a pediatric level I trauma center. J Urol. 178(1):246-50; discussion 250, 2007
4. Lee YJ et al: Renal trauma. Radiol Clin North Am. 45(3):581-92, 2007

IMAGE GALLERY

Typical

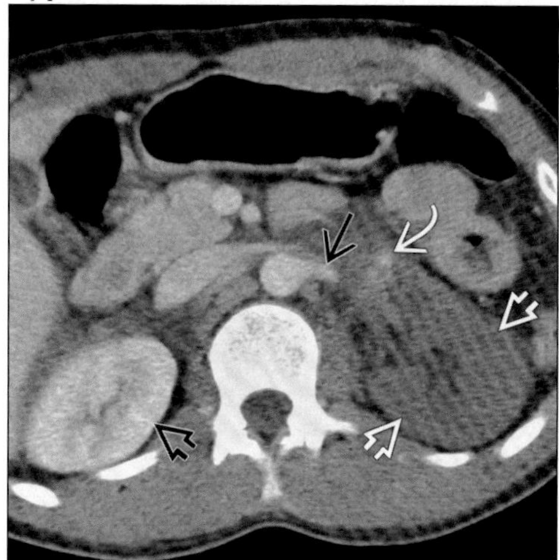

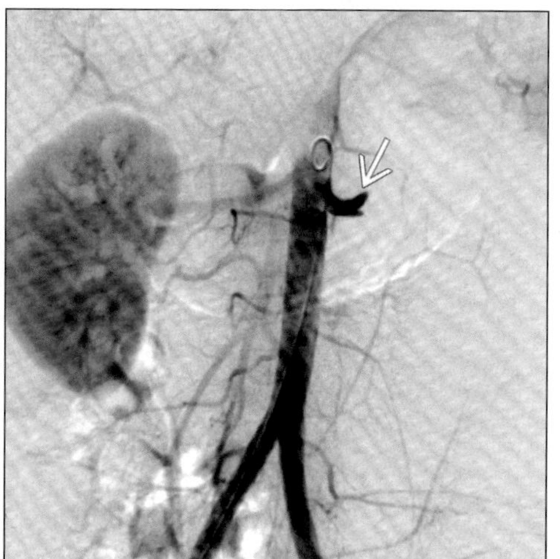

*(**Left**) Axial CECT shows nonperfusion of left kidney ➡. Proximal left renal artery ➡ is opacified but there is contrast extravasation ➡ at the renal hilum, suggesting vascular pedicle avulsion. Right kidney ➡ perfuses normally. (**Right**) Abdominal aortogram shows abrupt occlusion of the proximal left renal artery ➡ consistent with avulsion of the vascular pedicle in this class V injury. Transcatheter coil embolization successfully stabilized the patient.*

Typical

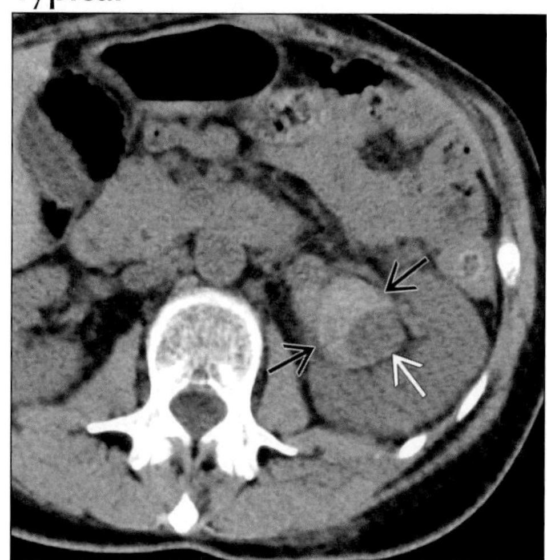

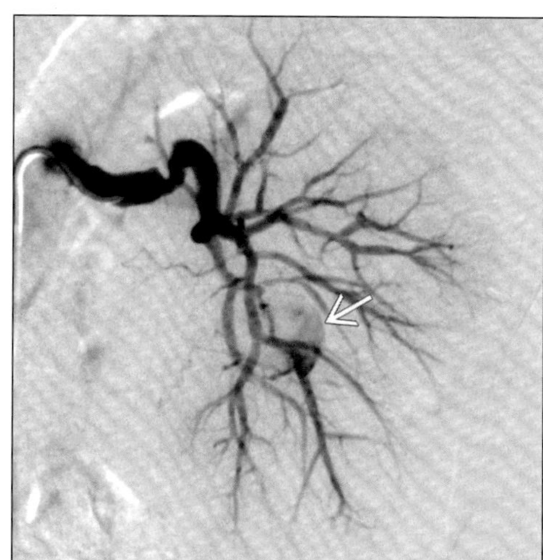

*(**Left**) Axial NECT in a patient who became hypotensive after renal biopsy, shows a high density collection ➡ with central filling defect ➡. This was felt to represent bleeding into either a thrombus-filled renal collecting system or pseudoaneurysm. (**Right**) Renal arteriogram in the same patient shows contrast extravasation ➡ into a pseudoaneurysm corresponding to the collection seen on NECT. This is the source of active hemorrhage in this patient.*

Typical

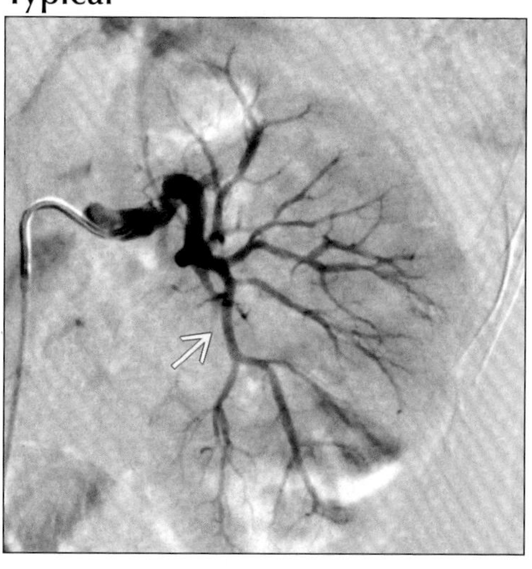

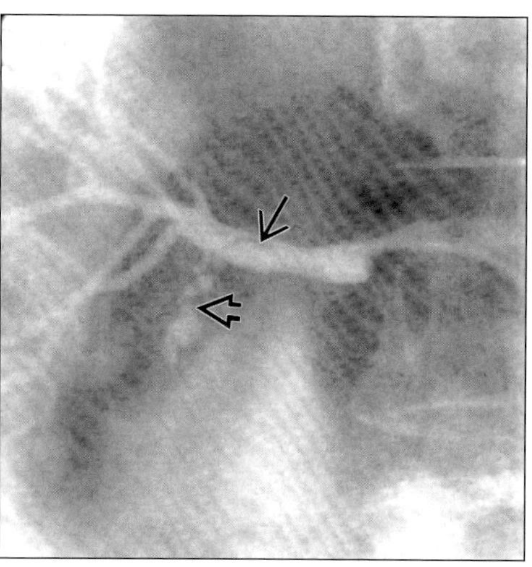

*(**Left**) Renal arteriogram (same patient as prior image) following Gelfoam embolization of the injured arterial branch ➡. Pseudoaneurysm no longer fills & patient became clinically stable, with no further signs of active bleeding. (**Right**) Right renal arteriogram in a different patient shows an iatrogenic arterial injury, with an intimal flap ➡ caused during selective catheterization. There is active extravasation ➡ of contrast indicating that perforation also occurred.*

RENAL TUMOR

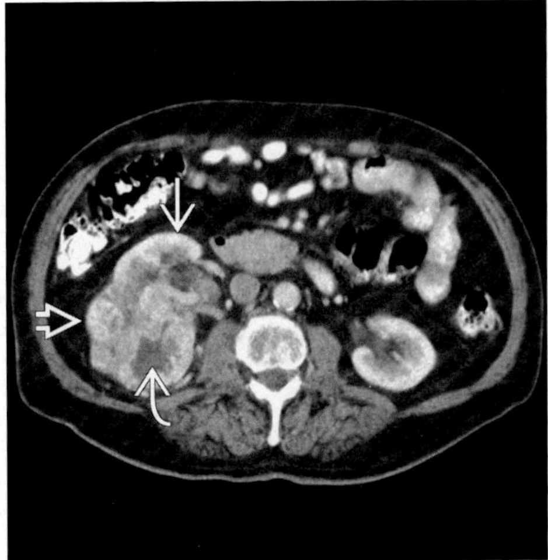

Axial CECT shows a hypervascular, complex renal cell carcinoma ➡ in the mid pole of the right kidney. The nonenhancing area ➡ represents necrosis. The kidney ➡ is enlarged and is displaced anteriorly by the mass.

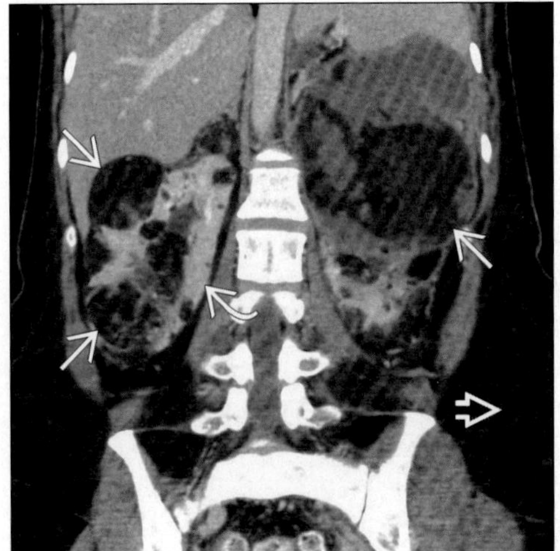

Coronal CECT shows bilateral angiomyolipomas ➡ in a patient with tuberous sclerosis. The fat content of these masses equals that of the subcutaneous tissue ➡. The remaining renal parenchyma ➡ enhances normally.

TERMINOLOGY

Abbreviations and Synonyms

- Renal cell carcinoma (RCC), hypernephroma, renal cell adenocarcinoma, nephrocarcinoma & Grawitz tumor
- Angiomyolipoma (AML), renal hamartoma
- Oncocytoma (OC), renal adenoma
- Multilocular cystic nephroma (MLCN)

Definitions

- Renal parenchymal neoplasm, benign or malignant

IMAGING FINDINGS

General Features

- Best diagnostic clue
  - RCC: Hypervascular renal cortical mass
  - AML: Mixed attenuation, containing fat
  - OC: Stellate, central scar
  - MLCN: Multiple various sized cysts with thick septa
- Morphology
  - RCC: Solid, round, focal ± hemorrhage or necrosis
    - May be cystic, unilocular or multilocular
  - AML: Muscle and fat present in variable quantities
    - Non-invasive; projects into perirenal space
  - OC: Large and homogeneous
    - Stellate central scar
  - MLCN: Multicystic with thick, enhancing septa
    - Cysts may herniate into renal pelvis

Radiographic Findings

- Radiography
  - Asymmetric renal enlargement or abnormal contour
  - Displaced bowel loops with large masses
  - Calcifications overlying renal parenchyma
    - RCC has irregular calcifications
    - MLCN has fine septal calcifications
  - Large AMLs with high fat content can appear lucent
- IVP
  - Asymmetric renal enlargement or abnormal contour
    - Large masses displace kidney; may alter renal axis
  - Mass effect on infundibula, calyces or renal pelvis
    - Increased distance between calyces and renal margin suggests tumor
    - Uretero-pelvic notching by venous collaterals seen with renal vein thrombosis

DDx: Renal Tumor

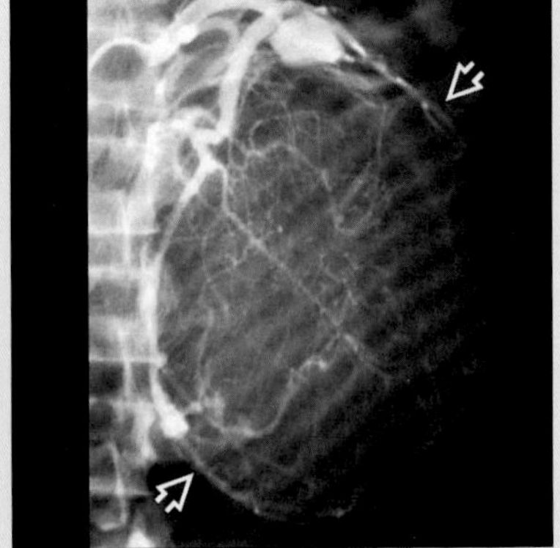

Oncocytoma

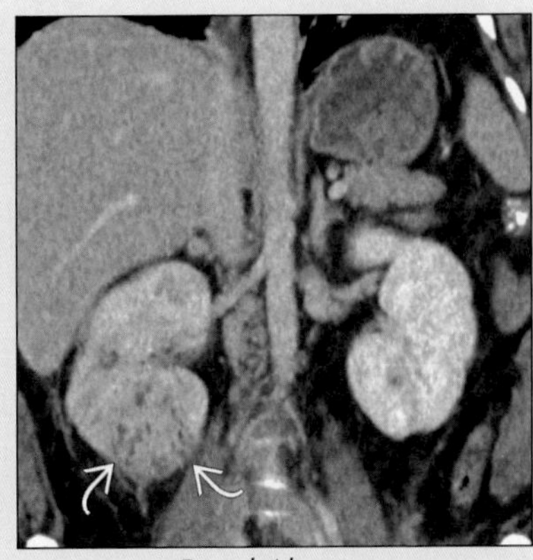

Renal Abscess

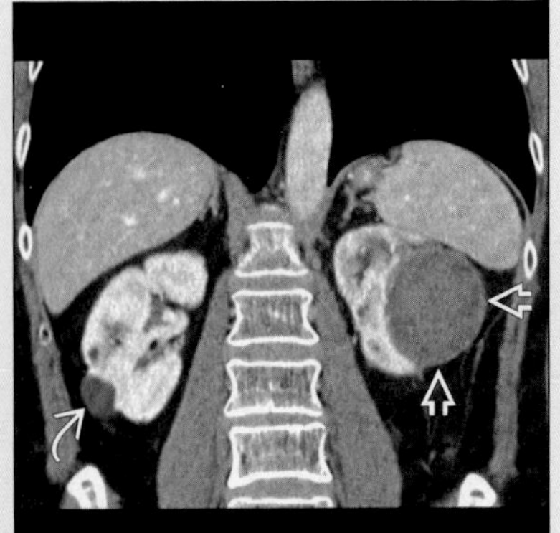

Simple Cyst and Hematoma

RENAL TUMOR

Key Facts

Terminology

- Renal parenchymal neoplasms, benign or malignant
  - Renal cell carcinoma (RCC), hypernephroma, renal cell adenocarcinoma, nephrocarcinoma & Grawitz tumor
  - Angiomyolipoma (AML), renal hamartoma
  - Oncocytoma (OC), renal adenoma
  - Multilocular cystic nephroma (MLCN)

Imaging Findings

- RCC: Hypervascular renal cortical mass
- AML: Mixed attenuation, containing fat
- OC: Stellate, central scar
- MLCN: Multiple varying sized cysts with thick septa
- Multiphase CECT with multiplanar reformations ideal for staging & treatment planning

Clinical Issues

- Hematuria, flank pain, palpable mass with all tumors
- Small lesions may be asymptomatic and found incidentally with imaging
- Treatments include
  - Arterial embolization for hemorrhage, pre-operative devascularization or palliation (RCC, AML)
  - Pre-surgical embolization of bony metastases (RCC)
  - Nephron-sparing procedures (all tumors)
  - Total nephrectomy (mainly RCC and MLCN)

Diagnostic Checklist

- All renal tumors can have similar appearances
- Enhancement, thickened septa, calcifications, solid components suggest malignancy
- Fat in renal tumor most indicative of AML

  - Lucent areas post-contrast suggest necrosis or hypoperfusion
  - RCC enhances in early nephrographic phase
    - Enhancing, irregular walls if cystic or necrotic
    - Delayed nephrogram with ureteral obstruction or renal vein thrombosis
  - Large MLCN can distort or obstruct collecting system
    - Well-defined filling defect in renal pelvis may represent herniated cysts

CT Findings

- NECT
  - Distorted renal contour or asymmetric enlargement
  - HU ≤ renal parenchyma: OC, metastases
  - HU ≥ renal parenchyma: RCC
  - Calcification present: RCC (course and irregular), MLCN (within septa), AML and OC (both very rare)
  - Hyperattenuating areas: RCC (hemorrhage)
  - Hypoattenuating areas: RCC (necrosis), OC (stellate area of ischemic fibrosis)
  - Cystic (uni- or multilocular): MLCN, cystic RCC
  - Contains fat: AML, rarely RCC
- CECT
  - RCC: Hypervascular on early arterial phase
    - Decreased attenuation relative to parenchyma in nephrographic phase
    - Necrosis does not enhance
    - Tumor may extend into adjacent structures, including renal vein or IVC
  - AML: Complex mass; fat and soft tissue attenuation
    - Soft tissue component enhances like renal parenchyma
  - OC: Focal, well-circumscribed, round; low attenuation pseudocapsule in large tumors
    - Homogeneous enhancement; less than renal parenchyma
  - MLCN: Well-circumscribed with multiple, variably-sized cysts
    - Hounsfield (HU) of cysts ≥ HU of water
    - Enhancing, thickened septa
    - Cysts can prolapse into renal pelvis

MR Findings

- RCC: Low signal intensity relative to renal parenchyma on T1WI; hemorrhage has increased signal intensity and necrosis has decreased signal intensity
  - Mildly increased signal intensity relative to renal parenchyma on T2WI; cystic areas have markedly increased signal intensity
  - Large masses heterogeneously and small masses homogeneously on T1 C+
    - Hemorrhage and necrosis do not enhance
- OC: Decreased signal intensity relative to renal parenchyma on T1WI; variable appearance on T2WI
  - Variable signal intensity of central scar on T1WI; enhancement less than remaining tumor on T1 C+
- AML: Increased signal intensity of acute hemorrhage mimics signal of fat on T1WI
  - Signal intensity of AML fat similar to that of retroperitoneal fat on all sequences
- MLCN: Multilocular with signal intensity of cysts like that of water on T1 and T2WI
  - Increased T1WI signal intensity if cysts contain elevated protein
  - T1 C+ shows septal enhancement

Ultrasonographic Findings

- Grayscale Ultrasound
  - RCC: Majority isoechoic to renal parenchyma; may be complex with necrosis
    - Cystic RCC will have thickened septations, nodularity and solid components
  - OC: Solid, homogeneous mass; central scar, if seen, may be echogenic
  - AML: Complex mass with areas of echogenicity similar to the perirenal fat
    - Mixed or decreased echogenicity with acute hemorrhage
  - MLCN: Multi-loculated, well-defined mass
    - Simple intracystic fluid; may have internal echoes

Angiographic Findings

- RCC: Hypervascular mass with enlarged renal artery

- Irregular, disorganized tumor neovascularity
- Arteriovenous shunting, contrast pooling
- OC: Spoke-wheel vessels with dense, homogeneous nephrogram
  - Stellate central scar is relatively hypovascular
- AML: Irregular, bizarre vascularity
  - Vessels circumferentially draped around tumor
  - May have arterial aneurysms within tumor
- MLCN: Irregular vessels delineating tumor margin and septae
  - Nephrographic phase: Septa radiodense and encircle radiolucent mass
- Intra-arterial epinephrine causes vasoconstriction of normal arteries but not tumor vascularity

Imaging Recommendations

- Best imaging tool: Multiphase CECT with multiplanar reformations
- Multiphase CECT ideal for staging & treatment planning
  - NECT, arterial, corticomedullary, nephrographic and excretory phases
  - Multiplanar reformations, volume rendering, MIPs
- Multiplanar MR useful for staging & pretreatment planning
- US used to determine cystic vs. solid mass

DIFFERENTIAL DIAGNOSIS

Renal Cyst

- Simple cysts: Nonenhancing, thin walls, low HUs
- Hemorrhagic cysts: Can have enhancing, thick walls and septa

Renal Abscess

- Focal abscess simulates necrotic RCC
- Has thickened, enhancing wall ± calcifications
- History and physical distinguish abscess from RCC

Transitional Cell Carcinoma

- Tends to have calyceal invasion

Hematoma

- May have hematocrit level; history of trauma

PATHOLOGY

General Features

- Genetics
  - RCC associated with von Hippel-Lindau
  - AML associated with tuberous sclerosis
- Epidemiology: RCC most common renal primary

Microscopic Features

- RCC: Adenocarcinoma of proximal tubular origin
- AML: Fat, smooth muscle and arteries with abnormal wall architecture
- OC: Large epithelial cells; eosinophilic cytoplasm with small, round nuclei and abnormal mitochondria
- MLCN: Loose connective tissue in the septae; cysts lined with cuboidal epithelium

Staging, Grading or Classification Criteria

- Bosniak classification of cystic renal masses
- TNM staging for malignancy

CLINICAL ISSUES

Presentation

- Most common signs/symptoms: Hematuria, flank pain and palpable mass with all tumors
- Other signs/symptoms
  - Small lesions may be asymptomatic and found incidentally with imaging
  - AMLs can present with acute hemorrhage

Demographics

- Age
  - RCC: Middle age (40-70 years)
  - AML: Young adulthood to 9th decade
  - OC: Similar to RCC
  - MLCN: Two peaks: Infants and toddlers, then middle-age
- Gender
  - RCC: M:F = 2:1
  - AML: Female predominance
  - OC: Similar to RCC
  - MLCN: Male predominance in pediatric group; female predominance in adults

Natural History & Prognosis

- Dependent on tumor type

Treatment

- Chemotherapy or biologic therapies (RCC)
- Arterial embolization for hemorrhage, pre-operative devascularization or palliation (RCC, AML)
  - Used for pre-surgical embolization of bony metastases (RCC)
- Radiation therapy for palliative and pre- or post-operative (RCC)
- Nephron-sparing procedures (all tumors)
  - Radiofrequency ablation or cryoablation
  - Partial nephrectomy
- Total nephrectomy (mainly RCC and MLCN)

DIAGNOSTIC CHECKLIST

Consider

- All renal tumors can have similar appearances

Image Interpretation Pearls

- Enhancement, thickened septa, calcifications, solid components suggest malignancy
- Fat in renal tumor most indicative of AML

SELECTED REFERENCES

1. Hartman DS et al: From the RSNA refresher courses: a practical approach to the cystic renal mass. Radiographics. 24 Suppl 1:S101-15, 2004
2. Davidson AJ et al: Radiologic assessment of renal masses: implications for patient care. Radiology. 202(2):297-305, 1997

RENAL TUMOR

IMAGE GALLERY

Typical

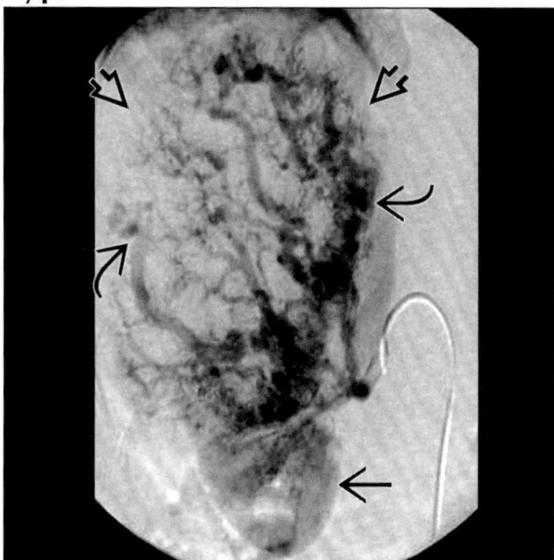

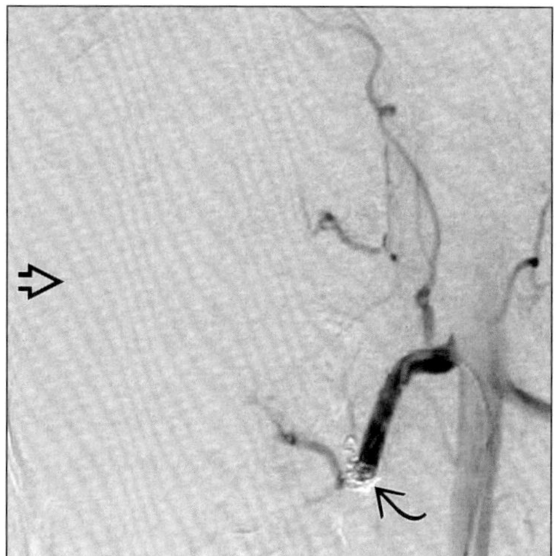

*(**Left**) Posteroanterior DSA shows a hypervascular renal cell carcinoma of the right kidney. The vessels are irregular and enlarged, with contrast pooling and arteriovenous shunting. The lower pole is normal. (**Right**) Posteroanterior DSA of same patient following pre-operative embolization shows no flow to the right kidney. The embolization was performed with particles followed by placement of coils in the renal artery, in preparation for a nephrectomy.*

Typical

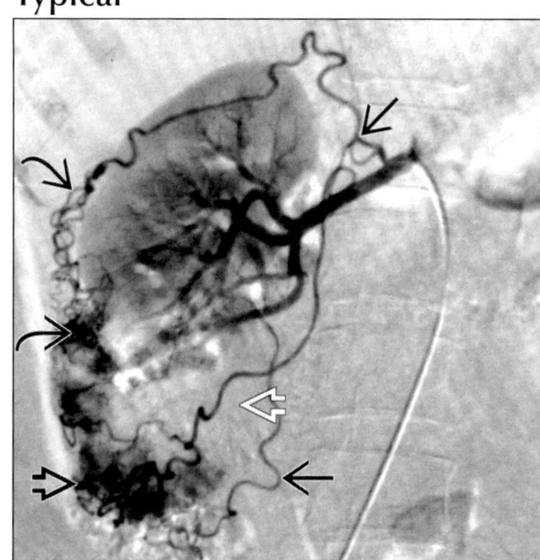

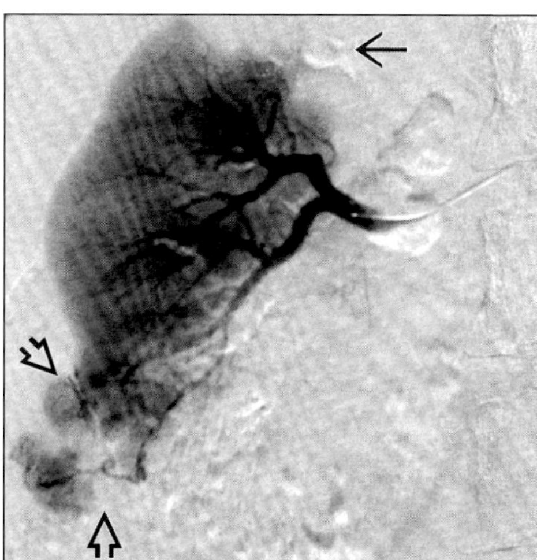

*(**Left**) Posteroanterior DSA shows an angiomyolipoma in the lower renal pole. The vessels are bizarre, with blood supply parasitized from other arteries. The mass is somewhat lucent, reflecting the fat content. (**Right**) Posteroanterior DSA in the same patient following embolization with particles shows markedly decreased vascularity of the lower pole angiomyolipoma. The upper pole is not seen due to the catheter position during contrast injection.*

Typical

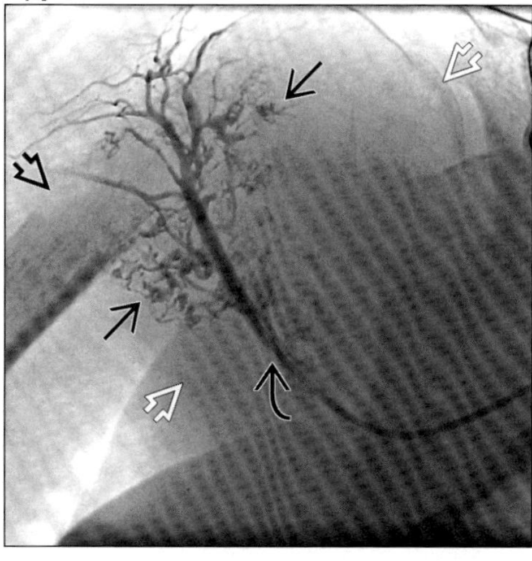

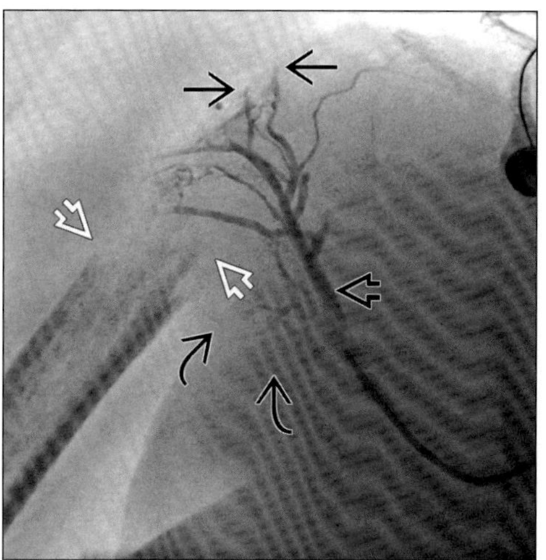

*(**Left**) Posteroanterior DSA of the posterior circumflex humeral artery shows tumor neovascularity and the tumor blush of a renal cell carcinoma osseous metastasis. Note the bony destruction and the associated soft tissue mass. (**Right**) Posteroanterior DSA (same patient) following embolization of the posterior circumflex humeral artery shows decreased tumor blush and pruned larger branches. Again note the cortical destruction by the metastasis.*

RENAL ARTERIOVENOUS FISTULA

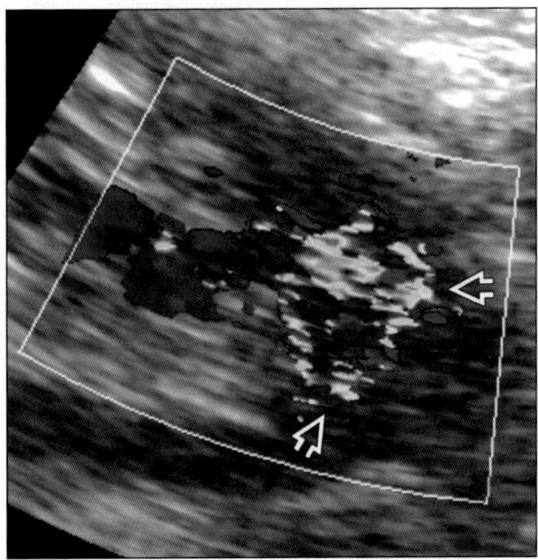

Sagittal color Doppler ultrasound obtained in a patient who sustained penetrating trauma shows mixed arterial and venous signal ➡ within the kidney, suggesting a pseudoaneurysm.

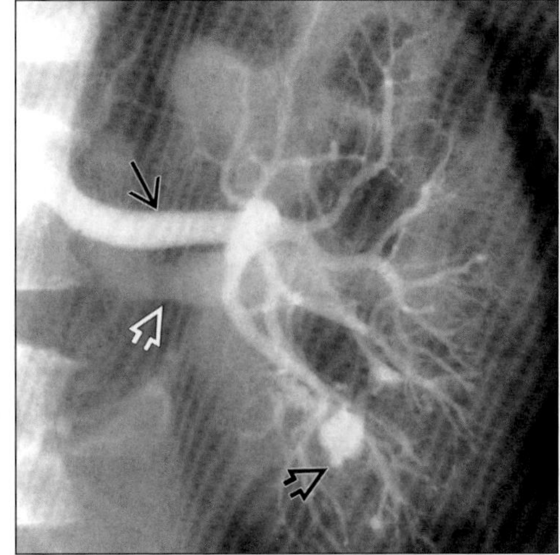

Arteriogram obtained in the same patient confirms the pseudoaneurysm ➡ in the lower renal pole, in association with an arteriovenous fistula. The renal artery → and vein ➡ are simultaneously opacified.

TERMINOLOGY

Abbreviations and Synonyms

- Renal arteriovenous fistula (AV fistula or AVF)
- Post-traumatic renal arteriovenous fistula

Definitions

- Renal arteriovenous fistula
  - Abnormal direct communication between an artery and a vein

IMAGING FINDINGS

General Features

- Best diagnostic clue
  - Simultaneous opacification of artery and vein during arterial injection phase of CECT or angiography
  - Intraparenchymal pseudoaneurysm connecting arterial and venous branches
- Location: Typically intraparenchymal, less frequently extraparenchymal
- Size: Variable; dependent upon size and location of arterial and venous branches involved in fistulous communication

CT Findings

- CECT
  - In addition to angiographic findings, may show intraparenchymal hematoma or infarct from post-traumatic AV fistula
  - May be useful following transcatheter embolization to assess for parenchymal infarcts
- CTA: Will have similar findings to catheter angiography

MR Findings

- MRA
  - Will have similar findings to angiography and CTA
  - Not frequently used in evaluation, treatment planning or follow-up of AV fistula

Ultrasonographic Findings

- Color Doppler
  - May show direct arterial to venous branch communication

DDx: Renal Arteriovenous Fistula

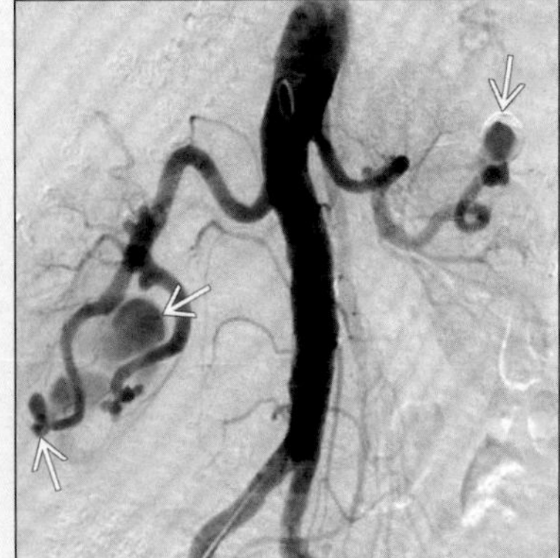

Renal Artery Aneurysms

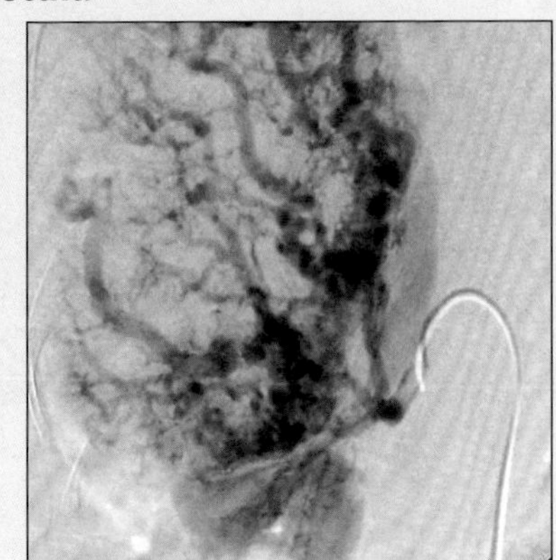

Renal Cell Carcinoma

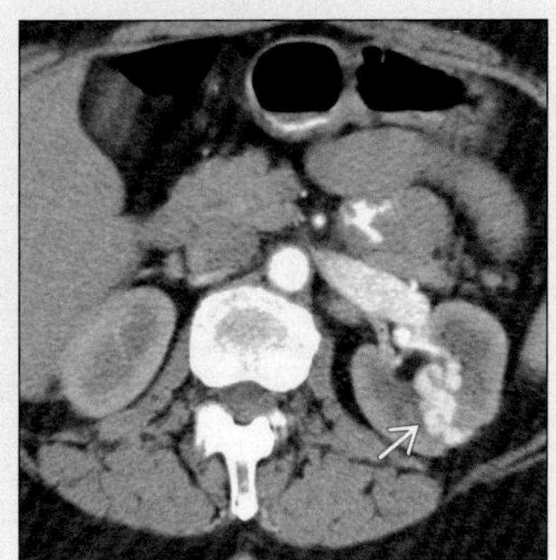

Renal Arteriovenous Malformation

RENAL ARTERIOVENOUS FISTULA

Key Facts

Terminology
- Renal arteriovenous fistula: Abnormal direct communication between an artery and a vein

Imaging Findings
- Angiography shows direct arterial to venous communication, often with pseudoaneurysm
  - Presence of early-draining vein
- Simultaneous opacification of artery and vein during arterial injection phase of CECT or angiography

Top Differential Diagnoses
- Renal Arteriovenous Malformation (AVM)
  - Similar to AV fistula but is congenital
- Renal Neoplasm
- Renal Artery Aneurysm

Pathology
- AV fistulas are almost always acquired
  - Penetrating and iatrogenic trauma are most common causes of renal AV fistula
  - Idiopathic renal AV fistulas have characteristics of acquired fistulas but no identifiable cause

Clinical Issues
- Most conservative treatment possible favored in management of renal injury such as AV fistula
  - Many post-traumatic renal AV fistulas may close spontaneously, particularly if small
  - Percutaneous transcatheter embolization is preferred treatment for symptomatic lesions; has high success rate (80-100%)
  - Gelatin sponge (Gelfoam) and coils are most commonly used embolic agents

    - When arteriovenous fistula is identified, draining vein may show arterialized flow pattern
  - May demonstrate any pseudoaneurysm and relationship to AV fistula
    - Pseudoaneurysm seen as anechoic mass with internal color flow

Angiographic Findings
- Direct arterial to venous branch communication
- Pseudoaneurysm may be present at site of arteriovenous communication
  - Extravascular contrast collection; delayed clearing
- Intrarenal hematoma, with vessel displacement or splaying may be present
- Presence of early-draining vein

Imaging Recommendations
- Best imaging tool
  - Angiography or CECT with CTA
  - Angiography used for guidance during transcatheter treatment of AV fistula

DIFFERENTIAL DIAGNOSIS

Renal Arteriovenous Malformation (AVM)
- Congenital abnormal communications between intrarenal arterial and venous systems, typically with a central vascular "nidus"
- Congenital renal AVM rare, with incidence of 0.004%
  - Congenital cirsoid AVMs have dilated, corkscrew appearance, much like varicose vein
    - Multiple communications exist between arteries and veins
    - Communications develop multiple coiled channels, forming mass within renal parenchyma
    - Arterial supply arises from one or more segmental or interlobar renal arteries
    - Proximity to collecting system may explain high prevalence of hematuria
  - Cavernous AVMs have with single dilated vessels
    - Much less common; has single artery feeding into single cystic chamber, with single draining vein
- Symptomatic patients present with hematuria, hypertension and flank pain
  - Gross hematuria is initial symptom in 75%, hypertension in 25%
  - Less common symptoms are high-output cardiac failure and spontaneous retroperitoneal hemorrhage
- Large lesions seen on CT and MR, but need angiography for definitive diagnosis and potential transcatheter treatment
- Preferred treatment is embolization; extremely large AVMs may require surgical resection

Renal Neoplasm
- Most are asymptomatic but may have symptoms of hematuria and flank pain
- Renal cell carcinoma can be highly vascular, with significant arteriovenous shunting
  - Very rarely can have sufficient arteriovenous shunting to produce high-output cardiac failure
  - Angiogenic tumor factors have been implicated in development of AVMs within renal neoplasms
- Treated with surgical resection; percutaneous ablation for smaller tumors

Renal Artery Aneurysm
- Rare lesions with incidence of approximately 0.1%
  - 20% bilateral and 30% multiple
  - Occur equally in men and women although ruptures more common during pregnancy
- Aneurysms from atherosclerosis, fibromuscular dysplasia and segmental arterial mediolysis typically involve extraparenchymal renal artery branches
  - Extraparenchymal aneurysms predominate, comprising approximately 85%
  - Of the extraparenchymal type, 70% saccular, 20% fusiform, and 10% dissecting
- Aneurysms associated with vasculitis (polyarteritis nodosa) or with hematogenous infection are typically intraparenchymal and located peripherally
  - Commonly are microaneurysms
- Symptomatic patients may have hematuria, hypertension and flank pain
  - Incidence of hypertension may be as high as 90%

- Treatment of symptomatic or ruptured aneurysms may be surgical or endovascular

Nutcracker Syndrome

- Compression of left renal vein between aorta and SMA causes left renal venous hypertension and hematuria
  - Intrarenal and perirenal varices caused by venous hypertension
    - May rupture into renal collecting system and cause hematuria
- May have abdominal, flank and pelvic pain in addition to hematuria
  - Recurrent or massive hematuria is indication for treatment
    - Surgical and endovascular treatments have been used, with varying degrees of success

PATHOLOGY

General Features

- Etiology
  - AV fistulas are almost always acquired
    - Idiopathic renal arteriovenous fistulas have characteristics of acquired fistulas, but no cause can be identified
    - Idiopathic arteriovenous fistulas may arise from spontaneous erosion or rupture of diseased renal arterial segment into nearby renal vein
  - Penetrating injuries such as gunshot and stab wounds may result in renal AV fistula
  - Iatrogenic trauma is a common cause of renal AV fistula
    - Occurs in 15% of percutaneous renal biopsies
    - Percutaneous nephrostomy and tract dilatation for percutaneous nephrostolithotomy are also causes
- Epidemiology
  - In patients with hypertension following renal trauma, renal AV fistulas be present in one third
  - In patients with penetrating trauma, arteriovenous fistulas may affect as many as 60-80%

CLINICAL ISSUES

Presentation

- Most common signs/symptoms
  - Majority are asymptomatic
    - Hematuria, hypertension and/or flank pain when symptomatic
- Other signs/symptoms: Less commonly may have high-output cardiac failure, bruit or spontaneous retroperitoneal hemorrhage

Natural History & Prognosis

- Many post-traumatic renal AV fistulas may close spontaneously, particularly if small
- New onset of hypertension may be seen in larger AV fistulas
- Large AV fistulas require corrective treatment
  - Very high success and typically low complication rates with endovascular treatment

Treatment

- Most conservative treatment possible favored in management of renal injury such as AV fistula
  - Percutaneous transcatheter embolization is preferred treatment for symptomatic lesions
    - Must determine whether vessel(s) can be sacrificed and alternative treatment methods
    - Occlusion of renal branch vessels causes infarction proportional to vessel size and vascular territory
    - Embolization should be as selective as possible, with catheter positioned close to fistula
    - Gelatin sponge (Gelfoam) and coils are most commonly used embolic agents
    - Extraparenchymal AV fistulas between renal artery and vein have been treated with covered stents
  - High success rate (80-100%) with transcatheter embolization
    - Low complication rate
    - Greatest concerns are nontarget embolization and large infarcts; small infarcts asymptomatic
    - Transient hypertension occasionally occurs
    - 10% incidence of postembolization syndrome: Transient pain, leukocytosis and fever
- Nephrectomy was past treatment for large AV fistulas
  - Variety of newer embolic agents (e.g., Amplatzer plug, covered stents) allow endovascular treatment of even very large renal AV fistulas

DIAGNOSTIC CHECKLIST

Consider

- Renal AV fistula in patient with hypertension or hematuria after renal intervention or trauma
  - Simultaneous arterial and venous opacification during injection phase of CECT or angiography
  - Pseudoaneurysm may be present at site of arteriovenous communication

SELECTED REFERENCES

1. Idowu O et al: Dual use of an amplatzer device in the transcatheter embolization of a large high-flow renal arteriovenous fistula. J Vasc Interv Radiol. 18(5):671-6, 2007
2. Kensella D et al: Transcatheter Embolization of a Renal Arteriovenous Fistula Complicated by an Aneurysm of the Feeding Renal Artery. Cardiovasc Intervent Radiol. 2007
3. Park BK et al: Arteriovenous Fistula after Radiofrequency Ablation of a Renal Tumor Located within the Renal Sinus. J Vasc Interv Radiol. 18(9):1183-5, 2007
4. Tam J et al: Acute traumatic renal artery to inferior vena cava fistula treated with a covered stent. Cardiovasc Intervent Radiol. 29(6):1129-31, 2006
5. Cakmak M et al: Congestive heart failure due to traumatic arteriovenous fistula--two case reports. Angiology. 54(5):625-9, 2003
6. Garcia-Schurmann JM et al: Spontaneous thrombosis of an iatrogenic arteriovenous fistula of the kidney. Urology. 58(1):106, 2001
7. Reilly KJ et al: Angiographic embolization of a penetrating traumatic renal arteriovenous fistula. J Trauma. 41(4):763-5, 1996
8. Corr P et al: Embolization in traumatic intrarenal vascular injuries. Clin Radiol. 43(4):262-4, 1991

IMAGE GALLERY

Typical

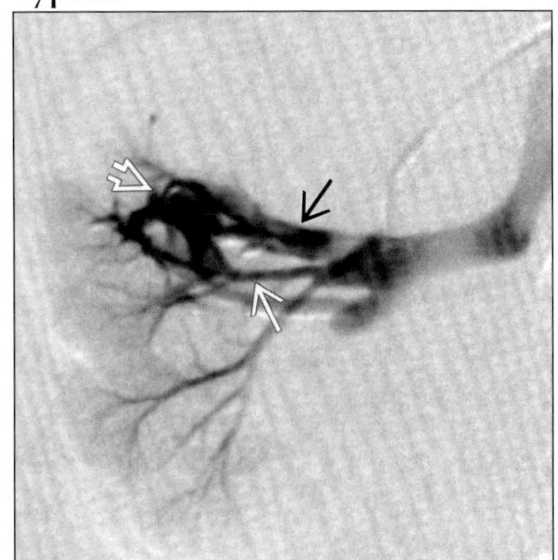

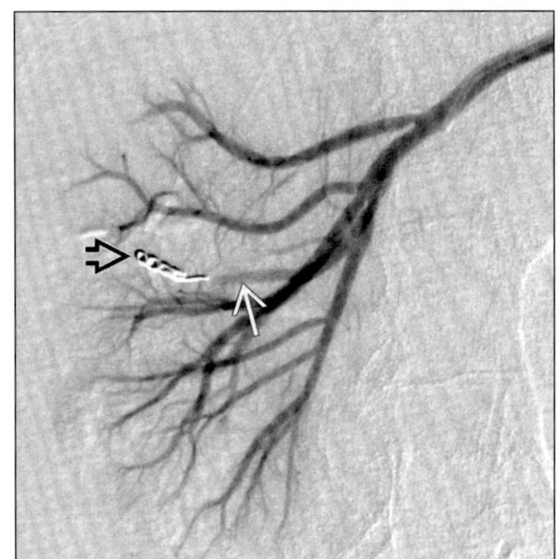

(Left) *Selective renal arteriogram shows an arteriovenous fistula ➡, with simultaneous opacification of the renal arterial ➡ and venous ➡ branches during the initial phase of the contrast injection.* ***(Right)*** *Renal arteriogram (same patient as previous image) following transcatheter embolization shows coils ➡ occluding distal portion of the renal arterial branch ➡ that previously supplied the arteriovenous fistula. There is a high success rate with embolization therapy.*

Variant

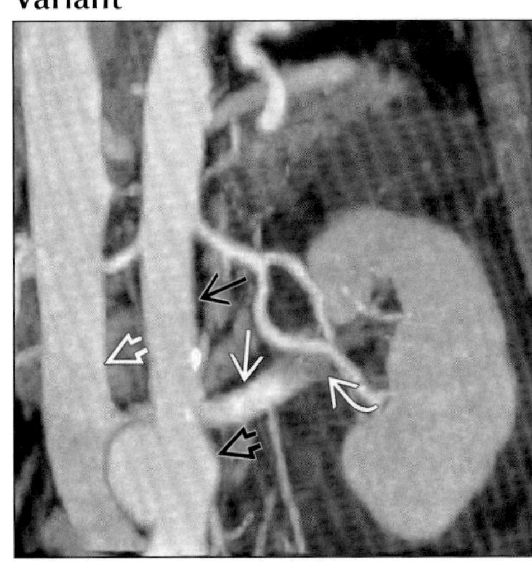

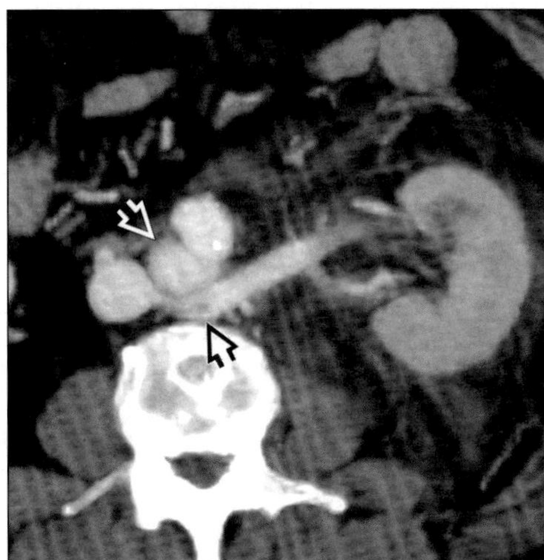

(Left) *CECT coronal MIP shows simultaneous opacification of aorta ➡ & IVC ➡ from erosion of distal AAA ➡ into left renal vein ➡, causing an AV fistula. The renal vein is nonopacified at the renal hilus ➡, because contrast is entering at the fistulous communication.* ***(Right)*** *CECT axial MIP (same patient) shows the left renal vein is retroaortic ➡ & is compressed by the AAA ➡. Aortic pulsation & this anatomic variant caused the aortorenal AV fistula.*

Typical

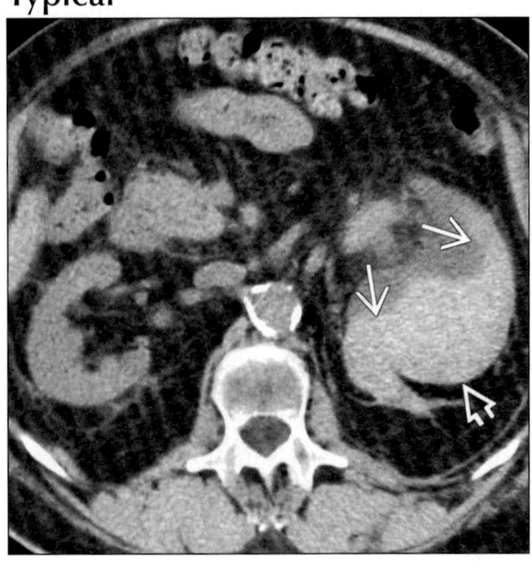

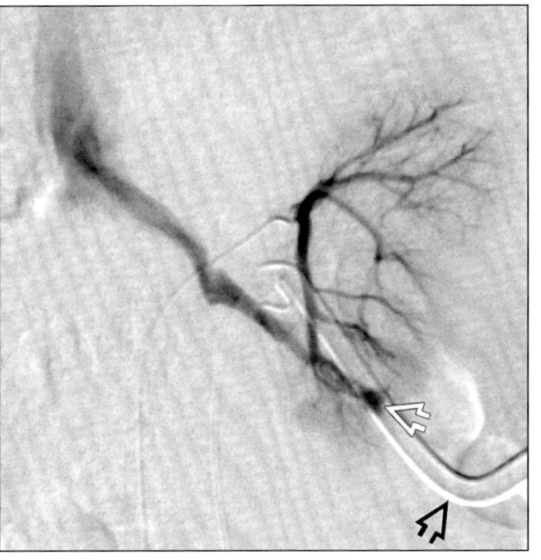

(Left) *Axial NECT shows left renal subcapsular hematoma ➡ in a patient who underwent placement of a percutaneous left nephrostomy tube. There is an interface ➡ between the normal renal parenchyma & higher density blood of the subcapsular hematoma.* ***(Right)*** *Selective left renal arteriogram (same patient as previous image) shows an AV fistula ➡ as the etiology for the renal subcapsular hematoma. Note indwelling percutaneous nephrostomy tube ➡.*

RENAL/ADRENAL VENOGRAPHY AND SAMPLING

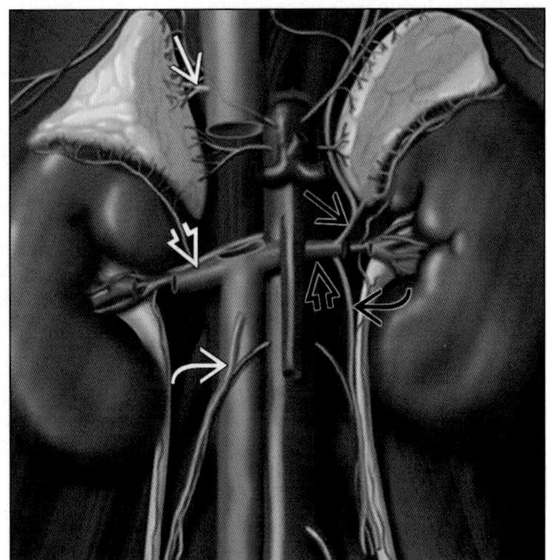

Graphic shows the right adrenal ➔, renal ➔ and gonadal ➔ veins drain directly into the IVC, while the left adrenal ➔ and gonadal ➔ veins drain into the left renal vein ➔, which courses anterior to the aorta.

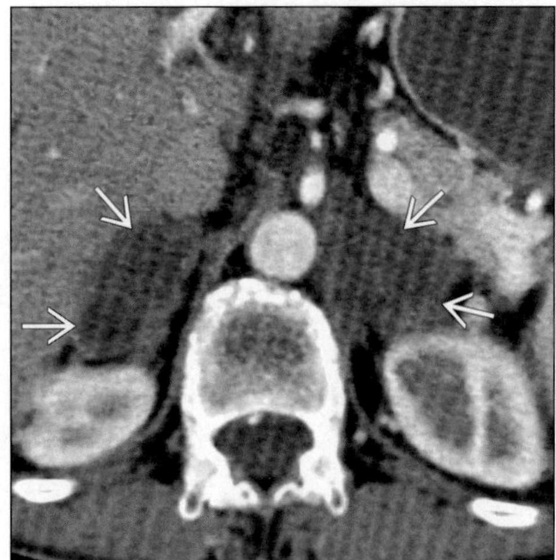

Axial CECT shows bilateral adrenal masses ➔ in a patient with hypokalemia and diastolic hypertension, suspected of primary aldosteronism. Bilateral adrenal vein sampling was performed for further evaluation.

TERMINOLOGY

Abbreviations

- Renal vein sampling (RVS)
- Adrenal vein sampling (AVS)

Synonyms

- Renal vein sampling (RVS) and renal vein renin sampling (RVRS)

Definitions

- Primary aldosteronism (Conn syndrome): Hypersecretion of aldosterone by adrenal glands
  - Hypersecretion by adrenal adenoma is cause in 2/3 of cases
  - Bilateral idiopathic adrenal hyperplasia is cause in remaining 1/3
- Cushing syndrome: Clinical complex resulting from prolonged, inappropriate exposure to glucocorticoids
  - Most frequently caused by administration of exogenous glucocorticoids or adrenocorticotrophic hormone (ACTH)
  - Endogenous causes include ACTH secreting pituitary tumor, adrenal neoplasm (benign or malignant) or ectopic ACTH secretion by tumor

PRE-PROCEDURE

Indications

- Adrenal sampling used when a confirmed endocrine disorder requires localization to guide treatment
- Adrenal venous sampling used to identify primary aldosteronism
  - Serum potassium < 3.5 mEq/L and diastolic hypertension suggest primary aldosteronism
  - Other laboratory data: Plasma renin and 24 hour urine collection for sodium, cortisol and aldosterone
  - Adrenal venous sampling may identify surgically correctable forms of primary aldosteronism
    - Aldosterone-producing adenoma and bilateral adrenal hyperplasia most common subtypes of primary aldosteronism
    - Bilateral adrenal hyperplasia treated medically
    - With aldosterone-producing adenoma, adrenalectomy may normalize blood pressure and correct primary aldosteronism
    - Most frequent form of secondary hypertension
  - Adrenal vein sampling currently superior to imaging for differentiation of primary hyperaldosteronism
    - Most accurate way of differentiating subtypes of primary aldosteronism
    - Diagnosing aldosterone-producing adenoma requires demonstration of lateralization of aldosterone hypersecretion
- Adrenal venous sampling sometimes used to confirm adrenal gland as source of excess ACTH in patient with Cushing syndrome and adrenal mass on imaging
  - Localization of cause of Cushing syndrome extremely important in directing therapy
    - In endogenous Cushing syndrome, urinary cortisol excretion elevated; plasma levels fail to drop in response to dose of dexamethasone
    - Pituitary or ectopic sources generally have elevated serum ACTH levels
    - With independently functioning adrenal masses, serum ACTH may be low, necessitating adrenal vein sampling to localize
    - Resection for functioning unilateral adrenal mass
- Adrenal venous sampling for pheochromocytomas and paraganglionomas
  - With advances in MR and CT, adrenal vein sampling infrequently needed
    - Used in localizing occult pheochromocytoma when imaging is equivocal or negative

RENAL/ADRENAL VENOGRAPHY AND SAMPLING

Key Facts

Pre-procedure

- Adrenal venous sampling used to identify primary aldosteronism
- Adrenal venous sampling sometimes used to confirm adrenal gland as source of excess ACTH in patient with Cushing syndrome and adrenal mass on imaging studies
- In majority of individuals, each adrenal gland drained by single adrenal vein
  - Right adrenal vein drains directly into IVC
  - Left adrenal vein drains into left renal vein
- Renal vein renin sampling in evaluation and treatment of renovascular hypertension now infrequently performed
  - Renal venography now usually associated with therapy (e.g., gonadal vein embolization)
- Usually each kidney drained by a single renal vein
  - Left renal vein courses anterior to aorta and posterior to SMA to join IVC opposite right renal vein, which is shorter and joins IVC at L-2

Procedure

- Introduction of two separate selective catheters, each from common femoral vein
- Simultaneous samples from both adrenal veins before and 15 minutes after administration of ACTH (primary hyperaldosteronism)
  - Adrenal adenoma has high aldosterone/cortisol ratio before and after ACTH, lateralizing to affected gland
- In endogenous Cushing syndrome, elevated ACTH lateralizing to adrenal vein in presence of adrenal mass on CT or MR is confirmatory

---

    - Detection of bilateral tumors in familial syndromes such as von Hippel-Lindau, when imaging shows only unilateral disease
- Use of renal vein renin sampling in evaluation and treatment of renovascular hypertension has decreased and now infrequently performed
  - Selective sampling of renin directly from each renal vein and from IVC above and below renal vein level
    - Renin levels from one kidney that are > 1.5 times that of the contralateral kidney is positive result
    - Rise in renin from infrarenal to suprarenal IVC is further evidence for renovascular hypertension
- Renal venography for diagnosis and/or treatment
  - Nutcracker syndrome
    - Compression of the left renal vein between the SMA and the abdominal aorta as it courses between the two vessels
    - Results in left renal venous hypertension and may produce chronic pain, hematuria and proteinuria
    - May result in male varicoceles and female pelvic congestion syndrome
    - Left renal venography, with measurement of pressure gradient (> 2 mm Hg significant) between renal vein and IVC to confirm diagnosis
    - Has been treated with left renal vein stent, with varying degrees of success
  - Pelvic congestion syndrome
    - Left ovarian (gonadal) vein drains directly into left renal vein
    - Left renal venography may demonstrate reflux into dilated ovarian vein, indicating venous valvular incompetency
  - Varicocele
    - Left internal spermatic (gonadal) vein drains directly into left renal vein
    - Left renal venography may demonstrate reflux into the gonadal vein and thus diagnose venous valvular incompetency

Contraindications

- Contrast allergy
- Renal dysfunction

Getting Started

- Angiographic sheaths and catheters
  - Two separate vascular sheaths (6 or 7 Fr.) for initial femoral venous access
  - Angiographic catheters
    - Selective catheters should have side-hole near tip
    - Simmons, Sos or Mickaelson catheters are typical choices for right adrenal vein
    - Cobra catheter is typical choice for left adrenal vein and for either renal vein
    - Pigtail or other nonselective catheter may be used for suprarenal or infrarenal IVC
- Iodinated contrast medium
- Medications
  - Cortisol for adrenal gland stimulation
- Laboratory vials for sample collection

Adrenal Venous Anatomy

- In majority of individuals, each adrenal gland drained by single adrenal vein
  - Multiple adrenal veins are exception but occasionally occur
  - Adrenal veins communicate with retroperitoneal and renal capsular veins
- Right adrenal vein drains directly into posterolateral aspect of IVC
  - Typically located 2-4 cm above right renal vein
  - Small accessory hepatic vein may rarely drain into right adrenal vein or vice versa
- Left adrenal vein drains into superior aspect of left renal vein
  - Typically located 3-5 cm from left renal vein orifice
  - May very rarely drain directly into IVC

Renal Venous Anatomy

- Usually each kidney is drained by a single renal vein
  - Renal veins rarely have valves
  - Communicate with other retroperitoneal veins (e.g., lumbar, azygos, gonadal veins)
- Left renal vein courses anterior to aorta and posterior to SMA to join IVC opposite right renal vein
  - Left renal vein drains somewhat anteriorly into IVC

RENAL/ADRENAL VENOGRAPHY AND SAMPLING

- Right renal vein is shorter and drains into IVC at approximately L-2 vertebral level
- Frequent variations in renal venous anatomy

PROCEDURE

Patient Position/Location

- For both renal and adrenal venography/sampling
  - Introduction of two selective catheters from common femoral vein, via separate vascular sheaths
  - Both sheaths may be introduced from same femoral vein or from bilateral femoral approach
    - Two catheters unnecessary for venography without sampling

Procedure Steps

- Adrenal venography and sampling
  - Obtain venous access from common femoral vein punctures, with introduction of two separate 6 or 7 French vascular sheaths
  - Introduce two separate selective catheters into IVC and cannulate left and right adrenal veins
    - Cobra catheter often used for left adrenal vein cannulation; may require use of Waltman loop
    - Simmons, Sos, or Mickaelson catheter often used for cannulation of right adrenal vein
  - Venous sampling from both adrenal veins and peripheral source (e.g., femoral vein)
    - Obtain simultaneously from both adrenal veins before and 15 minutes after administration of ACTH (0.25 mg bolus followed by infusion of 0.15-0.20 mg/hr)
  - Label all tubes, with attention to right vs. left
  - Submit samples for aldosterone and cortisol assays
    - Appropriate cortisol level confirms correct catheter position within adrenal vein

Findings and Reporting

- Adrenal vein sampling for primary aldosteronism
  - Appropriate cortisol level confirms correct catheter position within adrenal vein
    - Cortisol production should be same for both adrenal glands
  - Adrenal venous sampling may distinguish between functioning adrenal adenoma and idiopathic adrenal hyperplasia
    - Adrenal adenoma has high aldosterone/cortisol ratio before and after ACTH, lateralizing to affected gland
    - Lateralization generally considered > 4:1 ratio difference between glands
    - In bilateral hyperplasia, no lateralization of ratios before or after ACTH, but aldosterone/cortisol ratio is higher than in IVC
- Adrenal vein sampling for Cushing syndrome
  - Obtain samples from both adrenal veins, suprarenal and infrarenal IVC with no cortisol stimulation
    - Elevated ACTH lateralizing to one adrenal vein in presence of adrenal mass on CT or MR is confirmatory

Alternative Procedures/Therapies

- Radiologic
  - Adrenal vein sampling has been augmented with multiplanar C-arm CT images acquired during 180° C-arm rotation
    - Whenever C-arm CT images shows sampling catheter in wrong position, catheter repositioned
  - Do imaging and other tests obviate need for sampling?
    - In one study of sampling after equivocal CT, 22% would have had incorrect exclusion from surgery and 25% unnecessary adrenalectomy

POST-PROCEDURE

Things To Do

- When obtaining venous samples, note time obtained and label all tubes with attention to right vs. left
- Collect samples in appropriate containers for laboratory analysis; conform to lab requirements for accurate sample analysis (e.g., refrigerated sample)

Things To Avoid

- Adrenal veins are small, weak and prone to rupture; avoid forceful contrast injections
- Usually tenuous selective catheter positions in adrenal veins; avoid excessive catheter movement when obtaining samples to prevent dislodgement

PROBLEMS & COMPLICATIONS

Problems

- Most common difficulty is failure to cannulate right adrenal vein, due to challenging anatomy

Complications

- Most feared complication(s)
  - Contrast reaction or contrast-induced nephropathy
  - Adrenal vein dissection (0.5%), adrenal hemorrhage or infarction (0.5%)
- Other complications: Hematoma at puncture site, venous thrombosis, infection

SELECTED REFERENCES

1. Georgiades CS et al: Adjunctive use of C-arm CT may eliminate technical failure in adrenal vein sampling. J Vasc Interv Radiol. 18(9):1102-5, 2007
2. Mengozzi G et al: Rapid Cortisol Assay during Adrenal Vein Sampling in Patients with Primary Aldosteronism. Clin Chem. 2007
3. Rossi GP: New concepts in adrenal vein sampling for aldosterone in the diagnosis of primary aldosteronism. Curr Hypertens Rep. 9(2):90-7, 2007
4. Harvey A et al: Adrenal venous sampling in primary hyperaldosteronism: comparison of radiographic with biochemical success and the clinical decision-making with "less than ideal" testing. Surgery. 140(6):847-53; discussion 853-5, 2006
5. Nwariaku FE et al: Primary hyperaldosteronism: effect of adrenal vein sampling on surgical outcome. Arch Surg. 141(5):497-502; discussion 502-3, 2006
6. Hasbak P et al: Hypertension and renovascular disease: follow-up on 100 renal vein renin samplings. J Hum Hypertens. 16(4):275-80, 2002

IMAGE GALLERY

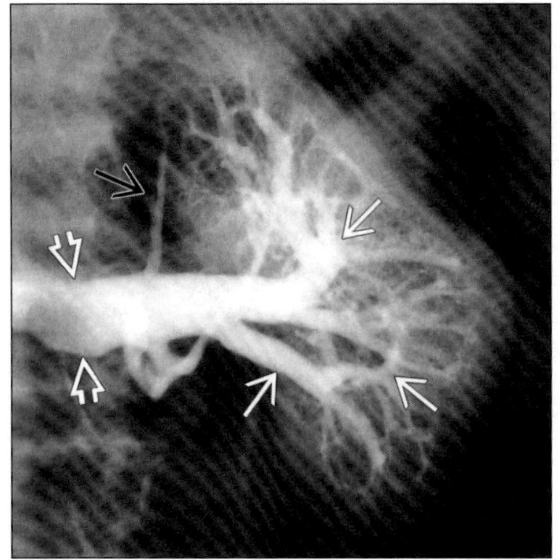

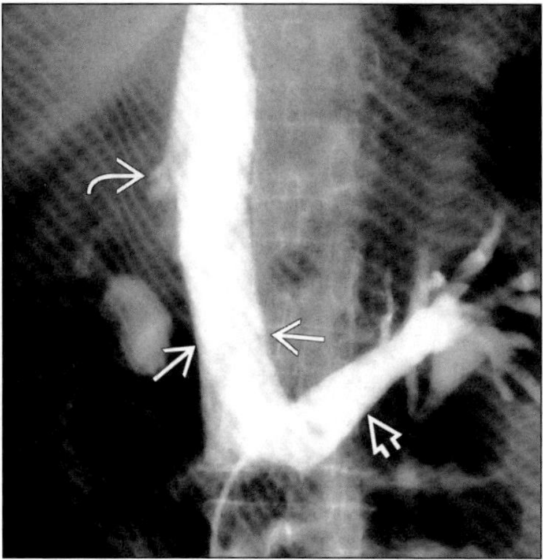

(Left) Left renal venogram shows multiple intrarenal branches ➡ draining into the main renal vein ➡, which courses anterior to the abdominal aorta to drain into the IVC. The left adrenal vein ➡ drains directly into the left renal vein. (Right) Venogram shows an unusual course of the left renal vein ➡ as it joins the IVC ➡. This appearance is typical of a retroaortic left renal vein, an anatomic variant. A small portion of the right renal vein ➡ is seen, entering the IVC at the expected location.

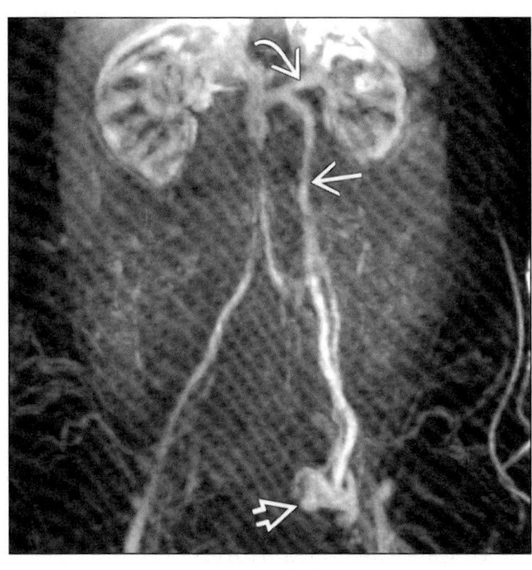

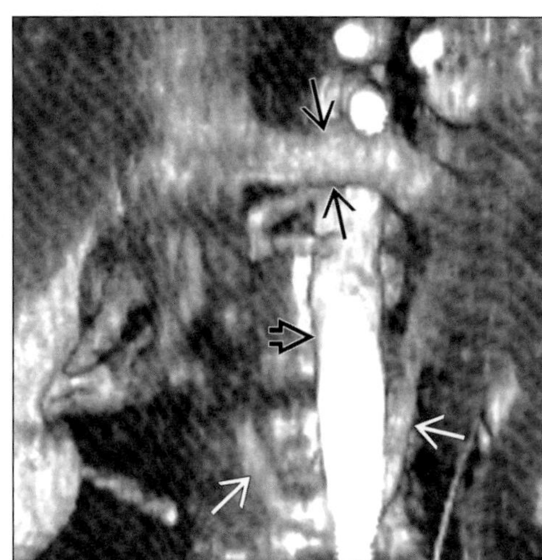

(Left) Coronal MRV of suspected "nutcracker syndrome" shows a dilated left gonadal vein ➡ and pelvic varicosities ➡. Compression of the left renal vein ➡ between the aorta and SMA causes renal venous hypertension and gonadal vein reflux. (Right) 3-D CTA of a circumaortic left renal vein shows a normal course of the superior vein ➡, anterior to the aorta ➡, and a retroaortic inferior vein ➡. This has implications for IVC filter placement.

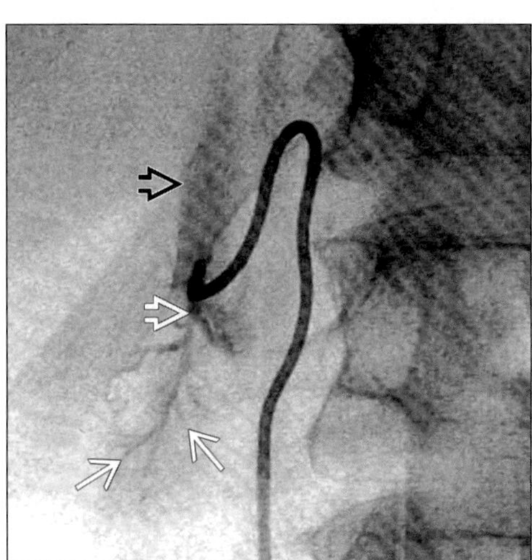

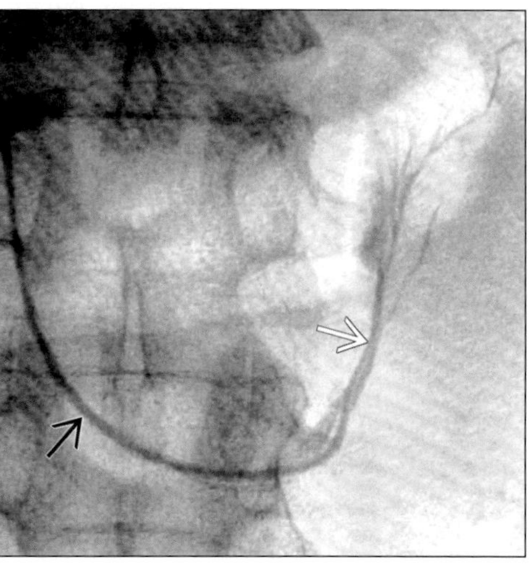

(Left) Right adrenal venogram shows filling of branches within the adrenal gland ➡ and the short main venous trunk ➡. The right adrenal vein drains directly into the IVC ➡ in most individuals. (Right) Left adrenal venogram shows a catheter ➡ coursing through the left renal vein, with the tip in the left adrenal vein ➡, which normally drains into the renal vein. After confirming a correct catheter tip position, venous sampling is performed before and after stimulation with cortisol.

RENAL VEIN THROMBOSIS

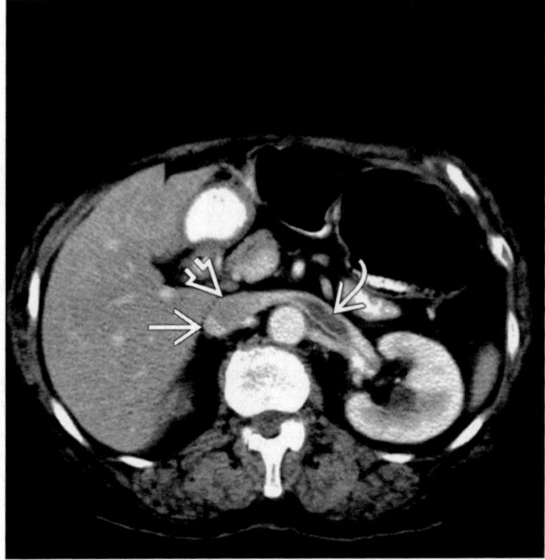

Axial CECT shows a low attenuation, smooth filling defect → in the left renal vein. The thrombus is not completely obstructing. Note the normal mixing of unopacified blood → and contrast → in the IVC.

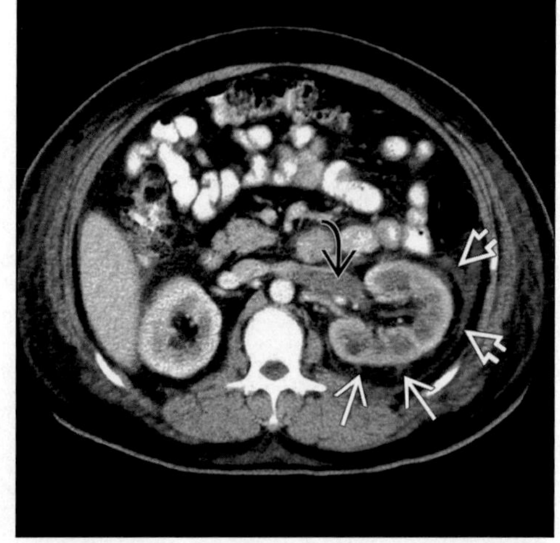

Axial CECT shows a filling defect → in an enlarged left renal vein, consistent with renal vein thrombosis. The kidney is slightly enlarged and there is perinephric stranding → and thickening of Gerota fascia →.

TERMINOLOGY

Abbreviations and Synonyms

- Renal vein thrombosis, renal vein occlusion

Definitions

- Thrombotic renal vein obstruction or occlusion

IMAGING FINDINGS

General Features

- Best diagnostic clue: Filling defect in renal vein, renal enlargement, delayed function
- Location
  - Unilateral > bilateral (more common in children)
  - Left renal vein > right renal vein
  - Thrombus extension to IVC, sometimes to right atrium
- Size
  - Renal enlargement (75% of cases)
  - Renal vein enlargement with acute thrombosis
  - Small shrunken kidney with chronic thrombosis
- Morphology
  - Acute or chronic (more common) thrombosis
    - Partial or complete venous obstruction

Radiographic Findings

- IVP
  - Delayed, hyperdense or prolonged nephrogram (partial obstruction)
  - Little or no nephrographic opacification (complete)
  - Poorly opacified renal collecting system
  - Notching of renal pelvis and ureter by collaterals
  - Enlarged or small kidney, depending on chronicity

CT Findings

- CECT
  - Low-attenuation filling defect within renal vein
  - Decreased nephrographic attenuation
  - Persistent parenchymal opacification
  - No corticomedullary differentiation
  - Delayed excretion into renal calyces and pelvis
  - Enlarged (acute) or shrunken (chronic) renal vein
  - Thickening of Gerota fascia and perinephric "whiskering" (edema or hemorrhage)
  - Opacified periureteral and perinephric ("cobwebs") venous collaterals
- CTA

DDx: Renal Vein Thrombosis

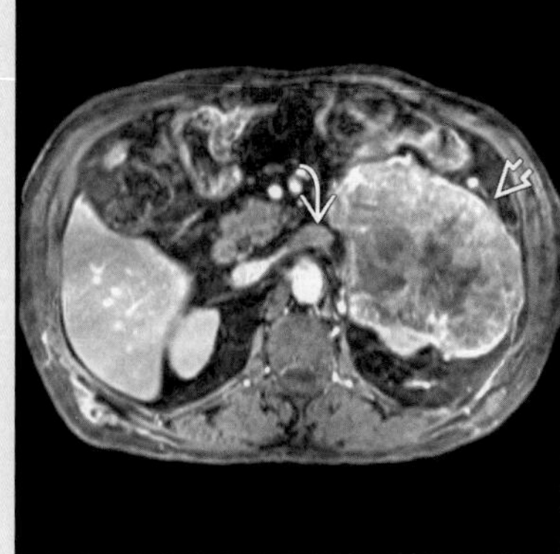

Renal Vein Tumor Extension

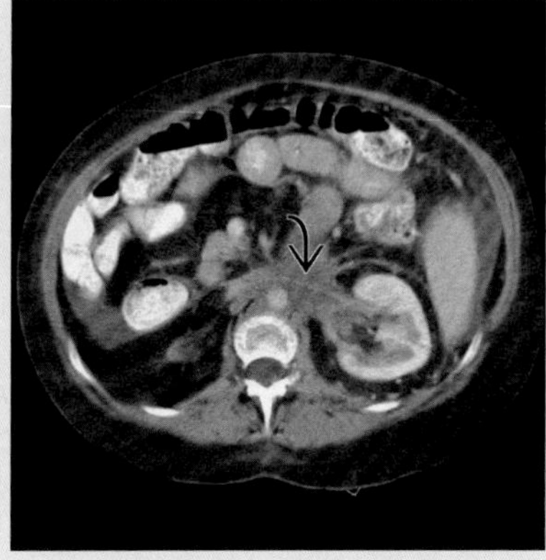

Lymphoma Encasing Renal Vein

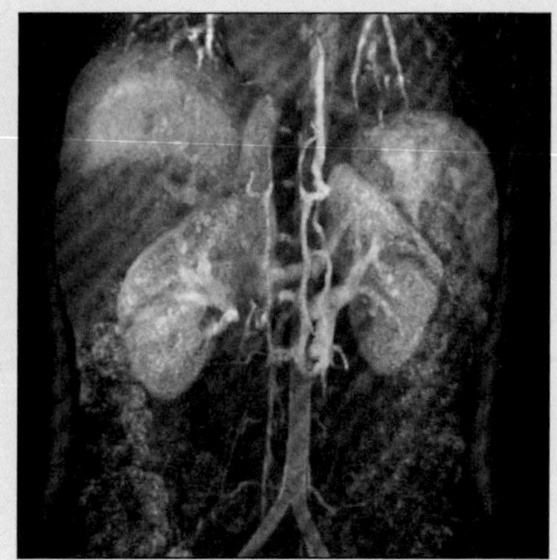

Nutcracker Syndrome

RENAL VEIN THROMBOSIS

Key Facts

Terminology
- Renal vein thrombosis: Renal vein obstruction or occlusion by thrombus

Imaging Findings
- Filling defect in renal vein with renal enlargement and delayed renal function (acute)
- Small shrunken kidney (chronic)
- Delayed, hyperdense or prolonged nephrogram (partial obstruction)
- Little or no nephrographic opacification (complete occlusion)
- Multiple collateral veins in perinephric space

Pathology
- Associated with nephrotic syndrome in adults
- Associated with dehydration and sepsis in children

Clinical Issues
- Primary medical therapy is anticoagulation
- Suprarenal IVC filter; protects from thromboembolism
- Mechanical thrombectomy rapidly improves renal vein outflow
- Surgical therapy with thrombectomy or nephrectomy if other management fails
- Sequelae of renal vein thrombosis depends on duration of occlusion, recanalization and collateralization

Diagnostic Checklist
- Clinical suspicion, rapid diagnosis and early intervention allows preservation of renal function
- Rapid return of venous outflow results in decreased mean serum creatinine and increased GFR

- Tortuous and dilated collateral veins near ureters
- Retrograde flow in dilated superficial epigastric veins

MR Findings
- MRA: Contrast-enhanced to delineate thrombus
- T1WI, T2WI
  - Filling defect in renal vein
  - Prolongation of renal cortex and medulla relaxation times, resulting in low signal intensity
  - Poor corticomedullary differentiation
  - Increased attenuation of renal veins
  - Multiple perinephric collateral veins

Nuclear Medicine Findings
- Delayed or absent renal perfusion
  - Accumulation of radiotracer mimics accumulation of contrast

Ultrasonographic Findings
- Grayscale Ultrasound
  - Acute: Renal enlargement from venous congestion and edema
    - Renal vein distended by faintly echogenic thrombus
    - Hypoechoic kidney; loss of corticomedullary differentiation
    - Heterogeneous kidney; areas of necrosis, hemorrhage
    - Echogenic thrombosed parenchymal veins radiating from hilum
  - Subacute: Improved corticomedullary differentiation; increased cortical echogenicity
    - Increased echogenicity of thrombus; decreased size of renal vein
  - Chronic: Varies with degree of renal injury
    - Normal appearance
    - Increased corticomedullary differentiation
    - Small, shrunken kidney with scarring
    - Echogenic thrombus with small, scarred renal vein
  - Thrombus or tumor in IVC (≤ 20%)
- Color Doppler
  - Absent flow in renal vein in acute complete occlusion
  - Renal vein filling defect in acute incomplete occlusion
    - "Tram track" sign of flow around thrombus
    - Increased flow velocity and turbulence
  - Chronic occlusion can recanalize
    - Multiple collateral veins if minimal or no recanalization
  - Absent duplex venous signal
  - Renal artery and proximal branches
    - Narrow, sharp systolic peaks from increased pulsatility
    - Continuous retrograde flow during diastole

Angiographic Findings
- Renal arteriogram with imaging into venous phase
  - Filling defect in main renal vein; possible extension into IVC
  - Non-visualized main renal vein
  - Multiple enlarged venous collaterals
- Renal venography
  - Intraluminal filling defect or venous occlusion
  - Venous collaterals if chronic

Imaging Recommendations
- Best imaging tool: US followed by CECT or C+ MR
- Protocol advice: CTA: Corticomedullary phase best; second helical acquisition performed at 90-120 seconds

DIFFERENTIAL DIAGNOSIS

Renal Vein Tumor Extension
- Large renal mass; usually renal cell carcinoma
- Vascular, enhancing tumor thrombus

Pyelonephritis
- Kidney has appearance of renal vein thrombosis, but with patent renal vein
- Differentiate by clinical history and urinalysis

Retroperitoneal Processes
- Lymphoma, other neoplasm, retroperitoneal fibrosis
  - Process narrows, encases or displaces renal vein

Gonadal Vein Thrombosis
- Usually bland thrombus; may extend into renal vein

Nutcracker Syndrome
- Compression of left renal vein as it crosses between aorta and SMA
- May cause left renal venous hypertension, hematuria
- May have extensive venous collaterals

PATHOLOGY

General Features
- General path comments
  - Associated with nephrotic syndrome in adults
  - Associated with dehydration and sepsis in children
- Genetics: Inherited hypercoagulable states (protein S, protein C deficiency)
- Etiology
  - Primary renal disease
    - Nephrotic syndrome, typically membranous glomerulonephritis
    - Pyelonephritis
  - Renal hypoperfusion by hypovolemia or vascular stasis (dehydration, sepsis, hemorrhage)
  - Hypercoagulable states (pregnancy)
  - Mechanical compression (tumor, nutcracker syndrome)
- Epidemiology
  - Incidence
    - Unknown in asymptomatic patients
    - Nephrotic syndrome: 16-42% of patients

Gross Pathologic & Surgical Features
- Acute: Congested and edematous kidney
  - Total occlusion leads to hemorrhagic infarction followed by necrosis and fibrosis
- Chronic: Small, scarred kidney
  - Fibrosis leading to renal atrophy

Microscopic Features
- Acute: Edema, hemorrhage, infarction
- Subacute: Necrosis
- Chronic: Fibrosis, scarring, dystrophic calcification

CLINICAL ISSUES

Presentation
- Most common signs/symptoms
  - Acute (more common in children)
    - Flank pain, nausea, vomiting
    - Palpable kidney, hypertension
    - Hematuria, proteinuria if renal function persists
    - Acute renal failure
  - Chronic
    - Asymptomatic
    - Renal failure
    - Hypertension
- Other signs/symptoms: Thromboembolic disease, particularly pulmonary embolus

Demographics
- Age: Adults (more common) or < 2 years of age

Natural History & Prognosis
- Sequelae of renal vein thrombosis depends on duration of occlusion, recanalization and collateralization
- Complications
  - Recurrent thromboemboli, particularly to pulmonary circulation
  - Renal failure
  - Renal hemorrhage
- Good prognosis; frequent spontaneous recovery

Treatment
- Primary medical therapy is anticoagulation
  - Intravenous heparin, then oral warfarin
  - Low molecular weight heparin
  - Systemic thrombolytic administration
    - Consider with: Bilateral renal vein thrombosis, IVC extension, massive clot burden, pulmonary emboli, severe flank pain or failed anticoagulation
- Endovascular therapy
  - Suprarenal IVC filter placement if thrombus extends into IVC
    - Recurrent pulmonary embolism or thromboembolic disease
    - Risk of embolization during mechanical thrombectomy
  - Mechanical thrombectomy improves renal vein outflow rapidly
  - Catheter-directed thrombolysis can be used primarily or to "clean up" residual thrombus after mechanical thrombectomy
  - Following endovascular therapy, patient chronically anticoagulated
- Surgical therapy with thrombectomy or nephrectomy if other management fails

DIAGNOSTIC CHECKLIST

Consider
- Clinical suspicion, rapid diagnosis and early intervention allows preservation of renal function
- Rapid return of venous outflow yields decreased serum creatinine; increased glomerular filtration rate (GFR)

Image Interpretation Pearls
- Look for filling defect in renal vein and multiple venous collaterals

SELECTED REFERENCES

1. Kim HS et al: Catheter-directed thrombectomy and thrombolysis for acute renal vein thrombosis. J Vasc Interv Radiol. 17(5):815-22, 2006
2. Kawashima A et al: CT evaluation of renovascular disease. Radiographics. 20(5):1321-40, 2000
3. Tempany CM et al: MRI of the renal veins: assessment of nonneoplastic venous thrombosis. J Comput Assist Tomogr. 16(6):929-34, 1992
4. Jeffrey RB et al: CT and ultrasonography of acute renal abnormalities. Radiol Clin North Am. 21(3):515-25, 1983

RENAL VEIN THROMBOSIS

IMAGE GALLERY

Typical

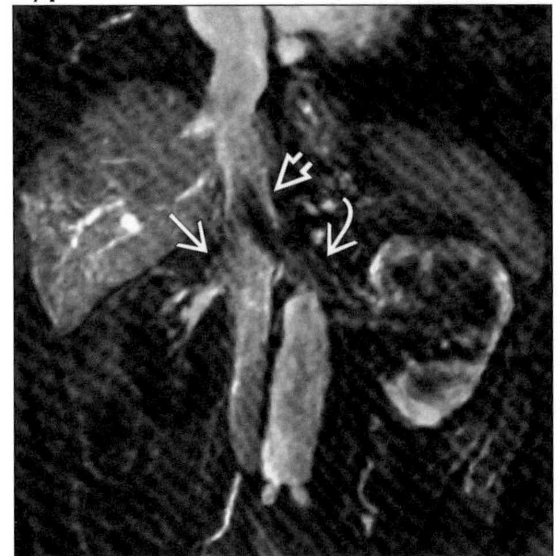

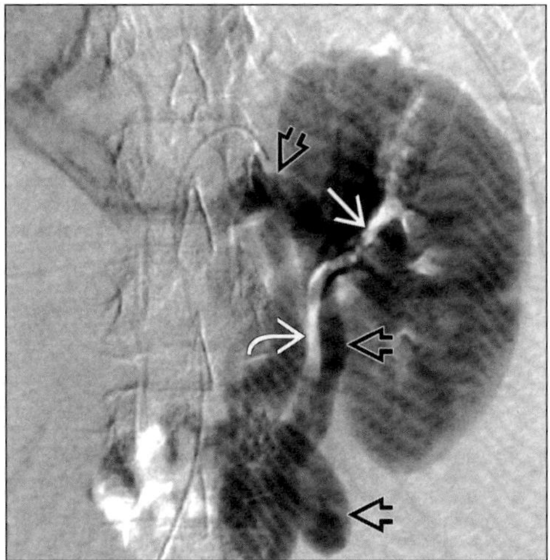

(Left) *Coronal MR cine shows a decreased signal filling defect in the left renal vein, extending into the inferior vena cava, consistent with renal vein thrombosis. The right renal vein is patent. The shrunken left kidney suggests this is chronic.* ***(Right)*** *Venous phase of a right renal arteriogram (different patient) shows enlarged venous collaterals and no main left renal vein. Note the proximity of the collaterals to the renal pelvis and proximal ureter.*

Typical

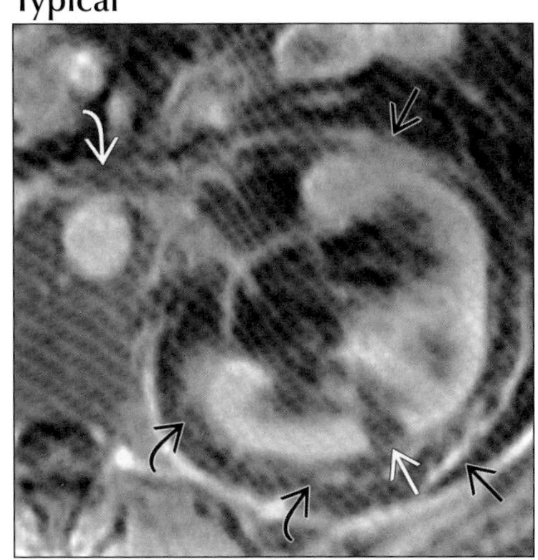

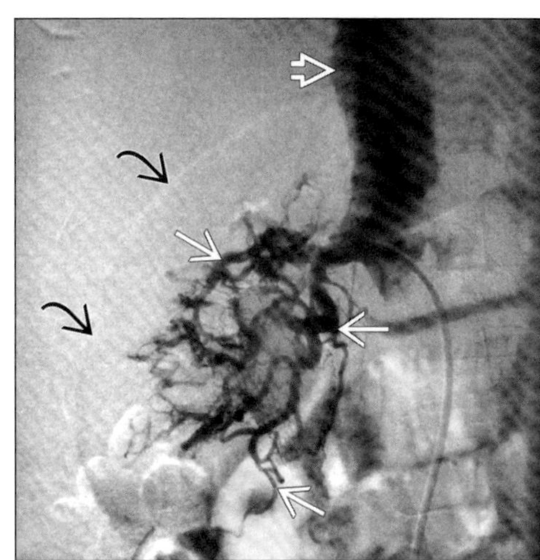

(Left) *Axial T1 C+ FS MR shows a filling defect in the renal vein and a renal hematoma from renal vein thrombosis. The left kidney is edematous, with perinephric stranding and thickening of Gerota fascia.* ***(Right)*** *Renal venogram (different patient) shows no visible main right renal vein. Multiple collateral veins drain into the IVC. The right kidney has a normal size and contour. The findings are consistent with chronic right renal vein thrombosis.*

Typical

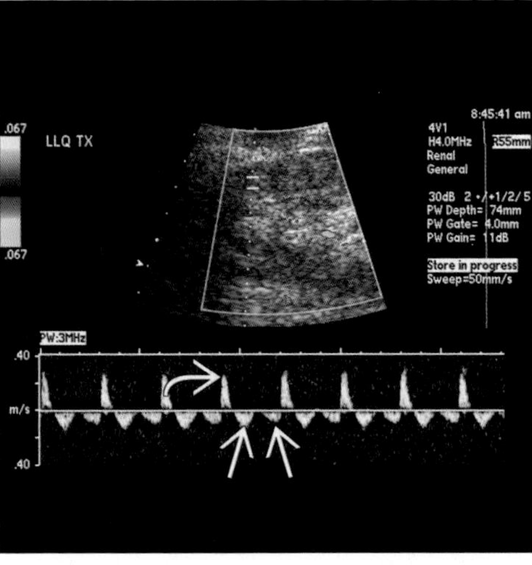

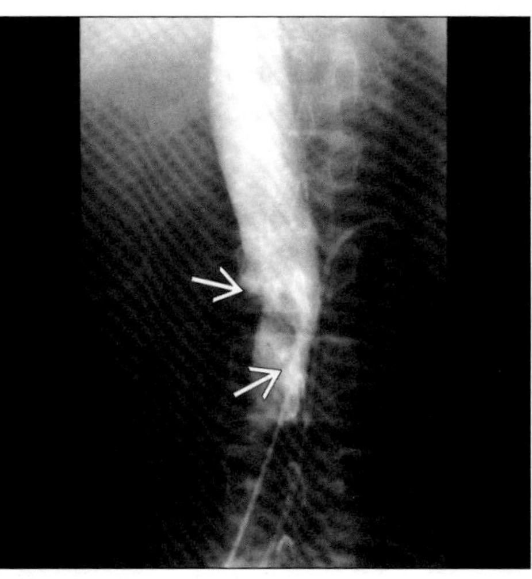

(Left) *Color Doppler ultrasound of a parenchymal renal artery in a transplanted kidney with known renal vein thrombosis shows a sharp, narrow systolic upstroke with persistent retrograde flow during diastole.* ***(Right)*** *Posteroanterior inferior vena cavagram (different patient) shows an intraluminal filling defect consistent with right renal vein thrombus extension into the IVC. Extension from the right renal vein is more common, due to its shorter length.*

RENAL VEIN TUMOR EXTENSION

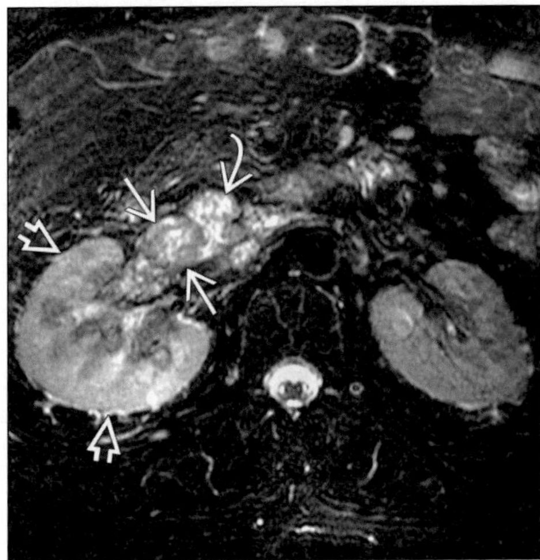

Axial T2WI MR shows an enlarged right kidney ⇨ with a heterogeneous mass ➡ extending into the renal vein and the IVC ➡. Increased signal in the right renal parenchyma relative to the left suggests edema.

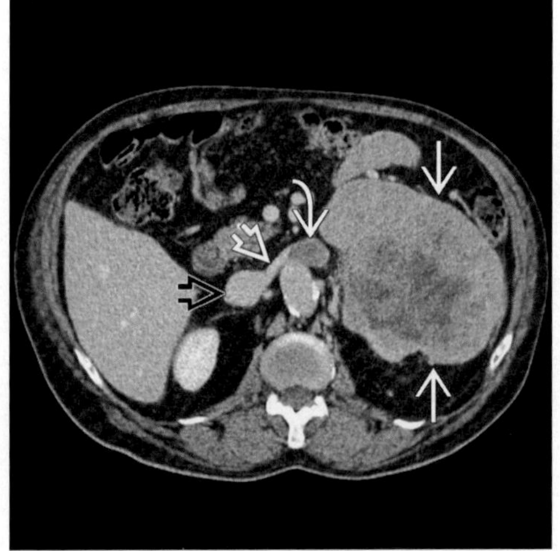

Axial CECT shows a low attenuation filling defect ➡ in the left renal vein ➡ caused by extension of tumor from a large heterogeneous renal cell carcinoma ➡ in the left kidney. The IVC ⇨ is free of tumor in this patient.

TERMINOLOGY

Abbreviations and Synonyms

- Extension of tumor into renal vein (RV), renal vein tumor thrombus

Definitions

- Extension of renal neoplasm into renal vein, inferior vena cava (IVC), and occasionally right atrium

IMAGING FINDINGS

General Features

- Best diagnostic clue
  - Distended renal vein, tumor vessels on color Doppler, tumor enhancement on CECT or T1 C+
    - Bland thrombus is non-enhancing
- Location
  - Renal vein with possible extension into IVC or as far centrally as right atrium
  - IVC extension involves right renal vein more than left due to shorter vein length of former

Radiographic Findings

- Radiography
  - Enlarged kidney or irregular contour suggests mass
    - Renal vein thrombosis can cause renal enlargement if acute, or renal atrophy if chronic
  - Mass effect of renal tumor on adjacent structures
    - Displaced bowel loops
- IVP
  - Abnormal renal contour consistent with mass
  - Enlarged kidney
  - Delayed or hyperdense nephrogram
  - Delayed excretion of contrast
  - Notching of renal pelvis and sometimes proximal ureter by large venous collaterals

CT Findings

- NECT
  - Enlarged kidney or abnormal renal contour with large renal cell carcinoma
  - Enlarged renal vein
  - Tumor within renal vein may not be visible
    - Hounsfield units (HU) of thrombus ~ HU of blood
- CECT
  - Filling defect in contrast-filled renal vein

DDx: Renal Vein Occlusion

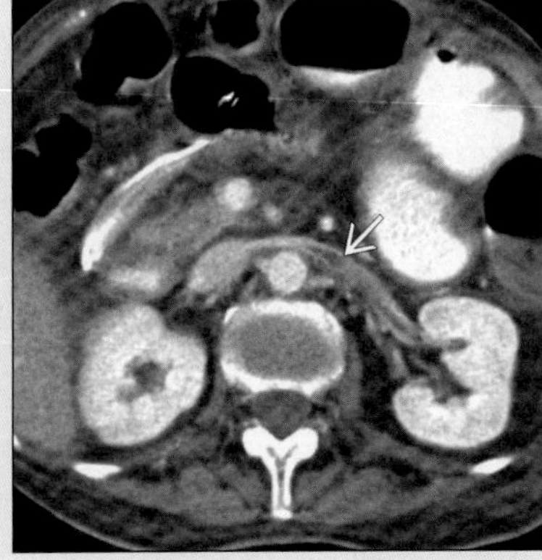

Renal Vein Thrombosis

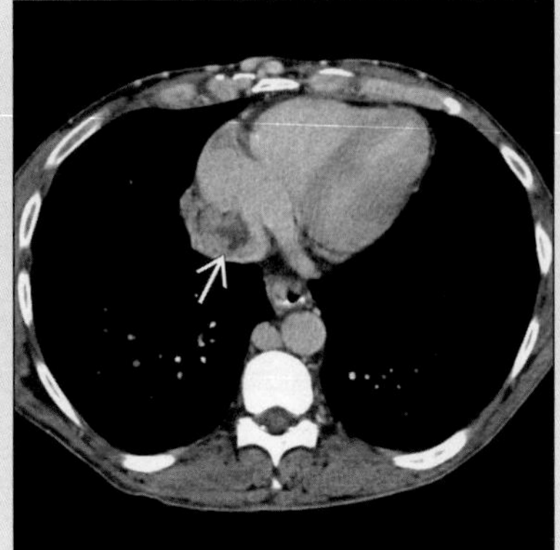

Hepatoma Extension into Rt Atrium

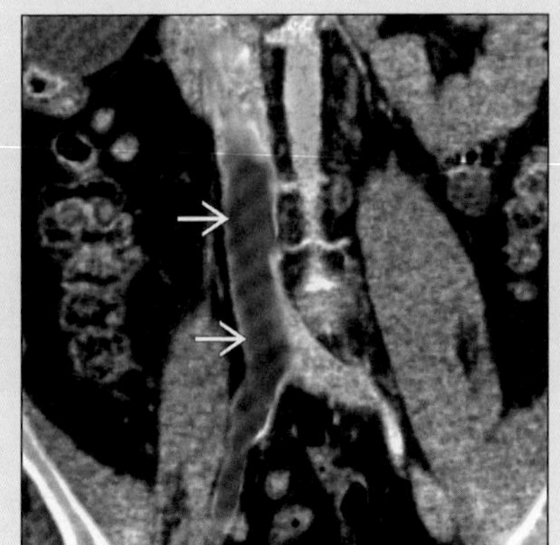

IVC Thrombosis

RENAL VEIN TUMOR EXTENSION

Key Facts

Terminology

- Extension of renal neoplasm into renal vein, inferior vena cava (IVC), and occasionally right atrium

Imaging Findings

- Distended renal vein, tumor vessels on color Doppler, tumor enhancement on CECT or MR C+
- Bland thrombus non-enhancing
- Abnormal renal contour consistent with mass
- Delayed or hyperdense nephrogram
- Mass effect on renal pelvis and sometimes proximal ureter by venous collaterals
- Vessel striations extending into renal vein and IVC
- May see "tram-track" sign of contrast flowing around non-occlusive thrombus
- Venous phase shows venous collaterals around kidney with eventual flow into IVC

Pathology

- Renal cell carcinoma extension to renal vein and IVC graded as Robson stage IIIa, TNM stage III or T3bNXMX

Clinical Issues

- 5-year survival of ~ 60% for stage III tumors
- Treatment depends on TNM stage at diagnosis
- Presenting symptoms are those of renal primary
- Can be asymptomatic in patient with known RCC
- Radical nephrectomy can be curative

Diagnostic Checklist

- Renal vein invasion in patients with renal mass worsens TNM staging
- Tumor thrombus shows enhancement on CT or MR; variable vascularity on US

        - "Tram track" sign of contrast flow around non-occlusive thrombus
        - Tumor thrombus may enhance in arterial phase
        - Non-enhancing thrombus is bland
        - Tumor thrombus may not be visible in venous/equilibrium phase; tumor HU ~ contrast HU
    - Renal vein may be distended
    - With significant renal vein obstruction or occlusion
        - Absent or decreased renal vein flow
        - Delayed or hyperdense nephrogram
        - Delayed excretion
        - Mass effect on renal pelvis and sometimes proximal ureter by venous collaterals
    - Primary renal tumor clearly demonstrated
        - Hypervascular mass visible in arterial phase
        - Renal enlargement or contour abnormality

MR Findings

- T1WI: Lower signal intensity in renal vein thrombus than renal primary
- T2WI: Signal intensity of renal vein thrombus less than renal primary
- T1 C+
    - Arterial phase enhancement of large primary renal cell carcinoma
    - Tumor thrombus enhancement in arterial phase
    - Contrast may decrease tumor thrombus conspicuity
- MRA
    - MRA C+ may obscure enhancing tumor thrombus
        - Bland thrombus can be visible
- MRV
    - Absent visualization of renal vein
    - Multiple venous collaterals in chronic obstruction
- Black Blood SE: Soft tissue signal intensity easily seen when flowing blood is black
- 2-D time-of-flight (TOF)
    - Decreased signal intensity of tumor with increased signal intensity of flowing blood
- Phase-contrast
    - Hypointense renal vein filling-defect
- Renal vein may be distended
- Cardiac motion may interfere with visualization of tumor high in IVC or right atrium

Ultrasonographic Findings

- Grayscale Ultrasound
    - Renal vein may be distended
    - RCC primary and renal vein tumor echogenicity ≤ parenchymal echogenicity
- Color Doppler
    - Decreased, turbulent or absent renal vein flow
    - Tumor vascularity in renal vein thrombus
    - Low resistance Doppler waveforms in tumor vessels
    - Renal primary readily seen, including tumor vessels
    - Color Doppler US can visualize superior extent of IVC tumor through liver "window"
    - Enlarged, anechoic renal vein suggests high flow from hypervascular mass and A-V shunting

Angiographic Findings

- DSA
    - Arteriography
        - Primary tumor: Large hypervascular mass
        - Fine vessel striations extending into renal vein and IVC
        - Linear, striated tumor blush "cast" of renal vein
        - Thrombus without vascularity is bland thrombus
        - Enlarged or unopacified renal vein
        - Venous phase shows venous collaterals around kidney with eventual flow into IVC
        - Collateral veins (lumbar, gonadal, adrenal, intercostal, capsular, ureteric) drain kidney
    - Venography
        - Filling defect in main renal vein and intrarenal branches
        - Filling defect protruding into or occluding IVC
        - May see "tram-track" sign of contrast flowing around non-occlusive thrombus
        - Filling defects may be tumor or bland thrombus; cannot be definitive with venography

Imaging Recommendations

- Best imaging tool

- CT or MR are best modalities for determining presence and extent of renal vein tumor
- MRA superior to CT for IVC tumor extent (CT compromised by flow artifact from renal veins)

- Protocol advice
  - Multiphase CECT with multiplanar reformations useful for diagnosis and treatment planning
  - Tumor thrombus may be obscured on T1 C+ MR
    - Confirm tumor invasion with more than one sequence (black blood, TOF, phase contrast)
  - Use Doppler ultrasound to evaluate renal vein

DIFFERENTIAL DIAGNOSIS

Bland Renal Vein Thrombosis

- Considerable overlap in CT, MR and US findings
  - CECT and T1 C+ MR: Non-enhancing filling defect
  - US: No thrombus hypervascularity
- Renal primary can cause bland or tumor thrombus

Sluggish Flow in Renal Vein

- Can mimic renal vein occlusion on US and MRA C-
- Etiology includes extrinsic renal vein or IVC compression or IVC obstruction
  - Imaging evidence of mass, lymphadenopathy

Mixing of Unopacified Renal Venous Return

- More likely to be seen with CT; may mimic thrombus

Tumor Invasion of Renal Vein or IVC

- Tumor invades and grows into vessel wall
  - Sarcomas, hepatic, pancreatic and duodenal tumors
- Tumor thrombus extension does not invade vessel

PATHOLOGY

General Features

- General path comments
  - Renal cell carcinoma primary tends to be large (> 4.5 cm) with renal vein invasion
  - Renal vein tumor extension into IVC more common on right
    - Right renal vein shorter than left
  - Renal cell carcinoma extension incidence: Renal vein 21-35%, IVC 5-10%
- Etiology
  - Renal cell carcinoma most common tumor with renal vein extension
  - Wilms tumor can extend into renal vein and IVC
  - Primary leiomyosarcoma extension from renal vein to IVC or vice versa
  - Can be seen with transitional cell Ca or lymphoma

Gross Pathologic & Surgical Features

- Tumor and bland thrombus present in most specimens

Staging, Grading or Classification Criteria

- Renal cell carcinoma extension to renal vein and IVC graded as Robson stage IIIa, TNM stage III or T3bNXMX

CLINICAL ISSUES

Presentation

- Most common signs/symptoms
  - Presenting symptoms are those of renal primary
    - Classic triad of renal cell carcinoma: Gross hematuria, flank pain, palpable abdominal mass
  - Can be asymptomatic in patient with known renal cell carcinoma
- Other signs/symptoms: Constitutional symptoms

Demographics

- Age: Most commonly seen in middle age (40-70 years)
- Gender: M > F with a ratio of 2-3:1

Natural History & Prognosis

- Prognosis depends on tumor stage at time of diagnosis
- 5-year survival of ~ 60% for stage III tumors

Treatment

- Options, risks, complications: Treatment depends on TNM stage at diagnosis
- Surgery determined by tumor stage
  - Stage T3N0M0: Radical nephrectomy is treatment of choice; can be curative
    - Kidney, renal vein, adrenal gland, perirenal fat, Gerota's fascia resected ± local lymphadenectomy
    - Non-invasive renal vein and IVC thrombus easily shelled out; partial resection of IVC as indicated
  - T3bN1M0: Surgery curative in very small minority
  - Nephron-sparing procedure in appropriate setting
- Pre- or post-operative external beam radiation therapy
  - Efficacy not proven compared with surgery alone
  - Used for palliation in non-surgical candidates
- Endovascular therapy
  - Pre-operative embolization of renal tumor can decrease intra-operative blood loss
    - Can use particulates, alcohol and/or coils
  - Palliative embolization in non-surgical candidates
- Cytokine therapy with adjuvant interferon-α
- Chemotherapy has < 10% efficacy

DIAGNOSTIC CHECKLIST

Consider

- Renal vein invasion in patients with renal mass worsens TNM staging

Image Interpretation Pearls

- Look for clearly visible, large primary tumor
- Tumor thrombus shows enhancement on CT or MR; variable vascularity on US

SELECTED REFERENCES

1. Kawashima A et al: CT evaluation of renovascular disease. Radiographics. 20(5):1321-40, 2000
2. Motzer RJ et al: Renal-cell carcinoma. N Engl J Med. 335(12):865-75, 1996
3. Weyman PJ et al: Comparison of computed tomography and angiography in the evaluation of renal cell carcinoma. Radiology. 137(2):417-24, 1980

RENAL VEIN TUMOR EXTENSION

IMAGE GALLERY

Typical

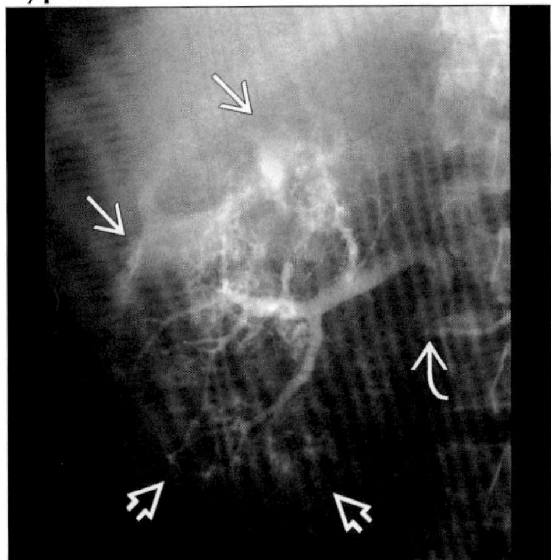

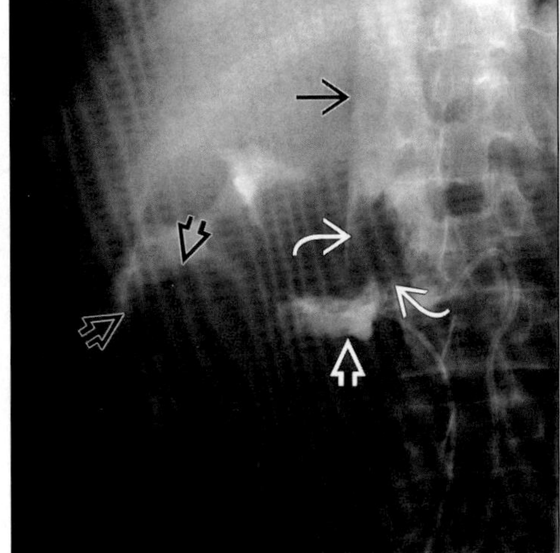

(Left) *Posteroanterior catheter angiography of the right renal artery shows neovascularity and extensive tumor blush. Note the distortion of the renal collecting system. The renal size is increased as a result of the mass.* ***(Right)*** *Posteroanterior catheter angiography of the right renal vein, in the same patient, shows a filling defect extending into the IVC and distortion of the renal collecting system by a lower pole renal cell carcinoma.*

Typical

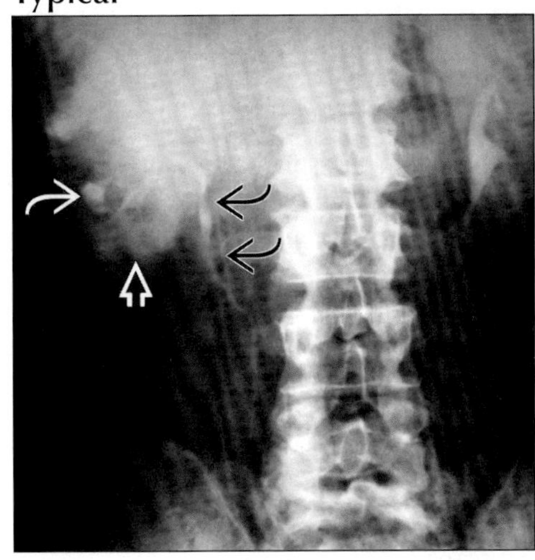

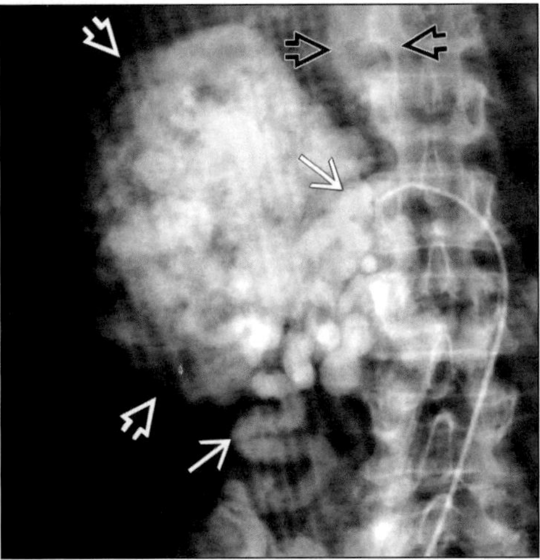

(Left) *Posteroanterior conventional IVP shows an enlarged right kidney. There is notching and lateral displacement of the proximal ureter, with distortion of the collecting system.* ***(Right)*** *Posteroanterior catheter angiography in the venous phase shows an enlarged kidney with large venous collaterals draining into the IVC as a result of right renal vein occlusion by tumor thrombus. The renal enlargement suggests renal cell carcinoma.*

Typical

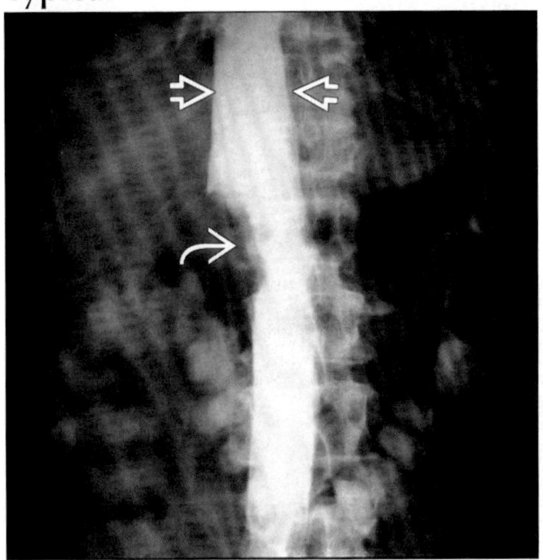

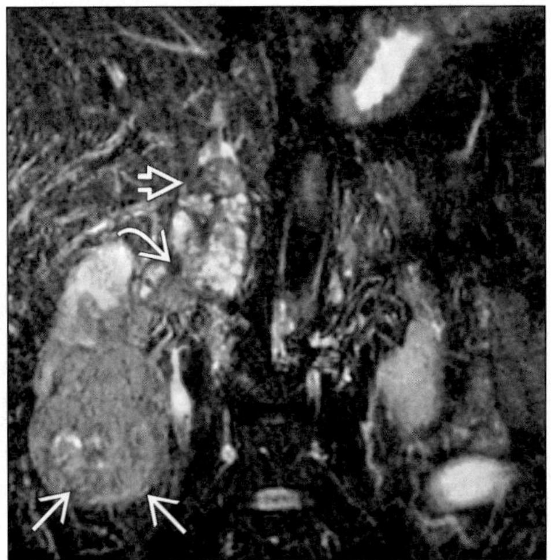

(Left) *Posteroanterior conventional inferior venacavagram shows a large irregular filling defect extending into the inferior vena cava from the right renal vein. This thrombus can contain bland and/or tumor thrombus.* ***(Right)*** *Coronal T2WI FSE MR shows a large renal mass extending into the right renal vein and the IVC. The mass in the renal vein and the IVC has mixed signal intensity, consistent with mixed bland and tumor thrombus.*

RENAL TRANSPLANT DYSFUNCTION

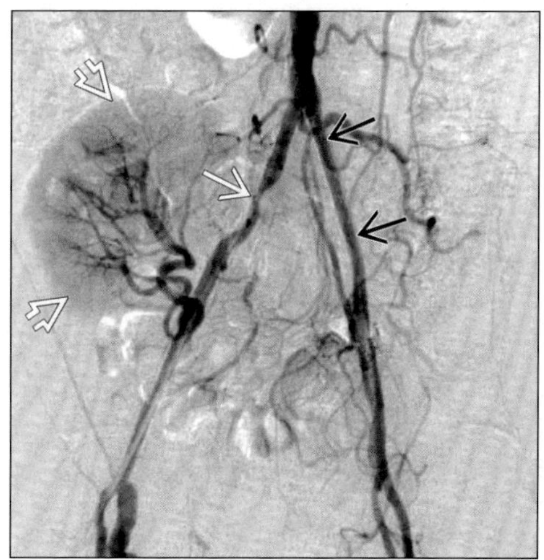

Arteriogram shows a right common iliac artery stenosis ➔, clinically causing diminished perfusion to the transplanted kidney ➔. A stent ➔ has been previously placed in the left common iliac artery.

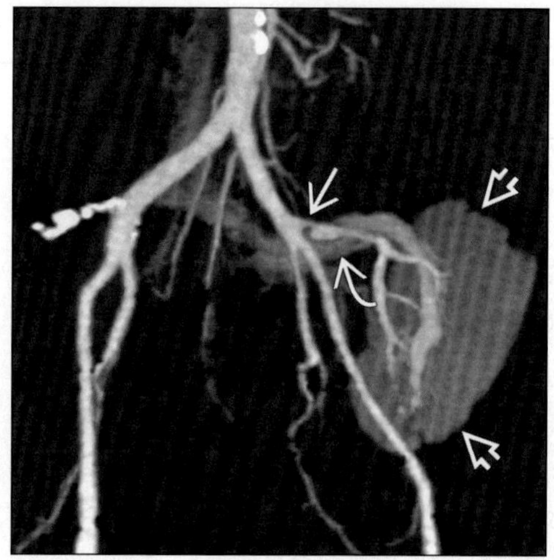

CTA shows a high grade stenosis ➔ of the renal artery of the transplant kidney ➔ and a patent renal vein ➔. CTA is infrequently used for renal transplant evaluation because of the large contrast volumes required.

TERMINOLOGY

Definitions

- Dysfunction of renal transplant as a result of hydronephrosis, infection, vascular pathology or parenchymal abnormality
  - Parenchymal pathology includes rejection, acute tubular necrosis and immunosuppressive toxicity from agents such as cyclosporine
  - Vascular pathology includes arterial thrombosis, anastomotic or inflow stenosis or occlusion, pseudoaneurysm, AV fistula and venous thrombosis

IMAGING FINDINGS

General Features

- Best diagnostic clue: Ultrasound demonstrating narrowing of transplant renal artery and high peak systolic velocity (> 200-250 cm/s) waveform
- Location
  - Transplanted kidney placed heterotopically in pelvis in extraperitoneal space (i.e., right kidney placed in left iliac fossa and vice versa)
    - Right iliac fossa preferred, since right iliac vein has more superficial and horizontal course than left, allowing easier creation of vascular anastomoses

CT Findings

- Not usually applicable in transplants because large contrast volumes required

MR Findings

- MRI/MRA can be used to evaluate transplant
  - Diffusion-weighted and functional imaging sequences currently being investigated
- 3D MRA, MIP and/or MPVR techniques useful
- Presence of surgical clips may compromise imaging

Nuclear Medicine Findings

- Assesses function; Tc-99m MAG for acute tubular necrosis
- Captopril renal scans may be helpful

Ultrasonographic Findings

- Color Doppler
  - Excellent modality for evaluation of renal transplant
    - Absence of arterial or venous signal prompts further evaluation with angiography or surgery

DDx: Renal Transplant Dysfunction

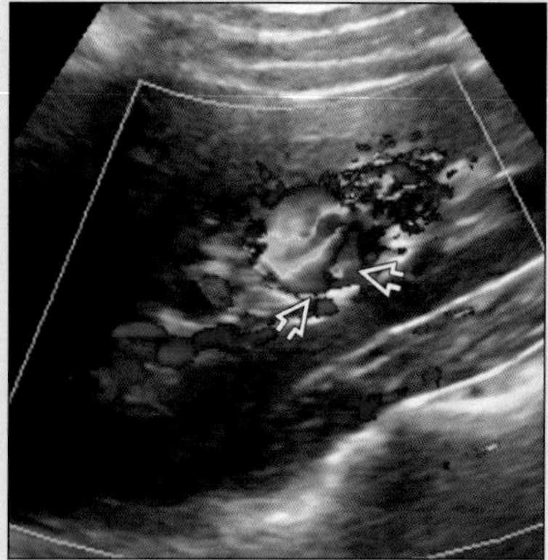

Post-Biopsy AV Fistula

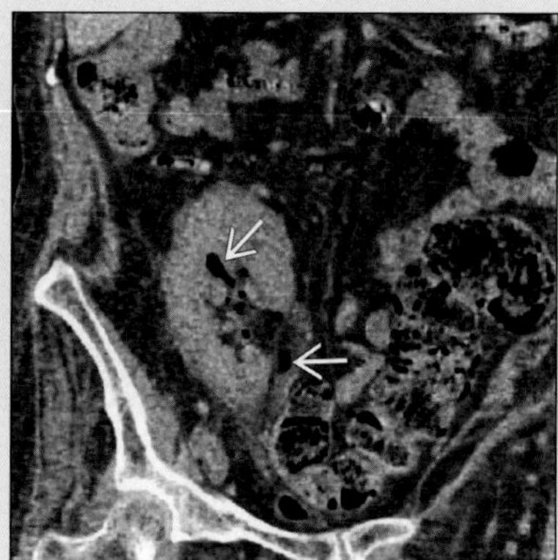

Infected Transplant Kidney

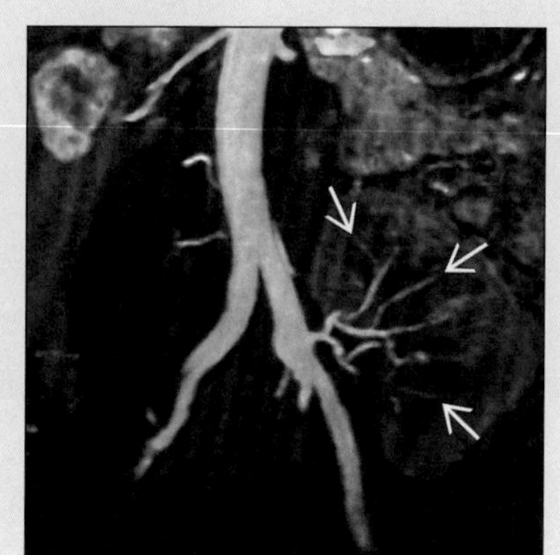

Transplant Rejection

RENAL TRANSPLANT DYSFUNCTION

Key Facts

Terminology

- Dysfunction of renal transplant as a result of hydronephrosis, infection, vascular pathology or parenchymal abnormality

Imaging Findings

- Best diagnostic clue: Doppler ultrasound showing narrowed transplant renal artery and high peak systolic velocity (> 200-250 cm/sec) waveform
- Turbulence, flow reversal and spectral broadening are secondary findings

Pathology

- Renal artery stenosis most common vascular complication, venous stenosis may also be responsible for renal dysfunction
  - Stenosis in arteries proximal to transplant may also cause dysfunction
- Arteriovenous fistula from biopsy may cause renal transplant dysfunction
- Must differentiate anatomic dysfunction from rejection

Clinical Issues

- Progressive renal insufficiency and/or accelerated hypertension refractory to multiple drug regimens suggests transplant dysfunction
- Angioplasty is first line of therapy for arterial stenosis and has high technical success rate
  - Stent placement may improve restenosis rate
- For treatment of ureteral obstruction, nephrostomy catheter placed to permit recovery of renal function and provide access for subsequent intervention

---

- High peak systolic velocity waveform (200-250 cm/s) on Doppler examination indicates arterial stenosis
  - Turbulence, flow reversal and spectral broadening are secondary findings
- Reversed diastolic flow in main renal artery suggests venous obstruction
  - Renal vein thrombosis will exhibit intraluminal echoes and lack of venous flow
- Arteriovenous fistulas and/or pseudoaneurysms demonstrated with color flow ultrasound
  - Draining vein of arteriovenous fistula shows arterialized flow pattern
  - Biopsy-related pseudoaneurysm appears as anechoic mass with internal color flow
- Intrarenal arterial evaluation for resistive index (RI)
  - Value of 0.8 or greater suggests parenchymal pathology such as rejection, acute tubular necrosis or cyclosporine toxicity

Angiographic Findings

- Confirms ultrasound findings of arterial/venous stenosis or occlusion and demonstrates anatomy
  - Living donor kidney renal artery is anastomosed either end-to-end to hypogastric artery or end-to-side to recipient external iliac artery
  - Cadaveric transplant donor renal artery along with portion of aorta (Carrel patch) anastomosed end-to-side to external iliac artery
    - Demonstrates arterial stenosis or occlusion
    - Used to guide subsequent transcatheter therapy
  - Type of anastomosis determines optimal angiographic approach to transplant renal artery
    - Contralateral approach for end-to-end hypogastric artery anastomosis and ipsilateral for end-to-side external iliac artery anastomosis
  - Venous anastomoses almost always placed end-to-side to external iliac vein
- Gadolinium or CO_2 used as contrast agents when renal insufficiency is present

Imaging Recommendations

- Screening with duplex color-flow Doppler ultrasound
- MRI/MRA, particularly in obese patients

DIFFERENTIAL DIAGNOSIS

Rejection vs. Acute Tubular Necrosis

- Color Doppler can be useful, but histology is required
- Acute rejection: High resistive indices on ultrasound
  - Edematous kidney; "pruned" intrarenal branches

Venous Thrombosis

- Dilated vein containing thrombus
- Absent venous flow
- Reversed diastolic flow within infrarenal and transplant renal arteries

Arteriovenous Fistula

- Secondary to transplant biopsy, incidence 1-2%
- Increased systolic and diastolic flow
  - Arterialized flow pattern to draining vein of arteriovenous fistula
- Usually small and insignificant, maybe associated with hemorrhage
- If large may cause ischemia and transplant dysfunction; may require transcatheter intervention (e.g., embolization)

Obstruction

- Creation of a ureteroneocystostomy is most common method for implanting transplant ureter
  - Distal ureter, especially at ureterovesical junction, is most common location of ureteral obstruction
  - Some institutions prefer a ureteroureterostomy or ureteropyelostomy that connects recipient native ureter to donor renal pelvis
- Ultrasound used to diagnose hydronephrosis
  - Ultrasound also for diagnosis of post-operative fluid collections which may occlude ureter/vein

Infection

- Perirenal fluid may be present with pelvic abscess; pyonephrosis
- Urine leak is potentially life-threatening; requires prompt intervention because of infection risk
  - Most leaks occur at distal ureter, possibly from necrosis due to ischemia or rejection

RENAL TRANSPLANT DYSFUNCTION

PATHOLOGY

General Features

- General path comments
  - Vascular pathology (up to 15% of transplants)
    - Acute renal artery thrombosis usually occurs in 1st post-operative month; transplant loss in > 90%
    - Arterial thrombosis occurring later usually due to renal artery stenosis or rejection
    - Renal artery stenosis most common vascular complication
    - Stenosis involving inflow arteries proximal to transplant may cause dysfunction
    - Anastomotic pseudoaneurysm: Should raise suspicion of infection
    - Venous thrombosis usually occurs early in post-operative period; renal vein stenosis typically occurs later in post-transplant period
    - Arteriovenous fistula or intraparenchymal pseudoaneurysm: Usually secondary to percutaneous biopsy
  - Nonvascular urologic pathology (3-9% rate)
    - Transplant ureter tends to be involved in complications because of limited vascular supply originating only from renal hilum
    - Ureteral obstruction reported to occur in 2-10%; most common cause is ureteral ischemia
    - Urine leak with or without urinoma occurs in approximately 1-5% of renal transplant patients
  - Other nonvascular pathology
    - Perigraft fluid collections such as lymphocele, hematoma
- Etiology
  - Predisposing factors: Renal donor atherosclerosis, transplantation of pediatric kidneys into adults
  - Surgical: Trauma to donor or recipient arteries, clamp injury, traction on renal vessels, suture technique
    - Acute renal artery thrombosis usually stems from surgical technique; caused by torsion, angulation or kinking of anastomosis or arterial dissection
  - Atherosclerosis of recipient's iliac arteries
- Epidemiology: Renal artery stenosis occurs in up to 10% of renal transplants

Gross Pathologic & Surgical Features

- Intimal flaps, dissection, scarring and hyperplasia

Microscopic Features

- Histologic features of acute rejection include interstitial inflammation with or without hemorrhage, tubulitis, and arterial endotheliitis
- Chronic rejection (1° cause of late graft loss) characterized by sclerosing vasculitis and interstitial fibrosis

CLINICAL ISSUES

Presentation

- Most common signs/symptoms
  - Progressive renal insufficiency
    - Deterioration in renal function following ACE inhibitor therapy
  - Accelerated hypertension (sudden or insidious onset) refractory to multiple drug regimens
    - Renal ischemia causes activation of renin angiotensin system
- Other signs/symptoms: Flash pulmonary edema

Natural History & Prognosis

- Poor without therapy; eventual loss of transplant
- With angioplasty, good technical and clinical response

Treatment

- Medical therapy: Drug intolerance is common and may cause progressive renal failure
- Surgical therapy: Success 65-90%, risk of graft loss, ureteral injury, restenosis 12%
- Angioplasty is first line of therapy for arterial stenosis
  - Technical success rate > 80%, hypertension control > 75%, renal function stable or improved > 80%, restenosis 10-33%
    - Stent placement may improve restenosis rate
- For treatment of ureteral obstruction, nephrostomy catheter placed to permit recovery of renal function and provide access for subsequent intervention
  - Antegrade nephroureteral stent placed in patients with persistent obstruction after initial nephrostomy
  - Balloon ureteroplasty may be performed when high grade peri-anastomotic strictures are found
- Urinoma should be drained percutaneously to relieve extrinsic compression and prevent infection

DIAGNOSTIC CHECKLIST

Consider

- Differentiate anatomic dysfunction from rejection
  - Screening with ultrasound is excellent means for evaluation of renal transplant

SELECTED REFERENCES

1. Khurana A et al: Nephrogenic systemic fibrosis: a review of 6 cases temporally related to gadodiamide injection (omniscan). Invest Radiol. 42(2):139-45, 2007
2. Kobayashi K et al: Interventional radiologic management of renal transplant dysfunction: indications, limitations, and technical considerations. Radiographics. 27(4):1109-30, 2007
3. Gurkan A et al: Comparing two ureter reimplantation techniques in kidney transplant recipients. Transpl Int. 19(10):802-6, 2006
4. Libicher M et al: Interventional therapy of vascular complications following renal transplantation. Clin Transplant. 20 Suppl 17:55-9, 2006
5. Rajiah P et al: Renal transplant imaging and complications. Abdom Imaging. 31(6):735-46, 2006
6. Schwenger V et al: Real-time contrast-enhanced sonography in renal transplant recipients. Clin Transplant. 20 Suppl 17:51-4, 2006
7. Hohenwalter MD et al: Renal transplant evaluation with MR angiography and MR imaging. Radiographics. 21(6):1505-17, 2001
8. Spinosa DJ et al: Angiographic evaluation and treatment of transplant renal artery stenosis. Curr Opin Urol. 11(2):197-205, 2001

IMAGE GALLERY

Typical

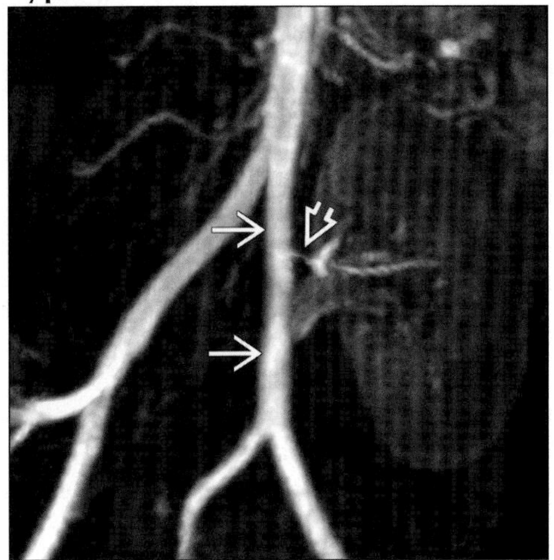

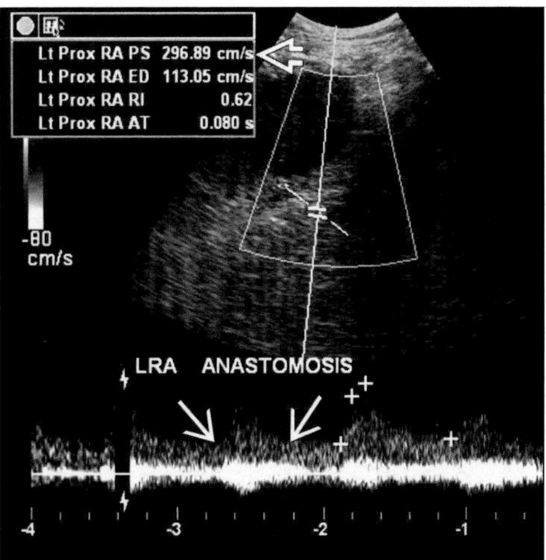

(Left) *MRA shows high grade stenosis of the transplant renal artery at the anastomosis to the left common iliac artery.* ***(Right)*** *Color Doppler ultrasound (same patient as previous image) shows elevated peak systolic velocity of 296.89 cm/sec at the anastomosis of the transplant kidney left renal artery. Turbulence & spectral broadening of arterial waveform are also present. These are typical ultrasonographic findings of renal artery stenosis.*

Typical

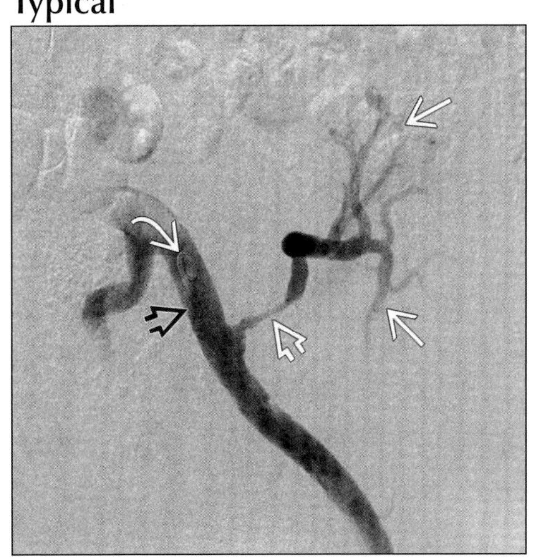

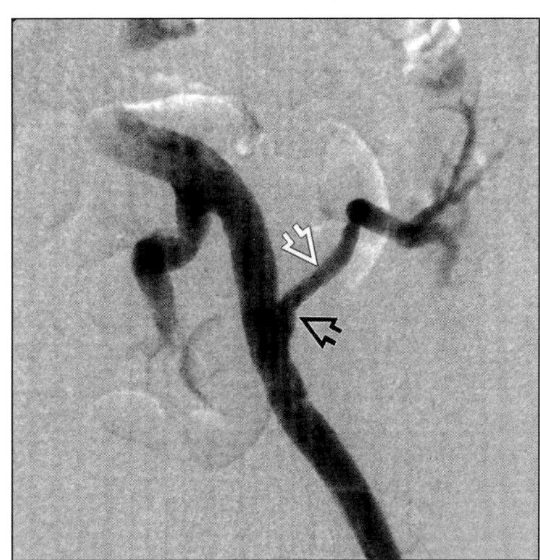

(Left) *DSA obtained with a catheter in the left external iliac artery, shows a severe stenosis in the transplant renal artery. The intrarenal branches of the transplant kidney are widely patent.* ***(Right)*** *DSA (same patient as previous image) following transcatheter intervention shows a widely patent renal artery following intravascular stent placement. Note the typical end-to-side configuration of the arterial anastomosis to the external iliac artery.*

Typical

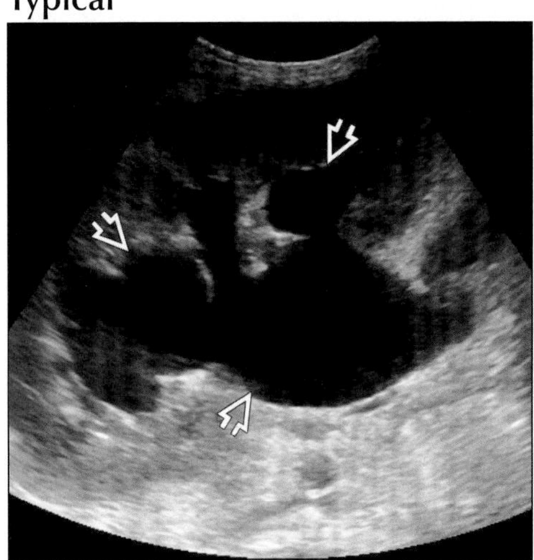

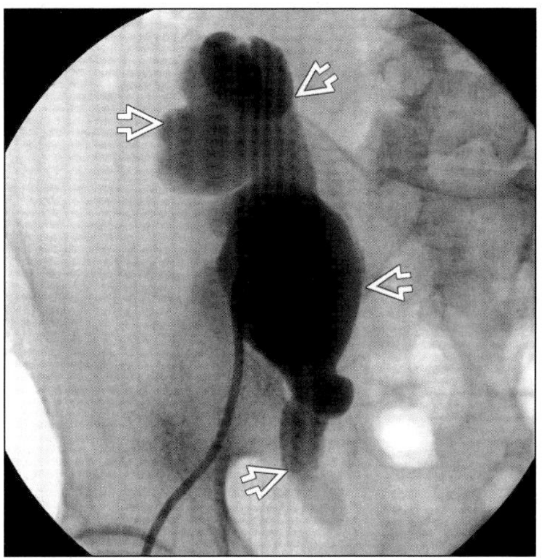

(Left) *Sagittal US of a transplant kidney shows marked hydronephrosis. Distal ureteral ischemia is the most common cause because of poor distal blood supply. Secondary infection may occur in these immunosuppressed patients.* ***(Right)*** *Nephrostogram after percutaneous catheter placement (same patient as previous) shows diffuse dilatation of renal collecting system. Nephrostomy can permit recovery of renal function & provide access for subsequent intervention.*

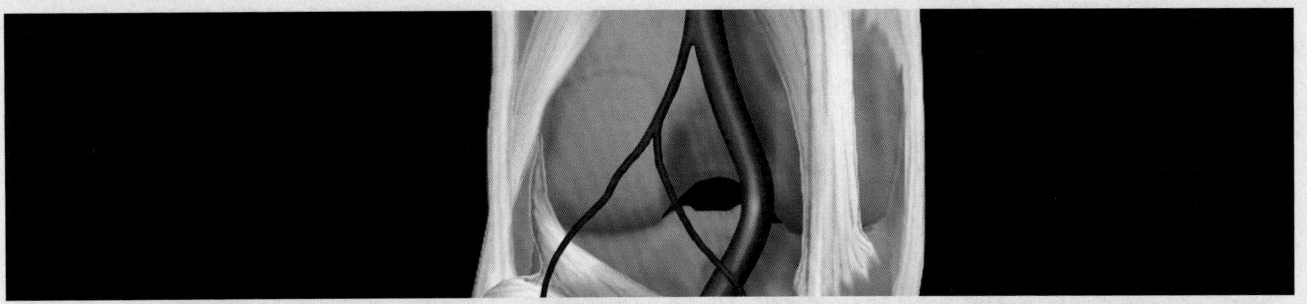

SECTION 7: Extremities

Upper Extremities

Pelvis

Lower Extremities

SUBCLAVIAN ARTERY STENOSIS/OCCLUSION

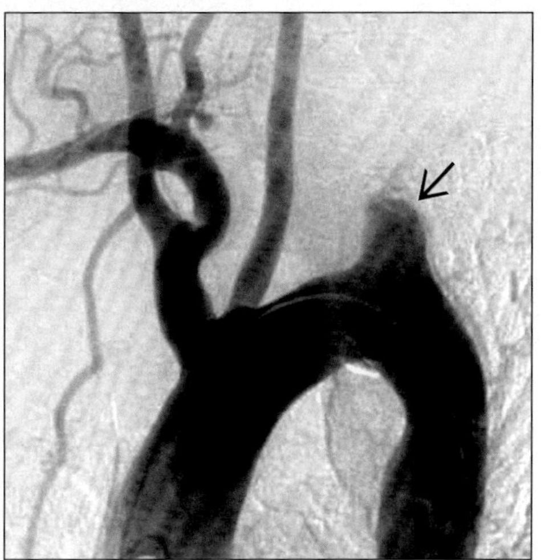

Conventional aortogram shows occlusion of the left subclavian artery ➔ proximal to the vertebral artery with absent filling of the ipsilateral vertebral artery and distal subclavian artery.

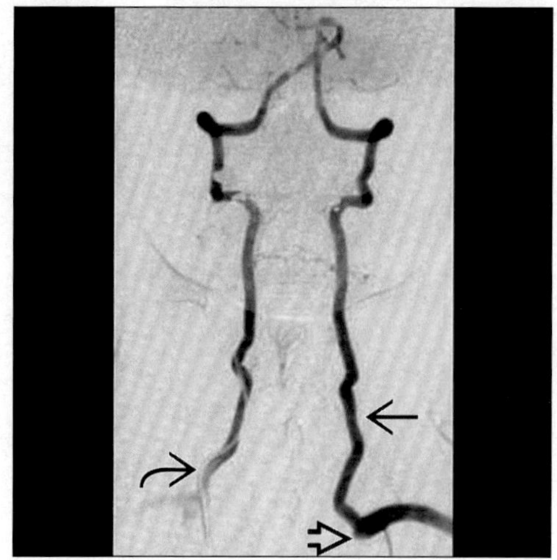

Right vertebral ➔ arteriogram (same patient) shows retrograde flow in the left vertebral artery ➔ and filling of the left subclavian artery distal to the occlusion ➔. This is typical of a subclavian steal phenomenon.

TERMINOLOGY

Abbreviations and Synonyms

- Subclavian artery stenosis or obstruction; subclavian occlusive disease; subclavian steal syndrome; thoracic outlet syndrome

Definitions

- Subclavian artery luminal narrowing or blockage

IMAGING FINDINGS

General Features

- Best diagnostic clue: Focal narrowing or occlusion of subclavian artery
- Location
  - 85% involve left subclavian artery (atherosclerosis)
  - Most common atherosclerosis locations: Subclavian artery origin proximal to vertebral artery origin
- Size: Stenosis graded as mild (< 50%), moderate (50-70%), high grade (> 70%)
- Morphology: Eccentric atherosclerotic plaque; may evolve to concentric stenosis or occlusion

CT Findings

- CTA
  - Eccentric irregularly calcified, noncalcified or mixed plaque with resulting stenosis/occlusion
    - Atherosclerotic ulcerated plaque shows irregular contrast filled outpouchings
  - Concentric mural soft tissue thickening in vasculitis
    - Delayed mural enhancement in active vasculitis
  - Low density intimal flap in dissection
    - Differential enhancement of true and false lumen
    - False lumen larger than true lumen

MR Findings

- T1WI
  - Pre-contrast T1 GRE shows mural thickening, dissection flap or atherosclerotic plaque
    - High signal intensity in intramural hematoma
- T2WI: SSFP (bright blood) may show low signal intimal flap, and intermediate signal intramural hematoma, mural thickening and plaque
- T1 C+
  - Shows mural thickening and any enhancement (vasculitis)

DDx: Subclavian Artery Stenosis/Occlusion

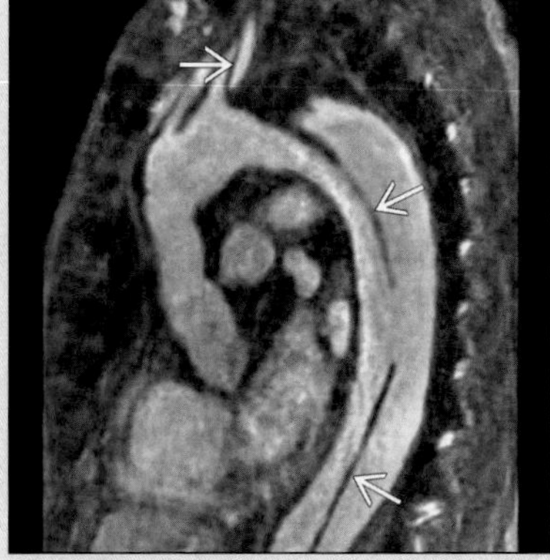

Aortic/Subclavian Dissection

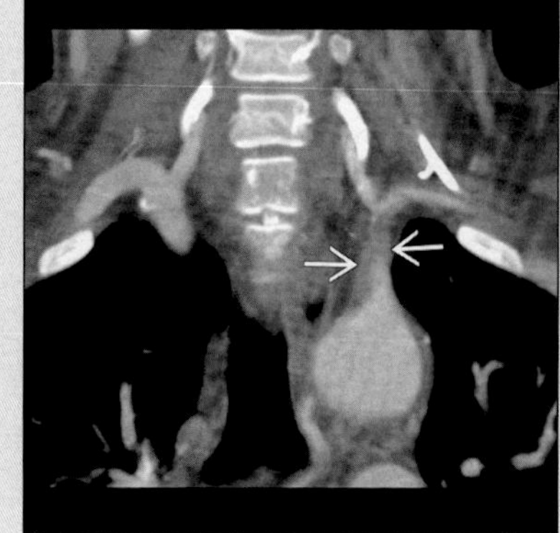

Vasculitis

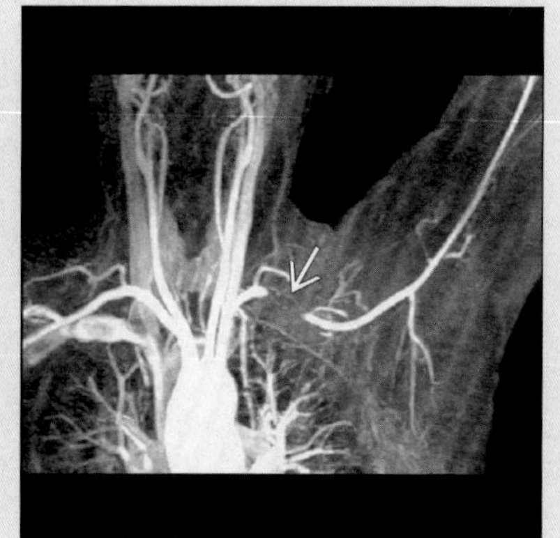

Thoracic Outlet Syndrome

SUBCLAVIAN ARTERY STENOSIS/OCCLUSION

Key Facts

Terminology
- Subclavian artery luminal narrowing or occlusion

Imaging Findings
- Luminal stenosis/occlusion (> 70% high grade)
  - Post-stenotic dilatation (severe stenosis)
- Collaterals in chest wall and shoulder
- Irregular outpouchings (ulcerated plaque)
- Intimal flap in dissection
- Mural thickening and enhancement in vasculitis (MR better)
- Compression of subclavian artery at thoracic outlet by mass, scar, clavicular fracture, or cervical rib
- Retrograde flow in vertebral artery with high grade stenosis/occlusion of proximal subclavian artery in "subclavian steal"
  - TE-MRA, PC-MRA , catheter angiogram and ultrasound show reverse flow
- Pre- and post-T1 GRE for mural thickening, dissection flap, thrombus or plaque
- US: Absence of flow in occluded segment; elevated peak systolic velocity

Top Differential Diagnoses
- Thoracic Outlet Syndrome
- Embolization (Cardiac Origin)/Iatrogenic
- Vasculitis

Clinical Issues
- Arm or hand pain, cold hand with delayed capillary refill, decreased/absent pulse, decreased BP, dizziness (subclavian steal)
- Treat with angioplasty or stenting if symptomatic

    - More sensitive in assessment of mural enhancement than CT
    - Ulcerated atherosclerotic plaque shows irregular contrast filled outpouching
- MRA
  - TE-MRA images mimic catheter angiogram: Assess real time flow dynamics
    - High grade proximal subclavian artery stenosis with retrograde flow in ipsilateral vertebral artery and distal subclavian artery in "subclavian steal"
  - CE MRA images demonstrate luminal stenosis, irregularities or occlusion
    - Limited evaluation of vessel wall, flow dynamics
  - Phase contrast MRA (PC MRA) confirms reverse flow (usually dark signal) in vertebral artery from steal

Ultrasonographic Findings
- Color Doppler: Turbulence and aliasing at stenosis
- Duplex ultrasound findings
  - Absence of flow in occluded segment
  - Elevated flow velocity in stenosis (peak systolic velocity ≥ 300 cm/sec)
    - Post-stenotic flow disturbance/reduced velocity
  - Damped or monophasic Doppler waveforms in arterial segment distal to stenosis (assuming no retrograde flow from ipsilateral vertebral artery)
  - Reversed or biphasic flow in ipsilateral vertebral artery in "subclavian steal"

Angiographic Findings
- Conventional
  - Thoracic arch aortogram prior to selective angiography; LAO projection
  - Luminal diameter reduced in focal stenosis or occlusion; ulcerated plaque with irregular web-like stenosis with contrast-filled outpouching
  - Acute thrombosis/embolus shows intraluminal filling defect or occlusion
  - CTA, MRA or DSA findings
    - Post-stenotic dilatation (severe stenosis)
    - Long, smoothly tapered stenosis with dissection
    - Reversed vertebral artery flow (subclavian steal)
    - Collaterals in chest wall and shoulder
    - Soft tissue masses, scar or clavicular fracture (if obstructed by extrinsic compression)
    - Vessel compression or occlusion at thoracic outlet; post-stenotic aneurysm (thoracic outlet syndrome)

Imaging Recommendations
- Best imaging tool
  - MRA and CTA with contrast
    - Catheter angiography "gold standard" but limited in assessing arterial wall
- MRA, CTA, or DSA for pre-treatment assessment
- MR/MRA: MRA with double dose (0.2 mmol/kg); timing bolus with ROI in ascending aorta; 2 passes (early arterial and venous)
  - TE- MRA (4-5 cc contrast at 3 cc/sec for flow pattern)
  - Axial and coronal pre- and post-T1 GRE to assess arterial wall
  - Phase contrast MR to determine flow direction
- CTA: Bolus tracking technique with ROI in aortic arch or ascending aorta; 80 cc of contrast at 3 cc/sec
  - Axial 0.75-1.5 mm collimated volumetric acquisitions
    - 3 mm coronal and sagittal reconstructions
- Inject contrast from asymptomatic side in CTA/MRA; right IV access for bilateral study
  - 30-40 mL saline flush (avoids artifact from contrast in veins)

DIFFERENTIAL DIAGNOSIS

Thoracic Outlet Syndrome
- Arm pain from compression of neurovascular bundle at thoracic outlet
  - Most symptoms from brachial plexus compression
    - Also from subclavian artery or vein compression
- Thoracic outlet boundaries: Clavicle and first rib, anterior and posterior scalene muscles
- Changes in Doppler waveforms or arm blood pressure during provocative maneuvers (e.g., Adson maneuver)
- Compression of subclavian artery at thoracic outlet, possible post stenotic aneurysm (diagnostic)
- Imaging in neutral & stress (abduction) positions

Embolization/Iatrogenic

- 30% upper extremity ischemia embolic
- 30% upper extremity ischemia iatrogenic (e.g., arterial puncture, hemodialysis access)

Vasculitis

- Luminal irregularity
- Presents at younger age
- Mural thickening with or without enhancement

Dissection

- Intimal flap separating "true" and "false" lumens can extend into great vessels
  - Can cause subclavian stenosis or occlusion

PATHOLOGY

General Features

- Etiology
  - Atherosclerosis (approximately 30% of upper extremity ischemia)
  - Emboli: Most commonly of cardiac origin
  - Other causes
    - Arterial dissection
    - Neoplasm (e.g., Pancoast tumor)
    - Trauma (blunt or penetrating, iatrogenic)
    - Scar (e.g., post radiation, fibrosing mediastinitis)
    - Thoracic outlet syndrome
    - Fibromuscular dysplasia
    - Vasculitis (e.g., Takayasu, giant cell arteritis)
    - Congenital absence of subclavian artery (rare)
- Epidemiology: 12-19% of subclavian artery stenoses occur in patients with peripheral vascular disease
- Associated abnormalities: Coronary artery disease, myocardial infarction, TIA, stroke

CLINICAL ISSUES

Presentation

- Most common signs/symptoms
  - Acute ischemia: Arm/hand pain, cold hand with delayed capillary refill, decreased/absent pulses
  - Chronic ischemia: Diminished pulses; differential arm pressures; dizziness if subclavian steal
  - Commonly asymptomatic
- Other signs/symptoms
  - Upper extremity claudication (exercise-induced ischemic pain), rest pain or tissue loss rare
  - Vertebrobasilar ischemia (subclavian steal)
    - Confluence of two vertebral arteries at foramen magnum enables retrograde ipsilateral vertebral collateral flow to subclavian artery
  - Distal embolization (from ulcerated atherosclerotic plaque or post-stenotic aneurysm)
  - Intermittent arm, shoulder and neck pain (thoracic outlet syndrome)
  - Chest pain (post left, internal mammary artery, coronary artery, bypass graft and subsequent subclavian artery origin stenosis)
  - Decreased pulses on side of subclavian stenosis
    - 20-30 mmHg arm BP difference diagnostic
  - Cold, blanched extremity with acute occlusion

Demographics

- Age: Usually > 65 years
- Gender: Males and females equally affected

Natural History & Prognosis

- Atherosclerotic subclavian artery occlusion usually asymptomatic
  - Arm claudication or posterior fossa symptoms may develop
- Symptomatic dissection: Requires angioplasty/stenting or bypass surgery
- Fibromuscular dysplasia and vasculitis progressive
- Persistent symptoms can progress with thoracic outlet syndrome

Treatment

- No treatment for asymptomatic cases
- Endovascular treatment for symptomatic patients
  - Angioplasty and/or stenting
- Arterial bypass surgery if endovascular treatment unsuccessful (e.g., axillo-axillary, or carotid-subclavian bypass), endarterectomy
- Decompression surgery for thoracic outlet syndrome
- Thoracic sympathectomy

DIAGNOSTIC CHECKLIST

Consider

- Subclavian steal syndrome in patients with vertebrobasilar insufficiency symptoms and exercised-induced upper extremity ischemia
- Coronary-subclavian syndrome in patients with internal mammary cardiac bypass surgery and angina

Image Interpretation Pearls

- Acute emboli appear as intraluminal filling defects

SELECTED REFERENCES

1. du Toit DF et al: Long-term results of stent graft treatment of subclavian artery injuries: Management of choice for stable patients? J Vasc Surg. 2008
2. Liava'a M et al: Progressive subclavian artery stenosis causing late coronary artery bypass graft failure as a result of coronary-subclavian artery steal. J Thorac Cardiovasc Surg. 135(2):438-9, 2008
3. Palchik E et al: Subclavian artery revascularization: an outcome analysis based on mode of therapy and presenting symptoms. Ann Vasc Surg. 22(1):70-8, 2008
4. Henry M et al: Percutaneous transluminal angioplasty of the subclavian arteries. Int Angiol. 26(4):324-40, 2007
5. Van Grimberge F et al: Role of magnetic resonance in the diagnosis of subclavian steal syndrome. J Magn Reson Imaging. 12(2):339-42, 2000
6. Taneja K et al: Occlusive arterial disease of the upper extremity: colour Doppler as a screening technique and for assessment of distal circulation. Australas Radiol. 40(3):226-9, 1996
7. Kaufman JA, Lee MJ: Vascular & Interventional Radiology: the requisites, 1st ed. Philadelphia, Mosby.

SUBCLAVIAN ARTERY STENOSIS/OCCLUSION

IMAGE GALLERY

Typical

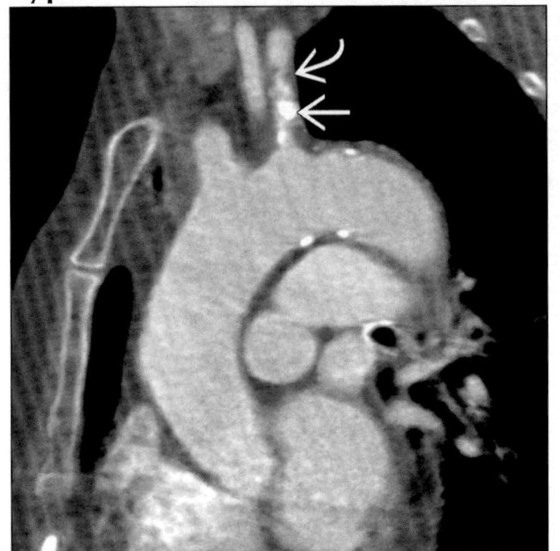

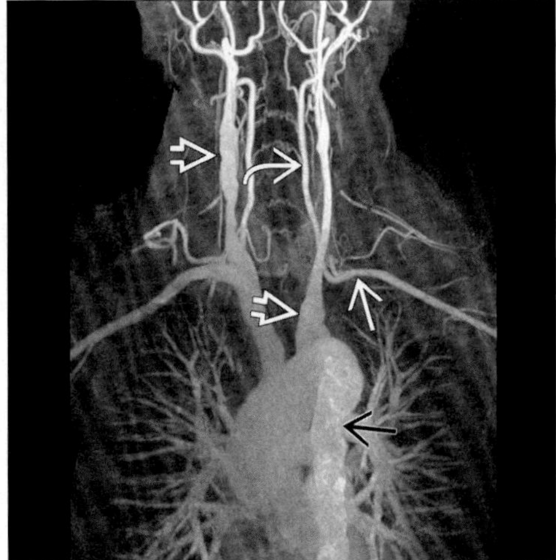

(Left) *CTA shows atherosclerotic noncalcified and calcified plaques of the proximal left subclavian artery with a resultant high grade stenosis.* **(Right)** *CE-MRA in a patient with vasculitis shows an irregular narrowing of the descending aorta, occlusion of the proximal left subclavian artery, and distal reconstitution of the left subclavian artery via the left vertebral artery. There is ectasia of both common carotid arteries.*

Typical

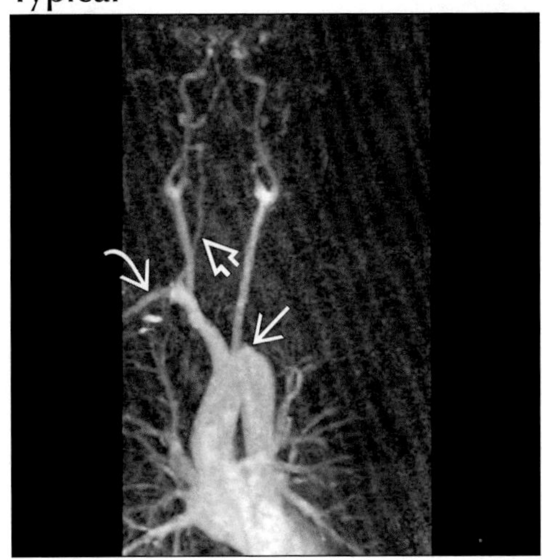

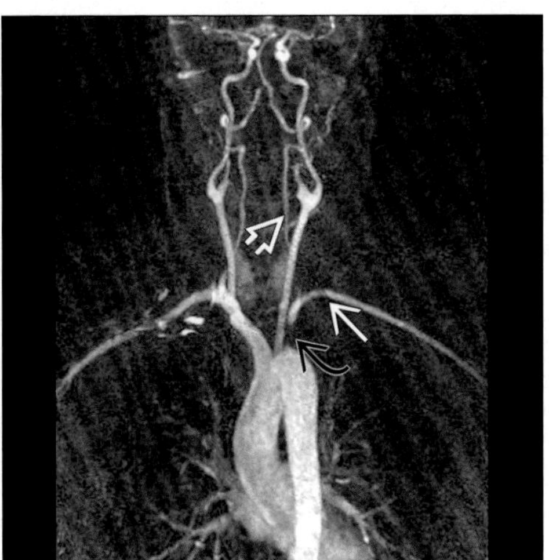

(Left) *Early phase TE-MRA shows occlusion of the left subclavian artery origin and absence of antegrade contrast flow in the left vertebral artery. The right vertebral and subclavian arteries are normal.* **(Right)** *Coronal later phase TR MRA in the same patient shows filling of the left subclavian artery by retrograde flow from the left vertebral artery and occlusion of proximal left subclavian artery, consistent with subclavian steal syndrome.*

Typical

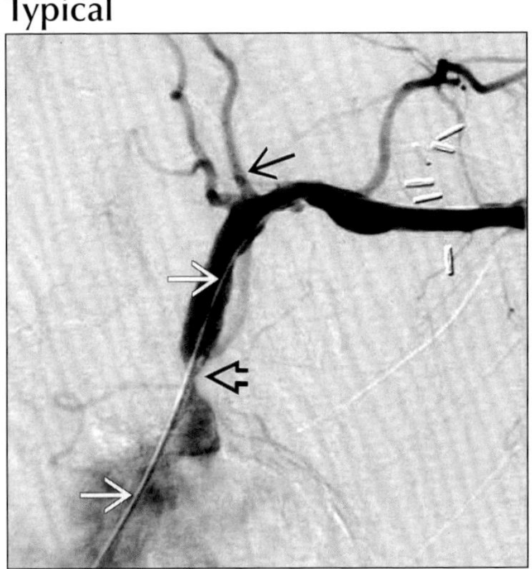

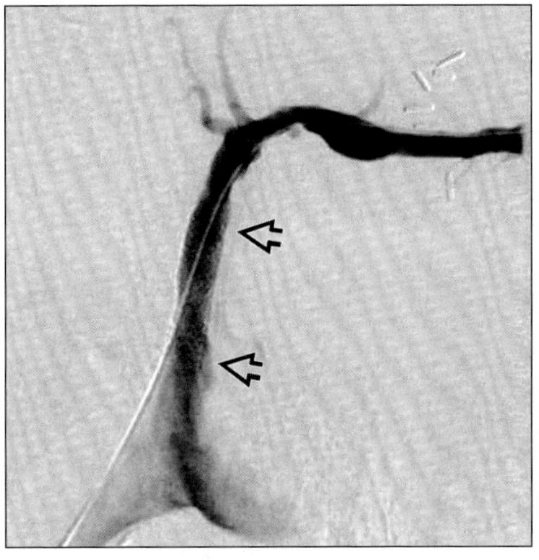

(Left) *DSA shows a severe left subclavian artery stenosis proximal to the left vertebral artery. A guidewire has been advanced across the stenosis in preparation for endovascular treatment. Most atherosclerotic stenoses of the left subclavian artery occur in this location.* **(Right)** *DSA shows an intravascular stent has been placed across the stenosis, restoring a normal luminal diameter to the artery. This intervention was performed using a brachial artery access.*

INNOMINATE ARTERY COMPRESSION

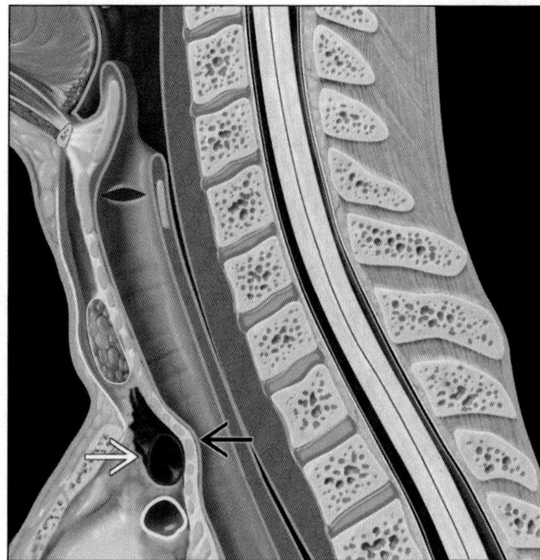

Graphic shows the innominate artery ➔ compressing the anterior wall of the trachea ⇨. The narrowing of the trachea causes the symptoms of dyspnea, stridor, and apnea.

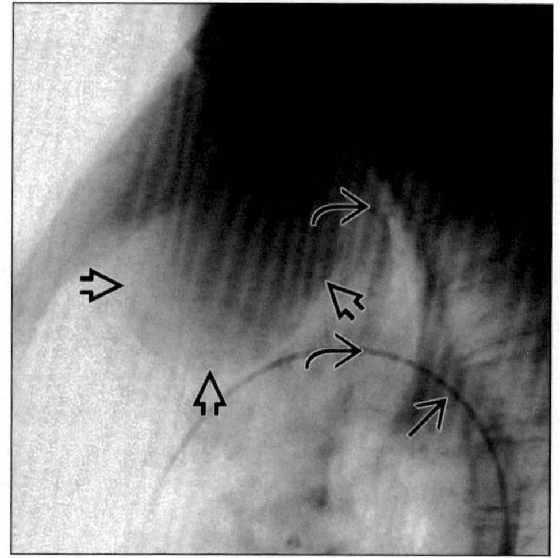

Sagittal radiograph shows a large mass ⇨ in the anterior mediastinum compressing the trachea ↷. An angiographic catheter ⇨ is in place. This mass is a large innominate artery aneurysm.

TERMINOLOGY

Abbreviations and Synonyms

- Innominate artery compression (IAC)
- Aneurysm of the innominate artery (AIA)

Definitions

- Innominate artery passes immediately anterior to anterior aspect of trachea and leads to tracheal compression

IMAGING FINDINGS

General Features

- Best diagnostic clue: Narrowing of trachea from anterior compression just below thoracic inlet - best seen on lateral radiograph

Radiographic Findings

- Radiography
  - On lateral radiography, compression from the anterior aspect of the trachea is present
  - Compression is at level of superior trachea just below thoracic inlet
  - Left sided aortic arch identified
  - Lung aeration not affected
  - If aneurysm is present, lateral neck image will show compression and posterior displacement of upper cervical trachea by anterior soft tissue mass

Fluoroscopic Findings

- Barium was an important study evaluating patients with a vascular ring, now supplanted by CT and MR

CT Findings

- Marked narrowing of trachea in superior mediastinum
- Tracheal narrowing confined to level at which innominate artery crosses anterior to trachea
- Innominate artery immediately abuts area of tracheal narrowing
- Trachea can be compressed between spine and innominate artery

MR Findings

- T1WI
  - Sagittal sections to identify innominate artery as it courses anterior to trachea

DDx: Innominate Artery Compression (Images Courtesy J. Donaldson, MD)

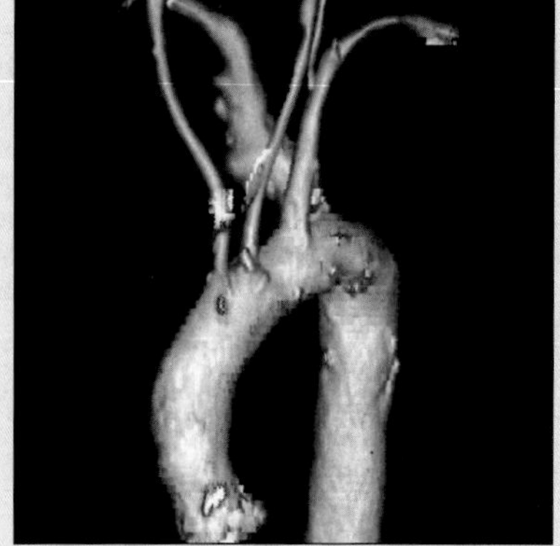

Kommerell Diverticulum

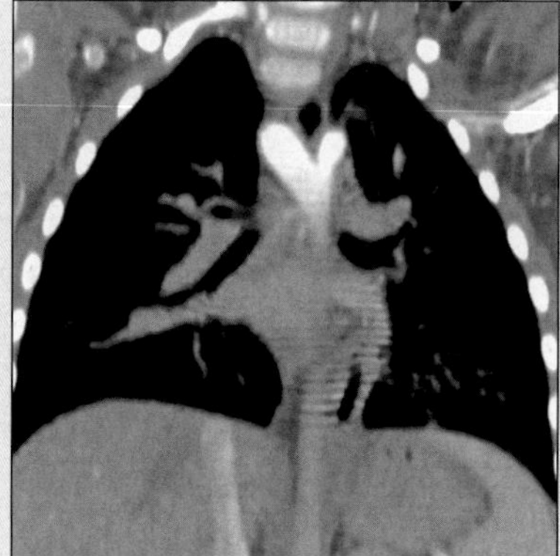

Right Aortic Arch/Vascular Ring

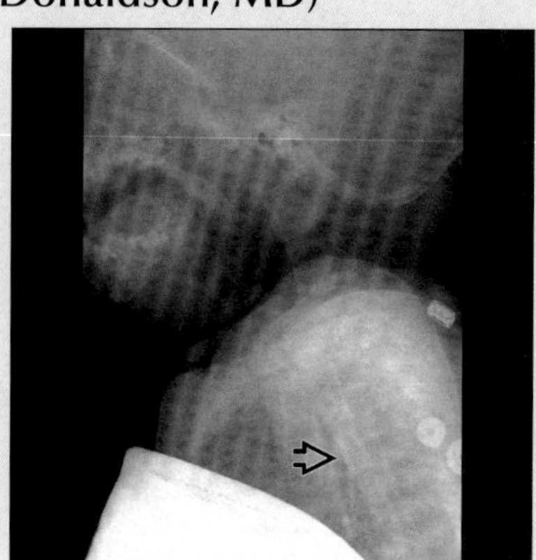

Tracheomalacia in Infant

INNOMINATE ARTERY COMPRESSION

Key Facts

Terminology
- Innominate artery passes immediately anterior to anterior aspect of trachea and leads to tracheal compression

Imaging Findings
- Narrow trachea from anterior compression just below thoracic inlet - seen on lateral radiograph, CT, MR
- Bronchoscopy shows compression of cervical trachea with pulsatile compression by innominate artery

Top Differential Diagnoses
- Vascular Rings
  - Double aortic arch is tight and results in stridor, and recurrent respiratory tract infections

Pathology
- In infants, innominate artery arises from aortic arch more to left of trachea than in adults
- In combination with "crowded" anterior mediastinum (thymus) leading to compression of trachea by innominate artery
- Presents in older patients if innominate artery is dilated or aneurysmal

Clinical Issues
- Presents in infancy with stridor, apnea, dyspnea
- Symptoms will typically resolve as child grows
- Tracheomalacia may be an important causative factor
- Surgical therapy is controversial, reserved for severe symptoms and failure of conservative management
- In adults presents with dyspnea and cough

  - Axial images perpendicular to trachea, imaging entire trachea
  - Innominate artery arises anterior and to left of trachea, then crosses from left to right in front of trachea
  - Narrowing of trachea in superior mediastinum
  - Tracheal narrowing confined to level at which innominate artery crosses anterior to trachea
  - Innominate artery immediately abuts area of tracheal narrowing
- MRA
  - Shows origin of innominate artery off aortic arch and its course in mediastinum
  - Good visualization in both children and adults without ionizing radiation

Echocardiographic Findings
- Echocardiogram: May identify innominate artery arising from a distal portion of aortic arch, but is commonly not diagnostic

Other Modality Findings
- Bronchoscopy shows a pulsatile indention or constriction of tracheobronchial wall
- Allows for evaluation of tracheomalacia and bronchomalacia

Angiographic Findings
- Conventional
  - In congenital type of innominate artery compression
    - Innominate artery arises from position on left side of trachea
    - Then crosses trachea anteriorly, compressing it
  - In acquired type of compression, innominate artery is aneurysmal and aneurysm is seen to be compressing trachea on lateral view

DIFFERENTIAL DIAGNOSIS

Vascular Rings
- Anomalies of aortic arch system and its branches
- Approximately 3% of general population will have a congential anomaly involving aortic arch system
- Only a small percentage of these will have symptomatic vascular compression of airway
- Double aortic arch is tight and results in stridor, and recurrent respiratory tract infections
- Right aortic arch with ligamentum arteriosum results in ring which can also cause tracheal compression and symptoms
- Right aortic arch with aberrant left subclavian (Kommerell diverticulum)
- Left aortic arch with aberrant right subclavian (Kommerell diverticulum) passes behind trachea and esophagus and commonly is asymptomatic
- Pulmonary artery sling is result of left pulmonary artery arising from right pulmonary artery and passing between trachea and esophagus
  - Results in significant airway compromise

Duplication Cyst Compressing Airway
- Three categories: Bronchogenic, intramural esophagus, and enteric
- Present with dyspnea, stridor or persistent cough

Lymphatic Malformation Compressing Airway
- Lymphangiomas: 5-6% of all benign soft tissue tumors in pediatrics
- May cause stridor and cyanosis

PATHOLOGY

General Features
- General path comments
  - Controversial topic
  - In infants, innominate artery arises from the aortic arch more to the left of the trachea than in adults
  - In theory, this can, in combination with "crowded" anterior mediastinum (thymus), lead to compression of trachea as innominate artery crosses obliquely rightward and ascends into neck

- Combination of these factors in theory leads to innominate artery compressing trachea as it passes rightward and anterior to trachea
- Crossing of the innominate artery over the trachea is seen in asymptomatic patients, so it maybe an intrinsic defect of the trachea causes symptoms
- May present in older patients if the innominate artery is dilated or aneurysmal
- In older symptomatic cases surgical therapy should be performed
- Tracheal necrosis has been reported in a patient with tracheal compression from an innominate artery aneurysm

- Etiology
  - Innominate artery aneurysms
    - Atherosclerosis
    - Infection - syphilis, bacterial
    - Takayasu disease, other collagen vascular diseases, trauma, chronic dissection

Staging, Grading or Classification Criteria

- Vascular ring hierarchy as defined by International Congenital Heart Surgery Nomenclature and Database Committee
  - Double aortic arch
    - Right arch dominant
    - Left arch dominant
    - Balanced arches
  - Right aortic arch-left ligamentum
    - Mirror-image branching
    - Retroesophageal left subclavian artery
    - Circumflex aorta
  - Innominate artery compression
  - Pulmonary artery sling

CLINICAL ISSUES

Presentation

- Most common signs/symptoms: Stridor, episodic apnea, dyspnea, wheezing, or recurrent pneumonia/bronchitis
- Other signs/symptoms
  - In older patients with an innominate aneurysm there may be a pulsatile mass
  - On bronchoscopy, trachea is posteriorly displaced, and right lateral wall is pulsatile just below thoracic inlet
- Usually presents during infancy
- Spectrum of severity from severe compromise of trachea to minimal indentation on trachea (normal variation)
- Symptoms will typically resolve as the child grows
- May present in older patients when the innominate artery is dilated or aneurysmal
- In adults presents with dyspnea and cough
- Very occasionally maybe seen in patients with severe scoliosis

Demographics

- Age
  - Very young patients who may outgrow the compression
  - Older patients who have tracheal compression due to innominate artery aneurysms

Natural History & Prognosis

- Compression and resultant symptoms decrease over time as child grows
- With aneurysms, patients may have strokes due to cerebral emboli, aneurysm may rupture, there maybe superior vena cava syndrome and dysphonia
- Erosion into mediastinum has been reported

Treatment

- Surgical therapy is controversial for children and reserved for those with severe symptoms and who fail conservative management
- With conservative management many patients will improve as they age
- Tracheomalacia resulting from primary weakness in tracheal wall may be an important causative factor
- Surgical aortopexy, innominate arteriopexy, or re-implantation of innominate artery origin more rightward from aortic arch
- Persistent symptoms may be present after surgery if tracheomalacia present
- In adults if patient is hypertensive, then hypertension should be controlled
- If innominate artery is aneurysmal then aneurysm will require resection
- In some cases stent-grafting of the innominate artery to exclude the aneurysm could be performed

DIAGNOSTIC CHECKLIST

Consider

- Vascular rings/slings causing dyspnea
- Tracheomalacia

SELECTED REFERENCES

1. Backer CL et al: Congenital Anomalies: Vascular Rings. In: Patterson GA (ed): Pearson's Thoracic and Esophageal Surgery. Philadelphia, Elsevier. 242-255, 2008
2. Malik TH et al: The role of magnetic resonance imaging in the assessment of suspected extrinsic tracheobronchial compression due to vascular anomalies. Arch Dis Child. 91(1):52-5, 2006
3. Park JG et al: Congenital stridor: unusual manifestation of coarctation of the aorta. Pediatr Cardiol. 27(1):137-9, 2006
4. Backer CL et al: Trends in vascular ring surgery. J Thorac Cardiovasc Surg. 129(6):1339-47, 2005
5. Friedman E et al: Innominate artery compression of the trachea: an unusual cause of apnea in a 12-year-old boy. South Med J. 96(11):1161-4, 2003
6. Kieffer E et al: Aneurysms of the innominate artery: surgical treatment of 27 patients. J Vasc Surg. 34(2):222-8, 2001
7. Montgomery PQ et al: Tracheal compression by an innominate artery aneurysm. Eur J Vasc Surg. 1(6):425-7, 1987
8. Strife JL et al: Tracheal compression by the innominate artery in infancy and childhood. Radiology. 139(1):73-5, 1981

IMAGE GALLERY

Typical

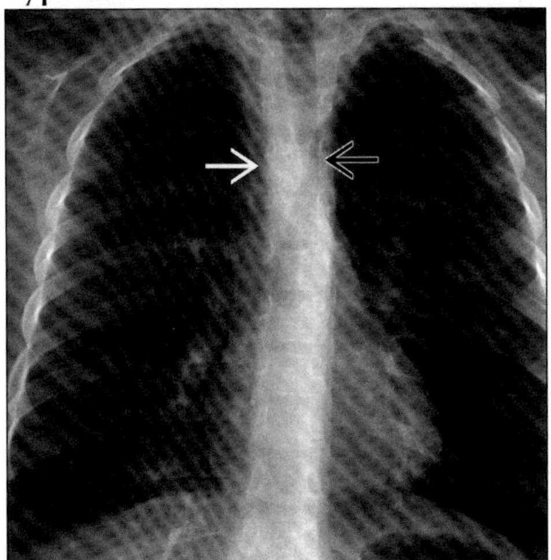

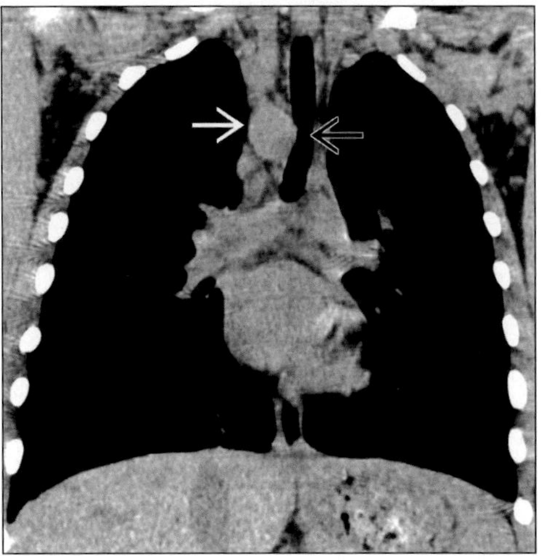

(Left) *Radiograph shows deviation of the trachea to the left ⇨ and a soft tissue mass ➡ which is causing the compression and deviation of the trachea. This mass represents a prominent innominate artery. Innominate artery compression maybe caused by a congenital or acquired abnormality.* ***(Right)*** *Coronal NECT shows the prominent innominate artery ➡ compressing the trachea ⇨ and deviating the trachea to the left.*

Typical

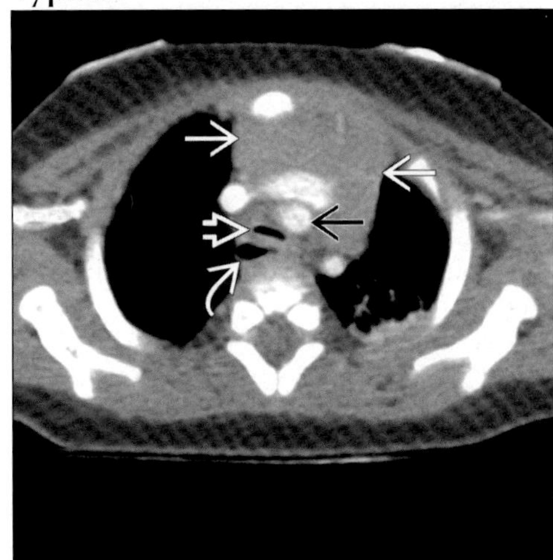

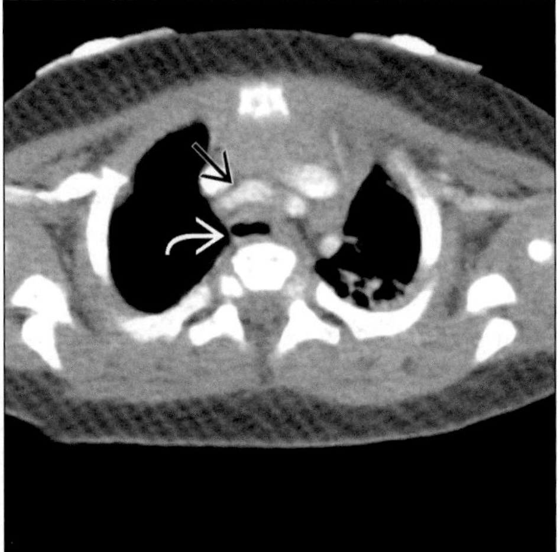

(Left) *Axial CECT shows compression of the trachea ➡ and esophagus, ➡ a 5 month old with severe stridor. The compression is caused by the innominate artery ⇨. The patient has a very prominent thymus ➡, which has been implicated in this syndrome.* ***(Right)*** *Axial CECT shows esophagus ➡, but trachea is not seen. Innominate artery ⇨ in front of the trachea. Infant underwent innominate arteriopexy. (Courtesy reference 1).*

Typical

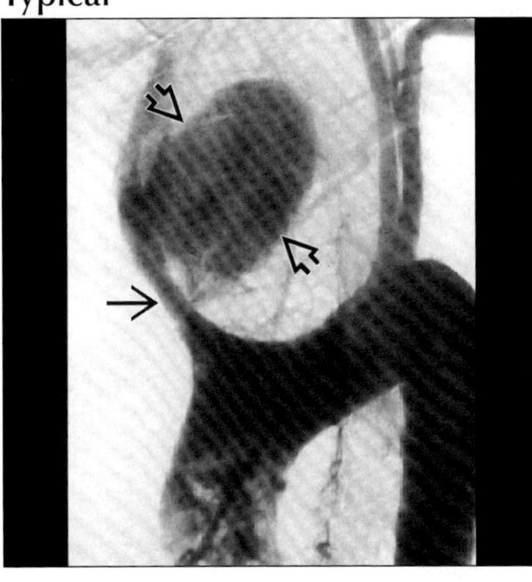

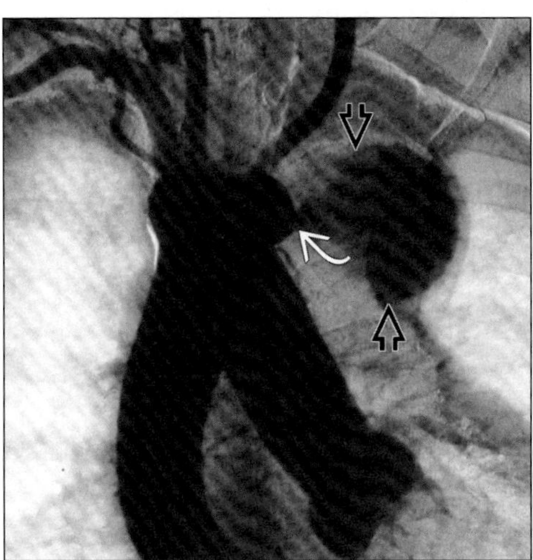

(Left) *Oblique catheter angiography shows a large pseudoaneurysm ⇨ originating from the innominate artery ⇨. Pseudoaneurysm was causing compression of the trachea causing the patient to be dyspneic, with stridor.* ***(Right)*** *Oblique catheter angiography shows the origin ➡ of the pseudoaneurysm ⇨. Etiology was a mycotic aneurysm. This required a surgical repair. If it was not mycotic it could be treated with a stent graft.*

RAYNAUD PHENOMENON

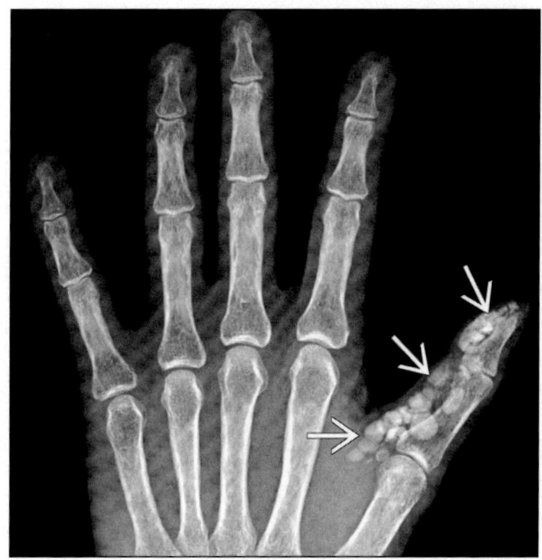
Radiograph in a patient with scleroderma shows soft tissue calcifications ➡. Digital ulcers often accompany calcinosis. Raynaud phenomenon may be the initial manifestation of scleroderma.

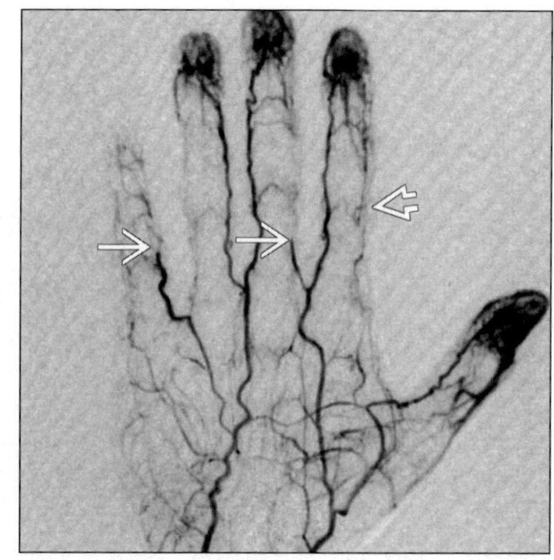
DSA in a patient with known scleroderma, who exhibits cyanosis of the fingers during cold exposure, shows occlusions ➡ and irregularity ⇨ of several digital arteries, typical of 2° Raynaud phenomenon.

TERMINOLOGY

Abbreviations and Synonyms

- Primary (1°) Raynaud phenomenon also termed Raynaud disease, idiopathic Raynaud phenomenon, or primary Raynaud syndrome
- Secondary (2°) Raynaud phenomenon also termed Raynaud syndrome

Definitions

- Raynaud phenomenon: Disorder characterized by episodic vasospasm and vasoconstriction of digital arteries; classified as primary or secondary
  - 1° Raynaud phenomenon (Raynaud disease): Exaggerated constriction of smooth muscle cells in otherwise normal artery, usually cold-induced
    - No identifiable underlying vascular abnormality
    - Environmental trigger causes primary vasospasm
  - 2° Raynaud phenomenon (Raynaud syndrome): Vasospastic digital ischemia associated with underlying arterial pathology
    - Patients have an underlying disease or condition that causes Raynaud phenomenon
    - Triggered by cold, nicotine, caffeine and stress
    - Most commonly associated with cutaneous disorders and connective tissue diseases

IMAGING FINDINGS

General Features

- Best diagnostic clue
  - Patient history, physical examination, and nailfold capillaroscopy
    - Nailfold capillaroscopy (study of skin at base of fingernail under a microscope) can help distinguish 1° and 2° Raynaud phenomenon
    - 1° Raynaud phenomenon has normal nailfold capillaroscopic pattern
    - 2° Raynaud phenomenon has abnormal nailfold capillaroscopy, with enlarged capillaries, hemorrhage and avascular areas
    - Fingertip rewarming time in response to local cold provocation also used for evaluation
  - Antinuclear antibody test (ANA) determines whether there is specific antibody production for connective tissue diseases or other autoimmune disorders

DDx: Digital Ischemia

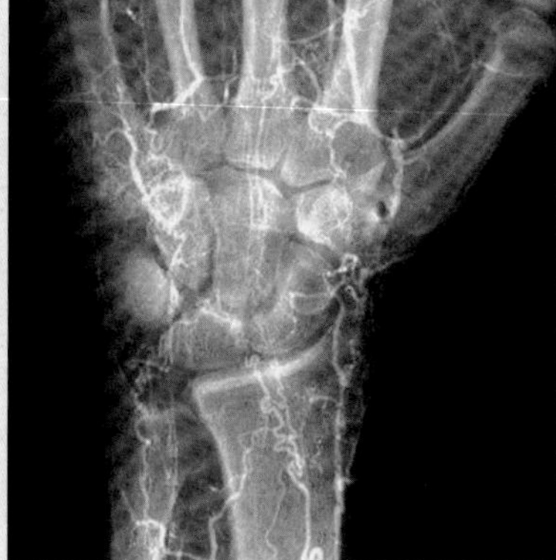
Buerger Disease

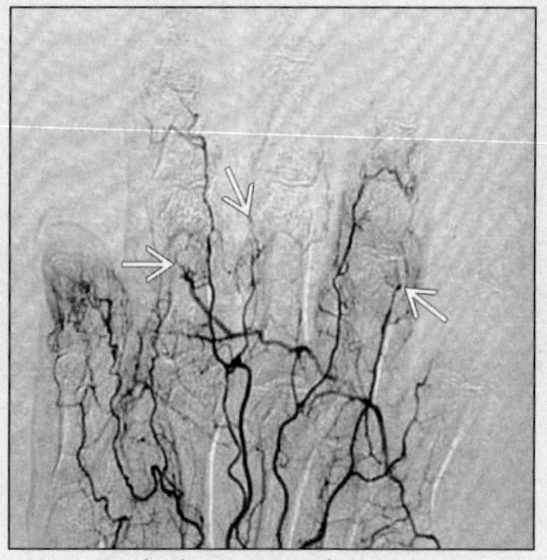
Emboli to Digital Arteries

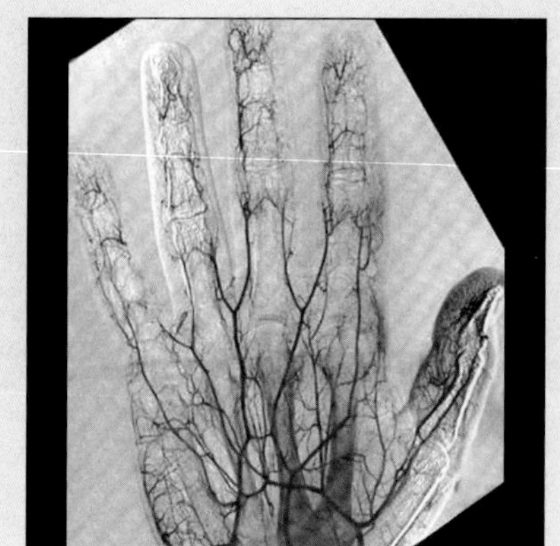
Lupus Erythematosus

RAYNAUD PHENOMENON

Key Facts

Terminology

- Raynaud phenomenon: Disorder characterized by episodic vasospasm and vasoconstriction of digital arteries; classified as primary or secondary
  - 1° Raynaud phenomenon (Raynaud disease): Exaggerated cold-induced constriction of smooth muscle cells in otherwise normal artery
  - 2° Raynaud phenomenon (Raynaud syndrome): Vasospastic digital ischemia associated with underlying arterial pathology

Imaging Findings

- Nailfold capillaroscopy (study of skin at base of fingernail under a microscope) can help distinguish 1° and 2° Raynaud phenomenon
  - 1° Raynaud phenomenon has normal nailfold capillaroscopic pattern
  - 2° Raynaud phenomenon has abnormal nailfold capillaroscopy: Enlarged capillaries, hemorrhages and avascular areas
- Ultrasound shows reduced vascularity in nail beds with 2° Raynaud phenomenon due to connective tissue diseases

Clinical Issues

- Treatment of 1° Raynaud phenomenon focuses on avoiding triggers
- Treatment of 2° Raynaud phenomenon involves therapy for underlying disease process
  - Calcium-channel blockers used to relax smooth muscle and dilate small blood vessels
  - Alpha blockers to counteract vasoconstrictive actions of norepinephrine

---

  - Erythrocyte sedimentation rate (ESR) is a nonspecific inflammatory indicator
    - Normal in 1° and elevated in 2° Raynaud phenomenon
- Location
  - Commonly affects digits of hands and feet
    - Can affect other areas of body including nose, cheeks, ears, and tongue

Radiographic Findings

- Radiographs of hands may demonstrate typical abnormalities of connective tissue disorders
  - Erosions, joint space narrowing, demineralization, acro-osteolysis, flexion contractures, and calcinosis
    - Calcinosis most often seen with digital ulcers
    - Calcinosis and acro-osteolysis both associated with vascular complications

MR Findings

- Gadolinium enhanced MRA has been investigated for assessment of digital vasculature in systemic sclerosis
  - Diffuse lesions involving small caliber arteries and veins and microcirculation have been demonstrated

Ultrasonographic Findings

- Reduced vascularity in nail beds with 2° Raynaud phenomenon from connective tissue diseases
  - Small digital arteries with decreased pulsation and frequent stenoses

Angiographic Findings

- Angiography rarely used in evaluation of Raynaud phenomenon
  - When employed, may show very poor opacification of digital arteries
  - Improved digital arterial perfusion after intra-arterial vasodilator administration in 1° form
    - Underlying arterial pathology in 2° form

Imaging Recommendations

- Best imaging tool: Nailfold capillaroscopy

DIFFERENTIAL DIAGNOSIS

Connective Tissue Disorders

- Lupus erythematosus
  - Raynaud phenomenon is earliest manifestation in 1/3 of patients with this disorder
  - IgG and IgM anticardiolipin antibodies are also common clinical manifestations in patients with systemic lupus erythematosus
    - Associated with thrombotic episodes involving small arteries
- Rheumatoid arthritis
  - Endothelial cell activation is a common pathway in rheumatoid arthritis associated systemic vasculitis
    - May cause inflammatory arterial necrosis
- Scleroderma
  - 90% of patients present with Raynaud phenomenon as earliest manifestation
  - Microcirculation undergoes structural and functional changes that are interdependent
    - Microangiopathy characterized by capillary rarefaction, development of megacapillaries and vascular obliteration
  - Intimal hyperplasia caused mainly by collagen overproduction
    - Causes narrowing of smaller digital arteries
  - Endothelial cells seem to play role in pathogenesis via impaired endothelium-dependent vasodilation
    - Impaired early in disease process, mainly through an diminished ability to release nitric oxide
- Other connective tissue disorders
  - Dermatomyositis
  - Polymyositis
  - Sjögren syndrome

Obstructive Arterial Diseases

- Atherosclerosis
- Arterial emboli
- Buerger disease (thromboangiitis obliterans)
  - Inflammatory occlusive disorder affecting small and medium-sized arteries and veins of young, predominantly male, smokers

- Autoimmune response triggered by nicotine
- Total tobacco abstinence to halt disease progression
- Thoracic outlet syndrome

Occupational Related

- Vibration injury
  - Hypothenar hammer syndrome
- Vinyl chloride exposure
  - Plastics industry workers may develop illness similar to scleroderma

Medication Related

- Beta-blocking antihypertensive agents
- Chemotherapeutic agents (particularly bleomycin)
- Ergotamine preparations for migraine headache
- Over-the-counter cold medications

PATHOLOGY

General Features

- Genetics: Possible familial component to 1° Raynaud phenomenon
- Etiology
  - 1° Raynaud phenomenon has no underlying arterial pathology
    - Triggered by cold, emotions (e.g., stress, anxiety)
    - Possible acquired adrenoreceptor hypersensitivity
  - 2° Raynaud phenomenon has underlying arterial pathology
    - Connective tissue disorders most common cause
    - Carpal tunnel syndrome
    - Obstructive arterial disease
    - Medication induced
- Epidemiology: 5-10% of US population affected with Raynaud phenomenon (both forms combined)

Microscopic Features

- Microvascular damage is typical of scleroderma as underlying etiology for 2° Raynaud phenomenon
  - > 95% have architectural disorganization, giant capillaries, hemorrhages, capillary loss, avascular areas and neovascularization
  - Found in other systemic diseases such as systemic lupus erythematosus, antiphospholipid syndrome and Sjögren syndrome

CLINICAL ISSUES

Presentation

- Most common signs/symptoms
  - Numbness and loss of tactile perception in response to cold/emotional stress
  - Demarcated pallor/cyanosis
- Other signs/symptoms
  - Hyperemic throbbing during rewarming
  - Small painful ulcers at tips of digits

Demographics

- Age: Presentation typically before age 30; usually earlier presentation in 1° form than in 2° form
- Gender: 80% females
- More common in colder climates

Natural History & Prognosis

- Initially during an episode, affected areas of skin develop pallor in response to the arterial vasospasm
- These areas subsequently become cyanotic and develop numbness and loss of tactile perception
- As circulation improves, affected areas redden, with accompanying throbbing, tingling or swelling
  - An episode may last from minutes to hours

Treatment

- Treatment options dependent on type of Raynaud phenomenon
  - Treatment of 1° Raynaud phenomenon
    - Conservative management and reassurance that digital ischemia and tissue loss rarely occur
    - Avoidance of environmental triggers (e.g., cold, nicotine, caffeine)
    - Warm clothing for extremities
  - Treatment of 2° Raynaud phenomenon
    - Therapy for underlying disease process
    - More often treated with medication than 1° form
    - Calcium-channel blockers used to relax smooth muscle and dilate small blood vessels
    - Alpha blockers to counteract vasoconstrictive actions of norepinephrine
    - Nonspecific vasodilator (e.g., nitroglycerin paste) application to fingers to help heal skin ulcers
- Rarely sympathectomy

DIAGNOSTIC CHECKLIST

Consider

- Evaluation for underlying connective tissue disorder in patient presenting with Raynaud phenomenon

SELECTED REFERENCES

1. Cherkas LF et al: Heritability of Raynaud's phenomenon and vascular responsiveness to cold: a study of adult female twins. Arthritis Rheum. 57(3):524-8, 2007
2. Dobrev H: In vivo study of skin mechanical properties in Raynaud's phenomenon. Skin Res Technol. 13(1):91-4, 2007
3. Gayraud M: Raynaud's phenomenon. Joint Bone Spine. 74(1):e1-8, 2007
4. Gunawardena H et al: Maximum blood flow and microvascular regulatory responses in systemic sclerosis. Rheumatology (Oxford). 46(7):1079-82, 2007
5. Pope JE: The diagnosis and treatment of Raynaud's phenomenon: a practical approach. Drugs. 67(4):517-25, 2007
6. Suter LG et al: Smoking, alcohol consumption, and Raynaud's phenomenon in middle age. Am J Med. 120(3):264-71, 2007
7. Carpentier PH et al: Incidence and natural history of Raynaud phenomenon: A long-term follow-up (14 years) of a random sample from the general population. J Vasc Surg. 44(5):1023-8, 2006
8. Tangri N et al: Soft-tissue infection and underlying calcinosis of CREST syndrome. CMAJ. 175(9):1059, 2006
9. Wang WH et al: Peripheral sympathectomy for Raynaud's phenomenon: a salvage procedure. Kaohsiung J Med Sci. 22(10):491-9, 2006

RAYNAUD PHENOMENON

IMAGE GALLERY

Typical

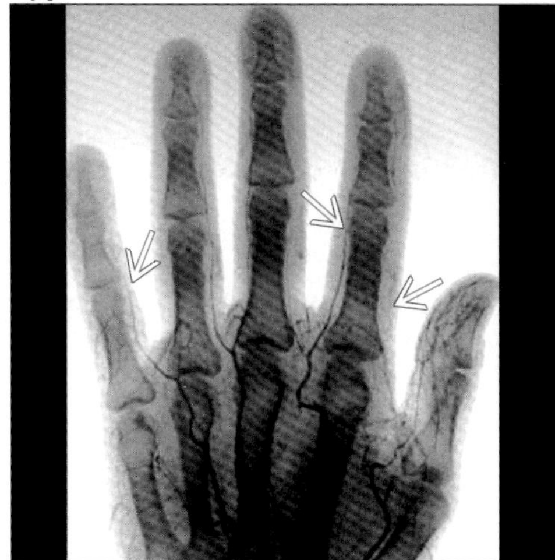

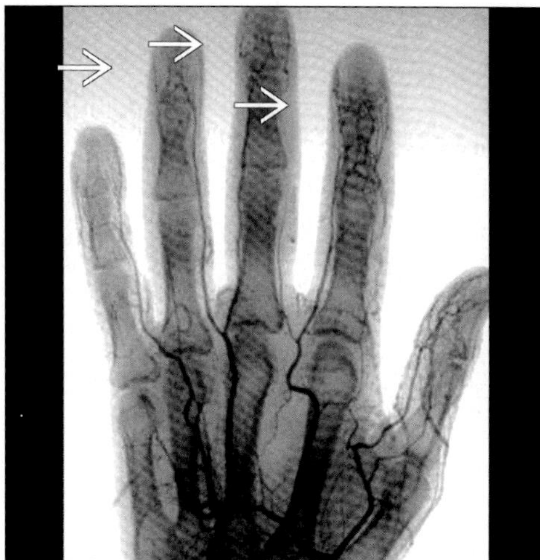

(Left) *Arteriogram shows very poor opacification of the digital arteries ➡, particularly distal to the proximal phalanges, in a patient with a history of numbness and pallor of the fingers during cold exposure.* ***(Right)*** *Arteriogram obtained after intra-arterial vasodilator administration shows greatly improved perfusion of the digital arteries ➡, confirming that the poor digital circulation was non-occlusive. This is typical of primary Raynaud phenomenon.*

Typical

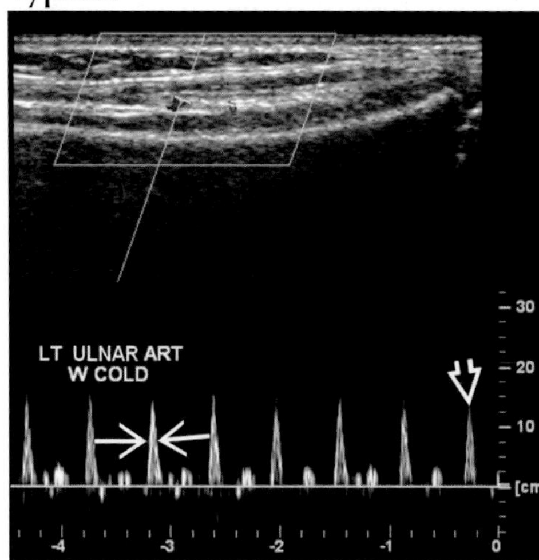

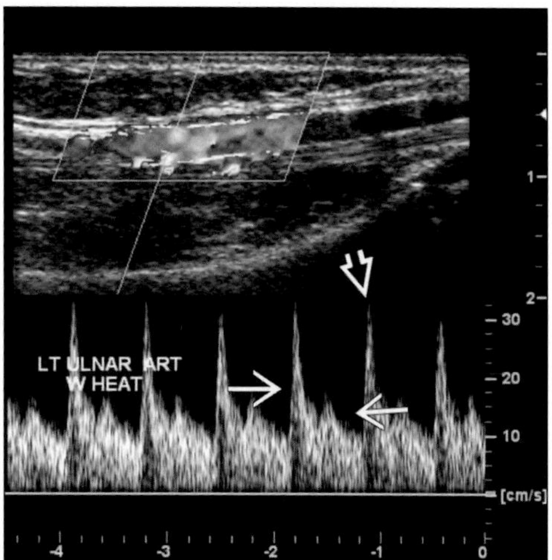

(Left) *Doppler US of the ulnar artery in a patient with Raynaud phenomenon, obtained during cold stimulation of the hand, shows a narrowed monophasic arterial waveform ➡ with ↓ amplitude ⇨.* ***(Right)*** *Doppler US (same patient as previous image) after hand warming shows a normal triphasic arterial waveform ➡ in the ulnar artery, with significantly stronger amplitude ⇨. This is a positive cold stimulation test for Raynaud phenomenon.*

Typical

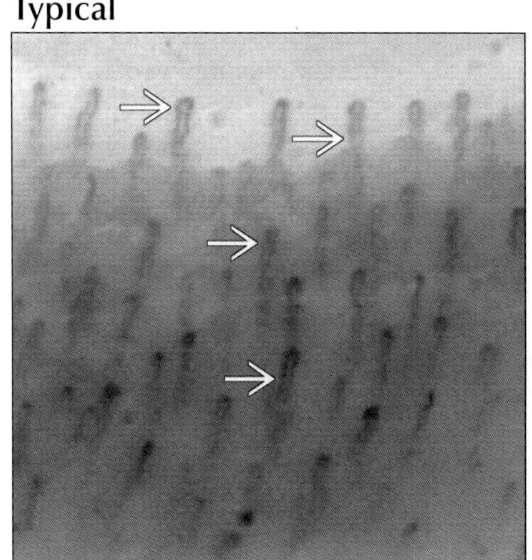

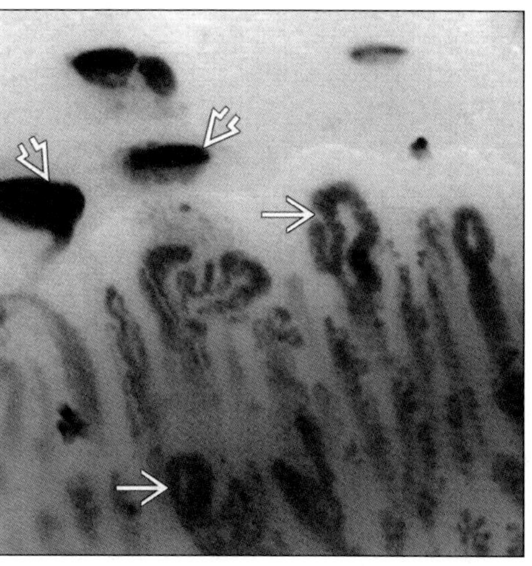

(Left) *Normal nailfold capillaroscopy shows a regular arrangement of the capillary loops ➡. There are no areas of architectural distortion, avascularity or hemorrhage. Primary Raynaud phenomenon, in the absence of cold exposure, has the same appearance.* ***(Right)*** *Nailfold capillaroscopy in a patient with secondary Raynaud phenomenon and known scleroderma shows architectural disorganization with giant capillaries ➡ and hemorrhages ⇨.*

COLLAGEN VASCULAR DISEASES

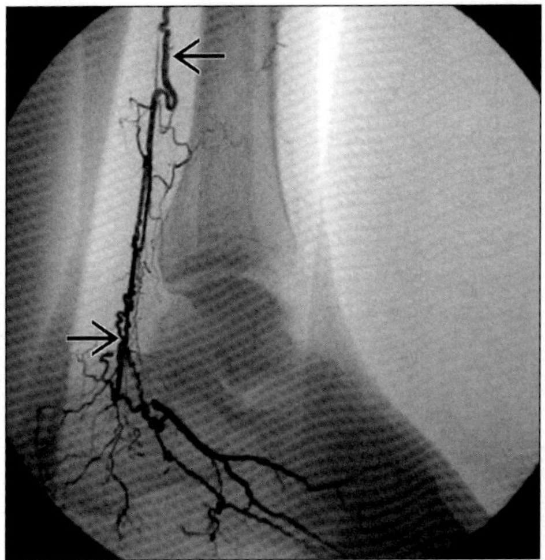

DSA shows involvement of the medium and small arteries of the leg and foot. There are characteristic "corkscrew" collaterals ⇒ None of the tibial arteries are seen. Patient with Buerger disease.

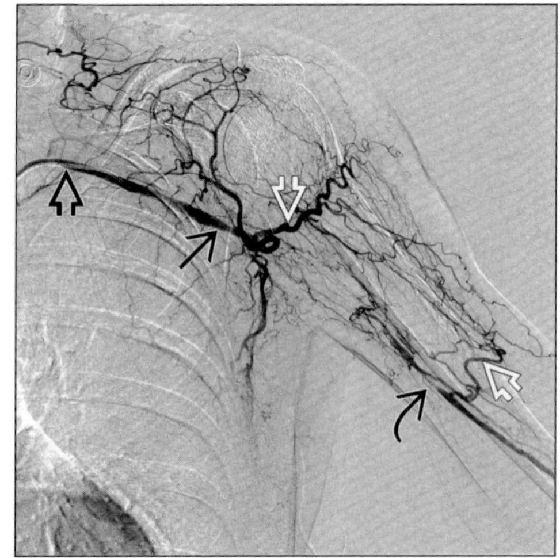

DSA shows irregularity, narrowing and occlusions of subclavian ⇨, axillary → and brachial arteries ⇨. Multiple collaterals ➡ refill the brachial artery. Patient with giant cell arteritis.

TERMINOLOGY

Abbreviations and Synonyms

- Collagen vascular disease (CVD)
- Connective tissue disorder (CTD)

Definitions

- CVDs include CTDs with associated blood vessel abnormalities due to inflammation or weakness of collagen
- Describes vast & heterogeneous group of vasculitides; result of a number of different underlying conditions
  - Primary vasculitides
    - Takayasu, Buerger, giant cell arteritis, polyarteritis nodosa, Behçet disease
  - Vasculitis secondary to systemic autoimmune diseases
    - Systemic lupus erythematosus, rheumatoid arthritis, psoriatic arthritis, Sjögren syndrome, scleroderma, dermatomyositis, polymyositis, mixed connective tissue disease, juvenile rheumatoid arthritis, relapsing polychondritis, ankylosing spondylitis, Reiter disease
  - Radiation vasculitis

IMAGING FINDINGS

General Features

- Best diagnostic clue: Multiple stenoses and occlusions of medium to small arteries in extremities, particularly hands
- Location
  - CTDs can affect blood vessels anywhere
  - Small and medium caliber vessels are affected
    - Peripheral arteries of hands often affected with sparing of forearm and upper arm
  - Concomitant visceral microaneurysms suggest CVD
- Size
  - CTDs can involve vessels of any size, but small vessel involvement predominates
  - Some CTDs, such as Takayasu arteritis, will primarily affect large and medium caliber vessels
- Morphology
  - CVD occlusions are usually tapered, and multiple, often with poor collateralization
    - Look for absence of intraluminal filling defects that would suggest embolic disease
- Disease specific findings
  - Takayasu arteritis (pulseless disease)

DDx: Collagen Vascular Disease

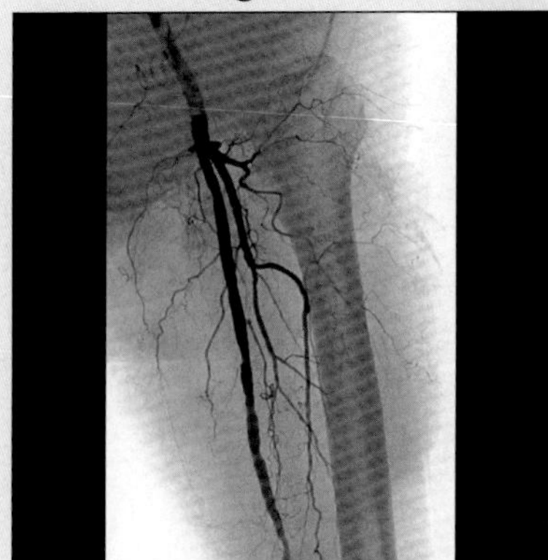

Atherosclerotic Disease

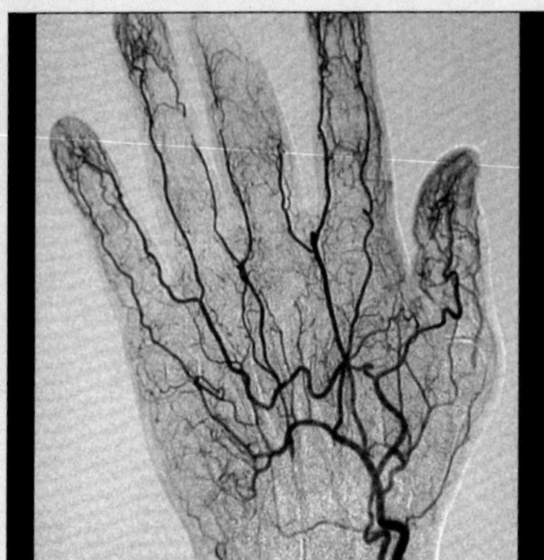

Emboli to the Hand

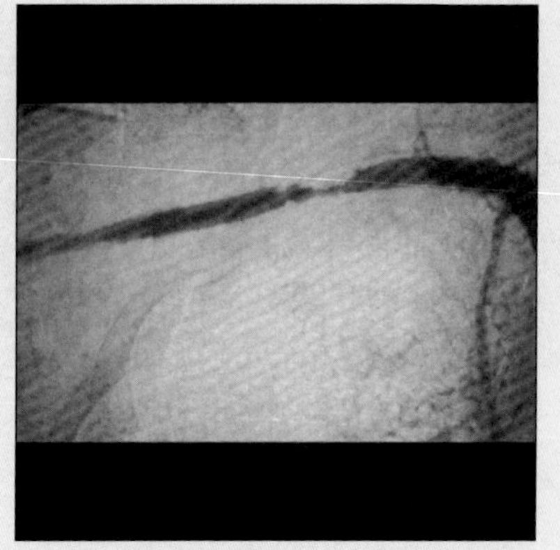

Trauma, Stretch Injury

COLLAGEN VASCULAR DISEASES

Key Facts

Terminology

- CVDs include CTDs with associated blood vessel abnormalities due to inflammation or collagen weakness
- Vast, heterogeneous group of vasculitides
- Primary vasculitides
  - Takayasu, Buerger, giant cell arteritis, polyarteritis nodosa, Behçet disease
- Vasculitis secondary to systemic autoimmune diseases
  - Systemic lupus erythematosus, rheumatoid arthritis, psoriatic arthritis, Sjögren syndrome, scleroderma, dermatomyositis, polymyositis, mixed connective tissue disease, juvenile rheumatoid arthritis, relapsing polychondritis, ankylosing spondylitis, Reiter disease
- Radiation vasculitis

Imaging Findings

- Multiple stenoses and occlusions of medium to small arteries in the extremities, particularly the hands
- CTDs can affect blood vessels anywhere
- CTDs can involve vessels of any size, but small vessel involvement predominates
- Angiography is often needed to evaluate CVD
- Buerger disease (thromboangiitis obliterans)

Pathology

- Although biopsy is gold standard for vasculitis, definitive diagnosis is rare
- Histology can confirm presence of vasculitis, but pathognomonic histopathological findings for specific diseases are uncommon

---

    - Wall-enhancement with CECT or MR
    - Long stenoses in aorta, common carotid, and subclavian arteries are common
    - Patients also commonly have aortic aneurysms
  - Giant cell arteritis (temporal arteritis)
    - Multiple, long, irregular stenoses & occlusions of distal subclavian, axial, & proximal brachial arteries
    - Patients sometimes have thoracic or abdominal aortic aneurysms and/or dissection
  - Polyarteritis nodosa
    - Multiple microaneurysms involving extremities, renal or other visceral arteries
    - Stenoses and occlusions of digital arteries
  - Buerger disease (thromboangiitis obliterans)
    - Distal small to medium vessels of upper and lower extremities
    - With angiography, occlusion of vessels below knee and/or elbow will be seen
    - Corkscrew appearance of collaterals
    - Migratory thrombophlebitis in a third of cases
  - Behçet disease
    - Thrombosis of venules or small veins
    - Rarely, aortic and pulmonary artery aneurysms, arterial occlusive disease, or central venous thrombosis
  - Vasculitis secondary to systemic CVD (SLE, scleroderma)
    - Angiographic findings of focal occlusions and irregular stenoses of palmar and digital arteries
    - Stenoses & occlusions variable in length & tapered
  - Rheumatoid arthritis, ankylosing spondylitis, Reiter syndrome, & psoriatic arthritis (HLA-B27 positive)
    - Patients develop ascending aortic dilatation and aortic valve insufficiency
  - Radiation vasculitis: Limited to area of treatment
    - Stenoses and occlusions with limited collaterals
    - Susceptible to increased atherosclerotic changes

Imaging Recommendations

- Best imaging tool
  - Initiate imaging with CT or MR to evaluate wall thickening that enhances with contrast, central stenoses, and central aneurysms
    - More effective with larger vessels
  - Angiography often needed to evaluate CVD: Differentiates from atherosclerotic or embolic causes

DIFFERENTIAL DIAGNOSIS

Atherosclerotic Disease

- Angiography typically shows irregularity of vessel walls and abundant collateralization
- History of atherosclerotic risk factors: Hypertension, hypercholesterolemia, smoking, diabetes, family history of heart disease, sedentary lifestyle

Embolic Disease

- Angiography shows abrupt occlusion with filling defect, poor collateralization, with multiple downstream vessels involved
- Embolic disease often recurrent, and unpredictable

Vascular Infection

- Mycotic destruction of vessel walls can result in multilobulated aneurysmal changes
- Majority of infections occur in lower extremity peripheral arteries and aorta
- Patients present with constitutional symptoms and pain in affected area

PATHOLOGY

General Features

- Etiology
  - Often result of autoimmune collagen destruction leading to blood vessel wall breakdown & necrosis
  - Primarily type II (antibody to self antigens) & type III (immune complex deposition) mediated
- Epidemiology: Depends on primary systemic disease process causing vasculitis
- Associated abnormalities

COLLAGEN VASCULAR DISEASES

- In general, CVDs are systemic diseases
  - Degree of damage depends on patient's specific autoimmune disease

Gross Pathologic & Surgical Features

- Although biopsy is gold standard for vasculitis, definitive diagnosis are rare
- Histology can confirm presence of vasculitis, but pathognomonic histopathological findings for specific diseases are uncommon
- Histopathology can be modulated by immunosuppressive therapy & often complicates diagnosis

Microscopic Features

- Histologic appearance varies depending on immunologic process involved
- A few disease specific appearances include
  - Takayasu arteritis: Thickened intima and media from granulomatous changes
  - Giant cell arteritis: Giant cell infiltration throughout vessel wall
  - Buerger disease: Occlusion of vessel from inflammatory cellular debris
  - Systemic CVDs: Often show immune complex deposition in vessel wall

CLINICAL ISSUES

Presentation

- Most common signs/symptoms: Patient who is too young for atherosclerotic disease with constitutional symptoms such as arthralgias, myalgias, or skin rashes
- Other signs/symptoms: Disease specific, often presents with upper extremity claudication, diminished upper extremity pulses, digital ulceration or evidence of Raynaud syndrome
- Disease specific presentations
  - Takayasu arteritis
    - Predominately affects 20-40 year old females
    - Results in occlusions and stenoses in upper extremity proximal arteries, "pulseless disease"
    - May develop hypertension from renal stenoses
  - Giant cell arteritis
    - Common in elderly females
    - Present with weeks of headaches, fever, & tender temporal arteries, "temporal arteritis"
  - Polyarteritis nodosa
    - M:F = 2:1; age: 40-60 years
    - Small to medium-sized arteries in the viscera, heart, hands & feet affected
    - Associated with Hepatitis B, C, and IVDU
  - Buerger Disease
    - M:F = 4:1; young smokers
    - Patients present with evidence of small-vessel occlusive disease in distal extremities
  - Behçet disease
    - M:F = 2:1; age: 20-40 years
    - Present with recurrent oral and genital ulcers, ocular inflammation, arthritis, skin lesions, GI symptoms, and epididymitis
  - Patients with vasculitis secondary to systemic CVDs often present with digital ischemia & ulcerations
  - Rheumatoid arthritis, ankylosing spondylitis, Reiter syndrome, & psoriatic arthritis patients can develop ascending aortic dilatation with aortic valve insufficiency
  - Radiation vasculitis localized to treatment area
    - Symptoms due to arterial thrombosis can occur within five years of treatment
    - Stenoses & occlusions tend to occur at 5-10 years; sequela such as accelerated atherosclerosis & periarterial fibrosis occur much later
- Laboratory work-up includes
  - CRP, ESR, and rheumatoid factor: Elevated levels suggest autoimmune disorder
  - Eosinophilia can be indicative of Churg-Strauss disease
  - C-ANCA titers: Wegener granulomatosis-associated
  - Hepatitis B and C titers: Associated with polyarteritis nodosa and cryoglobulinemia respectively

Demographics

- Age: Can occur at any age; patients often younger than those presenting with atherosclerotic disease
- Gender: Depends on the specific disease process causing the vasculitis

Natural History & Prognosis

- Disease involvement and progression depends on underlying disorder
  - Ranges from isolated cutaneous involvement to life threatening cardiovascular compromise

Treatment

- Treatments vary with disease process
- Early diagnosis important to limit progression
- Autoimmune causes: Goal to limit autoimmune destruction
- Examples of treatments include
  - NSAIDs such as aspirin or ibuprofen
  - Corticosteroids such as prednisone or methylprednisolone for systemic disease
  - For more severe disease, cytotoxic drugs such as azathioprine and cyclophosphamide
  - Other medications include: Mycophenolate mofetil, tumor necrosis factor blockers, & rituximab

DIAGNOSTIC CHECKLIST

Consider

- When multiple stenoses and occlusions are present in small vessels, with microaneurysms

SELECTED REFERENCES

1. Amezcua-Guerra LM et al: Imaging studies in the diagnosis and management of vasculitis. Curr Rheumatol Rep. 9(4):320-7, 2007
2. Doyle MK: Vasculitis associated with connective tissue disorders. Curr Rheumatol Rep. 8(4):312-6, 2006
3. Hellmich B et al: Difficult to diagnose manifestations of vasculitis: does an interdisciplinary approach help? Best Pract Res Clin Rheumatol. 19(2):243-61, 2005
4. Herrick AL et al: Vascular imaging. Best Pract Res Clin Rheumatol. 18(6):957-79, 2004

IMAGE GALLERY

Typical

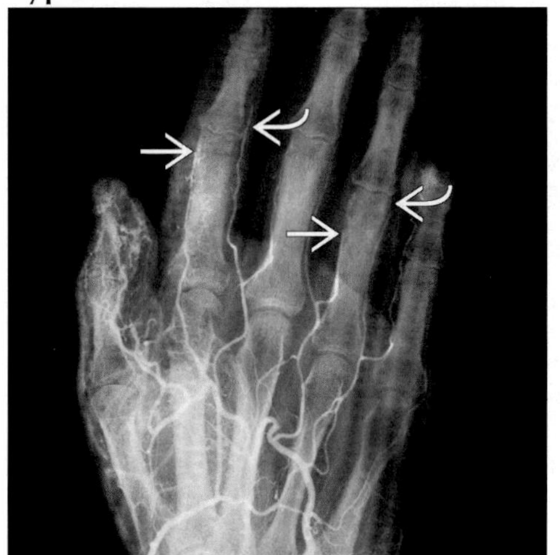

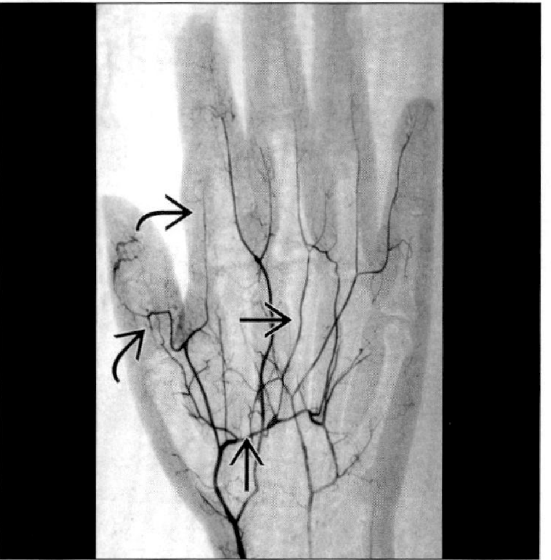

(Left) *DSA shows small vessel involvement in the hand. The ulnar artery and radial artery are relatively normal. In the fingers there are multiple arteries that are occluded. Other arteries show evidence of stenosis and tapered narrowing. Patient with SLE.* ***(Right)*** *DSA shows multiple arteries with narrowing. The digital arteries are stenotic and have areas of occlusion or severe narrowing. These are findings of CVD, in this case, scleroderma.*

Typical

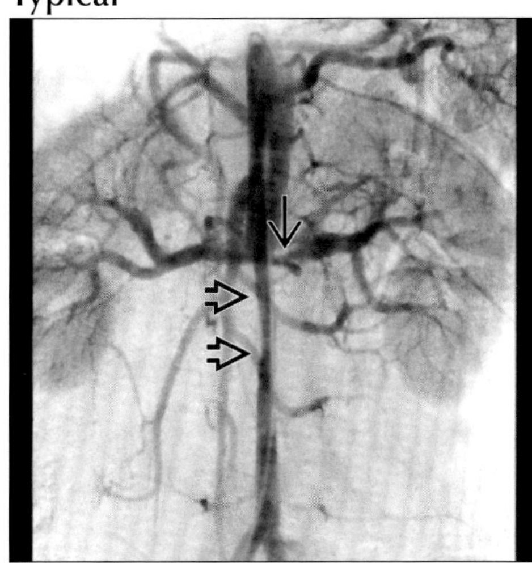

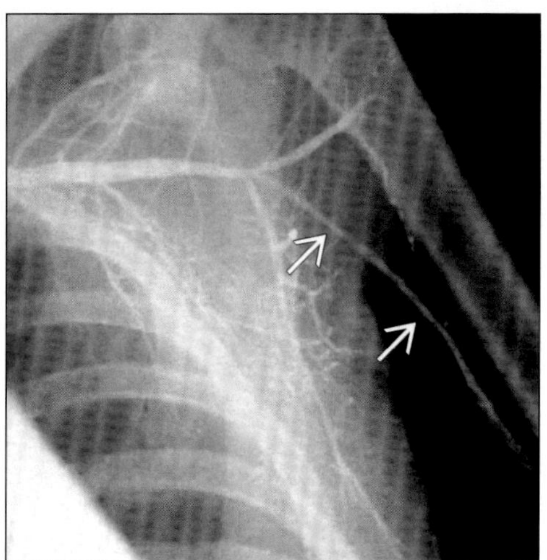

(Left) *Catheter angiography shows renal artery stenosis and aortic stenosis in a patient with Takayasu arteritis with aortic involvement. In some patients aneurysms develop, in others stenoses predominate.* ***(Right)*** *Catheter angiography shows severe, long narrowing of brachial artery. In Takayasu arteritis, narrowing is due to thickening of intima & media from granulomatous changes. Involvement of upper extremity leads to "pulseless disease".*

Typical

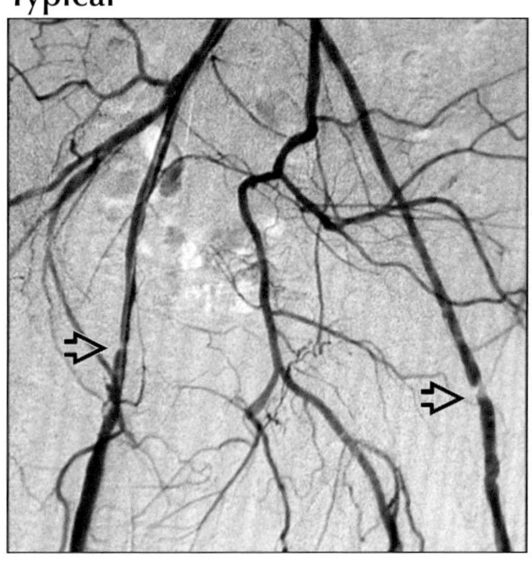

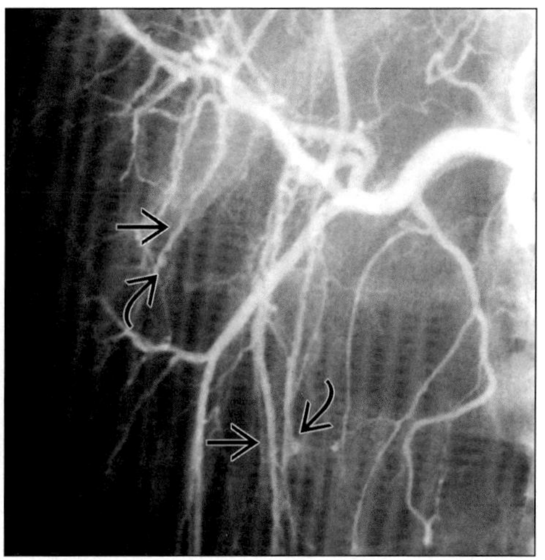

(Left) *DSA shows external iliac arteries w/focal stenoses. Patient with no risk factors for atherosclerotic disease & previous radiation therapy to the pelvis. Radiation vasculitis results in stenoses and occlusions, & accelerated atherosclerotic changes result from radiation exposure.* ***(Right)*** *Catheter angiography shows irregularity of multiple arteries with microaneurysms; a typical appearance of polyarteritis nodosa with microaneurysms.*

MUSCULOSKELETAL HEMANGIOMA

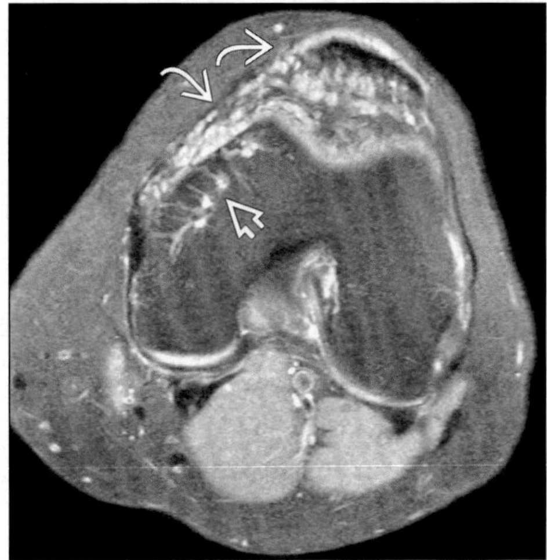

Axial T2WI FSE MR shows an extensive hemangioma involving both the bones and soft tissues around the knee, as well as the peripheral edges of the femur. (Courtesy M. Pathria, MD).

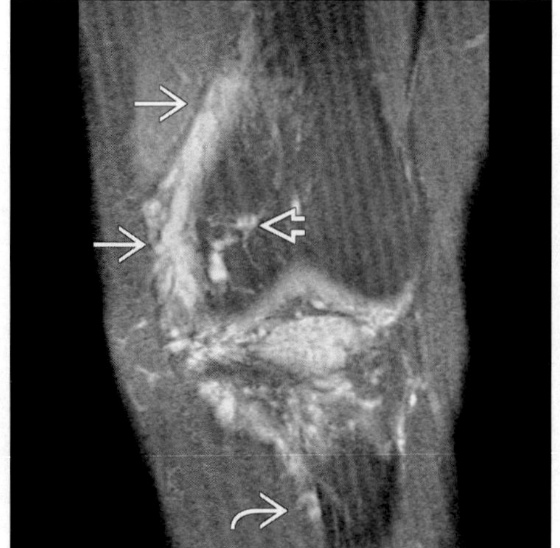

Coronal T2WI FSE MR shows the hemangioma involving the soft tissues medial to the femur and the distal femur bone with extension into the proximal calf. (Courtesy T. Hughes, MD).

TERMINOLOGY

Abbreviations and Synonyms

- Vascular malformation or cavernous hemangioma

Definitions

- Hemangiomas are benign vascular tumors, most often seen at birth or infancy

IMAGING FINDINGS

General Features

- Best diagnostic clue
  - Lobulated blue or blue-black subcutaneous lower extremities mass that is readily compressible
    - Mass varies in size with posture
- Location: Involves soft tissue (striated muscle, skin, subcutaneous tissue and synovial tissue), bone
- Size: Different sizes
- Morphology: Rounded and lobulated masses

Radiographic Findings

- Radiography
  - Soft tissue mass or prominence containing phleboliths (small calcifications)
  - Medullary hemangiomas: "Soap bubbles" or coarsely loculated appearance
  - Periosteal hemangiomas: Shallow, cup-shaped depression underlined by sclerotic margins
  - Cortical hemangiomas: Intracortical nidus surrounded by sclerotic reaction

CT Findings

- CECT
  - Serpentine vascular structures surrounded by fatty tissue
  - Characteristic centripetal enhancement seen in liver does not always occur peripherally
  - Calcifications, phleboliths

Nuclear Medicine Findings

- Tc-99m Labeled Red Cell Scintigraphy
  - Non invasive, low radiation dose exposure, no complications, multiple views
  - Sensitivity of 89% and specificity of 100%
  - Uptake of radiotracer is progressive over time, delayed blood pool imaging is necessary
  - Accurate determination of size of lesions

DDx: Manifestations of Hemangioma

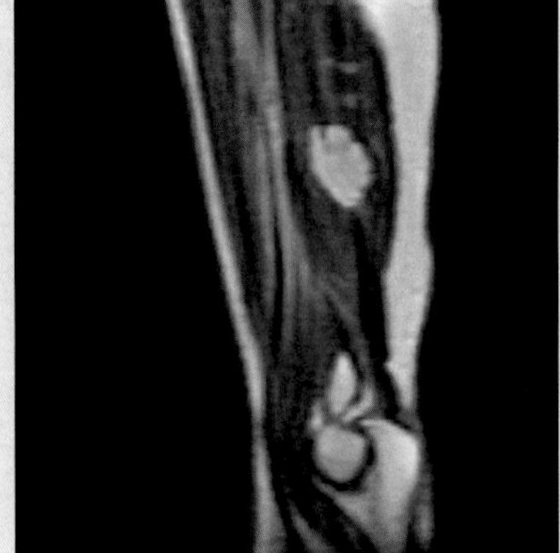

Intramuscular Hemangioma

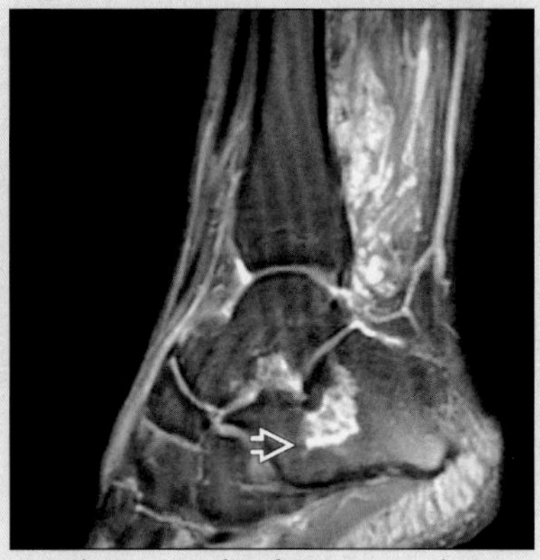

Involvement of Soft Tissue and Bone

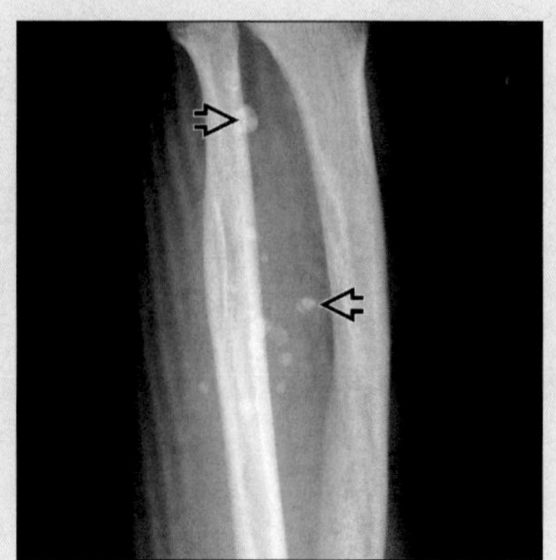

Soft Tissue Mass and Phleboliths

MUSCULOSKELETAL HEMANGIOMA

Key Facts

Terminology

- Hemangiomas are benign vascular tumors, most often seen at birth or infancy

Imaging Findings

- Involves soft tissue (striated muscle, skin, subcutaneous tissue and synovial tissue), bone
- MR imaging
- T1 weighted images: Low to intermediate signal intensity masses with high signal adipose tissue most prominent along the circumference of vascular complex
- T2 weighted images: Central angiomatous core shows high signal intensity
- Prominent enhancement of mass after administration of gadolinium
- Angiography: Unless feeding vessel is injected there may be no flow of contrast into cavernous hemangioma
  - Can usually be avoided and replaced by CT or MR unless used as a pre-embolization procedure
- Tc-99m Labeled RCS: Sensitivity of 89% and specificity of 100%

Pathology

- Incidence of these tumors in the extremities varies from 4.9% to 28.5%

Clinical Issues

- Cavernous hemangiomas occur later in life compared to capillary hemangiomas (diagnosed during first two years of life)

  - Best investigation for diagnosis and post-treatment follow up of lesions

Ultrasonographic Findings

- Grayscale Ultrasound: Lack of definition of entire periphery of lesion also typical of inflammatory and malignant lesions
- Color Doppler: Low resistance arterial flow with forward flow during both systole and diastole

Angiographic Findings

- Angiography: Unless feeding vessel is injected there may be no flow of contrast into cavernous hemangioma
- Can usually be avoided and replaced by CT or MR unless used as a pre-embolization procedure

Imaging Recommendations

- Best imaging tool
  - MR imaging
    - All sequences show heterogeneous mass even if lesions under 2 cm tend to be homogeneous
- Protocol advice
  - T1WI: Low to intermediate signal intensity masses with high signal adipose tissue most prominent along the circumference of vascular complex
  - T2WI: Central angiomatous core shows high signal intensity
  - Prominent enhancement of mass after administration of gadolinium
  - Rapid flow can cause signal voids
  - Lobulated appearance, with septations

DIFFERENTIAL DIAGNOSIS

Lymphatic Malformations

- MR imaging: Enhancement is more patchy and central than in venous malformations, minimal or no enhancement is seen in periphery of lesion

Lipoma-Angiolipoma

- If the fat overgrowth is very prominent hemangiomas can be mistaken for lipomas
- Angiolipomas are variants of lipoma or hemangioma
- MR imaging: Intensity similar to that of subcutaneous fat on both T1 and T2

Spindle Cell Hemangioendothelioma

- Rare vascular neoplasm characterized by cavernous spaces, thrombi, phleboliths and spindle cells
- It may arise at sites of vascular injury

Pigmented Villonodular Synovitis (PVNS)

- Benign proliferative lesions of the synovium
- MR: Low or intermediate signal on T1WI and low signal intensity on T2WI and gradient echo images

Osteoid Osteoma

- Benign bone tumor, usually less than 1.5 cm
- Radiographically can be confused for cortical hemangioma (central nidus with adjacent new bone sclerotic reaction)
- Uncommon in children younger than 5 and adults older than 40
- Pain at site exacerbated by exercise; worsen at night

Arteriovenous Malformation (AVM)

- Abnormal connection between arteries and veins
- Arterial blood is shunted to venous system through a central tortuous "nidus" of vessels
- Even if congenital they are always discovered later in life

PATHOLOGY

General Features

- General path comments
  - Five categories of soft tissue hemangioma
    - Capillary, cavernous, arteriovenous, venous, and mixed variations
    - Capillary: Superficial lesion; diagnosed in first few years of life and spontaneously involutes
    - Cavernous: Develops later in life; dilated blood-filled spaces lined by endothelium; does not involute

  - Arteriovenous: Persistent fetal capillary bed leads to abnormal communication/shunting
  - Venous: Thicker walled vessels with smooth muscle cells
- Can contain thrombus, calcification, hemosiderin, fat, smooth muscle, fibrous tissue
- Soft tissue types most often arise in skin and subcutaneous tissue; skeletal muscle and synovial membrane less frequent sites of origin
  - Intramuscular hemangiomas very rare (0.8%) not usually suspected clinically
  - Quadriceps is most affected muscle
- Intraosseous hemangioma accounts for less than 1% of bone neoplasms
  - Most cases are located in metadiaphysis or diaphysis
  - Vertebrae and skull account for more than 75% of cases; long tubular bones least affected
  - Hemangiomas of long tubular bones are mainly medullary
- Genetics: Most hemangiomas not familial conditions
- Etiology: Infection, trauma and pregnancy are associated with lesion's formation and development
- Epidemiology: Incidence of these tumors in the extremities varies from 4.9-28.5%
- Associated abnormalities: If soft tissue mass is in close proximity to adjacent bone, osseous changes, periosteal reaction and cortical thickening can occur

Gross Pathologic & Surgical Features

- Several classifications of hemangiomas have been described ranging from four to nine categories based on depth, clinical appearance, histology and location
  - Categories: Capillary hemangiomas, cavernous hemangiomas, combined or mixed types and diffuse or systemic hemangiomas
- Phlebolites are associated with cavernous hemangiomas in approximately 50% of cases
- Cavernous hemangiomas are larger and deeper than capillary hemangiomas

Microscopic Features

- Cavernous hemangiomas are masses of dilated, thin-walled vessels or sinuses, lined with endothelium and surrounded by a fibrous connective tissue stroma

CLINICAL ISSUES

Presentation

- Most common signs/symptoms
  - Pain with no trauma and swelling; a mass is present in almost all cases (98%)
    - Pain due to compression of nerves and fibers by surrounding edema
- Other signs/symptoms
  - Restriction of movement if they involve the deep fascia and muscles
  - Pain especially with physical exertion which results in retrograde flow in arterial segment distal to hemangioma; therefore ischemia of surrounding tissue (steal phenomenon)
  - Limb-length discrepancy especially if large
  - Bone hemangiomas can cause structural weakening of the osseous shaft and pathologic fractures
  - Involvement of a joint may result in hemosiderin-arthropathy due to repeated intraarticular bleeding (typically seen in the knee)
  - Maffucci syndrome: Multiple soft tissue cavernous hemangiomas are associated with multiple enchondromas
    - Malignant transformation may occur in both hemangiomas and enchondromas

Demographics

- Age: Cavernous hemangiomas occur later in life compared to capillary hemangiomas (diagnosed during first two years of life)
- Gender
  - Female > Male
  - Most often seen in Caucasians

Natural History & Prognosis

- Cavernous hemangiomas do not spontaneously involute and therefore may require surgical intervention
- Large connections exist with the general circulation, explaining frequent recurrence rate after surgical removal
- Intramuscular types progressively enlarge locally but never metastasize

Treatment

- Options, risks, complications
  - Sclerosing agents (alcohol, Sotradecol) injected into feeding vascular tributaries of the hemangioma
    - Glue (cyanoacrylate) maybe used, very rarely coils will be used
  - With vascular supplies interrupted, hemangiomas shrink and may involute; risk of tissue necrosis
  - Hemangiomas are radioresistant
- Radiofrequency ablation: Early experience

DIAGNOSTIC CHECKLIST

Consider

- Vascular malformations are a complex group of entities ranging from capillary hemangiomas which can spontaneously involute to very aggressive high-flow arterial malformations which can cause congestive heart failure and limb loss

SELECTED REFERENCES

1. Downey-Carmona FJ et al: Acute compartment syndrome of the foot caused by a hemangioma. J Foot Ankle Surg. 45(1):52-5, 2006
2. Haroon N et al: Intramuscular cavernous hemangioma with juxta-articular swelling. CMAJ. 175(9):1059, 2006
3. Sheldon PJ et al: Imaging of intraarticular masses. Radiographics. 25(1):105-19, 2005
4. Olsen KI et al: Soft-tissue cavernous hemangioma. Radiographics. 24(3):849-54, 2004
5. Llauger J et al: MR imaging of benign soft-tissue masses of the foot and ankle. Radiographics. 18(6):1481-98, 1998

IMAGE GALLERY

Typical

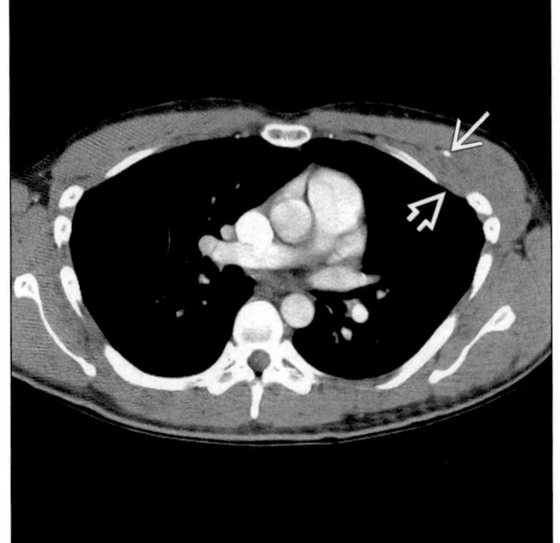

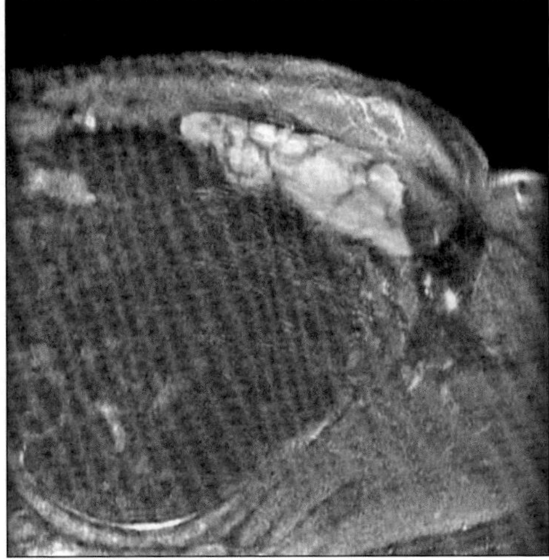

*(**Left**) Axial CECT shows asymmetry of the left chest wall ⇨ compared with the right. There is a focal area of calcification ➡ in the soft tissue that represents a phlebolith and no enhancement of the soft tissues is evident. (**Right**) Axial T2WI FS MR shows a mass in the subpectoral region which is very bright. The mass contains lobules and septations which are characteristic of hemangiomas. (Courtesy S. Ferrara, MD).*

Typical

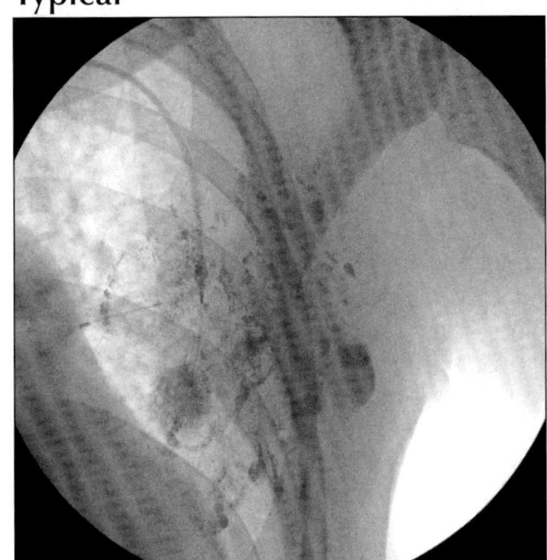

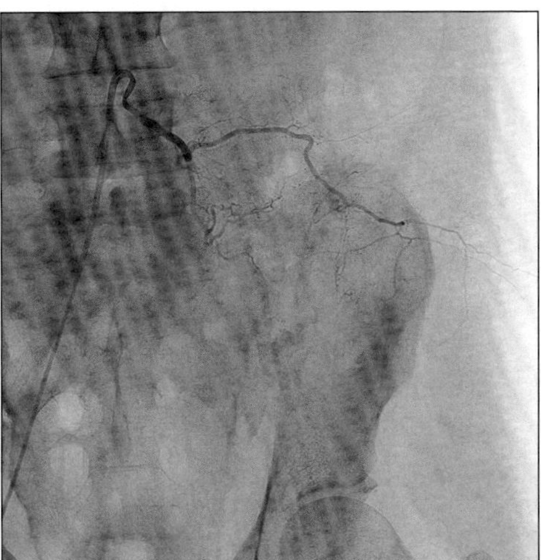

*(**Left**) Radiograph taken during an embolization procedure for treatment of the hemangioma. Relatively low flow in the lesion makes catheter embolization difficult. Direct puncture with administration of a sclerosing agent such as alcohol or Sotradecol can be performed. The sclerosing agent is mixed with Ethiodol for better visualization. (**Right**) DSA shows the catheterization of the left iliac hemangioma (see following images). The lesion is quite hypovascular.*

Typical

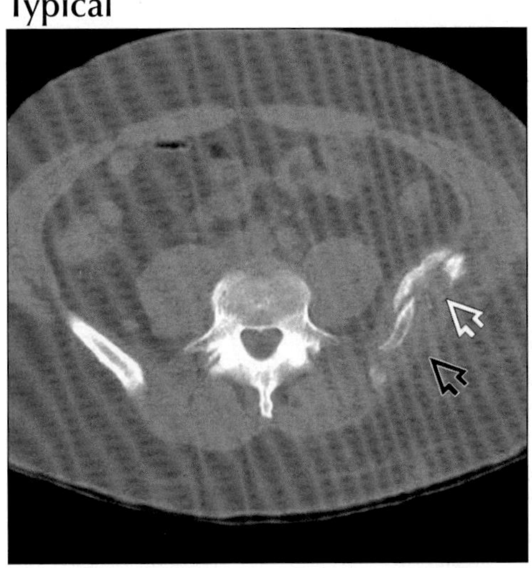

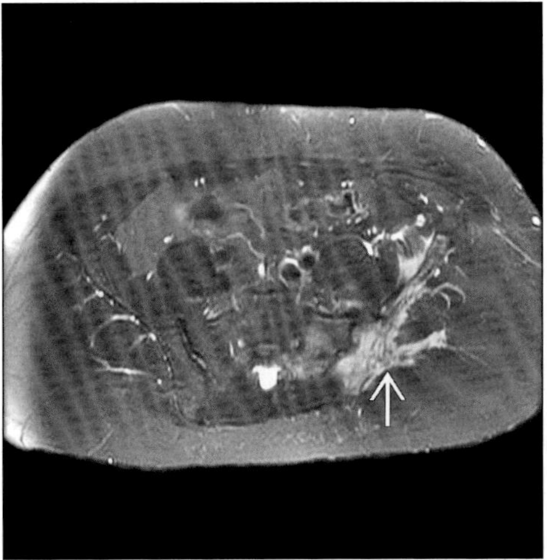

*(**Left**) Axial CECT shows a bony deformity of the left iliac bone ⇨, with an associated soft tissue mass ⇨. Hemangioma will commonly directly cause deformation of bony structures. (**Right**) Axial T2WI FSE MR shows an enhancing mass ➡ which appears more infiltrative. It involves the iliac bone, with some involvement of the sacrum, and extending out into the soft tissue posterior and lateral to the pelvis.*

CAVERNOUS HEMANGIOMA

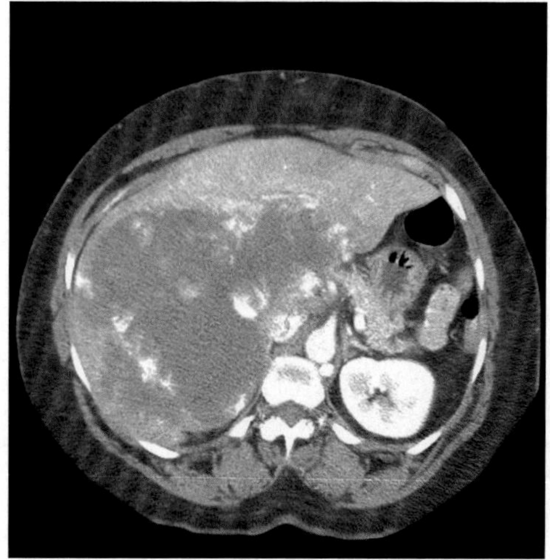

Axial CECT shows a giant hemangioma in the right lobe of the liver. In the arterial phase, most of the enhancement is in the periphery of the lesion. The enhancement is discontinuous and patchy.

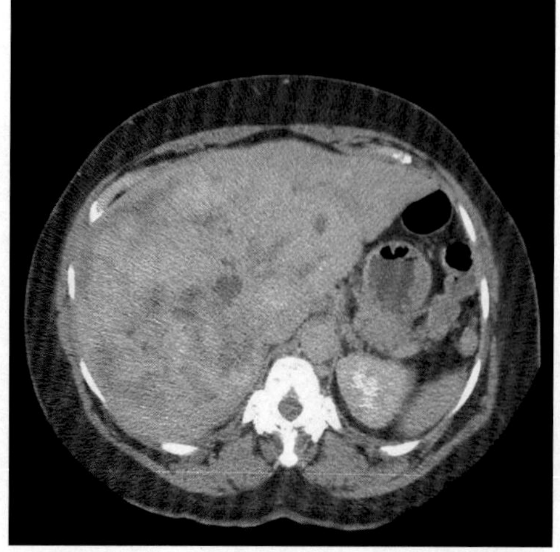

Axial CECT shows a later phase. On delayed imaging, there has been progressive centripetal filling in of the lesion. However, typically the very large hemangiomas do not have uniform enhancement.

TERMINOLOGY

Abbreviations and Synonyms

- Hepatic cavernous hemangioma (CH), hepatic hemangioma, giant hemangioma of the liver

Definitions

- Cavernous hemangioma is the most common benign hepatic tumor

IMAGING FINDINGS

General Features

- Best diagnostic clue: Most hemangiomas are incidentally detected on imaging studies
- Location: No lobar predilection exists but frequently are located peripherally or adjacent to a large hepatic vein branch
- Size: Hemangiomas typically measure less than 5 cm; those larger than 4-5 cm are sometimes called giant hemangiomas
- Morphology: Focal, often rounded lesions

CT Findings

- NECT
  - Lesions are usually relatively hypoattenuating when compared with adjacent liver
  - Calcifications are uncommon, if present they can be central or marginal, spotty or chunky
- CECT
  - Small hemangiomas in arterial phase show intense and uniform contrast-enhancement; the lesion retains enhancement during portal phase
  - Pathognomonic pattern: Peripheral, discontinuous, intense nodular enhancement during arterial dominant phase with progressive centripetal fill
    - Nodular areas consist of small vascular spaces more densely packed than the rest of the lesion
  - Atypical features: Arterio-portal shunts and capsular retraction

MR Findings

- Strong "light bulb"-like signal on heavily T2-weighted images
- Dynamic CT findings can be more clearly detected with dynamic MR imaging

DDx: Hepatocellular Carcinoma

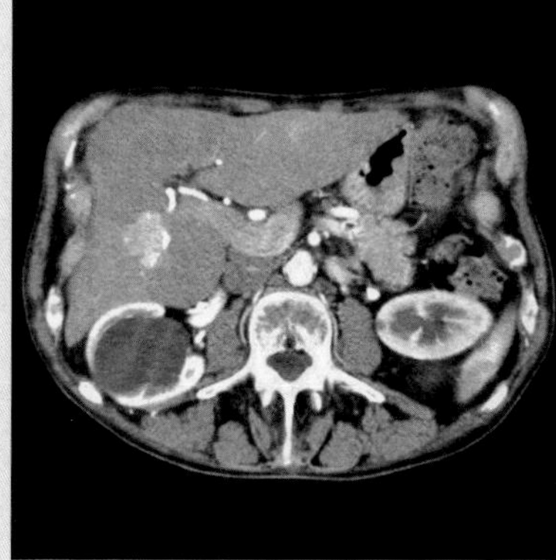

CECT: Arterial Phase

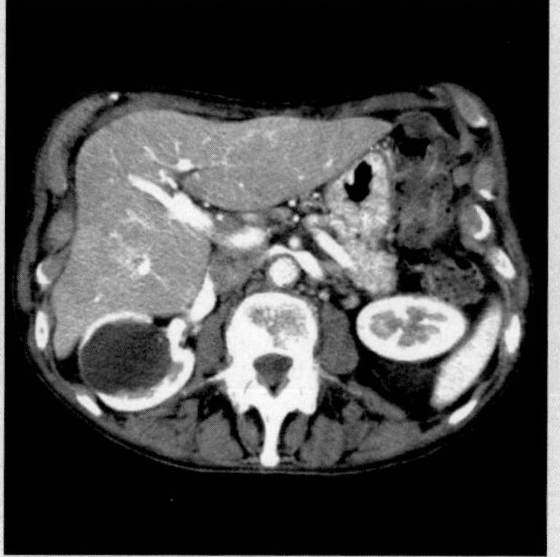

CECT: Portal Phase

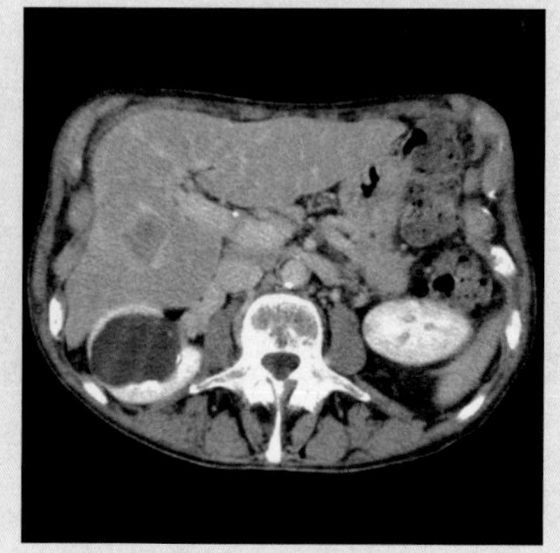

CECT: Late Phase

CAVERNOUS HEMANGIOMA

Key Facts

Terminology
- Cavernous hemangioma is the most common benign hepatic tumor

Imaging Findings
- Most hemangiomas are incidentally detected on imaging studies
- US is a cost-effective modality for diagnosis
  - However CT and MR may be required for a more specific diagnosis
- Lesion relatively hypoattenuating when compared with adjacent liver
- Pathognomonic pattern: Peripheral, discontinuous, intense nodular enhancement during arterial dominant phase with progressive centripetal fill
- Strong light bulb-like signal on heavily T2-weighted images

Top Differential Diagnoses
- Focal Nodular Hyperplasia (FNH)
- Hepatocellular Carcinoma (HCC)
- Liver Metastasis

Pathology
- Probably congenital in origin; their natural history is not completely understood
- Occurrence in general population: 0.4-20%

Clinical Issues
- Surgical treatment of hepatic hemangiomas is required in case of complications such as platelet sequestration (KMS), Budd-Chiari syndrome and rupture

  - Highly concentrated contrast agent injected over short period of time and fast image acquisition in arterial dominant phase
- On basis of liver hemangiomas detection with T2WI MR has sensitivity of 100% and specificity of 92%

Ultrasonographic Findings
- Grayscale Ultrasound
  - Homogeneously hyperechoic focal lesion
    - In a patient with a low risk for malignancy this feature is usually sufficient for a confident diagnosis
- Contrast-enhancement US: Early arterial nodular enhancement with delayed centripetal fill-in
  - Real time nature of contrast enhancement US is useful in diagnosing small and rapidly perfusing (flash-filling) hemangiomas
  - Complete enhancement does not usually occur in larger (> 3 cm) hemangiomas because of central thrombosis or fibrosis

Angiographic Findings
- DSA
  - Feeding vessels of hemangioma are of normal caliber, except those in the large tumors
  - During late arterial/hepatic parenchymal phases, a dense, nodular pattern of opacification of dilated vascular spaces persists into the venous phase
  - Angiography is not frequently used for diagnosis because of availability of accurate non invasive technique
  - Angiography is usually only performed prior to embolization

Imaging Recommendations
- Best imaging tool
  - US is a cost-effective modality for diagnosis of CH
    - However, CT and MR may be required for a more specific diagnosis
- Protocol advice: Combined interpretation of hemodynamic studies and sonographic findings may provide more reliable information concerning diagnosis of CH in liver

DIFFERENTIAL DIAGNOSIS

Focal Nodular Hyperplasia (FNH)
- FNH is the second most common solid benign hepatic lesion
- Prevalence: 0.9-3%
- Incidence: Women > man; 3rd-5th decade of life
- US findings: Homogeneous, near isoechoic lesion with central hypoechoic scar detected in 20-45% of cases

Hepatocellular Carcinoma (HCC)
- Most common primary malignant tumor of liver
- Early detection crucial for curative treatment; small HCC (< 2 cm) treated with liver transplantation have survival rate of about 80% while 5-year survival of untreated HCC less than 5%
- Non invasive diagnosis of HCC based on dynamic CT and MR detection of hypervascular masses in patients with chronic liver disease
- 83-97% of HCCs have contrast washout and appear as a defect during late phase, however lack of washout does not guarantee the lesion is benign

Liver Metastasis
- Liver is a frequent site of metastases
- Accuracy of US in detection of liver metastases in lower than that of CT or MR
- Regardless of behavior during early phase, metastases show rapid, complete washout of contrast and appear as enhancement defects on late phase scans
- With second generation US contrast media 85% of metastases show some arterial enhancement more pronounced in periphery

Hepatocellular Adenoma (HA)
- Rare hepatocellular neoplasm
- 90% of HAs occur in young women; 90% of young females with HAs have reported the use of oral contraceptives
- CECT shows homogeneous enhancement in smaller lesions and heterogeneous enhancement in larger lesions due to previous intramural hemorrhage or necrosis

- Management is by surgical resection because of risk of malignant degeneration and hemorrhage
- Rim-like enhancement and early and complete washout of the lesion are typical of metastasis

PATHOLOGY

General Features

- Genetics
  - Probably congenital in origin; their natural history not completely understood
  - Possibly abnormal angiogenesis and vasculogenesis may be involved
- Etiology: Hereditary factors influence pathogenesis of familial forms
- Epidemiology
  - Occurrence in general population: 0.4-20%
  - Incidence of CH in female > male has been reported in surgical series; female to male ratio is 5:1 to 6:1
  - In children and autopsy series CH affects males and females equally
- Associated abnormalities: They may occur in association with multiple cutaneous hemangiomas or without cutaneous lesions

Gross Pathologic & Surgical Features

- Mass not encapsulated and made up of vascular spaces of various size and supported by collagenous wall

Microscopic Features

- Vascular spaces separated by walls of various thickness but endothelial cells (EC) arranged in single layer

CLINICAL ISSUES

Presentation

- Most common signs/symptoms
  - CH often asymptomatic (85%)
  - Symptoms caused by compression of adjacent structures, thrombosis, rupture
- Other signs/symptoms
  - Abdominal pain, nausea and vomiting can be created by compression of the stomach by CH
  - Compression of the inferior vena cava can cause Budd-Chiari syndrome
  - Rupture can occur in 1-4% of hemangiomas and mortality rate can be as high as 60%
  - Kasabach-Merritt syndrome (KMS) is a combination of hemangioma, thrombocytopenia and coagulopathy
    - KMS is an infrequent but potentially fatal complication of rapidly growing hemangiomas in infant
  - Hemangiomas may become fibrotic and shrink in patients with progressive cirrhosis (more difficult radiological and pathological characterization
    - Changes in blood flow as a result of hepatic fibrosis may influence the regression of hemangiomas

Demographics

- Age: Middle age women
- Gender: Female > male

Natural History & Prognosis

- Hemangiomas may become fibrotic and shrink in patients with progressive cirrhosis (more difficult radiologic and pathologic diagnosis)

Treatment

- Surgical treatment of hepatic hemangiomas is required in case of complications such as platelet sequestration (KMS), Budd-Chiari syndrome and rupture
- In pregnancy a conservative approach with serial ultrasound monitoring is indicated
- Transcatheter arterial embolization (TAE) can be a less invasive approach in treatment of CH but may result in complications such as biliary damage
  - Performed for pain control in symptomatic patients or as an emergency with rupture
  - Performed prior to surgical resection to decrease risk of bleeding
- Percutaneous radiofrequency ablation (RFA)
  - Needle electrode inserted directly into hepatic tumor percutaneously under local anesthesia and conscious sedation by US or CT guidance
  - Local tissue is heated creating 3.5-5.0 cm area of thermal coagulative necrosis

DIAGNOSTIC CHECKLIST

Image Interpretation Pearls

- Large hemangiomas have very heterogeneous enhancement while small hemangioma are much more homogeneous
- CT should be done with delayed imaging to assess continued enhancement centrally

SELECTED REFERENCES

1. Morin SH et al: Use of second generation contrast-enhanced ultrasound in the assessment of focal liver lesions. World J Gastroenterol. 13(45):5963-70, 2007
2. Srinivasa Prasad MD et al: Cavernous Hemangioma, Liver; eMedicine. Aug 29, 2007
3. Berloco P et al: Giant hemangiomas of the liver: surgical strategies and technical aspects. HPB (Oxford). 8(3):200-1, 2006
4. Zhang WJ et al: Morphologic, phenotypic and functional characteristics of endothelial cells derived from human hepatic cavernous hemangioma. J Vasc Res. 43(6):522-32, 2006
5. Cui Y et al: Ultrasonography guided percutaneous radiofrequency ablation for hepatic cavernous hemangioma. World J Gastroenterol. 9(9):2132-4, 2003
6. Yu JS et al: Hepatic cavernous hemangioma in cirrhotic liver: imaging findings. Korean J Radiol. 1(4):185-90, 2000
7. Yu JS et al: Hepatic cavernous hemangioma: sonographic patterns and speed of contrast enhancement on multiphase dynamic MR imaging. AJR Am J Roentgenol. 171(4):1021-5, 1998

IMAGE GALLERY

Typical

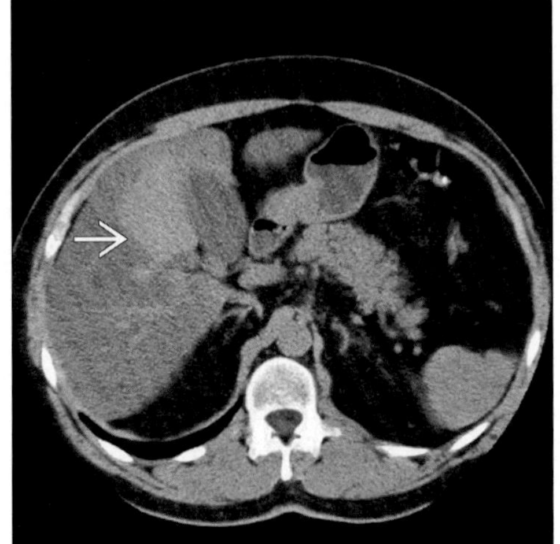

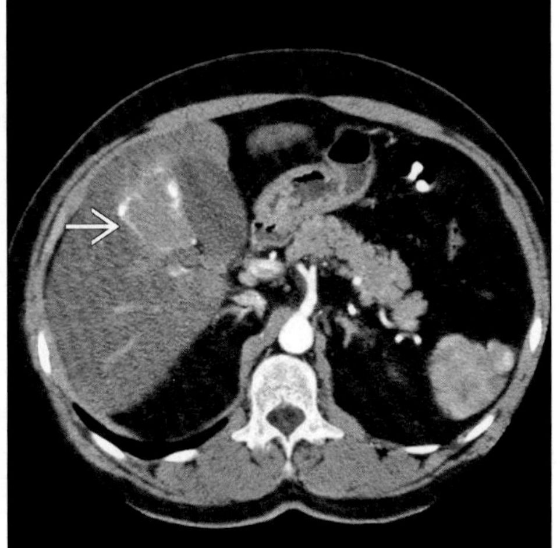

*(**Left**) Axial NECT shows a pericholecystic lesion which is hyperattenuated when compared with surrounding liver parenchyma ➡. This appearance is less usual. They are usually hypoattenuated. (**Right**) Axial CECT shows same lesion in early arterial phase of CT. Lesion shows a typical early peripheral rim enhancement of a cavernous hemangioma ➡. Enhancement pattern is discontinuous and slightly nodular, which is typical. (Courtesy G. Bonenti, MD).*

Typical

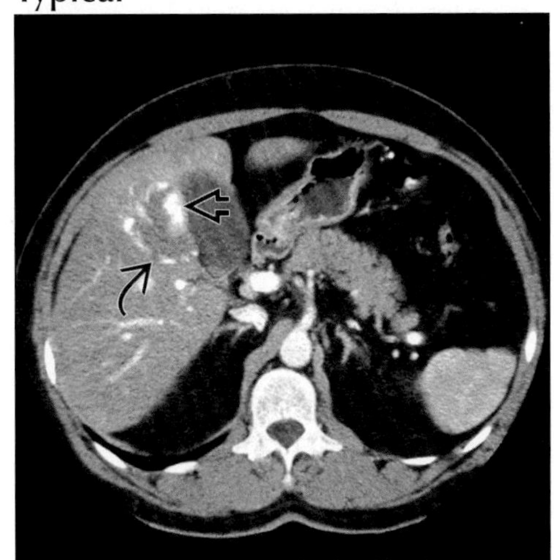

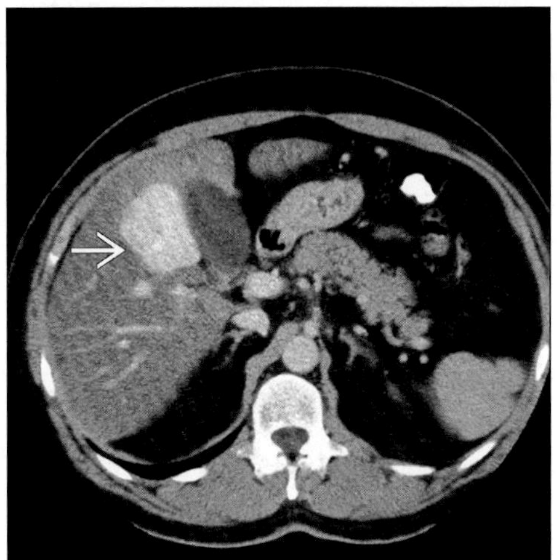

*(**Left**) Axial CECT shows, in a later phase of injection, gradual centripetal enhancement of same lesion. Enhancement is still discontinuous in the periphery ↗ and also nodular in its appearance ⇨ but with quite intense enhancement. (**Right**) Axial CECT shows with further delayed imaging, same lesion completely enhanced and hyperattenuating compared to surrounding parenchyma consistent with diagnosis of cavernous hemangioma ➡. (Courtesy G. Bonenti, MD).*

Typical

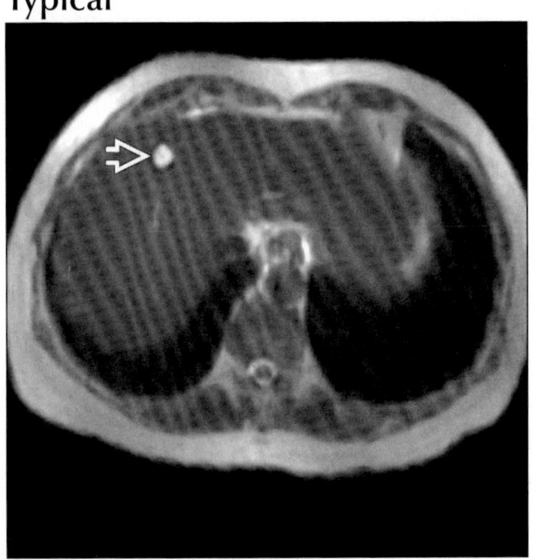

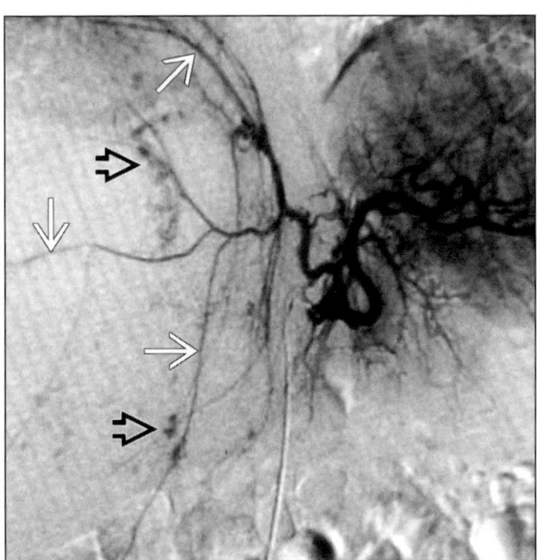

*(**Left**) Axial T2WI FS MR shows a very focal area of hyperintensity ➡. "Light-bulb" like signal which is very characteristic of a small hemangioma. (**Right**) DSA shows splaying of the vessels ➡ around a large, relatively hypovascular mass in the liver. The vessels appear stretched but are not enlarged. In this early phase of the injection there are the beginning of vascular enhancement "puddling" of contrast ⇨ characteristic of a cavernous hemangioma.*

HYPOTHENAR HAMMER SYNDROME

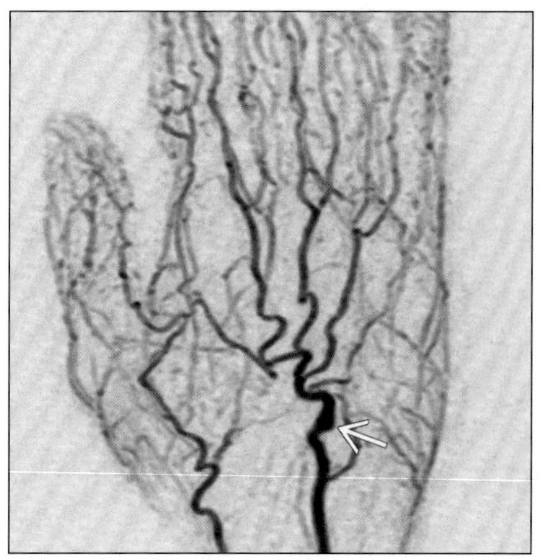

Coronal MRA shows a focal ulnar artery aneurysm ➡ at the level of the hook of the hamate bone. This has occurred from repetitive trauma and may progress to occlusion or be a source of emboli to the digital arteries.

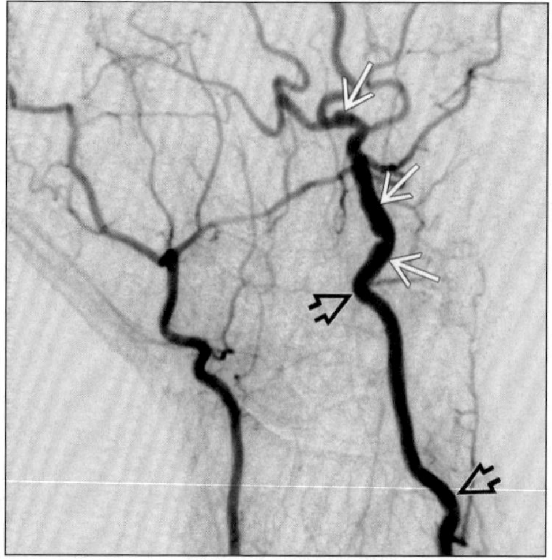

DSA shows "corkscrew" elongation ⇨ and ectasia ➡ of the ulnar artery, which is another characteristic appearance in this entity. Associated areas of alternating stenoses may sometimes also be present.

TERMINOLOGY

Abbreviations and Synonyms

- Hypothenar hammer syndrome (HHS)

Definitions

- Occlusion or focal aneurysm of ulnar artery at level of hamate bone due to repetitive trauma to hypothenar eminence, often with emboli to digital arteries

IMAGING FINDINGS

General Features

- Best diagnostic clue: Focal ulnar artery aneurysm, ectasia or occlusion at level of hamate bone associated with history of repetitive trauma to heel of hand
- Location: Distal ulnar artery at level of hook of hamate bone, where vessel courses through the Guyon canal and is relatively superficial and unprotected
- Morphology
  - Formation of an ulnar artery aneurysm, thrombotic occlusion of distal ulnar artery with extension to superficial palmar arch
    - Occasional occlusion of palmar arch
  - Occlusive emboli to digital arteries

MR Findings

- T1WI
  - Isointense to hyperintense signal in the arterial lumen indicative of thrombus within a partially patent or occluded ulnar artery aneurysm
  - May better demonstrate true size of a thrombus-filled aneurysm than MRA or DSA
- MRA: Findings similar to conventional angiography

Ultrasonographic Findings

- Color Doppler
  - Ulnar artery aneurysm, ectasia, endoluminal thickening or arterial occlusion
  - Digital artery or palmar arch occlusion

Angiographic Findings

- DSA
  - Focal ulnar artery aneurysm at hamate level, segmental palmar ulnar artery occlusion
    - May have characteristic "corkscrew" elongation, with alternating stenoses and ectasia

DDx: Hypothenar Hammer Syndrome

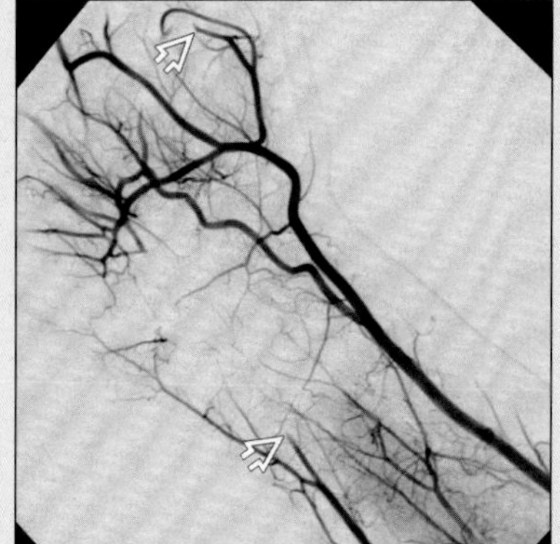

Scleroderma

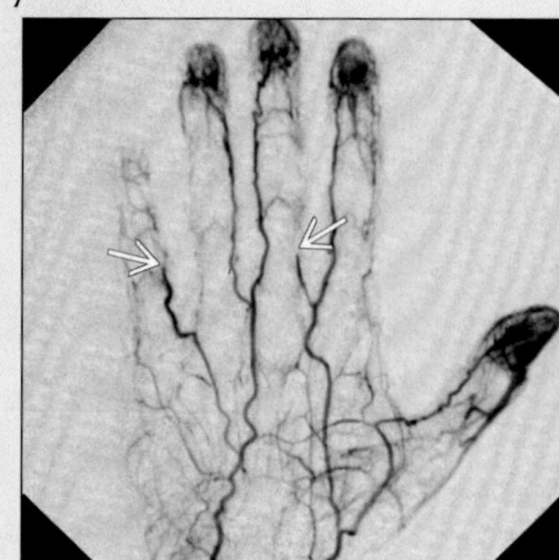

Raynaud Disease

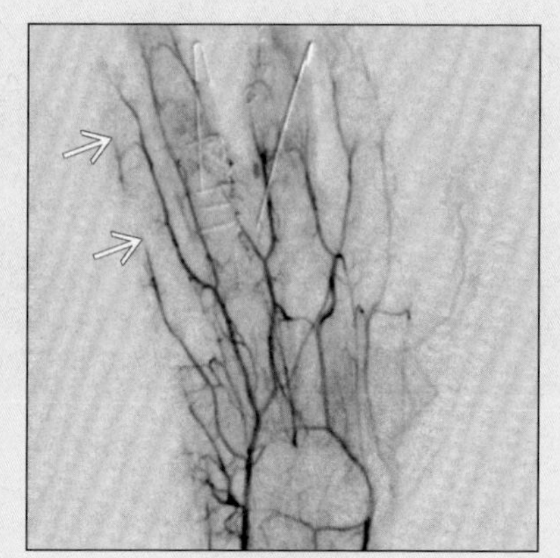

Acute Trauma

HYPOTHENAR HAMMER SYNDROME

Key Facts

Terminology
- Occlusion or focal aneurysm of ulnar artery at level of hamate bone due to repetitive trauma to hypothenar eminence, often with emboli to digital arteries

Imaging Findings
- Best imaging tool: DSA
- Focal ulnar artery aneurysm at hamate level, segmental palmar ulnar artery occlusion
  - May have characteristic "corkscrew" elongation, with alternating stenoses and ectasia
- Multiple digital artery occlusions in symptomatic hand

Top Differential Diagnoses
- Raynaud Syndrome
- Vasculitis
- Buerger Disease
- Atherosclerosis with Secondary Thrombosis
- Arterial Emboli from Cardiac Source

Pathology
- Histology compatible with fibromuscular dysplasia with superimposed trauma

Clinical Issues
- Conservative treatment for thrombotic form unless symptoms persist or progress, then surgical intervention required
- Surgical segmental excision of palmar ulnar artery and primary end-to-end anastomosis or vein grafting in aneurysmal form of syndrome
  - Two year surgical patency rate of 84%

  - Multiple digital artery occlusions in symptomatic hand
  - Palmar arches may also be occluded
  - Superficial palmar arch more often affected than deep palmar arch
  - May be difficult to distinguish incomplete superficial palmar arch from a segmental arterial occlusion
  - Similar changes in contralateral, asymptomatic (and less traumatized) hand

Imaging Recommendations
- Best imaging tool: DSA
- Protocol advice: Selective subclavian, axillary or brachial DSA with magnification views of wrist and digits

DIFFERENTIAL DIAGNOSIS

Raynaud Syndrome
- Raynaud disease
  - Primary vasospasm with no identifiable underlying cause
- Raynaud phenomenon
  - Vasospastic digital ischemia in response to cold
  - Vasospasm also associated with nicotine, stress and caffeine
  - Associated with connective tissue diseases and cutaneous disorders
    - Scleroderma
    - Systemic lupus erythematosus (SLE)
    - Rheumatoid arthritis
    - Polyarteritis nodosa

Vasculitis
- Often associated with connective tissue diseases and cutaneous disorders when vasculitis involves digits

Buerger Disease
- Type of vasculitis (thromboangiitis obliterans) in young, mostly male subjects strongly linked to smoking
- Affects small and medium-sized arteries and veins of extremities
- Absence of systemic signs and symptoms

Atherosclerosis with Secondary Thrombosis
- Systemic and somewhat symmetrical atherosclerotic disease typically
- Diabetes associated atherosclerosis has predilection for smaller caliber arteries as in hands and feet

Arterial Emboli from Cardiac Source
- Multiple emboli to multifocal sites usually evident
- Consider septic emboli with IV drug abuser

Thoracic Outlet Syndrome
- Can be complicated by local subclavian artery aneurysm with mural thrombus and distal embolization

Acute Trauma
- Acute mechanical trauma to hand and digits may result in arterial injury with resultant occlusions

PATHOLOGY

General Features
- Etiology
  - Frequent blunt trauma to the hypothenar eminence compresses unprotected segment of ulnar artery within Guyon canal against hook of hamate
    - Arterial vasospasm is triggered by repetitive trauma
  - Underlying intrinsic abnormality of ulnar artery (fibromuscular dysplasia) renders it susceptible to repetitive trauma
  - Chronic trauma to arterial media results in aneurysm formation
  - Injury to arterial intima often results in thrombotic occlusion
  - Aneurysm or intimal irregularity may become source of emboli to digits
- Epidemiology: Considered rare, but is frequently underdiagnosed

- Associated abnormalities: Striking incidence of bilateral arterial abnormalities in patients with unilateral symptoms

Gross Pathologic & Surgical Features

- Focal ectasia or aneurysm of ulnar artery, often with multifocal stenoses
- Thickened arterial wall
- Distal occlusion of ulnar artery, extending to palmar arch

Microscopic Features

- Histology compatible with fibromuscular dysplasia with superimposed trauma

CLINICAL ISSUES

Presentation

- Most common signs/symptoms
  - Occupational or avocational exposure to repetitive palmar trauma, e.g., carpenter, mechanic
  - Unilateral ischemic symptoms involving the 3rd through 5th digits
- Other signs/symptoms
  - May present with intolerance to cold as in Raynaud syndrome
  - Palmar pain or tender mass in the hypothenar eminence

Demographics

- Age: Usually found in working-aged individuals
- Gender: Male preponderance

Natural History & Prognosis

- Ulnar arterial wall damage may lead to aneurysm formation with or without vessel thrombosis
- Intimal irregularity or aneurysm may result in formation of occlusive microemboli to digits
- Ectatic or aneurysmal ulnar artery may compress sensory branch of ulnar nerve
- Often incorrectly diagnosed as it may be confused with Raynaud phenomenon
- May be diagnosed at a stage where irreversible consequences have already occurred
- Severe cases may progress to digital gangrene requiring amputation

Treatment

- Often diagnosed too late for recanalization to be a viable therapeutic option
- Conservative treatment for thrombotic form unless symptoms persist or progress, then surgical intervention required
  - Cessation of the offending activity and avoidance of exacerbating factors such as smoking
  - Consider anticoagulant and antiplatelet therapy
- Regional thrombolysis can be successful in fresh thrombotic occlusions
- Surgical segmental excision of palmar ulnar artery and primary end-to-end anastomosis or vein grafting in aneurysmal form of syndrome
  - Two year surgical patency rate of 84%
- No recurrences of ischemia in patients with patent bypass grafts

DIAGNOSTIC CHECKLIST

Consider

- Hypothenar hammer syndrome in differential diagnosis of a male patient presenting with unilateral digital ischemic symptoms
  - May mimic Raynaud syndrome, Buerger disease or arterial emboli from cardiac or unknown source

Image Interpretation Pearls

- If distal ulnar artery aneurysm, ectasia or luminal irregularity is identified, must further evaluate for digital emboli
  - Consider surgical intervention so as to avoid potentially irreversible complications

SELECTED REFERENCES

1. Aleksic M et al: Occupation-related vascular disorders of the upper extremity--two case reports. Angiology. 57(1):107-14, 2006
2. Blum AG et al: Pathologic conditions of the hypothenar eminence: evaluation with multidetector CT and MR imaging. Radiographics. 26(4):1021-44, 2006
3. Buda SJ et al: Brachial, radial, and ulnar arteries in the endovascular era: choice of intervention. Semin Vasc Surg. 18(4):191-5, 2005
4. Dethmers RS et al: Surgical management of hypothenar and thenar hammer syndromes: a retrospective study of 31 instances in 28 patients. J Hand Surg [Br]. 30(4):419-23, 2005
5. Drape JL et al: Vascular lesions of the hand. Eur J Radiol. 56(3):331-43, 2005
6. Stone JR: Intimal hyperplasia in the distal ulnar artery; Influence of gender and implications for the hypothenar hammer syndrome. Cardiovasc Pathol. 13(1):20-5, 2004
7. Coulier B et al: Colour duplex sonographic and multislice spiral CT angiographic diagnosis of ulnar artery aneurysm in hypothenar hammer syndrome. JBR-BTR. 86(4):211-4, 2003
8. Taylor LM Jr: Hypothenar hammer syndrome. J Vasc Surg. 37(3):697, 2003
9. Lorelli DR et al: Hypothenar hammer syndrome: an uncommon and correctable cause of digital ischemia. J Cardiovasc Surg (Torino). 43(1):83-5, 2002
10. Winterer JT et al: Diagnosis of the hypothenar hammer syndrome by high-resolution contrast-enhanced MR angiography. Eur Radiol. 12(10):2457-62, 2002
11. Velling TE et al: Sonographic diagnosis of ulnar artery aneurysm in hypothenar hammer syndrome: report of 2 cases. J Ultrasound Med. 20(8):921-4, 2001
12. Ferris BL et al: Hypothenar hammer syndrome: proposed etiology. J Vasc Surg. 31(1 Pt 1):104-13, 2000
13. Liskutin J et al: Hypothenar hammer syndrome. Eur Radiol. 10(3):542, 2000
14. Dean Okereke C et al: Hypothenar hammer syndrome diagnosed by ultrasound. Injury. 30(6):448-9, 1999
15. Bakhach J et al: Hypothenar hammer syndrome: management of distal embolization by intra-arterial fibrinolytics. Chir Main. 17(3):215-20, 1998

IMAGE GALLERY

Typical

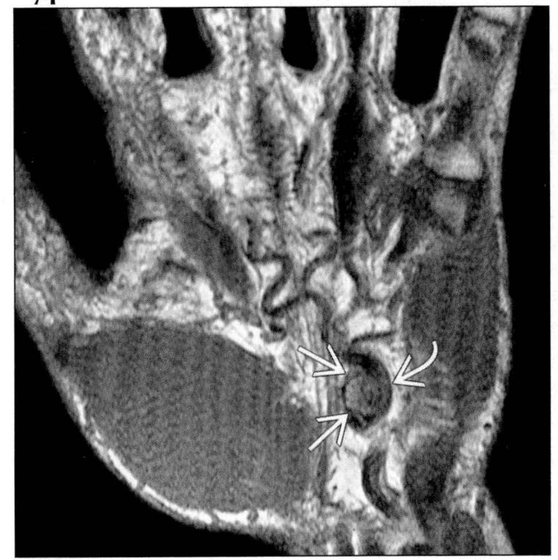

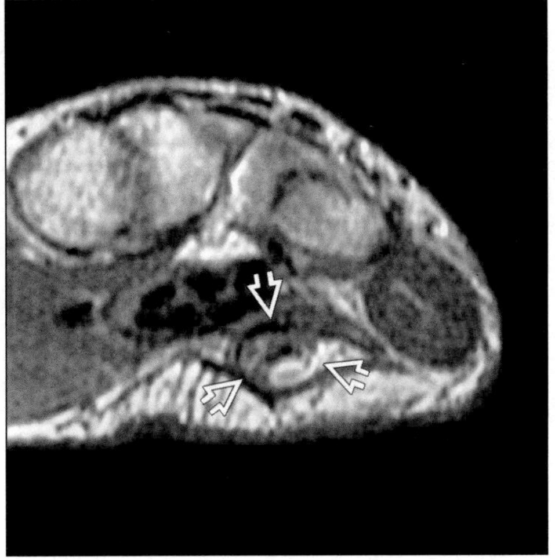

(Left) Coronal T1WI MR shows a large focal ulnar artery aneurysm ➢ at the level of the hook of the hamate bone. Note the thrombus ➔ within the aneurysm. This serves as a potential source for emboli to the digital arteries. *(Right)* Axial T1WI MR (same patient as previous image) shows the ulnar artery aneurysm ➔ within the Guyon canal. Note the superficial location of the aneurysm, where the ulnar artery is susceptible to repetitive trauma.

Typical

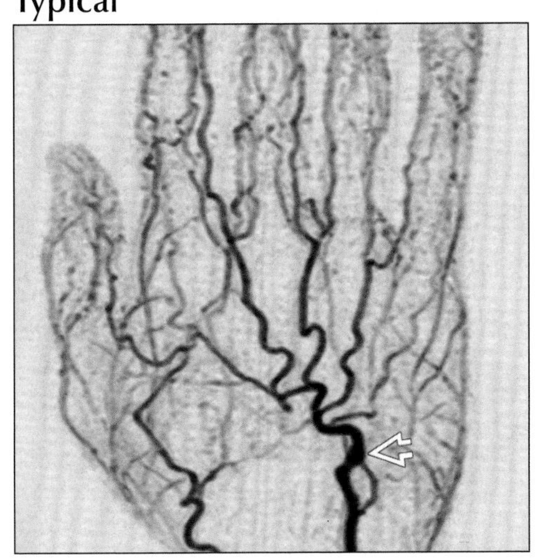

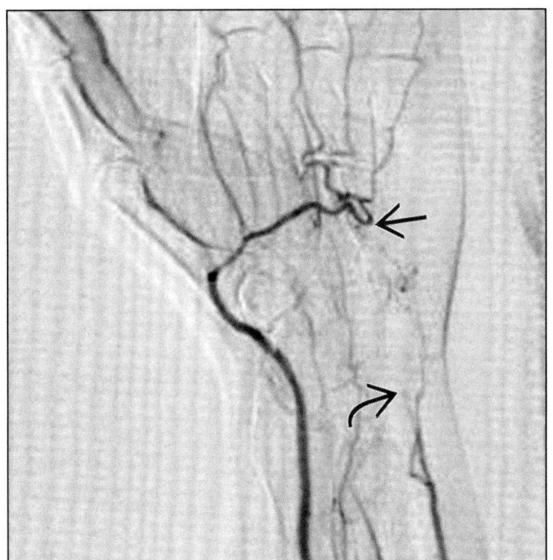

(Left) Coronal MRA (same patient as previous image) shows ulnar artery aneurysm ➔ but fails to demonstrate actual aneurysm size, as the thrombus-filled portion seen on T1WI is not seen on MRA. DSA would also underestimate the aneurysm size. *(Right)* DSA in a different patient shows ulnar artery occlusion ➢ beginning at hamate level & extending to the palmar arch ➔, which is characteristic of the thrombotic form of hypothenar hammer syndrome.

Typical

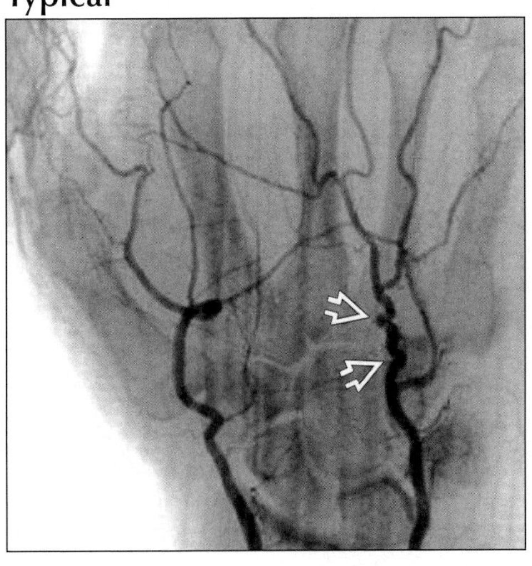

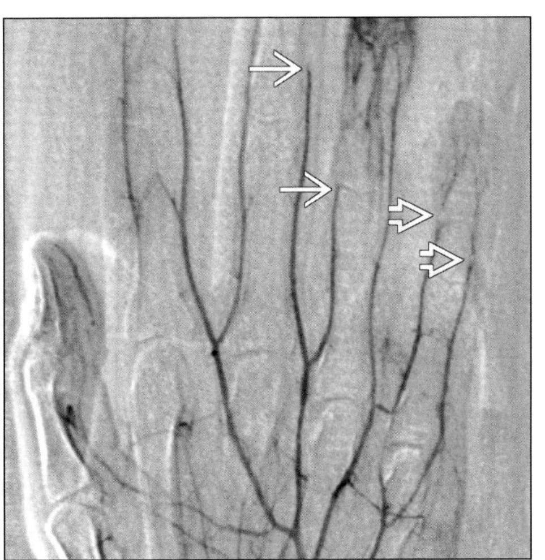

(Left) DSA shows "corkscrew" appearance to the ulnar artery ➔, representing alternating stenoses and ectasia. This may eventually cause ulnar artery thrombosis, or distal emboli to the digital arteries. *(Right)* DSA shows filling defects ➔ and abrupt occlusions ➔ in the proper digital arteries of the fingers. These findings are typical of distal embolization, a complication that can occur with the aneurysmal form of hypothenar hammer syndrome.

SUBCLAVIAN VEIN THROMBOSIS

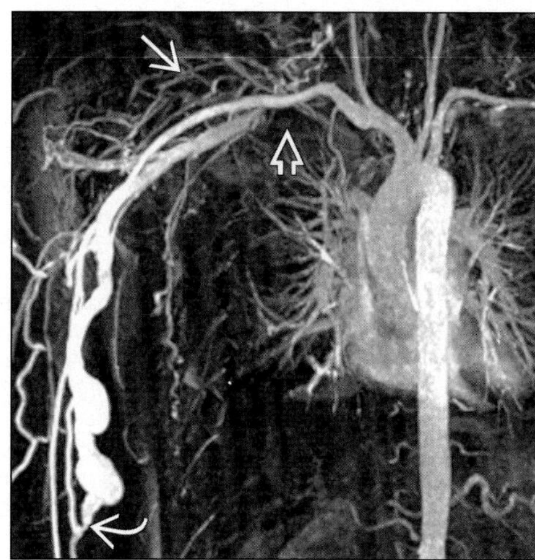

Coronal thin MIP MRA in a patient with a right arm AV fistula ➔ and a swollen right upper extremity, shows complete occlusion of the proximal subclavian vein ➔ and extensive collaterals ➔.

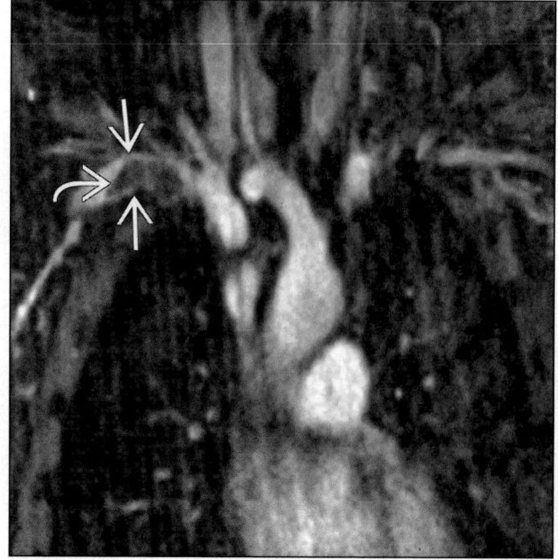

Coronal post-contrast T1 GRE (same patient) shows a dilatated right subclavian vein with a central filling defect ➔ consistent with subclavian vein thrombosis. This appearance ➔ is the "tram track" sign.

TERMINOLOGY

Abbreviations and Synonyms

- Subclavian thrombophlebitis, subclavian thrombosis, upper extremity deep vein thrombosis (DVT)

Definitions

- Occlusive or partially occlusive thrombus formation in subclavian vein, with collateralization

IMAGING FINDINGS

General Features

- Best diagnostic clue: Subclavian vein occlusion with extensive collaterals; intraluminal thrombus
- Location: Right subclavian vein involved in 2/3 cases

Radiographic Findings

- Radiography: Mass or cervical rib at thoracic outlet

CT Findings

- CECT and CT venography
  - Thrombus avascular, seen as very low density filling defect
    - Contrast flows around periphery of thrombus and outlines as "tram-track" sign on coronal and sagittal images; "polo mint" sign on axial images
  - Dilated vein, collaterals
  - Post-thrombotic changes in chronic DVT of severe venous narrowing with barely visible lumen (stricture), eccentric linear filling defect, occasional calcification
  - Tumor thrombus may show partial enhancement
  - May show surrounding structures (e.g., cervical rib, mass lesion)

MR Findings

- T1WI: Acute thrombus may appear as high signal
- T2WI: Bright blood SSFP shows thrombus as low signal
- MRV
  - TR-MRA mimics contrast venogram; shows absent contrast opacification and collateral flow pattern
    - Intraluminal thrombus difficult to appreciate
  - CE MRA: Acute - dark signal thrombus within distended subclavian vein
  - CE MRA: Chronic - vein may be markedly narrowed, strictured or occluded
    - Lack of contrast opacification of vein

DDx: Subclavian Vein Thrombosis

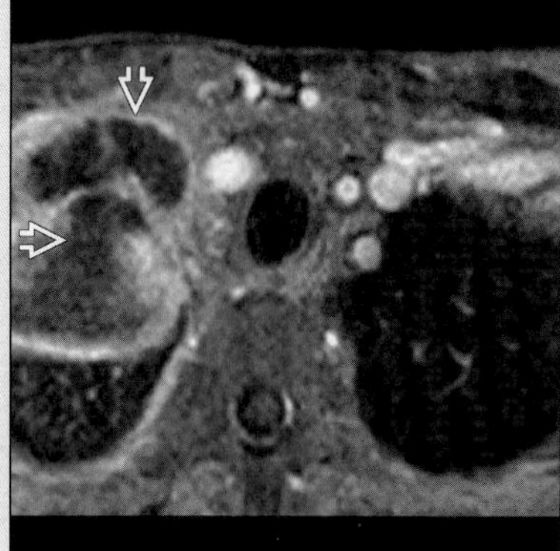

Tumor Thrombus

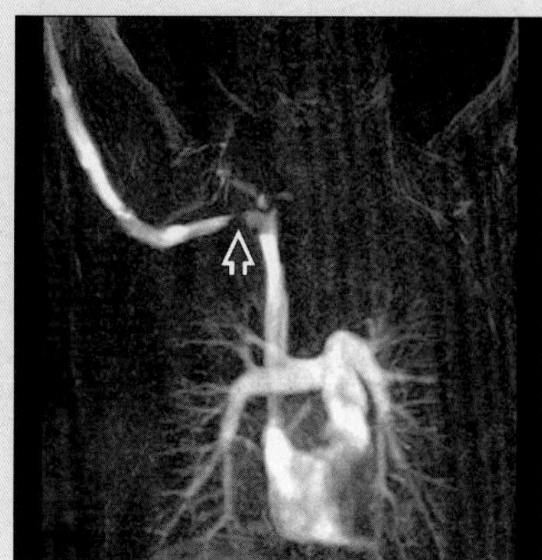

Thoracic Outlet Syndrome

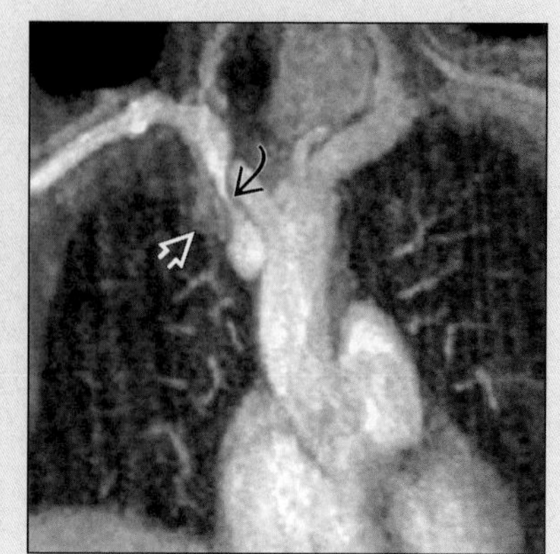

Extrinsic Compression by Tumor

SUBCLAVIAN VEIN THROMBOSIS

Key Facts

Imaging Findings

- Intraluminal thrombus, dilated vein, occlusion, collaterals; thrombus is avascular
- CT/MRV: Thrombus very low density/signal
- Acute thrombus: Near occlusive central filling defect
  - Acute thrombus may be high signal on T1WI
- Chronic DVT: Narrowed, strictured or occluded vein, eccentric non-occlusive thrombus, calcification
  - TR-MRA shows dynamic absent contrast opacification and collateral pathways
  - Post-contrast T1WI shows low signal hypovascular thrombus and inflammation
- US: Echogenic thrombus or non-compressible vein
  - Dilated collateral may be mistaken for normal vein
  - Limited to distal subclavian vein
- Venography/DSA remains "gold standard"

Top Differential Diagnoses

- Extrinsic Venous Compression
- Thoracic Outlet Syndrome
- Tumor Thrombus (Partial Internal Enhancement)

Clinical Issues

- Clinical presentation of upper extremity nonpitting edema
- Catheter-related thrombosis more common than other etiologies
- Treatment options: Anticoagulation, fibrinolysis, endovascular intervention, surgery

Diagnostic Checklist

- Consider effort thrombosis in young patient presenting with sudden upper extremity swelling following physical activity

---

    - Eccentric, linear, wall-adherent, filling defect (thrombus, organized fibrotic plaque)
    - Web-like stenosis
    - Extensive dilated tortuous collaterals: Chest wall, paravertebral, cervical and axillary
  - Post-contrast T1 2D GRE or 3D GRE (VIBE) shows low signal hypovascular thrombus; high signal contrast around thrombus
    - Better demonstrate thrombus and vessel wall
    - Shows perivascular inflammatory soft tissue thickening and enhancement
    - Tumor thrombus may enhance internally

Ultrasonographic Findings

- Visible thrombus or non-compressibility of vein diagnostic of vein thrombosis
- Compressibility of suspected vein excludes thrombosis
  - Dilated collateral may be mistaken for normal vein
- Abnormal flow pattern on Duplex scan only suggests thrombosis
  - With Valsalva maneuver, vein size normally increases with reduced flow
  - With sniff test, vein size normally decreases with increased flow
  - Need further imaging to confirm thrombosis, stenosis, or obstruction
- Acute
  - Vein markedly distended
  - Hypo/isoechoic thrombus
- Subacute
  - Increased thrombus echogenicity/heterogeneity
  - Shrinkage of thrombus, decreased vein size
- Chronic stage
  - Possible return to normal appearance
  - Scarred veins, variable vein caliber, focal or diffuse wall thickening, plaque-like scars, webs

Angiographic Findings

- Conventional
  - Contrast venography/DSA not feasible in 20% due to edematous arm
    - Thrombus seen as central filling defect; peripheral luminal contrast flow ("tram track")
    - Venous occlusion with extensive collaterals
    - Pericatheter thrombus/fibrin
    - Image in neutral and stress (arm abduction) positions
    - Pitfall: Absent opacification of normal cephalic vein

Imaging Recommendations

- Best imaging tool: Contrast venography/DSA remains "gold standard" but not as versatile as MR
- Protocol advice
  - Duplex ultrasound: First line of imaging but limited to distal subclavian vein and arm veins
  - MR: Pre & post-contrast, fat-saturated T1 GRE
  - MRV: Double dose gadolinium, 2-3 passes, 40 sec delay between 2nd and 3rd pass, coronal acquisition
  - TR-MRA: Less than 5 cc of contrast, temporal resolution 1.2 sec, ipsilateral injection
  - Neutral & stress positions in thoracic outlet syndrome
  - CT venography: 120-140 mL of contrast injected from unaffected site
    - Arterial phase (ROI-pulmonary artery) and 2 min delayed venous phase from C3 to heart or simultaneous bilateral antecubital injections
  - Contrast venography: 20 mL contrast injected from ipsilateral antecubital vein access
    - Separate injection to see SVC (rarely bilateral injections)
    - Dynamic images in neutral and stress positions for thoracic outlet syndrome

DIFFERENTIAL DIAGNOSIS

Extrinsic Venous Compression

- Thrombosis (due to stasis) may present
- Causes: Lymphadenopathy, Pancoast lung cancer, scarring (e.g., post radiation)
- MR is better modality to assess

Thoracic Outlet Syndrome (TOS)

- Vein pinched by 1st rib, clavicle & scalene muscles

SUBCLAVIAN VEIN THROMBOSIS

- Intermittent arm pain/swelling
- Possible arterial ischemia & brachial plexus neuropathy
- May be associated with subclavian vein thrombosis

Tumor Thrombus

- Local extension of malignant tumor into vein
- Dilated vein with filling defect
- Partial enhancement of thrombus on delayed scan

PATHOLOGY

General Features

- Etiology
  - Usually underlying cause; often multifactorial
  - Primary subclavian vein thrombosis, rare
    - Causes: Effort induced, traumatic, thoracic outlet abnormality or unknown
    - No underlying hypercoagulable state
    - Repeated venous microtrauma and stasis predisposes to thrombosis
    - Majority (> 75%) of patients present within 24 hrs after strenuous effort
    - Cervical rib and other variants can contribute to thoracic outlet obstruction and effort thrombosis
    - Medical urgency to prevent debilitation from permanent subclavian occlusion
  - Secondary subclavian vein thrombosis, common
    - Systemic hypercoagulability from dehydration, surgery, heart failure, nephrotic syndrome
    - Hypercoagulability also from oral contraceptives, immobility, pregnancy, protein C, S, and antithrombin deficiencies, cancer
    - Intimal injury from IV drug abuse (e.g., heroin, cocaine) pacemaker wires
    - 12-30% incidence of central venous catheter related thrombosis; larger polyvinyl catheters more thrombogenic than small silicone catheters
    - Obstruction from tumor, lymphadenopathy, scar
    - Insidious onset of symptoms
- Epidemiology
  - 1° subclavian vein thrombosis: Young adult male
  - 2° subclavian vein thrombosis: M = F, older patients
- Associated abnormalities
  - Often associated with axillary vein thrombosis
    - Palpable tender axillary "cord"
  - Occasional thoracic outlet abnormality

CLINICAL ISSUES

Presentation

- Most common signs/symptoms: Upper extremity swelling (nonpitting edema)
- Other signs/symptoms
  - Arm pain - dull ache to severe discomfort
  - Visible collaterals in shoulder and thorax

Natural History & Prognosis

- Post thrombotic syndrome (4-22%) - venous hypertension due to outflow obstruction
  - After effort thrombosis, 40-70% incidence of venous insufficiency
- Without treatment, may fail to recanalize, resulting in chronic occlusion
  - Organized fibrotic tissue eventually replaces vein
  - Extensive collaterals provide central venous return

Treatment

- Standard anticoagulation therapy
  - Heparin followed by warfarin
- Fibrinolysis (urokinase or r-tPA) has better chance of recanalization through lysis of thrombi; risk of bleeding: Major 0-4%, minor 0-40%
  - Young patients with effort thrombosis, within 1 week of thrombus formation, < 2 cm thrombus, patients on dialysis or TPN
  - Time to achieve total lysis may be up to 72 hrs
- Interventional: Mechanical thrombectomy yields rapid debulking and restoration of vein patency
  - Chronic thrombus > 1 week may not benefit
  - Angioplasty and stent - for catheter related stenosis
- Surgery: First rib, clavicle and anterior scalene resections (thoracic outlet or Paget-Schroetter syndromes)
  - Vein patch angioplasty: Chronic stenosis or occlusion > 2 cm; failed fibrinolytics in 1° subclavian vein thrombosis

DIAGNOSTIC CHECKLIST

Consider

- Effort thrombosis in young patient with sudden upper extremity swelling following physical activity
- Intermittent nonthrombotic subclavian vein obstruction or lymphedema if patient has
  - Normal-sized patent vein in neutral position and absent thrombus

Image Interpretation Pearls

- Acute thrombus near occlusive; chronic nonocclusive and eccentric
- Always look for associated PE

SELECTED REFERENCES

1. Chin EE et al: Sonographic evaluation of upper extremity deep venous thrombosis. J Ultrasound Med. 24(6):829-38; quiz 839-40, 2005
2. Baarslag HJ et al: Diagnosis and management of deep vein thrombosis of the upper extremity: a review. Eur Radiol. 14(7):1263-74, 2004
3. Sharafuddin MJ et al: Endovascular management of venous thrombotic diseases of the upper torso and extremities. J Vasc Interv Radiol. 13(10):975-90, 2002
4. Thornton MJ et al: A three-dimensional gadolinium-enhanced MR venography technique for imaging central veins. AJR Am J Roentgenol. 173(4):999-1003, 1999
5. Haire WD et al: Limitations of magnetic resonance imaging and ultrasound-directed (duplex) scanning in the diagnosis of subclavian vein thrombosis. J Vasc Surg. 13(3):391-7, 1991

SUBCLAVIAN VEIN THROMBOSIS

IMAGE GALLERY

Typical

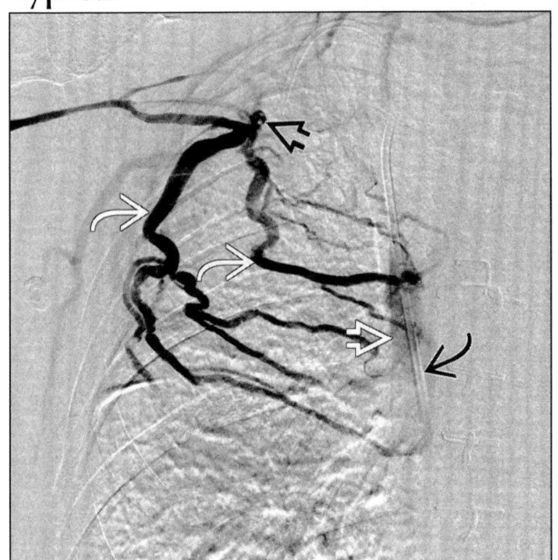

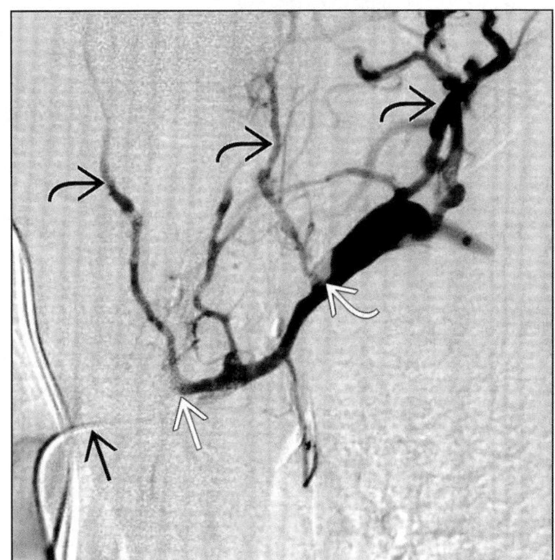

(Left) *Digital subtraction venogram shows right subclavian vein occlusion. Chest wall collateral veins provide blood return to the SVC. A right internal jugular catheter is seen.* ***(Right)*** *Digital subtraction venogram shows a partially occlusive thrombus in the left subclavian vein extending into and occluding the left brachiocephalic vein. A pacemaker wire is the etiology of the occlusion. Extensive collateral veins are present.*

Typical

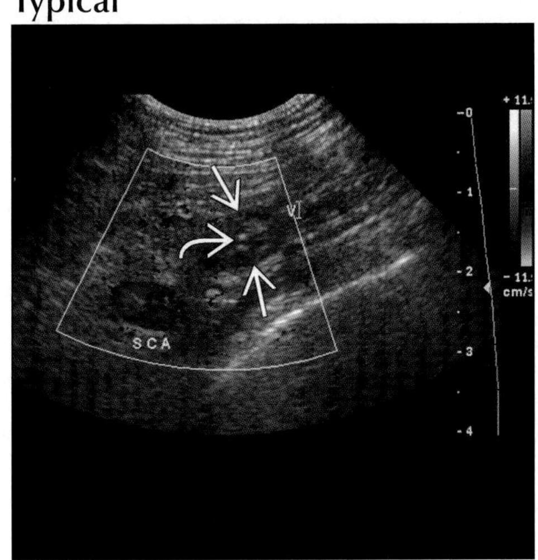

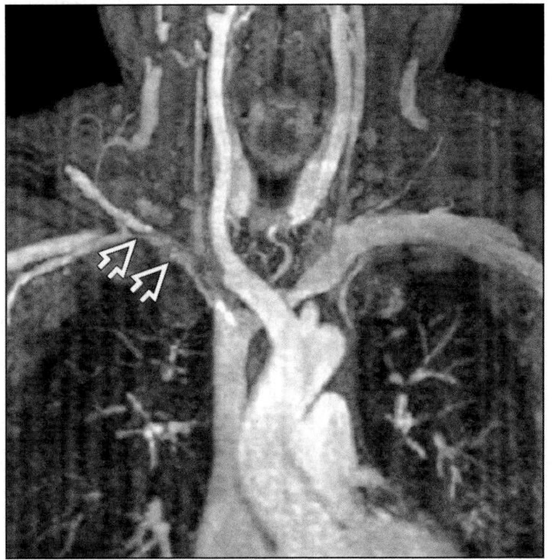

(Left) *Axial color Doppler ultrasound in a patient with left arm edema shows echogenic thrombus and absent flow in the dilated and noncompressible subclavian vein. Two small hyperechoic foci represent a PICC line.* ***(Right)*** *Coronal MRV shows decreased contrast opacification and marked narrowing of the proximal right subclavian and brachiocephalic veins, represent post-thrombotic stricture due to prior central line placements.*

Typical

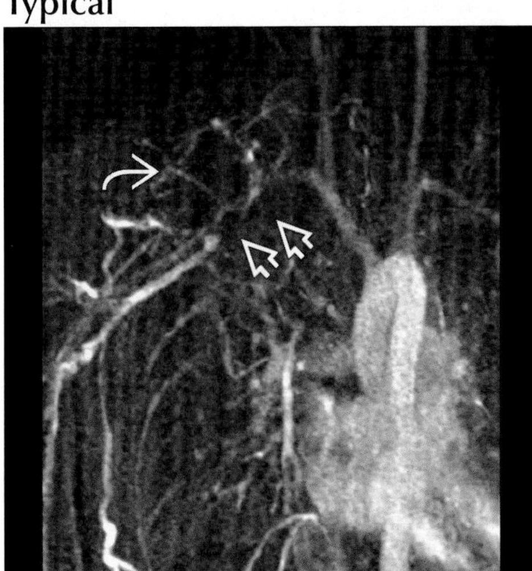

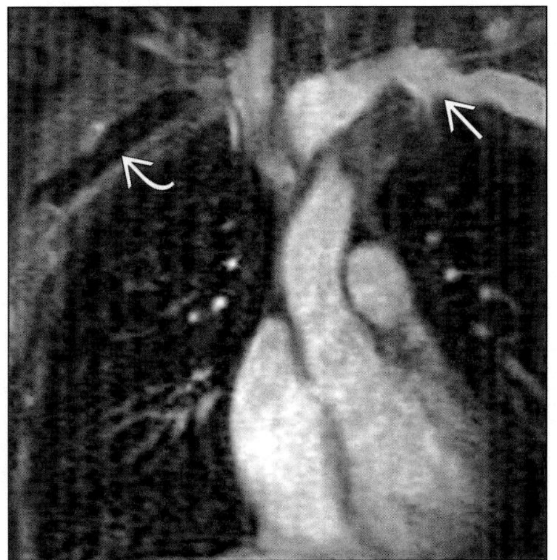

(Left) *Coronal TE-MRA during 4 cc of contrast injection via the right antecubital vein shows absent contrast filling of the right subclavian vein with dynamic collateral flow, consistent with complete subclavian vein occlusion.* ***(Right)*** *Coronal CE MRV (same patient) shows a large low signal filling defect in the right subclavian and axillary veins, representing an occlusive thrombus and consistent with acute DVT. The left subclavian vein is normal.*

THORACIC OUTLET SYNDROME, VENOUS

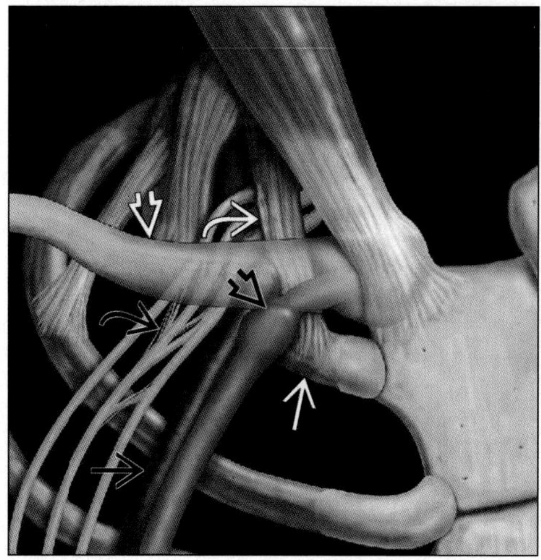

Graphic shows the subclavian vein crossing over anterior scalene muscle and being compressed between the 1st rib and the clavicle. The subclavian artery and brachial plexus.

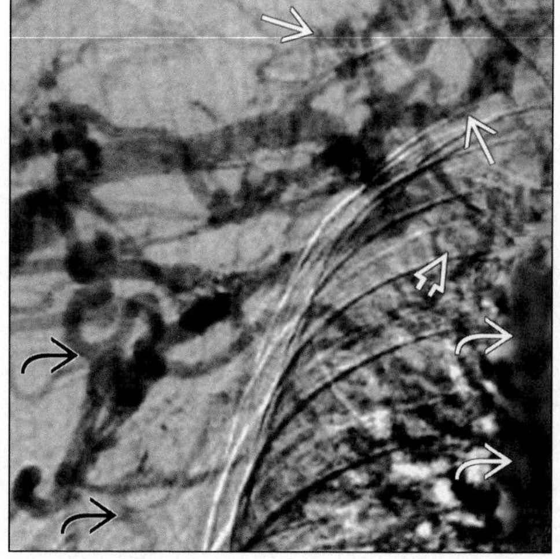

DSA upper extremity venogram shows subclavian vein occlusion at junction of clavicle and 1st rib, with extensive neck and chest wall collateral veins providing venous return to the patent SVC.

TERMINOLOGY

Abbreviations and Synonyms

- Venous or vascular thoracic outlet syndrome
- Paget-von Schroetter syndrome (effort thrombosis)
- Scalenus anticus syndrome
- Costo-clavicular syndrome

Definitions

- Musculoskeletal compression of axillary or subclavian vein as it crosses thoracic outlet
- Thoracic outlet boundaries
  - Posterior boundary: First thoracic vertebra
  - Lateral boundary: First rib and costal cartilage
  - Anterior boundary: Superior border of manubrium
- Clinically "thoracic outlet" refers to exit site of neurovascular bundle going to upper extremity
  - Also "thoracic inlet" or "superior thoracic aperture"

IMAGING FINDINGS

General Features

- Best diagnostic clue
  - Venographic narrowing of axillary and/or subclavian vein with stress/provocative maneuvers
  - Collateral veins develop with significant narrowing or thrombosis
- Location
  - Subclavian vein at junction of first rib and clavicle
  - Dominant upper extremity involved in 70% of cases
    - < 4% bilateral and requiring intervention

Radiographic Findings

- Radiography
  - Supernumerary cervical rib
    - Arises from C7, but also from C6 or rarely C5
  - Prominent C7 transverse process or straight 1st rib
  - Clavicular deformity or previous trauma

CT Findings

- NECT
  - Abnormal insertion of anterior scalene muscle
  - Cervical rib or straight first rib
  - Prior clavicle fracture; prominent callous
  - Lymphadenopathy or supraclavicular mass
- CECT
  - Demonstrates site of venous compression
    - Shows osseous and soft tissue relationships to vein

DDx: Venous Thoracic Outlet Syndrome

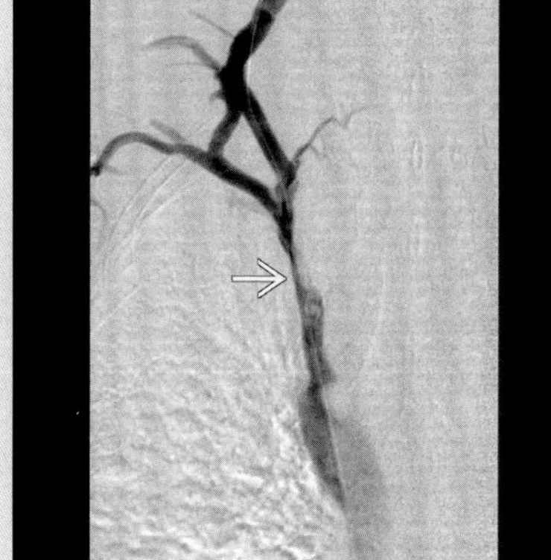

Superior Vena Cava Syndrome

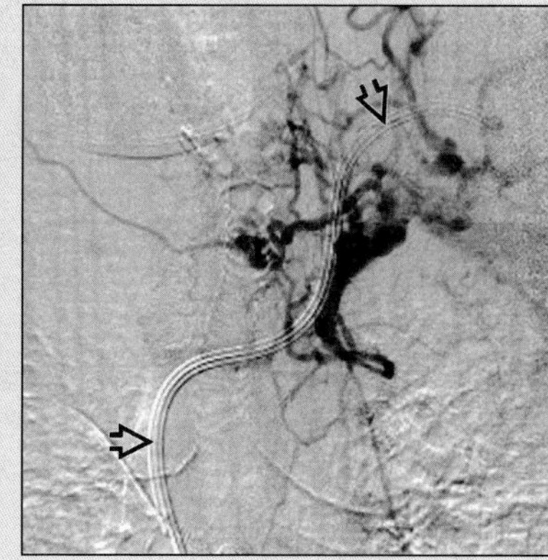

Central Venous Catheters

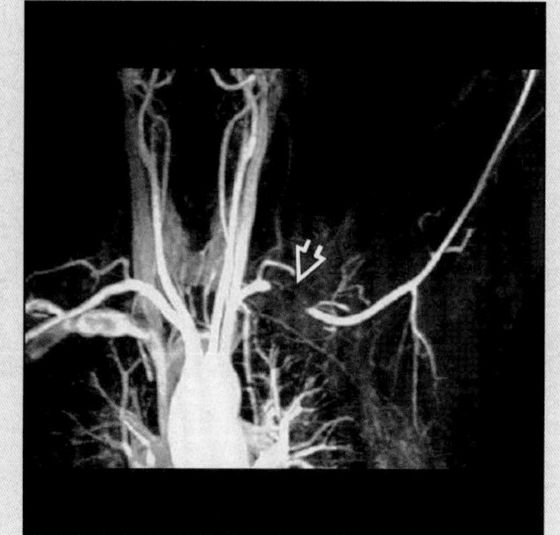

Arterial Thoracic Outlet Syndrome

THORACIC OUTLET SYNDROME, VENOUS

Key Facts

Terminology

- Paget-von Schroetter syndrome, venous or vascular thoracic outlet syndrome, effort thrombosis, scalenus anticus syndrome
- Musculoskeletal compression of axillary or subclavian vein as it crosses thoracic outlet

Imaging Findings

- Venographic narrowing of axillary and/or subclavian vein with stress/provocative maneuvers
- Collateral veins develop with significant narrowing and/or thrombosis
- Involves subclavian vein at junction of first rib and clavicle
- Venography used for anatomic evaluation and treatment planning
- If vein appears normal with arm in neutral position, perform provocative maneuvers
- MR and CT demonstrate structures causing venous compression

Clinical Issues

- Medical therapy is systemic anticoagulation
- Catheter directed or mechanical thrombolysis in acute occlusion, then anti-coagulation
- Surgical decompression necessary for correction of anatomic abnormality

Diagnostic Checklist

- Subclavian vein occlusion or stenosis at junction of 1st rib and clavicle virtually pathognomonic
- Thoracic outlet syndrome can involve vein, artery or nerve

        - Requires venous stress views, 3D reconstruction
    - Cervical and chest wall collaterals may be present
        - Highly concentrated contrast in these veins suggests occlusion or high grade stenosis

MR Findings

- T1WI: Demonstrates soft tissue structures causing venous compression
- MRV
    - Requires stress views of subclavian vein
    - Demonstrates occlusion, stenosis or obstruction
        - Venous collaterals bypassing venous abnormality

Ultrasonographic Findings

- Grayscale Ultrasound
    - Non-invasive, available and easy to perform
    - Evaluates visible axillary, subclavian, brachiocephalic and internal jugular vein segments
        - Central veins difficult to evaluate
    - Echogenic intraluminal filling defect
    - Multiple cervical and upper trunk collateral veins
    - Venous occlusion or stenosis
- Color Doppler
    - Absent or decreased axillary/subclavian vein flow
        - Absent respiratory variation or atrial pulsations with stress views
    - Asymmetric examination of upper extremity veins

Angiographic Findings

- Venography evaluates anatomy, plans treatment
- Antecubital or brachial vein access for venogram
    - Evaluate veins from access site to right atrium
- Filling defect in vein represents thrombus
    - Thrombus may be occlusive or non-occlusive
- Short/long segment stenosis or occlusion at costoclavicular junction
    - Stenosis may be visible only after thrombolysis
- Multiple cervical and chest wall collaterals
- If normal vein with arm in neutral position, perform provocative maneuvers
    - Upper extremity abduction rotates clavicle toward first rib
    - Adson maneuver tests compression by anterior scalene muscle: Deep inspiration, neck extended and rotated to contralateral side
    - Costoclavicular maneuver tests compression between 1st rib and clavicle: Shoulders pulled posteriorly and inferiorly
    - Hyperabduction maneuver tests compression between humeral head and pectoralis minor: Arm abducted from neutral to 180° above head
    - Recreate position that reproduces symptoms
    - Low sensitivity (72%) and specificity (53%) for provocative maneuvers
    - Highest positive predictive value with Adson (85%) and hyperabduction (92%) maneuvers
- Superior vena cava widely patent

Imaging Recommendations

- Best imaging tool
    - CECT with multiplanar reformations
        - Contrast-filled veins readily seen
        - Adjacent osseus and soft tissue structures well seen
- Protocol advice: Perform provocative maneuvers described above with all imaging

DIFFERENTIAL DIAGNOSIS

Arterial Thoracic Outlet Syndrome

- Normal subclavian venography, no venous collaterals
- Multiple arterial collaterals
- Arterial stenoses, occlusions, aneurysms
    - May have distal embolization from aneurysms

Neurological Thoracic Outlet Syndrome

- Normal subclavian arteriography and venography

Superior Vena Cava Syndrome

- SVC stenosis or occlusion
- Azygos vein and multiple collaterals opacified

Previous Central Line or Pacemaker

- Long segment, smooth narrowing; venous occlusion
- Same side as central line or pacemaker

THORACIC OUTLET SYNDROME, VENOUS

Malignant Encasement of Vein

- Not always associated with costoclavicular junction
- Extrinsic lesion on cross-sectional imaging

Trauma

- Exuberant bony callus at site of venous abnormality

PATHOLOGY

General Features

- General path comments
  - Anatomy
    - Subclavian vein compression as it passes anteriorly between clavicle and subclavius muscle and first rib and anterior scalene muscle posteriorly
    - Compression by cervical rib
  - Least common variant of thoracic outlet syndrome
- Etiology
  - Congenital predisposition aggravated by hypertrophy of subclavius and anterior scalene muscles or their insertions
    - Injury with repetitive activities involving arm elevation
  - Costal or clavicular abnormality
  - Hypercoagulable states predispose to thrombosis
  - Postural effects altering normal relationship between 1st rib and adjacent soft tissues
  - Slow flow or stasis from chronic intimal injury
- Epidemiology
  - 10/100,000 people/year
  - 2nd most common cause of axillary and subclavian vein thrombosis

Gross Pathologic & Surgical Features

- Organized, fibrotic thrombus with scarred vein wall

CLINICAL ISSUES

Presentation

- Most common signs/symptoms
  - Upper extremity pain, edema, cyanosis
  - Strenuous or repetitive upper extremity activity prior to sudden onset of symptoms
- Other signs/symptoms
  - Prominent superficial veins over arm and chest wall
  - Rapid extremity fatigue, particularly after exercise
  - Cool upper extremity
  - In extremely rare cases, extensive thrombus can cause phlegmasia cerulea dolens
    - Venous outflow impaired and arterial inflow decreased causing arterial insufficiency
- Clinical Profile
  - Young, highly functional, physically active
  - > 80% are asymptomatic before 1° presentation

Demographics

- Age: 20-50 years; average = 31 years
- Gender: Male > female

Natural History & Prognosis

- May progress to thrombosis
- Symptoms persist, made worse with activity
- Reported 3 year post-surgical patency rate: 93%

Treatment

- Medical therapy: Systemic anticoagulation
  - Limits thrombus propagation
  - Allows collateral formation
  - Recanalization of thrombosis uncommon
  - Thrombus organizes with vein wall scarring
- Endovascular therapy: Venography for diagnosis
  - Catheter-directed thrombolysis and/or mechanical thrombectomy in acute occlusion, then anti-coagulation
  - If extrinsic compression persists, surgical decompression performed
  - If narrowing persists post surgical decompression, consider angioplasty and/or stenting
  - Patient with acute thrombosis and no prior symptoms most likely to respond
  - Early treatment of acute thrombosis ↓ intimal injury
  - Stenting contraindicated until after surgery
    - Stent cannot withstand osseous compression
    - Increased risk of re-thrombosis with stent deformity
    - Pre-surgical stenting can affect future surgeries
  - If thrombolysis unsuccessful, consider surgical decompression to improve space for collaterals and decrease nerve and arterial involvement
  - Angioplasty without surgical decompression fails due to recurrent injury and thrombosis
    - May prolong patency in interim between thrombolysis and surgery
- Surgical therapy: Correction of anatomic abnormality
  - First rib resection, scalenectomy, or combination
    - Similar long term outcomes
  - Perform decompression after initial successful thrombolysis or after period of anti-coagulation
- Conservative therapy can be considered in absence of occlusion or significant stenosis
  - Consider early surgical intervention if symptoms persist with conservative management

DIAGNOSTIC CHECKLIST

Consider

- Thoracic outlet syndrome involves vein, artery or nerve
- History and physical with relevant tests aids diagnosis

Image Interpretation Pearls

- Subclavian vein occlusion/stenosis at junction of 1st rib and clavicle virtually pathognomonic

SELECTED REFERENCES

1. Molina JE et al: Paget-Schroetter syndrome treated with thrombolytics and immediate surgery. J Vasc Surg. 45(2):328-34, 2007
2. Kommareddy A et al: Upper extremity deep venous thrombosis. Semin Thromb Hemost. 28(1):89-99, 2002
3. Sharafuddin MJ et al: Endovascular management of venous thrombotic diseases of the upper torso and extremities. J Vasc Interv Radiol. 13(10):975-90, 2002

THORACIC OUTLET SYNDROME, VENOUS

IMAGE GALLERY

Typical

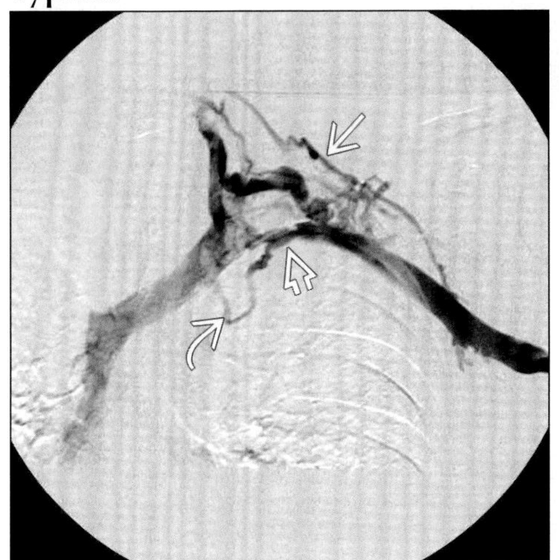

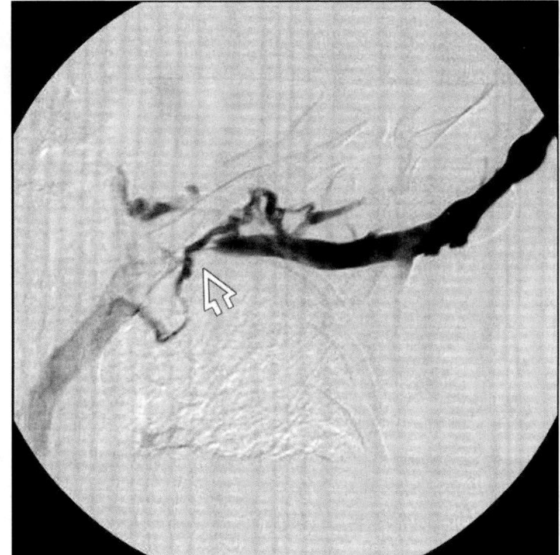

(Left) *Posteroanterior DSA with the left shoulder in neutral position shows the subclavian vein is patent but narrowed and irregular at the 1st rib/clavicular junction. Chest wall and cervical venous collaterals are present.* ***(Right)*** *DSA (same patient) shows the left shoulder in abduction. Subclavian vein occlusion occurs at the junction of the 1st rib and clavicle during this maneuver. Provocative maneuvers are used to accentuate the abnormality.*

Typical

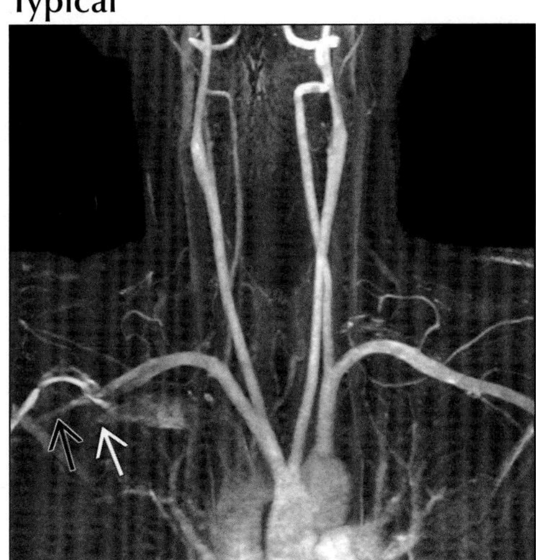

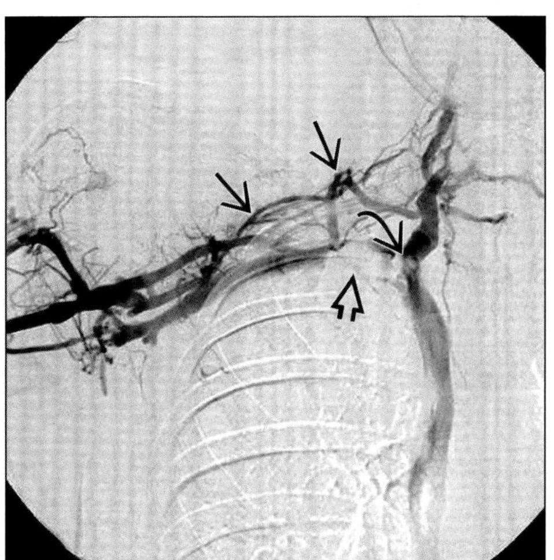

(Left) *Coronal FSPGR CE-MRA shows occlusion of the right subclavian vein and narrowing of the right subclavian artery at the thoracic outlet in a patient with right arm pain and edema.* ***(Right)*** *Posteroanterior DSA shows a filling defect in the central segment of the right subclavian vein. The thrombus extends into the junction of the subclavian vein and the SVC. Multiple venous collaterals are present.*

Typical

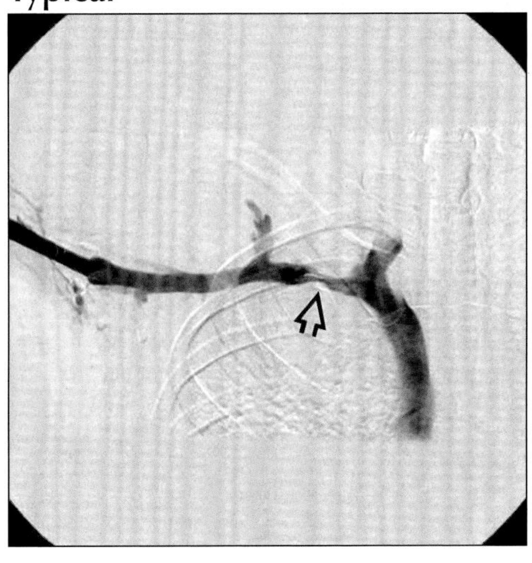

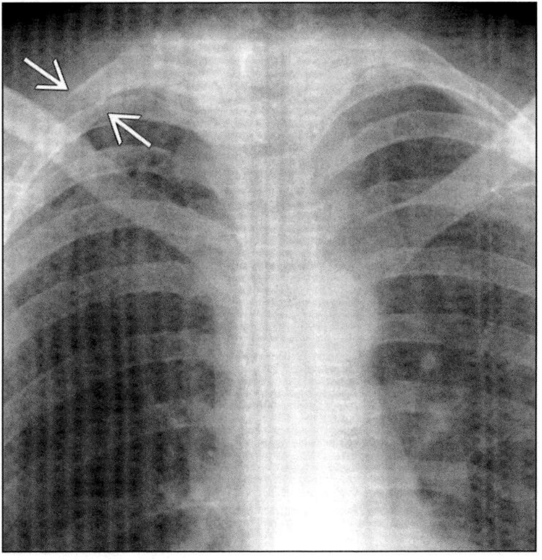

(Left) *Posteroanterior DSA with the arm abducted, obtained in the same patient 3 months after thrombolysis and angioplasty, shows that the subclavian vein is patent, but is narrowed. The likelihood of recurrence is high unless there is surgical decompression.* ***(Right)*** *Posteroanterior radiograph shows that following the successful thrombolysis there has been surgical decompression of the thoracic outlet. The first rib has been resected as was the anterior scalene muscle.*

CATHETER INDUCED VENOUS OCCLUSION

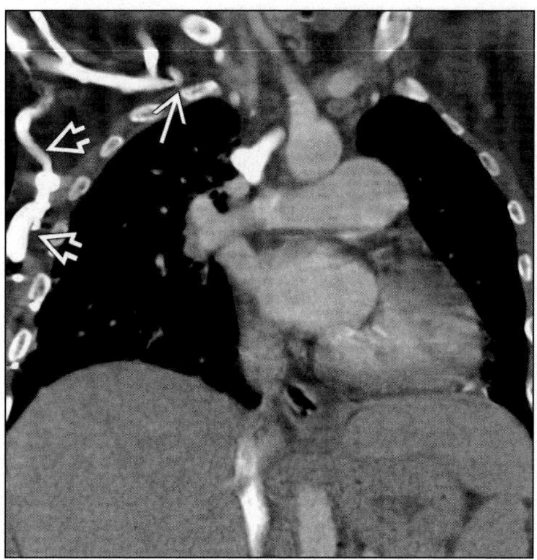

Coronal reformatted CECT shows occlusion of the proximal right subclavian and brachiocephalic veins ➡ and extensive collaterals ⇨ in a patient who previously had a right internal jugular dialysis catheter.

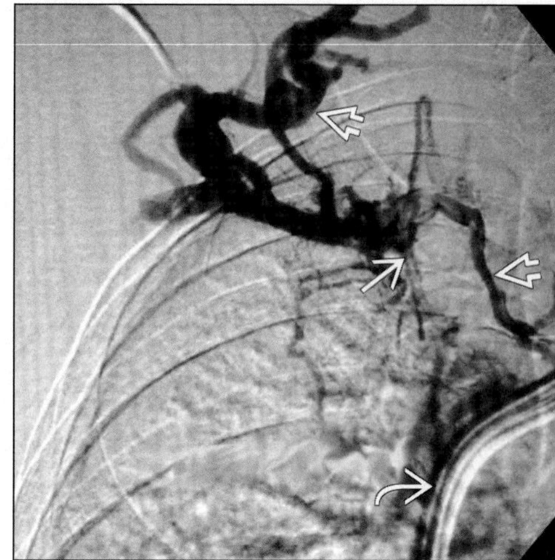

Venogram in the same patient as previous image shows occlusion of the right brachiocephalic vein ➡ and extensive collaterals ⇨. A new dialysis catheter has been placed on the left ➦.

TERMINOLOGY

Abbreviations and Synonyms

- Iatrogenic superior vena cava (SVC) syndrome
  - Occurs if SVC is involved with catheter induced occlusive process

Definitions

- Catheter induced venous occlusion: Thrombosis and subsequent occlusion of major venous structures caused by presence of an indwelling venous catheter
  - Seen primarily in upper extremities
  - May also occur in lower extremities if catheter placed via femoral vein

IMAGING FINDINGS

General Features

- Best diagnostic clue
  - Venous occlusion
    - Thrombosis occurs initially in acute occlusion
    - Stenosis, segmental occlusion or recanalization with mural irregularity if more chronic
  - Extensive collateral venous pathways
    - Axillary or subclavian vein occlusion results in collaterals around shoulder, scapula, chest wall
    - Key collateral pathways include ipsilateral internal and external jugular veins, ipsilateral intercostal veins and contralateral jugular or subclavian veins
    - Dilated subcutaneous veins over upper chest and shoulder may be visible

CT Findings

- CECT
  - Excellent for evaluating jugular, proximal subclavian and brachiocephalic veins, as well as SVC
    - Nonopacified venous lumen in acute occlusion
    - String-like or stenotic vessel may be seen with chronic thrombosis and partial recanalization
  - Demonstrates collateral venous return involving chest wall, shoulder, scapula and neck
    - Reveals extrinsic causes of venous obstruction (adenopathy, neoplasm)
  - Thrombus in major vein where catheter placed
  - Presence of indwelling venous catheter

MR Findings

- MRV

DDx: Central Venous Occlusion

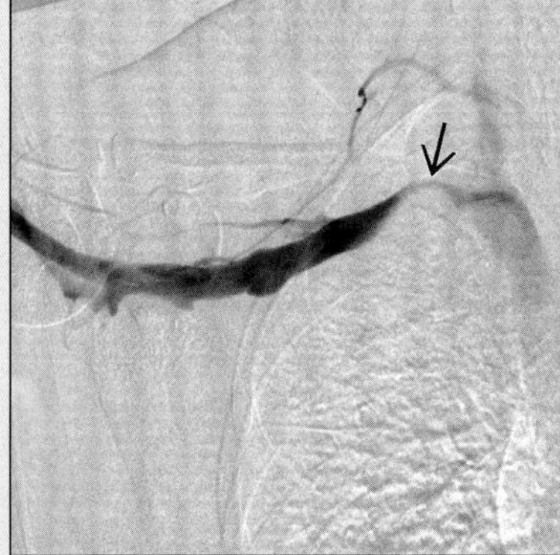

Thoracic Outlet Syndrome

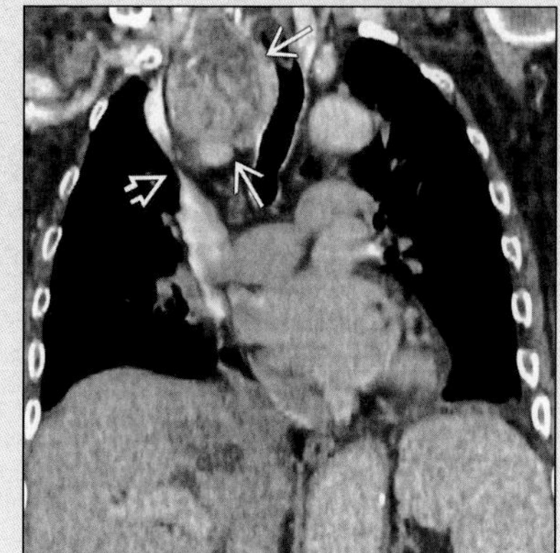

Tumor

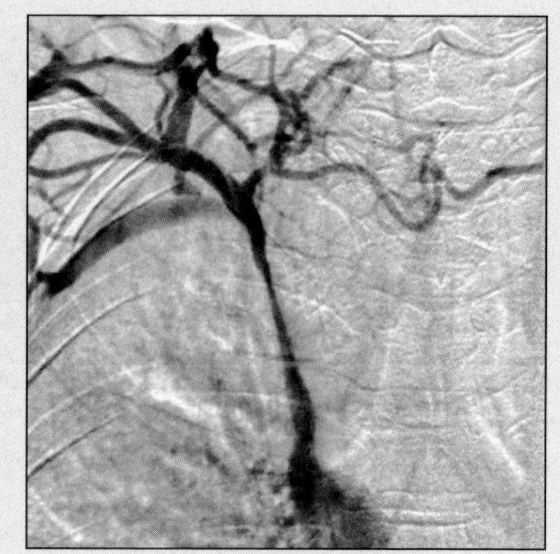

SVC Syndrome from Radiation

CATHETER INDUCED VENOUS OCCLUSION

Key Facts

Terminology

- Catheter induced venous occlusion: Thrombosis and subsequent occlusion of major venous structures caused by presence of an indwelling venous catheter

Imaging Findings

- Venous occlusion is the best diagnostic clue and is best demonstrated by CECT or venography
- Ultrasound good for diagnosis of peripheral thrombosis but limited evaluation of central veins
    - Demonstrates hypoechoic to echogenic intraluminal thrombus acutely; hyperechoic intraluminal focus in chronic occlusion
    - Central veins (brachiocephalic and SVC) poorly imaged because of surrounding bone and lung
- If intervention planned, obtain venogram
    - May demonstrate intraluminal filling defect, mural irregularity, stenoses and/or stringlike vessel lumen

Pathology

- Venous occlusion usually caused by large catheters
- May be caused by smaller catheters, particularly with underlying mild thoracic outlet pathology

Clinical Issues

- As venous collaterals develop, arm and neck swelling may improve or resolve
- Conservative management if catheter still required
    - Anticoagulation and arm elevation
- Catheter removal if no longer required
    - Venous angioplasty and intravascular stents have been used to re-establish patency to occluded central veins following catheter removal

---

- Excellent modality for evaluation of extremity, neck and central venous structures
    - Absent signal in lumen on flow sequences where venous occlusion is present
    - Thrombosis in major vein where catheter placed
    - Large collaterals in chest, shoulder, neck
- Signal suppression from structures such as bone and soft tissues renders excellent vascular anatomy
- Gadolinium enhanced imaging with 2-D time of flight technique used with great success
- Conventional T1WI for adjacent soft tissues
- If osseous etiology for venous obstruction suspected, CECT is better imaging choice

Ultrasonographic Findings

- Grayscale Ultrasound
    - Noncompressible vessel
    - Hypoechoic to echogenic intraluminal thrombus acutely; hyperechoic intraluminal focus in chronic occlusion
- Color Doppler
    - Central veins (brachiocephalic and SVC) poorly imaged because of surrounding bone and lung
        - Vessel patency can be inferred through subclavian and internal jugular vein Doppler waveforms at rest and in response to respiration and Valsalva
    - Even if thrombus is not identified, Doppler studies will show lack of flow or respiratory variation

Angiographic Findings

- Venography findings
    - Intraluminal filling defects in acute thrombosis
    - Linear intraluminal webs, mural irregularity, stenoses and/or stringlike vessel lumen may be present in chronic thrombosis or recanalization
    - Best way to visualize venous flow, and collaterals
    - Provides guidance for percutaneous procedures

Imaging Recommendations

- Best imaging tool
    - Initial evaluation with ultrasound
        - Ultrasound good for diagnosis of peripheral thrombosis but limited evaluation of central veins
    - CECT or MR to diagnose extent of central occlusion
    - If intervention is contemplated, contrast venography to guide therapy
- Protocol advice
    - With CECT evaluation, contrast injection into extremity on side of interest provides best opacification of unobstructed and collateral veins
        - If bilateral obstruction suspected, may require bilateral contrast injections
    - Intervention may require dual evaluation of venous anatomy of affected extremity with venography
        - Venography catheter or sheath introduced peripherally in affected extremity
        - Second venography catheter introduced into SVC

DIFFERENTIAL DIAGNOSIS

Defibrillator/Pacemaker

- Transvenous leads may induce venous thrombosis

Drug Induced Venous Thrombosis

- Chemical irritation of venous endothelium from IV injection may lead to thrombosis
    - Antibiotics, chemotherapy, hyperalimentation
- Oral agents such as contraceptives may predispose to venous thrombosis

Hypercoagulable States

- Disorders may induce arterial or venous thrombosis
    - Heparin-induced thrombocytopenia (HIT), antithrombin III deficiency, antiphospholipid syndrome (lupus anticoagulants and anticardiolipin antibodies), factor V Leiden, malignancy

Thoracic Outlet Syndrome

- Also known as effort thrombosis or Paget-Schroetter syndrome
    - Young, healthy, athletic patient presenting with unexplained acute subclavian vein thrombosis
- Etiology of < 5% of upper extremity thrombosis
- Mechanical compression causes intimal hyperplasia, then axillary or subclavian vein stenosis or occlusion

- Causes of compression
  - Cervical rib
  - Clavicle and subclavius muscle
  - Hypertrophied scalene muscles
  - Osseous exostosis
- Initial management with anticoagulation and catheter directed thrombolysis
  - Improves arm swelling and delineates pathology
- Surgical decompression is definitive treatment
  - Stent deformity or fracture will occur if placed without decompression
  - Poor long term stent patency in this location

Tumor

- Pancoast (superior sulcus) or thoracic inlet tumors may compress or invade vein, with eventual occlusion

Trauma

- Blunt trauma, stab wounds or projectiles may cause venous injury, thrombosis and occlusion

Superior Vena Cava (SVC) Syndrome

- Most common etiology is extrinsic compression or invasion of SVC by thoracic neoplasm, adenopathy
  - Additional causes are central venous catheter, trauma, mediastinal fibrosis, sarcoid, radiation
- Characteristic facial and upper extremity edema, superficial venous distension and cyanosis
  - Patient discomfort when supine
  - Acute SVC syndrome can be medical emergency
- Level of obstruction important, as occlusion below azygos vein may be well-tolerated
- CECT is best modality for initial evaluation followed by venography for intervention
- May be managed with angioplasty and/or intravascular stent; thrombolysis if necessary

PATHOLOGY

General Features

- General path comments: Indwelling catheter causes irritation of venous endothelium
- Etiology
  - Intimal hyperplasia from chronic irritation
    - Stenosis develops as a result of intimal hyperplasia followed by thrombosis when stenosis becomes severe enough to restrict flow
  - Usually caused by large catheters such as dialysis or pheresis catheters
  - May be caused by smaller catheters, particularly with underlying mild thoracic outlet pathology
- Epidemiology
  - Patients with indwelling catheters
    - Occlusion more likely with larger catheters
    - Dialysis catheters have higher risk than smaller catheters such as PICC lines or ports
  - Subclavian catheters are most problematic
    - Problems occur in left subclavian catheters > right subclavian catheters > left internal jugular catheter > right internal jugular catheters
    - Left internal jugular catheters are problematic because of relatively tortuous course of left brachiocephalic vein compared to right
    - Should place all catheters via right internal jugular vein whenever possible
  - Hypercoagulable patients more prone to thrombosis

CLINICAL ISSUES

Presentation

- Relatively acute swelling of the arm and neck
- Bilateral swelling with SVC involvement
  - Bilateral neck and arm swelling
  - Facial swelling
  - Mental status changes due to brain edema

Natural History & Prognosis

- As venous collaterals develop, arm and neck swelling may improve or resolve
  - Swelling commonly recurs if arm actively used
- Collaterals commonly will form, improving symptoms and allowing catheter to remain in place
- Thrombolysis generally successful in removing clot and improving symptoms

Treatment

- Conservative management when catheter still required
  - Anticoagulation and arm elevation
  - Consider low-dose Coumadin in patients with malignancy
- Catheter removal if no longer required
  - Removing catheter and placing it in another vein puts a second vein at risk
- If very symptomatic, consider course of catheter directed thrombolysis followed by anticoagulation
- If severely symptomatic, initiate thrombolysis if possible and catheter will likely require removal
  - Venous angioplasty and intravascular stents have been used to re-establish patency to occluded central veins following catheter removal
    - Predominantly used to alleviate severe symptoms of arm, neck and facial swelling by restoring patency to central venous drainage
    - Generally poor long term patency for subclavian and brachiocephalic venous stents
    - SVC stents have slightly better long term patency

DIAGNOSTIC CHECKLIST

Consider

- Venogram to evaluate venous drainage in patient with venous occlusion, particularly if intervention planned

SELECTED REFERENCES

1. Kommareddy A et al: Upper extremity deep venous thrombosis. Semin Thromb Hemost. 28(1):89-99, 2002
2. Ratcliffe M et al: Thrombosis, markers of thrombotic risk, indwelling central venous catheters and antithrombotic prophylaxis using low-dose warfarin in subjects with malignant disease. Clin Lab Haematol. 21(5):353-7, 1999
3. Trerotola SO: Interventional radiology in central venous stenosis and occlusion. Semin in Interv Radiol. 11: 291-304, 1994

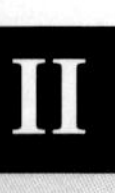

CATHETER INDUCED VENOUS OCCLUSION

IMAGE GALLERY

Typical

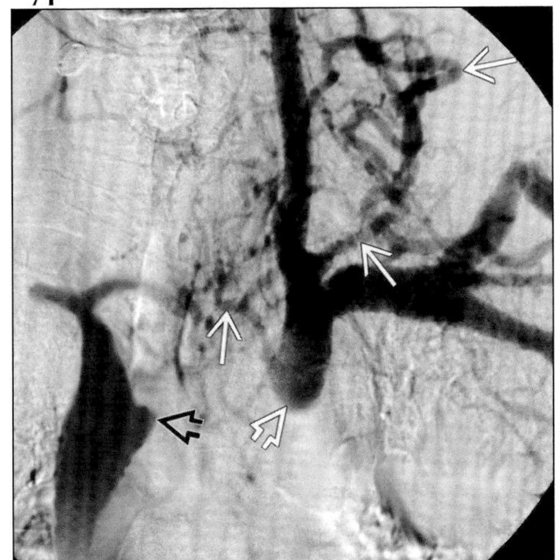

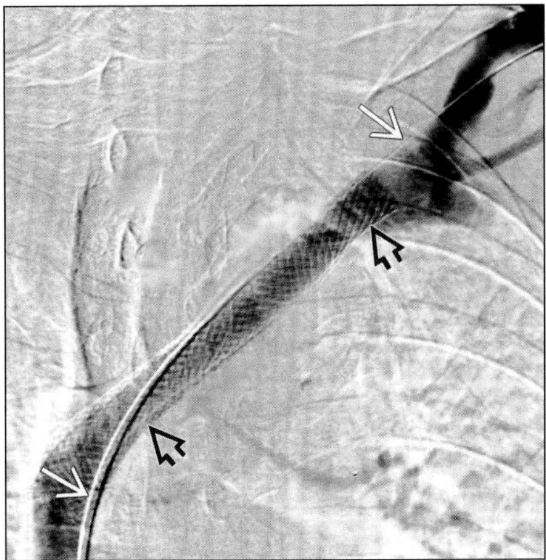

(Left) *Left subclavian venogram shows occluded left brachiocephalic vein & extensive collaterals communicating with the SVC. A left-sided dialysis catheter had been removed because of arm swelling.* ***(Right)*** *Venogram (same patient as previous image) shows intravascular stent has established patency to the previously occluded brachiocephalic vein. A guidewire is still in place. Stent placement was for persistent arm swelling despite catheter removal.*

Typical

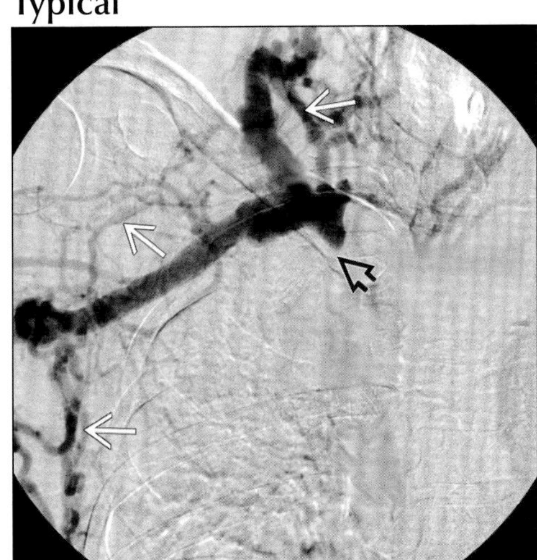

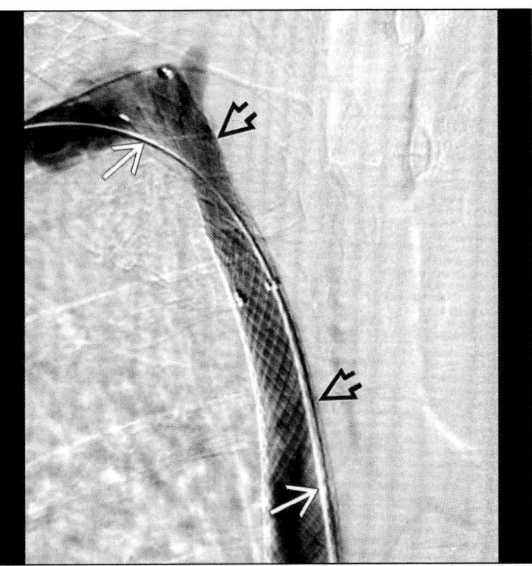

(Left) *Right subclavian venogram shows occlusion of the SVC and extensive collaterals in the neck, shoulder and lateral chest wall. A right internal jugular dialysis catheter had been removed because of severe arm and facial swelling.* ***(Right)*** *Venogram in the same patient with iatrogenic SVC syndrome, shows intravascular stents re-establishing patency to the SVC. A guidewire is still in place. The patient's symptoms rapidly resolved following stent placement.*

Typical

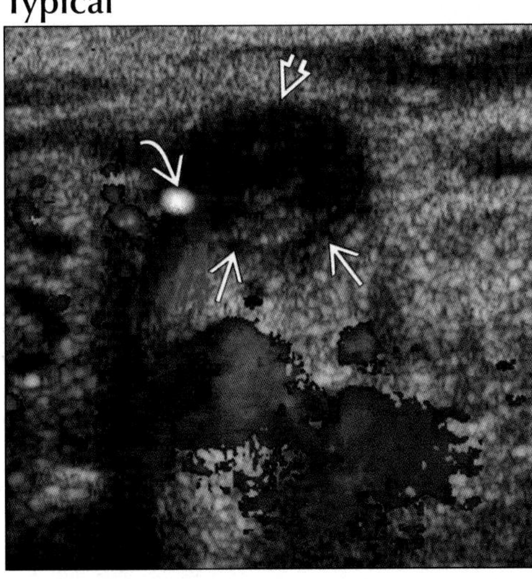

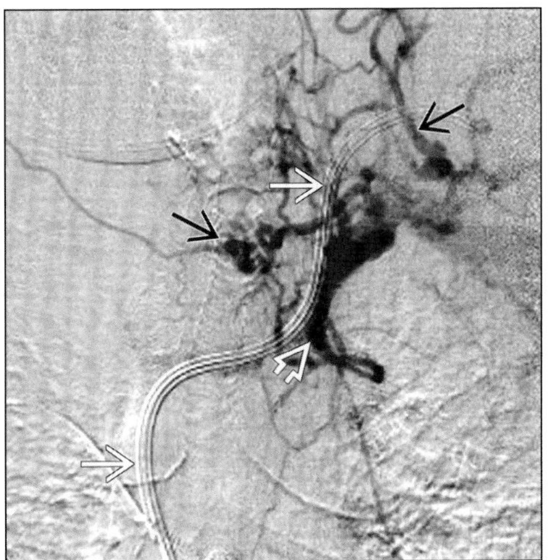

(Left) *Axial color Doppler ultrasound of the neck shows an occluded left internal jugular vein filled with echogenic thrombus caused by an indwelling dialysis catheter. The catheter is seen as an echogenic focus with acoustic shadowing.* ***(Right)*** *Venogram in the same patient as previous image, shows the dialysis catheter also caused occlusion of the left brachiocephalic vein. There are extensive venous collaterals.*

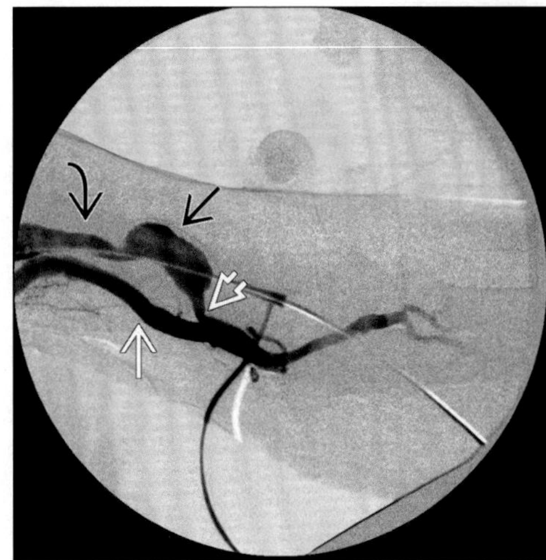

Oblique DSA Brachio-cephalic fistula: Side-to-end anastomosis ➡ of brachial artery ➡ to cephalic vein ➡; pseudoaneurysm formation due to upstream stenosis ➡.

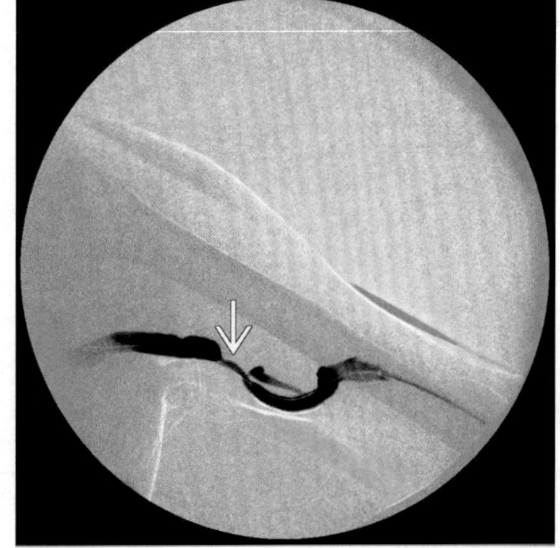

Axial DSA Same patient as previous: Main draining vein has severe stenosis ➡ further upstream causing pseudoaneurysm as well as venous pulsatility further downstream.

TERMINOLOGY

Abbreviations and Synonyms

- Autogenous arteriovenous (AV) fistula, radio-cephalic (Brescia-Cimino) AV fistula, brachiobasilic AV fistula, brachiocephalic (Kaufman) fistula

Definitions

- Surgically constructed fistula between an artery and vein for dialysis access

IMAGING FINDINGS

General Features

- Best diagnostic clue
  - Non-anatomic, surgically created arterio-venous connection usually above level of wrist, just below level of elbow or at upper arm
  - Surgical clips usually present at site of anastomosis
- Location: Connection between artery and vein usually in forearm, but fistulas also placed in proximal upper extremity, or less commonly in upper thigh
- Size: Vein must have minimum diameter of 3-4 mm after dilatation for access
- Morphology
  - Anastomotic connection with partial arterial flow diversion into main draining vein
  - Main draining vein usually exceeds adjacent veins in caliber and carries rapid, arterialized flow centrally

CT Findings

- Evaluation of arterial inflow (atherosclerotic stenoses)
- Evaluation of central venous outflow to evaluate for stenoses, particularly in patients with previous dialysis catheters

MR Findings

- MRV
  - May be used to image central veins to evaluate for central venous stenosis or occlusion
    - Evaluate size and patency of upper extremity veins prior to fistula creation

Ultrasonographic Findings

- Grayscale Ultrasound
  - May be used in pre-operative planning to evaluate the size and patency of forearm and upper arm veins

DDx: Forearm Loop Graft

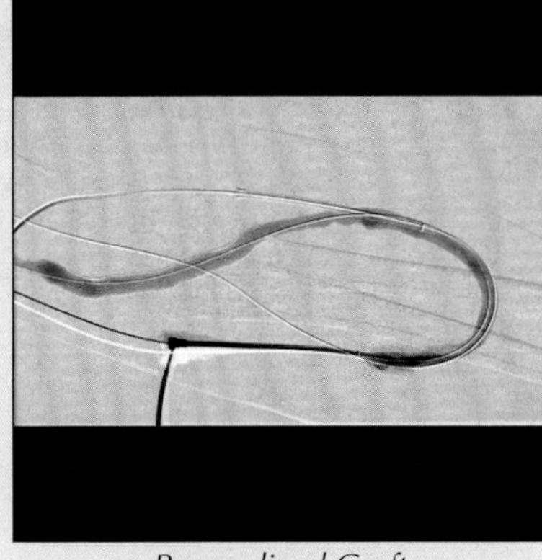

Recanalized Graft

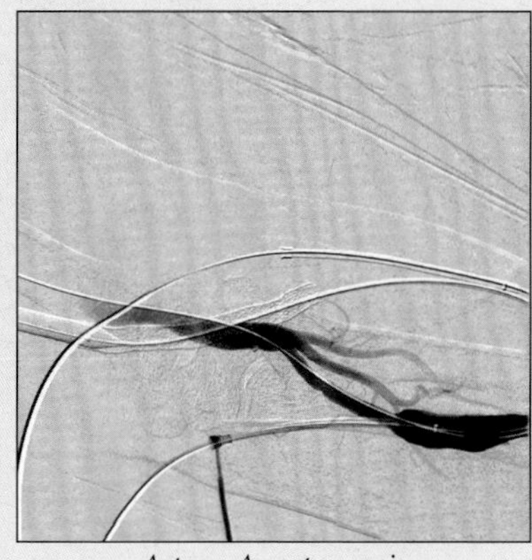

Artery Anastomosis

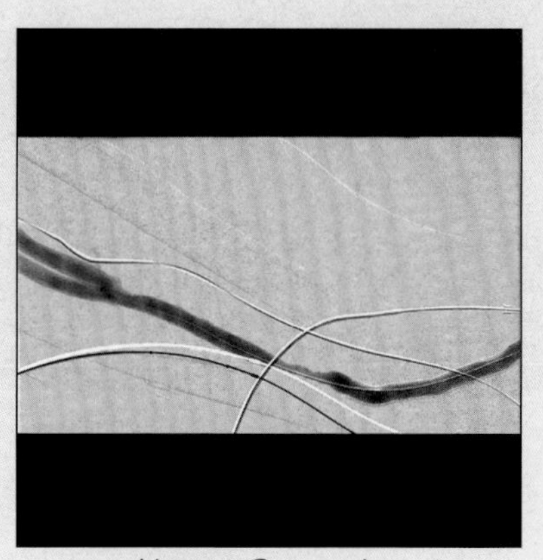

Venous Connection

DIALYSIS AVF

Key Facts

Terminology

- Surgically constructed fistula between an artery and vein for dialysis access

Imaging Findings

- Non-anatomic, iatrogenic, surgically created arterio-venous connection usually above level of wrist, just below level of elbow or at upper arm

Clinical Issues

- Most common signs/symptoms: Normally matured fistula has palpable thrill at anastomosis that fades along course of distended but non-pulsatile main draining vein
- Longest lasting and most dependable type of dialysis access if it can be established
- Unfortunately difficult to construct, not possible in up to 65% of patients
- Failures common in elderly and diabetic patients
- Once established has a primary patency of 70% at one year, and 75% patency rate at 4 years
- In US, ~ 20% have AV fistula, goal is ≥ 50%
- Dysfunctional dialysis/impending fistula failure
- Venous stenosis: Most commonly just beyond the anastomosis, less common a few cm upstream from anastomosis at dialysis access or in central venous system (usually due to prior dialysis catheter insertion)
- Clinical signs of early fistula failure: Arm swelling, increased urea recirculation, increased venous pressures with dialysis

---

- ○ Not ideal for examining central veins though may suggest significant central venous stenosis or occlusion due to abnormal Doppler waveforms
- Color Doppler: Non-invasive assessment of venous flow & evaluation for stenoses within venous outflow

Angiographic Findings

- Venography findings
  - ○ Gold standard for pre-operative planning of AVF
    - ▪ Evaluates size, position and patency of venous system of forearm, upper arm and central veins
    - ▪ Important for patients with previously failed access or in obese patients
  - ○ Primary evaluation of poorly maturing fistula or previous fistula access thrombosis
    - ▪ Evaluation for fistulae showing signs of early failure (arm swelling, venous pulsatility etc.)
    - ▪ Clinical signs of failure: Decrease flows in fistula, elevated venous pressure, increased recirculation
    - ▪ Signs of early failure usually followed by intervention (venoplasty) if stenosis causing > 50% luminal compromise is found in setting of early fistula failure

Imaging Recommendations

- Best imaging tool: Angiographic evaluation to include evaluation of main draining vein, arterio-venous anastomosis and central venous system
- Protocol advice
  - ○ If flow is adequate, fistulogram and central venogram may be performed
  - ○ Arterial approach: Brachial artery puncture with small access system
    - ▪ Venous approach: Inflow evaluation by contrast injection with blood pressure cuff inflation or manual compression of the outflow
  - ○ Main draining vein access allows interventions on the venous side such as venoplasty of main draining vein or within central venous system
  - ○ Diagnostic angiographic imaging often followed by intervention: Venoplasty (rarely stent placement) of flow limiting main draining or central vein stenosis
  - ○ Removal of clot within fistula or venous system or embolization of flow diverting competitive outflow veins
- Ultrasound is least expensive way to evaluate venous system pre-operatively; suboptimal for evaluating central veins
- MR venography excellent for central veins & can be used to evaluate upper extremity venous system
  - ○ Useful in patients with allergic reactions to contrast
- Contrast venography allows pre-operative evaluation of the arm and central venous system (venous mapping)

DIFFERENTIAL DIAGNOSIS

Dialysis Graft

- Synthetic tube placement between artery and vein, usually polytetrafluoroethylene (PTFE, Gore-Tex)
  - ○ Graft is placed between artery and vein either as a straight or loop graft at the forearm or upper arm; a loop graft may also be placed in the upper thigh
    - ▪ Unusual access sites: Graft placement between axillary artery and ipsilateral axillary vein
- Axillary artery to ipsilateral jugular vein (Gore-Tex loop shunt)
- Axillary artery to contralateral axillary vein (necklace shunt)

PATHOLOGY

General Features

- General path comments
  - ○ With connection between the artery and the vein, the arterial pressure/flow is transmitted into the vein
  - ○ Dilatation of the vein, hypertrophy of the vein wall
  - ○ Anatomy
    - ▪ Brescia-Cimino: Connection between radial artery and cephalic vein; side-to-side (most common), side of artery to end of vein
    - ▪ End-to-end or end-to-side fistula creation at wrist: Initial & most common choice for access creation

    - Below elbow or at upper arm (brachio-cephalic or brachio-basilic fistula)
    - Second choice and performed if more distal access creation not possible or prior distal non-salvageable access failure
- Etiology
  - Leading cause of ESRD is diabetes, followed by arterial hypertension and glomerulonephritis
  - Less common causes are hereditary renal disease, obstructive uropathy and interstitial nephritis
- Epidemiology
  - Prevalence of ESRD was 336,000 in 2004 (3.4 times higher than in 2003)
    - Incidence of new patients with ESRD was 104,000
    - 15% of patients with ESRD treated by renal transplantation, 85-90% by hemodialysis

Gross Pathologic & Surgical Features

- Arteriovenous fistula results in venous distension and wall thickening of main draining vein due to increased pressure from arterialized flow

CLINICAL ISSUES

Presentation

- Most common signs/symptoms: Normally matured fistula has palpable thrill at anastomosis that fades along course of distended but non-pulsatile main draining vein
- Clinical Profile
  - Longest lasting and most dependable type of dialysis access if it can be established
    - Unfortunately difficult to construct, not possible in up to 65% of patients
    - Failures common in elderly and diabetic patients
    - Once established has a primary patency of 70% at one year, and 75% patency rate at 4 years
    - US goal is ≥ 50% AV fistulas
  - Dysfunctional dialysis/impending fistula failure
- Venous stenosis: Most commonly just beyond the anastomosis, less common a few cm upstream from anastomosis at dialysis access or in central venous system (usually due to prior dialysis catheter insertion)
  - Clinical signs of early fistula failure: Arm swelling, increased urea recirculation, increased venous pressures with dialysis
  - Prolonged bleeding post dialysis needle removal, main draining vein pulsatile downstream and collapsed upstream from venous stenosis
  - Failure to mature: Typically thrill at anastomosis but collapsed outflow vein
    - Main reasons: Discontinuous or too small main draining vein, inadequate inflow or additional competing outflow veins
  - Aneurysms and pseudoaneurysms: Usually clinically insignificant unless causing skin erosion
    - Puncture site pseudoaneurysms often related to upstream stenosis & angiographic evaluation indicated
    - Arterial flow diversion into main draining vein may cause hand ischemia secondary to steal

Demographics

- Age: Incidence of ESRD generally increases with age, but point prevalence is highest in the 40-64 age group
- Gender: ESRD: M > F
- Ethnicity: ↑ Incidence for ESRD in African Americans

Natural History & Prognosis

- If becomes functional may last for years
- If inflow problem or venous stenosis develops, the fistula may be treated with percutaneous methods
- Main draining vein or outflow problems much more common than inflow problems
- Venous stenosis recurrence post treatment is common and usually requires re-intervention

Treatment

- Angioplasty for venous stenoses
  - Stents rarely used and indicated for venous rupture during angioplasty
    - For aneurysm exclusion (covered stents), early restenosis (> 2 interventions in 3 months period), primary elastic stenosis
    - If fistula doesn't mature because of flow diverting competitive outflow veins, embolization/surgical ligation of competing veins can be performed

DIAGNOSTIC CHECKLIST

Consider

- Distinguish native fistula from graft
  - Grafts are characterized by presence of synthetic material, fairly inelastic on physical exam; grafts appear in straight or looped configurations
  - Fistula are created by utilization of native vein that carries arterialized flow centrally; main draining vein is distended on physical exam and elastic

Image Interpretation Pearls

- Fistula evaluation: Visualization of arterial inflow, main draining vein and central venous system
- Is flow limiting (> 50%) stenosis present in main draining vein or central venous system?
- Is arterial inflow adequate or compromised by presence of stenosis or clot at AV-fistula or atherosclerotic disease of inflow artery?
- Are there competitive outflow veins that may divert outflow from the main draining vein?

SELECTED REFERENCES

1. Rayner HC et al: Vascular access results from the Dialysis Outcomes and Practice Patterns Study (DOPPS): performance against Kidney Disease Outcomes Quality Initiative (K/DOQI) Clinical Practice Guidelines. Am J Kidney Dis. 44(5 Suppl 2):22-6, 2004
2. Turmel-Rodrigues L: Stenosis and thrombosis in haemodialysis fistulae and grafts: the radiologist's point of view. Nephrol Dial Transplant. 19(2):306-8, 2004
3. Weiswasser JM et al: Strategies of arteriovenous dialysis access. Semin Vasc Surg. 17(1):10-8, 2004

IMAGE GALLERY

Typical

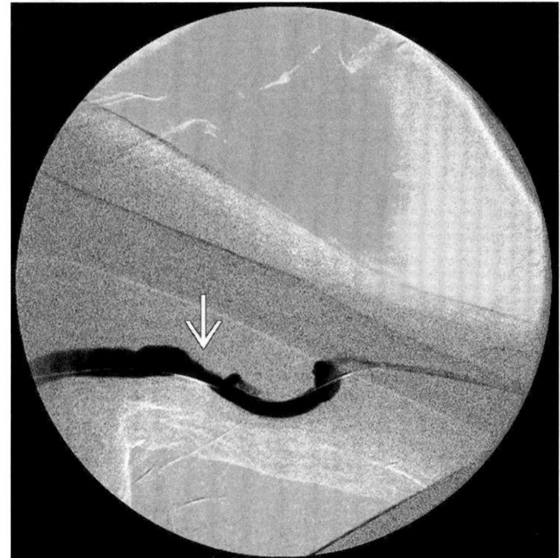

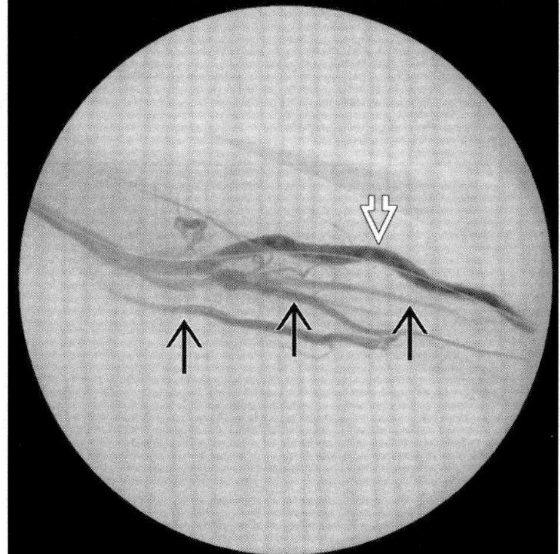

*(**Left**) Axial DSA in the same patient as previous image shows satisfactory result ➔ after treatment with venoplasty. Flow rates during dialysis increased from < 400 to > 400 cc/min and venous pulsatility disappeared. (**Right**) Axial catheter angiography fistula outflow evaluation: Many collateral veins ➔ compete for outflow with main draining cephalic vein ➔ causing dysfunctional dialysis fistula.*

Typical

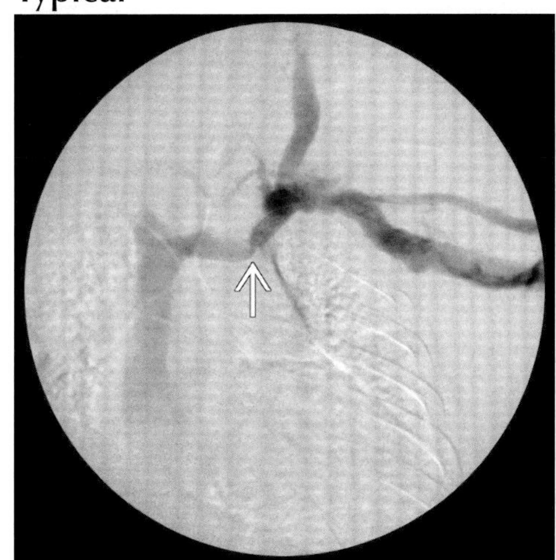

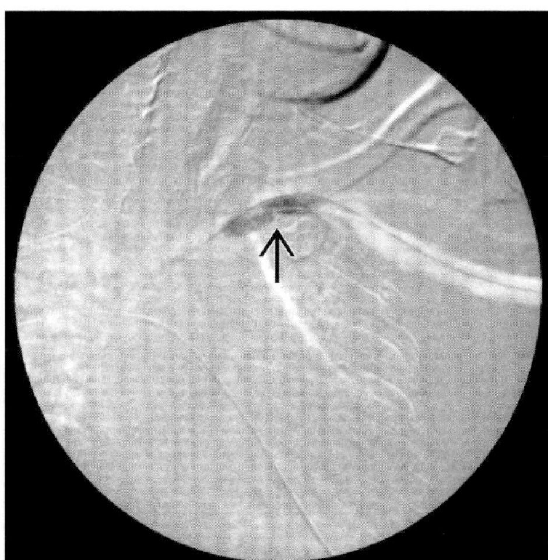

*(**Left**) Coronal catheter angiography central venogram shows severe focal stenosis of left innominate vein ➔ as cause of increased venous pressure during dialysis (note reflux into IJV). (**Right**) Coronal DSA of the same central venous stenosis as previous image, which was properly treated with balloon venoplasty. Balloon waist ➔ during balloon inflation was overcome with higher inflation pressures.*

Typical

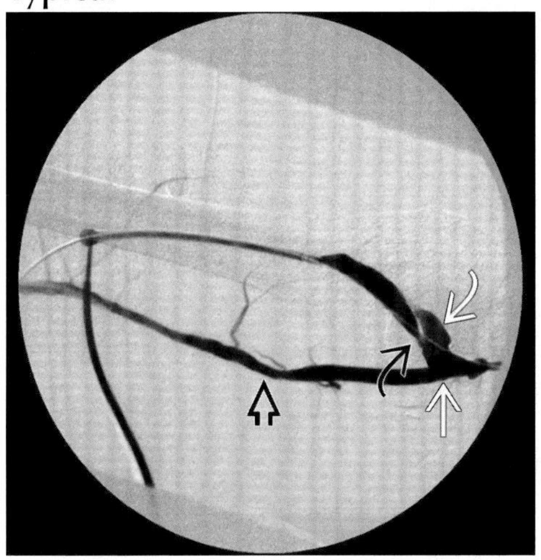

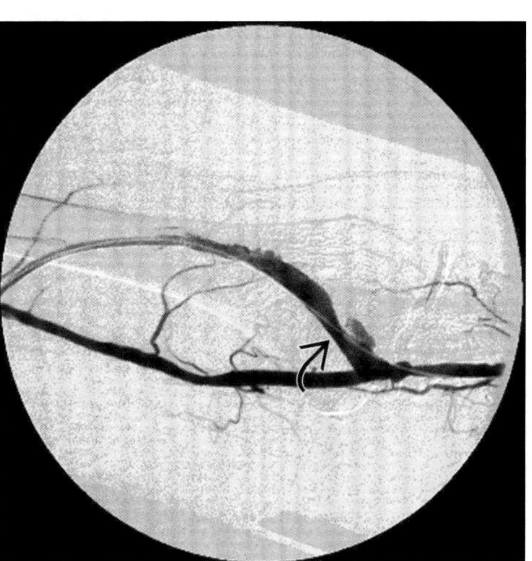

*(**Left**) Axial DSA shows brachial artery ➔ and AV anastomosis ➔. There is severe stenosis ➔ just upstream of anastomosis in a typical location with small pseudoaneurysm ➔ downstream from the stenosis. (**Right**) Axial DSA of the same fistula as previous image. Angioplasty of the prior site of the stenosis ➔ results in substantial caliber improvement and restoration of full fistula function.*

DIALYSIS AV GRAFT

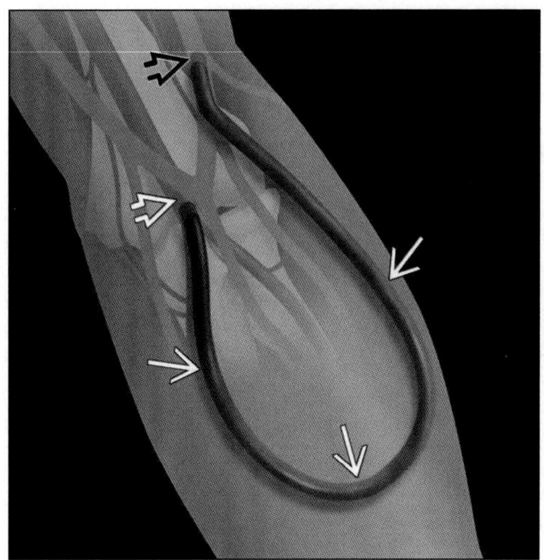

Graphic of left forearm AV dialysis graft shows a prosthetic loop ➡ that has been surgically anastomosed to the brachial artery ➡ and the cephalic vein ⇨ to provide access for hemodialysis.

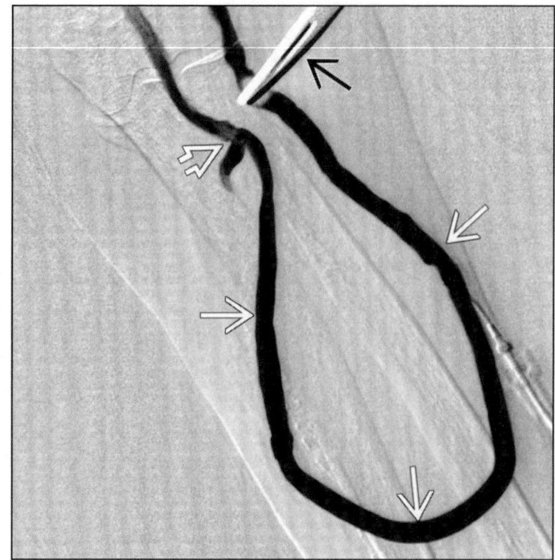

DSA shows an AV graft ➡ coursing from the arterial anastomosis ➡ to the venous outflow. A surgical clamp → was used to extrinsically compress the venous limb and allow opacification of the graft and arterial inflow.

TERMINOLOGY

Abbreviations and Synonyms

- Dialysis arteriovenous graft (AV graft)
- Dialysis arteriovenous fistula (AV fistula)

Definitions

- Surgically created communication between arterial and venous systems using prosthetic material to form connection, constructed for purpose of dialysis access
  - Unlike fistulas, grafts do not need to mature and may be used 4-6 weeks after placement
  - Used in patients with unsuitable arterial and venous anatomy for fistula

IMAGING FINDINGS

General Features

- Location
  - More options for graft placement sites than fistulas
    - Graft can be placed without mobilizing artery and vein
    - Grafts can have variable lengths
    - Typically located in forearm or upper arm
    - Occasionally placed in upper thigh; rarely in upper chest or neck

MR Findings

- 3-D CE-MRA may be used as an imaging modality in complicated AV graft evaluation
  - Can demonstrate stenoses in arterial inflow, AV graft segment or venous outflow
- Infrequently used in AV graft evaluation

Ultrasonographic Findings

- Color Doppler
  - Provides accurate imaging and flow volume measurement of hemodialysis vascular access
  - Decreased blood flow can be measured by color flow Doppler
    - Can readily identify subsets of patients at high risk for future thrombosis
    - Relative risk of graft failure increases 40% when blood flow in graft decreases to < 500 mL/min and risk doubles when blood flow < 300 mL/min

Angiographic Findings

- Venous or arterial anastomotic stenoses

DDx: Arteriovenous Communication

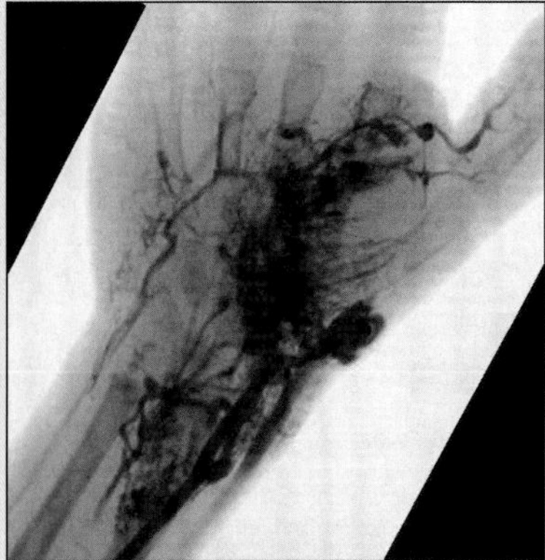

Arteriovenous Malformation (AVM)

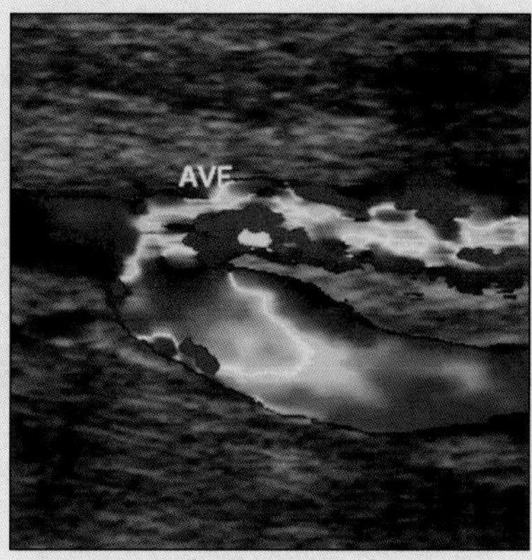

Dialysis AV Fistula

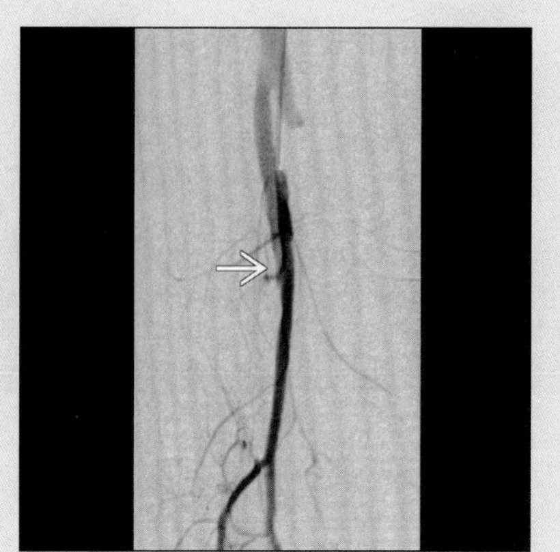

Iatrogenic Arteriovenous Fistula

DIALYSIS AV GRAFT

Key Facts

Terminology

- AV graft: Surgically created communication between arterial and venous systems using prosthetic material to form connection for dialysis access
  - Unlike fistulas, grafts do not need to mature and may be used 4-6 weeks after placement
  - Used in patients with unsuitable arterial and venous anatomy for fistula

Imaging Findings

- Venous or arterial anastomotic stenoses well-demonstrated by angiography
  - Intimal hyperplasia at venous anastomosis is most frequently occurring underlying pathology
  - Thrombotic occlusion of AV graft (results from diminished flow within graft)
- Color Doppler ultrasound provides accurate imaging and flow volume measurements

Clinical Issues

- More options for graft placement sites than fistulas
- AV grafts typically have shorter lifespan than fistulas
  - AV grafts are at high risk for developing stenosis and resultant thrombosis
  - Because of foreign material, greater risk for becoming infected
- Thrombotic graft occlusion requires use of thrombolytic agents or mechanical devices for restoration of patency
  - Ancillary angioplasty usually required since thrombosis typically caused by outflow or inflow stenosis

  - Intimal hyperplasia at venous anastomosis is most frequently occurring underlying pathology

- Thrombotic occlusion of AV graft
  - Results from diminished flow within graft (secondary to anastomotic stenosis)
- Diffuse intimal hyperplasia within graft
- Stenosis involving central venous structures (e.g., axillary, subclavian or brachiocephalic veins)
- Atherosclerotic disease or focal stenosis of inflow artery from which AV graft arises
- Pseudoaneurysm involving prosthetic of AV graft

Imaging Recommendations

- Best imaging tool
  - DSA angiography required for confirmation of stenosis or occlusion in poorly functioning AV graft
    - Used to guide endovascular treatment of failing graft
  - Color Doppler ultrasound can be used to assess and quantify flow volumes

DIFFERENTIAL DIAGNOSIS

Dialysis AV Fistula

- Direct surgically created native communication between arterial and venous systems for dialysis access; does not use prosthetic to form communication
  - Usually located in forearm or upper arm; less commonly in upper thigh
  - Surgical anastomosis between artery and vein results in arterialization and resultant enlargement of vein draining fistula
- Fistulas preferred to grafts, as constructed with native vessels only
  - More durable and resistant to infection than grafts
- Access patency and longevity with AV fistulas is much better than with venous catheters or AV grafts

Arteriovenous Malformation (AVM)

- Congenital abnormal communications between arterial and venous systems, typically with a central vascular "nidus"
- Large lesions seen on CT and MR, but need angiography for definitive diagnosis and potential transcatheter treatment
  - Preferred treatment is embolization; extremely large AVMs may require surgical resection

Congenital or Acquired AV Fistula

- AV fistulas are almost always acquired
  - Idiopathic arteriovenous fistulas have characteristics of acquired fistulas, but no cause can be identified
  - Idiopathic arteriovenous fistulas may arise from spontaneous erosion or rupture of diseased arterial segment into nearby renal vein
- Penetrating injuries such as gunshot and stab wounds may result in acquired AV fistula
- Iatrogenic trauma can be a cause of AV fistula
  - Catheterization and surgical procedures can inadvertently result in arteriovenous fistulas

PATHOLOGY

General Features

- Etiology
  - Intimal hyperplasia at venous anastomosis results in venous stenosis at outflow of AV graft
    - Venous stenosis will cause decreased flow within graft, with eventual graft thrombosis
  - AV graft pseudoaneurysm results from repetitive punctures with resultant thinning and weakening of prosthetic
    - With chronic hemodialysis, ultimately leads to pseudoaneurysm (incidence of 2-10%)
    - May also result from poor puncture technique of graft before fully mature
- Associated abnormalities: Infection occurs much more frequently in AV grafts than in AV fistulas

Microscopic Features

- Absence of a functional endothelial monolayer lining prosthetic grafts is an important stimulus for intimal hyperplasia

DIALYSIS AV GRAFT

CLINICAL ISSUES

Presentation

- Most common signs/symptoms: Acute AV graft thrombosis with resultant loss of graft patency and inability to dialyze patient
- Other signs/symptoms
  - High venous pressures during dialysis predictive of underlying venous stenosis
  - "Steal syndrome": Cool, painful and sometimes ischemic extremity distal to fistula
    - Results from arterial stenosis distal to arterial anastomosis of graft, with resultant preferential arterial flow into graft

Natural History & Prognosis

- AV grafts are created when native vasculature does not permit fistula
  - AV grafts typically have shorter lifespan than fistulas
    - AV graft failure usually due to intimal hyperplasia at venous anastomosis, resulting in graft flow decline, ultimately causing thrombosis
  - Graft infection results in substantial morbidity, prolonged dependence on dialysis catheters, and multiple vascular-access procedures
    - Because of foreign material, greater infection risk
- AV grafts can be constructed from various materials
  - Bovine vein graft
    - Several studies show this has better patency than other materials used in graft construction
  - Polytetrafluoroethylene (PTFE) graft
    - Most frequently used material in AV graft construction
  - Diastat graft (Gore-Tex)
    - Has poorer patency rate than other materials
- Recent U.S. Renal Data System now shows about 50% of hemodialysis patients use arteriovenous fistulae (AVF), falling short of goal of 60% AVF use

Treatment

- Few technologies have exceeded balloon angioplasty for treating venous anastomotic stenosis, which is most common cause of AV graft failure
  - Intravascular stent placement has applications in treatment of failing AV grafts
    - Longevity improved in older grafts that would have been abandoned or revised, when venous anastomotic stenoses are treated with stents
    - Stent implantation is safe and effective treatment of residual or recurrent AV graft venous stenoses
    - Investigational studies underway evaluating drug eluting stents to minimize intimal hyperplasia
- Thrombotic graft occlusion requires use of thrombolytic agents or mechanical devices for restoration of patency
  - Ancillary angioplasty usually required since thrombosis typically caused by outflow or inflow stenosis
- Pseudoaneurysm treatment with surgical revision or placement of covered endovascular stent graft
- Treatment of "steal syndrome" involves correction of arterial stenosis, bypass of arterial anastomosis or ligation of AV graft
- Surgical revision of failing AV graft generally has disappointing long-term patency
- Tunneled AV dialysis catheter placement when failed AV graft unresponsive to endovascular or surgical intervention

DIAGNOSTIC CHECKLIST

Consider

- Venous anastomotic stenosis is usual cause of AV graft failure
  - Evaluate for underlying venous stenosis in all cases of thrombotic AV graft occlusion
    - Venous angioplasty to correct any significant stenosis (arterial or venous)
- Intravascular stent placement in cases of recurrent stenosis, failed angioplasty or pseudoaneurysm
  - May improve AV graft longevity

Image Interpretation Pearls

- Color Doppler ultrasound can provide accurate imaging and flow volume measurement of hemodialysis vascular access
  - Can readily identify subsets of patients at high risk for future thrombosis
    - When blood flow in graft decreases to < 500 mL/min there is 40% risk of AV graft failure
    - Risk of AV graft failure doubles when blood flow < 300 mL/min

SELECTED REFERENCES

1. Englesbe MJ et al: Single center review of femoral arteriovenous grafts for hemodialysis. World J Surg. 30(2):171-5, 2006
2. Haage P et al: Radiological intervention to maintain vascular access. Eur J Vasc Endovasc Surg. 32(1):84-9, 2006
3. Inrig JK et al: Relationship between clinical outcomes and vascular access type among hemodialysis patients with Staphylococcus aureus bacteremia. Clin J Am Soc Nephrol. 1(3):518-24, 2006
4. McGill RL et al: AV fistula rates: changing the culture of vascular access. J Vasc Access. 6(1):13-7, 2005
5. Ponikvar R: Surgical salvage of thrombosed arteriovenous fistulas and grafts. Ther Apher Dial. 9(3):245-9, 2005
6. Roca-Tey R et al: [Study of vascular access (VA) by color Doppler ultrasonography (CDU). Comparison between delta-H and CDU methods in measuring VA blood flow rate] Nefrologia. 25(6):678-83, 2005
7. Rotmans JI et al: Hemodialysis access graft failure: time to revisit an unmet clinical need? J Nephrol. 18(1):9-20, 2005
8. Scher LA et al: Alternative graft materials for hemodialysis access. Semin Vasc Surg. 17(1):19-24, 2004
9. Tynan-Cuisiner G et al: Advances in endovascular techniques to treat failing and failed hemodialysis access. J Endovasc Ther. 11 Suppl 2:II134-9, 2004
10. Senkaya I et al: The graft selection for haemodialysis. Vasa. 32(4):209-13, 2003
11. Sands JJ et al: The role of color flow Doppler ultrasound in dialysis access. Semin Nephrol. 22(3):195-201, 2002
12. Bay WH et al: Predicting hemodialysis access failure with color flow Doppler ultrasound. Am J Nephrol. 18(4):296-304, 1998

IMAGE GALLERY

Typical

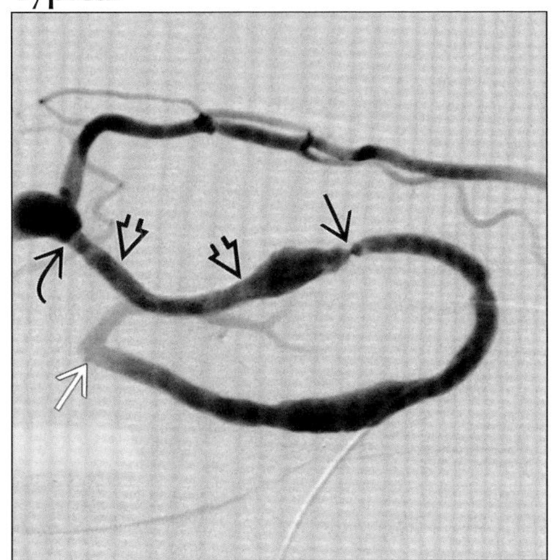

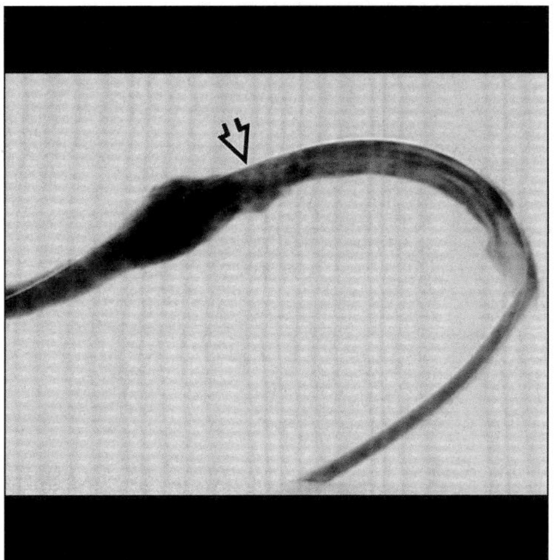

(Left) *DSA of a failing AV graft shows a high grade stenosis . A covered stent , extending to the venous anastomosis from within the graft, had been previously placed to treat a graft pseudoaneurysm. The arterial anastomosis is patent.* ***(Right)*** *DSA (same patient) shows a normal caliber to the graft lumen after venous angioplasty. This treatment salvaged the failing AV graft. Multiple interventions are often necessary to maintain graft patency, as in this patient.*

Typical

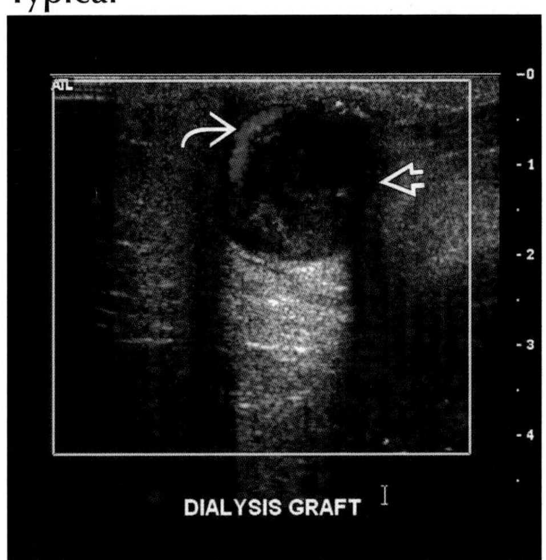

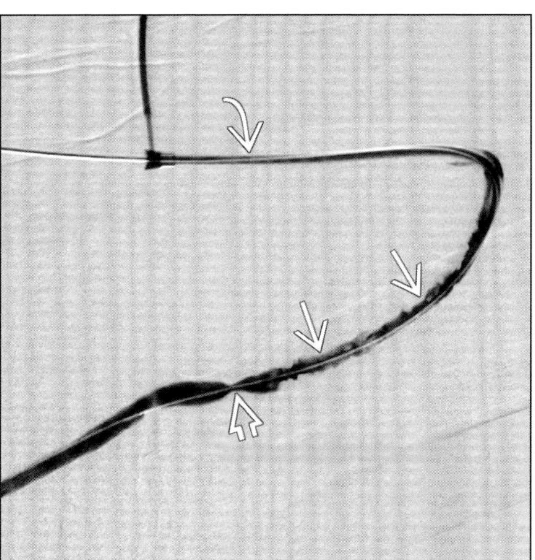

(Left) *Axial color Doppler ultrasound shows thrombus almost completely filling the lumen of an AV graft. There is still very minimal flow in the periphery of the graft lumen .* ***(Right)*** *DSA obtained through vascular sheath (same patient as previous) shows diffuse thrombus within lumen of occluded graft . Graft occlusion occurred because of a venous anastomotic stenosis . AV graft venous stenoses are typically caused by intimal hyperplasia at the venous anastomosis.*

Typical

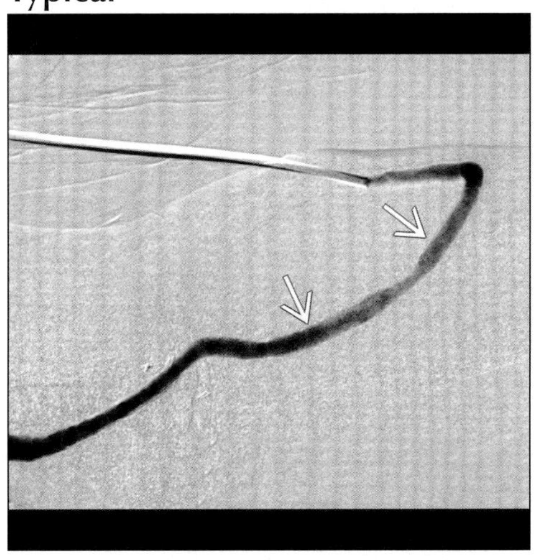

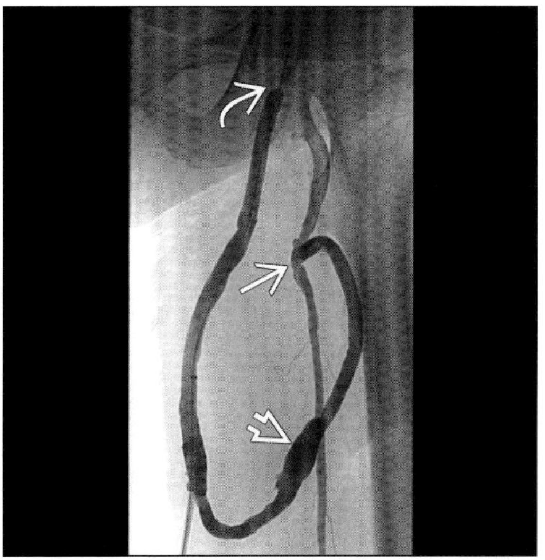

(Left) *DSA obtained after intervention (same patient as previous image) shows that patency has been restored to the AV graft following thrombolysis. Additionally, the venous stenosis has been treated with angioplasty.* ***(Right)*** *Arteriogram of a left thigh dialysis AV graft (different patient) shows the arterial anastomosis is to the SFA and the venous anastomosis is to the common femoral vein. A pseudoaneurysm in the graft was later successfully treated with a covered stent.*

ILIAC ARTERY OCCLUSIVE DISEASE

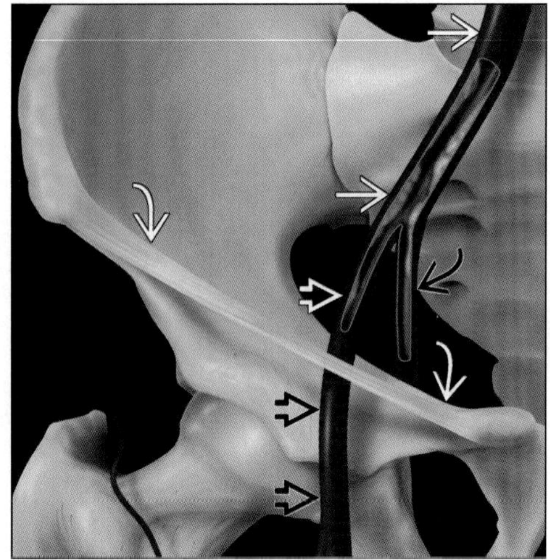

Graphic shows the course, within the pelvis, of the common →, internal → and external → iliac arteries. The inguinal ligament → delineates the transition to the common femoral artery →.

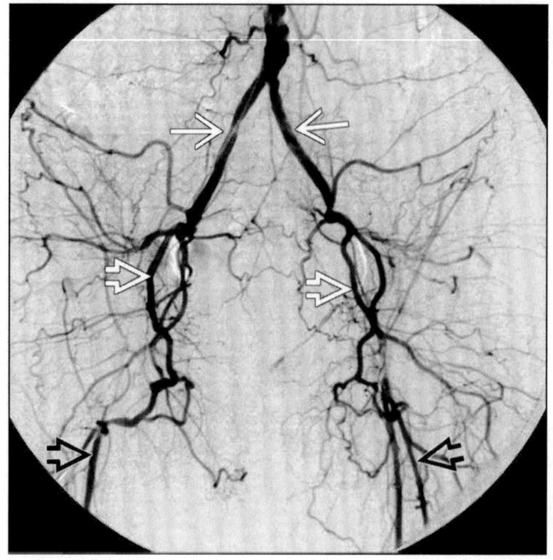

Pelvic arteriogram shows patent common iliac arteries → and occluded external iliac and common femoral arteries. The anterior divisions → of the internal iliac arteries reconstitute both profunda femoral arteries →.

TERMINOLOGY

Abbreviations and Synonyms

- Common iliac artery (CIA)
- Internal iliac artery (hypogastric artery)
- External iliac artery (EIA)

Definitions

- Stenosis or occlusion of major pelvic arteries

IMAGING FINDINGS

General Features

- Best diagnostic clue
  - Arterial stenoses, usually at bifurcations
  - Collateral vessels imply chronic rather than acute obstruction
  - Post-stenotic dilatation distal to severe stenoses
  - Severe stenosis may progress to occlusion
    - Thrombosis of lesion propagates proximally and distally to first patent outflow vessel
- Location
  - Common iliac arteries extend from aortic bifurcation to terminate as bifurcation into internal and external iliac arteries
  - Internal iliac arteries extend from common iliac artery bifurcation to terminate as bifurcation into anterior and posterior divisions
  - External iliac arteries extend from common iliac artery bifurcation to terminate at inguinal ligament
  - Origins of deep circumflex iliac and inferior epigastric arteries angiographically define beginning of common femoral artery
    - Anatomically corresponds to inguinal ligament

CT Findings

- CTA
  - Accurately depicts stenoses, occlusions and collateral vasculature in format similar to angiography
    - CECT combined with CTA also depicts adjacent nonvascular anatomic structures, unlike conventional angiography
  - Multidetector scanner, high contrast dose, rapid bolus injection, and sophisticated post-processing
    - Potential for contrast induced renal dysfunction or allergic reaction

DDx: Iliac Artery Occlusive Disease

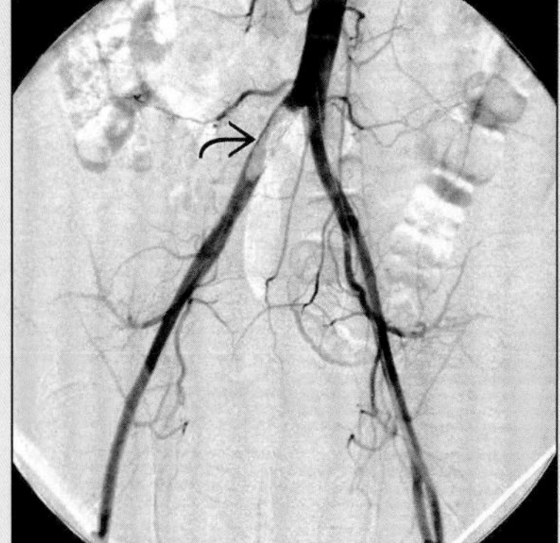

Embolic Disease

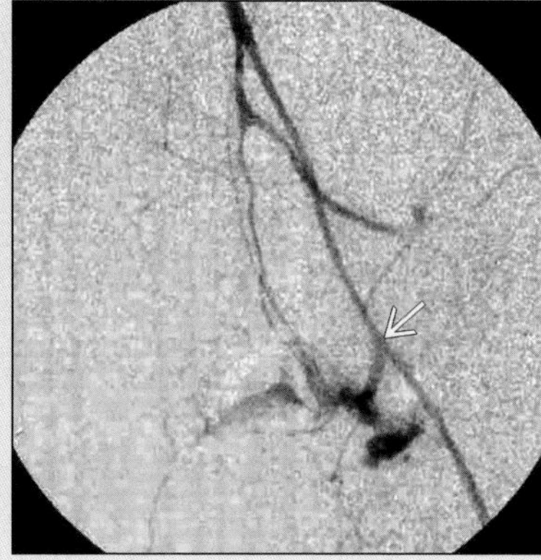

Traumatic Arterial Perforation

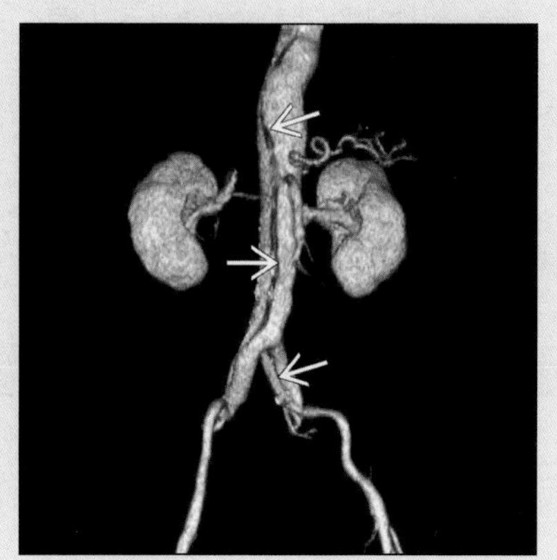

Aortoiliac Dissection

ILIAC ARTERY OCCLUSIVE DISEASE

Key Facts

Terminology

- Stenosis or occlusion of one or more major pelvic arterial vessels

Imaging Findings

- Arterial stenoses, usually at bifurcations
- Collateral vessels imply chronic rather than acute obstruction
- Post-stenotic dilatation distal to severe chronic stenoses
- Severe stenosis may progress to occlusion
  - Thrombus forms at lesion and propagates proximally and distally to first patent outflow vessel
- CTA accurately depicts stenoses, occlusions and collateral vasculature in similar format to conventional angiography

Clinical Issues

- Disease manifests as pain or muscle cramping that worsens with activity and improves with rest
- Endovascular treatment of iliac stenotic disease
  - Focal (< 5 cm length): Angioplasty with stent 97% primary patency, 80-90% 5-year patency
  - Diffuse (> 5 cm length): May attempt angioplasty and stent placement, poorer long-term patency than bypass
- Surgical treatment of iliac stenotic or occlusive disease
  - Endovascular therapy can be attempted as first line therapy; may have inferior long-term patency compared to vascular bypass surgery
  - Surgical bypass performed as aortobifemoral graft or extra-anatomic bypass (e.g., axillofemoral graft)

    - Heavily calcified plaque may limit usefulness of rendered images; include source images for accurate interpretation
  - High resolution iliac images may be obtained with CTA and contrast-enhanced MRA, but technology not universally available

MR Findings

- MRA
  - Time-of-flight MRA technique inaccurate due to flow-related artifacts
    - Gadolinium enhanced MRA for more accuracy
    - Similar findings to those of angiography or CTA, but may inaccurately estimate severity of stenoses

Ultrasonographic Findings

- Color Doppler
  - Visible luminal narrowing on color Doppler, with post-stenotic turbulent flow
  - Hemodynamically significant stenosis
    - Peak systolic velocity in stenosis ≥ 2x velocity proximal to stenosis
    - Monophasic waveforms in stenosis
    - Damped waveforms distal to stenosis
  - Iliac artery duplex assessment often limited by obesity, bowel gas etc.
- Non-invasive vascular evaluation; pulse volume recording (PVR)
  - Pneumatic cuff is wrapped around extremity
  - Standardized volume of air injected, achieving standardized cuff pressure (65 mmHg)
    - Allows volume changes to be detected by a transducer and displayed as arterial waveforms
  - Ratio between arterial pressures at ankle and brachial levels calculated and reported as ankle/brachial index (ABI)

Angiographic Findings

- Current gold standard for vessel characterization
  - Accurately demonstrates arterial anatomy, stenoses, occlusions and collateral arterial pathways
  - Invasive procedure but allows for percutaneous endovascular therapies

DIFFERENTIAL DIAGNOSIS

Atherosclerosis

- Aneurysmal disease
  - May involve common and/or internal iliac arteries, with or without aortic involvement
- Dissection
  - Iatrogenic dissection secondary to diagnostic angiography or intervention
  - Spontaneous iliac dissection usually an extension from thoracoabdominal aortic dissection
    - Characteristic intimal flap separating "true" and "false" lumens
- Occlusive disease
  - Distal aortic occlusion or stenosis may extend into common iliac arteries
  - Isolated stenoses of common iliac arteries
    - Usually involves common iliac artery origins
  - Internal iliac artery origin stenoses common
  - Extensive collateralization

Embolic Disease

- Acute or subacute symptoms
- Smooth abrupt occlusions, usually at bifurcations
  - Often multifocal areas of occlusion
- Lack of collateral vessels
- Etiologies include proximal aneurysm, irregular atherosclerotic plaque, cardiac arrhythmia with intra-cardiac thrombus

Fibromuscular Dysplasia (FMD)

- Iliac arteries are 3rd most common location
- Typically female, but older age than with renal FMD
- Occlusive symptoms or spontaneous dissection

Iliac Artery Endofibrosis

- Rare entity seen in young athletes
- Linked to repetitive hip joint motion such as cycling
  - Fibrotic lesion often symptomatic only during exercise

Traumatic Occlusion

- Common cause of iliac occlusion in young patients

ILIAC ARTERY OCCLUSIVE DISEASE

- Blunt or penetrating pelvic trauma
- Catheterization related (iatrogenic) injury (e.g. dissection, hematoma, perforation, rupture)

Vasculitis

- More frequent in younger patients
- Aortic involvement in Takayasu arteritis may extend from aortic root to include common iliac arteries
- Usually pseudoaneurysmal iliac arteries in Behçet disease; adjacent arteries are highly inflammatory

PATHOLOGY

General Features

- General path comments
  - Younger patients: Trauma, vasculitis, tumor encasement, dissection more frequent etiologies
  - Older patients: Atherosclerosis most common
- Etiology
  - Atherosclerotic intimal plaques
    - From smooth muscle proliferation, extracellular lipid/collagen deposition, and inflammation
    - Plaque projects into lumen causing stenosis/occlusion
  - Risk factors for atherosclerotic vascular disease
    - Family history
    - Diabetes
    - Hypercholesterolemia
    - Smoking
- Epidemiology
  - Atherosclerotic obstruction
    - Males > > Females
    - Incidence increases with age: 3% age 45-54 yrs, 6% age 55-64 yrs

CLINICAL ISSUES

Presentation

- Most common signs/symptoms
  - Intermittent claudication
    - Typically involves buttocks and thighs with iliac occlusive disease
    - Symptoms vary with extent of arterial collaterals
- Other signs/symptoms: Impotence
- Assessment of lower extremity arterial insufficiency
  - History and physical examination focused on vasculature, including evaluation of arterial pulses
  - Non-invasive arterial assessment (e.g., PVR, ABI)
  - If strong clinical evidence of pelvic arterial disease
    - Limited imaging assessment may be satisfactory
    - Use CTA or MRA to confirm localized iliac disease
    - Proceed to endovascular intervention or surgery
  - If uncertain extent of disease, based on clinical findings, or evidence of multilevel occlusive disease
    - Comprehensive assessment of lower extremity arteries required; include PVR, ABI
    - CTA/MRA if appropriate equipment available
    - Catheter angiography if CTA/MRA unavailable
- Intermittent claudication
  - Exercise-related pain or muscle cramping, worsening with activity, and subsiding after rest
  - Graded by distance patient is able to walk
  - Location of pain may indicate level of obstruction
    - Buttock: Aorta, common or internal iliac artery
    - Thigh: External iliac, common femoral artery
- Impotence
  - Diseased internal iliac, pudendal, obturator arteries
- Leriche syndrome
  - Bilateral claudication, absent femoral pulses, impotence
    - Aortic or bilateral common iliac artery obstruction

Treatment

- Endovascular
  - Iliac stenosis
    - Focal (< 5 cm length): Angioplasty with stent 97% primary patency, 80-90% 5-year patency
    - Diffuse (> 5 cm length): May attempt angioplasty and stent placement, poorer long-term patency
    - Bilateral common iliac artery origin stenoses may require "kissing angioplasties" or "kissing stents"
  - Acute occlusive thrombus
    - Thrombolytic therapy followed by secondary endovascular or surgical procedure
    - Angioplasty may be successful; may be combined with covered or noncovered intravascular stent
    - Surgical thrombectomy
- Surgical
  - Iliac occlusion, diffuse multifocal iliac disease, or aortic stenosis/occlusion
    - Endovascular therapy can be attempted as first line treatment; may have inferior long-term patency compared to vascular bypass surgery
    - Surgical bypass or endarterectomy (gold standard)
  - Surgical bypass
    - Aorto-bifemoral or extra-anatomic bypass (e.g., axillofemoral bypass graft)

DIAGNOSTIC CHECKLIST

Consider

- Endovascular therapy as first line treatment for iliac stenosis or occlusion; may have inferior long-term patency compared to vascular bypass surgery

SELECTED REFERENCES

1. De Roeck A et al: Long-term results of primary stenting for long and complex iliac artery occlusions. Acta Chir Belg. 106(2):187-92, 2006
2. Kropman RH et al: Long-term results of percutaneous transluminal angioplasty for symptomatic iliac in-stent stenosis. Eur J Vasc Endovasc Surg. 32(6):634-8, 2006
3. Castelli P et al: Hybrid treatment for juxtarenal aortic occlusion: successful revascularization using iliofemoral semiclosed endarterectomy and kissing-stents technique. J Vasc Surg. 42(3):559-63, 2005
4. Rubin GD et al: Multi-detector row CT angiography of lower extremity arterial inflow and runoff: initial experience. Radiology. 221(1):146-58, 2001
5. Lenhart M et al: [Contrast media-enhanced MR angiography of the lower extremity arteries using a dedicated peripheral vascular coil system. First clinical results] Rofo. 172(12):992-9, 2000

ILIAC ARTERY OCCLUSIVE DISEASE

IMAGE GALLERY

Typical

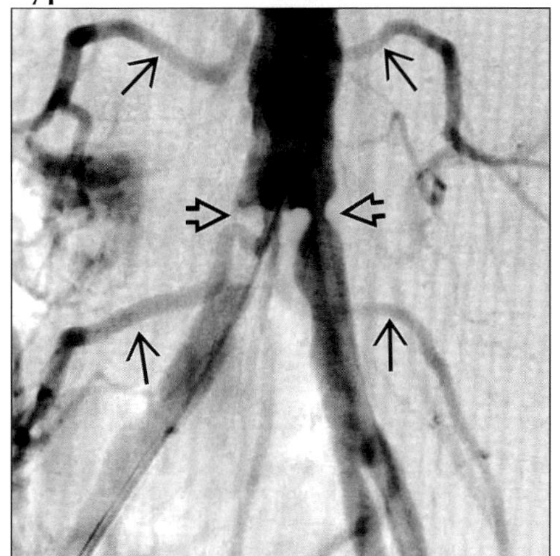

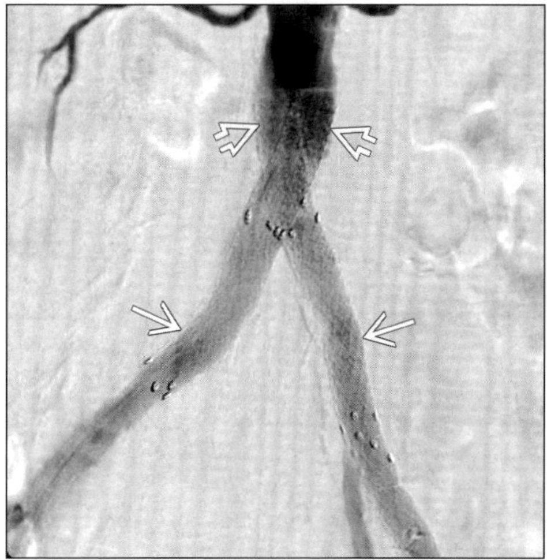

(Left) *Pelvic arteriogram shows high grade stenoses of both common iliac arteries. Prominent lumbar arteries provide collateral circulation in the presence of the stenoses.* ***(Right)*** *Pelvic arteriogram (same patient as previous) shows intravascular stents in both CIAs, eliminating the stenoses. Stents extend proximally into the distal abdominal aorta. This "kissing stent" technique is used in bifurcation lesions such as bilateral CIA stenoses.*

Typical

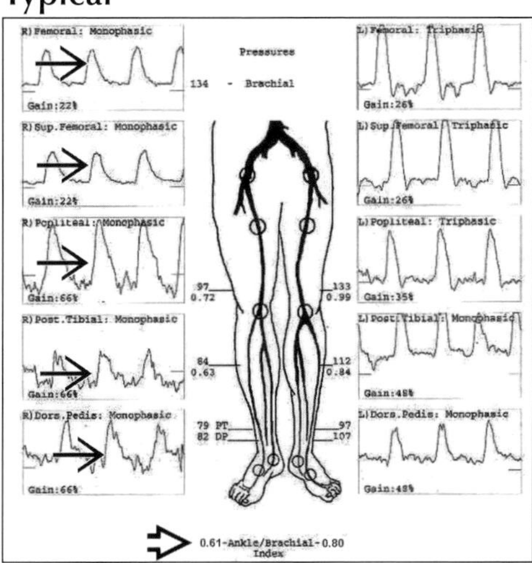

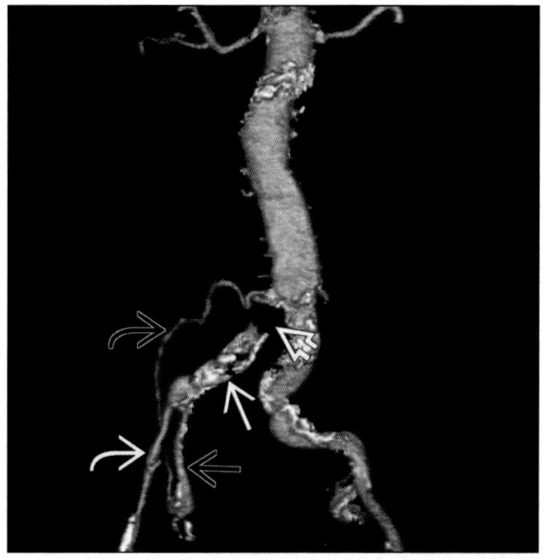

(Left) *Non-invasive vascular evaluation with pulse volume recording (PVR) and ankle/brachial index (ABI) shows monophasic waveforms at all levels in the right lower extremity, and an abnormal ABI of 0.61. Findings suggest pelvic arterial inflow disease.* ***(Right)*** *3-D CTA shows right CIA occlusion with circumferential calcification. A large lumbar arterial collateral reconstitutes the right internal and external iliac arteries.*

Typical

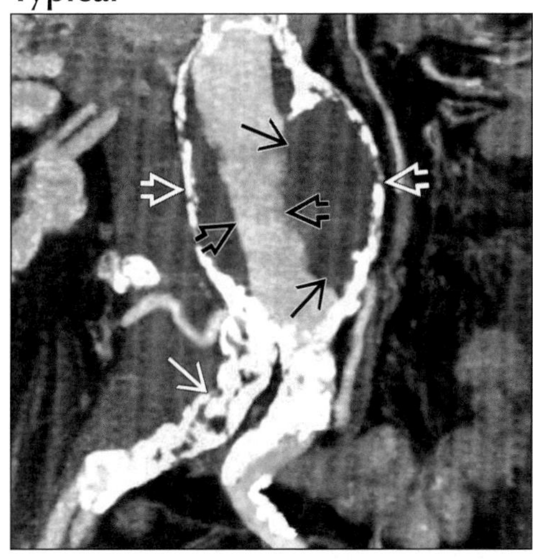

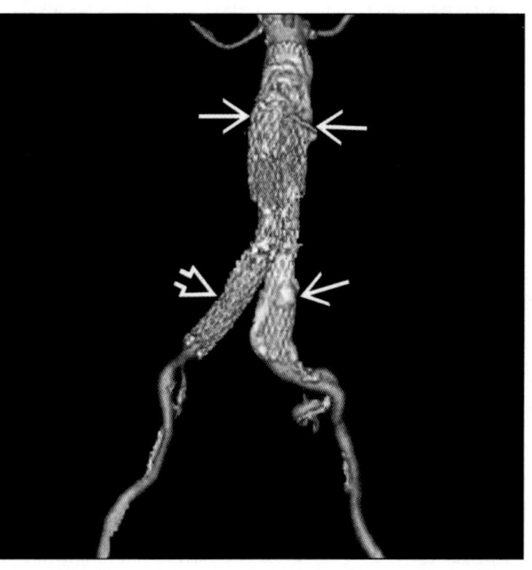

(Left) *Coronal CECT (same patient as previous) shows an abdominal aortic aneurysm (AAA) in addition to the CIA occlusion. The aneurysm has laminar thrombus & a normal caliber lumen centrally.* ***(Right)*** *3-D CTA (same patient as previous) after endovascular repair of the AAA shows an aortic stent graft has been placed. The occluded right CIA was recanalized during the procedure, with placement of the right iliac limb of the graft.*

ILIAC ARTERY ANEURYSMAL DISEASE

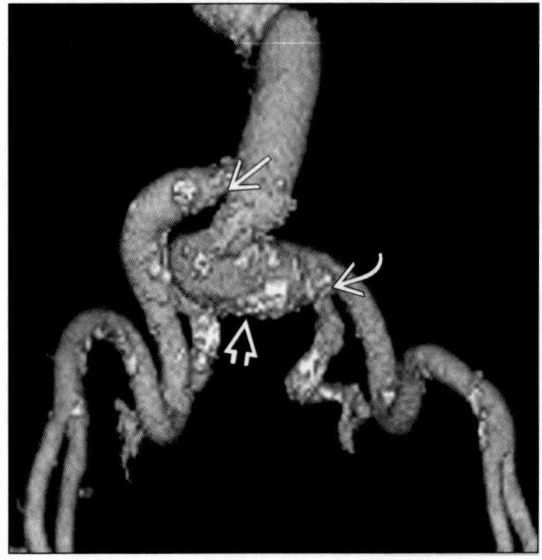

Right anterior oblique CTA shows a large left common iliac artery aneurysm ➡ extending from the aortic bifurcation ➡ to the left iliac bifurcation ➡. Aneurysm repair is recommended if the diameter exceeds 3 cm.

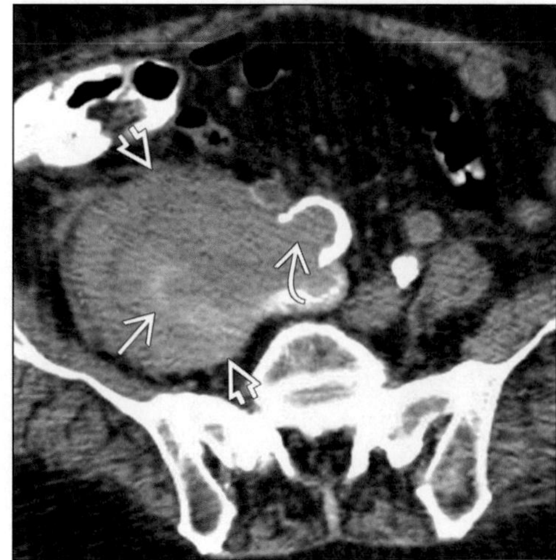

Axial CECT shows rupture ➡ of a right common iliac artery aneurysm with layering of contrast ➡ dependently. There is a defect ➡ in the calcified wall of the iliac artery aneurysm at the site of the rupture.

TERMINOLOGY

Abbreviations and Synonyms

- Iliac artery aneurysm (IAA)
- Common iliac artery (CIA)
- Internal iliac artery (hypogastric artery)
- External iliac artery (EIA)
- Abdominal aortic aneurysm (AAA)

Definitions

- Iliac artery aneurysm: Focal or diffuse dilatation more than 1.5 times normal iliac artery diameter
  - Regarded as aneurysmal if ≥ 25 mm in diameter
- Fusiform aneurysm diffusely and circumferentially involves lengthy arterial segment
- Saccular aneurysm focally involves arterial segment; appears as focal outpouching or bulge
- "True" aneurysm contains all three arterial wall layers
  - Most commonly due to atherosclerosis
- "False" aneurysm (pseudoaneurysm) does not contain all three layers of arterial wall
  - Focal or diffuse disruption of arterial wall
  - Causes include iatrogenic or penetrating trauma, contained rupture, vascular infection (mycotic)

IMAGING FINDINGS

General Features

- Best diagnostic clue: Focal or diffuse iliac arterial enlargement; mural calcification may define margins
- Location
  - Aneurysms involve common and internal iliac arteries > external iliac arteries
    - Common iliac arteries extend from aortic bifurcation to terminate as bifurcation into internal and external iliac arteries
    - Internal iliac arteries extend from common iliac artery bifurcation to terminate as bifurcation into anterior and posterior divisions
    - External iliac arteries extend from common iliac bifurcation to terminate at inguinal ligament
- Size
  - Enlargement greater than 1.5 times normal iliac artery diameter
    - If diameter exceeds 25 mm considered aneurysm
- Morphology: May be fusiform or saccular; may be continuous with abdominal aortic aneurysm (most common) or may be isolated

DDx: Iliac Artery Aneurysmal Disease

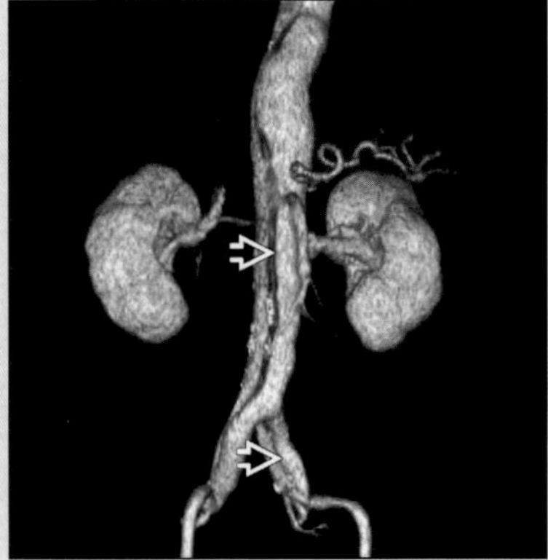

Aortoiliac Dissection

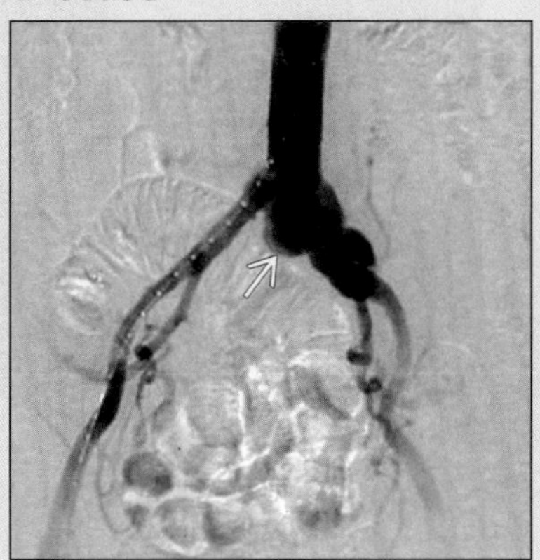

Anastomotic Pseudoaneurysm

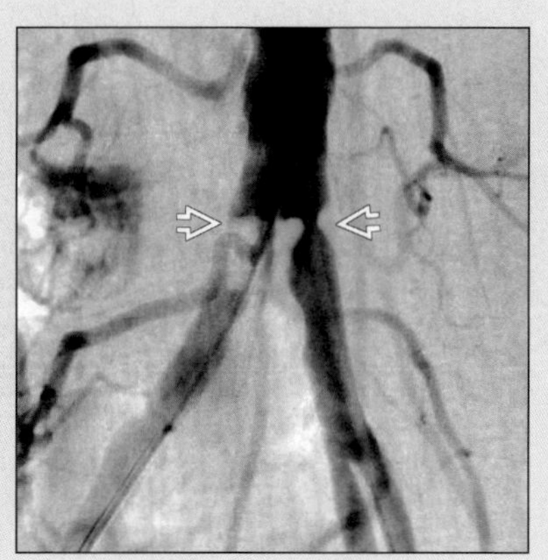

Iliac Artery Stenosis

ILIAC ARTERY ANEURYSMAL DISEASE

Key Facts

Imaging Findings

- Aneurysms involve common and internal iliac arteries > external iliac arteries
  - Iliac artery aneurysm defined as vessel diameter > 1.5 times normal iliac artery diameter or ≥ 25 mm in diameter
- CECT with CTA provides excellent information for surveillance and/or treatment planning
  - Maximum aneurysm diameter and length
  - Aneurysm relationship to aortic and iliac artery bifurcations
- Angiography with calibrated catheter may allow both diagnosis and therapy

Pathology

- Most common cause is atherosclerosis
- Isolated iliac artery aneurysms rare; 0.03% incidence

Clinical Issues

- Most iliac artery aneurysms incidentally found
  - More than 65% asymptomatic
- Natural history of progressive expansion, rupture
  - Rupture associated with up to 80% mortality risk
- Repair iliac artery aneurysm > 3 cm in diameter
  - Conventional treatment is open surgery
  - Endovascular aneurysm repair (EVAR) with stent graft increasing as primary therapy
  - Aortoiliac EVAR necessary if common iliac artery origin aneurysmal; inadequate proximal "landing zone" for graft seal and endoleak prevention
  - Common iliac artery aneurysm involving iliac bifurcation requires graft extension into external iliac artery; embolization of internal iliac artery

CT Findings

- CECT with CTA provides excellent information for surveillance and/or treatment planning
  - Maximum aneurysm diameter and length
  - Aneurysm relationship to aortic and iliac artery bifurcations
  - Anatomy of access arteries (common femoral, external iliac) if endovascular repair (EVAR) planned
    - Diameter, tortuosity, stenoses, heavy calcification
  - Presence or absence of adequate proximal/distal "landing zones" for EVAR graft fixation
    - Evaluation for endoleak following EVAR

MR Findings

- T1WI
  - High signal intensity lumen
  - Relatively low, heterogeneous signal intensity mural thrombus
- MRA: Useful for evaluation pre-EVAR anatomy, similar finding to CTA
- Calcification in aneurysm walls difficult to evaluate
- Artifact from stents or embolization coils limits evaluation of stented/coiled vessels

Ultrasonographic Findings

- Good for monitoring AAA; less reliable in iliac arteries
- Inadequate information for treatment planning
  - Shows luminal diameter, intraluminal thrombus; aneurysm diameter better measured than length
- May be limited by body habitus and overlying bowel gas

Angiographic Findings

- Pre-operative angiography usually unnecessary in majority of patients
  - Shows intraluminal diameter, relationship of aneurysm to aortic and iliac bifurcations
  - Inaccurate for aneurysm size because of mural thrombus
  - Calibrated catheter used for length measurements
- Pre-operative internal iliac artery coil embolization prior to EVAR if stent-graft is to extend beyond iliac bifurcation
  - Prevents retrograde perfusion of aneurysm sac following EVAR
  - May serve as 1° treatment for internal iliac artery aneurysm
  - Risk of buttock claudication, impotence with internal iliac artery embolization

Imaging Recommendations

- Best imaging tool
  - Noninvasive imaging modalities
    - CECT and CTA with 3D reconstruction
    - MRI/MRA: Gated SE T1, enhanced 3D GE
  - Angiography with calibrated catheter may allow both diagnosis and therapy

DIFFERENTIAL DIAGNOSIS

Atherosclerotic Stenosis or Occlusion

- Luminal narrowing secondary to laminar thrombus in aneurysm may mimic stenosis
- Thrombosed aneurysm may mimic atherosclerotic occlusion
- Distal aortic occlusive disease usually extends to involve common iliac arteries
  - With severe stenosis may have post-stenotic dilatation in adjacent arterial segment

Iliac Artery Dissection

- Extension from thoracoabdominal or abdominal aortic dissection most common etiology
  - Iliac and/or femoral artery extension in 50% of abdominal aortic dissections
- Intimal flap divides into "true" and "false" lumens
  - True lumen circumferentially lined with intima
  - False lumen lies outside of intima
    - May thrombose and/or compress true lumen

Anastomotic Pseudoaneurysm

- Associated with AAA repair in 0.5-5%

- Due to suture line disruption, graft or arterial wall failure, infection, technical error
- Repair if symptomatic (e.g., rupture, thrombosis, embolus), or diameter twice aortic graft diameter

Fibromuscular Dysplasia

- Iliac arteries third most common location for FMD
- Typically female, older age than in renal artery FMD
- May have occlusive symptoms, occasional spontaneous dissection

PATHOLOGY

General Features

- Etiology
  - Most common cause is atherosclerosis
  - Other causes include
    - Chronic dissection
    - Inflammatory (unknown etiology; younger patient; enhancing circumferential rim of tissue)
    - Vasculitis (e.g., Behçet disease, Takayasu arteritis)
    - Infectious (mycotic aneurysm)
    - Connective tissue disorders (e.g., Ehlers-Danlos, Marfan syndrome)
    - Anastomotic or traumatic pseudoaneurysm
- Epidemiology
  - Isolated iliac artery aneurysms rare; 0.03% incidence
    - Represent 2-7% of all intra-abdominal aneurysms
  - Iliac artery aneurysms seen in 10-20% of patients with abdominal aortic aneurysms

CLINICAL ISSUES

Presentation

- Most common signs/symptoms
  - Most incidental findings during noninvasive imaging
    - More than 65% asymptomatic
  - When symptomatic, similar to AAA
    - Abdominal pain in 32% of symptomatic patients
    - Neurologic, genitourologic, gastrointestinal symptoms due to external compression
    - Occasional groin, hip or buttock pain
- Other signs/symptoms: Present with rupture in 40%, leading to rapid death if untreated

Demographics

- Age: Commonly occur in elderly men, similar to AAA
- Gender: Males > females

Natural History & Prognosis

- Reported overall death rate of 31% for isolated iliac artery aneurysms
- Progressive expansion with eventual rupture most common
  - Rupture associated with up to 80% mortality risk
  - Risk of rupture increases with aneurysm size
    - Repair recommended for aneurysm > 3 cm in diameter
- Occasionally may spontaneously thrombose or cause distal embolization

Treatment

- Conventional treatment is open surgery
  - Iliac artery aneurysms with compressive symptoms (neurologic or urologic) treated with open surgery
    - Endovascular treatment cannot rapidly reduce aneurysm size
  - Mortality rates after rupture and emergency treatment as high as 33%
- Endovascular aneurysm repair (EVAR) with stent grafts and/or coil embolization
  - Long term results of EVAR still unknown but EVAR playing increasing role
  - Specific strategy for treatment depends on aneurysm location and morphology
    - Aortoiliac EVAR necessary if common iliac artery origin aneurysmal; inadequate proximal "landing zone" for graft seal and endoleak prevention
    - Common iliac artery aneurysm involving iliac bifurcation requires graft extension into external iliac artery; embolization of internal iliac artery
  - Regular post-procedure follow-up imaging necessary to document aneurysm thrombosis, reduction of aneurysm sac size and lack of endoleak
    - Excellent long-term outcomes reported with regard to delayed rupture or death; few secondary interventions required

SELECTED REFERENCES

1. Dorigo W et al: The Treatment of Isolated Iliac Artery Aneurysm in Patients with Non-aneurysmal Aorta. Eur J Vasc Endovasc Surg. 2008
2. Gabrielli R et al: Classic and endovascular surgical management of isolated iliac artery aneurysms. Minerva Cardioangiol. 55(2):133-48, 2007
3. LaganÃ D et al: Endovascular treatment of isolated iliac artery aneurysms: 2-year follow-up. Radiol Med (Torino). 112(6):826-36, 2007
4. Mofidi R et al: Endovascular repair of a ruptured mycotic aneurysm of the common iliac artery. Cardiovasc Intervent Radiol. 30(5):1029-32, 2007
5. Pitoulias GA et al: Isolated iliac artery aneurysms: endovascular versus open elective repair. J Vasc Surg. 46(4):648-54, 2007
6. Stroumpouli E et al: The endovascular management of iliac artery aneurysms. Cardiovasc Intervent Radiol. 30(6):1099-104, 2007
7. van Kelckhoven BJ et al: Ruptured internal iliac artery aneurysm: staged emergency endovascular treatment in the interventional radiology suite. Cardiovasc Intervent Radiol. 30(4):774-7, 2007
8. Boules TN et al: Endovascular management of isolated iliac artery aneurysms. J Vasc Surg. 44(1):29-37, 2006
9. Tielliu IF et al: Endovascular treatment of iliac artery aneurysms with a tubular stent-graft: mid-term results. J Vasc Surg. 43(3):440-5, 2006
10. Dix FP et al: The isolated internal iliac artery aneurysm--a review. Eur J Vasc Endovasc Surg. 30(2):119-29, 2005
11. Sakamoto I et al: Endovascular treatment of iliac artery aneurysms. Radiographics. 25 Suppl 1:S213-27, 2005
12. Sandhu RS et al: Isolated iliac artery aneurysms. Semin Vasc Surg. 18(4):209-15, 2005

IMAGE GALLERY

Typical

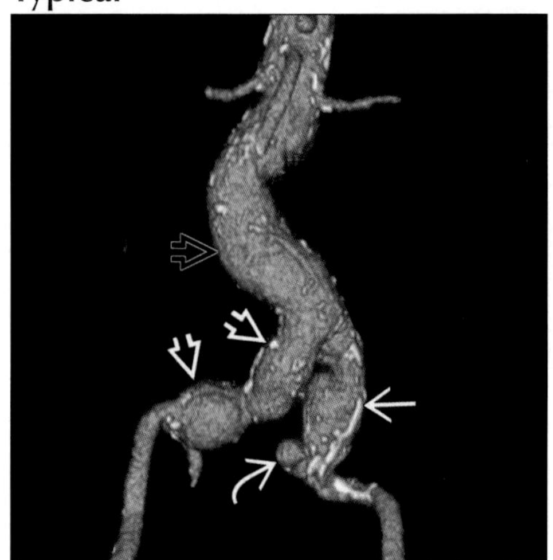

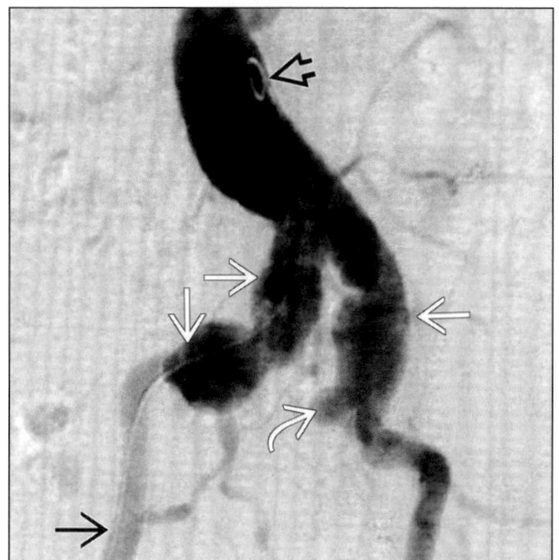

(Left) *Right anterior oblique CTA shows aneurysms of both the right ➡ & left ➡ common iliac arteries & of the left internal iliac artery ➡. There is also a small infrarenal aortic aneurysm ➡. Up to 20% of patients with AAA also have iliac artery aneurysms.* ***(Right)*** *Catheter angiography (same patient as previous) shows the fusiform aneurysms of both common iliac arteries ➡ & the left internal iliac artery ➡. A pigtail catheter ➡ enters via the right common femoral artery →.*

Typical

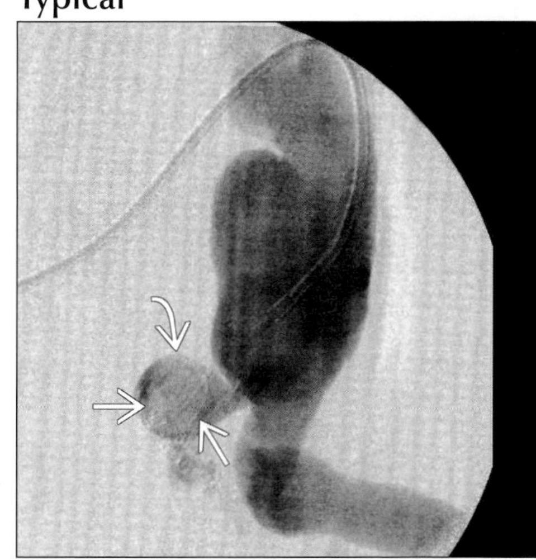

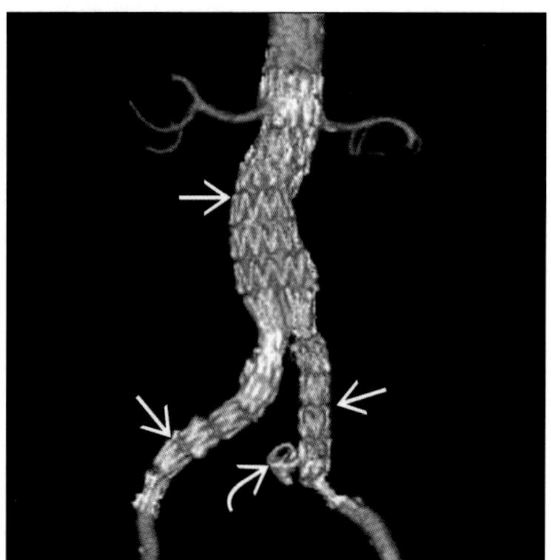

(Left) *Catheter angiography shows embolization coils ➡ in the left internal iliac artery aneurysm ➡, placed prior to endovascular repair (EVAR) of the aortic and iliac artery aneurysms.* ***(Right)*** *CTA shows exclusion of the aortic and iliac artery aneurysms following placement of an aorto-iliac stent graft ➡ and embolization coils ➡ in the left internal iliac artery aneurysm. Aortoiliac EVAR was indicated because of the combination of AAA and fusiform common iliac artery aneurysms.*

Typical

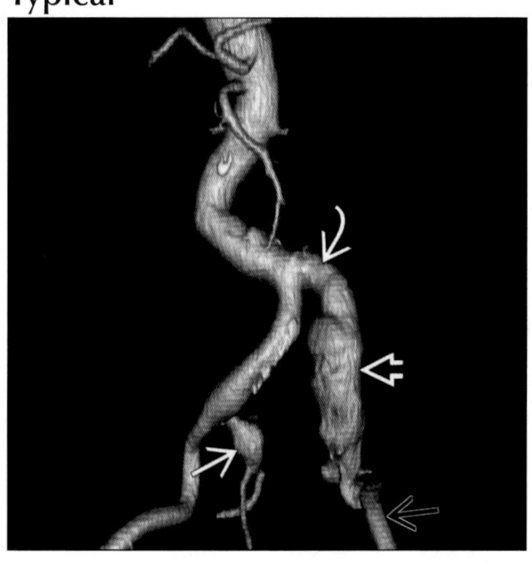

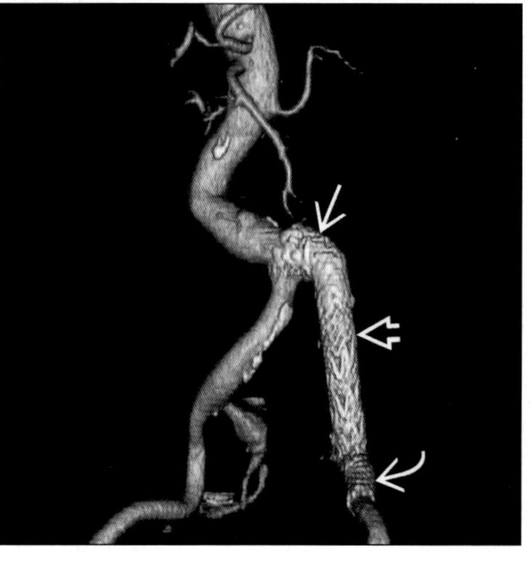

(Left) *CTA shows aneurysms of the left common iliac ➡ and proximal right internal iliac ➡ arteries. The proximal left common iliac ➡ and the external iliac → arteries are normal in caliber, allowing for EVAR with a single stent-graft.* ***(Right)*** *CTA shows EVAR of the left common iliac artery aneurysm with the stent-graft ➡ extending from the normal caliber "landing zone" of the proximal common iliac artery ➡ to the normal caliber external iliac artery ➡.*

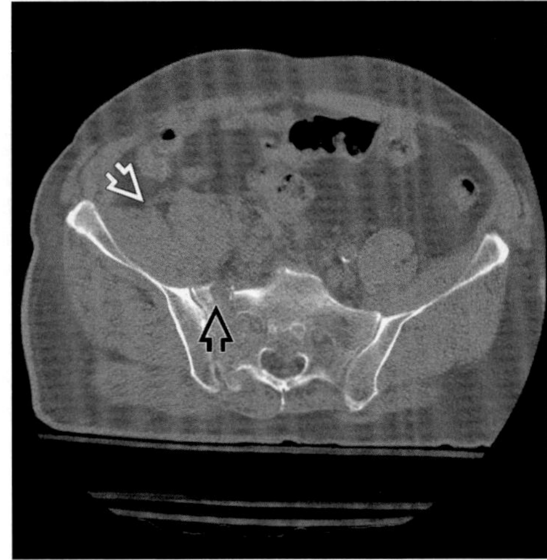

Axial NECT shows fracture in right sacrum ⇨ with a hematoma ➡ in the right iliopsoas, but no evidence of extravasation. The patient became hemodynamically unstable and the following angiogram was performed.

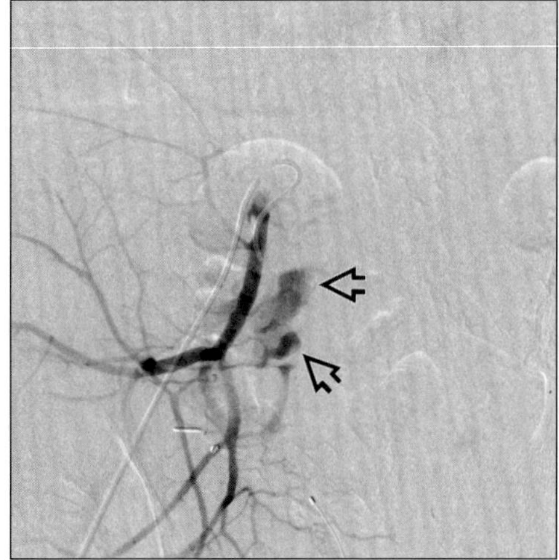

DSA shows the anterior division of the internal iliac artery. There is significant extravasation of contrast ⇨ from a branch of the anterior division. Always treat the patient not the images.

TERMINOLOGY

Abbreviations and Synonyms

- Blunt pelvic trauma, pelvic fracture

Definitions

- Injury to the pelvic area, which may result in damage to musculoskeletal, vascular, nervous, and visceral structures

IMAGING FINDINGS

General Features

- Best diagnostic clue
  - Extravasation of contrast on pelvic CT in region of bony fracture
  - Fractures of the pelvic ring on AP radiograph
  - Blood and fluid accumulation within the pelvis and peritoneum
  - Extravasation of contrast during retrograde urethrogram
- Location
  - Pelvic ring composed of the ilium, ischium, and pubis
    - Joined together anteriorly at pubic symphysis
    - Posteriorly connected to sacrum at sacroiliac joints

Radiographic Findings

- Radiography
  - Gross pathologic fractures and dislocations, can detect up to 90% of fractures
  - Hemoperitoneum
    - Classic signs such as "dog ears" and "bladder ears" represent accumulations of blood within dependent portions of pelvis
- IVP
  - Extravasation of contrast material; renal injury is commonly associated with pelvic trauma
    - Extravasation of contrast along the ureter is indicative of a site of ureteral injury

CT Findings

- Best evaluation of bony pelvis and evaluation of pelvic organs that may be injured
- Contrast CT will show areas of extravasated contrast material in areas of active hemorrhage

DDx: Pelvic Trauma

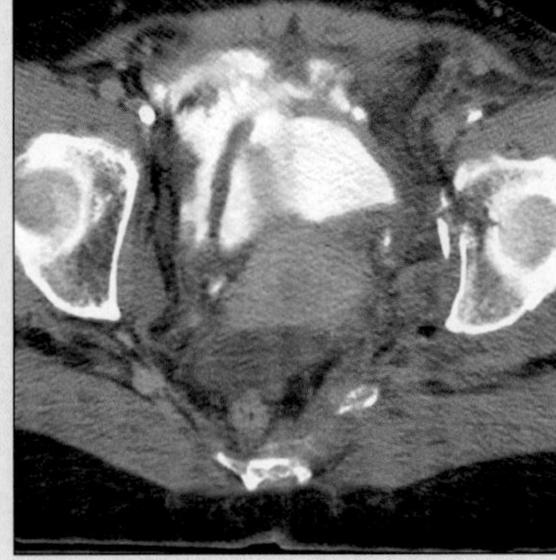

Bladder Extravasation

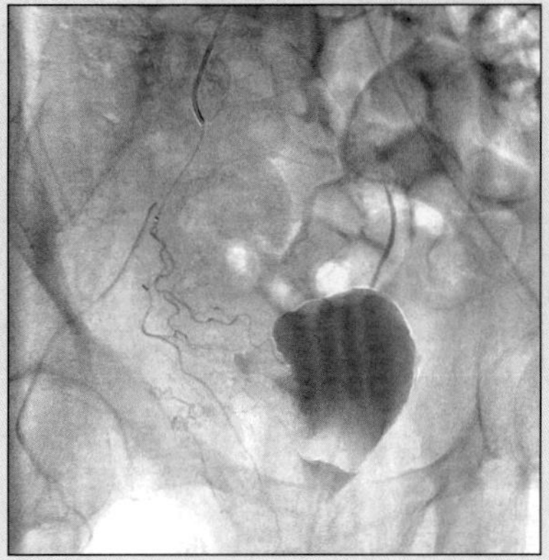

Bladder Displacement by Hematoma

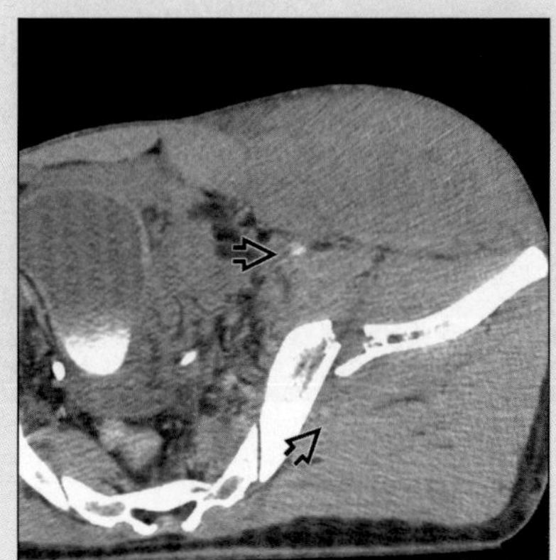

Iliac Fracture: Massive Hematoma

PELVIC TRAUMA

Key Facts

Imaging Findings

- Extravasation of contrast on pelvic CT in region of bony fracture
- Fractures of the pelvic ring on AP radiograph
- Contrast CT will show areas of extravasated contrast material in areas of active hemorrhage
- Angiography is indicated when CT shows active extravasation, a large pelvic hematoma, or in a hemodynamically unstable patient with pelvic fracture
- Retrograde urethrograms for suspected urethral injury
- Cystography detects bladder rupture, indicated when gross hematuria is present

Pathology

- Closed head injury, long bone fracture, spleen and liver trauma, kidney trauma, thoracic trauma, and peripheral nerve injury

Clinical Issues

- Patients > 60 years old have a high likelihood of active bleeding (94% compared to 52% of younger patients)
- Mortality rate ranges from 15-50%
- Interventional radiology is first choice for stabilization of patients with hemorrhage - allows selective embolization
- Early angiography and embolization to avoid development of coagulopathy and multisystem organ dysfunction
- Pelvic binding, MAST-suit, to help stabilize pelvis

  - Identify site of hemorrhage, useful adjunct in planning for angiography (embolization) and surgery
- Pelvic, intra-abdominal and retroperitoneal bleeding
- Occult intra-abdominal injuries

MR Findings

- Limited value in imaging acute trauma of pelvis
- Most valuable in confirmation or exclusion of radiographically occult fractures

Ultrasonographic Findings

- Grayscale Ultrasound
  - FAST can rapidly detect free intraperitoneal fluid
  - Less accurate in patients with major pelvic injury

Other Modality Findings

- Retrograde urethrograms for suspected urethral injury
  - Will show extravasation of contrast if urethra is disrupted
- Cystography detects bladder rupture, indicated when gross hematuria is present
  - Exclude urethral injury prior to this intervention
  - Extraperitoneal rupture: Contrast will remain next to the bladder within the perivesical space
  - Intraperitoneal rupture: Contrast will flow freely in the peritoneal cavity

Angiographic Findings

- Indicated when CT shows active extravasation, a large pelvic hematoma, or hemodynamically unstable patient with pelvic fracture
- Active arterial contrast extravasation
- Injuries to arterial branches are an indication for embolization, whereas larger artery injury may require surgery

Imaging Recommendations

- Best imaging tool: Computed tomography demonstrates fractures, may demonstrate bleeding site
- Protocol advice
  - Unstable patient
    - Focused abdominal sonogram for trauma (FAST) and/or diagnostic peritoneal lavage (DPL) and AP radiograph of pelvis to localize fractures
    - If patient remains unstable, consider angiography and embolization to diagnose and treat hemorrhage
    - Pelvic fixation first if angiography not available
  - Stable patient
    - CT of pelvis; fully evaluate and manage patients, particularly for acetabular and sacral fractures

DIFFERENTIAL DIAGNOSIS

Visceral Injuries

- Urinary bladder, urethra, ureter and bowel, all maybe damaged with pelvic injury

PATHOLOGY

General Features

- General path comments
  - Bony pelvis is a ring (ilium, ischium, and pubis) and significant force is required to disrupt the ring
    - Three basic vectors of force contribute to pelvic fracture: Anteroposterior (AP) compression, lateral compression, and vertical shear, or combination
  - Ligaments stabilize the pelvis, with separation of the pubic symphysis and SI joints, ligaments have been disrupted
  - Internal and external iliac vessels and branches are anatomically connected to the bony pelvis
    - Because of extensive vascular supply in pelvis, trauma and fracture can produce significant bleeding
    - Most bleeding venous; about 10-15% arterial
    - Arteries most likely to be injured: Superior gluteal, internal pudendal, obturator, inferior gluteal, lateral sacral, iliolumbar, external iliac, deep circumflex iliac, inferior epigastric
  - Organs enclosed within pelvis susceptible to injury

    - Extraperitoneal (80%) and intraperitoneal bladder rupture (20%), ureters and urethra injury; bowel injury
  - Sacral plexus and sciatic nerve can be injured with pelvic ring fracture
  - Soft tissue injury may occur and can be detected with imaging
    - Pelvic hematomas may displace ureters and bladder
    - Loss of obturator internus, iliopsoas, and gluteal fat planes
  - With open fractures, risk of bleeding much higher, as is risk of infection
  - Male genitalia are susceptible to injury in pelvic trauma
    - Testicular and scrotal injuries are best evaluated with US and CT
    - Suspected penile fracture may be evaluated with US or caversonography
- Etiology: Motor vehicle accident, motorcycle accident, auto-pedestrian accident, falls, crush injuries
- Epidemiology
  - Pelvic injuries account for nearly 10% of injuries in blunt trauma
  - Mortality rate 15-50%
  - Causes of death include: Uncontrolled hemorrhage, associated head injury, and multiple organ failure
- Associated abnormalities: Closed head injury, long bone fracture, spleen and liver trauma, kidney trauma, thoracic trauma, and peripheral nerve injury

CLINICAL ISSUES

Presentation

- Most common signs/symptoms
  - Pain in the groin, hip, or lower back
  - Signs of urethral injury-blood at the meatus
  - Vaginal or rectal bleeding
  - Palpable fracture line
- Other signs/symptoms
  - Pelvic instability and severe shock
  - Pelvic and perineal edema, lacerations, deformities, and ecchymoses
  - Delayed recognition of a ureteric injury includes fever, flank mass, fistula, or a renal obstruction resulting in pain and hydronephrosis
  - Irregularities, crepitus, and movement of the iliac crests, pubic rami, and ischial rami
  - Rectal exam - palpation of a bony prominence, hematoma, displacement of prostate, tenderness along the fracture line
  - Decrease in anal sphincter tone may suggest serious neurologic injury

Demographics

- Age
  - Children tend to sustain a higher number of intraabdominal injuries
  - Because young adults, particularly males, more often involved in MVAs, they have higher incidence of pelvic fractures
  - Elderly patients more often sustain osteoporotic fractures, particularly isolated pubic rami fractures
  - Patients > 60 years old have a high likelihood of active bleeding (94% compared to 52% of younger patients)
- Gender
  - In men, the bladder neck, prostatic urethra, and prostate are anchored to pelvis
    - Males have higher incidence of urethral injury (15%) compared to women (6%)
  - Special consideration in women is pregnancy
    - Assess fetal well-being with ultrasound; amniotic fluid volume and placental integrity should be examined to rule out placental abruption

Natural History & Prognosis

- Mortality rate ranges from 15-50%

Treatment

- Pelvic binding, MAST-suit, to help stabilize pelvis
- Interventional radiology is first choice for stabilization of patients with hemorrhage - allows selective embolization
  - Call interventional radiology for patient with pelvic fracture with hemodynamic instability poorly responsive to fluid, no hemoperitoneum
  - Hemodynamic stability, little hemoperitoneum, and more than 4 unit transfusion in 24 hours, or 6 units in 48 hours
  - Large or expanding retroperitoneal hematoma or active bleed on CT
  - Embolization is usually with Gelfoam pledglets; particles or occasionally coils may be used
  - Early angiography and embolization to avoid development of coagulopathy and multisystem organ dysfunction
  - Success rate (assessed on hemodynamic criteria) for arterial embolization 80-100%
- External fixation of the pelvis

DIAGNOSTIC CHECKLIST

Consider

- If one fracture is present there is usually a second fracture

SELECTED REFERENCES

1. Geeraerts T et al: Clinical review: initial management of blunt pelvic trauma patients with haemodynamic instability. Crit Care. 11(1):204, 2007
2. Rice PL Jr et al: Pelvic fractures. Emerg Med Clin North Am. 2007
3. Durkin A et al: Contemporary management of pelvic fractures. Am J Surg. 192(2):211-23, 2006
4. Dyer GS et al: Review of the pathophysiology and acute management of haemorrhage in pelvic fracture. Injury. 37(7):602-13, 2006

IMAGE GALLERY

Typical

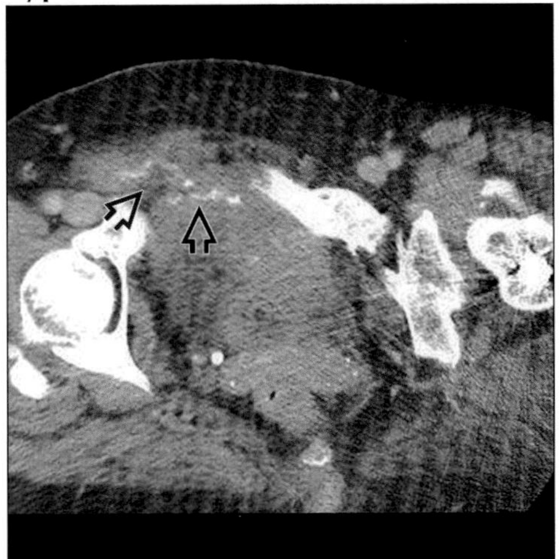

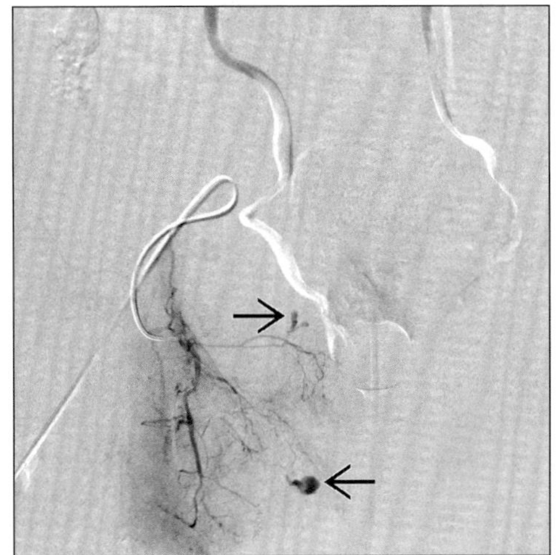

*(**Left**) Axial CECT shows pelvic ramus fracture with extravasation of contrast ➩ extending into the soft tissues of the anterior abdominal wall. This patient fell from about 30 feet and needed significant fluids to maintain her blood pressure. (**Right**) DSA shows catheter in a branch of the common femoral artery. No bleeding was seen from the internal iliac. Bleeding can arise from multiple vessels in pelvic trauma. There are two branches → involved.*

Typical

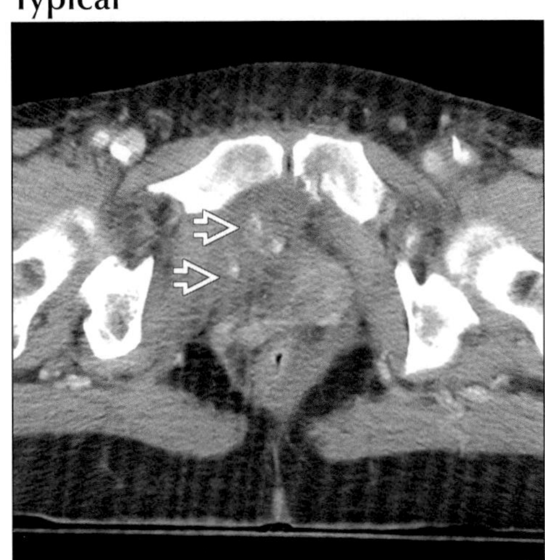

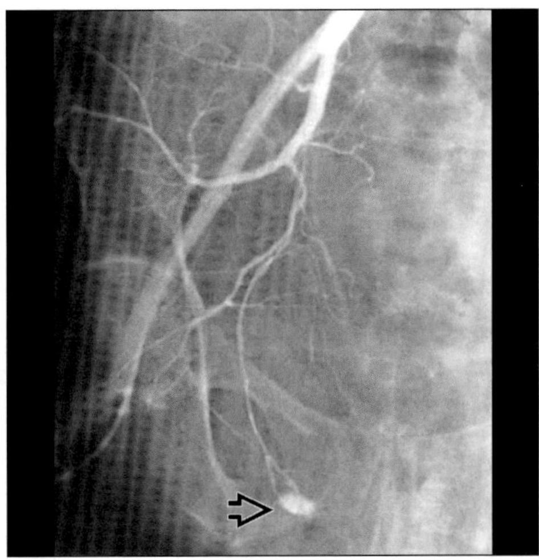

*(**Left**) Axial CECT shows contrast extravasation ➩ with a hematoma involving the right-sided soft tissues. The patient was becoming hemodynamically unstable and was taken to angiography. (**Right**) Catheter angiography shows a non-selective injection with the catheter in the distal aorta. Extravasation can be easily identified ➩. The internal iliac branches are quite small, suggesting shock.*

Typical

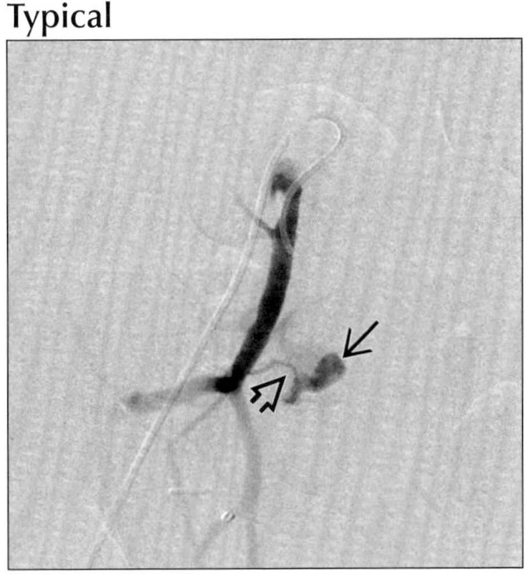

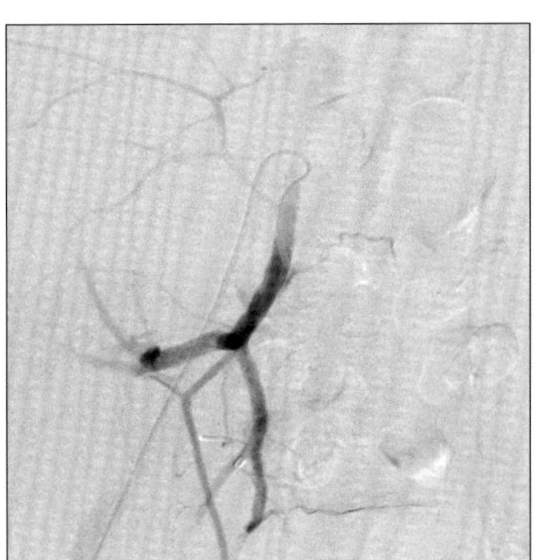

*(**Left**) DSA shows angiogram, with the catheter selectively in anterior division of internal iliac artery. An oblique view clearly demonstrates the small, damaged branch ➩, and extravasation →. Embolization can now be performed. (**Right**) DSA (same view as previous image), following selective Gelfoam embolization. Bleeding was stopped. In most cases of pelvic trauma Gelfoam is embolization material of choice. Occasionally coils will be used.*

UTERINE ARTERY EMBOLIZATION

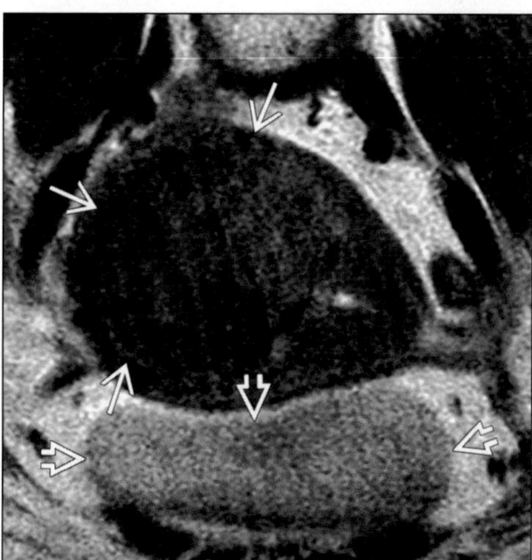

Coronal T1WI MR shows a large intramural fibroid ➡ within the uterine fundus. In addition to menorrhagia and pelvic discomfort, the patient had urinary frequency as a result of pressure on the urinary bladder ➡.

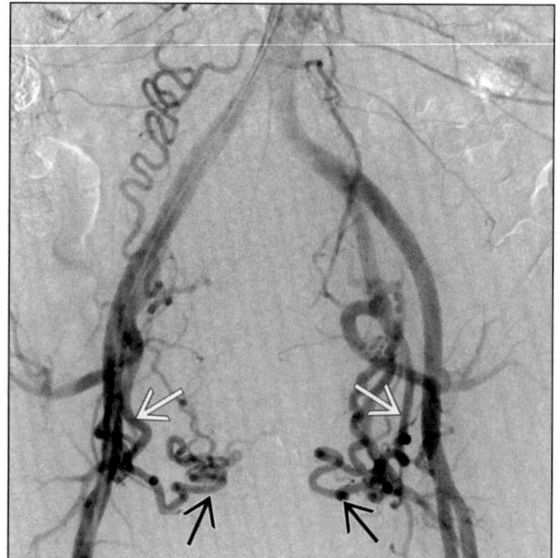

Pelvic arteriogram (same patient as previous image) shows enlarged uterine arteries ➡ with hypertrophied distal branches ➡ supplying the fibroid. After uterine artery embolization her symptoms resolved.

TERMINOLOGY

Abbreviations and Synonyms

- Uterine artery embolization (UAE)
- Uterine fibroid embolization (UFE)

Definitions

- Uterine fibroid (myoma, leiomyoma): Benign muscular tumor occurring in the female uterus
- Uterine artery embolization: A therapy in which uterine arteries are catheterized and embolic material is injected to occlude arterial supply to uterine fibroid

IMAGING FINDINGS

General Features

- Location
  - Fibroids named according to position in uterus, with center of fibroid dictating the location
    - Submucosal: Protruding into endometrial cavity
    - Intramural: Within myometrium
    - Subserosal: Based in myometrium, but covered by parietal peritoneum
    - Transmural: Extending from serosal to endometrial surface
    - Pedunculated: Attached to uterus by stalk
    - Cervical: Within uterine cervix

MR Findings

- Dominant tumor signal classified as hypointense, isointense or hyperintense compared to myometrium
- On post-embolization MR, degree of fibroid shrinkage does not correlate with outcome but incomplete infarction predicts regrowth and symptom recurrence

Ultrasonographic Findings

- Grayscale Ultrasound: Well-defined hypoechoic masses that are typically poorly reflective with relatively poor through transmission
- Color Doppler
  - Flow in dominant fibroid graded as hypovascular, normal or hypervascular compared to myometrium
  - Typically have marked peripheral blood flow (perifibroid plexus) and decreased central flow

Angiographic Findings

- Uterine arteries arise from anterior division of hypogastric arteries

DDx: Painful Pelvic Processes

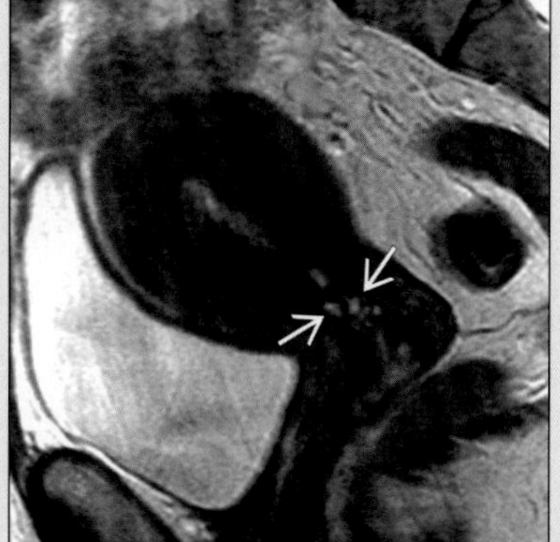

Uterine Adenomyosis

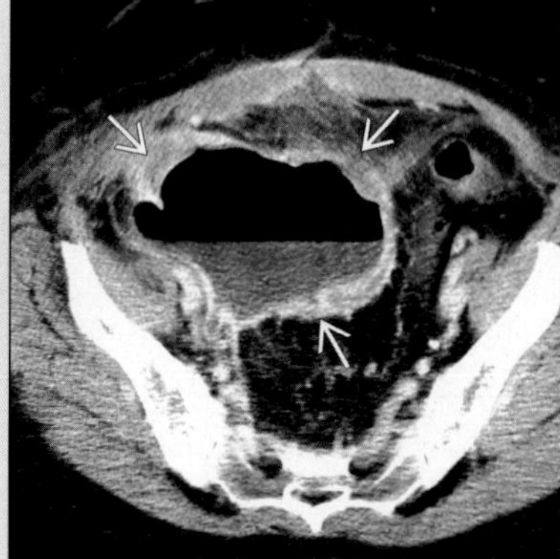

Tubo-Ovarian Abscess

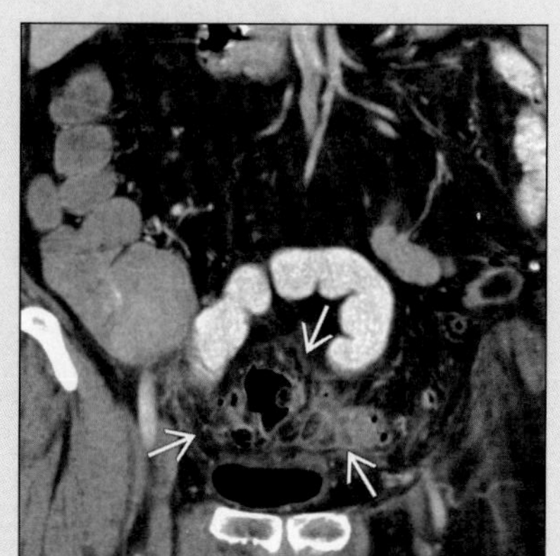

Diverticulitis

UTERINE ARTERY EMBOLIZATION

Key Facts

Terminology
- Uterine fibroid (myoma, leiomyoma): Benign muscular tumor occurring in the female uterus
- Uterine artery embolization: A therapy in which uterine arteries are catheterized and embolic material is injected to occlude arterial supply to uterine fibroid

Imaging Findings
- Fibroids named according to position in uterus, with center of fibroid dictating the location
- MR shows fibroid vascularity and architecture
- Angiography shows vascular fibroid tumor blush

Pathology
- Most common female reproductive tract tumor

Clinical Issues
- Most common signs/symptoms
  - Heavy menstrual bleeding, anemia, pelvic pressure, vague discomfort, bloating or pain
  - Bulk symptoms: Pressure on adjacent structures
- Incidence of fibroids increases with age (40-60)
- Fibroids present in 40% of women still menstruating beyond age 50
- Uterine fibroid embolization
  - Selective bilateral uterine artery catheterization
  - Embolization with microspheres until complete occlusion of flow to fibroids and slow flow in main uterine arteries
- Significant improvement in pelvic pain or discomfort in 83% and improvement in urinary problems in 69% of patients in large series

- Prominent uterine artery with vascular tumor blush
  - Catheter advanced sufficiently into uterine artery so embolic material does not reflux into other vessels
  - Embolization until sluggish flow in uterine artery and elimination of fibroid blush

Imaging Recommendations
- Best imaging tool
  - MR for preprocedural imaging
    - Best anatomic detail of fibroid size and location
    - Demonstrates internal architecture of fibroids, enabling determination of fibroid degeneration
    - Evaluates vascularity of fibroid
    - Sensitive and specific for alternate diagnosis of adenomyosis
  - Angiography for imaging during embolization
- Protocol advice: Sagittal T1WI and T2WI FS oblique coronal, axial and sagittal sequences with gadolinium

DIFFERENTIAL DIAGNOSIS

Uterine
- Adenomyosis/endometriosis
- Other neoplasms: Adenocarcinoma, leiomyosarcoma

Adnexal
- Ovarian cyst
- Ovarian neoplasms: Adenocarcinoma, germ cell tumor, metastatic, sex cord-stromal tumors
- Ectopic pregnancy
- Tubo-ovarian abscess

Bladder
- Neoplasm
- Neurogenic

Bowel
- Inflammatory: Appendicitis, diverticulitis, abscess
- Neoplasm

Pelvic Congestion Syndrome
- Reflux in incompetent ovarian veins results in dilated pelvic varicosities

PATHOLOGY

General Features
- General path comments
  - Fibroids unicellular in origin; growth influenced by estrogen, growth hormone, and progesterone
  - Arise during reproductive years, may enlarge during pregnancy and regress after menopause
- Etiology: Risk factors include nulliparity, obesity, family history, black race, and hypertension
- Epidemiology
  - Most common female reproductive tract tumor
  - Higher incidence of uterine fibroid tumors in African-American women
  - Some evidence that African-American women more likely to have larger and more symptomatic tumors

CLINICAL ISSUES

Presentation
- Most common signs/symptoms: Heavy menstrual bleeding, anemia, pelvic pressure, vague discomfort, bloating or pain
- Other signs/symptoms
  - Bulk symptoms: Pressure on adjacent structures
    - Urinary bladder: Frequency, urgency, nocturia; occasionally incontinence, hydronephrosis
    - Bowel: Rectal pain or pressure, constipation
    - Endometrium: Infertility, repeated miscarriages, complicated pregnancies

Demographics
- Age
  - Incidence of fibroids increases with age (40-60)
  - Fibroids present in 40% of women still menstruating beyond age 50

Treatment
- Uterine fibroid embolization
  - Preprocedural evaluation and patient selection
    - Clinical examination, pelvic MR and ultrasound

UTERINE ARTERY EMBOLIZATION

  - Premenopausal patient aged 30-50 with symptomatic fibroids, usually with menorrhagia
  - Postmenopausal women should rarely undergo UFE for fibroids as most fibroids shrink after menopause and become asymptomatic
  - Exclusion of malignancy with biopsy if necessary
  - Size of largest fibroid shown to be inversely related to success of UFE; may have suboptimal results if one or more fibroids larger than 10 cm
- Selective bilateral uterine artery embolization from a femoral arterial approach
  - Catheter selection based on operator preference
  - Typically a 4 or 5 Fr cobra catheter with Waltman loop technique employed to selectively catheterize uterine arteries, with optional microcatheter use
  - Initial embolic agents were polyvinyl alcohol particles (PVA) or gelatin sponge (Gelfoam)
  - Tris-acryl gelatin microspheres (embospheres) now agent of choice: Uniform particles in various sizes, with 500-700 or 700-900 micron particles used
  - Preferred endpoint is complete occlusion of flow to fibroids, with slow flow in main uterine artery
  - Patient admitted for overnight care, with pain management according to local practice
- Causes of failure of uterine fibroid embolization
  - Failure to successfully catheterize one or both uterine arteries
  - Blood supply to fibroids from sources other than uterine arteries, most commonly ovarian arteries
  - Uterine artery spasm, with poor flow into perifibroid plexus and insufficient delivery of embolic material
  - Clumping of embolic agent yields false endpoint, with appearance of occlusion; later redistribution restores flow (less problematic with embospheres)
  - Incomplete fibroid infarction on post-procedure imaging; regrowth over time, with symptom recurrence
- Treatment results
  - Postprocedural MR at 3 months if bulk symptoms persist and at 6 months if clinical success
  - Complete infarction of all fibroids by follow-up MR predicts excellent long-term outcome
  - Significant improvement in pelvic pain or discomfort in 83% and improvement in urinary problems in 69% of patients in large series
- Complications
  - Prolonged pain, fever, groin hematoma, sudden transient hypertension, infection
  - Necrotic pedunculated submucosal fibroid expulsion
  - Uterine ischemia and necrosis

- Alternate treatment options for uterine fibroids
  - Gonadotropin-releasing hormone agonists
    - Pre-operative treatment to decrease size of tumors before hysterectomy, myomectomy, or myolysis
    - Costly long-term therapy; bone loss, menopausal symptoms, recurrence risk with myomectomy
  - Hysterectomy
    - Surgical removal of the uterus (transabdominal, transvaginal, or laparoscopic)
    - Definitive treatment for women who do not wish to preserve fertility
    - Substantially improves symptoms and quality of life in women with multiple and severe symptoms
  - Myomectomy
    - Surgical or endoscopic excision of fibroids
    - Resolution of symptoms with preserved fertility; perioperative morbidity similar to hysterectomy
    - 5 year recurrence rate of 15-30%; success determined by number and extent of fibroids
  - Myolysis
    - In situ destruction of tumors by heat, laser, focused ultrasound or cryotherapy
    - Minimal blood loss; rapid recovery time
    - Delayed uterine size reduction; unknown recurrence risk

DIAGNOSTIC CHECKLIST

Consider

- Uterine fibroid embolization as primary therapy in premenopausal patient with symptomatic fibroids
- Alternative treatment modalities if multiple extremely large fibroids (> 10 cm)
- Blood supply to fibroids from sources other than uterine arteries during embolization procedure

Image Interpretation Pearls

- If fibroid avascular on preprocedural imaging, embolization not beneficial
- After successful uterine fibroid embolization, there should no longer be gadolinium enhancement on MR

SELECTED REFERENCES

1. Borghese B et al: Treatment of symptomatic uterine fibroids. N Engl J Med. 356(21):2218-9; author reply 2219, 2007
2. Chrisman HB et al: Uterine artery embolization: a treatment option for symptomatic fibroids in postmenopausal women. J Vasc Interv Radiol. 18(3):451-4, 2007
3. Edwards RD et al: Uterine-artery embolization versus surgery for symptomatic uterine fibroids. N Engl J Med. 356(4):360-70, 2007
4. Evans P et al: Uterine fibroid tumors: diagnosis and treatment. Am Fam Physician. 75(10):1503-8, 2007
5. Jacobson GF et al: Changes in rates of hysterectomy and uterine conserving procedures for treatment of uterine leiomyoma. Am J Obstet Gynecol. 196(6):601, 2007
6. Justesen P: [Embolization for treatment of symptomatic uterine fibroma] Ugeskr Laeger. 169(17):1548-50, 2007
7. Radeleff BA et al: [Clinical 3-year follow-up of uterine fibroid embolization] Rofo. 179(6):593-600, 2007
8. Spies JB et al: Long-term outcome from uterine fibroid embolization with tris-acryl gelatin microspheres: results of a multicenter study. J Vasc Interv Radiol. 18(2):203-7, 2007
9. White AM et al: Uterine fibroid embolization: the utility of aortography in detecting ovarian artery collateral supply. Radiology. 244(1):291-8, 2007

IMAGE GALLERY

Typical

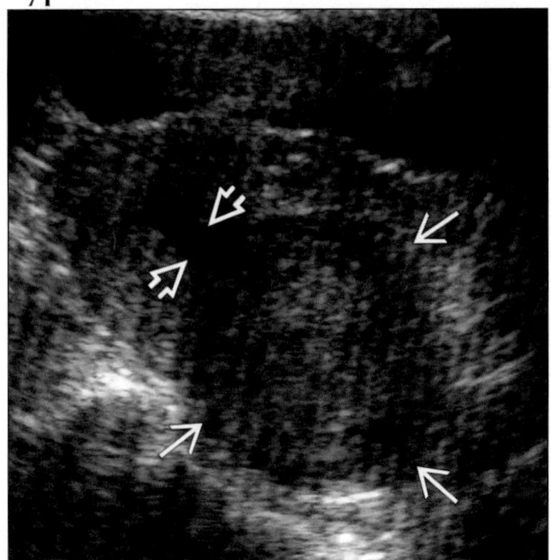

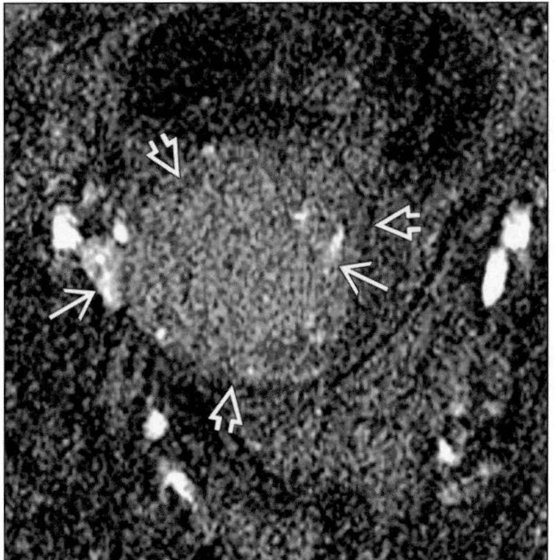

(Left) *Sagittal transabdominal pelvic US in a patient with menorrhagia & pelvic discomfort shows a large intramural uterine fibroid ➡, with submucosal margin deforming the endometrial canal ➡.* ***(Right)*** *Coronal gadolinium-enhanced T1 GRE MR (same patient as previous image) shows that the large uterine fibroid ➡ diffusely enhances & has a rich vascular supply ➡. Tumor size & vascularity are appropriate for transcatheter uterine fibroid embolization.*

Typical

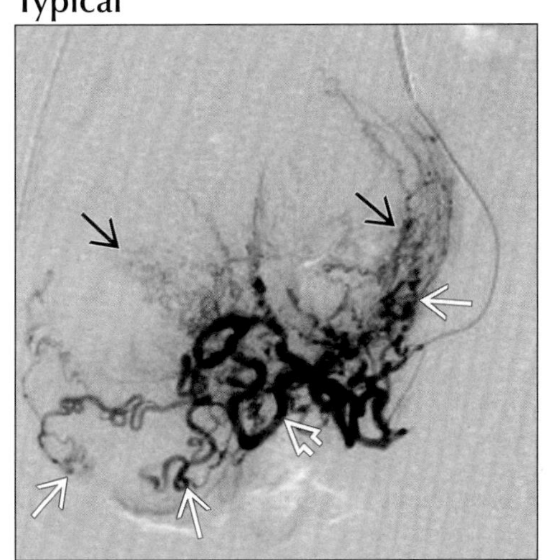

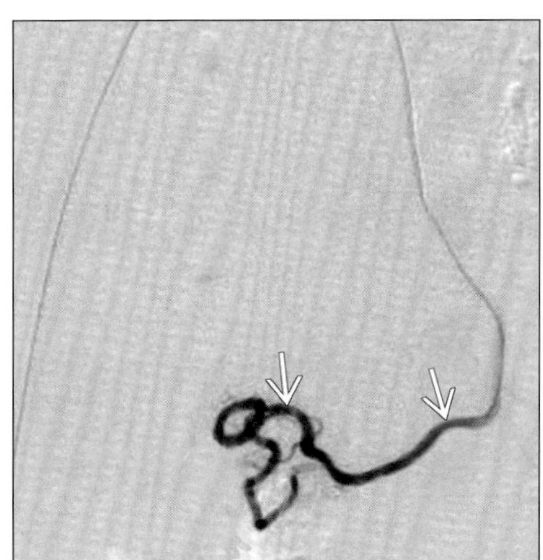

(Left) *Left uterine arteriogram (same patient as previous image) shows an extensive arterial supply ➡ to the fibroid from the main uterine artery ➡. There is a diffuse tumor blush ➡, corresponding to the enhancement on MR.* ***(Right)*** *Uterine arteriogram after transcatheter embolization with 500-700 micron particle embospheres shows slow flow in the main uterine artery ➡ but distal occlusion of flow to the fibroid. This is the preferred endpoint for optimal fibroid embolization.*

Variant

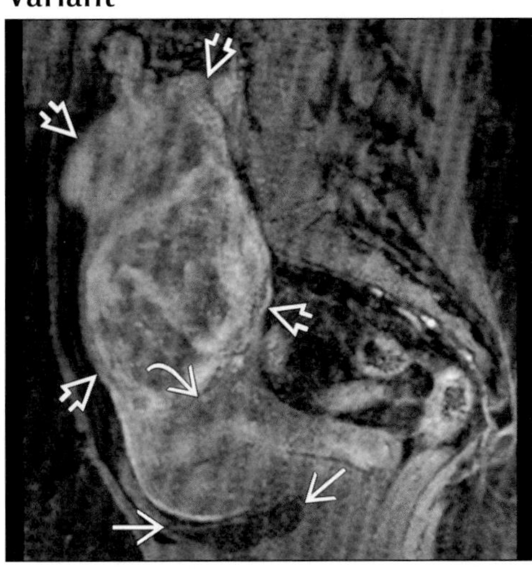

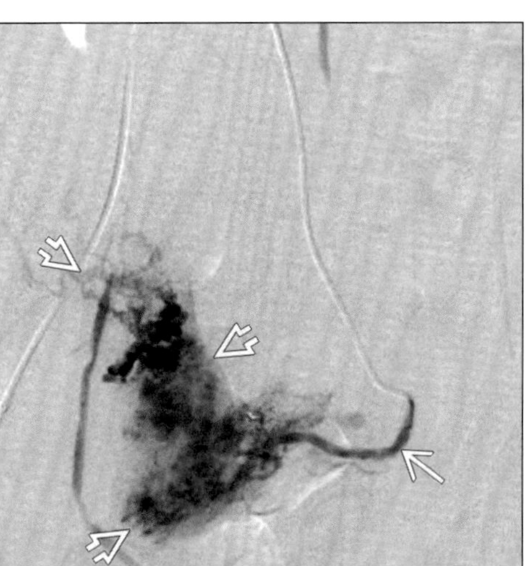

(Left) *Sagittal gadolinium-enhanced T1WI Vibe MR shows a massive exophytic subserosal fibroid ➡ arising from the uterus ➡. There were marked bulk symptoms from pressure on the urinary bladder ➡ and abdominal contents.* ***(Right)*** *Left uterine arteriogram ➡ shows an intense vascular tumor blush ➡, correlating with the enhancement and hyperintense signal on MR. Despite the massive fibroid size, the patient opted for UAE, and had relief of symptoms.*

HIGH-FLOW PRIAPISM

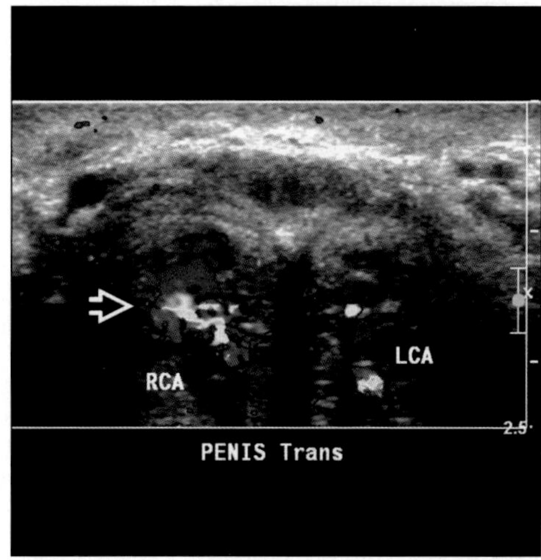

Axial color Doppler ultrasound shows high velocity turbulent flow in the right cavernosal artery ⇨. The left cavernosal artery has normal flow.

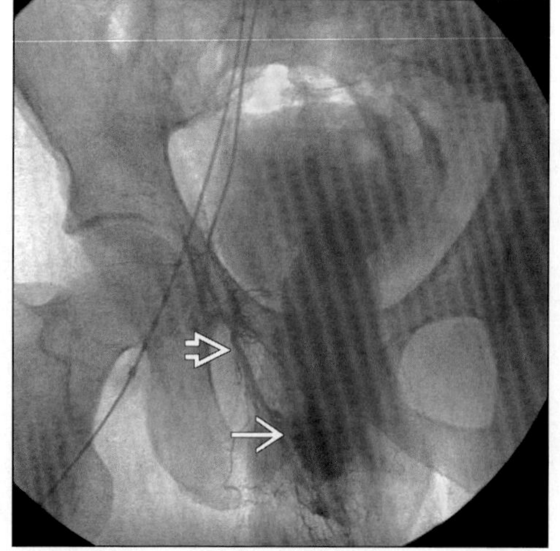

DSA with selective injection of the internal pudendal artery ⇨ shows extravasation of contrast material from the injured right cavernosal artery →.

TERMINOLOGY

Abbreviations and Synonyms

- High-flow priapism (HFP)

Definitions

- Persistent erection for greater than 6 hours not accompanied by sexual desire
  - Caused by unregulated cavernous arterial inflow
  - Most commonly caused by trauma resulting in laceration of cavernous artery
- First described by Burt et al in 1960

IMAGING FINDINGS

General Features

- Best diagnostic clue: Ultrasound in conjunction with blood gas and physical exam
- Location: Majority of fistulas are of the internal pudendal artery and its branches

Ultrasonographic Findings

- Grayscale Ultrasound
  - Irregular hypoechoic region within echogenic cavernous tissues
    - Increased blood flow with distention of lacunar spaces and tissue injury
    - May appear regular and circumscribed in long standing priapism and mimic a pseudoaneurysm
- Color Doppler
  - Demonstrates extravasated blood from lacerated cavernosal artery as area of high velocity, turbulent flow
    - Can identify feeding vessels
    - As sensitive as angiography
  - Provides lesion lateralization and localization essential before radiological embolization or surgical intervention
  - Can confirm successful or unsuccessful microvascular therapy
    - Successful cases demonstrate disappearance or reduction of fistula
    - Unsuccessful cases demonstrate patency of collateral feeding vessels or early recanalization of embolized artery
  - Combination of intraoperative color Doppler US with therapeutic angiography

DDx: High-Flow Priapism

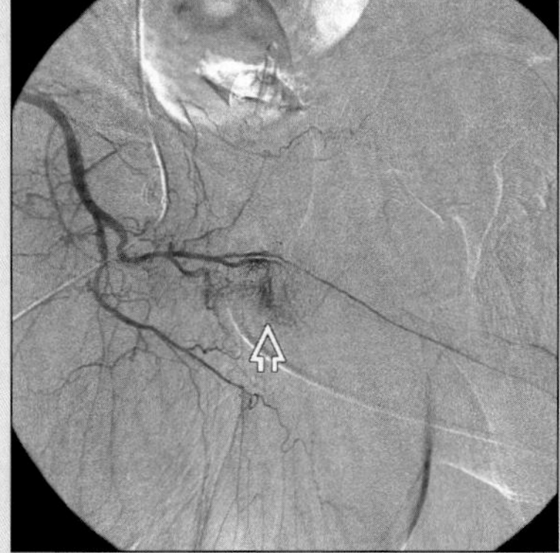

Normal Bulbous Spongiosum

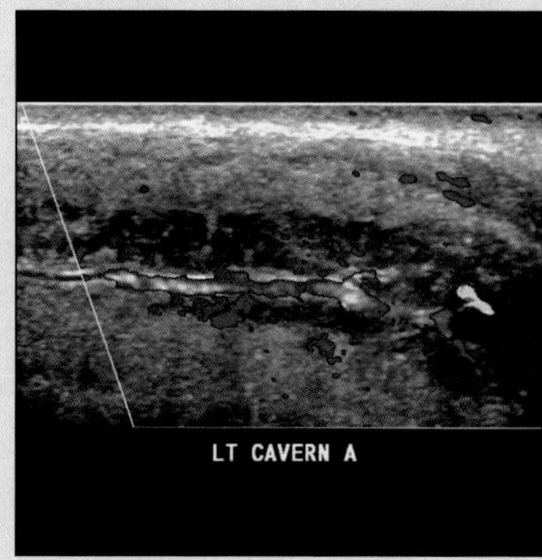

Normal Cavernosal Artery

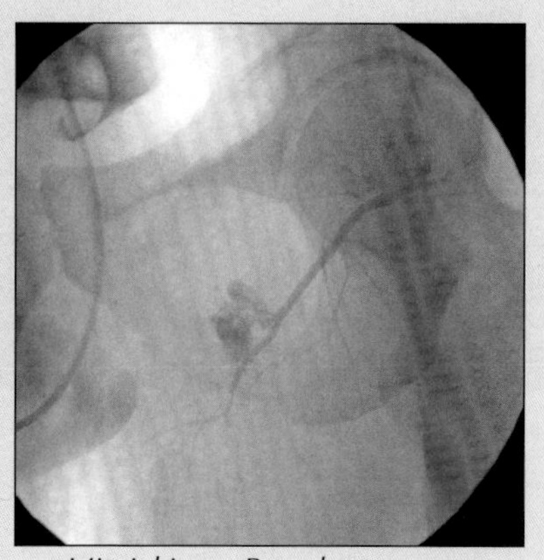

Mimicking a Pseudoaneurysm

HIGH-FLOW PRIAPISM

Key Facts

Terminology

- Persistent erection for greater than 6 hours not accompanied by sexual desire

Imaging Findings

- Color Doppler
  - Demonstrates extravasated blood from lacerated cavernosal artery as area of high velocity, turbulent flow
  - Can differentiate from ischemic priapism, which demonstrates little or no blood flow in cavernosal arteries
  - Highly sensitive for arterial fistula, noninvasive, and widely available

Top Differential Diagnoses

- Low-Flow Priapism
  - Inadequate venous outflow leading to hypoxia, acidosis, and ischemia
  - Prolonged ischemia results in corpora fibrosis and permanent erectile dysfunction

Pathology

- Arteriocavernous fistula from perineal or penile blunt trauma
- Venous outflow is maintained, preventing complete erection, stasis, and hypoxia

Clinical Issues

- All patients with priapism should be evaluated immediately to intervene early on ischemic priapism
- Transcatheter embolization of internal pudendal arteries is therapy of first choice

---

    - US used to achieve optimal position of catheter
    - May reduce radiation exposure to genitourinary tract and reduce volume of contrast infused
  - Can differentiate from ischemic priapism, which demonstrates little or no blood flow in cavernosal arteries
  - Can be used after embolization to investigate erectile dysfunction
    - Induce erection pharmacologically (prostaglandin E1)
    - Search for arterial insufficiency or veno-occlusive dysfunction

Angiographic Findings

- Conventional
  - Demonstrates fistula when contrast medium injected in pudendal artery and spreads into cavernous body
  - Usually only performed as part of embolization procedure

Imaging Recommendations

- Best imaging tool: Color Doppler is highly sensitive for arterial fistula, noninvasive, and widely available

DIFFERENTIAL DIAGNOSIS

Low Flow (Ischemic) Priapism

- History and physical
  - Painful erection
  - Corpora are rigid and painful to exam
- Inadequate venous outflow leading to hypoxia, acidosis, and ischemia
  - Commonly seen after injection of vasoactive drugs or in men with sickle cell disease
  - May result from blockage of draining venules in sickle cell crisis and leukemia
  - Blood gas is hypoxic, acidotic, and hypercarbic
- Urologic emergency
  - Prolonged ischemia results in corpora fibrosis and permanent erectile dysfunction
- Important clues to differentiate from high-flow priapism; in high-flow priapism
  - Corpora cavernosa are rarely fully rigid
  - Pain is seldom present
  - Cavernous blood gas is often normal
  - Blood abnormalities and hematologic malignancy are seldom present
  - Intracavernous vasoactive drug injection rarely precedes symptoms
  - Priapism is seldom chronic
  - Symptoms are often seen after trauma

Stuttering Priapism

- Recurrent ischemic priapism with repeated painful erections and intervals of detumescence
- Clinician should be prompted to evaluate for prevention of future ischemic episodes

Medication Effect

- Intracavernous agents: Papaverine, phentolamine, prostaglandin E1
- Antihypertensives: Vasodilators, alpha-antagonists
- Psychotropics: Phenothiazine, hypnotics, SSRI
- Anticoagulants: Heparin, warfarin
- Recreational drugs: Cocaine, marijuana, ethanol
- Hormones: Gonadotropin-releasing hormone, tamoxifen, testosterone

PATHOLOGY

General Features

- General path comments: Venous outflow is maintained, preventing complete erection, stasis, and hypoxia
- Etiology
  - Arteriocavernous fistula from perineal or penile blunt trauma
    - Often laceration of cavernosal artery or one of its branches
    - Results in uncontrolled arterial inflow to the penile sinusoidal spaces

HIGH-FLOW PRIAPISM

- Epidemiology: Rare, approximately 200 cases in the literature

CLINICAL ISSUES

Presentation

- Most common signs/symptoms
  - Penis is neither fully rigid nor painful
    - May present several days or even months after trauma
    - Cavernous bodies erect with corpus spongiosum remaining flaccid
  - Cavernous blood gases are not hypoxic or acidotic
- Clinical Profile
  - All patients with priapism should be evaluated immediately to intervene early on ischemic priapism
  - Blood gas
    - Ischemic priapism: PO2 < 30 mmHg, PCO2 > 60 mmHg, pH < 7.25
    - High-flow priapism: PO2 > 30 mmHg, PCO2 < 60 mmHg, pH > 7.25
  - Only 2/3 of patients exhibit penile erection immediately following trauma; often develops over 1-15 hours

Demographics

- Age: Often children and adults < 55 years old

Treatment

- Treatment is not emergent
  - Spontaneous resolution in up to 62% of cases
  - O2 sat is normal and risk of ischemic injury is low
  - However, watchful waiting not recommended due to rare reports of reduced potency in longstanding disease
- Conservative therapy
  - Observation, external compression of perineum, and application of ice
  - Many patients remain potent after spontaneous resolution
  - Intracavernosal injection of phenylephrine and methylene blue with limited success
  - Aspiration with injection of vasoconstrictive agents has little therapeutic benefit compared to low-flow priapism
- Transcatheter embolization of internal pudendal arteries is therapy of first choice
  - First described by Wear et al in 1977
  - Goal is closing of arteriocavernous fistula without jeopardizing erectile function
  - Priapism often disappears immediately after embolization
  - Restoration of erectile potency 80-89%
  - Temporary and permanent occlusive agents
    - Temporary occlusive agents, such as blood clot and gelatin sponge, allow eventual recanalization
    - Temporary agents may increase likelihood of maintaining erectile function
    - Permanent agents, such as microcoils, have also been successfully used
    - Permanent agents may maintain erectile function by collateral formation from contralateral cavernosal artery, dorsal penile artery, and external pudendal artery
  - Embolization may fail when collateral circulation develops from contralateral corpora in long-standing disease
- Surgery is therapy of last resort
  - Resection of fistula and ligation of internal pudendal or cavernous arteries
  - High success with detumescence in 70-100% but potency from 10-50%
  - Scarring of tunica albuginea places patients at high risk for ED

DIAGNOSTIC CHECKLIST

Consider

- Diagnosis often begins with color Doppler, followed by cavernous blood analysis
- Angiography of pudendal arteries often reserved for difficult cases or intervention

SELECTED REFERENCES

1. Kim KR et al: Treatment of high-flow priapism with superselective transcatheter embolization in 27 patients: a multicenter study. J Vasc Interv Radiol. 18(10):1222-6, 2007
2. O'Sullivan P et al: Treatment of "high-flow" priapism with superselective transcatheter embolization: a useful alternative to surgery. Cardiovasc Intervent Radiol. 29(2):198-201, 2006
3. Savoca G et al: Sexual function after highly selective embolization of cavernous artery in patients with high flow priapism: long-term followup. J Urol. 172(2):644-7, 2004
4. Bertolotto M et al: Color Doppler imaging of posttraumatic priapism before and after selective embolization. Radiographics. 23(2):495-503, 2003
5. Montague DK et al: American Urological Association guideline on the management of priapism. J Urol. 170(4 Pt 1):1318-24, 2003
6. Wilkins CJ et al: Colour Doppler ultrasound of the penis. Clin Radiol. 58(7):514-23, 2003
7. Ciampalini S et al: High-flow priapism: treatment and long-term follow-up. Urology. 59(1):110-3, 2002
8. Volkmer BG et al: High-flow priapism: a combined interventional approach with angiography and colour Doppler. Ultrasound Med Biol. 28(2):165-9, 2002

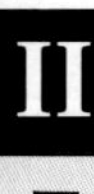

IMAGE GALLERY

Typical

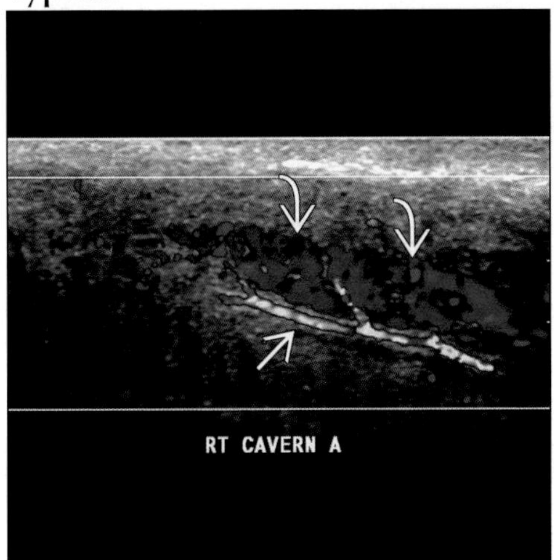

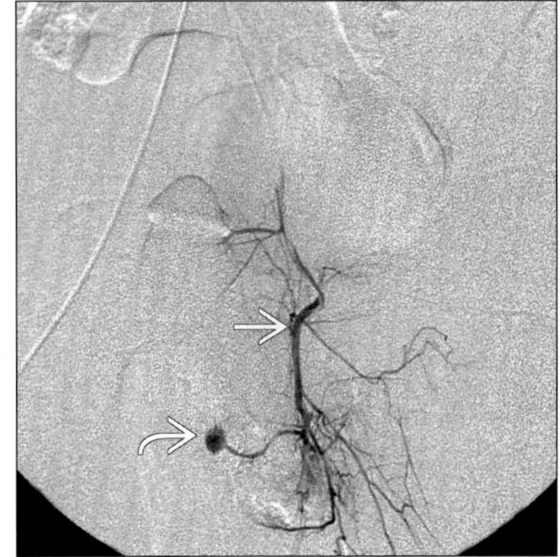

(Left) Color Doppler ultrasound shows the cavernosal artery ➔ with rapid flow of blood into the corpus cavernosum ➔. The arterial color blush in the corpus cavernosum is characteristic. *(Right)* DSA subselective angiogram of the right internal pudendal artery ➔ with the penis in an oblique position demonstrates an appearance of extravasation ➔ from the cavernosal artery.

Typical

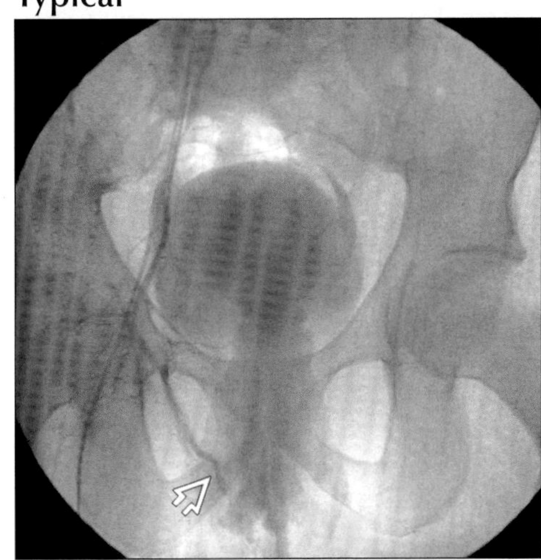

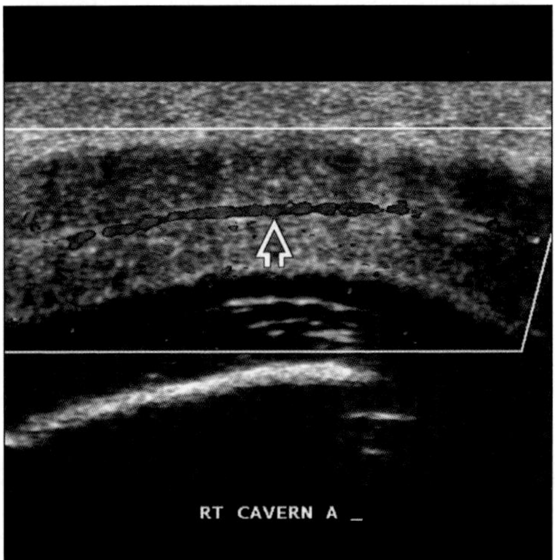

(Left) DSA shows embolization of the cavernosal artery with Gelfoam ➔. Gelfoam has the advantage of possibly recanalizing which may allow revascularization of the artery. *(Right)* Color Doppler ultrasound shows appearance of the right cavernosal artery ➔ 3 months following embolization. Artery is of normal caliber, no arterial blush seen in the corpus cavernosum.

Typical

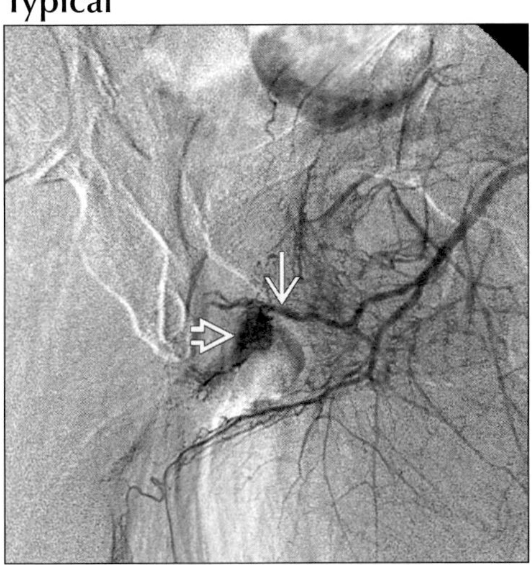

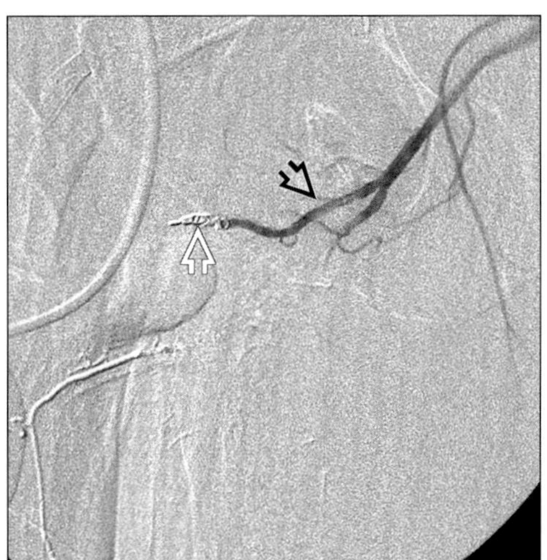

(Left) DSA shows extravasation from the dorsal penile artery ➔ with contrast extravasation ➔ in the region of the bulbous spongiosum of the penis. *(Right)* DSA shows microcoils ➔ which have been placed into the dorsal penile artery ➔ with cessation of extravasation. Transcatheter embolization is the therapy of first choice in high-flow priapism.

LOWER EXTREMITY VASCULATURE

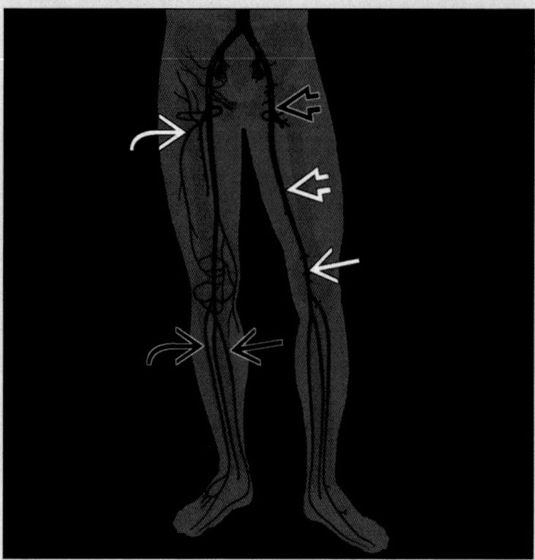

Graphic shows the common ➾, superficial ➡, and profunda ➡ femoral arteries. The popliteal ➡, peroneal, anterior ➚, and posterior ➡ tibial arteries provide circulation to the knee, calf and foot.

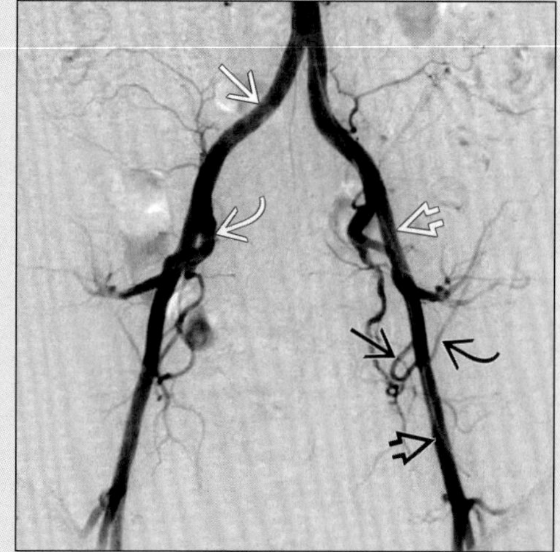

Pelvic arteriogram shows common ➡, internal ➚ and external ➡ iliac arteries. The deep circumflex iliac ➚ and inferior epigastric ➡ arteries mark the inguinal ligament and the level of the common femoral artery ➾.

TERMINOLOGY

Abbreviations

- Common femoral artery (CFA)
- Superficial femoral artery (SFA)
- Profunda femoral artery (PFA)
- Greater saphenous vein (GSV)
- Small saphenous vein (SSV)

Synonyms

- Internal iliac, hypogastric artery
- Small saphenous vein, lesser saphenous vein

IMAGING ANATOMY

Anatomic Relationships

- Abdominal aorta bifurcates into common iliac arteries
- Common iliac arteries 3-6 cm long, 8-10 mm diameter
  - Divide into internal/external iliac arteries
    - Internal iliac arteries bifurcate into anterior and posterior divisions; supply pelvic muscles, viscera
    - Anterior division yields inferior gluteal, obturator, internal pudendal, vesicle, uterine arteries
    - Posterior division gives off superior gluteal, iliolumbar, lateral sacral arteries
- External iliac arteries become CFA at inguinal ligament
  - Ligament delineated by origins of inferior epigastric and deep circumflex iliac arteries
- CFA usually 5-7 cm long; 5-9 mm in diameter
  - CFA and vein within femoral sheath; continuation of abdominal wall fascia; femoral nerve outside
  - Bifurcates into SFA and PFA
- PFA origin posterolateral to SFA origin
  - Supplies proximal hip (medial and lateral femoral circumflex arteries)
  - Main trunk has deep course adjacent to femur
    - Anastomoses with SFA/popliteal branches
  - Important collateral pathway in proximal SFA occlusion or stenosis
- SFA dominant in-line arterial supply in thigh
  - Courses beneath sartorius anterior to femoral vein
  - Exits Hunter canal at adductor hiatus; becomes popliteal artery
  - Multiple muscular branches; largest branch, supreme geniculate (medial)
- Popliteal artery extends from adductor hiatus to calf
  - Knee joint delineates above-/below-knee segments
    - Levels influence intervention choices, outcomes
  - Yields superior and inferior (medial/lateral); middle geniculate arteries
  - Bifurcates into anterior tibial, tibioperoneal trunk
    - Tibioperoneal trunk divides into posterior tibial, peroneal arteries
- Three calf runoff arteries
  - Anterior tibial artery
    - Courses to foot in anterior compartment of calf
    - Continues into foot as dorsalis pedis artery
  - Posterior tibial artery
    - Extends from upper calf to medial malleolus
    - Contained in deep posterior calf compartment
    - Terminates as medial and lateral plantar arteries; form plantar arch of foot
  - Peroneal artery
    - Descends posteromedial to fibula in deep posterior calf compartment
    - Ends in characteristic "forked" anterior and posterior perforating branches

PATHOLOGIC ISSUES

Lower Extremity Vascular Pathology

- Atherosclerotic occlusive disease
  - Acute limb ischemia
    - Embolic vs. thrombotic occlusion
    - Endovascular or surgical treatment
  - Chronic limb ischemia
    - Symptoms relate to level of occlusion, presence and quality of collaterals, comorbidities
    - Medical, endovascular and surgical management
- Aneurysms
  - "True" or "false" (pseudoaneurysm)
  - Common femoral artery aneurysm

LOWER EXTREMITY VASCULATURE

Normal Lower Extremity Venous Anatomy

Deep Venous System

- Common femoral vein
  - Confluence of femoral and deep femoral veins
- Femoral vein (superficial femoral vein)
  - Deep and lateral to SFA; often duplicated
  - Extends from groin to adductor hiatus
- Popliteal vein
  - Formed by confluence of tibial veins in upper calf; extends proximally to adductor hiatus
- Tibial veins
  - Paired anterior and posterior tibial, peroneal veins

Superficial Venous System

- Greater saphenous vein (GSV)
  - Courses from ankle to common femoral vein
- Small (lesser) saphenous vein (SSV)
  - Courses in posterior calf; joins popliteal vein
- Perforating veins
  - Direct blood from superficial into deep system

    - Most frequent site for pseudoaneurysm; 2° to catheterization, surgical anastomosis
  - Popliteal artery aneurysm
    - Most common lower extremity aneurysm
    - Presents with limb ischemia in > 50%
    - Thromboembolic complications common
- Arteriovenous malformations
  - Lower extremities most common location
- Congenital abnormalities
  - Persistent sciatic artery
    - Internal iliac artery continues as sciatic artery, then as popliteal artery
    - May have hypoplastic SFA; sciatic artery dominant blood supply to lower extremity (complete form)
- Cystic adventitial disease
  - Focal cystic mucin accumulation in adventitia
  - Cysts cause vascular compression, claudication
  - Popliteal artery most often affected
- Ergotism
  - Ergot alkaloids cause diffuse vasospasm
  - Arterial constriction may progress to occlusion
- Fibromuscular dysplasia
  - Common and external iliac arteries
- Popliteal artery entrapment
  - Artery deviates around gastrocnemius muscle or compressed between muscular structures
  - Claudication; may progress to occlusion
- Peripheral vascular surgical reconstruction
  - Vascular conduit bypass of diseased arterial segment
- Trauma
  - 1/3 cases vascular trauma involves extremities
    - Penetrating or blunt trauma
  - Arterial injury with 30-40% of knee dislocations
- Vasculitis
  - Most common is Buerger disease; others uncommon
- Venous diseases
  - Chronic venous insufficiency
    - Chronic swelling, pigmentation, venous stasis ulcers; 2° to DVT (post-thrombotic syndrome)
    - Varicose veins, incompetent perforators
  - Deep vein thrombosis (DVT)
    - Blood clots in deep veins of lower extremity
    - Risk of embolism to pulmonary arteries
    - May result in chronic venous insufficiency
  - Klippel-Trenaunay syndrome: Congenital disorder
    - Capillary malformations (port wine stain), soft tissue or bone hypertrophy, varicose veins or venous malformations affecting extremity
  - Venous malformations
    - Congenital abnormality; deep or superficial malformations; sclerotherapy for treatment

RELATED REFERENCES

1. Fragomeni G et al: A haemodynamic model of the venous network of the lower limbs. Conf Proc IEEE Eng Med Biol Soc. 2007:1002-5, 2007
2. FIGLEY MM et al: The arteries of the abdomen, pelvis, and thigh. I. Normal roentgenographic anatomy. II. Collateral circulation in obstructive arterial disease. Am J Roentgenol Radium Ther Nucl Med. 77(2):296-311, 1957

IMAGE GALLERY

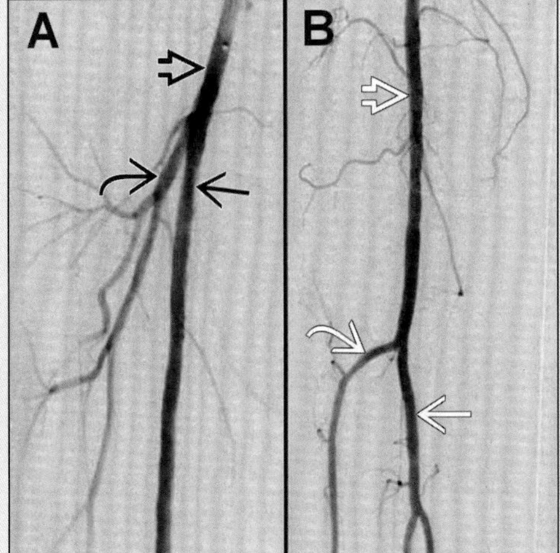

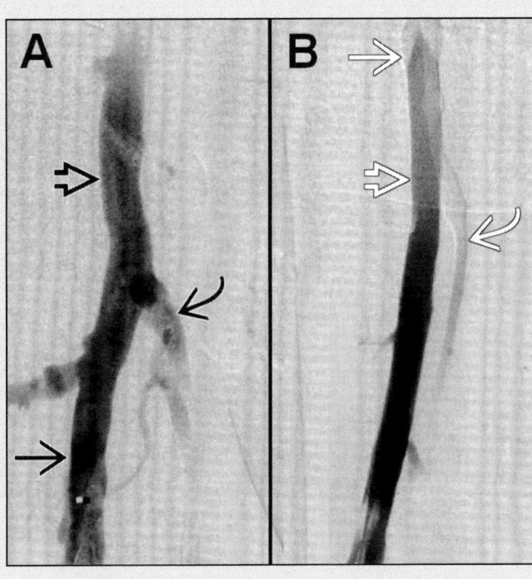

(Left) *DSA shows (A) the common femoral artery bifurcates into the profunda and superficial femoral arteries. The SFA exits the adductor hiatus in the thigh to become (B) the popliteal artery, which divides into the anterior tibial artery and the tibioperoneal trunk.* ***(Right)*** *Venogram shows (A) the femoral and greater saphenous veins join at the saphenofemoral junction to become the common femoral vein. (B) The small saphenous vein drains into the popliteal vein. Note the well-defined venous valve.*

LOWER EXTREMITY ANEURYSMS

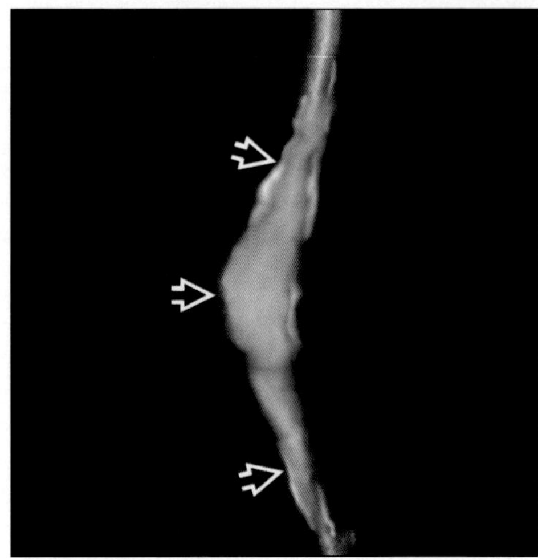

Coronal 3-D CTA shows a diffuse fusiform left popliteal artery aneurysm ⇨. CTA can provide excellent anatomic detail of peripheral arterial aneurysms, while CECT can show thrombus and perivascular anatomy.

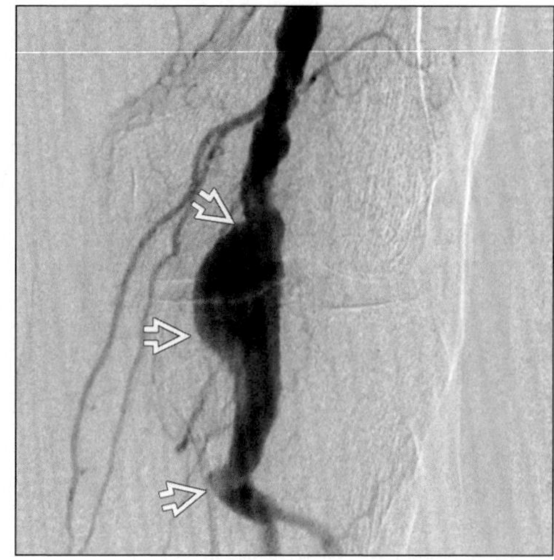

DSA arteriogram also shows a fusiform left popliteal artery aneurysm ⇨. Angiography can underestimate the true diameter of a peripheral aneurysm if there is considerable intraluminal thrombus.

TERMINOLOGY

Definitions

- Aneurysm ("true" aneurysm): Focal enlargement of vascular lumen caused by intrinsic abnormality of arterial wall
  - All three layers of arterial wall remain intact
- Pseudoaneurysm ("false" aneurysm): Focal enlargement of vascular lumen caused by disruption of arterial wall integrity
  - Less than normal three layers of arterial wall

IMAGING FINDINGS

General Features

- Location
  - Popliteal artery aneurysms are most common lower extremity aneurysm, with common femoral artery aneurysms second most frequent of peripheral artery aneurysms
    - Common femoral artery aneurysms associated with abdominal aortic aneurysms (AAA) and with popliteal artery aneurysms
    - 1/3 of patients with common femoral aneurysms also have popliteal aneurysm
    - Must be distinguished from pseudoaneurysms, which are common in femoral location
  - Profunda femoral artery aneurysms rare (0.5% of all peripheral aneurysms)
    - High complication rate at presentation and significant incidence of other aneurysms
  - Superficial femoral artery aneurysms also rare
  - Popliteal artery aneurysms, although uncommon, account for > 70% of all peripheral aneurysms
    - Incidence is higher in patients with AAA, occurring in 6-12% of these patients
  - Tibial artery aneurysms are very infrequent
    - Usually are pseudoaneurysms associated with trauma or iatrogenic injury such as catheterization

CT Findings

- Similar findings to angiography with CTA; provides 3-D arterial and perivascular anatomy
- Will demonstrate thrombus and true luminal diameter

MR Findings

- Similar findings to catheter angiography and CTA with MRA

DDx: Lower Extremity Vascular Mass

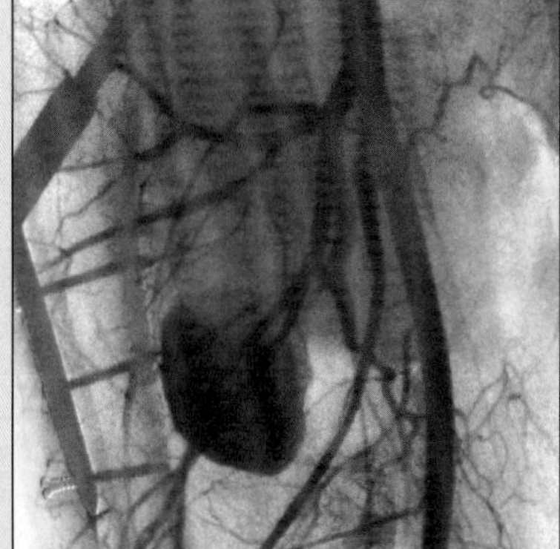

Iatrogenic Pseudoaneurysm

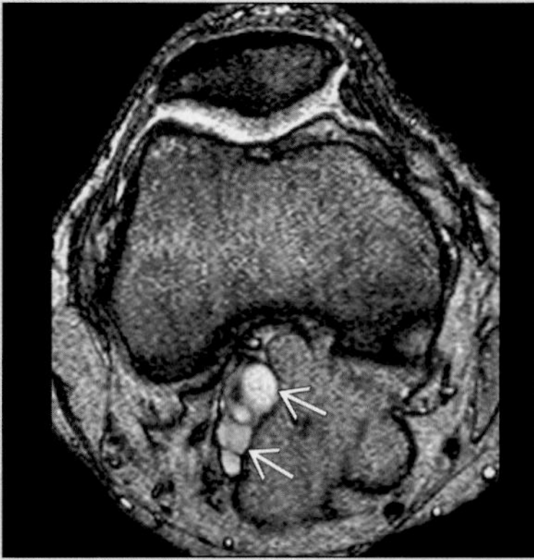

Cystic Adventitial Disease

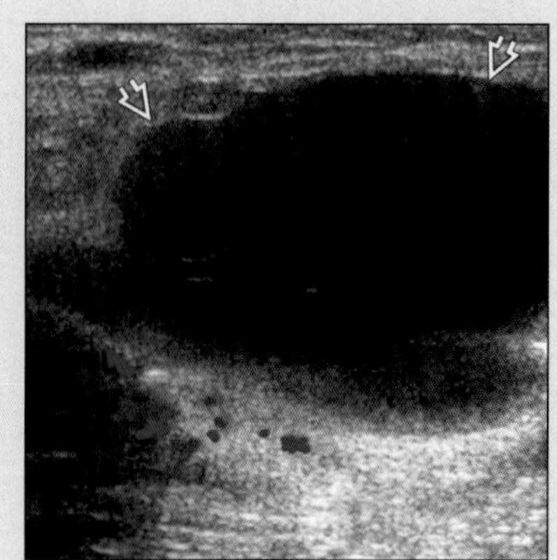

Post-Operative Seroma

LOWER EXTREMITY ANEURYSMS

Key Facts

Terminology

- Aneurysm ("true" aneurysm): Focal enlargement of vascular lumen caused by intrinsic abnormality of arterial wall
- Pseudoaneurysm ("false" aneurysm): Focal enlargement of vascular lumen caused by disruption of arterial wall integrity

Imaging Findings

- Ultrasound or CECT may show fusiform or saccular enlargement of artery, often with laminar thrombus within
- Consider thrombosed aneurysm with popliteal artery occlusion, particularly if there are other aneurysms
  - Absent side branches clue to presence of aneurysm

Pathology

- Pathogenesis of peripheral arterial aneurysms usually due to same mechanisms involved in AAA
- > 70% of patients with peripheral aneurysms also have AAA
- Common femoral artery aneurysms associated with abdominal aortic aneurysms (AAA) and with popliteal artery aneurysms
  - 1/3 of patients with common femoral aneurysms also have popliteal aneurysm
- Popliteal artery aneurysms are most common lower extremity aneurysm, with common femoral artery aneurysms second most frequent

Diagnostic Checklist

- Angiography may underestimate size of aneurysm if there is significant thrombus within

- Will also demonstrate thrombus and true luminal diameter, as well as perivascular anatomy

Ultrasonographic Findings

- Grayscale Ultrasound: Fusiform or saccular arterial enlargement, often with laminar thrombus within

Angiographic Findings

- Saccular or tortuous fusiform arterial enlargement
  - Occasional normal diameter if significant thrombus
    - Absent side branches clue to presence of aneurysm
  - Always consider thrombosed aneurysm with popliteal artery occlusion, particularly if there are other aneurysms
- Shows status of arteries distal to aneurysm; embolization common and is an outcome determinant

DIFFERENTIAL DIAGNOSIS

Atherosclerotic Occlusive Disease

- Chronic claudication, often bilateral
- Involvement of multiple arterial levels or segments
  - Stenoses or occlusions
    - Acute symptoms similar to distal embolization from, or acute occlusion of peripheral aneurysm
- Well developed collateral circulation

Cystic Adventitial Disease

- Unilateral "scimitar-shaped" stenosis of popliteal artery caused by cystic mucinous fluid within adventitia
- Sudden onset of claudication in young patient
- Ultrasound or MR will demonstrate cysts adjacent to arterial stenosis
- Rarely thrombose or cause distal embolization

Ehlers-Danlos Syndrome

- Rare inherited disorder with defect in collagen synthesis; multiple types within classification
- Autosomal dominant defect in type 3 collagen synthesis affects vascular system
- Spontaneous dissection, aneurysms and vessel rupture are most common vascular symptoms
- 70% angiography complication rate due to abnormal arterial wall

Embolus

- Intraluminal filling defect(s) on CTA or angiogram
- Meniscus at margin of occlusion on angiogram
- Poorly formed collaterals
- Acute symptoms similar to distal embolization from, or acute occlusion of peripheral aneurysm

Extravascular Collection

- Hematoma, seroma or lymphocele can produce palpable mass adjacent to artery
- Close proximity of collection to artery may result in transmitted pulsation, and thus mimic aneurysm, pseudoaneurysm or AV fistula

Neoplasm

- Inguinal adenopathy may produce palpable mass that mimics hematoma, thrombosed aneurysm or pseudoaneurysm
- Soft tissue neoplasms may mimic aneurysms if highly vascular, e.g. hemangioma

Popliteal Artery Entrapment

- Aberrant relationship of artery to gastrocnemius muscle with resultant arterial compression
- Eventual adventitial thickening and fibrosis followed by aneurysm formation, thrombosis and distal embolization

Pseudoaneurysm

- Disruption in arterial wall continuity resulting from inflammation, trauma, or iatrogenic (surgical or interventional procedures)
- Contains less than three normal layers of arterial wall
- Higher rupture risk than same size "true" aneurysm
- Often associated with vascular surgical anastomoses or catheterization sites
  - Pseudoaneurysms resulting from catheterization procedures may be treated with ultrasound compression or with thrombin injection
  - Vascular anastomotic pseudoaneurysms require surgical revision

LOWER EXTREMITY ANEURYSMS

Trauma

- Repetitive, blunt, penetrating or iatrogenic trauma may cause aneurysm, AV fistula or pseudoaneurysm
- Hematoma may mimic pseudoaneurysm, particularly at anastomosis or catheterization site

PATHOLOGY

General Features

- Etiology
  - Pathogenesis of peripheral arterial aneurysms usually due to same mechanisms involved in AAA
    - Degenerative process affecting elastin fibers and inflammatory infiltrative changes affecting arterial media and adventitia
    - Proteolytic enzymatic degradation of collagen and elastin in arterial wall
  - Popliteal artery aneurysms can also result from popliteal artery entrapment syndrome
  - Other etiologies for peripheral aneurysms
    - Iatrogenic (catheterization, surgical bypass, intervention)
    - Trauma
    - Infection
    - Bechet disease
    - Ehlers-Danlos syndrome
- Associated abnormalities
  - High association of peripheral arterial aneurysms with AAA
    - > 70% of patients with peripheral aneurysms also have AAA
  - Popliteal aneurysms associated with arteriomegaly

CLINICAL ISSUES

Presentation

- Most common signs/symptoms
  - Common femoral artery aneurysms
    - Asymptomatic groin swelling or occasional compression of femoral vein (edema) or nerve (pain, paresthesia)
    - Rarely complications of thrombosis, distal embolization or rupture
  - Profunda femoral artery aneurysms
    - Greater rupture rate than peripheral aneurysms
  - Superficial femoral artery aneurysms
    - Present with limb-threatening ischemia or rupture
  - Popliteal artery aneurysms
    - Symptom occurrence related to aneurysm diameter as larger aneurysms (> 2 cm) contain more thrombus
    - Limb ischemia is presenting symptom in > 50%
    - 1/3 are asymptomatic at time of diagnosis but 50% develop distal ischemia within 5 years
  - Tibial artery aneurysms
    - Usually absent symptoms; occasional calf swelling

Natural History & Prognosis

- Thromboembolic complications, often with irreversible ischemia are most serious complication of lower extremity aneurysms
  - Complication rate highly dependent upon aneurysm diameter, with almost all complications occurring with aneurysm diameters > 2 cm
  - Patients in whom popliteal aneurysms remain untreated have 35% thromboembolic complication rate and 25% amputation rate
    - Complication rate increases to 74% after 5 years
  - Rupture of "true" lower extremity aneurysms is much less common than with pseudoaneurysms or aortic and iliac artery aneurysms

Treatment

- Surgical resection and bypass is the accepted standard treatment for lower extremity aneurysms
  - Treatment results are far superior in asymptomatic patients (85-100% patency at 5 years) than symptomatic patients (54-72% patency)
  - High mortality rate (5-8%) with emergency treatment
- Endovascular repair of lower extremity arterial aneurysms now performed with significantly increasing frequency
  - Endovascular treatment lacks long-term follow-up
    - Early mid-term results of elective endovascular repair of popliteal artery aneurysms are encouraging, with some studies showing similar patency rates to open repair

DIAGNOSTIC CHECKLIST

Image Interpretation Pearls

- Angiography may underestimate size of aneurysm if there is significant thrombus within
- Consider thrombosed aneurysm with popliteal artery occlusion, particularly if there are other aneurysms

SELECTED REFERENCES

1. Curi MA et al: Mid-term outcomes of endovascular popliteal artery aneurysm repair. J Vasc Surg. 45(3):505-10, 2007
2. Davies RS et al: Long-term Results of Surgical Repair of Popliteal Artery Aneurysm. Eur J Vasc Endovasc Surg. 2007
3. Kropman RH et al: Surgical and endovascular treatment of atherosclerotic popliteal artery aneurysms. J Cardiovasc Surg (Torino). 48(3):281-8, 2007
4. Ravn H et al: Nationwide study of the outcome of popliteal artery aneurysms treated surgically. Br J Surg. 94(8):970-7, 2007
5. Ravn H et al: Surgical technique and long-term results after popliteal artery aneurysm repair: results from 717 legs. J Vasc Surg. 46(2):236-43, 2007
6. Watelet J: Popliteal aneurysms. J Cardiovasc Surg (Torino). 48(3):263-5, 2007
7. Corriere MA et al: True and false aneurysms of the femoral artery. Semin Vasc Surg. 18(4):216-23, 2005
8. Edgerton JR et al: Obliteration of femoral artery pseudoaneurysm by thrombin injection. Ann Thorac Surg. 74(4):S1413-5, 2002
9. Cappendijk VC et al: A true aneurysm of the tibioperoneal trunk. Case report and literature review. Eur J Vasc Endovasc Surg. 18(6):536-7, 1999
10. Marmorale A et al: Aneurysms of the infrapopliteal arteries. J R Coll Surg Edinb. 40(5):324-6, 1995

LOWER EXTREMITY ANEURYSMS

IMAGE GALLERY

Typical

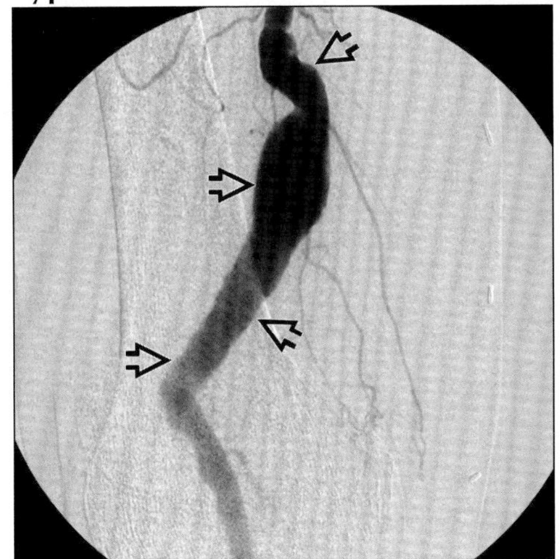

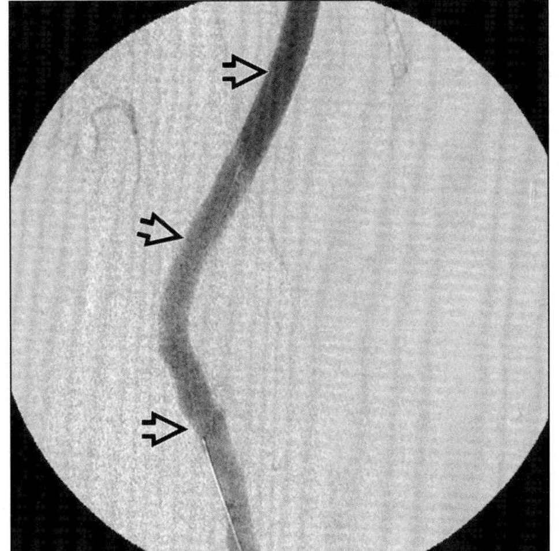

(Left) *DSA arteriogram shows a fusiform right popliteal artery aneurysm ⇨ in a patient who previously underwent endovascular repair of an AAA. Popliteal artery aneurysms are present in up to 12% of patients with AAA, and are frequently bilateral.* ***(Right)*** *Arteriogram in the same patient shows there has been endovascular repair ⇨ with successful exclusion of the aneurysm. Endovascular repair results are encouraging, with some studies showing similar patency rates to open repair.*

Typical

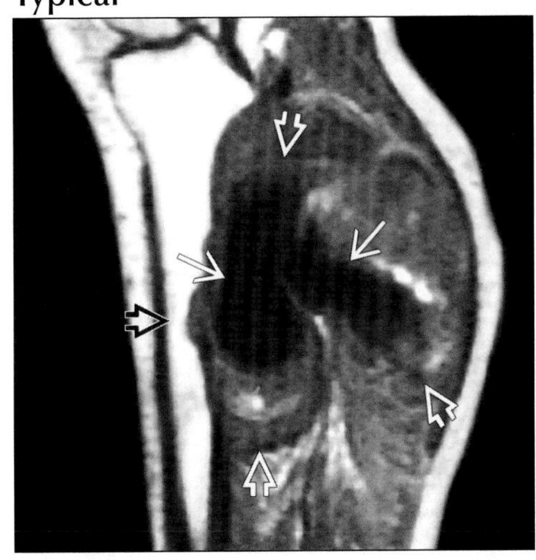

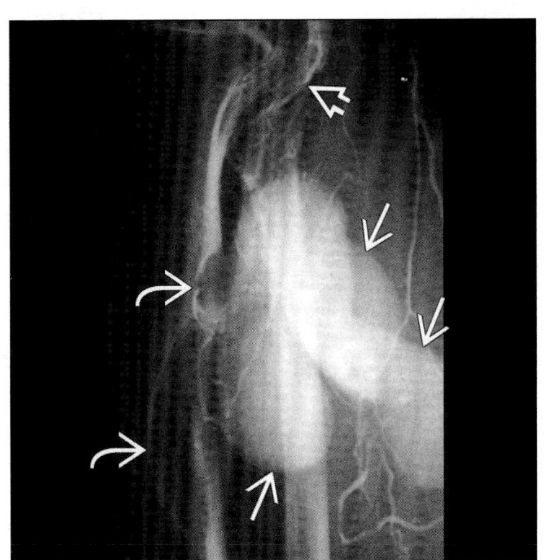

(Left) *Sagittal T1WI MR in a patient with longstanding history of a pulsatile calf mass shows a lobulated soft tissue mass ➡ posterior to the tibia ⇨, with bone erosion. Within the mass are central signal voids ➡.* ***(Right)*** *Arteriogram in the same patient shows a large tri-lobed aneurysm of the tibial arteries ➡, arising from the below-knee popliteal artery segment ➡, which is still partially contrast filled. The associated adjacent bone erosion ↪ is an unusual finding.*

Typical

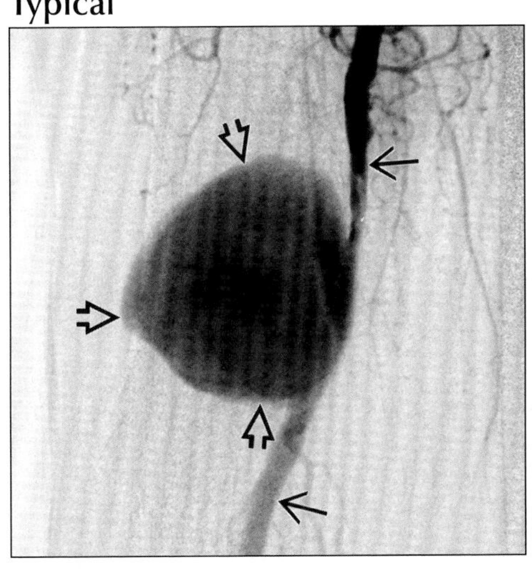

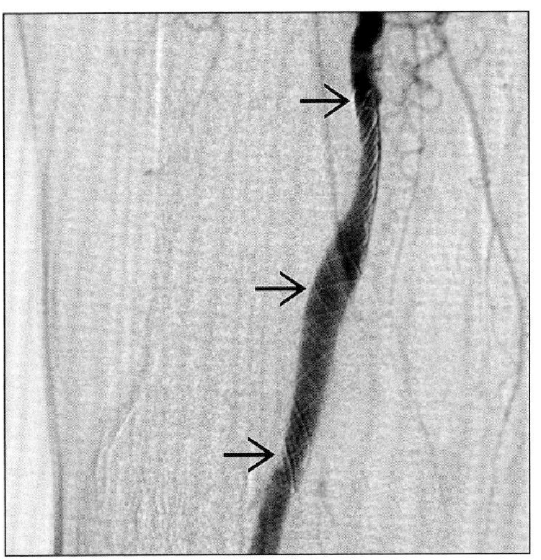

(Left) *Arteriogram shows an eccentric contrast collection ⇨ arising from the popliteal artery → in a patient with history of trauma and a pulsatile popliteal fossa mass. This was felt to represent a traumatic pseudoaneurysm.* ***(Right)*** *DSA following endovascular treatment of the post-traumatic popliteal artery pseudoaneurysm with covered stent-graft endoprosthesis → shows successful pseudoaneurysm exclusion. The patient had complete resolution of his symptoms.*

ACUTE LOWER EXTREMITY ISCHEMIA

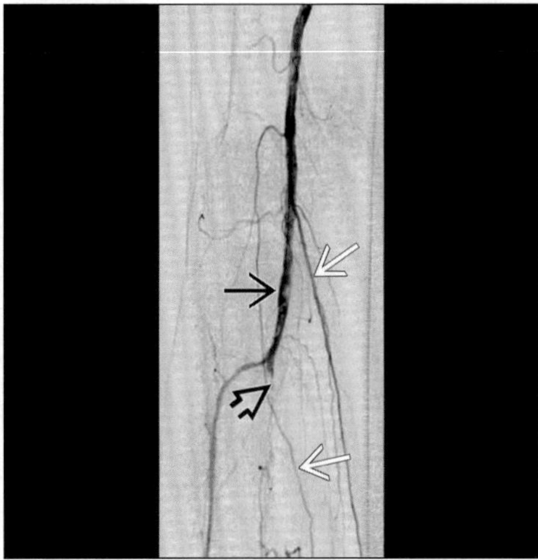

DSA shows occlusion of the tibioperoneal trunk and intraluminal filling defects in the popliteal artery, with filling of several very small collateral branches, consistent with acute thromboembolic occlusion.

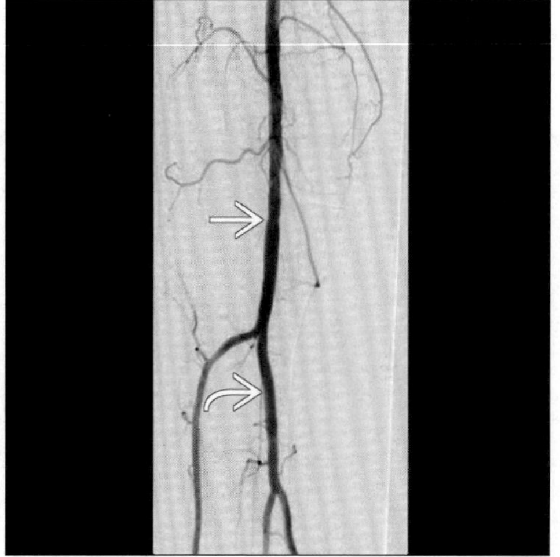

Catheter angiography of the same patient after 24 hrs of transcatheter tPA infusion shows recanalization of the popliteal artery and of the tibioperoneal trunk with complete lysis of the thromboembolic material.

TERMINOLOGY

Definitions

- Sudden decrease in tissue perfusion of lower extremity from arterial occlusive disease; may threaten limb viability

IMAGING FINDINGS

General Features

- Best diagnostic clue: Abrupt termination of distal femoral, popliteal or trifurcation arteries
- Location: Peripheral arterial bifurcations

CT Findings

- CTA: Abrupt occlusion ± filling defect; similar findings to angiography

MR Findings

- MRA
  - Embolus: Low signal focal occlusive filling defect with "meniscus" sign; similar to angiography
  - Thrombotic occlusion: Low signal focal filling thrombus defect; no "meniscus" sign
  - T1 post-contrast GRE
    - Thromboemboli seen as low signal intra-arterial filling defect
    - Arterial wall better evaluated than CE MRA
    - Low signal mural thrombus in aneurysm
    - Thrombosed popliteal artery aneurysms better demonstrated
    - Peripheral enhancement of perigraft collections

Ultrasonographic Findings

- Grayscale Ultrasound
  - Vessel wall thickening; luminal narrowing from plaque
  - Echogenic luminal filling defect, intimal flap, aneurysm with thrombus, non-visualization
- Pulsed Doppler
  - Very elevated peak systolic velocity ratio indicates high grade stenosis
  - Absent, dampened or monophasic distal waveform suggests more proximal occlusion
- Ankle-brachial indices (ABI)
  - Normal: > 0.97 (usually 1.10)

DDx: Acute Lower Extremity Ischemia

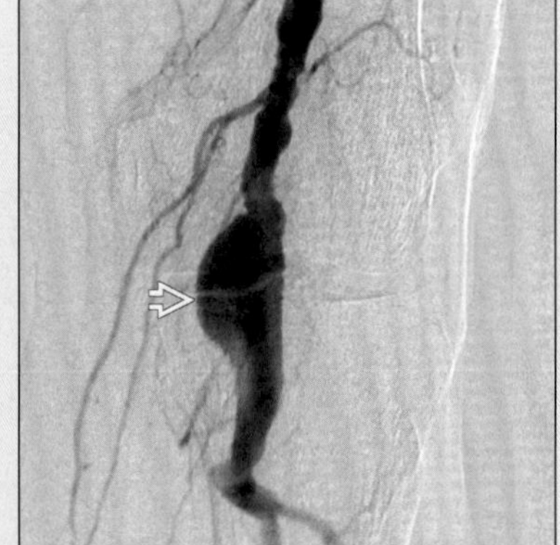

Popliteal Artery Aneurysm

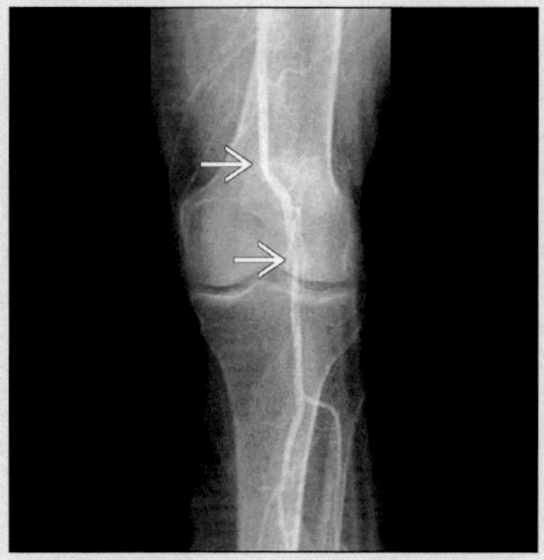

Popliteal Artery Entrapment

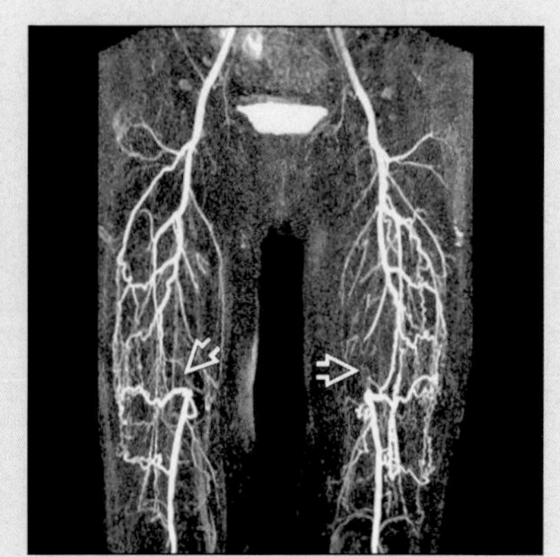

Chronic Atherosclerotic Occlusions

ACUTE LOWER EXTREMITY ISCHEMIA

Key Facts

Terminology
- Sudden decreased perfusion of lower extremity from arterial occlusive disease

Imaging Findings
- Best imaging tool: Catheter angiography
- CTA/MRA/DSA: Abrupt termination of femoral, popliteal or trifurcation arteries
- Embolus: Low signal or low density filling defect
  - "Meniscus" sign indicates embolus
  - Absence of collaterals
  - Shaggy, ulcerated atherosclerosis in microembolization
- Thrombotic occlusion
  - Significant atherosclerotic disease elsewhere
  - Popliteal aneurysm with associated thrombosis
- Post C+ T1 GRE shows arterial wall better
  - Perigraft collections show peripheral enhancement
- DSA: Gold standard for diagnosing acute occlusion

Top Differential Diagnoses
- Embolization, acute thrombosis, traumatic arterial injury
- Vasculitis, popliteal artery entrapment, aneurysm

Pathology
- Thrombosis 85% and embolism in 15%, majority have atherosclerosis
- Other causes of acute limb ischemia: Dissection

Clinical Issues
- Ankle pressure < 70 mm Hg in severe lower extremity ischemia
- Surgical therapy or Interventional radiology

  - Claudication: 0.40-0.80
  - Rest pain: 0.20-0.40
  - Ulceration, gangrene: 0.10-0.40
  - Acute ischemia: Usually < 0.10

Angiographic Findings
- DSA: "Gold standard" for diagnosing acute occlusion
  - Embolic occlusion
    - Macroemboli usually lodge in distal femoral or popliteal artery
    - Total occlusion with presence of "meniscus" indicating embolus
    - Absence of collaterals
    - In microembolization syndromes, shaggy, ulcerated atherosclerotic disease found in proximal vessels
  - Thrombotic occlusion
    - Presence of significant atherosclerotic disease elsewhere
    - Abrupt termination of vessel with or without collateral formation
- Diagnostic catheter angiography may be combined with intervention (e.g., thrombolysis)
  - Can diagnose and treat significant inflow stenoses or occlusions

Imaging Recommendations
- Best imaging tool
  - Catheter angiography
  - CE MRA or CTA
    - Sensitivities/specificities: 88% & 95% for US; 92-100% & 93-100% for CTA ; 97% & 96% for CE MRA (using angiography as "gold standard")
- Protocol advice
  - Multislice CTA: Bolus tracking, ROI lower abdominal aorta, 120-140 cc contrast at 3-4 cc/sec, 30-40 ml of saline chaser to keep compact bolus
    - 0.6, 0.75 or 1 mm thin collimation volumetric acquisition with axial reconstructions at 0.75-1 mm thickness with 0.5 mm overlap
    - Coronal and sagittal multiplanar reformats and if needed volume rendered images
- MRA: 3D high resolution CEMRA with timing bolus injection
  - Double dose contrast with dual injection technique on moving table MR scanner
    - 1st injection for calves (1st station, 2 passes); 2nd injection for combined aortoiliac (2nd station, 1 pass) and thighs (3rd station, 2 passes)
    - Nonenhanced mask images for subtraction to increase vessel to background contrast
    - Overlapping MIP and rotational MIP post-processing
  - Immediate axial post T1 GRE to assess arterial wall, veins, bypass grafts, luminal thrombus, aneurysm
  - Pre-contrast targeted T2 or STIR in suspected cystic lesions, and osteomyelitis

DIFFERENTIAL DIAGNOSIS

Embolization
- Macroembolization
  - Cardiac source (left atrium or left ventricular thrombus)
  - Proximal atherosclerotic plaque
  - Abdominal or thoracic aortic aneurysm
- Microembolization
  - Cholesterol embolization from prior catheterization
  - Blue toe syndrome: Subacute or chronic microembolization

Acute Thrombosis
- Thrombosis due to pre-existing arterial stenosis or obstruction
- Arterial bypass graft thrombosis
- Thrombosis at site of aneurysm

Traumatic Arterial Injury
- Associated bone fractures
- May be iatrogenic (arterial catheterization)

Vasculitis
- Young patient
- Abnormal narrowing or occluded digital arteries

ACUTE LOWER EXTREMITY ISCHEMIA

Popliteal Entrapment Syndrome

- Young individuals, bilateral in 60-70%
- Medial deviation of popliteal artery, which courses under medial head of gastrocnemius
- Aneurysmal, thrombosed/occluded with poor distal run off
- Stress (plantar flexion) position increases arterial angulation and deviation

Popliteal Artery Aneurysm

- Unilateral trifurcation disease; thromboemboli or decreased run off
- Peripheral thrombus, rim calcification
- Symptoms typically related to distal embolization or acute thrombosis; rupture least common complication

PATHOLOGY

General Features

- General path comments
  - Acute arterial occlusion consequences multifactorial
    - Tibial compartment pressure, degree of collateral circulation, reperfusion injury
    - Occlusion duration; presence of oxygen-free radicals
    - Cellular edema causing microvascular obstruction with "no-reflow" phenomenon
- Etiology
  - Acute embolic or thrombotic arterial occlusion
  - Thrombosis in 85% and embolism in 15% of patients; majority have atherosclerotic disease
    - Source of emboli are cardiac (most common), aneurysm, atherosclerotic plaque, or upstream critical stenosis
  - Thrombosis usually superimposed on chronic atherosclerotic disease
    - Typically 2° to atherosclerotic stenosis in native vessel; anastomotic stenosis or distal progression of disease in bypass graft
    - Bypass graft can develop de novo thrombosis
    - Thrombosed aneurysm (popliteal)

Microscopic Features

- Microscopic embolization
  - From ulcerated plaques or aneurysms
  - Cholesterol crystals, fibrin-platelet deposits, cellular thrombi

Staging, Grading or Classification Criteria

- Rutherford Criteria of Acute Limb Ischemia
  - Class 1: Viable; non-threatened extremity
    - No rest pain, neurologic deficit or compromised skin circulation
    - Audible Doppler flow signals
  - Class 2: Threatened viability; reversible ischemia, salvageable limb if arterial obstruction relieved
    - 2A: Limb not immediately threatened
    - 2B: Severely threatened; urgent revascularization necessary for salvage
    - Rest pain, mild neurologic deficits; Doppler arterial signals absent; venous signals present
  - Class 3: Major, irreversible ischemic change: Frequently requires major amputation
    - Absent capillary or skin perfusion, muscle rigor, sensory loss, muscle paralysis; completely absent Doppler signals

CLINICAL ISSUES

Presentation

- Most common signs/symptoms
  - Pain, pallor, paresthesias, pulselessness, paralysis, cold sensation
    - Ankle pressure < 70 mm Hg in severe lower extremity ischemia

Demographics

- Age: Elderly
- Gender: Severe ischemia more common in women

Natural History & Prognosis

- Limb loss, sepsis or death

Treatment

- Initial anticoagulation followed by imaging
  - Typically requires angiography if intervention planned
- Thrombolytic therapy with transcatheter infusion
- Mechanical thrombectomy, thromboaspiration
- Surgical therapy; thromboembolectomy, vascular bypass graft, amputation

DIAGNOSTIC CHECKLIST

Consider

- Cardiac and aortic source of thromboemboli in patients with acute limb ischemia

Image Interpretation Pearls

- Protruding aortic mural thrombus and floating intraluminal aortic thrombus hypovascular; appear as irregular low attenuation or signal on CTA/MRA
- Suspect acute thromboembolism in abrupt occlusion, occlusive filling defect, unilateral disease, meniscus sign, and absent collaterals

SELECTED REFERENCES

1. Heijenbrok-Kal MH et al: Lower extremity arterial disease: multidetector CT angiography meta-analysis. Radiology. 245(2):433-9, 2007
2. Moore Wesley S et al: Acute Arterial and Graft Occlusion. In: Vascular and Endovascular Surgery A Comprehensive Review, 7th edition. Philadelphia, Saunders Elsevier. 732-54, 2006
3. Costantini V et al: Treatment of acute occlusion of peripheral arteries. Thromb Res. 106(6):V285-94, 2002
4. Visser K et al: Peripheral arterial disease: gadolinium-enhanced MR angiography versus color-guided duplex US--a meta-analysis. Radiology. 216(1):67-77, 2000
5. Wagner HJ et al: Acute embolic occlusions of the infrainguinal arteries: percutaneous aspiration embolectomy in 102 patients. Radiology. 182(2):403-7, 1992

IMAGE GALLERY

Typical

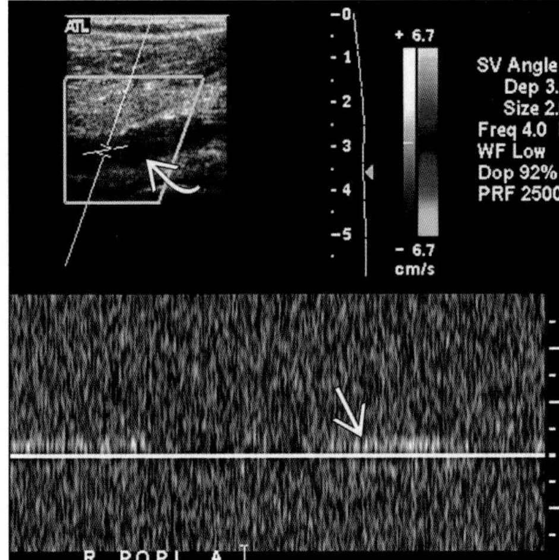

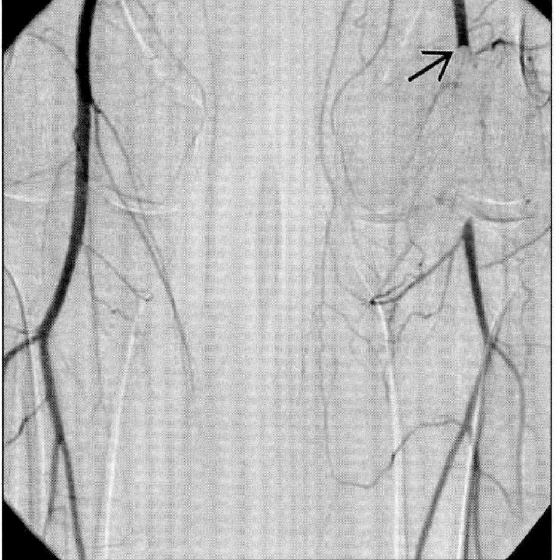

(Left) *Spectral and color Doppler ultrasound shows occlusive intraluminal hypoechoic thrombus with absence of color Doppler signal and of the expected triphasic waveform , consistent with thromboembolic occlusion.* ***(Right)*** *Catheter angiography of a different patient shows segmental occlusion of the left popliteal artery with proximal meniscoid filling defect consistent with acute embolic occlusion. The poor collaterals indicate this is an acute process.*

Typical

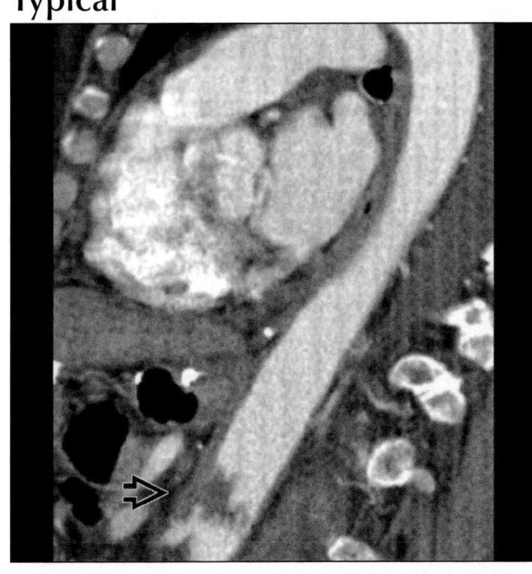

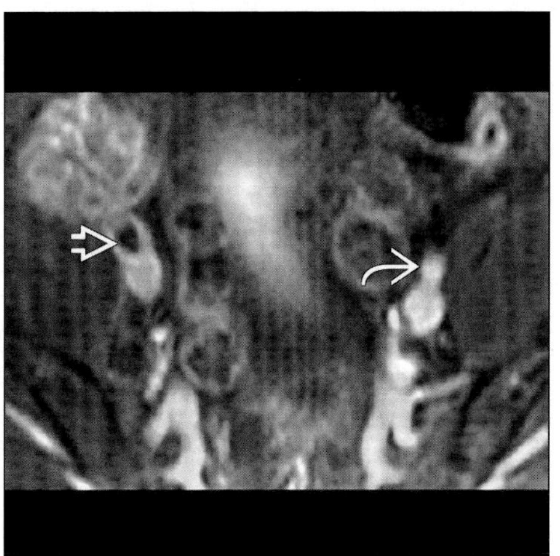

(Left) *Sagittal CTA in a patient with acute leg ischemia shows eccentric, irregular noncalcified low density thrombus protruding into the supraceliac aortic lumen; there is a high likelihood of distal embolization from this source.* ***(Right)*** *Post-contrast axial T1 GRE (same patient) shows a central occlusive filling defect in the dilated right external iliac artery, typical of an acute arterial embolus . The left external iliac artery is normal.*

Typical

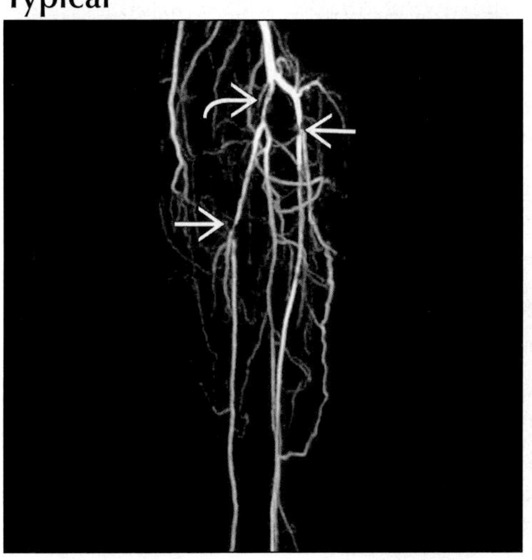

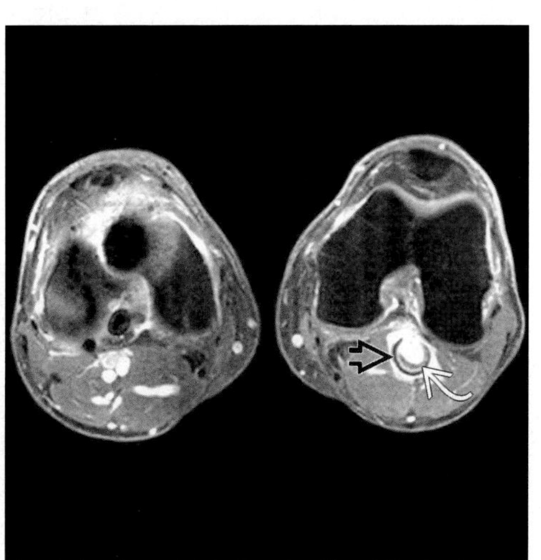

(Left) *Anteroposterior MIP image from high resolution CEMRA shows multifocal stenoses and irregularities of left tibioperoneal trunk and proximal trifurcation arteries due to multiple emboli.* ***(Right)*** *Axial GRE fat-saturation post-contrast image (same patient as previous image) shows a left popliteal artery aneurysm with eccentric low signal mural thrombus within the lumen. The popliteal artery aneurysm is the likely source of the distal emboli.*

LOWER EXTREMITY ARTERIAL TRAUMA

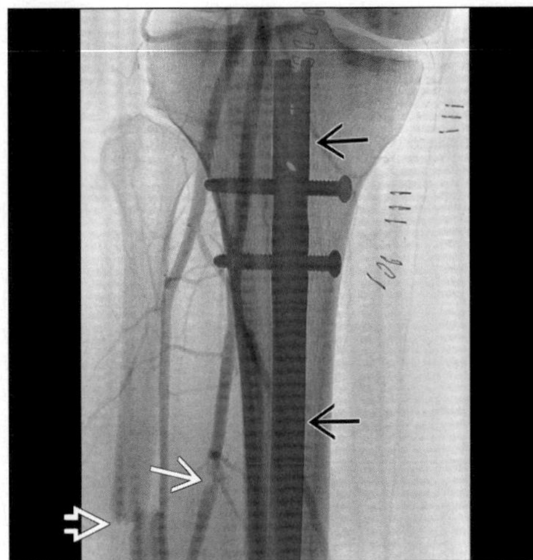

Catheter angiography shows a defect ➔ in the peroneal artery where there has been a shearing injury associated with a fibular fracture ➔. A tibial fracture was treated with an intramedullary rod ➔.

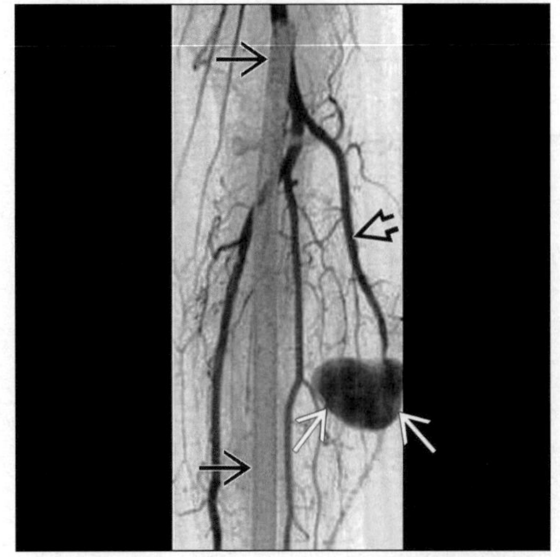

Catheter angiography in a different patient who sustained a tibial fracture requiring an intramedullary rod ➔, shows a large pseudoaneurysm ➔ of the anterior tibial artery ➔ located in the mid-calf.

TERMINOLOGY

Abbreviations and Synonyms

- Traumatic peripheral arterial injury

Definitions

- Peripheral, lower extremity, arterial injury from blunt or penetrating trauma

IMAGING FINDINGS

General Features

- Best diagnostic clue
  - Arterial laceration, dissection, occlusion or abrupt narrowing
  - Mural hematoma, pseudoaneurysm, or arteriovenous fistula (AVF)
  - Soft tissue hematoma and bone fractures
- Location
  - Superficial femoral or profunda femoral artery in penetrating trauma
  - Common femoral artery following instrumentation
  - Anterior and posterior tibial arteries in blunt trauma
- Size
  - Usually small-sized laceration or pseudoaneurysm
  - Small mural hematoma
  - Long segment narrowing can occur

CT Findings

- NECT: Not useful
- CTA
  - Fast, reliable and accurate initial diagnostic tool for traumatic peripheral arteries
  - Multidetector CTA has high sensitivity (90-95%) and specificity (> 98%) for lower extremity arterial injury
  - Simultaneous depiction of soft-tissue, osseous and vascular structures
  - Review of source axial images recommended but coronal reformation very helpful
  - Findings
    - Focal enlargement or irregularity of lumen suggests laceration
    - Stenosis/narrowing could be due to arterial dissection, spasm, extrinsic compression
    - Eccentric lumen or tapered stenosis with dissection; may visualize occluded false lumen (long, eccentric filling void) in larger vessels

DDx: Lower Extremity Arterial Injury

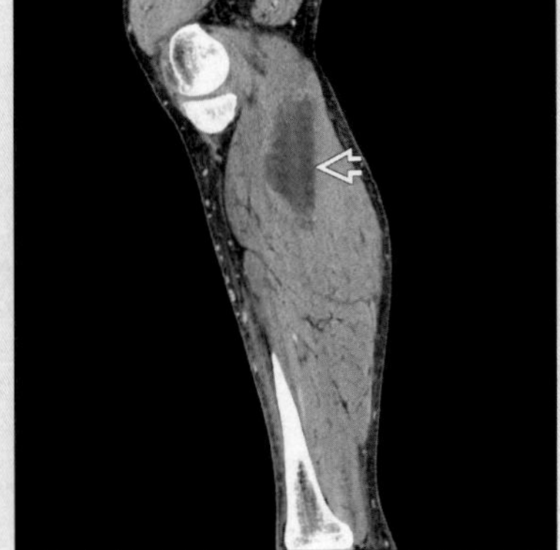

Soft Tissue Hematoma

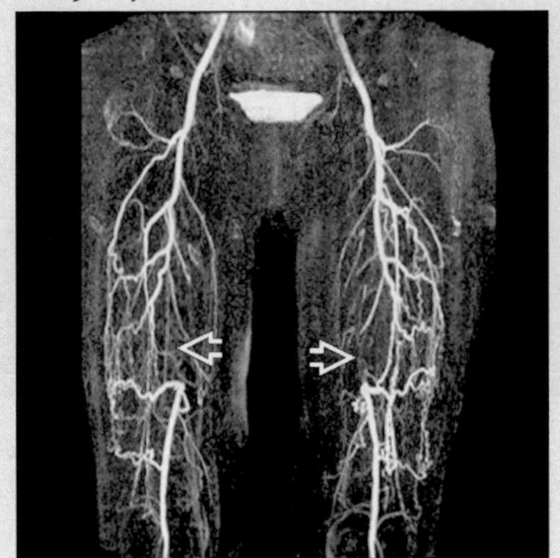

Atherosclerotic SFA Occlusions

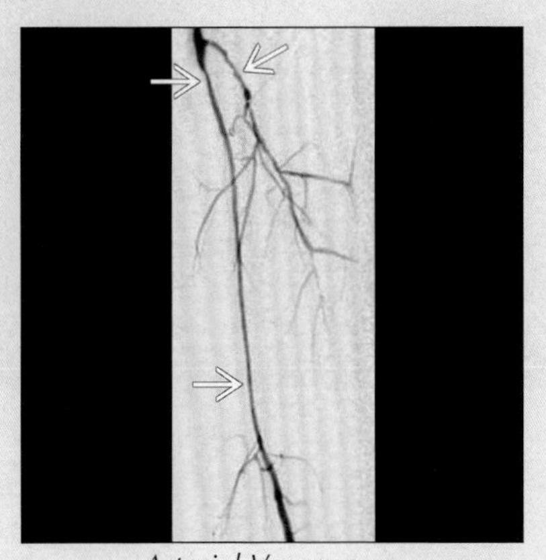

Arterial Vasospasm

LOWER EXTREMITY ARTERIAL TRAUMA

Key Facts

Terminology

- Lower extremity arterial injury from blunt or penetrating trauma

Imaging Findings

- CTA for initial assessment of arterial integrity
  - Sensitivity 90-95%; specificity > 98% for lower extremity arterial injury
  - Superficial femoral or profunda femoral artery in penetrating trauma
  - Axial source images more useful than multiplanar reformatted images
  - Arterial laceration, dissection, occlusion or abrupt narrowing
  - Mural hematoma, pseudoaneurysm, or AVF
  - Soft tissue hematoma and bone fractures
- MRA more time consuming and limited in trauma
- Ultrasound: Dampened Doppler waveforms distal to stenosis or occlusion; used to monitor arterial spasm
- DSA: Images not limited by metallic streak artifacts

Top Differential Diagnoses

- Hematoma/Contusion without Arterial Injury
- Atherosclerotic Peripheral Vascular Disease
- Arterial Spasm

Clinical Issues

- Cold, pale extremity: Major arterial occlusion
- Radiologic intervention is preferred over surgery

Diagnostic Checklist

- In trauma, consider CTA or angiography to exclude arterial injury in presence of diminished or absent peripheral pulses and absent audible Doppler

---

- Intimal flap seen as focal intraluminal linear filling defect
- Occlusion 2° to arterial injury or extrinsic compression
- Localized extraluminal contrast in transection and pseudoaneurysm
- Early draining vein and arteriovenous tract with AV fistula
- Extravasation of contrast into soft-tissue indicates active bleeding
- Severe arterial spasm simulates occlusion (pitfall)
- Hematoma/soft tissue edema, possible fracture or joint injury
- Intimal flap may be difficult to see on earlier generation MDCT scanners, DSA is better

MR Findings

- MRA
  - Contrast-enhanced, 3D MRA
    - Accurate, but more time consuming than CTA
    - More prone to artifacts
    - May be cumbersome in acute trauma setting
    - More suitable for subacute examination

Ultrasonographic Findings

- Color Doppler
  - Accurate, convenient, cost effective
    - Requires technical competence and experience
    - Cannot be used in areas of soft-tissue destruction/laceration or bone injury
  - Useful to assess arterial segments distal to injury
  - Direct visualization of arterial defects, pseudoaneurysm, AVF
  - High-velocity flow in stenosis, no flow in occlusion
    - Dampened Doppler waveforms distal to severe stenosis or occlusion
    - Focal, severe arterial turbulence with intimal flap
  - Turbulent, high-velocity venous flow in AVF
  - Useful for continuous monitoring of arterial spasm to differentiate from occlusion, thereby avoids unnecessary vascular surgery
    - Absence of normal audible sound needs further evaluation

Angiographic Findings

- Conventional
  - "Gold standard" for imaging traumatized vessels
    - Image quality not limited by streak artifacts due to metallic bullet fragments as in CTA
    - Direct visualization of arterial lumen, revealing laceration, transection, stenosis, occlusion, dissection, pseudoaneurysm, AVF
  - Inherent delay in treating arterial injury; lower extremity ischemic time prolonged
  - Excellent spatial resolution to depict intimal flap injuries and below ankle tibial arteries
  - Spasm can be reliably assessed after intraarterial vasodilator injection

Imaging Recommendations

- Best imaging tool
  - Multidetector CTA for initial assessment of arterial integrity
  - Catheter angiography for patients with extensive soft tissue metallic fragments or high index of suspicion and planned catheter-based intervention
  - Doppler for rapid bedside evaluation of artery distal to injury site and for follow-up
- Protocol advice
  - Strong indication of acute arterial injury, especially if unstable
    - DSA with radiologic intervention (preferred) or surgical exploration
  - Uncertain arterial injury, acute but stable
    - Investigate with CTA, US
  - Uncertain arterial injury, subacute or chronic
    - Investigate with CTA, US or MRA
  - CTA: 16 slice scanner; 1.5 mm thin slice volumetric acquisition with 2 x 1.5 mm reconstructed images
    - 64 slice 0.6 mm thin collimation volumetric acquisition with 2 x 1.5 mm reconstructed images
    - 120-150 mL of contrast at 3 cc/sec, ROI lower abdominal aorta
    - Coronal reformatted and volume rendered images useful

LOWER EXTREMITY ARTERIAL TRAUMA

DIFFERENTIAL DIAGNOSIS

Hematoma/Contusion without Arterial Injury

- Intact arteries
- No extraluminal blood flow (pseudoaneurysm/AVF)
- Soft tissue swelling

Atherosclerotic Peripheral Vascular Disease

- Older patients, vascular insufficiency by history
- Evidence of atherosclerotic disease
- Acute occlusion may be 2° to
  - Thrombosis of atherosclerotic stenosis or aneurysm
  - Acute embolic occlusion
- Collaterals present in chronic occlusive disease

Arterial Spasm

- Difficult to differentiate from occlusion
- False negative arterial occlusions on CTA due to severe spasm
- Continuous pulse monitoring and Doppler can help differentiate spasm vs. occlusion
- DSA can be performed following intraarterial vasodilator to open the artery

PATHOLOGY

General Features

- General path comments
  - Suspect arterial injury with any penetrating trauma within 5 cm of major thigh vessels or at any location below knee or in calf
  - Vascular trauma much more frequent with penetrating injury (36%) than with blunt trauma, contusion (1%)
  - Common femoral artery: Frequent site of iatrogenic injury; most common access site for catheterization procedures
  - Delayed recognition of arterial trauma may have serious consequences
- Associated abnormalities: Skin wound, soft tissue and osseous injuries, joint dislocation, soft tissue emphysema, rhabdomyolysis

CLINICAL ISSUES

Presentation

- Most common signs/symptoms: Expanding hematoma, loss of pulses, pulsatile mass
- Clinical Profile: Normal peripheral pulses and ABI usually exclude lower extremity arterial injury, if there are no other findings (e.g., bruit)
- Acute iatrogenic trauma
  - Ecchymosis
  - Post-procedural hematoma
  - Pulsatile mass: Pseudoaneurysm
  - Audible bruit: Stenosis, intimal flap, dissection, AVF
  - Palpable thrill: AVF
  - Diminished peripheral pulses or decreased ABI: Stenosis or occlusion, AVF
  - Cold, pale extremity: Major arterial occlusion
- Acute violent trauma
  - Above findings; also may include
    - Open lower extremity wound
    - Expanding hematoma
- Subacute, chronic trauma
  - Findings as in acute trauma but stable
  - Possible claudication, delayed arterial rupture (pseudoaneurysm), high output heart failure or chronic venous congestion (AVF)
- Acute lower extremity fractures
  - Infrequent cause of vascular injury
  - Arterial imaging needed for diminished peripheral pulses, abnormal ankle brachial index (ABI), or severe soft tissue crush/contusion

Natural History & Prognosis

- Good prognosis for vasospasm
- Limb ischemia is imminent for severe arterial injury

Treatment

- Radiologic intervention preferred over surgical arterial repair (less traumatic, faster recovery, lower cost)
- Focal intramural hematoma and intimal dissection without flow compromise, needs no urgent treatment
- Intimal flap with thrombosed obstructed lumen needs immediate intervention; arterial injuries with complete obliteration need surgery

DIAGNOSTIC CHECKLIST

Consider

- In trauma, consider CTA or angiography to exclude arterial injury in presence of diminished or absent peripheral pulses and absent audible Doppler

Image Interpretation Pearls

- Metallic streak artifact, motion artifact, and poor contrast opacification results non diagnostic CTA
- Axial source images of CTA are most useful dataset; volume rendered are more useful than MIP
- Good quality CTA with normal appearing peripheral arteries rules out significant arterial injury
  - With absent pulses and acutely ischemic extremity, angiography indicated, even if negative CTA
- Severe spasm may simulate occlusion

SELECTED REFERENCES

1. Rieger M et al: Traumatic arterial injuries of the extremities: initial evaluation with MDCT angiography. AJR Am J Roentgenol. 186(3):656-64, 2006
2. Miller-Thomas MM et al: Diagnosing traumatic arterial injury in the extremities with CT angiography: pearls and pitfalls. Radiographics. 25 Suppl 1:S133-42, 2005
3. Soto JA et al: Focal arterial injuries of the proximal extremities: helical CT arteriography as the initial method of diagnosis. Radiology. 218(1):188-94, 2001
4. Anderson RJ et al: Penetrating extremity trauma: identification of patients at high-risk requiring arteriography. J Vasc Surg. 11(4):544-8, 1990

IMAGE GALLERY

Typical

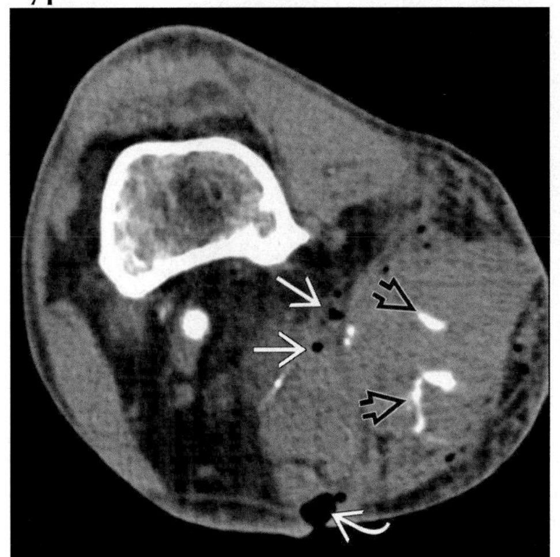

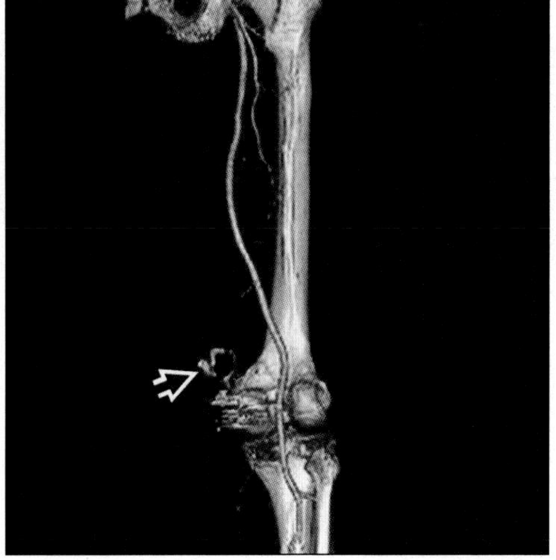

*(**Left**) Axial CECT shows contrast extravasation within soft tissues posteromedial to the femur in a patient who suffered penetrating injury to the lower extremity. Findings are compatible with an arterial laceration. Note air in the soft tissues and open skin wound. (**Right**) Posteroanterior CTA volume rendered image (same patient as previous) shows contrast extravasation in the soft tissues, without direct communication with SFA or popliteal artery.*

Typical

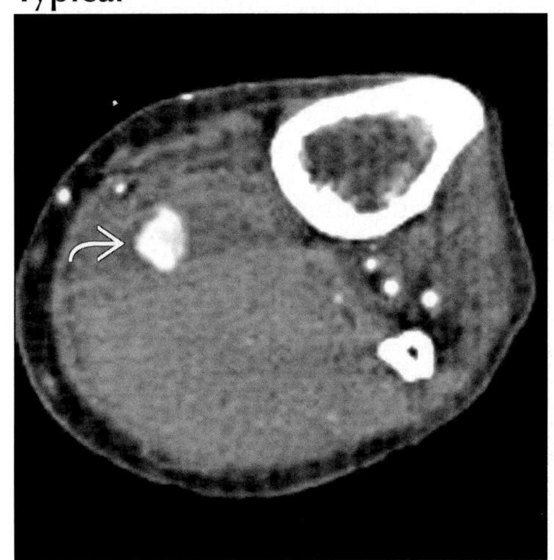

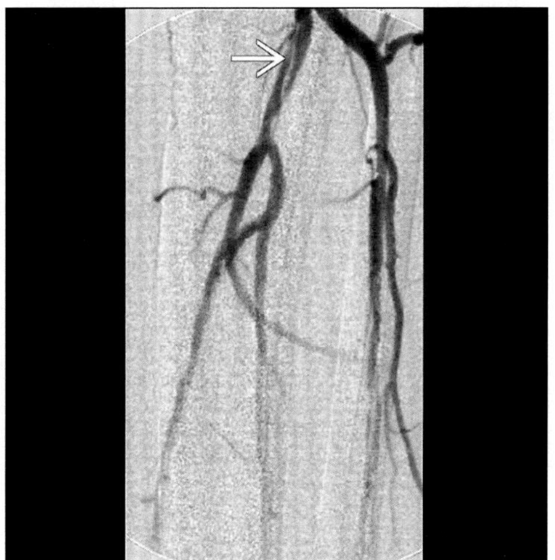

*(**Left**) Axial CTA shows a focal well-defined contrast collection in the left posteromedial calf consistent with a pseudoaneurysm. Active extravasation from an arterial laceration is also a consideration. (**Right**) Anteroposterior DSA image of the arteries of the calf (different patient) shows a linear filling defect in the tibioperoneal trunk consistent with an intimal flap or dissection. This patient sustained blunt trauma to the posterior aspect of the upper calf.*

Typical

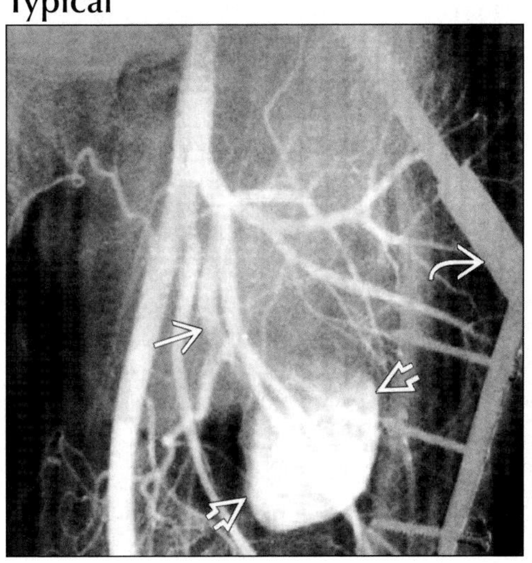

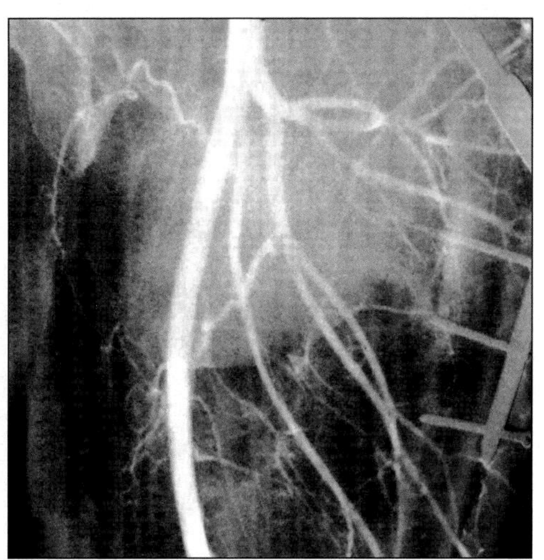

*(**Left**) Femoral arteriogram shows a pseudoaneurysm arising from a profunda femoral arterial branch. Iatrogenic injury occurred during orthopedic left hip fracture repair (note surgical hardware). (**Right**) Arteriogram following transcatheter embolization with coils & thrombin injection shows the pseudoaneurysm no longer opacifies & has been successfully occluded. Arterial branch supplying pseudoaneurysm was sacrificed.*

FEMOROPOPLITEAL ARTERY OCCLUSIVE DISEASE

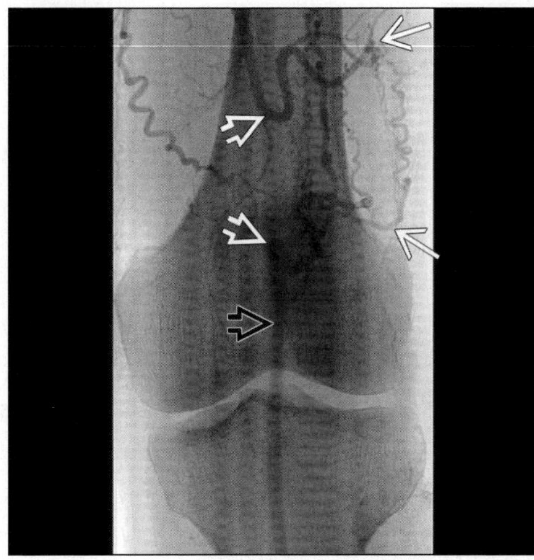

Catheter angiography shows a short chronic total occlusion ➡ of the above-knee segment of the popliteal artery. Extensive collateral vessels ➡ reconstitute the popliteal artery ⇨ at the patellar level.

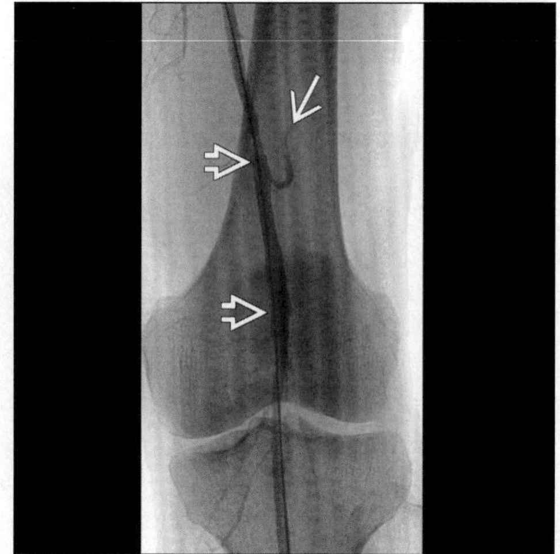

Catheter angiography (same patient) after intervention, shows patency has been restored to the popliteal artery via angioplasty and covered stent placement ➡. Note that there is no longer filling of the collaterals ➡.

TERMINOLOGY

Abbreviations and Synonyms

- Common femoral artery (CFA)
- Superficial femoral artery (SFA)
- Ankle-brachial index (ABI)
- Chronic total occlusion (CTO)

Definitions

- Stenosis or occlusion of common femoral, superficial femoral, or popliteal artery(ies)

IMAGING FINDINGS

General Features

- Best diagnostic clue
  - Arterial stenoses and occlusions, common at CFA bifurcation, adductor hiatus, popliteal artery
  - Well-developed collaterals imply chronic, rather than acute obstruction
  - Post-stenotic dilatation distal to severe stenoses
  - Segmental occlusions with distal reconstitution
- Location
  - CFA extends from inguinal ligament to bifurcation into superficial and profunda femoral arteries
  - SFA courses beneath sartorius muscle to pass through adductor (Hunter) canal
    - SFA emerges at adductor hiatus in distal thigh to become popliteal artery
  - Popliteal artery continues from adductor hiatus to terminate at origins of tibial vessels below knee
    - Popliteal described as above and below-knee segments; these divisions influence interventions

CT Findings

- CTA
  - Accurately depicts stenoses, occlusions and collaterals in format similar to angiography
    - CECT combined with CTA also depicts adjacent nonvascular structures, unlike angiography
  - Multidetector scanner, high contrast dose, rapid bolus injection, and sophisticated post-processing
    - Potential for contrast-induced renal dysfunction, allergic reaction
    - Heavily calcified plaque may limit usefulness of rendered images with CTA; include source images for accurate interpretation

DDx: Femoropopliteal Artery Occlusive Disease

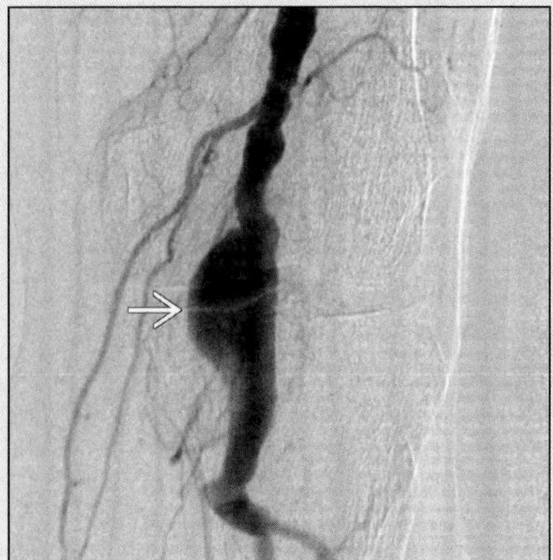

Popliteal Artery Aneurysm

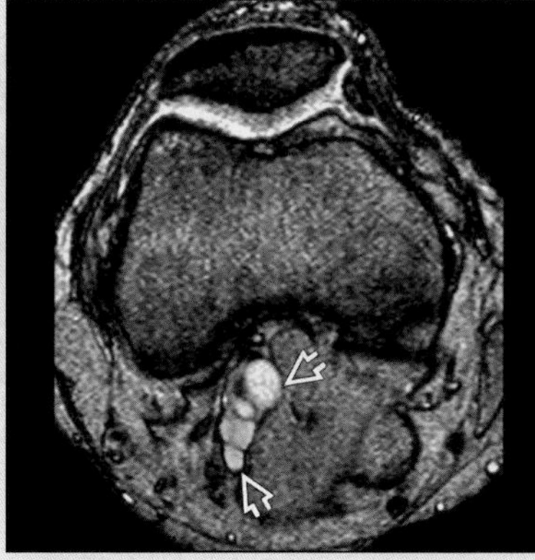

Popliteal Cystic Adventitial Disease

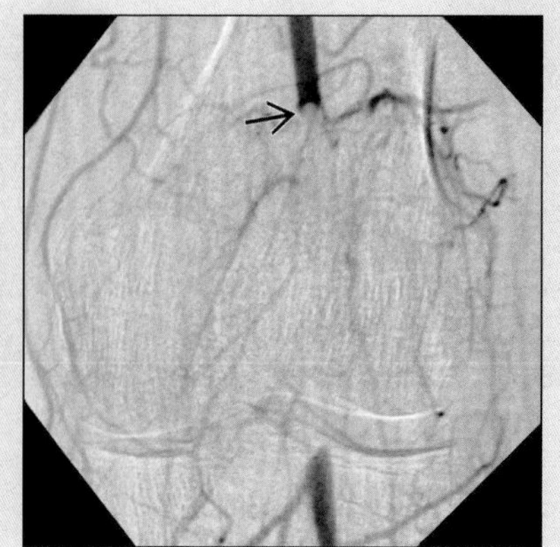

Acute Embolic Occlusion

FEMOROPOPLITEAL ARTERY OCCLUSIVE DISEASE

Key Facts

Terminology
- Stenosis or occlusion of common femoral (CFA), superficial femoral (SFA), or popliteal artery

Imaging Findings
- MRA and CTA are excellent imaging modalities
- Angiography may be initial imaging, particularly if endovascular therapy planned
- MRA, CTA and angiography findings
  - Arterial stenoses, common at CFA bifurcation, adductor canal region or popliteal artery
  - Collateral flow-implies chronic, rather than acute obstruction
  - Post-stenotic dilatation distal to severe stenoses
- Severe stenosis may progress to occlusion
  - Thrombus forms at lesion and propagates

Pathology
- Atherosclerotic intimal plaques
  - Smooth muscle proliferation, extracellular lipid/collagen deposition, and inflammation
  - Plaque projects into vessel lumen causing stenosis/occlusion

Clinical Issues
- Endovascular treatment
  - For acute thrombotic occlusion, thrombolysis trial; angioplasty/stent if necessary
  - Angioplasty/stent (covered and non-covered) for stenotic disease
- Surgical bypass
  - Long-term durability; remains "gold standard"
  - Reversed or in situ saphenous vein bypass

  - High-resolution images possible with CTA; rivals angiography; not universally available

MR Findings
- MRA
  - High-resolution images with contrast-enhanced MRA; rivals angiography; not universally available
  - Time-of-flight MRA technique inaccurate due to flow-related artifacts; use contrast-enhanced MRA

Ultrasonographic Findings
- Color Doppler
  - Visible lumen narrowing on color Doppler, with post-stenotic turbulence
  - Hemodynamically significant stenosis
    - Peak systolic velocity in stenosis ≥ 2 x velocity proximal to stenosis
    - Monophasic waveforms in stenosis
    - Damped waveforms distal to stenosis with high-grade obstruction
- Non-invasive vascular evaluation; pulse volume recording (PVR)
  - Pneumatic cuff is wrapped around extremity
  - Standardized volume of air injected, achieving standardized cuff pressure (65 mm Hg)
    - Allows volume changes to be detected with a transducer and displayed as arterial waveforms
  - Ratio between arterial pressures at ankle and brachial levels calculated and reported as ankle/brachial index (ABI)
    - Normal ≥ 0.96; mild disease = 0.81-0.95; moderate disease = 0.51-0.80; moderate to severe disease = 0.3 -0.50; severe disease ≤ 0.30

Angiographic Findings
- Conventional
  - Angiography is current gold standard for characterization of arterial disease
    - Vascular stenoses, occlusions, collateral pathways, aneurysms
  - Invasive but relatively low risk
    - Potential for hematoma, vessel injury, pseudoaneurysm, contrast allergy, renal failure

Imaging Recommendations
- Best imaging tool
  - MRA and CTA are excellent imaging modalities
  - Angiography may be initial imaging, particularly if endovascular therapy planned
- Protocol advice
  - Detailed vascular history and physical examination
  - ABI, segmental limb pressures, PVR, treadmill test
  - If clinical evidence of inflow (iliac artery) disease
    - Use CTA or MRA to confirm localized iliac disease
    - Proceed to percutaneous intervention or surgery
  - If extent of disease uncertain clinically, or evidence of femoropopliteal or severe multilevel disease
    - Comprehensive arterial assessment required
    - CTA/MRA if available or catheter angiography

DIFFERENTIAL DIAGNOSIS

Atherosclerosis
- Occlusive disease
  - Irregular, eccentric narrowing; occurs at CFA, popliteal artery or tibioperoneal trunk bifurcations
  - Extensive collateralization
- Aneurysmal disease
  - Popliteal artery aneurysm
    - Spontaneous thrombosis rather than rupture
    - Distal embolization may occur

Embolic Disease
- Abrupt occlusion with "meniscus", usually at bifurcations
- Lack of collateral vessels
- Search for etiology: Proximal aneurysm, cardiac vegetations, atrial thrombus

Traumatic Occlusion
- Common cause in young
  - Extremity fracture, penetrating injury

Vasculitis
- Uncommon in femoral and popliteal arteries

- Typically affects tibial and peroneal arteries and foot arteries (e.g., Buerger disease, Raynaud phenomenon)

Cystic Adventitial Disease

- Focal cystic fluid accumulation in arterial adventitia
  - Affects popliteal artery in 85% of cases
  - Also external iliac and common femoral arteries
- Causes smoothly tapered "spiral" stenosis or occlusion
  - Symptoms of intermittent claudication

Popliteal Artery Entrapment

- Aberrant arterial relationship to gastrocnemius muscles
  - Arterial compression, thickening and fibrosis
  - Aneurysm, thrombosis, distal embolization

PATHOLOGY

General Features

- General path comments
  - Younger patients: Vasculitis, trauma more likely
  - Older patients: Atherosclerosis more likely
- Etiology
  - Atherosclerotic intimal plaques
    - Smooth muscle proliferation, extracellular lipid/collagen deposition, and inflammation
    - Plaque projects into vessel lumen causing stenosis/occlusion

Staging, Grading or Classification Criteria

- Trans Atlantic Inter-Societal Consensus (TASC)
  - Classification system for treatment of peripheral arterial disease, based upon response to intervention
  - TASC A lesion (endovascular treatment)
    - Single stenosis ≤ 10 cm, or occlusion ≤ 5 cm long
  - TASC B lesion (endovascular treatment)
    - Multiple stenoses or occlusions, each ≤ 5 cm
    - Single stenosis or occlusion ≤ 15 cm (not involving infra-geniculate popliteal)
    - Heavily calcified occlusions ≤ 5 cm long
    - Single popliteal stenosis
  - TASC C lesion (surgery preferred; good-risk patients)
    - Multiple stenoses or occlusions totaling > 15 cm (with or without heavy calcification)
    - Recurrent stenoses or occlusions requiring re-treatment after two endovascular interventions
  - TASC D lesion (surgical treatment)
    - CTO of SFA > 20 cm, involving popliteal artery
    - CTO of popliteal artery and proximal trifurcation

CLINICAL ISSUES

Presentation

- Most common signs/symptoms
  - Atherosclerosis: Gradual evolution of symptoms most common
  - Intermittent claudication
    - Definition: Exercise-related pain worsening with activity, and subsiding after several minutes rest
    - Graded by distance patient is able to walk
    - Location of pain may indicate level of obstruction
- Other signs/symptoms: Embolic occlusion: Abrupt onset arterial insufficiency symptoms
- Intermittent claudication
  - Definition: Exercise-related pain worsening with activity, and subsiding after several minutes rest
  - Graded by distance patient is able to walk
  - Location of pain may indicate level of obstruction
    - Thigh pain: External iliac, common femoral artery
    - Calf pain: Femoropopliteal occlusive disease

Demographics

- Age
  - Atherosclerotic disease
    - Incidence increases with age: 45-54 yrs (3%), 55-64 yrs (6%)
- Gender: Males > > females

Natural History & Prognosis

- Untreated severe atherosclerotic stenoses may progress to occlusion
  - More complex interventions/surgery required for occlusion vs. stenosis

Treatment

- Acute occlusive thrombus
  - Thrombolysis trial; angioplasty/stent if necessary
  - Surgical thrombectomy
- Atherosclerosis
  - Angioplasty/stent (covered and non-covered)
    - Originally temporizing measure
    - Now often primary treatment of choice
    - Can delay or avoid bypass surgery
  - Atherectomy
    - Catheter based treatment allowing plaque excision
  - Laser
    - Remains primarily investigational
  - Surgical bypass
    - Long-term durability; remains "gold standard"
    - Reversed or in situ saphenous vein bypass
    - Distal revascularization to tibial and peroneal vessels, if needed

DIAGNOSTIC CHECKLIST

Consider

- Thrombosed popliteal artery aneurysm in patient with acute onset of leg pain and popliteal artery occlusion

SELECTED REFERENCES

1. Sun Z: Diagnostic accuracy of multislice CT angiography in peripheral arterial disease. J Vasc Interv Radiol. 17(12):1915-21, 2006
2. Rubin GD et al: Multi-detector row CT angiography of lower extremity arterial inflow and runoff: initial experience. Radiology. 221(1):146-58, 2001
3. Lenhart M et al: [Contrast media-enhanced MR angiography of the lower extremity arteries using a dedicated peripheral vascular coil system. First clinical results] Rofo. 172(12):992-9, 2000
4. Kadir S: Teaching atlas of interventional radiology: Diagnostic and therapeutic angiography. Thieme, New York, 1999

FEMOROPOPLITEAL ARTERY OCCLUSIVE DISEASE

IMAGE GALLERY

Typical

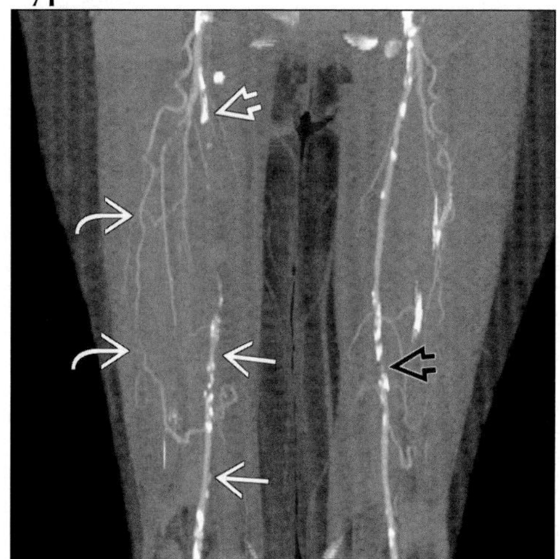

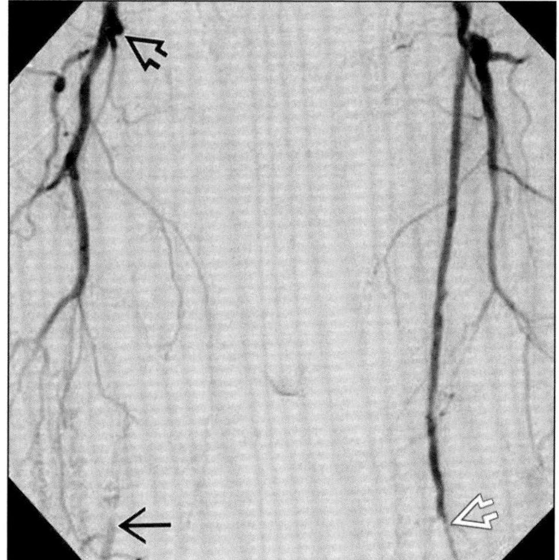

*(**Left**) 3D CTA MIP of the thighs shows proximal occlusion of the right SFA with distal reconstitution via collateral vessels from the profunda femoral artery. There is a left SFA stenosis at the adductor hiatus level. (**Right**) DSA of the proximal thighs in another patient with a similar disease pattern, shows a right SFA occlusion with distal reconstitution and a stenosis of the distal left SFA. These images were obtained during endovascular treatment of the right SFA occlusion.*

Typical

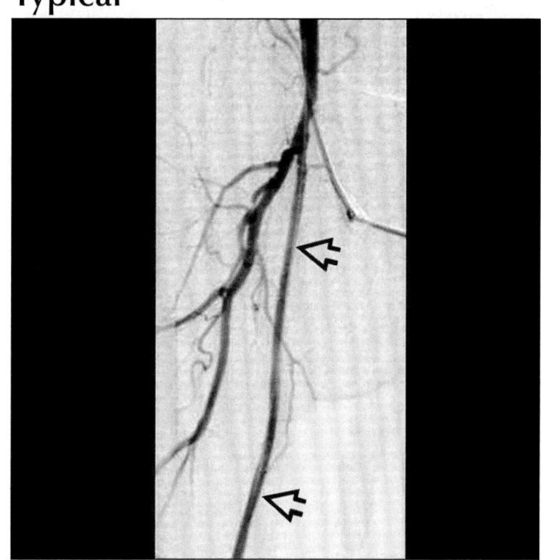

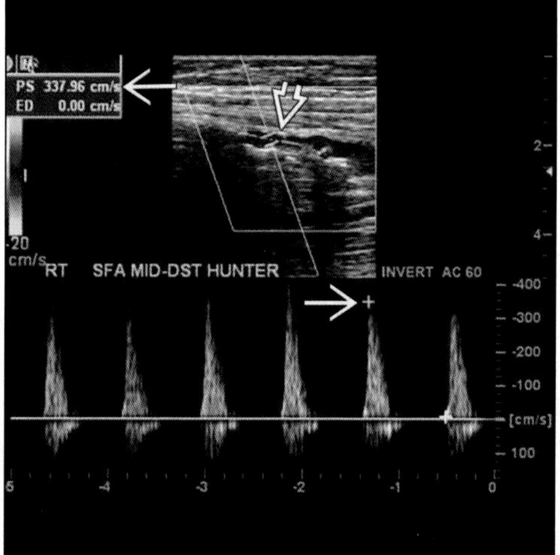

*(**Left**) DSA (previous patient) after endovascular treatment, shows that the right SFA is patent. The vessel was recanalized, angioplastied and then treated with placement of multiple covered stents. (**Right**) Color Doppler ultrasound of the right superficial femoral artery (different patient) shows marked elevation of the peak systolic velocity to 337.96 cm/sec within an area of narrowing sampled by the Doppler. This is consistent with a high grade stenosis.*

Typical

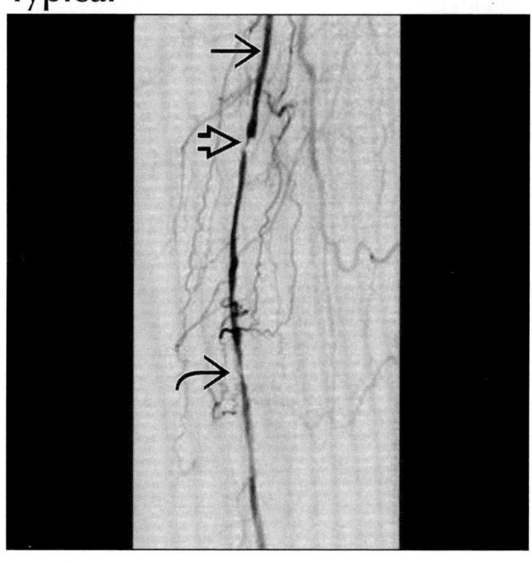

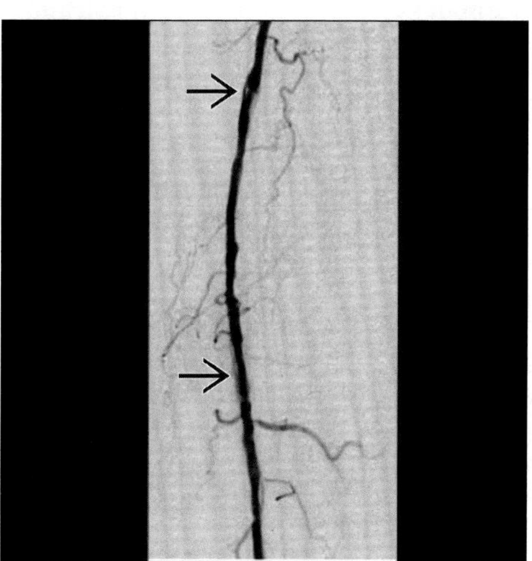

*(**Left**) DSA of the distal right SFA (same patient) shows a severe stenosis, corresponding to the ultrasound findings. The stenosis is at the adductor hiatus, a common location for a lesion. There is a second lesion in the popliteal artery. (**Right**) DSA following angioplasty of both lesions shows irregularity at each angioplasty site, corresponding to intimal fissures that occur during the procedure. Normal luminal calibers have been restored at each level of treatment.*

PERIPHERAL VASCULAR SURGICAL RECONSTRUCTION

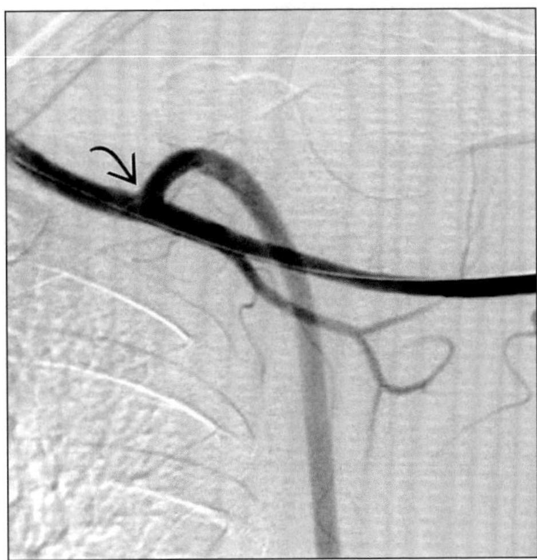

DSA shows the proximal anastomosis ➔ of an axillofemoral bypass graft. Extra-anatomic grafts such as this may be necessary in patients with aortoiliac disease who are a poor risk for aortofemoral bypass surgery.

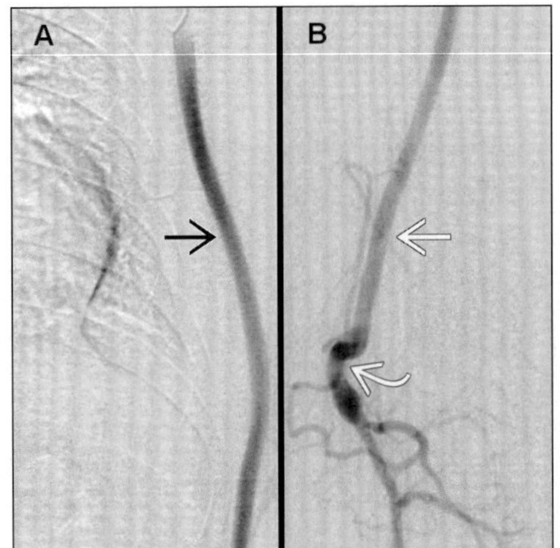

DSA (same patient as previous image) shows the course of the thoracic ➔ (A) and abdominal ➔ (B) portions of the axillofemoral bypass graft. The distal anastomosis is to the left common femoral artery ➔.

TERMINOLOGY

Abbreviations

- Femoral-popliteal bypass graft (FPBPG)
- Common femoral artery (CFA); superficial femoral artery (SFA)

Synonyms

- Cross-femoral bypass, fem-fem bypass
- Femoral-popliteal bypass, femoropopliteal bypass, fem-pop bypass
  - In-situ saphenous vein graft
  - Reversed saphenous vein graft
- Femoral-tibial bypass, femorotibial bypass, fem-tib bypass
- Extra-anatomic bypass: Axillo-femoral bypass, axillo-bifemoral bypass, ax-fem bypass

Definitions

- Vascular bypass surgery: Insertion of vascular conduit for replacement or bypass of diseased arterial segment
- Infrainguinal bypass: Arterial reconstruction using vascular conduit originating at or below inguinal ligament
  - Inflow sites include common, deep or superficial femoral arteries; popliteal and tibial arteries
  - Distal anastomosis sites: SFA, above- or below-knee popliteal, tibial, peroneal or pedal arteries
  - Available choices for conduits
    - Autogenous (native) vein: Greater saphenous vein preferred; other veins include short saphenous, femoral (superficial femoral), basilic, cephalic
    - Prosthetics: Include expanded polytetrafluoroethylene (ePTFE), externally supported ePTFE (xPTFE) and Dacron
    - Non-native biologic conduits: Human umbilical vein, arterial or venous homografts
- Autogenous vein grafts subdivided into
  - In-situ greater saphenous vein graft
    - Proximal and distal ends of vein anastomosed to artery, leaving remainder of vein in place
    - Venous side branches ligated and valves incised
  - Reversed saphenous vein graft
    - Vein carefully harvested from thigh
    - Venous side branches ligated; vein reversed allowing unobstructed flow through venous valves

PRE-PROCEDURE

Indications

- Arterial bypass remains standard for revascularization; infrainguinal bypass indicated in symptomatic patients with
  - Long-segment chronic total SFA occlusion
  - Diffuse multiple stenoses or occlusions of entire SFA
  - Chronic total occlusion of popliteal and/or proximal trifurcation arteries
  - Recurrent stenoses or occlusions that have failed after two or more prior endovascular treatments
- Extra-anatomic bypass indications
  - Appropriate for patients at high risk for aortofemoral bypass; unsuccessful endovascular intervention
  - Femorofemoral bypass
    - Unilateral symptomatic iliac artery occlusion
  - Axillofemoral bypass
    - Infected native aorta or aortic prosthesis

Contraindications

- Arterial bypass surgery contraindicated if
  - Inadequate inflow or outflow to maintain patency
    - Uncorrected inflow disease or no target vessel for distal anastomosis results in poor outcomes
  - Conduit to be placed in actively infected tissue bed
    - Aggressively treat infection to resolution

PERIPHERAL VASCULAR SURGICAL RECONSTRUCTION

Key Facts

Terminology

- Vascular bypass surgery: Insertion of vascular conduit for replacement or bypass of diseased arterial segment
- Infrainguinal bypass: Arterial reconstruction using vascular conduit originating at or below inguinal ligament
- Available choices for conduits
  - Autogenous (native) vein: Greater saphenous vein preferred; other veins include short saphenous, femoral (superficial femoral), basilic, cephalic
  - Prosthetics: Include expanded polytetrafluoroethylene (ePTFE) and Dacron
  - Non-native biologic conduits: Human umbilical vein, arterial or venous homografts

Pre-procedure

- Arterial bypass remains standard for revascularization
- Prior to bypass perform some type of imaging (CTA, MRA or catheter angiography)
  - Delineate arterial anatomy and identify appropriate target artery for distal anastomosis
- Attempt to bypass all hemodynamically significant disease when selecting target vessel

Procedure

- Endovascular revascularization alternative to surgical bypass; stents/angioplasty often initial therapy

Common Problems & Complications

- Graft infection
- Progression of disease distal to graft resulting in inadequate outflow
- Development of anastomotic stenoses or pseudoaneurysms; may cause distal ischemia

---

- If insufficient vascularity for healing, consider extra-anatomic bypass or amputation

Getting Started

- Things to Check
  - Imaging (CTA, MRA or angiography) prior to bypass
    - Delineate arterial anatomy and identify appropriate target artery for distal anastomosis
    - Identify and correct significant arterial inflow lesions prior to infrainguinal bypass
    - Identify and correct disease involving origin and proximal portion of profunda femoral artery
    - Attempt to bypass all hemodynamically significant disease when selecting target vessel; need single continuously patent runoff artery
  - Pre-operative duplex imaging to identify optimal vein; avoid segments with occlusion, sclerosis, poor caliber or calcifications
    - Attempt to perform infrainguinal bypass with autogenous vein whenever possible; conduit of choice
- Medications: Heparin 5,000 units; maintain appropriate level of therapeutic anticoagulation intra-procedurally

PROCEDURE

Patient Position/Location

- Best procedure approach
  - Vertical incision over common femoral artery allows access to CFA, profunda, SFA for bypass anastomosis
  - Medial leg incisions for exposure of popliteal and below-knee arteries

Findings and Reporting

- Completion assessment following bypass surgery
  - Pulse palpation and Doppler flow assessment
  - Completion arteriogram
  - Intraoperative duplex scanning or angioscopy

Alternative Procedures/Therapies

- Conservative nonoperative/non-interventional management for claudication
  - Trial of smoking cessation, exercise, risk-factor modification and possible medical therapy indicated prior to intervention
  - Surgical or endovascular treatment only if high risk-benefit ratio and satisfactory anatomy
  - Chronic limb ischemia generally requires surgery or endovascular intervention
- Endovascular revascularization
  - Angioplasty
    - 1° mechanism: Controlled fracture of plaque; fissures accompanied by stretching of media
    - Subsequent remodeling; lumen normalizes
  - Stents
    - Provides intravascular scaffold for vessel lumen; employed as 1° therapy or adjunct to angioplasty
    - Mechanism differs from angioplasty; plaque & vessel wall displaced by stent to enlarge lumen
    - Non-covered and covered stents used
  - Atherectomy
    - Catheter-mounted, tiny rotating blade used to shave away and remove intra-arterial plaque
  - Cryoplasty
    - Liquid nitrous oxide inflates angioplasty balloon
    - Lowers balloon surface temperature to -10 C
    - Theoretically causes altered plaque response, decreased elastic recoil, cellular apoptosis
  - Laser
    - Primarily investigational
- Lumbar sympathectomy
  - Increases blood flow to extremity; abolishes basal and reflex constriction at arteriolar and precapillary levels
  - Severe multilevel occlusions, ischemic rest pain and tissue loss generally have marginal if any improvement following sympathectomy
  - Used infrequently and in selected patients

POST-PROCEDURE

Expected Outcome

- 1° reported endpoints for revascularization procedures are long-term graft patency, limb salvage, mortality
  - Patency described as 1°, assisted 1° and 2°
    - 1° patency: No additional procedures have been performed that involve vascular conduit
    - Assisted 1° patency: Any minor revisions or endovascular treatments of lesions threatening graft patency
    - 2° patency: Restoration of patency to thrombosed graft by thrombolysis, thrombectomy, revision
- 3 year 1° patency for above- and below-knee FPBPG
  - Reversed saphenous vein graft: 73% (above-) 79% (below-knee)
  - In-situ vein graft: 73% (below-knee)
  - Prosthetic (ePTFE): 66% (above-) 44% (below-knee)
- 3 year 1° patency for extra-anatomic bypass grafts
  - Femorofemoral bypass: 60%
    - Better patency in claudication than rest pain
    - Questionable ability of femorofemoral bypass to adequately perfuse both legs with exercise
  - Axillofemoral bypass: From 39-76% (various series)
    - Thrombosis more often than aortofemoral bypass
    - Slightly better results with externally supported prosthetic conduits compared with unsupported

Things To Do

- Post-operatively maintain patient on antiplatelet therapy or anticoagulation
  - Anticoagulation used selectively in patients at greatest risk of graft thrombosis; increased bleeding risk for anticoagulation vs. antiplatelet therapy
- Vein graft surveillance important to good long-term outcomes
  - ABI determination and duplex graft imaging on regular schedule
- Prosthetic graft surveillance not shown beneficial
- Wound care to insure healing of any ischemic ulcers following bypass
  - Delay debridement/amputation several days following bypass; allows for maximum reperfusion and demarcation of persistently ischemic zones

PROBLEMS & COMPLICATIONS

Problems

- Poor conduit quality
  - Do not use compromised conduit for bypass, as quality of conduit highly important for good result
- Failure to incise all valves or ligate all venous side branches within in-situ bypass graft

Complications

- Most feared complication(s)
  - Graft infection
    - Result from hospital-acquired organisms in early period; increased in presence of hematoma, lymphocele or wound infection
    - Occurring > three months after bypass usually from microorganisms such as normal skin flora
- Other complications
  - Hemorrhage
    - Usually related to anastomotic problem such as suture line disruption or poorly ligated arterial or venous side branch
  - Progression of disease distal to graft resulting in inadequate outflow
    - May result in graft thrombosis or distal ischemia
  - Anastomotic stenoses or pseudoaneurysms
    - May lead to graft thrombosis or distal ischemia
  - Graft degeneration or graft intimal hyperplasia
  - Failing graft manifests as recurrent symptoms, decreased pulses, deteriorating non-invasive examination
    - If 1° procedure originally justified then 2° procedure mandated to maintain graft patency
    - Pre-operative imaging before any 2° procedure
    - Identify and correct underlying cause of graft failure

SELECTED REFERENCES

1. Bosiers M et al: Endovascular therapy as the primary approach for limb salvage in patients with critical limb ischemia: experience with 443 infrapopliteal procedures. Vascular. 14(2):63-9, 2006
2. Chung J et al: Wound healing and functional outcomes after infrainguinal bypass with reversed saphenous vein for critical limb ischemia. J Vasc Surg. 43(6):1183-90, 2006
3. Yancey AE et al: Peripheral atherectomy in TransAtlantic InterSociety Consensus type C femoropopliteal lesions for limb salvage. J Vasc Surg. 44(3):503-9, 2006
4. Albers M et al: Meta-analysis of alternate autologous vein bypass grafts to infrapopliteal arteries. J Vasc Surg. 42(3):449-55, 2005
5. Trocciola SM et al: Comparison of results in endovascular interventions for infrainguinal lesions: claudication versus critical limb ischemia. Am Surg. 71(6):474-9; discussion 479-80, 2005
6. Alcocer F et al: Early results of lower extremity infrageniculate revascularization with a new polytetrafluoroethylene graft. Vascular. 12(5):318-24, 2004
7. Goshima KR et al: A new look at outcomes after infrainguinal bypass surgery: traditional reporting standards systematically underestimate the expenditure of effort required to attain limb salvage. J Vasc Surg. 39(2):330-5, 2004
8. Nehler MR et al: Is revascularization and limb salvage always the treatment for critical limb ischemia? J Cardiovasc Surg (Torino). 45(3):177-84, 2004
9. Nguyen LL et al: Infrainguinal vein bypass graft revision: factors affecting long-term outcome. J Vasc Surg. 40(5):916-23, 2004
10. Curi MA et al: Conduit choice for above-knee femoropopliteal bypass grafting in patients with limb-threatening ischemia. Ann Vasc Surg. 16(1):95-101, 2002
11. Landry GJ et al: Long-term outcome of revised lower-extremity bypass grafts. J Vasc Surg. 35(1):56-62; discussion 62-3, 2002
12. Singh S et al: The costs of managing lower limb-threatening ischaemia. Eur J Vasc Endovasc Surg. 12(3):359-62, 1996
13. DE CAMP PT: Surgical reconstruction for arterial occlusive disease. Postgrad Med. 23(4):378-84, 1958

PERIPHERAL VASCULAR SURGICAL RECONSTRUCTION

IMAGE GALLERY

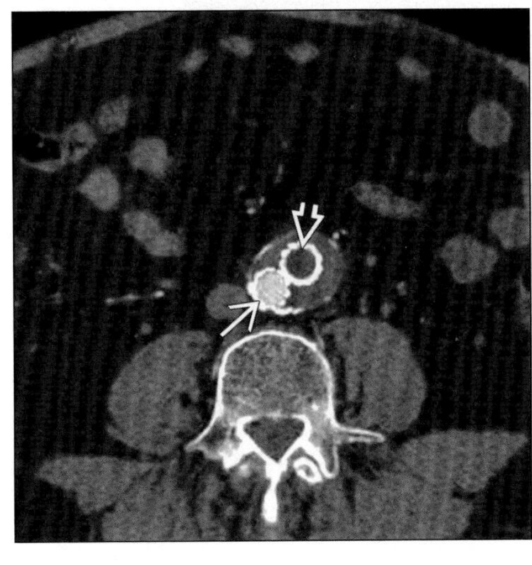

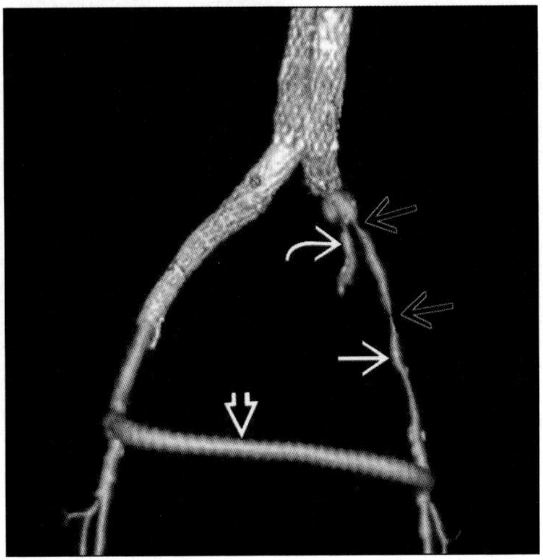

(Left) *Axial CECT in a patient who previously underwent EVAR for AAA and now has new left leg ischemia shows an opacified right graft limb, but a nonopacified occluded left graft limb.* ***(Right)*** *CTA following bypass surgery shows a right-to-left, cross-femoral graft providing antegrade perfusion to the left leg and retrograde perfusion of the left external and internal iliac arteries. The external iliac artery stenotic disease was likely the cause of the left limb thrombosis.*

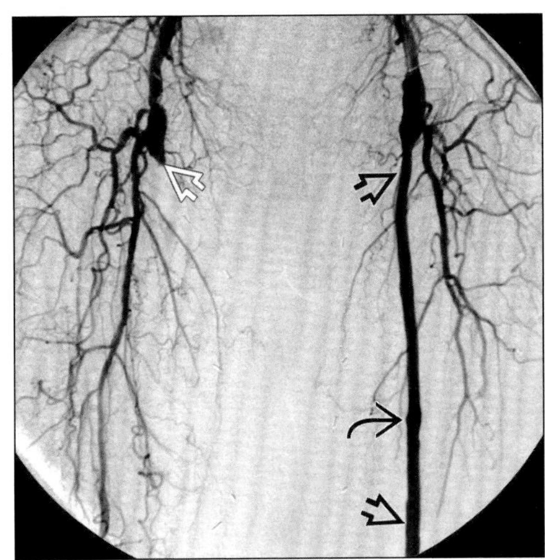

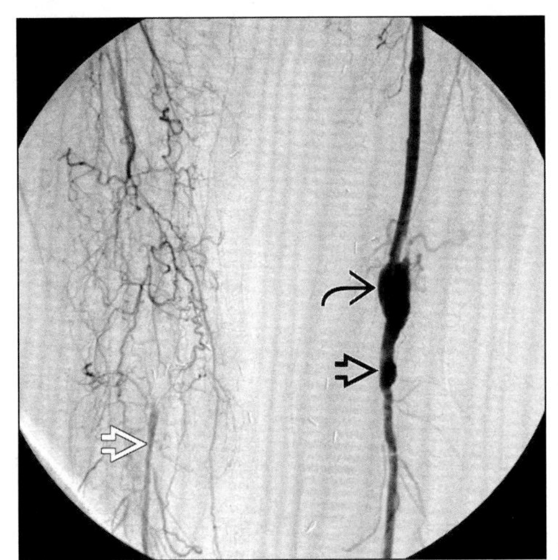

(Left) *DSA shows a patent left and an occluded right femoropopliteal bypass graft. The focal bulge in the right graft is where a venous valve was previously present, consistent with a saphenous vein conduit.* ***(Right)*** *DSA (same patient as previous image) shows that the distal anastomosis of the left femoropopliteal bypass graft is to the above-knee popliteal artery. On the right, only the tibioperoneal artery is seen as a result of graft thrombosis.*

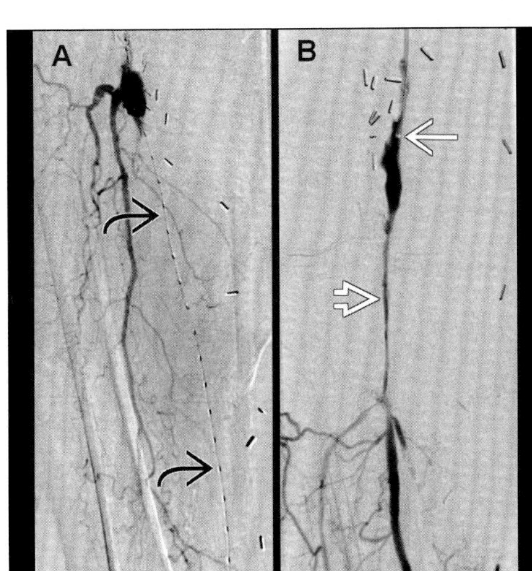

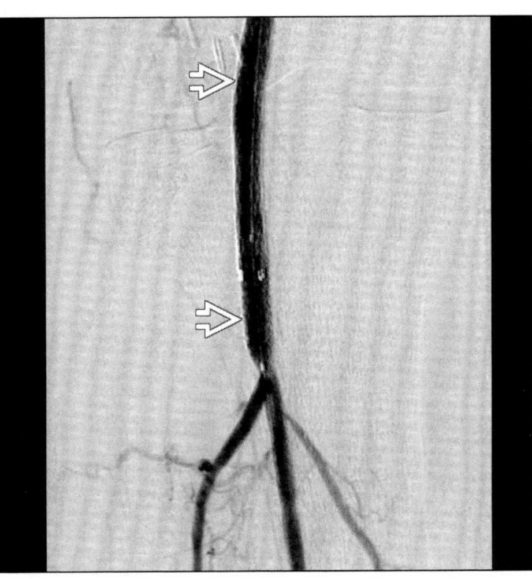

(Left) *DSA in the same patient (image A) shows a thrombolysis infusion catheter in the occluded right femoropopliteal bypass graft. Image B shows the catheter tip distally in the bypass graft. The graft has thrombosed as a result of progression of disease in the below-knee popliteal artery.* ***(Right)*** *DSA shows stents have been placed in the below-knee popliteal artery to correct the distal disease that caused bypass graft thrombosis. This is an example of 2° patency.*

FIBROMUSCULAR DYSPLASIA, EXTREMITY

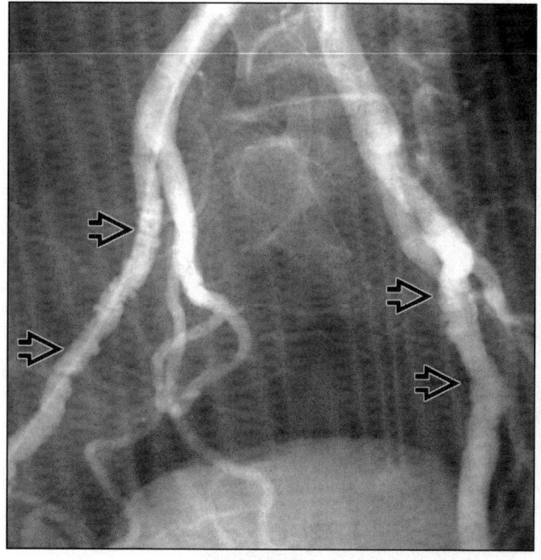

Catheter angiography shows "beaded" appearance of the external iliac arteries bilaterally ⇨. Characteristic appearance of the medial fibroplasia subtype of FMD.

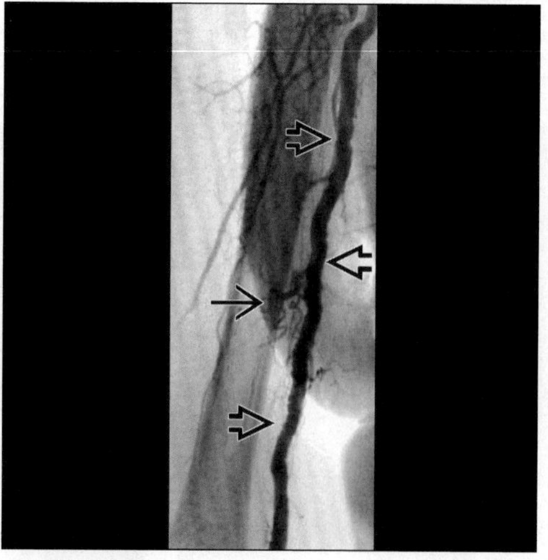

Catheter angiography shows an irregular corrugated appearance of the brachial artery ⇨. Collaterals are present →, indicating hemodynamically significant stenoses.

TERMINOLOGY

Abbreviations and Synonyms

- Fibromuscular dysplasia, extremity (FMD)

Definitions

- Noninflammatory, nonatherosclerotic arterial disease of unknown etiology

IMAGING FINDINGS

General Features

- Best diagnostic clue: "String of beads" appearance on diagnostic imaging
- Location
  - Renal is most common 60-70%
  - Internal carotid 20-30%
  - Vertebral, mesenteric, extremity arteries less commonly involved
    - Most common upper extremity artery: Brachial; also seen in subclavian, and axillary arteries
    - Most common lower extremity artery: External iliac; also seen in femoral, popliteal, and tibial arteries
  - 28% of cases involve multiple arteries

CT Findings

- CTA
  - Lower sensitivity than angiography
  - Maximum-intensity projection reconstruction and transverse sections are more definitive
  - Limited by allergic reactions to iodinated contrast and radiation exposure
  - Rapid acquisition time

MR Findings

- MRA
  - Lower sensitivity than angiography
  - Important in multisystem disease to assess for intracranial aneurysms
  - No radiation, limited nephrotoxicity, noninvasive
  - Sensitive to motion artifact

Ultrasonographic Findings

- Color Doppler
  - Lower sensitivity than angiography

DDx: Fibromuscular Dysplasia, Extremity

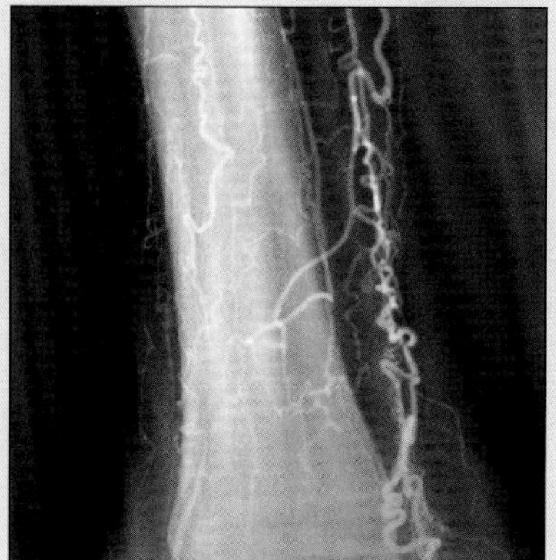

Buerger-Corkscrew Collateral

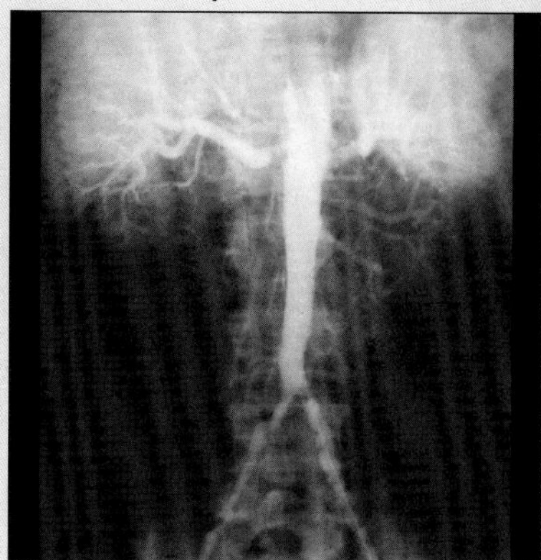

Atherosclerosis of Iliacs

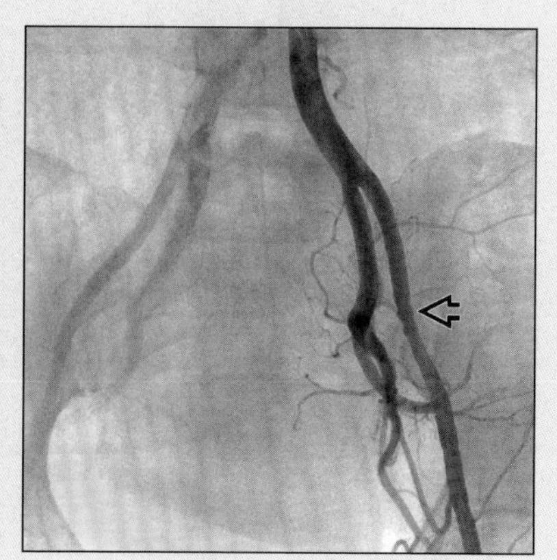

Iliac Artery Endofibrosis

FIBROMUSCULAR DYSPLASIA, EXTREMITY

Key Facts

Terminology
- Noninflammatory, nonatherosclerotic arterial disease of unknown etiology

Imaging Findings
- Most common upper extremity artery: Brachial; also seen in subclavian, and axillary arteries
- Most common lower extremity artery: External iliac; also seen in femoral, popliteal, and tibial arteries
- DSA is traditional "gold standard"
- Angiography offers the option of simultaneous therapeutic intervention

Pathology
- Unknown
- FMD rarely affects extremities: Less than 5% of cases
- 5 categories of FMD based on arterial layer involved (intima, media, or adventitia)
- Medial fibroplasia (70-80%)
  - Classic "string of beads"
  - Diameter of beading larger than diameter of normal artery
- Perimedial fibroplasia (< 10%)
  - Multiple "beads", less numerous and smaller than in medial fibroplasia
- Intimal fibroplasia (< 10%) and medial hyperplasia (1-2%)
  - Concentric smooth stenosis
  - Intimal fibroplasia may also present as long, smooth narrowing referred to as tubular stenosis
- Adventitial fibroplasia (< 1%)
  - Sharply localized tubular areas of stenosis

  - Provides arterial flow and hemodynamic information
    - Dysplasia leads to decrease in luminal diameter and increase in turbulence leading to altered flow
    - Commonly see alternating dilation and constriction
  - May demonstrate typical "beading" appearance
  - Excellent modality to access restenosis after intervention

Angiographic Findings
- DSA
  - "Gold standard" offers simultaneous therapeutic interventions: Percutaneous revascularization with balloon angioplasty and/or stenting
  - Media fibroplasia subtype
    - Classic "string of beads"
    - Diameter of beading larger than diameter of normal artery
  - Perimedial fibroplasia subtype
    - Multiple "beads", less numerous and smaller than in medial fibroplasia
    - Collateral arteries often seen around areas of stenosis
  - Media hyperplasia and intimal fibroplasia
    - Concentric smooth stenosis
    - Intimal fibroplasia may also present as long, smooth narrowing called tubular stenosis
  - Adventitial fibroplasia
    - Sharply localized tubular areas of stenosis

Imaging Recommendations
- Best imaging tool
  - DSA is still the gold standard, and is also used in cases suitable for percutaneous intervention
  - US, CTA, MRA may demonstrate the lesions, although mild disease maybe missed

DIFFERENTIAL DIAGNOSIS

Atherosclerotic Vascular Disease
- Usually older patients with typical risk factors
- Lesions often at origin of artery, bifurcations, and areas of mechanica stress
- "String of beads" appearance not seen

Vasculitis
- Inflammatory disease with anemia, thrombocytopenia, and elevated acute phase reactants
- Angiographic microaneurysms and strictures may appear similar to FMD

Ehlers-Danlos Syndrome
- Associated with medial fibroplasia
- Multiple aneurysms in addition to typical angiographic findings of FMD

Type I Neurofibromatosis
- Autosomal dominant multisystem disease with cutaneous, neurologic, and orthopedic manifestations
- Associated with arterial ectasia, aneurysms, stenosis, and arteriovenous malformations
- Most commonly involves renal artery and presents with hypertension

Takayasu Disease
- Granulomatous vasculitis of thoracic and abdominal aorta
- Intimal fibroplasia may result in stenosis, occlusions, and aneurysms
- May be mistaken for FMD when involving the renal arteries

Standing Waves
- Corrugated luminal contour of artery
- Very regular periodicity which is different from fibromuscular disease where artery more irregular
- Unclear etiology: Originally thought to be caused by contrast injection, but can be seen in MRA images and on ultrasound
  - Postulated they are due to oscillations resulting from retrograde flow in an artery during pulse cycle
- With vasodilatation they tend to disappear, unlike fibromuscular dysplasia; also may change from one injection to the next

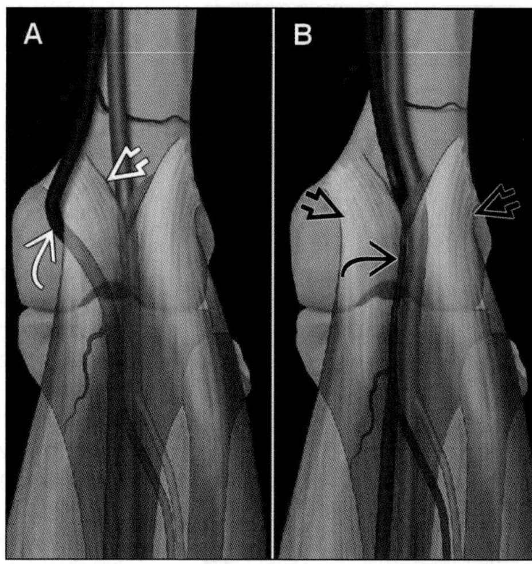

Graphic of (A) Type I anomaly: The popliteal artery deviates around medial head of the gastrocnemius muscle. (B) Type VI anomaly: The gastrocnemius muscles compress the popliteal artery.

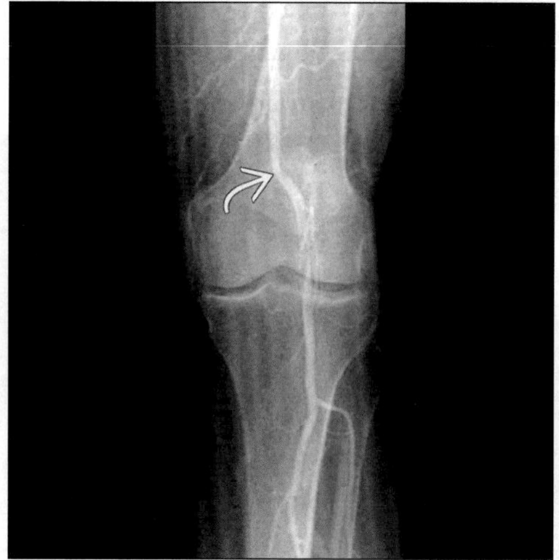

Catheter angiography of a type I anomaly shows that the popliteal artery is deviated medially by the medial head of the gastrocnemius muscle during a plantar flexion stress maneuver.

TERMINOLOGY

Abbreviations and Synonyms

- Popliteal artery entrapment syndrome (PAES)

Definitions

- Intermittent claudication induced by compression of popliteal artery between musculoskeletal structures

IMAGING FINDINGS

General Features

- Best diagnostic clue
  - Medial deviation and deformation of popliteal artery
  - Stenosis/compression of mid popliteal artery during stress maneuvers, such as plantar flexion; sometimes dorsiflexion
- Location
  - Popliteal artery may become entrapped in several locations
    - Popliteal artery deviates medially around medial head of gastrocnemius muscle
    - Medial head of gastrocnemius muscle arises laterally from femoral condyle
    - Popliteal artery may be trapped by a lateral slip of medial head of gastrocnemius muscle
    - Popliteal muscle or deep fibrous band compresses popliteal artery

CT Findings

- NECT: Limited role due to difficulty in identifying popliteal artery
- CECT
  - CTA useful for delineating popliteal artery
  - Soft tissue contrast less well-suited for demonstrating muscular anatomy than MR

MR Findings

- T1WI: Well-suited for demonstrating anatomic variants of gastrocnemius muscle and popliteal muscle
- T2WI: May be helpful for identifying and characterizing other masses that may occur in popliteal fossa
- MRA
  - Valuable non-invasive study with capacity to demonstrate vessel lumen with/without stress maneuvers

DDx: Popliteal Artery Entrapment Syndrome

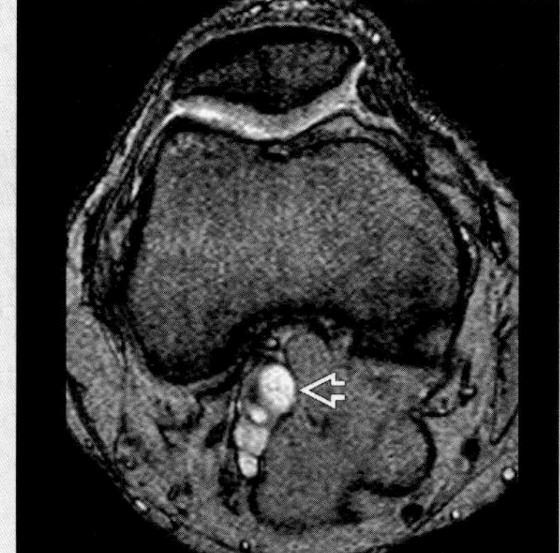

Cystic Adventitial Disease

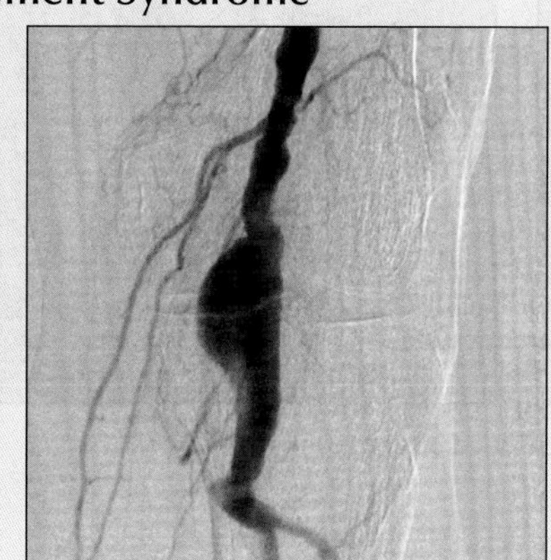

Popliteal Artery Aneurysm

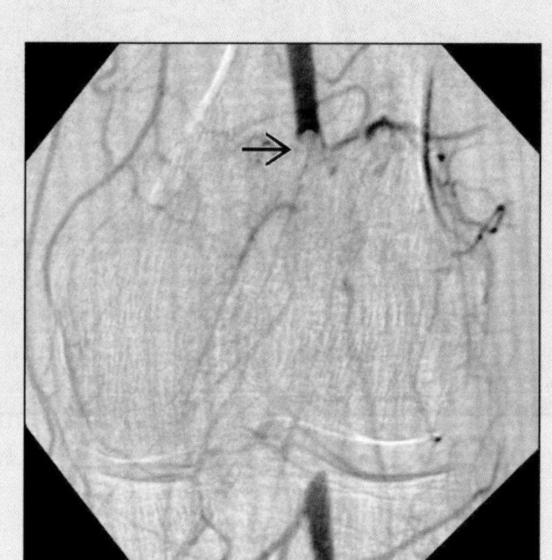

Popliteal Artery Embolism

II 7 94 II 7 96

POPLITEAL ENTRAPMENT

Key Facts

Terminology
- Intermittent claudication induced by compression of popliteal artery between musculoskeletal structures

Imaging Findings
- Medial deviation and deformation of popliteal artery
- Stenosis/compression of mid popliteal artery during stress maneuvers, such as plantar flexion
- MR to evaluate anatomic relationship of popliteal artery with gastrocnemius muscle
- MR angiography in neutral, plantar flexion, and dorsiflexion positions to look for dynamic changes in caliber of popliteal artery

Top Differential Diagnoses
- Cystic Adventitial Disease (CAD)
- Popliteal Artery Aneurysm
- Popliteal Artery Embolism

Pathology
- Most commonly caused by compression from medial head of gastrocnemius muscle (74%)

Clinical Issues
- Usually presents in healthy, athletic males complaining of claudication syndrome in the absence of atherosclerosis

Diagnostic Checklist
- Combined functional and anatomic imaging required to make diagnosis
- Diagnosis may be missed unless provocative maneuvers are performed

---

  - Evaluates artery-muscle relationship in popliteal fossa
  - Evaluates for post-stenotic dilatation involving popliteal artery
  - In neutral position popliteal artery may appear normal, narrowed, or medially deviated in midportion
  - During prolonged plantar flexion, deformation of popliteal artery lumen with narrowing or obliteration

Ultrasonographic Findings
- Evaluates patency and narrowing of popliteal artery
  - Increased velocity seen in narrowed portion
  - Exam in neutral and during provocative maneuvers
- Anatomic relationships not as well-evaluated as MR
- Requires skilled sonographer
- Not considered reliable for diagnosis

Angiographic Findings
- Conventional
  - Initial exam performed in neutral position
  - Perform provocative maneuver with foot until symptoms are reproduced
    - This is generally in plantar flexion but in some patients it may occur during dorsiflexion
    - Manually check for decrease in foot pulses
  - Re-inject while patient is symptomatic
  - MRA has largely replaced conventional angiography for diagnosis

Imaging Recommendations
- MR to evaluate anatomic relationship of popliteal artery with gastrocnemius muscle
- MR angiography in neutral, plantar flexion, and dorsiflexion positions to look for dynamic changes in caliber of popliteal artery

DIFFERENTIAL DIAGNOSIS

Cystic Adventitial Disease (CAD)
- Rare condition; mucin collects in cysts within adventitial layer of popliteal artery that compress vessel lumen
- Relatively sudden onset of intermittent claudication
  - Decrease or loss of distal pulses
- MRA appearance of smooth, eccentric, extrinsic "hour-glass", or "scimitar sign" narrowing of popliteal artery in neutral position
  - Classic angiographic appearance of "spiral" or "scimitar-shaped" stenosis
- Cysts hyperintense on T2-weighted MR images
- Treatment with surgical cyst resection or bypass; cyst aspiration ineffective due to high recurrence rate

Popliteal Artery Embolism
- Abrupt onset of claudication
- Patient with history of embolic source
- Angiographic findings (MRA/CTA/angiography) demonstrate abrupt "cutoff" of popliteal artery with "meniscus" associated with embolus
- Emboli tend to lodge at bifurcation into tibioperoneal trunk and anterior tibial artery
- Collateral vessels typically seen with chronic obstruction are not present

Popliteal Artery Aneurysm
- Patients with history of atherosclerotic and/or aneurysmal disease
- MRA/CTA/angiography demonstrates aneurysmal dilatation of popliteal artery (> 0.7 cm)
- Can be complicated by thrombosis, distal embolization of thrombotic material, & rarely, rupture

PATHOLOGY

General Features
- General path comments
  - Generally regarded as congenital condition, or developmental abnormality

POPLITEAL ENTRAPMENT

- Most commonly caused by compression from the medial head of the gastrocnemius muscle (74%)

- Epidemiology
  - Male > > female, 15:1
    - Some recent publications suggest ratio less skewed (M:F = 2:1)
  - Age 12-65 years, most less than 30 years
  - Incidence unknown, estimated at 0.165% of 20,000 in Greek army patients
  - Bilateral in 22-67%

Microscopic Features

- Exam of arterial segment demonstrates abundant longitudinal muscle fibers in tunica media
- Internal elastic lamina disrupted, with fibrous thickening of intima

Staging, Grading or Classification Criteria

- Type I
  - Popliteal artery (PA) deviates medially around medial head of gastrocnemius muscle that arises at or close to its normal location
- Type II
  - Medial head of gastrocnemius muscle arises more laterally on femoral condyle
  - Artery passes medial to and beneath muscle
- Type III
  - Popliteal artery trapped by lateral slip of medial gastrocnemius muscle
- Type IV
  - Popliteus muscle or deep fibrous band compresses popliteal artery
- Type V
  - Any four preceding types that includes popliteal vein
- Type VI
  - Functional popliteal artery entrapment syndrome; may be due to hypertrophy of gastrocnemius muscles

CLINICAL ISSUES

Presentation

- Most common signs/symptoms
  - Athletic male complaining of claudication symptoms in absence of atherosclerosis, and absence of risk factors for atherosclerosis
  - Not unusual for onset of symptoms to be sudden
  - Patients typically have normal pulses that decrease or disappear with plantar or dorsiflexion of foot
- Other signs/symptoms
  - Nocturnal cramps
  - Numbness
  - Paresthesias (14%)
  - Rest pain or ulcer (11%)

Natural History & Prognosis

- Excellent with timely diagnosis and treatment
- If left untreated, popliteal artery entrapment may progress to permanent popliteal artery narrowing 2° to repeated vascular microtrauma
  - Subsequent fibrosis may narrow vessel increasing susceptibility to thrombosis and eventual occlusion
  - Some cases may progress to popliteal artery aneurysm formation
  - Once thrombosis or aneurysm occurs, such advanced degeneration that artery cannot be salvaged; bypass required

Treatment

- Transection of muscle or fibrous band with mobilization of popliteal artery
- Condition of popliteal artery dictates need for vascular intervention
  - Poor medium term patency with thrombolysis, angioplasty or thrombectomy
  - Surgical entrapment release and saphenous vein interposition graft
    - If arterial wall degeneration or thrombosis
    - If stenosis 2° to fibrosis; aneurysm formation
    - Excellent long-term patency for bypass

DIAGNOSTIC CHECKLIST

Consider

- Popliteal artery entrapment as possible diagnosis in young healthy individuals with claudication
  - Also consider in young healthy individuals with palpable popliteal artery aneurysm

Image Interpretation Pearls

- Combined functional and anatomic imaging required to make diagnosis
  - MRI for anatomic definition of gastrocnemius, soleus, and popliteus muscles
  - MRA or angiography in neutral position, dorsiflexion, and plantar flexion
- Diagnosis may be missed unless provocative maneuvers are performed
  - More commonly associated with strong plantar flexion but may occur with dorsiflexion

SELECTED REFERENCES

1. Kim HK et al: Popliteal artery entrapment syndrome: morphological classification utilizing MR imaging. Skeletal Radiol. 35(9):648-58, 2006
2. Alvarez Rey I et al: Popliteal artery entrapment syndrome in an elite rower: sonographic appearances. J Ultrasound Med. 23(12):1667-74, 2004
3. Henry MF et al: Popliteal Artery Entrapment Syndrome. Curr Treat Options Cardiovasc Med. 6(2):113-120, 2004
4. Wright LB et al: Popliteal artery disease: diagnosis and treatment. Radiographics. 24(2):467-79, 2004
5. Elias DA et al: Clinical evaluation and MR imaging features of popliteal artery entrapment and cystic adventitial disease. AJR Am J Roentgenol. 180(3):627-32, 2003
6. Forster BB et al: Comparison of two-dimensional time-of-flight dynamic magnetic resonance angiography with digital subtraction angiography in popliteal artery entrapment syndrome. Can Assoc Radiol J. 48(1):11-8, 1997
7. Hoelting T et al: Entrapment of the popliteal artery and its surgical management in a 20-year period. Br J Surg. 84(3):338-41, 1997
8. Collins PS et al: Popliteal artery entrapment: an evolving syndrome. J Vasc Surg. 10(5):484-9; discussion 489-90, 1989

IMAGE GALLERY

Typical

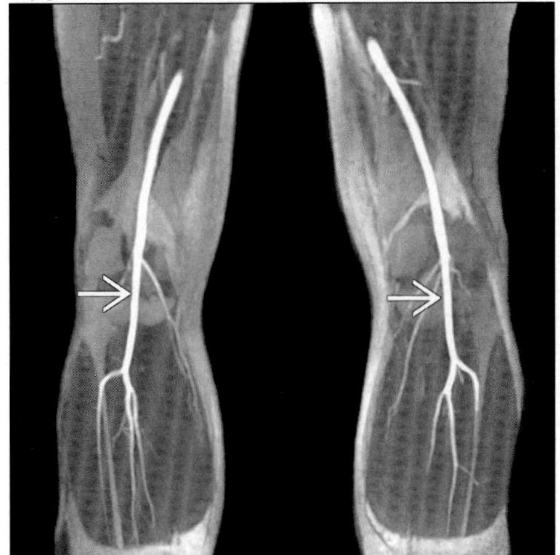

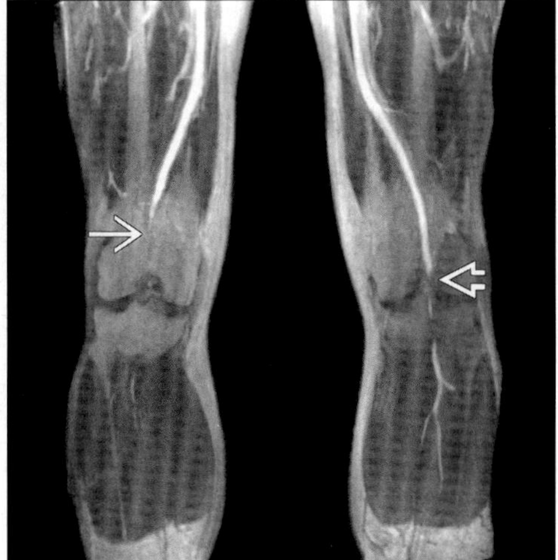

(Left) *Coronal post-gadolinium T1WI MIP image of the lower extremities shows normal caliber popliteal arteries ➔ with normal anatomic vessel course.* ***(Right)*** *With forceful plantar flexion, there is near complete occlusion of the right popliteal artery ➔ and significant narrowing of the left popliteal artery ➔. This demonstrates the importance of provocative maneuvers in making the diagnosis of popliteal artery entrapment syndrome.*

Typical

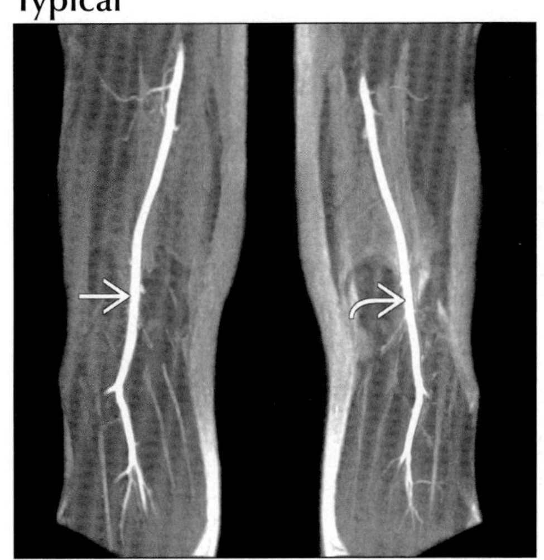

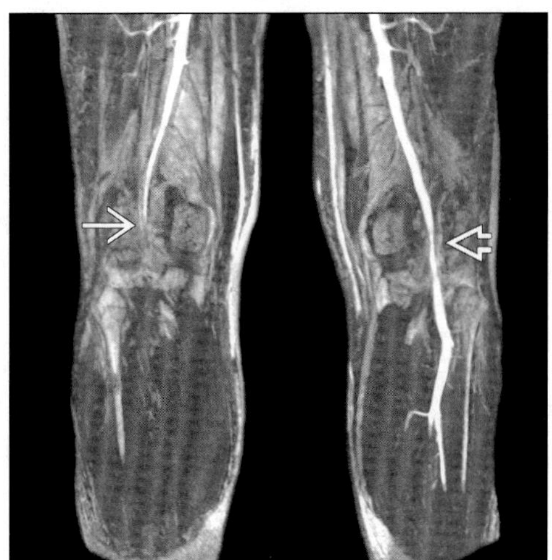

(Left) *Coronal, T1WI, post-gadolinium, MIP images shows another patient who exhibits normal anatomy of the lower extremity arterial blood supply and normal calibers to the right ➔ and left ➔ popliteal arteries.* ***(Right)*** *During plantar flexion (same patient as previous image) there is nearly complete occlusion of the right popliteal artery ➔ and segmental narrowing of the left popliteal artery ➔ adjacent to the heads of the gastrocnemius muscles.*

Typical

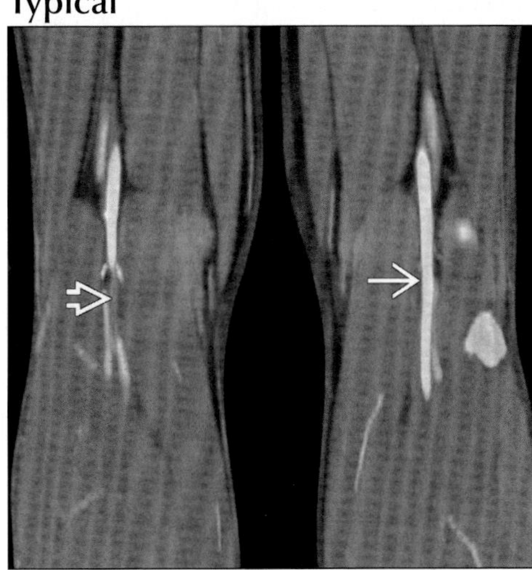

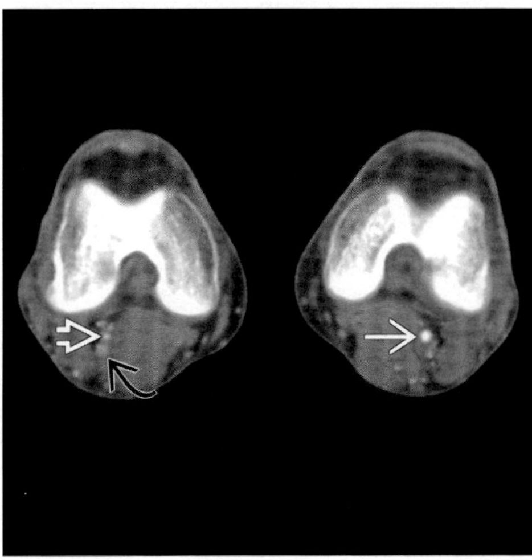

(Left) *Coronal CTA MIP image during a provocative maneuver with plantar flexion, shows significant narrowing of the right popliteal artery ➔. The left popliteal artery ➔ is normal.* ***(Right)*** *Axial CECT (same patient) at the level of the popliteal arteries shows the narrowed segment of the right popliteal artery ➔. The right popliteal vein ➔ is seen superficial to the artery. The left popliteal artery ➔ is normal. Stenoses are shown to better advantage on the coronal MIP images.*

CYSTIC ADVENTITIAL DISEASE

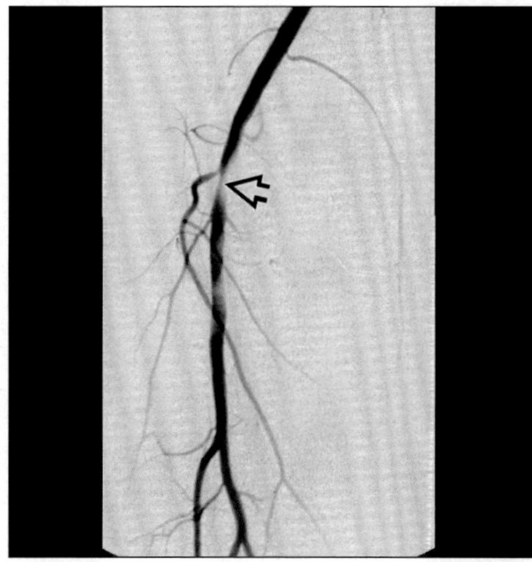

Oblique DSA shows spiral popliteal artery stenosis ➢ and multifocal areas of extrinsic arterial compression distal to the stenosis, all resulting from adventitial cysts.

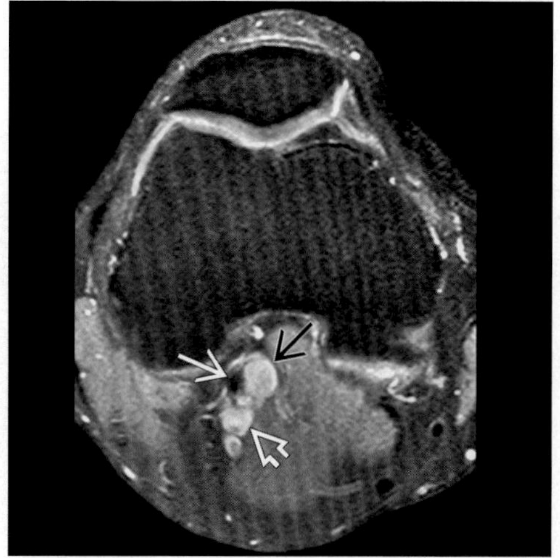

Axial PD MR shows popliteal arterial lumen ➡ compressed by cysts ➡ within the adventitia. Popliteal vein and lesser saphenous vein ➢ are seen posteriorly.

TERMINOLOGY

Abbreviations and Synonyms

- Cystic adventitial disease (CAD)
- Adventitial cystic disease (ACD)

Definitions

- Rare vascular disorder characterized by focal cystic accumulation of mucinous fluid within the adventitia of larger arteries adjacent to joints

IMAGING FINDINGS

General Features

- Best diagnostic clue: Solitary unilateral scimitar-shaped stenosis of above-knee segment of popliteal artery causing sudden onset of intermittent claudication in young male patient
- Location
  - Always located adjacent to joints, within adventitia of larger arteries
  - Popliteal artery most commonly affected (85%)
  - External iliac/common femoral artery level next most frequent site
  - Brachial, radial and ulnar artery involvement has been reported but exceedingly rare
- Size: Cysts may be multiloculated and extend over several centimeters

CT Findings

- CECT: Compressed or narrowed popliteal artery with adjacent low attenuation, smoothly marginated mass(es)
- CTA: Appearance of popliteal artery and characteristics of stenosis similar to angiographic findings

MR Findings

- T1WI
  - Cysts have variable signal intensity on T1WI depending upon amount of mucoid material
  - Compression of arterial lumen produced by cysts in arterial wall visible on axial images
  - Gadolinium enhancement and fat-suppression sequences useful
- T2WI: Cysts are hyperintense
- MRA: Arterial stenosis of popliteal artery above or at the knee joint

DDx: Cystic Adventitial Disease

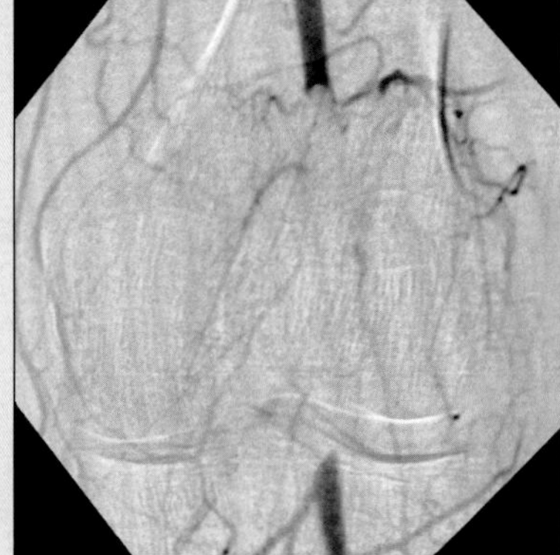

Popliteal Embolus

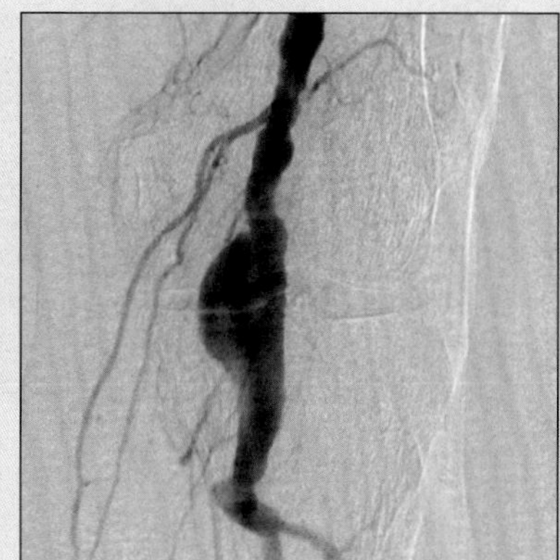

Popliteal Aneurysm

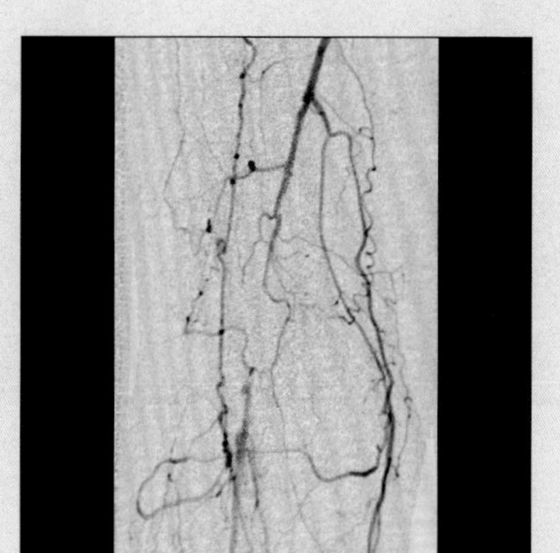

Peripheral Vascular Disease

CYSTIC ADVENTITIAL DISEASE

Key Facts

Terminology

- Rare vascular disorder characterized by focal cystic accumulation of mucinous fluid within the adventitia of larger arteries adjacent to joints

Imaging Findings

- Best diagnostic clue: Solitary unilateral scimitar-shaped stenosis of above-knee segment of popliteal artery causing sudden onset of intermittent claudication in young male patient
- Always located adjacent to joints, within adventitia of larger arteries
- Popliteal artery most commonly affected (85%)
- Size: Cysts may be multiloculated and extend over several centimeters
- Initial evaluation with ultrasound
- Cysts have variable signal intensity on T1WI depending upon amount of mucoid material
- T2WI: Cysts are hyperintense
- Duplex US depicts an arterial stenosis with adjacent surrounding cysts
- Smoothly tapered, curvilinear or spiral stenosis or a nonspecific complete occlusion, usually involving popliteal artery above the knee joint

Clinical Issues

- Intermittent claudication and/or limb pain, mostly involving the popliteal artery
- Surgical evacuation of the cysts with maintenance of native artery is preferred
- Vascular bypass with vein graft may be required if native artery cannot be preserved

Ultrasonographic Findings

- Color Doppler
  - Duplex US depicts an arterial stenosis with adjacent surrounding cysts
  - Anechoic or hypoechoic masses within arterial wall
- Arterial non-invasive ultrasound
  - Decreased ankle-brachial index
  - Segmental pressure and pulse volume drop across the affected popliteal artery

Angiographic Findings

- DSA
  - Smoothly tapered, curvilinear or spiral stenosis or a nonspecific complete occlusion, usually involving popliteal artery above the knee joint
  - If cysts are concentric, stenosis will have "hourglass" appearance
  - Eccentric stenoses are more common and will produce a classic scimitar-shaped stenosis
  - Post-stenotic dilatation usually absent
  - Poorly developed collateral vessels
  - May be normal

Imaging Recommendations

- Best imaging tool
  - Initial evaluation with ultrasound
  - MR/MRA may better characterize findings on ultrasound
  - Angiography may be useful in surgical planning or occasionally for intervention such as thrombolysis

DIFFERENTIAL DIAGNOSIS

Popliteal Artery Aneurysm

- Partially thrombosed popliteal artery aneurysm with patent central luminal channel and surrounding laminar thrombus may mimic cystic adventitial disease on ultrasound and angiography
- MR should distinguish from cystic adventitial disease, as signal characteristics of thrombus will differ from adventitial cysts
- Frequently thrombose or cause distal embolization; the latter is atypical for cystic adventitial disease

Popliteal Artery Entrapment

- Aberrant relationship of artery to gastrocnemius muscles, with resultant arterial compression
- Eventually causes adventitial thickening & fibrosis followed by aneurysm formation, thrombosis & distal embolization
- MR reveals an abnormal artery with aberrant relationship to muscles
- Conventional angiography sensitive for entrapment but lacks information regarding muscular abnormality

Peripheral Arterial Disease

- Chronic claudication, often bilateral
- Rest pain may be present with severe stenoses
- Spiral or scimitar-shaped stenosis atypical for atherosclerotic stenosis
- Involvement of multiple arterial levels or segments
- Well-developed collateral circulation usually present

Popliteal Artery Embolus

- Filling defect(s) within popliteal artery found on CTA or angiogram
- Meniscus at margin of occlusion on angiogram
- Poorly formed collaterals
- Involvement of multiple arterial levels or segments
- Acute onset of symptoms similar to cystic adventitial disease

Popliteal Fossa Mass

- In popliteal fossa
- Symptoms of arterial insufficiency if significant arterial compromise from mass
- May have associated popliteal venous thrombosis

Trauma

- May result in acute popliteal artery occlusion

CYSTIC ADVENTITIAL DISEASE

PATHOLOGY

General Features

- Etiology
  - Four theories concerning the causes of cystic adventitial disease
    - Embryologic theory in which cysts arise from mucin-producing mesenchymal cell that rests incorporated into the vessel wall during development
    - Cysts arise from synovial or ganglion cysts that migrate or herniate into the adventitia from an adjacent joint
    - Myxomatous systemic degenerative condition associated with a systemic disease
    - Repeated trauma
- Epidemiology
  - Rare, accounting for 0.1% of all vascular disease
  - Solitary unilateral lesion
  - Single case report of bilateral popliteal artery cystic adventitial disease

Gross Pathologic & Surgical Features

- Unilocular or multilocular mucin containing cysts within arterial adventitial layer causing luminal compression, with intact endothelium

Microscopic Features

- Cysts found in the adventitia, but also located in media
- Media shows decrease of smooth muscle cells and prominent mucinous degeneration circumferentially, suggesting that medial degeneration precedes cyst formation

CLINICAL ISSUES

Presentation

- Most common signs/symptoms
  - Intermittent claudication and/or limb pain, mostly involving the popliteal artery
  - Claudication may be acute in onset with intervals of exacerbation and remission but rarely rest pain
  - As cyst enlarges, can lead to vascular compression with stenosis or occlusion
- Other signs/symptoms
  - Decrease in or loss of pulses and, rarely, a popliteal bruit
  - Cyst rarely palpable, but distal pulses may diminish or become absent with leg flexion

Demographics

- Age: Young to middle aged in 3rd to 5th decades
- Gender: Male

Natural History & Prognosis

- Persistent claudication that rarely progresses to rest pain or limb-threatening ischemia
- Distal embolization rare, as arterial intima remains intact
- Occlusion without thrombosis may occur

Treatment

- Treatment methods derived anecdotally due to rarity of entity
- Cyst aspiration alone always results in recurrence
- Surgical evacuation of the cysts with maintenance of native artery is preferred
- Vascular bypass with vein graft may be required if native artery cannot be preserved
- Angioplasty not beneficial as it will not affect the cystic compression of the artery
- If arterial thrombosis has occurred, thrombolytic therapy may be instituted prior to surgical correction

DIAGNOSTIC CHECKLIST

Consider

- Cystic adventitial disease in differential diagnosis of a young male presenting with new onset of unilateral claudication and diminished distal pulses

Image Interpretation Pearls

- Popliteal ultrasound showing narrowed popliteal artery with adjacent hypoechoic or anechoic mass should be supplemented with MR or contrast-enhanced CT for exclusion or confirmation of cystic adventitial disease

SELECTED REFERENCES

1. Papas TT et al: Adventitial cystic disease of the popliteal artery: a potential cause of intermittent claudication. Wien Klin Wochenschr. 119(5-6):186-188, 2007
2. Tsilimparis N et al: Cystic adventitial disease of the popliteal artery: An argument for the developmental theory. J Vasc Surg. 45(6):1249-1252, 2007
3. Buijsrogge MP et al: "Intermittent claudication intermittence" as a manifestation of adventitial cystic disease communicating with the knee joint. Ann Vasc Surg. 20(5):687-9, 2006
4. Ortiz M WR et al: Bilateral adventitial cystic disease of the popliteal artery: a case report. Cardiovasc Intervent Radiol. 29(2):306-10, 2006
5. Cassar K et al: Cystic adventitial disease: a trap for the unwary. Eur J Vasc Endovasc Surg. 29(1):93-6, 2005
6. Fox CJ et al: Cystic adventitial disease of the popliteal artery. J Vasc Surg. 39(6):1351, 2004
7. Wright LB et al: Popliteal artery disease: diagnosis and treatment. Radiographics. 24(2):467-79, 2004
8. Elias DA et al: Clinical evaluation and MR imaging features of popliteal artery entrapment and cystic adventitial disease. AJR Am J Roentgenol. 180(3):627-32, 2003
9. Tsolakis IA et al: Cystic adventitial disease of the popliteal artery: diagnosis and treatment. Eur J Vasc Endovasc Surg. 15(3):188-94, 1998
10. Inoue Y et al: A case of popliteal cystic degeneration with pathological considerations. Ann Vasc Surg. 6(6):525-9, 1992

IMAGE GALLERY

Typical

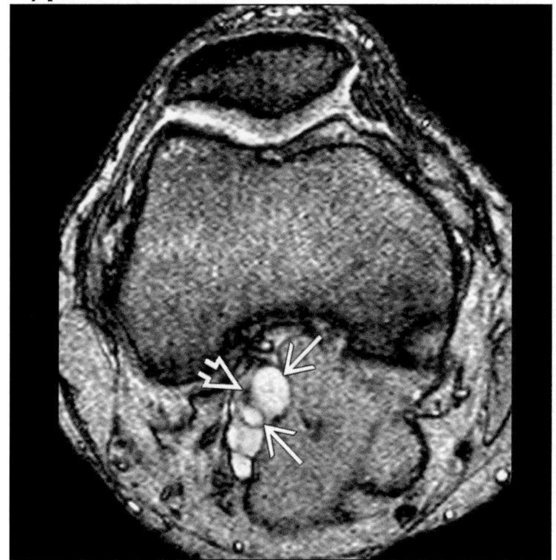

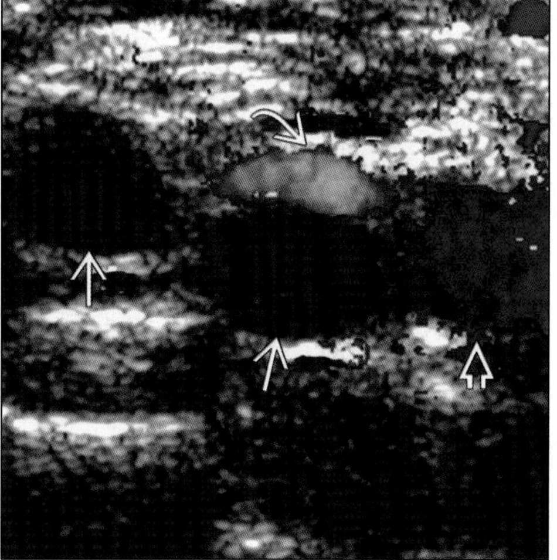

(Left) *Axial T2WI MR shows popliteal arterial lumen ➡ compressed by adventitial cysts ➡. The hyperintense appearance of the cysts on T2WI MR is the typical appearance in cystic adventitial disease.* ***(Right)*** *Axial color Doppler ultrasound shows two anechoic adventitial cysts ➡ compressing the popliteal arterial lumen ➡. The popliteal vein ➡ is seen adjacent to the artery.*

Typical

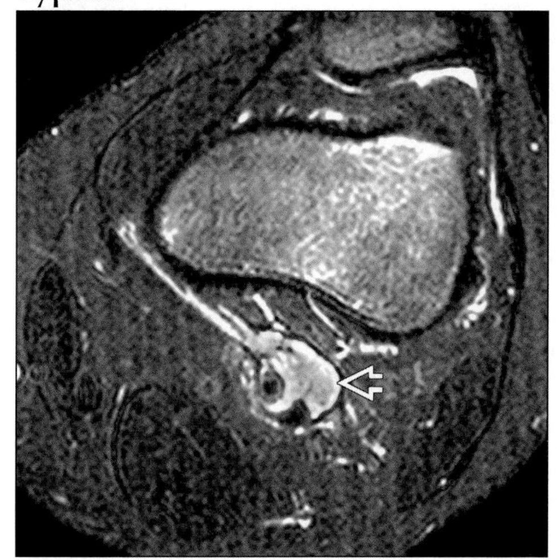

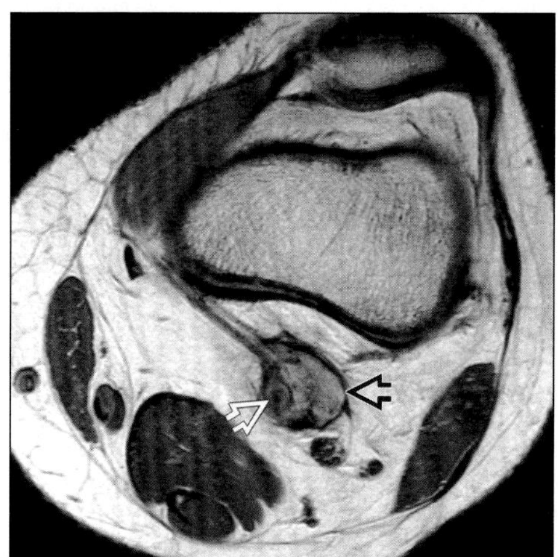

(Left) *Axial T2WI MR shows cyst ➡ surrounding popliteal artery. Note that the cysts are hyperintense while the partially compressed artery exhibits a typical signal void.* ***(Right)*** *Axial T1WI MR shows cystic mass ➡ surrounding and partially compressing popliteal artery ➡. The variable signal of the cyst is a typical finding of T1WI MR of cystic adventitial disease.*

Typical

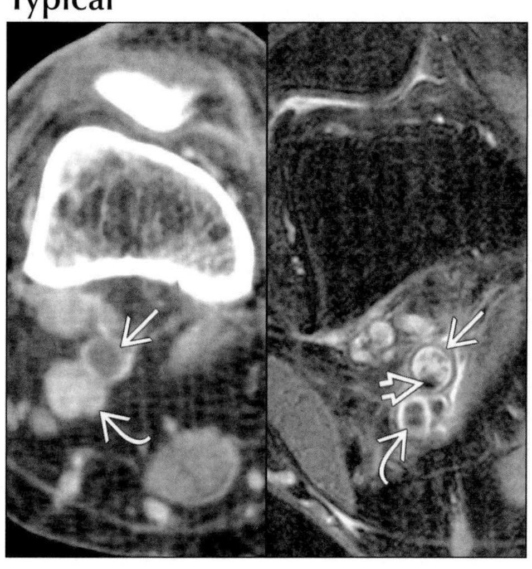

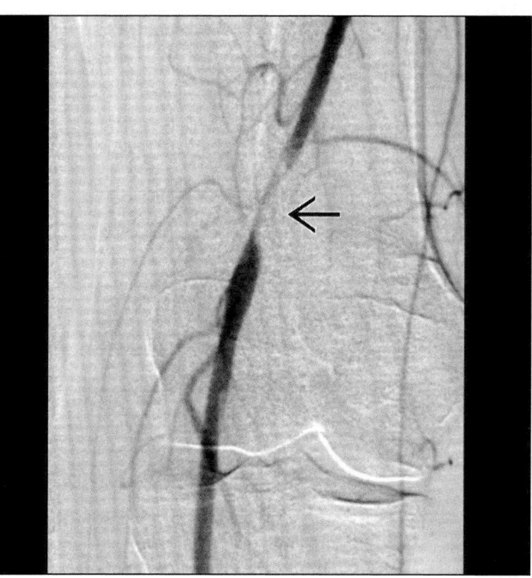

(Left) *Axial CECT (left) and T2WI FS MR (right) shows cystic mass ➡ compressing popliteal artery ➡ with veins seen posteriorly ➡.* ***(Right)*** *Oblique DSA shows smoothly tapered stenosis ➡ of the above-knee popliteal arterial segment. The scimitar shape of the stenosis is the classic angiographic appearance of cystic adventitial disease.*

BUERGER DISEASE

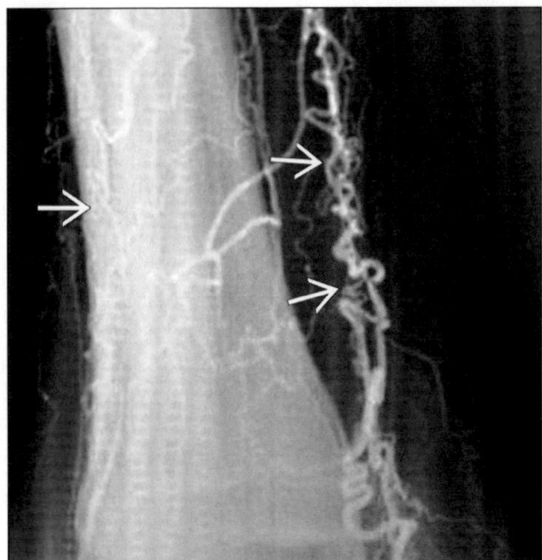

Arteriogram shows "corkscrew" collaterals ➡ that have developed in the vasa vasorum of occluded distal calf arteries in a 38 year old patient with a history of heavy tobacco use. This pattern is typical of Buerger disease.

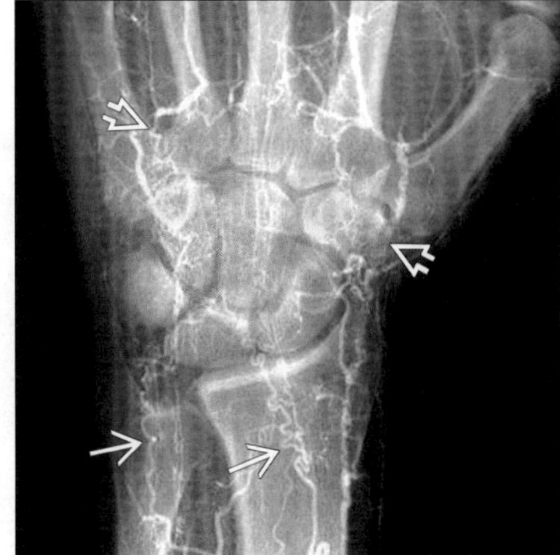

Arteriogram of the wrist also shows distinctive "corkscrew" collateral vessels ➡ as well as multiple segmental occlusions ⇨ involving small and medium-sized arteries in a patient with Buerger disease.

TERMINOLOGY

Abbreviations and Synonyms

- Thromboangiitis obliterans

Definitions

- Nonatherosclerotic segmental inflammatory disease affecting small and medium-sized arteries and veins in the upper and lower extremities, strongly associated with heavy tobacco use
- Known as "thromboangiitis obliterans" because of the inflammatory cellular debris that occludes vessel lumen

IMAGING FINDINGS

General Features

- Best diagnostic clue
  - Stenoses and occlusions of multiple small to medium-sized vessels
  - Bilateral multifocal segmental occlusions or severe stenoses
- Location: Arteries and veins of calf, foot, forearm, wrist and hands commonly involved
- "Corkscrew" collaterals

CT Findings

- CTA
  - Not commonly performed
  - Similar findings to DSA or conventional angiography

MR Findings

- MRA: If performed, findings are similar to those seen with DSA or conventional angiography

Ultrasonographic Findings

- Color Doppler
  - Not commonly performed
  - Thickening of the arterial or venous walls; multiple collaterals
  - Occlusions and stenoses

Angiographic Findings

- DSA
  - Normal non-atherosclerotic proximal arteries with more severe disease distally

DDx: Buerger Disease

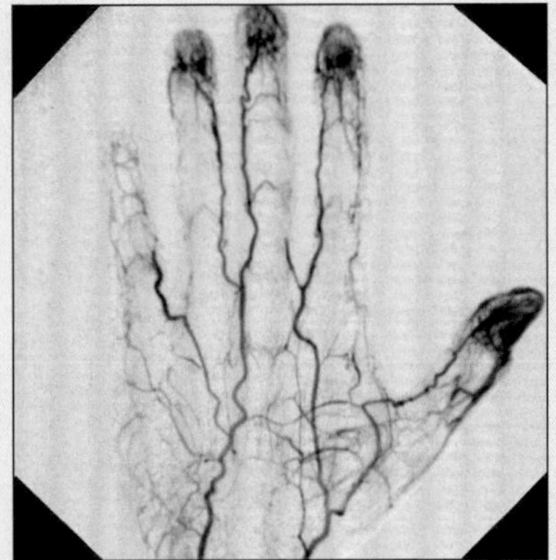

Raynaud Disease

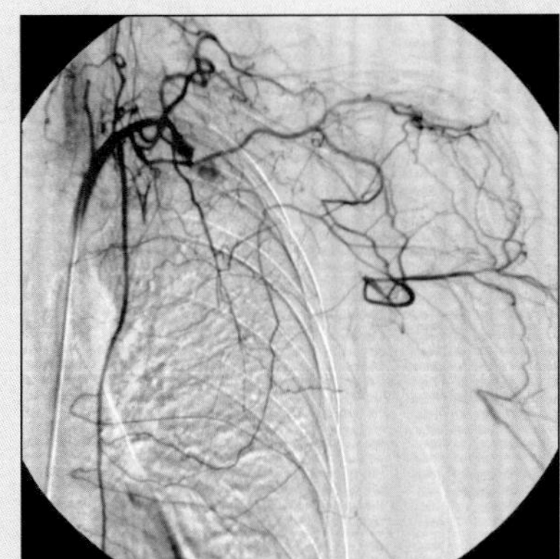

Thoracic Outlet Syndrome

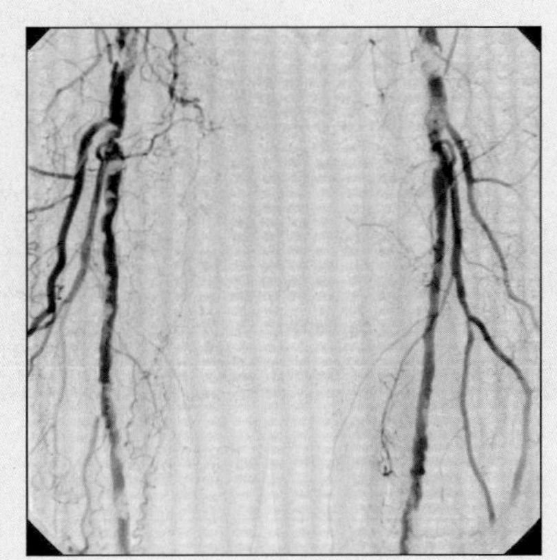

Atherosclerosis

BUERGER DISEASE

Key Facts

Terminology
- Also known as thromboangiitis obliterans
  - Nonatherosclerotic segmental inflammatory disease affecting small and medium-sized arteries and veins in the upper and lower extremities
  - Strongly associated with heavy tobacco use

Imaging Findings
- Stenoses and occlusions of multiple small to medium-sized vessels
- Best imaging tool: DSA or conventional angiography

Top Differential Diagnoses
- Atherosclerosis
- Other Vasculitides
- Raynaud Phenomenon
- Thoracic Outlet Syndrome

Pathology
- Segmental in distribution, with "skip" areas of normal vessel between diseased segments common
- Varies with chronology of disease but all phases have highly cellular thrombus that contains inflammatory infiltrate

Clinical Issues
- Classic initial presentation of young male smoker with foot and lower leg claudication
- Common for disease to progress to amputation with continued smoking
- Total smoking cessation imperative and is cornerstone of therapy
- Surgical revascularization or angioplasty usually poor options due to diffuse segmental involvement and extreme distal distribution

  - Involvement of small and medium-sized vessels
    - Lower extremities: Tibial, peroneal, plantar and digital arteries; popliteal artery involvement infrequent
    - Upper extremities: Radial, ulnar, palmar and digital arteries; rarely brachial artery
  - Bilateral, focal or multifocal severe stenoses or segmental occlusions with abrupt transitions
  - Extensive "corkscrew" collaterals around areas of occlusion
    - Because vessel wall architecture is preserved, collaterals develop in vasa vasorum of occluded arteries, resulting in the distinctive "corkscrew" appearance
    - Not pathognomonic for Buerger disease and may be seen in other entities with diffuse arterial narrowing and occlusions
  - No source of emboli

Imaging Recommendations
- Best imaging tool: DSA or conventional angiography
- Angiography should be diagnostic procedure of choice, although MRA may be performed with contrast allergy

DIFFERENTIAL DIAGNOSIS

Atherosclerosis
- Usually involves older patients
- Large and medium-sized arteries more commonly affected
- May have significant smoking history, but have additional risk factors
  - Hypertension
  - Diabetes
  - Family history
  - Hypercholesterolemia

Other Vasculitides
- Upper extremity distribution more common
- Small, medium and larger arteries commonly involved
- Association with multiple collagen vascular disorders

Raynaud Phenomenon
- Primary Raynaud phenomenon
  - Primary vasospasm without identifiable underlying cause; environmental trigger causes primary vasospasm
- Secondary Raynaud phenomenon
  - Vasospastic digital ischemia associated with underlying arterial pathology
  - Associated with cutaneous disorders and connective tissue diseases
    - Polyarteritis nodosa
    - Rheumatoid arthritis
    - Scleroderma
    - Systemic lupus erythematosus (SLE)
  - Vasospasm triggered by cold exposure; also nicotine, caffeine and stress

Thoracic Outlet Syndrome
- Can be complicated by localized subclavian artery aneurysm with mural thrombus and distal embolization

PATHOLOGY

General Features
- General path comments
  - Classified as vasculitis but with unique characteristics
    - Often has highly inflammatory thrombus with relative sparing of vessel wall
    - Acute phase reactant levels are normal except in presence of acute infarction
    - Markers of immunoactivation are absent
  - Biopsy indicated only for unusual features such as
    - Onset at age > 45 years
    - Disease in unusual location such as large proximal arteries
    - Inconsistent history of tobacco use
- Genetics: No identifiable gene to date
- Etiology
  - Extremely strong association with tobacco use

- Smoking or tobacco use in some form required for diagnosis
- Smoking central to initiation and progression of disease
  - Possibly an abnormal sensitivity or allergy to some tobacco component triggers inflammatory small vessel disease
- Epidemiology: Most prevalent medium vessel inflammatory-type disease of the lower extremities
- Associated abnormalities: Endothelial dysfunction, hypercoagulability, and immunologic mechanisms may be involved in disease process

Gross Pathologic & Surgical Features

- Segmental in distribution with "skip" areas of normal vessel between diseased segments common

Microscopic Features

- Varies with chronology of disease but all phases have highly cellular thrombus that contains inflammatory infiltrate
  - Acute phase of transmural panarteritis with highly cellular, occlusive thrombus containing characteristic microabscesses, particularly involving veins
  - Intermediate phase has progressive organization of occlusive thrombus in arteries and veins
  - Chronic phase characterized by organization of occlusive thrombus with extensive recanalization and perivascular fibrosis

CLINICAL ISSUES

Presentation

- Most common signs/symptoms
  - More than 60% of patients will present with intermittent claudication
  - Classic initial presentation of young male smoker with foot and lower leg claudication
    - Foot or arch claudication may initially be mistaken for orthopedic problem
  - Occasionally claudication initially involves arms and hands
- Other signs/symptoms
  - Ischemic distal ulcers in toes and fingers later in disease course, reported in 40-50% of patients
  - Cold sensitivity is common, with Raynaud phenomenon reported in 40% of patients
  - Migratory thrombophlebitis, usually of superficial veins, seen in up to 30% of patients
- Clinical Profile
  - Young male smoker with onset of symptoms before age 40-45
    - Bilateral claudication
    - Usually normal femoral pulses
    - Pedal pulses may be present, but are usually diminished or absent
    - Rest pain, ulceration and gangrene may be present
    - Superficial migratory phlebitis

Demographics

- Gender
  - Young adult males
  - Originally rare in females (1-2%), but rising incidence probably due to increasing number of women smokers
- Ethnicity: Worldwide distribution but more prevalent in Middle East and Asia than in North America and Europe

Natural History & Prognosis

- Patients have extreme difficulty with smoking cessation
- Poor prognosis, with progression of disease unless patients stop smoking
- Common for disease to progress to amputation with continued smoking

Treatment

- Total smoking cessation imperative and is cornerstone of therapy
  - With successful smoking cessation, amputation rarely required if diagnosed prior to onset of gangrene
- Meticulous hand and foot care
- If significant vasospasm present, trial of dihydropyridine calcium channel blocker such as nifedipine
- Antibiotics for cellulitis and nonsteroidal anti-inflammatory agents for superficial thrombophlebitis
- Surgical revascularization or angioplasty usually poor options due to diffuse segmental involvement and extreme distal distribution
- Limited data on intra-arterial thrombolytic therapy
- Sympathectomy may occasionally help in healing superficial ischemic ulcerations
- Last resort prior to amputation
  - Implantable spinal cord stimulator
  - Entry into therapeutic angiogenesis trial
- Treatment failure may ultimately require amputation

DIAGNOSTIC CHECKLIST

Consider

- Buerger disease in a young patient (< 45 years) presenting with symptoms of peripheral vascular small-vessel occlusive disease in the absence of diabetes

SELECTED REFERENCES

1. Batsis JA et al: Thromboangiitis obliterans (Buerger disease). Mayo Clin Proc. 82(4):448, 2007
2. Paraskevas KI et al: Thromboangiitis obliterans (Buerger's disease): searching for a therapeutic strategy. Angiology. 58(1):75-84, 2007
3. Puechal X et al: Thromboangiitis obliterans or Buerger's disease: challenges for the rheumatologist. Rheumatology (Oxford). 46(2):192-9, 2007
4. Lazarides MK et al: Diagnostic criteria and treatment of Buerger's disease: a review. Int J Low Extrem Wounds. 5(2):89-95, 2006
5. Diehm C et al: Thromboangiitis obliterans (Buerger's disease). N Engl J Med. 344(3):230-1, 2001
6. Olin JW: Thromboangiitis obliterans (Buerger's disease). N Engl J Med. 343(12):864-9, 2000

BUERGER DISEASE

IMAGE GALLERY

Typical

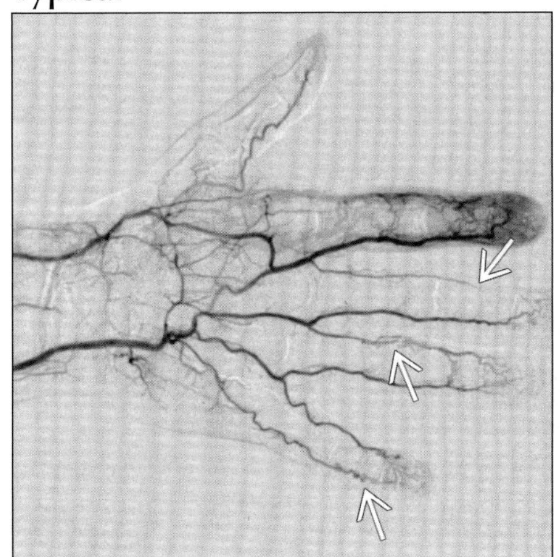

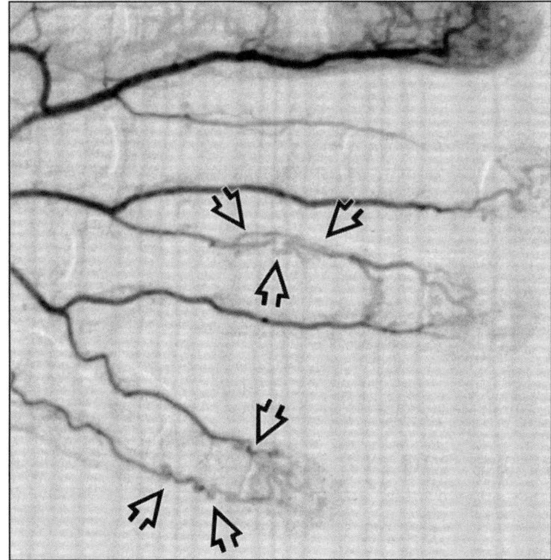

(Left) *DSA in a young male patient with a long-standing history of smoking shows several focal occlusions of the digital arteries. This clinical history and the disease distribution is typical of Buerger disease.* ***(Right)*** *Magnified DSA of the digital arteries in the same patient as previous image, shows the "corkscrew" collateral vessels within the vasa vasorum of the occluded segments of the digital arteries, serving to bypass the occlusions.*

Typical

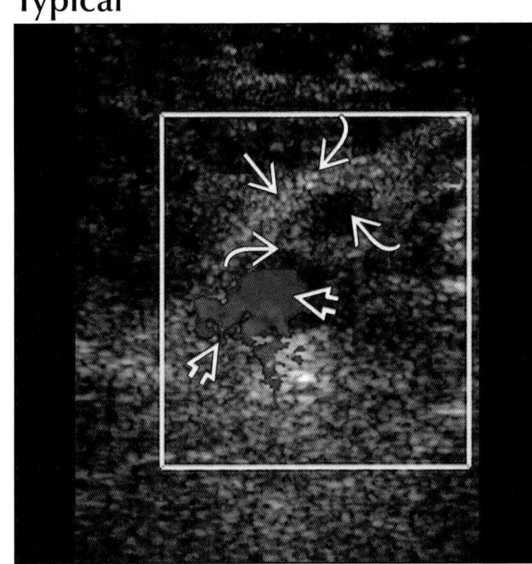

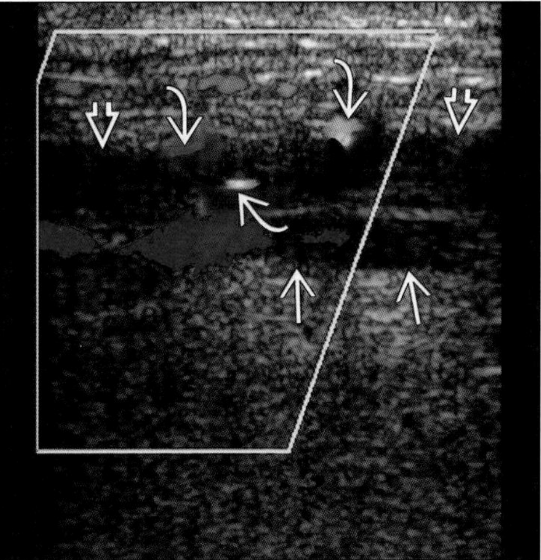

(Left) *Axial color Doppler ultrasound shows patent thick-walled vein adjacent to occluded posterior tibial artery. Small arterial collateral vessels course within the vasa vasorum of the occluded artery.* ***(Right)*** *Sagittal color Doppler ultrasound (same patient as previous image) shows occluded artery & partially occluded vein. Small collaterals adjacent to occluded artery will have a "corkscrew" appearance angiographically.*

Typical

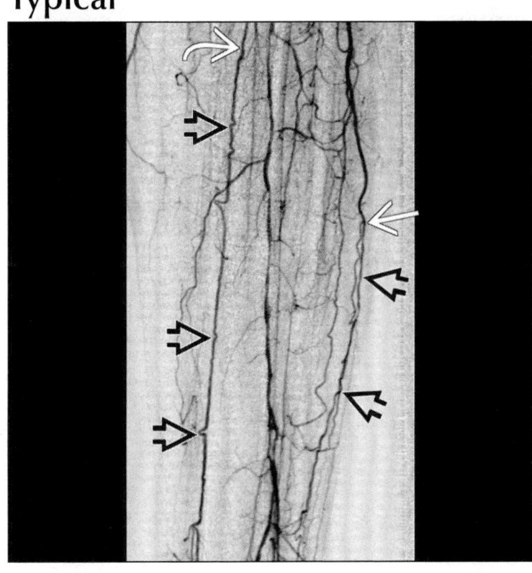

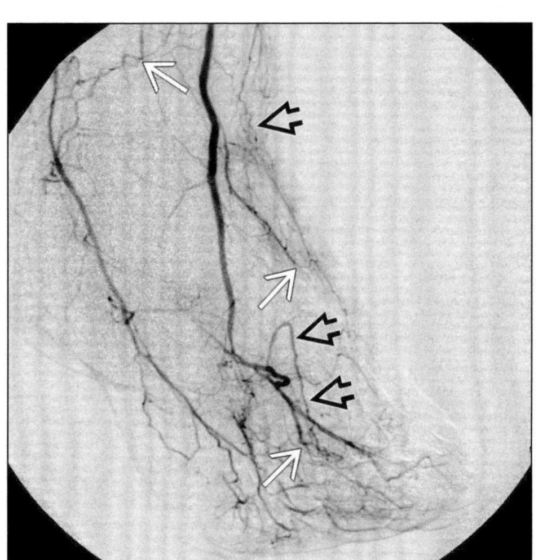

(Left) *DSA of the lower leg in the patient evaluated with the previous ultrasound shows the "corkscrew" collaterals along the course of the occluded anterior tibial & posterior tibial arteries.* ***(Right)*** *DSA of the ankle & foot (same patient as previous) shows multiple occlusions of small & medium-sized arteries, typical of Buerger disease. Again note "corkscrew" collaterals at multiple levels. This 42 year old male had a long-standing smoking history.*

ERGOTISM

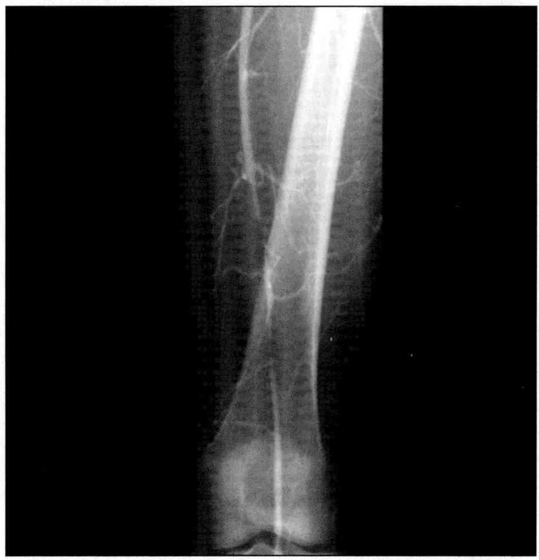

Catheter angiography shows diffuse narrowing of the distal superficial femoral and popliteal arteries. Patient taking an ergot alkaloid for treatment of migraine headaches, developed ischemic symptoms.

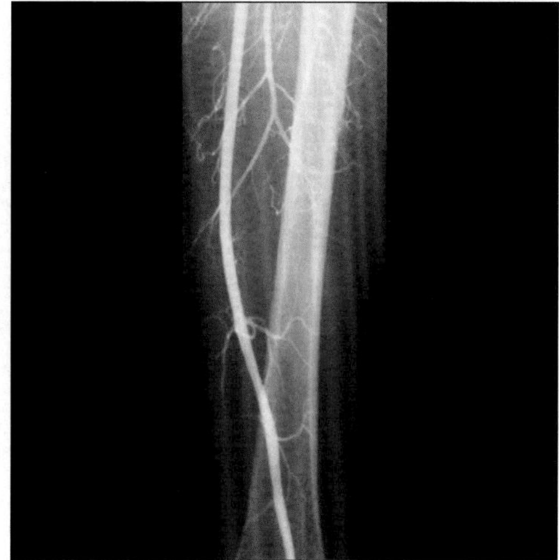

Catheter angiography shows the same patient after cessation of the ergot preparation. The arteries became of normal caliber, and the ischemic symptoms resolved.

TERMINOLOGY

Abbreviations and Synonyms

- St. Anthony's fire; holy fire

Definitions

- Vasoconstriction from overdose or sensitivity to ergot compounds

IMAGING FINDINGS

General Features

- Best diagnostic clue: Arterial constriction with tapering or total occlusion in a patient consuming ergot compounds
- Location
  - May affect any artery but most common in lower extremities
  - Typically begins in superficial femoral arteries and progresses distally

CT Findings

- CTA
  - May demonstrate arterial narrowing and occlusion
  - Less sensitive than angiography
  - Rapid acquisition time

MR Findings

- MRA
  - May demonstrate arterial narrowing and occlusion
  - Less sensitive than angiography
  - Avoids radiation and ionizing contrast

Ultrasonographic Findings

- May demonstrate vasospasm in the lower extremities
- Often useful to follow resolution of symptoms

Angiographic Findings

- Tapering, thread-like narrowing or total occlusion in lower extremities
- Extensive collaterals seen with chronic ergot consumption
- Thrombus may appear as small filling defect within the vascular lumen
- Vascular changes often completely resolve once the drug is discontinued

DDx: Egotism

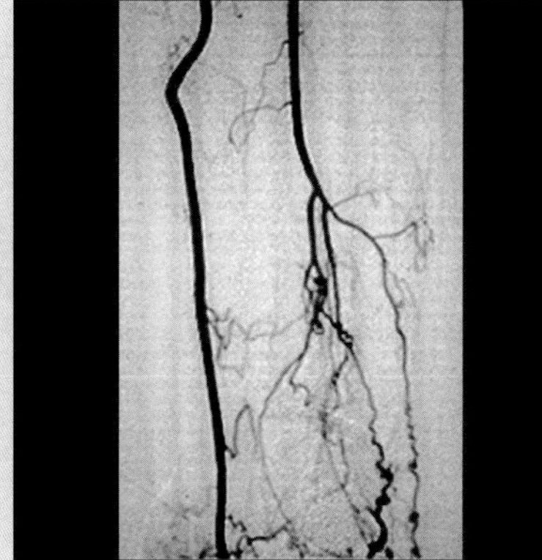

Buerger Disease

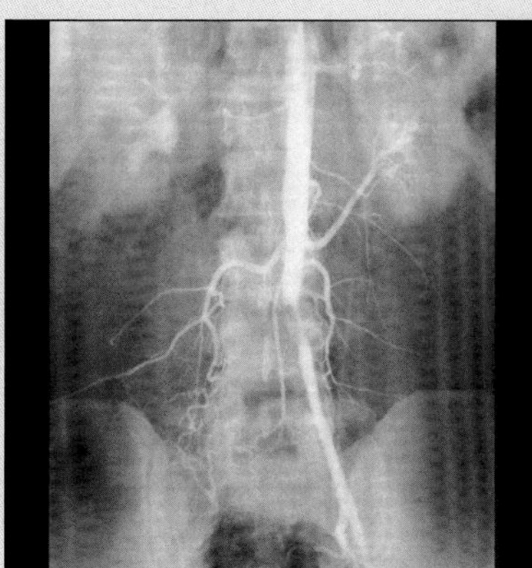

Atherosclerotic Disease

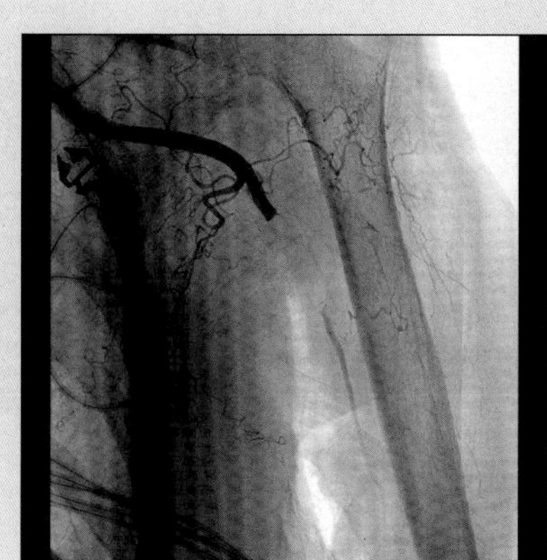

Giant Cell Arteritis - Emboli

ERGOTISM

Key Facts

Terminology

- Vasoconstriction from overdose or sensitivity to ergot derivatives

Imaging Findings

- Arterial constriction with tapering or total occlusion in a patient consuming ergot compounds
- May affect any artery but most common in lower extremities

Pathology

- Now seen almost exclusively with consumption of ergot for migraine headache
- Ergot induces smooth muscle stimulation (vasoconstriction and uterine constriction), central sympatholytic activity, and peripheral alpha-adrenergic blockade
- Outbreaks of gangrene in Middle Ages described as "holy fire" from burning pain of gangrenous limbs
- Most effective treatment provided at hospitals of St. Anthony, resulting in the name "St. Anthony's fire"
- In 1767, Claviceps purpura, an ergot producing fungus, was identified as the cause of epidemic gangrene

Clinical Issues

- Vasospasm presents as pallor, coolness, numbness, claudication, rest pain, and dry gangrene
- Convulsive ergotism: Grand mal seizures, formication, contractions, paresis, hallucinations
- Rapidly reversible vasospasm often resolves with discontinuation of ergotamine containing compounds

Imaging Recommendations

- Best imaging tool
  - Noninvasive imaging for screening
  - Angiography for increased sensitivity and treatment planning

DIFFERENTIAL DIAGNOSIS

Thromboangiitis Obliterans

- Nonatherosclerotic vascular disease
- May present with vasoocclusion: Rest pain, ulceration, and gangrene
- Correlated with smoking
- Angiography demonstrates segmental occlusive lesions with small-vessel collaterals

Raynaud Disease

- Reversible ischemia of peripheral arterioles
- Intermittent attacks of pallor or cyanosis
- Most commonly affects fingers, toes, nose, and ears

Lupus Anticoagulant

- Presents with vascular thrombosis and thrombocytopenia
- Lower extremity symptoms similar to ergotism

Takayasu Arteritis

- Chronic inflammatory disease of aorta and major branches
- Stenosis and thrombosis may lead to lower extremity claudication
- Angiography demonstrates smooth, tapered narrowing of affected vessels

PATHOLOGY

General Features

- Etiology
  - Sensitivity to, or overdose of, ergot-containing compounds
    - Now seen almost exclusively with consumption of ergot for migraine headache
    - Decrease in vasodilation of cranial arteries results in headache relief
  - Ergot induces
    - Smooth muscle stimulation causing vasoconstriction and uterine constriction
    - Central sympatholytic activity
    - Peripheral alpha-adrenergic blockade
  - Three groups of Ergot alkaloids
    - Amino acid alkaloids: Ergotamine, the most potent vasoconstrictor
    - Dihydrogenated amino acid alkaloids: Dihydroergotamine, dihydroergotoxine
    - Amine alkaloids: Ergonovine, methylergonovine; potent oxytocics
  - Erythromycin/clarithromycin and certain HIV protease inhibitors (ritonavir) inhibit liver cytochromes and enhance ergotamine toxicity
  - Other drugs that may be responsible for an increase in side effects - oral contraceptives, xanthine derivatives
- Epidemiology
  - Outbreaks of gangrene in Middle Ages described as "holy fire" from burning pain of gangrenous limbs
    - Most effective treatment provided at hospitals of St. Anthony, resulting in the name "St. Anthony's fire"
    - In 1767, Claviceps purpura, an ergot producing fungus, was identified as the cause of epidemic gangrene
  - Epidemics typically present as purely gangrenous or purely convulsive forms
    - Gangrenous form common in France and other European countries
    - Convulsive form common in eastern Europe and Scandinavia
  - Ergot derivatives were described in 1582 as a uterine stimulant
    - Used by midwives to accelerate labor
    - Later used after delivery as strong stimulant of contraction to prevent hemorrhage

- Earliest reference as treatment for migraine in 1883
- In 1918 Stoll isolated ergotamine; the first pure alkaloid to be isolated from ergot
- Ergot toxicity seen in less than 0.01% of ergot users
- 60-70% of toxicity manifest in lower extremities

Microscopic Features

- Direct, irreversible damage to vascular endothelium may occur with subsequent thrombosis of vessels

CLINICAL ISSUES

Presentation

- Most common signs/symptoms
  - Toxicity seen with short-term doses, excessive doses, and therapeutic doses with chronic use
    - Typical dose 1 mg orally or 2 mg rectally
    - Absorption is erratic, therapeutic levels difficult to predict
  - 3 classes of side effects
    - Neurologic: Headache, vertigo, psychosis, convulsions, coma
    - Alimentary: Nausea, vomiting, diarrhea, cramping
    - Vascular: Vasospasm, thrombosis
  - Vasospasm presents as pallor, coolness, numbness, claudication, rest pain, and dry gangrene
  - Gangrenous ergotism
    - Pulseless limbs, burning pain; usually symmetric
    - Intestinal infarction, acute renal failure, acute MI, blindness; due to systemic arterial involvement
    - Lower extremities are the most frequently involved, but the upper extremities can also be affected
  - Convulsive ergotism
    - Grand mal seizures, formication, contractions, pseudotabes dorsalis, paresis, hallucinations
    - Similar presentation to serotonin syndrome
  - Gangrenous and convulsive forms rarely occur in the same patient

Demographics

- Age: 30's (high correlation with migraine therapy)
- Gender: Women (high correlation with migraine therapy)

Treatment

- Rapidly reversible vasospasm often resolves with discontinuation of ergotamine containing compounds
  - Caffeine also discontinued due to vasoconstrictive effects
  - Resolution as soon as 10 days, may take several months with chronic use
  - Rebound headache after discontinuation may lead to further abuse
- Several medical therapies tried with limited success
  - Sodium nitroprusside infusion reported to relieve spasm in a few cases
  - Nifedipine, prazosin, and prostacyclin with limited success
  - Corticosteroids, anticoagulation, and prostaglandin inhibitors with mixed results
- Thrombolysis and hydrostatic dilation also tried with some success
- Anticoagulation may be beneficial in preventing thrombosis

DIAGNOSTIC CHECKLIST

Consider

- In patients with treatment of migraine headache and ischemia
- When angiogram shows long, smooth narrowing without evidence of atherosclerotic disease, and without the irregularities usually seen with collagen vascular disease

SELECTED REFERENCES

1. Molkara AM et al: Chronic ergot toxicity presenting with bilateral external iliac artery dissection and lower extremity rest pain. Ann Vasc Surg. 20(6):803-8, 2006
2. Kim MD et al: Ergotamine-induced upper extremity ischemia: a case report. Korean J Radiol. 2005
3. Eadie MJ: Convulsive ergotism: epidemics of the serotonin syndrome? Lancet Neurol. 2(7):429-34, 2003
4. De Costa C: St Anthony's fire and living ligatures: a short history of ergometrine. Lancet. 359(9319):1768-70, 2002
5. Garcia GD et al: Chronic ergot toxicity: A rare cause of lower extremity ischemia. J Vasc Surg. 31(6):1245-7, 2000
6. Salvesen R et al: Limb-threatening ischemia due to ergotamine: case report with angiographic evidence. Headache. 40(4):320-3, 2000
7. Tfelt-Hansen P et al: Ergotamine in the acute treatment of migraine: a review and European consensus. Brain. 123 (Pt 1):9-18, 2000
8. Merhoff GC et al: Ergot intoxication: historical review and description of unusual clinical manifestations. Ann Surg. 180(5):773-9, 1974

IMAGE GALLERY

Typical

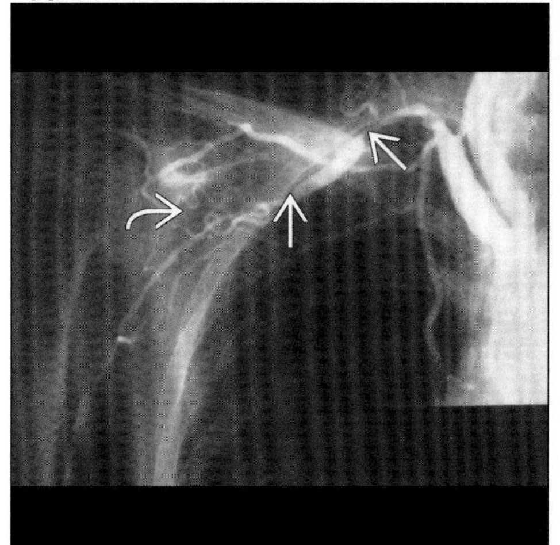

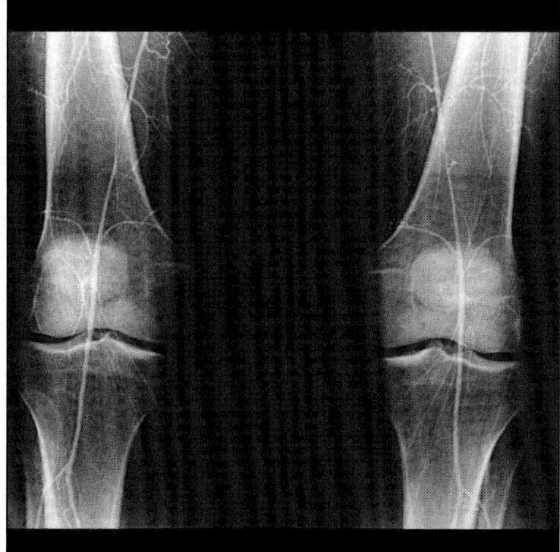

(Left) *Catheter angiography shows areas of narrowing in the subclavian and axillary arteries →. The brachial artery is diffusely narrowed. The arteries appear relatively smooth, unlike atherosclerotic disease. The differential diagnosis would include giant cell or Takayasu arteritis. Collaterals are present ↷.* ***(Right)*** *Catheter angiography shows bilateral diffuse narrowing of the distal SFA and popliteal arteries. The lower extremities are more likely to be affected.*

Typical

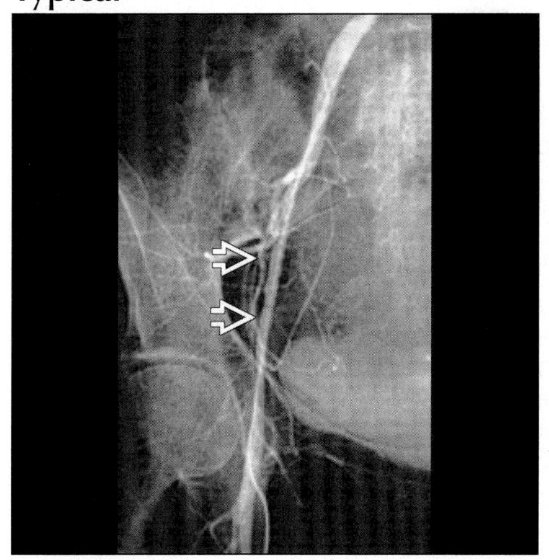

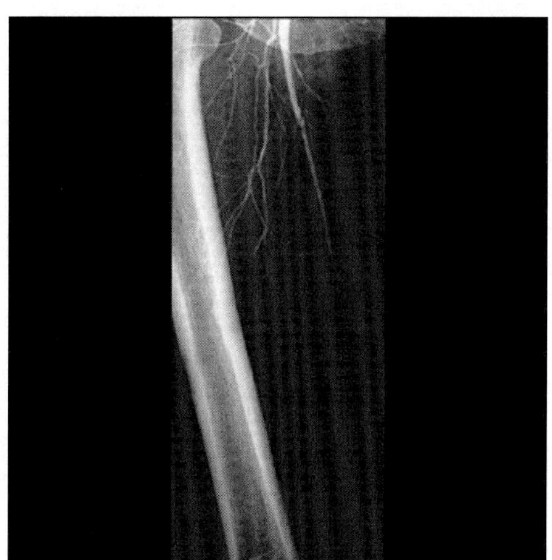

(Left) *Catheter angiography shows relatively normal size of the distal common iliac artery with diffuse narrowing of the external iliac artery ⇨. This type of narrowing can been seen with spasm around the catheter. The patient had been given an ergot preparation for DVT prophylaxis.* ***(Right)*** *Catheter angiography shows the same patient, now with diffuse narrowing, and occlusion of the SFA in the mid thigh.*

Typical

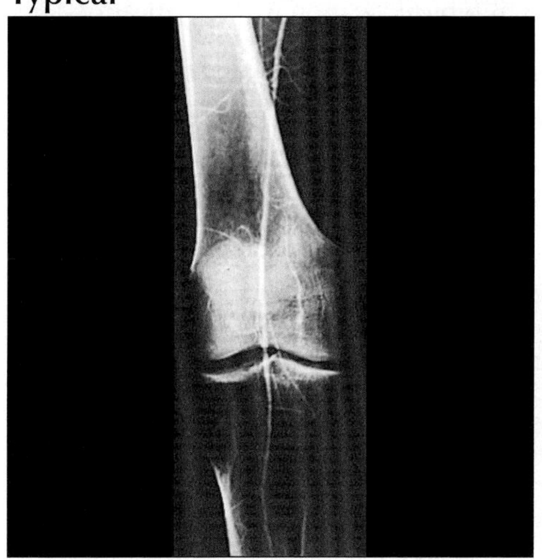

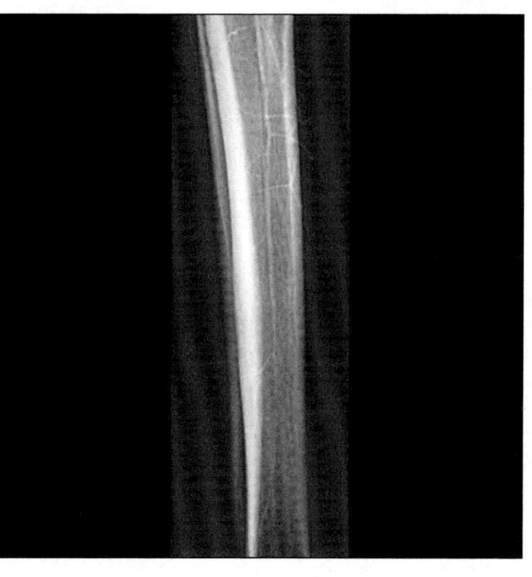

(Left) *Catheter angiography shows slightly better caliber of the popliteal artery, although it is still diffusely narrowed. The more severe the vasospasm, the more likelihood that there will be less recovery of the vasculature.* ***(Right)*** *Catheter angiography shows very poor flow in the tibial vessels. One vessel is seen, but the other two are not visualized. The overall poor flow makes severe ischemia very likely. The best treatment is stopping the ergot medication.*

PERSISTANT SCIATIC ARTERY

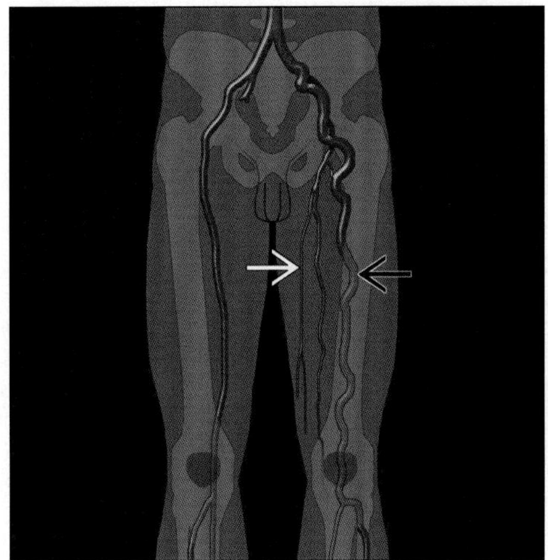

Graphic shows an artistic depiction of a persistent sciatic artery ⇒. The superficial femoral artery ➡ is atretic and ends in a fork like configuration.

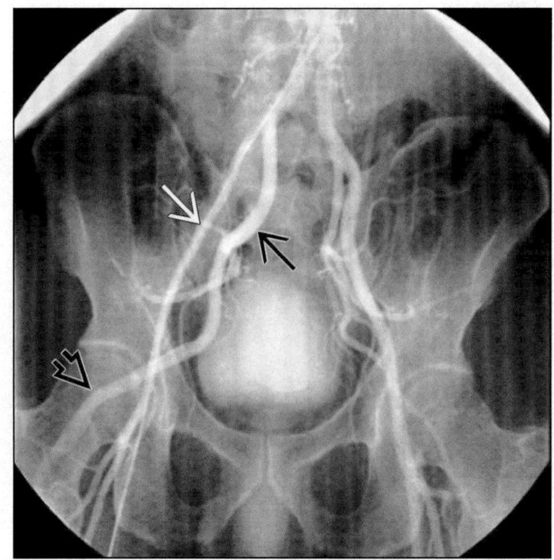

Anteroposterior pelvic angiography shows enlarged right internal iliac artery ⇒ that continues as the persistent sciatic artery ⇨. Note the small right external iliac ➡ and femoral arteries.

TERMINOLOGY

Definitions

- Persistence of embryonic sciatic or axial artery as major arterial channel to lower leg

IMAGING FINDINGS

General Features

- Best diagnostic clue
  - Internal iliac artery continues as sciatic artery and then as popliteal artery
  - Hypoplastic external iliac, common femoral and superficial femoral arteries
- Location
  - Courses through greater sciatic foramen below piriformis to enter thigh
  - Accompanies posterior cutaneous nerve or lies within or adjacent to sheath of sciatic nerve
  - Runs on posterior aspect of adductor magnus, inferior to gluteus maximus
  - Enters popliteal fossa to continue as popliteal artery
- Size
  - Varies, 6-15 mm
  - Arteriomegaly common
- Morphology
  - Two types based on degree of hypoplasia of femoral arterial system
  - Complete form: Superficial femoral artery is grossly hypoplastic or absent and persistent sciatic artery forms dominant supply to leg
  - Incomplete form: Femoral artery is the dominant supply to leg and persistent sciatic artery is small; may or may not communicate with popliteal artery
  - Tortuous course common
  - Early atherosclerotic disease with plaques, calcification
  - Aneurysm formation in 25%
  - Aneurysms typically occur under the gluteus maximus muscle at the level of greater trochanter
- CTA and MRA
  - Shows the typical course of the artery
  - Aneurysms at typical location with calcification and thrombus
  - Large internal iliac artery and small external iliac artery, common femoral arteries

DDx: Aneurysmal Persistent Sciatic Artery

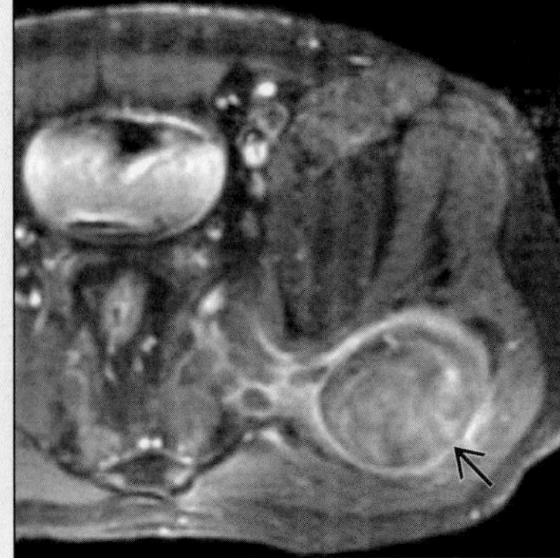

Neurogenic Mass

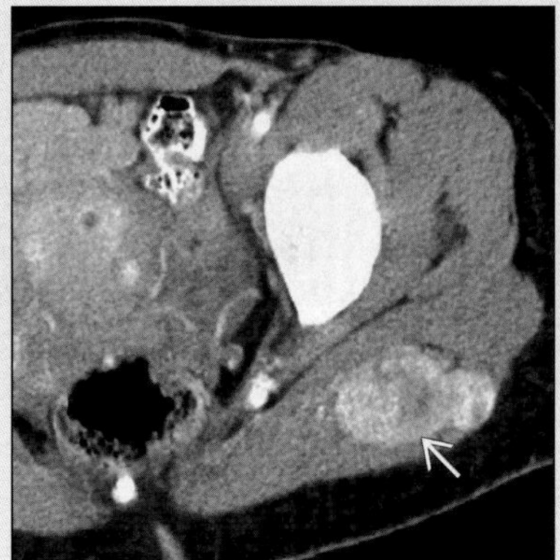

Soft Tissue Sarcoma

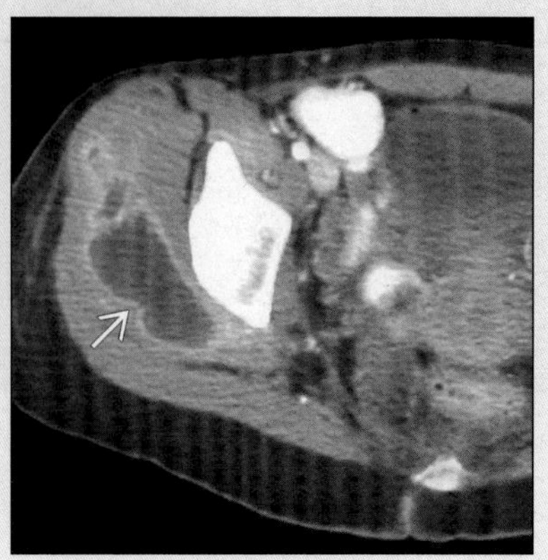

Abscess

PERSISTANT SCIATIC ARTERY

Key Facts

Terminology
- Persistence of embryonic sciatic or axial artery as major arterial channel to lower leg

Imaging Findings
- Internal iliac artery continues as sciatic artery and then as popliteal artery
- Hypoplastic external iliac, common femoral and superficial femoral arteries
- Two types, based on degree of hypoplasia of femoral arterial system
- Aneurysms typically occur under the gluteus maximus muscle at the level of greater trochanter

Top Differential Diagnoses
- Neurogenic Mass
- Soft Tissue Sarcoma
- Aneurysms of Inferior Gluteal Artery
- Gluteal Abscess

Pathology
- Incidence 0.25 per 1,000
- Bilateral in 12-50%

Clinical Issues
- Pulsatile mass in the buttock with absent common femoral pulse but palpable popliteal pulse
- Ligation/resection of aneurysm with femoropopliteal bypass

Diagnostic Checklist
- Demonstrate continuation of the inferior gluteal artery in to thigh and communication with popliteal artery

  - Distal superficial femoral artery terminates in a forked configuration
- Angiography
  - Internal iliac artery larger and non-tapering; courses laterally at the level of the femoral head
  - Oblique views helpful to ascertain posterior location of the artery
  - Tortuous, ectatic artery with irregular walls with or without aneurysm
  - Continues as popliteal artery
- Ultrasound
  - Useful to detect flow in the aneurysm in patients with pulsatile buttock mass

Imaging Recommendations
- Best imaging tool: Angiography; CTA; MRA
- Protocol advice
  - Delayed images on CTA and MRA as slow flow is common
  - During catheter angiography, tip of the catheter should be placed in common iliac artery

DIFFERENTIAL DIAGNOSIS

Neurogenic Mass
- Soft tissue mass with variable vascularity
- Hyperintense on T2WI
- Enhancement on contrast studies

Soft Tissue Sarcoma
- Soft tissue mass with variable attenuation/intensity
- Variable enhancement

Aneurysms of Inferior Gluteal Artery
- No continuation of artery in to thigh
- Normal sized external iliac and femoral arteries

Gluteal Abscess
- Fluid collection, hyperintense on T2WI
- Rim-enhancement
- No continuity with the artery

PATHOLOGY

General Features
- Etiology: Congenital
- Epidemiology
  - Incidence 0.25 per 1,000
  - No predilection for race
  - Equal sex incidence
  - Bilateral in 12-50%
  - Aneurysms in 25%
  - If unilateral, symptoms more common on right
- Associated abnormalities
  - Hemihypertrophy of the leg
  - Hypoplasia of the leg
  - Arteriovenous malformation
  - Multiple angiomas
  - Neuromas
  - Neurofibromatosis
- Embryology
  - At 6 mm stage embryo, primitive sciatic artery (axial limb artery) arises from umbilical artery and supplies the lower limb bud
  - At 12 mm stage, external iliac artery, femoral arteries develop
  - At 18 mm stage, femoral artery communicates with popliteal artery
  - At 22 mm stage, continuity of sciatic artery interrupted, femoropopliteal system becomes the main supply to the lower extremity
  - Segments of primitive sciatic artery persist as inferior gluteal, companion artery to sciatic nerve, arteria comitans nervi ischiadici, popliteal artery and distal part of peroneal artery
  - Failure of development of femoral arterial system leads to persistence of sciatic artery

Gross Pathologic & Surgical Features
- Ectatic, tortuous artery
- Early atherosclerotic disease with plaques, calcification
- Aneurysm formation with thrombosis, distal embolism
- Subject to repetitive trauma

Microscopic Features

- Atherosclerotic changes with plaques, calcification
- Hypoplasia of elastic components of arterial wall

CLINICAL ISSUES

Presentation

- Most common signs/symptoms
  - Pain in buttock and thigh
  - Mass in the buttock
  - Pulsatile mass in the buttock
  - Acute ischemia of leg due to thromboembolism
  - Chronic ischemic symptoms of leg due to repeated distal microemboli
  - Incidental findings on CT or MR
- Other signs/symptoms
  - Pulsatile mass in buttock with absent common femoral pulse but palpable popliteal pulse
  - Rupture leading to sudden death
  - Incomplete forms usually asymptomatic

Demographics

- Age: Average age at presentation 60 years (range: 42-82 years)
- Gender: Equal sex predominance

Natural History & Prognosis

- Early atherosclerotic disease
- Aneurysm formation with distal thromboemboli

Treatment

- Ligation/resection of aneurysm with femoropopliteal bypass
- Endoaneurysmorrhaphy
- Aneurysm resection, interposition graft
- Endovascular stenting
- Endovascular coiling with or without femoropopliteal bypass graft

DIAGNOSTIC CHECKLIST

Image Interpretation Pearls

- Demonstrate continuation of the inferior gluteal artery into thigh and communication with popliteal artery
- Demonstrate absent or hypoplastic superficial femoral artery; this is complete form

SELECTED REFERENCES

1. Hayashi H et al: Minimally invasive diagnosis of persistent sciatic artery by multidetector-row computed tomographic angiography. Heart Vessels. 21(4):267-9, 2006
2. Kritsch D et al: Persistent sciatic artery: an uncommon cause of intermittent claudication. Int Angiol. 25(3):327-9, 2006
3. Mazet N et al: Bilateral persistent sciatic artery aneurysm discovered by atypical sciatica: a case report. Cardiovasc Intervent Radiol. 29(6):1107-10, 2006
4. Sindel T et al: Persistent sciatic artery. Radiologic features and patient management. Saudi Med J. 27(5):721-4, 2006
5. Erturk SM et al: Persistent sciatic artery aneurysm. J Vasc Interv Radiol. 16(10):1407-8, 2005
6. Fearing NM et al: Endovascular stent graft repair of a persistent sciatic artery aneurysm. Ann Vasc Surg. 19(3):438-41, 2005
7. Ishida K et al: A ruptured aneurysm in persistent sciatic artery: a case report. J Vasc Surg. 42(3):556-8, 2005
8. Jung AY et al: Role of computed tomographic angiography in the detection and comprehensive evaluation of persistent sciatic artery. J Vasc Surg. 42(4):678-83, 2005
9. Maldini G et al: Combined percutaneous endovascular and open surgical approach in the treatment of a persistent sciatic artery aneurysm presenting with acute limb-threatening ischemia--a case report and review of the literature. Vasc Endovascular Surg. 36(5):403-8, 2002
10. Parry DJ et al: Persistent sciatic vessels, varicose veins, and lower limb hypertrophy: an unusual case or discrete clinical syndrome? J Vasc Surg. 36(2):396-400, 2002
11. Gabelmann A et al: Endovascular interventions on persistent sciatic arteries. J Endovasc Ther. 8(6):622-8, 2001
12. Kubota Y et al: Coil embolization of a persistent sciatic artery aneurysm. Cardiovasc Intervent Radiol. 23(3):245-7, 2000
13. Sultan SA et al: Endovascular management of rare sciatic artery aneurysm. J Endovasc Ther. 7(5):415-22, 2000
14. Lin CW et al: MR angiography of persistent sciatic artery. J Vasc Interv Radiol. 10(8):1119-21, 1999
15. Madson DI et al: Persistent sciatic artery in association with varicosities and limb length discrepancy: an unrecognized entity? Am Surg. 61(5):387-92, 1995
16. Ikezawa T et al: Aneurysm of bilateral persistent sciatic arteries with ischemic complications: case report and review of the world literature. J Vasc Surg. 20(1):96-103, 1994
17. Brantley SK et al: Persistent sciatic artery: embryology, pathology, and treatment. J Vasc Surg. 18(2):242-8, 1993
18. Wolf YG et al: Surgical treatment of aneurysm of the persistent sciatic artery. J Vasc Surg. 17(1):218-21, 1993
19. Johansson G: Intermittent claudication in adolescence due to incomplete persistent sciatic artery. Vasa. 19(1):72-4, 1990
20. Noblet D et al: Persistent sciatic artery: case report, anatomy, and review of the literature. Ann Vasc Surg. 2(4):390-6, 1988

PERSISTANT SCIATIC ARTERY

IMAGE GALLERY

Typical

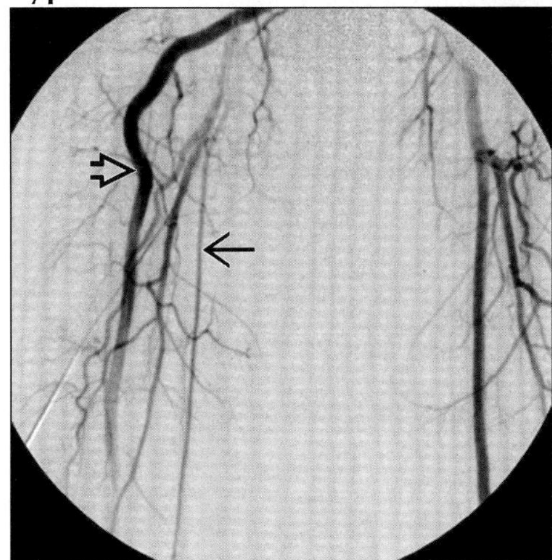

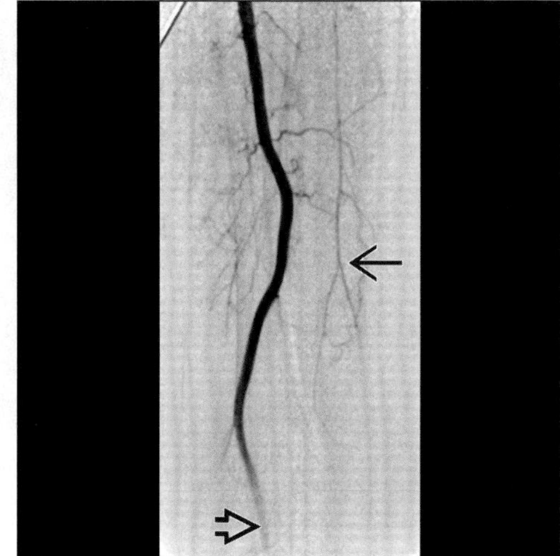

(Left) *Anteroposterior run off shows persistent sciatic artery ➪ that is ectatic and tortuous. Note the small, hypoplastic superficial femoral artery →.* ***(Right)*** *Anteroposterior runoff shows persistent sciatic artery continuing as the popliteal artery ➪. Note the typical forked appearance of the superficial femoral artery → at its termination.*

Typical

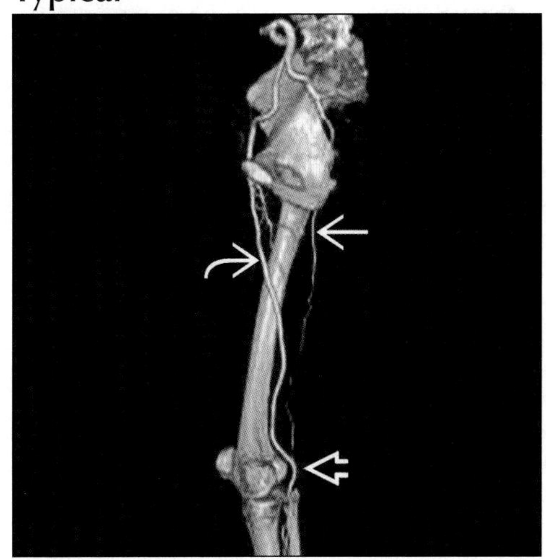

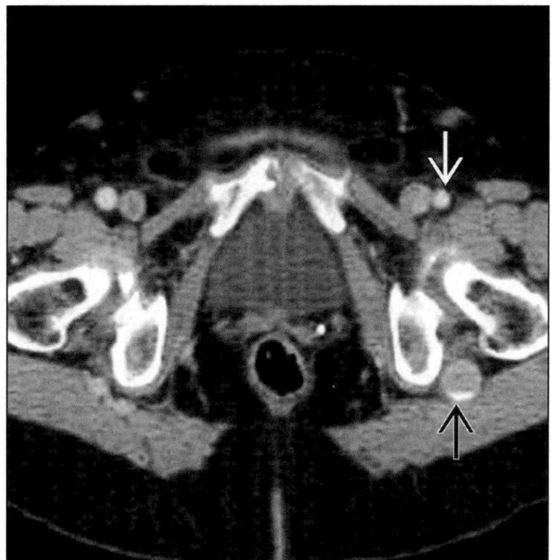

(Left) *Oblique CTA shows incomplete form of the persistent sciatic artery → that communicates with the popliteal artery ➪. The superficial femoral artery ↷ is normal.* ***(Right)*** *Axial CECT shows aneurysm → from persistent left sciatic artery. Note ipsilateral hypoplastic common femoral artery → compared to the contralateral side.*

Typical

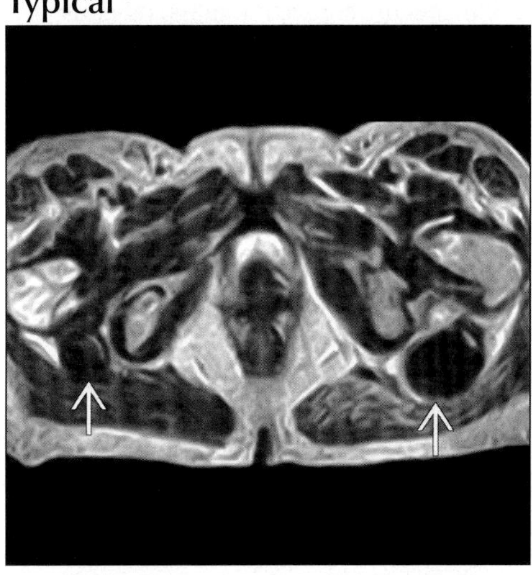

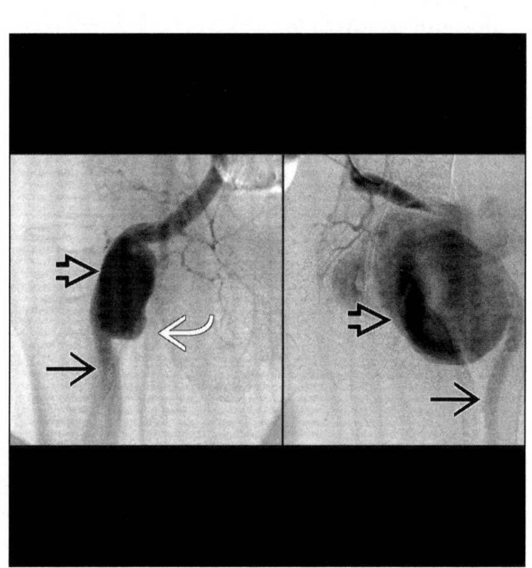

(Left) *Axial T2WI FS MR shows aneurysms → arising from persistent sciatic artery on either side. (Courtesy M. Cherian, MD).* ***(Right)*** *Anteroposterior radiograph (fused image from two separate angiograms) shows bilateral persistent sciatic arteries → with aneurysms ➪. Hypoplastic right SFA ↷ is also seen. (Courtesy M. Cherian, MD).*

ARTERIOVENOUS MALFORMATION, EXTREMITY

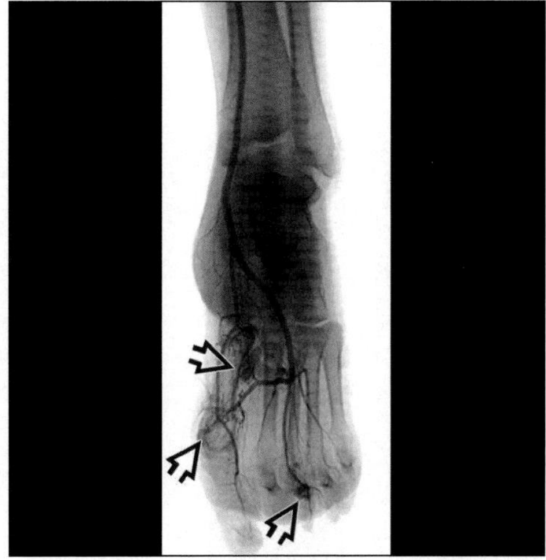

Anteroposterior catheter angiography shows the presence of multiple arteriovenous malformations ⇨ involving the left forefoot. AVMs may have high or low flow hemodynamics, depending upon the vascularity.

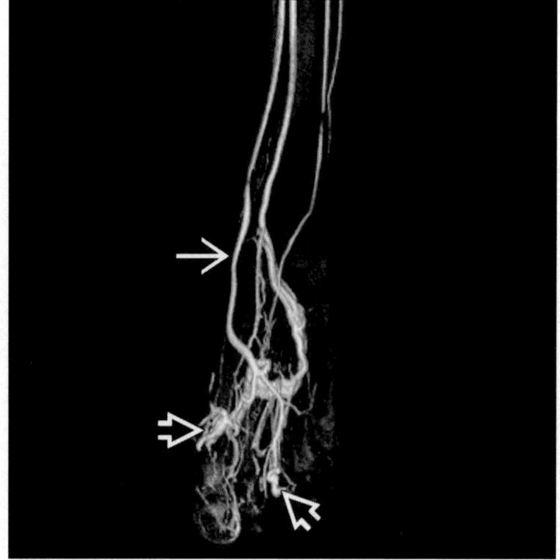

Coronal CE-MRA MIP in the same patient, again shows multiple arteriovenous malformations ⇨. Note the presence of venous contamination ➡ owing to rapid arterial venous shunting, indicating "high flow" AVMs.

TERMINOLOGY

Abbreviations and Synonyms

- High flow arteriovenous malformation (AVM), low flow AVM, vascular malformation, mixed venous and arterial malformation

Definitions

- Congenitally abnormal communication between dilated tortuous arteries and veins

IMAGING FINDINGS

General Features

- Best diagnostic clue
  - Diffuse mass of dilated tortuous serpiginous vessels involving both arteries and veins
  - "Bag of black worms" (flow voids) on spin-echo MR
- Location: Skin, soft tissues, fascia, nerve, muscle, tendon, cartilage or bone
- Size
  - Variable: Ranges from focal vascular ectasia to multinodular or diffuse limb-deforming anomaly
  - Extent of soft tissue and osseous involvement often underestimated on clinical examination
- Morphology
  - Dependent upon degree of arterial-venous shunting
    - Spectrum from "low flow" venous to "high flow'"arterial shunting
  - Venous malformations (50-70%)
    - Often blue; darken and enlarge with advancing age from repeated engorgement
    - Soft, may contain phleboliths
  - Arterial malformations (10%)
    - Presents often in puberty, may cause deforming limb hypertrophy
    - Palpable thrill, bruit, often visible pulsation
    - May cause ipsilateral "steal syndrome" (adjacent tissue ischemia)
    - High-output cardiac failure with severe shunting

Radiographic Findings

- Radiography: Nonspecific soft tissue mass, osseous deformity, periosteal reaction and/or phleboliths

CT Findings

- NECT: Calcification in 30%, tissue deformity, skeletal hypertrophy, muscle atrophy, limb contractures

DDx: Arteriovenous Malformation

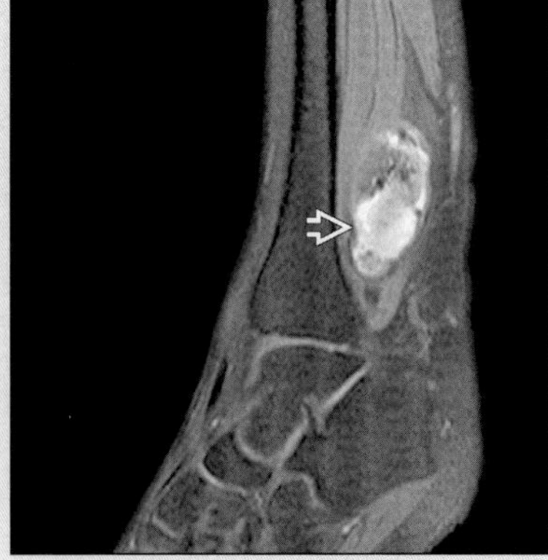

Soft Tissue Sarcoma

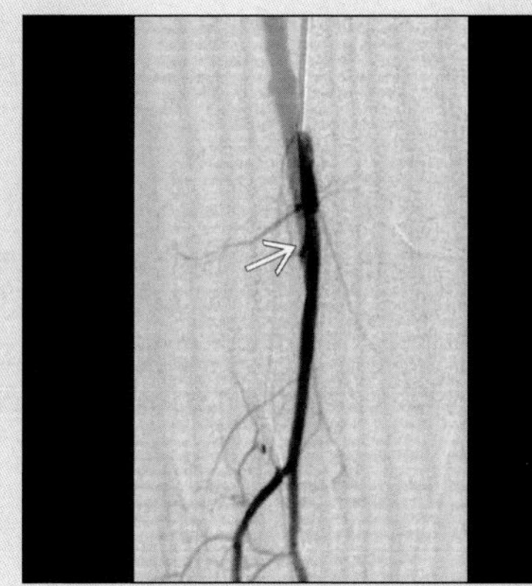

Arteriovenous Fistula

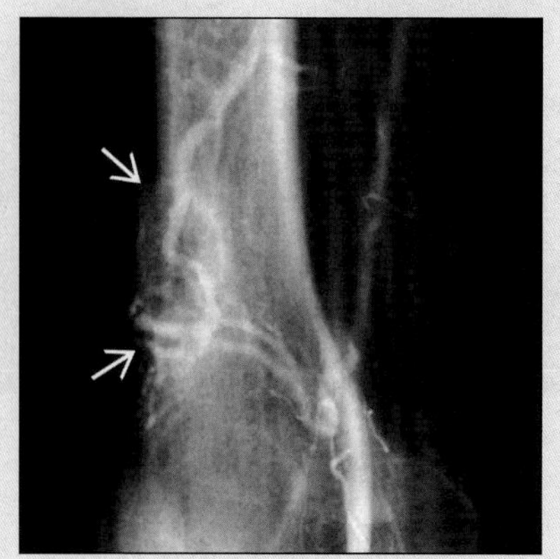

Vascular Metastasis

ARTERIOVENOUS MALFORMATION, EXTREMITY

Key Facts

Terminology

- High flow arteriovenous malformation (AVM), low flow AVM, vascular malformation
- Congenitally abnormal communication between dilated tortuous arteries and veins

Imaging Findings

- Contrast MR is best non-invasive imaging tool
  - Diffuse mass of dilated tortuous serpiginous vessels involving both arteries and veins
  - Contrast filling of dilated feeding arteries and draining veins in arterial phase (early frames of TR MRA images) in high flow AVMs
  - TE MRA (for flow dynamics, high vs. low), high resolution CE-MRA (to assess vascular details), and post-contrast T1WI GRE (to assess for extent and intraluminal filling defects of AVM)
- Best diagnostic clue: "Bag of black worms" (flow voids) on spin-echo MR

Top Differential Diagnoses

- Arteriovenous Fistula (AVF)
- Vascular Neoplasm
  - Hemangioma, sarcoma, vascular metastasis
- Lymphangioma

Pathology

- Communication of abnormally dilated arteries and veins

Clinical Issues

- AVMs neither proliferate nor involute spontaneously
- No tumoral transformation
- Multidisciplinary approach for treatment

- CTA
  - Variable enhancement depending on morphology of AVM and phase of imaging performed
    - High flow AVMs seen during arterial phase, but low flow AVMs seen on delayed venous phase

MR Findings

- T1WI
  - "Honeycomb" appearance of "flow voids" in high flow AVM
  - Increased luminal signal in low flow lesions
  - Predominantly iso- to low-signal intensity on T1WI
  - High signal intensity foci associated with stromal fat
- T2WI
  - High signal intensity on fat-suppressed T2WI : Bright "bag of worms"
  - Low T2WI signal intensity foci may reflect phleboliths, scars or hemosiderin deposition
  - Muscular high T2WI signal in presence of atrophy
- STIR
  - Complementary to T2 fat-saturated imaging
    - Assesses soft tissue and bone involvement of AVM
- T2* GRE: Susceptibility artifact indicates presence of hemosiderin from previous leakage/hemorrhage
- T1 C+
  - Tubular nodular enhancement (dynamic curve depends on lesion arterial/venous composition)
    - Enhancement of arterial/venous components
  - Allows concomitant evaluation of deep venous system of limb, to exclude stenosis or hypoplasia
  - Intraluminal filling defects due to clot, phlebolith, or post embolization material
  - AVM extension into soft tissue and bone well seen
- MRA
  - 3D time-resolved contrast-enhanced MRA
    - Contrast fills dilated feeding arteries and draining veins during arterial phase in high flow AVMs
    - Early venous drainage
    - Varying degrees of enhanced venous washout
    - Low flow malformations may show blush in soft tissue during delayed phase (late frames TE-MRA)
    - Delineates arterial feeders and draining veins
  - High-resolution 3D MRA assesses vascular details
    - Feeding artery(ies), draining vein(s)
    - Enhancing tangle of vessels in first pass
    - Difficulty separating arteries/veins in high flow
    - Slow flow AVMs enhance in delayed venous phase

Ultrasonographic Findings

- Color Doppler
  - Often initial evaluation of soft tissue pathology
  - Hypoechoic, serpiginous compressible vascular mass

Angiographic Findings

- For pre-operative planning; used for interventions
- Enlarged feeding artery and numerous arterial venous connections around nidus
- Early venous drainage, rapid venous washout
- No contrast retention/pooling in AVMs
- Delineates internal architecture (superselective best)

Imaging Recommendations

- Best imaging tool
  - Contrast MR is best non-invasive imaging tool
  - Allows differentiation of low flow vascular lesions from high flow, evaluation of true extent of lesion
- Protocol advice
  - Non contrast TI, T2 and STIR sequences insufficient to reliably evaluate and characterize an AVM
  - Time resolved MRA (temporal resolution 1.2 sec)
    - Assesses flow dynamics (e.g., high vs. low flow)
  - High-resolution CE-MRA to assess vascular details
  - Post-contrast T1WI fat-saturated (FS) GRE images
    - Assesses intraluminal filling defects; AVM extent

DIFFERENTIAL DIAGNOSIS

Arteriovenous Fistula

- Direct connection between adjacent artery and vein
- Usually acquired abnormalities (trauma, iatrogenic)
- Lack of multiple feeders; high flow communication

Vascular Neoplasm

- Hemangioma
  - Benign vascular neoplasms, present in infancy, then proliferate and usually involute during adulthood

- Cutaneous or mucosal low flow malformation
- Normal-caliber feeding vessels
- Early nodular filling of vascular spaces that persists through venous phase (contrast pooling)

- Soft tissue sarcoma
  - Enhancing mass; no feeding or draining vessels
- Metastasis
  - Melanoma, neuroendocrine, renal cell carcinoma

Lymphangioma

- Low flow malformation; cystic chyle-filled spaces
- T1 hypo- and T2 high intensity; rarely fluid level
- No venous enhancement, feeders or draining vessels
- Common in childhood; rare in adults and extremities

PATHOLOGY

General Features

- General path comments
  - Communication of abnormally dilated arteries and veins with multiple dilated ectatic vessels
  - Persistent fetal capillaries
- Etiology
  - Inborn error of vascular morphogenesis between 4th and 10th weeks of intrauterine life
  - Persistence of vascular embryonal elements
- Epidemiology: 1.5% prevalence
- Associated abnormalities
  - Klippel-Trenaunay syndrome (limb overgrowth, cutaneous capillary stains, low flow capillary-lymphatic-venous malformation)
  - Parkes-Weber syndrome (limb overgrowth, high flow capillary arteriovenous malformation)
  - Servelle-Martorell syndrome (limb deformity, low flow capillary-lymphatic-venous malformation)

Gross Pathologic & Surgical Features

- Central nidus with arterial feeding vessels, single or multiple efferent venous channels

Microscopic Features

- Feeding arteries, draining veins have thick walls from subintimal fibrosis and smooth muscle hypertrophy
- AVMs arise from mesenchymal tissue: Therefore high recurrence rate after treatment
- May have focal nidus, comprising
  - Thin-walled dysplastic vessels (no capillary bed)
  - Conglomeration of numerous AV shunts

Staging, Grading or Classification Criteria

- Multiple classifications
  - Low flow (venous, lymphatic, mixed malformations) vs. high flow (A-V malformations and fistulas)
    - Determines therapeutic approach (transdermal for low flow vs. transarterial for high flow lesions)
  - Mulliken and Glowacki classification (kinetics, histology, natural history, physical characteristics)
  - International Society for the Study of Vascular Anomalies classification (ISSVA), 1996
  - Hamburg classification

CLINICAL ISSUES

Presentation

- Most common signs/symptoms
  - May be completely asymptomatic
  - Skin discoloration
  - Pain and localized swelling exacerbated by exercise
- Other signs/symptoms
  - Limb hypertrophy
  - Ulceration or bleeding with "steal" phenomenon
  - May have high-output cardiac failure
- Clinical Profile
  - Usually located in extremities, head, neck, pelvis
  - Significant shunting is less frequent in extremities

Demographics

- Age: Usually detected in late childhood
- Gender: No sex predilection

Natural History & Prognosis

- AVMs neither proliferate nor involute spontaneously since 2° to abnormal vascular morphogenesis
- No tumoral transformation; size may increase with age
- High recurrence rate due to mesenchymal cell origin

Treatment

- Multidisciplinary approach
  - Adjuncts to conventional surgical resection
    - Embolotherapy (coils, gelatin sponge, polyvinyl alcohol, spherical or liquid embolics)
    - Sclerotherapy (alcohol, sotradecol)
  - Transarterial, transvenous or percutaneous access
    - Transdermal approach for low flow lesions whereas transarterial for high flow lesions
- Stereotactic radiosurgery
- Amputation if AVM causes total loss of limb function

DIAGNOSTIC CHECKLIST

Consider

- AVM in patient with skin discoloration and swelling

Image Interpretation Pearls

- "High flow" AVM has multiple vessels; dilated feeding artery and draining vein

SELECTED REFERENCES

1. Fayad LM et al: Vascular malformations in the extremities: emphasis on MR imaging features that guide treatment options. Skeletal Radiol. 35(3):127-37, 2006
2. Yu GV et al: Arteriovenous malformation of the foot: a case presentation. J Foot Ankle Surg. 43(4):252-9, 2004
3. Mulliken JB et al: Vascular anomalies. Curr Probl Surg. 37(8):517-84, 2000
4. Fellows KE: What is an arteriovenous malformation? Cardiovasc Intervent Radiol. 10(2):53-4, 1987
5. Cohen JM et al: Arteriovenous malformations of the extremities: MR imaging. Radiology. 158(2):475-9, 1986

IMAGE GALLERY

Typical

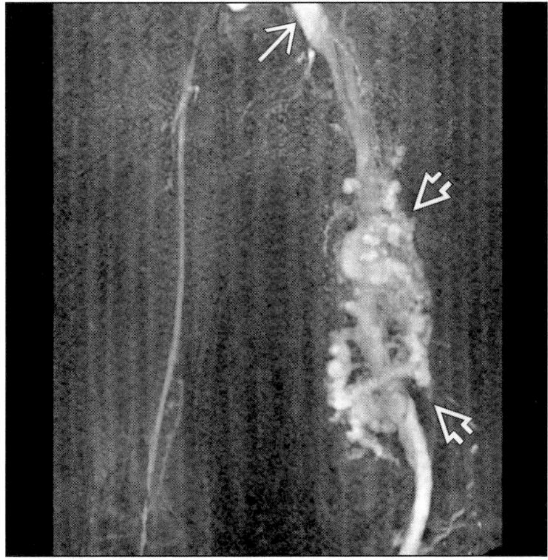

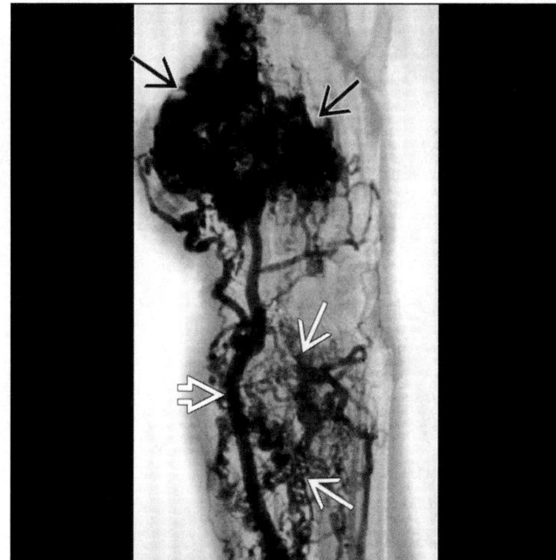

(Left) *Coronal arterial-phase TR-MRA image shows massively dilated left leg veins ➡ from rapid arterial venous shunting in an extensive AVM ➡. "High flow" AVMs can cause limb hypertrophy, ischemia of the adjacent soft tissues or high-output CHF.* ***(Right)*** *Catheter angiography (different patient) shows a very large high flow AVM ➡ of the right hand. Note the hypertrophy of the radial artery ➡ supplying the AVM and the numerous arterial venous connections ➡.*

Typical

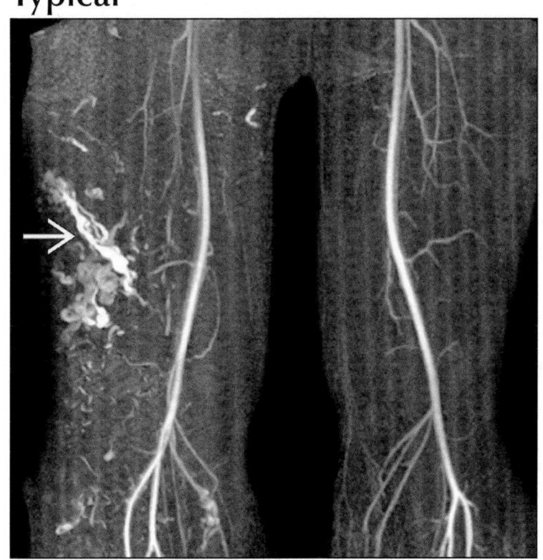

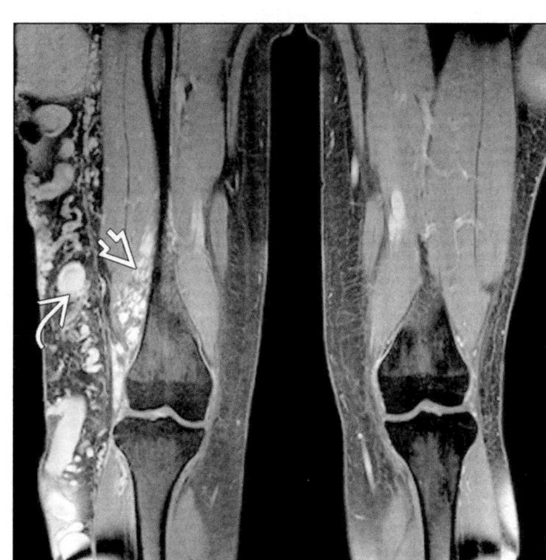

(Left) *Coronal CE-MRA MIP shows a tangle of dilated right thigh superficial veins ➡ in a patient with no apparent arterial feeder and no dominant draining vein. This is consistent with a "low flow" AVM.* ***(Right)*** *Coronal GRE MR following administration of gadolinium shows significant right lower extremity enlargement relative to the left. This is due to a "low flow" arteriovenous malformation with both superficial ➡ and deep ➡ intramuscular extension of the AVM.*

Typical

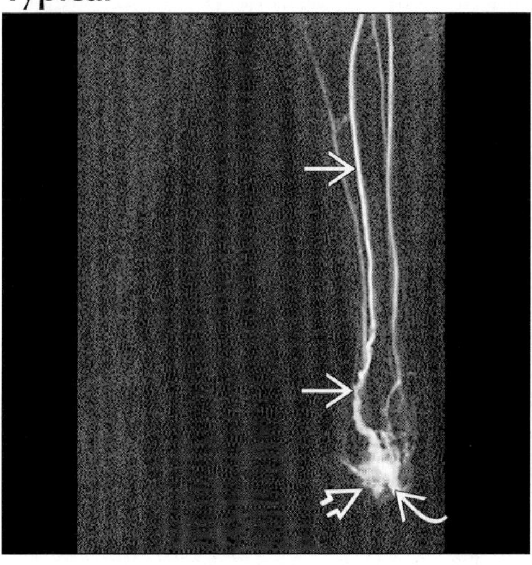

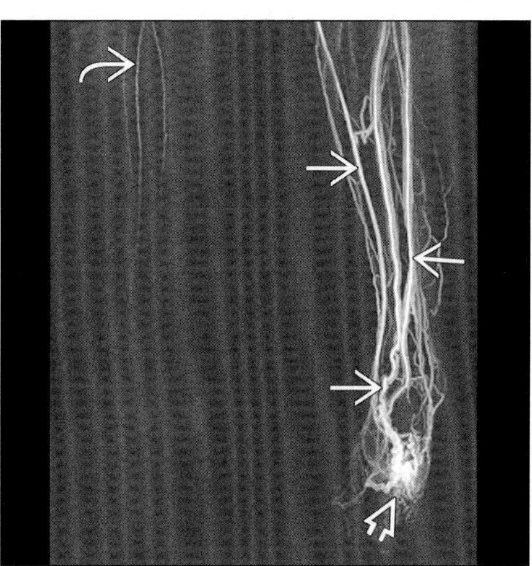

(Left) *Coronal arterial-phase TR-MRA simultaneous imaging over both lower extremities shows more rapid arterial flow on the left compared to the right, with vascular blushing ➡ and venous shunting ➡ due to a "high flow" AVM ➡ in the left foot.* ***(Right)*** *Coronal CE-MRA MIP (same patient as previous image) confirms the left foot AVM ➡ with venous contamination ➡ owing to "high flow" arterial venous shunting. Arterial enhancement on the right ➡ is just beginning.*

KLIPPEL-TRENAUNAY SYNDROME

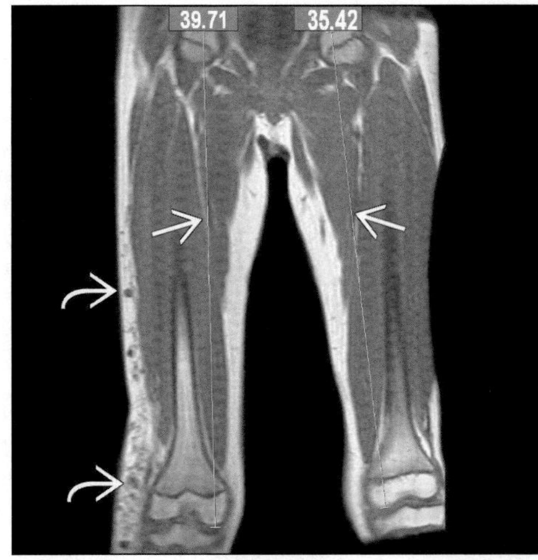

Coronal T1WI MR shows length discrepancy between the right and left legs → of this pediatric patient. There are superficial varicosities in the right thigh and calf ↪. There was an extensive port wine stain over the thigh.

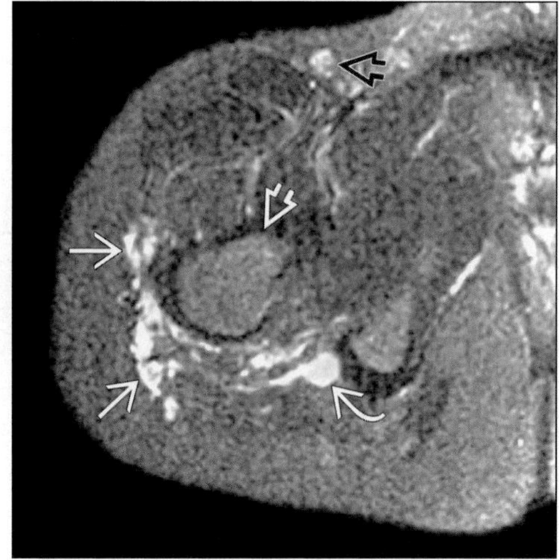

Axial T2WI FS MR shows dilated varicose veins → surrounding the proximal femur ⇨ and draining into the right hemipelvis through a persistent sciatic vein ↪ rather than via the common femoral vein ⇨.

TERMINOLOGY

Abbreviations and Synonyms

- Angio-osteohypertrophy syndrome
- Capillary-lymphatic-venous malformation (CLVM)
- Elephantiasis Congenita Angiomatosa
- Klippel-Trenaunay-Parkes-Weber syndrome

Definitions

- Klippel-Trenaunay syndrome, also known as capillary-lymphatic-venous malformation
  - Combination of capillary malformations (port wine stain), soft-tissue or bone hypertrophy, and varicose veins or venous malformations of affected extremity
- Klippel-Trenaunay-Parkes-Weber syndrome (more commonly Parkes-Weber syndrome)
  - More rare than Klippel-Trenaunay syndrome
  - Similar findings of limb hypertrophy, atypical varicosities and capillary malformations (port wine stains)
  - Critical difference is presence of high-flow arteriovenous malformation (AVM)
  - AVM may cause major complications such as bleeding, ulceration and high output cardiac failure

IMAGING FINDINGS

Radiographic Findings

- Radiography
  - Phleboliths in a very young patient are pathognomonic for venous malformations and are manifestations of prior hemorrhage or thrombus
  - Barium studies can show luminal narrowing and scalloped mucosa of affected bowel, caused by varicosities or submucosal vascular malformations

CT Findings

- CECT: Assessment of visceral vascular malformations

MR Findings

- Hypoplasia or absence of deep venous system
- Persistent sciatic vein
- Persistent subcutaneous lateral embryonic vein
  - "Marginal vein of Servelle" in lateral calf and thigh; multiple communications with deep system
  - May carry bulk of venous return from leg
- Marked hypertrophy of varicose superficial veins

Ultrasonographic Findings

- Grayscale Ultrasound

DDx: Klippel-Trenaunay Syndrome

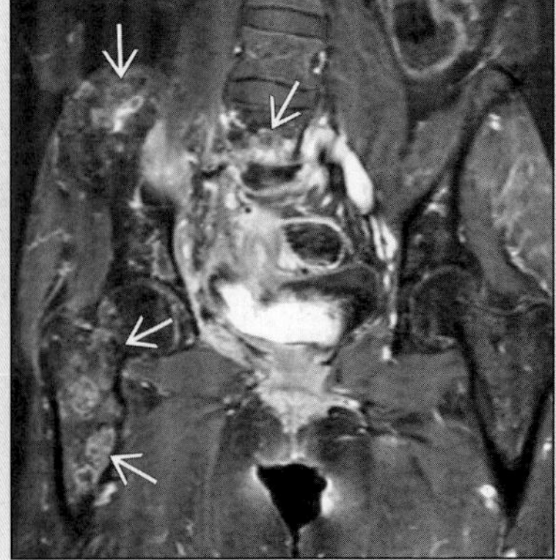

Mafucci Syndrome

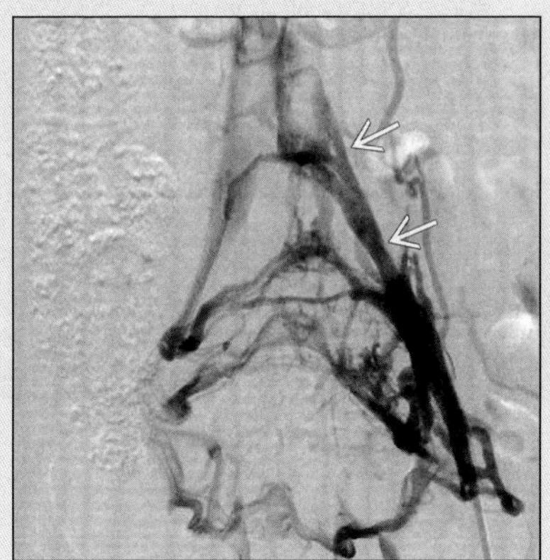

May-Thurner Syndrome

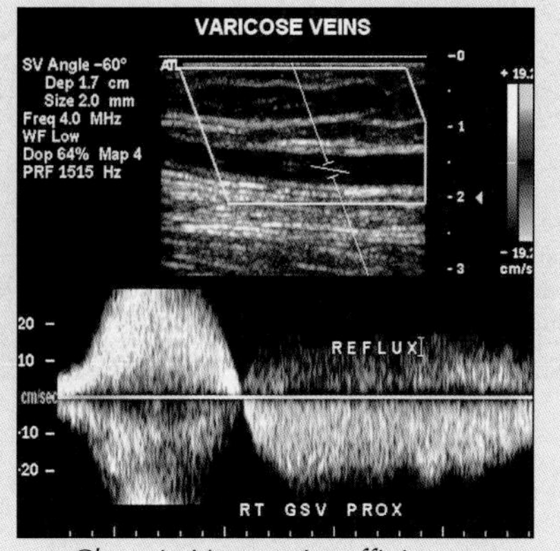

Chronic Venous Insufficiency

KLIPPEL-TRENAUNAY SYNDROME

Key Facts

Terminology

- Klippel-Trenaunay, or capillary-lymphatic-venous malformation syndrome
  - Defined as a combination of capillary malformations (port wine stain), soft-tissue or bone hypertrophy, and varicosities or venous malformations of an affected extremity
- Klippel-Trenaunay-Parkes-Weber syndrome (more commonly Parkes-Weber syndrome)
  - More rare than Klippel-Trenaunay syndrome, with similar findings of limb hypertrophy, atypical varicosities and capillary malformations
  - Critical difference is presence of high-flow arteriovenous malformation (AVM)

Imaging Findings

- MRV to determine extent of venous abnormalities
- Conventional contrast venography may demonstrate hypoplastic or atretic deep venous system if other imaging inconclusive
- Documentation of status of deep veins necessary prior to intervention for varicosities

Clinical Issues

- Capillary malformations are most common cutaneous manifestation (large irregular birthmark)
- Varicose veins are present in a majority of patients
- Hypertrophy is most variable of three classic features of Klippel-Trenaunay syndrome
- Complications include stasis dermatitis, thrombophlebitis and cellulitis
- More serious sequelae are thrombosis, coagulopathy, pulmonary embolism, and bleeding from abnormal vessels in the gut, kidney, and genitalia

  - May identify abnormal veins and varicosities
  - Hypoplastic or absent deep venous system
- Color Doppler: Soft, nonpulsatile and compressible venous malformations

Angiographic Findings

- Conventional contrast venography may demonstrate hypoplastic or atretic deep venous system if other imaging inconclusive
  - Documentation of status of deep veins necessary prior to intervention for varicosities
- For gastrointestinal (GI) hemorrhage requiring surgery, pre-operative angiography may be necessary to define anatomy and extent of intestinal involvement

Imaging Recommendations

- Best imaging tool
  - MRV to determine extent of venous abnormalities
  - Contrast venography if other studies inconclusive

DIFFERENTIAL DIAGNOSIS

Proteus Syndrome

- Sporadic progressive vascular, skeletal and soft tissue condition with asymmetry and variable expression
  - Asymmetric limbs, partial foot and hand gigantism, cerebriform plantar thickening ("moccasin feet")
- Vascular anomalies (capillary, venous or lymphatic)
- Patients at risk for thromboembolism

Mafucci Syndrome

- Coexisting vascular anomalies with bony exostoses and enchondromas
- Childhood osseous lesions and vascular lesions later
  - Venous malformations occur in subcutaneous tissue and bone; may be unilateral or bilateral
- Development of spindle cell hemangioendotheliomas
- Malignant transformation of bone lesions, usually into chondrosarcoma, occurs in 20-30%

Blue Rubber Bleb Nevus Syndrome

- Rare disorder of venous malformations in skin, GI tract and other internal organs
- Characteristic cutaneous lesions consist of deep-blue, soft, rubbery blebs, which are easily compressible
- Subcutaneous venous malformations may occasionally be sole presenting finding in this unusual syndrome
- A serious complication is gastrointestinal bleeding

Sturge-Weber Syndrome

- Meningeal angioma, cutaneous capillary malformation of the face, and glaucoma
- Often accompanied by hemiparesis and hemiatrophy contralateral to meningeal angioma

May-Thurner Syndrome

- Extrinsic compression of left common iliac vein by right common iliac artery
- Unilateral left leg pain and swelling, often with accompanying DVT or venous stasis changes
- Significant stenosis has gradient > 2 mm Hg at rest
- Intraluminal web or "spur" in left common iliac vein by venography or intravascular ultrasound (IVUS)

Chronic Venous Insufficiency

- Incompetent valves allow venous reflux and stasis
- Extensive superficial varicosities
- May respond to sclerosis or ablation

Congenital Lymphatic Obstruction

- Autosomal dominant form of primary lymphedema also known as Milroy Disease
- Hypoplasia, dilation, and tortuosity of lymphatics

PATHOLOGY

General Features

- Genetics
  - Congenital but not heritable
  - Mutation E133K changes properties of angiogenic protein VG5Q to stimulate angiogenesis more strongly than normal; present in less than 4%
- Etiology
  - Vascular changes are congenital

- Vascular malformations have normal numbers of endothelial cells but improperly formed vessels, whereas tumors of vascular origin have excessive numbers of endothelial cells
- Lesions do not respond to agents used to treat hemangiomas, and thus term should be avoided in description of cutaneous findings in this entity
- Epidemiology: Clinically is most frequently encountered major venous malformation

CLINICAL ISSUES

Presentation

- Most common signs/symptoms
  - Capillary malformations are most common cutaneous manifestation (large irregular birthmark)
    - Typically involve enlarged limb, although skin changes may be seen on any body part
    - Lower limb is site of malformations in approximately 95% of patients
    - If large enough, cutaneous lesions may sequester platelets, possibly leading to Kasabach-Merritt syndrome, a type of consumptive coagulopathy
  - Varicose veins are present in a majority of patients
    - Venous malformations can occur in both superficial and deep venous systems
    - Superficial venous abnormalities range from ectasia of small veins to persistent embryologic veins and large venous malformations
    - Deep venous abnormalities include aneurysmal dilatation, aplasia, hypoplasia, duplications, and venous incompetence
    - Changes of long-standing venous hypertension (hyperpigmentation, skin thickening, edema, ulceration and superficial phlebitis)
  - Hypertrophy is most variable of three classic features of Klippel-Trenaunay Syndrome
    - Extremity enlargement consists of bone elongation, circumferential soft-tissue hypertrophy, or both
    - Hypertrophy often manifests as leg-length discrepancy, although any limb may be affected
    - Significant limb-length discrepancy requiring intervention relatively uncommon (< 14%)
- Other signs/symptoms
  - Involvement of GI tract may be more common than previously believed, occurring in up to 20%
    - May go unrecognized if no overt symptoms
    - Bleeding is most common GI symptom
    - GI involvement mostly in distal colon and rectum
    - Symptoms range from occult bleeding to massive hemorrhage and consumptive coagulopathy
  - Lymphatic hypoplasia and lymphedema in 50%

Demographics

- Gender: Equal incidence in males and females

Natural History & Prognosis

- Often present with severe pain, orthostatic hypotension or pulmonary emboli from insufficiency of anomalous subcutaneous veins
- Vascular malformations of GI and genitourinary (GU) tracts can be source of morbidity and mortality
- Vascular malformations of bladder frequently have associated rectosigmoid involvement
- Rectal and bladder hemorrhage reported in 1% of cases

Treatment

- Options, risks, complications
  - Complications include stasis dermatitis, thrombophlebitis and cellulitis
  - More serious sequelae are thrombosis, coagulopathy, pulmonary embolism, and bleeding from abnormal vessels in gut, kidney, and genitalia
  - Patients with AVM may have high output CHF and major local complications (bleeding, ulceration)
- Most patients best managed conservatively
  - Support stockings, leg elevation at night, symptomatic treatment for superficial phlebitis
  - Some patients may worsen after surgical treatment
    - With hypoplastic deep venous system, removal of superficial veins or varicosities may result in acute venous insufficiency and intractable leg swelling
    - If appropriate, localized symptomatic veins may be stripped, sclerosed or ablated
- Pulmonary emboli treated with appropriate anticoagulation and IVC filter
- Cavernous lesions may respond to embolization
- Management of GI and GU vascular malformations depends on extent and severity of blood loss
  - Transfusion dependency and life-threatening GI bleeding episodes necessitate definitive surgical therapy, which involves resection of diseased bowel
  - Both partial cystectomy and conservative treatment have been successful in treating gross hematuria
- Symptoms may be controlled by AVM embolization in Klippel-Trenaunay-Parkes-Weber Syndrome

DIAGNOSTIC CHECKLIST

Consider

- Venogram if inconclusive noninvasive imaging
- Documentation of status of deep venous system prior to any surgical or endovenous intervention

Image Interpretation Pearls

- Lateral embryonic vein (marginal vein of Servelle) located in subcutaneous fat of lateral calf and thigh; communicates with deep system at various levels
- Venography may depict route of drainage and feasibility of resecting or sclerosing varicosities

SELECTED REFERENCES

1. Steven M et al: Haemangiomas and vascular malformations of the limb in children. Pediatr Surg Int. 23(6):565-9, 2007
2. Barker KT et al: Is the E133K allele of VG5Q associated with Klippel-Trenaunay and other overgrowth syndromes? J Med Genet. 43(7):613-4, 2006
3. Cha SH et al: Visceral manifestations of Klippel-Trenaunay syndrome. Radiographics. 25(6):1694-7, 2005
4. Timur AA et al: Biomedicine and diseases: the Klippel-Trenaunay syndrome, vascular anomalies and vascular morphogenesis. Cell Mol Life Sci. 62(13):1434-47, 2005
5. Jih MH: Klippel-Trenaunay syndrome. Dermatol Online J. 9(4):31, 2003

KLIPPEL-TRENAUNAY SYNDROME

IMAGE GALLERY

Typical

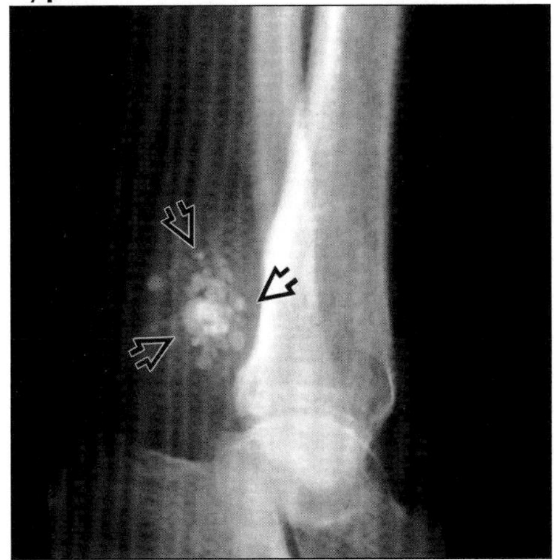

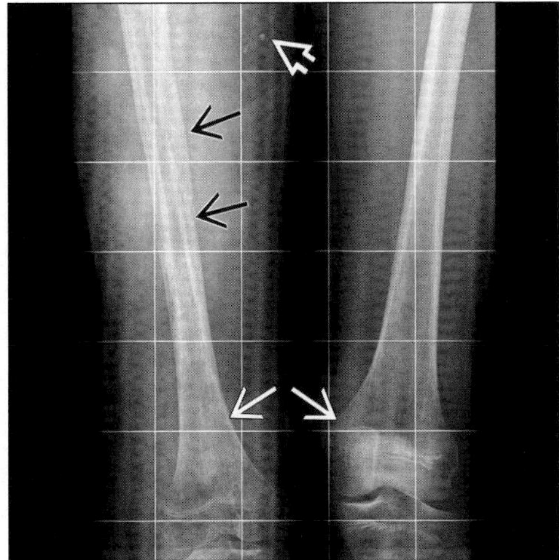

(Left) *Right ankle radiograph shows multiple phleboliths in the posterolateral soft tissues. In a young patient these are pathognomonic for a venous malformation and are indicative of prior hemorrhage or thrombosis.* ***(Right)*** *Anteroposterior radiograph (same patient as previous image) shows leg length discrepancy, with cortical thickening and soft tissue hypertrophy of the right lower extremity. A phlebolith is also present in the medial thigh.*

Typical

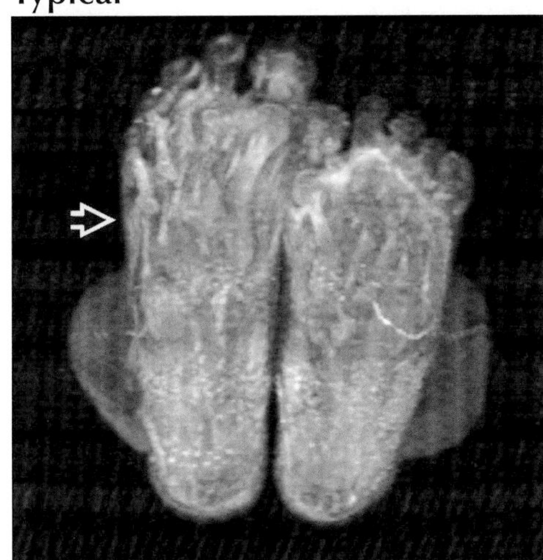

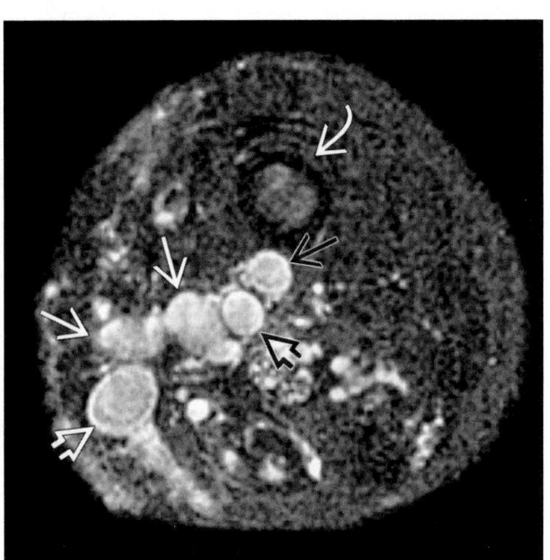

(Left) *MR MIP image of plantar aspects of both feet (same patient as previous image) shows hypertrophy of the right foot relative to the left foot.* ***(Right)*** *Axial Gadolinium-enhanced T2WI FS MR shows an aneurysmal venous malformation communicating with a marginal vein of Servelle in the posterolateral distal right thigh. This embryonal vein has numerous connections to the deep system. The popliteal artery and vein are seen posterior to the femur.*

Typical

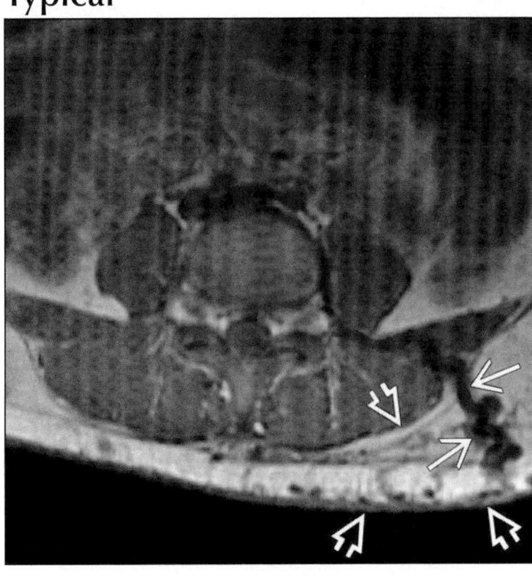

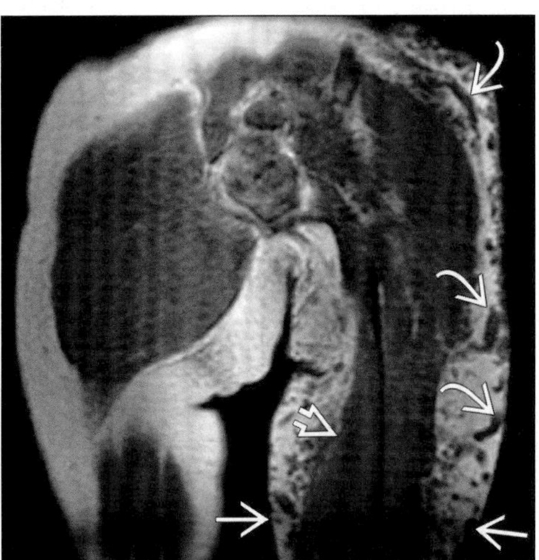

(Left) *Axial T2WI MR shows a dilated serpiginous vein coursing anteriorly into the pelvis from the thickened superficial soft tissues. Vein drains directly into the ascending lumbar plexus. Left external & common iliac veins were hypoplastic.* ***(Right)*** *Coronal T2WI MR in the same patient as previous image, shows hypertrophy of the subcutaneous tissues & muscles, as well as numerous superficial varicosities of the left lower extremity relative to the right.*

ARTERIOVENOUS FISTULA

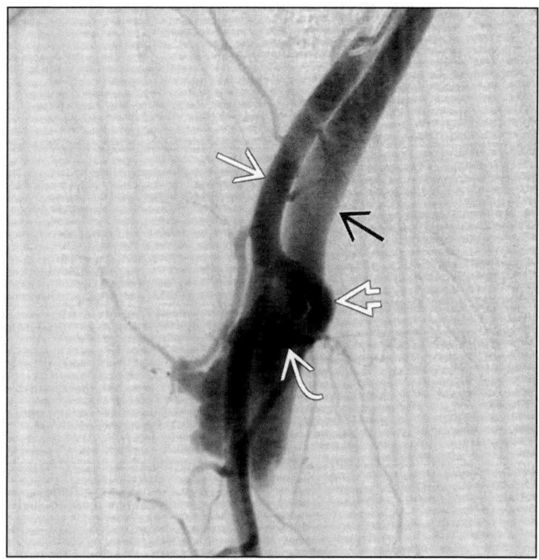

Right femoral arteriogram shows an arteriovenous fistula → between an enlarged branch → of the common femoral artery → and vein →. This was an iatrogenic injury that resulted from a catheterization procedure.

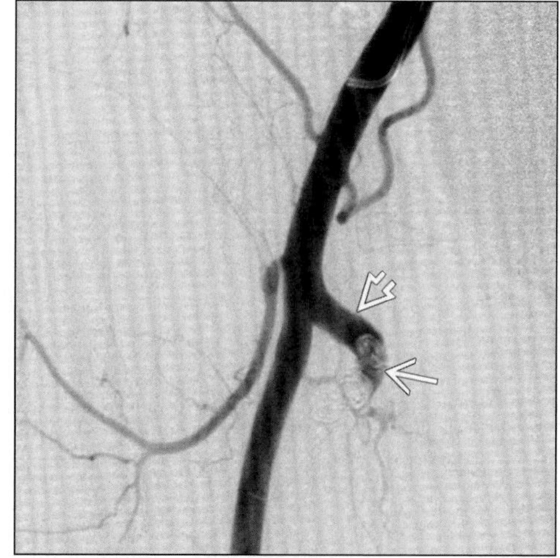

Arteriogram (same patient) following treatment shows embolization coils → occluding the arterial branch → involved in the arteriovenous fistula. The vein is no longer opacified, indicating a successful result.

TERMINOLOGY

Abbreviations and Synonyms

- Arteriovenous fistula (AVF)

Definitions

- Acquired abnormal communication between an adjacent artery and vein

IMAGING FINDINGS

General Features

- Best diagnostic clue
  - Focal "high-flow" arterial to venous shunting
  - Simultaneous opacification of artery and vein in initial phase of contrast injection during angiography and CECT
- Location: Occurs most frequently where arteries and veins are adjacent to each other, often in extremities
- Size
  - Variable; dependent upon size and location of arterial and venous branches involved in fistulous communication
    - Venous dilatation from arterialization through fistula

CT Findings

- NECT: May see indications of prior trauma (foreign bodies, shrapnel)
- CECT
  - Simultaneous arterial and venous opacification
  - Opacification of venous structures during arterial injection phase
- CTA: Will have similar findings to catheter angiography

MR Findings

- T1WI
  - Large vessels have "flow void"
  - Evidence of prior trauma
- MRA
  - Large "inflow" vessel
  - Enlarged, aneurysmal venous outflow
  - Rapid arterial to venous transit time
  - Will have similar findings to angiography and CTA

Ultrasonographic Findings

- Color Doppler

DDx: Arteriovenous Communication

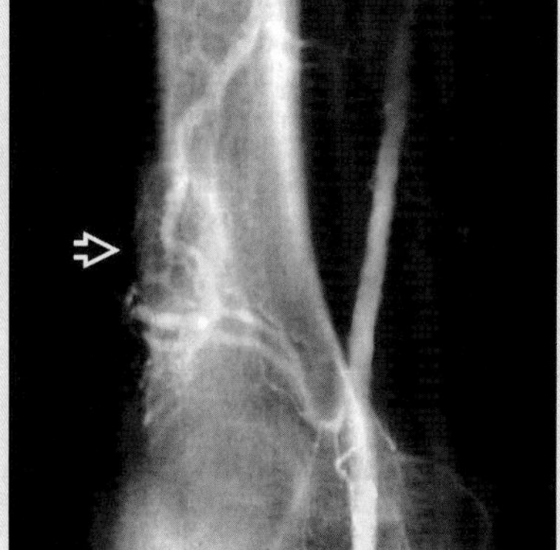

Vascular Neoplasm

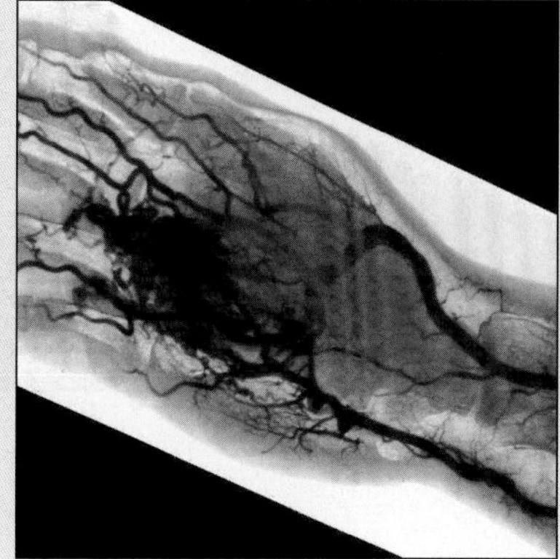

Arteriovenous Malformation

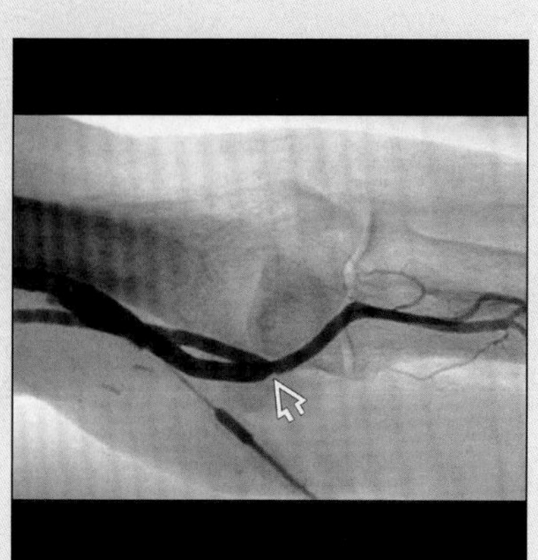

Dialysis AV Fistula

Key Facts

Terminology

- Arteriovenous fistula (AVF)
  - Acquired abnormal communication between an adjacent artery and vein

Imaging Findings

- Occurs most often where superficial arteries and veins are adjacent to each other, often in extremities
- On ultrasound of AV fistula, draining vein shows arterialized flow pattern
- DSA demonstrates focal communication between enlarged feeding arteries and draining veins with rapid shunting

Pathology

- Almost always acquired post-traumatic abnormalities
  - Lower extremities more frequently involved due to proximity of arteries and veins and increased likelihood for trauma

Clinical Issues

- Large AVF may have marked increase in cardiac venous return, with associated high cardiac output and rapid heart rate
  - "High output cardiac failure"
- High success rate (80-100%) with transcatheter embolization as primary treatment
  - Must determine whether vessel(s) can be sacrificed and alternative treatment methods
  - Variety of newer embolic agents (e.g., Amplatzer plug, covered stents) allow endovascular treatment of even very large AV fistulas

---

  - May show direct arterial to venous branch communication
    - When arteriovenous fistula is identified, draining vein may show arterialized flow pattern
  - May demonstrate any pseudoaneurysm and relationship to AV fistula
    - Pseudoaneurysm seen as anechoic mass with internal color flow

Angiographic Findings

- DSA may be used to evaluate more complex cases and may demonstrate
  - Direct focal arterial to venous communication
  - Enlarged feeding arteries and draining veins
    - Rapid shunting with hypertrophy of involved vessels
  - Additional recruited vessel involvement in chronic and enlarged arteriovenous fistula
  - Dilated venous circulation distal to fistula
    - Venous aneurysm may be present as a result of chronic arterialization of vein through fistula
  - Pseudoaneurysm may be present at site of arteriovenous communication
    - Extravascular contrast collection with delayed clearing

Imaging Recommendations

- Best imaging tool
  - Angiography or CECT with CTA
  - Angiography used for guidance during transcatheter treatment of AV fistula

DIFFERENTIAL DIAGNOSIS

Vascular Neoplasm

- Hemangioma
  - Benign vascular tumors, present in infancy, proliferate over time, usually involute during adulthood
    - Vascular malformation that occurs in capillary stage of development
  - Usually cutaneous or mucosal lesion; also found in brain, liver, spleen, pancreas and kidneys
  - Normal caliber feeding vessels
  - Early filling of vascular spaces that persists through venous phase, without venous shunting
  - MR features
    - Low signal T-1; very bright signal T-2; normal arteries and veins
- Other vascular neoplasms
  - Adrenal carcinoma
  - Angiomyolipoma
  - Germ cell tumors
  - Hepatocellular carcinoma
  - Melanoma
  - Neuroendocrine tumors
  - Primary vascular neoplasm
    - Angiosarcoma, liposarcoma, venous leiomyosarcoma
  - Renal cell carcinoma
  - Thyroid carcinoma
  - Vascular metastases from primary neoplasms

Vascular Malformations

- Arteriovenous malformation (AVM)
  - Congenital abnormal communications between arterial and venous systems, typically with central vascular "nidus"
    - Approximately 60% occur in lower extremities
    - Enlarge through recruitment of additional feeding arteries and draining veins
  - Often have slower flow than AV fistula, therefore bright signal intensity on T2-weighted imaging, and incomplete flow void on T1-weighted imaging
  - Large lesions seen on CT and MR, but need angiography for definitive diagnosis and potential transcatheter treatment
  - No history of trauma
- Venous malformation
  - Congenital low-flow lesion
    - Normal feeding arteries
    - Localized dilated venous structures
    - Slow flow and delayed opacification on CECT and angiography

- Soft, nonpulsatile, without bruit
- Large lesions can be painful if thrombosis occurs
  - May cause disfigurement
- Sclerotherapy often used for treatment

Dialysis Arteriovenous Fistula

- Surgically created communication between artery and vein, typically located in upper extremity
  - After allowing for maturation of the fistula, provides access for hemodialysis
- Surgically created fistula has same imaging characteristics as acquired or post-traumatic AV fistula
  - Rapid arteriovenous shunting through focal communication
  - Dilated, arterialized draining vein

PATHOLOGY

General Features

- General path comments: Lower extremities more frequently involved due to proximity of arteries and veins and increased likelihood for trauma
- Etiology
  - Almost always acquired, post-traumatic abnormalities
  - Gunshot wound in 50% of cases
  - Less commonly iatrogenic (disk surgery, balloon thrombectomy, percutaneous catheterization or biopsy)

Gross Pathologic & Surgical Features

- Direct communication between artery and vein
- Often have multiple arteriovenous communications, particularly in large chronic fistulas
- Dilatation of venous channels distal to fistula because of increased flow from direct exposure to arterial pressure

Microscopic Features

- Absence of proliferative cellular elements

CLINICAL ISSUES

Presentation

- Most common signs/symptoms
  - Localized, pulsatile soft tissue mass
  - Audible bruit and palpable thrill
  - Venous dilatation
  - Lymphedema in chronic fistulas
  - Branham sign: Onset of bradycardia after temporary digital compression of arterial venous fistula
- Other signs/symptoms: Marked increase in cardiac venous return; associated high cardiac output and rapid heart rate: "High output cardiac failure"

Natural History & Prognosis

- Spontaneous resolution is rare except in very small AV fistulas
  - Fistulas of all sizes can gradually enlarge
  - With enlargement, additional arteries and veins may be recruited into fistula
- Often difficult to control

Treatment

- Surgical
  - Ligation of fistula and associated branches
- Transcatheter occlusion
  - Must determine whether vessel(s) can be sacrificed and alternative treatment methods
  - Embolization should be as selective as possible, with catheter positioned close to fistula
  - Gelatin sponge (Gelfoam) and coils are most commonly used embolic agents
- High success rate (80-100%) with embolization
  - Low complication rate
  - Greatest concerns are nontarget embolization and large infarcts; small infarcts asymptomatic
    - Risk for nontarget embolization increases with larger fistulous communications
  - Variety of newer embolic agents (e.g., Amplatzer plug, covered stents) allow endovascular treatment of even very large AV fistulas

DIAGNOSTIC CHECKLIST

Consider

- Transcatheter embolization as primary treatment modality for acquired AV fistula
  - Perform embolization as selectively as possible
- Multiple arteriovenous communications may be present in large, chronic acquired AV fistulas
  - All points of communication must be closed in order to achieve complete treatment

Image Interpretation Pearls

- With large or longstanding AV fistula, venous aneurysm may be present from chronic arterialization of vein through fistula
- Pseudoaneurysm may be associated with AV fistula at point of communication and may require treatment

SELECTED REFERENCES

1. Spirito R et al: Endovascular treatment of a post-traumatic tibial pseudoaneurysm and arteriovenous fistula: case report and review of the literature. J Vasc Surg. 45(5):1076-9, 2007
2. Ray CE Jr et al: Endovascular repair of a large post-traumatic calf pseudoaneurysm and arteriovenous fistula. Mil Med. 171(7):659-61, 2006
3. Durakoglugil ME et al: High output heart failure 8 months after an acquired arteriovenous fistula. Jpn Heart J. 44(5):805-9, 2003
4. Li JC et al: Diagnostic criteria for locating acquired arteriovenous fistulas with color Doppler sonography. J Clin Ultrasound. 30(6):336-42, 2002
5. Sigler L et al: Aortocava fistula: experience with five patients. Vasc Surg. 35(3):207-12, 2001
6. Chen L et al: Surgical treatment of post-traumatic pseudoaneurysms and arteriovenous fistulas. Chin J Traumatol. 3(3):163-165, 2000
7. Parodi JC et al: Endovascular stent-graft treatment of traumatic arterial lesions. Ann Vasc Surg. 13(2):121-9, 1999
8. Picus D et al: Iatrogenic femoral arterial fistulae: evaluation by digital vascular imaging. AJR. 142(3):567-70, 1984
9. Holman E: Reflections on arteriovenous fistulas. Ann Thorac Surg. 11(2):176-86, 1971

ARTERIOVENOUS FISTULA

IMAGE GALLERY

Typical

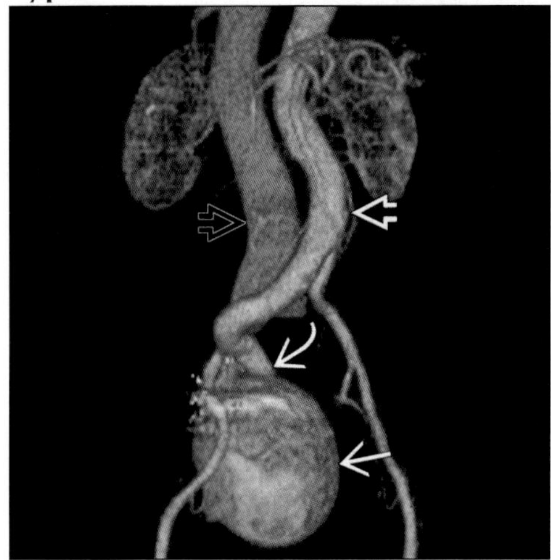

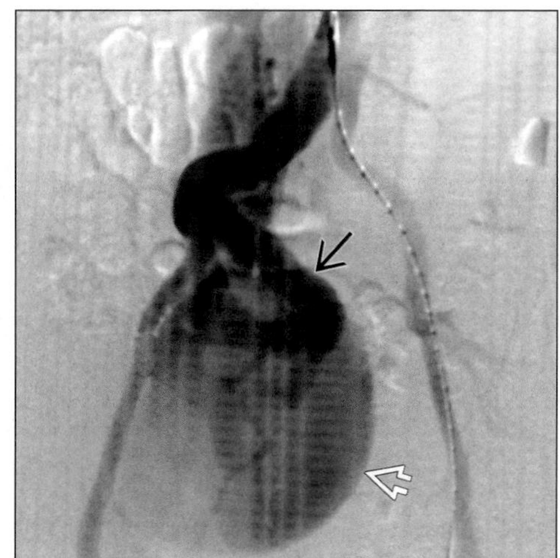

(Left) *3-D CTA shows simultaneous opacification of aorta & IVC, & a large pelvic venous aneurysm in a patient with a chronic acquired AV fistula. The chronic arterialization of the vein from the fistula with the right internal iliac artery has caused the aneurysm.* ***(Right)*** *Arteriogram (same patient as previous image) shows the AV fistula between the right internal iliac artery & vein & the resultant venous aneurysm. The patient had high output CHF.*

Typical

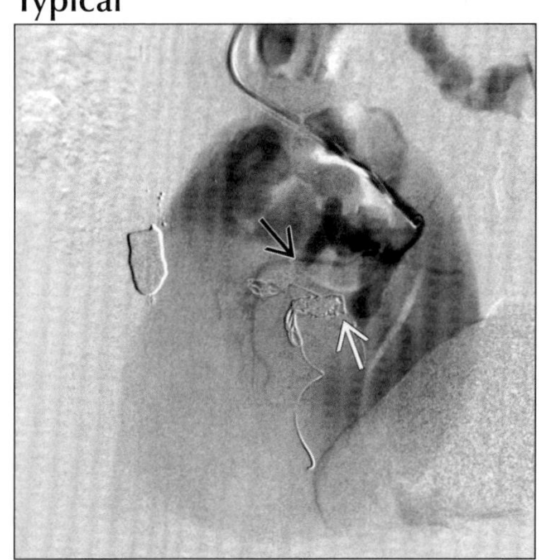

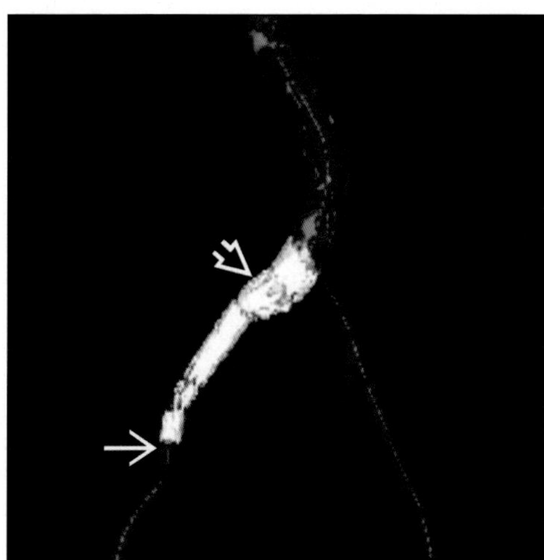

(Left) *The AV fistula in the previous patient was treated in staged procedures. This arteriogram shows the initial coil embolization of the anterior and posterior divisions of the hypogastric artery, to prevent retrograde perfusion of the fistula through pelvic collaterals.* ***(Right)*** *3-D CTA shows a stent-graft was placed from the right common iliac artery into the external iliac artery, occluding the origin of the right hypogastric artery and eliminating arterial flow into the AV fistula.*

Typical

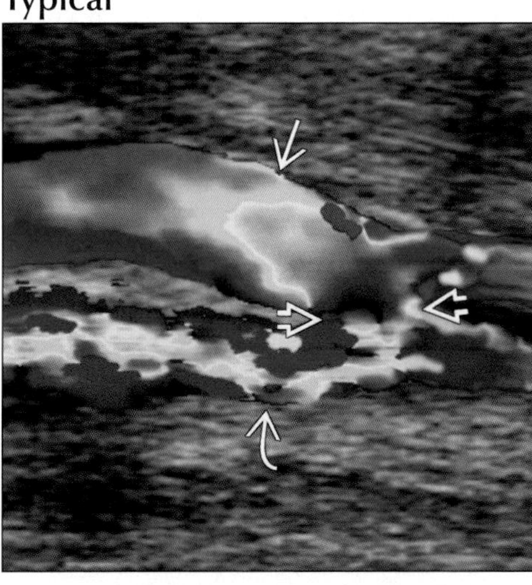

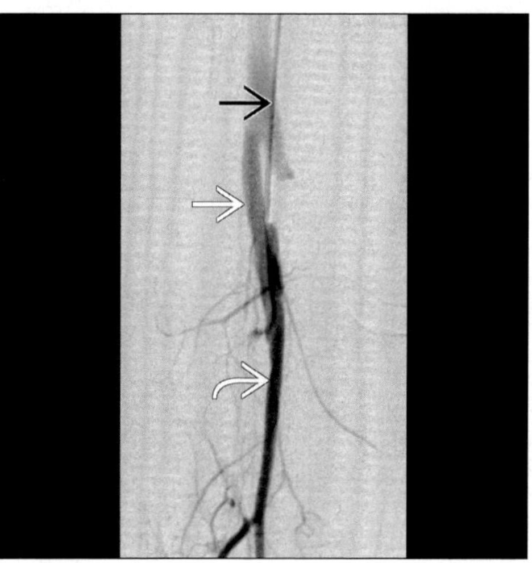

(Left) *Sagittal color Doppler ultrasound shows arteriovenous fistula between popliteal artery & vein. This iatrogenic fistula occurred during US guided popliteal artery puncture for an arterial intervention.* ***(Right)*** *DSA (same patient as previous image) with catheter in the popliteal artery shows simultaneous opacification of popliteal artery & vein, confirming AV fistula. A covered stent placed in the popliteal artery eliminated the fistula.*

DEEP VEIN THROMBOSIS

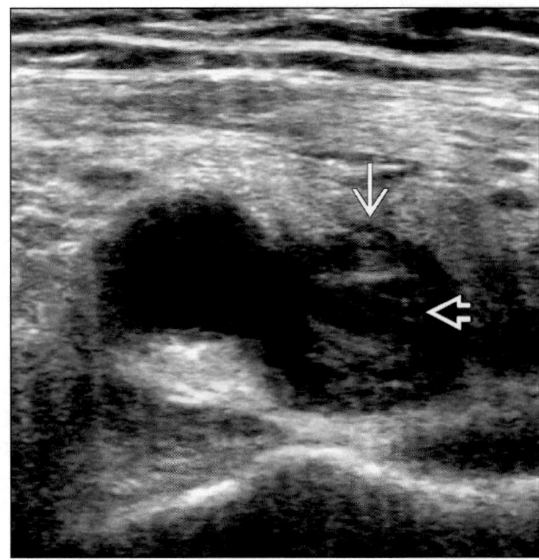

Transverse ultrasound shows subacute DVT of the right common femoral vein ➡, which is filled with echogenic thrombus ➡. Additionally, the vein is non-compressible with transducer pressure.

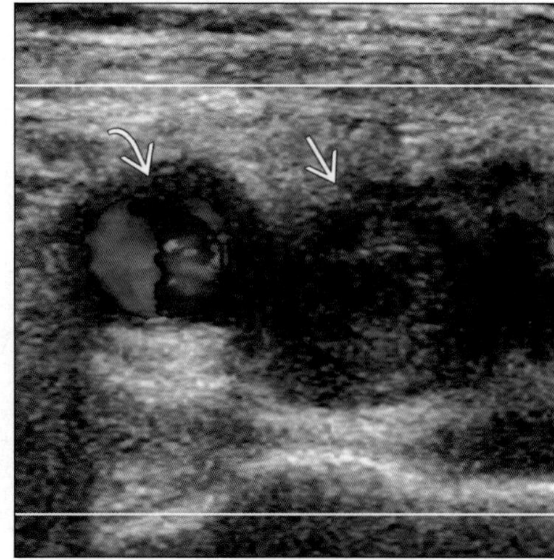

Corresponding color Doppler ultrasound shows normal color flow in the more lateral right common femoral artery ➡ and no flow in the thrombus-filled right common femoral vein ➡, located medially.

TERMINOLOGY

Abbreviations and Synonyms

- Deep vein thrombosis (DVT), pulmonary embolism (PE), venous thromboembolic disease (VTE)

Definitions

- Deep vein thrombosis: Condition where blood solidifies, producing blood clot (thrombus) within deep venous system, typically in lower limbs
- Can also be seen in upper limbs (especially related to central venous catheters)
- Pulmonary embolism: Obstruction of pulmonary artery or one of its branches by embolus, usually blood clot derived from leg vein thrombosis
- Venous thromboembolic disease: Combined deep vein thrombosis and pulmonary embolism

IMAGING FINDINGS

General Features

- Best diagnostic clue
  - Filling defect in deep veins or pulmonary arteries
    - CT, MR or contrast venogram, pulmonary CTA
  - Noncompressible vein, with intraluminal echoes on ultrasound examination
- Location
  - Iliac veins extend from inguinal ligament and join to form IVC
  - Common femoral vein extends proximally from junction of femoral vein (superficial femoral vein) and greater saphenous vein to inguinal ligament
  - Femoral vein (superficial femoral vein) courses through Hunter canal in thigh to junction with greater saphenous vein proximally
  - Popliteal vein extends proximally from paired tibial veins to Hunter canal
  - Calf veins: Paired anterior tibial, posterior tibial and peroneal veins

Ultrasonographic Findings

- Grayscale Ultrasound
  - Acute thrombosis (~ 14 days)
    - Low echogenicity or nearly anechoic thrombus
    - Venous distension: Recently thrombosed veins distended; substantially larger than adjacent artery

DDx: Deep Vein Thrombosis

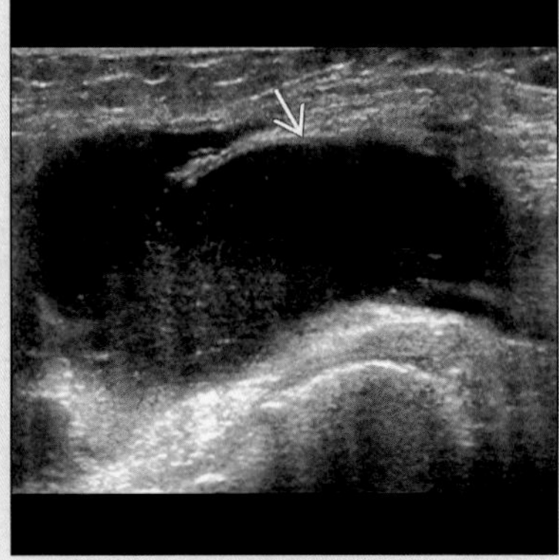

Baker Cyst

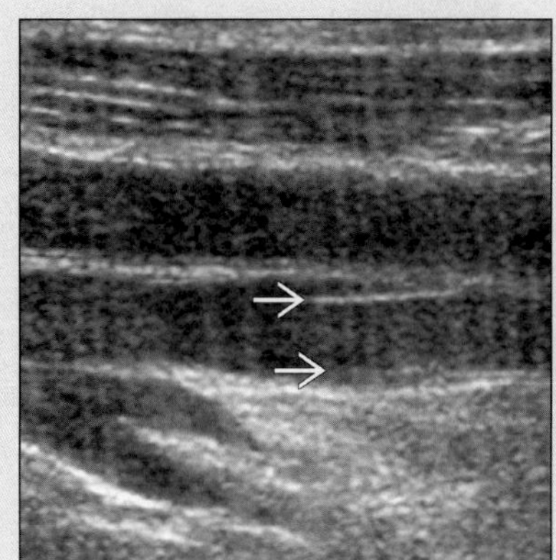

Thickened Valves

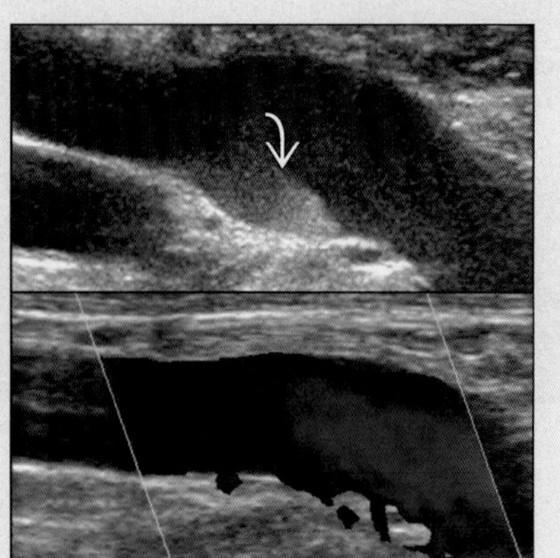

Artifactual "Echocontrast"

DEEP VEIN THROMBOSIS

Key Facts

Imaging Findings

- Acute thrombosis (~ 14 days)
  - Low echogenicity or nearly anechoic thrombus; flow may be seen within recanalized thrombus
  - Venous distension: Recently thrombosed veins distended; substantially larger than adjacent artery
  - Loss of compressibility: Thrombus excluded if vein can be completely compressed
  - Free floating thrombus: Most recently formed clot may not adhere to vein wall
  - Collateralization: Tortuous collateral veins, usually smaller than normal vein
- Duplex Doppler ultrasound first line imaging tool; 90-100% sensitivity and specificity for acute DVT
- Color Doppler: Useful to detect low echo or anechoic thrombus which may be missed on grayscale US
- CT and MR venography good non-invasive imaging tools for assessment of pelvic veins and IVC and for exclusion of pelvic and abdominal causes of DVT
- Contrast venography was once "gold standard"
  - Now infrequently used for diagnosis of DVT

Clinical Issues

- Acute DVT: Swollen and tender lower limb (extent of swelling depends on site of DVT), increased temperature
- Chronic DVT: Chronic leg swelling, ankle pigmentation, ulceration in lower calf and ankle
- Anticoagulation therapy for above knee DVT and PE; treatment for calf vein DVT controversial
- Catheter-directed thrombolysis reduces prevalence and severity of post thrombotic syndrome

---

- Loss of compressibility: Thrombus excluded if vein can be completely compressed
- Free floating thrombus: Most recently formed clot may not adhere to vein wall
- Collaterals: Tortuous veins bypassing occlusion, usually smaller than normal veins

- Subacute thrombosis (~ 2 weeks to 6 months)
  - Thrombus becomes more echogenic, variable
  - Decreased thrombus and vein size: Retraction and lysis may reduce vein size
  - Adherence of thrombus: Free floating thrombus becomes attached to vein wall
  - Resumption of flow: Luminal flow may be restored; but vein may remain occluded
  - Collateralization: Collateral venous channel continues to develop
- Chronic phase (≥ 6 months)
  - Post-thrombotic scarring: Fibroblasts invade non-lysed thrombus; organizes as fibrous tissue
  - Wall thickening: Scarred veins thick-walled with reduced luminal diameter
  - Echogenic intraluminal material: Post thrombotic fibrous scars appear as plaque-like areas along vein; may occasionally calcify
  - Synechiae: Formed from non-lysed thrombus attached to one side of vein wall; gradually transformed into fibrous band
  - Fibrous cord: In veins which fail to recanalize, vein may be reduced to echogenic cord; smaller than normal vein
  - Valve abnormalities: Valve damage associated with venous thrombosis; valve cusp thickening and restricted motion leads to reflux and stasis

- Pulsed Doppler
  - Spontaneous flow (any waveform present)
    - Expected in medium to large veins, but often not spontaneous in smaller calf veins
  - Phasic flow (variation in flow velocity with respiration)
    - When phasic pattern absent, flow described as continuous, indicating obstruction closer to heart
  - Valsalva maneuver
    - Causes blood flow cessation in large and medium size veins, documenting venous patency from point of examination to thorax
  - Augmentation (increased flow velocity with distal compression)
    - Absent response indicates obstruction further from heart and close to site of examination
- Color Doppler
  - Color Doppler: Detects low echo or anechoic thrombus that may be missed on grayscale US
  - Demonstration of recanalized lumen in thrombus, collateralization
  - Demonstration of reflux in valvular incompetence
- Power Doppler: Particularly useful in demonstration of slow flow through recanalized lumen and collaterals

Angiographic Findings

- Contrast venography was once "gold standard"
  - Now infrequently used for diagnosis of DVT
- Filling defect in deep veins
  - Contrast outlines incompletely occlusive thrombus
    - "Tram track" sign of flow around thrombus
- Venography used in combination with percutaneous intervention such as catheter-directed thrombolysis
  - Used in extensive ilio-femoral venous thrombosis, phlegmasia cerulea dolens
  - Lysis may reduce incidence of chronic venous insufficiency

Imaging Recommendations

- Best imaging tool
  - Duplex Doppler ultrasound first line imaging tool; 90-100% sensitivity and specificity for acute DVT
  - CECT and CT/MR venography good non-invasive imaging tools
    - Assessment of pelvic veins and IVC; exclusion of pelvic and abdominal causes of DVT
  - Conventional venography has 11% false negative rate
    - Reserved for use as problem solving aid
    - Used in combination with catheter-directed or mechanical thrombolysis

DEEP VEIN THROMBOSIS

DIFFERENTIAL DIAGNOSIS

Interpretation Errors

- Baker cyst
- Artifactual "echocontrast" from slow flow
- Thickened valve mistaken for thrombus in chronic venous obstruction
- Failure to identify duplicated vein

Technical Errors

- Inadequate compression
- Improper use of color flow imaging
- Poor venous distension
- Misidentification of deep vs. superficial veins

Cellulitis

- Clinically may mimic DVT; swollen, tender extremity

Superficial Thrombophlebitis

- Also clinically similar to DVT

PATHOLOGY

General Features

- Genetics
  - Number of inherited prothrombotic disease states
    - Antithrombin III deficiency
    - Protein C and protein S deficiency
    - Factor V Leiden, factor II G20210A
    - Primary hyperhomocysteinemia
    - Dysfibrinogenemias and hypofibrinolysis
- Etiology
  - Acquired prothrombotic states associated with DVT
  - Immobilization, stroke, recent surgery (especially orthopedic), paralysis, DVT history (risk factor 2.5)
  - Obesity (risk factor 1.5), malignancy (risk factor 2.5)
  - Cigarette smoking, hypertension
  - Oral contraceptives, hormone replacement therapy, pregnancy, 2° homocystinemia
  - Antiphospholipid syndrome, CHF, myeloproliferative disorders, nephrotic syndrome
  - Inflammatory bowel disease, sickle cell anemia, polycythemia, age > 40 (risk factor 2.2)
- Epidemiology
  - VTE: 70-113 cases/100,000/year; DVT: 48/100,000; PE: 23/100,000 in clinical studies in Caucasians with no post mortem data
  - Race/ethnicity: 2.5-4x lower risk of development of VTE amongst Hispanics and Asian-Pacific islanders compared with Caucasians and African-Americans
  - Seasonal variation: Occurs in winter > summer
  - About 25-50% idiopathic

CLINICAL ISSUES

Presentation

- Most common signs/symptoms
  - Acute DVT: Swollen, tender lower limb (swelling extent depends on DVT site), increased temperature
  - Post thrombotic syndrome: Sequelae of DVT resulting from chronic venous obstruction and/or acquired incompetence of valves
    - Chronic leg swelling, ankle pigmentation, ulceration in lower calf and ankle (gaiter zone)
- Other signs/symptoms: With associated pulmonary embolus: Shortness of breath, pleuritic chest pain, tachycardia, hypoxia, hypotension

Demographics

- Age: Exponential increase in VTE with age > 40 yrs; 25-30 yr old ~ 30 cases/100,000; 70-79 yr old ~ 300-500 cases/100,000
- Gender: M = F

Natural History & Prognosis

- Tibial/peroneal thrombi resolve spontaneously in 40%, stabilize in 40%, propagate proximally in 20%
- Likelihood for pulmonary embolism: Iliac veins (77%), femoropopliteal veins (35-67%), calf veins (0-46%)
- Post thrombotic syndrome in 20% of DVT
- Death after treated VTE: 30 day incidence ~ 6% after incident DVT; 30 day incidence ~ 12% after PE; death associated with cancer, age and cardiovascular disease

Treatment

- Anticoagulation therapy for above knee DVT and PE; treatment for calf vein DVT controversial
- Heparin anticoagulation (unfractionated or low molecular weight) initial treatment for acute DVT
- Oral warfarin begun once therapeutic heparinization achieved; follow International Normalized Ratio (INR)
- Warfarinization for DVT usually 3 months; generally longer for PE; maybe life-long for recurrent DVT/PE or prothrombotic tendencies
- IVC filter considered for patients with high PE risk
  - Patients with fresh iliac vein or IVC thrombus
  - Unsuitable patients for anticoagulation
    - Recent surgery, bleeding peptic ulcer, bleeding diatheses, vascular neoplasm
- Catheter-directed thrombolysis reduces prevalence and severity of post thrombotic syndrome
  - Considered in extensive ilio-femoral venous thrombosis and venous gangrene
  - Use limited by contraindications
    - Increased major bleeding risk (11%), stroke (3%)
- Surgery for managing chronic venous obstruction
  - Valve repair or transplantation, venous bypasses
  - Perforator interruption, stripping of superficial venous system if deep venous system patent

DIAGNOSTIC CHECKLIST

Image Interpretation Pearls

- Thrombus excluded if vein completely compressible

SELECTED REFERENCES

1. Zwiebel WJ et al: Introduction to Vascular Sonography. 5th edition. Philadelphia, Elsevier Saunders. 403-78, 2005
2. White RH. Related Articles et al: The epidemiology of venous thromboembolism. Circulation. 107(23 Suppl 1):I4-8, 2003
3. Dähnert W: Deep vein thrombosis. In: Radiology Review Manual. 3rd edition. Baltimore, William & Wilkins. 462-3, 1996

DEEP VEIN THROMBOSIS

IMAGE GALLERY

Typical

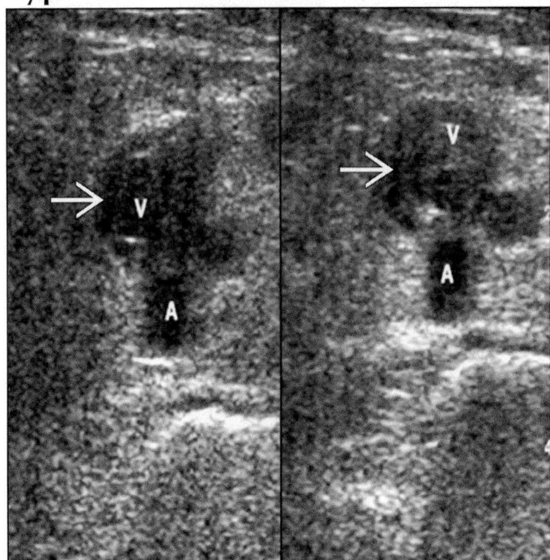

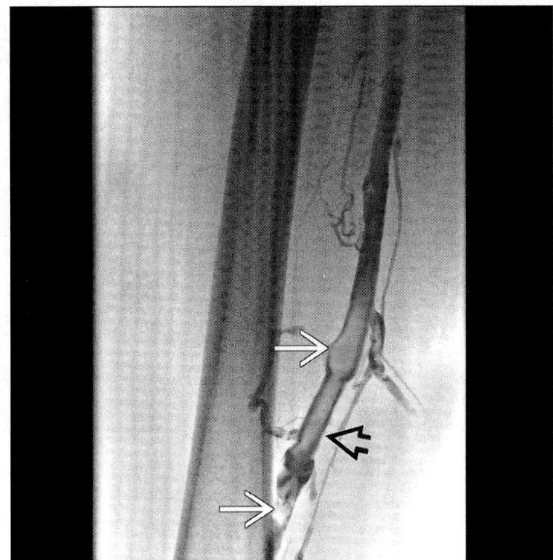

(Left) *Transverse ultrasound shows acute DVT of the popliteal vein (V) filled with hypoechoic thrombus (right) and noncompressible with transducer pressure (left).* ***(Right)*** *Corresponding venogram shows extensive intraluminal filling defects in the superficial femoral vein of the thigh. A small amount of contrast outlines the thrombus, with a resultant "tram track" sign. An intravenous catheter was subsequently introduced for catheter-directed thrombolytic therapy.*

Typical

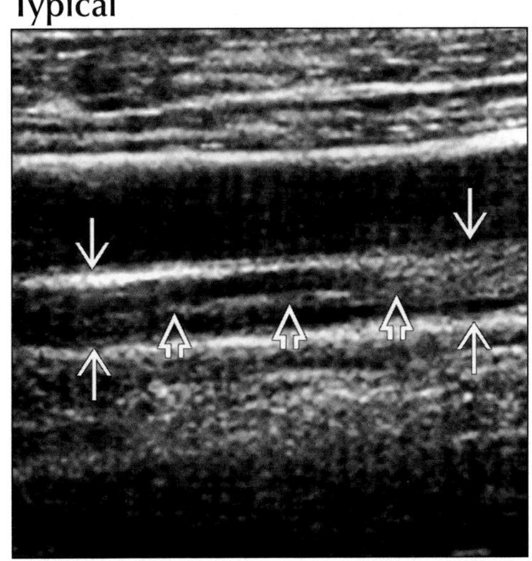

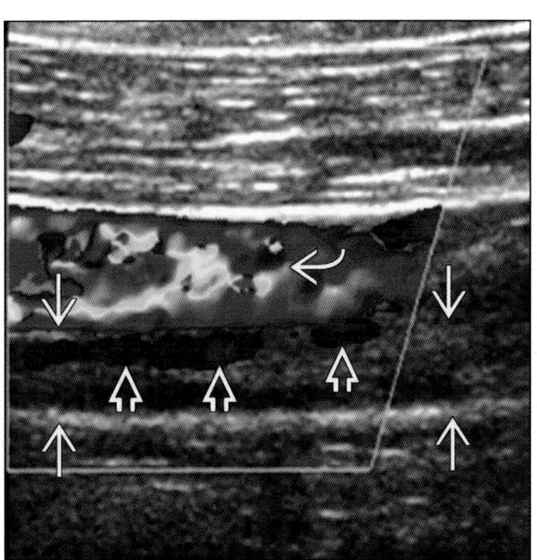

(Left) *Longitudinal grayscale ultrasound shows chronic deep vein thrombosis in the superficial femoral vein of the thigh with an echogenic intraluminal post-thrombotic fibrous scar.* ***(Right)*** *Corresponding longitudinal color Doppler ultrasound shows color flow in the normal superficial femoral artery and limited venous flow in the recanalized channel of the superficial femoral vein. Post-thrombotic fibrous scars appear as plaque-like areas along the vein wall.*

Typical

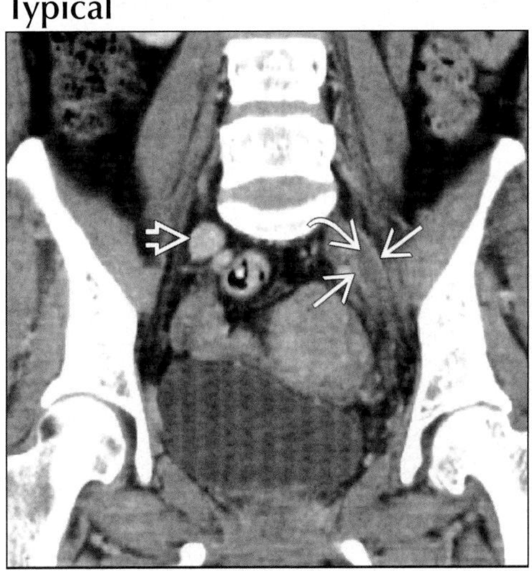

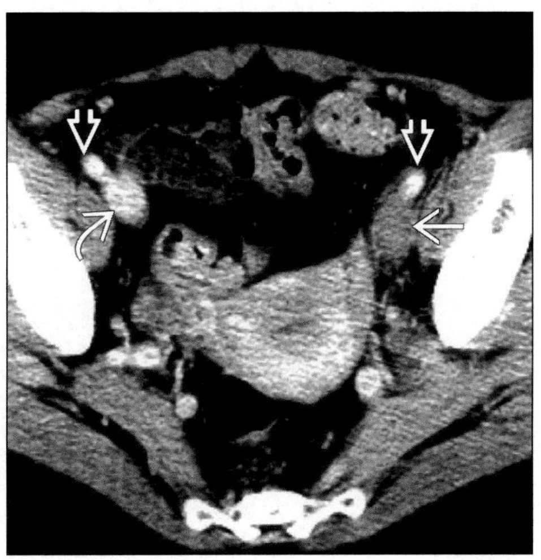

(Left) *Coronal CECT shows expansion of the left external iliac vein by hypodense non-enhancing thrombus. Note the normal contrast-enhancement in the patent right external iliac vein.* ***(Right)*** *Axial CECT in the same patient as previous image, shows expansion of the left external iliac vein by the hypodense thrombus. Note the normal contrast-enhancement in the right external iliac vein and in both the right and left external iliac arteries.*

VARICOSE VEINS/INCOMPETENT PERFORATORS

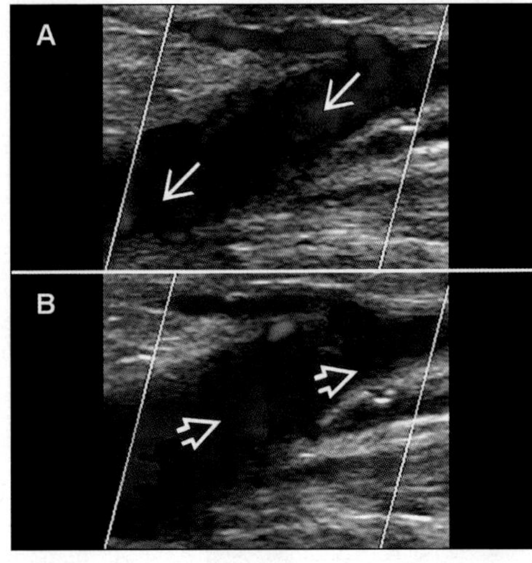

Color Doppler ultrasound (A) shows normal flow in the greater saphenous vein depicted in blue ➔. GSV reflux ⇨ is seen (B) during Valsalva maneuver. The blue to red color change is due to flow reversal.

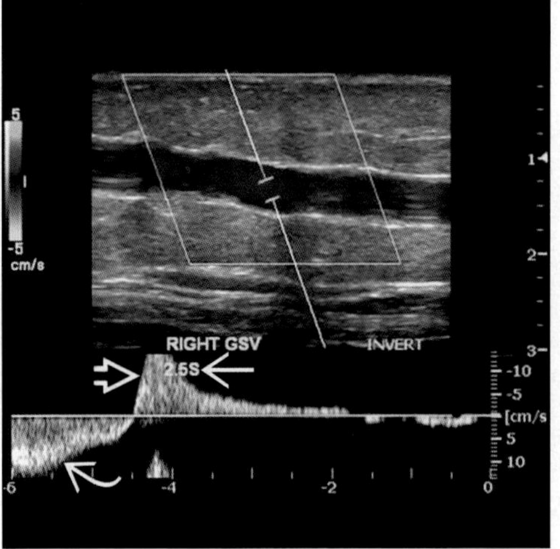

Color Doppler ultrasound in the same patient shows reflux ⇨ in the right greater saphenous vein below the saphenofemoral junction, persisting for 2.5 seconds ➔ following a venous augmentation maneuver ↩.

TERMINOLOGY

Definitions

- Lower extremity veins divided into superficial and deep systems, connected by perforating veins
  - Perforating veins normally drain blood from superficial into deep veins
    - Incompetent perforating veins allow blood to abnormally drain from deep to superficial veins as result of faulty valves
- Varicose veins are enlarged, painful, serpiginous, superficial veins that distend when patient is standing
  - Greater saphenous vein valvular incompetence causes > 75% of varicose veins, with remainder caused by incompetent perforators
- Chronic venous insufficiency refers to venous valvular incompetence in superficial, deep, or perforating veins
- "Proximal" and "distal" in venous system refers to vein segment position relative to cardiac position (rather than blood flow direction)

IMAGING FINDINGS

Ultrasonographic Findings

- Grayscale Ultrasound
  - Defines vein lumen, valve leaflets and vein wall
  - Assesses vein compressibility, acoustic properties of thrombus (evaluates age of thrombus)
- Pulsed Doppler
  - Differentiates venous from arterial flow
  - Documents venous flow pattern and flow direction
  - Timing of duration of venous reflux
    - Venous reflux > 0.5 sec clinically abnormal
  - Normal venous flow signal
    - Spontaneous and phasic with respiration
    - Normal augmentation with distal compression
  - Abnormal venous signal in presence of thrombotic obstruction or extrinsic compression
    - Doppler waveforms are continuous and nonphasic
    - Augmentation with distal limb compression diminished (contralateral limb used as reference)
- Color Doppler
  - Differentiates partial thrombosis from occlusion
  - Distinguishes deep from superficial venous reflux at saphenofemoral and saphenopopliteal junctions

DDx: Varicose Veins

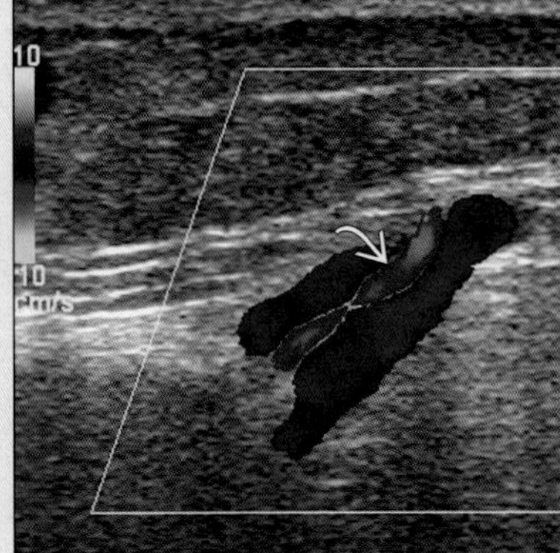

Arterial Perforator

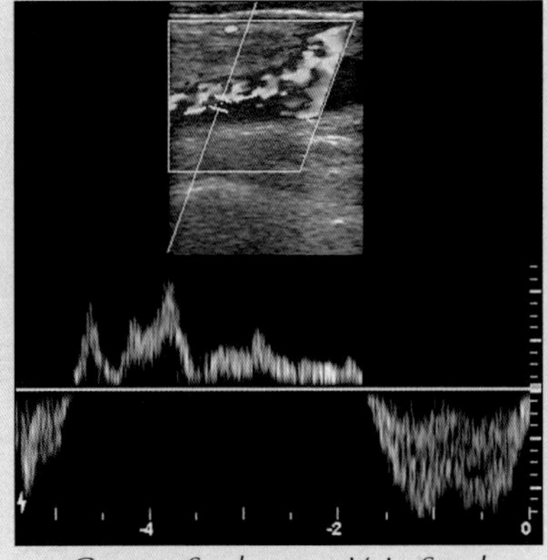

Greater Saphenous Vein Steal

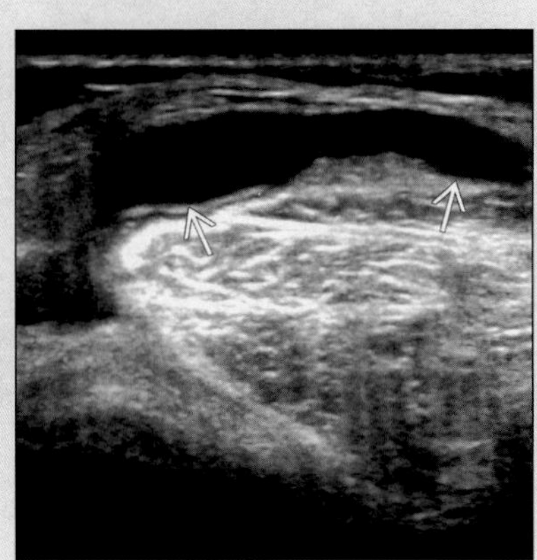

Baker Cyst

VARICOSE VEINS/INCOMPETENT PERFORATORS

Key Facts

Imaging Findings

- Grayscale ultrasound: Allows definition of vein lumen, vein valve leaflets and vein wall morphology
  - Assesses vein compressibility, acoustic properties of thrombus (evaluates age of thrombus)
- Pulsed Doppler: Differentiates venous from arterial flow
  - Documents venous flow pattern and flow direction
  - Allows timing of duration of venous reflux through incompetent valves (> 0.5 sec abnormal)
- Color Doppler: Differentiates partial thrombosis from venous occlusion
  - Distinguishes deep from superficial venous reflux at saphenofemoral and saphenopopliteal junctions
  - Identifies incompetent perforating veins
  - Demonstrates recanalization of chronically thrombosed venous segment and collateralization
- Best imaging tool: Combination of grayscale, pulsed Doppler and color Doppler ultrasound

Top Differential Diagnoses

- Calf Arterial Perforator
- GSV Steal
- Baker Cyst

Clinical Issues

- Several minimally invasive therapies available

Diagnostic Checklist

- When venous insufficiency suggested during recumbent ultrasound examination, confirm findings by moving patient to standing position

  - Identifies incompetent perforating veins
  - Demonstrates recanalization of chronically thrombosed venous segment and collateralization

Imaging Recommendations

- Best imaging tool
  - Grayscale, pulsed and color Doppler ultrasound
    - High-resolution ultrasound with 3-10 MHz pulsed and color Doppler transducers
- Patient positioning
  - Supine position
    - Head slightly elevated, feet lower than heart (if tilt table available); maximizes venous pooling
    - Hips externally rotated; knees slightly flexed
    - Permits easy access to common femoral vein (CFV), superficial femoral vein (SFV), deep femoral vein (DFV), posterior tibial vein (PTV) and greater saphenous vein (GSV)
  - Lateral decubitus position
    - Permits easy access to common iliac vein (CIV), external iliac vein (EIV), popliteal vein (Pop V) and short saphenous vein (SSV)
  - Prone position with feet slightly elevated
    - Useful for examination of Pop V and SSV
- Technique
  - Examination of venous system includes deep and superficial venous systems and perforator veins
  - Longitudinal imaging to assess flow direction, reflux
  - Transverse imaging for assessing compressibility
  - Evaluate deep venous system for DVT and reflux
  - Superficial venous system examination starts with saphenofemoral junction and includes GSV, saphenopopliteal junction and SSV
  - Perforator veins examination includes mid-thigh, medial calf and lateral thigh perforators
    - In thigh, medially located perforators best identified by beginning at CFV level
    - Perforators connect GSV to deep veins
    - Hunterian perforator(s) (proximal thigh); Dodd perforator(s) (distal thigh)
    - Incompetent perforator veins larger than competent perforator veins
    - Perforator veins > 4 mm usually incompetent
    - Perforator veins < 3 mm usually competent
    - Cockett perforators (distal medial calf); Boyd perforators (proximal medial calf)
    - Location of lateral perforators in calf vary: 2 perforators connect SSV to gastrocnemius vein proximally; 2 distal perforators above ankle
  - Examination at each level should include
    - Confirmation of flow by placing spectral Doppler sample volume over vein lumen
    - Flow occurs in forward cephalad direction when limb compressed distal to probe
    - Should be no retrograde flow with release of distal compression, with Valsalva maneuver or with limb compression proximal to probe
    - Recognition of flow direction with color Doppler
    - Identification of anatomy and flow patterns
    - Detection of morphologic and hemodynamic abnormalities
  - Color flow imaging parameters should be optimized for detection of low velocity flow
    - Decrease velocity scale and wall filters
    - Use appropriately angled, narrow color box
    - When venous insufficiency suggested during recumbent ultrasound examination, confirm findings by moving patient to standing position

DIFFERENTIAL DIAGNOSIS

Calf Arterial Perforator

- Flow direction opposite to perforator vein; may mimic reflux in calf perforators
  - Important to assess flow with spectral Doppler

Greater Saphenous Vein Steal

- Flow regurgitation in external iliac and/or common femoral vein due to blood stealing from significant GSV reflux
  - Common association with GSV incompetence

Baker Cyst

- May mimic large varicose veins

VARICOSE VEINS/INCOMPETENT PERFORATORS

PATHOLOGY

General Features

- Genetics: Positive family history of varicose veins increases risk twofold
- Etiology
  - Primary valvular incompetence
    - Hereditary, hormonal factors and endothelial damage may affect vein wall
    - Intrinsic weakness of smooth muscle media layer of vein wall causes dilatation of valve ring and resultant lack of valve apposition
  - Secondary valvular incompetence
    - Post-thrombotic damage to valve leaflets
    - Extrinsic compression of vein
    - Venous hypertension from AV communications
  - Vascular malformations
- Epidemiology: Prevalence of 30-60% adult population

Staging, Grading or Classification Criteria

- Varicose veins classified as telangiectasias, venulectasias, reticular veins, non-saphenous and saphenous varicose veins; depends on size, location
- Clinical, etiologic, anatomic, pathophysiologic (CEAP) classification of venous insufficiency
  - C1 Telangiectasias
  - C2 Varicose veins
  - C3 Edema without skin changes
  - C4 Pigmentation
  - C5 Skin changes with healed ulceration
  - C6 Active ulceration

CLINICAL ISSUES

Presentation

- Most common signs/symptoms
  - Edema, dilated veins, leg pain
  - Changes in skin around ankle region
    - Pigmentation
    - Skin-thickening
    - Ulceration (venous stasis ulcers)
  - Incompetent superficial, perforating and deep veins may cause full spectrum of symptoms
  - Segmental incompetence less symptomatic

Demographics

- Age
  - Visible tortuous varicose veins
    - 10-15% of males; 20-25% of females > 15 yrs old
  - Moderate or chronic venous insufficiency
    - 2-5% of adult males; 3-7% of adult females
- Gender: Females affected fourfold more than males

Natural History & Prognosis

- Without treatment, a cycle of worsening valvular incompetence and venous reflux may occur
  - Leads to venous hypertension, vein distension and additional valvular incompetency

Treatment

- Indicated for venous insufficiency attributable to GSV incompetence
- Several minimally invasive procedures performed as outpatient or day case procedure
  - Foam sclerosant ablation of GSV and/or varicosities
    - Sodium tetradecyl sulphate 3% can be used
    - Ultrasound used to guide treatment and compression of saphenofemoral junction
  - Radiofrequency ablation (RFA) or laser ablation (EVLT) of GSV
    - Conscious sedation and IV analgesia may be given
    - Ultrasound used to guide catheter placement and injection of tumescent local anesthesia in perivenous fascia around GSV
    - Tumescent anesthesia compresses vein around laser or RFA probe to maximize contact; provides thermal barrier to protect adjacent structures
    - RF or laser energy heats and contracts vein wall
    - Catheter withdrawn from 1.5 cm below saphenofemoral junction to knee level or below
    - Vein contracts, narrows and forms fibrous scar
  - Ambulatory phlebectomy
    - Tiny incisions made and varicose veins removed
  - Transilluminated powered phlebectomy (TIPP)
    - Minimally invasive surgical procedure for removing varicose veins
    - Transillumination of vein allows surgeon to accurately identify and remove varicose veins
  - Conventional surgery
    - Usually performed under general anesthesia
    - GSV stripping and phlebectomy of varicosities
    - Involves tying off cephalad end of GSV followed by complete surgical removal

DIAGNOSTIC CHECKLIST

Image Interpretation Pearls

- When venous insufficiency suggested during recumbent ultrasound examination, confirm findings by moving patient to standing position

SELECTED REFERENCES

1. Merchant RF et al: Long-term outcomes of endovenous radiofrequency obliteration of saphenous reflux as a treatment for superficial venous insufficiency. J Vasc Surg. 42(3):502-9; discussion 509, 2005
2. Neumyer MM: Ultrasound diagnosis of venous insufficiency. In: Zwiebel et al: Introduction to Vascular Sonography, 5th ed. Philadelphia, Elsevier Saunders. 479-510, 2005
3. Perala J et al: Radiofrequency endovenous obliteration versus stripping of the long saphenous vein in the management of primary varicose veins: 3-year outcome of a randomized study. Ann Vasc Surg. 2005
4. Min RJ et al: Endovenous laser treatment of saphenous vein reflux: long-term results. J Vasc Interv Radiol. 14(8):991-6, 2003

IMAGE GALLERY

Typical

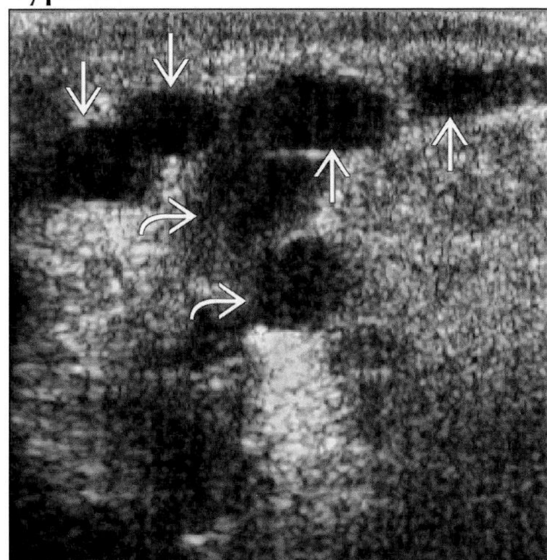

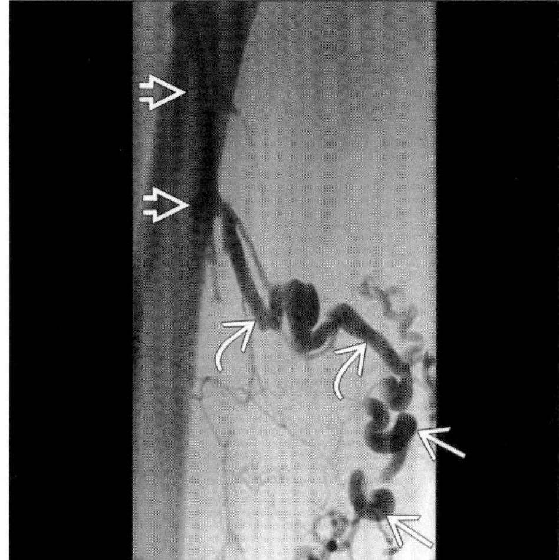

(Left) Longitudinal grayscale ultrasound shows superficial varicosities → connected to a large venous perforator → in the thigh. *(Right)* Contrast venography in the same patient shows the varicose veins in the lateral thigh → communicating with the deep venous system → via a prominent incompetent perforating vein →. Normally the perforating veins drain blood from the superficial to the deep venous system. With valvular incompetence, the flow is reversed.

Typical

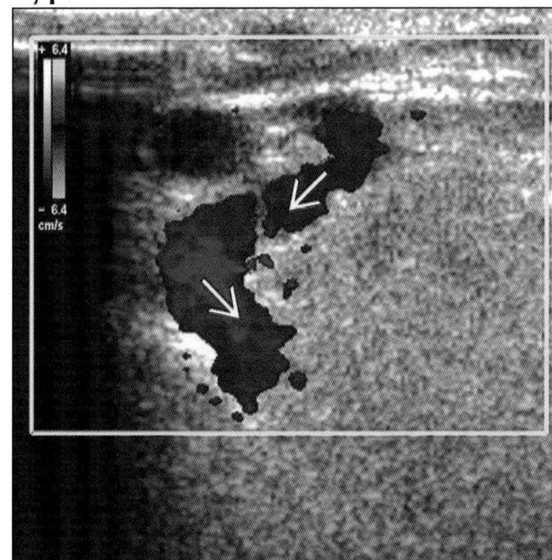

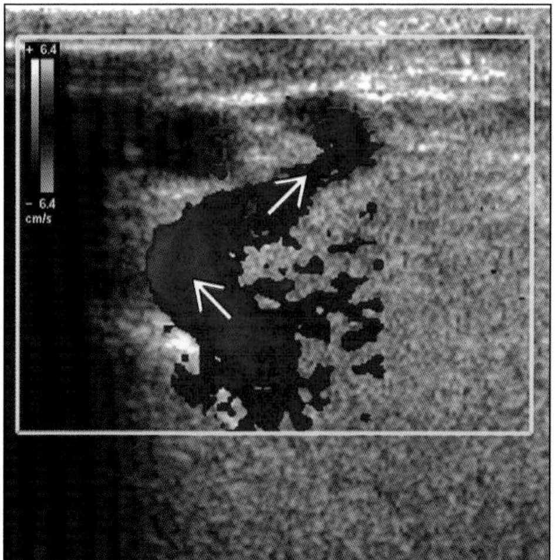

(Left) Longitudinal color Doppler ultrasound shows flow in a large calf perforator with antegrade flow → to the deep venous system depicted in red. *(Right)* Corresponding longitudinal color Doppler ultrasound shows flow in the large calf perforator with retrograde flow → to the superficial venous system after sudden cuff deflation. This indicates that the perforating vein is incompetent. Typically, incompetent perforators have a larger diameter than when competent.

Typical

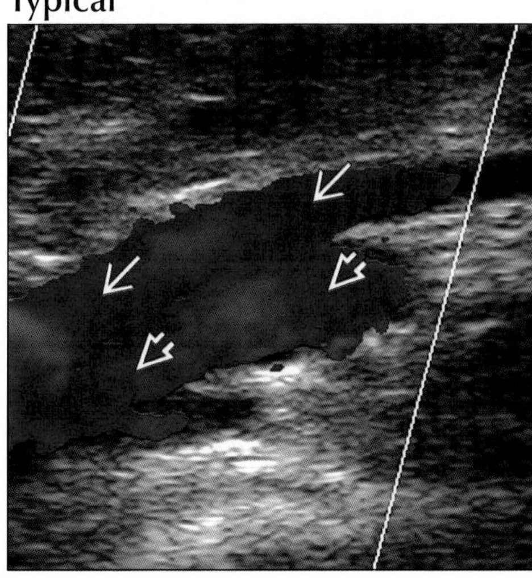

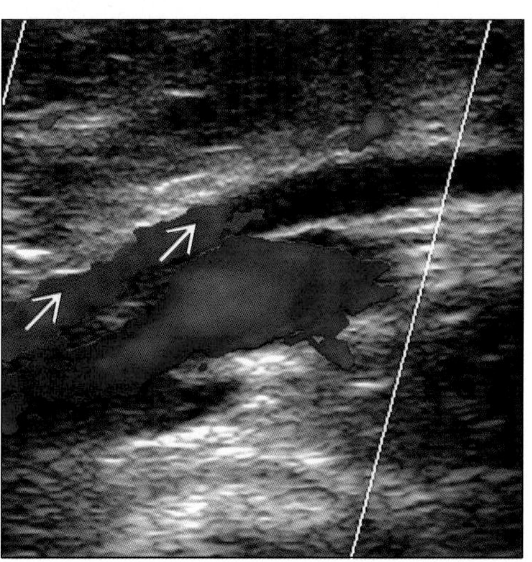

(Left) Longitudinal color Doppler ultrasound shows normal antegrade flow in the short saphenous vein → and in the popliteal vein → both depicted in blue. *(Right)* Corresponding longitudinal color Doppler ultrasound (same patient) shows reflux in the short saphenous vein at the saphenopopliteal junction during a Valsalva maneuver. The reversed flow seen in the short saphenous vein is depicted in red →. Short saphenous venous insufficiency may cause posterior calf varicosities.

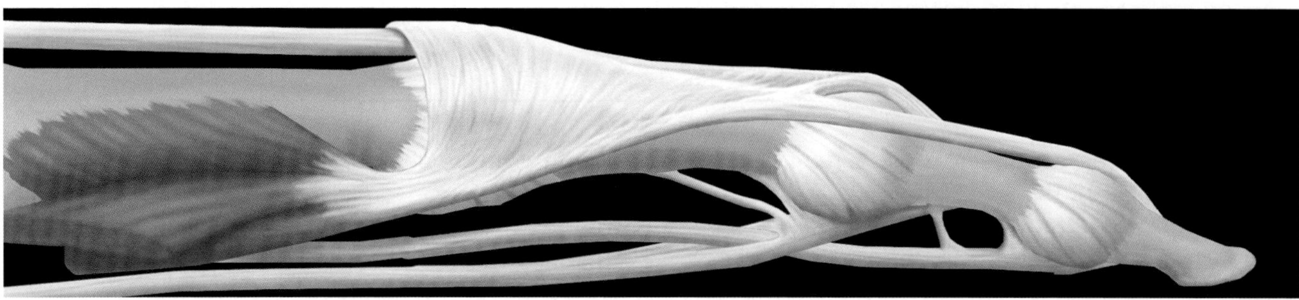

INDEX

A

INDEX

INDEX

INDEX

INDEX

B

INDEX

i

INDEX

C

INDEX

i

D

INDEX

E

F

INDEX

G

H

INDEX

INDEX

K

L

INDEX

INDEX

M

INDEX

N

INDEX

INDEX

i

INDEX

INDEX

i

R

S

INDEX

INDEX

T

INDEX

INDEX

U

V

W